IV Compatibilities

The IV compatibility table provides data when two or more medications are given into a Y-site of administration. The data in this table largely represent physical incompatibilities (e.g., haze, precipitate, change in color). Therapeutic incompatibilities have not been included, so when using the table, professional judgment should be exercised.

C Physically compatible via Y-site administration.
I Physically incompatible.

	amikacin	aminophylline	amiodarone	amphotericin B	aztreonam	bumetanide	calcium chloride	calcium gluconate	cefazolin	cefepime	ceftazidime	cimetidine	ciprofloxacin	cisatracurium	clindamycin	co-trimoxazole	dexamethasone	digoxin	diltiazem	diphenhydramine	dobutamine	dolasetron	dopamine	enalapril	epinephrine	esmolol	esomeprazole	famotidine	fluconazole	furosemide	gentamicin	heparin	hydrocortisone	hydromorphine	imipenem	insulin	labetalol	levofloxacin	lidocaine	linezolid	lorazepam	magnesium	meperidine	meropenem	methylprednisone	metoclopramide	metoprolol	metronidazole	midazolam	milrinone	morphine	multiple vitamin	nitroglycerin	nitroprusside	norepinephrine	ondansetron	pantoprazole	phenylephrine	piperacillin/tazobactam	potassium	procainamide	propofol	ranitidine	sodium bicarbonate	tobramycin	vancomycin	vecuronium
amikacin	-	C	C	I	C	-	C	C	-	-	-	C	C	C	C	-	C	-	C	C	-	-	-	C	C	C	-	-	C	-	-	I	C	C	-	-	C	C	C	-	C	C	C	-	-	-	-	-	C	C	C	-	C	C	C	-	-	C	-	C	-	I	C	C	-	-
aminophylline	C	-	I	-	C	-	I	C	-	I	-	-	I	-	I	-	C	C	-	C	I	-	C	I	C	-	C	C	C	C	C	-	-	-	-	I	C	C	C	C	-	-	I	C	-	-	C	-	-	C	-	C	-	C	-	I	-	C	C	C	C	C	C	C	-	I	C
amiodarone	C	I	-	-	-	-	-	-	-	I	-	-	-	-	-	-	-	-	C	-	C	-	C	-	C	-	-	C	-	-	C	-	C	C	C	-	C	C	-	-	-	-	-	-	-	I	-	-	-	I	C	-	-	C	C	-	C	-	C	-	C	-	-	-	-	-	-
amphotericin B	I	-	-	-	I	-	-	-	-	-	-	I	-	-	-	-	C	-	-	-	-	-	C	-	-	-	-	I	-	I	-	C	-	C	I	-	-	-	-	-	I	-	-	-	I	C	-	-	-	-	-	-	-	-	-	-	-	-	I	-	-	I	-	-	I	-	-
aztreonam	C	C	-	I	-	C	-	C	C	-	C	C	C	C	C	-	C	C	C	C	-	-	C	C	-	-	C	-	C	C	C	C	C	C	-	C	-	-	-	C	I	C	C	-	C	C	-	-	C	-	-	C	-	-	-	C	-	-	C	-	-	C	C	C	C	-	-
bumetanide	-	-	-	-	C	-	-	-	-	-	-	-	-	-	-	-	C	-	-	C	-	I	-	-	-	-	-	-	-	C	-	-	-	-	C	-	-	C	-	C	-	-	-	-	-	-	-	-	-	I	C	C	-	-	-	-	-	-	-	C	-	-	C	-	-	-	-
calcium chloride	C	I	-	-	-	-	-	-	-	-	-	-	-	-	-	-	-	-	C	-	-	-	C	-	-	-	-	C	-	-	-	-	C	-	-	-	-	C	C	-	-	I	-	-	-	-	C	C	-	C	C	-	-	C	-	-	-	-	-	-	-	I	-	-	-	-	-
calcium gluconate	C	C	-	-	C	-	-	-	-	-	C	-	C	C	-	-	C	-	C	-	C	-	-	-	C	-	C	-	-	C	-	-	C	-	-	C	C	C	C	-	-	-	-	-	-	-	C	C	-	-	C	C	-	-	-	C	-	-	C	C	C	-	C	-	-	-	-
cefazolin	-	-	I	-	C	-	-	-	-	-	C	-	-	C	C	-	C	-	C	C	-	-	C	-	C	-	C	-	C	C	-	C	-	-	I	-	C	C	C	C	-	-	C	C	-	-	C	C	C	C	-	-	-	-	-	C	-	-	C	-	-	C	C	-	C	-	C
cefepime	-	I	-	-	-	-	-	-	-	-	-	-	-	-	-	-	-	-	-	-	-	-	-	-	-	-	I	-	-	-	-	-	-	-	-	-	-	-	-	-	-	-	-	-	-	-	-	C	-	-	-	-	-	-	-	-	-	-	-	-	-	-	-	-	I	I	I
ceftazidime	-	-	-	-	C	-	-	C	-	-	-	-	C	-	-	C	-	-	C	-	C	-	C	-	-	-	C	-	C	I	-	-	C	C	-	I	-	-	-	-	C	-	C	C	-	-	C	-	-	C	I	C	-	C	-	C	-	-	C	-	-	-	C	-	C	C	C
cimetidine	C	-	-	I	C	-	-	-	C	-	-	-	C	C	C	C	C	-	-	C	C	-	C	-	-	-	C	-	C	C	C	C	C	-	C	C	C	C	C	C	C	C	-	C	C	C	C	C	C	C	C	C	-	C	C	C	-	C	C	-	C	C	C	C	C	-	-
ciprofloxacin	C	I	-	-	C	-	-	-	C	C	C	C	-	-	I	-	C	C	C	C	C	-	C	-	-	-	C	-	C	I	-	-	C	I	-	-	-	-	C	-	-	C	C	-	-	I	I	-	C	-	C	C	-	I	C	C	-	-	C	-	-	C	C	-	C	C	C
cisatracurium	C	-	-	-	C	C	-	C	C	-	-	C	-	-	C	-	C	-	C	C	-	-	C	-	C	C	C	-	-	C	C	C	C	-	C	C	C	C	C	-	-	C	C	-	-	C	C	C	C	C	C	C	-	C	C	-	-	C	C	C	C	C	C	C	-	C	-
clindamycin	C	I	C	-	C	-	-	-	C	-	-	-	I	C	-	C	C	-	C	-	-	-	C	-	C	-	C	-	C	C	C	C	C	C	-	-	C	C	C	-	C	-	C	C	-	-	C	-	C	C	C	C	-	C	C	C	-	-	C	-	-	C	C	-	C	C	C
co-trimoxazole	-	-	-	-	C	-	-	-	-	-	C	-	-	-	-	-	C	-	-	C	-	-	C	-	-	-	-	-	-	-	I	-	-	C	-	-	C	-	C	-	C	-	-	-	-	-	C	-	-	-	-	-	C	-	-	-	-	-	C	-	-	-	-	-	-	-	C
dexamethasone	C	C	-	-	C	-	-	-	C	-	C	C	C	C	-	-	-	-	C	-	-	-	C	-	-	-	C	-	C	C	-	-	C	C	-	C	C	-	C	C	C	C	-	-	-	C	C	-	C	C	C	C	-	-	-	C	-	-	C	-	-	C	-	-	C	C	-
digoxin	-	C	-	-	C	-	-	-	-	-	-	-	C	C	C	-	-	-	C	-	C	-	-	-	C	-	C	-	-	C	-	-	C	-	-	-	C	-	C	-	-	-	-	-	-	-	C	C	C	-	-	C	-	-	-	C	-	-	C	-	-	-	-	-	C	-	-
diltiazem	C	-	C	C	C	-	C	C	C	-	C	-	C	C	C	C	C	C	-	C	C	-	C	-	C	C	C	C	C	-	C	C	C	C	C	C	C	C	C	C	C	C	C	C	-	C	C	C	C	C	C	C	C	C	C	C	-	C	C	C	C	C	C	C	C	C	C
diphenhydramine	C	C	-	-	C	C	-	-	C	-	-	-	C	C	-	C	-	-	C	-	C	-	C	-	C	-	C	C	C	I	C	C	C	-	C	-	C	C	C	C	I	-	C	C	I	-	C	C	C	-	C	-	C	-	-	C	-	-	C	-	-	C	C	-	C	C	C
dobutamine	-	I	C	-	C	I	-	-	-	-	C	-	C	C	C	-	-	C	C	C	-	-	-	-	-	-	C	-	C	-	C	C	C	C	C	-	C	C	C	-	-	C	C	-	C	C	C	-	C	C	C	-	C	-	C	C	-	C	C	-	C	I	-	C	C	C	C
dolasetron	-	-	-	-	-	-	-	-	-	-	-	-	-	-	-	-	-	-	-	-	-	-	-	-	-	-	-	-	-	-	-	-	-	-	-	-	-	-	-	-	-	-	-	-	-	-	-	-	-	-	-	-	-	-	-	-	-	-	-	-	-	-	-	-	-	-	-
dopamine	-	C	C	C	C	-	C	-	C	-	C	-	C	C	C	C	C	-	C	C	-	-	-	-	C	C	C	-	C	-	-	C	C	C	-	-	C	C	C	C	C	-	C	-	C	C	C	-	C	C	C	-	C	-	C	C	C	C	C	C	C	C	C	C	C	-	C
enalapril	C	C	-	C	C	-	C	-	C	-	-	-	C	C	C	C	C	-	C	-	C	-	-	-	C	C	C	-	C	C	-	C	C	C	-	-	C	C	C	-	C	-	C	C	-	-	C	-	C	-	C	C	-	C	C	C	-	-	C	C	C	-	C	C	-	C	-	C
epinephrine	C	I	C	-	-	-	-	C	C	-	-	-	-	C	C	-	-	C	C	-	-	-	C	C	-	C	C	-	-	-	-	C	C	-	-	C	C	C	C	-	C	-	C	C	-	C	-	C	C	-	-	C	C	C	C	-	-	-	C	C	C	-	C	-	I	C
esmolol	C	C	C	-	-	-	-	-	C	-	-	C	-	C	C	C	-	C	-	C	-	-	C	-	C	-	-	-	I	C	C	-	C	C	-	C	C	-	C	C	C	-	C	C	-	C	C	-	C	C	C	-	C	C	-	C	-	-	C	-	-	C	C	C	C	C	C
esomeprazole	-	-	-	-	-	-	-	-	-	-	-	-	-	-	-	-	-	-	-	-	-	-	-	-	-	-	-	-	-	-	-	-	-	-	-	-	-	-	-	-	-	-	-	-	-	-	-	-	-	-	-	-	-	-	-	-	-	-	-	-	-	-	-	-	-	-	-
famotidine	-	C	-	-	C	C	-	-	C	C	-	-	C	-	-	C	-	C	C	-	C	-	C	-	C	C	C	-	C	C	C	C	C	C	C	C	C	C	C	C	-	C	-	C	-	C	C	-	C	C	C	C	C	-	C	C	-	C	-	I	C	C	C	C	C	-	-
fluconazole	C	C	-	-	C	-	-	-	C	-	-	I	C	-	C	I	-	-	I	C	-	-	C	-	-	-	-	-	C	C	-	-	-	-	I	-	-	-	-	-	C	-	C	-	-	-	C	-	-	C	C	-	-	C	-	C	-	-	C	-	-	C	C	C	C	C	C
furosemide	C	C	C	I	C	C	-	-	C	-	I	C	I	-	C	-	-	C	I	I	-	-	-	-	-	C	-	I	C	C	C	C	-	-	-	I	I	I	-	-	-	I	-	I	-	C	C	-	-	C	C	-	I	-	C	C	C	-	-	-	-	-	C	C	C	C	-
gentamicin	-	C	C	I	C	-	-	-	-	-	-	C	-	C	C	C	-	-	C	C	C	-	-	-	I	I	C	C	C	C	-	-	C	-	-	C	-	-	-	-	-	-	C	C	-	-	C	-	C	C	C	-	-	C	-	-	-	-	-	-	-	-	I	-	C	-	C
heparin	I	-	-	-	C	-	C	-	C	-	-	C	-	C	-	-	-	-	C	C	C	-	C	C	C	-	C	C	-	C	-	-	-	C	-	-	-	I	C	C	C	-	C	C	C	-	-	-	C	C	-	-	C	C	C	-	-	C	C	C	C	-	-	C	C	I	C
hydrocortisone	C	-	C	-	C	-	C	C	-	-	C	C	C	C	C	-	C	C	C	C	C	-	C	C	C	C	-	C	-	-	C	-	-	-	-	C	C	C	C	C	-	-	C	C	C	-	C	-	C	-	-	C	C	C	C	-	-	C	C	C	-	-	C	C	C	-	I	C
hydromorphine	C	-	-	-	C	-	-	-	-	-	C	-	C	-	C	C	C	-	-	C	-	-	C	-	-	-	-	-	C	-	-	C	-	-	-	C	-	-	C	C	C	C	-	-	-	-	C	C	C	-	-	C	-	C	-	-	C	-	-	C	-	-	C	-	I	C	C

From Hodgson BB, Kizior RJ: *Saunders nursing drug handbook 2007*, Philadelphia, 2007, WB Saunders.

IV Compatibilities *(continued)*

The IV compatibility table provides data when two or more medications are given into a Y-site of administration. The data in this table largely represent physical incompatibilities (e.g., haze, precipitate, change in color). Therapeutic incompatibilities have not been included, so when using the table, professional judgment should be exercised.

C Physically compatible via Y-site administration.
I Physically incompatible.

	amikacin	aminophylline	amiodarone	amphotericin B	aztreonam	bumatanide	calcium chloride	calcium gluconate	cefazolin	cefepime	ceftazidime	cimetidine	ciprofloxacin	cisatracurium	clindamycin	co-trimoxazole	dexamethasone	digoxin	diltiazem	diphenhydramine	dobutamine	dolasetron	dopamine	enalapril	epinephrine	esmolol	esomeprazole	famotidine	fluconazole	furosemide	gentamicin	heparin	hydrocortisone	hydromorphine	imipenem	insulin	labetalol	levofloxacin	lidocaine	linezolid	lorazepam	magnesium	meperidine	meropenem	methylprednisone	metoclopramide	metoprolol	metronidazole	midazolam	milrinone	morphine	multiple vitamin	nitroglycerin	nitroprusside	norepinephrine	ondansetron	pantoprazole	phenylephrine	piperacillin/tazobactam	potassium	procainamide	propofol	ranitidine	sodium bicarbonate	tobramycin	vancomycin	vecuronium
imipenem	-	-	-	-	C	-	-	-	-	-	-	-	-	C	-	-	-	-	C	-	-	-	-	-	-	-	-	C	I	-	-	C	-	-	-	C	-	-	-	C	I	-	I	-	-	-	-	-	I	I	-	-	-	-	-	C	-	-	-	-	-	C	-	-	-	-	-
insulin	-	I	C	-	C	C	-	-	C	-	-	C	-	-	-	-	-	-	-	-	-	-	I	-	-	C	-	C	-	-	C	-	C	-	C	-	I	I	-	-	-	C	C	C	-	C	-	-	C	C	C	-	C	C	I	-	-	-	-	C	-	C	-	-	C	C	-
labetolol	C	C	C	-	-	-	-	C	C	-	C	C	-	-	C	C	-	-	-	-	C	-	C	C	-	C	-	C	-	I	C	-	-	-	-	I	-	-	C	C	-	C	C	-	-	-	-	C	C	-	C	-	C	C	C	-	-	-	-	C	-	C	C	I	C	C	-
levofloxacin	C	C	-	-	-	-	-	-	-	-	-	C	-	-	C	-	C	-	-	-	C	-	C	-	C	-	-	-	-	I	C	I	-	-	-	I	-	-	C	C	C	-	-	-	-	C	-	-	-	-	C	-	I	I	-	-	-	C	-	-	-	-	-	C	-	C	-
lidocaine	C	C	C	-	-	-	C	C	-	-	-	C	C	C	-	-	C	C	C	C	C	-	C	C	-	C	-	C	-	-	-	C	C	C	-	-	C	C	-	C	-	C	C	-	C	C	-	C	-	C	C	-	C	C	-	-	-	C	-	C	C	-	C	-	-	-	-
linezolid	C	C	-	I	C	-	-	C	C	-	C	C	-	C	C	C	C	C	-	C	C	-	C	C	-	C	-	C	C	C	C	C	C	C	C	-	C	C	C	C	-	C	C	C	C	C	-	C	C	-	C	-	C	-	-	C	-	-	C	C	-	-	C	C	C	C	C
lorazepam	C	-	-	-	I	C	-	-	-	-	-	C	C	C	-	-	-	-	C	I	-	-	-	-	-	-	-	C	C	C	C	C	C	C	I	-	C	C	-	-	C	-	-	-	-	C	-	C	-	C	C	-	-	-	-	-	-	-	C	C	-	C	C	-	-	C	C
magnesium	C	-	-	-	C	-	I	-	C	-	-	-	I	C	-	-	-	-	-	-	-	-	-	C	-	C	-	C	-	-	C	C	-	C	-	C	C	-	-	C	-	-	C	C	-	C	-	C	-	C	C	-	-	C	-	C	-	-	C	C	-	C	-	I	C	C	-
meperidine	C	I	-	-	C	C	-	-	C	-	C	C	-	C	C	C	C	C	C	C	C	-	C	-	-	-	-	C	C	-	C	-	-	-	I	C	C	-	C	C	-	C	-	-	C	C	C	C	C	-	I	-	-	-	-	C	-	-	C	C	-	C	C	I	C	C	-
meropenem	-	C	-	I	-	-	-	-	-	-	-	C	-	-	-	-	C	C	-	C	C	-	C	C	-	-	-	-	C	C	C	C	-	-	-	C	-	-	-	C	-	C	-	-	-	C	-	-	-	C	C	I	-	-	C	I	-	-	-	-	-	-	C	-	-	C	-
methylprednisone	-	-	-	C	C	-	-	C	-	-	-	C	I	-	C	-	-	-	-	I	-	-	C	C	-	-	-	C	-	-	-	C	-	-	-	-	-	-	-	C	-	-	C	-	-	C	-	C	-	C	C	-	-	-	-	-	-	-	C	-	-	I	C	-	-	-	-
metoclopramide	-	-	C	-	C	-	-	-	-	-	-	C	C	C	C	-	-	-	C	-	-	-	-	-	-	-	-	C	C	I	-	-	-	-	-	C	-	C	C	C	-	C	C	C	C	-	-	-	-	-	C	C	-	-	-	C	-	C	C	C	-	C	C	I	-	-	-
metoprolol	-	-	-	-	-	-	-	-	-	-	-	-	-	-	-	-	-	-	-	-	-	-	-	-	-	-	-	-	-	-	-	-	-	-	-	-	-	-	-	-	-	-	C	-	-	-	-	-	-	-	C	-	-	-	-	-	-	-	-	-	-	-	-	-	-	-	-
metronidazole	C	C	C	-	I	-	-	-	-	-	C	C	C	C	C	-	-	-	C	-	-	-	-	C	-	C	-	-	C	-	C	C	C	C	-	-	C	-	-	C	C	C	C	-	C	-	-	-	C	C	C	-	-	-	-	-	-	-	C	-	-	-	-	-	C		-
midazolam	C	-	C	-	-	I	-	C	C	-	I	C	C	C	C	-	-	C	-	-	-	-	C	-	-	C	-	C	C	-	C	C	-	C	I	C	C	-	-	C	-	-	C	-	-	-	-	C	-	C	C	-	C	C	C	C	I	-	-	C	-	-	C	-	C	C	C
milrinone	C	-	-	-	-	C	C	C	C	C	C	C	C	-	C	-	C	C	C	-	C	-	C	-	C	-	-	-	-	I	C	C	-	-	I	C	-	-	C	-	C	C	-	C	C	-	-	C	C	-	C	-	C	C	C	-	-	-	C	C	-	C	C	C	C	C	C
morphine	C	C	C	-	C	C	C	-	C	-	C	C	-	C	C	C	C	C	C	C	C	-	C	C	-	C	-	C	C	I	C	-	C	-	-	C	C	C	C	C	C	C	I	C	C	C	C	C	C	C	-	-	-	C	C	C	-	-	C	C	-	-	C	-	C	C	C
multiple vitamin	-	-	-	-	-	-	-	-	-	-	-	-	-	-	-	-	C	-	C	-	C	C	C	-	C	-	-	-	-	-	C	-	-	-	-	-	-	-	-	-	-	-	-	I	-	C	-	-	-	-	-	-	-	-	-	-	-	-	-	-	-	-	-	-	-	-	-
nitroglycerin	-	C	C	-	-	-	-	-	-	-	-	-	-	C	-	-	-	-	C	-	C	-	C	-	-	C	-	C	C	C	-	-	-	-	-	C	C	I	C	C	-	-	-	-	-	-	-	-	C	C	-	-	-	C	-	-	-	-	-	-	-	C	C	-	-	-	-
nitroprusside	-	-	-	-	-	-	C	-	-	-	-	C	-	-	-	-	-	-	C	-	C	-	C	C	C	-	-	C	-	C	-	C	-	-	-	C	C	I	C	-	-	C	-	-	-	-	-	-	C	C	C	-	C	-	C	-	-	-	-	C	C	C	C	-	-	-	-
norepinephrine	-	-	C	-	-	-	-	-	-	-	-	-	-	C	-	-	-	-	C	-	C	-	C	-	-	C	-	C	-	-	-	-	-	-	-	I	C	-	-	-	-	-	-	C	-	-	-	-	C	C	C	-	-	C	-	-	-	-	-	-	-	C	C	-	-	-	-
ondansetron	C	I	-	I	C	-	-	-	C	-	C	C	-	C	C	-	-	-	-	C	-	-	C	-	-	-	-	C	C	I	C	C	C	C	C	-	-	-	-	C	-	C	C	I	-	C	-	-	C	-	C	-	-	-	-	-	-	-	C	C	-	C	C	I	-	-	-
pantoprazole	-	-	-	-	-	-	-	-	-	-	-	-	-	-	-	-	-	-	-	-	-	-	-	-	-	-	-	-	-	-	-	-	-	-	-	-	-	-	-	-	-	-	-	-	-	-	-	-	I	-	-	-	-	-	-	-	-	-	-	-	-	-	-	-	-	-	-
phenylephrine	-	C	C	-	-	-	-	C	-	-	-	-	-	C	-	-	-	-	-	C	C	-	-	-	-	-	-	C	-	-	-	C	-	-	-	-	-	C	C	-	-	-	-	-	-	C	-	-	-	-	-	-	-	-	-	-	-	-	-	-	-	-	-	-	C	C	-
piperacillin/tazobactam	-	C	-	I	C	C	-	C	-	-	-	C	-	-	C	-	C	-	-	C	I	-	C	C	-	C	-	I	C	C	-	C	C	C	-	-	-	-	-	C	C	C	C	-	C	C	-	C	-	C	C	-	-	-	-	C	-	-	-	C	-	-	C	C	-	-	-
potassium	C	C	C	-	C	-	-	C	C	-	C	C	C	C	-	-	C	C	C	-	-	-	C	C	-	C	-	C	C	-	-	C	-	C	-	C	C	-	C	C	C	C	C	-	-	C	-	-	C	C	C	-	-	C	-	C	-	-	C	-	C	C	C	C	-	-	-
procainamide	-	C	C	-	-	-	-	C	-	-	-	-	-	C	-	-	-	-	-	C	C	-	-	-	-	C	-	C	-	-	-		C	-	-	-	-	-	C	-	-	-	-	-	-	-	-	-	-	-	-	-	-	C	-	-	-	-	-	C	-	C	C	-	-	C	-
propofol	I	C	-	I	C	C	I	C	C	-	C	C	C	-	C	-	C	C	-	C	C	-	C	C	C	C	-	C	C	C	I	C	C	C	C	C	C	-	-	-	C	C	C	-	I	C	-	-	-	C	-	-	C	C	C	C	-	-	-	C	C	-	C	C	I	C	-
rantidine	C	C	-	I	C	-	-	-	C	-	C	-	C	C	C	-	C	C	C	-	C	-	C	C	C	C	-	-	C	C	C	C	-	-	-	-	C	-	C	C	C	-	C	C	C	C	-	-	C	C	C	-	C	C	C	C	-	-	C	C	C	C	-	-	-	C	-
sodium bicarbonate	C	C	I	-	C	-	I	I	-	-	I	-	-	-	-	-	-	-	-		I	-	I	-	-	-	-	C	-	C	-	C	C	I	-	-	I	C	-	C	-	I	I	-	-	I	-	-	-	C	-	-	-	-	-	I	-	-	C	C	-	C	-	-	-	I	-
tobramycin	-	-	C	-	C	-	-	C	C	I	-	-	C	C	-	-	-	-	C	-	-	-	-	C	-	C	-	-	C	C	-	I	-	C	-	C	C	-	-	C	-	C	C	-	-	-	-	C	C	C	C	-	-	-	-	-	-	-	-	-	-	I	-	-	-	-	-
vancomycin	C	I	C	-	-	-	I	C	-	I	-	C	-	C	-	-	I	-	C	C	-	-	-	C	I	C	-	C	C	-	-	-	I	C	-	C	C	C	-	C	C	C	C	C	-	-	-	-	C	C	C	-	-	-	-	C	-	C	-	-	C	C	C	I	-	-	C
vecuronium	-	C	-	-	-	-	-	-	C	-	-	C	-	-	-	C	-	-	-	-	C	-	C	-	C	C	-	-	C	-	C	C	C	-	-	-	-	-	-	C	C	-	-	-	-	-	-	-	C	C	C	-	C	C	-	-	-	-	-	-	-	C	C	-	-	C	-

methylprednisolone

Companion CD Contents*

NCLEX® Examination Review Questions

450 NCLEX questions cover key pharmacology concepts, cardiovascular drugs, antiinfective and antiinflammatory drugs, gastrointestinal drugs, and more!

Pharmacology Animations

- Acute Myocardial Infarction
- Adenosine Infusion, Cardiac Effects
- Agonists/Antagonists
- Amiodarone, Antidarrhythmic Drug; Treatment of Ventricular Fibrillation
- Amiodarone Treatment for Ventricular Tachycardia
- Atropine Therapy for Sinus Bradycardia
- Cytochrome P-450 Drug Metabolism
- Diltiazem Injection, Cardiac Effects
- Distribution: Fat- vs. Water-Soluble Drugs
- Drug Movement Through the Body
- Epinephrine and CPR
- Half-Life of Intravenously Administered Ampicillin
- Heparin for Acute Coronary Syndrome
- Heparin for Atrial Fibrillation
- Impact of Surface Area
- Normal Electrophysiology
- Nursing, Medical, and Pharmacology Domains
- Overview of Pharmacokinetics: Oral Administration
- Passive Diffusion
- Patient Noncompliance
- Pharmacokinetic Profiles: Normal, Renal Failure, and Hemodialysis
- Receptor Interaction
- Renin-Angiotensin in Control of Blood Pressure
- Thrombolytic Drugs; Clot Dissolving Drugs
- Time to Steady State
- Time to Steady State: Starting and Stopping Drug

Medication Errors Checklists

- Administering Medications
- Appropriate Documentation of Medication Administration
- Assessing Patient Response
- Interpreting Medication Orders
- Preparing Medications
- Procedural Safeguards
- Reporting Medication Errors
- Reviewing Medication Orders
- Transcribing Medication Orders

IV Therapy Checklists

- Adding Medication to an Intravenous Bag, Bottle, or Volume Control Set
- Administering Bolus Medication Through a Continuous IV
- Administering Medication Through an Intermittent IV (Saline Lock)
- Administering Medication via a Piggyback or Secondary Set
- Changing the Container of an Existing Intravenous Solution

Category Catchers

- ACE Inhibitors
- Aminoglycoside Antibiotics
- Angiotensin II Receptor Blockers
- Beta Adrenergic Blocking Drugs
- Beta Agonist (Sympathomimetic) Bronchodilators
- Beta Lactam Antibiotics
- Calcium Channel Blockers
- Cardiac Glycosides
- HMG-CoA Reductase Inhibitors
- Hydantoin Antiepileptic Drugs
- Insulin Therapy
- Loop Diuretics
- NSAIDs
- Opioid Analgesics
- Oral Anticoagulant Drugs
- Parenteral Anticoagulant Drugs
- Sodium Channel Blockers
- SSRIs
- Sulfonamide Antibiotics
- Thrombolytic Drugs

1 oz = 30 ml

1 ml = 1 cc

Calculators

- Absolute Neutrophil Count (ANC)
- Body Mass Index (BMI)
- Body Surface Area (BSA)
- Body Surface Area—Pediatric
- Calculated Serum Osmolality
- Corrected Phenytoin
- Corrected QT
- Corrected Serum Calcium
- Corrected Serum Sodium
- Creatinine Clearance—Estimated (Cockroft-Gault)
- Creatinine Clearance—Measured
- Fluid Deficit
- Glomerular Filtration Rate (MDRD)
- Heart Rate
- Ideal Body Weight (IBW)—Females
- Ideal Body Weight (IBW)—Males
- IV Infusion Rate
- LDL
- Predicted Peak Flow (PPF)—Females
- Predicted Peak Flow (PPF)—Males
- Risk Assessment Tool for Falls
- Six-Item Cognitive Impairment Test
- Sodium Deficit

Answer Key

- Answers to Critical Thinking Activities in the book
- Answers to Case Studies in the book

Audio Glossary

- Chapter-by-chapter pronunciations for many key terms in the book

---

*Companion CD content prepared by Dorothy Mathers, RN, MSN. Selected pharmacology animations prepared by Ed Tessier, PharmD, MPH, BCPS.

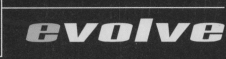

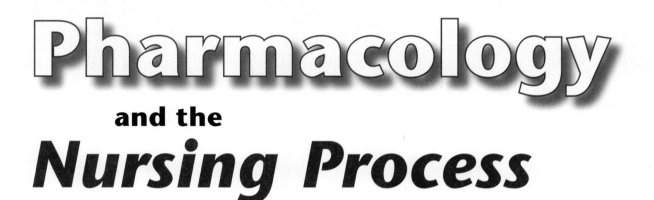

Pharmacology
and the
Nursing Process

Pharmacology
and the
Nursing Process

Fifth Edition

Linda Lane Lilley, RN, PhD

Associate Professor Emeritus and University Professor
Old Dominion University
School of Nursing
Norfolk, Virginia

Scott Harrington, PharmD

Harrington Health Informatics, LLC
Tucson, Arizona
Director of Pharmacy, Northern Cochise Community Hospital
Willcox, Arizona

Julie S. Snyder, MSN, RN, BC

Adjunct Faculty
Old Dominion University
School of Nursing
Norfolk, Virginia

With Study Skills content by

Diane Savoca

Coordinator of Student Transition
St. Louis Community College at Florissant Valley
St. Louis, Missouri

With special thanks to

Richard E. Lake, BS, MS, MLA

for his contribution to the first edition Study Skills content

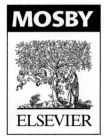

MOSBY

ELSEVIER

MOSBY
ELSEVIER

11830 Westline Industrial Drive
St. Louis, MO 63146

PHARMACOLOGY AND THE NURSING PROCESS,   ISBN: 978-0-323-04486-8
FIFTH EDITION
Copyright © 2007 by Mosby, Inc., an affiliate of Elsevier Inc.

Previous editions copyrighted 2005, 2001, 1999, and 1996.

Library of Congress Control Number: 2007921015

Acquisitions Editor: Kristin Geen
Developmental Editor: Jamie Horn
Publishing Services Manager: Jeff Patterson
Senior Project Manager: Clay S. Broeker
Text Designer: Paula Ruckenbrod
Cover Design Direction: Paula Ruckenbrod

Printed in Canada

Last digit is the print number: 9   8   7   6   5   4   3   2

About the Authors

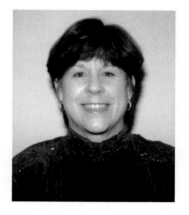

Linda Lane Lilley, RN, PhD

Linda Lilley received her diploma from Norfolk General School of Nursing, her BSN from the University of Virginia, her Master of Science (Nursing) from Old Dominion University, and her PhD in Nursing from George Mason University. As an Associate Professor Emeritus and University Professor at Old Dominion University, her teaching experience in nursing education spans over 25 years, including almost 20 years at Old Dominion University. Linda's teaching expertise includes drug therapy and the nursing process, adult nursing, physical assessment, fundamentals in nursing, oncology nursing, nursing theory, and trends in health care. The awarding of the University's most prestigious title of University Professor reflects her teaching excellence as a tenured faculty member. She has also been a two-time university nominee for the State Council of Higher Education in Virginia award for excellence in teaching, service, and scholarship. While at Old Dominion University, Linda mentored and taught undergraduate and graduate students as well as registered nurses returning for their BSN. She continues to serve as a member on dissertation committees with the College of Health Sciences. Since retirement in 2005, Linda has continued to be active in nursing, with involvement in the American Nurses Association, Virginia Nurses Association, Sigma Theta Tau International, Phi Kappa Phi, and other professional organizations. Linda's research interests include the identification of factors affecting recruitment and retention of minority students in baccalaureate schools of nursing. Dr. Lilley's professional service varies, having served as a consultant with school nurses in the city of Virginia Beach and as a member on the City of Virginia Beach's Health Advisory Board. Linda was also an appointed member on the national advisory panel on medication errors prevention with the U.S. Pharmacopeia in Rockville, Maryland. Linda currently serves as a member of the Community Health Services Advisory Board, City of Virginia Beach. She continues to educate nursing students and professional nurses about drug therapy and the nursing process and offers educational sessions about medication safety to the elderly.

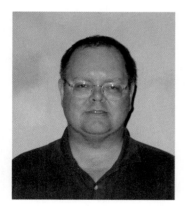

Scott Harrington, PharmD

Scott Harrington received his Associate of Science in Pharmacy Technology with High Honors from Pima Community College, Tucson, Arizona, in 1991. He then worked as both an outpatient and inpatient pharmacy technician while completing his Doctor of Pharmacy degree at the University of Arizona College of Pharmacy, which he received in 1997. He then completed two postdoctoral residency training programs. The first was a specialty residency in Pharmacocybernetics at Creighton University in Omaha, Nebraska, which he completed in 1998. The second was an additional specialty residency in Drug Information and Pharmaceutical Informatics at the University of California—San Francisco medical center and First DataBank in San Bruno, California, which he completed in 1999. Since that time he has worked in a variety of settings, including outpatient retail pharmacy where he also compounded customized prescriptions. He has since worked in hospital pharmacy and has served as a proofreader and content reviewer for Elsevier since 1999. He is now Director of Pharmacy for Northern Cochise Community Hospital in Willcox, Arizona, and most recently a staff pharmacist for Walgreens Pharmacy. Scott also regularly offers public education regarding medication use in mental illness during public outreach support groups at the office of the National Alliance for the Mentally Ill of Southern Arizona in Tucson. Scott's professional affiliations include the American Society of Health-System Pharmacy, the American Society for Consultant Pharmacists, the American Pharmacists Association, the Society for Technical Communicators, the American Medical Informatics Association, and the American College of Clinical Pharmacy. Scott is also a member of American MENSA.

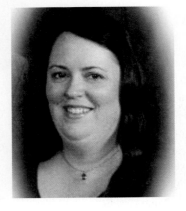

Julie S. Snyder, MSN, RN, BC

Julie Snyder received her diploma from Norfolk General Hospital School of Nursing and her BSN and MSN from Old Dominion University. After working in medical-surgical nursing for over 10 years, she began working in nursing staff development and community education. After 8 years, she transferred to teaching in a school of nursing, and over the past 10 years she has taught fundamentals of nursing, pharmacology, physical assessment, gerontologic nursing, and adult medical-surgical nursing. She has been certified by the ANCC in Nursing Continuing Education and Staff Development and currently holds ANCC certification in Medical-Surgical Nursing. She is a member of Sigma Theta Tau International and was inducted into Phi Kappi Phi as Outstanding Alumni for Old Dominion University. She has worked for Elsevier as a reviewer and ancillary writer since 1997. Julie's professional service has included serving on the Virginia Nurses' Association Continuing Education Committee, serving as Educational Development Committee chair for the Epsilon Chi chapter of Sigma Theta Tau, serving as an item writer for the ANCC, working with a regional hospital educators' group, and serving as a consultant on various projects for local hospital education departments.

Reviewers

Julie Painter, RN, MSN, OCN
Clinical Nurse Specialist/Adult Nurse
  Practitioner
Clinical Practice Education and
  Research
Community Health Network
Indianapolis, Indiana

Brenda Pavill, RN, PhD
Associate Professor of Nursing
College Misericordia
Dallas, Pennsylvania

*Kim L. Paxton, MSN, ANP,
APRN-BC*
Assistant Professor
College of Nursing
Cardinal Stritch University
Milwaukee, Wisconsin

Joan Reale, PhD, RN
Professor of Nursing
Carlow University
Pittsburgh, Pennsylvania

Randolph Regal, BS, PharmD
Clinical Assistant Professor/Clinical
  Pharmacist
College of Pharmacy, Department of
  Pharmacy Services
University of Michigan
Ann Arbor, Michigan

*Bruce Austin Scott, MSN,
APRN, BC*
Nursing Instructor
San Joaquin Delta College
Stockton, California

Roberta Secrest, PhD, PharmD
Global Media Communications
Eli Lilly and Company
Indianapolis, Indiana

Sarah Steele, BSN, MSN
Assistant Professor
Allen College
Waterloo, Iowa

Darlene Thomay, RN, BA, DNC
Medical Specialties Clinics
Metrohealth
Cleveland, Ohio

Sarah Reidunn Tvedt, MS, RN
Nursing Education Specialist of Cardiac
  Surgery
Mayo Clinic
Rochester, Minnesota

*Kathleen Dorman Wagner RN,
MSN, EdD (c)*
Lecturer
College of Nursing
University of Kentucky
Lexington, Kentucky

Angela S. Wilson, PhD, RN, BC
Associate Professor and Department
  Chair
Nursing Department
University of Virginia College at Wise
Wise, Virginia

Derek Wood, RN, BC, MS
Instructor of Nursing
Aims Community College
Greeley, Colorado

Thomas Worms, RN, MSN
Professor of Nursing
Truman College
Chicago, Illinois

Preface

Now in its fifth edition, *Pharmacology and the Nursing Process* provides the most current and clinically relevant information in an appealing, understandable, and practical format. The accessible size, readable writing style, and full-color design are ideal for today's busy nursing student. This text takes a unique approach to the study of pharmacology by presenting study skills content that will help students understand and learn the particularly demanding subject of pharmacology. Each part begins with a Study Skills Tips section, which features a discussion of researched and proven study skills and applies the discussion to the content in that part. Students are encouraged to use research-based study skills to enhance their study of pharmacology and nursing.

MARKET RESEARCH

This text incorporates many suggestions from focus group participants composed of nursing instructors from 2-, 3-, and 4-year degree programs in Chicago, Philadelphia, and Los Angeles. The focus groups assessed changes that have occurred in the teaching of pharmacology and determined what was needed to better teach pharmacology to nursing students. Based on faculty descriptions of their courses and students, these general recommendations were made:

- Accommodate the reading styles and abilities of the growing number of nontraditional nursing students.
- Increase the use of tables, boxes, illustrations, graphics, and other visually oriented approaches.
- Use color to increase interest and highlight important drug interactions and processes.

We have taken a truly collaborative approach with this text. The concerns raised by faculty members in market research have been addressed, as have additional improvements suggested by faculty members who served as reviewers or consultants, either formally or informally, throughout the manuscript's development and by the authors and editors of this text.

ORGANIZATION

This book includes 59 chapters presented in 10 parts and organized by body system. The 9 concepts chapters in Part 1 lay a solid foundation for the subsequent drug units and address the following topics:

- Study skills tips applied to learning pharmacology
- The nursing process and drug therapy
- Pharmacologic principles
- Life span considerations related to pharmacology
- Cultural, legal, and, ethical considerations
- Preventing and responding to medication errors
- Patient education and drug therapy
- Over-the-counter drugs and herbal and dietary supplements
- Substance abuse
- Photo atlas of drug administration techniques, including over 100 illustrations and photographs

Parts 2 through 10 present pharmacology and nursing management in a traditional body systems/drug function framework. This approach facilitates learning by grouping functionally related drugs and drug groups. It provides an effective means to integrate the content into medical-surgical or adult health nursing courses or for teaching pharmacology in a separate course.

The 50 drug chapters in these parts constitute the main portion of the book. Drugs are presented in a consistent format with an emphasis on drug groups and key similarities and differences among the drugs in each group. Each chapter is subdivided into two discussions, beginning with a complete discussion of pharmacology and a brief review of pathophysiology of disease processes, followed by a comprehensive yet succinct discussion of the nursing process. Pharmacology is presented for each drug group in a consistent format:

- Mechanism of Action and Drug Effects
- Indications
- Contraindications
- Adverse Effects (often including Toxicity and Management of Overdose)
- Interactions
- Dosages

Drug group discussions are followed by Drug Profiles, or brief narrative capsules of individual drugs in the class or group, including Pharmacokinetics tables for each drug. Key drugs, or prototypical drugs within a class, are identified with the ▶ symbol for easy identification. These individual drug profiles are followed by a Nursing Process discussion relating to the entire drug group. The nursing content is covered in the following functional nursing process format:

- Assessment
- Nursing Diagnoses
- Planning (including Goals and Outcome Criteria)
- Implementation
- Evaluation

At the end of each nursing process section is a Patient Teaching Tips box that summarizes key points for nursing students and/or nurses to include in the education of patients about their medications, with attention to how the drugs work, possible interactions, adverse effects, and other information related to the safe and effective use of the drug(s). The role of the nurse as patient educator and advocate continues to grow in importance in professional practice; thus there is emphasis of this key content in each chapter in this edition.

Additionally, each part begins with a Study Skills Tips section that presents a study skills topic and relates it to the unit being discussed. Topics include time management, note taking, studying, test taking, and others. This unique approach to teaching pharmacology is intended to aid students who find pharmacology difficult and to provide a tool that may prove beneficial throughout their nursing school careers. Coverage of this study skills content is limited to the beginning of each part so that instructors who choose not to require their students to read this material can easily eliminate it. However, this arrangement of content may be beneficial to faculty members who teach pharmacology through an integrated approach because it helps the student identify key content and concepts. This arrangement also facilitates location of content for either required or optional reading.

NEW TO THIS EDITION

Most importantly, the pharmacology and nursing content has been thoroughly revised to reflect the latest drug information and research. This includes:

- A new focus on the **role of prioritization** in nursing care
- An **increased focus on drug classes** to help students acquire a better knowledge of how various drugs work in the body, allowing them to apply this knowledge to individual drugs
- The **antibiotics and antineoplastics chapters divided** into smaller chapters to help make the complex content easier to grasp
- **Expanded coverage of biochemical and terrorism agents and cultural aspects** of drug therapy
- **Improved readability** throughout the text to make the content more understandable than ever
  New features include:
- **Pharmacokinetic Bridge to the Nursing Process** sections that transition from the pharmacology content into the nursing process content by applying key pharmacokinetic information to nursing practice
- **State-of-the-art animations** on the companion CD and Evolve website to help students understand and retain information more easily by depicting important pharmacologic concepts visually (topics include agonists/antagonists, cytochrome P-450 drug metabolism, drug movement through the body, medication administration techniques, and much more)
- **Evidence-Based Practice** boxes that summarize current research and emphasize findings relevant to professional nursing practice and safe and effective drug therapy
- **Laboratory Values Related to Drug Therapy** boxes that highlight specific laboratory tests applicable to drug therapy
- **Preventing Medication Errors** boxes that reinforce concepts introduced in the medication errors chapter and relate them to specific common errors that occur in clinical practice
- **NCLEX® Examination Review Questions** at the end of each chapter that now include examples of Alternate Item questions, feature a new focus on application and analysis, and incorporate prioritization
- **Answers to the NCLEX® Examination Review Questions** now included in the book to facilitate student review
- **Companion CD** updated and including the following:
  - 450 NCLEX examination review questions
  - 26 State-of-the-art animations (*10 NEW!*)
  - IV therapy and medication errors checklists
  - Category Catcher handouts with the need-to-know information about each drug category (*NEW!*)
  - An audio glossary
  - Various calculators
  - Answers to critical thinking activities and case studies from the book

FEATURES

This book includes various pedagogic features that prepare the student for important content covered in each chapter and encourage review and reinforcement of that content. Chapter opener pedagogy includes the following:

- Learning Objectives
- e-Learning Activities boxes listing related content and exercises on the Companion CD and Evolve website
- Summary boxes listing the Drug Profiles in the chapter with page number references
- Glossaries of key terms with definitions and page number references (glossary terms are bolded in the narrative to emphasize this essential terminology)
  The following features appear at the end of each chapter:
- Patient Teaching Tips related to drug therapy
- Points to Remember boxes summarizing key points
- NCLEX Examination Review Questions, with answers provided upside-down at the bottom of the section for quick and easy review
- Critical Thinking Activities, with answers provided on the Evolve website
  Special features that appear throughout the text include the following:
- Cultural Implications boxes
- Herbal Therapies and Dietary Supplements boxes
- Legal and Ethical Principles boxes
- Life Span Considerations boxes for The Pediatric Patient and also The Elderly Patient
- Case Studies, with answers provided on the Companion CD and Evolve website, as well as in the Instructor's Manual
- Dosages tables listing generic and trade names, pharmacologic class, usual dosage ranges, and indications for the drugs
  For a more comprehensive listing of the special features, please see the last page and inside back cover of the book.
  Additional special features in this book include the following:
- A tear-out IV Compatibilities Chart that provides students with a portable reference on incompatible drugs administered intravenously
- A Bibliography listing references for more information

COLOR

The first edition of this book was the first full-color pharmacology text for nursing students. Faculty members suggested that color be used in both a functionally and visually appealing manner to more fully engage students in this typically demanding yet important content. Full color is used throughout to do the following:

- Highlight important content
- Illustrate how drugs work in the body in numerous anatomic and drug process color figures
- Improve the visual appearance of the content to make it more engaging and appealing to today's more visually sophisticated reader

We believe that the use of color in these ways significantly improves students' involvement and understanding of pharmacology.

SUPPLEMENTAL RESOURCES

A comprehensive ancillary package is available to students and instructors using *Pharmacology and the Nursing Process.* The following supplemental resources have been thoroughly revised for this edition and can significantly assist teaching and learning of pharmacology:

Study Guide

The carefully prepared student workbook includes the following:
- Study Tips Guide that reinforces the study skills explained in the text and provides a "how to" guide to applying test-taking strategies
- Worksheets for each chapter with multiple-choice questions, critical thinking and application questions, case studies, and other activities
- In-depth case studies followed by related critical thinking questions
- A new focus on prioritization to help students identify the most important nursing diagnoses and interventions
- A special, updated Overview of Dosage Calculations with helpful tips for calculating doses, sample drug labels, practice problems, and a quiz
- Answers to all questions provided in the back of the book to enable self-study

Instructor's Electronic Resource

This CD product includes the following main components:
- **Instructor's Manual** that features overview summaries, key terms, learning objectives, chapter outlines, teaching strategies, critical thinking activities, learning activities, additional resources listing, case studies, quizzes, and answer key
- **ExamView Test Bank** that features approximately 625 NCLEX-format test questions (including Alternate Item questions) with text page references, rationales (*NEW!*), and answers coded for NCLEX Client Need category, nursing process, and cognitive level; the ExamView program allows instructors to create new tests; edit, add, and delete test questions; sort questions by NCLEX category, cognitive level, and nursing process step; and administer and grade online tests
- **Image Collection** with approximately 220 full-color images from the book for instructors to use in lectures
- **PowerPoint Lecture Slides** containing more than 2200 customizable text slides for instructors to use in lectures; the presentations include applicable illustrations from the Image Collection
- **i-Clicker Question Suite** developed especially for use with audience response systems

Evolve Website

Located at *http://evolve.elsevier.com/Lilley*, the Evolve website for this book includes the following:
For students:
- Printable Nursing Care Plans related to drug therapy and the nursing process
- A variety of supplemental resources, including a list of Canadian trade names and generic equivalents; a list of common formulas, weights, and equivalents; and a summary of the nonpharmacologic treatment of cardiac dysrhythmias
- Content Updates
- Frequently Asked Questions

- An updated library of WebLinks for each chapter
- Bonus medication administration animations
- Access to *Elsevier ePharmacology Update*, an online newsletter updated twice each semester and featuring the latest drug news, warnings, precautions, and more

For instructors:
- Course Management System
- Teaching Tips
- Access to all student resources listed above
- Online access to the Instructor's Manual, Test Bank, PowerPoint Lecture Slides, Image Collection, and i-Clicker Question Suite

Pharmacology Online

This dynamic, three-part online course resource is designed to accompany *Pharmacology and the Nursing Process.* It includes the following:
- **16 self-study modules**, including 12 modules covering the basic principles of pharmacology, a concise *Drug Calculation Review* module, and three new *Drug Content Review* modules; the self-study modules include an integrated *Online Drug Handbook* and *Audio Glossary,* with pronunciations for more than 1400 drug names and terms; they also include a rich variety of interactive activities and animations, as well as a quiz to ensure content mastery
- **Unit resources,** including:
  - **26 case studies** using true-to-life clinical scenarios to promote "learning by doing," with consequences for both correct and incorrect choices, plus feedback for incorrect choices
  - **220 interactive learning activities,** offering a challenging, game-like review of drug essentials
  - **20 care planning activities** that challenge you to create complete care plans
  - **Practice quizzes for the NCLEX-RN® examination** in each chapter that help you prepare for the NCLEX exam with its increased emphasis on pharmacology
  - **Flashcards** that offer a handy, easy-to-use way to memorize information about major drugs, drug classes, and pharmacologic principles
- **Library of Supplemental Resources** includes unique *Roadside Assistance* video clips, all of the animations from the self-study modules, a complete audio glossary, and more; the *Roadside Assistance* video clips use humor, analogy, and memorable visuals to help clarify core pharmacology concepts in a way you'll never forget!

Evolve Select

This exciting new program is available to faculty who adopt a number of Elsevier texts, including *Pharmacology and the Nursing Process.* Evolve Select is an integrated electronic study center consisting of a collection of textbooks made available electronically in CD format. It is carefully designed to "extend" the textbook for an easier and more efficient teaching and learning experience. It includes study aids such as highlighting, e-note taking, and cut and paste capabilities. Even more importantly, it allows students and instructors to do a comprehensive search within the specific text or across a number of titles. Please check with your Elsevier sales representative for more information.

Acknowledgments

This book truly has been a collaborative effort. We wish to thank the instructors who provided input on an ongoing basis throughout the development of the first, second, third, and fourth editions. In addition, we would like to thank the following people: Rick Brady, Dottie Mathers, Chuck Dresner, Judith Myers, Ted Huff, Donald O'Connor, Linda Wendling, Ken Turnbough, Greg McVicar, Anthony Saranita, and Susan Orf. We thank Carolyn Duke and the Saint Louis University School of Nursing for their assistance and cooperation. Thanks also to Chesapeake General Hospital for assistance with the fourth edition photo shoot.

We thank Kristin Geen and Jamie Horn for their contributions and support throughout the fourth edition. We are also grateful to Jeff Patterson and Clay Broeker for very capably guiding the project through to publication and to Paula Ruckenbrod for her effective design. Diane Savoca lent her study skills expertise and has updated the unique and appropriate feature for students, and for her collaboration we are most grateful. Finally we thank Joe Albanese for his contributions to the first edition and Bob Aucker for his contributions to the first three editions of the book.

Linda thanks her husband Les, daughter Karen, and mother-in-law Mary Anne Lilley for their constant support and encouragement. Long hours and time spent researching and writing has preempted time with family, but they have been there through all five editions. Linda wishes to dedicate this book to her parents, John and Thelma Lane, who passed away during the fourth edition, and to her father-in-law, J.C. Lilley, who passed away during the last drafts of the fifth edition. Their memory continues to serve as inspiration and motivation for Linda's work with this book. Students and graduates of Old Dominion University School of Nursing have been eager to provide feedback and support, beginning with the Class of 1990 and continuing through the class of 2005. Without their participation, the book would not have been so user-friendly and helpful to students beginning the study of drug therapy and subsequently applying this knowledge to nursing practice. Linda attributes her successes and accomplishments to a strong sense of purpose, faith, family and appreciation for the light-hearted side of life. To Jibby Baucom, Linda offers many thanks because without her recommendation to Mosby, Inc., the book would never have been developed. Robin Carter and Kristin Geen have been constant resources and more than just editors with Elsevier; they have been sources of strength and encouragement. Working with Jamie Horn has been positive, and her calming nature and vision to succeed will forever be appreciated. The fifth edition also involved Clay Broeker, who has been a tremendous resource with editorial issues; his contributions to this edition have been strong and forward-thinking. Elsevier has shared some of its best employees with Linda beginning with day one of the first edition; for that, Linda is most thankful.

Scott extends his thanks to his fellow staff members at Northern Cochise Community Hospital. Thank you for all of your consultations and questions that continuously help make me a better pharmacist. Thanks to both hospital staff and citizens of Willcox and Tucson, Arizona, as well as family and friends, who have been kind enough to show interest in this project and ask me how it was coming along. Your interest and enthusiasm helped me down the long road to completion. Thank you also to the staff and volunteers of the National Alliance for the Mentally Ill of Southern Arizona (NAMISA), where I continue to grow and learn through volunteer work, for your continued support and encouragement for this and other endeavors and for allowing me to be a part of your team as well. Very special thanks to my dear friend Gerry Bovell who allowed me to work on this project for many months at his home and congratulated me as I finished each chapter. Both he and my other friend Ed Thorpe also sometimes brought me food. Thanks to both of them for their support and encouragement. Lastly, I offer heartfelt thanks to my mother and father Bonnie and John Harrington who granted me this life to begin with. My mother has an amazing heart and my father has an amazing mind. I believe that I was fortunate enough to inherit some of the best of both.

Julie thanks her husband, Jonathan, her daughter Emily, and her parents, Willis and Jean Simmons, for their unfailing support and encouragement. They were all patient despite the long hours spent "at the computer" for revisions. Thanks also to those who participated in the fourth edition photo shoot. At Chesapeake General Hospital, Doug Crowe in the Pharmacy Department has been an unending source of answers and support. Thanks to Kristin Geen, Jamie Horn, and others at Elsevier for keeping the project organized and on track, as well as for providing all the support needed for such a project. Thanks also to each student who has provided feedback and comments on the text and study aids. Deep appreciation goes to Dr. Linda L. Lilley for her encouragement and mentoring over the years. Lastly, the support and encouragement of family and friends is vital to projects like this, so thanks and gratitude to all.

Finally, to those who teach, although your work may seem to go unnoticed or unappreciated, your impact will always be remembered in the accomplishments of your students. Your inspiration and motivation shape the future.

We always welcome comments from instructors and students who use this book so that we may continue to make improvements and be responsive to your needs in future editions. Please send any comments you may have in care of the publisher.

Contents

PART 3

PART 4

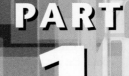

Pharmacology Basics

STUDY SKILLS TIPS

- *Introduction to Study Skills Concepts*
- *PURR*
- *Pharmacology Basics*

INTRODUCTION TO STUDY SKILLS CONCEPTS

What to study? When to study? How much to study? How to study? In the best of worlds, every student would have all the skills necessary to be effective in all academic areas. Unfortunately, many students do not know how to study effectively or have developed techniques that work well in some circumstance but not in others. The purpose of this Study Skills Tips is to introduce you to the steps to follow in learning text and maintaining focus on the appropriate material. This section also offers some specific examples for selected chapters in Part 1 to help you apply the study techniques and strategies discussed here.

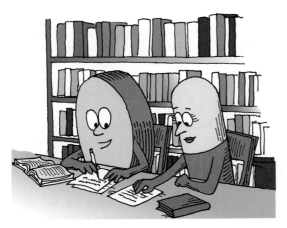

Extensive study skills covering time management, lecture note taking, mastering of the text, preparation for and taking of examinations, establishing effective study groups and development of vocabulary are presented in the *Study Guide* that accompanies this text. These tools are important to any student, but in challenging technical areas such as nursing and pharmacology, they become even more valuable. The techniques described here

and in the *Study Guide* will not necessarily make learning easy, but they will help you achieve your goals as a student.

PURR

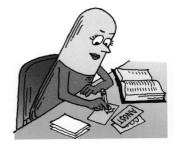

PURR is a handy mnemonic device representing a four-step process that will lead to mastery of material. These steps are as follows:

- *Prepare*
- *Understand*
- *Rehearse*
- *Review*

PURR has positive and negative aspects. The negative is that it requires that you go through every chapter four times. The good news is that you are not going to actually *read* the chapter four times. You are only going to *go through* it four times. Only one of those times is a slow, careful, intensive reading. The other trips through the chapter are much quicker. The first time you go through the chapter should only take 5 or 10 minutes. Each time you go through the chapter, you are processing the information in distinctly different ways. The PURR approach will enhance your learning, and if you use it from the first assignment on, you will find that it takes you less time than you were spending before you adopted the PURR approach to learn what you need.

Prepare

Reading the text, like any complex process, is not something to dive into without thought and planning. *Pharmacology and the Nursing Process* is organized to help you learn the material, but you have to take advantage of what the authors have done for you to facilitate this. Preparing to read means setting goals and objectives for your own learning, but the tools you need to help you do this are already in place. Look at the opening pages of any chapter in the text and you will see a standard structure.

Every chapter begins with a **title.** Learn to use the title as the first step in preparing to learn. Chapter 4 is entitled Cultural, Legal, and

Ethical Considerations. This instantly identifies what the chapter is about. Do not start reading immediately; instead think about the title for a few seconds. Are there any unfamiliar terms? If your answer is "no," great. If it is "yes," then you already have some focus for your reading because you know you will need to learn the unfamiliar terms and their meanings.

The next feature of every chapter is the **objectives.** You need objectives for learning, and the authors have anticipated this. Read the objectives actively. Do not just look at the words; think about the objectives. Ask yourself the following questions: What do I already know about this material? How do these objectives relate to earlier assignments? How do they relate to objectives the instructor has given? The chapter objectives identify things you should be able to do after you have read the material. Do not wait until you have read the chapter to start trying to respond. *Prepare* means getting the brain engaged from the beginning. Studying the chapter objectives establishes a direction and purpose for your reading. This will enable you to maintain concentration and focus while you read.

Another feature in the opening pages of each chapter is the **glossary.** This is one of the most valuable tools the authors have provided. They know that there are many terms to learn and are giving you a head start on learning them. Spend a few minutes with the glossary. Notice the terms that are also used in the chapter objectives and are bolded in the text. Go back and look at the objectives and think about what you have learned from the glossary. As you study the glossary, look for shared root words, prefixes, or suffixes. If words share such common word elements, these words also have a shared meaning. Learning the meaning of common word elements can simplify the whole process of learning vocabulary. Perhaps you remember in elementary school being told to "look for the little words in the big word." This is essentially the same technique—one that worked then and one that will work now.

Now make a quick pass through the chapter or the assigned pages from the chapter. Focus on the text conventions, which are described later in this chapter. Look for anything that stands out in the chapter, such as boldfaced text, boxed material, and tables. This provides a quick overview of the chapter, which will make the next steps in the PURR process much more effective and efficient.

The **chapter headings** show the major points to be covered. Study them and notice the major headings (topics) and the subordinate headings (subtopics). This is essentially a picture of the chapter, and using the picture is an essential step in preparing to read. As you read through the chapter headings, turn the topic and subtopics into a series of questions that you want to be able to answer when you finish reading. Think about the objectives and how these headings relate to them. Finally, in the headings devoted to specific classes of drugs, notice there are elements that are common to every one. The last two headings are always "Implementation" and "Evaluation." This tells you that these are two common elements you will be expected to know at the end of every chapter. The minutes you spend *preparing* will pay off in a big way when you start to read.

Preparing makes the whole approach to learning an active one. It may not make the chapters the most exciting reading you will ever do, but it will help you accomplish your personal learning objectives as well as those set by the authors.

On-the-Run Action. Preparing is great to do during "found" time. It should not take more than 5 or 10 minutes. Time between classes, time spent waiting for the coffee water to boil, or any other small block of time that usually just slips away can be used to accomplish this step.

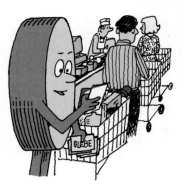

Understand

Now read the assignment. Go to your desk, the library, or wherever you have chosen for serious study. Reading the assignment is where all your preparation pays off. If you did the *Prepare* step earlier in the day, it is not a bad idea to spend a minute or two going through the chapter features again to get your focus. As you read the assignment, remember the chapter objectives and notice the chapter headings in the body of the chapter. As you read, rephrase the chapter headings as questions to help keep you focused on the task at hand. Because this is the first time you are really focusing on the concepts and the details, this is not the time to do any text notations. Read and, as you read, think. Terms from the glossary are repeated, and their meanings are often expanded and clarified in the body of the text. Pay attention to these terms as you read. Think about what they mean and how you would define them to someone else. Read for meaning. Read to *understand.* Do not read just to get to the end of the assignment. That is a passive action. Ask yourself questions. Analyze, respond, and react as you read.

Often, reading assignments are too long to be read with complete understanding in one session. If you find that your concentration is flagging or you do not remember anything you read on the previous page, it is time to take a break. All too often students have only one objective—to finish the assignment. You might be able to force yourself to continue reading, but you will not learn much. Mark your place and take a 5- or 10-minute break. Take a walk, read the daily comic strips, get a soda or a cup of coffee, and then go back to reading. When you come back to the assignment, spend the first 3 or 4 minutes reviewing. Look back at the previous chapter heading and think about what you were reading before the break. The chapter can be broken down into many small reading sessions, but it is critical that you do not lose sight of the chapter as a whole. Spending these minutes in review may seem like time that could be better spent continuing with the reading, but this quick review will save time in the long run.

There is no quick way to read a chapter. You will not find an "on-the-run action" for this step because it cannot be done in this way. However, if you do the *Prepare* step first, you will be surprised at how much more easily you get the reading done and how much more learning you have achieved in the process.

Rehearse

Rehearsing is the third step in the process. It starts the process of consolidating your learning and establishing a basis for long-term memory. Rehearsal accomplishes two things. First, it helps you find out what you understand from the reading. Knowing what you know is really important. Second, it identifies what you do not understand, and this may be an even more important benefit. Knowing what you do not know before it comes to light during an examination is critical.

How to Rehearse. Everything you do in the *Prepare* and *Understand* steps comes into play in the *Rehearse* step. Rehearsal should begin with the features at the beginning of the chapter. Open the text to the beginning of the chapter. Start with the chapter title and begin to quiz yourself on what you have read. Compose three or four questions pertaining to the chapter title, and then try to answer them to your satisfaction. The questions you ask yourself should be both literal (asking for specific information presented in the chapter) and interpretive (testing your comprehension of concepts and relationships). An example of a literal question using the Chapter 4 title might be, "What are the definitions of *cultural, legal,* and *ethical?*" This question would help you determine whether you can satisfactorily define these terms in your own words. Asking and answering such questions as this always serves to move learning from short-term to long-term memory. Literal questions are very important to help you grasp the factual information and terminology contained in the reading assignment. However, it is also necessary to ask questions that stimulate thought about the concepts and the relationships between the facts and concepts presented in the chapter. An example of an interpretive question regarding the Chapter 4 title might be: "What are the most important *cultural, legal,* and *ethical* concepts pertaining to the use of drugs?" Sometimes you will find that, even though the question is interpretive, the authors have anticipated the question and the text does contain the direct answer to your question. Other times you will need to formulate your own response by pulling together bits and pieces of information from the entire reading assignment.

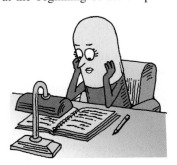

Once you have exhausted the question potential for the chapter title, move on to the chapter objectives. Use the same process here. Rephrase the objectives as questions and try to answer them. Remember that the object of rehearsal is to reinforce what you have learned and to identify areas where you need to spend additional time (review).

Go to the glossary. Cover the definitions, and try to define each term in your own words. Another method is to cover the term, and on the basis of the definition, name the term. Do not just memorize the definition, because you may find the information presented differently on an examination, and you will then be unable to respond.

Now proceed to the chapter or assigned pages. The chapter headings are the main tools for rehearsal. Apply the same question-and-answer technique used for the title and objectives to test what you may already know about the chapter content. Turn the headings into questions and answer them. Look at the text for boldfaced and italicized items, lists, and other text conventions. These too can become the basis for questions. The tables and diagrams should also be used for this purpose. Keep in mind the importance of asking both literal and interpretive questions. Some of the questions you ask yourself should also tie different topic headings together. Ask yourself how topic A relates to topic B.

As you proceed through the chapter, do not worry if you cannot answer the questions you ask. As stated earlier, one of the goals of the rehearsal process is to identify what you need to spend more time on. If you can give no response to a particular question, put a mark in the margin of the pertinent place in the text to remind

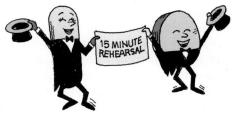

yourself to come back and spend more time on this material, but move on at this point. Rehearsal should be a relatively quick procedure. Once you become accustomed to the PURR method, it should take no more than 15 or 20 minutes to rehearse 15 pages after doing the *Prepare* and *Understand* steps.

As you reach the end of the chapter, skim the *Implementation* and *Evaluation* sections. Make sure that the relationship between these sections and the information in the rest of the chapter is clear. If you have questions or concerns, note them in the margins and ask your instructor to clarify these points. Although the objective is to master the chapter content as an independent learner, sometimes it is essential to ask questions of the instructor to facilitate the process.

When to Rehearse. Ideally rehearsal should take place almost immediately after you finish reading the material. Take a 10- to 15-minute break, and then start the process. The longer the gap between reading and rehearsal, the more you will forget and the longer it will take to rehearse. If you are breaking a reading assignment down into smaller segments, do the rehearsal for each segment before you begin reading the new material. This helps maintain the sense of continuity in the chapter. This seems like a lot of work to do in a study session, but with practice it will go quickly and you will be pleasantly surprised at the quality and quantity of your learning.

Review

Review is the fourth and final step in the PURR process, and it is an essential step. No matter how well you have learned material in the preceding steps, forgetting will always occur. Reviewing is the only way to store what you have learned in long-term memory. The good news is that, using the PURR model, the review can be done for small segments of material and can be done relatively quickly.

How to Review. The basic review process is essentially the same as the rehearsal process, with some limited rereading as the only difference. When you cannot immediately answer a question, read the pertinent material again. *This does not mean you should read the entire chapter again.* Often the answer to the question will pop into your mind after you have read only a few lines. When this happens, stop reading and go back to responding to your question. The idea is to reread only as much material as is necessary to make the answer clear. One or two words or one or two sentences may trigger personal recall, but it may also take two or three paragraphs for this to happen.

Frequency of Review. How many times should you review material in this way? This actually depends on many factors, such as the difficulty of the material, the length of the assignment, and your personal background. Only you can determine how often you need to review, but there are some guidelines that will help you decide this for yourself.

First, consider the difficulty of the material. If it is very complex, contains many new terms and difficult concepts, and seems difficult to grasp, then you should review very frequently. On the other hand, if the material is straightforward and you are able to relate it well to what you have already learned, then less frequent reviews will serve to keep the material in your memory.

Second, consider how well the review went. If you had difficulty answering many questions to your satisfaction or had to do a lot of rereading, you should schedule another review soon (a day or two later at most).

The success of each review session should be used to help you determine when to schedule another session. The review step is a means of monitoring the success of the learning process. If reviews go well, limited rereading is necessary, and you are able to give clear answers to your questions, this tells you that you can wait several days (4 or 5) before reviewing this material again. A mediocre review, more extensive rereading, and poor answers indicate that you should only let 2 or 3 days go by before reviewing the material again. If the review goes very poorly, you should plan to review the material again the next day. It is up to you to judge the success of each review and to decide how often you need to review. The nice thing about PURR is that it enables you to monitor your success and to easily regulate the learning process.

Techniques for Rehearsal and Review. Both rehearsal and review foster active learning, which helps you maintain interest in the material and strengthens your memory. For these benefits to occur, it is essential that the review and rehearsal processes be done orally. Talking to yourself is one way to accomplish this but working with a study group is another and sometimes more interesting way to rehearse and review. Strategies for establishing and maintaining effective study groups can be found in the *Study Guide* that accompanies this text, You can find a short overview in Part three in this text. Study groups are not for everyone. The key is to do what works for you. If studying alone gets the results you want then continue. If not, you may want to try a study group.

When you ask questions and give your answers out loud this forces you to think about the material. It helps you organize it and translate it into your own words. The object is not to memorize everything you have read but to understand and be able to explain it. Eventually you will need to answer questions on an examination. Framing questions as a part of the learning process is a way to anticipate examination questions. The more questions you ask yourself during study time, the more likely some of the questions on the examination will be ones you have asked yourself. When you work with a study group you have several brains anticipating test questions. Further, by doing the rehearsal and review orally, you will find it easier to recall the

answers during the examination, because this oral model requires more than just remembering seeing the material; you will actually be able to hear the rehearsed answers in your mind. Another advantage of doing the rehearsal and review processes orally is, as stated earlier, that it helps to identify what needs further study. When your oral answer is fragmentary, contains many "uhs," and is really disorganized, then you know that you need to devote more time to learning this term, fact, or concept.

The PURR system may seem like a lot of work at first. The idea of going through a chapter four times understandably seems daunting. Add to this the need for several review sessions, and the first reaction is likely to be: "This won't work," or "I don't have the time to do this." Don't take that attitude. This system does work. It cultivates interest, aids concentration, fosters mastery of the material, and ensures long-term memory of the material, which is important not just for doing well on examinations but also for doing well as a nurse with the safe care of patients at stake. The PURR system will work if you use it. It may take 3 or 4 weeks to get comfortable with the system, but if you keep at it, pretty soon it will become a good habit. After a while you will not be able to imagine studying in any other way.

Like all study systems, the PURR method is a model. As you use it, you may discover ways of changing it that work better for you. That is okay. Do not hesitate to make adjustments that better suit your learning style and strategies. Just remember as you start out that *Preparation, Understanding, Rehearsal,* and *Review* are solid learning principles and cannot be ignored.

Study skills tips are included on the pages at the beginning of each part of the book. These hints are directly applied to the content found within the chapters of the following unit. Detailed information on specialized study skills, such as time management, note taking, examination preparation, and vocabulary building, are present in the *Study Guide* that accompanies this text.

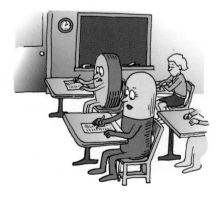

PHARMACOLOGY BASICS

Prepare

As you begin to work with individual chapters, consider how the first step in the PURR system can be used to help you set a purpose and become an active learner.

Chapter 1 Objectives

Consider Objective 1. *List the five phases of the nursing process.* Now turn the objective into a question. What are the five phases of the nursing process? Now move to Objective 2 and make it a question. What are the components of the assessment process for patients receiving medications, including collection and analysis of subjective and objective data? You might recognize that this question relates to Objective 1 because assessment is one phase of the nursing process. By putting Objective 2 into a question format you will begin to expand and extend on the focus of the first objective, and you will begin to focus on active learning with a clear purpose.

When you begin to read Chapter 1 you will discover that the five phases of the nursing process are repeated as topic headings, and you have the Objective 2 question on which to focus your reading. Begin now to develop the habit of applying this strategy to the objectives in every chapter assigned before you begin to read. Remember to look at the chapter headings at this point as well. It is amazing how much can be learned by using the text structures provided.

Vocabulary Development

Turn to Chapter 2. Objective 1 makes an important point. *Define the common terms used in pharmacology.* Success depends heavily on knowledge of the "language." The objective makes it clear that this chapter contains a number of terms that the author views as important to be mastered. This is only Chapter 2, and now is the time to begin to apply yourself to mastering the language of this content. Look at the glossary. There are six terms that share the common element *pharmaco.* Although each of these six words will have different meanings, they will have something in common. *Pharmaco* is an example of a group word. No matter what prefixes, group words, and/or suffixes are added to it, a part of the meaning of any word containing *pharmaco* will be "drug" or "medicine." Look up a word containing *pharmaco* in any dictionary and you will find that its definition pertains to "drug" or "medicine" in some way. Although you probably already knew that, it is always beneficial to start working on a new technique with something that is familiar. Look at four of the words that begin with *pharmaco,* and consider the rest of the word:

| dynamics | genetics | gnosy | kinetics |

What do each of these word parts mean? The meaning of *pharmacodynamics* is simply the combination of the meaning of *pharmaco* and *dynamics.* The definition, according to the glossary begins, "the study of the biochemical and physiologic interactions of drugs." You could simply memorize this definition, which would seem to accomplish Objective 1. However, memorization does not always equal understanding. Try another approach. What does *dynamics* mean? Think about the word, and relate it to your own experience and background. It appears to deal with movement or action. After looking it up in the dictionary, all the meanings given seem to relate in some fashion to the idea of motion and/or action. A simplistic defini-

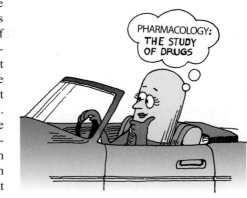

tion of *pharmacodynamics* would be "drugs in action." Certainly this is not a technical or medical definition, but it contributes a great deal to an understanding of the definition provided in the glossary. This is the object of learning vocabulary. Do not m e m o r i z e words without understanding. Apply a little thought, and relate the term and definition in a way that makes the meaning personal for you. When you do that, you will find that you understand the glossary definition better, and your ability to retain the meaning will be significantly improved. This means that the test item that asks you to select the definition for *pharmacodynamics* from a list of similar definitions will be much easier, because you will remember action and movement and look for the choice that best represents that concept.

Apply this same strategy to genetics. You already know what genetics means. Now you must determine how to connect that to the meaning in the text. After you have the definitions of *gnosy* and *kinetics,* you can apply the same procedure. When you have done this with all four words, you will discover that you will not need to spend a great amount of time trying to memorize esoteric definitions. You will have personalized the meanings. Those meanings will stay with you much more readily than those learned by rote memorization. By the way, do you know what *biochemical* and *physiologic* mean? These terms are used in the glossary definition of *pharmacodynamics.* You need to know what they mean to fully understand pharmacodynamics.

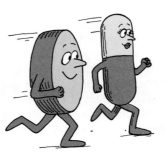

The Nursing Process and Drug Therapy

Objectives

When you reach the end of this chapter, you should be able to do the following:

1. List the five phases of the nursing process.
2. Identify the components of the assessment process for patients receiving medications, including collection and analysis of subjective and objective data.
3. Discuss the process of formulating nursing diagnoses for patients receiving medications.
4. Identify goals and outcome criteria for patients receiving medications.
5. Discuss the evaluation process as it relates to the administration of medications and as reflected by goals and outcome criteria.
6. Develop a nursing care plan with use of the nursing process and medication administration.
7. Briefly discuss the Five Rights of drug administration and the related professional responsibility for safe medication practice.
8. Discuss the additional rights of drug administration that are ensured in safe medication practice.

e-Learning Activities

Companion CD

* NCLEX Review Questions: see questions 1-4
* Animations
* Audio Glossary
* Category Catchers
* Medication Errors Checklists
* IV Therapy Checklists

evolve Website (http://evolve.elsevier.com/Lilley)

* Nursing Care Plans • Frequently Asked Questions • Content Updates • WebLinks • Supplemental Resources • Elsevier ePharmacology Update • Medication Administration Animations

Glossary

Goals Statements that are time specific and describe generally what is to be accomplished to address a specific nursing diagnosis. Goals are developed in collaboration with the patient and are objective, verifiable, realistic, and measureable statements about changes in behavior that are to be achieved through nursing care within an established time frame. Behavior-based goals fall into the physiologic, psychologic, spiritual, sexual, cognitive, motor, and/or other domains. (p. 6)

Medication error Any preventable adverse drug event involving inappropriate medication use by a patient or health care professional; it may or may not cause the patient harm. (p. 12)

Nursing process An organizational framework for the practice of nursing. It encompasses all steps taken by the nurse in

caring for a patient: assessment, nursing diagnoses, planning (with goals and outcome criteria), implementation of the plan (with patient teaching), and evaluation. (p. 6)

Outcome criteria Descriptions of specific patient behaviors or responses that demonstrate meeting of or achievement of goals related to each nursing diagnosis. These statements, like goals, should be verifiable, framed in behavioral terms, measurable, and time specific. Outcome criteria are considered to be specific, whereas goals are broad. (p. 6)

OVERVIEW OF THE NURSING PROCESS

The **nursing process** is a well-established, research-supported framework for professional nursing practice. It is a flexible, adaptable, and adjustable five-step process consisting of assessment, nursing diagnoses, planning (including establishment of **goals** and **outcome criteria**), implementation (including patient education), and evaluation. As such, the nursing process ensures the delivery of thorough, individualized, and quality nursing care to patients, regardless of age, gender, medical diagnosis, or setting. Through use of the nursing process combined with knowledge and skills, the professional nurse will be able to develop effective solutions to meet patient's needs. The nursing process is usually discussed within nursing courses and/or textbooks about the fundamentals of nursing practice, nursing theory, physical assessment, adult and pediatric nursing and other nursing specialty areas. However, because of the importance of nursing process in the care of patients, the process with all five phases will be included in each chapter as related to specific drug groups/classifications.

Critical thinking is a major part of the nursing process and involves the use of the mind to develop conclusions, make decisions, draw inferences, and reflect upon all aspects of the patient.

Box 1-1   Sample Nursing Care Plan Related to Drug Therapy and the Nursing Process

This sample presents information useful for developing a nursing process–focused care plan for patients receiving medications. Brief listings and discussions of what should be presented in each phase of the nursing process are included. This sample may be used as a template for formatting nursing care plans in a variety of patient care situations. Only one nursing diagnosis will be presented with each care plan throughout the book.

Assessment
Objective Data
Objective data include information available through the senses, such as what is seen, felt, heard, and smelled. Among the sources of data are the chart, laboratory test results, reports of diagnostic procedures, health history, physical assessment, and examination findings. Other examples include age, height, weight, allergies, medication profile, and health history.

Subjective Data
Subjective data include all spoken information shared by the patient, such as complaints, problems, or stated needs (e.g., patient complains of "dizziness, headache, vomiting, and feeling hot for 10 days").

Nursing Diagnoses
Once the assessment phase has been completed the nurse analyzes objective and subjective data about the patient and the drug and formulates nursing diagnoses. The following is a sample of a nursing diagnosis statement: "Deficient knowledge related to lack of experience with medication regimen and second-grade reading level as an adult as evidenced by inability to perform a return demonstration and inability to state adverse effects." This statement of the nursing diagnosis can be broken down into three parts, as follows:

- **Part 1**—"Deficient knowledge" This is the statement of the human response of the patient to illness, injury, medications, or significant change. This can be an actual response, an increased risk, or an opportunity to improve the patient's health status.
- **Part 2**—"Related to lack of experience with medication regimen and second-grade reading level as an adult." This statement identifies factors related to the response; it often includes multiple factors with some degree of connection between them. The nursing diagnosis statement does not necessarily claim that there is a cause-and-effect link between these factors and the response, only that there is a connection.
- **Part 3**—"As evidenced by inability to perform a return demonstration and inability to state adverse effects to report to the physician." This statement lists clues, cues, evidence, and/or data that support the nurse's claim that the nursing diagnosis is accurate.

Nursing diagnoses are prioritized in order of criticality based on patient needs or problems. The ABCs of care (airway, breathing, and circulation) are often used as a basis for prioritization. Prioritizing always begins with the most important, significant, or critical need of the patient. Nursing diagnoses that involve actual responses are always ranked above nursing diagnoses that involve only risks.

Planning: Goals and Outcome Criteria
The planning phase includes the identification of goals and outcome criteria, provides time frames, and is patient oriented. Goals are objective, verifiable, realistic, and measurable patient-centered statements with time frames and are broad, whereas outcome criteria are more specific descriptions of patient goals. See the Insulin Therapy nursing care plan available at http://evolve.elsevier.com/Lilley for examples of goal and outcome criteria statements.

Implementation
In the implementation phase, the nurse intervenes on behalf of the patient to address specific patient problems and needs. This is done through independent nursing actions; collaborative activities such as physical therapy, occupational therapy, and music therapy; and implementation of medical orders. Family, significant others, and other caregivers assist in carrying out this phase of the nursing care plan. Specific interventions that relate to particular drugs (e.g., giving a particular cardiac drug only after monitoring the patient's pulse and blood pressure), nonpharmacologic interventions that enhance the therapeutic effects of medications, and patient education are major components of the implementation phase. See the previous discussion of the nursing process for more information on nursing interventions.

Evaluation
Evaluation is the part of the nursing process that includes monitoring whether patient goals and outcome criteria related to the nursing diagnoses are met. Monitoring includes observing for therapeutic effects of drug treatment as well as for adverse effects and toxicity. Many indicators are used to monitor these aspects of drug therapy as well as the results of appropriately related nonpharmacologic interventions. If the goals and outcome criteria are met, the nursing care plan may or may not be revised to include new nursing diagnoses; such changes are made only if appropriate. If goals and outcome criteria are not met, revisions are made to the entire nursing care plan with further evaluation.

These aspects include the physical, emotional, spiritual, sexual, financial, cultural, and cognitive parts of a patient. Attention to these many aspects allows a more *holistic* approach to patient care. For example, a cardiologist may focus on cardiac functioning and pathology, a physical therapist on movement, and a chaplain on the spiritual aspects of patient care. However, it is the professional nurse who critically thinks, processes, and incorporates all these aspects and points of information about the patient and develops and coordinates patient care. Therefore, the nursing process remains a central process and framework for nursing care. Box 1-1 provides a sample nursing care plan as related to drug therapy and the nursing process. Other more specific nursing care plans are located online at http://evolve.elsevier.com/Lilley.

ASSESSMENT

During the initial assessment phase of the nursing process, data are collected, reviewed, and analyzed. Performing a comprehensive assessment allows the nurse to formulate a nursing diagnosis related to the patient's needs and, for the purposes of this textbook, specifically needs related to drug administration. Information about the patient may come from a variety of sources, including the patient; the patient's family, caregiver, or significant other; and the patient's chart. Methods of data collection include interviewing, direct and indirect questioning, observation, medical records review, and head-to-toe physical examination (nursing assessment). Data are categorized into objective and subjective data. Objective data may be defined as any information gathered through the senses (that which is seen, heard, felt or smelled). Objective data may also be obtained through a nursing physical assessment, nursing history, past and present medical history, laboratory reports, results of diagnostic studies/procedures, vital signs, weight, height, and medication profile. A comprehensive medication profile should include, but not be limited to, collection about the following: (1) Any and all drug use; (2) use of home or folk remedies, herbal or homeopathic treatments, plant or animal extracts, and dietary supplements; (3) intake of alcohol, tobacco, and caffeine; (4) current or past history of illegal drug use; (5) use of over-the-counter (OTC) medications, including, but not limited to, aspirin or acetaminophen products, vitamins, laxatives, cold preparations, sinus medications, antacids, acid reducers, antidiarrheals, minerals, and elements; (6) use of hormonal drugs (e.g., testosterone, estrogens, progestins and oral contraceptives); (7) past and present health history and associated drug regimen; (8) family history, racial, ethnic, and/or cultural differences with attention to specific and/or different responses to medications; (9) any unusual responses to medications; and (10) growth and developmental stages (e.g., Erikson's Developmental Tasks) and related issues to the patient's age and medication use. A *holistic* nursing assessment would include gathering of data about religious preference, health beliefs, sociocultural profile, race, ethnicity, lifestyle, stressors, socioeconomic status, educational level, motor skills, cognitive ability, support systems, lifestyle, and use of any alternative/complimentary therapies. Subjective data includes information shared by the spoken word from any reliable source (e.g., patient, spouse, family member, significant other, and/or caregiver).

Assessment of the drug is also important including specific information about prescribed, OTC, and herbal drug use including signs and symptoms of allergic reaction; administration routes; recommended dosages; actions; contraindications; drug incompatibilities; drug-drug, drug-food, and drug–laboratory test interactions; and adverse effects and toxic effects. Nursing pharmacology textbooks provide a more nursing-specific knowledge base regarding drug therapy (and the nursing process) and use of current references (e.g., references dated within the last 5 years). Some examples of authoritative references include the *Physicians' Desk Reference*, the drug manufacturer's insert, drug handbooks, references such as *Mosby's Drug Consult,* and/or a licensed pharmacist. Reliable online resources include the following (although not a comprehensive listing): U.S. Pharmacopeia (USP) (www.usp.org), U.S. Food and Drug Administration (FDA) (www.fda.gov), and www.WebMD.com.

Data gathering about the patient and drug may be done through asking simple questions, such as the following: (1) What is the patient's oral intake? Tolerance of fluids? Swallowing ability for pills, tablets, capsules, liquids? If there is difficulty swallowing, what is the degree of difficulty and are there solutions to the problem (e.g., "thickening" of fluids for some patients) or are other dosage forms needed? (2) What are laboratory and other diagnostic test values related to organ functioning and drug therapy? What do renal studies such as blood urea nitrogen level or serum creatinine level show? What are the results of hepatic function tests such as total protein level and serum levels of bilirubin, alkaline phosphatase, creatinine phosphokinase, and other liver enzymes? What is the patient's red blood cell count, hemoglobin level, hematocrit, and white blood cell count? (3) What have been the patient's previous and current experiences with health, illness, prescription drug use, and use of herbal substances and alternative medications? Previous relationships with health care professiona ls and/or previous experience with hospitalization? (4) What are past and present values for blood pressure, pulse rate, temperature, and respiratory rate? (5) In addition to the medication profile, how is the patient taking medications and how is the patient tolerating them? Compliance/adherence issues? Any use of folklore? (6) What emotional, physical, cognitive, cultural, and socioeconomic factors are influencing drug therapy and the nursing process for the patient (for a holistic framework)? (7) What are a given drug's adverse effects, contraindications, appropriate dosages, routes of administration, therapeutic levels, and toxicity and any antidotes? (8) What does the given drug do? Is it really helping the patient? What is the patient's understanding of this information? and, (9) Are there any age-specific medication concerns? These are just a few sample questions that may be posed to patients, family members, significant others, and/or caregivers.

Once assessment of the patient and the drug has been completed, the specific prescription or medication order from a physician or other professional licensed/certified prescriber must be checked for the following six elements:
1. Patient's name
2. Date order was written
3. Name of medications
4. Dosage (includes size, frequency, and number of doses)
5. Route of delivery
6. Signature of the prescriber

It is also important during assessment to consider the traditional, non-traditional, expanded, and collaborative roles of the nurse. Physicians and dentists are no longer the only health care professionals prescribing and writing medication orders. Nurse practitioners and physician assistants have gained the professional privilege to legally prescribe medications. Nurses should always be aware of these roles and be familiar with the specific state nurse practice acts and standards of care.

Analysis of Data

Once data about the patient and drug have been collected and reviewed, the nurse must critically analyze and synthesize the information. All information should be verified and documented appropriately and, it is at this point, that the sum of the information about the patient and drug are used in the development of nursing diagnoses.

NURSING DIAGNOSES

Nursing diagnoses are developed by professional nurses and are used as a means of communicating and sharing information about the patient and the patient experience. Nursing diagnoses are the result of critical thinking, creativity, and accurate data collection about the patient and drug. Nursing diagnoses related to drug therapy will most likely develop out of data associated with the following: deficient knowledge; risk for injury; noncompliance; and various disturbances, deficits, excesses, impairments in bodily functions and/or other problems or concerns as noted by the North American Nursing Diagnosis Association (NANDA). NANDA is the formal organization recognized by professional nursing groups, such as the American Nurses Association (ANA), as being the major contributor to the development of nursing knowledge and is considered to be the leading authority in the development and classification of nursing diagnoses. The purpose of NANDA is to increase the visibility of nursing's contribution to the care of patients and to further develop, refine, and classify the information and phenomena related to nurses and professional nursing practice. See Box 1-2 for more information about NANDA.

Formulation of nursing diagnoses is usually a three step process and stated as follows: (1) The first part of the nursing diagnosis statement is the human response of the patient to illness, injury, or significant change. This response can be an actual problem, an increased risk of developing a problem, or an opportunity or intent to increase the patient's health; (2) the second part of the nursing diagnosis statement identifies the factor or factors related to the response, and more than one factor is often named. The nursing diagnosis statement does not necessarily claim a cause-and-effect link between these factors and the response but only indicates that there is a connection between them; and (3) the third part of the nursing diagnosis statement lists clues, cues, evidence, or other data that support the nurse's claim that this diagnosis is accurate. Some *tips* for writing nursing diagnoses are as follows: (1) Start with a statement of a *human response;* (2) connect the first part of the statement or the human response with the second part, the cause, using the phrase *related to;* (3) be sure that the first two parts are not restatements of one another; (4) several factors may be included in the second part of the statement (i.e., the etiology); (5) select a cause for the second part of the statement that can be changed by nursing interventions; (6) avoid negative wording or language; and (7) list clues or cues that led to the nursing diagnosis in the third part of the statement, which may also include more defining characteristics (e.g., *as evidenced by*). A listing of NANDA-approved nursing diagnoses is provided in Box 1-3. These nursing diagnoses, as well as all other phases of the nursing process, will be presented in the chapters to follow because of the framework of practice that the nursing process provides to all professional nurses.

PLANNING

After data are collected and nursing diagnoses formulated, the planning phase begins; this includes identification of goals and outcome criteria. The major purposes of the planning phase are to prioritize the nursing diagnoses and specify goals and outcome criteria, including time frame for their achievement. The planning phase provides time to obtain special equipment for interventions, review the possible procedures or techniques to be used and gather information for oneself (the nurse) or for the patient. This step leads to the provision of safe care if professional judgment is combined with the acquisition of knowledge about the patient and the medications to be given.

Box 1-2   A Brief Look at NANDA and the Nursing Process

NANDA is characterized by the following: (1) It increases visibility of nursing's contribution to patient care; (2) it develops, refines, and classifies information and phenomena related to professional nursing practice; (3) it remains the working organization for development of evidence-based nursing diagnoses; and (4) it continues to provide support to the improvement of quality nursing care through evidence-based practice and through use of a global network of professional nurses. In 1987, NANDA and ANA endorsed a framework for establishing nursing diagnoses and in 1990, *Nursing Diagnoses* became the official journal of NANDA with the most current resource titled *The International Journal of Nursing Terminologies and Classifications*. In 2001 and 2003, NANDA modified and updated the listing of nursing diagnoses, and nursing diagnoses continue to be submitted for consideration to the AdHoc Research Committee of NANDA with some of the more recent changes noted as follows: The phrase *potential for* has been replaced with *risk for,* and the terms *impaired, deficient, ineffective, decreased, increased,* and *imbalanced* have replaced outdated terms of *altered* and *alteration* (though the outdated terms may still be in use).

Box 1-3   Selected NANDA-Approved Nursing Diagnoses

Activity intolerance
Acute pain
Anxiety
Caregiver role strain
Constipation
Deficient fluid volume
Deficient knowledge
Diarrhea
Disturbed body image
Disturbed energy field
Disturbed sensory perception
Disturbed thought processes
Dysfunctional family processes: alcoholism
Excess fluid volume
Fatigue
Grieving
Imbalanced nutrition: less than or more than body requirements
Impaired gas exchange
Impaired urinary elimination
Ineffective airway clearance
Ineffective breathing pattern
Ineffective coping
Ineffective health maintenance
Ineffective therapeutic regimen management
Ineffective tissue perfusion
Noncompliance
Powerlessness
Risk for aspiration
Risk for disuse syndrome
Risk for falls
Risk for impaired skin integrity
Risk for infection
Risk for injury
Sexual dysfunction
Situational low self-esteem
Sleep deprivation
Urinary retention

From NANDA International: *NANDA nursing diagnoses: definitions and classification, 2005-2006,* Philadelphia, 2005, NANDA.
NANDA, North American Nursing Diagnosis Association.

Goals and Outcome Criteria

Goals are objective, measurable, and realistic, with an established time period for achievement of the outcomes, which are specifically stated in the outcome criteria. Patient goals reflect expected changes through nursing care. The outcome criteria (concrete descriptions of patient goals) should be succinct, well thought out, and patient focused. They should include expectations for behavior (something that can be changed) that are to be met by certain deadlines. The ultimate aim of these criteria is the safe and effective administration of medications, and they should relate to each nursing diagnosis and should guide the implementation of nursing care. Formulation of outcome criteria begins with the analysis of the judgments made about all of the patient data and subsequent nursing diagnoses and ends with the development of a nursing care plan. Outcome criteria provide a standard for measuring movement toward goals. They may address special storage and handling techniques, administration procedures, equipment needed, drug interactions, adverse effects, and contraindications. In this textbook, specific time frames are *not* provided in the discussion of the nursing process in each chapter because each patient care situation is individualized.

Patient-oriented outcome criteria must apply to any medications the patient will receive. For example, the outcome criteria for a 43-year-old male with diabetes mellitus might be focused on the administration of insulin and general aspects of insulin therapy. In this situation, the patient-oriented outcome criteria revolve around specific patient education regarding insulin, adverse effects, contraindications, and injection techniques (see the Insulin Therapy nursing care plan at http://evolve.elsevier.com/ Lilley). It is also during the planning phase that planning for the unexpected must occur as well as planning to allow the nurse to be ready for any status or order changes.

IMPLEMENTATION

Implementation is guided by the preceding phases of the nursing process (e.g., assessment, nursing diagnoses, planning). Implementation requires constant communication and collaboration with the patient and with members of the health care team involved in the patient's care, as well as with any family members, significant others, or other caregivers. Implementation consists of initiation and completion of specific actions by the nurse as defined by nursing diagnoses, goals, and outcome criteria. Implementation of nursing actions may be independent, collaborative, or dependent upon a physician's order. Interventions should include frequency, specific instructions, and any other pertinent information. With medication administration, the nurse needs to know and understand all of the information about the patient and about each medication prescribed (see assessment questions). The nurse must also adhere to the "Five Rights" of medication administration: right drug, right dose, right time, right route, and right patient (discussed in the next section of this chapter). In addition, the nurse needs to be aware of these additional patient rights:

- The right to patient safety, ensured by use of the correct procedures, equipment, and techniques of medication administration and documentation
- The right to individualized, holistic, accurate, and complete patient education

- The right to a double-check and constant analysis of the system (i.e., the process of drug administration, including everyone involved, such as the doctor, the nurse, the nursing unit, and the pharmacy department, as well as patient education)
- The right to proper drug storage
- The right to accurate calculation and preparation of the dose of medication and proper use of all types of medication delivery systems
- The right to careful checking of the transcription of medication orders
- The right to accurate use of the various routes of administration and awareness of the specific implications of their use
- The right to close consideration of special situations (e.g., patient difficulty in swallowing, use of a nasogastric tube, unconsciousness of the patient, advanced patient age)
- The right to have all appropriate measures taken to prevent and report medication errors
- The right to accurate and cautious patient monitoring for therapeutic effects, adverse effects, and toxic effects
- The right to continued safe application of the nursing process, with accurate documentation in electronic form, narrative form, SOAP (*s*ubjective, *o*bjective, *a*ssessment, *p*lanning) notes format, or other form
- The right to correct use of computer/electronic documentation
- The right to refuse medication with proper documentation

Right Drug

The "right drug" begins with the registered nurse's valid license to practice. (Some states allow licensed practical nurses to administer medications; they should also hold a current license.) The registered nurse should check all medication orders and/or prescriptions. To ensure that the correct drug is given, the nurse must check the specific medication order against the medication label/profile three times prior to giving the medication beginning with the first check of the right drug/drug name while preparing the medications for administration. At this time, the nurse should also consider whether the drug is appropriate for the patient and, if in doubt or an error is deemed possible, the physician should be contacted immediately. It would be appropriate, at this time, to also note the drug's indication and be aware that a drug may have multiple indications. This textbook will present a particular drug's indication as appropriate to its main indication but may also cross-reference the drug in another chapter or other chapters because of multiple uses.

All medication orders or prescriptions should be signed by the physician, physician's assistant, nurse practitioner, or other health care provider. If there is a verbal order, the prescriber should sign the order within 24 hours or as per facility protocol. Verbal and/or telephone orders are often used in emergency or time-sensitive patient care situations. To ensure that the right drug is given, the nurse must obtain information about the patient and drug (see previous discussion of the assessment phase) to ensure that all factors have been considered. Information about prescribed drugs should come from authoritative sources (see previous discussion). Relying upon knowledge from peers is discouraged. The professional nurse should be familiar with the generic (nonproprietary) drug name as well as the trade name (proprietary name that is registered by a specific drug manufacturer);

however, use of the drug's generic name is now preferred in clinical practice to reduce the risk of medication errors. Trade names for one drug are often numerous and similarly-spelled names occur across drug classes leading to possible medication errors. If the nurse has any questions at any time in the process, the nurse should contact the physician to clarify the order. The nurse should never *assume* anything when it comes to drug administration and, as previously emphasized in this chapter, the nurse should check for compliance with *all* of the Five Rights at least three times *before* giving the medication.

Right Dose

Whenever a medication is ordered, a dosage is identified from the doctor's order. The nurse must always check the dose and confirm that it is appropriate to the patient's age and size and check the prescribed dose against what is available and against what is the normal dosage range. Always *recheck* any mathematical calculations and pay careful attention to decimal points which could lead to a tenfold or even greater overdose. Leading zeros, or zeros placed before a decimal point, are allowed but trailing zeros, or zeros following the decimal point, should not be used. For example, 0.2 milligrams is allowed, but 2.0 milligrams is not acceptable. Patient variables, (e.g., vital signs, age, gender, weight, height) should be noted because of the need for dosage change due to specific parameters. Remember that pediatric and elderly patients are more sensitive to medications than younger and middle adult-aged patients; thus, there is a need for extra caution with drug dosage amounts in these patients.

Right Time

Each health care agency or institution has a policy regarding routine medication administration times; therefore, the nurse must always check this policy. However, when giving a medication at the prescribed time, the nurse may be confronted with a dilemma between the timing suggested by the physician and specific pharmacokinetic/pharmacodynamic drug properties, concurrent drug therapy, dietary influences, laboratory and/or diagnostic testing, and specific patient variables. For example, the prescribed right time for administration of antihypertensive drugs may be four times a day, but for an active, professional, 42-year-old male patient working 13 to 14 hours a day, taking a medication four times daily may not be feasible and lead to noncompliance and subsequent complications. The nurse should contact the physician and inquire about another drug with different dosing frequency (e.g., once or twice daily).

PREVENTING MEDICATION ERRORS

Right Dose?

The nurse is reviewing the orders for a newly admitted patient. One order reads: "Tylenol, 2 tablets PO, every 4 hours as needed for pain or fever."

The pharmacist calls to clarify this order, saying "The dose is not clear." What does the pharmacist mean by this? The order says "2 tablets." Isn't that the dose?

NO! If you look up Tylenol (acetaminophen) in a drug resource book, you will see that Tylenol tablets are available in strengths of both 325 mg and 500 mg. The order is missing the "Right Dose" and needs to be clarified. Never assume the dose of a medication order!

For routine medication orders, the medications must be given no more than $\frac{1}{2}$ hour before or after the actual time specified in the physician's order (i.e., if a medication is ordered to be given at 0900 every morning, it may be given anytime between 0830 and 0930); the exception is medications designated to be given stat (immediately), which must be administered within $\frac{1}{2}$ hour of the time the order is written. The nurse should always check the hospital or facility policy and procedure for any other specific information concerning the "$\frac{1}{2}$ hour before or after" rule. For medication orders with the annotation *prn* (pro re nata, or "as required"), the medication should be given at special times and under certain circumstances. For example, an analgesic is ordered every 4 to 6 hours as needed *prn* for pain; after one dose of the medication the patient complains of pain. After assessment, intervention with another dose of analgesic would occur, but only 4 to 6 hours after the previous dose. Military time is used when medication and other orders are written into a patient's chart (Table 1-1).

Nursing judgment may lead to some variations in timing, but the nurse should be sure to document any change and rationale for the change. If medications are ordered to be given once every day, twice daily, three times daily, or even four times daily, the times of administration may be changed if not harmful to the patient, if the medication/patient's condition does not require adherence to an exact schedule, and only if approved by the physician. For example, suppose that an antacid is ordered to be given three times daily at 0900, 1300, and 1700, but the nurse has misread the order and gives the first dose at 1100. Depending on the hospital or facility policy, the medication and the patient's condition, such an occurrence may not be considered an error, because the dosing may be changed, once the physician is contacted, so

Table 1-1	Conversion of Standard Time to Military Time
Standard Time	**Military Time**
1 AM	0100
2 AM	0200
3 AM	0300
4 AM	0400
5 AM	0500
6 AM	0600
7 AM	0700
8 AM	0800
9 AM	0900
10 AM	1000
11 AM	1100
12 PM (noon)	1200
1 PM	1300
2 PM	1400
3 PM	1500
4 PM	1600
5 PM	1700
6 PM	1800
7 PM	1900
8 PM	2000
9 PM	2100
10 PM	2200
11 PM	2300
12 AM (midnight)	2400

that the drug is given at 1100, 1500, and 1900 without harm to the patient and without incident to the nurse. If this were an antihypertensive medication, the patient's condition and well-being could be greatly compromised by one missed or late dose. Thus, falling behind in dosing times is not to be taken lightly or ignored. A change in the dosing or timing of medication should never be underestimated because one missed dose of certain medications can be life threatening.

Other factors must be considered in determining the right time. These include multiple-drug therapy, drug-drug or drug-food compatibility, scheduling of diagnostic studies, bioavailability of the drug (e.g., the need for consistent timing of doses around the clock to maintain blood levels), drug actions, and any biorhythm effects such as occur with steroids. It is also critical to patient safety to *avoid* using abbreviations for *any* component of a drug order (i.e., dose, time, route). The nurse should spell out *all* terms (e.g., "three times daily" instead of "tid"). The nurse must always be careful to write out all words and abbreviations, because the possibility of miscommunication or misinterpretation poses a risk to the patient.

Right Route

As previously stated, the nurse must know the particulars about each medication before administering it to ensure that the right drug, dose, and route are being used. A complete medication order includes the route of administration. If a medication order does not include the route, the nurse must ask the physician to clarify it. The nurse must never *assume* the route of administration.

Right Patient

Checking the patient's identity before giving each medication dose is critical to the patient's safety. The nurse should ask the patient to state their name and check the patient's identification band to confirm the patient's name, identification number, age, and allergies. With pediatric patients, the parents and/or legal guardians are often the ones who identify the patient for the purpose of giving prescribed medications. With newborns and in labor and delivery situations, the mother and baby have identification bracelets with matching numbers that should be checked before giving medications. With elderly patients or patients with altered sensorium/level of consciousness, asking them their names or having them state their name is not realistic, nor is it safe. Therefore, checking identification bands against the medication profile or medication order is important to avoiding errors.

System Analysis

Although the standard Five Rights of medication administration promote safe nursing practice, they do not include all of the variables that affect medication administration. A possible sixth right—the Right to an appropriate medication process from start to end—should also be considered. The medication administration process looks at more than just the Five Rights because it also examines the entire system such as ordering, dispensing, preparing, administering, and documenting. The pharmacist is responsible for his or her own actions; however, the nurse has to be aware of all facets of medication administration process, check the actions of other health care providers, never assume that all is correct and appropriate, and be responsible for his or her own actions.

Medication Errors

When the Five Rights (and other rights) of drug administration are discussed, medication errors must be considered. Medication errors are a major problem for all of health care, regardless of the setting. The National Coordinating Council for Medication Error Reporting and Prevention defines a **medication error** as any *preventable* event that may cause or lead to inappropriate medication use or patient harm while the medication is in the control of the health care professional, patient, or consumer. Such events may be related to professional practice, health care products, procedures, and systems, including prescribing; order communication; product labeling, packaging, and nomenclature; compounding; dispensing; distribution; administration; education; monitoring; and use (www.nccmerp.org/aboutMedErrors.html).

It is important for the nurse to understand the definition of medication error because the term emphasizes that, in evaluating contributors to a medication error, the nurse must look at the Five Rights of medication administration as well as the entire system involved in the medication administration process. For further discussion of medication errors and their prevention, see Chapter 5.

EVALUATION

Evaluation occurs after the nursing care plan has been implemented. It is systematic, ongoing, and a dynamic phase of the nursing process as related to drug therapy. It includes monitoring of goals and outcome criteria, as well as monitoring the patient's therapeutic response to the drug and its adverse effects and toxic effects. Documentation is also a very important component of evaluation and consists of clear, concise, abbreviation-free charting as related to the meeting of goals and outcome criteria as well as documenting therapeutic effects versus adverse effects and toxic effects of anything related to the medication administration process (see the Legal and Ethical Principles box on this page).

LEGAL AND ETHICAL PRINCIPLES
Charting Don'ts

- Don't record staffing problems (don't mention them in a patient's chart but instead talk with the nurse manager).
- Don't record a peer's conflicts, such as charting possible disputes between a patient and a nurse.
- Don't mention incident reports in charting because they are confidential and are filed separately and not in the patient's chart. The facts of an incident may be documented, but don't mention the terms (e.g., that it was an error).
- Don't use the following terms: "by mistake," "by accident," "accidentally," "unintentional," or "miscalculated."
- Don't chart other patients' names because this is a violation of confidentiality.
- Don't chart anything but facts.
- Don't chart casual conversations with peers, physicians, or other members of the health care team.
- Don't use abbreviations as a general rule of thumb. Some agencies or facilities may still use a list of approved abbreviations, but overall they are discouraged.
- Don't use negative language because it may come back to haunt you!

Data from Institute for Safe Medication Practices: *ISMP medication safety alert,* Huntingdon Valley, Penn, Feb 20, 2003, The Institute; and *Medication and prescription errors.* Available at www.injuryboard.com.

Evaluation also includes the process of monitoring the practice of standards of care. Several standards are in place to help in the evaluation of outcomes of care, such as those established by state nurse practice acts and by the Joint Commission on Accreditation of Healthcare Organizations (JCAHO). Guidelines for nursing services policies and procedures are established by the JCAHO. There are even specific standards regarding medication administration to protect both the patient and the nurse. The ANA Code of Ethics and Patient Rights statement are also used in establishing and evaluating standards of care.

In summary, the nursing process is an ongoing and constantly evolving process (see Box 1-1). The nursing process, as it relates to drug therapy, involves the way in which a nurse gathers, analyzes, organizes, provides, and acts upon data about the patient within the context of prudent nursing care and standards of care. The nurse's ability to make astute assessments, formulate sound nursing diagnoses, establish goals and outcome criteria, correctly administer drugs, and continually evaluate patients' responses to drugs increases with additional experience and knowledge.

Points to Remember

- Nurses are entrusted with confidential information and with the lives of their patients during all facets of patient care, including drug therapy.
- Safe, therapeutic, and effective medication administration is a major responsibility of professional nurses in their care of patients of all ages and in a wide variety of facilities.

- Nurses are responsible for safe and prudent decision making in the nursing care of their patients, including the provision of drug therapy; in accomplishing this task, they attend to the Five Rights and adhere to legal and ethical standards related to medication administration and documentation.
- Nurses need to document in clear, concise language and avoid the use of abbreviations.

NCLEX Examination Review Questions

1. An 86-year-old patient is being discharged to home on digitalis therapy and has very little information regarding the medication. Which of the following statements best reflects a realistic goal or outcome of patient teaching activities?
   a. The patient and patient's daughter will state the correct dosing and administration of the drug.
   b. The nurse will provide teaching about the drug's adverse effects.
   c. The patient will state all the symptoms of digitalis toxicity.
   d. The patient will call the physician if adverse effects occur.
2. What is the most appropriate response to a patient who informs the nurse that he or she does not want to share information about the drugs he or she takes at home?
   a. "It sounds like you are taking something that you don't want us to know about."
   b. "The information about the drugs you take at home, including herbal products, is important for safe administration of drugs while you are here and will be kept confidential."
   c. "We're just asking to make sure you don't have any drug allergies."
   d. "This information will not become part of your medical record, but we need to know so that we can monitor your responses to therapy while you are here."

3. A patient's chart includes an order that reads as follows: "Lanoxin 250 mcg once daily at 0900." Which statement regarding the dosage route for this drug is correct?
   a. The drug should be given via the transdermal route.
   b. The drug should only be given orally.
   c. The drug should be given intravenously.
   d. The dosage route should never be assumed when an order does not specify the route.
4. Which of the following questions is most helpful in compiling a drug history for a patient?
   a. "Do you depend on sleeping pills to get to sleep?"
   b. "Do you have a family history of heart disease?"
   c. "When you take your pain medicine, does it relieve the pain?"
   d. "What childhood diseases did you have?"
5. A 77-year-old man who has been diagnosed with an upper respiratory tract infection tells the nurse that he is allergic to penicillin. Which of the following is the most appropriate response?
   a. "That's to be expected—lots of people are allergic to penicillin."
   b. "This allergy is not of major concern because the drug is given so commonly."
   c. "What type of reaction did you have when you took penicillin?"
   d. "Drug allergies don't usually occur in older individuals because they have built up resistance."

1. a, 2. b, 3. d, 4. c, 5. c.

Critical Thinking Activities

1. What are the crucial responsibilities of the nurse when implementing drug therapy?
2. When medications were administered during the night shift, a patient refused to take his 0200 dose of an antibiotic, claiming that he had just taken it. What actions by the nurse would ensure sound decision making and maintain patient safety?

3. During a busy shift, you note that the chart of your newly admitted patient has a few orders for various medications and diagnostic tests, taken by telephone by another nurse. You were on the way to the patient's room to do your assessment when the unit secretary tells you that one of the orders reads as follows: "Lasix, 20 mg, stat." What should you do first? How do you go about giving this drug? Explain.

For answers, see http://evolve.elsevier.com/Lilley.

Pharmacologic Principles

Objectives

When you reach the end of this chapter, you should be able to do the following:

1. Define the common terms used in pharmacology (see the listing of terms in the Glossary).
2. Understand the role of pharmaceutics, pharmacokinetics, and pharmacodynamics in medication administration and the application of the nursing process.
3. Discuss the application of the four principles of pharmacotherapeutics to everyday nursing practice as they relate to drug therapy for a variety of patients in different health care settings.
4. Discuss the use of natural drug sources in the development of new drugs.
5. Develop a nursing care plan that considers the phases of pharmacokinetics in carrying out drug therapy as related to the nursing process.

e-Learning Activities

Companion CD
- NCLEX Review Questions: see questions 5-17
- Animations
- Audio Glossary
- Category Catchers
- Medication Errors Checklists
- IV Therapy Checklists

evolve Website (http://evolve.elsevier.com/Lilley)
- Nursing Care Plans • Frequently Asked Questions • Content Updates • WebLinks • Supplemental Resources • Elsevier ePharmacology Update • Medication Administration Animations

Glossary

Additive effects Drug interactions in which the effect of a combination of two or more drugs with similar actions is equivalent to the sum of the individual effects of the same drugs given alone (compare with *synergistic effects*). (p. 29)

Adverse drug event (ADE) Any undesirable occurrence related to administering or failing to administer a prescribed medication. (p. 30)

Adverse drug reaction (ADR) Any unexpected, unintended, undesired, or excessive response to a medication given at therapeutic dosages (as opposed to overdose). (p. 30)

Adverse effects Any undesirable bodily effects that are a direct response to one or more drugs. These effects may include *side effects,* which are generally considered to be relatively minor adverse effects that are expected to occur in a percentage of the population receiving a given drug. However, the severity of such effects exists on a continuum. More severe adverse effects may result in changes in prescribed drug therapy after weighing the risk-to-benefit ratio of a drug in a specific clinical situation. The term *adverse effects* is a more general term and will be used in this book to connote any undesirable drug effects. (p. 29)

Agonist A drug that binds to and stimulates the activity of one or more biochemical receptor types in the body. (p. 27)

Allergic reaction An immunologic hypersensitivity reaction resulting from the unusual sensitivity of a patient to a particular medication; a type of ADE. (p. 31)

Antagonist A drug that binds to and inhibits the activity of one or more biochemical receptor types in the body. Antagonists are also called *inhibitors.* (p. 27)

Antagonistic effects Drug interactions in which the effect of a combination of two or more drugs is less than the sum of the individual effects of the same drugs given alone; it is usually caused by an antagonizing (blocking or reducing) effect of one drug on another. (p. 29)

Bioavailability A measure of the extent of drug absorption for a given drug and route (from 0% to 100%). (p. 18)

Biotransformation One or more biochemical reactions involving a *parent* drug. Biotransformation occurs mainly in the liver and produce a metabolite that is either inactive or active. Also known as *metabolism.* (p. 23)

Chemical name The name that describes the chemical composition and molecular structure of a drug. (p. 16)

Contraindication Any condition, especially one related to a disease state or other patient characteristic, including current or recent drug therapy, that renders a particular form of treatment improper or undesirable. (p. 28)

Cytochrome P-450 General name for a large class of enzymes (found especially in the liver) that play a significant role in drug metabolism. (p. 23)

Dissolution The process by which solid forms of drugs disintegrate in the gastrointestinal tract, become soluble, and are absorbed into the circulation. (p. 17)

Drug Any chemical that affects the physiologic processes of a living organism. (p. 16)

Drug actions The cellular processes involved in the interaction between a drug and body cells (e.g., the action of a drug on a receptor protein); also called *mechanism of action.* (p. 17)

Drug effects The physiologic reactions of the body to a drug. They can be *therapeutic* or *toxic* and constitute how the function of the body is affected as a whole by the drug. The terms *onset, peak,* and *duration* are used to describe drug effects (most often referring to therapeutic effects). (p. 26)

Drug-induced teratogenesis The development of congenital anomalies or defects in the developing fetus caused by the toxic effects of drugs. (p. 31)

Drug interaction Alteration in the pharmacologic activity of a given drug caused by the presence of one or more additional drugs; it is usually related to effects on the enzymes required for metabolism of the involved drugs. (p. 29)

Duration of action The length of time the concentration of a drug in the blood or tissues is sufficient to elicit a therapeutic response. (p. 26)

Enzymes Protein molecules that catalyze one or more of a variety of biochemical reactions, including those related to the body's own physiologic processes as well as those related to drug metabolism. (p. 27)

First-pass effect The initial metabolism in the liver of a drug absorbed from the gastrointestinal tract before the drug reaches systemic circulation through the bloodstream. (p. 18)

Generic name The name given to a drug by the United States Adopted Names Council. Also called the *nonproprietary name.* The generic name is much shorter and simpler than the chemical name and is not protected by trademark. (p. 16)

Half-life In *pharmacokinetics,* the time required for half of an administered dose of drug to be eliminated by the body (also called *elimination half-life*). (p. 26)

Idiosyncratic reaction An abnormal and unexpected response to a medication, other than an allergic reaction, that is peculiar to an individual patient. (p. 31)

Incompatibility The quality of two parenteral drugs or solutions that leads to a reaction resulting in the chemical deterioration of at least one of the drugs when the two substances are mixed. (p. 30)

Medication error (ME) Any *preventable* ADE involving inappropriate medication use by a patient or health care professional; it may or may not cause patient harm. (p. 30)

Medication use process The prescribing, dispensing, and administering of medications, and the monitoring of their effects. (p. 30)

Metabolite A chemical form of a drug that is the product of one or more biochemical (metabolic) reactions involving the *parent drug* (see below). Active metabolites are those that have pharmacologic activity of their own, even if the parent drug is inactive (see *prodrug*). Inactive metabolites lack pharmacologic activity and are simply drug waste products awaiting excretion from the body (e.g., via the urinary, gastrointestinal, or respiratory tract). (p. 16)

Onset of action The time required for a drug to elicit a therapeutic response after dosing. (p. 26)

Parent drug The chemical form of a drug that is administered before it is metabolized by the body's biochemical reactions into its active or inactive metabolites (see *metabolite*). A parent drug that is not pharmacologically active itself is called a *prodrug.* A prodrug is then metabolized to pharmacologically active metabolites. (p. 18)

Peak effect The time required for a drug to reach its maximum therapeutic response in the body. (p. 26)

Peak level The maximum concentration of a drug in the body after administration, usually measured in a blood sample for *therapeutic drug monitoring.* (p. 27)

Pharmaceutics The science of preparing and dispensing drugs, including dosage form design (e.g., tablets, capsules, injections, patches, etc.). (p. 16)

Pharmacodynamics The study of the biochemical and physiologic interactions of drugs at their sites of activity. It examines the physicochemical properties of drugs and their pharmacologic interactions with body receptors. (p. 16)

Pharmacogenetics The study of the influence of genetic factors on drug response, including the nature of genetic aberrations that result in the absence, overabundance, or insufficiency of drug-metabolizing enzymes (also called *pharmacogenomics;* Chapter 50). (p. 31)

Pharmacognosy The study of drugs that are obtained from natural plant and animal sources. This science was formerly called *materia medica* (medicinal materials) and is concerned with the botanical or zoologic origin, biochemical composition, and therapeutic effects of *natural* drugs, their derivatives, and their constituents. (p. 17)

Pharmacokinetics The rate of drug distribution among various body compartments after a drug has entered the body. It includes the phases of absorption, distribution, metabolism, and excretion of drugs. (p. 16)

Pharmacology Broadest term for the study or science of drugs. (p. 16)

Pharmacotherapeutics The treatment of pathologic conditions through the use of drugs. (p. 17)

Prodrug An inactive drug dosage form that is converted to an active metabolite by various biochemical chemical reactions once it is inside the body. Often a prodrug is more readily absorbable than is its active metabolite, hence the need for its development. (p. 23)

Receptor A molecular structure within or on the outer surface of a cell. Receptors bind specific substances (e.g., drug molecules), and one or more corresponding cellular effects (drug effects) occurs as a result of this drug-receptor interaction. (p. 16)

Steady state The physiologic state in which the amount of drug removed via elimination is equal to the amount of drug absorbed with each dose. (p. 26)

Substrate A substance (e.g., drug or natural biochemical in the body) on which an enzyme acts. (p. 24)

Synergistic effects Drug interactions in which the effect of a combination of two or more drugs with similar actions is *greater than* the sum of the individual effects of the same drugs given alone (compare with *additive effects*). (p. 29)

Therapeutic drug monitoring The process of measuring drug *peak* and *trough levels* to gauge the level of a patient's drug exposure and allow adjustment of dosages with the joint goals of maximizing *therapeutic effects* and minimizing *toxicity.* (p. 27)

Therapeutic effect The desired or intended effect of a particular medication. (p. 27)

Therapeutic index The ratio between the toxic and therapeutic concentrations of a drug. If the index is low, the difference between the therapeutic and toxic drug concentrations is small, and use of the drug is more hazardous. (p. 29)

Toxic   The quality of being poisonous (i.e., injurious to health or dangerous to life). (p. 17)

Toxicity   The condition of producing adverse bodily effects due to poisonous qualities. (p. 27)

Toxicology   The study of poisons. It deals with the effects of drugs and other chemicals in living systems, their detection, and treatments to counteract their poisonous effects. (p. 17)

Trade name   The commercial name given to a drug product by its manufacturer; also called the *proprietary name.* The presence of a trade name indicates that a particular drug is registered and that its production is restricted to the owner of the patent for that drug until the patent expires. (p. 16)

Trough level   The lowest concentration of drug reached in the body after it falls from its *peak level,* usually measured in a blood sample for *therapeutic drug monitoring.* (p. 27)

OVERVIEW

Any chemical that affects the physiologic processes of a living organism can broadly be defined as a **drug.** The study or science of drugs is known as **pharmacology.** Pharmacology encompasses a variety of topics, including the following:

- Absorption
- Biochemical effects
- Biotransformation (metabolism)
- Distribution
- Drug history
- Drug origin
- Excretion
- Mechanisms of action
- Physical and chemical properties
- Physical effects
- Drug receptor mechanisms
- Therapeutic (beneficial) effects
- Toxic (harmful) effects

Knowledge of these various areas of pharmacology enables the nurse to better understand how drugs affect humans. Without a sound understanding of basic pharmacologic principles, the nurse cannot fully appreciate the therapeutic benefits and potential toxicity of drugs.

Pharmacology is an extensive science that incorporates several interrelated areas: pharmaceutics, pharmacokinetics, pharmacodynamics, pharmacotherapeutics, pharmacognosy, and toxicology. The various drugs discussed in each chapter of this text are described from the standpoint of one or more of these five areas.

Throughout the process of development, a drug will acquire at least three different names. The **chemical name** describes the drug's chemical composition and molecular structure. The **generic name,** or nonproprietary name, is given to the drug by the United States Adopted Names (USAN) Council. It is often much shorter and simpler than the chemical name. The generic name is used in most official drug compendiums to list drugs. The **trade name,** or proprietary name, is the drug's registered trademark and indicates that its commercial use is restricted to the owner of the patent for the drug. The owner is usually the manufacturer of the drug. Trade names are generally created by the manufacturer with marketability in mind. For this reason, they are usually shorter and easier to pronounce and remember than generic drug names. The *patent life* of a newly discovered drug molecule is normally 17 years. This is the length of time from patent approval until patent expiration. Because the research processes for new drug development normally require about 10 years, a drug manufacturer generally has the remaining 7 years for sales profits before patent expiration. A significant amount of these profits serves merely to offset the multimillion-dollar costs for research and development of the drug. After the patent expires for a given drug, other manufacturers may legally begin to manufacturer *generic* drugs with the same active ingredient. At this point, the drug price usually falls substantially, which offers many patients and third-party payers the benefit of savings on the generic (vs. the original brand name) drug (Figure 2-1).

Three basic areas of pharmacology—pharmaceutics, pharmacokinetics, and pharmacodynamics—describe the relationship between the dose of a drug given to a patient and the activity of that drug in treating the patient's disorder. **Pharmaceutics** includes the study of how various dosage forms (e.g., injection, capsule, controlled-release tablet) influence the way in which the body metabolizes a drug and the way in which the drug affects the body. **Pharmacokinetics** is the study of what the body does to the drug molecules. Pharmacokinetics involves the processes of absorption, distribution, metabolism, and excretion. These four phases and their relationship to drug and drug **metabolite** concentrations are determined for various body sites over specified periods. The onset of action, the peak effect of a drug, and the duration of action of a drug are all part of the drug's pharmacokinetics. **Pharmacodynamics,** on the other hand, is the study of what the drug does to the body. Pharmacodynamics involves drug-receptor interactions. *Receptor theory* assumes that all drugs perform their unique actions at chemically specific **receptor** sites in various tissues. Receptors are usually specialized protein molecules on the outer surfaces of cells or within cells to which drug molecules bind to exert their effects. It must be

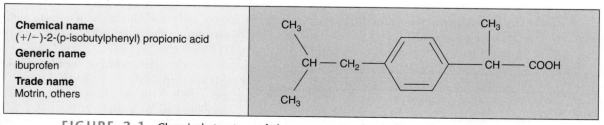

Chemical name
(+/−)-2-(p-isobutylphenyl) propionic acid

Generic name
ibuprofen

Trade name
Motrin, others

FIGURE 2-1   Chemical structure of the common analgesic ibuprofen and the chemical, generic, and trade names for the drug.

noted, however, that not all mechanisms of action have been identified for all drugs. Thus, a drug may be said to have an unknown or unclear mechanism of action, even though it has observable therapeutic effects in the body. Figure 2-2 illustrates the three phases that affect drug activity, starting with the pharmaceutical phase, proceeding to the pharmacokinetic phase, and finishing with the pharmacodynamic phase.

Pharmacotherapeutics (also called *therapeutics*) focuses on the use of drugs and the clinical indications for administering drugs to prevent and treat diseases. It defines the principles of **drug actions**—the cellular processes that change in response to the presence of drug molecules. Therefore, an understanding of pharmacotherapeutics is essential for nurses when implementing drug therapy. *Empirical therapeutics* refers to drug therapy that is effective but for which the mechanism of drug action is unknown. *Rational therapeutics* is drug therapy in which specific evidence has been obtained for the mechanisms of drug action. Some drug mechanisms of action are more clearly understood than others.

The study of the adverse effects of drugs and other chemicals on living systems is known as **toxicology. Toxic** effects are often an extension of a drug's therapeutic action. Therefore, toxicology often involves overlapping principles of both pharmacotherapy and toxicology. The study of *natural* (vs. *synthetic*) drug sources (both plants and animals) is called **pharmacognosy.**

In summary, pharmacology is a very dynamic science incorporating several different disciplines (as mentioned earlier). Tra-ditionally, chemistry has been seen as the primary basis of pharmacology, but pharmacology also relies heavily on physiology and biology.

PHARMACEUTICS

Different drug dosage forms have different pharmaceutical properties. Dosage form design determines the rate at which drug **dissolution** (dissolving of solid dosage forms and their absorption [e.g., from gastrointestinal (GI) tract fluids]). A drug to be ingested orally may be taken in either a solid form (tablet, capsule, or powder) or a liquid form (solution or suspension). Table 2-1 lists various oral drug preparations and the relative rate at which they are absorbed. Oral drugs that are liquids (e.g., elixirs, syrups) are already dissolved and are usually absorbed more quickly than solid dosage forms. Enteric-coated tablets, on the other hand, have a coating that prevents them from being broken down in an acidic pH environment and therefore are not absorbed until they reach the higher (more alkaline) pH of the intestines. This pharmaceutical property results in slower dissolution and therefore slower absorption. Sometimes the size of the particles within a capsule can make different capsules containing the same drug dissolve at different rates, become absorbed at different rates, and thus have different times to onset of action. A prime example is the difference between micronized glyburide and nonmicronized glyburide. Micronized glyburide reaches a maximum concentration peak faster than does the nonmicronized formulation because of how the dosage form is pharmaceutically engineered.

A variety of dosage forms exist to provide both accurate and convenient drug delivery systems (Table 2-2). These delivery systems are designed to achieve a desired therapeutic response with minimal adverse effects. Many dosage forms have been de-

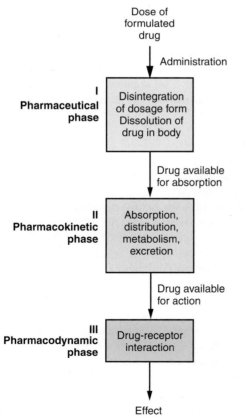

FIGURE 2-2   Phases of drug activity. *(From McKenry LM, Tessier E, Hogan M: Mosby's pharmacology in nursing, ed 22, St Louis, 2006, Mosby.)*

Table 2-1	Drug Absorption of Various Oral Preparations
Liquids, elixirs, and syrups	Fastest
Suspension solutions	
Powders	
Capsules	
Tablets	
Coated tablets	
Enteric-coated tablets	Slowest

Table 2-2	Dosage Forms
Route	**Forms**
Enteral	Tablets, capsules, pills, timed-release capsules, timed-release tablets, elixirs, suspensions, syrups, emulsions, solutions, lozenges or troches, rectal suppositories (rectal)
Parenteral	Injectable forms, solutions, suspensions, emulsions, powders for reconstitution, sublingual or buccal tablets
Topical	Aerosols, ointments, creams, pastes, powders, solutions, foams, gels, transdermal patches, inhalers, vaginal suppositories

veloped to encourage patient compliance with the medication regimen. Convenience of administration correlates strongly with medication compliance. Many of the extended-release oral dosage forms were designed with this in mind, as they often require fewer daily doses.

The specific characteristics of various dosage forms have a large impact on how and to what extent the drug is absorbed. If a drug is to work at a specific site in the body, either it must be applied directly at that site in an active form or it must have a way of getting to that site. Oral dosage forms rely on gastric and intestinal enzymes and pH environments to break the medication down into particles that are small enough to be absorbed into the circulation. Once absorbed through the mucosa of the stomach or intestines, the drug is then transported to the site of action by blood or lymph.

Many topically applied dosage forms work directly on the surface of the skin. Therefore, when the drug is applied, it is already in a dosage form that allows it to act immediately. With other topical dosage forms, the skin acts as a barrier through which the drug must pass to get into the circulation; once there, the drug is then carried to its site of action (e.g., fentanyl transdermal patch for pain).

Dosage forms that are administered via injection are called *parenteral* forms. They must have certain characteristics to be safe and effective. The arteries and veins that carry drugs throughout the body can easily be damaged if the drug is too concentrated or corrosive. The pH of injections must be very similar to the blood to be safely administered. Parenteral dosage forms that are injected intravenously or intraarterially are immediately placed into solution in the bloodstream and do not have to be dissolved in the body. Therefore, 100% absorption is assumed to occur immediately upon intravenous or intraarterial injection. The intraarterial route is used much less commonly than the intravenous route but is commonly used in intensive care unit and oncology care settings.

PHARMACOKINETICS

A particular drug's onset of action, peak effect, and duration of action are all characteristics defined by pharmacokinetics. Pharmacokinetics is the study of what actually happens to a drug from the time it is put into the body until the **parent drug** and all metabolites have left the body. Thus, drug absorption into, distribution and metabolism within, and excretion from a living organism represent the combined focus of pharmacokinetics.

Absorption

Absorption is the movement of a drug from its site of administration into the bloodstream for distribution to the tissues. A term used to express the extent of drug absorption is **bioavailability.** For example, a drug that is absorbed from the intestine must first pass through the liver before it reaches the systemic circulation. If the drug is metabolized in the liver or excreted in the bile, some of the active drug will be inactivated or diverted before it can reach the general circulation and its intended sites of action. This is known as the **first-pass effect,** and it reduces the bioavailability of the drug to less than 100%. Many drugs administered by mouth have a bioavailability of less than 100%, whereas drugs administered by the intravenous route are 100% bioavailable, as noted earlier. If two medications have the same bioavailability and same concentration of active ingredient, they are said to be *bioequivalent* (e.g., a brand-name drug and the same generic drug).

Various factors affect the rate of drug absorption. These include the presence of food or fluids ingested with the drug, the dosage formulation, the status of the absorptive surface, the rate of blood flow to the small intestine, the acidity of the stomach, and GI motility. How a drug is administered, or its *route of administration*, also affects the rate and extent of absorption of that drug. Although a number of dosage formulations are available for delivering medications to the body, they can all be categorized into three basic routes of administration: enteral (GI tract), parenteral, and topical. Various administration routes and their effects on absorption are examined in detail in the following sections. Drug distribution, metabolism, and excretion are then discussed.

Enteral

In enteral drug administration, the drug is absorbed into the systemic circulation through the mucosa of the stomach or small intestine. The rate of absorption of enterally administered drugs can be altered by many factors. Depending on the particular drug, it may be extensively metabolized in the liver before it reaches the systemic circulation. Normally, orally administered drugs are absorbed from the intestinal lumen into the mesenteric blood system and conveyed by the portal vein to the liver. Once the drug is in the liver, the hepatic enzyme systems metabolize it, and the remaining active ingredients are passed into the general circulation. As noted previously, this initial metabolism of a drug and its passage from the liver into the circulation is called the *first-pass effect* (Figure 2-3). If a large proportion of a drug is chemically processed into inactive metabolites in the liver, then a much smaller amount of drug will pass into the circulation (i.e., will be bioavailable). Such a drug is said to have a high first-pass effect (e.g., oral nitrates).

The same drug given intravenously will bypass the liver. This prevents the first-pass effect from taking place, and therefore more of the drug reaches the circulation. For this reason, paren-

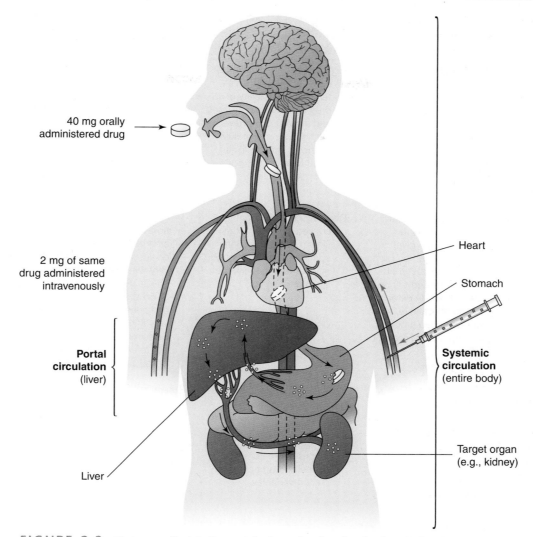

40 mg orally
administered drug

2 mg of same
drug administered
intravenously

**Portal
circulation**
(liver)

Liver

Heart

Stomach

**Systemic
circulation**
(entire body)

Target organ
(e.g., kidney)

FIGURE 2-3   First-pass effect is the metabolism of a drug by the liver before its systemic availability.

teral doses of drugs with a high first-pass effect are often much smaller than enterally administered (oral) doses, yet they produce the same pharmacologic response. See Table 2-3 for further discussion of the advantages, disadvantages, and nursing considerations related to the various routes of administration.

Many factors can alter the absorption of enterally administered drugs, including acid changes within the stomach, absorption changes in the intestines, and the presence or absence of food and fluid. Various factors that affect the acidity of the stomach include the time of day; the age of the patient; and the presence and types of any medications, foods, or beverages. If food is in the stomach during the dissolution of an orally administered medication, this may interfere with the drug's dissolution and absorption and delay its transit from the stomach to the small intestine, where most drugs are absorbed. On the other hand, food may enhance the absorption of some fat-soluble drugs (depending on the fat content of the food) or drugs that are more easily broken down in an acidic environment. (Food in the stomach increases gastric acid production.)

Before orally administered drugs are passed into the portal circulation of the liver, they are absorbed in the small intestine,

which has an enormous surface area. Drug absorption may be altered in patients who have had portions of the small intestine removed because of disease. Anticholinergic drugs may slow the GI *transit time* or the time it takes for substances in the stomach to be dissolved and absorbed into the intestines. This may allow more time for an acid-susceptible drug to be in contact with the acid in the stomach and subsequently to be broken down, which reduces drug absorption. Examples of drugs to be taken on an empty stomach and those to be taken with food are provided in Box 2-1. The stomach and small intestine are highly vascularized. When blood flow to that area is decreased, absorption may also be decreased. Sepsis and exercise are examples of circumstances under which blood flow to the GI tract is often reduced. In both cases, blood tends to be routed to the heart and other vital organs. In the case of exercise, it is also routed to the skeletal muscles.

Sublingual and Buccal

Drugs administered by the *sublingual* route are absorbed into the highly vascularized tissue under the tongue—the oral mucosa. Sublingual nitroglycerin is an example. Sublingually administered drugs are absorbed rapidly because the area under the

Table 2-3	Routes of Administration and Related Nursing Considerations		
Route	**Advantages**	**Disadvantages**	**Nursing Considerations**
Intravenous (IV)	Provides rapid onset (drug delivered immediately to bloodstream), allows more direct control of drug level in blood, gives option of larger fluid volume therefore diluting irritating drugs; avoids first-pass metabolism	Higher cost; inconvenience (e.g., not self-administered); irreversibility of drug action in most cases and inability to retrieve medication; risk of fluid overload; greater likelihood of infection; possibility of embolism	Continuous IV infusions require frequent monitoring to be sure that the correct volume and amount are administered and that drug reaches safe, therapeutic blood levels. IV drugs and solutions should be checked for compatibilities. IV sites should be monitored for redness, swelling, heat, and drainage—all indicative of complications, such as thrombophlebitis. If intermittent IV infusions are used, clearing or flushing of the line with normal saline before and after is generally indicated to keep the IV site patent and minimize incompatibilities.
Intramuscular (IM); subcutaneous (SC)	IM injections are good for poorly soluble drugs, which are often given in "depot" preparation form and are then absorbed over a prolonged period; onsets of action differ depending on route (e.g., IM injections often produce more rapid onset than SC injections)	Discomfort of injection; inconvenience; bruising; slower onset of action compared to IV, although quicker than oral in most situations	Using landmarks to identify correct IM and SC sites is always required and is recommended as a nursing standard of care. Ventral gluteal site is IM site of choice with use of 1½-inch (sometimes 1-inch in very thin or emaciated patients) and 21-25 gauge needle. SC injections are recommended to be given at 90-degree angle with proper size syringe and needle (½- to ⅝-inch needle); in emaciated or very thin patients, SC angle should be 45 degrees. Selection of correct size of syringe and needle is key to safe administration by these routes and is based on thorough assessment of the patient as well as drug characteristics.
Oral	Usually easier, more convenient, and less expensive; safer than injection, dosing more likely to be reversible in cases of accidental ingestion (e.g., through induction of emesis, administration of activated charcoal)	Variable absorption; inactivation of some drugs by stomach acid and/or pH; problems with first-pass effect or pre-systemic metabolism; greater dependence of drug action on patient variables	Enteral routes include oral administration and involve a variety of dosage forms, e.g., liquids, solutions, tablets, and enteric-coated pills or tablets. Some medications should be taken with food and some should not be taken with food; oral forms should always be taken with at least 6-8 oz of fluid, such as water. Other factors to consider include other medicines being taken at the same time and concurrent use of dairy products or antacids. If oral forms are given via nasogastric tube or gastrostomy tube, tube should be assessed for placement in stomach and head should remain elevated; at least 30-60 mL of water or carbonated fluids should be used to flush tube prior to and after drug has been given to keep tube patent.
Sublingual, buccal (subtypes of oral, but more parenteral than enteral)	Absorbed more rapidly from oral mucosa and leads to more rapid onset of action; avoids breakdown of drug by stomach acid; *avoids* first-pass metabolism because gastric absorption is bypassed	Patients may swallow pill instead of keeping under tongue until dissolved; pills often smaller to handle	Drugs given via sublingual route should be placed under tongue; once dissolved, drug may then be swallowed. In buccal route, medication is placed between cheek and gum. Both of these dosage forms are relatively nonirritating; drug is usually without flavor and water soluble.
Rectal	Provides relatively rapid absorption; good alternative when oral route not feasible; useful for local or systemic drug delivery; usually leads to mixed first-pass and non–first-pass metabolism	Possible discomfort and embarrassment to patient; often higher cost than oral route	Absorption via this route is erratic and unpredictable, but it provides a safe alternative whenever nausea or vomiting prevents oral dosing of drugs. Patient should lie on left side for insertion of rectal dosage form. Suppositories are inserted using gloved hand or index finger and water-soluble lubricant. Drug should be administered exactly as ordered.

Table 2-3	**Routes of Administration and Related Nursing Considerations—cont'd**		
Route	**Advantages**	**Disadvantages**	**Nursing Considerations**
Topical	Delivers medication directly to affected area; decreases likelihood of systemic drug effects	Sometimes awkward to self-administer (e.g., eyedrops); can be messy; usually higher cost than oral route	Most dermatologic drugs are given via topical route in form of a solution, ointment, spray, or drops. Skin should be clean and free of debris; if measurement of ointment is necessary—such as with topical nitroglycerin—it should be done carefully and per instructions (e.g., apply 1 inch of ointment). Nurse should wear gloves to minimize cross contamination and prevent absorption of drug into his or her skin. If patient's skin is not intact, sterile technique is needed.
Transdermal (subtype of topical)	Provides relatively constant rate of drug absorption; one patch can last 1-7 days, depending on drug; avoids first-pass metabolism	Rate of absorption can be affected by excessive perspiration and body temperature; patch may peel off; cost is higher; used patches must be disposed of safely	Transdermal drugs should be placed on alternating sites, on a clean and nonirritating area, and only after previously applied patch has been removed and area cleansed and dried. Transdermal drugs generally come in a single-dose, adhesive-backed drug application system.

Box 2-1 **Drugs to Be Taken on an Empty Stomach and Drugs to Be Taken with Food**

Many medications are taken on an empty stomach with at least 6 oz of water. The nurse must give patients specific instructions regarding those medications that are not to be taken with food and should be taken on an empty stomach. Examples include alendronate sodium and risedronate sodium.

Medications that are generally taken with food include carbamazepine, iron and iron-containing products, hydralazine, lithium, propranolol, spironolactone, nonsteroidal antiinflammatory drugs, and theophylline.

Erythromycins, tetracyclines, and theophylline are often taken with food (even though they are specified to be taken with a full glass of water and on an empty stomach) to minimize the gastrointestinal irritation associated with these drugs. If doubt exists, a licensed pharmacist or a current authoritative drug resource should be consulted. An Internet source to use is http://www.usp.org.

---

tongue has a large blood supply. These drugs bypass the liver and yet are systemically bioavailable. The same concepts apply for drugs administered by the *buccal* route (the oral mucosa between the cheek and the gum). Through these routes, drugs such as nitroglycerin are absorbed rapidly into the bloodstream and delivered to their site of action (e.g., coronary arteries).

Parenteral

For most medications, the parenteral route is the fastest route by which a drug can be absorbed, followed by the enteral and topical routes. *Parenteral* is a general term meaning any route of administration other than the GI tract. Most commonly it refers to injection by any method, although topical and transdermal medications can also be considered parenteral dosage forms (see later), as can sublingual and buccal medications. Intravenous injection delivers the drug directly into the circulation, where it is distributed with the blood throughout the body. An intravenous drug formulation is thus absorbed the fastest. At the other end of the spectrum are transdermal patches, intramuscular injections, and

subcutaneous injections. These drug formulations are usually absorbed over a period of several hours, days, or weeks.

Drugs can be injected intradermally, subcutaneously, intraarterially, intramuscularly, intrathecally, intraarticularly, or intravenously. Medications given by the parenteral route also have the advantage of bypassing the first-pass effect of the liver. The parenteral route of administration offers an alternative route of delivery for those medications that cannot be given orally. The problems posed by acid changes in the stomach, absorption changes in the intestines (e.g., following intestinal surgery), and the presence or absence of food and fluid are no longer a concern. There are fewer obstacles to absorption with parenteral administration than with enteral administration of drugs. However, drugs that are administered by the parenteral route must still be absorbed into cells and tissues before they can exert their pharmacologic effect. (See Table 2-3.)

Subcutaneous, Intradermal, and Intramuscular
Parenteral injections into the fatty subcutaneous tissues under the dermal layer of skin are referred to as *subcutaneous injections*, whereas injections under the more superficial skin layers immediately underneath the epidermal layer of skin and into the dermal layer are known as *intradermal injections*. Parenteral injections given into the muscle beneath the subcutaneous fatty tissue are referred to as *intramuscular injections*. Muscles have a greater blood supply than does the skin; therefore, drugs injected intramuscularly are typically absorbed faster than drugs injected subcutaneously. Absorption from either of these sites may be increased by applying heat to the injection site or by massaging the site. Both increase blood flow to the area, thereby enhancing absorption. Most intramuscularly injected drugs are absorbed over several hours. However, specially formulated long-acting intramuscular dosage forms known as *depot* drugs are designed for slow absorption and may be absorbed over a period of several days to a few months or longer. The intramuscular corticosteroid known as methylprednisolone acetate (Kenalog injection) can provide antiinflammatory effects for several weeks. The intramuscular contraceptive medroxyprogesterone acetate (Depo-Provera) normally

prevents pregnancy for 3 months per dose. The subcutaneously administered drug insulin glargine (Lantus) is a long-acting insulin product that is now in common use.

In contrast, the presence of cold, hypotension, or poor peripheral blood flow compromises the circulation, reducing drug activity by reducing drug delivery to the tissues.

Topical

Topical routes of drug administration involve the application of medications to various body surfaces. Several different topical drug delivery systems exist. Topically administered drugs can be applied to the skin, eyes, ears, nose, lungs, rectum, or vagina. As with the enteral and parenteral routes, there are benefits and drawbacks to use of the topical route of administration. Topical application delivers a more uniform amount of drug over a longer period of time, but the effects of the drug are usually slower in their onset and more prolonged in their duration of action. This can be a problem if the patient begins to experience adverse effects from the drug and a considerable amount of drug has already been absorbed into the subcutaneous or mucosal tissues. All topical routes of drug administration also avoid first-pass effects of the liver, with the exception of rectal drug administration. Because the rectum is part of the GI tract, some drug will be absorbed into the capillaries that feed the portal vein to the liver. However, some drugs will also be absorbed locally into the perirectal tissues. Therefore, rectally administered drugs are said to have a mixed first-pass and non–first-pass absorption and metabolism. Box 2-2 lists the various drug routes and indicates whether they are associated with first-pass effects in the liver.

Topical ointments, gels, and creams are common types of topically administered drugs. Examples include sunscreens, antibiotics, and nitroglycerin ointment. The drawback to their use is that their systemic absorption is often erratic and unreliable. Generally, these medications are used for local effects, but some are used for systemic effects (e.g., nitroglycerin ointment for maintenance treatment of angina). Topically applied drugs can also be used in the treatment of various illnesses of the eyes, ears, and sinuses. Eye, ear, and nose drops are administered primarily for local and not systemic effects, whereas nasal sprays may be used for both (e.g., oxymetazoline for nasal sinus congestion, sumatriptan for migraine headaches). Rectally administered drugs are often given for systemic effects (e.g., antinausea, analgesia), but they are also used to treat disease within the rectum or adjacent bowel (e.g., antiinflammatory ointment for hemorrhoids, corticosteroid enemas for colitis). Vaginal medications may also be given for systemic effects (e.g., progestational hormone therapy) but are more commonly used for local effects (e.g., treatment of vaginal infection).

Transdermal

Transdermal drug delivery through adhesive drug patches is a more elaborate topical route of drug administration that is commonly used for systemic drug effects. Some examples of drugs administered by this route are fentanyl (for pain), nitroglycerin (for angina), nicotine (for smoking cessation), estrogen (for menopausal symptoms), and clonidine (for hypertension). Transdermal patches are usually designed to deliver a constant amount of drug per unit of time for a specified time period. For example, a nitroglycerin patch may deliver 0.1 or 0.2 mg of drug in a 24-hour period, whereas a fentanyl patch may deliver 25 to 100 mcg/hr of fentanyl for a 72-hour period. Transdermal drug delivery also offers the advantage of bypassing the liver and its first-pass effects. It is suitable for patients who cannot tolerate orally administered medications and in other situations provides a practical and convenient method for drug delivery. The design of the drug delivery system in a specific transdermal patch determines its duration of action.

Inhaled

Inhalation is another type of topical drug administration. Inhaled drugs are delivered to the lungs as micrometer-sized drug particles. This small drug size is necessary for the drug to be transported to the small air sacs within the lungs (alveoli). Once the small particles of drug are in the alveoli, drug absorption is fairly rapid. At this site the thin-walled pulmonary alveolus is in contact with the capillaries, where the drug can be absorbed quickly. Many pulmonary and other types of diseases can be treated with such topically applied (inhaled) drugs. Examples of inhaled drugs are pentamidine, which is used to treat *Pneumocystis jirovecii* (formerly *Pneumocystis carinii*) infections in the lung; albuterol, which is used to treat bronchial constriction in individuals with asthma; and vasopressin, which is used to treat diabetes insipidus.

Distribution

Distribution refers to the transport of a drug in the body by the bloodstream to its site of action (Figure 2-4). The areas to which the drug is distributed first are those that are most extensively supplied with blood. Areas of rapid distribution include the heart, liver, kidneys, and brain. Areas of slower distribution include muscle, skin, and fat. Once a drug enters the bloodstream (circulation), it is distributed throughout the body. At this point it is also beginning to be eliminated by the organs that metabolize and excrete drugs—primarily the liver and the kidneys. Drug molecules can be freely distributed to *extravascular* tissue (outside the blood vessels) to reach their site of action only if they are not bound to plasma proteins. If a drug is bound to plasma proteins, the drug-protein complex is generally too large to pass through

---

Box 2-2	**Drug Routes and First-Pass Effects**

First-Pass Routes
Hepatic arterial
Oral
Portal venous
Rectal*

Non–First-Pass Routes
Aural (instilled into the ear)
Buccal
Inhaled
Intraarterial
Intramuscular
Intranasal
Intraocular
Intravaginal
Intravenous
Subcutaneous
Sublingual
Transdermal

*Leads to both first-pass and non–first-pass effects.

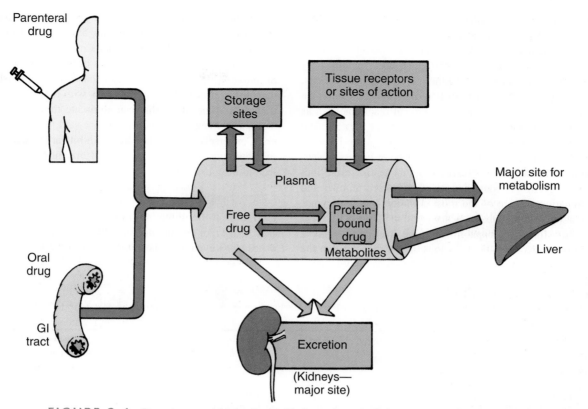

FIGURE 2-4   Drug transport in the body. *GI,* Gastrointestinal. *(From McKenry LM, Salerno E: Mosby's pharmacology in nursing, ed 19, St Louis, 1995, Mosby.)*

the walls of blood capillaries into tissues. There are three primary proteins that bind to and carry drugs in the bloodstream throughout the body: *albumin,* α_1-acid glycoprotein, and *corticosteroid-binding globulin.* By far the most important of these is albumin. As the most common blood protein, albumin carries the majority of protein-bound drug molecules. If a given drug binds to plasma proteins as part of its chemical attributes, then there is only a limited amount of drug that is *not* bound to protein. This unbound portion is pharmacologically active and is considered "free" drug, whereas "bound" drug is pharmacologically inactive. Certain conditions that cause low albumin levels, such as extensive burns, malnourished states, and negative nitrogen balance, result in the presence of a larger fraction of free (unbound and active) drug. This can raise the risk of drug toxicity.

When an individual is taking two medications that are highly protein bound, the medications may compete for binding sites on plasma proteins. Because of this competition, less of one or both of the drugs binds to the proteins. Consequently, there is more free, unbound drug. This can lead to an unpredictable drug response called a *drug-drug interaction.* A drug-drug interaction occurs when the presence of one drug decreases or increases the actions of another drug administered concurrently (given at the same time).

A theoretical volume, called the *volume of distribution,* is sometimes used to describe the various areas in which drugs may be distributed. These areas, or *compartments,* may be the blood (*intravascular space*), total body water, body fat, or other body tissues and organs. Typically a drug that is highly water soluble will have a small volume of distribution and high blood concentrations. In other words, the drug tends to stay within the blood

because of its high water content. The opposite is true for drugs that are highly fat soluble. Fat-soluble drugs have a large volume of distribution and low blood concentrations. This is because they tend to be chemically repelled by the high water content of the blood and more attracted by the relatively low water content and higher fat content of the tissues. Drugs that are water soluble and highly protein bound are more strongly bound to proteins in the blood and are less likely to be absorbed into tissues. Because of this, their distribution and onset of action can be slow. Drugs that are highly lipid soluble and poorly bound to protein are more easily taken up into tissues and distributed throughout the body. They may also be reabsorbed back into the circulation from tissue.

There are some sites in the body into which it may be very difficult to distribute a drug. These sites typically either have a poor blood supply (e.g., bone) or have physiologic barriers that make it difficult for drugs to pass through (e.g., the brain due to the blood-brain barrier).

Metabolism

Metabolism is also referred to as **biotransformation** because it involves the biochemical alteration of a drug into an inactive metabolite, a more soluble compound, or a more potent active metabolite (as in the conversion of an inactive **prodrug** to its active form). Metabolism is the next step after absorption and distribution. The organ most responsible for the metabolism of drugs is the liver. Other metabolic tissues include skeletal muscle, kidneys, lungs, plasma, and intestinal mucosa.

Hepatic biotransformation involves the activity of a very large class of enzymes known as **cytochrome P-450** enzymes (or simply P-450 enzymes), also known as *microsomal* enzymes. These enzymes control a variety of biochemical reactions that aid in the metabolism of medications and are largely targeted against lipid-soluble, nonpolar (no charge) drugs, which are typically very difficult to eliminate. These include the majority of medications. Those medications with water-soluble (polar) molecules may be more easily metabolized by simpler chemical reactions such as hydrolysis (splitting by water molecules). Some of the chemical reactions by which the liver can metabolize drugs are listed in Table 2-4. Drug molecules that are the metabolic targets of specific enzymes are said to be **substrates** of those enzymes. Specific P-450 enzymes are identified by standardized number and letter designations. Some of the most common P-450 enzymes and corresponding drug substrates are listed in Table 2-5.

The biotransformation capabilities of the liver can vary considerably from patient to patient. Various factors that can alter the biotransformation of a drug, including genetics, diseases, and the concurrent use of other medications, are listed in Table 2-6.

Delayed drug metabolism results in the accumulation of the drug and prolongation of the effects of or responses to the drug. Stimulating drug metabolism can thus cause diminishing pharmacologic effects. This often occurs with the repeated administration of some drugs that can stimulate the formation of new microsomal enzymes. Such drugs are said to be enzyme *inducers*. Conversely, many other drugs inhibit various classes of drug-metabolizing enzymes and are called enzyme *inhibitors*. This can lead to drug toxicity.

Excretion

Excretion is the elimination of drugs from the body. Whether they are parent compounds or active or inactive metabolites, all drugs must eventually be removed from the body. The primary

Table 2-4 Mechanisms of Biotransformation

Type of Biotransformation	Mechanism	Result
Oxidation Reduction Hydrolysis	Chemical reactions	Increase polarity of chemical, making it more water soluble and more easily excreted. Often this results in a loss of pharmacologic activity.
Conjugation (e.g., *glucuronidation, glycination, sulfation methylation, alkylation*)	Combination with another substance (e.g., glucuronide, glycine, sulfate, methyl groups, alkyl groups)	

Table 2-5 Common Liver Cytochrome P-450 Enzymes and Corresponding Drug Substrates

Enzyme	Common Drug Substrates
1A2	acetaminophen, caffeine, theophylline, warfarin
2C9	ibuprofen, phenytoin
2C19	diazepam, naproxen, omeprazole, propranolol
2D6	clozapine, codeine, fluoxetine, haloperidol, hydrocodone, metoprolol, oxycodone, paroxetine, propoxyphene, risperidone, selegiline, tricyclic antidepressants
2E1	acetaminophen, enflurane, halothane, ethanol
3A4	acetaminophen, amiodarone, cocaine, cyclosporine, diltiazem, ethinyl estradiol, indinavir, lidocaine, macrolides, progesterone, spironolactone, sulfamethoxazole, testosterone, verapamil

Table 2-6 Examples of Conditions and Drugs That Affect Drug Metabolism

Category	Example	Drug Metabolism Increased	Drug Metabolism Decreased
Diseases	Cardiovascular dysfunction		X
	Renal insufficiency		X
Conditions	Starvation		X
	Obstructive jaundice		X
	Genetic constitution		
	Fast acetylator	X	
	Slow acetylator		X
Drugs	Barbiturates	X	
	rifampin (P-450 inducer)	X	
	erythromycin (P-450 inhibitor)		X
	ketoconazole (P-450 inhibitor)		X

organ responsible for this elimination is the kidney. Two other organs that play an important role in the excretion of drugs are the liver and the bowel. Most drugs are metabolized in the liver by various glucuronidases and by hydroxylation and acetylation. Therefore, by the time most drugs reach the kidneys, they have been extensively metabolized, and only a relatively small fraction of the original drug is excreted as the original compound. Other drugs may circumvent metabolism and reach the kidneys in their original form. Drugs that have been metabolized by the liver become more polar and water soluble. This makes their elimination by the kidneys much easier, because the urinary tract is water based. The kidneys themselves are also capable of forming glucuronides and sulfates from various drugs and their metabolites, although usually to a lesser extent than the liver.

The actual act of renal excretion is accomplished through *glomerular filtration, active tubular reabsorption,* and *active tubular secretion.* Free (unbound) water-soluble drugs and metabolites go through passive glomerular filtration, which takes place between the blood vessels of the afferent arterioles and the glomeruli. Many substances present in the nephrons go through active reabsorption at the level of the tubules, where they are taken back up into the systemic circulation and transported away from the kidney. This process is an attempt by the body to retain needed substances. Some substances may also be secreted into the nephron from the vasculature surrounding it. For urinary elimination, the processes of filtration, reabsorption, and secretion are shown in Figure 2-5.

The excretion of drugs by the intestines is another common route of elimination. This process is referred to as *biliary excretion.* Drugs that are eliminated by this route are taken up by the liver, released into the bile, and eliminated in the feces. Once certain drugs, such as fat-soluble drugs, are in the bile, they may be reabsorbed into the bloodstream, returned to the liver, and again secreted into the bile. This process is called *enterohepatic recirculation.* Enterohepatically recirculated drugs persist in the body for much longer periods. Less common routes of elimination are the lungs and the sweat, salivary, and mammary glands. Depending on the drug, these organs and glands can be highly effective eliminators.

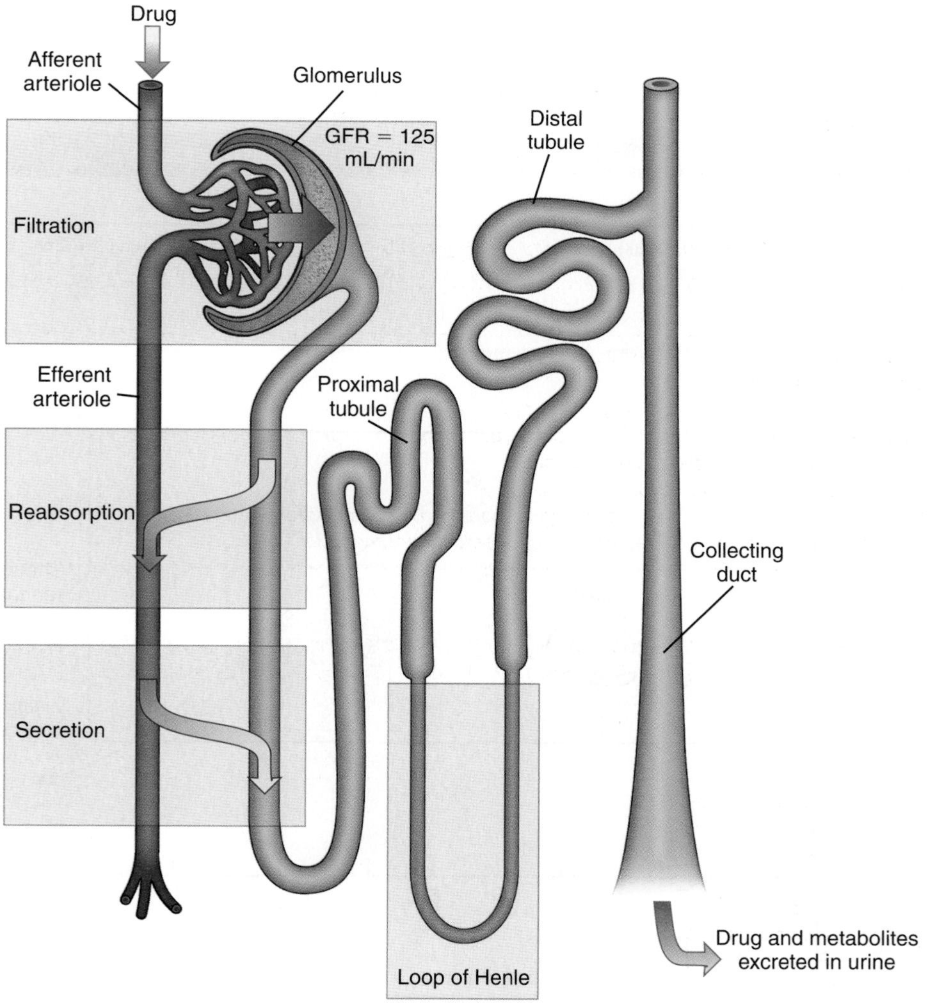

FIGURE 2-5 Renal drug excretion. The primary processes involved in drug excretion and the approximate location where these processes take place in the kidney are illustrated. *GFR,* Glomerular filtration rate.

Half-Life

Another pharmacokinetic variable is the **half-life** of the drug. The half-life is the time required for one half of a given amount of drug in the body to be removed and is a measure of the rate at which the drug is eliminated from the body. For instance, if the maximum level that a particular dosage could achieve in the body is 100 mg/L, and in 8 hours the measured drug level is 50 mg/L, the estimated half-life of that drug is 8 hours. The concept of drug half-life viewed from several different perspectives is shown in Table 2-7.

After about five half-lives, most drugs are considered to be effectively removed from the body. At that time approximately 97% of the drug has been eliminated, and what little amount remains is usually too small to have either therapeutic or toxic effects.

The concept of half-life is clinically useful for determining when a patient taking a particular drug will be at steady state. **Steady state** with regard to blood levels of a drug refers to the physiologic state in which the amount of drug removed via elimination (e.g., renal clearance) is equal to the amount of drug absorbed with each dose. This physiologic plateau phenomenon typically occurs after four to five half-lives of administered drug. Therefore, if a drug has an extremely long half-life, it will take much longer for the drug to reach steady-state blood levels. This commonly occurs, for example, when patients are started on cer-

tain antidepressants such as fluoxetine (Chapter 15). Once steady-state blood levels have been reached, there are consistent levels of drug in the body that correlate with maximum therapeutic benefits.

Onset, Peak, and Duration

The pharmacokinetic terms *absorption, distribution, metabolism,* and *excretion* are all used to describe the movement of drugs through the body. Drug actions are the cellular processes involved in the interaction between a drug and a cell (e.g., a drug's action on a receptor). In contrast, **drug effects** are the physiologic reactions of the body to the drug. The terms *onset, peak, duration,* and *trough* are used to describe drug effects. *Peak* and *trough* are also used to describe drug concentrations, which are usually measured from blood samples.

A drug's **onset of action** is the time required for the drug to elicit a therapeutic response. A drug's **peak effect** is the time required for a drug to reach its maximum therapeutic response.

Physiologically, this corresponds to increasing drug concentrations at the site of action. The **duration of action** of a drug is the length of time that the drug concentration is sufficient (without more doses) to elicit a therapeutic response. These concepts are illustrated in Figure 2-6.

Table 2-7	**Example of Drug Half-Life Viewed from Different Perspectives**					
Metric	**Changing Values**					
Drug concentration (mg/L)	100 (peak)	50	25	12.5	6.25	3.125 (trough)
Hours after peak concentration	0	8	16	24	32	40
Number of half-lives	0	1	2	3	4	5
Percentage of drug removed	0	50	75	88	94	97

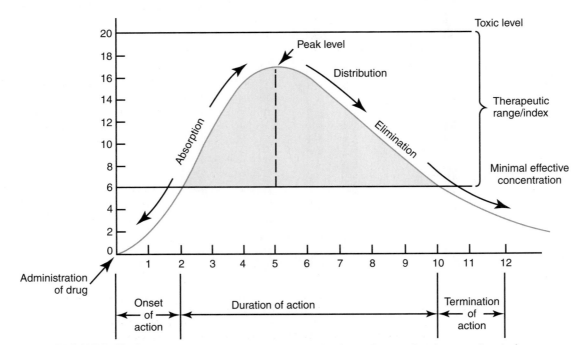

FIGURE 2-6 Characteristics of drug effect and relationship to the therapeutic window. *(From McKenry LM, Tessier E, Hogan M:* Mosby's pharmacology in nursing, *ed 22, St Louis, 2006, Mosby.)*

The amount of time of the onset and peak of action and the duration of action often play an important part in determining the **peak level** (highest blood level) and **trough level** (lowest blood level) of a drug. If the peak blood level is too high, then drug **toxicity** may occur; that is, the drug may become poisonous. The toxicity may be mild, such as extension of the effects of the given drug (e.g., excessive sedation resulting from overdose of a drug with sedative properties). However, it can also be severe (e.g., damage to vital organs or cessation of vital signs due to excessive drug exposure). If the trough blood level is too low, then the drug may not be at therapeutic levels. (A common example is antibiotic drug therapy with aminoglycoside antibiotics [Chapter 37].) Therefore, peak and trough levels are important parameters and are used in **therapeutic drug monitoring** of some medications. In therapeutic drug monitoring, peak and trough values are measured to verify adequate drug exposure, maximize therapeutic effects, and minimize drug toxicity. This monitoring is often carried out by a clinical pharmacist working with other members of the health care team.

PHARMACODYNAMICS

Pharmacodynamics is concerned with the mechanisms of drug action in living tissues. Anatomy and physiology are the study of how the body is structured and why the body functions the way it does. Drug-induced alterations in normal physiologic functions are explained by the principles of pharmacodynamics. A positive change in a faulty physiologic system is called a **therapeutic effect** of a drug. Such an effect is the goal of drug therapy. Understanding the pharmacodynamic characteristics of a drug can aid in assessing the drug's therapeutic effect.

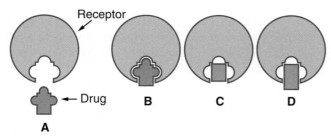

FIGURE 2-7   **A**, Drugs act by forming a chemical bond with specific receptor sites, similar to a key and lock. **B**, The better the "fit," the better the response. Drugs with complete attachment and response are called *agonists*. **C**, Drugs that attach but do not elicit a response are called *antagonists*. **D**, Drugs that attach, elicit some response, and also block other responses are called *partial agonists* or *agonist-antagonists*. (From Clayton BD, Stock YN: Basic pharmacology for nurses, ed 13, St Louis, 2004, Mosby.)

Mechanism of Action

Drugs can produce actions (therapeutic effects) in several ways. The effects of a particular drug depend on the cells or tissue targeted by the drug. Once the drug is at the site of action, it can modify (increase or decrease) the rate at which that cell or tissue functions, or it can modify the strength of function itself of that cell or tissue. A drug cannot, however, cause a cell or tissue to perform a function that is not part of its natural physiology.

Drugs can exert their actions in three basic ways: through *receptors,* through *enzymes,* and through *nonselective interactions.* These mechanisms are discussed in the following sections.

Receptor Interactions

If the mechanism of action of a drug involves a receptor interaction, then the molecular structure of the drug is critical. Drug-receptor interaction entails the selective joining of the drug molecule with a reactive site on the surface of a cell or tissue. Most commonly, this site is a macromolecular protein structure within the cell membrane. This binding of the drug molecule to the receptor molecule in turn elicits a biologic effect. Therefore, a receptor can be defined as a reactive site on the surface or inside of a cell. Once a drug binds to and interacts with the receptor, a pharmacologic response is produced (Figure 2-7). The degree to which a drug attaches to and binds with a receptor is called its *affinity*. The drug with the best "fit" and strongest affinity for the receptor will elicit the greatest response from the cell or tissue. A drug becomes bound to the receptor through the formation of chemical bonds between the receptor on the cell and the *active site* on the drug molecule. Drugs that bind to receptors interact with receptors in different ways either to elicit or to block a physiologic response. Table 2-8 describes the different types of drug-receptor interaction. The drugs that are most effective at eliciting a response from a receptor are those drugs that most closely resemble the endogenous substances in the body (e.g., hormones, neurotransmitters) that normally bind to that receptor.

Enzyme Interactions

Enzymes are the substances that catalyze nearly every biochemical reaction in a cell. The second way drugs can produce effects is by interacting with these enzyme systems. For a drug to alter a physiologic response in this way, it may either inhibit (more common) or enhance (less common) the action of a specific enzyme. This process is called *selective interaction.* Drug-enzyme interaction occcurs when the drug chemically binds to an enzyme molecule in such a way that alters (inhibits or enhances) the enzyme's interaction with its normal target molecules in the body. For example, angiotensin-converting enzyme (ACE) causes a chemical reaction that results in the production of a substance

Table 2-8 **Drug-Receptor Interactions**	
Drug Type	**Action**
Agonist	Drug binds to the receptor; there is a response.
Partial agonist (agonist-antagonist)	Drug binds to the receptor; the response is diminished compared with that elicited by an agonist.
Antagonist	Drug binds to the receptor; there is no response. Drug prevents binding of agonists.
Competitive antagonist	Drug competes with the agonist for binding to the receptor. If it binds, there is no response.
Noncompetitive antagonist	Drug combines with different parts of the receptor and inactivates it; agonist then has no effect.

known as *angiotensin II,* which is a potent vasoconstrictor and mediator of several other processes. The group of drugs called *ACE inhibitors* attract ACE to bind to them rather than to angiotensin I, the usual substrate of ACE, and thereby prevent the formation of angiotensin II. This in turn causes vasodilation and helps reduce blood pressure.

Nonselective Interactions

Drugs with nonspecific mechanisms of action do not interact with receptors or enzymes to alter a physiologic or biologic function of the body. Instead, cell membranes and various cellular processes such as metabolic activities are their main targets. Such drugs can either physically interfere with or chemically alter these cellular structures or processes. Some cancer drugs and antibiotics have this mechanism of action. By incorporating themselves into the normal metabolic process, they cause a defect in the final product or state. This defect may be an improperly formed cell wall that results in cell death through cell lysis or it may be the lack of a necessary energy substrate, which leads to cell starvation and death.

PHARMACOTHERAPEUTICS

Before drug therapy is initiated, an end point or expected outcome of therapy should be established. This desired therapeutic outcome should be patient specific, should be established in collaboration with the patient, and, if appropriate, should be determined with other members of the health care team. Outcomes must be clearly defined and must be either measurable or observable by the patient or caregiver. A time line for these outcomes should also be specified. The progress being made toward the targeted objective should be monitored. Goal outcomes should be realistic and should be prioritized so that drug therapy begins with interventions that are essential to the patient's acute well-being or interventions that the patient perceives to be important. Examples of such outcomes are curing a disease, eliminating or reducing a preexisting symptom, arresting or slowing a disease process, preventing a disease or other unwanted condition, or otherwise improving the quality of life. These goals and outcomes are not the same as nursing goals and outcomes.

Patient therapy assessment is the process by which a practitioner integrates his or her knowledge of medical and drug-related facts with information about a specific patient's medical and social history. Items that should be considered in the assessment are drugs currently used (prescription, over-the-counter, and illicit or street drugs), pregnancy and breast-feeding status, and concurrent illnesses that could contraindicate starting a given medication. A **contraindication** to a medication is any characteristic of the patient, especially a disease state, that makes the use of a given medication dangerous for the patient. Careful attention to this assessment process helps to ensure an optimal therapeutic plan for the patient. The implementation of a treatment plan can involve delivery of several types and combinations of therapies. The type of therapy can be categorized as acute, maintenance, supplemental (or replacement), palliative, supportive, prophylactic, or empiric.

Acute Therapy

Acute therapy often involves more intensive drug treatment and is implemented in the acutely ill (those with rapid onset of illness) or even the critically ill. It is often needed to sustain life or treat disease. Examples are the administration of vasopressors to maintain blood pressure and cardiac output after open-heart surgery, the use of volume expanders in a patient who is in shock, the use of antibiotics in a trauma patient at high risk of infection, and intensive chemotherapy for a patient with newly diagnosed cancer.

Maintenance Therapy

Maintenance therapy typically does not eradicate problems the patient may have but does prevent progression of a disease or condition. It is used for the treatment of chronic illnesses such as hypertension. In the latter case, maintenance therapy maintains the patient's blood pressure within given limits, which prevents certain end-organ damage. Another example of maintenance therapy is the use of oral contraceptives for birth control.

Supplemental Therapy

Supplemental or replacement therapy supplies the body with a substance needed to maintain normal function. This substance may be needed either because it cannot be made by the body or because it is produced in insufficient quantity. Examples are the administration of insulin to diabetic patients and of iron to patients with iron-deficiency anemia.

Palliative Therapy

The goal of palliative therapy is to make the patient as comfortable as possible. It is typically used in the end stages of an illness when all attempts at curative therapy have failed. Examples are the use of high-dose opioid analgesics to relieve pain in the final stages of cancer and the use of oxygen in end-stage pulmonary disease.

Supportive Therapy

Supportive therapy maintains the integrity of body functions while the patient is recovering from illness or trauma. Examples are provision of fluids and electrolytes to prevent dehydration in a patient with influenza who is vomiting and has diarrhea, and administration of fluids, volume expanders, or blood products to a patient who has lost blood during surgery.

Prophylactic Therapy and Empiric Therapy

Prophylactic therapy is drug therapy provided to *prevent* illness or other undesirable outcome. Its use is based on scientific knowledge often acquired during years of observation of a disease and its causes. For example, a surgeon knows that when he or she makes an incision through the skin there is the possibility that skin bacteria are present that can later infect the incision. The surgeon therefore administers an antibiotic before making the incision. Prophylactic therapy is also used when dental procedures are performed in patients with mitral valve prolapse and in patients with prosthetic valves or joints or Teflon grafts.

Unlike most prophylactic therapy, empiric therapy does not have a scientific basis but instead is based on experience. It is the administration of a drug when a certain pathologic process is suspected based on the patient's symptoms because the drug has been found in the past to be beneficial in such cases. For example, acetaminophen is given to a patient who has a fever. The cause of the fever may not be known, but empirically the patient is given acetaminophen because it has been demonstrated to lower the body temperature.

Monitoring

Once the appropriate therapy has been implemented, the effectiveness of that therapy—that is, the clinical response of the patient to the therapy—must be evaluated. Evaluating the clinical response requires that the evaluator be familiar with both the drug's intended therapeutic action (beneficial effects) and its unintended possible **adverse effects** (predictable adverse drug reactions). It should be noted that this text generally highlights only the most common adverse effects of a given drug; the drug may have many other less commonly reported adverse effects. One must always keep in mind that patients may sometimes experience less common, and therefore less readily identifiable, adverse drug effects. The nurse should consult comprehensive references, pharmacists, or poison and drug information center staff whenever there is uncertainty regarding adverse effects that a patient may be experiencing.

All drugs are potentially toxic and can have cumulative effects. Recognizing these toxic effects and knowing their manifestations in the patient are integral components of the monitoring process. A drug accumulates when it is absorbed more quickly than it is eliminated or when it is administered before the previous dose has been metabolized or cleared from the body. Knowledge of the function of the organs responsible for metabolizing and eliminating a drug, combined with knowledge of how a particular drug is metabolized and excreted, enables the nurse to anticipate problems and treat them appropriately if they occur.

Therapeutic Index

The ratio of a drug's toxic level to the level that provides therapeutic benefits is referred to as the drug's **therapeutic index.** The safety of a particular drug therapy is determined by this index. A low therapeutic index means that the difference between a therapeutically active dose and a toxic dose is small. A drug with a low therapeutic index has a greater likelihood than other drugs of causing an adverse reaction, and therefore its use requires closer monitoring. Examples of such drugs are warfarin and digoxin.

Drug Concentration

Drug concentration in patients can be an important tool for evaluating the clinical response to drug therapy. Certain drug levels are associated with therapeutic responses, whereas other drug levels are associated with toxic effects. Toxic drug levels are typically seen when the body's normal mechanisms for metabolizing and excreting drugs are compromised. This commonly occurs when liver and kidney functions are impaired or when the liver or kidneys are immature (as in neonates). Dosage adjustments should be made in these patients to appropriately accommodate their impaired metabolism and excretion.

Patient's Condition

Another patient-specific factor to be considered when monitoring drug therapy is the patient's concurrent diseases or other medical conditions. A patient's response to a drug may vary greatly depending on physiologic and psychologic demands. Disease of any kind, infection, cardiovascular function, and GI function are just a few of the physiologic elements that can alter a patient's therapeutic response. Stress, depression, and anxiety are some of the psychologic factors affecting response.

Tolerance and Dependence

The monitoring of drug therapy requires a knowledge of tolerance and dependence and an understanding of the difference between the two. *Tolerance* is a decreasing response to repeated drug doses. *Dependence* is a physiologic or psychologic need for a drug. *Physical dependence* is the physiologic need for a drug to avoid physical withdrawal symptoms (e.g., tachycardia in an opioid-addicted patient). *Psychologic dependence* is also known as *addiction* and is the obsessive desire for the euphoric effects of a drug. Addiction typically involves the recreational use of various drugs such as benzodiazepines, narcotics, and amphetamines. See Chapter 8 for further discussion of dependence.

Interactions

Drugs may interact with other drugs, with foods, or with agents administered as part of laboratory tests. Knowledge of drug interactions is vital for the appropriate monitoring of drug therapy. The more drugs a patient receives, the more likely that a drug interaction will occur. This is especially true in older adults, who typically have an increased sensitivity to drug effects and are receiving several medications. In addition, over-the-counter medications and herbal therapies can interact significantly with prescribed medications.

Alteration of the action of one drug by another is referred to as **drug interaction.** A drug interaction can either increase or decrease the actions of one or both of the involved drugs and can be either beneficial or harmful. Drug interactions increase in frequency with the number of drugs taken by the patient. Careful patient care combined with knowledge of all drugs being administered can decrease the likelihood of a harmful drug interaction.

Understanding the mechanisms by which drug interactions occur can help prevent them. Concurrently administered drugs may interact with each other and alter the pharmacokinetics of one another during any of the four phases of pharmacokinetics discussed previously: absorption, distribution, metabolism, or excretion. Table 2-9 provides examples of drug interaction during each of these phases. It also indicates how some drug interactions can be beneficial.

Many terms are used to categorize drug interactions. When two drugs with similar actions are given together, they can have **additive effects.** Examples are the many combinations of analgesic products, such as aspirin and opioid combinations (e.g., aspirin and codeine) and acetaminophen and opioid combinations (e.g., acetaminophen and oxycodone). Often drugs are used together for their additive effects so that smaller doses of each drug can be given; toxic effects are thus avoided while adequate drug action is maintained.

Synergistic effects are different from simple additive effects and occur when two drugs administered together interact in such a way that their combined effects are greater than the sum of the effects for each drug given alone. The combination of hydrochlorothiazide with enalapril for the treatment of hypertension is an example.

Drug effects that are almost the opposite of synergistic effects are known as **antagonistic effects.** Antagonistic effects are said to occur when the combination of two drugs results in drug effects that are less than the sum of the effects for each drug given separately. Such an interaction is seen when antacids are given

Table 2-9	Examples of Drug Interactions and Their Effects on Pharmacokinetics		
Pharmacokinetic Phase	**Drug Combination**	**Mechanism**	**Result**
Absorption	Antacid with ketoconazole	Increases gastric pH, preventing the breakdown of ketoconazole	Decreased effectiveness of ketoconazole, resulting from decreased blood levels (harmful)
Distribution	warfarin with amiodarone	Both drugs compete for protein-binding sites	Higher levels of free (unbound) warfarin and amiodarone, which increases actions of both drugs (harmful)
Metabolism	erythromycin with cyclosporine	Both drugs compete for the same hepatic enzymes	Decreased metabolism of cyclosporine, possibly resulting in toxic levels of cyclosporine (harmful)
Excretion	amoxicillin with probenecid	Inhibits the secretion of amoxicillin into the kidneys	Elevates and prolongs the plasma levels of amoxicillin (can be beneficial)

with tetracycline, which results in decreased absorption of the tetracycline.

Incompatibility is a term most commonly used to describe parenteral drugs. Drug incompatibility occurs when two parenteral drugs or solutions are mixed together and the result is a chemical deterioration of one or both of the drugs. The combination of two such drugs usually produces a precipitate, haziness, or color change in the solution. An example of incompatible drugs is the combination of parenteral furosemide and heparin.

Adverse Drug Events

The recognition of the potential hazards and actual detrimental effects of medication use is a topic that continues to receive much attention in the literature. This focus has contributed to an increasing body of knowledge regarding this topic as well as the development of new terminology. Health care institutions are also under increasing pressure to put into practice effective strategies for preventing adverse effects of drugs and addressing them when they do occur.

Adverse drug event (ADE) is a broad term for any undesirable occurrence involving medications. A similarly broad term also seen in the literature is *drug misadventure*. Patient outcomes associated with ADEs vary from no effects to mild discomfort to life-threatening complications, permanent disability, disfigurement, or death. ADEs can be preventable (see discussion of medication errors later) or nonpreventable. Fortunately, many ADEs result in no measurable patient harm. For example, a nurse may mistakenly give a single dose of an unprescribed drug (medication error) that is simply metabolized and excreted by the patient's body with no resultant injury. The most common causes of ADE *external* to the patient are errors by caregivers (both professional and nonprofessional) and malfunctioning equipment (e.g., intravenous infusion pumps). However, an ADE can also be *patient induced*, such as when a patient fails to take medication as prescribed or drinks alcoholic beverages that he or she was advised not to consume while taking a given medication. In such situations as well, the patient may experience no ill effects or may suffer varying degrees of harm. An ADE that is noticed before it actually occurs should be considered a *potential* ADE (and appropriate steps should be taken to avoid such a "near miss" in the future). A less common situation, but one still worth mentioning, is an *adverse drug withdrawal event*. This is an adverse outcome associated with discontinuation of drug therapy, such as hypertension caused by abruptly discontinuing blood pressure

medication or return of infection caused by stopping antibiotic therapy too soon. Of course, these situations can also result from either patient or caregiver actions.

The two most common broad categories of ADE are medication errors and adverse drug reactions. A **medication error (ME)** is a *preventable* situation in which there is a compromise in the *Five Rights* of medication use: *right patient, right drug, right time, right route,* and *right dose.* MEs are more common than adverse drug reactions but can also be the direct cause of such reactions. MEs occur during the *prescribing, dispensing, administering,* or *monitoring* of drug therapy. These four phases are collectively known as the **medication use process.** MEs are discussed in more detail in Chapter 5.

An **adverse drug reaction (ADR)** is any reaction to a drug that is unexpected and undesirable and occurs at therapeutic drug dosages. ADRs may or may not be caused by MEs. ADRs may result in hospital admission, prolongation of hospital stay, change in drug therapy, initiation of supportive treatment, or complication of a patient's disease state. ADRs are caused by processes inside the patient's body. They may or may not be preventable, depending on the situation. Milder ADRs (e.g., drug *adverse effects*—see later) usually do not require a change in the patient's drug therapy or other interventions. More severe ADRs, however, are likely to require changes to a patient's drug regimen. Severe ADRs can be permanently or significantly disabling, life threatening, or fatal. They may require or prolong hospitalization, lead to organ damage (e.g., to the liver, kidneys, bone marrow, skin), cause congenital anomalies, or require specific interventions to prevent permanent impairment or tissue damage.

ADRs that are specific to particular drug groups are discussed in the corresponding drug chapters in this book. Four general categories of ADR are discussed here: pharmacologic reaction, hypersensitivity (allergic) reaction, idiosyncratic reaction, and drug interaction.

A pharmacologic reaction is an extension of the drug's normal effects in the body. For example, a drug that is used to lower blood pressure in a patient with hypertension causes a pharmacologic ADR when it lowers the blood pressure to the point at which the patient becomes unconscious.

Pharmacologic reactions also include adverse effects. Adverse effects are predictable, well-known ADRs resulting in minor or no changes in patient management. They have predictable frequency and intensity, and their occurrence is related to the dose. They also usually resolve upon discontinuation of drug therapy.

An **allergic reaction** (also known as a *hypersensitivity reaction*) involves the patient's immune system. Immune system proteins known as *immunoglobulins* (Chapters 46 and 49) recognize the drug molecule, its metabolite(s), or another ingredient in a drug formulation as a dangerous foreign substance. At this point, an *immune response* may occur in which immunoglobulin proteins bind to the drug substance in an attempt to neutralize the drug. Various chemical mediators, such as *histamine,* as well as *cytokines* and other inflammatory substances (e.g., *prostaglandins* [Chapter 44]) usually are released during this process. This response can result in reactions ranging from mild (e.g., skin erythema or mild rash) to severe, even life-threatening reactions such as constriction of bronchial airways and tachycardia.

An **idiosyncratic reaction** is not the result of a known pharmacologic property of a drug or of a patient allergy but instead occurs unexpectedly in a particular patient. Such a reaction is a genetically determined abnormal response to normal dosages of a drug. Genetically inherited traits that result in the abnormal metabolism of drugs are distributed throughout the population. The study of such traits, which are solely revealed by drug administration, is called **pharmacogenetics** (Chapter 50). Idiosyncratic drug reactions are usually caused by a deficiency or excess of drug-metabolizing enzymes. Many pharmacogenetic disorders exist. A more common one is glucose-6-phosphate dehydrogenase (G6PD) deficiency. This pharmacogenetic disease is transmitted as a sex-linked trait and affects approximately 100 million people. People who lack proper levels of G6PD have idiosyncratic reactions to a wide range of drugs. There are more than 80 variations of the disease, and all produce some degree of drug-induced hemolysis. Drugs capable of inducing hemolysis in such patients are listed in Box 2-3.

The final type of ADR is due to drug interaction. As described earlier, drug interaction occurs when the simultaneous presence of two (or more) drugs in the body produces an unwanted effect. This unwanted effect can result when one drug either accentuates or reduces the effects of another drug to an undesirable degree. As previously mentioned, in some instances drug interactions are intentional and beneficial (see Table 2-9).

Other Drug Effects

Other drug-related effects that must be considered during drug therapy are teratogenic, mutagenic, and carcinogenic effects. These can result in devastating patient outcomes and can be prevented in many instances by appropriate monitoring.

Teratogenic effects of drugs or other chemicals result in structural defects in the fetus. Compounds that produce such effects are called *teratogens.* Viral diseases (e.g., measles) and radiation can also have teratogenic effects. Prenatal development involves a delicate programmed sequence of interrelated embryologic events. Any significant disruption in this process of *embryogenesis* can have a teratogenic effect. Drugs that are capable of crossing the placenta can act as teratogens and cause **drug-induced teratogenesis.** Drugs administered during pregnancy can produce different types of congenital anomalies. The period during which the fetus is most vulnerable to teratogenic effects begins with the third week of development and usually ends after the third month. Chapter 3 describes the Food and Drug Administration safety classification for drugs used by pregnant women.

Mutagenic effects are permanent changes in the genetic composition of living organisms and consist of alterations in chromosome structure, the number of chromosomes, or the genetic code of the deoxyribonucleic acid (DNA) molecule. Drugs capable of inducing mutations are called *mutagens.* Radiation, viruses, chemicals, and drugs can all act as mutagenic agents in human beings. The largest genetic unit that can be involved in a mutation is a *chromosome* (large DNA strand in all cells) the smallest is a base pair in a DNA molecule. Drugs that affect genetic processes are active primarily during cell reproduction (*mitosis*).

Carcinogenic effects are the cancer-causing effects of drugs, other chemicals, radiation, and viruses. Entities that produce such effects are called *carcinogens.* Some exogenous causes of cancer are listed in Box 2-4.

CULTURAL IMPLICATIONS

Glucose-6-Phosphate Dehydrogenase Deficiency

Glucose-6-phosphate dehydrogenase (G6PD) is an enzyme found in abundant amounts in the tissues of most individuals. It reduces the risk of hemolysis of red blood cells when they are exposed to oxidizing drugs such as aspirin. Approximately 13% of African American men and 20% of African American women carry the gene that results in G6PD deficiency. Approximately 14% of Sardinians and more than 50% of the Kurdish Jewish population also show G6PD deficiencies. When exposed to drugs such as sulfonamides, antimalarials, and aspirin, patients with this deficiency may suffer life-threatening hemolysis of the red blood cells, whereas individuals with adequate quantities of the enzyme have no problems in taking these drugs.

Box 2-3 Drugs to Avoid in Patients with Glucose-6-Phosphate Dehydrogenase Deficiency

aspirin
chloramphenicol
chloroquine
furazolidone
nitrofurantoin
Oxidants (all)
paraaminosalicylic acid
phenacetin
primaquine
probenecid
Sulfonamides
Sulfones

Box 2-4 Exogenous Causes of Cancer

Dietary customs
Drug abuse
Carcinogenic drugs
Workplace chemicals
Radiation
Environmental pollution
Food-processing procedures
Food production procedures
Oncogenic viruses
Smoking

PHARMACOGNOSY

The source of all early drugs was nature, and the study of these natural drug sources (plants and animals) is called pharmacognosy. Although many drugs in current use are synthetically derived, most were first isolated in nature. By studying the composition of natural substances and their physiologic effects in living systems, researchers can identify the chemical features of a substance that produce a desired clinical response. Once identified and isolated, these natural substances are often synthesized in a laboratory for mass production of synthetic drugs. Isolation of a specific natural compound may also alleviate undesirable effects that may occur from other compounds in the natural source (e.g., a plant). Although most new drug products are synthetic, the underlying principle of pharmacognosy is that an understanding of the actions and effects of natural drug sources is essential to new drug development. As one important example, pharmacognosy enabled the isolation of the naturally occurring hormone insulin from animal sources, determination of its exact genetic sequence, modification of this sequence to "humanize" the insulin, and large-scale synthesis of that modified product in the laboratory. This led to the commercial production of synthetic human insulin, one of the world's most widely used drugs.

The four main sources for drugs are plants, animals, minerals, and laboratory synthesis. An example of a plant from which a drug is derived is foxglove. Foxglove is the source of cardiac glycosides and has yielded the present-day drug digoxin. Plants provide many weak acids and weak bases (*alkaloids*) that are very useful and potent drugs. Alkaloids are more common. Examples include atropine (belladonna plant), caffeine (coffee bean), and nicotine (tobacco leaf). Animals are the source of many hormone drugs. Conjugated estrogen is derived from the urine of pregnant mares (hence the drug trade name Premarin). Insulin comes from three sources: cows (beef), pigs (pork), and humans. Human insulin is either semisynthetic (pork insulin is converted to human insulin by changing one amino acid) or is made from human sources. Both types are now mass-produced using recombinant DNA techniques. Heparin is another commonly used drug that is derived from cows and pigs (bovine and porcine heparin). Some common mineral sources of currently used drugs are salicylic acid, aluminum hydroxide, and sodium chloride. Recombinant DNA techniques provide many other synthetic drug products, such as erythropoietin, granulocyte-macrophage colony-stimulating factor (sargramostim), and granulocyte colony-stimulating factor (filgrastim), all used to stimulate formation of various blood components (Chapter 49).

TOXICOLOGY

The study of poisons and unwanted responses to both drugs and other chemicals is known as toxicology. Toxicology is the science of the adverse effects of chemicals on living organisms. Clinical toxicology deals specifically with the care of the poisoned patient. Poisoning can result from a variety of causes, ranging from prescription drug overdose to ingestion of household cleaning agents to snakebite. Poison control centers (PCCs) are health care institutions equipped with sufficient personnel and information resources to recommend appropriate treatment for the poisoned patient. They are usually staffed by specially trained pharmacists and/or nurses who triage incoming calls and refer complex cases to clinical toxicologists. Telephone contact with a PCC is usually an important early step in aiding the poisoned patient. Computerized drug and chemical information databases are often searched to determine quickly the most effective known treatment for a particular cause of poisoning. Many cases can be handled over the telephone with advice from the PCC pharmacist or nurse. As noted, treatment of more severe poisonings is overseen by clinical toxicologists, who are usually specially trained physicians.

Effective treatment of the poisoned patient is based on a system of priorities, the first of which is to preserve the patient's vital functions by maintaining the airway, ventilation, and circulation. The second priority is to prevent absorption of the toxic substance and/or speed its elimination from the body using one or more of the variety of clinical methods available. These methods include administering syrup of ipecac (to induce vomiting to clear the stomach), giving activated charcoal to adsorb the substance in the stomach, and administering cathartics (laxatives) to speed fecal elimination of the charcoal-toxin complex. Syrup of ipecac has been employed for several decades. However, there is currently a clinical trend away from its use in favor of other treatments for most types of poisoning because of frequent misuse by patients and caregivers and limited efficacy. Whole-bowel irrigation, using solutions of polyethylene glycol (e.g., Golytely) for example, may also be helpful in eliminating some drugs. In more severe cases, hemodialysis or peritoneal dialysis may be effective in removing certain types of drugs that have already been absorbed into the bloodstream. Hemoperfusion is similar to dialysis

---

CASE STUDY

Pharmacokinetics

Four patients with angina are receiving a form of nitroglycerin, as follows:

Mrs. A., age 88, takes 9 mg twice a day to prevent angina.
Mr. B., age 63, takes a form that delivers 0.2 mg/hr, also to prevent angina.
Mrs. C., age 58, takes 0.4 mg only if needed for chest pain.
Mr. D., age 62, is in the hospital with severe, unstable angina and is receiving 20 mcg/hr.

You may refer to the section on nitroglycerin in Chapter 23 or to a nursing drug handbook to answer the following questions.

1. State the route or form of nitroglycerin that each patient is receiving. In addition, specify the *trade* name(s) for each particular form.
2. For each patient, state the rationale for the route or form of drug that was chosen. Which forms have immediate action? Why would this be important?
3. Which form or forms are most affected by the first-pass effect? Explain.
4. What would happen if Mrs. A. chewed her nitroglycerin dose? If Mrs. C chewed her nitroglycerin dose?

and involves pumping the patient's blood through a charcoal column, which clears certain drugs from the blood by adsorption (as when charcoal is used in the GI tract). Diuretic drugs may also be administered to force renal elimination of the toxic substance. In this instance, acid or alkaline diuresis involves administering weak acids or bases to speed renal elimination of basic or acidic drugs, respectively, by altering the chemistry of the urine. Oral or intravenous solutions of ascorbic acid (vitamin C) or sodium bicarbonate (a base) are often used for this purpose. In the case of snakebite, a drug product known as *antivenin* (also called *antivenom*) is often administered intravenously. This compound chemically binds to venom molecules to reduce tissue damage. Radiation poisoning requires decontamination using specially trained personnel and equipment. Several common poisons and their specific antidotes are listed in Table 2-10.

CONCLUSION

A thorough understanding of the interrelated pharmacologic principles of pharmacokinetics, pharmacodynamics, pharmacotherapeutics, pharmacognosy, and toxicology is essential to the implementation of drug therapy in the nursing process and to safe, quality nursing practice. Medications may be very helpful in treating disease, but without an adequate, up-to-date knowledge base and clinical skills combined with critical thinking and good decision making, this very useful treatment modality may become a very harmful one in the nurse's hands. Application of pharmacologic principles enables the nurse to provide safe and effective drug therapy while always acting on behalf of the patient and respecting the patient's rights. Nursing considerations associated with various routes of drug administration are summarized in Table 2-3.

Table 2-10 **Common Causes of Poisoning and Antidotes**	
Substance	**Antidote**
acetaminophen	acetylcysteine
Organophosphates (e.g., insecticides)	atropine
Tricyclic antidepressants, quinidine	sodium bicarbonate
Calcium channel blockers	Intravenous calcium
Iron salts	deferoxamine
digoxin and other cardiac glycosides	digoxin antibodies
ethylene glycol (e.g., automotive antifreeze solution), methanol	ethanol (same as alcohol used for drinking), given intravenously
Benzodiazepines	flumazenil
β-blockers	glucagon
Opiates, opioid drugs	naloxone
Carbon monoxide (by inhalation)	Oxygen (at high concentration), known as bariatric therapy

Points to Remember

- The following definitions related to drug therapy are important to remember: pharmacology—the study or science of drugs; pharmacokinetics—the study of drug distribution among various body compartments after a drug has entered the body, including the phases of absorption, distribution, metabolism, and excretion; pharmaceutics—the science of dosage form design.
- The nurse's role in drug therapy and the nursing process as it relates to pharmacologic treatment is more than just the memorization of the names of drugs, their uses, and associated interventions. It involves a thorough comprehension of all aspects of

pharmaceutics, pharmacokinetics, and pharmacodynamics and the sound application of this drug knowledge to a variety of clinical situations. Refer to Chapter 1 for more detailed discussion of drug therapy in relation to the nursing process.
- Drug actions are related to the pharmacologic, pharmaceutical, pharmacokinetic, and pharmacodynamic properties of a given medication, and each of these has a specific influence on the overall effects produced by the drug in a patient.
- Selection of the route of administration is based on patient variables and the specific characteristics of a drug.

NCLEX Examination Review Questions

1. An elderly woman took a prescription medicine to help her to sleep; however, she felt restless all night and did not sleep at all. Which term below best describes this patient's response to the drug?
   a. Allergic reaction
   b. Idiosyncratic reaction
   c. Mutagenic effect
   d. Synergistic effect

2. Patients with cirrhosis or hepatitis may have abnormalities in which phase of pharmacokinetics?
   a. Absorption
   b. Distribution
   c. Metabolism
   d. Excretion

3. A patient who has advanced cancer is receiving opioid medications around the clock to "keep him comfortable" as he nears the end of his life. Which term best describes this type of therapy?
   a. Palliative therapy
   b. Maintenance therapy
   c. Supportive therapy
   d. Supplemental therapy

4. The nurse is giving medications to a patient in cardiogenic shock. The intravenous route is chosen instead of the intramuscular route. Which factor most influences this decision? The patient's:
   a. altered biliary function
   b. increased glomerular filtration
   c. reduced liver metabolism
   d. diminished circulation

5. A patient has just received a prescription for an enteric-coated stool softener. Which of the following statements is most important to include when teaching the patient?
   a. "Take the tablet with 2 to 3 oz of orange juice."
   b. "Avoid taking all other medications with any enteric-coated tablet."
   c. "Crush the tablet before swallowing if you have problems with swallowing."
   d. "Be sure to swallow the tablet whole without chewing it."

1. b, 2. c, 3. a, 4. d, 5. d.

Critical Thinking Activities

1. Your patient relates to you during the nursing assessment that he experiences some "strange" problem with drug metabolism that he was born with, so he is not to take certain medications. What type of disorder do you think this patient is referring to, and what are the problems it can cause in the patient when specific medications are taken?

2. Mr. L. is admitted to the trauma unit with multisystem injuries from an automobile accident. He arrived at the unit with multiple abnormal findings, including shock, decreased cardiac output, and urinary output of less than 30 mL/hr. Which route of administration would be indicated for any medications for this patient? Explain your reasoning.

3. Explain the difference between a medication's action and its effect.

4. Explain the importance of each phase of pharmacokinetics.

For answers, see http://evolve.elsevier.com/Lilley.

Life Span Considerations

Objectives

When you reach the end of this chapter, you should be able to do the following:

1. Discuss the influences of the patient's age on the effects of drugs and drug responses.
2. Identify drug-related concerns during pregnancy and lactation and provide an explanation of the physiologic basis for these concerns.
3. Discuss the process of pharmacokinetics and associated changes in various patient age groups, such as in pediatrics, pregnancy, and the elderly.
4. Summarize the impact of age-related changes on pharmacokinetics in drug therapy.
5. Calculate a drug dose for a pediatric patient using a variety of formulas.
6. Identify the importance of a body surface area nomogram for pediatric patients.
7. Develop a nursing care plan for drug therapy and the nursing process for patients across the life span.

e-Learning Activities

Companion CD

- NCLEX Review Questions: see questions 18-22
- Animations
- Audio Glossary
- Category Catchers
- Medication Errors Checklists
- IV Therapy Checklists

evolve Website (http://evolve.elsevier.com/Lilley)

• Nursing Care Plans • Frequently Asked Questions • Content Updates • WebLinks • Supplemental Resources • Elsevier ePharmacology Update • Medication Administration Animations

Glossary

Active transport The active (energy-requiring) movement of a substance between different tissues via biomolecular pumping mechanisms contained within cell membranes. (p. 36)

Diffusion The passive movement of a substance (e.g., a drug) between different tissues from areas of higher concentration to areas of lower concentration. (Compare with *active transport*.) (p. 36)

Elderly Pertaining to a person who is 65 years of age or older. (NOTE: Some sources consider "elderly" to be 55 years of age or older.) (p. 39)

Nomogram A graphical tool for estimating drug dosages using various body measurements. (p. 38)

Pediatric Pertaining to a person who is 12 years of age or younger. (p. 37)

Polypharmacy The use of many different drugs concurrently in treating a patient, who often has several health problems. (p. 39)

Most of the experience with drugs and pharmacology has been gained from the adult population, and by far the great majority of drug studies and articles on drugs have focused on the population between the ages of 13 and 65 years. It has also been estimated that 75% of currently approved drugs lack U.S. Food and Drug Administration (FDA) approval for pediatric use and therefore lack specific dosage guidelines for use in neonates and children. Drug usage, however, extends far beyond patients between the ages of 13 and 65 years. Most drugs are also effective in younger and older patients, but drugs often behave very differently in these patients at the opposite ends of the age spectrum. It is therefore vitally important from the standpoint of safe and effective drug administration to understand what these differences are and how to adjust for them.

During the time from the beginning to the end of life, the human body changes in many ways. These changes have a dramatic effect on the four phases of pharmacokinetics—drug absorption, distribution, metabolism, and excretion. Newborn, pediatric, and elderly patients each have special needs, which are discussed in this chapter. Drug therapy at the two ends of the spectrum of life is more likely to result in adverse effects and toxicity. This is especially true if certain basic principles are not understood and followed. However, response to drug therapy changes in a reasonably predictable manner in younger and older patients. Knowing the effect that age has on the pharmacokinetic characteristics of drugs helps predict these changes.

DRUG THERAPY DURING PREGNANCY

Exposure to drugs occurs across the entire life span, which begins before birth. A fetus is exposed to many of the same substances as the mother, including any drugs that she takes—prescription, nonprescription, or street drugs. Therefore, it is important to know and understand drug effects during gestational life. The first trimester of pregnancy is generally the period of

Table 3-1	Pregnancy Safety Categories
Category	**Description**
Category A	Studies indicate no risk to human fetus.
Category B	Studies indicate no risk to animal fetus; information for humans is not available.
Category C	Adverse effects reported in animal fetus; information for humans is not available.
Category D	Possible fetal risk in humans reported; however, consideration of potential benefit vs. risk may, in selected cases, warrant use of these drugs in pregnant women.
Category X	Fetal abnormalities reported and positive evidence of fetal risk in humans available from animal and/or human studies. These drugs should not be used in pregnant women.

greatest danger of drug-induced developmental defects. Also of importance is the fact that an average of at least four drugs are taken by the typical pregnant patient.

Transfer of both drugs and nutrients to the fetus occurs primarily by **diffusion** across the placenta, although not all drugs cross the placenta. **Active transport** plays a lesser role. Recall from chemistry studies that diffusion is a passive process based on differences in concentration between different tissues, whereas active transport requires the expenditure of energy to move a substance between different areas and often involves some sort of cell-surface protein pump. The factors that contribute to the safety or potential harm of drug therapy during pregnancy can be broadly broken down into three areas: drug properties, fetal gestational age, and maternal factors.

Factors that impact drug transfer to the fetus include drug chemical properties, drug dosage, and concurrently administered drugs. Examples of relevant chemical properties include molecular weight, protein binding, lipid solubility, and chemical structure. Important drug dosage variables include dose and duration of therapy.

Fetal gestational age is an important factor in determining the potential for harmful drug effects to the fetus. As noted earlier, the fetus is at greatest risk for drug-induced developmental defects during the first trimester of pregnancy. During this period the fetus undergoes rapid cell proliferation, and the skeleton, muscles, limbs, and visceral organs are developing at their most rapid rate. Self-treatment of any minor illness should be strongly discouraged anytime during pregnancy, but especially during the first trimester. Gestational age is also important in determining when a drug can most easily cross the placenta to the fetus. During the last trimester the greatest percentage of maternally absorbed drug gets to the fetus.

Maternal factors can also play a role in determining drug effects on the fetus. Any change in the mother's physiology that could impact the pharmacokinetic characteristics of drugs (absorption, distribution, metabolism, and excretion) can affect the amount of drug to which the fetus may be exposed. Maternal kidney and liver function play a major role in drug metabolism and excretion and are critical factors, especially if the drug crosses the placenta. Impairment in either kidney or liver function may result in higher drug levels than normal and/or prolonged drug exposure. Maternal genotype may also affect how and to what extent certain drugs are metabolized (pharmacogenetics), which in turn affects drug exposure of the fetus. The lack of certain enzyme systems, as seen in the pharmacogenetic disease glucose-6-phosphate dehydrogenase deficiency, may result in adverse drug effects to the fetus when the mother is exposed

to a drug that is normally metabolized by this enzyme, including the commonly used over-the-counter (OTC) drug aspirin.

Although exposure of the fetus to drugs is most detrimental during the first trimester, drug transfer to the fetus is more likely during the last trimester. This is the result of enhanced blood flow to the fetus, increased fetal surface area, and increased amount of free drug in the mother's circulation.

As important as it is to judiciously use drugs during pregnancy, there are certain situations that require their use. Without drugs, such maternal conditions as hypertension, epilepsy, diabetes, and infection could seriously endanger both the mother and the fetus.

The FDA classifies drugs according to their safety for use during pregnancy. This system of drug classification is based primarily on animal studies and limited human studies. This fact is due in part to ethical dilemmas surrounding the study of potential adverse effects on fetuses. We have also learned from some unfortunate mistakes, such as the maternal use of thalidomide, which induces birth defects, and diethylstilbestrol (DES), which causes a high incidence of gynecologic malignancy in female offspring. Currently the best method for determining the potential fetal risk of a drug is to note the FDA's pregnancy safety category for the drug. The five safety categories are described in Table 3-1.

DRUG THERAPY DURING BREAST-FEEDING

Breast-fed infants are also at risk for exposure to drugs consumed by the mother. A wide variety of drugs easily cross from the mother's circulation to the breast milk and subsequently to the breast-feeding infant. Drug properties similar to those discussed in the previous section on drug therapy during pregnancy influence the exposure of infants to drugs that are taken by mothers who breast-feed. The primary drug characteristics that increase the likelihood that a drug given to a breast-feeding mother will end up in the breast milk include fat solubility, low molecular weight, nonionization, and high concentration.

Fortunately, breast milk is not the primary route for maternal drug excretion. Drug levels in breast milk are usually lower than those in the maternal circulation. The actual amount of drug to which a breast-feeding infant is exposed depends largely on the volume of milk consumed. The ultimate decision as to whether a breast-feeding mother should take a particular drug depends on the risk-to-benefit ratio. The risks of transfer of maternal medication to the infant in relation to the benefits of continuing breast-feeding and the therapeutic benefits to the mother must be considered on a case-by-case basis.

CONSIDERATIONS FOR NEONATAL AND PEDIATRIC PATIENTS

In terms of age, a *child* is defined differently from a *neonate* or an *infant*. Therefore, the term *child* should not be mistakenly used to refer to a patient younger than 1 year of age. The age ranges that correspond to the various terms applied to young patients are shown in Table 3-2. This classification is used throughout this chapter.

Physiology and Pharmacokinetics

The anatomic and physiologic characteristics unique to **pediatric** patients account for most of the differences in the pharmacokinetic and pharmacodynamic behavior of drugs in their bodies (as is the case with other age-related anatomic and physiologic differences between neonates and adults). The immaturity of organs is the physiologic factor most responsible for these differences. The various physiologic characteristics of the neonatal population are also seen in the overall pediatric population, but to a lesser extent. In both groups, anatomic structures and physiologic systems and functions are still in the process of developing. The Life Span Considerations: The Pediatric Patient box on this page lists those physiologic factors that alter the pharmacokinetic properties of drugs in young patients.

Pharmacodynamics

As previously mentioned, drug actions (or pharmacodynamics) are altered in young patients, and the maturity of various organs plays a role in how drugs act in the body. In young patients, certain drugs may be more toxic and others less toxic than they are in adult patients. Drugs that are more toxic in children include phenobarbital, morphine, and aspirin. Drugs that children tolerate as well as or better than adults include atropine, codeine, digoxin, and phenylephrine. The sensitivity of receptor sites may also vary with age; thus, higher or lower dosages may be required depending on the drug. In addition, rapidly developing tissues may be more sensitive to certain drugs and therefore smaller dosages may be required. Because of this, certain drugs are generally contraindicated during the growth years. For instance, tetracycline may discolor a young person's teeth; corticosteroids may suppress growth if given systemically (but not when delivered via asthma inhalers, for example); and fluoroquinolone antibiotics may damage cartilage, which can lead to deformities in gait.

Dosage Calculations for Pediatric Patients

Many drugs commonly used in adults have not been sufficiently investigated to ensure their safety and effectiveness in children. Most drugs administered in pediatrics are given on an empirical

Table 3-2   Classification of Young Patients

Age Range	Classification
Younger than 38 wk gestation	Premature or preterm infant
Younger than 1 mo	Neonate or newborn infant
1 mo to younger than 1 yr	Infant
1 yr to younger than 12 yr	Child

NOTE: The meaning of the term *pediatric* may vary with the individual drug and clinical situation. Often the maximum age for a pediatric patient may be identified as 16 years of age. Consult manufacturer's guidelines for specific dosing information.

basis. Because pediatric patients (especially premature infants and neonates) are small and have immature organs, they are very susceptible to many drug interactions, toxicity, and unusual drug responses and therefore require very different dosage calculations. Characteristics of pediatric patients that play a significant role in dosage calculation include the following:

- Skin is thinner and more permeable.
- Stomach lacks acid to kill bacteria.
- Lungs have weaker mucus barriers.
- Body temperature is less well regulated and dehydration occurs easily.
- Liver and kidneys are immature and so drug metabolism and excretion are impaired.

Many formulas for pediatric dosage calculation have been used throughout the years. Formulas involving age, weight, and body surface area (BSA) are most commonly employed as the basis for calculations. BSA is the most accurate of these dosage formulas.

For the BSA method, the nurse needs the following information:

- Drug order with drug name, dose, route, time, and frequency
- Information regarding available dosage forms

Life Span Considerations: The Pediatric Patient

Pharmacokinetic Changes in the Neonate and Pediatric Patient

Absorption
- Gastric pH is less acidic because acid-producing cells in the stomach are immature until approximately 1 to 2 years of age.
- Gastric emptying is slowed because of slow or irregular peristalsis.
- First-pass elimination by the liver is reduced because of the immaturity of the liver and reduced levels of microsomal enzymes.
- Intramuscular absorption is faster and irregular.

Distribution
- Total body water is 70% to 80% in full-term infants, 85% in premature newborns, and 64% in children 1 to 12 years of age.
- Fat content is lower in young patients because of greater total body water.
- Protein binding is decreased because of decreased production of protein by the immature liver.
- More drugs enter the brain because of an immature blood-brain barrier.

Metabolism
- Levels of microsomal enzymes are decreased because the immature liver has not yet started producing enough.
- Older children may have increased metabolism and require higher dosages once hepatic enzymes are produced.
- Many variables affect metabolism in premature infants, infants, and children, including the status of liver enzyme production, genetic differences, and what the mother has been exposed to during pregnancy.

Excretion
- Glomerular filtration rate and tubular secretion and resorption are all decreased in young patients because of kidney immaturity.
- Perfusion to the kidneys may be decreased and results in reduced renal function, concentrating ability, and excretion of drugs.

- Pediatric patient's height in centimeters (cm) and weight in kilograms (kg)
- BSA **nomogram** for children (e.g., West nomogram, shown in Figure 3-1,
- Recommended adult drug dosage

The West nomogram (see Figure 3-1) uses a child's height and weight to determine the child's BSA. This information is then inserted into the BSA formula to obtain a drug dosage for a specific pediatric patient. Consider the following example:

$$\frac{\text{BSA of child}}{\text{BSA of adult}} \times \text{adult dose} = \text{estimated child's dose}$$

$$\text{BSA of child (m}^2) \times \frac{\text{manufacturer recommended dose}}{\text{m}^2} = \text{estimated child's dose}$$

Calculating the drug dosage according to the body weight method is appropriate when the child is of usual stature for his or her age and gender, and most drug references recommend

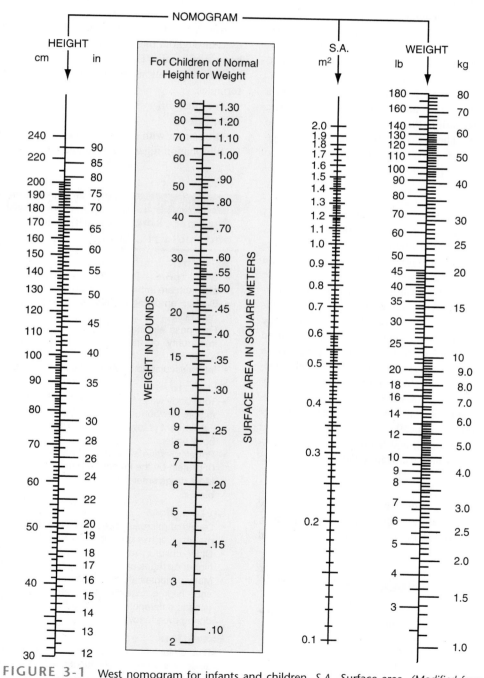

FIGURE 3-1   West nomogram for infants and children. *S.A., Surface area. (Modified from data by E. Boyd and C. D. West. In Behrman RE, Kliegman RM, Jensen HB: Nelson textbook of pediatrics, ed 17, Philadelphia, 2004, Saunders.)*

dosages based on milligrams per kilogram of body weight. The following information is needed to calculate the pediatric dosage:

- Drug order (as discussed previously)
- Pediatric patient's weight in kilograms (1 kg = 2.2 lb)
- Pediatric dosage as per manufacturer or drug formulary guidelines
- Information regarding available dosage forms

When using either of the previous methods, the nurse does the following:

- Determines the pediatric patient's weight in kilograms
- Uses a current drug reference to determine the usual dosage range per 24 hours in milligrams per kilogram
- Determines the dose parameters by multiplying the weight by the minimum and maximum daily doses of the drug (the safe range)
- Determines the total amount of the drug to administer per dose and per day
- Compares the drug dosage prescribed with the calculated safe range
- If the drug dosage raises any concerns or varies from the safe range, contacts the health care provider or prescriber immediately—does not give the drug!

The nurse should never underestimate the importance of organ maturity, along with BSA, age, and weight, in calculating pediatric dosage. If all of these physical developmental factors are considered, the likelihood of safe and effective drug administration is increased. Emotional developmental considerations must also be a part of the decision-making process in drug therapy with pediatric patients (see Life Span Considerations: The Pediatric Patient box on p. 37).

CONSIDERATIONS FOR ELDERLY PATIENTS

The **elderly** patient has special needs due to decline in organ function, which contributes to various pharmacokinetic changes. Therefore, drug therapy is much more likely to result in adverse effects and toxicity at this end of the life span than that at other times.

In this book, the word *elderly* is used instead of the word *geriatric;* however, these terms are synonymous. An elderly patient is defined as a person who is 65 years of age or older. (However, *Healthy People 2010* categorizes a person as elderly at 55 years of age.) This segment of the population is growing at a dramatic pace (see the Life Span Considerations: The Elderly Patient box on this page). At the beginning of the twentieth century, the elderly constituted a mere 4% of the total population. At that time more people died of infections than of degenerative, chronic illnesses such as heart disease, cancer, and diabetes. As medical and health care

technology has advanced, so has the ability to prolong life, often by treating and controlling, or even curing, illnesses from which people commonly died in the past. This has resulted in a growing population of older adults. Today patients over 65 years of age constitute 13% of the population. At any given time, an elderly patient takes four or five prescription drugs as well as two OTC medications. In addition, the estimated incidence of drug interactions increases from 6% in patients taking two drugs daily to 50% in patients taking five medications. Life expectancy is currently approximately 74.9 years, and it is estimated that by the year 2020, 20% of the population will be 65 years of age or older. Older adults represent the fastest growing segment of the population, increasing by about 2% a year. These trends are expected to continue as new disease prevention and treatment methods are developed.

Polypharmacy and Drug Use

The growing elderly population consumes a larger proportion of all medications than other population groups (30% of all prescription drugs and over 40% of OTC drugs). Commonly prescribed drugs for the elderly include antihypertensives, β-blockers, digitalis, diuretics, insulin, and potassium supplements. The most commonly used OTC drugs are analgesics, laxatives, and nonsteroidal antiinflammatory drugs (NSAIDs). Elderly patients, especially those of certain ethnicities, may use various folk remedies of unknown composition that are unfamiliar to their health care providers.

Not only do elderly patients consume a greater proportion of prescription and OTC medications, they commonly take multiple medications on a daily basis. One in three elderly patients takes more than 8 different drugs each day, and some take as many as 15 or more. One reason for patients' use of so many medications is the occurrence of more chronic diseases, which now have even more drug options for treatment. More than 80% of patients taking eight or more drugs have one or more chronic illness. In this age of medical specialization, patients may see several physicians for their many illnesses. These specialists may all prescribe medications for the disorder(s) they are treating, which explains why a patient can be taking 8 to 15 drugs plus OTC medications. This situation is called **polypharmacy.** Polypharmacy leads to what is known as the "prescribing cascade," in which an elderly

Lifespan Considerations: The Elderly Patient
Percentage of Population over 65 Years of Age

Year	Percentage over Age 65
1900	4%
2000	12%
2020	20%

Life Span Considerations: The Elderly Patient
Alzheimer's Disease

- Alzheimer's disease affects approximately 4 million Americans, and the figure may reach 14 million by the middle of the twenty-first century. It is presently the fourth leading cause of death in adults, preceded by heart disease, cancer, and stroke. Unfortunately, approximately 1 in 10 families in the United States has a loved one with Alzheimer's disease.
- The disease process has a major impact on the patient's mental and physical abilities. Due to deterioration of mental status and chronic physical decline, these patients need assistance in performing the activities of daily living, including assistance with medication administration.
- Caregivers and family members need to be informed of the short-term and long-term characteristics of the illness, and resources need to be provided in either a private care setting or through special needs units in assisted living settings or nursing homes.

patient develops adverse effects from one or more of the medications he or she is taking and the health care provider then prescribes yet another drug, which creates the potential for even more adverse effects. The risk of drug interactions, adverse effects, and potentially a hospitalization (possibly prolonged) is far greater in this situation. As the number of medications a person takes increases, so does the risk of drug interaction. For example, the chance of a drug interaction is approximately 6% for a patient receiving two medications. This risk dramatically increases as the number of drugs the patient is taking increases. For a patient taking five medications, the chance of a drug interaction is 50%. This likelihood rises to 100% if the patient is taking eight medications. Some drugs in a regimen may even be given specifically to counteract the adverse effects of other drugs (e.g., a potassium supplement to counteract the potassium loss caused by certain diuretic medications). In one study encompassing more than 150,000 elderly patients, nearly 30% received at least 1 of 33 drugs that were identified as often inappropriately prescribed for patients in this age group (see more discussion in Chapter 4). A study of almost 30,000 Medicare patients documented more than 1500 adverse drug events in 1 year.

Along with the risk of drug interaction come other risks. More hospitalizations for the treatment of adverse drug effects, greater likelihood of drug-induced falls that lead to hip fractures, and heightened risk of addiction are just a few. Many of these are preventable. Recognizing polypharmacy in a patient and taking steps to reduce it whenever possible by decreasing the number and/or dosages of drugs taken can dramatically reduce the incidence of these undesirable drug effects and adverse outcomes.

Physiologic Changes

The physiologic changes associated with aging also affect how many drugs act. Having an understanding of these physiologic changes and how they affect pharmacokinetics and pharmacodynamics in elderly patients helps ensure the provision of safe and effective drug therapy. The body ages, and the function of several organ systems slowly deteriorates after many years of wear and tear. The collective physiologic changes associated with the aging process have a major effect on the disposition of drugs. Table 3-3 lists some of the body systems most affected by the aging process.

These and other physiologic changes that take place in older adults directly affect drug action. The sensitivity of the elderly

Table 3-3	**Physiologic Changes in the Elderly Patient**
System	**Physiologic Change**
Cardiovascular	↓ Cardiac output = ↓ absorption and distribution
	↓ Blood flow = ↓ absorption and distribution
Gastrointestinal	↑ pH (alkaline gastric secretions = altered absorption)
	↓ Peristalsis = delayed gastric emptying
Hepatic	↓ Enzyme production = ↓ metabolism
	↓ Blood flow = ↓ metabolism
Renal	↓ Blood flow = ↓ excretion
	↓ Function = ↓ excretion
	↓ Glomerular filtration rate = ↓ excretion

patient to many drugs is altered as a result of these physiologic changes; therefore, drug usage should be adjusted to accommodate these changes. For instance, with aging there is a general decrease in body weight. However, the drug dosages administered to elderly patients are often the same as those administered to younger adults. The criteria for drug dosages in older adults therefore should include consideration of kilograms of body weight and organ functioning, with emphasis on liver, renal, cardiovascular, and central nervous system function (similar to the criteria for pediatric dosages).

It is important for the nurse to monitor the results of laboratory tests that have been ordered for elderly patients. These values serve as a gauge of organ function. The most important organs from the standpoint of the breakdown and elimination of drugs are the liver and the kidneys. Kidney function is assessed by measuring serum creatinine and blood urea nitrogen levels. A more thorough but also more cumbersome and expensive test that is sometimes ordered is creatinine clearance. This test involves collecting a patient's entire urine output for 24 hours and measuring the actual amount of creatinine excreted. The test is usually only ordered for more complicated clinical cases. Liver function is assessed by testing the blood for liver enzymes such as aspartate aminotransferase (AST) and alanine aminotransferase (ALT). These laboratory values can help in the assessment of an older patient's ability to metabolize and eliminate medications and can aid in anticipating the risk of toxicity and/or drug accumulation. Laboratory assessments should ideally be conducted at least annually for most elderly patients, both for preventive health monitoring and for screening for possible toxic effects of drug therapy. Such assessments may be indicated more frequently (e.g., every 1, 3, or 6 months) in those patients requiring higher-risk drug regimens.

Pharmacokinetics

What happens during the pharmacokinetic phases of absorption, distribution, metabolism, and excretion may be different in the older adult than in the younger adult. Awareness of these differences helps the nurse ensure appropriate administration of drugs and monitoring of elderly patients taking medications. The Life Span Considerations: The Elderly Patient box on page 41 lists the four pharmacokinetic phases and summarizes how they are altered by the aging process.

Absorption

Absorption in the older person can be altered by many mechanisms. Advancing age results in reduced absorption of both dietary nutrients and drugs. Several physiologic changes account for this. There is a gradual reduction in the ability of the stomach to produce hydrochloric acid, which results in a decrease in gastric acidity and may alter the absorption of weakly acidic drugs such as barbiturates and aspirin. In addition, the combination of decreased cardiac output and advancing atherosclerosis results in a general reduction in the flow of blood to major organs, including the stomach. By 65 years of age, there is an approximately 50% reduction in blood flow to the gastrointestinal (GI) tract. Absorption, whether of nutrient or drug, is dependent on good blood supply to the stomach and intestines. The absorptive surface area of an elderly person's GI tract is often reduced by flattening and blunting of the villi. These age-related changes reduce overall GI

Life Span Considerations: The Elderly Patient
Pharmacokinetic Changes

Absorption
- Gastric pH is less acidic because of a gradual reduction in the production of hydrochloric acid in the stomach.
- Gastric emptying is slowed because of a decline in smooth muscle tone and motor activity.
- Movement throughout the gastrointestinal (GI) tract is slower because of decreased muscle tone and motor activity.
- Blood flow to the GI tract is reduced by 40% to 50% because of decreased cardiac output and decreased perfusion.
- The absorptive surface area is decreased because the aging process blunts and flattens villi.

Distribution
- In adults 40 to 60 years of age, total body water is 55% in males and 47% in females; in those over 60 years of age, total body water is 52% in males and 46% in females.
- Fat content is increased because of decreased lean body mass.
- Protein (albumin) binding sites are reduced because of decreased production of proteins by the aging liver and reduced protein intake.

Metabolism
- The levels of microsomal enzymes are decreased because the capacity of the aging liver to produce them is reduced.
- Liver blood flow is reduced by approximately 1.5% per year after 25 years of age, which decreases hepatic metabolism.

Excretion
- Glomerular filtration rate is decreased by 40% to 50% primarily because of decreased blood flow.
- The number of intact nephrons is decreased.

absorptive capabilities, including drug absorption. Once absorbed, drugs must be carried by the bloodstream to their eventual site of action (i.e., to receptors in various tissues). The speed and intensity with which this happens depends on the quality of the circulation, which, in turn, depends on cardiac output, blood pressure, and patency of both central and peripheral blood vessels.

GI motility is important not only for moving substances out of the stomach but also for moving them throughout the GI tract. Muscle tone and motor activity in the GI tract are reduced in older adults. This often results in constipation, for which older adults frequently take laxatives. This use of laxatives may accelerate GI motility enough to actually reduce the absorption of drugs. One particular category of laxatives, bulk-forming laxatives, has been shown to reduce the absorption of certain medications such as cardiac glycosides (e.g., digoxin). Bran and high-fiber foods may have the same effect on this group of medications.

Distribution

The distribution of medications throughout the body is vastly different in older adults than it is in younger adults. There seems to be a gradual reduction in the total body water content with aging. Therefore, the concentrations of highly water-soluble drugs may be higher in elderly patients because they have less body water in which the drugs can be diluted. The composition of the body also changes with aging. The lean muscle mass decreases, which results in increased body fat. In both men and women

there is an approximately 20% reduction in muscle mass between the ages of 25 and 65 years and a corresponding 20% increase in body fat. Drugs such as hypnotics and sedatives that are primarily distributed to the fat will therefore have a prolonged effect.

Many drugs distributed by means of the blood are carried by proteins. By far the most important of these proteins is albumin. Reduced protein concentrations are seen with aging, due in large part to reduced liver function. In addition, reduced dietary intake, or poor GI protein absorption even with adequate dietary intake, also contributes to reduced blood protein levels. Whatever the cause, the reduced number of protein-binding sites for highly protein-bound drugs results in higher levels of unbound drug in the blood. Drugs that are not bound to proteins are active. Therefore, the effects of highly protein-bound drugs may be enhanced if their dosages are not adjusted to accommodate any reduced serum albumin concentrations, as measured in blood samples. Highly protein-bound drugs include warfarin and phenytoin, among many others.

Metabolism

Metabolism declines with advancing age. The transformation of active drugs into inactive metabolites is primarily performed by the liver, but the liver slowly loses its ability to metabolize drugs effectively because the production of microsomal enzymes is reduced. There is also a reduction in blood flow to the liver because of reduced cardiac output and atherosclerosis. A reduction in the hepatic blood flow of approximately 1.5% per year occurs after 25 years of age. All of these factors contribute to prolonging the half-life of many drugs (e.g., warfarin), which can potentially result in drug accumulation if serum drug levels are not closely monitored.

Excretion

The excretion of drugs is reduced in the elderly population. A reduction in the glomerular filtration rate of 40% to 50% in older adults, combined with a reduction in blood flow (for the same reasons as in the liver), can result in extremely delayed drug excretion and hence drug accumulation. Renal function should be monitored frequently in elderly patients through laboratory studies such as measurement of serum creatinine level, blood urea nitrogen level, or creatinine clearance to prevent drug accumulation. Appropriate dose and interval adjustments may be determined based on results of a patient's renal and liver function studies as well as the presence of therapeutic levels of the drug in the serum. If a decrease in renal and liver function is a known variable, the drug dosage should be altered—as ordered—so that accumulation of the drug and possible toxicity may be minimized.

Problematic Medications for the Elderly

- Drugs in certain classes are more likely to cause problems in elderly patients because of many of the physiologic alterations and pharmacokinetic changes already discussed. Table 3-4 lists some of the more common medications that are problematic. Knowledge of the physiologic changes in older adults and understanding of accompanying pharmacokinetic changes is extremely useful in optimizing drug therapy for elderly patients. Some of the drugs that should be avoided in the elderly have been identified by various professional organizations such as the American Nurses Association, as well as by various other authoritative sources. Since the 1990s, a very

Table 3-4 Problematic Medications and Conditions to Consider for the Elderly Patient

Medication	Common Complications
Analgesics Opioids	Confusion, constipation, urinary retention, nausea, vomiting, respiratory depression, decreased level of consciousness, falls
Nonsteroidal antiinflammatory drugs	Edema, nausea, abdominal distress, gastric ulceration, bleeding, renal toxicity
Anticoagulants (heparin, warfarin)	Major and minor bleeding episodes, many drug interactions, dietary interactions
Anticholinergics	Blurred vision, dry mouth, constipation, confusion, urinary retention, tachycardia
Antidepressants	Sedation and strong anticholinergic adverse effects (see above)
Antihypertensives	Nausea, hypotension, diarrhea, bradycardia, heart failure, impotence
Cardiac glycosides (e.g., digoxin)	Visual disorders, nausea, diarrhea, dysrhythmias, hallucinations, decreased appetite, weight loss
CNS depressants (muscle relaxants, narcotics)	Sedation, weakness, dry mouth, confusion, urinary retention, ataxia
Sedatives and hypnotics	Confusion, daytime sedation, ataxia, lethargy, forgetfulness, increased risk of falls
Thiazide diuretics	Electrolyte imbalance, rashes, fatigue, leg cramps, dehydration

Condition	Common Drugs to Avoid
Bladder flow obstruction	Anticholinergics, anithistamines, decongestants, antidepressants
Clotting disorders	NSAIDs, aspirin, antiplatelet drugs
Chronic constipation	Calcium channel blockers, tricyclic antidepressants, anticholinergics
COPD	Long-acting sedatives/hypnotics, narcotics, β-blockers
Depression	Some anithypertensives: methyldopa, reserpine, quanethidine
Heart failure and hypertension	Sodium, decongestants, amphetamines, OTC cold products
Insomnia	Decongestants, bronchodilators, MAO inhibitors
Parkinson's disease	Antipsychotics, phenothiazines
Syncope/falls	Sedatives, hypnotics, narcotics, CNS depressants, muscle relaxants, antidepressants, antihypertensives

effective tool, the Beers criteria, has been used to identify drugs that may be inappropriately prescribed, ineffective, or cause adverse drug reactions in elderly patients (see the Evidence-Based Practice box on p. 43). Research has been conducted using these criteria and was updated in 2002. The Beers criteria are very useful and help determine risk-associated situations for the elderly and specific drugs that may be problematic.

◆ NURSING PROCESS

◆ ASSESSMENT

Before any medication is administered to a *pediatric* patient, a health history and medication history should be obtained with assistance from parents, caregivers, or legal guardian; these include the following:

- Age
- Age-related concerns about organ functioning
- Age-related fears
- Allergies to drugs and food
- Baseline vital signs
- Head-to-toe physical assessment findings
- Height in feet/inches and centimeters
- Weight in kilograms and pounds
- Level of growth and development and related developmental tasks
- Medical and medication history (including adverse drug reactions); current medications and related dosage forms and routes and the patient's tolerance of the forms and/or routes

- State of anxiety of the patient and/or family members or caregiver
- Use of prescription and OTC medications in the home setting
- Usual method of medication administration, such as use of a calibrated spoon or needleless syringe
- Usual response to medications
- Motor and cognitive responses and their age appropriateness
- Resources available to the patient and family

In addition, the prescriber's orders should be checked and rechecked by the nurse, because there is no room for error when working with pediatric patients (or any patients). The medication dosage should be calculated and rechecked several times for accuracy. Calculations for dosages should take into account a variety of information and variables that may affect patient response and should use BSA formulas and body weight formulas (milligrams per kilogram). If any doubts exist regarding the calculation, time should always be taken to have the calculations rechecked. In addition to an assessment of the patient, an assessment of the drug should be performed, focusing specifically on information about the drug's purpose, dosage ranges, routes of administration, and cautions and contraindications. The saying that pediatric patients are just "small adults" is incorrect, because in these patients every organ is anatomically and physiologically immature and not fully functioning. As pediatric patients grow older, their body surface areas and weights are still smaller; thus, pediatric patients must be treated with extreme caution. Organ function may be determined through laboratory testing. Hepatic and renal function studies, red and white blood cell counts, and measurement of hemoglobin levels, hematocrit, and protein

EVIDENCE-BASED PRACTICE

The Beers Criteria for Drug Use in the Elderly

Review

The Beers criteria establish basic guidelines for identifying medications that may be inappropriate for the elderly. These criteria define drugs that have been determined by a panel of experts to have "potential risks" that outweigh the possible benefits of their use in this age group. Chang and colleagues (2005) applied criteria to evaluate drug therapy in patients 65 years or older with the purpose of predicting adverse drug reactions (ADRs) in elderly individuals managed in an outpatient clinic.

Type of Evidence

The research method was a prospective study of some 500 or more participants through use of a follow-up telephone survey. Statistical analysis focused on the possible relationship between ADRs and inappropriate drug prescribing in the elderly. The Beers criteria have been published since the 1990s, being one of the first tools to suggest a positive association between ADRs and drug prescribing policies in elderly patients, especially in those who take fewer than five drugs.

Results of Study

The study provided evidence that the Beers criteria may be used to predict ADRs among elderly outpatients and to examine the possible impact of potentially inappropriate drug prescribing. Of the 500+ patients, 64 had potentially inappropriate drugs prescribed and 126 experienced ADRs. Statistical analysis confirmed an association between ADRs and potentially inappropriate drug prescribing. The results of this study have been extremely beneficial because few studies have focused on investigation of drug-related problems experienced by the elderly.

Link of Evidence to Nursing Practice

This study showed a positive association between potentially inappropriate drug prescriptions as defined by the Beers criteria and ADRs. This study alerts clinicians of the possibility of ADRs in the elderly and raises concerns specific to certain medications. Developing and publishing these criteria for professional nursing practice is important because of the increase in serious problems and concerns caused by inappropriate drug use in elderly patients, as well as with other age groups. With education, awareness, more research, and subsequent evidenced-based nursing practice, medication-related risks may be decreased and safety may be increased. The Beers criteria may be applied to other patient care and medication-related issues as well.

Based on Chang CM, Liu PY, Yang YH, et al: Use of the Beers criteria to predict adverse drug reactions among first-visit elderly outpatients, *Pharmacotherapy* 25(6):831-838, 2005. Available at www.medscape.com/viewarticle/507059; Molony S: Beers criteria for potentially inappropriate medication use in the elderly, *Dermatol Nurs* 16(6):547-548, 2004. Available at www.medscape.com/viewarticle/496383; Sloane PD et al: Inappropriate medication prescribing in residential care/assisted living facilities, *J Am Geriatr Soc* 50:1001-1011, 2002.

levels are just a few examples of tests needed before initiation of drug therapy. Immature organ and system development will influence pharmacokinetics and thus affect the way the patient responds to a drug.

Assessment data to be gathered on the *elderly* patient include the following:

- Age
- Allergies to drugs and food
- Dietary habits
- Sensory, visual, hearing, cognitive, and motor skill deficits
- Financial status and any limitations
- List of all health-related care providers, including physicians, dentists, optometrists and ophthalmologists, podiatrists, alternative medicine health care practitioners such as osteopathic physicians, chiropractors, and nurse practitioners
- Past and present medical history
- Listing of medications, past and present, including prescription drugs, OTC medications, herbals, nutritional supplements, vitamins, and home-remedies
- Polypharmacy
- Self-medication practices
- Laboratory testing results, especially those indicative of renal and liver function
- History of smoking and use of alcohol with notation of amount, frequency, and years of use
- Risk situations related to drug therapy identified by the Beers criteria (see the Evidence-Based Practice box on p. 43)

One way to collect data about the various medications or drugs being taken is to obtain that information from the patient and/or caregiver using the brown-bag technique. It is an effective means of identifying various drugs the patient is taking, regardless of the patient's age, and should be used in conjunction with a complete review of the patient's medical history or record. The brown-bag technique requires the patient or caregiver to collect all medications in a bag and bring them to the health care provider. All medications should be kept within their original containers. A list of medications with generic names, dosages, routes of administration, and frequencies is compiled. The list of medications should be compared with what is prescribed or with what the patient states he or she is actually taking. In addition, the patient's insight into his or her medical problems is very beneficial in developing a plan of care. It is also important for the nurse to realize that although elderly patients may be able to provide the required information themselves, many may be confused or poorly informed about their medications. In such cases, a more reliable historian, such as a significant other, family member, or caregiver, should be used. Elderly patients may also have sensory deficits that require the nurse to speak slowly, loudly, and clearly while facing the patient.

With the elderly patient—as with a patient of any age—the nurse should always assess support systems and the patient's ability to take medications safely. Whenever possible, with the elderly and various age groups, health care providers should always opt to use a nonpharmacologic approach to treatment first if appropriate. Other data the nurse should gather include information about acute or chronic illnesses, nutritional problems, cardiac problems, respiratory illnesses, and GI tract disorders. Laboratory tests related to life span considerations that should be completed include the following: hemoglobin and hematocrit levels, red and white blood cell counts, blood urea nitrogen level, serum and urine creatinine levels, urine specific gravity, serum electrolyte levels, and protein and serum albumin levels.

◆ NURSING DIAGNOSES

- Risk for injury related to adverse effects of medications or to the method of drug administration
- Imbalanced nutrition: less than body requirements, related to age or drug therapy and possible drug adverse effects
- Risk for injury related to idiosyncratic reactions to drugs due to age-related drug sensitivity
- Deficient knowledge related to information about drugs and their adverse effects or about when to contact the physician

◆ PLANNING

Goals

- Patient states measures to minimize complications and adverse effects associated with the drugs taken during the therapeutic regimen.
- Patient states the importance of adhering to the prescribed drug therapy (or takes medication as prescribed with assistance).
- Patient contacts the physician when appropriate (such as when unusual effects occur) during drug therapy.

Outcome Criteria

- Patient (or the parent, legal guardian, or caregiver) states the importance of taking the medication as prescribed (e.g., improved condition, decreased symptoms) for the duration of the recommended drug therapy.
- Patient (or the parent, legal guardian, or caregiver) follows instructions specific to the administration of the medication ordered (e.g., special application of an ointment, proper administration of a liquid, correct dosage) for the duration of treatment.
- Patient (specifically the elderly patient) states why he or she is taking a specific medication and identifies what the drug looks like and when the drug is to be taken during the duration of drug treatment.
- Patient shows improvement in the condition being treated that is related to compliance with the medication regimen and successful medication therapy during the treatment period.
- Patient takes or receives medications safely and without injury to self over the duration of therapy.
- Patient (or the parent, legal guardian, or caregiver) states specific situations in which the physician must be contacted (e.g., occurrence of fever, pain, vomiting, rash, or diarrhea; worsening of the condition being treated; bronchospasm; dyspnea; intolerable adverse effects; signs of major adverse effects).

◆ IMPLEMENTATION

In general, it is always important to emphasize and practice the Five Rights of medication administration (Chapter 1) and follow the physician's order and/or medication instructions. All drugs should be checked three times against the Five Rights and the physician's order before giving the drug to the patient (for inpatient situations). For the pediatric patient, some specific nursing actions are as follows: (1) If necessary, mix medications in a substance or fluid other than essential foods such as milk, orange juice, or cereal, because the child may develop a dislike for the food in the future. Instead of such foods, find a liquid or food item that can be used to make the medications taste better, such as sherbet or another form or flavor of ice cream. This intervention should be used only if the patient is not able to swallow the dosage form. (2) Do not add drug(s) to the fluid in a cup or bottle, because the amount consumed is difficult to calculate if the entire amount is not taken. (3) Always document special techniques of drug administration so that others involved in the care of the patient may use the same technique. For example, if having the child eat a frozen Popsicle before giving an unpleasant-tasting pill, liquid, or tablet helps to get the medication administered, then share that information. (4) Unless contraindicated, add small amounts of water or fluids to elixirs so that the child may tolerate the medication. Remember, however, that it is essential that the child take the entire volume, so be very cautious with this practice. (5) Avoid using the word *candy* in place of *drug* or *medication*. Medications should be called medicines and their dangers made known to children, and no games should be played with this information. (6) Keep all medications out of the reach of children of all ages and be sure that parents and other family members understand this information and know to request child-protective lids or tops for medication containers. (7) Always ask about how the pediatric patient is used to taking medications (e.g., liquid vs. pill or tablet dosage forms) and if there are any methods that the family or caregiver have found to be helpful in administering distasteful drugs. See the Life Span Considerations: The Pediatric Patient box on page 45 for recommendations regarding medication administration in pediatric patients from infancy through adolescence.

Elderly patients should be encouraged to take medications as directed and not to discontinue them or double up on doses. Regardless of the patient's age, the nurse should ensure that the patient, parent, legal guardian, or caregiver understands treatment- and/or medication-related instructions and understands safety measures related to drug therapy, such as keeping all medications out of the reach of children. Written and oral instructions should be provided concerning the drug name, action, purpose, dose, time of administration, route, adverse effects, safety of administration, storage, interactions, and any cautions about or contraindications to its use. Remember that simple is always best! Always try to find ways to simplify the patient's therapeutic regimen and be especially alert to polypharmacy. If a nurse advocate or a nurse practitioner with prescription privileges has the opportunity to review the patient's chart, he or she should take the time to simplify and write down the use or purpose of the drug, how to best take the drug, and a list of adverse effects. Provide this information on paper in bold, large print. Some specific interventions proving to be helpful in promoting medication safety in the elderly include use of the Beers criteria (see the Evidence-Based Practice box on p. 43). These criteria provide a systematic way of identifying prescription medications that are potentially harmful to elderly patients. The prescriber and nurse must constantly remember that clinical judgment and knowledge base are important in making critical decisions about a patient's care and drug therapy. In addition, evidence-based nursing practice, as seen with the Beers criteria, is important for the nurse to remain current in clinical nursing practice. Specific guidelines for medication administration by various routes are presented in detail in Chapter 9.

In summary, drug therapy across the life span must be well-thought out, with full consideration to the patient's age, gender, cultural background, ethnicity, medical history, and medication profile. With inclusion of all phases of the nursing process and the specific life span considerations discussed in this chapter, there is a better chance of decreasing adverse effects and a better chance of reducing risks to the patient and increasing drug safety.

◆ EVALUATION

In general, when the nurse is dealing with life span issues and drug therapy, the nurse's observation and monitoring for therapeutic effects as well as adverse effects is critical to safe and effective therapy. The nurse must know the patient's profile and history just as well as the nurse knows the drug and related information. The drug's purpose, specific use in the patient, simply stated action, dose, frequency of dosing, adverse effects, cautions, and contraindications should be listed and kept on the nurse's person. This information will allow more comprehensive monitoring of drug therapy, regardless of the age of the patient.

Life Span Considerations: The Pediatric Patient

Age-Related Considerations for Medication Administration from Infancy to Adolescence

General Interventions

- Always come prepared for the procedure (e.g., prepare for injections with needleless syringe and gather all needed equipment).
- Ask the parent and/or child (if age appropriate) if the parent should or should not remain for the procedure (for in-hospital administration).
- Assess comfort methods that are appropriate before and after drug administration.

Infants

- While maintaining safe and secure positioning of the infant (e.g., with parent holding, rocking, cuddling, soothing), perform the procedure (e.g., injection) swiftly and safely.
- Allow self-comforting measures as age appropriate (e.g., use of pacifier, fingers in mouth, self-movement).

Toddlers

- Offer a brief, concrete explanation of the procedure but with realistic expectations of the child's actual understanding of the information. Parents, caregivers, or other legal guardians have to be part of the process. Hold the child securely while administering the medication.
- Accept aggressive behavior as a healthy response, but only within reasonable limits.
- Provide comfort measures immediately after the procedure (e.g., touching, holding).
- Help the child understand the treatment and his or her feelings through puppet play or play with stuffed animals or hospital equipment such as empty, needleless syringes.
- Provide for healthy ways to release aggression such as age-appropriate, supervised playtime.

Preschoolers

- Offer a brief, concrete explanation of the procedure at the patient's level and with the parent or caregiver.
- Provide comfort measures after the procedure (e.g., touching, holding).

- Identify and accept aggressive responses and provide age-appropriate outlets.
- Make use of magical thinking (e.g., using ointments or "special medicines" to make discomfort go away).
- Note that the role of the parent is very important for providing comfort and understanding.

School-Aged Children

- Explain the procedure, allowing for some control over body and situation.
- Provide comfort measures.
- Explore feelings and concepts through the use of therapeutic play. Art may be used to help the patient express fears. Use of age-appropriate books and realistic hospital equipment may also be helpful.
- Set appropriate behavior limits (e.g., okay to cry or scream, but not to bite).
- Provide activities for releasing aggression and anger.
- Use the opportunity to teach about the relationship between getting medication and body function and structure (e.g., what a seizure is and how medication helps prevent the seizure).
- Offer the complete picture (e.g., need to take medication, relax with deep breaths; medication will help prevent pain).

Adolescents

- Prepare the patient in advance for the procedure but without scare tactics.
- Allow for expression in a way that does not cause losing face, such as giving the adolescent time alone after the procedure (e.g., once a seizure is controlled) and giving the adolescent time to discuss his or her feelings.
- Explore with the adolescent any current concepts of self, hospitalization, and illness, and correct any misconceptions.
- Encourage self-expression, individuality, and self-care.
- Encourage participation in procedures and as appropriate.

Modified from McKenry LM, Salerno E: *Mosby's pharmacology in nursing,* ed 22, St Louis, 2006, Mosby; Blaber M: Related to nursing intervention in pain. *Newington's Children's Hospital manual for global pediatric nursing assessment* (unpublished).

Points to Remember

- There are many age-related pharmacokinetic effects that lead to dramatic differences in drug absorption, distribution, metabolism, and excretion. At one end of the life span is the pediatric patient and at the other end is the elderly patient, both of whom are very sensitive to the effects of drugs.
- Most common dosage calculations use the milligrams per kilogram formula related to age; however, BSA is also used for drug calculations, as is consideration of organ maturity. It is important for the nurse to know that many variables besides the mathematical calculation itself contribute to safe dosage calculations. Safety should be the number one concern,

with full consideration of the Five Rights of medication administration.
- The percentage of the population over the age of 65 years continues to grow; therefore, nurses will continue to be exposed to an increasing number of elderly patients. Polypharmacy raises many concerns for the elderly; thus, there is a need for a current listing of all medications with the patient at all times!
- The nurse's responsibility is to act as a patient advocate as well as to be informed about growth and development principles and the effects of various drugs during the life span and in various phases of illness.

NCLEX Examination Review Questions

1. Which of the following factors influencing pharmacokinetics puts the neonatal patient at risk with regard to drug therapy?
   a. Immature renal system
   b. Hyperperistalsis in the GI tract
   c. Irregular temperature regulation
   d. Smaller circulatory capacity
2. The physiologic differences in the pediatric patient compared with the adult patient affect the amount of drug needed to produce a therapeutic effect. One of the main differences is that infants have the following:
   a. Increased protein in circulation
   b. Fat composition lower than 0.001%
   c. More muscular body composition
   d. Water composition of approximately 75%
3. While teaching a 76-year-old patient about the adverse effects of his medications, the nurse encourages him to keep a journal of the adverse effects he experiences. This intervention is important for the elderly patient because of alterations in pharmacokinetics, such as the following:
   a. Increased renal excretion of protein-bound drugs
   b. More alkaline gastric pH, resulting in more adverse effects
   c. Decreased blood flow to the liver with altered metabolism
   d. Less adipose tissue to store fat-soluble drugs

4. When the nurse is reviewing a list of medications taken by an 88-year-old patient, the patient notes that she gets "dizzy when I stand up" and has nearly fainted in the afternoon. Her systolic blood pressure drops 15 points when she stands up. Which of the following types of medications may be responsible for these effects?
   a. NSAIDs
   b. Cardiac glycosides
   c. Anticoagulants
   d. Antihypertensives
5. A patient who is at 32 weeks' gestation has a cold and calls the office to ask about taking an OTC medication that is rated as pregnancy category A. Which answer by the nurse is correct?
   a. "This drug causes problems in the human fetus, so you should not take this medication."
   b. "This drug may cause problems in the human fetus, but nothing has been proven in clinical trials. It is best not to take this medication."
   c. "This drug has not caused problems in animals, but no testing has been done in humans. It is probably safe to take."
   d. "Studies indicate there is no risk to the human fetus, so it is okay to take this medication, as directed, if you need it."

1. a, 2. d, 3. c, 4. d, 5. d.

Critical Thinking Activities

1. Select either phenytoin or tetracycline and discuss its potential risks to the fetus or breast-feeding newborn in relation to the benefits to the mother.
2. A 73-year-old nursing home resident is experiencing problems that you, as the nurse, think are indicative of absorption problems with his oral medications (he is currently taking warfarin sodium). Specifically, you notice that he has been experiencing unusual bleeding tendencies over the past few days; however, he has tolerated the medication "very well" over the "last 3 years." Which of the following physiologic changes is *most* likely to be the basis of his untoward reaction to the warfarin?

   a. Increased cardiac output and cardiac volume
   b. Increased glomerular filtration rate and renin excretion
   c. Decreased GI pH with increased peristalsis
   d. Decreased hepatic enzyme production and altered liver perfusion
3. List at least three medications that have a high risk for causing problems (e.g., adverse effects, toxicity) in the elderly patient. Discuss the problems or complications associated with these drugs or drug groups.

For answers, see http://evolve.elsevier.com/Lilley.

Cultural, Legal, and Ethical Considerations

Objectives

When you reach the end of this chapter, you should be able to do the following:

1. Discuss the various cultural, genetic, and racial or ethnic factors that may influence an individual's response to medications.
2. Identify various cultural phenomena affecting health care and use of medications.
3. List the various drugs more commonly affected by cultural, racial, and ethnic factors.
4. Develop a nursing care plan that addresses the cultural care of patients in drug therapy and the nursing process.
5. Briefly discuss the important components of drug legislation at the state and federal levels.
6. Identify the impact of drug legislation on drug therapy and the nursing process.
7. Discuss the various categories of controlled substances and provide specific drug examples.
8. Identify the process involved in the development of new drugs, including the investigational new drug application, phases of investigational drug studies, and process for informed consent.
9. Discuss the nurse's role in the development of new and investigational drugs and the informed consent process.
10. Discuss the ethical aspects of drug administration as they relate to drug therapy and the nursing process.
11. Identify the ethical principles involved in making an ethical decision.
12. Develop a nursing care plan that addresses the legal and ethical care of patients, drug therapy, and the nursing process.

e-Learning Activities

Companion CD
* NCLEX Review Questions: see questions 23-26
* Animations
* Audio Glossary
* Category Catchers
* Medication Errors Checklists
* IV Therapy Checklists

evolve Website (http://evolve.elsevier.com/Lilley)
* Nursing Care Plans • Frequently Asked Questions • Content Updates • WebLinks • Supplemental Resources • Elsevier ePharmacology Update • Medication Administration Animations

Glossary

Blinded investigational drug study A research design in which the subjects are purposely unaware of whether the substance they are administered is the drug under study or a placebo. This method eliminates bias on the part of the subject in reporting the substance's effects. (p. 50)

Controlled substances Any drugs listed on one of the "schedules" of the Controlled Substance Act (also called *scheduled drugs*). (p. 48)

Double-blind, investigated drug study A research design in which both the investigator(s) and the subjects are purposely unaware of whether the substance administered to a given subject is the drug under study or a placebo. This method eliminates bias on the part of both the investigator and the subject. (p. 50)

Drug polymorphism Variation in response to a drug because of a patient's age, gender, size, and/or body composition. (p. 53)

Expedited drug approval A speeding of the usual investigational new drug approval process by the U.S. Food and Drug Administration (FDA) and pharmaceutical companies in response to a public health threat (e.g., acquired immunodeficiency syndrome). Drugs showing promise in phase I and phase II clinical trials are given to qualified patients, and the drug approval process is shortened if the drug continues to show promise. (p. 51)

Informed consent Permission obtained from a patient consenting to the performance of a specific test or procedure. Informed consent is required before most invasive procedures can be performed and before a patient can be admitted into a research study. The document must be written in a language understood by the patient and must be dated and signed by the patient and at least one witness. Included in the document are clear, rational descriptions of the procedure or test. Should the patient decide *not* to participate in the research at any time, the patient should be informed that this decision will not have a negative effect on his or her nursing or health care. Informed consent is voluntary. By law, informed consent must be obtained more than a given number of days or hours before certain procedures are performed and must always be obtained when the patient is fully mentally competent. (p. 49)

Investigational new drug (IND) A drug not approved for marketing by the FDA but available for use in experiments to determine its safety and efficacy; also, the actual name of the category of application that the drug manufacturer submits to the FDA to obtain permission for human *(clinical)* studies following successful completion of animal *(preclinical)* studies. (p. 49)

Legend drugs   Another name for prescription drugs. (p. 48)

Narcotic   A drug that produces insensibility or stupor; the term is applied especially to the opioids (e.g., morphine). (p. 48)

New drug application (NDA)   The type of application that a drug manufacturer submits to the FDA following successful completion of required human research studies. (p. 50)

Orphan drugs   A special category of drugs that have been identified to help patients with rare diseases. (p. 48)

Over-the-counter (OTC) drugs   Drugs that are available to consumers without a prescription. Also called *nonprescription drugs*. (p. 54)

Placebo   An inactive (inert) substance (e.g., saline, distilled water, starch, sugar). In some drug studies (termed *placebo controlled*) a placebo is given to some subjects so that the effects of this inactive substance can be compared with the effects of the experimental drug. Placebos may also be prescribed to satisfy the requests of patients who cannot be given the medication they desire or who, in the judgment of the health care provider, do not need that medication. (p. 50)

U.S. DRUG LEGISLATION

Until the beginning of the twentieth century there were no federal rules and regulations in the United States to protect consumers from the dangers of medications. The various legislative interventions that have occurred were often prompted by large-scale serious adverse drug reactions. One example is the sulfanilamide tragedy of 1937. Over 100 deaths occurred in the United States when people ingested a diethylene glycol solution of sulfanilamide that had been marketed as a therapeutic drug. Diethylene glycol is a component of automobile antifreeze solution, and the drug containing it was never tested for its toxicity. Another prominent example is the thalidomide tragedy that occurred in Europe between the 1940s and 1960s. Many pregnant women who took this sedative-hypnotic drug gave birth to seriously deformed infants. Originally, the first piece of legislation related to safety of medicinal rugs to be passed by the federal government was the Food and Drugs Act of 1906. Since 1906, several other acts have been passed to further ensure the safe and effective use of drugs. This federal legislation protects the public from drugs that are impure, toxic, or ineffective or that have not been tested before public sale. The primary purpose of this federal legislation is to ensure the safety and efficacy of new drugs. Table 4-1 provides a timeline summary of major U.S. drug legislation.

Table 4-1   Summary of Major U.S. Drug Legislation

Name of Legislation (Year)	Provisions/Comments
Federal Food and Drugs Act (FFDA, 1906)	Required drug manufacturers to list on the drug product label the presence of dangerous and possibly addicting substances; recognized the *U.S. Pharmacopeia* and *National Formulary* as printed references standards for drugs
Sherley Amendment (1912) to FFDA	Prohibited fraudulent claims for drug products
Harrison Narcotic Act (1914)	Established the legal term **narcotic** and regulated the manufacture and sale of habit-forming drugs
Federal Food, Drug, and Cosmetic Act (FFDCA, 1938; amendment to FFDA)	Required drug manufacturers to provide data proving drug safety, with FDA review; established the investigational new drug application process (prompted by sulfanilamide elixir tragedy)
Durham-Humphrey Amendment (1951) to FFDCA	Established **legend drugs** or prescription drugs; drug labels must carry the legend, "Caution—Federal law prohibits dispensing without a prescription"
Kefauver-Harris Amendments (1962) to FFDCA	Required manufacturers to demonstrate both therapeutic efficacy *and* safety of new drugs (prompted by thalidomide tragedy)
Controlled Substance Act (1970)	Established "schedules" for **controlled substances** (Tables 4-2 and 4-3); promoted drug addiction education, research, and treatment
Orphan Drug Act (1983)	Enabled FDA to promote research and marketing of **orphan drugs** used to treat rare diseases
Accelerated Drug Review Regulations (1991)	Enabled faster approval by the FDA of drugs to treat life-threatening illnesses (prompted by HIV/AIDS epidemic)

AIDS, Acquired immunodeficiency syndrome; *FDA,* Food and Drug Administration; *HIV,* human immunodeficiency virus.

Table 4-2   Controlled Substances: Schedule Categories

Schedule	Abuse Potential	Medical Use	Dependency
C-I	High	None	Severe physical and psychologic
C-II	High	Accepted	Severe physical and psychologic
C-III	Less than C-II	Accepted	Moderate to low physical or high psychologic
C-IV	Less than C-III	Accepted	Limited physical or psychologic
C-V	Less than C-IV	Accepted	Limited physical or psychologic

Table 4-3 Controlled Substances: Categories, Dispensing Restrictions, and Examples

Schedule	Dispensing Restrictions	Examples
C-I	Only with approved protocol	Heroin, lysergic acid diethylamide (LSD), marijuana, mescaline, peyote, psilocybin, and methaqualone
C-II	• Written prescription only (if telephoned in, written prescription required within 72 hr) • No prescription refills • Container must have warning label	Codeine, cocaine, hydromorphone, meperidine, morphine, methadone, secobarbital, pentobarbital, oxycodone, amphetamine, methylphenidate, and others
C-III	• Written or oral prescription that expires in 6 mo • No more than five refills in 6-mo period • Container must have warning label	Codeine with selected other medications (e.g. acetaminophen), hydrocodone, pentobarbital rectal suppositories, and dihydrocodeine combination products
C-IV	• Written or oral prescription that expires in 6 mo • No more than five refills in 6-mo period • Container must have warning label	Phenobarbital, chloral hydrate, meprobamate, the benzodiazepines (e.g., diazepam, temazepam, lorazepam), dextropropoxyphene, pentazocine, and others
C-V	Written prescription or over the counter (varies with state law)	Medications generally for relief of coughs or diarrhea containing limited quantities of certain opioid controlled substances

NEW DRUG DEVELOPMENT

The research into and development of new drugs is an ongoing process. The pharmaceutical industry is a multibillion-dollar industry, and pharmaceutical companies must continuously develop new and better drugs to maintain a competitive edge. The research required for the development of these new drugs may take several years. Hundreds of substances are isolated that never make it to market. Once a potentially beneficial drug has been identified, the pharmaceutical company must follow a very regulated, systematic process before the drug can be sold in the open market. This highly sophisticated process is regulated and carefully monitored by the Food and Drug Administration (FDA). The primary purpose of the FDA is to protect the patient and ensure drug effectiveness.

This system of drug research and development is one of the most stringent in the world, and there are many benefits and drawbacks to it. It was developed out of concern for patient safety and drug efficacy. To ensure that these two very important objectives are met with some degree of certainty requires much time and paperwork. This is the downside of the system. Many drugs are marketed and used in foreign countries long before they receive approval for use in the United States. However, drug-related calamities are more likely to be avoided by this more stringent drug approval system. The thalidomide tragedy mentioned earlier, which resulted from the use of a drug that was marketed in Europe but not in the United States, is an illustrative example. A balance must be achieved between making new life-saving therapies available and protecting consumers from potential drug-induced adverse effects. Historically, the FDA has had markedly less regulatory authority over vitamin, herbal, and homeopathic preparations because they are designated as dietary supplements rather than drugs. In 1994, however, Congress passed the Dietary Supplement Health and Education Act, which requires manufacturers of such products at least to ensure their safety (though not necessarily their efficacy) and prohibits them from making any unsubstantiated claims in the product labeling. For example, a product label may read "For depression" but cannot read "Known to cure depression." Reliable, objective information about these kinds of products is limited but is growing as more formal research studies are conducted. In 1998, Congress

established the National Center for Complementary and Alternative Medicine as a new branch of the National Institutes of Health. The function of this center is to conduct rigorous scientific studies of alternative medical treatments and to publish the data from such studies. Consumer demand for and interest in these alternative medicine products continues to drive this process. Patients should be advised to exercise caution in using such products and to communicate regularly with their health care providers regarding their use.

Investigational New Drug Application

A pharmaceutical company must prove both the safety and the efficacy of a newly isolated drug before it can be used in the general population. It has been noted that on average 10 to 12 years is needed for a drug to move from application for testing in humans to actual availability for prescribing. Testing begins in animal subjects. The new medication must be tested for its pharmacologic effects, dosage ranges, and possible toxic effects. After extensive animal testing that proves the safety and efficacy of the new drug, the pharmaceutical company can then submit an application to have it accepted as an **investigational new drug (IND).** Only after the FDA reviews and approves this application can the pharmaceutical company proceed with investigational studies of the drug in human subjects.

Informed Consent

Informed consent involves the careful explanation to the human test patient or *research subject* of the purpose of the study in which he or she is being asked to participate, the procedures to be used, the possible benefits, and the risks involved. The principles of medical ethics dictate that participants in experimental drug studies be informed volunteers and not be uninformed or coerced to participate in a given study in any way. Therefore, informed consent must be obtained from all patients (or their legal guardians) before they can be enrolled in an IND study. Some patients may have unrealistic expectations of the IND's usefulness. Often they have the misconception that because an investigational drug is new it must automatically be better than existing forms of therapy. Other volunteers may be reluctant to enter the study because they think they will be treated as "guinea pigs."

Whatever the circumstances of the study, the research subjects must be informed of all potential hazards as well as the possible benefits of the new therapy. It should be stressed that involvement in IND studies is truly voluntary and that the individual can quit the study at any time.

U.S. Food and Drug Administration Drug Approval Process

The FDA is responsible for approving drugs for clinical safety and efficacy before they are brought to the market. The approval process begins with *preclinical* testing phases, which include *in vitro* studies (using tissue samples and cell cultures) and animal studies. *Clinical* (human) studies follow the preclinical phase. There are four clinical phases. The drug is put on the market after phase III is completed if a **new drug application (NDA)** submitted by the manufacturer is approved by the FDA. Phase IV consists of postmarketing studies. The collective goal of these phases is to provide information on the safety, toxicity, efficacy, potency, bioavailability, and purity of the IND.

For many years the FDA remained probably one of the most trusted of U.S. government agencies. However, the agency has come under increasing scrutiny from consumers, health providers, and even some of its own staff members. Criticisms include ineffective leadership and compromise of patient safety to appease pharmaceutical manufacturers. One of the most recent examples concerns the recall of the prescription arthritic pain medication rofecoxib (Vioxx), which has been associated with cardiovascular complications, including stroke. Some critics have accused the FDA leadership of ignoring adverse drug reaction data obtained before this drug was marketed and allowing the manufacturer to sell the medication despite such data.

Preclinical Investigational Drug Studies

Current medical ethics still require that all new drugs undergo laboratory testing using both *in vitro* (cell or tissue) and animal studies before any testing in human subjects can be done. *In vitro* studies include testing of the response of various types of mammalian (including human) cells and tissues to different concentrations of the investigational drug. Various types of cells and tissues used for this purpose are collected from living or dead animal or human subjects (e.g., surgical or autopsy specimens). These cell samples may then be grown synthetically in the laboratory for several generations of continuous research. These *in vitro* studies help researchers to determine early on if a substance might be too toxic for human patients. Many prospective new drugs are ruled out for human use during this preclinical phase of drug testing. However, a small percentage of the many drugs tested in this manner are referred on for further clinical testing in human subjects.

Four Clinical Phases of Investigational Drug Studies

Phase I

Phase I studies usually involve small numbers of healthy subjects rather than those who have the disease or ailment that the new drug is intended to treat. An exception might be a study involving a very toxic drug used to treat a life-threatening illness. In this case the only study subjects might be those who already have the illness and for whom other viable treatment options may not be available. The purpose of phase I studies is to determine the optimal dosage range and the pharmacokinetics of the drug (i.e., absorption, distribution, metabolism, and excretion) and to ascertain if further testing is needed. Blood tests, urinalyses, assessments of vital signs, and specific monitoring tests are also performed.

Phase II

Phase II studies involve small numbers of volunteers who have the disease or ailment that the drug is designed to diagnose or treat. Study participants are closely monitored for the drug's effectiveness and any side effects. This is also the phase during which therapeutic dosage ranges are refined. If no serious side effects occur, the study can progress to phase III.

Phase III

Phase III studies involve large numbers of patients who are followed by medical research centers and other types of health care facilities. The patients may be treated at the center itself or may be spread over a wider geographic area and be followed at a local inpatient or outpatient facility. The purpose of this larger sample size is to provide information about infrequent or rare adverse effects that may not yet have been observed during previous smaller studies. Information obtained during this clinical phase helps identify any risks associated with the new drug. To enhance objectivity, many studies are designed to incorporate a placebo. A **placebo** is an inert substance that is not a drug (e.g., normal saline). The rationale for administering a placebo to a portion of the research subjects is to separate out the real benefits of the investigational drug from the apparent benefits arising out of researcher or subject bias regarding expected or desired results of the drug therapy. A study incorporating a placebo is called a *placebo-controlled study.* If the study subject does not know whether the drug he or she is administered is a placebo or the IND, but the investigator does know, the study is referred to as a **blinded investigational drug study.** In most studies neither the research staff nor the subjects being tested know which subjects are being given the real drug and which are receiving the placebo. This further enhances the objectivity of the study results and is known as a **double-blind, investigated drug study** because both the researcher and the subject are "blinded" to the actual identity of the substance administered to a given subject. Both drug and placebo dosage forms given to patients often look identical except for a secret code that appears on the medication itself and/or its container. At the completion of the study, this code is revealed or broken to determine which study patients received the drug and which were given the placebo. The code can also be broken before study completion by the principle investigator in the event of a clinical emergency that requires a determination of what individual patients received. The three objectives of phase III studies are to establish the drug's clinical effectiveness, safety, and dosage range. After phase III is completed, the FDA receives a report from the manufacturer, at which time the drug company submits an NDA. The approval of an NDA paves the way for the pharmaceutical company to market the new drug exclusively until the patent for the drug molecule expires. This is normally 17 years after discovery of the molecule and includes the 10- to 12-year period generally required to complete drug research. Therefore, a new drug manufacturer typically has 5 to 7 years after drug marketing to recoup research costs, which are usually in the hundreds of millions of dollars for a single drug.

Phase IV

Phase IV studies are postmarketing studies voluntarily conducted by pharmaceutical companies to obtain further proof of the therapeutic effects of the new drug. Data from such studies are usually gathered for at least 2 years after the drug's release. Often these studies compare the safety and efficacy of the new drug with that of another drug in the same therapeutic category. An example would be a comparison of a new nonsteroidal antiinflammatory drug with ibuprofen in the treatment of osteoarthritis. Some medications make it through all phases of clinical trials without causing any problems among study patients. When they are used in the larger general population, however, severe adverse effects may appear for the first time. If a pattern of severe reactions to a newly marketed drug begins to emerge, the FDA may request that the manufacturer of the drug issue a voluntary recall. If the drug manufacturer refuses to recall the medication, and if the number and/or severity of reactions reaches a certain level, then the FDA may seek court action to condemn the product and allow it to be seized by legal authorities. Such an action, in effect, becomes an involuntary recall on behalf of the manufacturer. There are three designated classes of drug recall based on FDA response to postmarketing data for a given drug:

- **Class I:** The most serious type of recall—use of the drug product carries a reasonable probability of serious adverse health effects or death
- **Class II:** Less severe—use of the drug product may result in temporary or medically reversible health effects, but the probability of lasting major adverse health effects is low
- **Class III:** Least severe—use of the drug product is not likely to result in any significant health problems
  Notification by the FDA of a drug recall may take the form of press releases, website announcements (www.fda.gov), or letters to health professionals.

Expedited Drug Approval

The FDA has attempted to make lifesaving investigational drug therapies available to the population sooner by offering an **expedited drug approval** process. The public health threat posed by acquired immunodeficiency syndrome (AIDS) has motivated the FDA and pharmaceutical companies to shorten the IND approval process to allow physicians to give medications that have shown promise during early phase I and phase II clinical trials to qualified patients with AIDS. If the drug then continues to show favorable results, the overall process of drug approval is hastened as much as possible.

LEGAL ISSUES AND NURSING IMPLICATIONS

The standards, scope, and role of professional nursing practice are well defined by federal, state, and local legislation. In addition to these laws and standards, there are specific institutional policies and procedures with which nurses must be familiar to fulfill their legal obligations and responsibilities to their patients. Federal and state legislation, standards of care, and nurse practice acts provide the legal framework for safe nursing practice, including drug therapy and medication administration. In addition, as discussed in Chapter 1, the standard "Five Rights" of medication administration are another measure for ensuring safety and adherence to laws necessary for protecting the patient. Other rights were also discussed in Chapter 1 that should become a part of the practice of every licensed, registered nurse and every student studying the art and science of nursing. These rights should all be examined within the context of the nursing philosophy of a given institution and within an ethical framework, and they should be applied through critical thinking in the care of patients, and specifically in drug therapy and the nursing process.

LEGAL AND ETHICAL PRINCIPLES
Use of Placebos

Use of placebo therapy may be one of the legal-ethical dilemmas within the context of research studies and clinical trials and should never be taken lightly. All aspects of research studies (e.g., drug trials) are to be clearly identified within the informed consent documents. Informed consent should clearly identify the patient's rights, such as the right to (1) leave the study at any time without any pressure or coercion to stay, (2) leave the study without consequences to medical care, (3) have full and complete information about the study, and (4) be aware of all alternative options, with information on all options, including placebo therapy, made available in the study. It is important to know that placebo therapy is randomly assigned and that even the researchers have no say in the decision or assignment of patients. Use of randomization does not guarantee what a person will get when entering a drug trial; however, if patients inquire about the specifics of the drug(s) offered—including use of a placebo—the information must be shared truthfully but within the confines of the trial or research study.

LEGAL AND ETHICAL PRINCIPLES
Ethical Terms Related to Nursing Practice

Autonomy: Self-determination and the ability to act on one's own; related nursing actions include promoting a patient's decision making, supporting informed consent, and assisting in decisions or making a decision when a patient is posing harm to himself or herself.

Beneficence: The ethical principle of doing or actively promoting good; related nursing actions include determining how the patient is best served.

Confidentiality: The duty to respect privileged information about a patient; related nursing actions include not talking about a patient in public or outside the context of the health care setting.

Justice: The ethical principle of being fair or equal in one's actions; related nursing actions include ensuring fairness in distributing resources for the care of patients and determining when to treat.

Nonmaleficence: The duty to do no harm to a patient; related nursing actions include avoiding doing any deliberate harm while rendering nursing care.

Veracity: The duty to tell the truth; related nursing actions include telling the truth with regard to placebos, investigational new drugs, and informed consent.

Box 4-1   American Nurses Association Code of Ethics for Nurses

The American Nurses Association (ANA) *Code of Ethics for Nurses* was revised in 1985, and further revisions were made by the ANA House of Delegates in 2001. The *Code of Ethics* continues to serve as an integral part of the foundation of professional nursing and is applicable to contemporary nursing practice. The *Code* draws on a broad knowledge base of ethical principles and theories, humanist perspectives, and ethics of care.

Provisions of the *Code*

- The nurse, in all professional relationships, practices with compassion and respect for the inherent dignity, worth, and uniqueness of every individual, unrestricted by considerations of social or economic status, personal attributes, or the nature of health problems.
- The nurse's primary commitment is to the patient, whether an individual, family group, or community.
- The nurse promotes, advocates for, and strives to protect the health, safety, and rights of the patient.
- The nurse is responsible and accountable for individual nursing practice and determines the appropriate delegation of tasks consistent with the nurse's obligation to provide optimum patient care.
- The nurse owes the same duty to self as to others, including the responsibility to preserve integrity and safety, to maintain competence, and to continue personal and professional growth.
- The nurse participates in establishing, maintaining, and improving health care environments and conditions of employment conducive to the provision of quality health care and consistent with the values of the profession through individual and collective action.
- The nurse participates in the advancement of the profession through contributions to practice, education, administration, and knowledge development.
- The nurse collaborates with other health professionals and the public in promoting community, national, and international efforts to meet health needs.
- The profession of nursing, as represented by associations and their members, is responsible for articulating nursing values, for maintaining the integrity of the profession and its practice, and for shaping social policy.

Reprinted with permission from American Nurses Association: *Code of ethics for nurses with interpretive statements,* copyright 2001, Nursebooks.org, American Nurses Association, Washington, DC.

Ethical Practice

Ethical nursing practice is based on fundamental principles such as beneficence, autonomy, justice, veracity, and confidentiality. The American Nurses Association *Code of Ethics for Nurses* (Box 4-1) and the International Council of Nurses *ICN Code of Ethics for Nurses* (Box 4-2) should be familiar frameworks of practice for all nurses and serve as ethical guidelines for nursing care. These ethical principles and codes of ethics ensure that the nurse is acting on behalf of the patient and with the patient's best interests at heart. As a professional, the nurse has the responsibility to provide safe nursing care to patients regardless of the setting, person, group, community, or family involved. Although it is not within the nurse's realm of ethical and professional responsibility to impose his or her own values or standards on the patient, it *is* within the nurse's realm to provide information and to assist the patient in facing decisions regarding health care.

Box 4-2   Legal-Ethical Considerations in Nursing Practice: *The ICN Code of Ethics for Nurses*

The International Council of Nurses (ICN) first adopted the *ICN Code of Ethics for Nurses* in 1953; the *Code* has been revised several times since then, most recently in 2000. The 2000 revision is available in English, French, Spanish, and German. The Preamble identifies the four fundamental responsibilities of nurses—promoting health, preventing illness, restoring health, and alleviating suffering—and points out that the need for nursing is universal. The Preamble also notes that inherent in nursing is respect for human rights, including the right to life, the right to dignity, and the right to be treated with respect. Nursing care is provided without regard to age, color, creed, culture, disability, illness, gender, nationality, politics, race, or social status. Nurses render services to the individual, family, and community. The *Code* describes four principal elements that provide a framework for the standards of ethical conduct it defines: nurses and people, nurses and practice, nurses and the profession, and nurses and co-workers. The *ICN Code of Ethics for Nurses* should serve as a guide for action based on social values and needs and should be understood, internalized, and applied by nurses in all aspects of their work. Nurses can obtain assistance in translating these standards into conduct by discussing the *Code* with co-workers and collaborating with their national nurses' associations in the application of ethical standards in nursing practice, education, management, and research.

Copyright 2000 by the International Council of Nurses, 3 Place Jean-Marteau, CH-1201 Geneva, Switzerland. ISBN: 92-95005-16-3.

The nurse also has the right to refuse to participate in any treatment or aspect of a patient's care that violates the nurse's personal ethical principles. However, this should be done without deserting the patient, and in some facilities the nurse may be transferred to another patient care assignment only if the transfer is approved by the nurse manager or nurse supervisor. The nurse must always remember, however, that the *Code of Ethics* and professional responsibility and accountability require the nurse to provide nonjudgmental nursing care from the start of the patient's treatment until the time of the patient's discharge. If transferring to a different assignment is not an option because of institutional policy and because of the increase in the acuteness of patients' conditions and the high patient-to-nurse workload, the nurse must always act in the best interest of the patient while remaining an objective patient advocate. It is always the nurse's responsibility to provide the highest quality nursing care and to practice within the professional standards of care. The ANA *Code of Ethics for Nurses,* the *ICN Code of Ethics for Nurses,* nurse practice acts, federal and state codes, ethical principles, and the previously mentioned legal principles and legislation are readily accessible and provide nurses with a sound, rational framework for professional nursing practice.

CULTURAL CONSIDERATIONS

The United States is a tremendously culturally diverse nation. Because the health care system emphasizes cure, prescribed drugs are often a major part of a patient's therapeutic regimen. The U.S. health care system often advocates a "one size fits all" treatment approach; however, a more multicultural, holistic approach to alterations in health status would help in meeting the needs of such a diverse patient population. The demographics of the United States continue to change. It is estimated that at least until 2010 the diversity will only continue to increase. For example, in 2000, the U.S. Census Bureau reported that the national population was about 281,422,000, and of this total 12.5% were self-identified as Hispanic or Latino, 12.3% as black or African American, 3.6% as Asian, and about 1% as American Indian or Alaskan Native. The most recent data show that some population groups are growing at a more rapid rate than others. Between April of 2000 and July of 2003, the rates of growth for Hispanic and Asian Americans were 13% and 12.5%, respectively, compared with 3.3% for the population as a whole.

The new and expanding field of ethnopharmacology holds much promise for understanding the specific impact of ethnicity on drug effects and responses. It is hampered, however, by the lack of clarity in terms such as *race, ethnicity,* and *culture.* Although some researchers have used the term *Hispanic* to encompass groups as diverse as Puerto Ricans, Mexicans, and Peruvians, other researchers have used it to denote a specific racial group. This lack of clarity in terminology and lack of consistency in the use of terms in research raises questions about the validity of the data collected. One thing is certain, however: it is impossible to know a patient's genotype by looking at the patient or at his or her health care history and documentation.

The ever-changing national demographics demand that the nurse be culturally competent while administering holistic and individualized nursing care involving both nonpharmacologic and pharmacologic therapies. To ensure this competence, the nurse must be up to date in his or her basic knowledge of the nursing process and understanding of the art and science of professional nursing practice. Acknowledgment and acceptance of the influences of a patient's cultural beliefs, values, and customs is necessary to promote optimal health and wellness. Some related terms and examples of cultural influences are presented in the Cultural Implications boxes on page 53.

Influence of Ethnicity and Genetics

The important concept of polymorphism is critical to an understanding of how the same drug may result in very different responses in different individuals. For example, why does a Chinese patient require lower dosages of an antianxiety drug than a white patient? Why does an African American patient respond differently to antihypertensives than a white patient? **Drug polymorphism** refers to the effect of a patient's age, gender, size, body composition, and other characteristics on the pharmacokinetics of specific drugs. Factors contributing to drug polymorphism may be loosely categorized into environmental factors (e.g., diet and nutritional status), cultural factors, and genetic (inherited) factors.

With regard to cultural influences on drug therapy, consider that medication response depends greatly on the level of the patient's compliance with the therapy regimen. Yet compliance may vary depending on the patient's cultural beliefs, experiences with medications, personal expectations, family expectations, family influence, and level of education. Compliance is not the only issue, however. Health care providers must also be aware that some patients use alternative therapies, such as herbal and homeo-

---

CULTURAL IMPLICATIONS
Cultural Terms Related to Nursing Practice

Culture: An integrated system of beliefs, values, and customs that are associated with a particular group of people and are generally handed down from generation to generation.

Cultural competence: The ability to work with patients with proper consideration for the cultural context, which includes patients' belief systems and values regarding health, wellness, and illness. It also involves learning about different patients and their specific responses to treatment, including drug therapies.

Ethnicity: Ethnic affiliation based on shared culture or genetic heritage or both.

Ethnopharmacology: The study of the effect of ethnicity on drug responses, specifically drug absorption, metabolism, distribution, and excretion (i.e., pharmacokinetics; see Chapter 2) as well as the study of genetic variations to drugs (i.e., pharmacogenetics).

Race: Often defined as a class of individuals with a common lineage. In genetics, a race is considered to be a population having a somewhat different genetic composition or gene frequencies. Race is also used to refer to geographical origins of ancestry.

CULTURAL IMPLICATIONS
Common Practices of Selected Cultural Groups

Cultural Group	Common Practices
African	Practice folk medicine; employ "root workers" as healers
Asian	Believe in traditional medicine; use physicians and herbalists in their health care
Hispanic	View health as a result of good luck and living right, and illness as a result of doing a bad deed; use heat and cold as remedies
European	Hold traditional health beliefs; some still practice folk medicine
Native American	Believe in harmony with nature; view ill spirits as causing disease
Western	Show increased participation in health care; demand more explanation about diseases and treatment, as well as the prevention of diseases

---

pathic remedies, that can inhibit or accelerate drug metabolism and therefore alter a drug's response.

Environmental considerations that play an important part in drug responses and their variability include factors such as diet. For example, a diet high in fat has been documented to increase the absorption of the drug griseofulvin (an antifungal drug). Malnutrition with deficiencies in protein, vitamins, and minerals may modify the functioning of metabolic enzymes, which may alter the body's ability to absorb or eliminate a medication.

Genetic factors also influence how different racial or ethnic groups respond to drugs. Some patients of European and African descent are slow acetylators and metabolize drugs at a slower rate, which results in elevated drug concentrations. Some patients of Japanese and Inuit descent are more rapid acetylators and metabolize drugs more quickly, which leads to decreased drug concentrations. Chinese, Japanese, Malaysians, and Thais are poor metabolizers of debrisoquine; therefore, drugs such as codeine are likely to be *more* effective at lower dosages in these patients than in those of European descent. Several major drug classifications are relatively well researched with regard to differential responses in different cultural groups; two of these are outlined in Table 4-4.

Individuals throughout the world share many common views and beliefs regarding health practices and medication use. However, specific cultural influences, beliefs, and practices related to medication administration do exist. Awareness of cultural differences is critical for the care of patients in the United States today because U.S. demographics are constantly changing. As previously mentioned, the minority composition of the United States is expected to continue to change drastically between now and 2010. In addition, the white majority not only is shrinking but also is aging, whereas the Asian, Native American, and Hispanic populations not only are growing but also are young. As a result of these changes, nurses need to attend to and be concerned with each patient's cultural background to ensure safe and quality nursing care, including medication administration.

For example, some African Americans have health beliefs and practices that include an emphasis on proper diet and rest; the use of herbal teas, laxatives, and protective bracelets; and the use of folk medicine, prayer, and the "laying on of hands." Reliance on various home remedies can also be an important component of their health practices. Some Asian American patients, especially the Chinese, believe in the concepts of yin and yang. Yin and yang are opposing forces that lead to illness or health, depending on which force is dominant in the individual and whether the forces are balanced, which produces healthy states. Yin represents the female and the negative energies of darkness and cold; yang represents the male and the positive energies of light and warmth. Beliefs regarding yin and yang must be respected by all who participate in the care of Chinese patients. Other common health practices of Asian Americans include acupuncture, use of herbal remedies, and use of heat. All such beliefs and practices need to be considered—especially when the patient values their use more highly than the use of medications. Many of these be-

liefs are strongly grounded in religion. The Asian and Pacific Islander racial-ethnic group also includes Thais, Vietnamese, Filipinos, Koreans, and Japanese, among others.

Some Native Americans believe in preserving harmony with nature or keeping a balance between the body and mind and the environment to maintain health. Ill spirits are seen as the cause of disease. The traditional healer for this culture is the medicine man, and treatments vary from massage and application of heat to acts of purification. Some individuals of Hispanic descent view health as a result of good luck and living right and illness as a result of bad luck or committing a bad deed. To restore health, these individuals seek out a balance between the body and mind through use of cold remedies or foods for "hot" illnesses (of blood or yellow bile) and hot remedies for "cold" illnesses (of phlegm or black bile). Hispanics may use a variety of religious rituals for healing (e.g., lighting of candles), which may also be practiced by adherents of other religions and/or belief systems. It is very important to remember that these beliefs vary from patient to patient; therefore, the nurse should always consult with the patient rather than assuming that the patient holds certain beliefs.

Barriers to adequate health care for the culturally diverse U.S. patient population include language, poverty, access, pride, and beliefs regarding medical practices. Medications may have a different meaning to different cultures, as would any form of medical treatment. Therefore, before any medication is administered, a thorough cultural assessment should be completed, which should include questions regarding the following:

- Health beliefs and practices
- Past uses of medicine
- Use of folk remedies
- Use of home remedies
- Use of **over-the-counter drugs** and herbal products
- Usual responses to illness
- Responsiveness to medical treatment
- Religious practices and beliefs (e.g., many Christian Scientists believe in taking no medications at all)
- Dietary habits

The Cultural Implications box on page 53 provides further information on cultural considerations related to the nursing process and drug therapy. It provides a quick reference to important patient care issues related to drug therapy and culturally competent care. In addition, the legal and ethical guidelines and principles men-

Table 4-4	**Examples of Varying Drug Responses in Different Racial or Ethnic Groups**	
Racial or Ethnic Group	**Drug Classification**	**Response**
African Americans	Antihypertensive drugs	African-Americans respond better to diuretics than to β-blockers and angiotensin-converting enzyme inhibitors.
		African-Americans respond less effectively to β-blockers.
		African-Americans respond best to calcium channel blockers, especially diltiazem.
		African-Americans respond less effectively to single-drug therapy.
Asians and Hispanics	Antipsychotic and antianxiety drugs	Asians need lower dosages of certain drugs such as haloperidol.
		Japanese and Chinese are more prone to rapid buildup of mephenytoin and so are at risk for sedation and overdosage.
		Asians and Hispanics respond better to lower dosages of antidepressants.
		Chinese require lower dosages of antipsychotics.
		Japanese require lower dosages of antimanic drugs.

NOTE: The comparative group for all responses is whites.

tioned earlier must be taken into account in developing and implementing each patient's nursing care plan and drug therapy.

◆ NURSING PROCESS

✦ ASSESSMENT

A thorough cultural assessment is needed for the provision of culturally competent nursing care. A variety of assessment tools and resources are available for the professional nurse to incorporate into nursing care including Madeline Leininger's *Transcultural nursing: concepts, theories, research, and practice* (ed 3, New York, 2002, McGraw-Hill) and the following online resources: www.ac.wwu.edu/~culture, www.xculture.org, www.diversityrx.org, http://gucchd.georgetown.edu/ncc, www.transculturalcare.net, and www.tcns.org.

Areas to assess to identify different racial, ethnic, and cultural influences include the following. The questions provided are only examples of those that can be used to identify the patient's methods for maintaining, protecting, and restoring physical, mental, and spiritual health.

Maintaining Health
- *For physical health:* Where are special foods and clothing items purchased? What types of health education are of the patient's culture? Where does the patient usually obtain information about health and illness? Folklore? Where are health services obtained? Who are health care providers (e.g., physicians, nurse practitioners, community services, health departments, healers)?
- *For mental health:* What are examples of culturally specific activities for the mind and for maintaining mental health, as well as beliefs about reducing stress, rest, and relaxation?
- *For spiritual health:* What are resources for meeting spiritual needs?

Protecting Health
- *For physical health:* Where are special clothing and everyday essentials? What are examples of the patient's symbolic clothing, if any?
- *For mental health:* Who within the family and community teaches the roles in the patient's specific culture? Are there rules about avoiding certain persons or places? Are there special activities that must be performed?
- *For spiritual health:* Who teaches spiritual practices and where can special protective symbolic objects such as crystals or amulets be purchased? Are they expensive and how available are they for the patient when needed?

Restoring Health
- *For physical health:* Where are special remedies purchased? Can individuals produce or grow their own remedies, herbs, etc.? How often are traditional and nontraditional services obtained?
- *For mental health:* Who are the traditional and nontraditional resources for mental health? Are there culture-specific activities for coping with stress and illness?
- *For spiritual health:* How often and where are traditional and nontraditional spiritual leaders or healers accessed? (From Spector RE: *Cultural care: guides to heritage assessment and health traditions,* Upper Saddle River, NJ, ed 2, 2000, Pearson/Prentice Hall, pp 24-25.)

✦ NURSING DIAGNOSES
- Risk for injury related to interruption of daily activities and cultural patterns of health and wellness
- Risk for injury and falls related to decreased sensorium and confusion caused by unfamiliar hospital environment
- Insomnia related to a lack of adherence to cultural practices for encouraging stress release and sleep induction
- Risk for injury to self and/or adverse drug reactions related to drug therapy and impact of cultural, racial, and/or ethnic factors on pharmacokinetics (ethnopharmacology)
- Deficient knowledge related to lack of experience with and information about drug therapy

✦ PLANNING
Goals
- Patient states the need for assistance while in the hospital or while health status is altered.
- Patient requests assistance in implementing cultural practices.
- Patient states specific needs related to performance of activities of daily living (ADLs), relaxation, healing, sleep, or rest.
- Patient states the importance of racial, ethnic, and cultural influences on nonpharmacologic and pharmacologic treatment regimens.

Outcome Criteria
- Patient experiences minimal or no difficulty in obtaining assistance with special needs and ADLs.
- Patient identifies specific cultural practices such as use of herbal teas and other herbal preparations, yin and yang balancing, aromatherapy, crystal therapy, and healing bracelets that will help with healing during illness.
- Patient is able to implement cultural practices as an integral part of a holistic nursing care plan and treatment regimen.

✦ IMPLEMENTATION

There are numerous interventions for implementation of culturally competent nursing care, but one very important requirement is that the nurse remain current in the knowledge of various cultures and related ADL practices, health beliefs, and emotional and spiritual health practices and beliefs. With regard to drug therapy, the nurse's knowledge about drugs that may elicit varied responses in specific racial and ethnic groups must remain current, and critical thinking must be used in applying the concepts of culturally competent care and ethnopharmacology to each patient care situation. Important principles include the following: One group of enzymes, cytochrome P-450 or CYP enzymes, are responsible for certain phases of the metabolism of many drugs, including antipsychotics and antidepressants. Genetic differences in certain CYP enzymes affect the rate of drug metabolism and thus influence drug levels and dosages. People with more than two functioning copies of CYP2D6 genes have faster than normal enzyme activity and are very quick metabolizers, which results in lower serum drug concentrations; those with two nonfunctional copies of CYP2D6 genes have slower enzyme activity and are slow metabolizers, which results in higher serum concentrations of certain drugs. Some examples are as follows: Hispanic patients may be treated effectively using lower dosages of antipsychotics than usual. African American patients taking lithium need closer monitoring for toxicity, and Japanese and Taiwanese patients may also require lower dosages of lithium. In treatment for hypertension, African Americans have been found to respond less favorably to some angiotensin-converting enzyme inhibitors, such as captopril, than do whites. Thiazide diuretics have been found to be more effective in African Americans than in whites. Additional factors to consider during implementation are lifestyle and health belief systems. For example, with regard to compliance with the treatment regimen, Hispanics with hypertension have been found in some studies to be less likely than African Americans or whites to continue to take medication as prescribed, a finding that may reflect the patients' health belief systems. Other lifestyle decisions (e.g., use of tobacco or alco-hol) may also affect responses to drugs and must be considered during drug administration.

◆ **EVALUATION**

The impact of cultural, legal, and ethical factors on the therapeutic effects of drug therapy should be evaluated for the duration of therapy. Evaluation should also include monitoring of goals and outcome criteria as well as therapeutic versus side effects and toxic effects.

Points to Remember

- Various pieces of federal legislation, as well as state law, state practice acts, and institutional policies, have been established to help ensure the safety and efficacy of drug therapy and the nursing process.
- The Controlled Substance Act of 1970 provides nurses and other health care providers with information on drugs that cause little to no dependence versus those with a high level of abuse and dependency.
- Informed consent should always be obtained as needed, and nurses must thoroughly understand their role and responsibilities as patient advocates in obtaining such consent.

- The nurse's role in the IND process should be one of adhering to the research protocol while also acting as a patient advocate and honoring the patient's right to safe, quality nursing care.
- Adherence to legal guidelines, ethical principles, and the ANA *Code of Ethics for Nurses* ensures that the nurse's actions are based on a solid foundation.
- There are a variety of culturally based assessment tools available for use in patient care and drug therapy.
- In relation to racial and ethnic variables, drug therapy and subsequent patient responses may be affected by specific enzymes and metabolic pathways of drugs.

NCLEX Examination Review Questions

1. During a home visit, an elderly patient tells the home health nurse that she has been taking six or more aspirin per day for her "bad bones." The nurse continues with a thorough assessment and makes the decision to double the prescribed dose to help minimize this patient's "bad bones." Which of the following statements correctly describes this scenario?
   a. The nurse is planning to give medications within the guidelines of professional autonomy, such as deciding on a dosage not ordered.
   b. The nurse should make his or her own decision to change the specific dosage of the drug.
   c. The nurse is following one of the Five Rights of drug administration; specifically, the right to fairly safe standards of care.
   d. The "right" of the right dosage of drug is being violated in this situation.

2. Cultural influences on health care for a 59-year-old female Chinese patient would most likely include which of the following?
   a. Radiographs are seen as a break in the soul's integrity.
   b. Hospital diets are interpreted as being healing and healthful.
   c. The use of heat may be an important practice for this patient.
   d. Being hospitalized is a source of peace and socialization for this culture.

3. A patient is being counseled for possible participation in a clinical trial for a new medication. After meeting with the physician, the nurse is asked to obtain the patient's signature on the consent forms. This "informed consent" indicates which of the following?
   a. Once therapy has begun, the patient cannot withdraw from the clinical trial.

   b. The patient has been informed of all potential hazards and benefits of the therapy.
   c. The patient has received only the information that will help to make the clinical trial a success.
   d. No matter what happens, the patient will not be able to sue the researchers for damages.

4. A new drug has been approved for use and the drug manufacturer has made it available for sale. During the first 6 months, the FDA receives reports of severe side effects that were not discovered during the testing and considers whether to withdraw the drug. This illustrates which phase of investigational drug studies?
   a. Phase I
   b. Phase II
   c. Phase III
   d. Phase IV

5. A patient of Japanese descent describes a family trait that manifests frequently: she says that members of her family often have "strong reactions" after taking certain medications, but her white friends have no problems with the same dosages of the same medications. Because of this trait, which of the following statement applies?
   a. She may need lower dosages of the medications prescribed.
   b. She may need higher dosages of the medications prescribed.
   c. She should not receive these medications because of potential problems with metabolism.
   d. These situations vary greatly, and her accounts may not indicate a valid cause for concern.

1. d, 2. c, 3. b, 4. d, 5. a.

Critical Thinking Activities

1. Discuss the impact of cultural practices as they relate to safe and effective drug therapy.
2. Choose at least two of the terms in the Legal and Ethical Principles box on page 51 and apply the concepts to an example of drug administration and nursing.

3. Interview someone who is not in your racial or ethnic group about cultural practices and drug therapy, using the suggestions given on page 54. Compare them with your family's practices.

For answers, see http://evolve.elsevier.com/Lilley.

Medication Errors: Preventing and Responding

Objectives

When you reach the end of this chapter, you should be able to do the following:

1. Compare the following terms related to drug therapy in the context of professional nursing practice: *adverse drug event, adverse drug reaction, medication error,* and the new term *medication reconciliation.*
2. Discuss the importance of the 100,000 Lives Campaign as related to drug therapy.
3. Describe the medication errors that are most common among professional nurses and other health care professionals.
4. Develop a framework for professional nursing practice that includes specific measures to prevent medication errors in patients of all ages.
5. Identify the possible consequences of a medication error on a patient's physiologic and psychologic well-being.
6. Discuss the impact of medication errors in patients of different ages and cultural backgrounds.
7. Analyze the various ethical dilemmas associated with medication errors as related to the nursing process.
8. Distinguish the various needs of patients in different age groups for political action related to drug therapy and the prevention of medication errors.

e-Learning Activities

Companion CD

- NCLEX Review Questions: see questions 27-29
- Animations
- Audio Glossary
- Category Catchers
- Medication Errors Checklists
- IV Therapy Checklists

evolve Website (http://evolve.elsevier.com/Lilley)

• Nursing Care Plans • Frequently Asked Questions • Content Updates • WebLinks • Supplemental Resources • Elsevier ePharmacology Update • Medication Administration Animations

Glossary

100,000 Lives Campaign A 2005-2006 campaign of the Institute for Healthcare Improvement to radically reduce morbidity and mortality in American health care, including preventing as many as 100,000 avoidable patient deaths, through specific improvements in the operations of health care facilities. (p. 61)

Adverse drug event (ADE) Any undesirable occurrence related to administration of or failure to administer a prescribed medication. (p. 59)

Adverse drug reactions (ADRs) Unexpected, unintended, undesired, or excessive responses to medications given at therapeutic dosages (as opposed to overdose); one type of ADE. (p. 59)

Adverse effects Any undesirable bodily effects that are a direct response to one or more drugs. These effects may include *side effects,* which are generally considered to be rela-

tively minor adverse effects that are expected to occur in a percentage of the population receiving a given drug. However, the severity of such effects exists on a continuum. More severe adverse effects may result in changes in prescribed drug therapy after weighing the risk-to-benefit ratio of a drug in a specific clinical situation. (p. 59)

Allergic reaction Immunologic hypersensitivity reaction resulting from an unusual sensitivity of a patient to a particular medication; a type of ADE and a subtype of ADR. (p. 59)

Idiosyncratic reaction Abnormal and unexpected response to a medication, other than an allergic reaction, that is peculiar to an individual patient. (p. 59)

Medical error Broad term commonly used to refer to any error in any phase of clinical patient care that causes or has the potential to cause patient harm; the error may involve incorrect actions related to medication, medical or surgical procedures, patient monitoring, and so on (error of commission), or it may involve failure to implement an intervention when it would normally be indicated (error of omission). (p. 59)

Medication errors (MEs) Any *preventable* ADEs involving inappropriate medication use by a patient or health care professional; they may or may not cause the patient harm. (p. 59)

Medication reconciliation A procedure implemented by health care providers to continually maintain an accurate and up-to-date list of medications for all patients at every phase of health care that is communicated in a timely manner to all applicable members of the health care team, with the overall goal of dramatically reducing the rate of medication errors; a key strategy of the *100,000 Lives Campaign.* (p. 62)

INTRODUCTION

General Impact of Errors on Patients

According to a 1999 report of the Institute of Medicine, the number of patient deaths in the United States attributable to errors in hospital care ranged from 44,000 to 98,000 annually based on data from two large-scale studies. Although **medical error** is often used as an umbrella term in the published literature, errors can occur during all phases of health care delivery and involve errant actions by all categories of health professionals. Some of the more common types of error include misdiagnosis, patient misidentification, wrong-site surgery, and medication errors. Intangible losses resulting from such adverse outcomes include patient dissatisfaction with and loss of trust in the health care system. This chapter focuses on the issues related to medication errors and ways to prevent and respond to these errors. Included is an overview of various institutional, educational, and sociologic factors that may contribute to such errors.

Medication Errors

As mentioned in Chapter 2, **adverse drug event (ADE)** is a general term that includes *all* types of clinical problems encountered regarding medications. These include **medication errors (MEs)** and **adverse drug reactions (ADRs).** The various subsets of ADEs and their interrelationships are illustrated in Figure 5-1. Two major types of ADR are **allergic reaction** (often predictable) and **idiosyncratic reaction** (usually unpredictable). **Adverse effects** are ADRs that are usually predictable and generally are not viewed as severe ADRs (i.e., serious enough to warrant discontinuation of the given drug).

It is important to consider the medication administration and system analysis processes when discussing MEs. Identifying, responding to, and ultimately preventing MEs requires more than implementing the "Five Rights" of drug administration or considering the actions of the nurse. Attention must be focused on all persons involved in the medication administration process, including the prescriber, the transcriber of the order to the chart, nurses, pharmacy staff, and any other ancillary staff involved in this process. A system analysis takes the Five Rights one step further and examines the entire health care system, the health care professionals involved, and any other factor that has an impact on the error.

MEs are a particularly important segment of ADEs because, by definition, any error is potentially preventable. MEs are a common cause of adverse health care outcomes and can range in severity from having no significant effect on the patient to directly causing patient disability or death. A study of 447 cases of fatal ADEs recorded the classes of medications associated with the highest likelihood of fatal outcomes. The majority of these errors (68%) were classified as preventable; 40% occurred in healthy patients. A second study of 227 cases of drug-induced permanent disability found chemotherapeutic drugs, central nervous system drugs, antibiotics, and vaccines to be the top causative drugs. Some of the more common categories of such "high-alert" medications are listed in Box 5-1. Many of these errors result from the fact that there are an increasing number of drugs on the market and, therefore, an increasing number of drug names to keep track of, some of which have similarities in spelling and/or pronunciation (i.e., look-alike or sound-alike names).

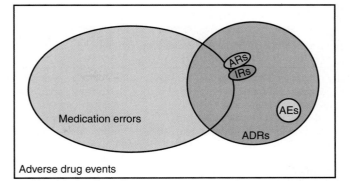

FIGURE 5-1   Diagram illustrating the various classes and subclasses of adverse drug events. *ADRs,* Adverse drug reactions; *ARs,* allergic reactions; *IRs,* idiosyncratic reactions; *SEs,* side effects.

Box 5-1	Common Classes of Medications Involved in Serious Errors

- Antibiotics
- Anticoagulants
- Antidiabetic drugs (particularly insulin)
- Antineoplastic (anticancer) drugs
- Cardiovascular drugs
- Central nervous system–active drugs (e.g., opiates, anesthetics)
- Vaccines

Most dangerous is when two drugs from very different therapeutic classes have similar names. This can result in effects on the patient that are grossly different from those intended as part of the drug therapy. The Preventing Medication Errors box on page 60 lists examples of commonly confused drug names.

It is widely recognized that the majority of medication errors result from weaknesses in the systems within health care organizations rather than from individual shortcomings. Such weaknesses include failure to create a "just culture" or nonpunitive work atmosphere for reporting errors, excessive workload with minimal time for staff preventive education, and lack of interdisciplinary communication and collaboration.

PSYCHOSOCIAL ISSUES THAT CONTRIBUTE TO ERRORS

Organizational Issues

One study noted that half of all preventable ADRs begin at the medication ordering (prescribing) stage. A 2003 study published in the *Archives of Internal Medicine* also stated that prescribers are involved in "most" errors. This particular study focused on cardiovascular medications, the most commonly used general category of prescription drugs. It concluded that the presence of a pharmacist during medical rounds reduced the incidence of errors. This finding illustrates an important issue in modern health care practice: namely, both nurses and pharmacists have a vested interest in rational drug therapy, yet neither normally acts independently in health care delivery. This points up the value of developing collaborative relationships between these two groups of

PREVENTING MEDICATION ERRORS

Selected Examples of Commonly Confused Drug Names

Names of Medications	Comments
Accupril vs. Monopril	Two different antihypertensive drugs (though both are ACE inhibitors)
Avandia vs. Amaryl	Two different antidiabetic drugs
Cardura vs. Coumadin	Antihypertensive vs. anticoagulant (very different pharmacologic effects)
Celebrex vs. Celexa vs. Cerebyx	Antiinflammatory drug vs. antidepressant vs. anticonvulsant drug
chlorpromazine vs. prochlorperazine	Antipsychotic drug vs. antiemetic drug
Claritin-D 24-Hour vs. Claritin-D	24-hr vs. 12-hr duration of action
Cytovene vs. Cytosar	Antiviral drug vs. antineoplastic (anticancer) drug
daunorubicin vs. doxorubicin	Two different antineoplastic drugs with possibly different indications for use
Depo-Estradiol vs. Depo-Testadiol	Female vs. male hormonal injection
Elavil vs. Plavix	Antidepressant vs. antiplatelet drug
Epivir vs. Combivir	Single-drug anti-HIV drug vs. double-drug combination anti-HIV drug
fentanyl vs. sufentanil	Both are injectable anesthetics but with a significant difference in potency and duration of action
glipizide vs. glyburide	Two different antidiabetic drugs
Glucotrol vs. Glucotrol XL	Immediate-release vs. sustained-release antidiabetic drug (different duration of action and thus different effect on blood sugar levels)
Lacri-Lube vs. Surgilube	Ophthalmic lubricant vs. skin or orifice lubricant
Micronase vs. Micro-K	Antidiabetic drugs vs. potassium supplement
Narcan vs. Norcuron	Opiate antidote vs. skeletal muscle paralyzing drug for OR use
Ocuflox vs. Ocufen	Ophthalmic antibiotic vs. ophthalmic antiinflammatory drug
paclitaxel vs. Paxil	Antineoplastic drug vs. antidepressant
Paxil vs. Plavix	Antidepressant vs. antiplatelet drug
Quinine vs. quinidine	Antimalarial drug vs. cardiac antidysrhythmic drug
Soma Compound vs. Soma	Combination muscle relaxant with aspirin vs. muscle relaxant alone
Tamiflu vs. Theraflu	Prescription antiviral drug vs. nonprescription (OTC) cold remedy
Tegretol vs. Toradol	Anticonvulsant vs. antiinflammatory drug
TobraDex vs. Tobrex	Combination ophthalmic antibiotic and antiinflammatory drug vs. ophthalmic antibiotic alone
Vancenase vs. Vanceril	Nasal steroid inhaler vs. oral steroid inhaler
Viagra vs. Allegra	Male sexual stimulant vs. antihistamine allergy drug
Xanax vs. Zantac vs. Zyrtec	Antianxiety drug vs. anti–stomach acid drug vs. antihistamine allergy drug
Zocor vs. Cozaar vs. Zoloft	Anticholesterol drug vs. antihypertensive drug vs. antidepressant
Zofran vs. Zosyn	Antiemetic drug vs. antibiotic

ACE, Angiotensin-converting enzyme; *HIV,* human immunodeficiency virus; *OR,* operating room; *OTC,* over the counter.

professionals and between these groups and all other health care professionals in the health care system. Such relationships can be especially helpful when approaching prescribers regarding questionable orders or when advocating for workplace improvements that benefit both patients and staff.

Effective use of technologies such as computerized prescriber order entry and bar coding of medication packages has also been shown to reduce MEs. Computerized order entry eliminates handwriting and standardizes many prescribing functions, especially dosage specifications. Bar coding of medications has allowed the use of electronic devices by nurses for verification of correct medication at the patient's bedside. Computer programs are often used in the pharmacy to screen for potential drug interactions when prescriber orders are being entered into the patient's computer profile. As noted previously, however, the workload at many institutions may prevent adequate staff education regarding the use of such technology. Also, technology that is difficult to use may itself present a barrier to medication safety. This often happens when patient care staff have insufficient input into the design of patient care–related technology. Interestingly, self-medication by patients (e.g., patient-controlled analgesia) has been shown to reduce errors, provided patients have adequate cognitive ability and mental alertness.

Educational System Issues and Their Potential Impact on Medication Errors

Because of the rigorous cognitive and even physical challenges of health care study and practice, the health professions tend to attract strong-willed, intelligent people. However, the constant expectation that one be "smart" and "on top of things" with regard to clinical knowledge often leads to denial, fear, or shame about being wrong or simply not remembering a piece of information while on duty. Instead of making guesses about medications in clinical situations, nurses need to stop and check the medication orders and be sure to have a thorough knowledge of the given drug and its route, dosage, and indications *before* administering the drug. Authoritative sources for information about drugs include current drug reference guides (less than 5 years old) such as *Mosby's Drug Consult, Physicians' Desk Reference, Drug Formulary,* and others written by legitimate experts. Even the most capable health care provider cannot know everything or have immediate recall of every fact ever read. This is especially true given the increasing complexity of health care practice. Forward-thinking faculty members recognize that learning is a lifelong process. Adopting a philosophy of "no question is a stupid question" helps clinical instructors teach error prevention habits to their students as they begin their careers. In contrast, berating or otherwise penalizing a student for not immediately recalling a given fact, or for simply asking questions, instills fear and shame. It also discourages dialogue that would otherwise promote and enhance student learning and mastery of concepts. In general, it is also important to endorse routine competency evaluation of professional registered nurses and their knowledge of drugs and measures to reduce medication errors. The level of nurses' knowledge and understanding of drugs must be boosted to ensure safety and prevent harm to patients.

Medication Errors and Related Sociologic Factors

Health care practice has a long and ingrained tradition of disparate social and economic class structures among different categories of professionals. The most recognized differences are those among nurses, physicians, and administrators. At their worst, these differences have fostered maltreatment of nurses, especially by physicians, whose behavior often has not been challenged or corrected by administrators. A 2002 study published in the *American Journal of Nursing* identified disruptive physician behavior and lack of institutional response to it as significant factors affecting nurse job satisfaction and nursing staff retention. Such behavior was defined in this study as "any inappropriate behavior ranging from rudeness, intimidating manner, shouting, to physical or sexual harassment." This type of behavior, when not met with corrective action by the institution, is felt to contribute strongly to nursing shortages in health care facilities. Thirty percent of surveyed nurses stated that they know of one or more colleagues who had resigned their positions because of this problem. With regard to possible impact on MEs, this study pointed out that the quality of nurse-physician communication was one of the strongest predictors of patient outcomes. This issue has since been recognized by both the American Medical Association and the Joint Commission on Accreditation of Healthcare Organizations (JCAHO) as having harmful effects on the quality of patient care and staff morale. In fact, JCAHO accreditation guidelines now include a requirement for institutional policies to deal with disruptive physician behavior.

Fortunately, communication between prescribers and other members of the health care team has improved somewhat over the years with newer generations of physicians. This is due in large part to more progressive approaches in medical education that emphasize a team orientation, which is recognized as more realistic given the ever-increasing complexities of health care delivery and the undeniable fact that no one team member can master every fact and skill.

PREVENTING AND RESPONDING TO ERRORS

Reporting and Responding to Medication Errors

Reporting MEs is a professional responsibility that is shared by nurses and all members of the health care team. Steps for the nurse to take to prevent and respond to MEs include the following:

- Checking the patient by assessing all relevant parameters (e.g., vital signs, latest laboratory values) and documenting accordingly
- Assessing the patient for effects of the drug and consulting reference materials or colleagues as needed

- Performing medication reconciliation to verify all of the patient's correct medications at each point of care (e.g., transfer from intensive care unit to general nursing unit) and preparing a complete list of medications for the next provider upon patient discharge
- Taking a "time-out" when appropriate for all staff to collectively verify medications, especially during high-risk procedures
- Regularly asking the patient to verify his or her identity and date of birth
- Completing ME reporting forms after contacting the physician, charge nurse, or nurse supervisor or, for a student nurse, contacting the patient's nurse and the instructor
- Monitoring the progress of the patient's condition closely
- Thinking and acting critically and modifying nursing practice to prevent further errors
- Conducting detailed root cause analyses to learn from errors and avoid error repetition
- Analyzing methods to reduce the complexity of drug administration and develop consistent, easy-to-read procedures related to medication administration
- Suggesting needed changes in policy and procedures related to safe medication administration and the provision of simple medication error–related policies
- Participating in the development of user-friendly technology such as computerized prescriber order entry systems and systems for bar coding of medications to allow nurses to verify medications at bedside before administering them
- Joining political efforts to advocate for safer nurse-patient staffing ratios and for improved quality assurance protocols in the handling of MEs

Error reporting systems that offer the option of anonymity can also help to foster improved practice safety. Internal, facility-based systems of error tracking may generate data to help customize policy and procedure development. All institutional pharmacy departments are required to have an ADE monitoring program. Nurses should be aware of and comfortable in reporting suspected ADEs to this department for evaluation and follow-up. In addition, there are nationwide confidential reporting programs that collect and disseminate safety information on a larger scale. One such program is the U.S. Pharmacopeia Medication Errors Reporting Program (USPMERP). The U.S. Pharmacopeia (USP) has created a nationwide database of MEs and their causes, as well as potential errors. Any health care professional can report an ME by contacting the USPMERP at 800-23-ERROR. Many important institutional changes have been made based on the data collected by this program.

MedWatch is another useful error and adverse event reporting program provided by the U.S. Food and Drug Administration (FDA). Any member of the public can report problems with medications or medical devices via telephone or mail, or online at the FDA website. The Institute for Safe Medication Practices and JCAHO also provide useful information and reporting services to health care providers aimed at safety enhancement. See the Evolve website for addresses of these and other helpful organizations.

Medication Reconciliation

In 2005, the Institute for Healthcare Improvement (IHI) (www. ihi.org) launched its **100,000 Lives Campaign.** This campaign is an educational initiative that promotes specific strategies by which health care facilities can dramatically improve their patient safety records. The overall goal of this initiative is to prevent the approximately 100,000 avoidable deaths that have been reported to occur annually in U.S. health care facilities. One of the strategies focuses on preventing medication errors through medication reconciliation. Since 2006, implementation of this procedure has been required by both Medicare and the JCAHO (http://www.jcaho.org) for all health care facilities that receive Medicare reimbursement and/or JCAHO accreditation. Driving implementation of this procedure is the fact that poorly communicated medical information is the cause of up to 50% of hospital medication errors. In addition to being a key strategy of the IHI's 100,000 Lives Campaign, medication reconciliation is also one of JCAHO's 2006 national patient safety goals. **Medication reconciliation** is a procedure that seeks to prevent medication errors through the ongoing assessment and updating of every patient's list of medications throughout the health care process and the timely communication of such information to both patients and their health care providers. This procedure involves three steps (additional information can be found on either of the websites mentioned previously):

1. Verification—Collection of the patient's medication information with a focus on medications currently used (including prescription drugs as well as over-the-counter medications and supplements)
2. Clarification—Professional review of this information to ensure that medications and dosages are appropriate for the patient
3. Reconciliation—Further investigation of any discrepancies and documentation of relevant communications and changes in medication orders

To ensure ongoing accuracy of medication use, the steps listed should be repeated at each stage of health care delivery:
a. Admission
b. Status change (e.g., from critical to stable)
c. Patient transfer within or between facilities or provider teams
d. Discharge (the latest medication list should be provided to the patient to take to his or her next health care provider or this information should be otherwise forwarded to the provider; applicable confidentiality guidelines should be followed)

Some applicable assessment and education tips regarding medication reconciliation are the following:

1. Ask the patient open-ended questions and gradually move to yes-no questions to help determine specific medication information. (Details are important, maybe even critical!)
2. Avoid the use of medical jargon unless it is clear that the patient understands and is comfortable with such language.
3. Prompt the patient to try to remember all applicable medications (e.g., patches, creams, eyedrops, inhalers, professional samples, injections, dietary supplements). If the patient does provide a medication list, make a copy for the patient's chart as part of this process.
4. Clarify unclear information to the extent possible (e.g., by talking with the home caregiver or the outpatient pharmacist who fills the patient's prescriptions, if needed).
5. Record the aforementioned information in the patient's chart as the first step in the medication reconciliation process.
6. Emphasize to the patient the importance of always maintaining a current and complete medication list and bringing it to each health care encounter (e.g., as a wallet card or other list).

OTHER ETHICAL ISSUES

Notification of Patients Regarding Errors

An article published in the *Journal of Clinical Outcomes Management* in 2001 recognized the obligation of institutions and health care providers to notify patients when errors have occurred in their care. The article not only emphasized the ethical basis for this practice but also addressed the legal implications and was a starting point for understanding the issue of notification of patients regarding medication errors. The point was made that patients who seek attorney services are often motivated primarily by a perceived imbalance in power between themselves and their health care providers and by fear of financial burden. Health care organizations can choose to apologize and accept responsibility for obvious errors and even offer needed financial support (e.g., for travel expenses, temporary loss of wages). Research indicates that such actions help health care organizations to avoid litigation and potentially much larger financial settlements.

Whistle-Blowing

In clinical settings, whistle-blowing refers to a disclosure made outside a health care facility regarding patient care errors when an organization's internal chain of command has failed to correct significant problems within the facility. Such a disclosure may be made to a regulatory or investigative agency or to the public through the news media. One view is that whistle-blowing results from a failure of organizational ethics. Virtually all practicing nurses will eventually witness situations involving excessive lapses in patient care. Although a student or otherwise inexperienced nurse may not realistically be in a viable position to challenge an institution's hierarchy, every nurse should consider, preferably in advance, how he or she might choose to respond to such a situation. The *Code of Ethics for Nurses* published by the American Nurses Association (ANA) is described in Box 4-1 on page 52. Among other things, this document makes clear several moral imperatives for the practicing nurse that may ultimately justify a whistle-blowing action, even in the face of termination of employment. All health care providers should familiarize themselves with their institution's usual procedures for error reporting, including how and when to approach levels of leadership above their immediate supervisor. When the usual systems fail, a whistle-blowing disclosure may be the most ethical course of action.

NURSING MEASURES TO PREVENT MEDICATION ERRORS

Nurses may reduce the likelihood of medication errors by taking the following precautions—with awareness that the first step to defend against errors is assessing and documenting information about drug allergies:

- Minimize the use of verbal and telephone orders; if such an order must be taken, repeat the order to confirm it with the prescriber, spelling the drug name aloud and speaking slowly and clearly.
- List the indication (reason for use) next to each drug order on the medication administration record, patient materials, and any other educational materials.

- Avoid the use of abbreviations, medical shorthand, and acronyms, because they can lead to confusion, miscommunication, and risk for error (see the Legal and Ethical Principles table).
- Never assume anything about any drug order or prescription, including medication route.
- If a medication order is questioned for any reason (e.g., dose, drug, indication), never assume that the prescriber is correct. Always act as the patient's advocate.
- Do not try to decipher illegibly written orders. Instead, contact the prescriber for clarification. Illegible orders fall below applicable standards for quality medical care and can endanger patient well-being.
- If in doubt about the correctness of a legibly written order, always double-check with the prescriber, pharmacist, or other acceptable, authoritative source.
- Compare the medication order against what is on hand by checking the Five Rights of medication administration.
- *Never* use trailing zeros (e.g., 1.0 mg) in writing and/or transcribing medication orders. *Do* use a leading zero for decimal dosages (e.g., 0.25 mg). Use of trailing zeros is associated with increased occurrence of overdose. For example,

  1.0 mg warfarin sodium could be misread as 10 mg warfarin, a tenfold dose increase. Instead, use 1 mg.

  Failure to use leading zeros can also lead to overdose. For example,

  .25 mg digoxin could be misread as 25 mg digoxin, a potentially lethal dose that is 100 times the dose ordered. Instead, write 0.25 mg.

Other measures to prevent medication errors include the following:

- Carefully read all labels for accuracy, expiration dates, and dilution requirements.
- Be familiar with new techniques of administration and new equipment (e.g., use of the Diskus inhaled dosage forms or transdermal and transbuccal forms of drugs).
- Encourage the use of both trade and generic names in drug orders and prescriptions and include purpose whenever possible. Relying too heavily on trade names especially increases the likelihood of medication errors because many trade names sound alike and have similar spellings and syllabic structure.
- Listen to and honor any concerns expressed by patients. Should the patient state that he or she is allergic to a medication, that a pill has already been taken, or that the medication is not what the patient usually takes, stop, listen, and investigate.
- Remain alert, in good health, and educated, and never be too busy to stop, learn, and inquire.
- If working conditions are problematic, join organizations with other nurses to advocate for improved working conditions (see Political Action on p. 65) and to stand up for nurses' and patients' rights.
- Always double-check a medication's product labeling because often there are different formulations of the same active ingredient.
- Remember that generic names are preferred.
- Never crush, open, or allow the patient to chew extended-released or long-release dosage forms.
- Safeguard any medications that the patient had on admission or transfer so that additional doses are not given. In such situations, safeguarding is accomplished by compiling a current medication history and resolving any discrepancies rather than ignoring them.

There are other significant interventions that may help to decrease the risk of medication errors. The following measures address aspects of the system in order to prevent errors:

- Always verify new medication administration records if they have been rewritten or reentered for any reason. Make sure that all nurses and staff are alerted to carry out this process.
- Always compare the pharmacy label against the initial medication administration record before giving the first dose.
- Use computerized prescriber order entry and have that order entry system integrated with the computer in the pharmacy, because this can help eliminate the need for yet another person (pharmacist, technician, etc.) to enter an order. Fewer entries mean fewer errors!

LEGAL AND ETHICAL PRINCIPLES
Use of Abbreviations

Medication errors often occur as a result of misinterpretation of abbreviations. Therefore, the National Coordinating Council for Medication Error Reporting and Prevention recommends that the following abbreviations be written out *in full* and the abbreviations avoided. The U.S. Pharmacopeia and Institute of Safe Medication Practices endorse the avoidance of abbreviations whenever possible. Most hospitals and nursing care units are adopting this significant change in documentation.

Abbreviation	Intended Meaning	Common Error
U	Units	Mistaken for a zero (0), a four (4), or cc.
mcg (μg)	Micrograms	Mistaken for mg (milligrams).
Q.D.	Latin abbreviation for "every day"	The period after the "Q" can be mistaken for an "I" so that a medication is given "QID" (four times daily) instead of once daily.
Q.O.D.	Latin abbreviation for "every other day"	Misinterpreted as "QD" (daily) or QID. If "O" is poorly written it may look like a period or "I."
D/C	Discharge or discontinue	Medications have been prematurely discontinued when D/C (intended to mean "discharge") was misinterpreted as "discontinue" because it was followed by a list of drugs.
HS	Half strength	Misinterpreted as the Latin abbreviation "HS" (hour of sleep).
cc	Cubic centimeters	Mistaken for "U" (units) when written poorly.
AU, AS, AD	Both ears, left ear, right ear	Misinterpreted as the Latin abbreviation "OU" (both eyes), "OS" (left eye), "OD" (right eye).

- Provide for mandatory entry of the weight of every patient into the medication administration record before the first medication order goes to the pharmacy; this practice can help reduce dosage errors.
- Provide for mandatory recalculation of every drug dosage for patients taking high-risk drugs, pediatric patients, and elderly patients and in any other situation in which there is a narrow margin between therapeutic serum drug levels and toxic levels (e.g., administration of chemotherapeutic drugs or digitalis drugs, presence of altered liver or kidney function in an elderly or any other patient).
- Always suspect an error whenever an adult dosage form is dispensed for a pediatric patient.
- Be sure to provide a translator for patients who speak a language other than English.

See the Life Span Considerations boxes on pages 64 and 65 for information on drug therapy and medication errors in elderly and pediatric patients.

Possible Consequences of Medication Errors for Nurses

As mentioned earlier, the possible effects of medication errors on a patient range from no significant effect to permanent disability and even death in the most extreme cases. However, medication errors may also affect health care professionals, including nurses and student nurses, in a number of ways. An error that involves significant patient harm or death may take an extreme emotional toll on the nurse involved in the error. Nurses may be named as defendants in malpractice litigation, with possibly serious financial consequences. Many nurses choose to carry personal malpractice insurance for this reason, although nurses working in institutional settings are usually covered by the institution's liability insurance policy. Nurses should obtain clear written documentation of any provided institutional coverage before deciding whether to carry individual malpractice insurance.

Administrative responses to medication errors vary from institution to institution and depend on the severity of the error. One possible response is a directive to the nurse involved to obtain continuing education or refresher training. Disciplinary action, including suspension or termination of employment, may also occur depending on the specific incident. Nurses who have violated regulations of their state's nurse practice act may also be counseled or disciplined by their state nursing board, which may suspend or permanently revoke their nursing license. Student nurses, given their lack of clinical experience, should be especially careful to avoid medication errors, as well as errors in general. When in doubt about the correct course of action, students should consult with clinical instructors or more experienced staff nurses. Nonetheless, if a student nurse realizes that he or she has committed an error, the student should notify the responsible clinical instructor immediately. The patient may require additional monitoring or medication, and the prescriber may also need to be notified. Although such events are preferably avoided, they can ultimately be useful, though stressful, learning experiences for the student nurse. However, student nurses who commit sufficiently serious errors or display a pattern of errors can expect more severe disciplinary action. This may range from a requirement for extra clinical time or repeating of a clinical course to suspension or expulsion from the nursing school program (see the earlier section Educational System Issues and Their Potential Impact on Medication Errors).

Life Span Considerations: The Elderly Patient
Medication Errors

Approximately one third of medication errors in hospitals involve patients older than 65 years of age. Generally speaking, the majority of medication errors that occur are not considered harmful; those errors that are fatal are most likely to occur in seniors. The fourth annual report of MEDMARX, the national medication error reporting database operated by the U.S. Pharmacopeia (USP), indicated that 192,477 medication errors were voluntarily reported by 482 hospitals and other health care facilities across the United States in 2002. The USP is calling for more action to help reduce these medication errors in the highly vulnerable elderly population. The MEDMARX report revealed the following findings:

- Of all fatal hospital medication errors, approximately 55% involved seniors.
- 35% of medical errors involve medication errors that were not caught before the drugs were given to the patient.
- Approximately 4% of medication errors involved administration of the wrong medication to the patient.
- In 43% of medication errors, patients failed to receive their prescribed drugs.
- Some 18% of medication errors were related to drug dosage or quantity.

The annual report revealed the following findings regarding the 192,477 medication errors reported to the USP in 2002:

- The majority of the medication errors were corrected before injury occurred.

- Some 3213 of the errors resulted in patient injury; 47 required life-sustaining interventions and 20 resulted in death.
- Health care facilities cited many reasons for the drug errors, but frequently mentioned workplace distractions (43%), staffing issues (36%), and workload increases (22%).

Diane Cousins of the USP stated that hospitals will need to identify and track any trends and problem areas related to medication errors to help prevent and reduce errors in the future.

The USP recommends the following interventions for prevention of drug errors in the elderly:

- Make sure all health care professionals have full knowledge about the drugs they are giving.
- Use the brown bag technique (asking patients to bring in all medications in a paper bag) to identify drugs patients are taking (Chapter 3).
- Ensure that all allergies and adverse effects are recorded.
- Ensure that all prescription containers are labeled in a large font and clear print.

In addition, it is important to remember the lines of defense in medication error prevention. The first line of defense is the prescribing health care professional (e.g., physician, nurse practitioner); the second line of defense is the individual who dispenses the drug (pharmacist); and the third line of defense is the individual who actually administers the drug to the patient.

Data from www.WebMD.com; http://www.USP.org (Cousins D), Nov 18, 2003.

It is critical to the process of safe medication administration and the prevention of medication errors to boost the consumer's (i.e., patient's) knowledge and right to safe and quality nursing care, including drug therapy. Newer forms of drug administration and drug dispensing, such as automated dispensing cabinets and bar coding, and new forms of accessing drug information, such as personal digital assistants and other hand-held devices, also add more challenges in ensuring safe and effective drug therapy.

POLITICAL ACTION

An Ounce of Prevention: Nurse Advocacy for Safer Health Care Organizations

The ANA was founded in 1897, and from the beginning one of its objectives has been legislative advocacy on behalf of nurses and their patients. In a 2001 ANA staffing survey, 75% of nurses felt that the quality of patient care has declined, largely due to poorer nurse-patient staffing ratios. This is a major reason that nurses choose to leave the profession or practice setting. According to a 2002 report, 84% of hospitals indicate that they have nursing staff shortages.

One of the earliest studies to address the modern problem of hospital nursing shortages was published in 1989 in the *New England Journal of Medicine.* The significance of the study, which has implications regarding nursing care, is that it correlated rising patient mortality rates in hospitals with the presence of relatively fewer registered nurses on staff.

Life Span Considerations: The Pediatric Patient
Medication Errors

Of all the ways a pediatric patient may be harmed during medical treatment, medication errors are the most common. As with elderly patients, when medication errors occur, there is a higher risk of death. The findings of several studies indicate that medication errors involving inpatient pediatric patients occur at a rate of 4.5 to 5.7 errors per 100 drugs used. The most common medication errors in pediatrics are dosing errors. Research has begun to identify some of the groups of pediatric patients who are at highest risk of medication errors, and these include the following:

- Patients younger than 2 years of age
- Patients in intensive care units (ICUs) and specifically the neonatal ICU
- Patients who are in the emergency department between the hours of 4 AM and 8 AM or on the weekend and who are seriously ill
- Patients receiving intravenous drugs
- Patients receiving chemotherapy
- Patients whose weight has not been determined or recorded

Mathematical dosage calculations for pediatric patients are also problematic. In determination of the correct dosage once the drug has been ordered, the problems of most concern are the following:

- Inability of the nurse to understand and perform the correct mathematical calculation and carry out the dilution process
- Infrequent use of calculations in nursing practice
- Misplacement of the decimal point, which is a common dosing mistake and can lead to a tenfold error and subsequent overdosing or underdosing; the consequences can range from renal or respiratory failure to cardiac arrest

The following are some of the actions that can be taken to prevent pediatric medication errors:

- Report all medication errors, because this information is part of the practice of professional nursing and helps in identifying causes of medication error.
- Know the drug thoroughly, including its on- and off-label uses, action, adverse effects, dosage ranges, routes of administration, high-alert drug status,* cautions, and contraindications (e.g., is it recommended for use in pediatric patients?).
- Confirm information about the patient each and every time a dose is given and check three times before giving the drug by comparing the drug order with the patient's medication profile and verifying the Five Rights (right drug, right dose, right route, right time, and right patient).
- Double-check and verify information in handwritten orders and verbal orders that may be incomplete, unclear, or illegible.
- Avoid distractions while giving medications.
- Communicate with anyone (parent, caregiver) involved in patient care.
- Make sure all orders are clear and understood when the shift changes.
- Use authoritative resources such as drug handbooks, *Physicians' Desk Reference,* or information from the Food and Drug Administration website (www.fda.gov). For off-label use of drugs, see www.fda.gov/cder/pediatric/labelchange.htm.

*High-alert drugs include adrenal drugs (corticosteroids), analgesics (acetaminophen), antiinfectives and antibiotics, antihistamines, antineoplastics, asthma drugs, bronchodilators, cardiac drugs, electrolytes, vitamins, minerals, insulin, opioids, and sedatives.

CASE STUDY
Medication Errors

During your busy clinical day as a student nurse, the staff nurse assigned to your patient comes to you and says, "Would you like to give this injection? We have a 'now' order for Sandostatin (octreotide) 200 mcg subcutaneously. I've already drawn it up; 200 mcg equals 2 mL. It needs to be given as soon as possible, so I drew it up to save time." She hands you a syringe that has 2 mL of a clear fluid in it, and the patient's medication administration record (MAR).

1. Should you give this medication "now," as ordered? Why or why not?

You decide to check the order that is handwritten on the MAR with the order written on the chart. The physician wrote, "Octreotide, 200 mcg now, SC, then 100 mcg every 8 hours as needed." Before you have a chance to find your instructor, the nurse returns and says, "Your instructor probably won't let you give the injection unless you can show the medication ampules. Here are the ampules I used to draw up the octreotide. Be quick—your patient needs it now!"

You take the order, the MAR, the two ampules, and the syringe to your instructor. Together you read the order, then check the ampules. Each ampule is marked "Sandostatin (octreotide) 500 mcg/mL."

2. If the nurse drew up 2 ml from those two ampules, how much octreotide is in the syringe? How does that amount compare with the order?

The nurse is astonished when you point out that the ampules read "500 mcg/mL." She goes into the automated medication dispenser and sees two identical boxes of Sandostatin next to each other in the refrigerated section. One box is labeled "100 mcg/mL" and the other box is labeled "500 mcg/mL." She then realizes she chose an ampule of the wrong strength of drug and drew up an incorrect dose.

3. What would have happened if you had given the injection?
4. What should be done at this point? What contributed to this potential medication error, and how can it be prevented in the future?

Currently there is a new and growing advocacy movement among several groups of nurses in various regions of the United States. One of the newest professional associations for nurses is the American Association of Registered Nurses (AARN). This organization was founded in April 2002 by members of the California Nurses Association. Other state-based groups that have joined with the AARN include the Massachusetts Nurses Association, the Maine State Nurses Association, the Pennsylvania Association of Staff Nurses and Allied Professionals, the New York Professional Nurses Union, the United Health Care Workers of Missouri, and the Southern Arizona Nurses Coalition. The AARN makes a continuous effort to publicize its mission and to recruit members from other state groups.

The primary focus of the AARN thus far has been aggressive legislative advocacy at the state level for improved working conditions and patient care. Major issues include legally mandated safe nurse-patient ratios in acute and long-term care facilities, elimination of mandatory overtime, equitable wage and retirement benefits, and meaningful reform in the way the nation's health care system operates.

SUMMARY

The increasing complexity of nursing practice also increases the risk for medication errors. Widely recognized and common causes of error include misunderstanding of abbreviations, illegibility of prescriber handwriting, miscommunication during verbal or telephone orders, and confusing drug nomenclature. The structure of various organizational, educational, and sociologic systems involved in health care delivery may also contribute directly or indirectly to the occurrence of medication errors. Understanding these influences can help the nurse take proactive steps to improve these systems. Such actions can range from fostering improved communication with other health care team members, including students, to advocating politically for safer conditions for both patients and staff. The first priority when an error does occur is to protect the patient from further harm whenever possible. All errors should serve as red flags that warrant further reflection, detailed analysis, and future preventive actions on the part of nurses, other health care professionals, and possibly even patients themselves.

Points to Remember

- *Medical error* is a broad term used to designate any error that occurs in any phase of clinical patient care. Medical errors *may* involve medications.
- MEs may or may not lead to ADRs. MEs include giving the drug to the wrong patient, confusing sound-alike and look-alike drugs, administering the wrong drug or wrong dose, giving the drug by the wrong route, and giving the drug at the wrong time.
- There are many measures that nurses can take to help prevent MEs. Being prepared and knowledgeable and taking the time always to triple-check the Five Rights of medication administration are very important. It is also important for nurses always to be aware of the entire medication administration process and to take a system analysis approach to looking at MEs and their prevention.

- Nurses should always encourage patients to ask questions about their medications and to let their health care providers know if they are questioning the drug or any component of the medication administration process.
- Nurses should encourage patients always to keep drug allergy information on their person and a current list of medications in their wallet or purse and on their refrigerator. This list should include the following information:
- Drug name
- Reason the drug is being used
- Usual dosage range and the dosage the patient is taking
- Expected adverse effects and toxic effects of the drug
- Physician's name and phone number

NCLEX Examination Review Questions

1. Nursing measures to reduce the risk of medication errors include which of the following?
   a. If you are questioning a drug order, assume that the prescriber is correct.
   b. Be careful about questioning the drug order a board-certified surgeon has written for a patient.
   c. Always double-check the many drugs with sound-alike and look-alike names because of the high risk of error.
   d. Always go with your gut reaction, and if you think a drug route has been incorrectly prescribed, use the oral route.

2. It is important in the medication administration process to remember which of the following?
   a. When in doubt about an order, ask a colleague about the drug.
   b. Contact the patient and ask what the patient knows about the drug, and whether it was taken prior to this hospitalization.
   c. If you are too busy, ask the charge nurse about the drug, then research the drug once you have given it to the patient at the right time.
   d. Stop, listen, and investigate any concerns expressed by the patient.

NCLEX Examination Review Questions—cont'd

3. If a student nurse realizes that he or she has committed a drug error, which of the following should be emphasized to the student?
   a. The student bears no legal responsibility when giving medications.
   b. The major legal responsibility lies with the health care institution at which the student is placed for clinical experience.
   c. The major legal responsibility for drug errors lies with the faculty members.
   d. Once the student has committed a medication error, his or her responsibility is to the patient and to being honest and accountable.
4. The nurse is giving medications to a newly admitted patient who is to receive nothing by mouth (NPO status) and finds an order written as follows: "Digoxin, 250 mcg stat." Which action is appropriate?
   a. Give the medication immediately (stat) by mouth because the patient has no intravenous (IV) access at this time.

   b. Clarify the order with the prescribing physician before giving the drug.
   c. Ask the charge nurse what route the physician meant to use.
   d. Start an IV line, then give the medication IV so that it will work faster, because the patient's status is NPO at this time.
5. Which of the following is the best authoritative resource for information about medications?
   a. The faculty person supervising the student during clinical rotations
   b. Drug information obtained from Internet sites for lay persons
   c. Drug information obtained from Internet sites such as www. usp.org and www.fda.gov
   d. An experienced professional nurse colleague

1. c, 2. d, 3. d, 4. b, 5. c.

Critical Thinking Activities

1. Medication errors have been occurring with increasing frequency on the unit on which you are employed. A committee has been appointed to investigate why the medication errors occur and how to resolve the problem. Considering this situation and the drug administration process, is it always safe to follow only the guideline of checking the Five Rights of drug administration? Why or why not?
2. You are a charge nurse at a small community hospital. The physician ordered a STAT IV vancomycin infusion, but when the bag comes up from the pharmacy, you notice that the dose is incor-

rect. It takes 2 hours for the pharmacy to send up an IV bag with the correct dose. As you check the medication, you note that it is the right drug, right dose, and so on, yet it has been 2 hours since it was ordered STAT. What, if anything, should you do before you give this medication?
3. List several Internet sources for information on medication safety and briefly discuss how this information could be shared with patients in a community outpatient setting where mostly indigent patients are served.

For answers, see http://evolve.elsevier.com/Lilley.

Patient Education and Drug Therapy

Objectives

When you reach the end of this chapter, you should be able to do the following:

1. Discuss the importance of patient education in the safe and efficient administration of drugs (e.g., prescription drugs, over-the-counter drugs, herbal preparations, dietary supplements).
2. Discuss some of the teaching and learning principles related to patient education and drug therapy across the life span that are applicable to any health care setting or to home care.
3. Identify the impact of the various developmental phases (as described by Erikson) on patient education and drug therapy.
4. Develop a complete patient teaching plan as part of a comprehensive nursing care plan for drug therapy.

e-Learning Activities

Companion CD

- NCLEX Review Questions: see questions 30-32
- Animations
- Audio Glossary
- Category Catchers
- Medication Errors Checklists
- IV Therapy Checklists

evolve Website (http://evolve.elsevier.com/Lilley)

- Nursing Care Plans • Frequently Asked Questions • Content Updates • WebLinks • Supplemental Resources • Elsevier ePharmacology Update • Medication Administration Animations

Given the continual change in health care today and the increasing emphasis on consumer awareness, the role of nurses as educators is expanding. Because the frequency with which patients are being managed in the home setting is also increasing, patient education is an essential component of health care. Without it, high-quality patient care cannot be provided. Patient education is crucial for helping patients adapt to illness, prevent illness, maintain wellness, and provide self-care. Patient education is a process similar to the nursing process in which patients are assisted in learning healthy behaviors and assimilating these behaviors into their lifestyle. Learning is defined as a change in behavior and teaching as a sharing of knowledge. Although nurses can never be certain that patients will take medications as prescribed, they can be sure to carefully assess, plan, implement, and evaluate the teaching they provide to patients about their medications. Although the use of the nursing process is seen as controversial in some educational and health care institutions, it is still the major systematic framework for professional nursing practice. It is a strength of this textbook and is applied in the chapters as it relates to drug therapy and, in this chapter, patient education. The nursing process (discussed in Chapter 1) is presented and applied in this chapter using the following format: assessment; nursing

diagnoses; planning, including goals and outcome criteria; implementation; and evaluation.

ASSESSMENT OF LEARNING NEEDS RELATED TO DRUG THERAPY

The patient education process is similar to the nursing process. A very important facet of the patient education process is a thorough assessment of learning needs, and this assessment must be completed before patients begin any form of drug therapy, whether it involves a prescription drug, over-the-counter (OTC) drug, herbal preparation, or dietary supplement. Performing a thorough assessment includes gathering subjective and objective data about the following variables and factors:

- Adaptation to any illnesses
- Cognitive abilities
- Coping mechanisms
- Cultural background
- Developmental status for age group with attention to cognitive and mental processing abilities
- Emotional status
- Environment at home and work
- Family relationships
- Financial status
- Psychosocial growth and development level according to Erikson's stages (Box 6-1)
- Health beliefs
- Information the patient understands about past and present medical conditions, medical therapy, and medications
- Language(s) spoken
- Level of education (including literacy level)
- Level of knowledge about any medications being taken
- Limitations (physical, psychologic, cognitive, and motor)
- Medications currently taken (including OTC drugs, prescription drugs, and herbal products)
- Mobility
- Motivation
- Nutritional status

Box 6-1 Erikson's Stages of Development

Infancy (birth to 1 year of age): Trust versus mistrust. Infant learns to trust himself or herself, others, and the environment; learns to love and be loved.

Toddlerhood (1 to 3 years of age): Autonomy versus shame and doubt. Toddler learns independence; learns to master the physical environment and maintain self-esteem.

Preschool age (3 to 6 years of age): Initiative versus guilt. Preschooler learns basic problem solving; develops conscience and sexual identity; initiates activities as well as imitates.

School age (6 to 12 years of age): Industry versus inferiority. School-age child learns to do things well; develops a sense of self-worth.

Adolescence (12 to 18 years of age): Identity versus role confusion. Adolescent integrates many roles into self-identity through imitation of role models and peer pressure.

Young adulthood (18 to 45 years of age): Intimacy versus isolation. Young adult establishes deep and lasting relationships; learns to make commitment as a spouse, parent, and/or partner.

Middle adulthood (45 to 65 years of age): Generativity versus stagnation. Adult learns commitment to the community and world; is productive in career, family, and civic interests.

Older adulthood (over 65 years of age): Integrity versus despair. Older adult appreciates life role and status; deals with loss and prepares for death.

CULTURAL IMPLICATIONS
Patient Education

The nurse must research various cultures to enhance an individualized approach to nursing care. For example, with Mexican American patients, aspects of nursing care must be approached in a sensitive manner with strong consideration for the family, communication needs, and religion. Approximately 90% of native Mexicans are Roman Catholic. To help meet the needs of these patients more effectively, the nurse should consider speaking with them about their desire for clergy visits while in the hospital. Family members are generally involved, and Mexican Americans often have large extended families; therefore, the nurse should take the time to include family members in the patient's care and when providing discharge instructions and medication instructions.

Modified from McKenry LM, Salerno E: *Mosby's pharmacology in nursing,* ed 22, St Louis, 2006, Mosby.

- Past and present health behaviors
- Past and present experience with drug regimens and other forms of therapy
- Race and/or ethnicity
- Readiness to learn
- Self-care ability
- Sensory status
- Social support

In addition, the assessment is an appropriate time to probe for any misinformation regarding drug or related health care and to identify practices that might be contraindicated given the current drug regimen (e.g., use of certain folk medicine or home remedies, or alternative therapies such as chiropractic and osteopathic medicine and aromatherapy). Other questions posed to the patient may need to focus on the patient's belief system about health, wellness, and/or illness state as well as any experiences with health care regimens and therapies and history of compliance with drug and other therapies. Other barriers to learning may include language, finances, cultural beliefs, previous negative or limited experiences with the health care system or team, and denial of illness or need for health care intervention.

During the assessment of learning needs, the nurse must be astutely aware of the patient's verbal and nonverbal communication. Often a patient will not tell the nurse how he or she truly feels. A seeming discrepancy is an indication that the patient's emotional or physical state may need to be further assessed in relation to his or her readiness for learning and/or motivation to learn. The nurse should use open-ended questions when assessing patients, because this type of question encourages greater clarification and more discussion from the patient. Closed-ended questions that require only a yes or no answer provide limited information and insight about the patient. Level of anxiety must also be assessed, because a mild anxiety level is usually motivating, but a moderate or severe level may be an obstacle.

NURSING DIAGNOSES RELATED TO LEARNING NEEDS AND DRUG THERAPY

Some of the most commonly used nursing diagnoses related to patient education and drug therapy include the following: deficient knowledge, ineffective health maintenance, ineffective therapeutic regimen management, risk for injury, impaired memory, and noncompliance. *Deficient knowledge* refers to a situation in which the patient (or caregiver or significant other) has a limited knowledge base or skills with regard to the medication. A nursing diagnosis of deficient knowledge grows out of collected data which indicate that the patient has limited or no understanding of the medication and its action, adverse effects, or cautions and any related administration techniques. Deficient knowledge may also pertain to the lack of motor skills needed to safely self-administer the medication. Deficient knowledge differs from noncompliance in that the latter occurs when the patient does not take the medication as prescribed or at all—in other words, the patient does not adhere to the instructions given about the medication. Noncompliance is the patient's choice. A nursing diagnosis of noncompliance is made when data collected from the patient show that the condition or symptoms for which the patient is taking the medication have recurred or were never resolved because the patient did not take the medication per the physician's orders or did not take the medication at all. Other nursing diagnoses as listed by the North American Nursing Diagnosis Association (NANDA) (see Chapter 1) may also be used in relation to medication administration, when applicable.

PLANNING RELATED TO LEARNING NEEDS AND DRUG THERAPY

The planning phase of the teaching-learning process occurs as soon as a learning need has been identified in a patient or caregiver. With mutual understanding, the nurse and patient identify goals and outcome criteria that are associated with the identified nursing diagnosis and relate to the specific medication the patient is taking. The following is an example of a measurable goal with outcome criterion related to a nursing diagnosis of deficient knowledge for a patient who is self-administering an oral antidiabetic drug and has many questions about the medication therapy: *Sample goal:* The patient safely self-administers the prescribed oral antidiabetic drug. *Sample outcome criterion:* The patient remains without signs and symptoms of overmedication with an oral antidiabetic drug, such as hypoglycemia with tachycardia, palpitations, diaphoresis, hunger, and fatigue. When drug therapy goals and outcome criteria are developed, appropriate time frames for meeting outcome criteria should also be identified (see Chapter 1 for more information on the nursing process). Goals and outcome criteria should be realistic, based on patient needs, stated in patient terms, and include terms that are measurable, such as *list, identify, demonstrate, self-administer, state, describe,* and *discuss.*

IMPLEMENTATION RELATED TO PATIENT EDUCATION AND DRUG THERAPY

After the nurse has completed the assessment phase, identified nursing diagnoses, and created a plan of care, he or she begins the implementation phase of the teaching-learning process, which includes conveying specific information about the medication to the patient. Teaching-learning sessions should incorporate clear, simple, concise written instructions; oral instructions; and pamphlets, films, or any other learning aids that will help ensure patient learning. The nurse may have to conduct several short teaching-learning sessions with multiple strategies, depending on the needs of the patient. (Table 6-1 lists educational strategies for accommodating changes related to aging that may influence learning.) The nurse may also need to identify aids to help the patient in the safe administration of medications at home, such as the use of medication day and time calendars, pill reminder stickers, daily medication containers with alarms, and/or a method of

Table 6-1   Educational Strategies to Address Common Changes Related to Aging That May Influence Learning

Change Related to Aging	Educational Strategy
Disturbed Thought Processes	
Slowed cognitive functioning	Slow the pace of the presentation and attend to verbal and nonverbal patient cues to verify understanding.
Decreased short-term memory	Provide smaller amounts of information at one time. Repeat information frequently. Provide written instructions for home use.
Decreased ability to think abstractly	Use examples to illustrate information. Use a variety of methods, such as audiovisuals, props, videos, large-print materials, materials with vivid color, return demonstrations, and practice sessions.
Decreased ability to concentrate	Decrease external stimuli as much as possible.
Increased reaction time (slower to respond)	Always allow sufficient time and be patient. Allow more time for feedback.
Disturbed Sensory Perception *Hearing*	
Diminished hearing	Perform a baseline hearing assessment. Use tone- and volume-controlled teaching aids; use bright, large-print material to reinforce.
Decreased ability to distinguish sounds (e.g., words beginning with S, Z, T, D, F, and G)	Speak distinctly and slowly, and articulate carefully.
Decreased conduction of sound	Sit on side of the patient's best ear.
Loss of ability to hear high-frequency sounds	Do not shout; speak in a normal voice but lower voice pitch.
Partial to complete loss of hearing	Face the patient so that lip-reading is possible. Use visual aids to reinforce verbal instruction. Reinforce teaching with easy-to-read materials. Decrease extraneous noise. Use community resources for the hearing impaired.
Vision	
Decreased visual acuity	Ensure that the patient's glasses are clean and in place and that the prescription is current.
Decreased ability to read fine detail	Use printed material with large print that is brightly and clearly colored.
Decreased ability to discriminate among blue, violet, and green; tendency for all colors to fade, with red fading the least	Use high-contrast materials, such as black on white. Avoid the use of blue, violet, and green in type or graphics; use red instead.
Thickening and yellowing of the lenses of the eyes, with decreased accommodation	Use nonglare lighting and avoid contrasts of light (e.g., darkened room with single light).
Decreased depth perception	Adjust teaching to allow for the use of touch to gauge depth.
Decreased peripheral vision	Keep all teaching materials within the patient's visual field.
Touch and Vibration	
Decreased sense of touch	Increase the time allowed for the teaching of psychomotor skills, the number of repetitions, and the number of return demonstrations.
Decreased sense of vibration	Teach the patient to palpate more prominent pulse sites (e.g., carotid and radial arteries).

Modified from Weinrich SP, Boyd M, Nussbaum J: Continuing education: adapting strategies to teach the elderly, *J Gerontol Nurs* 15(11):17-21, 1989; McKenry LM, Salerno E: *Mosby's pharmacology in nursing,* ed 22, St Louis, 2006, Mosby.
NOTE: These strategies may also be appropriate for younger patients.

documenting doses taken to avoid overdosage or omission of doses.

Special considerations arise when the patient speaks limited or no English. The nurse should communicate with the patient in the patient's native language if at all possible. If the nurse is not able to speak the patient's native language, a translator should be made available if possible to prevent communication problems, minimize errors, and help boost the patient's level of trust and understanding of the nurse. In practice this translator is often either a lay family member (maybe even a child) or a nonclinical staff member, and the nurse should keep in mind that these individuals may not be competent at or comfortable with communicating technical clinical information.

In response to the rapidly growing population of non–English-speaking Hispanics in the United States, a number of publications have appeared containing patient education materials printed in both English and Spanish. Similar materials for other languages may also be available. These publications may enable the nurse to speak a sufficient amount of the patient's language to effectively educate the patient and can be given to the patient and family members to read on their own. The publishers of these patient education materials have generally granted permission to photocopy them for educational purposes.

Health care professionals who work in a geographic area where a variety of non-English languages are widely spoken should consider learning one or more of these languages. Adult foreign language education is available in many U.S. cities, often at 2- and 4-year colleges or universities. Many classes are designed for working professionals and are scheduled at a variety of convenient times during the day and evening to accommodate demanding work schedules. Many employers will pay for job-related courses, and some courses may be used as professional continuing education credits. Language courses provide a means of networking and developing quality friendships with other highly motivated, empathic individuals both within and outside of the health care profession. It should be noted that patients who are native English speakers may also have problems learning about their medications and treatment regimens because of learning deficits or difficulties, hearing and speech deficits, lack of education, or minimal previous exposure to treatment regimens and medication use.

The teaching of manual skills for specific medication administration is also part of the teaching-learning session. Sufficient time (each patient has different needs) should be allowed for the patient to become familiar with any equipment and to perform several return demonstrations to the nurse or other health care provider. Family members, significant others, or caregivers should also be included in this session or sessions for reinforcement purposes. Audiovisual aids may be incorporated and based on assessment findings. Resources for information about medications include the *USP Drug Information* volume II, *Advice for the Patient,* which is published annually (along with the *Health*

EVIDENCE-BASED PRACTICE

The Impact of Better Education of Nurses on Patient Outcomes

Patient education has proven its value in all aspects of the nursing care of patients in and out of the hospital setting. Management of various regimens, drug therapies, and other aspects of care is enhanced when patients and their families, significant others, and/or other support system members are informed and educated as well. The study examined the relationship between the level of educational preparation of the registered nurses at these hospitals and risk-adjusted patient mortality after surgery.

Type of Evidence
Clinical outcome data were obtained for 232,342 surgical patients at some 168 hospitals. Some 10,000 questionnaires were mailed to nurses who worked at these hospitals for the purpose of determining the educational backgrounds and professional nursing experience of the nurses.

Results of Study
The complex data analysis adjusted for hospital size and level of technology as well as patient characteristics. The survey of nurses revealed that the nurses had an average of 14 years experience, with a patient workload average of six patients per shift, and that in 20% of the hospitals, fewer than 20% of the nurses had a bachelor of science in nursing degree or higher. Other results included the following: (1) In 11% of the hospitals surveyed, 50%+ nurses had BSN or higher degrees; (2) in these 11%, nurses were more educated but slightly less experienced and had significantly fewer patients under their care; and (3) high-technology hospitals had more nurses with a BSN or master of science in nursing (MSN) degree. Other significant findings included the fact that the number of pa-

tient deaths was 19% lower in the 11% of hospitals with more educated nurses than in the other hospitals. A negative association was also found between the percentage of nurses in a hospital with either a BSN or MSN degree and the risk of death for patients within 30 days of admission, meaning that the greater the number of nurses with at least a bachelor's degree, the lower the patient mortality. Nurses' number of years of experience was *not* found to have a significant impact on patient death rates.

Link of Evidence to Nursing Practice
The findings of this study provide some very sobering evidence that there is an imbalance in staffing of hospitals that may be harming patient outcomes. Overall, the study indicated that greater emphasis should be placed on ensuring nurses' education at the BSN level to produce improvements in patient care and minimize poor patient outcomes. Nurses must look to nursing research to further their knowledge and understanding of significant issues and concerns related to patient care. Although the sample size in this study was fairly large, more research is required to provide support for the conclusion that nurses need to further their nursing education by obtaining a BSN, MSN, or other appropriate degree. In addition, use of a random sample that includes a larger number of patients, hospitals, and nurses can improve the reliability of the results and lend more support to existing findings as well as generate ideas for new research. The study reported here could be replicated with an emphasis on patient education and drug therapy and could examine the educational levels of nurses and determine which ones are better prepared to conduct accurate and efficient patient teaching.

Based on Aiken L et al: Educational levels of hospital nurses and surgical patient mortality, *JAMA* 290:1617-1623, 2003.

Box 6-2   General Teaching and Learning Principles

- Make learning patient centered and individualized to each patient's needs, including his or her learning needs. This includes assessment of the patient's cultural beliefs, educational level, previous experience with medications, level of growth and development (to best select a teaching-learning strategy), age, gender, family support system, resources, ability to learn and way he or she learns best, and level of sophistication with regard to health care and own health care treatment.
- Assess the patient's motivation and readiness to learn.
- Assess the patient's ability to use and interpret label information on medication containers.
- Remember that a patient's ability to interpret drug instructions is culturally based and therefore somewhat consistent regardless of age, gender, or educational background.
- Some studies have shown that as much as 20% of the U.S. population is functionally illiterate. Therefore, ensure that educational strategies and materials are at a level that the patient is able to understand, while taking care to not embarrass the patient.
- If a patient is illiterate, he or she still needs to be instructed on safe medication administration. Use pictures, demonstrations, and return demonstrations to emphasize instructions.
- Consider, assess, and appreciate language and ethnicity during patient teaching. Make every effort to educate non–English-speaking patients in their native language. Ideally the patient should be instructed by a health professional familiar with the patient's clinical situation who also speaks the patient's native language. At the very least, provide the patient detailed written instructions in his or her native language.
- Assess the family support system for adequate patient teaching. Family living arrangements, financial status, resources, communication patterns, the roles of family members, and the power and authority of different family members should always be considered.
- Make the teaching-learning session simple, easy, fun, thorough, effective, and not monotonous. Make it applicable to daily life and schedule it at a time when the patient is ready to learn.
- Remember that learning occurs best with repetition and periods of demonstration and with the use of audiovisuals and other educational aids.
- Patient teaching should focus on the various processes/actions within the cognitive, affective, or psychomotor domains (see previous discussion).
- Consult online resources for help in obtaining the most up-to-date and accurate patient teaching materials and information.

LEGAL AND ETHICAL PRINCIPLES
Discharge Teaching

The safest practices for discharge teaching include the following:
- Always follow the health care facility's policy on discharge teaching regarding how much information to impart to the patient.
- Do not assume that any patient has received adequate teaching before interacting with you.
- Always begin discharge teaching as soon as possible when the patient is ready.
- Minimize any distractions during the teaching session.
- Evaluate any teaching of the patient and/or significant others by having the individuals repeat the instructions you have given them.
- Contact the institution's social services department or the discharge planner if there are any concerns regarding the learning capacity of the patient.
- Document what you taught, who was present with the patient during the teaching, what specific written instructions were given, what the responses of the patient and significant other or caregiver were, and what your own nursing actions were, such as specific demonstrations or referrals to community resources.
- Document teaching-learning strategies, such as the use of videos and pamphlets.

Modified from the U.S. Pharmacopeia Safe Medication Use Expert Committee Meeting, Rockville, Md, May 2003. Available at http://www.usp.org.

- Complete a medication calendar that includes medications to take and dosage schedule
- Use audiovisual aids
- Involve family members or significant others
- Keep the teaching on a level that is most meaningful to the given patient; general research on reading skills has shown that materials should be written at an eighth-grade reading level

Box 6-2 lists some general teaching and learning principles for the nurse to keep in mind.

Documentation of learning, including specific information about what was taught (content), strategies used, patient response, and evaluation of learning, should be carried out after the teaching-learning process has been completed. The nurse also should remember that patient teaching should begin upon admission to the health care setting and should be documented in the nurse's notes in the patient's chart. (For information on discharge teaching, see the Legal and Ethical Principles box on this page.) Throughout this textbook, patient education is integrated into each chapter in the Implementation subsection under Nursing Process.

EVALUATION OF PATIENT LEARNING RELATED TO DRUG THERAPY

Evaluation of patient learning is critical to safe patient drug administration. Nurses should always verify whether learning has occurred by asking the patient questions related to the teaching session and having the patient provide a return demonstration of any skills taught. The patient's behavior—such as adherence to the schedule for medication administration with few or no complications of therapy—is the key to determining whether the teaching was successful and learning occurred. If a patient's behavior evi-

Care Professional volume) by Thomson Microdex; this information would be appropriate to share with the patient. This type of resource may be helpful to the patient when he or she seeks information about a medication (e.g., purpose, adverse effects, method of administration, drug interactions) and helpful to the nurse in developing a patient teaching plan. The nurse should be sure to create a safe, nonthreatening, nondistracting environment for learning and to be receptive to the patient's questions.

The nurse should do the following to ensure the effectiveness of the teaching-learning session:
- Individualize the teaching session
- Provide positive rewards or reinforcement for accurate return demonstration of the procedure and/or technique during the teaching session

dences noncompliance or an inadequate level of learning, a new plan of teaching should be developed and implemented.

SUMMARY

Patient education is a critical part of patient care, and medication administration is no exception. From the time of initial contact with the patient throughout the time the nurse works with the patient, the patient is entitled to all information about the medications prescribed as well as other aspects of his or her patient care. Evaluation of patient learning and compliance with the medication regimen should be a continual process, and the nurse should always be willing to listen to the patient about any aspect of his or her drug therapy. The U.S. Pharmacopeia is an advocate for patient safety and medications, and a new Center for the Advancement of Patient Safety is taking on the challenging goal of zero deaths due to medication errors. This organization is also a tremendous resource for patient information for the health care professional so that quality patient education can be provided. The U.S. Pharmacopeia values patient education as a means of enhancing patient safety as well as a means of decreasing medication errors in the hospital setting or at home. Health care professionals must continue to be patient advocates and take the initiative to plan, design, create, and implement discharge teaching for drug therapy and other parts of the therapy regimen.

Patient Teaching Tips

- Teaching may need to focus on either the cognitive, affective, or psychomotor domain or a combination of all three. The cognitive domain includes thought processes and problem-solving abilities and may involve recall for synthesis of facts. The affective domain includes values and beliefs and involves behaviors such as responding, valuing, and organizing. The psychomotor domain includes gross motor movements, speech, and nonverbal communication and involves behaviors such as learning how to perform a procedure.

- A thorough assessment of the patient and/or the patient's spouse, significant other, family members, and caregivers and their readiness to learn is crucial to effective patient education.
- Realistic patient teaching goals should be established, and the patient should be involved in setting these goals.
- The importance to the patient of knowing about his or her medications to prevent errors and maximize therapeutic benefits should be emphasized to the patient.

Points to Remember

- Patient teaching is an important and very necessary part of the nursing function during the implementation phase of the nursing process to ensure safe and effective drug therapy.
- Patient teaching should occur after the nurse has thoroughly assessed the patient's readiness to learn, and a comprehensive, holistic approach should be adopted.
- Patients need to receive information through as many senses as possible, such as aurally and visually (as with pamphlets, videos, diagrams), to maximize learning. Information should also be on the patient's reading level, in the patient's native language (if possible), and suitable for the patient's level of cognitive development (see Erikson's stages in Box 6-1).
- Both the patient and any significant others should always be involved in the teaching process.

NCLEX Examination Review Questions

1. A 47-year-old patient with diabetes is being discharged to home and must take insulin injections twice a day. Which of the following statements is most accurate regarding proper teaching for this patient?
   a. Teaching should begin at the time of diagnosis or admission and should be individualized to the patient's reading level.
   b. The nurse can assume that because the patient is in his forties he will be able to read any written or printed documents provided.
   c. The majority of the teaching can be done with pamphlets that the patient can share with family members.
   d. A thorough and comprehensive teaching plan designed for an eleventh-grade reading level should be developed.
2. Which statement about discharge teaching and medications is correct? It should:
   a. be done right before the patient leaves the hospital or doctor's office.
   b. be reserved for when the patient is comfortable or after narcotics are administered.
   c. include videos, demonstrations, and instructions written at least at the fifth-grade level.
   d. be individualized and based on the patient's level of cognitive development.
3. The nurse is responsible for the preoperative teaching for a patient who is mildly anxious about receiving narcotics postoperatively. As a nurse, you acknowledge that this level of anxiety may
   a. impede learning because no anxiety is helpful.
   b. lead to major unsteadiness of emotional status.
   c. result in learning by increasing the patient's willingness to learn.
   d. reorganize the patient's thoughts and lead to inadequate potential for learning.
4. What action by the nurse is the best way to assess a patient's learning needs?
   a. Quiz the patient daily on all medications
   b. Begin with validation of the patient's present level of knowledge
   c. Assess family members' knowledge of the prescribed medication even if they are not involved in the patient's care
   d. Question other caregivers about their level of experience with the drug regimen and assume lack of interest if no answers are given
5. Which of the following techniques would be most appropriate for teaching a patient with a potential language barrier?
   a. Obtain an interpreter who can speak in the patient's native tongue for teaching sessions
   b. Use detailed and lengthy explanations, speaking slowly and clearly
   c. If the nurse notes that there are no questions, it can be assumed that the patient is understanding the information
   d. Provide only written instructions

1. a, 2. d, 3. c, 4. b, 5. a.

Critical Thinking Activities

1. Your patient is a 65-year-old woman with diabetes mellitus who is to begin treatment with insulin injections. Develop a 10-minute teaching plan on the basics of subcutaneous self-administration of insulin.
2. Formulate a teaching plan for a 69-year-old male patient who has experienced a left-sided stroke, is aphasic, and is paralyzed on the right side. He is going to be returning home, where his wife will care for him. Your discharge teaching will be directed at the patient and his wife, and you are to teach them about safety measures for the patient, who has slight difficulty in swallowing and will be taking oral medications after he is sent home. He tolerates liquids, soft foods, and thickened liquids fairly well.
3. Your patient does not speak English or understand any of your communication techniques thus far. Develop a plan of care that addresses the patient's need for medication information on the cardiac drug digoxin and also focuses on the potential for toxicity. (Note that you may need to look up the drug in the textbook if you are not familiar with it.)

For answers, see http://evolve.elsevier.com/Lilley.

Over-the-Counter Drugs and Herbal and Dietary Supplements

Objectives

When you reach the end of this chapter, you should be able to do the following:

1. Discuss the differences between prescription drugs, over-the-counter (OTC) drugs, herbals, and dietary supplements.
2. Briefly discuss the differences between the federal legislation governing the promotion and sale of prescription drugs and that governing OTC drugs, herbals, and dietary supplements.
3. Describe the advantages and disadvantages of the use of OTC drugs, herbals, and dietary supplements.
4. Explain the proper use of OTC drugs, herbals, and dietary supplements.
5. Discuss the potential dangers associated with the use of OTC drugs, herbals, and dietary supplements.
6. Develop a nursing care plan for the patient who uses OTC drugs, herbals, and/or dietary supplements.

e-Learning Activities

Companion CD

- NCLEX Review Questions: see questions 33-36
- Animations
- Audio Glossary
- Category Catchers
- Medication Errors Checklists
- IV Therapy Checklists

evolve Website (http://evolve.elsevier.com/Lilley)

• Nursing Care Plans • Frequently Asked Questions • Content Updates • WebLinks • Supplemental Resources • Elsevier ePharmacology Update • Medication Administration Animations

Glossary

Alternative medicine Herbal medicine, chiropractic, acupuncture, reflexology, and any other therapies not taught in a medical school but used for health care. (p. 78)

Commission E Monographs Comprehensive published herbal recommendations from the German equivalent of the U.S. Food and Drug Administration. (p. 78)

Complementary medicine *Alternative medicine,* when used simultaneously with, as opposed to instead of, standard Western medicine. (p. 78)

Conventional medicine The practice of medicine as taught in a Western medical school. (p. 78)

Dietary supplement A product taken by mouth that contains an ingredient intended to supplement the diet, including vitamins, minerals, herbs or other botanicals, amino acids, and substances such as enzymes, organ tissues, glandular preparations, metabolites, extracts, and concentrates. (p. 77)

Herbal medicine The practice of using herbs to heal. (p. 78)

Herbs Herbaceous plants as well as the bark, roots, leaves, seeds, flowers, and fruit of trees, shrubs, and woody vines, and extracts of these plants and materials that are valued for their savory, aromatic, or medicinal qualities. (p. 78)

Iatrogenic effects Unintentional adverse effects that are caused by the actions of a physician or other health care professional or by a specific treatment. (p. 78)

Legend drugs Medications that are not legally available without a prescription from a licensed prescriber (e.g., physician, nurse practitioner, physician assistant; also called *prescription drugs*). (p. 79)

Over-the-counter drugs Medications that are legally available without a prescription. (p. 75)

Phytochemicals The pharmacologically active ingredients in herbal remedies. (p. 80)

OVER-THE-COUNTER DRUGS

Health care consumers are becoming increasingly involved in the diagnosis and treatment of common ailments. This has led to a great increase in the use of nonprescription or **over-the-counter drugs** (OTC drugs). OTC medications now account for about 60% of all medications used in the United States. Health care consumers use OTC drugs to treat or cure more than 400 different ailments. About 30% of the new OTC drugs marketed between 1975 and 1994 were products that had been changed from prescription to OTC status.

For nurses to understand current OTC classification, it is helpful for them to have some background on the U.S. Food and Drug Administration (FDA) approval process for OTC medications. Box 7-1 lists major legislative changes affecting the drug approval process. The purpose of the 1972 OTC Drug Review was to ensure the safety and effectiveness of the OTC products available at that time as well as appropriate labeling standards for these drugs. As a result of this review, approximately one third of the more than 500 OTC products then available were determined to be safe and effective for their intended uses and one third were found to be ineffective. A small number were considered to be unsafe, and the remainder required submission of additional data before their safety and effectiveness could be established. Products determined to be unsafe were removed from the market. Some established products that were found to be ineffective but not unsafe were "grandfathered in" and allowed to remain on the market. Many of these have gradually slipped into obscurity and are no longer sold.

Another result of the OTC Drug Review was the reclassification from prescription to OTC status of more than 40 primary product ingredients. The FDA's Nonprescription Drugs Advisory Committee is responsible for the reclassification of prescription drug products to OTC status. A drug must meet the criteria listed in Box 7-2 to be considered for reclassification. The required information is obtained from clinical trial results and postmarketing safety surveillance data, which are submitted to the FDA by the manufacturer of the product. Although this reclassification procedure has been criticized as overly time-consuming, it is structured to ensure that products reclassified to OTC status are safe and effective when used by the average consumer.

OTC status has many advantages over prescription status. Patients can conveniently and effectively self-treat many minor ailments. Some professionals argue that allowing patients to self-treat minor illnesses enables physicians to spend more time caring for patients with serious health problems. Others argue that it delays patients from seeking medical care until they are very ill. The financial effect of this status change is enormous: by the year 2010, OTC sales in the United States will reach an estimated $22 billion.

Manufacturers often benefit as well by prolonging market exclusivity without competition from generic products.

Reclassification of a prescription drug as an OTC drug may increase out-of-pocket costs for many patients. The reason is that third-party health insurance payers refuse to pay for OTC products. However, overall health care costs tend to decrease when reclassification occurs due to a direct reduction in drug costs, elimination of physician office visits, and avoidance of pharmacy dispensing fees. A case in point is the reclassification of cough and cold products to OTC status. This reclassification resulted in annual consumer health care savings of approximately $1 billion. Some examples of drugs that have recently been reclassified as OTC products appear in Box 7-3.

The importance of patient education cannot be overstated. Many patients are inexperienced in the interpretation of medication labels, which results in misuse of the products (Figure 7-1). The lack of experience and possibly deficient knowledge about the medication may lead to adverse events or drug interactions with prescription medications or even other OTC medications. Small print on the label often complicates the problem, especially for elderly patients. Another common problem associated with OTC drugs is that their use may postpone effective management of chronic disease states and may delay treatment of serious and/or life-threatening disorders. This is because the OTC medication may relieve symptoms without necessarily addressing the cause of the disorder.

Normally, OTC medications should be used only for short-term treatment of common minor illnesses. An appropriate medical evaluation should be sought for all chronic health conditions, even if the final decision is to prescribe OTC medications. Patient

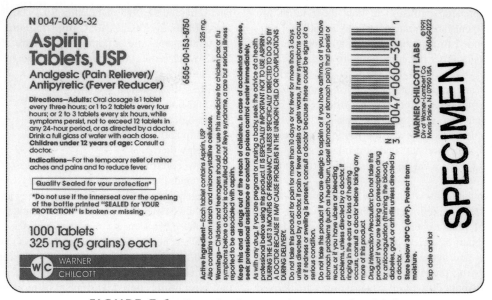

FIGURE 7-1   Example of an over-the-counter drug label.

Table 7-1   Common Over-the-Counter (OTC) Drugs

Type of OTC Drug	Examples	Where Discussed in This Book
Acid-controlling drugs (H₂ blockers) and antacids	cimetidine (Tagamet), famotidine (Pepcid), nizatidine (Axid), ranitidine (Zantac); aluminum- and magnesium-containing products (Maalox, Mylanta); calcium-containing products (Tums)	Chapter 51: Acid-Controlling Drugs
Antiasthma drugs, including mast cell stabilizers	cromolyn (Nasalcrom), epinephrine (Primatene Mist)	Chapter 36: Bronchodilators and Other Respiratory Drugs
Antifungal drugs (topical)	butoconazole (Femstat), clotrimazole (Lotrimin), miconazole (Monistat)	Chapter 57: Dermatologic Drugs
Antihistamines and decongestants	brompheniramine (Dimetapp), chlorpheniramine (Contac, Theraflu), clemastine (Tavist), diphenhydramine (Benadryl), guaifenesin (Robitussin), loratadine (Claritin), pseudoephedrine (Sudafed)	Chapter 35: Antihistamines, Decongestants, Antitussives, and Expectorants
Eyedrops	Artificial tears (Moisture Eyes, Murine)	Chapter 58: Ophthalmic Drugs
Hair growth drugs (topical)	minoxidil (Rogaine)	Chapter 57: Dermatologic Drugs
Pain-relieving drugs		
Analgesics	acetaminophen (Tylenol)	Chapter 10: Analgesic Drugs
NSAIDs	aspirin, ibuprofen (Advil, Motrin)	Chapter 44: Antiinflammatory, Antirheumatoid, and Related Drugs

NSAID, Nonsteroidal antiinflammatory drug.

assessment should definitely include questions regarding OTC drug use, including what conditions OTC medications are being used to treat. Such questions may help uncover more serious ongoing medical problems that require further evaluation. Patients should be informed that OTC medications, including herbal products, are still medications. Because of this, their use may have associated risks depending on the specific OTC drugs used, concurrent prescription medications, and the patient's overall health status and disease states.

Health care professionals have an excellent opportunity to prevent common problems associated with the use of reclassified drugs. Up to 60% of patients consult a health care professional when selecting an OTC product. Patients should be provided with verbal information about choice of an appropriate product, correct dosing, common adverse effects, and drug interactions with other medications.

For specific information on various OTC drugs, see the appropriate drug chapters later in this text (see Table 7-1 for cross-references to these chapters).

HERBALS AND DIETARY SUPPLEMENTS

History

Dietary supplement is a broad term for orally administered alternative medicines and includes the category of herbal supplement. Basic definitions are provided here to ensure complete understanding and to prevent confusion in how these terms are used. Dietary supplements are products taken by mouth that contain ingredients intended to augment the diet and include vitamins, minerals, herbs or other botanicals, amino acids, and substances such as enzymes, organ tissues, glandular products, metabolites, extracts, and concentrates. Dietary supplements may also be extracts or concentrates and may be produced in many forms, such as tablets, capsules, softgels, gelcaps, liquids, or powders. These supplements may also be found in nutritional, breakfast, snack, or health food bars and/or drinks or shakes. Labeling must be provided but must *not* represent the product to be a conventional food item.

Herbs come from nature and include the leaves, bark, berries, roots, gums, seeds, stems, and flowers of plants. They have been used for thousands of years to help maintain good health. Herbs have been an integral part of society because of their culinary and medicinal properties, and herbs have made numerous contributions to commercial drug preparations that are currently manufactured (Table 7-2). About 30% of all modern drugs are derived from plants. In the early nineteenth century, scientific methods became more advanced and became the preferred means of healing. At this time, the practice of botanical healing was dismissed as quackery. **Herbal medicine** lost ground to new synthetic medicines as the development of patent medicines grew during the early part of the twentieth century. These new synthetically derived medicines were touted by scientists and physicians as more effective and reliable.

In the 1960s, concerns were expressed over the **iatrogenic effects** of **conventional medicine.** These concerns, along with a desire for more self-reliance, led to a renewed interest in "natural health," and as a result the use of herbal products increased. In 1974 the World Health Organization encouraged developing countries to use traditional plant medicines to "fulfill a need unmet by modern systems." In 1978 the German equivalent of the FDA published a series of herbal recommendations known as the **Commission E Monographs.** These monographs focus on herbs whose effectiveness for specific indications is supported by the research literature. Worldwide use of herbal medicines again became popular. Recognition of the rising use of herbal products and other nontraditional remedies, known as **alternative medicine,** led to the establishment of the Office of Alternative Medicine by the National Institutes of Health in 1992. This office was

later renamed the National Center for Complementary and Alternative Medicine (NCCAM). **Complementary medicine** refers to the simultaneous use of both traditional and alternative medicine. NCCAM classifies complementary and alternative medicine into five categories:

1. Alternative medical systems
2. Mind-body interventions
3. Biologically based therapies
4. Manipulative and body-based methods
5. Energy therapies

Many controversies remain about the safety and control of herbals and dietary supplements, but they continue to be used in the United States and abroad. Because they are freely available in the United States and their uses and advantages are widely publicized, these products are marketed and placed in grocery stores, pharmacies, health food stores, and fitness gyms and can even be ordered through television and radio and over the Internet. With greater use, their therapeutic effects have been acknowledged, and they have been believed by some to be more beneficial than existing synthetic and natural prescription drugs. Adverse effects are considered to be minimal by the public as well as by the companies and businesses that sell these supplements. A false sense of security has been created by their widespread use, however, and the view of the public tends to be that if a product is "natural," then it is safe. Federal legislation and the FDA still do not provide safeguards and monitoring of dietary supplements. Currently, only the manufacturing companies are responsible for ensuring that their products are safe before they are put on the market. Unlike prescription drugs, dietary supplements do not have to be proven safe and effective for their intended use before marketing. In fact, the law contains no provisions for the FDA to approve herbals and dietary supplements for safety and effectiveness before these products reach the consumer.

A review of the last decade's legislation shows the controversy that persists about these drugs. Important to mention is the landmark event that occurred in the early 1990s. In 1993, FDA Commissioner David Kessler threatened to remove dietary supplements from the market. In addition, he proposed to change the law to ensure the safety and efficacy of herbals before any more consumers sustained injury or harm. The American public responded with a massive letter-writing campaign to Congress, and the 103rd Congress responded by passing the Dietary Supplement and Health Education Act (DSHEA) of 1994. One of the responsibilities of DSHEA is to define dietary supplements and provide the regulatory framework for their sale.

In June of 2000, Kessler continued his crusade against herbals and dietary supplements and publicly stated that these "natural" products were not without major concerns. In Kessler's view, Congress showed little interest in protecting consumers from the hazards of dietary supplements, and the public did not completely understand how potentially dangerous these products were. Congress showed little interest in protecting consumers from the hazards of dietary supplements, and the public did not completely understand how potentially dangerous these products were. Kessler's continued concern about herbal and dietary supplements was prompted by information showing that a Chinese herb, *Aristolochia fang-chi,* could damage the kidneys of individuals who were taking it. Kessler argued that change was needed in the controversial DSHEA, which he declared had allowed the $15-billion-dollar

Table 7-2	**Conventional Medicines Derived from Plants**
Medicine*	**Plant**
atropine	*Atropa belladonna*
capsaicin	*Capsicum frutescens*
cocaine	*Erythroxylon coca*
codeine	*Papaver somniferum*
ipecac	*Cephaelis ipecacuanha*
quinine	*Cinchona officinalis*
scopolamine	*Datura fastuosa*
senna	*Cassia acutifolia*
paclitaxel	*Taxis brevifolia*
vincristine	*Catharanthus roseus*

*Includes both over-the-counter and prescription drugs.

supplement industry to escape regulation. Kessler's position reflected his basic belief that the current method of handling herbals and dietary supplements was not working. In 2002, the U.S. Pharmacopeia (USP), an independent organization that is the government's official standard-setting authority for dietary supplements, announced that it had begun to issue certification for hundreds of products that it had independently tested as part of its Dietary Supplement Verification Program.

A major difference between **legend drugs** (prescription drugs) and dietary supplements is that DSHEA requires no proof of efficacy or safety and sets no standards for quality control for products labeled as supplements. The FDA has specific and stringent requirements for manufacturers of legend drugs; manufacturers of supplements may claim effect but cannot promise a specific cure on the label. However, DSHEA, which amended the Federal Food, Drug, and Cosmetic Act, created a new regulatory framework for the safety and labeling of dietary supplements.

Under DSHEA, a supplement manufacturer is responsible for determining the safety of its products and must be able to substantiate any claims regarding product efficacy for specific conditions. This means that dietary supplements do not need approval from the FDA before they are marketed. Except in the case of a new dietary ingredient, for which premarket safety data and other information are required by law, a manufacturer does not have to provide the FDA with the evidence on which it relies to substantiate the safety or effectiveness of a product before or after it markets the product. In fact, there are currently no FDA regulations that establish a minimum standard of practice for manufacturing dietary supplements. At present, the manufacturer is responsible for setting its own manufacturing practice guidelines to ensure that the dietary supplements it produces are safe and contain the ingredients listed on the label. In contrast, regulating agencies in Germany, France, the United Kingdom, and Canada require manufacturers to meet standards of herbal quality and safety assessment.

The FDA posts recent warnings on herbal products on its website (http://www.fda.gov).

Consumer Use of Dietary Supplements

In general, consumers use dietary supplements therapeutically for the treatment and cure of diseases and pathologic conditions, prophylactically for long-term prevention of disease, and proactively to preserve health and wellness and boost the immune system (e.g., reduce cardiovascular risk factors, increase liver and immune system functions, increase feelings of wellness). In addition, herbs and phytomedicinals can be used as adjunct therapy to support conventional pharmaceutical therapies. Such use is seen especially in societies in which phytotherapy, or the use of herbal medicines in clinical practice, is considerably more integrated with conventional medicine, such as in Germany.

Some herbal products may be used to treat minor conditions and illnesses (e.g., coughs, colds, stomach upset) in much the same way that conventional FDA-approved OTC nonprescription drugs are used. As the number of herbal products on the market increases, nurses will have more opportunities for patient education about these products.

Safety

Dietary supplements, and especially herbal medicines, are often perceived as being natural and therefore harmless; however, this is not the case. Many examples exist of allergic reactions, toxic reactions, and adverse effects caused by herbs. Some herbs have been shown to have possible mutagenic effects and to interact with drug (see the Herbal Therapies and Dietary Supplements box for drug interactions with herbal and dietary supplements). Cases have also been reported in which whole plants or parts of plants have not been identified properly and thus are mislabeled. Because of underreporting, present knowledge may represent but a small fraction of potential safety concerns. Also, as mentioned previously, the FDA has limited

---

HERBAL THERAPIES AND DIETARY SUPPLEMENTS

Selected Herbs and Dietary Supplements and Their Possible Drug Interactions

Herb or Dietary Supplement	Possible Drug Interaction
Chamomile	Increased risk for bleeding with anticoagulants
Cranberry	Decreased elimination of many drugs that are renally excreted
Echinacea	Possible interference with or counteraction to immunosuppressant drugs
Evening primrose	Possible interaction with antipsychotic drugs
Garlic	Possible interference with hypoglycemic therapy
Ginger root	At high dosages, possible interference with cardiac, antidiabetic, or anticoagulant drugs
Grapefruit	Decreases metabolism of drugs used for erectile dysfunction
	Decreases metabolism of estrogens, some psychotherapeutic drugs (sertraline)
	Increases risk of toxicity of immunosuppressants and some psychotherapeutic drugs (pimozide, escitalopram)
	Increases intensity and duration of effects of caffeine
Hawthorn	May lead to toxic levels of cardiac glycosides (e.g., digitalis)
Kava	May increase the effect of barbiturates and alcohol
Saw palmetto	May change the effects of hormones in oral contraceptive drugs, patches, or hormonal replacement therapies
St. John's wort	If other serotonergic drugs are also used (such as selective serotonin reuptake inhibitors [Chapter 15]), may lead to serotonin syndrome
Valerian	Increases central nervous system depression if used with sedatives

Modified from Huang SM et al: Drug interactions with herbal products and grapefruit juice, *Clin Pharmacol Ther* 75(1):1-12, 2004; Wolinsky I, Williams L: *Nutrition in pharmacy practice,* Washington, DC, 2003, APHA Publications.

oversight of how dietary supplements are prepared, whether herbal or not.

There are certainly fewer published scientific data regarding the relative safety of dietary supplements than regarding the safety of synthetic drug treatments. Two recent examples of some of the growing concerns about herbal remedies include the FDA warnings about possible liver toxicity with the use of kava and possible cardiovascular and stroke risks with the use of ephedra. Ephedra was officially banned by the FDA in April of 2004. Kava remains on the market despite a 2002 FDA consumer warning letter regarding the risk of liver toxicity. Health care providers should be on constant watch for literature about the safe and effective use of dietary supplements as well as reported adverse effects or problems. For some dietary supplements, the risk may be lower than that for conventional drugs. The discriminate and proper use of some dietary supplements is safe and may provide some therapeutic benefits, but the indiscriminate or excessive use of dietary supplements can be dangerous. The FDA has established MedWatch, which has a toll-free number (800-332-1088) consumers can call to report adverse effects of dietary supplements or of any drugs or medical devices.

Epidemiology

The FDA estimates that over 29,000 different dietary supplements are currently used in the United States, with approximately 1000 new products introduced annually. The many different herbs in these preparations contain a wide variety of active **phytochemicals** (plant compounds). A great deal of public interest in the use of dietary supplements remains. Estimates of the prevalence of dietary supplement use differ greatly, with various studies concluding that between 3% and 93% of the U.S. population, including nearly 16% of those taking prescription drugs, use these products. The wide disparity in these estimates is most likely due to the use of varying terminology (e.g., "herbs" vs. "dietary supplements") and differences in the wording of questions regarding length of use (e.g., "have you ever used" vs. "have you used in the last 12 months"). One recent estimate of the amount spent on dietary supplements was $17.8 billion annually in the United States. Although this figure is high, the use of botanical medicines is generally greater in other parts of the world (e.g., Europe) than it is in the United States.

Herbal medicine is based on the premise that plants contain natural substances that can promote health and alleviate illness. Some of the more common ailments and conditions treated with herbs are anxiety, arthritis, colds, constipation, cough, depression, fever, headache, infection, insomnia, intestinal disorders, premenstrual syndrome, menopausal symptoms, stress, ulcers, and weakness.

Herbal products constitute the largest growth area in retail pharmacy. Their use is increasing at a rate of 20% to 25% a year, which far exceeds the growth in the use of conventional drugs. Insurance plans and managed care organizations are beginning to offer reimbursement for alternative treatments. One managed care organization made the decision to cover herbal remedies based on a survey showing that 33% of its 1.5 million members had sought alternative treatments in the previous 2 years. The most commonly used herbal remedies are aloe, echinacea, feverfew, garlic, ginkgo, ginseng, goldenseal, hawthorn, St. John's wort, saw palmetto, and valerian. These products are covered in more detail in the Herbal Therapies and Dietary Supplements boxes that appear in various drug chapters (see inside back cover for a complete listing of these boxes with page numbers).

◆ NURSING PROCESS

◆ ASSESSMENT

Over-the-Counter Drugs

Assessment of patients taking any type of OTC drug should include consideration of allergies to any of the ingredients. A medication history must be taken that documents *all* medications and substances used (including prescription drugs, OTC drugs, herbal products, and vitamins and minerals, plus alcohol and tobacco). Also needed is a past and present medical history so that possible drug interactions, contraindications, and cautions may be identified. Patients should be screened carefully before an OTC drug is recommended, because patients may assume that if a drug is sold OTC then it must be completely safe and without negative consequences. This is not true; OTC drugs can be just as lethal or problematic as prescription drugs if they are not taken properly or are taken in high dosages and without regard to directions. Consumer safety begins with education, and the best way for patients to help themselves as consumers is for them to learn how to assess each situation, weigh all the factors, and find out all they can about any OTC product they consider using. Nursing assessments should be performed if the situation arises, but in most situations the patient is self-medicating. Reading level, cognitive level, motor abilities, previous use of OTC drugs, successes versus failures with drug therapies and self-medication, and caregiver support are just a few of the variables to be assessed as the nurse deems appropriate for the given situation.

Assessment of the patient's knowledge about the components of self-medication, including the positive or negative consequences of the use of a given OTC drug, is important to include. Assessment of the patient's (or caregiver's or family member's) level of knowledge and experience with OTC self-medication is critical to patient's safety, as is assessment of attitudes toward and beliefs about drug therapy, such as too casual an attitude or a lack of respect for and concern about the use OTC drugs. Such a belief system may very easily result in overuse, overdosage, and potential complications. The patient's level of readiness and developmental stage must also be assessed to allow individualized teaching.

Generally speaking, laboratory tests are not ordered before OTC drugs are taken because they are self-administered and self-monitored. However, there are situations in which patients may be taking certain medications that react adversely with OTC drugs and in which such testing may be deemed necessary. Certain patient groups are also at higher risk for adverse reactions to OTC drugs (as well as to all drugs), including elderly patients, pediatric patients, patients with single and/or multiple acute and chronic illnesses, those who are frail or in poor health, debilitated and nutritionally deficient patients, and those who are immuno-compromised. Other groups for which there may be cautions and contraindications for OTC drug use are patients with a history of renal, hepatic, cardiac, or vascular disorders. More assessment information for OTC drugs, herbals, and dietary supplements is provided in chapters that have corresponding drug/pharmacology content (see Table 7-1). The patient should be aware of contraindications, cautions, and drug interactions.

Herbal Products and Dietary Supplements

Many herbal products and dietary supplements are readily available in drug, health food, and grocery stores as well as in gardens, kitchens, and medicine cabinets. The most commonly used herbal and dietary supplements discussed in this book are aloe, echinacea, garlic, ginkgo, ginseng, St. John's wort, saw palmetto, and valerian. Although patients generally self-administer these products and do not perform an assessment, the nurse in various settings may be able to assess the patient through a head-to-toe physical examination, medical and nursing history, and medication history. Assessment data and factors and variables to consider should be shared with the patient for the patient's safety. This sharing of assessment information allows the health care provider to be sure that the patient who is taking herbal products is taking them in as safe a manner as possible. Many herbals and dietary supplements can potentially cause a variety of side effects. For example, some cause dermatitis when used topically and others are associated with nephritis. Therefore, for example, patients with existing skin problems or kidney dysfunction should seek medical advice before using certain herbal products. Contraindications, cautions, and drug interactions should be considered by the patient and nurse. See the Herbal Therapies and Dietary Supplements box on page 79 for drug interactions with herbals and dietary supplements.

✦ NURSING DIAGNOSES

Nursing diagnoses appropriate for the patient who is taking OTC drugs, herbals, and/or dietary supplements include the following:

- Acute pain related to various disease processes
- Chronic pain related to tissue injury
- Impaired physical mobility related to disease processes or injury
- Deficient knowledge related to first-time drug therapy with an OTC and/or herbal product
- Risk for injury related to potential drug interactions and adverse reactions of OTC and herbal products
- Risk for injury to self related to possible nicotine withdrawal (applies to patients using a smoking deterrent system)

✦ PLANNING

Goals

- Patient is able to describe the use of the drug in relation to symptoms or complaints.
- Patient experiences pain relief or relief of the symptoms of the disease process or injury within the expected time period.
- Patient reports both adverse effects and therapeutic responses to the appropriate health care professional.

- Patient states the rationale for and proper use of the drug.
- Patient states the adverse effects, cautions, and contraindications associated with the use of the drug.
- Patient has minimal complaints and experiences minimal side effects related to the use of the drug.
- Patient remains free from injury related to the possible improper use of the drug.
- Patient avoids adverse effects from improper self-administration (e.g., properly applies a transdermal patch).

Outcome Criteria

- Patient states the actions of the OTC drug, herbal, or dietary supplement as well as methods to minimize side effects and enhance therapeutic effects.
- Patient identifies factors that aggravate or alleviate symptoms for which the drug is being taken.
- Patient describes nonpharmacologic approaches to the treatment of symptoms, such as the use of hot or cold packs, physical therapy, massage, relaxation therapy, biofeedback, imagery, and hypnosis.
- Patient states the importance of immediately reporting any severe side effects or complications associated with the OTC drug, herbal, or dietary supplement, such as changes in blood pressure, clotting, or lack of clotting.
- Patient experiences relief of symptoms (the actual indication for the use of the OTC, herbal, or dietary supplement), such as a decrease in itching, pain, swelling, cold symptoms, or cough.
- Patient takes the OTC drug, herbal, or dietary supplement product as indicated, using proper dosage and technique (using no more than is directed) and knows when to stop medication if certain untoward effects occur.
- Patient contacts a health care provider or local poison control hotline should toxicity or complications occur.
- Patient demonstrates the correct technique for using the transdermal route or any other route of administration, including the specific steps required.

✦ IMPLEMENTATION

With OTC drugs, the most important determinant of safe patient self-administration is whether the patient receives thorough and individualized patient education. Patients need to receive as much information as possible and should understand that although these drugs are nonprescription they are *not* completely safe and without toxicity. Instructions should include information about safe use, frequency of dosing and dose, specifics of how to take the medication (e.g., with food or at bedtime), and steps the patient may take to prevent complications and toxic effects. Another consideration is the dosage form, because a variety of dosage forms are available, from liquids, tablets, and enteric-coated tablets to patches and gum. Instructions must be provided and the need to recheck dosage emphasized. With many of the patches used today for smoking cessation and for other indications, it is crucial to emphasize the proper use and application of the transdermal patch systems. For patients using herbal products (as for those using OTC drugs and other dietary supplements), education is of utmost importance for safe and effective use. The health care provider must inform the patient that the companies manufacturing herbals and dietary supplements are not required to provide

Drug Responses and Cultural Factors

Responses to drugs—including over-the-counter (OTC) drugs, herbals, and dietary supplements—may be affected by beliefs, values, and genetics as well as by culture, race, and ethnicity (see Chapter 4 for more discussion of cultural considerations). As one example of cultural impact on drug response and use, if patients who are Japanese experience nausea, vomiting, and bowel changes as side effects of OTC drugs, herbals, and/or dietary supplements, these often are not mentioned. The reason is that this culture finds it unacceptable to complain about gastrointestinal symptoms, and so they may go unreported to the point of causing risk to the patient.

Herbal and alternative therapies may also be used more extensively in some cultures than in others. Wide acceptance of herbal use without major concern for the effects on other therapies may be very problematic because of the many interactions of conventional drugs with herbals and dietary supplements. For example, the Chinese herb ginseng may inhibit or accelerate the metabolism of a specific medication and significantly affect the drug's absorption or elimination.

Genetic factors that have an influence on drug response include acetylation polymorphism; that is, prescription drugs, OTC drugs, herbals, and dietary supplements may be metabolized in different ways that are genetically determined and vary with race or ethnicity. For example, populations of European or African descent have approximately equal numbers of individuals showing rapid and slow acetylation (which affects drug metabolism), whereas Japanese and Inuit populations may contain more rapid acetylators. See Chapter 4 for a more in-depth discussion of these specific genetic attributes.

Modified from Munoz C, Hilgenberg C: Ethnopharmacology, *Am J Nurs* 105(8):40-49, 2005.

evidence of safety and effectiveness. Unfortunately, many patients believe that no risks exist if a medication is herbal and "natural." It is important for patients to realize that even if a product is natural, it must be taken as cautiously as any other medication. The health care provider must also emphasize that herbals are not FDA-approved drugs; therefore, their labeling cannot be relied on to provide adequate instructions for use or even warning information. The fact that a drug is an herbal or a dietary supplement does not mean that it can be safely administered to children, infants, pregnant or lactating women, or patients with certain health conditions that put them at risk.

◆ EVALUATION

Patients taking OTC drugs, herbals, or dietary supplements should carefully monitor themselves for unusual or adverse reactions and therapeutic responses to the medication to prevent overuse. The range of therapeutic responses will vary, depending on the specific drug and the indication for which it is used. These responses may include decreased pain; decreased stiffness and swelling in joints; increased ability to carry out the activities of daily living; the ability to move around with greater ease; increased hair growth; decreased asthma-related, gastrointestinal, or allergic symptoms; decreased vaginal itching and discharge; increased healing; increased sleep; decreased fatigue; improved energy; and others. For specific nursing diagnoses, planning, outcome criteria, nursing implementation, and evaluation information related to various OTC drugs, see the appropriate drug chapters later in this text (see Table 7-1 for cross-references to these chapters).

Patient Teaching Tips

- Provide verbal and written information about how to choose an appropriate OTC drug or herbal or dietary supplement as well as information about correct dosing, common side effects, and possible interactions with other medications.
- Many patients believe that no risks exist if a medication is herbal and "natural" or if it is sold OTC, so provide adequate education about the drug or product as well as all the pros and cons of its use, because this is crucial to patient safety.
- Provide instructions on how to read OTC drug, herbal, and dietary supplement labels.
- Emphasize the importance of taking all OTC drugs, herbals, and dietary supplements with extreme caution, being aware of all the possible interactions and/or concerns associated with the use of these products, and informing all health care providers about their use.

- Encourage journaling of any improvement of symptoms noted with the use of a specific OTC drug, herbal, and/or dietary supplement.
- Encourage the use of appropriate and authoritative resources for patient information.
- Instruct that all medications, whether OTC drug, herbal, dietary supplement, or prescription drug, should be kept out of the reach of children and pets.
- Provide thorough instructions for the various dosage forms of OTC drugs, herbals, and dietary supplements, such as how to mix powders and how to properly use transdermal patches, inhalers, ointments, lotions, nose drops, ophthalmic drops, elixirs, suppositories, vaginal suppositories or creams, and all other dosage forms (Chapter 9); also provide information about proper storage and cleansing of any equipment.

Points to Remember

- Consumers use herbal products therapeutically for the treatment and cure of diseases and pathologic conditions, prophylactically for long-term prevention of disease, and proactively for the maintenance of health and wellness.
- The FDA has established the MedWatch program to track adverse events and/or problems related to drug therapy. The toll-free number for reporting adverse effects of prescription drugs, OTC drugs, herbals, and dietary supplements is 800-332-1088. Nurses may report adverse events anonymously and without consequence.
- Some of the more commonly used herbal remedies are aloe, echinacea, garlic, ginkgo, ginseng, grapefruit extract, grapefruit juice,

St. John's wort, saw palmetto, and valerian. The nurse needs to be informed about these products so that adequate patient education can be provided regarding potential risks and adverse drug reactions, and drug interactions can be prevented or minimized.
- Herbal products are not FDA-approved drugs, and therefore their labeling cannot be relied on to provide consumers and patients with adequate instructions for use or even information about warnings.
- The fact that a drug is an herbal product, dietary supplement, or OTC medication is no guarantee that it can be safely administered to children, infants, pregnant or lactating women, or patients with certain health conditions that may put them at risk.

NCLEX Examination Review Questions

1. When reviewing a list of OTC drugs taken by a patient, the nurse recalls that the most commonly used OTC products currently available include which types of drugs?
   a. Mild antihypertensives
   b. Diuretics
   c. Acid-controlling drugs
   d. Drugs for bladder control
2. For the safe use of herbal products, it is important to educate patients that
   a. herbal and OTC products are approved by the FDA and under strict regulation.
   b. these products are tested for safety by the FDA and the USP.
   c. no side effects are associated with these products because they are natural and may be purchased without a prescription.
   d. labeling is not reliable in providing proper instructions or warnings, and the products should be taken with caution.
3. When taking a patient's drug history, the nurse asks about use of OTC drugs. The patient responds by saying, "Oh, I frequently take something for my headaches, but I didn't mention it because aspirin is nonprescription." What is the best response from the nurse?
   a. "That's true, over-the-counter drugs are generally not harmful."
   b. "Aspirin is one of the safest drugs out there."
   c. "Although aspirin is over the counter, it's still important to know why you take it, how much you take, and how often."
   d. "We need you to be honest about the drugs you are taking— are there any others that you haven't told us about?"

4. When making a home visit to a patient who was recently discharged from the hospital, the nurse notes that she has a small pack over her chest and that the pack has a strong odor. She also is drinking herbal tea. When asked about the pack and the tea, she says, "Oh, my grandmother never used medicines from the doctor. She told me that this plaster and tea were all I would need to fix things." Which of the following responses by the nurse is most appropriate?
   a. "You really should listen to what the doctor told you if you want to get better."
   b. "What's in the plaster and the tea? When do you usually use them?"
   c. "These herbal remedies rarely work, but if you want to use them, then it is your choice."
   d. "It's fine if you want to use this home remedy, as long as you use it with your prescription medicines."
5. Which of the following is true of current legislation regarding herbal products?
   a. Herbals were regulated in the early 1900s with regard to efficacy and toxicity.
   b. DSHEA permits the sale of herbal remedies as dietary supplements.
   c. The Kefauver-Harris Amendment was passed to help prevent carcinogenic effects related to herbal products.
   d. The Durham-Humphrey Amendment was specifically designed to regulate the safety and efficacy of OTC drugs and herbal agents.

1. c, 2. d, 3. c, 4. b, 5. b.

Critical Thinking Activities

1. Is the following statement true or false? Explain your answer.

   OTC drugs and herbal products may be safely taken in the recommended amounts without concern for adverse effects.

2. From which law have current laws regulating OTC medications evolved?
3. Discuss some important points to include when teaching patients about analgesia and pain control at home using OTC products.

4. Your neighbor, who tells you that he has been taking warfarin, a "blood thinner," for several months, calls you to ask your opinion about taking ginkgo to prevent memory loss. He says his sister uses it and it "works wonders." He also thinks it is safe because he can buy it at the local grocery store. What should you tell him? (You may need to look up the drug warfarin and the herbal product elsewhere in the text.)

For answers, see http://evolve.elsevier.com/Lilley.

Substance Abuse

Objectives

When you reach the end of this chapter, you should be able to do the following:

1. Define substance abuse.
2. Discuss the significance of the problem of substance abuse in the United States and in health care settings.
3. Identify the drugs that are most frequently abused and their drug classifications.
4. Contrast the signs and symptoms of drug abuse for specific drugs.
5. Compare the various symptoms of and treatments for drug withdrawal for the most commonly abused narcotics and opioids, amphetamines, other stimulants, and depressants, as well as alcohol and nicotine.
6. Describe alcohol abuse syndrome, its signs and symptoms, its withdrawal symptoms (mild to severe), and its treatment regimen.
7. Develop a nursing care plan encompassing all phases of the nursing process for a patient undergoing treatment for substance abuse and dependency.

e-Learning Activities

Companion CD
- NCLEX Review Questions: see questions 37-40
- Animations
- Audio Glossary
- Category Catchers
- Medication Errors Checklists
- IV Therapy Checklists

evolve Website (http://evolve.elsevier.com/Lilley)
- Nursing Care Plans • Frequently Asked Questions • Content Updates • WebLinks • Supplemental Resources • Elsevier ePharmacology Update • Medication Administration Animations

Glossary

Addiction Strong psychologic or physical dependence on a drug or other psychoactive substance. (p. 85)

Amphetamine A drug that stimulates the central nervous system. (p. 86)

Enuresis Urinary incontinence. (p. 87)

Habituation Development of a tolerance to a substance following prolonged medical use, but without psychologic or physical dependence (addiction). (p. 85)

Illicit drug use The use of a drug or substance in a way that it is not intended to be used or the use of a drug that is not legally approved for human administration. (p. 86)

Intoxication Stimulation, excitement, or stupefaction produced by a chemical substance. (p. 85)

Korsakoff's psychosis A syndrome of anterograde and retrograde amnesia with confabulation (making up of stories) associated with chronic alcohol abuse; it often occurs together with *Wernicke's encephalopathy*. (p. 90)

Micturition Urination, the desire to urinate, or the frequency of urination. (p. 87)

Narcolepsy A sleep disorder characterized by sleeping during the day, disrupted nighttime sleep, cataplexy, sleep paralysis, and hypnagogic hallucinations. (p. 88)

Narcotics Drugs that produce insensibility or stupor (narcosis); the term is applied most commonly to the opioid analgesics. (p. 85)

Opioid analgesics Synthetic pain-relieving substances that were originally derived from the opium poppy. Naturally occurring opium derivatives are called *opiates*. (p. 85)

Physical dependence A condition characterized by physiologic reliance on a substance, usually indicated by tolerance to the effects of the substance and development of withdrawal symptoms when use of the substance is terminated. (p. 85)

Psychoactive properties Drug properties that affect mood, behavior, cognitive processes, and mental status. (p. 87)

Psychologic dependence A condition characterized by strong desires to obtain and use a substance. (p. 85)

Raves Increasingly popular all-night parties that typically involve dancing, drinking, and the use of various illicit drugs. (p. 87)

Roofies Pills that are classified as benzodiazepines. They have recently gained popularity as a recreational drug; chemically known as flunitrazepam. (p. 88)

Substance abuse The use of a mood- or behavior-altering substance in a maladaptive manner that often compromises health, safety, and social and occupational functioning, and causes legal problems. (p. 85)

Wernicke's encephalopathy A neurologic disorder characterized by apathy, drowsiness, ataxia, nystagmus, and ophthalmoplegia; it is caused by thiamine (vitamin B₁) deficiency secondary to chronic alcohol abuse. (p. 90)

Withdrawal   A substance-specific mental disorder that follows the cessation or reduction in use of a psychoactive substance that has been taken regularly to induce a state of intoxication. (p. 85)

Substance abuse affects people of all ages, sexes, and ethnic and socioeconomic groups. **Physical dependence** and **psychologic dependence** on a substance are chronic disorders with remissions and relapses, such as occur with any other chronic illness. Exacerbations should not be seen as failures but as indications to intensify treatment. Recognizing physical or psychologic dependence and understanding the basis and various guidelines for treatment are important skills for the individual caring for these patients. **Habituation** refers to situations in which a patient becomes accustomed to a certain drug (develops tolerance) and may have mild psychologic dependence on it, but does not show compulsive dose escalation, drug-seeking behavior, or major withdrawal symptoms upon drug discontinuation. This might occur, for example, in a postsurgical patient who receives opioid pain therapy regularly for only a few weeks.

Nearly 50% of the adult patients seen in many family practice clinics have an alcohol or drug disorder. Some 25% to 40% of hospital admissions are related to substance abuse and its sequelae. Of outpatients seen in a general medicine practice, 10% to 16% are seeking treatment for problems related to substance abuse. Substance abuse is also strongly associated with many types of mental illness. Treatment of both disorders concurrently is often very difficult, in part because of the much greater risk of drug interactions with the abused substances (Chapter 15). Assessment, intervention, prescription of medications, collaboration in implementing specific **addiction** treatment strategies, and monitoring of recovery are essential to the care of this patient population.

This chapter focuses on three major classes of commonly abused substances and two commonly abused individual drugs. A description of the category or the individual drug, possible effects, signs and symptoms of **intoxication** and **withdrawal,** peak period and duration of withdrawal symptoms, and drugs used to treat withdrawal are discussed. The list of substances of abuse in Box 8-1 is not all inclusive, but it contains some of the substances most commonly abused at this time.

The specific drugs used to treat withdrawal symptoms are discussed in the sections covering the major drug category or the individual drug whose withdrawal symptoms they are intended to treat. Pharmacologic therapies are indicated for patients with ad-

---

Box 8-1   Categories of Abused Substances

Major Categories
Opioids
Stimulants
Depressants

Individual Drugs
Alcohol
Methamphetamine
Methylenedioxymethamphetamine (MDMA, ecstacy)
Nicotine

---

dictive disorders to prevent life-threatening withdrawal complications, such as seizures and delirium tremens, and to increase compliance with psychosocial forms of addiction treatment.

OPIOIDS

Opioid analgesics are synthetic pain-relieving substances that were originally derived from the opium poppy plant. Similar substances that occur in nature are called *opiates.* More than 20 different alkaloids are obtained from the unripe seed of the opium poppy plant, only a few of which are clinically useful. Morphine and codeine are the only two that are useful as analgesics. The multitude of other opioid analgesics that are currently used in medical practice are synthetic or semisynthetic derivatives of these two drugs.

Diacetylmorphine (better known as *heroin*) and opium are also opioids. Heroin and opium are classified as Schedule I drugs and are not available in the United States for therapeutic use. Heroin is a potent analgesic whose use is allowed for medical pain control purposes in Europe, where governmental programs also exist to provide addicts with the drug to reduce crime. Heroin was banned in the United States in 1924 because of its high potential for abuse and the increasing number of heroin addicts. Heroin is one of the most commonly abused opioids. Some of the other commonly abused substances in the opioid category are codeine, hydrocodone, hydromorphone, meperidine, morphine, opium, oxycodone, and propoxyphene.

Currently heroin remains one of the top 10 most abused drugs in the United States and often is used in combination with the stimulant drug cocaine (discussed later in the section on stimulants). When heroin is injected (mainlining or skin-popping), sniffed (snorting), or smoked, it binds with opiate receptors found in many regions of the brain. The result is intense euphoria, often referred to as a "rush." This rush lasts only briefly and is followed by a relaxed, contented state that lasts a couple of hours. In large doses, heroin, like other opioids, can reduce or stop respiration.

Mechanism of Action and Drug Effects

Opioids work by blocking receptors in the central nervous system (CNS). When these receptors are blocked, the perception of pain is blocked. There are three main receptor types to which opioids bind. These receptors and their physiologic effects when stimulated are discussed in Chapter 10. The unique mixture of receptor affinities that a specific opioid possesses determines its therapeutic and toxic effects. One of the reasons that opioids are abused is their ability to produce euphoria, which is mediated by the μ (mu) subset of opioid receptors in the brain.

The drug effects of opioids are primarily centered in the CNS. However, these drugs also act outside the CNS, and many of their unwanted effects stem from these actions. In addition to analgesia, opioids produce drowsiness, euphoria, tranquility, and other alterations of mood. The mechanism by which opioids produce these latter effects is not entirely clear. The effects of opioids can be collectively referred to as *narcosis* or *stupor,* which involves reduced sensory response, especially to painful stimuli. For this reason, opioid analgesics, along with other classes of drugs that produce similar effects, are also referred to as **narcotics,** especially by law enforcement authorities. Areas outside the CNS that are affected by opioids include the skin, gastrointestinal (GI) tract, and genitourinary tract.

Indications

The intended drug effects of opioids are to relieve pain, reduce cough, relieve diarrhea, and induce anesthesia. Many have a high potential for abuse and are therefore classified as Schedule II controlled substances. Relaxation and euphoria are the most common drug effects that lead to abuse and psychologic dependence. Sustained-release oxycodone is one example of an opioid narcotic that is controversial because it is often overprescribed, misused, and grossly abused.

Certain opioid drugs are themselves used to treat opioid dependence. Historically, methadone has been used most commonly for this purpose. Its long half-life of up to 12 to 24 hours allows patients to be dosed once daily at federally approved methadone maintenance clinics. Other drugs used for the same purpose include levomethadyl and buprenorphine. In theory, the ultimate goal of such programs is to reduce the patient's dosage gradually so that eventually the patient can live permanently drug free. Unfortunately, relapse rates are often high in these programs. However, patients who remain on long-term opioid maintenance therapy in a medical setting still benefit by avoiding the hazards associated with obtaining and using illegal street drugs.

Contraindications

Contraindications to the therapeutic use of opioid medications include known drug allergy, pregnancy (high dosage or prolonged use is contraindicated), respiratory depression or severe asthma without available resuscitative equipment, and paralytic ileus (bowel paralysis).

Adverse Effects

The adverse effects of opioids can be broken down into two groups: CNS and non-CNS. The primary adverse effects of opioids are related to their actions in the CNS. The major CNS-related adverse effects are diuresis, miosis, convulsions, nausea, vomiting, and respiratory depression. Many of the non-CNS adverse effects are secondary to the release of histamine caused by opioids. This histamine release can cause vasodilation leading to hypotension; spasms of the colon leading to constipation; increased contractions of the ureter resulting in decreased urine flow; and dilation of cutaneous blood vessels leading to flushing of the skin of the face, neck, and upper thorax. The release of histamine is also thought to cause sweating, urticaria, and pruritus.

Management of Withdrawal, Toxicity, and Overdose

Box 8-2 lists the signs and symptoms of opioid drug withdrawal. The box also indicates the time when these symptoms are most likely to occur and their duration. See Chapter 10 for a detailed discussion of physical dependence and the management of acute intoxication. Withdrawal symptoms include nausea, dysphoria, muscle aches, lacrimation, rhinorrhea, pupillary dilation, piloerection (hair standing on end) or sweating, diarrhea, yawning, fever, and insomnia. The medications listed in Box 8-3 are intended to help decrease the desire for the abused opioid and reduce the severity of these withdrawal symptoms.

Medications are sometimes used to prevent relapse to drug use once an initial remission is achieved. These medications are useful only when concurrent counseling is provided and offer additional insurance against return to **illicit drug use.** For opioid

---

| Box 8-2 | **Signs and Symptoms of Opioid Withdrawal** |

Peak Period
1-3 days
Duration
5-7 days
Signs
Drug seeking, mydriasis, piloerection, diaphoresis, rhinorrhea, lacrimation, diarrhea, insomnia, elevated blood pressure, and pulse rate
Symptoms
Intense desire for drugs, muscle cramps, arthralgia, anxiety, nausea, vomiting, malaise

---

| Box 8-3 | **Medications for Treatment of Opioid Withdrawal** |

Clonidine (Catapres) Substitution
Clonidine, 0.1 or 0.2 mg orally, is given every 4-6 hr as needed for signs and symptoms of withdrawal for 5-7 days. Days 2-4 are typically the toughest days in detoxification. Check blood pressure before each dose, and do not give medication if patient is hypotensive.
Methadone Substitution
Methadone test dose of 10 mg is given orally in liquid or crushed tablet. Additional 10-20 mg doses are given for signs and symptoms of withdrawal every 4-6 hr for 24 hr after initial dose. Range for daily dose is 15-30 mg. Repeat total first day dose in two divided doses (stabilization dose) for 2-3 days, then reduce dosage by 5-10 mg/day until medication is completely withdrawn.

---

abuse or dependence, naltrexone, an opioid antagonist, is administered (50 mg/day). Naltrexone works by blocking the opioid receptors so that use of opioid drugs does not produce euphoria. When euphoria is eliminated, the reinforcing effect of the drug is lost. The patient should be free from opioids for at least 1 week before beginning this medication, because naltrexone can produce withdrawal symptoms if given too soon. Naltrexone is also approved for use by alcohol-dependent patients. The same dose of naltrexone given to opioid-dependent patients, 50 mg/day, decreases craving for alcohol and reduces the likelihood of a full relapse if a slip occurs. Refer to Chapter 10 for information on management of toxicity and overdose.

STIMULANTS

Some of the effects of stimulants that have led to their abuse are elevation of mood, reduction of fatigue, a sense of increased alertness, and invigorating aggressiveness. One stimulant drug that produces strong CNS stimulation and is commonly abused is **amphetamine.** Chemically, three classes of amphetamine exist: salts of racemic amphetamine, dextroamphetamine, and methamphetamine. These classes vary with respect to their potency and peripheral effects. Another stimulant drug of abuse is cocaine, which also produces strong CNS stimulation. Cocaine was originally classified as a narcotic with the passage of the Harrison Narcotic Act of 1914. Since then it has continued to be considered a narcotic by the penal system and has been treated as a narcotic in terms of secured storage in health care facilities. However, unlike the opioid analge-

Table 8-1	**Various Forms of Amphetamine and Cocaine with Street Names**

Chemical Name	Street Names
dimethoxymethylamphetamine	DOM, STP
methamphetamine (crystallized form)	Ice, crystal, glass
methamphetamine (powdered form)	Speed, meth, crank
methylenedioxyamphetamine	MDA, love drug
methylenedioxymethamphetamine	MDMA, ecstasy
cocaine (powdered form)	Coke, dust, snow, flake, blow, girl
cocaine (crystallized form)	Crack, crack cocaine, freebase rocks, rock

sics, cocaine does not normally induce a state of narcosis or stupor and is therefore more correctly categorized as a stimulant drug, which is its current classification. Other commonly abused substances in this category include benzedrine, benzphetamine, butyl nitrite, methylphenidate, and phenmetrazine.

There is currently widespread abuse of the CNS stimulant methamphetamine. Multiple slight chemical variants of methamphetamine exist. Table 8-1 lists commonly abused forms of amphetamine and cocaine and their street names.

These "designer drugs" have **psychoactive properties** along with their stimulant properties, which further enhances their abuse potential. Cocaine and amphetamine are two of the most commonly abused stimulants. Although these drugs have many therapeutic benefits, they are often abused and can lead to physical and psychologic dependence. As noted earlier, methamphetamine is a chemical class of amphetamine, but it has a much stronger effect on the CNS than the other two classes of amphetamine.

Methamphetamine is generally used orally in pill form or in powder form by snorting or injecting. It has 15 to 20 times the potency of amphetamine sulfate, the original drug in this class. Crystallized methamphetamine, known as "ice," "crystal," or "crystal meth," is a smokable and more powerful form of the drug. Methamphetamine users who inject the drug and share needles are at risk for acquiring human immunodeficiency virus (HIV) infection and acquired immunodeficiency syndrome (AIDS), as well as hepatitis B and C. Marijuana and alcohol are commonly listed as additional drugs of abuse in those admitted for treatment of methamphetamine abuse. Most (92%) of the methamphetamine-related deaths reported in 1994 involved methamphetamine used in combination with at least one other drug, most often alcohol (30%), heroin (23%), or cocaine (21%). The over-the-counter (OTC) decongestant pseudoephedrine is now commonly used to synthesize methamphetamine in clandestine drug laboratories, often in private homes. This practice has lead to dramatic increases in the abuse of this drug. For these reasons, many retail pharmacies now sell pseudoephedrine tablets only from behind the pharmacy counter and in limited quantities.

Another synthetic amphetamine derivative is methylenedioxymethamphetamine (MDMA, "Ecstasy," or "E"), which is also usually prepared in secret home laboratories. This drug tends to have more calming effects that other amphetamine drugs. It is usually taken in pill form but can also be snorted or injected. Users often feel a strong sense of social bonding with and acceptance of other people, hence the nickname "love drug." The drug can also be very energizing, which makes it popular at **raves** (all-night dance parties). Originally synthesized by Merck Pharma-

ceuticals in 1914, it was studied by the U.S. Army as a "brain-washing" drug in the 1950s. Its popularity has grown widely since the Drug Enforcement Administration classified it as a Schedule I controlled substance in 1985.

Another illicit drug use problem is cocaine use. Cocaine is a white powder that is derived from the leaves of the South American coca plant. Cocaine is either snorted or injected intravenously. Cocaine tends to give a temporary illusion of limitless power and energy and afterward leaves the user feeling depressed, edgy, and craving more. Crack is a smokable form of cocaine that has been chemically altered. Cocaine and crack are highly addictive. The psychologic and physical dependence can erode physical and mental health and can become so strong that these drugs dominate all aspects of the addict's life.

Mechanism of Action and Drug Effects

Stimulants work by releasing *biogenic amines* from their storage sites in the nerve terminals. The primary biogenic amine released is norepinephrine. This release results in stimulation of the CNS. One drug effect of stimulants is typically cardiovascular stimulation, which results in increased blood pressure and heart rate and possibly cardiac dysrhythmias. The effect on smooth muscle is primarily seen in the urinary bladder and results in contraction of the sphincter. This is helpful in treating **enuresis** (urinary incontinence) but results in painful and difficult **micturition** (voiding or urination) otherwise. Stimulants, particularly amphetamines, are very potent CNS stimulants. This CNS stimulation commonly results in wakefulness, alertness, and a decreased sense of fatigue; elevation of mood, with increased initiative, self-confidence, and ability to concentrate; often elation and euphoria; and an increase in motor and speech activity. Physical performance in athletes may be improved due to both enhanced alertness and reduction of fatigue. This quality leads to abuse of these drugs by many athletes, especially those under intense pressure to perform. However, these performance enhancement effects may reach a plateau and even result in a personal or professional crisis for an athlete who abuses these drugs on a long-term basis.

Indications

Many therapeutic uses of stimulants exist. Currently their most common use is in the treatment of attention deficit disorder or attention deficit hyperactivity disorder. Stimulants may be used to prevent or reverse fatigue and sleep, such as when they are used to treat **narcolepsy** (episodes of acute sleepiness). They also have a slight analgesic effect and may be used to enhance the analgesic effects and limit the CNS-depressant effects of stronger analgesics such as opioids. Another therapeutic effect of amphetamines is their ability to stimulate the respiratory center. Occasionally they are used after anesthesia to stimulate the respiratory center in individuals whose respirations are slowed. Stimulants are also used to reduce food intake and treat obesity. This therapeutic effect is limited because of rapid development of tolerance.

Contraindications

Contraindications to the therapeutic use of stimulant medications include drug allergy, diabetes, cardiovascular disorders, states of agitation, hypertension, known history of drug abuse, and Tourette's syndrome.

Adverse Effects

The adverse effects of stimulants are commonly an extension of their therapeutic effects. The CNS-related adverse effects are restlessness, syncope (fainting), dizziness, tremor, hyperactive reflexes, talkativeness, tenseness, irritability, weakness, insomnia, fever, and sometimes euphoria. Confusion, aggression, increased libido, anxiety, delirium, paranoid hallucinations, panic states, and suicidal or homicidal tendencies occur, especially in mentally ill patients. Fatigue and depression usually follow the CNS stimulation. Cardiovascular effects are common and include headache, chilliness, pallor or flushing, palpitations, tachycardia, cardiac dysrhythmias, anginal pain, hypertension or hypotension, and circulatory collapse. Excessive sweating can also occur. GI effects include dry mouth, metallic taste, anorexia, nausea, vomiting, diarrhea, and abdominal cramps. A sometimes fatal hyperthermia can also occur, driven partly by excessive drug-induced muscular contractions.

Management of Withdrawal, Toxicity, and Overdose

Box 8-4 lists the signs and symptoms of withdrawal from stimulants. The box also indicates the peak period when these symptoms are most likely to occur and their duration. Death due to poisoning or toxic levels is usually a result of convulsions, coma, or cerebral hemorrhage and may occur during periods of intoxication or withdrawal.

Box 8-4 Signs and Symptoms of Stimulant Withdrawal

Peak Period
1-3 days

Duration
5-7 days

Signs
Social withdrawal, psychomotor retardation, hypersomnia, hyperphagia

Symptoms
Depression, suicidal thoughts and behavior, paranoid delusions

---

DEPRESSANTS

Depressants are drugs that relieve anxiety, irritability, and tension when used as intended. They are also used to treat seizure disorders and induce anesthesia. The two main pharmacologic classes of depressant are benzodiazepines and barbiturates. Both of these drug classes are also discussed further in Chapter 12. Benzodiazepines are relatively safe. They offer many advantages over older drugs used to relieve anxiety and insomnia. However, they are often intentionally and unintentionally misused. Ingestion of benzodiazepines together with alcohol can be lethal. Another depressant which is neither a benzodiazepine nor a barbiturate is marijuana. Derived from the cannabis plant ("pot," "grass," "weed"), marijuana is the most commonly abused drug worldwide. A 2001 survey revealed that more than 83 million Americans had used the drug at some time in their lives and many of these had used it recently. It is generally smoked as a cigarette ("joint") or in a pipe ("bong") but can be mixed in food or tea.

A benzodiazepine that has recently gained popularity as a recreational drug is flunitrazepam. Flunitrazepam is not legally available for prescription in the United States, but it is legal in over 60 countries for treatment of insomnia. The drug, known as **roofies** among young people, creates a sleepy, relaxed, drunken feeling that lasts 2 to 8 hours. A single dose costs from $1.50 to $5.00. Roofies are commonly used in combination with alcohol and other drugs. They are sometimes taken to enhance a heroin high or to mellow or ease the experience of coming down from a cocaine or crack high. Used with alcohol, roofies produce disinhibition and amnesia.

Roofies have recently gained a reputation as a "date rape" drug. Girls and women around the country have reported being raped after being involuntarily sedated with roofies, which were often slipped into their drinks by their attackers. The drug has no taste or odor so the victims do not realize what is happening. About 10 minutes after ingesting the drug, the woman may feel dizzy and disoriented, simultaneously too hot and too cold, and nauseous. She may experience difficulty speaking and moving and then pass out. Such a victim will have no memories of what happened while under the influence of the drug. Another popular date rape drug used in similar fashion is γ-hydroxybutyric acid (GHB). GHB works by mimicking the natural inhibitory brain neurotransmitter γ-aminobutyric acid (GABA). It is also known as "liquid Ecstasy." These drugs are also used simply for their depressant and hallucinogenic effects.

Flunitrazepam is sold under the trade name Rohypnol, from which the street name "rophy" was derived and modified to "roofy." In south Florida, street names include "circles," "Mexican Valium," "rib," "roach-2," "roofies," "roopies," "rope," "rop-ies," and "ruffies." Being under the influence of the drug is re-ferred to as being "roached out." In Texas, flunitrazepam is called "R-2" or "roaches."

Mechanism of Action and Drug Effects

Benzodiazepines and barbiturates work by increasing the action of GABA. GABA is an amino acid in the brain that inhibits nerve transmission in the CNS. The alteration of GABA action in the CNS results in relief of anxiety, sedation, and muscle relaxation. The ef-fects of depressants are primarily limited to the CNS. In addition to sedation, muscle relaxation, and reduced anxiety, their CNS effects include amnesia and unconsciousness. They have moderate effects outside the CNS, causing slight blood pressure decreases.

The active ingredients of the marijuana plant are known as cannabinoids, the most active of which is δ-9-trans-tetrahydro-cannabinol, abbreviated THC. THC exerts its effects on the body by chemically binding to and stimulating two cannabinoid recep-tors in the CNS (CB1 and CB2). Smoking the drug leads to acute sensorial changes that start within 3 minutes, peak in 20 to 30 minutes, and last for 2 to 3 hours. Effects are longer when the drug is taken via the oral route. Specific effects include mild eu-phoria, memory lapses, dry mouth, enhanced appetite, motor awkwardness, and distorted sense of time and space. THC also stimulates sympathetic receptors and inhibits parasympathetic re-ceptors in cardiac tissue, which leads to tachycardia. Other effects include hallucinations, anxiety, paranoia, and unsteady gait.

Indications

Many therapeutic uses of depressants exist. Benzodiazepines are more widely used and abused than barbiturates, and they are more commonly prescribed because they are felt by many to be safer than barbiturates. Benzodiazepines are used primarily to relieve anxiety, to induce sleep, to sedate, and to prevent seizures. Barbi-turates are used as hypnotics, sedatives, and anticonvulsants and to induce anesthesia. Controversial medical uses for marijuana include treatment of chronic pain, reduction of nausea and vomit-ing associated with cancer treatment, and appetite stimulation in those with wasting syndromes, such as patients with cancer or AIDS. Dronabinol is a synthetic FDA-approved THC prescription capsule used for these indications (see Chapter 53 for further dis-cussion of this drug). However, it is often not popular with those who claim it is not as effective as inhaled marijuana.

Contraindications

Contraindications to the therapeutic use of depressant medica-tions include known drug allergy, dyspnea or airway obstruction, narrow-angle glaucoma, and porphyria (a metabolic disorder).

Adverse Effects

The most common undesirable effect of benzodiazepines and barbiturates is an overexpression of their therapeutic effects. The CNS is the primary area of the body adversely affected by these drugs. Drowsiness, sedation, loss of coordination, dizziness, blurred vision, headaches, and paradoxical reactions (insomnia, increased excitability, hallucinations) are the primary CNS ad-verse effects. Occasional GI effects include nausea, vomiting, constipation, dry mouth, and abdominal cramping. Other possi-ble adverse effects include pruritus and skin rash. Long-term use of marijuana may result in chronic respiratory symptoms (similar

to those of tobacco abuse) and memory and attention deficit problems. A chronic, depressive "amotivational" syndrome has also been observed, especially among younger users.

Management of Withdrawal, Toxicity, and Overdose

Box 8-5 lists the signs and symptoms of withdrawal from depres-sants. The box also indicates the peak periods when these symp-toms are most likely to occur and their duration. Fatal poisoning is unusual with benzodiazepines when they are ingested alone. When benzodiazepines are ingested with alcohol or barbiturates, however, the combination can be lethal. Death is typically due to respiratory arrest. Abrupt withdrawal of benzodiazepines when they have been taken for several months to years has resulted in autonomic withdrawal symptoms, seizures, delirium, rebound anxiety, myoclonus (involuntary muscle contractions), myalgia, and sleep disturbances.

Table 8-2 shows the conversion from various barbiturates to phenobarbital, which is less addicting and from which withdrawal is easier. To use this table, the nurse determines the total dose of the barbiturate on which the patient is dependent, multiplies this dose by the conversion factor to get the equivalent dose of phenobarbital, and then tapers the phenobarbital as described in Box 8-5. Of course, a prescriber's order is required to implement this regimen.

Flumazenil can be used to acutely reverse the sedative effects of benzodiazepines. Flumazenil antagonizes the action of benzo-diazepines on the CNS by directly competing with them for bind-ing at the benzodiazepine receptor in the CNS. Flumazenil has a stronger affinity for the receptor, however, and knocks the benzo-diazepine off the receptor, which reverses the sedative action of

---

Box 8-5	Signs, Symptoms, and Treatment of Depressant Withdrawal

Peak Period
2-4 days for short-acting drugs
4-7 days for long-acting drugs

Duration
4-7 days for short-acting drugs
7-12 days for long-acting drugs

Signs
Increased psychomotor activity; agitation; muscular weakness; hyperpyrexia; diaphoresis; delirium; convulsions; elevated blood pressure, pulse rate, and temperature; tremors of eyelids, tongue, and hands

Symptoms
Anxiety; depression; euphoria; incoherent thoughts; hostility; grandiosity; disorientation; tactile, auditory, and visual halluci-nations; suicidal thoughts

Treatment of Benzodiazepine Withdrawal
A 7-10 day taper (10-14 day taper with long-acting benzodiaze-pines). Treat with diazepam (Valium) 10-20 mg orally qid on day 1, then taper until the dosage is 5-10 mg orally on last day. Avoid giving the drug "as needed." Adjustments in dosage according to the patient's clinical state may be indicated.

Treatment of Barbiturate Withdrawal
A 7-10 day taper or 10-14 day taper. Calculate barbiturate equiva-lence and give 50% of the original dosage (if actual dosage is known before detoxification); taper. Avoid giving the drug "as needed."

Table 8-2   Barbiturate Equivalencies

Drug	Dose (mg)	Phenobarbital Dose (mg)	Conversion Factor
Barbiturates			
butabarbital (Butisol)	600	180	0.3
phenobarbital (Nembutal)	600	180	0.3
phenobarbital	180	180	1.0
secobarbital (Seconal)	600	180	0.3
Others			
glutethimide (Doriden)	1500	180	0.12
meprobamate (Equanil)	2400	180	0.075
methaqualone	1800	180	0.1

the benzodiazepine. The dosage regimen to be followed for the reversal of conscious sedation or general anesthesia induced by a benzodiazepine and the management of suspected benzodiazepine overdoses are summarized in Table 12-7 on page 186.

Limiting depressant abuse is important. Barbiturates and benzodiazepines are commonly implicated in suicides, especially in combination with alcohol. Generally speaking, depressants should not be regularly prescribed over a long period. Relatively safe hypnotic drugs such as the benzodiazepines are preferred whenever possible, especially in emotionally disturbed patients. Combinations of sedative-hypnotic compounds and the use of a single drug with alcohol should be avoided. Long-term use of hypnotic drugs leads to ineffective control of insomnia, decrease in rapid eye movement sleep, dependence, and drug withdrawal symptoms.

Effects of marijuana use are usually self-limiting and resolve within a few hours.

ALCOHOL

Alcoholic beverages have been used since the beginning of human civilization. Individuals of Arab descent introduced the technique of distillation to Europe in the Middle Ages. Alcohol has been called the "elixir of life" and has been touted as a remedy for practically all diseases, which led to the use of the term *whisky,* Gaelic for "water of life." Over time, it has been determined that the therapeutic value of alcohol is extremely limited, and chronic ingestion of excessive amounts is a major social and medical problem.

Mechanism of Action and Drug Effects

Alcohol, more accurately known as *ethanol* (abbreviated as ETOH), causes CNS depression by dissolving in lipid membranes in the CNS. The latest hypothesis is that ethanol causes a local disordering in the lipid matrix of the brain. This has been termed *membrane fluidization.* Some also believe that ethanol may augment GABA-mediated synaptic inhibition and fluxes of chloride. This enhancement of the action of GABA, an inhibitory neurotransmitter in the brain, causes CNS depression. Ethanol has many effects. The CNS is continuously depressed in the presence of ethanol. Moderate amounts of ethanol may stimulate or depress respirations. Effects of ethanol on the circulation are relatively minor. In moderate doses, ethanol causes vasodilation, especially of the cutaneous vessels, and produces warm, flushed skin. Ingestion of ethanol causes a feeling of warmth because it enhances cutaneous and gastric blood flow. Increased sweating may also occur. Heat is therefore lost more rapidly, and the internal body temperature consequently falls. The acute (vs. chronic) ingestion

of ethanol, even in intoxicating doses, probably produces little lasting change in hepatic function. Ethanol exerts a diuretic effect by virtue of its inhibition of antidiuretic hormone secretion and the resultant decrease in renal tubular reabsorption of water.

Indications

Few legitimate uses of ethanol and alcoholic beverages exist. Ethanol is an excellent solvent for many drugs and is commonly employed as a vehicle for medicinal mixtures. When applied topically to the skin, ethanol acts as a coolant. Ethanol sponges are therefore used to treat fever. Ethanol may also be used in liniments (oily medications used on the skin). Applied topically, ethanol is the most popular skin disinfectant. More commonly, however, the type of alcohol used on the skin is isopropyl alcohol, which is similar in structure to ethanol but is more toxic and is not drinkable.

Ethanol is still widely employed for its hypnotic and antipyretic effects in various cold and cough products. Dehydrated alcohol is injected in the close proximity of nerves or sympathetic ganglia for the relief of the long-lasting pain that occurs in trigeminal neuralgia, inoperable carcinoma, and other conditions. Systemic uses of ethanol are primarily limited to the treatment of methyl alcohol and ethylene glycol intoxication (e.g., from drinking automotive antifreeze solution). However, small amounts of ethanol preparations (such as red wine) have been shown to have cardiovascular benefits.

Adverse Effects

Chronic excessive ingestion of ethanol is directly associated with serious neurologic and mental disorders. These neurologic disorders can result in seizures. Nutritional and vitamin deficiencies, especially of the B vitamins, can occur and can lead to **Wernicke's encephalopathy, Korsakoff's psychosis,** polyneuritis, and nicotinic acid deficiency encephalopathy.

Moderate amounts of ethanol may stimulate or depress respirations. Large amounts produce dangerous or lethal depression of respiration. Although circulatory effects of ethanol are relatively minor, acute severe alcoholic intoxication may cause cardiovascular depression. Long-term excessive use of ethanol has largely irreversible effects on the heart, such as cardiomyopathy.

When consumed on a regular basis in large quantities, ethanol produces a constellation of dose-related negative effects or serious sequelae, such as alcoholic hepatitis or its progression to cirrhosis. Teratogenic effects can be devastating and are caused by the direct action of ethanol, which inhibits embryonic cellular proliferation early in gestation. This often results in a condition known as *fetal alcohol syndrome,* which is characterized by craniofacial abnormalities, CNS dysfunction, and both prenatal and postnatal growth retardation in the infant. Pregnant women should therefore be strongly advised not to consume alcohol during pregnancy, and appropriate treatment and counseling should be arranged for pregnant women addicted to alcohol or any other drug of abuse.

Management of Withdrawal, Toxicity, and Overdose

Box 8-6 lists the common signs and symptoms of ethanol withdrawal. Signs and symptoms may vary depending on the individual's usage pattern, his or her preferred type of ethanol, and the presence of comorbidities.

Table 8-3 Acetaldehyde Syndrome	
Body System Affected	**Result**
Cardiovascular	Vasodilation over the entire body, hypotension, orthostatic syncope, chest pain
Central nervous	Intense throbbing of the head and neck leading to a pulsating headache, sweating, marked uneasiness, weakness, vertigo, blurred vision, confusion
Gastrointestinal	Nausea, copious vomiting, thirst
Respiratory	Difficulty breathing

Box 8-6   Signs, Symptoms, and Treatment of Ethanol Withdrawal

Mild Withdrawal
Signs and Symptoms
Systolic blood pressure higher than 150 mm Hg, diastolic blood pressure higher than 90 mm Hg, pulse rate higher than 110 beats/min, temperature above 37.7° C (100° F), tremors, insomnia, agitation

Treatment
- diazepam (Valium), 5-10 mg PO prn
- lorazepam (Ativan), 1-2 mg PO q4-6h prn for 1-3 days
- chlordiazepoxide (Librium), taper 5-25 mg PO q6-8h prn for 1-3 days

Moderate Withdrawal
Signs and Symptoms
Systolic blood pressure 150-200 mm Hg, diastolic blood pressure 90-140 mm Hg, pulse rate 110-140 beats/min, temperature 37.7°-38.3° C (100°-101° F), tremors, insomnia, agitation

Treatment
- diazepam (Valium)
  Day 1: 15-20 mg PO qid
  Day 2: 10-20 mg PO qid
  Day 3: 5-15 mg PO qid
  Day 4: 10 mg PO qid
  Day 5: 5 mg PO qid
- lorazepam (Ativan)
  Days 1 and 2: 2-4 mg PO qid
  Days 3 and 4: 1-2 mg PO qid
  Day 5: 1 mg PO bid
- chlordiazepoxide (Librium), taper 5-25 mg PO q6-8h prn for 1-3 days

Severe Withdrawal (Delirium Tremens)*
Signs and Symptoms
Systolic blood pressure higher than 200 mm Hg, diastolic blood pressure higher than 140 mm Hg, pulse rate higher than 140 beats/min, temperature above 38.3° C (101° F), tremors, insomnia, agitation

Treatment
- diazepam (Valium), 10-25 mg PO prn q1h while awake until sedation occurs
- lorazepam (Ativan), 1-2 mg IV prn q1h while awake for 3-5 days
- chlordiazepoxide (Librium), 50-100 mg IV prn q2-4h, maximum 300 mg/day

*Monitoring in an intensive care unit for cardiac and respiratory function, fluid and nutrition replacement, vital signs, and mental status is recommended. Restraints are indicated for a patient who is confused or agitated to protect the patient from self and to protect others (delirium tremens can be a terrifying and life-threatening state). Thiamine (100 mg IM or PO daily for 3-7 days), hydration, and magnesium replacement may be indicated depending on the severity of the withdrawal state.
IM, Intramuscularly; *IV*, intravenously; *PO*, orally.

One pharmacologic option for the treatment of alcoholism is disulfiram. Disulfiram is not a cure for alcoholism; it helps patients who have a sincere desire to stop drinking. The rationale for its use is that patients know that if they are to avoid the devastating experience of the *acetaldehyde syndrome,* they cannot drink for at least 3 or 4 days after taking disulfiram. Table 8-3 outlines the acetaldehyde syndrome. These adverse effects are obviously very uncomfortable and even potentially dangerous for someone with any other major illnesses. For this reason, disulfiram is usually reserved as the treatment of last resort for "hard core" alcoholic patients for whom other treatment options (e.g., Alcoholics Anonymous, psychotherapy) have failed but who still hope to avoid continued alcohol abuse. A less noxious drug therapy option is the use of naltrexone, as mentioned previously in the section on opioids earlier in this chapter.

Disulfiram works by altering the metabolism of alcohol. When ethanol is given to an individual previously treated with disulfiram, the blood acetaldehyde concentration rises 5 to 10 times higher than in an untreated individual. Within about 5 to 10 minutes of ingesting alcohol, the face feels hot, and soon afterward it is flushed and scarlet. After this, throbbing in the head and neck, nausea, copious vomiting, diaphoresis, dyspnea, hyperventilation, vertigo, blurred vision, and confusion appear. As little as 7 mL of alcohol will cause mild symptoms in a sensitive person. The effects last from 30 minutes to several hours. After the symptoms wear off, the patient is exhausted and may sleep for several hours. Most of the signs and symptoms observed after the ingestion of disulfiram plus alcohol are attributable to the resulting increase in the concentration of acetaldehyde in the body. There have even been a few published reports of localized disulfiram-alcohol skin reactions when alcohol preparations—even beer-containing shampoo—were placed on the skin. The usual dosage of disulfiram is 250 mg per day, or 125 mg per day in patients who experience adverse effects such as sedation, sexual dysfunction, and elevated liver enzyme levels.

NICOTINE

Nicotine was first isolated from the leaves of tobacco by Posselt and Reimann in 1828. The medical significance of nicotine grows out of its toxicity, presence in tobacco, and propensity for eliciting dependence in its users. The chronic effects of nicotine and the untoward effects of the chronic use of tobacco are considerable. Although many people smoke because they believe cigarettes calm their nerves, smoking releases epinephrine, a hormone that creates physiologic stress in the smoker rather than relaxation. The apparent calming effects may be related to the increased deep breathing associated with smoking. The use of tobacco is addictive. Most users develop tolerance for nicotine and need greater amounts to produce the desired effect. Smokers become physically and psychologically dependent and will suffer withdrawal symptoms. Smoking is particularly dangerous in adolescents because their bodies are still developing and changing. The 4000 chemicals, including 200 known poisons, present in cigarette smoke can adversely affect this maturation. Cigarettes are highly addictive. One third of young people who are just "experimenting" end up becoming addicted by the time they are 20 years of age.

Mechanism of Action and Drug Effects

Nicotine works by directly stimulating the autonomic ganglia of the nicotinic receptors. Its site of action is the ganglion itself rather than the preganglionic or postganglionic nerve fiber. The organs throughout the body that are innervated by nerves stimulated by nicotine actually contain nicotinic receptors. These receptors are so named because they were originally tested with nicotine to measure their responses. Nicotine can have multiple unpredictable and dramatic affects on the body because nicotinic receptors are found in several systems, including the adrenal glands, skeletal muscles, and CNS.

The major action of nicotine is transient stimulation, followed by more persistent depression of all autonomic ganglia. Small doses of nicotine stimulate the ganglion cells directly and facilitate the transmission of impulses. When larger doses of the drug are applied, the initial stimulation is followed quickly by a blockade of transmission.

Nicotine markedly stimulates the CNS. Respiratory stimulation is also common. This stimulation of the CNS is followed by depression. Nicotine can have dramatic effects on the cardiovascular system as well, resulting in increases in heart rate and blood pressure. The GI system is generally stimulated by nicotine, which produces increased tone and activity in the bowel. This often leads to nausea and vomiting and occasionally to diarrhea.

Indications

The nicotine found in nature (i.e., tobacco plants) has no known therapeutic uses. It is medically significant because of its addictive and toxic properties. However, nicotine that is formulated into various drug products to reduce cravings and promote smoking cessation can be considered a therapeutic drug. It is available for this purpose as chewing gum, transdermal patches, and nasal spray.

Adverse Effects

Nicotine primarily affects the CNS. Large doses can produce tremors and even convulsions. Respiratory stimulation is also common. The initial stimulation of the CNS induced by nicotine is quickly followed by depression. Death can even result from respiratory failure, which is thought to be due to both central paralysis and peripheral blockade of respiratory muscles.

The cardiovascular effects of nicotine are an increase in heart rate and blood pressure. Nicotine stimulates sympathetic ganglia with the discharge of catecholamines from the sympathetic nerve endings.

The effects of nicotine on the GI system are largely due to parasympathetic stimulation, which results in increased tone and motor activity of the bowel. Nicotine induces vomiting by both central and peripheral actions. Centrally, nicotine's emetic effects are due to stimulation of the *chemoreceptor trigger zone* in the brain.

Management of Withdrawal, Toxicity, and Overdose

Smoking cessation is the primary cause for nicotine withdrawal, although discontinuation of any tobacco product can lead to this syndrome. An important and often overlooked problem in hospitalized patients is nicotine withdrawal, which manifests largely as cigarette craving. Irritability, restlessness, and a decrease in heart rate and blood pressure occur. Cardiac symptoms resolve over 3 to 4 weeks, but cigarette craving may persist for months or even years.

The nicotine transdermal system (patch) and nicotine polacrilex (gum) can be used to provide nicotine without the carcinogens in tobacco and are now available OTC. The patch uses a stepwise reduction in subcutaneous delivery to gradually decrease the nicotine dose, and patient treatment compliance seems higher than with the gum. Acute relief from withdrawal symptoms is most easily achieved with the use of the gum, because rapid chewing releases an immediate dose of nicotine. The dose is approximately half the dose the average smoker receives in one cigarette, however, and the onset of action is 30 minutes versus 10 minutes or less from smoking. These pharmacologic changes in delivery minimize the immediate reinforcement and self-reward effects that are prominent with the rapid nicotine delivery of cigarette smoking.

A sustained-release form of the antidepressant bupropion, called Zyban, has been approved as first-line therapy to aid in smoking cessation treatment. Zyban is an innovative treatment because it is the first nicotine-free prescription medicine to treat nicotine dependence. Table 8-4 lists the currently available drugs for nicotine withdrawal therapy.

◆ NURSING PROCESS

◆ ASSESSMENT

The nurse's responsibility in substance abuse includes having excellent interpersonal communication skills and a strong knowledge base regarding the culture of abuse, drugs that are abused, abuse prevention, and development of an action plan that is individualized for the patient. A thorough patient assessment and history taking must be carried out that includes specific questions about the substance(s) being used, the duration of abuse, related physical and mental health concerns, and withdrawal potential. In patients with suspected or confirmed substance abuse, honesty—on the part of the patient as well as the family or significant other—may be problematic when it comes to answering questions about drug use. Therefore, the nurse should use open-ended questions and maintain a nonjudgmental approach during the nursing process and in all contacts with the patient. In taking a medication history, the nurse should also ask the patient about all drugs being used, including prescription drugs, OTC drugs, herbal products, dietary supplements, and illegal drugs. The names of the drugs, doses, and frequency and duration of use should be noted. The nurse must also be attentive to any clues the patient, family, or significant other may be sending, including behavioral and mood changes. A patient's reported use of multiple prescribed drugs as well as contact with multiple prescribers may well be a sign of drug abuse. Laboratory findings are important to assess, especially results of renal and liver function studies

Table 8-4 Nicotine Withdrawal Therapies

Drug	Dosage per Patch	Recommended Duration of Use
Transdermal Nicotine Systems		
Habitrol	7 mg/24 hr	2-4 wk
	14 mg/24 hr	2-4 wk
	21 mg/24 hr	4-8 wk
Nicoderm	7 mg/24 hr	2-4 wk
	14 mg/24 hr	2-4 wk
	21 mg/24 hr	4-8 wk
Nicotrol	5 mg/16 hr	2-4 wk
	10 mg/16 hr	2-4 wk
	15 mg/16 hr	4-12 wk
ProStep	11 mg/24 hr	2-4 wk
	22 mg/24 hr	4-8 wk
Nicotine Gum (Resin)	When the client has a strong urge to smoke, a stick of gum is chewed; use gradually reduced over a 2-3 mo period.	
Antidepressant		
bupropion (Zyban)	15 mg sustained-release tabs	15 mg on days 1-3, then 150 mg bid for 7-12 wk

and any drug screening studies. Baseline vital signs should also be measured and documented.

The most dangerous substances to be aware of in terms of withdrawal are CNS depressants such as alcohol, barbiturates, and benzodiazepines. Delirium tremens (DTs) may begin with tremors and agitation and progress to hallucinations and sometimes death. Careful assessment of mental status is critical to the safe care of the patient, because early withdrawal symptoms may begin with an increase in blood pressure and pulse rate, with subsequent altered mental status.

Assessment of opioid abuse, in addition to the assessment data mentioned earlier, includes determination of the route being used for drug delivery, such as oral versus intravenous. The use of some routes may give rise to other concerns (e.g., HIV/AIDS or hepatitis with needle use). Respiratory status and breathing rate and rhythm are important to assess because of the risk for respiratory depression. Assessment for marijuana use includes appraisal of cognitive and motor function and assessment for the inability to carry out minor tasks. Hallucinogen abuse requires assessment of neurologic status, cognitive dysfunction, bizarre changes in mood and demeanor, feelings of paranoia or dysphoria, and a feeling of unreality. The nurse should also assess for and document flashbacks, irrational behavior, psychosis, combativeness, and violent tendencies.

With alcohol abuse, the nurse should assess for interactions with other drugs, including other CNS depressants such as narcotics, sedatives, and hypnotics. Because alcohol use (long term) impacts the patient's nutritional status and liver function, assessment of vitamin/mineral levels, iron, clotting/platelet studies, and protein and albumin levels are needed. Also, blood alcohol levels should be obtained as ordered because the problems that appear are directly proportional to the blood alcohol level. If the blood alcohol level is less than 50 mg/dL, the patient may have euphoria, excitement, impaired judgment, lack of coordination, and loss of inhibitions. If the level is 50 to 100 mg/dL, the patient may show unstable gait, impaired cognitive and motor function, and further impairment of judgment and speech. At 100 to 140 mg/dL, ataxia, worsening cognitive and motor function, and worsening memory are seen. At 140 to 200 mg/dL, the patient is unable to drive a ve-

hicle. At 200 to 300 mg/dL, the patient will experience blackouts and possibly death if alcohol is mixed with other CNS depressants or the patient has altered health status. Finally, at more than 300 mg/dL, cardiac and respiratory arrest may occur. It is important to understand that chronic alcohol use is associated with the following health problems: cirrhosis, ascites, esophageal varices, portal hypertension, cardiac irregularities, enlarged heart (cardiomyopathy), GI bleeding, hepatic dysfunction, hypertension, impotence, malnutrition, ulcer disease, pancreatitis, and neurologic complications with neuropathies and seizures. This list is by no means complete, but these systems need thorough assessment.

Abuse of CNS depressants is manifested by confusion; decreased blood pressure, pulse rate, and respiration rate; poor concentration; and excessive sedation. Thus, assessment in these areas is necessary for a thorough history. Abuse of CNS stimulants, however, leads to increased blood pressure, increased pulse rate, and feelings of total exhilaration but with reduced appetite, GI problems, cardiac irregularities, and heart failure. Assessment should also include a head-to-toe physical examination (as for abuse of any drug) and documentation of any vomiting, agitation, tremors, seizures, hyperactive reflexes, flushing, headache, high temperatures, and mydriasis (pupil dilation). Nicotine is a CNS stimulant, so assessment in these areas is also appropriate for this substance. If the patient has a history of malnutrition, chronic lung disease, stroke, cancer, cardiac disease, or renal or liver dysfunction, associated laboratory test results must also be thoroughly examined.

◆ NURSING DIAGNOSES

- Risk for injury and falls related to substance abuse and/or abrupt withdrawal
- Self-concept disturbance with low self-esteem related to the influence of substance abuse
- Disturbed thought processes related to biochemical changes as a result of the chemical abuse
- Risk for other-directed violence related to drug abuse or alcohol abuse
- Ineffective health maintenance related to substance abuse
- Deficient knowledge related to lack of information about abusive, addictive behaviors and their long-term management

◆ PLANNING

Goals

- Patient remains without injury during treatment for substance abuse.
- Patient gains improved self-esteem during treatment.
- Patient discusses the drug abuse problem and its management openly with the health care team.
- Patient regains control of behavior with assistance from the health care team.
- Patient identifies any barriers to effective health maintenance and healthy self-image.

Outcome Criteria

- Patient is safely withdrawn from drug use with stabilization of the physical state that was aggravated by the substance abuse (see the specific drug and related signs and symptoms).
- Patient receives appropriate referrals and humane treatment for the substance abuse problem in a safe, nonthreatening, healthy environment.
- Patient has a decreased number of violent responses and identifies possible preventative measures.
- Patient has appropriate verbalization of increased positive feelings and healthy adaptation and coping skills.

◆ IMPLEMENTATION

Nurses working with substance abuse patients need a special understanding and empathy, beginning with knowledge of the substance abuse process and understanding of the patient's lifestyle. In general, nursing interventions involve maximizing all of the therapeutic plans and minimizing those factors contributing to the abusive behaviors. Once a therapeutic rapport has been established and a patient-nurse-physician contract has been agreed upon, maximizing recovery is the plan. Interventions will be based on the patient's specific physical and emotional problems and will be carried out accordingly and in order of priority of basic needs. For example, if the patient is experiencing hallucinations either from the substance or from withdrawal, the nurse must manage the ABCs of care (airway, breathing, circulation) and monitor vital signs and neurologic and mental status while providing a calm, quiet, nonjudgmental, and nonthreatening environment. Seizures may occur, so safety precautions are also necessary, with attention to airway, padding of side rails, and implementation of other seizure precautions.

Substance withdrawal symptoms may be treated with other drugs, and thorough knowledge of the abused substance and treatment is critical to patient safety. For example, with alcohol withdrawal, diazepam may be used to help ease the symptoms of withdrawal, but there are also concerns and specific interventions regarding its use; for example, diazepam given intravenously is compatible with NaCl and should be given slowly to prevent cardiovascular collapse. Clonidine is sometimes used to treat opioid or cocaine withdrawal, and disulfiram may be used to treat alcohol abuse. With abuse, the nurse and members of the health care team need to remain informed on all treatment approaches, pharmacologic and nonpharmacologic.

Family members and significant others should be encouraged to lend their support and assistance during treatment. Lifelong treatment is often indicated; the need for support during the long-term process of recovery should be emphasized and support recommended. Methods to encourage recovery and minimize relapse should be individualized for each patient and should draw on all available resources, whether private or public. Communication techniques must be reinforcing and firm, yet sensitive to the patient's values and beliefs. Family members must be an integral part of all treatment and must participate in all educational sessions.

◆ EVALUATION

The patient should experience a feeling of safety and security during treatment and should understand the symptoms that he or she may experience during withdrawal of the drug and associated substance abuse treatment. Any change in mental status or in any parameter (vital signs) should be reported.

Life Span Considerations: The Elderly Patient
Substance Abuse

- Alcohol remains the main substance of abuse among older adults, and admissions to substance abuse treatment centers continue to increase, with approximately 50% of older adults using alcohol.
- Alcohol abuse in people over 65 years of age leads to alcohol-related abuse hospitalization costs of over $230 million annually in the United States.
- Alcohol may alter the effects of other medications that elderly patients are taking (such as CNS depressants), leading to lethargy, confusion, hypotension, and dizziness. This interaction may occur even with over-the-counter alcohol-containing products such as cough and cold syrups.
- Adults aged 55 to 59 years were the largest group of older adults seeking substance abuse treatment, accounting for 59% of older adults in treatment in 2002.
- Opioid drugs are the second most abused substance in the elderly.
- Nicotine addiction from lifelong smoking is very problematic in older adults. It may alter drug metabolism and cause increased peripheral vasoconstriction, stimulation of antidiuretic hormone release, and increased gastric acid levels.
- Caffeine use is found in older adults and can result in gastrointestinal irritation, medication-induced changes in drug metabolism, increased lithium excretion, increased CNS stimulation, and cardiac irregularities.

Data from www.usdoj.gov/dea; Warner J: More older adults enter drug rehab centers: admissions for drug and alcohol abuse on the rise for older Americans, May 2005. Available at www.webmd.com.
CNS, Central nervous system.

Patient Teaching Tips

- The patient and family or significant other must receive current and accurate information about the treatment regimen to make a more informed and individualized decision about the treatment plan.
- Education of the family or significant other about support groups and community resources is important for success during and after a treatment program.

- The health care provider should include information about any medication the patient may be receiving, with an emphasis on timing of doses, consequences of missed doses, and adverse effects.
- The health care provider should emphasize the danger of multiple drug use and the combining of drugs with alcohol.

Points to Remember

- Nurses and all other health care providers continually encounter a variety of substance abuse problems in patients and may play a significant role in patient recovery.
- A thorough assessment of the patient's medical history, including medication history, is critical to the successful treatment of patients with substance abuse problems.
- Drug withdrawal symptoms vary with the class of drug and may even be the opposite of the drug's action, such as with alcohol (a

CNS depressant), which produces withdrawal symptoms that are typically characterized by hyperactivity.
- The nurse must understand the pathology of abuse and addictive behaviors and diseases and the way that these behaviors and diseases dominate all aspects of the patient's life as the patient "lives for the drug" every minute of the day.
- Including family members or other supportive persons in the treatment regimen results in more successful treatment.

NCLEX Examination Review Questions

1. A patient is experiencing withdrawal from opioids. Which of the following is most commonly associated with acute withdrawal from opioids and opioid-like drugs?
   a. Elevated blood pressure
   b. Decreased blood pressure
   c. Lethargy
   d. Constipation
2. During treatment for withdrawal from opioids, which medication may be used?
   a. amphetamine (Dexedrine)
   b. clonidine (Catapres)
   c. diazepam (Valium)
   d. disulfiram (Antabuse)
3. A patient being admitted from the emergency department is a young female adolescent of unknown age. She is being transferred to the intensive care unit after a suicide attempt. The initial assessment shows the following: blood pressure 80/40 mm Hg, pulse rate 118 beats/min, and respiratory rate 8 breaths/min; thought processes are altered, and she is responsive to only some verbal commands. The overdose probably involved which of the following drugs?
   a. Alcohol
   b. Marijuana

c. Barbiturates
d. Amphetamines
4. A patient taking disulfiram as part of an alcohol treatment program accidentally takes a dose of cough syrup that contains a small percentage of alcohol. What symptom may he experience as a result of acetaldehyde syndrome?
   a. Lethargy
   b. Copious vomiting
   c. Hypertension
   d. No ill effect because of the small amount of alcohol in the cough syrup
5. When a patient is assessed for possible substance abuse, which of the following would indicate possible use of amphetamines?
   a. Lethargy and fatigue
   b. Cardiovascular depression
   c. Talkativeness and euphoria
   d. Difficulty swallowing and constipation

1. a, 2. b, 3. c, 4. b, 5. c.

Critical Thinking Activities

1. Your patient has been admitted to the labor and delivery department. She has a history of heavy use of alcohol and appears to be intoxicated. What are the potential effects of alcohol use on a fetus, and what would be some concerns during the first few months of the newborn's life?
2. A friend of yours reveals that she has used crack cocaine often in the past few months and tells you that even though she enjoys the sensations she can "stop at any time." What should you do?

3. A patient is admitted to the hospital for major abdominal surgery, and the physician has ordered that a transdermal nicotine patch be used while the patient is hospitalized because the patient was a heavy smoker. While applying the patch, the patient asks, "Why in the world would you want to give me nicotine when I'm trying to stop smoking?" How do you answer him?

For answers, see http://evolve.elsevier.com/Lilley.

Photo Atlas of Drug Administration

PREPARING FOR DRUG ADMINISTRATION

NOTE: This photo atlas is designed to illustrate general aspects of drug administration. For detailed instructions, please refer to a nursing fundamentals or skills book.

When giving medications, remember safety measures and correct administration techniques to avoid errors and to ensure optimal drug actions. Keep in mind the basic "Five Rights":
1. Right drug
2. Right dose
3. Right time
4. Right route
5. Right patient

Refer to Chapter 1 for additional rights regarding drug administration. Other things to keep in mind when preparing to give medications are the following:

- Remember to wash your hands before preparing or giving medications.
- If you are unsure about a drug or dosage calculation, do not hesitate to double-check with a drug reference or with a pharmacist. **DO NOT** give a medication if you are unsure about it!
- Be punctual when giving drugs. Some medications must be given at regular intervals to maintain therapeutic blood levels.
- Figure 9-1 shows an example of a computer-controlled drug-dispensing system. To prevent errors, obtain the drugs for one patient at a time.
- Remember to check the drug at least three times before giving it. The nurse is responsible for checking medication labels against the transcribed medication order. In Figure 9-2, the nurse is checking the drug against the medication administration record (MAR) after taking it out of the dispenser drawer. The drug should also be checked before opening it and again after opening but before giving it to the patient.
- Health care facilities have various means of checking the MAR when a new one is printed, so be sure that you are working from a MAR that has been checked or verified before giving the oral medication. If the patient's MAR has a new drug order on it, the best rule of practice is to double-check that order against the patient's chart.
- Check the expiration date of all medications. Medications used past the expiration date may be less potent or even harmful.
- Before administering any medication, check the patient's identification bracelet. In addition, the patient's drug allergies should be assessed (Figure 9-3).
- Be sure to take the time to explain the purpose of each medication, its action, possible side effects, and any other pertinent information, especially drug-drug or drug-food interactions, to the patient and/or caregiver.

- Open the medication at the bedside into the patient's hand or into the medicine cup. Try not to touch the drugs with your hands. Leaving them in their packaging until you get to the patient's room helps to avoid contamination and waste should the patient refuse the drug.
- Discard any medications that fall to the floor or become contaminated by other means.
- Chart the medication on the MAR (see Figure 9-9 on p. 98) as soon as it is given and before going to the next patient. Be sure also to document therapeutic responses, adverse effects (if any), and other concerns in the nurse's notes.
- Return to evaluate the patient's response to the drug. Remember that the expected response time will vary according to the drug route. For example, responses to sublingual nitroglycerin or intravenous push medications should be evaluated within minutes, but it may take an hour for a response to be noted after an oral medication is given.
- See the Life Span Considerations: The Pediatric Patient box on page 37 for age-related considerations for medication administration for infants and children.

ENTERAL DRUGS

Administering Oral Drugs

Always begin by washing your hands and maintain Standard Precautions (Box 9-1). When administering oral drugs, keep in mind the following points:

Oral Medications
- Administration of some oral medications (and medications by other routes) requires special assessments. For example, the apical pulse should be auscultated for 1 full minute before any digitalis preparation is given (Figure 9-4). Administration of other oral medications may require blood pressure monitoring. Be sure to document all parameters on the MAR. In addition, do not forget to check the patient's identification and allergies before giving any oral medication (or medication by any other route).
- If the patient is experiencing difficulty swallowing (dysphagia), some types of tablets can be crushed with a clean mortar and pestle (or other device) (Figure 9-5) for easier administration. Crush one type of pill at a time, because if you mix together all of the medications before crushing (vs. crushing them one at a time) and then spill some, there is no way to tell which drug has been wasted. Also, if all are mixed together, you cannot check the Five Rights three times before giving the drug. Mix the crushed medication in a small amount of soft food, such as applesauce or pudding. Be sure that the pill-crushing device is clean before and after you use it.

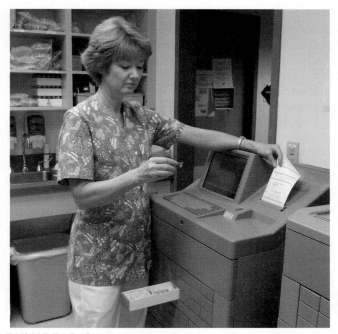

FIGURE 9-1   Using a computer-dispensing system to remove unit-dose medication.

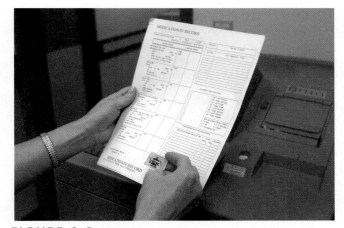

FIGURE 9-2   Checking the medication against the order on the medication administration record.

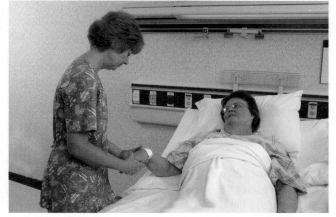

FIGURE 9-3   Always check the patient's identification and allergies before giving medications.

Box 9-1   Standard Precautions

Always adhere to Standard Precautions, including the following:
- Wear clean gloves when exposed to, or when there is potential exposure to, blood, body fluids, secretions, excretions, and any items that may contain these substances. Always wash hands immediately when there is direct contact with these substances or any item contaminated with blood, body fluids, secretions, or excretions. Gloves should always be worn when giving injections. Be sure to assess for latex allergies and use nonlatex gloves if indicated.
- Wash hands after removing gloves and between patient contacts.
- Wear a mask, eye protective gear, and face shield during any procedure or patient care situation with the potential for splashing or spraying of blood, body fluids, secretions, or excretions. Use of a gown may also be indicated for these situations.
- When administering medications, once the exposure or procedure is completed and exposure is no longer a danger, remove soiled protective garments or gear.
- Never remove, recap, cap, bend, or break any used needle or needle system. Be sure to discard any disposable syringes and needles in the appropriate puncture-resistant container.
- If, during drug administration, you are handling or transporting soiled and contaminated items from the patient, dispose of them in the appropriately labeled containers for contaminated wastes.

- **CAUTION:** Be sure to verify whether a medication can be crushed by consulting a drug reference book or a pharmacist. Some oral medications, such as capsules, enteric-coated tablets, and sustained-release or long-acting drugs, should *not* be crushed, broken, or chewed (Figure 9-6). These medications are formulated to protect the gastric lining from irritation or protect the drug from destruction by gastric acids, or are designed to break down gradually and slowly release the medication. If these drugs, designated with labels such as sustained release or extended release, are crushed or opened, then the intended action of the dosage form is destroyed. As a result, gastric irritation may occur, the drug may be inactivated by gastric acids, or the immediate availability of a drug that was supposed to be released slowly may cause toxic effects. Check with the health care provider to see if an alternate form of the drug is needed.
- Be sure to position the patient to a sitting or side-lying position to make it easier to swallow oral medications and to avoid the risk of aspiration (Figure 9-7). Always provide aspiration prevention measures as needed.
- Offer the patient a full glass of water; 4 to 6 oz of water or other fluid is recommended for the best dissolution and absorption of oral medications. Young patients and the elderly may not be able to drink a full glass of water but should take enough fluid to ensure that the medication reaches the stomach. If the patient prefers another fluid, be sure to check for interactions between the medication and the fluid of choice. If fluid restriction is ordered, be sure to follow the guidelines.
- If the patient requests, you may place the pill or capsule in his or her mouth with your gloved hand.
- Lozenges should not be chewed unless this is specifically instructed.

- Effervescent powders and tablets should be mixed with water and then given immediately after they are dissolved.
- Remain with the patient until all medication has been swallowed. If you are unsure whether a pill has been swallowed, ask the patient to open his or her mouth so that you can inspect to see if it is gone. Assist the patient to a comfortable position after the medication has been taken.
- Document the medication given on the MAR and monitor the patient for a therapeutic response as well as for adverse reactions.

Sublingual and Buccal Medications

The sublingual and buccal routes prevent destruction of the drugs in the gastrointestinal tract and allow for rapid absorption into the bloodstream through the oral mucous membranes. These routes are not often used. Be sure to provide instruction to the patient before giving these medications.

- Sublingual tablets should be placed under the tongue (Figure 9-8). Buccal tablets should be placed between the upper or lower molar teeth and the cheek.
- Be sure to wear gloves if you are placing the tablet into the patient's mouth. Adhere to Standard Precautions (see Box 9-1).
- Instruct the patient to allow the drug to dissolve completely before swallowing.
- Fluids should not be taken with these drug forms. Instruct the patient not to drink anything until the tablet has dissolved completely.
- Be sure to instruct the patient not to swallow the tablet.
- When using the buccal route, alternate sides with each dose to reduce possible oral mucosa irritation.
- Document the medication given on the MAR (Figure 9-9) and monitor the patient for a therapeutic response as well as for adverse reactions.

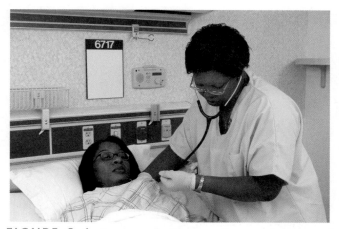

FIGURE 9-4   Some medications require special assessment before giving, such as taking an apical pulse.

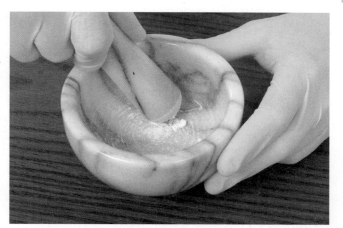

FIGURE 9-5   Crushing tablets with a mortar and pestle.

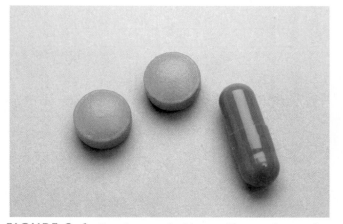

FIGURE 9-6   Enteric-coated tablets and long-acting medications should not be crushed.

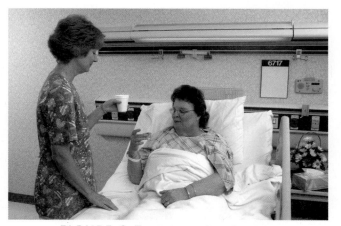

FIGURE 9-7   Giving oral medications.

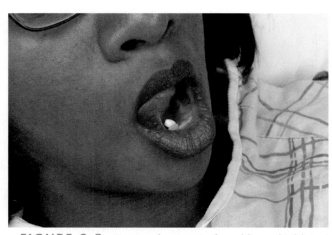

FIGURE 9-8   Proper placement of a sublingual tablet.

MEDICATION ADMINISTRATION RECORD

Effective: 11/04/03 at 0600	11/04/03 0600-2400	11/05/03 0001-0559
ROUTINE ORDERS	*Time/Initials*	*Time/Initials*
lansoprazole (Prevacid) 15 mg 1 CAPSULE AC BREAKFAST DOSE = 1 CAP = 15 mg ORD#: 5	0730 *LLL*	
nitroglycerin 2% ointment 1 pkt NITRO-BID 2% OINT(unit dose) 1 packet Q 6 H TP 1 inch = 1 packet ORD#: 6	0900 *JSS* 1500 __ 2100 __	0300 __
enoxaparin (Lovenox) 30 mg 30 mg DAILY SC DOSE = 30 mg = 0.3 ml (30 mg/0.3 ml premixed) DOCUMENT SITE ORD#: 7	0900 *JSS* Site: *RA*	
digoxin (Lanoxin) 0.125 mg ONE TABLET DAILY DOSE = 1 TAB = 0.125 MG CHECK & DOCUMENT APICAL PULSE ORD#: 8	0900 *JSS* AP = *90*	

PRN ORDERS		
acetaminophen 650 mg (Tylenol) 2 tablets Q 4 H prn PRN pain or headache DOSE = 650 mg = 2 TABLETS ORD #: 10		

ALLERGIES   INJECTION SITES

IVP DYE   Abdomen
PCN   LA = Left abdomen
SULFA   RA = Right abdomen

LT = Left thigh   RT = Right thigh

LB = Left buttock   RB = Right buttock

LA = Left arm   RA = Right arm

STAT and SINGLE DOSE MEDS

MED/DOSAGE/ROUTE	Date	Time	INITIALS
Lasix, 40 mg IV STAT	*11/04*	*1200*	*JSS*

INITIALS	MAR VERIFICATION/TIME
CTR	*Charles T. Ryan, RN/0500*

SIGNATURE LOG

INITIALS	FULL SIGNATURE / TITLE
JSS	*Julie S. Snyder, RN*
LLL	*Linda L. Lilley, RN*

Patient Name: *Rue, Jeannie*

MR#: *06121958*   DOB: *05/25/40*

Admitting Dr: *Keadle, Ralph*   Room: *6717*

MAYFIELD GENERAL HOSPITAL

Virginia Shores, VA

PAGE 1 of 1

FIGURE 9-9   Example of a medication administration record (MAR).

Liquid Medications

- Liquid medications may come in a single-dose (unit-dose) package, be poured into a medicine cup from a multidose bottle, or be drawn up in an oral-dosing syringe (Figure 9-10). For young children, liquid forms are preferred because children may aspirate pills.
- When pouring a liquid medication from a container, first shake the bottle gently to mix the contents if indicated. Remove the cap and place it on the counter, upside down. Hold the bottle with the label against the palm of your hand to keep any spilled medication from altering the label. Place the medication cup at eye level and fill to the proper level on the scale (Figure 9-11). Pour the liquid so that the base of the meniscus is even with the appropriate line measure on the medicine cup.
- If you overfill the medication cup, discard the excess in the sink. Do not pour it back into the multidose bottle. Before replacing the cap, wipe the rim of the bottle with a paper towel.
- For small doses of liquid medications, draw liquid into a calibrated oral syringe. Do not use a hypodermic syringe or a syringe with a needle or syringe cap. If hypodermic syringes are used, the drug may be inadvertently given parenterally, or the syringe cap or needle, if not removed from the syringe, may become dislodged and accidentally aspirated by the patient when the syringe plunger is pressed.

Oral Medications and Infants

- Because infants cannot swallow pills or capsules, liquids are usually ordered.
- A plastic disposable oral-dosing syringe is recommended for measuring small doses of liquid medications. Use of an oral-dosing syringe prevents the inadvertent parenteral administration of a drug once it is drawn up into the syringe.
- Position the infant so that the head is slightly elevated to prevent aspiration. Not all infants will be cooperative, and many may need to be partially restrained (Figure 9-12).
- Place the plastic dropper or syringe inside the infant's mouth, beside the tongue, and administer the liquid in small amounts while allowing the infant to swallow each time.
- An empty nipple may be used to administer the medication. Place the liquid inside the empty nipple and allow the infant to suck the nipple. Add a few milliliters of water to rinse any remaining medication into the infant's mouth, unless contraindicated.
- Take great care to prevent aspiration. A crying infant can easily aspirate medication.
- Do not add medication to a bottle of formula; the infant may refuse the feeding or may not drink all of it.
- Make sure that all of the oral medication has been taken, then return the infant to a safe, comfortable position.

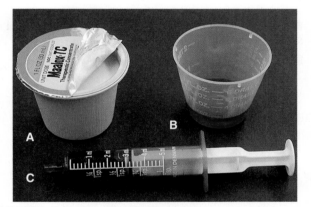

FIGURE 9-10 **A,** Liquid medication in a unit-dose package. **B,** Liquid measured into a medicine cup from a multidose container. **C,** Liquid medicine in an oral-dosing syringe.

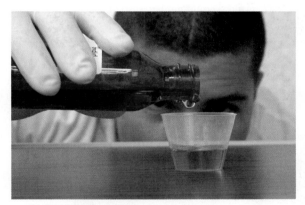

FIGURE 9-11 Measuring liquid medication.

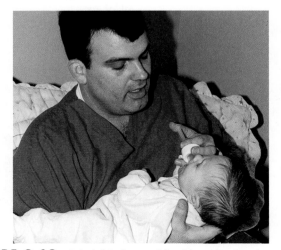

FIGURE 9-12 Administering oral liquid medication to an infant.

Administering Drugs Through a Nasogastric or Gastrostomy Tube

Always begin by washing your hands and maintain Standard Precautions (see Box 9-1). Gloves should be worn for these procedures. When administering drugs via these routes, keep in mind the following points:

- Before giving drugs via these routes, position the patient in a semi-Fowler's or Fowler's position and leave the head of the bed elevated for at least 30 minutes afterward to reduce the risk of aspiration (Figure 9-13).
- Assess whether fluid restriction or fluid overload is a concern. It will be necessary to give water along with the medications to flush the tubing.
- Check to see if the drug should be given on an empty or full stomach. If the drug should be given on an empty stomach, the feeding may need to be stopped before and/or after giving the medication. Follow the guidelines for the specific drug if this is necessary.
- Whenever possible, give liquid forms of drugs to prevent clogging the tube.
- If tablets must be given, crush the tablets individually into a fine powder. Administer the drugs separately (Figure 9-14). Keeping the drugs separate allows for accurate identification if a dose is spilled. Be sure to check whether the medication should be crushed; enteric-coated and sustained-release tablets or capsules should not be crushed. Check with a pharmacist if you are unsure.
- Before administering the drugs, follow the institution's policy for verifying tube placement and checking gastric residual.

Reinstill gastric residual per institutional policy, then clamp the tube.

- Dilute a crushed tablet or liquid medication in 15 to 30 mL of warm water. Some capsules may be opened and dissolved in 30 mL of warm water; check with a pharmacist.
- Remove the piston from an adaptable-tip syringe and attach it to the end of the tube. Unclamp the tube and pinch the tubing to close it again. Add 30 mL of warm water and release the pinched tubing. Allow the water to flow in by gravity to flush the tube, and then pinch the tubing closed again before all the water is gone to prevent excessive air from entering the stomach.
- Pour the diluted medication into the syringe and release the tubing to allow it to flow in by gravity. Flush between each drug with 10 mL of warm water (Figure 9-15). Be careful not to spill the medication mixture. Adjust fluid amounts if fluid restrictions are ordered, but sufficient fluid must be used to dilute the medications and to flush the tubing.
- If water or medication does not flow freely, you may apply gentle pressure with the plunger of the syringe or the bulb of an Asepto syringe. Do not try to force the medicine through the tubing.
- After the last drug dose, flush the tubing with 30 mL of warm water, then clamp the tube. Resume the tube feeding when appropriate.
- Have the patient remain in a high Fowler's or slightly elevated right-side-lying position to reduce the risk of aspiration.
- Document the medications given on the MAR, the amount of fluid given on the patient's intake and output record, and the patient's response.

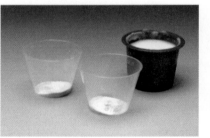

FIGURE 9-14 Medications given through gastric tubes should be administered separately. Dilute crushed pills in 15 to 30 mL of water before administration.

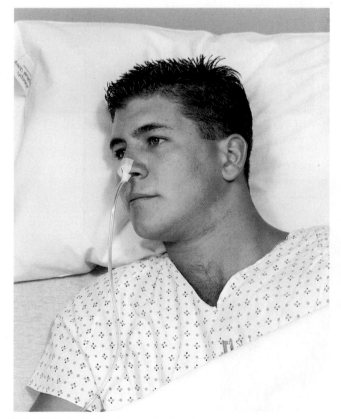

FIGURE 9-13 Elevate the head of the bed before administering medications through a nasogastric tube.

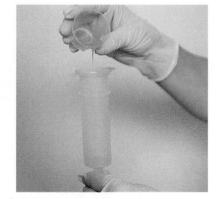

FIGURE 9-15 Pour liquid medication into the syringe, then unclamp the tubing and allow it to flow in by gravity.

Administering Rectal Drugs

Always begin by washing your hands and maintain Standard Precautions (see Box 9-1). Gloves should be worn for these procedures. When administering rectal drugs, keep in mind the following points:

- Assess the patient for the presence of active rectal bleeding or diarrhea, which generally are contraindications for the use of rectal suppositories.
- Suppositories should not be divided to provide a smaller dose. The active drug may not be evenly distributed within the suppository base.
- Position the patient on his or her left side, unless contraindicated. The uppermost leg should be flexed toward the waist (Sims' position). Provide privacy and drape.
- The suppository should not be inserted into stool. Gently palpate the rectal wall for the presence of feces. If possible, have the patient defecate. DO NOT palpate the patient's rectum if the patient has had rectal surgery.
- Remove the wrapping from the suppository and lubricate the rounded tip with water-soluble jelly (Figure 9-16).
- Insert the tip of the suppository into the rectum while having the patient take a deep breath and exhale through the mouth.

With your gloved finger, quickly and gently insert the suppository into the rectum, alongside the rectal wall, at least 1 inch beyond the internal sphincter (Figure 9-17).

- Have the patient remain lying on his or her left side for 15 to 20 minutes to allow absorption of the medication. With children it may be necessary to gently but firmly hold the buttocks in place for 5 to 10 minutes until the urge to expel the suppository has passed. Older adults with loss of sphincter control may not be able to retain the suppository.
- If the patient prefers to self-administer the suppository, the nurse should give specific instructions on the purpose and correct procedure. Be sure to tell the patient to remove the wrapper.
- Use the same procedure for medications administered by a retention enema, such as sodium polystyrene sulfonate (see Chapter 26). Drugs given by enemas are diluted in the smallest amount of solution possible. Retention enemas should be held for 30 minutes to 1 hour before expulsion, if possible.
- Document the medication on the MAR and monitor the patient for the therapeutic effects of the rectal medication.

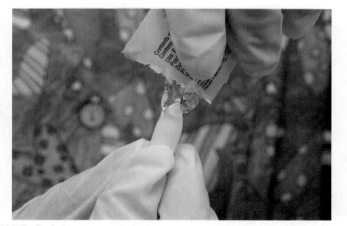

FIGURE 9-16   Lubricate the suppository with a water-soluble lubricant.

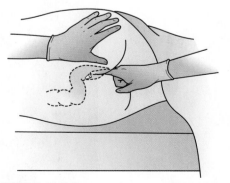

FIGURE 9-17   Inserting a rectal suppository.

PARENTERAL DRUGS

Preparing for Parenteral Drug Administration

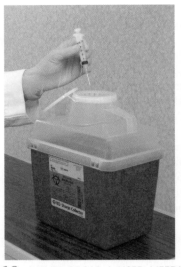

FIGURE 9-18 NEVER RECAP A USED NEEDLE! Always dispose of *uncapped* needles in the appropriate sharps container. Refer to Box 9-1 for Standard Precautions.

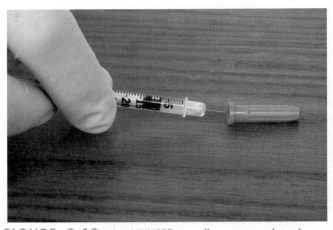

FIGURE 9-19 An UNUSED needle may need to be recapped before the medication is given to the patient. The "scoop method" is one way to recap an unused needle safely. Be sure not to touch the needle to the countertop or to the outside of the needle cap.

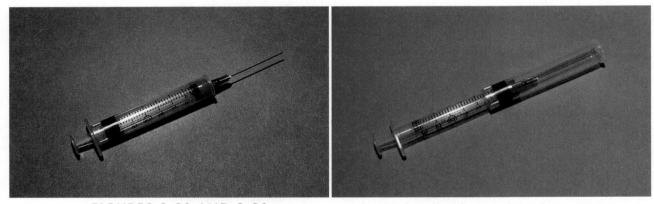

FIGURES 9-20 AND 9-21 There are several types of needlestick prevention syringes. This example (Figure 9-20) has a guard over the unused syringe. After the injection, the nurse pulls the guard up over the needle until it locks into place (Figure 9-21).

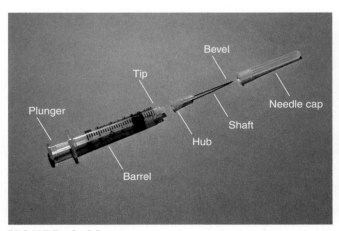

FIGURE 9-22 The parts of a syringe and hypodermic needle.

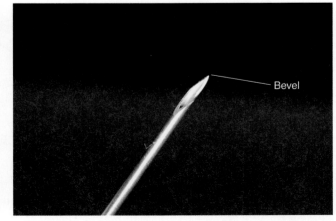

FIGURE 9-23 Close-up view of the bevel of a needle.

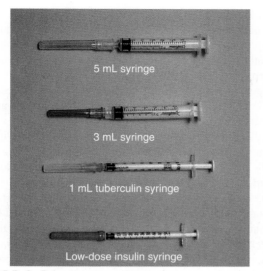

FIGURE 9-24 Be sure to choose the correct size and type of syringe for the drug ordered.

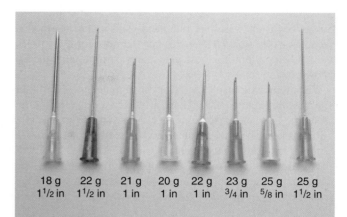

FIGURE 9-25 Needles come in various gauges and lengths. The larger the gauge, the smaller the needle. Be sure to choose the correct needle—gauge and length—for the type of injection ordered.

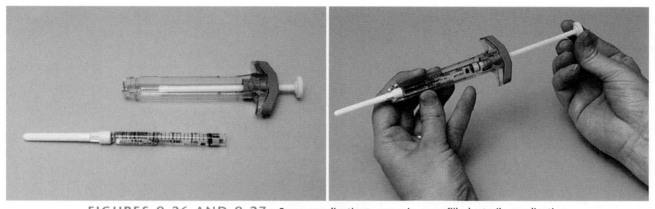

FIGURES 9-26 AND 9-27 Some medications come in a prefilled, sterile medication cartridge. Figures 9-26 and 9-27 show the Carpuject prefilled cartridge and syringe system. Follow the manufacturer's instructions for assembling prefilled syringes. After use, the syringe is disposed of in a sharps container; the cartridge is reusable.

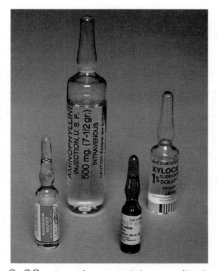

FIGURE 9-28 Ampules containing medications come in various sizes. The ampules must be broken carefully to withdraw the medication.

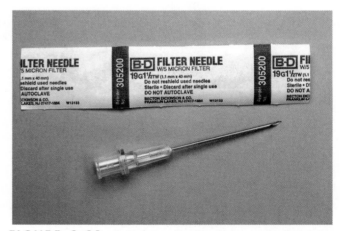

FIGURE 9-29 A filter needle should be used when withdrawing medication from an ampule. Filter needles help to remove tiny glass particles that may result from the ampule breakage. DO NOT USE A FILTER NEEDLE for injection into a patient! Some facilities may require the use of a filter needle to withdraw medications from a vial.

Removing Medications from Ampules

Always begin by washing your hands and maintain Standard Precautions (see Box 9-1). Gloves may be worn for these procedures. When performing these procedures, keep in mind the following points:

- When removing medication from an ampule, use a sterile filter needle (Figure 9-29). These needles are designed to filter out glass particles that may be present inside the ampule after it is broken. The filter needle IS NOT intended for administration of the drug to the patient.
- Medication often rests in the top part of the ampule. Tap the top of the ampule lightly and quickly with your finger until all fluid moves to the bottom portion of the ampule (Figure 9-30).
- Place a small gauze pad or dry alcohol swab around the neck of the ampule to protect your hand. Snap the neck quickly and firmly and break the ampule *away* from your body (Figures 9-31 and 9-32).
- To draw up the medication, either set the open ampule on a flat surface or hold the ampule upside down. Insert the filter needle (attached to a syringe) into the center of the ampule opening. Do not allow the needle tip or shaft to touch the rim of the ampule (Figure 9-33).
- Gently pull back on the plunger to draw up the medication. Keep the needle tip below the fluid within the vial; tip the ampule to bring all of the fluid within reach of the needle.
- If air bubbles are aspirated, do not expel them into the ampule. Remove the needle from the ampule, hold the syringe with the needle pointing up, and tap the side of the syringe with your finger to cause the bubbles to rise toward the needle. Draw back slightly on the plunger and slowly push the plunger upward to eject the air. Do not eject fluid.
- Excess medication should be disposed of in a sink. Hold the syringe vertically with the needle tip up and slanted toward the sink. Slowly eject the excess fluid into the sink, then recheck the fluid level by holding the syringe vertically.
- Remove the filter needle and replace with the appropriate needle for administration.
- Dispose of the glass ampule pieces and the used filter needle in the appropriate sharps container.

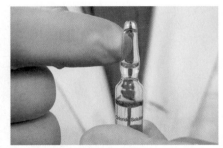

FIGURE 9-30 Tapping an ampule to move the fluid below the neck.

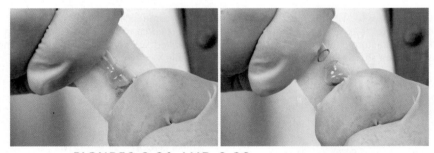

FIGURES 9-31 AND 9-32 Breaking an ampule.

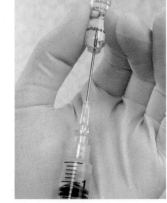

FIGURE 9-33 Using a filter needle to withdraw medication from an ampule.

Removing Medications from Vials

Always begin by washing your hands and maintain Standard Precautions (see Box 9-1). Gloves may be worn for these procedures. When performing these procedures, keep in mind the following points:

- Vials can contain either a single dose or multiple doses of medication. Follow the institution's policy for using opened multidose vials. Multidose vials should be marked with the date and time of opening and the discard date (per facility policy). If you are unsure about the age of an opened vial of medication, discard it and obtain a new one.
- Check institutional policies regarding which drugs should be prepared using a filter needle.
- If the vial is unused, remove the cap from the top of the vial.
- If the vial has been previously opened and used, wipe the top of the vial vigorously with an alcohol swab.
- Air must first be injected into a vial before fluid can be withdrawn. The amount of air injected into a vial should equal the amount of fluid that needs to be withdrawn.
- Determine the volume of fluid to be withdrawn from the vial. Pull back on the syringe's plunger to draw an amount of air into the syringe that is equivalent to the volume of medication to be removed from the vial. Insert the syringe into the vial,

preferably using a needleless system. Figure 9-34 shows a needleless system of vial access. Inject the air into the vial.

- While holding onto the plunger, invert the vial and remove the desired amount of medication (Figure 9-35).
- Gently but firmly tap the syringe to remove air bubbles. Excess fluid, if present, should be discarded into a sink.
- Some vials are not compatible with needleless systems and therefore require a needle for fluid withdrawals (Figure 9-36).
- When an injection requires two medications from two different vials, begin by injecting air into the first vial (without touching the fluid in the first vial), then inject air into the second vial. Immediately remove the desired dose from the second vial. Change needles (if possible), then remove the exact prescribed dose of drug from the first vial. Take great care not to contaminate the drug in one vial with the drug from the other vial.
- For injections, if a needle has been used to remove medication from a vial, always change the needle before administering the dose. Changing needles ensures that a clean and sharp needle is used for the injection. Medication that remains on the outside of the needle may cause irritation to the patient's tissues. In addition, the needle may become dull if used to puncture a rubber stopper.

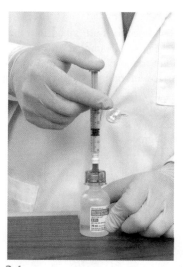

FIGURE 9-34 Insert air into a vial before withdrawing medication (needleless system shown).

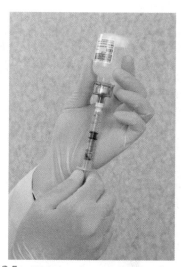

FIGURE 9-35 Withdrawing medication from a vial (needleless system shown).

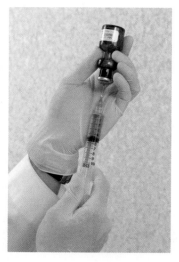

FIGURE 9-36 Using a needle and syringe to remove medication from a vial.

Injections Overview

Needle Insertion Angles for Intramuscular,
Subcutaneous, and Intradermal Injections

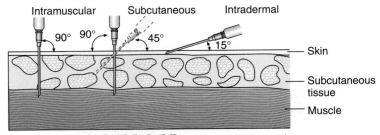

FIGURE 9-37   Various needle angles.

- For intramuscular (IM) injections, insert the needle at a 90-degree angle (Figure 9-37). Intramuscular injections deposit the drug deep into muscle tissue, where the drug is absorbed through blood vessels within the muscle. The rate of absorption of medication with the intramuscular route is slower than with the intravenous route but faster than with the subcutaneous route. Intramuscular injections generally require a longer needle to reach the muscle tissue, but shorter needles may be needed for older patients, children, and adults who are malnourished. The site chosen will also determine the length of the needle needed. In general, aqueous medications can be given with a 22- to 27-gauge needle, but oil-based or more viscous medications are given with an 18- to 25-gauge needle. Average needle lengths for children range from ⅝ to 1 inch, and needles for adults range from 1 to 1½ inches.
- For subcutaneous (SC or SQ) injections, insert the needle at either a 90- or 45-degree angle. Subcutaneous injections deposit the drug into the loose connective tissue under the dermis. This tissue is not as well supplied with blood vessels as is the muscle tissue; as a result, drugs are absorbed more slowly than drugs given intramuscularly. In general, use a 25-gauge, ½- to ⅝-inch needle. A 90-degree angle is used for an average-sized patient; a 45-degree angle may be used for thin, emaciated, and/or cachectic patients and for children. To ensure correct needle length, grasp the skinfold with thumb and forefinger, and choose a needle that is approximately half the length of the skinfold from top to bottom.
- Intradermal (ID) injections are given into the outer layers of the dermis in very small amounts, usually 0.01 to 0.1 mL. These injections are used mostly for diagnostic purposes, such as testing for allergies or tuberculosis, and for local anesthesia. Very little of the drug is absorbed systemically. In general, choose a tuberculin or 1-mL syringe with a 25- or 27-gauge needle that is ⅜ to ⅝ inch long. The angle of injection is 5 to 15 degrees.

Z-Track Method

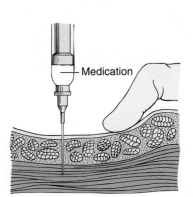

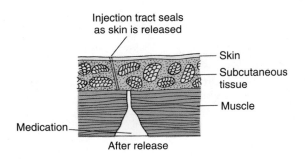

FIGURES 9-38 AND 9-39   The Z-track method for intramuscular injections.

- The Z-track method is used for injections of irritating substances such as iron dextran and hydroxyzine (Figures 9-38 and 9-39). The technique reduces pain, irritation, and staining at the injection site. Some facilities recommend this method for *all* intramuscular injections.
- After choosing and preparing the site for injection, use your nondominant hand to pull the skin laterally and hold it in this position while giving the injection. Insert the needle at a 90-degree angle, aspirate for 5 to 10 seconds to check for blood return, then inject the medication slowly. After injecting the medication, wait 10 seconds before withdrawing the needle. Withdraw the needle slowly and smoothly, and maintain the 90-degree angle.
- Release the skin immediately after withdrawing the needle to seal off the injection site. This technique forms a Z-shaped track in the tissue that prevents the medication from leaking through the more sensitive subcutaneous tissue from the muscle site of injection. Apply gentle pressure to the site with a dry gauze pad.

Air-Lock Technique

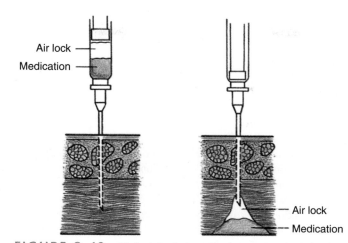

Air lock
Medication

Air lock
Medication

FIGURE 9-40 Air-lock technique for intramuscular injections.

- Some facilities recommend administering intramuscular injections using the air-lock technique (Figure 9-40). Check institutional policies.
- After withdrawing the desired amount of medication into the syringe, withdraw an additional 0.2 mL of air. Be sure

to inject using a 90-degree angle. The small air bubble that follows the medication during the injection may help prevent the medication from leaking through the needle track into the subcutaneous tissues.

Intradermal Injection

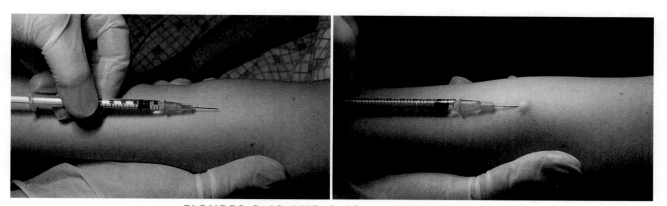

FIGURES 9-41 AND 9-42 Intradermal injection.

Always begin by washing your hands and maintain Standard Precautions (see Box 9-1). Gloves should be worn for these procedures. When giving an intradermal injection, keep in mind the following points:

- Be sure to choose an appropriate site for the injection. Avoid areas of bruising, rashes, inflammation, edema, or skin discolorations.
- Help the patient to a comfortable position. Extend and support the elbow and forearm on a flat surface.
- In general, three to four finger widths below the antecubital space and one hand width above the wrist are the preferred locations on the forearm. Areas on the back that are also suitable for subcutaneous injection may be used if the forearm is not appropriate.
- After cleansing the site with an alcohol swab and allowing it to dry, stretch the skin over the site with your nondominant hand.
- With the needle almost against the patient's skin, insert the needle, bevel UP, at a 5- to 15-degree angle until resistance is

felt, and then advance the needle through the epidermis, approximately 3 mm (Figures 9-41 and 9-42). The needle tip should still be visible under the skin.

- Do not aspirate. This area under the skin contains very few blood vessels.
- Slowly inject the medication. It is normal to feel resistance, and a bleb that resembles a mosquito bite (about 6 mm in diameter) should form at the site.
- Withdraw the needle slowly while gently applying a gauze pad at the site, but do not massage the site.
- Dispose of the syringe and needle in the appropriate container. DO NOT RECAP the needle. Wash your hands after removing gloves.
- Provide instructions to the patient as needed for a follow-up visit for reading the skin testing.
- Document in the MAR the date of the skin testing and the date that results should be read, if applicable.

Subcutaneous Injections

Always begin by washing your hands and maintain Standard Precautions (see Box 9-1). Gloves should be worn for these procedures. When giving a subcutaneous injection, keep in mind the following points:

- Be sure to choose an appropriate site for the injection. Avoid areas of bruising, rashes, inflammation, edema, or skin discolorations (Figure 9-43).
- Ensure that the needle size is correct. Grasp the skinfold between your thumb and forefinger and measure from top to bottom. The needle should be approximately half this length.
- Cleanse the site with an alcohol or antiseptic swab (Figure 9-44) and let the skin dry (occurs almost immediately).
- Tell the patient that he or she will feel a "stick" as you insert the needle.
- For an average-sized patient, pinch the skin with your nondominant hand and inject the needle quickly at a 90-degree angle (Figure 9-45).
- For an obese patient, pinch the skin and inject the needle at a 90-degree angle. Be sure the needle is long enough to reach the base of the skinfold.
- For a thin patient or a child, pinch the skin gently, then inject the needle at a 45-degree angle.
- Injections given in the abdomen should be given at least 2 inches away from the umbilicus because of the surrounding vascular structure (Figure 9-46).
- After the needle enters the skin, grasp the lower end of the syringe with your nondominant hand. Move your dominant hand to the end of the plunger—be careful not to move the syringe.
- Aspiration of medication to check for blood return is not necessary for subcutaneous injections, but some institutions may require it. Check institutional policy. Heparin injections and insulin injections are NOT aspirated before injection.

- With your dominant hand, slowly inject the medication.
- Withdraw the needle quickly and place a swab or sterile gauze pad over the site.
- Apply gentle pressure but do not massage the site. If necessary, apply a bandage to the site.
- Dispose of the syringe and needle in the appropriate container. DO NOT RECAP the needle. Wash your hands after removing gloves.
- Document the medication given on the MAR and monitor the patient for a therapeutic response as well as for adverse reactions.
- For injections of heparin or other subcutaneous anticoagulants, follow the manufacturer's recommendations for injection technique as needed. DO NOT ASPIRATE before injecting, and DO NOT massage the site after injection. These actions may cause a hematoma at the injection site.

Insulin Syringes

- Always use an insulin syringe to measure and administer insulin. When giving small doses of insulin, use an insulin syringe that is calibrated for smaller doses. Figure 9-47 shows insulin syringes with two different calibrations. Notice that in the 100-unit syringe, each line represents 2 units; in the 50-unit syringe, each line represents 1 unit. NOTE: A unit of insulin is NOT equivalent to a milliliter of insulin!
- Figure 9-48 shows several examples of devices that can be used to help the patient self-administer insulin. These devices feature a multidose container of insulin and easy-to-read dials for choosing the correct dose. The needle is changed with each use.
- When two different types of insulin are drawn up into the same syringe, always draw up the clear, rapid-acting insulin into the syringe first (Figure 9-49). See page 107 for information about mixing two medications in one syringe.

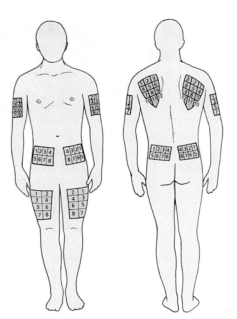

FIGURE 9-43 Potential sites for subcutaneous injections.

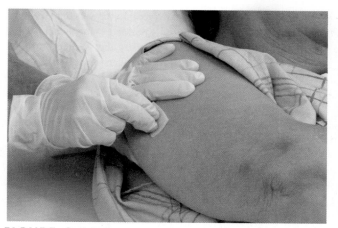

FIGURE 9-44   Before giving an injection, cleanse the skin with an alcohol or antiseptic swab.

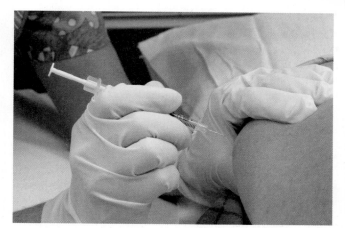

FIGURE 9-45   Giving a subcutaneous injection at a 90-degree angle.

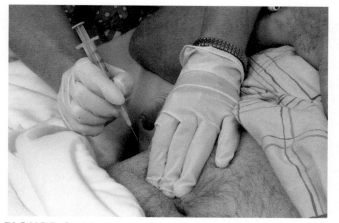

FIGURE 9-46   When giving a subcutaneous injection in the abdomen, be sure to choose a site at least 2 inches away from the umbilicus.

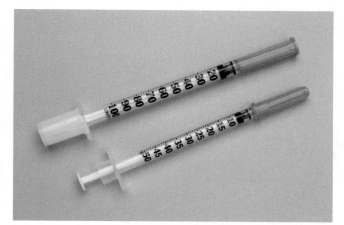

FIGURE 9-47   Insulin syringes are available in 100-unit and 50-unit calibrations.

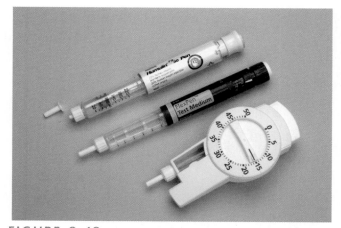

FIGURE 9-48   A variety of devices are available for insulin injections.

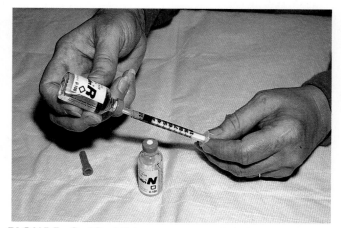

FIGURE 9-49   Mixing two types of insulin in the same syringe.

Intramuscular Injections

Always begin by washing your hands and maintain Standard Precautions (see Box 9-1). Gloves should be worn for these procedures. When giving an intramuscular injection, keep in mind the following points:

- Choose the appropriate site for the injection by assessing not only the size and integrity of the muscle but the amount and type of injection. Palpate potential sites for areas of hardness or tenderness and note the presence of bruising or infection.
- Assist the patient to the proper position and ensure his or her comfort.
- Locate the proper site for the injection and cleanse the site with an alcohol swab. Keep the swab or a sterile gauze pad nearby and allow the alcohol to dry before injection.
- With your nondominant hand, pull the skin taut. Follow the instructions for the Z-track method (p. 108) if appropriate.
- Grasp the syringe with your dominant hand as if holding a dart and hold the needle at a 90-degree angle to the skin. Tell the patient that he or she will feel a "stick" as you insert the needle.

- Insert the needle quickly and firmly into the muscle. Grasp the lower end of the syringe with the nondominant hand while still holding the skin back, to stabilize the syringe. With the dominant hand, pull back on the plunger for 5 to 10 seconds to check for blood return.
- If no blood appears in the syringe, inject the medication slowly, at the rate of 1 mL every 10 seconds. After the drug is injected, wait 10 seconds, then withdraw the needle smoothly while releasing the skin.
- Apply gentle pressure at the site and watch for bleeding. Apply a bandage if necessary.
- If blood does appear in the syringe, remove the needle, dispose of the medication and syringe, and prepare a new syringe with the medication.
- Dispose of the syringe and needle in the appropriate container. DO NOT RECAP the needle. Wash your hands after removing gloves.
- Document the medication given on the MAR and monitor the patient for a therapeutic response as well as for adverse reactions.

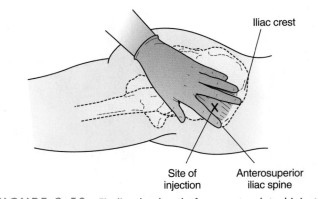

FIGURE 9-50 Finding landmarks for a ventrogluteal injection.

Ventrogluteal Site

- The ventrogluteal site is the *preferred* site for adults and children as well as infants. It is considered the safest of all sites because the muscle is deep and away from major blood vessels and nerves (Figure 9-50).
- The patient should be positioned on his or her side, with knees bent and upper leg slightly ahead of the bottom leg. If necessary, the patient may remain in a supine position.
- Palpate the greater trochanter at the head of the femur and the anterosuperior iliac spine. As illustrated in Figure 9-51, use the left hand to find landmarks when injecting into the patient's right ventrogluteal and use the right hand to find landmarks when injecting into the patient's left ventrogluteal site. Place the palm of your hand over the greater trochanter and your index finger on the anterosuperior iliac spine. Point your thumb toward the patient's groin and fingers toward the patient's head. Spread the middle finger back along the iliac crest, toward the buttocks, as much as possible.
- The injection site is the center of the triangle formed by your middle and index fingers (see arrow in Figure 9-51).
- Before giving the injection you may need to switch hands so that you can use your dominant hand to give the injection.
- Follow the general instructions for giving an intramuscular injection (Figure 9-52).

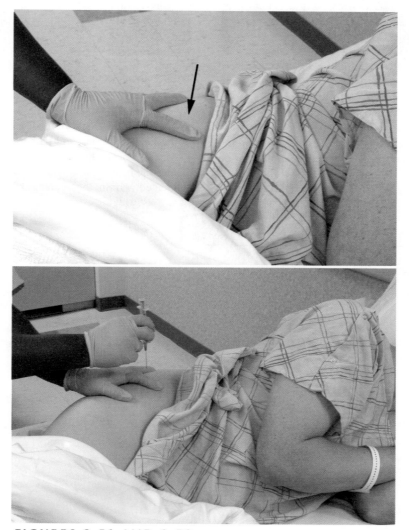

FIGURES 9-51 AND 9-52 Ventrogluteal intramuscular injection.

Vastus Lateralis Site

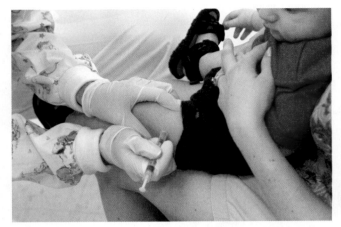

FIGURE 9-53   Vastus lateralis intramuscular injection in an infant.

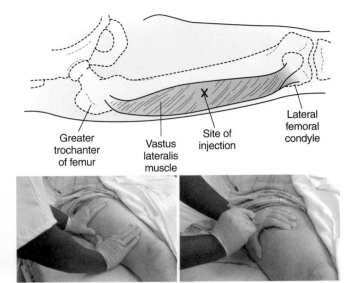

FIGURES 9-54, 9-55, AND 9-56   Vastus lateralis intramuscular injection.

- Generally the vastus lateralis muscle is well developed and not located near major nerves or blood vessels. It is the preferred site of injection of drugs such as immunizations for infants (Figure 9-53).
- The patient may be sitting or lying supine; if supine, have the patient bend the knee of the leg in which the injection will be given.

- To find the correct site of injection, place one hand above the knee and one hand below the greater trochanter of the femur. Locate the midline of the anterior thigh and the midline of the lateral side of the thigh. The injection site is located within the rectangular area (Figures 9-54, 9-55, and 9-56).

Dorsogluteal Site

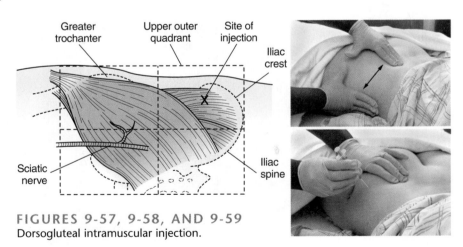

FIGURES 9-57, 9-58, AND 9-59
Dorsogluteal intramuscular injection.

- The dorsogluteal is *not* the preferred site for intramuscular injections because of the proximity of the sciatic nerve. It may be necessary to use this site, but extreme care should be taken when choosing the site for injection (Figure 9-57). If the sciatic nerve is hit during an injection, total or partial paralysis of the involved leg may occur.
- Have the patient lie on his or her abdomen with toes pointed in. Or, if preferred, the patient may lie on his or her side with the upper leg bent and anterior to the lower leg.

- Palpate the greater trochanter of the femur and the posterosuperior iliac spine. Draw an imaginary line between these landmarks (Figure 9-58).
- The injection should be given in the muscle above and outside this imaginary line (Figure 9-59).

Deltoid Site

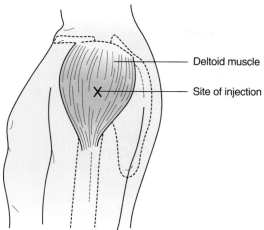

Deltoid muscle

Site of injection

FIGURES 9-60, 9-61, AND 9-62
Deltoid intramuscular injection.

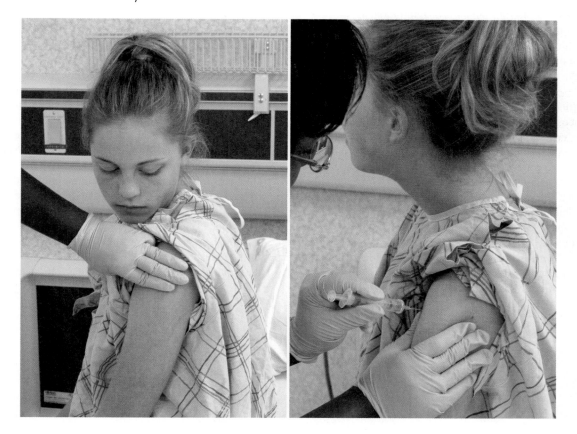

- The deltoid injection site is easily accessible but should be used only for small volumes of medication (0.5 to 1.0 mL). Assess the site carefully—this muscle may not be well developed in some adults (Figure 9-60). In addition, the axillary nerve lies beneath the deltoid muscle. Always check medication administration policies, because some facilities do not use deltoid intramuscular injections. The deltoid site is used for giving immunizations to toddlers, older children, and adults, but not to infants.
- The patient may be sitting or lying down. Remove clothing to expose the upper arm and shoulder. Tight-fitting sleeves should not be rolled up. Have the patient relax his or her arm and slightly bend the elbow.

- Palpate the lower edge of the acromion process. This edge becomes the base of an imaginary triangle (Figure 9-61).
- Place three fingers below this edge of the acromion process. Find the point on the lateral arm in line with the axilla. The injection site will be in the center of this triangle, three finger widths (1 to 2 inches) below the acromion process.
- In children and smaller adults it may be necessary to bunch the underlying tissue together before giving the injection and/ or use a shorter (⅝-inch) needle (Figure 9-62).
- To reduce anxiety, have the patient look away before giving the injection.

Preparing Intravenous Medications

Always begin by washing your hands and maintain Standard Precautions (see Box 9-1). Gloves should be worn for most of these procedures. When administering intravenous drugs, keep in mind the following points:

- The intravenous route for medication administration provides for rapid onset and faster therapeutic drug levels in the blood than other routes. However, the intravenous route is also potentially more dangerous. Once an intravenous drug is given, it begins to act immediately and cannot be removed. The nurse must be aware of the drug's intended effects and possible side or adverse effects. In addition, hypersensitivity (allergic) reactions may occur quickly.

- Since the passage of the Needle Safety and Prevention Act of 2001, many institutions now use a needleless system for all infusion lines.

- Before giving an intravenous medication, assess the patient's drug allergies, assess the intravenous line for patency, and assess the site for signs of phlebitis or infiltration.

- When more than one intravenous medication is to be given, check with the pharmacy for compatibility if the medications are to be infused at the same time.

- Check the expiration date of both the medication and infusion bags.

- In many institutions, the pharmacy is responsible for preparing intravenous solutions and intravenous piggyback (IVPB) admixtures under a special laminar air-flow hood. If you are mixing the IVPB medications, be sure to verify which type of fluid to use and the correct amount of solution for the dosage.

- Most IVPB medications are provided as part of a system that allows the intravenous medication vial to be attached to a small-volume minibag for administration. Figure 9-63 shows two examples of IVPB medications attached to small-volume infusion bags.

- These IVPB medication setups allow for mixing of the drug and diluent immediately before the medication is given. Remember that if the seals are not broken and the medication is not mixed with the fluid in the infusion bag, then the medication stays in the vial! As a result, the patient does not receive the ordered drug dose; instead, the patient receives a small amount of plain intravenous fluid.

- One type of IVPB system that needs to be activated before administration is illustrated in Figure 9-64. To activate this type of IVPB system, snap the connection area between the intravenous infusion bag and the vial (Figure 9-65). Gently squeeze the fluid from the infusion bag into the vial and allow the medication to dissolve (Figure 9-66). After a few minutes, rotate the vial gently to ensure that all of the powder is dissolved. When the drug is fully dissolved, hold the IVPB apparatus by the vial and squeeze the bag; fluid will enter the bag from the vial. Make sure that all of the medication is returned to the IVPB bag.

- When hanging these IVPB medications, take care NOT to squeeze the bag. This may cause some of the fluid to leak back into the vial and alter the dose given.

- Always label the IVPB bag with the patient's name and room number, the name of the medication, the dose, the date and time mixed, your initials, and the date and time the medication was given.

- Some intravenous medications must be mixed using a needle and syringe. After checking the order and the compatibility of the drug and the intravenous fluid, wipe the port of the intravenous bag with an alcohol swab (Figure 9-67).

- Carefully insert the needle into the center of the port and inject the medication (Figures 9-68 and 9-69). Note how the medication remains in the lower part of the intravenous infusion bag. To infuse an even concentration of medication, gently shake the bag after injecting the drug (Figure 9-70).

- Always label the intravenous infusion bag when a drug has been added (Figure 9-71). Label as per institution policy and include the patient's name and room number, the name of the medication, the date and time mixed, your initials, and the date and time the infusion was started. In addition, label all intravenous infusion tubing per institution policy.

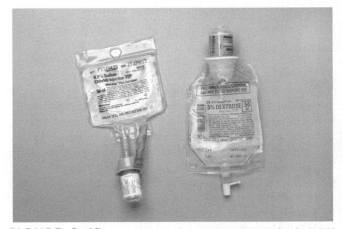

FIGURE 9-63 Two types of intravenous piggyback (IVPB) medication delivery systems. These IVPB medications must be activated before administration to the patient.

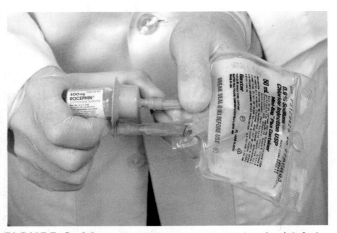

FIGURE 9-64 Activating an intravenous piggyback infusion bag (step 1).

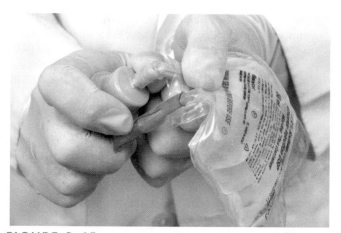

FIGURE 9-65 Activating an intravenous piggyback infusion bag (step 2).

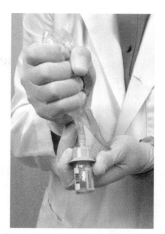

FIGURE 9-66 Activating an intravenous piggyback infusion bag (step 3).

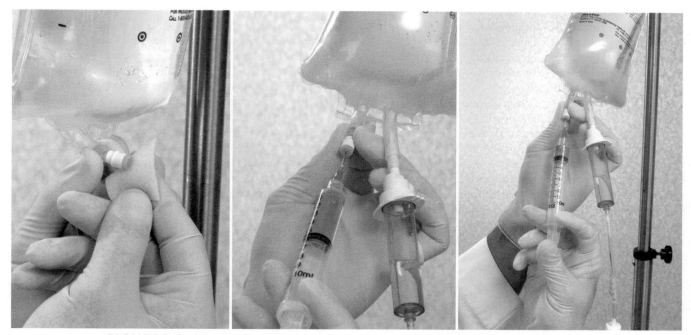

FIGURES 9-67, 9-68, AND 9-69 Adding a medication to an intravenous infusion bag with a needle and syringe.

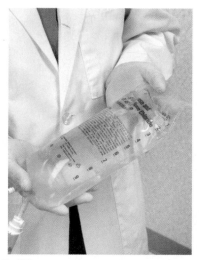

FIGURE 9-70 Mix the medication thoroughly before infusing.

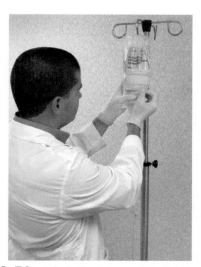

FIGURE 9-71 Label the intravenous infusion bag when medication has been added.

Infusions of Intravenous Piggyback Medications

Always begin by washing your hands and maintain Standard Precautions (see Box 9-1). Gloves should be worn for these procedures.

- Figure 9-72 shows an IVPB medication infusion with a primary gravity infusion. When the IVPB bag is hung higher than the primary intravenous infusion bag, the IVPB medication will infuse until empty, then the primary infusion will take over again.
- When beginning the infusion, attach the IVPB tubing to the upper port on the primary intravenous tubing. A back-check valve above this port prevents the medication from infusing up into the primary intravenous infusion bag.
- Fully open the clamp of the IVPB tubing and regulate the infusion rate with the roller clamp of the primary infusion tubing. Be sure to note the drip factor of the tubing and calculate the drops per minute to count in order to set the correct infusion rate for the IVPB medication.
- Monitor the patient during the infusion. Observe for hypersensitivity and for adverse reactions. In addition, observe the intravenous infusion site for infiltration. Have the patient report if pain or burning occurs.
- Monitor the rate of infusion during the IVPB administration. Changes in arm position may alter the infusion rate.
- When the infusion is complete, clamp the IVPB tubing and check the primary intravenous infusion rate. If necessary, adjust the clamp to the correct infusion rate.
- Figure 9-73 shows an IVPB medication infusion with a primary infusion that is going through an electronic infusion pump.
- When giving IVPB drugs through an intravenous infusion controlled by a pump, attach the IVPB tubing to the port on the primary intravenous tubing *above* the pump. Open the roller clamp of the IVPB bag. Make sure that the IVPB bag is higher than the primary intravenous infusion bag.

- Following the manufacturer's directions, set the infusion pump to deliver the IVPB medication. Entering the volume of the IVPB bag and the desired time frame of the infusion (such as over a 60-minute period) will cause the pump to automatically calculate the IVPB rate. Start the IVPB infusion as instructed by the pump.
- Monitor the patient during the infusion, as described earlier.
- When the infusion is complete, the primary intravenous infusion will automatically resume.
- Be sure to document the medication given on the MAR and continue to monitor the patient for adverse reactions and therapeutic effects.
- When giving IVPB medications through a saline (heparin) lock, follow the facility's guidelines for the flushing protocol before and after the medication is administered.
- Figure 9-74 illustrates a volume-controlled administration set that can be used to administer intravenous medications. The chamber is attached to the infusion between the intravenous infusion bag and the intravenous tubing. Fill the chamber with the desired amount of fluid, then add the medication via the port above the chamber, as shown in the photo. Be sure to cleanse the port with an alcohol swab before inserting the needle in the port. The chamber should be labeled with the medication's name, dose, and time added and your initials. Infuse the drug at the prescribed rate.
- In patient-controlled analgesia (PCA) a specialized pump is used to allow patients to self-administer pain medications, usually opiates (Figure 9-75). These pumps allow the patient to self-administer only as much medication as needed to control the pain by pushing a button for intravenous bolus doses. Safety features of the pump prevent accidental overdoses. A patient receiving PCA pump infusions should be monitored closely for his or her response to the drug, excessive sedation, hypotension, and changes in mental and respiratory status. Follow the facility's guidelines for setup and use.

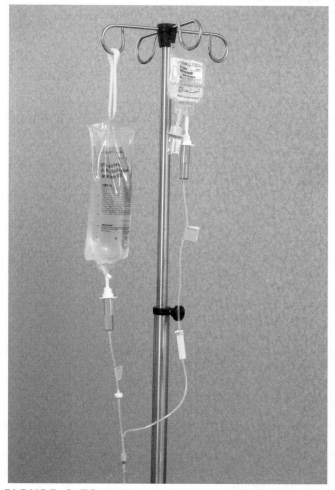

FIGURE 9-72   Infusing an intravenous piggyback medication with a gravity primary intravenous infusion.

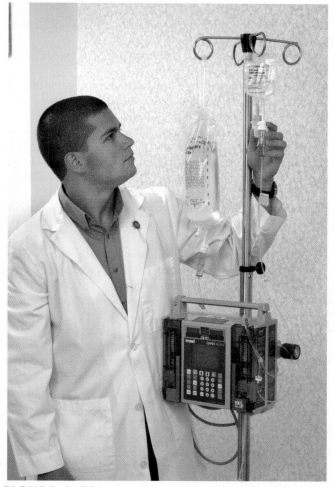

FIGURE 9-73   Infusing an intravenous piggyback medication with the primary intravenous infusion on an electronic infusion pump.

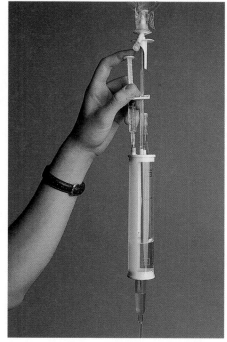

FIGURE 9-74   Adding a medication to a volume-controlled administration set.

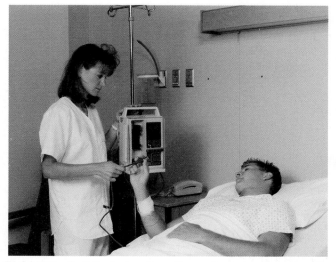

FIGURE 9-75   Instructing the patient on the use of a patient-controlled analgesia pump.

Intravenous Push Medications

Always begin by washing your hands and maintain Standard Precautions (see Box 9-1).

When administering intravenous push (or bolus) medications, keep in mind the following points:

- Registered nurses are usually the only nursing staff members, besides a nurse anesthetist, allowed to give intravenous push medications.
- Intravenous push injections allow for rapid intravenous administration of a drug. The term *bolus* refers to a dose given all at once. Intravenous push injections may be given through an existing intravenous line, through an intravenous (saline or heparin) lock, or directly into a vein.
- Because the medication may have an immediate effect, monitor the patient closely for adverse reactions as well as for therapeutic effects.
- Follow the manufacturer's guidelines carefully when preparing an intravenous push medication. Some drugs require careful dilution. Consult a pharmacist if you are unsure about the dilution procedure. Improper dilution may increase the risk of phlebitis and other complications.
- Most drugs given by intravenous push injection should be given over a period of 1 to 5 minutes to reduce local or systemic side effects. Always time the administration with your watch, because it is difficult to estimate the time accurately. Adenosine, however, must be given very rapidly, within 2 to 3 seconds, for optimal action. ALWAYS check packaging information for guidelines, because many errors and adverse effects have been associated with too-rapid intravenous drug administration.

Intravenous Push Medications Through an Intravenous Lock

- Prepare two syringes of 0.9% normal saline (NS); one should contain 3 mL and the other 5 mL. Prepare medication for injection. (Facilities may differ in the protocol for intravenous lock flushes—follow institutional policies.) If ordered, prepare a syringe with heparin flush solution.
- Follow the guidelines for a needleless system, if used.
- Cleanse the injection port of the intravenous lock with an antiseptic swab after removing the cap, if present (Figure 9-76).
- Insert the syringe of 3 mL NS into the injection port (Figure 9-77; needleless system shown). Open the clamp of the intravenous lock tubing, if present.

- Gently aspirate and observe for blood return. Absence of blood return does not mean that the intravenous line is occluded; further assessment may be required.
- Flush gently with saline while assessing for resistance. If resistance is felt, do not apply force. Stop and reassess the intravenous lock.
- Observe for signs of infiltration while injecting saline.
- Reclamp the tubing (if a clamp is present) and remove the NS syringe. Repeat cleansing of the port and attach the medication syringe. Open clamp again.
- Inject the medication over the prescribed length of time. Measure time with a watch or clock (Figure 9-78).
- When the medication is infused, clamp the intravenous lock tubing (if a clamp is present) and remove the syringe.
- Repeat cleansing of the port; attach the 5-mL NS syringe and inject the contents into the intravenous lock slowly. If a heparin flush is ordered, attach the syringe containing heparin flush solution and inject slowly (per the institution's protocol).

Intravenous Push Medications Through an Existing Infusion

- Prepare the medication for injection. Follow the guidelines for a needleless system, if used.
- Check compatibility of the intravenous medication with the existing intravenous solution.
- Choose the injection port that is closest to the patient.
- Remove the cap, if present, and cleanse the injection port with an antiseptic swab.
- Occlude the intravenous line by pinching the tubing just above the injection port (Figure 9-79). Attach the syringe to the injection port.
- Gently aspirate for blood return.
- While keeping the intravenous tubing clamped, slowly inject the medication according to administration guidelines. Be sure to time the injection with a watch or clock.
- After the injection, release the intravenous tubing, remove the syringe, and check the infusion rate of the intravenous fluid.

After Injection of an Intravenous Push Medication

- Monitor the patient closely for adverse effects. Monitor the intravenous infusion site for signs of phlebitis and infiltration.
- Document medication given on the MAR and monitor for therapeutic effects.

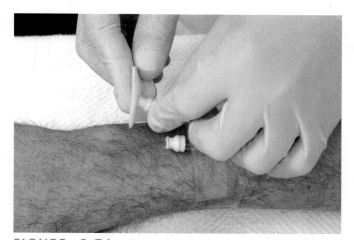

FIGURE 9-76 Cleanse the port before attaching the syringe.

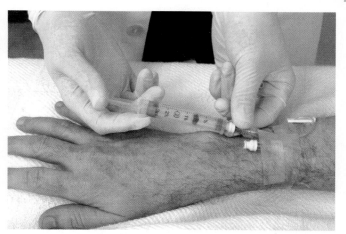

FIGURE 9-77 Attaching the syringe to the intravenous lock.

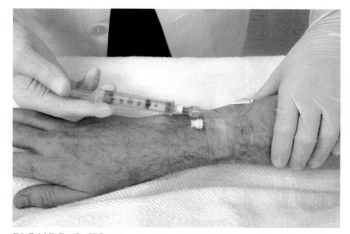

FIGURE 9-78 Slowly inject the intravenous push medication through the intravenous lock; use a watch to time the injection.

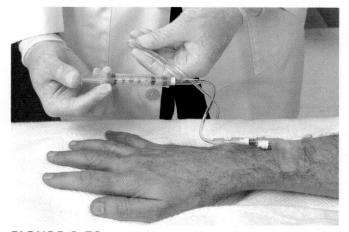

FIGURE 9-79 When giving an intravenous push medication through an intravenous line, pinch the tubing just above the injection port.

TOPICAL DRUGS

Administering Eye Medications

Always begin by washing your hands and maintain Standard Precautions (see Box 9-1). Gloves should be worn for these procedures. When administering eye preparations, keep in mind the following points:

- Assist the patient to a supine or sitting position. The patient's head should be tilted back slightly.
- Remove any secretions with a sterile gauze pad; be sure to wipe from the inner to outer canthus (Figure 9-80).
- Have the patient look up and, with your nondominant hand, gently pull the lower lid open to expose the conjunctival sac.

Eyedrops

- With your dominant hand resting on the patient's forehead, hold the eye medication dropper 1 to 2 cm above the conjunctival sac. Do not touch the tip of the dropper to the eye or with your fingers (Figure 9-81).
- Drop the prescribed number of drops into the conjunctival sac. Never apply eyedrops to the cornea.
- If the drops land on the outer lid margins (if the patient moved or blinked), repeat the procedure.
- Infants often clench the eyes tightly to avoid eyedrops. To give drops to an uncooperative infant, restrain the head gently and place the drops at the corner near the nose where the eyelids meet. When the eye opens, the medication will flow into the eye.

Eye Ointment

- Gently squeeze the tube of medication to apply an even strip of medication (about 1 to 2 cm) along the border of the conjunctival sac. Start at the inner canthus and move toward the outer canthus (Figure 9-82).

After Instillation of Eye Medications

- Ask the patient to close the eye gently. Squeezing the eye shut may force the medication out of the conjunctival sac. A tissue may be used to blot liquid that runs out of the eye, but the patient should be instructed not to wipe the eye.
- You may apply gentle pressure to the patient's nasolacrimal duct for 30 to 60 seconds with a gloved finger, wrapped in a tissue. This will help to reduce systemic absorption of the drug through the nasolacrimal duct and may also help to reduce the taste of the medication in the nasopharynx (Figure 9-83).
- Assist the patient to a comfortable position.
- Document the medication given on the MAR and check the patient for a therapeutic response or adverse reactions.

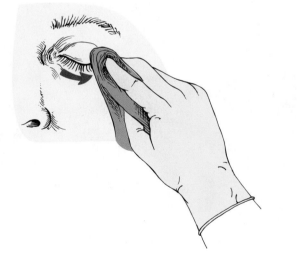

FIGURE 9-80 Cleanse the eye, washing from the inner to outer canthus, before giving eye medications.

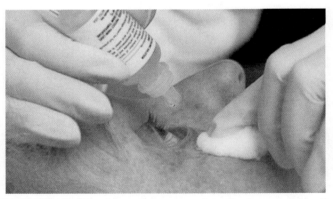

FIGURE 9-81 Insert the eyedrop into the lower conjunctival sac.

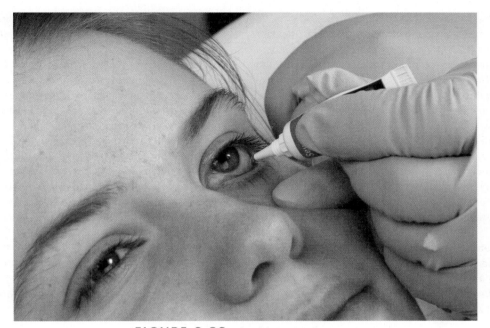

FIGURE 9-82   Applying eye ointment.

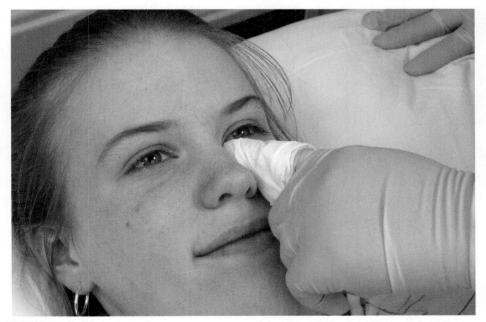

FIGURE 9-83   Applying gentle pressure against the nasolacrimal duct after giving eye medications.

Administering Eardrops

Always begin by washing your hands and maintain Standard Precautions (see Box 9-1). Gloves may be worn for these procedures. When administering ear preparations, keep in mind the following points:

- After explaining the procedure to the patient, assist the patient to a side-lying position with the affected ear facing up. If cerumen or drainage is noted in the outer ear canal, remove it carefully without pushing it back into the ear canal.
- Excessive amounts of cerumen should be removed before instillation of medication.
- If refrigerated, the ear medication should be warmed by taking it out of refrigeration for at least 30 minutes before administration. Instillation of cold eardrops can cause nausea, dizziness, and pain.
- For an adult (Figure 9-84) or a child older than 3 years of age, pull the pinna up and back.
- For an infant or a child younger than 3 years of age, pull the pinna down and back (Figure 9-85).

- Administer the prescribed number of drops. Direct the drops along the sides of the ear canal rather than directly onto the eardrum.
- Instruct the patient to lie on his or her side for 5 to 10 minutes. Gently massaging the tragus of the ear with a finger will help to distribute the medication down the ear canal.
- If ordered, a loose cotton pledget can be gently inserted into the ear canal to prevent the medication from flowing out. The cotton should still be loose enough to allow any discharge to drain out of the ear canal. To prevent the dry cotton from absorbing the eardrops that were instilled, moisten the cotton with a small amount of medication before inserting the pledget. Insertion of cotton too deeply may result in increased pressure within the ear canal and on the eardrum. Remove the cotton after about 15 minutes.
- If medication is needed in the other ear, wait 5 to 10 minutes after instillation of the first eardrops before administering.
- Document the medication given on the MAR and observe the patient for a therapeutic response or adverse reactions.

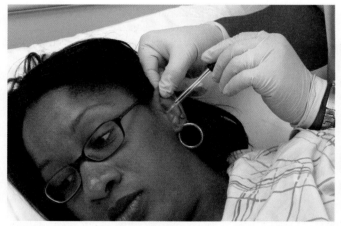

FIGURE 9-84   For adults, pull the pinna up and back.

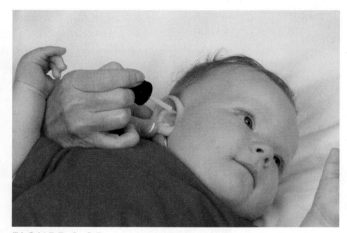

FIGURE 9-85   For infants and children younger than 3 years of age, pull the pinna down and back.

Administering Nasal Medications

Always begin by washing your hands and maintain Standard Precautions (see Box 9-1). Patients may self-administer some of these drugs after proper instruction. Gloves should be worn for these procedures. When administering nasal medications, keep in mind the following points:

- Before giving nasal medications, explain the procedure to the patient and tell him or her that temporary burning or stinging may occur. Instruct the patient that it is important to clear the nasal passages by blowing his or her nose, unless contraindicated (e.g., with increased intracranial pressure or nasal surgery), before administering the medication.
- Figure 9-86 illustrates various delivery forms for nasal medications: sprays, drops, and dose-metered sprays.
- Assist the patient to a supine position. Support the patient's head as needed.
- If specific areas are targeted for the medication, position as follows:
  - For the posterior pharynx, position the head backward.
  - For the ethmoid or sphenoid sinuses, place the head gently over the top edge of the bed or place a pillow under the shoulders and tilt the head back.
  - For the frontal or maxillary sinuses, place the head back and turned toward the side that is to receive the medication.

Nasal Drops

- Hold the nose dropper approximately ½ inch above the nostril. Administer the prescribed number of drops toward the midline of the ethmoid bone (Figure 9-87).

- Repeat the procedure as ordered, instilling the indicated number of drops per nostril.
- Keep the patient in a supine position for 5 minutes.
- Infants are nose breathers, and the potential congestion caused by nasal medications may make it difficult for them to suck. If nose drops are ordered, give them 20 to 30 minutes before a feeding.

Nasal Spray

- The patient should be sitting upright, with one nostril occluded. After gently shaking the nasal spray container, insert the tip into the nostril. Squeeze the spray bottle into the nostril while the patient inhales through the open nostril (Figure 9-88).
- Repeat the procedure as ordered, instilling the indicated number of sprays per nostril.
- Keep the patient in a supine position for 5 minutes.

After Administration of Nasal Medicines

- Offer the patient tissues for blotting any drainage, but instruct the patient to avoid blowing his or her nose for several minutes after instillation of the drops.
- Assist the patient to a comfortable position.
- Document the medication administration on the MAR and document drainage, if any. Monitor for adverse reactions and a therapeutic response.

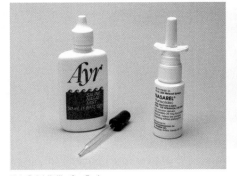

FIGURE 9-86 Nasal medications may come in various delivery forms.

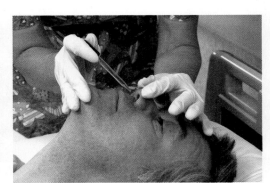

FIGURE 9-87 Administering nose drops.

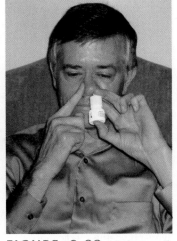

FIGURE 9-88 Before self-administering the nasal spray, the patient should occlude the other nostril.

Administering Inhaled Drugs

Always begin by washing your hands and maintain Standard Precautions (see Box 9-1). Gloves may be worn for these procedures. Patients with asthma should monitor their peak expiratory flow rates by using a peak flowmeter. A variety of inhalers are available (Figure 9-89). Be sure to check for specific instructions from the manufacturer as needed. Improper use will result in inadequate dosing. When administering inhaled preparations, keep in mind the following points.

Metered-Dose Inhalers

- Shake the metered-dose inhaler (MDI) gently before using.
- Remove the cap; hold the inhaler upright and grasp with the thumb and first two fingers.
- Tilt the patient's head back slightly.
- If the MDI is used without a spacer, do the following:
  1. Have the patient open his or her mouth; position the inhaler 1 to 2 inches away from the patient's mouth (Figure 9-90). For self-administration, some patients may measure this distance as 1 to 2 finger widths.
  2. Have the patient exhale, then press down once on the inhaler to release the medication; have the patient breathe in slowly and deeply for 5 seconds.
  3. Have the patient hold his or her breath for approximately 10 seconds, then exhale slowly through pursed lips.
- Spacers should be used with children and adults who have difficulty coordinating inhalations with activation of MDIs. If the MDI is used with a spacer, do the following:
  1. Attach the spacer to the mouthpiece of the inhaler after removing the inhaler cap (Figure 9-91).
  2. Place the mouthpiece of the spacer in the patient's mouth.
  3. Have the patient exhale.
  4. Press down on the inhaler to release the medication and have the patient inhale deeply and slowly through the spacer. The patient should breathe in and out slowly for 2

to 3 seconds, then hold his or her breath for 10 seconds (Figure 9-92).
- If a second puff of the same medication is ordered, wait 20 to 30 seconds between puffs.
- If a second type of inhaled medication is ordered, wait 2 to 5 minutes between medication inhalations or as prescribed.
- If both a bronchodilator and a steroid inhaled medication are ordered, the bronchodilator should be administered first so that the passages will be more open for the second medication.
- The patient should be instructed to rinse his or her mouth after inhaling a steroid medication to prevent the development of an oral fungal infection.
- Document the medication given on the MAR and monitor the patient for a therapeutic response as well as for adverse reactions.
- It is important to teach the patient how to calculate the number of doses in the inhaler and to keep track of uses. Simply shaking the inhaler to "estimate" whether it is empty is not accurate and may result in its being used when it is empty. The patient should be taught to count the number of puffs needed per day (doses) and divide this amount into the actual number of actuations (puffs) in the inhaler to estimate the number of days the inhaler will last. Then, a calendar can be marked a few days before this date with a note that it is time to obtain a refill. In addition, the date can be marked on the inhaler with a permanent marker. For example, an inhaler with 200 puffs, ordered to be used 4 times a day (2 puffs per dose, 8 puffs per day), would last for 25 days (200 divided by 8).
- Dry powder inhalers (DPIs) have varied instructions, and so the manufacturer's directions should be followed closely. Patients should be instructed to cover the mouthpiece completely with their mouths. Capsules that are intended for use with DPIs should NEVER be taken orally. Some DPIs have convenient built-in dose counters.

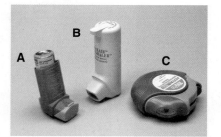

FIGURE 9-89 **A,** Metered-dose inhaler (MDI). **B,** Automated, or breath-activated, MDI. **C,** Dry powder inhaler that delivers powdered medication.

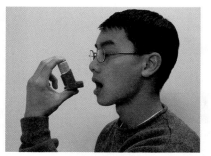

FIGURE 9-90 Using a metered-dose inhaler without a spacer.

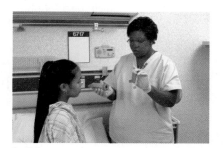

FIGURE 9-91 Instructing the patient on how to use a spacer device.

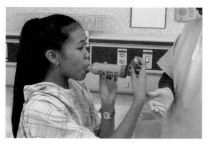

FIGURE 9-92 Using a spacer device with a metered-dose inhaler.

Small-Volume Nebulizers

- In some facilities, the air compressor is located in the wall unit of the room. In other facilities and at home, a small, portable air compressor is used. Be sure to follow the manufacturer's recommendations for use.
- Be sure to take the patient's baseline heart rate, especially if a β-adrenergic drug is used. Some drugs may increase the heart rate.
- After gathering the equipment, add the prescribed medication to the nebulizer cup (Figure 9-93). Some medications will require a diluent; others are premixed with a diluent. Be sure to verify before adding a diluent.
- Have the patient hold the mouthpiece between his or her lips (Figure 9-94). NOTE: A face mask should be used for a child or an adult who is too fatigued to hold the mouthpiece. Special adaptors are available if the patient has a tracheostomy.
- Before starting the nebulizer treatment, the patient should take a slow, deep breath, hold it briefly, then exhale slowly. Patients who are short of breath should be instructed to hold their breath every fourth or fifth breath.
- Turn on the small-volume nebulizer machine (or turn on the wall unit) and make sure that a sufficient mist is forming.

- Instruct the patient to repeat the breathing pattern mentioned previously during the treatment.
- Occasionally tap the nebulizer cup during the treatment and toward the end to move the fluid droplets back to the bottom of the cup.
- Monitor the patient's heart rate during and after the treatment.
- If inhaled steroids are given, instruct the patient to rinse his or her mouth afterward.
- After the procedure, clean and store the tubing per institutional policy.
- Document the medication given on the MAR and monitor the patient for a therapeutic response as well as for adverse reactions.
- If the patient will be using a nebulizer at home, instruct the patient to rinse the nebulizer parts after each use with warm, clear water and to air-dry. The parts should be washed daily with warm, soapy water and allowed to air-dry. Once a week, the nebulizer parts should be soaked in a solution of vinegar and water (four parts water and one part white vinegar) for 30 minutes; rinsed thoroughly with clear, warm water; and air-dried. Storing nebulizer parts that are still wet will encourage bacterial and mold growth.

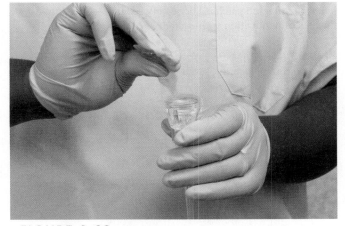

FIGURE 9-93 Adding medication to the nebulizer cup.

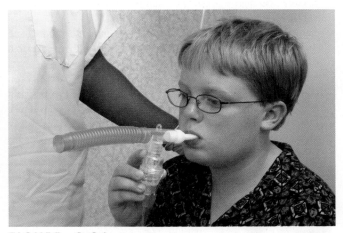

FIGURE 9-94 Administering a small-volume nebulizer treatment.

Administering Medications to the Skin

Always begin by washing your hands and maintain Standard Precautions (see Box 9-1). Gloves should be worn for these procedures. Avoid touching the preparations to your own skin. When administering skin preparations, keep in mind the following points.

Lotions, Creams, Ointments, and Powders

- Apply powder to clean, dry skin. Have the patient turn his or her head to the other side during application to avoid inhalation of powder particles.
- Apply lotion to clean, dry skin. Remove residual from previous applications with soap and water.
- Before administering any dose of a topical skin medication, ensure that the site is clean and dry. Thoroughly remove previous applications using soap and water, if appropriate for the patient's condition, and dry the area thoroughly. Also, rotate application sites.
- With lotion, cream, or gel, obtain the correct amount with your gloved hand (Figure 9-95). If the medication is in a jar, remove the dose with a sterile tongue depressor and apply to your gloved hand. Do not contaminate the medication in the jar.
- Apply the preparation with long, smooth, gentle strokes that follow the direction of hair growth (Figure 9-96). Avoid excessive pressure. Be especially careful with the skin of elderly persons, because age-related changes may result in increased capillary fragility and tendency to bruise.
- Some ointments and creams may soil the patient's clothes and linens. If ordered, cover the affected area with gauze or a transparent dressing.
- Nitroglycerin ointment in a tube is measured carefully on clean, ruled application paper before it is applied to the skin (Figure 9-97). Unit-dose packages should not be measured. Do not massage nitroglycerin ointment into the skin. Apply the measured amount onto a clean, dry site and then secure the application paper with a transparent dressing or a strip of tape. Always remove the old medication before applying a new dose.

Transdermal Patches

- Be sure that the old patch is removed as ordered. Some patches may be removed before the next patch is due—check the order. Clear patches may be difficult to find, and patches may be overlooked in obese patients with skinfolds. Cleanse the site of the old patch thoroughly. Observe for signs of skin irritation at the old patch site.
- Transdermal patches should be applied at the same time each day if ordered daily.
- The old patch can be pressed together, then wrapped in a glove as you remove the glove from your hand. Dispose in the proper container according to the facility's policy.
- Select a new site for application and ensure that it is clean and without powder or lotion. The site should be hairless and free from scratches or irritation. If it is necessary to remove hair, clip the hair instead of shaving to reduce irritation to the skin.
- Remove the backing from the new patch (Figure 9-98). Take care not to touch the medication side of the patch with your fingers.
- Place the patch on the skin site and press firmly (Figure 9-99). Press around the edges of the patch with one or two fingers to ensure that the patch is adequately secured to the skin. Rotate sites of application with each dose.

After Administration of Topical Skin Preparations

- Chart the medication given on the MAR and monitor the patient for a therapeutic response as well as for any adverse reactions.
- Provide instruction on administration to the patient and/or caregiver.

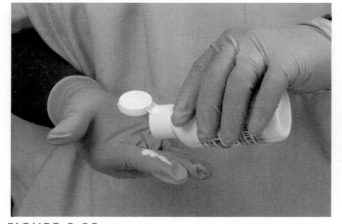

FIGURE 9-95 Use gloves to apply topical skin preparations.

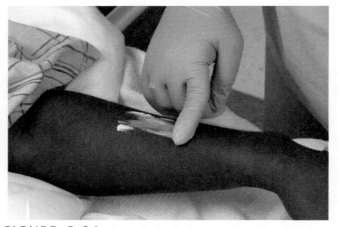

FIGURE 9-96 Spread the lotion on the skin with long, smooth, gentle strokes.

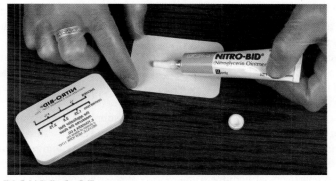

FIGURE 9-97   Measure nitroglycerin ointment carefully before application.

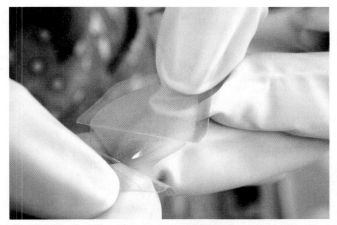

FIGURE 9-98   Opening a transdermal patch medication.

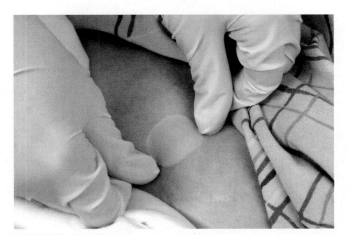

FIGURE 9-99   Ensure that the edges of the transdermal patch are secure after applying.

Administering Vaginal Medications

Always begin by washing your hands and maintain Standard Precautions (see Box 9-1). Gloves should be worn for these procedures. When administering vaginal preparations, keep in mind the following points:

- Vaginal suppositories are larger and more oval than rectal suppositories (Figure 9-100).
- Figure 9-101 shows examples of a vaginal suppository in an applicator and vaginal cream in an applicator.
- Before giving these medications explain the procedure to the patient and have her void.
- If possible, administer vaginal preparations at bedtime to allow the medications to remain in place as long as possible.
- Some patients may prefer to self-administer vaginal medications. Provide specific instructions if necessary.
- Position the patient in the lithotomy position and elevate the hips with a pillow, if tolerated. Be sure to drape the patient to provide privacy.

Creams, Foams, or Gels Applied with an Applicator

- Fit the applicator to the tube of the medication and then gently squeeze the tube to fill the applicator with the correct amount of medication.
- Lubricate the tip of the applicator with water-soluble lubricant.

- Use your nondominant hand to spread the labia and expose the vagina. Gently insert the applicator as far as possible into the vagina (Figure 9-102).
- Push the plunger to deposit the medication. Remove the applicator and wrap it in a paper towel for cleaning.

Suppositories

- For suppositories, remove the wrapping and lubricate the suppository with a water-soluble lubricant. Be sure that the suppository is at room temperature.
- Using the applicator, insert the suppository into the vagina, then push the plunger to deposit the suppository.
- If no applicator is available, use your dominant index finger to insert the suppository about 2 inches into the vagina (Figure 9-103).
- Have the patient remain in a supine position with hips elevated for 5 to 10 minutes to allow the suppository to melt and the medication to spread.
- If the patient desires, apply a perineal pad.
- If the applicator is to be reused, wash with soap and water and store in a clean container for the next use.
- Document the medication given and the patient's response on the MAR. Monitor for a therapeutic response and adverse reactions.

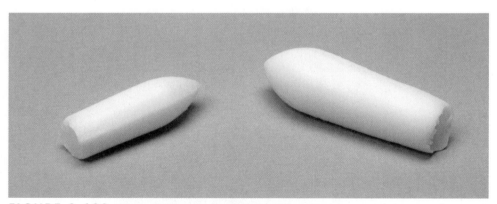

FIGURE 9-100 Vaginal suppositories *(right)* are larger and more oval than rectal suppositories *(left)*.

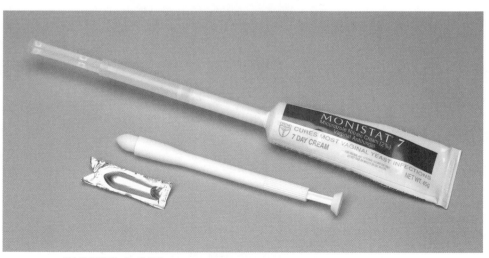

FIGURE 9-101 Vaginal cream and suppository, with applicators.

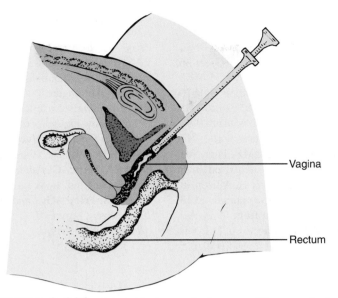

FIGURE 9-102   Administering vaginal cream with an applicator.

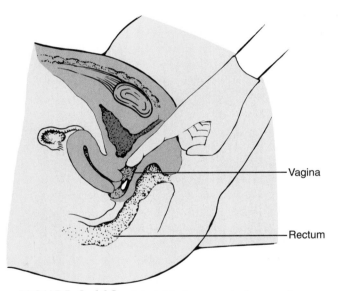

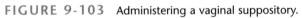

FIGURE 9-103   Administering a vaginal suppository.

ILLUSTRATION CREDITS

Figures 9-1, 9-2, 9-3, 9-4, 9-5, 9-6, 9-7, 9-8, 9-11, 9-14, 9-16, 9-18, 9-19, 9-25, 9-29, 9-30, 9-31, 9-32, 9-33, 9-34, 9-35, 9-36, 9-44, 9-45, 9-46, 9-47, 9-48, 9-51, 9-52, 9-53, 9-55, 9-56, 9-58, 9-59, 9-61, 9-62, 9-63, 9-64, 9-65, 9-66, 9-67, 9-68, 9-69, 9-70, 9-71, 9-72, 9-73, 9-76, 9-77, 9-78, 9-79, 9-82, 9-83, 9-84, 9-85, 9-86, 9-87, 9-89, 9-91, 9-92, 9-93, 9-94, 9-95, 9-96, 9-98, 9-99, 9-100, 9-101, from Rick Brady, Riva, MD. Figures 9-10, 9-15, 9-38, 9-40, 9-81, 9-90, 9-102, 9-103, from Elkin MK, Perry AG, Potter PA: *Nursing interventions and clinical skills,* ed 3, St Louis, 2004, Mosby. Figure 9-12, courtesy Oscar H. Allison, Jr. In Clayton BD, Stock YN: *Basic pharmacology for nurses,* ed 13, St Louis, 2004, Mosby. Figure 9-17, modified from Perry AG, Potter PA: *Clinical nursing skills and techniques,* ed 6, St Louis, 2006, Mosby. Figures 9-20, 9-21, 9-22, 9-23, 9-41, 9-42, 9-49, courtesy Chuck Dresner. Figures 9-24, 9-26, 9-27, from Potter PA, Perry AG: *Basic nursing: theory and practice,* ed 3, St Louis, 1995, Mosby. Figure 9-28, from Potter PA, Perry AG: *Fundamentals of nursing,* ed 5, St Louis, 2001, Mosby. Figure 9-37, courtesy Nadine Sokol. Figure 9-43, from Potter PA, Perry AG: *Fundamentals of nursing: concepts, process, and practice,* ed 4, St Louis, 1997, Mosby. Figures 9-50, 9-54, 9-60, modified from Potter PA, Perry AG: *Fundamentals of nursing: concepts, process, and practice,* ed 3, St Louis, 1993, Mosby. Figure 9-57, modified from Potter PA, Perry AG: *Fundamentals of nursing: concepts, process, and practice,* ed 4, St Louis, 1997, Mosby. Figure 9-74, from Potter PA, Perry AG: *Fundamentals of nursing,* ed 6, St Louis, 2005, Mosby. Figures 9-80, 9-97, from Perry AG, Potter PA: *Clinical skills and techniques,* ed 6, St Louis, 2006, Mosby

Drugs Affecting the Central Nervous System

STUDY SKILLS TIPS

- *Vocabulary*
- *Text Notation*
- *Language Conventions*

VOCABULARY

In any subject matter, mastering the vocabulary is essential to mastering the content. But in a complex, technical subject such as nursing pharmacology, if the vocabulary is not mastered, understanding the content will be almost impossible. Each chapter in this text contains a glossary of unfamiliar terms at the beginning and, as an independent learner, you should spend some time and energy on the vocabulary contained in the glossary. Do not expect to completely understand and master the terms from the glossary alone. The terms are further defined and explained in the body of the chapter, and it is when you read the chapter that you should expect to fully master the vocabulary. However, the time you spend working on the glossary will pay off when you read the chapter.

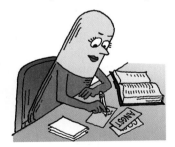

Consider the terms *agonist* and *antagonist* in the Chapter 10 glossary. These terms share a common word part, which means the words are related in meaning. This is an important first step in mastering them. What does *agonist* mean? What is the similarity between *agonist* and *antagonist?* What is the essential difference between the two? Asking these questions as you start to work on Chapter 10 is a valuable technique for beginning to master the language of the content. Do not simply memorize the terms. Learn what they mean, and link relationships between words with common elements. As you practice this technique it will become easier to retain the meaning.

The Chapter 10 glossary has another group of words that should be viewed as a group that shares an important relationship. The first of these words is *pain*. The definition provided is clear and relatively easy to understand, but your focus should be not just on that single word because there are 14 other words that relate to pain: *acute, cancer, central, chronic, neuropathic, phantom, psychogenic, referred, somatic, superficial, vascular,* and *visceral.* Each of these words defines and categorizes pain in very specific ways. As you go about setting up vocabulary cards, look at the opening pages in this chapter. You will find considerable discussion of these terms, which is useful in helping you obtain the fullest understanding of these terms. Do not simply focus on a meaning of each term, but also ask what the similarities and/or differences are and how these words relate to one another.

TEXT NOTATION

The Study Skills Tips for Part One discussed a method for text underlining. If it is done carefully, this strategy is particularly useful for later review of text material. The object of text underlining is to pick out important terms, ideas, and key information so you can come back to it later for quick review. The three key elements in successful text notation are as follows:

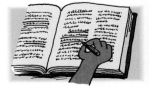

1. Read the material once before attempting any underlining.
2. Be acutely aware of the author's language.
3. Be selective in underlining. The most common fault in underlining is to mark too much material.

The following are two paragraphs from Chapter 10 that have been underlined. The underlining should be viewed as an example of what can be done. Each reader will mark the text somewhat differently based on his or her background and experience. As you study this example, think not only about what has been underlined but also about *why* that material was chosen.

A full understanding of how analgesics work requires knowledge of what pain is and what its characteristics are. **Pain** is most commonly defined as an unpleasant sensory and emotional experience associated with either actual or potential tissue damage. It is a very personal and individual experience. Pain can be defined as whatever the patient says it is, and it exists whenever the patient says it does. Although the mechanisms of pain and the nature of pain pathways are becoming better understood, an individual patient's perception of pain and appreciation of its meaning are complex processes. Pain involves physical, psychologic, and emotional factors. Because pain is a very individual experience and cannot be quantified, for a caregiver to effectively care for a patient suffering from pain he or she must cultivate a relationship with the patient that is built on trust and faith. There is no single approach to effective pain management. Instead, pain management has to be individualized and must take into account the cause of the pain, if known; the existence of concurrent medical conditions; the characteristics of the pain; and the psychologic and cultural characteristics of the patient (see the Cultural Implications box). It also requires ongoing reassessment of the pain and the effectiveness of treatment. Because pain is an individual experience, the emotional response depends on the psychologic experiences resulting from the physiologic stimulation (or nociception).

The physical impulses that signal pain activate various nerve pathways from the periphery to the spinal cord and to the brain. The level of stimulus needed to produce a painful sensation is referred to as the **pain threshold.** Because this is a measure of the physiologic response of the nervous system, it is similar for most persons. Variations in sensitivity to pain may be a result of genetic regulation. The μ receptors in the dorsal horn appear to play a crucial role. Pain perception—and, conversely, emotional well-being—is closely linked to the number of μ receptors. This number is controlled by a single gene, the μ opioid receptor gene. Pain sensitivity is diminished when the receptors are present in relative abundance. When the receptors are reduced in number or missing altogether, relatively minor noxious stimuli may be perceived as painful. The patient's emotional response to the pain is also molded by the patient's age, sex, culture, previous pain experience, and anxiety level. This psychologic element of pain is called **pain tolerance,** or the amount of pain a patient can endure without its interfering with normal function. Pain tolerance can vary from patient to patient because it is a subjective response to pain and can be modulated by the patient's individual personality, environment, culture, and ethnic background. Generally speaking, a constant pain threshold exists in all people under normal circumstances. However, pain tolerance varies widely. It can even vary within the same person depending on the circumstances involved. Table 10-1 lists the various conditions that can cause a person's pain threshold to be altered.

LANGUAGE CONVENTIONS

Certain words and phrases are like signal lights at an intersection. They serve to tell the reader that something special, important, or noteworthy is happening. To the attentive, active reader these conventions contribute significantly to understanding what the author is trying to convey. Whether you are highlighting, underlining, writing margin notes, or studying the material using the PURR model, it is important that you become sensitive to these conventions.

The text following the topic heading *Opioid Analgesics: Chemical Structure* in Chapter 10 contains several examples. The second sentence contains the phrase *classified by*. Whenever an author says that something is being classified it means there are at least two (and perhaps several more) elements of the term or idea that are being classified. This means that you should immediately ask a question about the reading, "What is being classified? How many classifications are there for this?" These questions will help you focus on what to learn and keep your attention firmly fixed on the process of learning.

As you read this chapter, or any other chapter, become aware of words and phrases like these that are intended to draw your attention to something the author especially wanted to emphasize. The more aware of language conventions you become, the easier it will be to become a selective reader. Selective readers do not try to remember everything they read, but they are able to select from the mass of information those concepts and/or terms that the writers tried to stress.

Analgesic Drugs

Objectives

When you reach the end of this chapter, you should be able to do the following:

1. Define analgesia.
2. Describe pharmacologic and non-pharmacologic approaches for the management and treatment of acute and chronic pain.
3. Discuss the use of nonopioids, nonsteroidal antiinflammatory drugs (NSAIDs), and opioids (opioid agonists and partial opioid agonists and antagonists) in the management of acute and chronic pain.
4. Identify the various drugs that are classified within the nonnarcotic and narcotic drug groups. (NSAIDs are discussed in Chapter 44.)
5. Discuss the difference between opioid agonist, agonist-antagonist, and antagonist drugs and their specific use in the management of acute and chronic pain.
6. Compare the mechanisms of action, drug effects, indications, adverse effects, cautions, contraindications, drug-drug and drug-food interactions, dosages, and routes of administration for nonnarcotic and narcotic drugs (agonist and partial agonist-antagonist narcotics).
7. Contrast the management of acute and chronic pain with the management of pain associated with cancer and pain experienced in terminal conditions.
8. Describe briefly the special pain situations as well as specific standards of pain management as defined by the World Health Organization and the Joint Commission on Accreditation of Healthcare Organizations.
9. Develop a nursing care plan related to the use of nonnarcotic and narcotic drugs and the nursing process for patients experiencing pain.
10. Identify various resources, agencies, and professional groups that are involved in establishing standards for the management of all types of pain and for a holistic approach to the care of patients with acute or chronic pain and those in special pain situations.

e-Learning Activities

Companion CD
- NCLEX Review Questions: see questions 50-64
- Animations
- Audio Glossary
- Category Catchers
- Medication Errors Checklists
- IV Therapy Checklists

evolve Website (http://evolve.elsevier.com/Lilley)
• Nursing Care Plans • Frequently Asked Questions • Content Updates • WebLinks • Supplemental Resources • Elsevier ePharmacology Update • Medication Administration Animations

Drug Profiles

▶ acetaminophen, p. 150
  codeine sulfate, p. 146
  fentanyl, p. 147
  meperidine hydrochloride,
    p. 148
  methadone hydrochloride,
    p. 148

▶ morphine sulfate, p. 144
▶ naloxone hydrochloride, p. 148
  naltrexone hydrochloride,
    p. 149
  oxycodone hydrochloride,
    p. 148
  tramadol hydrochloride, p. 150

▶ Key drug.

Glossary

Acute pain Pain that is sudden in onset, usually subsides when treated, and typically occurs over less than a 6-week period. (p. 136)

Addiction Psychologic dependence on a substance, usually resulting from habitual use, that is beyond normal voluntary control (same as *psychologic dependence*). (p. 139)

Adjuvant analgesic drugs Drugs that are added as a second drug for combined therapy with a primary drug and may have additive or independent analgesic properties, or both. (p. 142)

Agonist A substance that binds to a receptor and causes a response. (p. 141)

Agonist-antagonist A substance that binds to a receptor and causes a partial response that is not as strong as that caused by an agonist (also known as a *partial agonist*). (p. 144)

Analgesic ceiling effect What occurs when a given pain drug no longer effectively controls a patient's pain despite the administration of the highest safe dosages. (p. 140)

Analgesics Medications that relieve pain without causing loss of consciousness (sometimes referred to as *painkillers*). (p. 136)

Antagonist A drug that binds to a receptor and prevents (blocks) a response. (p. 141)

Cancer pain Pain resulting from any of a variety of causes related to cancer and/or the metastasis of cancer. (p. 138)

Central pain Pain resulting from any disorder that causes central nervous system damage. (p. 138)

Chronic pain Persistent or recurring pain that is often difficult to treat. Typically it is pain that lasts 3-6 months. (p. 136)

Gate theory The most common and well-described theory of pain transmission and pain relief. It uses a gate model to explain how impulses from damaged tissues are sensed in the brain. (p. 138)

Neuropathic pain Pain that results from a disturbance of function or pathologic change in a nerve. (p. 138)

Nonopiod analgesics Analgesics that are not classified as opioids. (p. 137)

Nonsteroidal antiinflammatory drugs (NSAIDs) A large, chemically diverse group of drugs that are analgesics and also possess antiinflammatory and antipyretic activity but are not steroids. (p. 136)

Opiate analgesic Natural narcotic drug containing or derived from opium that binds to opiate receptors in the brain to relieve pain. (p. 145)

Opioid analgesics Synthetic narcotic drugs that bind to opiate receptors to relieve pain but are not themselves derived from the opium plant. (p. 140)

Opioid-naive Describes patients who are receiving opioid analgesics for the first time and who therefore are not accustomed to their effects. (p. 143)

Opioid tolerance A normal physiologic condition that results from long-term opioid use, in which larger doses of opioids are required to maintain the same level of analgesia and in which abrupt discontinuation of the drug results in withdrawal symptoms (same as *physical dependence*). (p. 143)

Opioid-tolerant Opposite of opioid naive; describes patients who have been receiving opioid analgesics (legally or otherwise) for an extended period of time and who are therefore at greater risk of opioid withdrawal syndrome upon sudden discontinuation of opioid use. (p. 143)

Opioid withdrawal (opioid abstinence syndrome) The signs and symptoms associated with abstinence from or withdrawal of an opioid analgesic when the body has become physically dependent on the substance. (p. 144)

Pain An unpleasant sensory and emotional experience associated with actual or potential tissue damage. Pain is a subjective and individual experience; it can be defined as whatever the person experiencing it says it is, and it exists whenever he or she says it does. (p. 137)

Pain threshold The level of a stimulus that results in the perception of pain. (p. 137)

Pain tolerance The amount of pain a patient can endure without its interfering with normal function. (p. 137)

Partial agonist A drug that binds to a receptor and causes an activation response that is less than that caused by a full agonist. For all practical purposes, the terms *mixed agonist* and *agonist-antagonist* are synonymous with partial agonist, although a few advanced references distinguish further between these terms. (p. 141)

Phantom pain Pain experienced in the area of a body part that has been surgically or traumatically removed. (p. 138)

Physical dependence The physical adaptation of the body to the presence of an opioid or other addictive substance. (p. 143)

Psychogenic pain Pain that is of psychologic origin but is actual pain in the sense that pain impulses travel through nerve cells. (p. 138)

Psychologic dependence A pattern of compulsive use of opioids or any other addictive substance characterized by a continuous craving for the substance and the need to use it for effects other than pain relief (also called *addiction*). (p. 143)

Referred pain Pain occurring in an area away from the organ of origin. (p. 138)

Somatic pain Pain that originates from skeletal muscles, ligaments, or joints. (p. 137)

Special pain situation General term for a pain control situation that is complex and whose treatment typically involves multiple medications, various health care personnel, and nonpharmacologic therapeutic modalities (e.g., massage, chiropractic care, surgery). (p. 150)

Superficial pain Pain that originates from the skin or mucous membranes. (p. 137)

Vascular pain Pain that results from a pathology of the vascular or perivascular tissues. (p. 138)

Visceral pain Pain that originates from organs or smooth muscles. (p. 137)

World Health Organization (WHO) An international body of health care professionals, including clinicians and epidemiologists among many others, that studies and responds to health needs and trends worldwide. (p. 140)

The management of patients experiencing **acute pain** or **chronic pain** is a very important aspect of nursing care in a variety of settings and across the life span. Pain remains one of the more common reasons for patients to seek out the care of a physician and leads to some 70 million office visits annually in the United States. Surgical and diagnostic procedures often require pain management, and there are many diseases and pathologic conditions that also require pain management, such as arthritis, diabetes, multiple sclerosis, cancer, and acquired immunodeficiency syndrome (AIDS). Pain leads to much suffering and is a tremendous economic burden as a result of loss in productivity and workers' compensation and related health care costs. Because of the personal suffering involved and the prevalence and scope of the problem (e.g., overall, 30% to 45% of cancer patients have pain, and this figure increases to 75% of patients in advanced stages), it is critical that nurses be well informed about methods of pain management, including both nonpharmacologic (e.g., massage, acupuncture, therapeutic touch, spirituality, relaxation techniques, imagery) and pharmacologic, so that they can provide quality patient care.

Medications that relieve pain without causing loss of consciousness (commonly referred to as *painkillers*) are considered **analgesics.** There are various classes of analgesics. These classes are determined by the chemical structures and mechanisms of action of the drugs. This chapter focuses on those drugs commonly used to relieve moderate to severe pain—opioid analgesics. The next most common analgesic class consists of **nonsteroidal antiinflammatory drugs (NSAIDs),** which are discussed in Chapter 44.

PHYSIOLOGY AND PSYCHOLOGY OF PAIN

A full understanding of how analgesics work requires knowledge of what pain is and what its characteristics are. **Pain** is most commonly defined as an unpleasant sensory and emotional experience associated with either actual or potential tissue damage. It is a very personal and individual experience. Pain can be defined as whatever the patient says it is, and it exists whenever the patient says it does. Although the mechanisms of pain and the nature of pain pathways are becoming better understood, an individual patient's perception of pain and appreciation of its meaning are complex processes. Pain involves physical, psychologic, and emotional factors. Because pain is a very individual experience and cannot be quantified, for a caregiver to effectively care for a patient suffering from pain he or she must cultivate a relationship with the patient that is built on trust and faith. There is no single approach to effective pain management. Instead, pain management has to be individualized and must take into account the cause of the pain, if known; the existence of concurrent medical conditions; the characteristics of the pain; and the psychologic and cultural characteristics of the patient (see the Cultural Implications box). It also requires ongoing reassessment of the pain and the effectiveness of treatment. Because pain is an individual experience, the emotional response depends on the psychologic experiences resulting from the physiologic stimulation (or nociception).

CULTURAL IMPLICATIONS
The Patient Experiencing Pain

- Each culture has its own beliefs, thoughts, and ways of approaching, defining, and managing pain.
- Attitudes, meanings, and perceptions of pain vary with culture.
- Many African Americans believe in the power of healers, who rely strongly on the religious faith of people and often use prayer and the laying on of hands.
- Many Hispanic Americans believe in prayer, the wearing of amulets, and the use of herbs and spices to maintain health and wellness. Specific herbs are used in teas, and therapies often include religious practices, massage, and cleansings such as the passing of herbs over the body.
- Some traditional methods of healing for the Chinese include acupuncture, herbal remedies, yin and yang balancing, and cold treatment. Moxibustion, in which cones or cylinders of pulverized wormwood are burned on or near the skin over specific meridian points, is another form of healing.
- Asian and Pacific Islander patients are often reluctant to express their pain because they believe that the pain is God's will or punishment for past sins.
- For many Native Americans, treatments include massage, the application of heat, sweat baths, herbal remedies, and being in harmony with nature.
- In Arab culture, patients are expected to openly express their pain and anticipate immediate relief, preferably through injections or intravenous drugs.
- Nurses should be aware of all cultural influences on health-related behaviors and on patients' attitudes toward medication therapy and thus, ultimately, on its effectiveness. A thorough assessment that includes questions about the patient's cultural background and practices is important to the effective and individualized delivery of nursing care.

The physical impulses that signal pain activate various nerve pathways from the periphery to the spinal cord and to the brain. The level of stimulus needed to produce a painful sensation is referred to as the **pain threshold.** Because this is a measure of the physiologic response of the nervous system, it is similar for most persons. Variations in sensitivity to pain may be a result of genetic regulation. The μ receptors in the dorsal horn appear to play a crucial role. Pain perception—and, conversely, emotional well-being—is closely linked to the number of μ receptors. This number is controlled by a single gene, the μ opioid receptor gene. Pain sensitivity is diminished when the receptors are present in relative abundance. When the receptors are reduced in number or missing altogether, relatively minor noxious stimuli may be perceived as painful. The patient's emotional response to the pain is also molded by the patient's age, sex, culture, previous pain experience, and anxiety level. This psychologic element of pain is called **pain tolerance,** or the amount of pain a patient can endure without its interfering with normal function. Pain tolerance can vary from patient to patient because it is a subjective response to pain and can be modulated by the patient's individual personality, environment, culture, and ethnic background. Generally speaking, a constant pain threshold exists in all people under normal circumstances. However, pain tolerance varies widely. It can even vary within the same person depending on the circumstances involved. Table 10-1 lists the various conditions that can cause a person's pain threshold to be altered.

Pain can also be further classified in terms of its onset and duration as either acute or chronic. Acute and chronic pain differ not only in their onset and duration but also in the way they are treated. They are also associated with different diseases and conditions. Acute pain is sudden and usually subsides when treated. One example of acute pain is postoperative pain. Chronic pain is persistent or recurring, lasting 3-6 months. It is often more difficult to treat. This is because changes occur in the nervous system (tolerance) that often require increasing drug doses. Table 10-2 lists the different characteristics of acute and chronic pain and various diseases and conditions associated with each.

Pain can be further classified according to its source. The two most commonly mentioned sources of pain are somatic and visceral. **Somatic pain** originates from skeletal muscles, ligaments, and joints. **Visceral pain** originates from organs and smooth muscles. Sometimes pain is described as superficial. **Superficial pain** originates from the skin and mucous membranes. Pain treatment may be more appropriately selected when the source of the pain is known. For example, visceral and superficial pain usually requires opioids for relief, whereas somatic pain (including bone pain) usually responds better to **nonopioid analgesics** such as NSAIDs (Chapter 44).

Table 10-1	Conditions That Alter Pain Threshold
Pain Threshold	**Conditions**
Lowered	Anger, anxiety, depression, discomfort, fear, isolation, chronic pain, sleeplessness, tiredness
Raised	Diversion, empathy, rest, sympathy, medications (analgesics, antianxiety drugs, antidepressants)

Table 10-2   Acute Versus Chronic Pain

Type of Pain	Onset	Duration	Examples
Acute	Sudden (minutes to hours); usually sharp, localized; physiologic response (SNS: tachycardia, sweating, pallor, increased blood pressure)	Limited (has an end)	Myocardial infarction, appendicitis, dental procedures, kidney stones, surgical procedures
Chronic	Slow (days to months); long duration; dull, persistent aching	Persistent or recurring (endless)	Arthritis, cancer, lower back pain, peripheral neuropathy

SNS, Sympathetic nervous system.

Table 10-3   A and C Nerve Fibers

Type of Fiber	Myelin Sheath	Fiber Size	Conduction Speed	Type of Pain
A	Yes	Large	Fast	Sharp and well localized
C	No	Small	Slow	Dull and nonlocalized

Another type of pain is **vascular pain,** which possibly originates from some pathology of the vascular or perivascular tissues and is thought to account for a large percentage of migraine headaches. **Referred pain** occurs because visceral nerve fibers synapse at a level in the spinal cord close to fibers that supply specific subcutaneous tissues in the body. An example is the pain with cholecystitis, which is often referred to the back and scapula areas. **Neuropathic pain** results from injury or damage to peripheral nerve fibers or damage to the central nervous system (CNS) and is often present in the absence of disease or pathologic processes that generally result in pain. **Phantom pain** occurs in the area of a body part that has been removed—surgically or traumatically—and is characterized as burning, itching, tingling, or stabbing. It can also occur in attached limbs following spinal cord injury.

Cancer pain can be acute or chronic or both. It stems from various causes such as pressure on nerves, organs, or tissues. Other causes of cancer pain include hypoxia; blockage to an organ; metastasis; pathologic fractures; muscle spasms; and adverse effects of radiation, surgery, and chemotherapy. **Psychogenic pain** is pain that originates from psychologic factors, not physical conditions or disorders. However, this definition assumes that all physical causes of pain can be determined. Because the physical basis for many chronic pain syndromes is unknown, physiologic sources can never be completely ruled out. A diagnosis of psychogenic pain can lead to the assumption that the patient is not experiencing "real" pain, and the patient may receive a psychiatric diagnosis despite the presence of a medical cause for the pain. Another type of pain, **central pain,** occurs with tumors, trauma, or inflammation of the brain and may accompany any condition that causes CNS damage, such as cancer, diabetes, stroke, or multiple sclerosis.

Several theories attempt to explain pain transmission and pain relief. The most common and well described is the **gate theory.** This theory, proposed by Melzack and Wall in 1965, uses the analogy of a gate to describe how impulses from damaged tissues are sensed in the brain. First, the tissue injury causes the release of several substances, such as bradykinin, histamine, potassium, prostaglandins, and serotonin. Some current pain medications work by altering the actions and levels of these substances (e.g. NSAIDS ↔ prostaglandins; tricyclic antidepressants ↔ serotonin). Once these substances are released by the damaged tissue,

action potentials are initiated. These action potentials travel along a sensory nerve fiber and activate pain receptors in the spinal cord. There are two basic types of these nerve fibers: A and C. Table 10-3 summarizes the differences in the size and function of these two types of nerve fibers. The different types of pain experienced are believed to be related to the relative proportions of A and C fibers in particular areas of the body.

These pain fibers, along with other sensory nerve fibers, enter the spinal cord and travel up to the brain. The site where these fibers enter the spinal cord is referred to as the *dorsal (posterior) horn* of the spinal cord. It is here that the so-called gates are located. These gates regulate the flow of sensory impulses. If impulses are stopped by a gate at this junction, no impulses are transmitted to the higher centers of the brain. Because it is at these higher centers where impulses are consciously perceived by the patient, in this case there will be no perception of pain. Figure 10-1 depicts the gate theory of pain transmission.

Both the opening and the closing of this gate are influenced by the relative activation of the large-diameter A fibers and the small-diameter C fibers. The closing of the gate seems to be affected by the activation of A fibers. This causes the inhibition of impulse transmission to the brain and thus no pain is perceived. Opening of the gate is affected by the stimulation of the C fibers. This allows impulses to be transmitted to the brain and pain to be perceived. This gate is also innervated by nerve fibers that originate in the brain and modulate the pain sensation by sending impulses to the gate in the spinal cord. The nerve fibers that go from the brain to the gate allow the brain to have some control over this gate. They enable the brain to evaluate, identify, and localize the pain. Thus, the brain can control the gate, either keeping the gate closed or allowing it to open so that the brain is stimulated and pain is perceived. The cells that control the gate have a threshold. Impulses that reach these cells must rise above this threshold before an impulse is permitted to travel up to the brain.

The body is equipped with certain endogenous neurotransmitters known as *enkephalins* and *endorphins.* These substances are produced within the body to fight pain and are considered the body's painkillers. They are capable of binding with opioid receptors and inhibiting the transmission of pain impulses by closing the spinal cord gates, in a manner similar to that of opioid

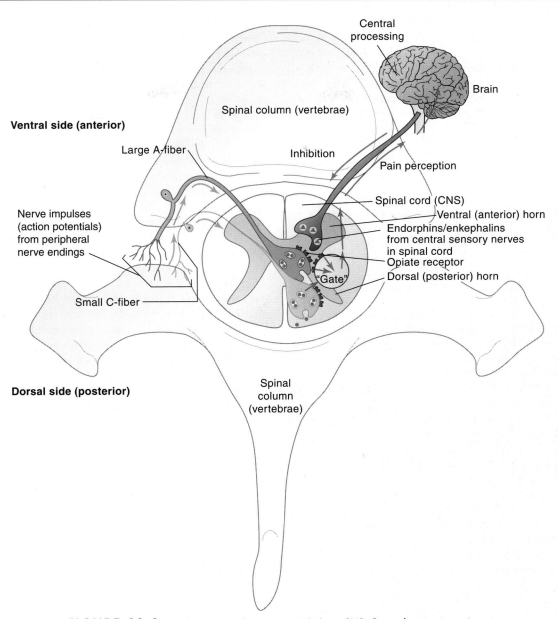

FIGURE 10-1 Gate theory of pain transmission. *CNS,* Central nervous system.

analgesic drugs.. These endogenous analgesic substances are released whenever the body experiences pain. They are responsible for the phenomenon of "runner's high." Figure 10-1 depicts this entire process.

Another phenomenon of pain relief that may be explained by the gate theory is the fact that massaging the affected area often decreases the pain. When rubbing or applying liniment to an area, large sensory "A" nerve fibers from peripheral receptors carry impulses to the spinal cord. This causes impulse transmission to be inhibited and the gate to be closed. This in turn reduces the recognition of the pain impulses arriving by means of the small fibers. This is the same pathway used by the opioid analgesics to alleviate pain.

Treatment of Pain in Special Situations

Estimates are that one of every three Americans experiences pain and that this pain is poorly understood and often undertreated. In addition to baseline chronic pain, patients with illnesses such as cancer, AIDS, and sickle cell anemia may also experience crisis periods of acute pain. Effective management of acute pain is often different from management of chronic pain in terms of medications and dosage used. Patients with complex pain syndromes often benefit from a holistic clinical approach and well-informed health care providers. Therapy in such situations may include use of opioid or nonopioid drugs (or both) as well as nonpharmacologic treatments such as transcutaneous electric nerve stimulation, massage, meditation, biofeedback, relaxation therapy, and psychologic counseling.

In situations such as pain associated with malignancies, the main consideration in pain management is patient comfort and not prevention of drug **addiction.** Often this means aggressive treatment with gradually increasing scheduled doses of opioid analgesics to relieve the pain and prevent it from recurring. As the disease progresses, the patient may require even larger doses and more frequent medication administration using oral, rectal, transdermal, and/or parenteral routes. This is due primarily to increasing pathology, but tolerance may also be a factor. For long-term use as in cancer patients, however, injectable forms are not the first choice because of the break in skin integrity and possible infections, especially with multiple intramuscular injections. Also, if a patient is taking long-acting narcotic analgesics, "breakthrough" pain may be problematic and must be treated with shorter-acting or fast-acting forms on a regular schedule. In this case, if the patient is requiring larger doses for breakthrough pain, the baseline dosage of the opioid

may need to be titrated upward (i.e., increased in increments). Other medications, such as adjuvants, may be added. Antiemetics and laxatives may also be needed to prevent or relieve associated constipation, nausea, and vomiting, because all of these adverse effects are commonly associated with opioid drugs (Box 10-1).

Before specific drug classes and recommended approaches to pain management in a variety of clinical situations are discussed, the standards established by the **World Health Organization (WHO)** should be mentioned. For safe and efficient use of analgesics, the health care practitioner should be knowledgeable about standards of pain management and should remain current on all forms of and protocols for pain management (for mild to severe pain). The three-step analgesic ladder defined by the WHO is often applied as the pain management standard for the use of nonopioid and opioid drugs. Step 1 is the use of nonopioids (with or without adjuvant medications) once the pain has been identified and assessed. If pain persists and/or increases, treatment moves to step 2, which is defined as the use of opioids with or without nonopioids and with or without adjuvants. Should pain persist or increase, management then rises to step 3, which is the use of opioids indicated for moderate to severe pain, administered with or without nonopioids or adjuvant medications. The ultimate goal for patients, as confirmed by the WHO, is freedom from pain. It is also important to understand that opioids and agonists are classified into mild agonists (codeine, hydrocodone, and propoxyphene) and strong agonists (morphine, hydromorphone, levorphanol, oxycodone, oxymorphone, meperidine, fentanyl, and methadone). Meperidine is not recommended for long-term use because of the accumulation of a neurotoxic metabolite, *normeperidine*. The opiate agonists-antagonists such as pentazocine and nalbuphine are associated with an **analgesic ceiling effect.** An analgesic ceiling effect means that once a specific dosage has been reached, the drug produces a maximal analgesic effect, and even if the dosage is increased, the analgesia will not improve; raising the dosage beyond this level is dangerous, has unpredictable effects, and provides no further therapeutic benefit for the patient (see drug profile). They are useful only in patients who have not been previously exposed to opioids and can be used for nonescalating moderate to severe pain. Finally, because of associated bruising and bleeding risks, as well as injection discomfort, there is now a strong trend away from intramuscular injections in favor of intravenous (IV), oral, and transdermal routes of drug administration.

Box 10-1 Potential Opioid Adverse Effects and Their Management

Constipation

Opioids decrease gastrointestinal (GI) tract peristalsis because of their central nervous system (CNS) depression, with subsequent constipation as an adverse effect. Stool becomes excessively dehydrated because it remains in the GI tract longer. **Preventative measures:** Constipation may be managed with increased intake of fluids; a regimen of stool softeners such as docusate sodium at the onset of treatment; possible use of mild osmotic drugs such as 70% sorbitol solution; use of bulk-forming laxatives (psyllium) with fluids; and use of mild cathartics such as senna.

Nausea and Vomiting

Opioids decrease GI tract peristalsis, and some also stimulate the vomiting center in the CNS, so nausea and vomiting are often experienced. **Preventative measures:** Nausea and vomiting may be managed with the use of antiemetics such as phenothiazines or metoclopramide.

Sedation and Mental Clouding

Always evaluate any change in mental status to be sure that causes other than drug-related CNS depression are ruled out. **Preventative measures:** Persistent drug-related sedation may be managed with a decrease in the dosage of opioid, and the physician may order various CNS stimulants.

Respiratory Depression

Long-term opioid use is generally associated with tolerance to respiratory depression. **Preventative measures:** For severe respiratory depression, narcotic antagonists may be used to improve respiratory status and, if titrated in small amounts, the respiratory depression may be reversed without analgesia reversal.

Subacute Overdose

Subacute overdose may be more common than acute respiratory depression and may progress slowly (over hours to days), with somnolence and respiratory depression. Before analgesic dosages are changed or reduced, advancing disease must be considered, especially in the dying patient. **Preventative measures:** Often, holding one or two doses of an opioid analgesic is enough to judge if the mental and respiratory depression are associated to the opioid. If there is improvement with this measure, the opioid dosage is often decreased by 25%.

Other Opioid Adverse Effects

Dry mouth, urinary retention, pruritus, myoclonus, dysphoria, euphoria, sleep disturbances, sexual dysfunction, and inappropriate secretion of antidiuretic hormone may occur but are less common than the aforementioned adverse effects. **Preventative measures:** Ongoing assessment is needed for each of the adverse effects so that appropriate measures may be implemented (e.g., sucking of sugar-free hard candy or use of artificial saliva drops or gum for dry mouth; use of diphenhydramine for pruritus).

OPIOID DRUGS

The pain-relieving drugs currently known as **opioid analgesics** originated from the opium poppy. The word *opium* is a Greek word that means "juice." More than 20 different alkaloids are obtained from the unripe seed of the opium poppy plant. The properties of opium and its many alkaloids have been known for centuries. As early as the third century BC, reference to poppy juice is found in the writings of Theophrastus. Arabian physicians were well versed in the uses of opium as well. It was Arabian traders who introduced the drug to East Asia. Opium-smoking immigrants brought opium to the United States, where unrestricted availability of opium prevailed until the early twentieth century.

Chemical Structure

Opioid analgesics are very strong pain relievers. They can be classified according to their chemical structure or their action at specific receptors. Of the 20 different natural alkaloids available from the opium poppy plant, only three are clinically useful: morphine, codeine, and papaverine. Of these three, only morphine and codeine are pain relievers; papaverine is a smooth muscle relaxant. Relatively simple synthetic chemical modifications of these opium alkaloids have produced the three different chemical classes of opioids: morphine-like drugs, meperidine-like drugs, and methadone-like drugs.

Table 10-4 lists the various opioid analgesics and their respective chemical categories.

Mechanism of Action and Drug Effects

Opioid analgesics can also be characterized according to their mechanism of action. They can be agonists, partial agonists, or antagonists (nonanalgesic). These same designations also apply to many other pharmacologic classes of medications and their respective sites of action (receptor proteins) in the various tissues. In the case of opioid analgesics, an **agonist** binds to an opioid pain receptor in the brain and causes an analgesic response—the reduction of pain sensation. A **partial agonist,** also called an *agonist-antagonist* or a *mixed agonist,* binds to a pain receptor but causes a weaker neurologic response than a full agonist. The latter three terms may present some confusion. For the purposes and scope of this textbook, they are essentially the same. Some very advanced references used by pharmacologic researchers further distinguish a mixed agonist as a drug with varying levels of agonist (not antagonist) potency among the different opiate receptor subtypes. These drugs are sometimes useful in pain management in opioid-addicted patients. An **antagonist** binds to a pain receptor but does not reduce pain signals. It also functions as a *competitive antagonist* because it competes with and reverses the effects of agonist and partial agonist drugs at the receptor sites. The nurse must keep in mind that the body also has its own internal biochemicals that stimulate various receptors. In the case of opioid receptors, these substances are known as *endorphins,* which stands for "endogenous morphine." The endorphins are a natural bodily mechanism of pain control.

The actual receptors to which opioids bind to relieve pain are listed and their characteristics are summarized in Table 10-5. Five types of opioid receptor have been identified to date: μ, κ, σ, δ, and ε. The μ, κ, and δ receptors are the most responsive to drug activity. Many of the characteristics of a particular opioid, such as its ability to sedate, its potency, and its ability to cause hallucinations, can be attributed to the particular opioid's relative affinity for these various receptors. Opioid analgesics achieve their beneficial effects by their actions in the CNS. However, they also act outside the CNS, and many of their unwanted effects stem from these actions.

Indications

The main use of opioids is to alleviate moderate to severe pain. The degree to which pain is relieved or unwanted adverse effects occur depends on the specific drug, the receptors to which it binds, and its chemical structure.

Strong opioid analgesics such as fentanyl, sufentanil, and alfentanil are commonly used in combination with anesthetics

Table 10-4	**Chemical Classification of Opioids**
Chemical Category	**Opioid Drugs**
meperidine-like drugs	meperidine, fentanyl, remifentanil, sufentanil, alfentanil
methadone-like drugs	methadone, propoxyphene
morphine-like drugs	morphine, heroin, hydromorphone, oxymorphone, levorphanol, codeine, hydrocodone, oxycodone
Other	tramadol

Table 10-5	**Opioid Receptors and Their Characteristics**	
Receptor Type	**Prototypical Agonist**	**Effects**
μ	Morphine	Supraspinal analgesia, respiratory depression, euphoria, ++ sedation
κ	ketocyclazocine	Spinal analgesia, ++++ sedation, miosis
δ	Enkephalins	Analgesia

during surgery. These drugs are used not only to relieve pain but also to maintain a balanced state of anesthesia. This practice of using combinations of drugs rather than a single drug to produce anesthesia is referred to as *balanced anesthesia* (Chapter 11). Use of fentanyl injection for postoperative and procedural pain has become more popular due to its rapid onset and short duration. Transdermal fentanyl comes in a patch formulation for use in long-term pain management, but this dosage form poses titration difficulties and should not be used for postoperative pain (see the Preventing Medication Errors box).

Similarly strong opioids such as morphine, meperidine, hydromorphone, and oxycodone are often used to control postoperative and other types of pain. Because morphine, meperidine, and hydromorphone are available in injectable forms, they are first-line analgesics in the immediate postoperative setting. All available oxycodone dosage forms are orally administered. The product OxyContin is a sustained-release form of oxycodone that is designed to last up to 12 hours. The "Contin" in the product name stands for "continuous-release," a synonym for long action in any drug product. There are also immediate-release forms of oxycodone in tablet, capsule, and liquid form. Similarly, the drug product MS Contin is a long-acting or sustained-release form of morphine that is also designed to provide about 12 hours of pain relief. The "MS" stands for the salt name, morphine sulfate. Morphine is also available in injectable forms and immediate-release tablets. Meperidine is available only in immediate-release dosage forms, both oral and injectable. The analgesic effects of immediate-release tablets of all three drugs typically last for about 4 hours. Sometimes a patient receiving doses of a long-acting dosage form every 12 hours will have what is known as *breakthrough pain*, when the long-acting drug does not quite provide pain relief for the entire 12-hour period. In this case, the patient's medication may be supplemented with immediate-release drugs (e.g., morphine, oxycodone). If the relief period for the long-acting drug continues to be inadequate, then the dosage of the long-acting drug may itself be increased.

Opioids also suppress the medullary cough center, which results in cough suppression. The most commonly used opioid for this purpose is codeine. Hydrocodone has also been used in many cough suppressants, either alone or in combination with other drugs. Sometimes the opioid-related cough suppressants have a depressant effect on the CNS and cause sedation. To avoid this problem, dextromethorphan, a nonopioid cough suppressant, is often given instead (see Chapter 35).

Constipation from decreased gastrointestinal (GI) motility is often an unwanted adverse effect of opioids related to their anticholinergic effects. However, these effects are sometimes helpful in treating diarrhea. Some of the most common opioid-containing antidiarrheal preparations are camphorated opium tincture (paregoric) and diphenoxylate/atropine tablets.

Often drugs from other chemical categories are added to the opioid regimen as **adjuvant analgesic drugs** (or *adjuvants*). These assist the primary drugs in relieving pain. Such adjuvant drug therapy may include NSAIDs, antidepressants, anticonvulsants, and corticosteroids, all of which are discussed further in their corresponding chapters. This allows the use of smaller dosages of opioids, which accomplishes two important functions. First, it diminishes some of the adverse effects that are seen with higher dosages of opioids, such as respiratory depression, constipation, and urinary retention. Second, it approaches the pain stimulus by another mechanism of drug action and has a beneficial synergistic effect in reducing the pain.

Contraindications

Contraindications to the use of opioid analgesics include known drug allergy and severe asthma. Although they are not absolute contraindications, extreme caution should be used in cases of respiratory insufficiency, especially when resuscitative equipment is not available; conditions involving elevated intracranial pressure (e.g., severe head injury); morbid obesity and/or sleep apnea; myasthenia gravis; paralytic ileus (bowel paralysis); and pregnancy, especially with long-term use or high dosages.

Adverse Effects

As previously mentioned, many of the unwanted effects of opioid analgesics are related to their effects on parts of the body other than the CNS. Some of these unwanted effects can be explained by the respective drug's selectivity for the receptors listed in Table 10-5. The various body systems that the opioids affect and their adverse effects and adverse effects are summarized in Table 10-6.

Opioids that have an affinity for μ receptors and have rapid onset of action produce marked euphoria. These are the opioids

---

PREVENTING MEDICATION ERRORS

Fentanyl Transdermal Patches

When giving fentanyl (Duragesic and other generic names) transdermal patches, the nurse needs to keep in mind several important points to avoid improper administration:

- These patches should only be used in patients who are considered opioid tolerant. To be considered opioid tolerant, a patient should have been taking, for a week or longer, morphine 60 mg daily, oral oxycodone 30 mg daily, or oral hydromorphone 8 mg daily (or an equianalgesic dose of another opioid). Giving fentanyl transdermal patches to non–opioid tolerant patients may result in severe respiratory depression. Thorough assessment is important.
- Patients should be taught that heat, such from a heating pad, should never be applied over a fentanyl transdermal patch. The increased circulation that results from the application of heat may result in increased absorption of medication, causing an overdose.
- Patients should be taught to dispose of patches properly. Children have pulled used patches from the trash, resulting in deaths due to exposure to the drug. Used patches should be folded with sticky sides together and flushed down the toilet.

The Institute for Safe Medication Practices describes examples of fatal patient incidents resulting from failure to follow the above three points. It is essential for the patient's safety to read the product labeling and follow instructions precisely.

For further information, visit www.ismp.org/Newsletters/acutecare/articles/20050811.asp. Accessed July 23, 2006.

Table 10-6	Opioid-Induced Adverse Effects by Body System
Body System	**Adverse Effects**
Cardiovascular	Hypotension, palpitations, flushing
Central nervous	Sedation, disorientation, euphoria, light-headedness, dysphoria, lowered seizure threshold, tremors
Gastrointestinal	Nausea, vomiting, constipation, biliary tract spasm
Genitourinary	Urinary retention
Integumentary	Itching, rash, wheal formation
Respiratory	Respiratory depression and aggravation of asthma

that are most likely to be abused and used recreationally. All opioid drugs have a strong abuse potential. They are common recreational drugs of abuse among the lay public and also among health care professionals, who often have relatively easy access to them. The person taking them to alter his or her mental status will soon become psychologically dependent on them.

Psychologic dependence is also known as addiction. It was defined by the American Pain Society, American Society of Addiction Medicine, and American Academy of Pain Medicine in 2006 as a primary, chronic, neurobiologic disease, with genetic, psychosocial, and environmental factors influencing its development and manifestations. Addiction is characterized by behaviors that include one or more of the following: impaired control over drug use, compulsive use, continued use despite harm, and craving.

In contrast, **physical dependence** is a state of physiologic adaptation that is manifested by a drug-class-specific withdrawal syndrome that can be produced by abrupt cessation, rapid dose reduction, decreasing blood level of the drug, and/or administration of an antagonist. Typical withdrawal symptoms include rebound pain, mental agitation, tachycardia, elevated blood pressure, and seizures. In severe cases, these symptoms can become life-threatening. Treatment of withdrawal is discussed in Chapter 8. A patient receiving opioid analgesics who does not normally take such medication is said to be **opioid-naive** and therefore not accustomed to the powerful effects of opioid drugs. Such a patient typically requires lower drug dosages for adequate therapeutic effects. In contrast, an **opioid-tolerant** patient is one who has been receiving opioid drugs (legally or otherwise) for an extended period of time. An opioid-tolerant patient is more likely to require higher drug dosages for desired therapeutic effects and is also at greater risk of opioid withdrawal syndrome upon dosage reduction or drug discontinuation.

Opioid tolerance is a state of adaptation in which exposure to a drug induces changes that result in a diminution of one or more of the drug's effects over time. This often leads to the need for progressively higher dosages to maintain the same analgesic effect. This is obviously a common problem in opioid-addicted patients, but it can also result from legitimate control of severe pain in patients with serious illnesses such as cancer. A patient who becomes addicted to pain medication under the latter circumstance is sometimes called a "medical addict." It should be noted, however, that patients who become addicted to opiate drug therapy most often have some initial predisposition to addiction in general. Nonetheless, fear of creating a medical addict may lead well-meaning prescribers to undertreat pain, which is generally considered inhumane and unethical. Under these circumstances, control of the patient's pain takes ethical and even clinical priority over concerns regarding drug addiction.

All opioids cause some histamine release. It is thought that this histamine release is responsible for many of the drugs' unwanted adverse effects, such as itching or pruritus, rash, and hemodynamic changes. The histamine release causes peripheral arteries and veins to dilate, which leads to flushing and orthostatic hypotension. The amount of histamine release that an opioid analgesic causes is related to its chemical class. The naturally occurring opiates elicit the most histamine release; the synthetic opioids (e.g., meperidine) elicit the least histamine release. (See Table 10-4 for a list of the various opioids and their respective chemical classes.)

The most serious adverse effect of opioid use is CNS depression, which may lead to respiratory depression. When opioids are given, care should be taken to titrate the dose so that the patient's pain is controlled without respiratory function's being affected. Individual responses to opioids vary, and patients may occasionally suffer respiratory compromise or the loss of airway reflexes despite careful dose titration. Respiratory depression can be prevented in part by using drugs with very short duration of action and no active metabolites. Respiratory depression seems to be more common in patients with a preexisting condition causing respiratory compromise, such as asthma or chronic obstructive pulmonary disease. Respiratory depression is strongly related to the degree of sedation. Stimulation of the patient may be adequate to reverse mild hypoventilation. If this is unsuccessful, ventilatory assistance using a bag and mask or endotracheal intubation may be needed to support respiration. Administration of naloxone, an opioid reversal drug, may also be necessary to reverse severe respiratory depression. However, the nurse should keep in mind that naloxone will not only reverse the patient's respiratory depression but will also reverse the pain control. Careful, slow titration of naloxone (until the patient is responding) will prevent an overreversal of the opioid-induced respiratory depression and pain relief. The effects of naloxone are short lived and usually last about 1 hour. With long-acting opioids the respiratory depressant effects can reappear after the naloxone has worn off, and redosing may be needed.

GI tract adverse effects are common in patients receiving opioids. Nausea, vomiting, and constipation are the most common adverse effects associated with opioid analgesics. Opioids can irritate the GI tract, stimulating the chemoreceptor trigger zone in the CNS, which in turn may cause nausea and vomiting. Opioids slow peristalsis and increase absorption of water from intestinal contents. These two actions combine to produce constipation.

LEGAL AND ETHICAL PRINCIPLES

The Impact of Nursing Assessment on Medication Administration–Related Errors

Over 600 pharmacists participated in a survey on pharmacy interventions by answering questions about what factors facilitated or decreased pharmacy interventions, what types of interventions were performed in their pharmacy departments, how information was sent out to physicians, and how the information was used. The findings focused strongly on pharmacy issues, but there are other results of the survey from which all health care providers may learn, especially nurses because they are often the first to assess a patient's need for pain medication or intervention. Assessing the patient's health history is an important component of safe care when any type of pain medication is administered. For example, the survey contained a scenario in which a patient who was not diabetic received an oral hypoglycemic drug, which resulted in a decrease in her blood glucose levels and led to her admission to the intensive care unit. Although the patient recovered without permanent injury, this case illustrates just one concern that health care professionals should have when administering medications (especially strong pain medications)—to consider any possible underlying disease processes such as diabetes or liver, kidney, or cardiac disease.

Modified from the Institute for Safe Medication Practices (ISMP): Pharmacy interventions can reduce clinical errors—part I of survey findings, *ISMP Medication Safety Alert!* 7(13):1-2, 2002.

Table 10-7 Opioid Antagonists (Reversal Drugs)			
Generic Name	**Trade Name**	**Dosage**	**Cautions**
nalmefene (IV)	Revex	0.5 mg/70 kg; if needed a second dose of 1.0 mg/70 kg 2-5 min later (for non–opioid-dependent patients)	Raised or lowered blood pressure, dysrhythmias, pulmonary edema, withdrawal
naloxone (IV)	Narcan	0.4-2 mg q2-3min (more than 10 mg); IV infusion: 2 mg in 500 mL (titrate to response)	Raised or lowered blood pressure, dysrhythmias, pulmonary edema, withdrawal
naltrexone (PO)	ReVia	25-50 mg daily	Nervousness, headache, nausea, vomiting, pulmonary edema, withdrawal

IV, Intravenous; *PO*, oral.

This is more pronounced in a hospitalized patient who is nonambulatory because of lack of daily activity.

Urinary retention, or the inability to void, is another unwanted adverse effect of opioid analgesics. They cause this by increasing bladder tone. This is sometimes prevented by giving low dosages of an opioid **agonist-antagonist** or an opioid antagonist. An alternative drug is a cholinergic agonist (Chapter 19) such as bethanechol.

Severe hypersensitivity or anaphylactic reaction to opioid analgesics is rare. Many patients will experience GI discomforts or histamine-mediated reactions to opioids and call these allergic reactions. However, true anaphylaxis is rare, even with intravenously administered opioids. Some patients may complain of flushing, itching, or wheal formation at the injection site, but this is usually local and histamine mediated. Box 10-1 provides additional information on opioid adverse effects and their management.

Toxicity and Management of Overdose

Opioid analgesics produce both beneficial effects and toxic or unwanted effects by means of receptors. These receptors and the positive and negative effects they bring about are listed in Table 10-5. The opioid antagonists naloxone and naltrexone bind to and occupy all of these receptor sites (μ, κ, and σ). They are competitive antagonists with a strong affinity for these binding sites. Through such binding they can reverse the adverse effects induced by the opioid drug, such as respiratory depression. These drugs are used in the management of both opioid overdose and opioid addiction. The commonly used opioid antagonists (reversal drugs) are listed in Table 10-7.

For effective management of opioid overdose or toxicity, it is important for the nurse to recognize the signs and symptoms of withdrawal. Opioid tolerance and physical dependence are expected in patients undergoing long-term opioid treatment and should not be confused with psychologic dependence, as seen with drug abuse behavior. Confusing these concepts in relation to opioid therapy sometimes leads to ineffective pain management and contributes to the problem of undertreatment. The extent of physical dependence on opioids is most visible to the nurse when an opioid drug is discontinued abruptly or when an opioid antagonist is administered. This physiologic response is referred to as **opioid withdrawal (opioid abstinence syndrome)** and is manifested by anxiety, irritability, chills and hot flashes, joint pain, lacrimation (tearing), rhinorrhea, diaphoresis, nausea, vomiting, confusion, and abdominal cramps and diarrhea. Drug therapy for acute withdrawal from opioids and other drugs of abuse is described in Chapter 8.

The timing of the onset of withdrawal symptoms is directly related to the half-life of the opioid analgesic being used. The withdrawal symptoms resulting from the discontinuance or reversal of short-acting opioid therapy (codeine, hydrocodone, morphine, and hydromorphone) will appear within 6 to 12 hours and peak at 24 to 72 hours. The withdrawal symptoms associated with the long half-life drugs (methadone, levorphanol, and transdermal fentanyl) may not appear for 24 hours or longer after drug discontinuation and may be milder. The appearance of abstinence syndrome indicates physical dependence on the opioid, which may occur after as little as 2 weeks of therapy. It does not, however, imply the existence of psychologic dependence or addiction. Most patients with cancer take opioid analgesics for longer than 2 weeks, and only very rarely do they exhibit the drug abuse behavior and psychologic dependence that characterize addiction. Gradual dosage reduction, when possible, after chronic opioid use generally helps to minimize the severity of withdrawal symptoms.

Interactions

Potential drug interactions with opioids are significant. Coadministration of opioids with alcohol, antihistamines, barbiturates, benzodiazepines, phenothiazine, and other CNS depressants can result in additive respiratory depressant effects. The combined use of opioids (such as meperidine) with monoamine oxidase inhibitors (MAOIs) can result in respiratory depression, seizures, and hypotension.

Laboratory Test Interactions

Opioids can cause an abnormal increase in the serum levels of amylase, alanine aminotransferase, alkaline phosphatase, bilirubin, lipase, creatinine kinase, and lactate dehydrogenase. Other abnormal results include a decrease in urinary 17-ketosteroid levels and an increase in the urinary alkaloid and glucose concentrations.

Dosages

For the recommended initial dosages of selected analgesic drugs in opioid-naive patients, see the Dosages table on page 145.

Drug Profiles

▶ **morphine sulfate**

Morphine, a naturally occurring alkaloid derived from the opium poppy, is the drug prototype for opioids and narcotics. Opium itself is the dried juice of the poppy plant *Papaver somniferum* and is a mixture of opioid and nonopioid alkaloids. As with other narcotics, there is a strong potential for misuse and abuse with morphine. For this reason, morphine is classified as a Schedule II controlled substance.

DOSAGES

Selected Analgesic Drugs and Related Drugs

Drug (Pregnancy Category)	Pharmacologic Class	Usual Dosage Range	Indications
Opioids			
codeine sulfate (D)	**Opiate analgesic;** opium alkaloid	**Pediatric** PO/SC/IM: 2.5 yr, 2.5-5 mg q4-6h—do not exceed 30 mg/day	Cough relief
		Pediatric (6-11 yr) 5-10 mg q4-6h	Cough relief
		Adult/pediatric (older than 12 yr) 10-20 mg q4-6h—do not exceed 120 mg/day	Cough relief
		Adult 15-60 mg tid-qid	Opioid analgesia
fentanyl citrate (Duragesic, Oralet, Actiq) (D)	Opioid analgesic	All doses titrated to response, starting with lowest effective dose IV/IM doses available in 50 mcg/mL ampule or premixed infusion of varying strengths **Pediatric** IV/IM: 0.5-3 mcg/kg/dose	Procedural sedation or adjunct to general anesthesia
		Adult IV/IM: 20-100 mcg/dose; or (pediatric and adult) titrated to response via continuous infusion Duragesic (transdermal patch): 12.5-200 mcg/hr q72h; Oralet, Actiq (buccal lozenges): begin with lowest dose (200 mcg) and titrate as needed Note that oral dosage forms are more commonly used in adults for safety due to high drug potency	Relief of moderate to severe acute pain; relief of chronic pain, including cancer pain
meperidine HCl (Demerol, Pethidine) (D)	Opioid analgesic	**Pediatric** PO/IM/SC: 1-1.5 mg/kg q2-3h prn (max 100 mg/dose) IM/SC: 0.5-1 mg/kg 30-90 min before anesthesia (max 100 mg/day)	Meperidine use should be restricted because of the unpredictable effects of neurometabolites at analgesic doses and risk for seizures
		Adult PO/IM/SC: 50-150 mg q2-3h prn IM/SC: 50-100 mg IM/SC: 50-100 mg 30-90 min before anesthesia IV: 50-150 mg q3-4h	Obstetric analgesia, preoperative sedation
methadone HCl (Dolophine) (D)	Opioid analgesic	**Adult** PO/IM/SC: 2.5-10 mg q3-4h; 40 mg or more daily, reduced doses every few days; 40-120 mg or more once daily	Opioid analgesia, relief of chronic pain, opioid detoxification, opioid addiction maintenance
▶morphine sulfate (Astramorph, Duramorph, Infumorph, MSIR, Oramorph, Roxanol, others) (D)	Opiate analgesic; opium alkaloid	**Pediatric** SC: 0.1-0.2 mg/kg dose—do not exceed a 15-mg single dose	Opioid analgesia
		Adult PO/IM/SC: 5-30 mg q4h PR: 10-20 mg q4h IV: 2.5-15 mg IV: 2.5-20 mg q2-6h PCA pump, epidural: titrate to effect	Opioid analgesia
morphine sulfate, continuous release (MS Contin) (D)	Opiate analgesic; opium alkaloid	**Adult only** PO: 15 mg q8h to 200 mg q12h	Relief of moderate to severe pain
oxycodone (D)	Opioid, synthetic	**Pediatric** PO: 1.25-2.5 mg q6h prn	Relief of moderate to severe pain
		Adult PO: 5-20 mg q4-6h prn	Relief of moderate to severe pain
oxycodone, continuous release (OxyContin) (D)	Opioid, synthetic	**Adult only** PO: 10-160 mg q12h	Relief of moderate to severe pain

IM, Intramuscular; *IV*, intravenous; *PCA*, patient-controlled analgesia; *PO*, oral; *PR*, rectal; *SC*, subcutaneous.

Continued

DOSAGES

Selected Analgesic Drugs and Related Drugs—cont'd

Drug (Pregnancy Category)	Pharmacologic Class	Usual Dosage Range	Indications
Opioid Antagonists			
▶naloxone HCl (Narcan)	Opioid antagonist	**Pediatric** IV 0.01 mg/kg IV followed by 0.1 mg/kg if needed; 0.0005-0.01 mg/kg IV—repeat at 2-3 min intervals	Treatment of opioid overdose, postoperative anesthesia reversal
		Adult IV 0.4-2 mg IV—repeat in 2-8 min if needed; 0.1-0.2 mg IV—repeat at 2-3 min intervals	Treatment of opioid overdose, postoperative anesthesia reversal
naltrexone HCl (Trexan)	Opioid antagonist	**Adult** PO: 50 mg q24h or 100 mg every other day	Maintenance of opioid-free state
Opioid/Acetaminophen* Combination Products			
NOTE: There are many others on the market, including combinations with aspirin			
Percocet (various strengths with OXY/APAP ratios of 2.5 mg/325 mg, 5 mg/325 mg, 7.5 mg/500 mg, 10 mg/650 mg) (D)	Opioid combination analgesic	PO: 1-2 tabs q4-8h (not to exceed 4000 mg APAP/24 hr, assuming normal liver function)	Combined opioid-nonopioid analgesia
Vicodin (HC 5 mg/APAP 500 mg) (D)	Opioid combination analgesic	PO: 1 tab q4h or 2 tabs q6h	Analgesia
Vicodin ES (HC 7.5 mg/APAP 750 mg) (D)	Opioid combination analgesic	PO: 1 tab q6-8h	Analgesia
Vicodin HP (HC 10 mg/APAP 660 mg) (D)	Opioid combination analgesic	PO: 1 tab q4h or 2 tabs q8h	Analgesia
Partial Agonists			
buprenorphine (Buprenex) (D)	Partial opioid agonist	**Pediatric (2-12 yr)** IV/IM: 2-6 mcg/kg q4-6h prn **Adult (older than 13 yr)** IV/IM: 0.3 mg q6-8h prn	Relief of moderate to severe pain; usually short-term postoperative or obstetric pain; tablets for opioid dependence only
butorphanol (Stadol) (D)	Partial opioid agonist	**Adult only** IV: 0.5-2 mg q3-4h prn IM: 1-4 mg q3-4h prn	Relief of moderate to severe pain; usually short-term postoperative or obstetric pain; also used as a premedication before procedure
nalbuphine (Nubain) (D)	Partial opioid agonist	**Pediatric (10 mo-14 yr)** IV/IM/SC: 0.2 mg/kg (for premedication) **Adult** IV/IM/SC: 10 mg/70 kg body weight q3-6h, max 160 mg/day	
pentazocine (Talwin) (D)	Partial opioid agonist	**Pediatric (1-16 yr)** IM: 0.5 mg/kg **Adult** IM: 30-60 mg q3-4h IV: 30 mg q3-4h	

APAP, Acetaminophen; *ES*, extra strength; *HC*, hydrocodone bitartrate; *HCL*, hydrochloride; *HP*, high potency; *OXY*, oxycodone HCl.
*The maximum recommended daily dose of acetaminophen for a typical adult patient with *normal* liver function is 4000 mg/24 hr. For hepatically compromised patients, this dosage may be 2000 mg or even lower. If in doubt, check with a pharmacist or prescriber regarding a particular patient. APAP is derived from the chemical name for acetaminophen: N-acetyl-*p*-aminophenol. It is a commonly used abbreviation for acetaminophen.

Morphine is also highly constipating, and stool softeners or laxatives are often required as adjunct medications. Although it is not as dangerous as meperidine, morphine also has a potentially toxic metabolite known as *morphine-6-glucuronide*. Accumulation of this metabolite is more likely to occur in patients with renal impairment. For this reason, other opioids such as hydromorphone (Dilaudid) and fentanyl may be safer analgesic choices for these patients. Drug profile information for hydromorphone is similar to that for morphine and meperidine. For dosage information, see the table on page 145.

Pharmacokinetics

Half-Life	Onset	Peak	Duration
IM: 1.7-4.5 hr	IM: Rapid	IM: 30-60 min	IM: 6-7 hr

▶ *codeine sulfate*

Codeine sulfate (methylmorphine) is another natural opiate alkaloid obtained from opium. The plant yield of this drug is too low to meet the high medical consumption needs for codeine. Therefore, it is most often prepared synthetically in the laboratory by methylation of

DOSAGES

Selected Analgesic Drugs and Related Drugs—cont'd

Drug (Pregnancy Category)	Pharmacologic Class	Usual Dosage Range	Indications
Nonopioid			
▶acetaminophen* (Tylenol, others) (B)	Nonopioid analgesic, antipyretic	**Pediatric** PO/PR: 0-3 mo, 40 mg q4-6h 4-11 mo, 80 mg q4-6h 1-2 yr, 120 mg q4-6h 2-3 yr, 160 mg q4-6h 4-5 yr, 245 mg q4-6h 6-8 yr, 320 mg q4-6h 9-10 yr, 400 mg q4-6h 11-12 yr, 480 mg q4-6h	Mild to moderate pain relief
		Adult PO/PR: 325-650 mg q4-6h; not to exceed 4 g/day In alcoholics, not to exceed 2 g/day	Relief of mild to moderate pain
Miscellaneous			
tramadol (Ultram)	Miscellaneous analgesic	**Adult** PO: 50-100 mg q4-6h; not to exceed 400 mg/day	Relief of moderate to moderately severe pain

morphine. Codeine is similar to morphine in terms of its pharmacokinetic and pharmacodynamic properties. However, codeine is less effective as an analgesic and is more widely used as an antitussive drug in an array of cough preparations. For example, codeine combined with acetaminophen (tablets or elixir) is classified as a Schedule III controlled substance and is commonly used for control of mild to moderate pain as well as cough. Codeine alone is still classified as a Schedule II controlled substance, which implies a high abuse and addiction potential. There is also an associated analgesic ceiling effect. For dosage information, see the table on page 145.

Pharmacokinetics

Half-Life	Onset	Peak	Duration
PO: 2.5-4 hr	PO: 15-30 min	PO: 35-45 min	PO: 4-6 hr

▶ fentanyl

Fentanyl is a synthetic opioid used to treat moderate to severe pain. Like other opioids, it also has a high abuse potential. It is available in several dosage forms: parenteral injections (Sublimaze), transdermal patches, buccal lozenges) (Duragesic), and, most recently, a "lollipop" lozenge on a stick (Actiq). The injectable form is used most commonly in perioperative settings (e.g., induction of general anesthesia) and in intensive care unit settings for sedation during mechanical ventilation. The oral and transdermal forms are used primarily for long-term control of both malignant and nonmalignant chronic pain. Fentanyl is a very potent analgesic. The equianalgesic doses of some of the more common opioids compared with both 10 mg of intramuscular and 30 mg of oral morphine are listed in Table 10-8. Fentanyl at a dose of 0.1 mg given intravenously is roughly equivalent to 10 mg of morphine given intravenously.

The transdermal delivery system (patch) has been shown to be highly effective in the treatment of various chronic types of pain syndrome such as cancer-induced pain, especially in patients who cannot take oral medications. This route should never be used in opiate-naive patients. Generally, fentanyl patches are best employed for nonescalating pain because of the difficulty of titrating doses. Table 10-9 is provided to aid in converting from morphine to fentanyl in treatment of pain. To perform the conversion using the table, first the daily (24-hour) opioid requirement of the patient should be determined. Second, if the opioid is not morphine, its dose should be converted to

Table 10-8 Equianalgesic Opioid Potencies (Based on Morphine 10 mg Intramuscularly and 30 mg Orally)

Opioid Analgesic	Equianalgesic Dose (mg)	
	Intramuscular	Oral
Codeine	130	75
Hydromorphone	1.5	7.5
Meperidine	75	300
Methadone	10	20
Morphine	10 (standard)	30 (standard)
Oxycodone	Injection not available	30
Oxymorphone	1	10 (rectal)

NOTE: Fentanyl is most commonly given intravenously, transdermally (patch), or orally (lollipop). See Table 10-9.

Table 10-9 Transdermal Fentanyl Dosages

Oral 24-Hr Morphine (mg/day)	Intramuscular 24-Hr Morphine (mg/day)	Transdermal Fentanyl (mcg/hr)
45-134	8-22	25
135-224	23-37	50
225-314	38-52	75
315-404	53-67	100
405-494	68-82	125
495-584	83-97	150
585-674	98-112	175
675-764	113-127	200
765-854	128-142	225
855-944	143-157	250
945-1034	158-172	275
1035-1124	173-187	300

the equianalgesic dose of morphine using Table 10-8. Finally, the equipotent transdermal fentanyl dosage can be calculated using Table 10-9. These tables are conservative in their dosages for achieving pain relief, and supplemental short-acting opioid analgesics should be added as needed. Nurses should be aware that after the first patch is applied it will take 6 to 12 hours to reach steady-state pain control again, so that supplemental short-acting therapy is required. Most patients will experience adequate pain control for 72 hours with this method of fentanyl delivery. A new patch should be applied every 72 hours.

The lollipop dosage form of fentanyl was approved by the U.S. Food and Drug Administration (FDA) in 1998. It was originally intended for prescription by either oncologists or pain medicine specialists for pain management in cancer patients. However, prescriptions of the drug increased by over 400% between 2001 and 2003, with many prescriptions written by general practice physicians for indications such as neck or back pain in workers' compensation cases. This has raised concern about misuse of this expensive drug, the cost of which can amount to $12,000 to $18,000 annually. Some insurance companies have refused to provide the drug except for treatment of documented cancer pain. There have also been reports of illegal sales of this drug.

Pharmacokinetics

Route	Half-Life	Onset	Peak	Duration
Intravenous	1.5-6 hr	Rapid	Minutes	30-60 min
Intramuscular	1.5-6 hr	7-15 min	20-30 min	1-2 hr
Transdermal	Delayed	12-24 hr	48-72 hr	13-40 hr
Oral (transmucosal)	5-15 hr	5-15 min	20-30 min	unknown

▶ meperidine hydrochloride

Meperidine hydrochloride (Demerol, Pethidine) is a widely used synthetic opioid analgesic. Meperidine should be used with caution, if at all, in elderly patients and in patients who require long-term analgesia or who have kidney dysfunction. A metabolite, normeperidine, can accumulate and lead to seizures. After 48 hours, meperidine accumulates in the body and is toxic. Use of the drug is contraindicated in patients showing a hypersensitivity to it and in patients currently or recently treated with MAOIs. The concurrent use of MAOIs and meperidine can lead to deep coma and death. Meperidine is available in tablet, oral liquid, and injectable form. For dosage information, see the table on page 145.

Pharmacokinetics

Half-Life	Onset	Peak	Duration
IM/PO: 3-5 hr	IM/PO: Rapid	IM/PO: 30-60 min	IM/PO: 2-4 hr

▶ methadone hydrochloride

Methadone hydrochloride (Dolophine) is a synthetic opioid analgesic. It is the opioid of choice for the detoxification treatment of opioid addicts in methadone maintenance programs. Use of agonist-antagonist opioids (e.g., pentazocine) in heroin-addicted patients or those in methadone maintenance programs can induce significant withdrawal symptoms. There has been renewed interest in the use of methadone for chronic (e.g., neuropathic) and cancer-related pain. Methadone is readily absorbed through the GI tract with peak plasma concentrations at 4 hours for single dosing. Multiple daily dosing (e.g., every 8 hours) slows down elimination of the drug, providing a longer duration of effect. However, 24-hour dosing is more common in methadone maintenance programs for addicted patients. Methadone is eliminated through the liver, which makes it a safer choice than some other opioids for renally impaired patients. For dosage information, see the table on page 145.

Pharmacokinetics

Half-Life	Onset	Peak	Duration
PO: 25 hr	PO: 30-60 min	PO: 1.5-2 hr	PO: 22-48 hr

▶ oxycodone hydrochloride

Oxycodone hydrochloride (OxyIR, OxyContin) is an analgesic drug that is structurally related to morphine and has comparable analgesic activity. Like morphine, it is a Schedule II drug. It is available in tablet, capsule, and oral solution form but not in injectable form. It is also commonly combined in tablets with acetaminophen (Percocet) and with aspirin (Percodan). A somewhat weaker but commonly used opioid is hydrocodone, which is available only in tablet form, most commonly in combination with acetaminophen (Vicodin, Lorcet, Lortab) but also with aspirin and ibuprofen. For dosage information, see the table on page 145.

Pharmacokinetics (Immediate Release)

Half-Life	Onset	Peak	Duration
PO: 2-3 hr	PO: 10-15 min	PO: 1 hr	PO: 3-6 hr

Opioids and Agonists-Antagonists

Opioids with mixed actions, often called *agonists-antagonists*, bind to the μ receptor and can therefore compete with other substances for these sites. However, they either exert no action (i.e., they are competitive antagonists) or have only limited action (i.e., they are partial agonists). The partial agonist opioid analgesics include buprenorphine (Buprenex), butorphanol (Staldol), nalbuphine (Nubain), and pentazocine (Talwin). These drugs are very similar to the agonist opioid drugs in terms of their therapeutic indications. They are potent synthetic analgesics, but their misuse potential and addiction risk are both lower than those of the pure agonist opioids. The antagonistic activity of this group can produce withdrawal symptoms in opioid-dependent patients. Their use is also contraindicated in patients who have shown hypersensitivity reactions to the drugs.

Partial Opioid Agonists

The partial opioid agonists—or, more simply, partial agonists—are a group of analgesic drugs that have varying degrees of agonistic and antagonistic effects on the different opioid receptor subtypes. These drugs are normally used in situations requiring short-term pain control, such as after surgery and for obstetric procedures. They are sometimes chosen for patients who have a history of opioid addiction. These medications can both help prevent overmedication and reduce posttreatment addictive cravings in these patients. These drugs are normally not strong enough for management of longer-term chronic pain (e.g., cancer pain, chronic low-back pain). They should also *not* be given concurrently with full opioid agonists, because they can both reduce analgesic effects and cause withdrawal symptoms in opioid-tolerant patients. Four partial agonists are currently available: buprenorphine, butorphanol, nalbuphine, and pentazocine. They are available in various oral, injectable, and intranasal dosage forms as indicated in the dosage table. All but butorphanol are also available in combination with the opioid antagonist naloxone to enhance their opioid antagonistic effects, which are usually weaker than the agonistic effects of these drugs.

Opioid Antagonists

Opioid antagonists are synthetic derivatives of oxymorphone, a potent semisynthetic opioid. They produce their opioid antagonistic activity by competing with opioids for CNS receptor sites.

▶ naloxone hydrochloride

Naloxone hydrochloride (Narcan) is a pure opioid antagonist because it possesses no agonistic morphine-like properties and works as a blocking drug to the opioid drugs. Accordingly, the drug does not produce analgesia or respiratory depression. Naloxone is the drug of choice for the complete or partial reversal of opioid-induced respiratory depression. It is also indicated in cases of suspected acute opioid overdose. Failure of its administration to significantly reverse the effects of the presumed opioid overdose indicates that the condition may be caused by an overdose of nonopioid drugs or the dosing process. Naloxone is available only in injectable dosage forms. Use of the drug is contraindicated in patients with a history of hypersensitivity to it. For dosage information, see the table on page 146.

Pharmacokinetics

Half-Life	Onset	Peak	Duration
IV: 64 min	IV: Less than 2 min	IV: Rapid	IV: Variable depending on dose and route

▸ naltrexone hydrochloride

Naltrexone hydrochloride (ReVia, Trexan) is an opioid antagonist used as an adjunct for the maintenance of an opioid-free state in former opioid addicts. The FDA has identified it as a safe and effective adjunct to psychosocial treatments of alcoholism. It is also recommended for reversal of postoperative opioid depression. It is available only in tablet form. Use of naltrexone hydrochloride is contraindicated in patients with hepatitis or liver dysfunction or failure and is also contraindicated in those with drug hypersensitivity. Nausea and tachycardia are the most common adverse effects and are related to reversal of the opioid effect. For dosage information, see the table on page 146.

Pharmacokinetics

Half-Life	Onset	Peak	Duration
PO: 3.9-12.9 hr	PO: Rapid	PO: 1 hr	PO: 24-72 hr

NONOPIOID ANALGESICS

The most widely used nonopioid analgesic is acetaminophen. All drugs in the NSAID class, which includes aspirin, and the cyclooxygenase-2 (COX-2) inhibitors (e.g., Celebrex) are also nonopioid analgesics, and these drugs are discussed in greater detail in Chapter 44. These medications are commonly used for management of pain, especially pain associated with inflammatory conditions such as arthritis, because they have significant antiinflammatory effects in addition to their analgesic effects. Acetaminophen is available in a variety of dosage formulations, both over the counter (OTC) and by prescription. It is also a component of many combination products with opioids.

Mechanism of Action and Drug Effects

The mechanism of action of acetaminophen is similar to that of the salicylates. It blocks peripheral pain impulses by inhibition of prostaglandin synthesis. Acetaminophen also lowers febrile body temperatures by acting on the hypothalamus, the structure in the brain that regulates body temperature. Heat is dissipated through resulting vasodilation and increased peripheral blood flow. In contrast to NSAIDs, acetaminophen has only weak antiinflammatory effects and thus is not used to treat inflammation (e.g., arthritic inflammation). Although acetaminophen shares the analgesic and antipyretic effects of the salicylates and other NSAIDs, it does not have many of the unwanted effects of these drugs. For example, acetaminophen products are not usually associated with cardiovascular effects (e.g., edema) or platelet effects (e.g., bleeding) and have no effect on platelets (such as a tendency to cause bleeding) as do aspirin and other NSAIDs). They cause none of the aspirin-related GI tract irritation or bleeding nor any of the aspirin-related acid-base changes.

Indications

Acetaminophen is indicated for the treatment of mild to moderate pain and fever. It is an appropriate substitute for aspirin because of its analgesic and antipyretic properties. Acetaminophen is a valuable alternative for those patients who cannot tolerate aspirin or for whom aspirin may be contraindicated.

Acetaminophen is also the antipyretic (antifever) drug of choice in children and adolescents with flu syndromes, because the use of aspirin in such populations is associated with a brain-wasting condition known as *Reye's syndrome.*

Contraindications

Contraindications to acetaminophen use include known drug allergy, severe liver disease, and the genetic disease known as *glucose-6-phosphate dehydrogenase (G6PD) deficiency.*

Adverse Effects

Acetaminophen is an effective and relatively safe drug. It is therefore available OTC and in many combination prescription drugs. Acetaminophen is generally well tolerated. Possible adverse effects include rash, nausea, and vomiting. Much less common but more severe are the adverse effects of blood disorders or dyscrasias (e.g., anemias) and nephrotoxicities, especially if the manufacturer's guidelines for dosage ranges are not followed.

Toxicity and Management of Overdose

Many people do not realize that acetaminophen, despite its OTC status, is a potentially lethal drug when taken in overdose. Depressed patients (especially adolescents) may intentionally overdose on the drug as an attention-seeking gesture without realizing the grave danger involved.

The ingestion of large amounts of acetaminophen, as in acute overdose, or even chronic unintentional misuse can cause hepatic necrosis. This is the most serious acute toxic effect. Acute ingestion of acetaminophen doses of 150 mg/kg or more may result in hepatic toxicity.

The standard maximum daily dose of acetaminophen for healthy adults is 4000 mg. Care should be exercised by nurses, physicians, and patients to avoid doses in excess of this amount for most patients. Excessive dosing may also occur inadvertently with the use of combination drug products such as tablets that include a fixed ratio of an opioid drug plus acetaminophen (e.g., hydrocodone plus acetaminophen).

The long-term ingestion of large doses of acetaminophen is more likely to result in nephropathy. Because the reported or estimated quantity of drug ingested is often inaccurate and not a reliable guide to the therapeutic management of the overdose, serum acetaminophen concentration should be determined for this purpose no sooner than 4 hours after the ingestion. If a serum acetaminophen level cannot be determined, it should be assumed that the overdose is potentially toxic and treatment with acetylcysteine (the recommended antidote for acetaminophen toxicity) should be started. Acetylcysteine works by preventing the hepatotoxic metabolites of acetaminophen from forming. The treatment regimen consists of an initial loading dose of 140 mg/kg orally, followed by 70 mg/kg every 4 hours for 17 additional doses. If the patient vomits within 1 hour of receiving a dose of acetylcysteine, that dose should be given again immediately. All 17 doses must be given to prevent hepatotoxicity, regardless of the subsequent acetaminophen serum levels.

Interactions

A variety of substances may interact with acetaminophen. Alcohol is potentially the most dangerous. Chronic heavy alcohol abusers may be at increased risk of liver toxicity from excessive acetaminophen use. The majority of reports are of cases in which individuals with severe chronic alcoholism took large doses of acetaminophen and exceeded recommended dosages, which led to possible overdose. Health care professionals should alert patients with regular intake of moderate to large amounts of alcohol not to exceed recommended doses of acetaminophen because of the risk of liver dysfunction and possible liver failure. Ideally, alcohol consumption should not exceed three drinks daily. Other hepatotoxic drugs should also be avoided. Other drugs that potentially can interact with acetaminophen include phenytoin, barbiturates, isoniazid, rifampin, β-blockers, and anticholinergic drugs, all of which are discussed in greater detail in later chapters.

Drug Profiles

Nonopioid Analgesics
▶ *acetaminophen*

Acetaminophen (Tylenol) is an effective and relatively safe nonopioid analgesic used for mild to moderate pain relief. It is contraindicated in patients with a hypersensitivity to it or an intolerance to tartrazine (yellow dye no. 5), alcohol, sugar, or saccharin. Its use should be avoided in patients who are anemic or who have renal or hepatic disease. Acetaminophen is provided in many oral and rectal dosage formulations. It is available in the form of capsules, solution, granules, suspension, tablets, chewable tablets, film-coated tablets, tablets for solution, and rectal suppositories and in numerous strengths, depending on whether it is intended for use in children or adults.

Pharmacokinetics

Half-Life	Onset	Peak	Duration
PO: 1-4 hr	PO: 10-30 min	PO: 0.5-2 hr	PO: 3-4 hr

tramadol hydrochloride

Tramadol hydrochloride (Ultram) is categorized as a miscellaneous analgesic due to its unique properties. It is a centrally acting analgesic with a dual mechanism of action. It creates a weak bond to the μ opioid receptors and inhibits the reuptake of both norepinephrine and serotonin. Both of these neurotransmitters are known as *monoamines* because they have a single amino group ($-NH_3$) as part of their chemical structure. In the spinal cord, their presence in the nerve synapses promotes what is known as *monoaminergic* inhibition of pain impulses. Although it does have weak opioid receptor activity, tramadol is not currently classified as a controlled substance. Tramadol is indicated for the treatment of moderate to moderately severe pain. Tramadol is rapidly absorbed and its absorption is unaffected by food. It is metabolized in the liver to an active metabolite (O-dimethyl tramadol) and eliminated via renal excretion. Adverse effects are similar to those of opioids and include drowsiness, dizziness, headache, nausea, constipation, and respiratory depression. Use of the drug is contraindicated in patients who have previously demonstrated hypersensitivity to tramadol, any other component of this product, or opioids. It is also contraindicated in cases of acute intoxication with alcohol, hypnotics, centrally acting analgesics, opioids, or psychotropic drugs. Seizures have been reported in patients taking tramadol. These seizures have occurred in patients taking normal dosages as well as dosages exceeding the normal recommended dosages. Patients who may be at risk are those taking tricyclic antidepressants, selective serotonin reuptake inhibitor antidepressants, MAOIs, neuroleptics, or other drugs that reduce the seizure threshold.

Pharmacokinetics

Half-Life	Onset	Peak	Duration
PO: 5-8 hr	PO: 30 min	PO: 2 hr	PO: Unknown

◆ NURSING PROCESS

Patients experiencing pain pose many challenges to the nurse and other health care providers who are involved in their health and nursing care, as well as to significant others or family members. This challenge requires astute nursing assessment with appropriate intervention based on the specific individual as well as the specific type of pain and related disease processes and health status. Adequate analgesia (providing pain relief without complications, toxicity, or a diminished level of consciousness) with thorough patient teaching is the goal of all those involved in the care of these patients. Nurses need to adequately and accurately assess the nature of the patient's pain (Box 10-2). Pain has been accepted as the fifth vital sign that must be assessed (along with blood pressure, pulse rate, temperature, and respirations) to ensure that pain management is adequate and effective. Pain assessment has also been established as a standard by the Joint Commission on Accreditation of Healthcare Organizations. Nurses also need to assess and reassess the patient's response to the pain management regimen, regardless of the medications involved—nonnarcotics, narcotics, a combination of both, and/or NSAIDs (Chapter 44).

There are several organizations and professional groups that establish standards for pain management (e.g., the Agency for Healthcare Research and Quality) or identify assessment tools such as the Numeric Pain Intensity Scale (a 0 to 10 pain rating scale) and the Visual Analog Scale. Other reliable resources include age-appropriate pain rating tools from the American Pain Society and the American Society for Pain Management Nursing. These tools have proved to be valid if the patient is capable of answering questions and is alert enough to participate in his or her care. With pediatric patients, use of the Visual Analog Scale as an ouch scale, along with other objective and subjective indicators, is helpful. On the opposite end of the age spectrum, the elderly also require special assessment and consideration of medications they are taking as well as pre-existing health problems. Because renal and hepatic function may be decreased in the elderly, lower doses of drugs may be needed/ordered. For analgesics, this may mean giving the lowest but most effective dosage amount ordered. In addition, drug accumulation and toxicity may occur with any patient with decreased renal/hepatic functioning.

◆ ASSESSMENT

Adequate analgesia, pain relief without complications, and patient teaching are goals of all health care providers. Nurses need to thoroughly assess the nature of the pain and to determine whether the pain occurring is acute or chronic, or represents a **special pain situation.** The management of acute or chronic pain in patients is a common part of clinical practice and a challenging part of nursing and health care.

Before the nurse administers *any* analgesic, a thorough health history, medication history, and nursing assessment must be obtained. This ensures that these medications are used safely—that is, that analgesic treatment is free of complications or injury to the patient. The nurse should obtain and document information regarding the following (also see Box 10-2):
- Allergies to nonopioids (acetaminophen, aspirin, and other NSAIDs) including COX-2 inhibitors (Chapter 44), opioids, and/or partial or mixed agonists.

Box 10-2   Assessment of Pain

- Assess factors influencing pain, such as individual reaction, pain tolerance, underlying cause, individual pain threshold, physical factors (e.g., stress), and psychologic factors (family roles, spiritual system, meaning of pain, stereotypes, stage of growth and development, motivations, personality, fatigue, anxiety, fear). Also assess age, gender, societal influences, and general state of health.
- Use an age-appropriate scale to assess pain (see the text).
- In children younger than 5 years of age, consider level of growth and development (e.g., Erikson's stages). Use pictures with happy faces (no pain with a rating of 0) and sad faces (bad pain with a rating of 5) and tools to which the pediatric patient can relate, such as a 6-inch ruler, to assess the level of pain.
- When assessing elderly patients, never assume that these patients do not feel pain the same way that they did when they were younger; although they may have barriers to verbal or nonverbal expression of pain (e.g., dementia, cognitive impairment), older adults still experience pain.
- When assessing for chronic pain, consider that pain can occur with or without evident tissue damage and serves no useful purpose. It is a complex and multifactorial problem that requires a holistic approach to patient care with consideration not only of physical factors but also of psychologic factors (insomnia, depression, withdrawal, anxiety, personality changes, and changes

in lifestyle), because chronic pain is generally characterized more by psychologic and functional ability changes rather than by physical changes.
- Assessing for chronic pain is challenging, but health care providers must go the extra mile to assess and then act. Remember that chronic pain is difficult to describe and manage and often is not responsive to conventional measures.
- When assessing for cancer pain, remember that management of this pain should be as individualized as all other aspects of patient care with full belief in the patient's pain and suffering. Treatment may include narcotics, possibly at high dosages; however, quality of life for the patient, rather than addiction, should be the concern in this situation.
- Ask the patient with acute or chronic pain (or any type of pain) to keep a daily journal of his or her pain experience, including information on precipitating and aggravating factors; measures that alleviate or help the pain; duration and intensity of pain; referred pain, character, onset, and pattern; the meaning of pain to the patient; and psychologic factors.
- Remember that chronic pain and cancer pain (in addition to the pain experience) may be perceived as an actual or potential loss to the patient, including a loss of control.

EVIDENCE-BASED PRACTICE

Strategies of Pain Assessment Used by Nurses on Surgical Units

Review

The purpose of this study was to identify various criteria that nurses use in the assessment of patients who are experiencing postoperative pain. In addition, the study looked at the kind of knowledge the nurses applied from previous experiences. Phenomenology was used to analyze the data from this more qualitative approach to studying pain assessment in an attempt to describe the differences and similarities in individual conceptions of the pain experience.

Type of Evidence

Ten nurses and 30 postsurgical patients were involved in this study, which was conducted at a large urban hospital in New England. Strategic sampling was used to identify five nurses with fewer than 6 years of experience (categorized as the least experienced group) and five nurses with more than 6 years of experience (the more experienced group). It was anticipated that the number of years of nursing experience on a surgical unit might be important in differentiating the types of criteria nurses used to assess pain. All patients had undergone surgery within the previous 24 hours and were experiencing pain but were not connected to a patient-controlled analgesia pump, had not been diagnosed with metastatic cancer, and were not experiencing confusion or an altered level of consciousness. The research method included a series of five highly interactive, semistructured, audiotaped interviews with each nurse. Interviews focused on what the nurse's conception of the patient's situation was and how and on what basis the nurse judged the patient's pain.

Results of Study

Data from 30 clinical pain assessments performed by the 10 nurses identified multiple criteria used in each nurse's assessment of a patient. These criteria related to the patient's appearance and other observational data as well as to the content of communication between the nurse and the patient. These criteria were used as the framework from which the nurses developed and implemented variations in pain

assessment. Nurses were also found to draw on their past experiences in several ways when working with their patients, including how to focus on listening to patients, what to look for, and what to do for the patient in pain. This study was one of the first to empirically identify criteria and types of past knowledge that nurses use when assessing patients for pain on a postoperative unit. Because it was a qualitative, descriptive study, the sample size was small, and the strategies identified were by no means exhaustive or representative. The criteria used by the nurses to assess pain were both objective and subjective. Objective criteria concerned how the patient looked, whereas subjective criteria were more concerned with what the patient said. The facility in which the research took place has now changed its pain assessment guidelines to provide a more subjective orientation and has identified the patient's self-report as one of the single most reliable indicators of the existence and intensity of pain.

Link of Evidence to Nursing Practice

This study had a major impact on the assessment of pain in the facility in which the data were collected, and major policy changes were made in the criteria to be used in assessing patients' pain. As a qualitative approach to studying pain assessment, this study provided significant data identifying the criteria and types of past knowledge nurses used while actually assessing patients for pain on a postoperative nursing unit. Questions that remain to be answered include the following: Does the strategy used for assessment influence the nurse's perception of the intensity of pain and the need for pain management? Does the assessment strategy used have an influence on pain management decisions? Quantification of the use of different pain assessment strategies in a large sample of nurses will allow the findings of this particular study to be extended to identify the strategies actually used in contemporary nursing practice and the resulting pain management techniques implemented by nurses.

Based on Kim HS et al: Strategies of pain assessment used by nurses on surgical units, *Pain Manag Nurs* 6(1):3-9, 2005.

- Drug history with identification of any interactions with other drugs, herbals, foods, and home remedies
- Underlying level of any CNS depression due to drug therapy and/or other physical conditions or diseases
- Adjunctive use of other nonopioids, NSAIDs, or opioids as well as their routes of administration, which should be assessed even more cautiously because of the risk of toxicity and overdosage
- Use of alcohol, street drugs, or any illegal drug or substance
- Pain intensity and character: onset; location; quality (stabbing, throbbing, dull ache, sharp, diffuse, localized, referred, or knifelike); intensity or severity (rated on a scale of 1 to 10 with 10 being the worst and/or assessed using validated age-appropriate tools); precipitating, aggravating, and relieving factors; previous treatment; and effect of pain on physical and social function
- Type of pain being experienced, such as acute pain, chronic pain, or pain due to cancer; each type of pain will require a different approach to treatment, with cancer pain and/or bone metastasis pain being most difficult to manage; various opioid drugs, along with NSAIDs or COX-2 inhibitors, and a variety of routes of administration and dosage forms (transdermal, parenteral [intramuscular, subcutaneous, IV, or patient-controlled analgesia], oral, transmucosal, lollipop, suppository, and epidural) may be used
- Other pain treatments (both pharmacologic and nonpharmacologic)
- Laboratory values reflective of liver function (levels of alanine aminotransferase, alkaline phosphatase, γ-glutamyl transferase, 5′-nucleotidase and bilirubin) and/or renal function (blood urea nitrogen and creatinine levels)
- Level of orientation, status of bowel sounds and urine output (e.g., possible confusion from narcotics and from CNS depression with resultant constipation and/or urinary retention)
- Cultural and religious beliefs about the experience of pain and its management; use of alternative measures to relieve pain by Asian and other cultural groups should be accepted

Objective and subjective findings of a thorough nursing assessment of patients who are being newly treated for pain or whose pain is being undermanaged are very important to efficient and effective therapy. Psychosocial assessment includes obtaining information regarding the following influences on the pain experience: family and occupational roles, past experiences with pain, spiritual beliefs, meaning of pain, cultural and societal influences, sexual identity, communication skills, level of growth and development in terms of Erikson's stages of development and related tasks, personality, attitude toward pain, level of anxiety, fatigue, motivations, and fears. Other factors or influences for which to assess include pain threshold, general state of health, sleep patterns and stressors, pain intensity and frequency, pain tolerance, prior experience of pain, CNS intactness, and age. The nurse should always remember, however, that each patient is an individual and should approach the patient from that perspective.

Vital signs (blood pressure, pulse rate, respirations, and temperature) should also be assessed and documented. The nurse should remember that during the acute pain response, stimulation of the sympathetic nervous system may result in elevated values for vital sign values (blood pressure over 120/80 mm Hg, pulse rate over 100 beats/min, respiration rate over 20 breaths/min), and use of analgesics, especially narcotics, will depress vital signs due to the central nervous system depressive effects. The nurse should always document all data and findings related to total system assessment and continue to monitor (and document) all basic system-related assessment parameters.

It is essential that the nurse check the route and time of administration of any previous analgesic and the patient's response before administering another analgesic dose, regardless of whether it is a nonopioid or opioid analgesic. The route of administration may also be dictated by considerations such as avoiding intramuscular dosage routes in chronic pain and cancer pain management. The nurse must always check the patient's chart, physician's order, nurses' notes, and medication administration record before administering any additional doses of analgesic. Patients taking *any* type of analgesic should be reassessed at regular intervals before and during treatment.

For *nonopioid analgesics,* specifically acetaminophen and tramadol hydrochloride (NSAIDs and COX-2 inhibitors are discussed in Chapter 44), assessment parameters are similar to those for opioids, but there are some differences because of the nonopioid status of the analgesics. With acetaminophen, assessment should include all of the parameters mentioned earlier as well as determination of whether the patient is pregnant or breast-feeding. There are no age-related precautions for children or the elderly and all other contraindications, cautions and drug interactions should also be thoroughly assessed. Liver and kidney function tests should be assessed, especially if long-term therapy is indicated. Once therapy has been initiated, the nurse must be cautious to assess for symptoms of chronic acetaminophen poisoning, such as rapid, weak pulse; dyspnea; and cold and clammy extremities. Chronic daily use of the drug may also lead to increased risk of permanent liver damage, and so liver function should continue to be monitored. Children rarely experience liver damage; however, adults who ingest more than 2.6 g within a 24-hour period may be at higher risk of varying degrees of loss of appetite, jaundice, nausea, and vomiting.

Use of tramadol hydrochloride requires assessment of contraindications, cautions, drug interactions, and liver/renal function (information presented previously). Elderly and pediatric patients may need age-related dosage adjustments (as for other nonnarcotic and narcotic analgesics). CNS stimulation may occasionally occur, so tramadol is not a drug of choice (analgesic) if there is a history of seizures.

For *narcotic analgesics,* assessment data include all the aforementioned information as well as respiratory status, renal status, and presence of head injury. Because narcotics are CNS depressants, respiratory depression is of major concern; therefore, assessing respiratory rate, depth, and pattern and listening to breath sounds is important. Decreased renal function can lead to possible drug accumulation and toxicity, and so the patient's blood urea nitrogen and creatinine levels should be assessed. Urinary output may need to be assessed as well because of possible urinary retention. With head injuries of undiagnosed cause, the administration of narcotics is not recommended because of the masking of changes in level of consciousness. Contraindications, cautions, and drug interactions also need to be assessed (as discussed previously in this chapter). The use of opioids in patients with disorders such as dementia, Alzheimer's disease, head injuries, increased intracranial pressure, multiple sclerosis, muscular dystrophy, myasthenia gravis, and cerebrovascular accident or a stroke may lead to an alteration of symptoms of the disease process with possible masking or worsening of the clinical presentation without actual pathologic changes. With opioids, it is also important to be aware that the elderly, although potentially more sensitive to the effects of these drugs, may also exhibit paradoxical excitement and excitatory behavior even though a CNS depressant drug has been given (thus the term *paradoxical*). Pediatric patients are also more susceptible to the CNS depressant effects, especially respiratory depression. See the Life Span Consideration boxes for both of these age groups.

In patients taking *partial agonists* such as buprenorphine hydrochloride, it is important to assess for pain and to assess for all of the parameters discussed earlier for opioids, because these drugs are still considered narcotics due to their effect at the opioid receptors. It is also very important in the assessment to remember that these drugs are still effective analgesics and still have CNS depressant effects. They are subject to the ceiling effect. The *ceiling effect* means that a drug has a maximal analgesic effect, even at higher doses of a drug. Increasing the dosage will not improve the analgesia beyond this maximal effect, and the higher dosage may have dangerous and unpredictable effects for the patient. (see drug profile).

For *opioid agonist-antagonist drugs,* it is also important for the nurse to determine whether the patient is in an addictive state or not, because if these drugs are given to a patient who is taking a narcotic (whether by self-administration or addiction or on an order from the physician), withdrawal will occur in the addicted patient, with reversal of the effects of the narcotic. Other assessment data includes vital signs, especially respirations (see the previous discussion). Use in children younger than 18 years of age is not recommended, and effects of these medications are more unpredictable in the elderly. These drugs also cause spasms of the sphincter of Oddi in the gallbladder and are not recommended for those who have biliary ductal disease or are scheduled for biliary surgery. (Morphine is usually indicated in this situation.)

If, during assessment, overdose, toxicity, and/or respiratory depression are suspected, *narcotic antagonists* are available for reversal of CNS depression. Analgesia will also be reversed. The pure opioid antagonists (e.g., naltraxone), will bind at opioid receptors and reverse the opioid's action.

The nurse must remember that the narcotic antagonists are effective *only* in reversing respiratory depression secondary to opioid overdosage. Naloxone may be used in patients of all ages, including neonates and children. Vital signs should be assessed and documented just before, during, and after the use of the antagonist so that the therapeutic effects can be further noted. Also, the nurse must remember that the antagonist drug

---

Life Span Considerations: The Pediatric Patient
Opioid Use

- Assessment of the pediatric patient is challenging, and all types of behavior that may indicate pain, such as muscular rigidity, restlessness, screaming, fear of moving, and withdrawn behavior, must be carefully considered.
- Pain management in children is complex because it is more difficult to determine their pain, especially in infants. Frequently the reason older pediatric patients do not verbalize their pain is their fear of the treatment, such as shots. Compassionate and therapeutic communication skills will help the nurse in these situations.
- The "ouch scale" is often used to determine the level of pain in children. This scale is used to obtain the child's rating of the intensity of pain from 0 to 5 by means of simple face diagrams, from a very happy face for level 0 (no pain) to a sad, tearful face for level 5 pain. Parents and caregivers play an important role in pain management in the pediatric patient and in noting any crying or whining.
- Assessment of pain is very important in pediatric patients because they are often undermedicated. The nurse should always thoroughly assess the pediatric patient and not underestimate the child's complaints.
- Always know the patient's age, weight and height, because drug calculations are often based on these variables. With the pediatric patient, *all* mathematical calculations should be checked and double-checked for accuracy to avoid excessive dosages; this is especially true for opioids.
- Always give analgesics before pain becomes severe, with use of oral dosage forms first if appropriate.
- If suppositories are used, the nurse must be careful to administer the exact dose and not to split, halve, or divide an adult dose into

a child's dose. This may result in the administration of an unknown amount of medication and possible overdose.
- When subcutaneous, intramuscular, and intravenous medications are used, the principle of atraumatic care in the delivery of nursing care is being followed. One method to ensure atraumatic care is the use of EMLA (eutectic mixture of local anesthetics) on the site before the actual injection. EMLA is a topical cream that anesthetizes the site of the injection if applied 1 to 2½ hours prior to the injection. Once the EMLA is applied to the site, the site is covered with a transparent dressing to keep the medication on the skin. A physician's order is needed.
- Distraction and creative imagery may be used for older children such as toddlers or preschool-aged children.
- Pediatric patients should always be monitored very closely for any unusual behavior while receiving opioids.
- The following signs and symptoms should be reported to the physician immediately if they occur: CNS changes such as dizziness, lightheadedness, drowsiness, hallucinations, changes in the level of consciousness, and sluggish pupil reaction. No further medication should be given until the nurse receives further orders from the physician.
- Always monitor and document vital signs before, during, and after the administration of opioid analgesics. Medication is withheld if respiration rate is less than 12 breaths/min or if there are any changes in the level of consciousness.
- Generally speaking, smaller doses of narcotics (with very close and frequent monitoring) are indicated for the pediatric patient.
- Give medications with meals to help decrease gastrointestinal upset.

Life Span Considerations: The Elderly Patient
Opioid Use

- The nurse should assess the patient carefully before administering narcotics, because a dose and interval adjustment may be necessary if undesirable adverse reactions such as confusion, decreased respirations, and excessive central nervous system (CNS) depression have developed.
- The nurse should note and record height and weight before the start of narcotic therapy.
- The nurse should carefully monitor and document any changes in elderly patients who are receiving opioids because they are generally more sensitive to these drugs. This includes frequent monitoring of vital signs, respiratory function, and CNS status.
- Many institutionalized elderly patients are very stoic about pain and may also have altered presentations of common illnesses so that the pain experience presents in a different manner. For example, the elderly may have silent myocardial infarctions or even painless abdominal or intraabdominal emergencies.
- It is a myth that aging increases the pain threshold. The problem is that cognitive impairment and dementia are often major barriers to pain assessment. Nevertheless, many elderly patients are still reliable in their reporting of pain, even with moderate to severe cognitive impairment.
- Over time, the elderly may lose reliability in recalling and accurately reporting chronic pain.
- The elderly, especially those older than 75 years of age—are at higher risk for too much or too little pain management, and it is important to remember that there is a higher peak and longer duration of action of drugs in these patients than in their younger counterparts.
- Smaller dosages of narcotics are generally indicated for elderly patients because of their increased sensitivity to the CNS depressant effects of the drugs as well as their diminished renal and hepatic function. Paradoxical (opposite) reactions and/or unexpected reactions may be more likely to occur in patients of this age group as well.

- In elderly male patients, benign prostatic hypertrophy or obstructive urinary diseases should be considered because of the urinary retention associated with the use of narcotics. Urinary outflow can become further diminished in these patients and result in adverse reactions or complications. Dosage adjustments may need to be made by the physician.
- Polypharmacy is often a problem in older adults; therefore, it is important for the nurse to have a complete list of all medications the patient is currently taking and to assess for drug interactions and treatment (drug) duplication.
- The nurse should conduct frequent assessments of patients for level of consciousness, alertness, and cognitive ability while ensuring that the environment is safe and keeping a call bell or light at the bedside; bed alarms are indicated where available.
- Decreased circulation causes variation in the absorption of intramuscular or intravenous dosage forms and often results in the slower absorption of parenteral forms of opioids.
- The nurse should encourage elderly patients to ask for medications if needed. They often hesitate to request pain medication because they do not want to bother the nurse or give in to pain.
- As stated by the American Geriatric Society on the Management of Pain, nonsteroidal antiinflammatory drugs should be used with caution because of their potential for renal and gastrointestinal toxicity. Acetaminophen is the drug of choice for relieving mild to moderate pain but with cautious dosing because of hepatic and renal concerns. The oral route of administration is preferred. The regimen should be as simple as possible to enhance compliance, and the nurse should be sure to note, report, and document any unusual reactions to the opioid drugs.
- Hypotension and respiratory depression may occur more often in elderly patients who are taking opioids for pain management, thus the need for even more astute vital sign monitoring.

may not work with just one dosing and that repeated doses are generally needed to reverse the effects of the opioid. This helps to ensure that effective treatment of the overdosage and CNS depression and safe patient recovery.

◆ NURSING DIAGNOSES

- Acute pain related to specific disease processes or conditions and other pathologies leading to various levels and types of pain (acute pain is pain of less than 3 months' duration)
- Chronic pain related to various disease processes, conditions, or syndromes causing pain (pain is usually considered chronic if it occurs over longer than 3 months; e.g., migraine headaches, rheumatoid arthritis)
- Risk for injury related to decreased sensorium or level of consciousness from analgesics with use of either nonnarcotic or narcotic or opioid drugs
- Risk for injury related to possible overdosage and severe adverse reactions and/or drug interactions associated with the various classes of analgesics
- Impaired gas exchange related to possible respiratory depression secondary to CNS depressive effects of narcotics or opioids
- Constipation related to the use of narcotics or opioids causing CNS depression and decreased peristalsis

- Risk for infection related to the adverse effect of urinary retention and subsequent urinary stasis from the use of narcotics or opioids
- Deficient knowledge related to lack of familiarity with opioids, their use, and their adverse effects

◆ PLANNING
Goals

- Patient states measures that will enhance the effectiveness of the analgesic regimen.
- Patient identifies the rationale for use, therapeutic effects, and adverse effects associated with all types of analgesics.
- Patient states various measures to help minimize the occurrence of common adverse effects of nonnarcotics as well as narcotics and opioids.

Outcome Criteria

- Patient demonstrates increased comfort levels as seen by decreased use of analgesics, increased activity and performance of activities of daily living (ADLs), decreased complaints of pain, and decreased levels of pain as rated on a scale of 0 to 10.
- Patient experiences minimal adverse effects and complications such as nausea, vomiting, and constipation associated with the use of analgesics, especially narcotics and opioids.

- Patient uses nonpharmacologic measures such as relaxation therapy, distraction, and music therapy to improve comfort and enhance any pharmacologic regimens.
- Patient manages adverse effects associated with analgesics through fluid intake and antiemetic therapy when necessary.

◆ IMPLEMENTATION

Once the cause of pain has been diagnosed, pain management should begin immediately and aggressively in conformity with each individual situation and the needs of each individual patient. Pain management is varied and multifaceted, and incorporates pharmacologic as well as nonpharmacologic approaches to pain relief (Box 10-3 and the Herbal Therapies and Dietary Supplements box). Pain management strategies should include an emphasis on the type of pain and its rating as well as pain quality, duration, precipitating factors, and interventions that help the pain. Some general principles of pain management include the following: (1) Management of mild to moderate pain often begins with the use of nonnarcotic drugs such as acetaminophen, tramadol, and NSAIDs (Chapter 44) unless contraindicated. (2) Moderate to severe pain is generally not managed with nonnarcotics but is usually treated with narcotics; such treatment requires a knowledge of the drugs used for acute versus chronic pain; drug action, adverse effects, and toxicity; and other drug- and patient-related information. (3) Drug selection for treatment of moderate to severe pain should be based on variables such as the characteristics of the individual patient, cultural influences (see the Cultural Implications box on p. 137), the disease process, and the use of other therapies such as homeopathic, folk, or herbal remedies. Nonpharmacologic measures for pain management should always be used, either as a beginning mode of treatment or as an adjuvant to pharmacologic therapy and include relaxation therapy, guided imagery, music distraction, exercise, transcutaneous electrical stimulation, and massage.

Nonopioid analgesics, such as acetaminophen, should be given as ordered or as indicated for fever or pain. Acetaminophen should be taken as prescribed by all patients, especially pediatric patients and the elderly. Patient teaching should emphasize taking the medication as indicated to avoid liver damage and acute toxicity. If a patient is taking other OTC medications with acetaminophen, the patient should read the labels very carefully to identify other drug-drug interactions. The patient should also be taught the signs of acetaminophen overdose, which include bleeding, malaise, fever, sore throat, and easy bruising (due to hepatotoxicity). The nurse should also instruct the patient to report pain lasting longer than 3 days, because further evaluation by a health care provider is indicated.

The wrapped suppository dosage forms of acetaminophen should be placed into a medicine cup of ice, and once the suppository is unwrapped, cold water should be run over it to moisten it for insertion into the rectum using a gloved finger and water-soluble lubricating gel if necessary. Tablets may be crushed if needed. Adult patients who take more than 2.6 g in 24 hours are at risk for mild liver damage; those taking 10 g or more (e.g., deliberate overdoses) are at high risk for severe liver damage, and death is possible after ingestion of more than 15 g. Liver damage from acetaminophen may be minimized by timely dosing with acetylcysteine (see p. 149). An important point to remember should acetylcysteine be ordered is that it has the flavor of rotten

---

Box 10-3 Nonpharmacologic Treatment Options for Pain

- Acupressure
- Acupuncture
- Art therapy
- Behavioral therapy
- Comfort measures
- Counseling
- Distraction
- Hot or cold packs
- Hypnosis
- Imagery
- Massage
- Meditation
- Music therapy
- Pet therapy
- Reduction of fear
- Relaxation
- Surgery
- Therapeutic baths
- Therapeutic communication
- Therapeutic touch
- Transcutaneous electric nerve stimulation
- Yoga

HERBAL THERAPIES AND DIETARY SUPPLEMENTS

Feverfew (*Chrysanthemum parthenium*)

Overview
A member of the marigold family known for its antiinflammatory properties

Common Uses
Treatment of migraine headaches, menstrual problems, arthritis, fever

Adverse Effects
Nausea and vomiting, anorexia, hypersensitivity reactions, muscle stiffness, muscle and joint pain

Potential Drug Interactions
Possible increase in bleeding with the use of aspirin, dipyridamole, and warfarin

Contraindications
Contraindicated in those allergic to ragweed, chrysanthemums, and marigolds, as well as those about to undergo surgery

---

eggs and is better tolerated if it is disguised by mixing with a drink such as cola or flavored water to increase its palatability. Use of a straw will help minimize contact with mucous membranes of the mouth and is recommended. This antidote may be given through a nasogastric or orogastric tube, if necessary.

Tramadol may cause nausea and vomiting, and the patient should be offered cola or dry crackers to help relieve the nausea. Taking with food or a snack may help to decrease gastrointestinal upset. If dizziness, blurred vision, or drowsiness occur, the nurse should be sure to assist the patient with ambulation (as with any analgesic that may lead to dizziness or lightheadedness). Educate the patient about injury prevention, such as the need to move and change positions slowly and to avoid any tasks that require mental clarity and alertness. The patient should be encouraged to report any heart palpitations, seizures, tremors, difficulty breathing, chest pain, and muscle weakness.

With use of *narcotics* (and other analgesics), the nurse should administer it as ordered after checking for the "Five Rights" of medication administration (right drug, right dose, right patient, right route, and right time) as with any medication. Documentation is stricter, however, with controlled substances such as opioids. Documents should be checked for the last time the medication was given before another dose is administered. The medication profile should always be double-checked against the original physician's order and signed with a full signature once the medication has been administered. The nurse should always return at the appropriate time (taking into consideration the onset and peak effect times of the drug and the route) and assess for the effects of the drug on the pain and the presence of any adverse effects. When administering analgesics, whether pure, mixed, or partial, the nurse must always be sure to give the patient the medication before the pain becomes severe or when the pain is beginning to return to provide adequate analgesia. With regard to the route of administration, it is recommended that oral forms of narcotics be used first, if ordered and if no nausea or vomiting. Taking the dose with food may help minimize gastrointestinal upset. Antiemetic therapy may be needed if nausea and vomiting from the narcotic occurs or is present prior to dosing. Safety measures such as keeping the side rails up (if used in the facility), turning the bed safety alarm on, and making sure the call bell is within the patient's reach are all crucial measures to prevent falls stemming from the use of narcotics (or other analgesics) and from the adverse effects of these drugs, including confusion, hypotension, and decreased sensorium. Elderly patients are at higher risk for falls and adverse effects (see Box 10-1).

When managing pain with morphine, meperidine, and similar *opioid drugs,* the nurse should withhold the dose and contact the physician if there is any decline in the patient's condition or if the vital signs are abnormal (see values given earlier), and especially if the respiratory rate is less than 12 breaths/min. Intramuscular injections should be used only if there is no other route available. Intramuscular injections of analgesics are rarely given because of the availability of newer dosage forms such as PCA pumps, transdermal patches, and constant subcutaneous or epidural infusions. For cancer patients, intramuscular injections may not be an option due to trauma at the site and possible thrombocytopenia and leucopenia with resulting bleeding and/or infection at the injection site.

For transdermal patches (e.g., transdermal fentanyl), two systems are used. The oldest type of patch contains a reservoir system consisting of four layers beginning with the adhesive layer and ending with the protective backing. Between these two layers are the permeable rate-controlling membrane and the reservoir layer, which holds the drug in a gel or liquid form. The newer patch has a matrix system consisting of two layers: one layer containing the active drug with the releasing and adhesive mechanisms plus the protective impermeable backing layer. The advantages of the matrix system over the reservoir system are that that patch is slimmer and smaller, it is more comfortable, it is worn for up to 7 days (the older reservoir system patch is worn for up to 3 to 4 days), and it appears to result in more constant serum drug levels. In addition, the matrix system is alcohol free; the alcohol in the reservoir system often irri-

tates the patient's skin. It is important for the nurse to know what type of delivery system is being used so that proper guidelines are followed to enhance the system's and drug's effectiveness.

Transdermal patches can be applied to any clean, nonhairy area. They should be changed as ordered and placed on a new site, but only after the old site has been cleansed of any residual medication. Rotation of sites helps to decrease irritation and enhance drug effects. Transdermal systems are beneficial for delivery of many types of medications, especially analgesics, and have the benefits of allowing multiday therapy with a single application, avoiding first-pass metabolism, improving patient compliance, and minimizing frequent dosing. However, the patient should be watched carefully for the development of any type of contact dermatitis caused by the patch (the physician or health care provider should be contacted immediately if this occurs) and should maintain his or her own pain journal when at home. Journal entries are a valid source of information for the nurse, other health care professionals, the patient, and family members to assess the patient's pain control and to monitor the effectiveness not only of transdermal analgesia but also any medication regimen.

With the intravenous administration of *narcotic agonists,* the nurse should always follow the manufacturer's guidelines and institutional policies regarding specific dilutional amounts and solution as well as the time period for infusion. When PCA is used, the amounts and times of dosing should be noted in the appropriate records and tracked by appropriate personnel. The fact that a PCA pump is being used, however, does not mean that it is 100% reliable. To be sure that all is stable, the nurse should monitor pain levels, response to medication, and vital signs just as frequently as with other parenteral opioid administration. The nurse should follow dosage ranges for all opioid agonists and agonists-antagonists and pay special attention to the dosages of morphine and morphine-like drugs. For intravenous infusions, the nurse is responsible for monitoring the intravenous needle site and infusion rates and documenting any adverse effects or complications. Another point for the nurse to remember when administering narcotic and nonnarcotic analgesics is that each medication has a different onset of action, peak, and duration of action. These differences apply to the route of administration as well; onset of action is immediate with intravenous administration (Table 10-10).

There are several important points to emphasize in discussing the use of opioids and related nursing interventions including watching for adverse effects. Urinary output and bowel status should be monitored. The patient should have a urinary output of at least 600 mL/24 hr and bowel movements of normal patterns and consistency for that patient—even if stool softeners must be ordered (see Box 10-1 for adverse effects related to chronic opioid use and related interventions). The patient's pupils should be monitored along with vital signs because pinpoint pupils may indicate overdosage. Naloxone should be kept available should respiratory depression or overdosage occur.

To reverse an opioid overdose or opioid-induced respiratory depression, an opioid antagonist such as naloxone must be administered. If naloxone is used, 0.4 to 2 mg should be given intravenously in undiluted form and should be administered over 15 seconds (or as ordered); if reconstitution is needed, 0.9% NaCl should be used (see Table 10-7). However, the guidelines in the package

Table 10-10   Opioid Administration Guidelines

Narcotic	Nursing Administration
buprenorphine and butorphanol	When giving IV, infuse over the recommended time (usually 3-5 min). Always assess respirations. Give IM butorphanol in deep gluteal muscle mass.
codeine	Give PO doses with food to minimize GI tract upset; ceiling effects with oral codeine.
dezocine	Mixed agonist-antagonist; short duration of action. Give IV or IM deep into gluteal muscle mass.
fentanyl	Administer parenteral doses as ordered and as per manufacturer guidelines in regard to mg/min to prevent CNS depression and possible cardiac or respiratory arrest. Transdermal patches come in a variety of dosages, and fentanyl lollipops are also available. Be sure to remove residual amounts of the old patch prior to application of a new patch. Dispose of patches properly to avoid inadvertent contact with children or pets.
hydromorphone	May be given SC, rectally, IV, PO, or IM.
levorphanol	May be given PO, SC, or IV; give IV forms over 5 min or adhere to manufacturer's guidelines; longer acting lasts 6-8 hours.
meperidine	Given by a variety of routes: IV, IM, or PO; highly protein bound, so watch for interactions and toxicity. Monitor elderly patients for increased sensitivity.
morphine	Available in a variety of forms: SC, IM, PO, IV, extended and immediate release, and morphine sulfate (Duramorph) for epidural infusion; morphine sulfate (MS Contin) now available in a 200-mg sustained-release tab. Always monitor respiratory rate.
nalbuphine	IV dosages of 10 mg undiluted over 5 min.
naloxone	Antagonist given for opioid overdose; 0.4 mg usually given IV over 15 sec or less. Reverses analgesia as well.
propoxyphene	PO dosing only; high abuse potential.
oxycodone	Often mixed with acetaminophen or aspirin; PO and suppository dosage forms. Now available in both immediate and sustained-release tabs.
oxymorphone	PO, IM, IV, SC, and rectal suppository dosage forms.
pentazocine	SC, IV, and IM forms; mixed agonist/antagonist; 5 mg IV to be given over 1 min.

GI, Gastrointestinal; *IM,* intramuscular; *IV,* intravenous; *PO,* oral; *SC,* subcutaneous.

insert should also be followed. Emergency resuscitative equipment should be nearby in the event of respiratory or cardiac arrest.

The nurse must remember when giving *agonists-antagonists* that they are effective analgesics when administered alone, but when they are given with other opioids or are given to a patient with long-term opioid use, their administration may lead to reversal of analgesia and acute withdrawal. If partial agonist drugs are given to a patient who is opioid naive and is not currently taking opioids in any form, the patient will experience effective analgesia, but analgesia reversal will occur with the coadministration of other opioids.

When opioid agonist-antagonist drugs, the nurse must be careful always to check the dosages and routes as well as to perform the aforementioned interventions. If a pure opioid is used with a mixed narcotic, the analgesic effects will be reversed; when a mixed narcotic is used alone, respirations and other vital signs must be monitored, just as with pure narcotic agonists. Patient education regarding mixed opiate agonists should emphasize the need for careful dosing to avoid CNS and respiratory depression and should include information on nonpharmacologic measures to manage pain. Patients should report any dizziness, constipation, difficulty with urination, blurred vision, hallucinations, or tachycardia. Mixed narcotic agonists also have the potential for misuse and addiction. The nurse should remember that withdrawal symptoms could manifest in individuals who are opioid dependent.

Regardless of whether nonopioid, opioid, or combination drug therapy is used, it is always important to be up to date on all forms and protocols of pain management, whether for moderate to severe pain or the management of cancer pain. The WHO's three-step analgesic ladder is often accepted as the standard for guiding the use of nonopioids and opioids and serves as a reminder for the stepped approach to pain management when this

is appropriate. Dosing of medications for pain management is very important to the treatment regimen. Once a thorough assessment has been performed, it is best to treat the patient's pain before it becomes severe, and thus, as noted earlier, pain needs to be added as the fifth vital sign. When pain is present, analgesic doses are best administered around the clock rather than as needed but always within dosage guidelines for each drug used. Around-the-clock (or scheduled) dosing maintains steady-state levels of the medication and prevents drug troughs and escalation of pain. No given dosage of an analgesic will provide the same level of pain relief for every patient, and so titration upward or even titration downward should be handled individually and should be implemented as long as the analgesic is needed. Aggressive titration may be necessary in difficult pain control cases and in cancer pain situations. Patients with severe pain, metastatic pain, or bone metastasis pain may need higher and higher doses of analgesic, and so an opiate such as morphine should be titrated until the desired response is achieved or until adverse effects occur. A patient-rated pain level of 4 out of 10 is considered to indicate effective pain relief. If pain is not managed adequately by monotherapy, other drugs or adjuvants may need to be added to enhance analgesic efficacy. This includes the use of NSAIDs (for analgesic, antiinflammatory effects), acetaminophen (for analgesic effects), corticosteroids (for mood elevation and antiinflammatory, antiemetic, and appetite stimulation effects), anticonvulsants (for treatment of neuropathic pain), tricyclic antidepressants (for treatment of neuropathic pain and for innate analgesic properties and opioid-potentiating effects), neuroleptics (for treatment of chronic pain syndromes), local anesthetics (for treatment of neuropathic pain), hydroxyzine (for mild antianxiety properties as well as sedating effects and antihistamine and mild antiemetic actions), psychostimulants (for reduction of opioid-induced sedation when opioid dosage adjustment is not effective). See Table 10-11 for a listing of drugs that should not be used in patients experiencing cancer pain.

Dosage forms are also important, especially with chronic pain and cancer pain. Oral administration is always preferred but is not always tolerated by the patient and may not even be a viable option for pain control. If oral dosing is not appropriate, less invasive routes of administration include rectal and transdermal routes. Rectal dosage forms are safe, inexpensive, effective, and helpful if the patient is experiencing nausea or vomiting or altered mental status; this route would not be suitable for those with diarrhea, stomatitis, and/or low blood cell counts. Transdermal patches may provide up to 72 hours of pain control but are not for rapid dose titration and are used only when stable analgesia has been previously achieved. In fact, long-acting forms of morphine and fentanyl may be delivered via transdermal patches when a longer duration of action is needed. Intermittent injections or continuous infusions via the intravenous or subcutaneous routes are often used for opioid delivery and may be administered at home in special pain situations, such as in hospice care and/or in chronic cancer pain management. Subcutaneous infusions are often used when there is no intravenous access. Patient-controlled analgesia (PCA) pumps may be used to help deliver opioids intravenously, subcutaneously, or even intraspinally and can be managed in home health care or hospice care for the patient at home. Use of the intrathecal or epidural route requires special skill and expertise, and delivery of pain medications using these routes is available only from certain home health care agencies for at-home care. The main reason for long-term intraspinal opioid administration is intractable pain. Transnasal dosage forms are approved only for butorphanol, an agonist-antagonist drug, and this dosage form is generally not used or recommended. Regardless of the specific drug or dosage form used, a fast-acting rescue drug should always be ordered for the patient with cancer pain and patients presenting other special challenges in pain management.

In summary, regardless of the drug(s) used for the pain management regimen, the nurse must always remember that individualization of treatment is one of the most important considerations for effective and quality pain control. The nurse should always do the following:

- At the initiation of pain therapy, conduct a review of all relevant histories, laboratory test values, and diagnostic study results in the patient's medical record.
- If there are underlying problems, be sure to consider them but do not forget to treat the patient. Do not let these problems overshadow the fact that there is a patient who is in pain.
- Always develop goals for pain management in conjunction with the patient and any family members or significant others.
- Collaborate with other members of the health care team to select a regimen that will be easy for the patient to follow while in the hospital and, if necessary, at home (e.g., with cancer patients and other patients with chronic pain).
- Be aware that most regimens for acute pain include management with short-acting opioids plus the addition of other medications such as NSAIDs.
- Be familiar with equianalgesic doses of opioids, because lack of knowledge may lead to inadequate analgesia or overdose.
- Use an analgesic appropriate for the situation (e.g., short-acting opioids for severe pain secondary to a myocardial infarction, surgery, or kidney stones). For cancer pain, the regimen usually begins with short-acting opioids with eventual conversion to sustained-release formulations. Preventative measures should be used to manage adverse effects. In addition, a switch is made to

Table 10-11 Drugs *Not* Recommended for Treatment of Cancer Pain

Class	Drug	Rationale for not Recommending
Opioids with dosing around the clock	meperidine	Short (2-3 hr) duration of analgesia; administration may lead to CNS toxicity (tremor, confusion, or seizures)
Miscellaneous	Cannabinoids	Adverse effects of dysphoria, drowsiness, hypotension, and bradycardia, which preclude its routine use as an analgesic; may be more appropriate for use in treating severe chemotherapy-induced nausea and vomiting
Opioid agonists-antagonists	pentazocine butorphanol nalbuphine	May precipitate withdrawal in opioid-dependent patients; analgesic ceiling effect; possible production of unpleasant psychologic adverse effects, including dysphoria, delusions, and hallucinations
Partial agonist	buprenorphine	Analgesic ceiling effect; can precipitate withdrawal if given with a narcotic
Antagonists	naloxone naltrexone	Reverses analgesia
Combination preparations	Brompton's cocktails	No evidence of analgesic benefit over use of single opioid analgesic
	DPT* (meperidine, promethazine, and chlorpromazine)	Efficacy poor compared with that of other analgesics; associated with a higher incidence of adverse effects
Anxiolytics (as monotherapy) or sedatives-hypnotics (as monotherapy)	Benzodiazepines (e.g., alprazolam)	Analgesic properties not associated with these drugs except in some situations of neuropathic pain; common risk of sedation, which may put some patients at higher risk for neurologic complications
	Barbiturates Benzodiazepines	Analgesic properties not demonstrated; sedation is problematic and limits use

*DPT is the abbreviation for the trade names Demerol, Phenergan, and Thorazine.

Pain Management in Terminal Illness

You are assigned to care for a patient who is in the terminal phases of breast cancer. As a home health care nurse, you have many responsibilities; however, you have not cared for many patients who are in the terminal phase of their illness. In fact, most of your patients are postoperative and have only required assessments, dressing changes, and wound care.

Ms. D. is 48 years of age and underwent bilateral mastectomy 4 years ago. She had lymph node involvement at the time of surgery, and recently metastasis to the bone has been diagnosed. She has been taking oxycodone (one 5-mg tab every 6 hours) at home but is not sleeping through the night and is now complaining of increasing pain to the point that her quality of life has decreased significantly. She wants to stay at home during the terminal phases of her illness but needs to have adequate and safe pain control. Her husband of 18 years is very supportive. They have no children. They are both college graduates and have medical insurance.

- Ms. D.'s recent increase in pain has been attributed to bone metastasis in the area of the lumbar spine. At this time the oxycodone is not beneficial, and you as the home health care nurse need to advocate for Ms. D. to receive adequate pain relief. When discussing her pain medications with her physician, what type of medication would you expect to be ordered to relieve the bone pain, and what is the rationale for this medication? (Provide references from within this chapter for the selection of the specific opioid drug.)
- Ms. D.'s husband confides in you that he is worried that she will become addicted to the new medication. He is not sure he agrees with around-the-clock dosing. How do you address his concerns?
- What should Mr. D. do if he feels that Ms. D. has had an overdose?

For answers, see http://evolve.elsevier.com/Lilley.

another opioid as soon as possible if the patient finds that the medication is not controlling the pain adequately.
- Consider the option of using adjuvants to analgesia, especially in cases of chronic pain or cancer pain; these might include other prescribed drugs such as corticosteroids, antidepressants, anticonvulsants, and muscle relaxants. OTCs, herbals, and NSAIDs are also helpful.
- Be alert to patients with special needs, such as patients with breakthrough pain. Generally, the drug used is one that is a short-acting form of the longer acting opioid (e.g., immediate release for breakthrough pain while also using sustained-release morphine).
- Identify community resources for assistance to the patient and any family members or significant others. These resources may include various web-based sites such as www.WebMD.com, www.pain.com, and www.mayohealth.org. Many other pain management sites may be found on the Internet by searching using the term *pain* or *pain clinic*.
- Because patient falls and the resulting injuries are the most common cause of litigation against nurses, when analgesics of any type—but especially opioids—are used, be sure to assess the patient's potential for falls. Make sure to take great care to prevent falls, whether by simply checking on the patient frequently after he or she has received analgesics, placing the patient on a frequent watch program, using bed alarms, or obtaining an order for restraints (but only in *extreme* circumstances).
- Restraints may cause many injuries; therefore, follow the appropriate procedures. Assess, monitor, evaluate, and document the reason for the restraint; also document the patient's behavior, type of restraint, and the assessment of the patient after the placement of restraints. Use of restraints has been replaced in most facilities by a bed watch system and the use of bed and/or wheelchair alarms as well as by instruction of the patient and family members regarding alternatives to restraints. Restraints are not used in long-term care facilities.

◆ EVALUATION

Positive therapeutic outcomes of acetaminophen use are decreased symptoms, fever, and pain. Adverse reactions for which the nurse should monitor include anemias and the previously mentioned liver problems with hepatotoxicity. In addition, abdominal pain and vomiting should be reported to the physician. During and after the administration of nonnarcotic analgesics, tramadol, opioids, and mixed narcotic agonists, the nurse should monitor the patient for both therapeutic effects and adverse effects. Therapeutic effects include decreased complaints of pain and increased periods of comfort, with improvements in performance of ADLs, appetite, and sense of well-being. Adverse effects vary with each drug (see discussion earlier in this chapter) but often consist of nausea, vomiting, constipation, dizziness, headache, blurred vision, decreased urinary output, drowsiness, lethargy, sedation, palpitations, bradycardia, bradypnea, dyspnea, and hypotension. Should vital signs change, the patient's condition decline, or pain continue, the physician should be contacted immediately and the patient closely monitored. Respiratory depression may be manifested by a rate of less than 12 breaths/min, dyspnea, diminished breath sounds, and/or shallow breathing.

Although many patients benefit from the administration of prescribed opioids alone, additional medications and complementary therapies may be needed to enhance comfort. During the evaluation process, the nurse should evaluate multimodal approaches to pain management such as relaxation, imagery, art therapy, pet therapy, massage, acupuncture, and music therapy. The nurse should evaluate the effectiveness of pain management by determining the degree, duration, and nature of pain experienced with drug therapy and by evaluating and reassessing for any new or different complaints of pain.

Patient Teaching Tips

- The nurse should emphasize to the patient that opioids should not be used with alcohol and/or other CNS depressants because of worsening of CNS depressant effects.
- A holistic approach to pain management may be appropriate, with the use of complementary modalities. Some complementary and alternative therapies include biofeedback, imagery, relaxation, deep breathing, humor, pet therapy, music therapy, massage, use of hot or cold compresses, and use of herbal products.
- The patient should report any dizziness, difficulty breathing, low blood pressure, excessive sleepiness (sedation), confusion, or loss of memory to their health care providers. Forcing fluids up to 3 L/day, unless contraindicated, and increasing fiber and bulk consumption and exercise as tolerated is recommended to prevent problems with constipation.
- The patient should report any nausea or vomiting, because these are adverse effects of opioids that may be prevented with the appropriate dosing of medications with food or use of antiemetics.
- The patient should avoid activities requiring mental clarity or alertness while he or she experiences any drowsiness or sedation.
- History of addiction is important to share with health care providers, but when such a patient experiences pain and is in need of opioid analgesia, the nurse must understand that the patient has a right to comfort. Any further issues with addiction may be managed during and after use of opioids. Keeping an open mind regarding the use of resources, counseling, and other treatment options is important in dealing with addictive behaviors.
- While the patient is taking an opioid drug, the patient should ambulate and perform ADLs with caution.

- The patient must understand that if pain is problematic and is not managed by monotherapy, then a combination of a variety of medications may be needed. It is not uncommon to see use of opioids, nonopioids, antianxiety drugs, sedatives or hypnotics, and NSAIDs. Most importantly, however, the patient must remain in communication with the physician or health care provider about alternative and combination drug therapy options.
- For the cancer patient, the health care provider will monitor pain control and the need for other options for therapy or dosing of drugs. For example, the use of transdermal patches, buccal tablets, and continuous infusions while the patient remains mobile or at home is often helpful in pain management. It is also important to understand that if morphine or morphine-like drugs are being used, the addictive potential is there; however, in specific situations, the concern for quality of life and pain management is more important than the concern for addiction.
- Should bone pain become moderate to severe with cancer patients, the physician may order NSAIDs or other antiinflammatory drugs.
- Most hospitals have inpatient and outpatient resources such as pain clinics. The patient should seek out these options and remain active in his or her care for as long as possible.
- Tolerance does occur with opioid use, so if the level of pain increases while the patient remains on the prescribed dosage, the patient should contact the physician or health care provider for assistance. The patient should never change dosages of or double up on medication of any type.
- Educate patients that narcotic agonists-antagonists work well as analgesics when given by themselves. Use with a pure narcotic agonist would lead to reversal of analgesia. CNS depression is also experienced.

Points to Remember

- Pain is individual and involves senses and emotions that are unpleasant. It is influenced by age, culture, race, spirituality, and all other aspects of the person.
- Pain is associated with actual or potential tissue damage and may be exacerbated or alleviated depending on the treatment and type of pain.
- Types of analgesics include the following:
  - Nonopioids, including acetaminophen and aspirin and other NSAIDs
  - Opioids, which are natural or synthetic drugs that either contain or are derived from morphine (opiates) or have opiate-like effects or activities (opioids); there are pure opioid agonists and partial opioid agonist-antagonist drugs

- Life span considerations are an important aspect in medication administration. A few examples are as follows:
  - Pediatric dosages of morphine should be calculated very cautiously with close attention to the dose and kilograms of body weight.
  - Elderly patients generally tolerate morphine well but seem less tolerant of other opioids such as meperidine.
  - In treating the elderly, the nurse should remember that these patients experience pain the same as does the general population, but they may be reluctant to report pain and metabolize opiates at a slower rate and thus are at increased risk for adverse effects such as sedation and respiratory depression. The best rule is to start with low dosages, reevaluate often, and go slowly during upward titration.

NCLEX Examination Review Questions

1. For best results when treating severe pain associated with patho-logic spinal fractures related to metastatic bone cancer, which type of dosage schedule should be used? Pain medication administered
   a. as needed.
   b. around the clock.
   c. on schedule during waking hours only.
   d. around the clock, with additional doses as needed for break-through pain.
2. A patient is receiving an opioid via a PCA pump as part of his postoperative pain management program. During rounds, the nurse notices that his respirations are 8 breaths/min and he is extremely lethargic. After stopping the opioid infusion, what should the nurse do next?
   a. Notify the charge nurse
   b. Administer oxygen
   c. Administer an opiate antagonist per standing orders
   d. Perform a thorough assessment, including mental status examination
3. Which of the following is a benefit of using transdermal fentanyl patches in the management of bone pain from the spread of cancer?
   a. More analgesia for longer time periods
   b. Less constipation and minimal dry mouth

   c. Greater CNS stimulation than with oral opioids
   d. Lower dependency potential and no major adverse effects
4. The nurse suspects that a patient is showing signs of respiratory depression. Which of the following drugs could be the cause of this complication?
   a. naloxone (Narcan)
   b. hydromorphone (Dilaudid)
   c. acetaminophen (Tylenol)
   d. naltrexone (ReVia)
5. Several patients have standard prn orders for acetaminophen as needed for pain. When the nurse reviews their histories and as-sessments, it is discovered that one of the patients has a contra-indication to acetaminophen therapy. Which patient is the one who should receive an alternate medication?
   a. A patient who has a fever of 39.7° C (103.4° F)
   b. A patient admitted with a deep vein thrombosis
   c. A patient admitted with severe hepatitis
   d. A patient who had abdominal surgery 1 week earlier

1. d, 2. c, 3. a, 4. b, 5. c.

Critical Thinking Activities

1. You administer 5 mg of morphine sulfate IV to a patient with se-vere postoperative pain, as ordered. What assessment data should be gathered before and after administering this drug? Ex-plain your answer.
2. Your patient complains that the drugs he is receiving for severe pain are not really helping. What would be the most appropriate response to this patient?

3. Compare and contrast the effectiveness of the following routes for opioid administration, including their ease of self-preparation and administration, onset of therapeutic serum concentrations, de-gree of sedation produced, adverse effects, and ease of manage-ment in the home setting: oral, intramuscular, transdermal.

For answers, see http://evolve.elsevier.com/Lilley.

General and Local Anesthetics

Objectives

When you reach the end of this chapter, you should be able to do the following:

1. Define anesthesia.
2. Describe the basic differences between general and local anesthesia.
3. List the most commonly used general and local anesthetics and their associated risks.
4. Discuss the differences between depolarizing neuromuscular blocking drugs and nondepolarizing blocking drugs.
5. Compare the mechanisms of action, indications, adverse effects, routes of administration, cautions, contraindications, and drug interactions of general and local anesthesia and for drugs used for moderate/conscious sedation.
6. Develop a nursing care plan for patients before anesthesia (preanesthesia), during anesthesia, and after anesthesia (postanesthesia) as related to general anesthesia.
7. Develop a nursing care plan for patients undergoing local anesthesia and/or moderate/conscious sedation.

e-Learning Activities

Companion CD

- NCLEX Review Questions: see questions 65-71
- Animations
- Audio Glossary
- Category Catchers
- Medication Errors Checklists
- IV Therapy Checklists

evolve Website (http://evolve.elsevier.com/Lilley)

• Nursing Care Plans • Frequently Asked Questions • Content Updates • WebLinks • Supplemental Resources • Elsevier ePharmacology Update • Medication Administration Animations

Drug Profiles

enflurane, p. 165
halothane, p. 166
isoflurane, p. 166
▶ lidocaine, p. 170
methoxyflurane, p. 166
nitrous oxide, p. 166

pancuronium, p. 172
▶ propofol, p. 166
sevoflurane, p. 167
▶ succinylcholine, p. 172
▶ vecuronium, p. 173

▶ Key drug.

Glossary

Adjunctive anesthetic drugs Drugs used in combination with anesthetic drugs to control the adverse effects of anesthetics or to help maintain the anesthetic state in the patient. (See *balanced anesthesia*.) (p. 163)

Anesthesia Loss of the ability to feel pain, resulting from the administration of an anesthetic drug or other medical intervention. (p. 163)

Anesthetics Drugs that depress the central nervous system (CNS) to produce diminution of consciousness, loss of responsiveness to sensory stimulation, or muscle relaxation. (p. 163)

Balanced anesthesia The practice of using combinations of drugs rather than a single drug to produce anesthesia. A common combination is a mixture of a sedative-hypnotic, an antianxiety drug, an analgesic, an antiemetic, and an anticholinergic. (p. 163)

General anesthesia A drug-induced state in which the CNS is altered to produce varying degrees of pain relief throughout the body as well as depression of consciousness, skeletal muscle relaxation, and diminished or absent reflexes. It is most commonly induced for performance of surgical procedures. (p. 163)

General anesthetic A drug that induces a state of anesthesia. Its effects are global in that they involve the whole body, with loss of consciousness being one of those effects. (p. 163)

Local anesthetics Drugs that render a specific portion of the body insensitive to pain at the level of the peripheral nervous system, normally without affecting consciousness. Also called *regional anesthetics*. (p. 167)

Malignant hyperthermia A genetically-linked major adverse reaction to general anesthesia, characterized by a rapid rise in body temperature, as well as tachycardia, tachypnea, and sweating. (p. 171)

Moderate sedation A form of anesthesia induced by combinations of parenteral benzodiazepines and an opiate. It reduces anxiety, sensitivity to pain, and recall of the procedure (also called *conscious sedation*). (p. 173)

Overton-Meyer theory A theory that describes the relationship between the lipid solubility of anesthetic drugs and their potency. It is often used to explain how anesthetic drugs are believed to work. (p. 164)

Parenteral anesthetics   Any anesthetic drugs that can be administered by injection via any route (e.g., intravenously, spinally/epidurally, as a local nerve block). Depending on the specific site of injection, the drug may anesthetize all or parts of the central or peripheral nervous system or both. (p. 167)

Topical anesthetics   A class of local anesthetics that are applied directly to the skin and mucous membranes. They consist of solutions, ointments, gels, creams, powders, ophthalmic drops, and suppositories. (p. 167)

Anesthetics are drugs that depress the central nervous system (CNS) and/or the peripheral nervous system (PNS), which in turn produces depression of consciousness, loss of responsiveness to sensory stimulation (including pain), or muscle relaxation. This state of depressed CNS or PNS activity is called **anesthesia.** There are many mechanisms by which anesthetics accomplish these responses, but in general they do so by interfering with nerve conduction. They can produce any or all of the actions just mentioned, depending on the drug. Anesthetics are most commonly classified as either general anesthetics or local anesthetics, depending on where in the CNS or PNS the particular anesthetic drug works. Functions of the autonomic nervous system, which is a branch of the PNS, may also be effected.

GENERAL ANESTHETICS

A **general anesthetic** is a drug that induces a state in which the CNS is altered so that varying degrees of pain relief, depression of consciousness, skeletal muscle relaxation, and reflex reduction are produced. This condition is known as **general anesthesia.** General anesthesia can be achieved by the use of one drug or a combination of drugs. Often a combination of drugs is used to produce general anesthesia, which allows less of each drug to be used and a more balanced, controlled state of anesthesia to be achieved. General anesthetic drugs are used most commonly to produce deep muscle relaxation and loss of consciousness during surgical procedures. For a historical perspective on general anesthesia, see Box 11-1.

There are two main categories of general anesthetics based on route of administration: inhaled and injectable. Inhaled anesthetics are volatile liquids or gases that are vaporized in oxygen and inhaled to induce anesthesia. Injectable anesthetics are administered intravenously. The different inhaled gases and volatile liquids used as general anesthetics are listed in Table 11-1.

Intravenously administered anesthetic drugs are used for induction or maintenance of general anesthesia, induction of amnesia, and as an adjunct to inhalation-type anesthetics. Common intravenous anesthetic drugs include the following:
- General anesthetics, such as etomidate and propofol
- Sedatives-hypnotics, such as barbiturates (e.g., thiopental, methohexital) and benzodiazepines (e.g., diazepam, midazolam)
- Narcotics (e.g., morphine sulfate, fentanyl, sufentanil, propofol)
- Neuromuscular blocking agents (NMBAs), both depolarizing (e.g., succinylcholine) and nondepolarizing, or competitive (e.g., pancuronium, d-tubocurarine, vecuronium).

The term for the practice of using such combinations of drugs is **balanced anesthesia,** which is the administration of minimal doses of multiple anesthetic drugs to achieve the desired level of

Box 11-1   General Anesthesia: A Historical Perspective

Until recently, general anesthesia was described as having several definitive stages. This was especially true with the use of many of the ether-based inhaled anesthetic drugs. Features of these distinctive stages were easily observable to the trained eye. They included specific physical and physiologic changes that progressed gradually and predictably with the depth of the patient's anesthetized state. Gradual changes in pupil size, progression from thoracic to diaphragmatic breathing, vital sign changes, and several other changes all characterized the various stages. Newer inhalational and intravenous general anesthetic drugs, however, often have a much more rapid onset of action and body distribution. As a result, the specific stages of anesthesia once observed with older drugs are no longer sufficiently well defined to be observable. Thus, the concept of stages of anesthesia is an outdated one in most modern surgical facilities. Registered nurses who pursue advanced training to become a certified registered nurse anesthetist often find this to be a rewarding and interesting area of nursing practice. Some nurses also find that this type of work offers greater flexibility in their work schedule than do other practice areas.

Table 11-1   Inhaled General Anesthetics

Generic Name	Trade Name
Inhaled Gas	
nitrous oxide ("laughing gas")	
Inhaled Volatile Liquid	
desflurane	Suprane
enflurane	Ethrane
halothane	Fluothane
isoflurane	Forane
methoxyflurane	Penthrane
sevoflurane	Ultane

anesthesia for the given surgical procedure. Other than the inhaled drugs, almost all of the drugs used in balanced anesthesia are administered intravenously. Although propofol is an example of a true general anesthetic in the sense that it is used not only to induce but also to maintain the state of anesthesia, most of the other drugs previously mentioned serve a more limited function, such as anesthesia induction, sedation, amnesia, and reduction of anxiety. These drugs are commonly called **adjunctive anesthetic drugs** because they are administered in addition to a general anesthetic drug. Common adverse effects include dry mouth, bradycardia, nausea, and vomiting. The combining of several different drugs makes it possible for general anesthesia to be accomplished using smaller amounts of anesthetic gases, which reduces the adverse effects. The general anesthetics and their usual dosages are presented in Table 11-2. Table 11-3 lists the adjunctive anesthetic drugs. These drugs are discussed in greater detail in the chapters covering the respective classes of drugs.

Mechanism of Action and Drug Effects

Many theories have been proposed to explain the actual mechanism of action of general anesthetics. The drugs vary widely in their chemical structures, however, and therefore their mechanism of action is not easily explained by a structure-receptor relationship. The concentrations of various anesthetics required to produce a given state of anesthesia also differ greatly. The **Overton-Meyer theory** explains some of the properties of anesthetic drugs that may make the mechanism of action of these drugs easier to understand. This theory states that there is a relationship between the lipid solubility of an anesthetic drug and its potency: the greater the solubility of the drug in fat, the greater the effect. Nerve cell membranes have a high lipid content, as does the blood-brain barrier. Lipid-soluble anesthetic drugs can therefore easily cross the blood-brain barrier and concentrate in nerve cell membranes. Initially this produces a loss of the senses of sight, touch, taste, smell, and hearing and a loss of awareness, and usually the patient becomes unconscious. Although the heart and lungs (the vital centers responsible for blood pressure and breathing) are controlled by the medulla, they usually can be spared because the medullary center is depressed last during anesthetic procedures.

The overall effect of general anesthetics is an orderly and systematic reduction of sensory and motor CNS functions. They produce a progressive depression of cerebral and spinal cord functions. Therapeutic (anesthetic) doses cause minimal depression of the medullary centers that govern vital functions. However, an anesthetic overdose paralyzes the medullary centers.

This can lead to death from circulatory and respiratory failure. The progressive paralysis of nervous system functions produced by general anesthetics and the level of decreased CNS functioning depends on the anesthetic used and the dosage and route of administration. The reactions of the CNS (and other systems) to these general anesthetics are presented in Table 11-4. The previously distinct and identifiable stages of anesthesia now exist more on a continuum with the newer generation of anesthetics discussed in this chapter. This is especially the case with the now standardized use of balanced anesthesia and moderate sedation. Therefore, rather than structuring patient assessment in terms of the older concept of "stages of anesthesia," the nurse should

Table 11-2   General Anesthetic Drugs

Drug		
Generic Name	**Trade Name**	**Dosage**
etomidate	Amidate	0.2-0.6 mg/kg IV
ketamine	Ketalar	1-4.5 mg/kg IV; 3-8 mg/kg IM
methohexital	Brevital	50-120 mg IV (induction); 20-40 mg IV (maintenance)
propofol*	Diprivan	1-2.5 mg/kg IV (induction); 50-200 mcg/kg/min IV (maintenance)
thiamylal	Surital	Titrate to response IV
thiopental	Pentothal	25-250 mg IV as needed

IV, Intravenous; *IM*, intramuscular.
*Dosages for propofol are typically 5-50 mg/kg/min for initiation and maintenance of sedation in the intensive care unit.

Life Span Considerations: The Elderly Patient
Anesthesia

- The elderly patient is affected more adversely by anesthesia than the young or middle-aged adult patient. With aging comes organ system deterioration. A decline in the function of the liver results in decreased metabolism of drugs. A decline in renal functioning leads to decreased drug excretion so that unsafe levels of the drug may be reached. If either of these organ systems are not functioning properly, drug toxicity may occur due to inadequate drug metabolism and excretion. Because of this decline in organ functioning, the elderly patient becomes more sensitive to the effects of anesthetics. In addition, the central nervous system is more sensitive to the effects of anesthetics and other drugs.
- The elderly patient's cardiac and respiratory systems are also affected by aging. These age-related changes make the elderly patient more susceptible to problems such as respiratory depression, atelectasis, pneumonia, and cardiac abnormalities.
- With the older individual, it is important to assess for the presence of any diseases of the cardiac, renal, hepatic, or respiratory systems, because these would put the patient at higher risk for complications related to the anesthesia and adjunct drugs.
- Another concern regarding anesthesia in the elderly patient is the practice of polypharmacy. Generally speaking, because of the presence of various age-related diseases, the older patient is generally taking more than one or two drugs. The more drugs a patient is taking, the higher the risk of adverse reactions and drug-drug interactions, including with anesthesia.

Table 11-3   Adjunctive Anesthetic Drugs

Drug	Pharmacologic Class	Usual Dosage Range	Indications
alfentanil (Alfenta)	Opioid analgesic	130-245 mcg/kg IV	Anesthesia induction
fentanyl (Sublimaze)		50-100 mcg/kg IV	
sufentanil (Sufenta)		8-30 mcg/kg IV	
diazepam (Valium)	Benzodiazepine	2-20 mg PO/IV/IM	Amnesia and anxiety reduction
midazolam (Versed)		0.05-0.35 mg/kg IV	
atropine	Anticholinergic	0.1-0.6 mg IV/IMSC	Drying up of excessive secretions
glycopyrrolate (Robinul)		0.0044 mg/kg IM	
scopolamine		0.3-0.6 mg SC/IM	
meperidine (Demerol)	Opioid analgesic	50-100 mg IM/SC	Pain prevention and pain relief
morphine		5-20 mg IM/SC	
hydroxyzine (Atarax, Vistaril)	Sedative-hypnotic	25-100 mg IM	Amnesia and sedation
pentobarbital (Nembutal)		150-200 mg IM	
promethazine (Phenergan)		25-50 mg IM	
secobarbital (Seconal)		100 mg PO	

IM, Intramuscularly; *IV*, intravenously; *PO*, orally; *SC*, subcutaneously.

focus on understanding each of the drug types used, including their characteristics, actions, adverse effects, and toxicities.

Indications

General anesthetics are used to produce unconsciousness, skeletal muscular relaxation, and visceral smooth muscle relaxation for surgical procedures.

Contraindications

Contraindications to the use of anesthetic drugs include known drug allergy and, depending on the drug type, may include pregnancy, narrow-angle glaucoma, and known susceptibility to malignant hyperthermia from prior experience with anesthetics.

Adverse Effects

The adverse effects of general anesthetics are dose dependent and vary with the individual drug. The heart, peripheral circulation, liver, kidneys, and respiratory tract are the sites primarily affected. Myocardial depression is a common adverse effect. All of the halogenated anesthetics are capable of causing hepatotoxicity, and methoxyflurane can cause significant respiratory depression.

With the development and use of newer drugs, many of the unwanted adverse effects characteristic of the older drugs (such as hepatotoxicity and myocardial depression) are now a thing of the past. In addition, many of the bothersome adverse effects such as nausea, vomiting, and confusion have become less common since balanced anesthesia has become more widely used. This practice prevents many of the unwanted dose-dependent adverse effects and toxicity associated with the anesthetic drugs while simultaneously achieving a more balanced general anesthesia. One medication with a long history of use for prevention or control of postoperative nausea and vomiting is droperidol. The common dosage range is 0.625 to 1.25 mg intravenously or intramuscularly every 4 to 6 hours as needed. It should also be noted that substance abuse (e.g., alcohol) can predispose a patient to anesthetic-induced complications (e.g., liver toxicity). A positive determination of substance abuse during the anesthetist's history-taking interview may lead to dosage adjustments in one or more of the drugs used. The anesthetist may reduce drug dosages in cases of known liver or kidney damage, whether or not a consequence of substance abuse. However, a drug abusing patient with a high tolerance for street drugs, may also require larger doses of anesthesia-related drugs (e.g., benzodiazepines) to achieve the desired sedative effects. Again, the anesthetist makes these decisions based on her/his best knowledge of each patient's social history.

Toxicity and Management of Overdose

In large doses all anesthetics are potentially life threatening, with cardiac and respiratory arrest as the ultimate causes of death. However, these drugs are almost exclusively administered in a very controlled environment by personnel trained in advanced cardiac life support. These drugs are also very quickly metabolized. In addition, as noted earlier the medullary center, which governs the vital centers, is the last area of the brain to be affected by anesthetics and the first to regain function if it is lost. These factors combined make an anesthetic overdose rare and easily reversible. Symptomatic and supportive therapy, primarily of circulatory and respiratory functions, is usually all that is needed in the event of an anesthetic overdose.

Interactions

Because general anesthetics produce both desired and adverse effects on so many body systems, they are associated with a wide array of drug interactions that also vary widely in severity. Some of the more common drug-drug interactions occur with antihypertensives, β-blockers, and tetracycline. These drugs have additive effects when combined with general anesthetics. When given with antihypertensives, general anesthetics may lead to increased hypotensive effects; with β-blockers, to increased myocardial depression; and with tetracycline, to increased renal toxicity. No significant laboratory test interactions have been reported.

Dosages

For the recommended dosages of selected general anesthetic drugs, see the Dosages table on page 166.

Drug Profiles

All of the drugs used for general anesthesia are, of course, prescription-only drugs. Desflurane, enflurane, sevoflurane, halothane, isoflurane, and methoxyflurane are all volatile liquids; nitrous oxide is a gas. The dose of each drug depends on the surgical procedure to be performed and the physical characteristics of the patient. All of the general anesthetics have a rapid onset of action, and action is maintained for the duration of the surgical procedure by continuous administration of the drug. Propofol is chemically unrelated to the other intravenous anesthetic drugs. Its favorable pharmacokinetics and the quick onset of anesthesia and quick recovery associated with it have popularized its use since its approval by the Food and Drug Administration in 1989.

enflurane

Enflurane (Ethrane) is a fluorinated ether that produces good muscular relaxation and minimal cardiac sensitivity to catecholamines. The drug can produce seizures in patients who develop hypocapnia (low

---

Table 11-4   Effects of Inhaled and Intravenous General Anesthetics

Organ/System	Reaction
Respiratory	Depressed muscles and patterns of respiration; altered gas exchange and impaired oxygenation; depressed airway-protective mechanisms; airway irritation and possible laryngospasms
Cardiovascular	Depressed myocardium; hypotension and tachycardia; bradycardia in response to vagal stimulation
Cerebrovascular	Increased intracranial blood volume and increased intracranial pressure
Gastrointestinal	Reduced hepatic blood flow and thus reduced hepatic clearance
Renal	Decreased glomerular filtration
Skeletal muscles	Skeletal muscle relaxation
Cutaneous circulation	Vasodilation
Central nervous system (CNS)	CNS depression; blurred vision; nystagmus; progression of CNS depression to decreased alertness and sensorium as well as decreased level of consciousness

DOSAGES

Selected General Anesthetic Drugs

Drug	Pharmacologic Class	Usual Dosage Range	Indications
enflurane (Ethrane)	Inhalation general anesthetic (halogenated ether)	0.5%-3% concentration	General anesthesia
halothane (Fluothane)	Inhalation general anesthetic (halogenated hydrocarbon)	0.5%-1.5% concentration	General anesthesia
isoflurane (Forane)	Inhalation general anesthetic (enflurane isomer)	0.1%-2% concentration with appropriate drugs	General anesthesia
methoxyflurane (Penthrane)	Inhalation general anesthetic (halogenated ether)	0.1%-2% concentration with appropriate drugs	General anesthesia
nitrous oxide ("laughing gas")	Inorganic inhalation general anesthetic	20%-40% with oxygen (e.g., 70% with 30% oxygen)	Analgesia Anesthesia

Life Span Considerations: The Pediatric Patient

Anesthesia

- Premature infants, neonates, and pediatric patients are more adversely affected by anesthesia than is the young or middle-aged adult patient. The reason for this difference in response is the increased sensitivity of the pediatric patient to anesthetics and related drugs. Immature functioning of the liver and kidneys leads to possible drug accumulation and toxicity and subsequent complications. The central nervous system of pediatric patients is more sensitive to the effects of anesthetics. Because of the risk of toxicity and complications with all forms of anesthesia, the nurse must take all precautions to ensure that the patient remains safe and free from harm.
- The pediatric patient's cardiac and respiratory systems are not fully developed or not yet fully functional, which makes those in this age group more susceptible to problems such as central nervous system depression accompanied by respiratory and cardiac depression, which can result in atelectasis, pneumonia, and cardiac abnormalities.
- Documentation of a thorough head-to-toe assessment with additional focus on the patient profile (such as results of various laboratory studies, chest radiography, and other tests of organ function) is key to preventing complications and also to identifying patients potentially at risk. Thorough assessment for the presence of any diseases of the cardiac, renal, hepatic, respiratory, and central nervous systems is important in identifying patients at risk and preventing complications during anesthesia.
- Neonates, in particular (see age-group definitions in Chapter 3), are at higher risk of upper airway obstruction during general anesthesia. During the anesthetic process, the risk of laryngospasm, which often occurs with intubation in patients of any age, may be increased for neonates because of the specific physical characteristics of the larynx and respiratory structures. Their higher metabolic rate and small airway diameter also put neonates at greater risk of experiencing complications during general anesthesia.
- All drugs used in preanesthesia and postanesthesia phases require careful checks of mathematical drug calculations. The patient's weight, body surface area, and laboratory test results that indicate organ function or dysfunction should always be taken into consideration.
- Resuscitative equipment should be readily available on any neonatal or pediatric nursing unit for postanesthesia care.

blood carbon dioxide levels) during anesthesia and therefore should not be used in patients with convulsive disorders. Dosage information is given in the table on this page.

halothane

Halothane (Fluothane) is a halogenated hydrocarbon (containing three atoms of fluorine and one each of chlorine and bromine) that is commonly used with nitrous oxide. It was a mainstay of general anesthesia for many years and is still on the U.S. market. However, it causes considerable cardiac sensitivity to catecholamines and produces poor muscular relaxation when used alone, and its high halogen content can result in significant liver toxicity. Because of these limitations and toxicities, halothane is now less commonly used than the newer, less toxic inhalational anesthetics. Dosage information is given in the table on this page.

isoflurane

Isoflurane (Forane) is very similar to enflurane in its chemical structure. However, the differences in its structure give it some favorable characteristics that distinguish it from its chemical relative. Isoflurane has a more rapid onset of action, causes less cardiovascular depression, and overall has been associated with little or no toxicity. Dosage information is given in the table on this page.

methoxyflurane

Methoxyflurane (Penthrane) is a fluorinated and chlorinated ether that produces excellent muscular relaxation without causing any significant cardiac sensitivity to catecholamines. However, the biotransformation of this drug produces free halogen ions that can cause significant liver toxicity, and its use is therefore contraindicated in patients with liver disease. In addition, methoxyflurane produces respiratory depression, which limits its use to patients undergoing short operations. Dosage information is given in the table on this page.

nitrous oxide

Nitrous oxide, also known as "laughing gas," is the only inhaled gas currently used as a general anesthetic. It is the weakest of the general anesthetic drugs and is primarily used for dental procedures or as a useful supplement to other, more potent anesthetics. Dosage information is given in the table on this page.

▶ propofol

Propofol (Diprivan) is an intravenous general anesthetic drug used for the induction and maintenance of anesthesia or sedation in the intensive care unit (ICU) and other critical care settings. Propofol has many favorable characteristics that have led to its widespread use. It produces its effects very rapidly, and when its delivery is halted, its effects subside very quickly. Propofol also is typically well tolerated, producing few undesirable effects. Propofol can be used to induce and maintain monitored-anesthesia-care sedation during diagnostic procedures in adults. It is also used in intubated, mechanically ventilated adult patients in the ICU to provide continuous sedation and control of stress responses. When used in the ICU, typical dosages are 5 to 50 mcg/kg/min. At higher dosages it can be used for induction and maintenance of general anesthesia. Dosage information is provided in Table 11-2 on page 164.

sevoflurane
Sevoflurane (Ultane) is another fluorinated ether that is now more widely used in the United States after several years of successful use in Japan. Its rapid onset and recovery pharmacokinetics make it especially useful in outpatient surgery settings. It is also nonirritating to the airway, which greatly facilitates induction of an unconscious state, especially in pediatric patients.

LOCAL ANESTHETICS

Local anesthetics are the second class of anesthetics. They are also called *regional anesthetics* because they render a specific portion of the body insensitive to pain without major reduction of CNS function and level of consciousness. They do this by interfering with nerve transmission in specific areas of the body, blocking nerve conduction only in the area in which they are applied without causing loss of consciousness. They are most commonly used in those clinical settings in which loss of consciousness, whole body muscle relaxation, and loss of responsiveness are either undesirable or unnecessary (e.g., during childbirth).

Other uses for local anesthetics include dental procedures, the suturing of skin lacerations, spinal anesthesia, and diagnostic procedures such as lumbar puncture or thoracentesis.

Most local anesthetics belong to one of two major groups of organic compounds, esters and amides, and are classified as either topical or parenteral (injectable) anesthetics. **Topical anesthetics** are applied directly to the skin and mucous membranes. They are available in the form of solutions, ointments, gels, creams, or powders, and their dosage strengths are listed in Table 11-5. **Parenteral anesthetics** can be administered intravenously or by various spinal injection techniques. The injection of certain anesthetic drugs into the area near the spinal cord is known as *spinal anesthesia*. This type of anesthesia is generally used to block all peripheral nerves that branch out below a selected level of the spinal cord. The result is temporary skeletal and smooth muscle paralysis and anesthesia within the anatomical areas of the body that are ultimately innervated by these nerve tracts lying between this selected spinal cord location and the affected organs and tissues. Because spinal anesthesia does not normally depress the CNS in a way that causes loss of consciousness, spinal anesthesia can be thought of as a large-scale type of *local* rather than general anesthesia. Some of the common types of local anesthesia are described in Box 11-2. The par-

---

Table 11-5   Topical Anesthetics

Drug	Route	Dose Strength
benzocaine (Dermoplast, Lanacane, Solarcaine)	Topical, aerosol, and spray	0.5%-20% ointment or cream
butamben (Butesin)	Topical	1% ointment
cocaine	Topical	4%-10% solution, jelly
dibucaine (Nupercainal)	Injection and topical	0.5%-1% solution, ointment, or cream
dibucaine	Topical	1% ointment
dyclonine (Dyclone, Sucrets)	Topical	0.5%-1% solution
ethyl chloride (Chloroethane)	Topical	Spray
Lidocaine (Lidoderm)	Topical	5% patch
proparacaine (Alcaine, Ophthetic)	Ophthalmic	0.5% solution
pramoxine (Tronolane)	Topical	1% jelly, cream, or lotion
prilocaine/lidocaine (EMLA)	Topical	2.5% prilocaine and 2.5% lidocaine cream
tetracaine (Pontocaine)	Injection, topical, and ophthalmic	0.5%-2% solution, ointment, or cream

EMLA, Eutectic mixture of local anesthetics.

Box 11-2   Types of Local Anesthesia

Central

Spinal or intraspinal anesthesia: Anesthetic drugs are injected into the area near the spinal cord within the vertebral column. Intraspinal anesthesia is commonly accomplished by one of two injection techniques: intrathecal and epidural.

- **Intrathecal** anesthesia involves injection of anesthetic into the subarachnoid space. Intrathecal anesthesia is commonly used for patients undergoing major abdominal or limb surgery for whom the risks of general anesthesia are too high or patients who prefer this technique instead of complete loss of consciousness during their surgical procedure. More recently, intrathecal injection of anesthetics through implantable drug pumps is even being used on an outpatient basis in patients with severe chronic pain syndromes, such as those resulting from occupational injuries.
- **Epidural** anesthesia involves injection of anesthetic via a small catheter into the epidural space without puncturing the dura. Epidural anesthesia is commonly used to reduce maternal discomfort during labor and delivery and to manage postoperative acute pain management after major abdominal or pelvic

surgery. This route is becoming more popular for the administration of opioids for pain management.

Peripheral

Infiltration: Small amounts of anesthetic solution are injected into the tissue that surrounds the operative site. This approach to anesthesia is commonly used for such procedures as wound suturing and dental surgery. Often drugs that cause constriction of local blood vessels (e.g., epinephrine, cocaine) are also administered to limit the site of action to the local area.

Nerve block: Anesthetic solution is injected at the site where a nerve innervates a specific area such as a tissue. This allows large amounts of anesthetic drug to be delivered to a very specific area without affecting the whole body. This method is often reserved for more difficult-to-treat pain syndromes such as cancer pain and chronic orthopedic pain.

Topical anesthesia: The anesthetic drug is applied directly onto the surface of the skin, eye, or any other mucous membrane to relieve pain or prevent it from being sensed. It is commonly used for diagnostic eye examinations and skin suturing.

enteral anesthetic drugs and their pharmacokinetics are summarized in Table 11-6.

Intraspinal anesthesia is accomplished by the insertion of a needle into the subarachnoid space to achieve intrathecal dose administration. The subarachnoid space surrounds the spinal cord and is filled with cerebrospinal fluid that continually bathes the spinal cord. The dura mater membrane separates the epidural space from the subarachnoid space. The epidural space is filled with a network of nerve extensions. Analgesic and/or anesthetic drugs are injected into the epidural space into the twelfth thoracic vertebral space or through the first lumbar space in the vertebral column. If the needle is aimed at the subarachnoid space, then it is termed *intrathecal* administration. Distinguishing between these terms and understanding the spinal column and spinal nerves is very important for the nurse. If the epidural space is the desired site of administration, then the needle must stop before penetrating the dura; otherwise, it will enter into the subarachnoid space and free-flowing cerebrospinal fluid may be aspirated. Some of the medications that may be used for intraspinal anesthesia and analgesia include morphine, hydromorphone (Dilaudid), fentanyl, and meperidine (Demerol).

Finally, anesthesia of specific areas of the peripheral nervous system is accomplished either by injecting the drugs adjacent to major nerves (to produce anesthesia in a large body area) or by infiltrating the area with multiple small injections (for a more limited area of anesthesia). Like spinal anesthesia described earlier, this type of anesthesia is also a local (rather than a general) type of anesthesia, but unlike spinal anesthesia, it is focused on a much smaller ("local") region of the body (e.g., hand, part of face, teeth, skin wound). For this reason, it is what is usually meant by the term *local anesthesia*. Some of the common types of local anesthesia are described in Box 11-2. Yet another option is the injection or topical application of a local anesthetic (e.g., lidocaine) near the most distal peripheral nerves at a surgical site (e.g., eye, mucous membrane) as needed to further enhance patient comfort.

Mechanism of Action and Drug Effects

Local anesthetics work by rendering a specific portion of the body insensitive to pain by interfering with nerve transmission in that area. Nerve conduction is blocked only in the area in which the anesthetic is applied, and there is no loss of consciousness. Local anesthetics block both the generation and conduction of impulses through all types of nerve fibers (sensory, motor, and autonomic) by blocking the movement of certain ions (sodium, potassium, and calcium) important to this process. They do this by making it more difficult for these ions to move in and out of the nerve fiber. For this reason, some of these drugs are also described as *membrane-stabilizing* because they alter the cell mem-

brane of the nerve so that the free movement of ions is inhibited. The membrane-stabilizing effects occur first in the small fibers, then in the large fibers. In terms of paralysis, usually autonomic activity is affected first, then pain and other sensory functions are lost. Motor activity is the last to be lost. When the effects of the local anesthetic wear off, recovery occurs in reverse order: motor activity returns first, then sensory functions, and finally autonomic activity.

Possible systemic effects of the administration of local anesthetics include effects on circulatory and respiratory function. The systemic adverse effects depend on where and how the drug is administered (e.g., injection at a certain level in the spinal cord or topical application of a drug that gains access to the circulation). Such adverse effects are somewhat unlikely unless large quantities of a drug are injected, which increases the likelihood of significant systemic absorption. Local anesthetics produce sympathetic blockade; that is, they block the action of the two neurotransmitters of the sympathetic nervous system, norepinephrine and epinephrine. The cardiac effects of such a sympathetic blockade include a decrease in stroke volume, cardiac output, and peripheral resistance. The respiratory effects include reduced respiratory function and altered breathing patterns, but complete paralysis of respiratory function is unlikely because of the large amount of drug that would have to be absorbed. Some local anesthetics used for either infiltration or nerve block anesthesia are combined with vasoconstrictors such as epinephrine, phenylephrine, and norepinephrine to help confine the local anesthetic to the injected area and prevent systemic absorption.

Indications

Local anesthetics are used for surgical, dental, or diagnostic procedures, as well as for the treatment of various types of chronic pain. They are administered by two techniques: infiltration anesthesia and nerve block anesthesia. Infiltration anesthesia is commonly used for minor surgical and dental procedures. It involves injection of the local anesthetic solution by intradermal, subcutaneous, or submucosal routes and across the path of nerves supplying the area to be anesthetized. The local anesthetic may be administered in a circular pattern around the operative field. Nerve block anesthesia is used for surgical, dental, and diagnostic procedures and for the therapeutic management of chronic pain. It involves injection of the local anesthetic directly into or around the nerve trunks or nerve ganglia that supply the area to be numbed.

Contraindications

Contraindications for local anesthetics include known drug allergy. Only specially designed dosage forms are intended for ophthalmic use.

Table 11-6   Selected Parenteral Anesthetic Drugs*

Generic Name	Trade Name	Potency	Onset	Duration	Dose
lidocaine	Xylocaine	Moderate	Immediate	60-90 min	0.5%-4% injection
mepivacaine	Carbocaine	Moderate		120-150 min	1%, 1.5%, 2%, 3% injection
procaine	Novocain	Lowest	2-5 min	30-60 min	1%, 2%, 10% injection
tetracaine	Pontocaine	Highest	5-10 min	90-120 min	0.2%, 0.3%, 1% injection

*Other common parenteral anesthetic drugs include bupivacaine (Marcaine, Sensorcaine), chloroprocaine (Nesacaine), etidocaine (Duranest), propoxycaine (Ravocaine), and ropivacaine (Naropin).

Adverse Effects

The adverse effects of the local anesthetics are limited and of little clinical importance in most circumstances. The undesirable effects usually occur with high plasma concentrations of the drug, which result from inadvertent intravascular injection, an excessive dose or rate of injection, slow metabolic breakdown, or injection into a highly vascular tissue. When a local anesthetic is absorbed into the circulation, it may lead to adverse reactions similar to those produced by general anesthetics. One complication of note regarding spinal anesthesia is "spinal headache," which occurs in varying numbers of patients. Spinal headache is most often self-limiting with bedrest and conventional analgesic medications. However, severe cases may be treated by the anesthetist injecting a small volume (roughly 15 mL) of a venous blood sample from the same patient into the patient's epidural space. The exact mechanism of this "epidural blood patch" is unknown, but it has shown efficacy against spinal headache in over 90% of cases.

True allergic reactions to local anesthetics are rare. However, allergic reactions can occur. They may appear as skin lesions, urticaria, or edema, or they may be acutely anaphylactic. These rare allergic reactions are generally limited to a particular chemical class of anesthetics called the *ester type*. Box 11-3 categorizes the local anesthetic drugs into these two chemical families. Different enzymes are responsible for the breakdown of these two groups of anesthetics in the body. Anesthetics belonging to the ester family are metabolized by cholinesterase in the plasma and liver. They are converted into a paraaminobenzoic acid (PABA) compound. This compound is mainly responsible for the allergic reactions. The amide type of anesthetics is metabolized in the liver by other enzymes to active and inactive metabolites. Often when an individual has an undesirable experience after the administration of one of the local anesthetics, changing from one chemical class to another helps to decrease the chance of future problems.

Toxicity and Management of Overdose

Local anesthetics have little opportunity to cause toxicity under most circumstances. As mentioned, however, they can become just as toxic as the general anesthetics if they become systemically absorbed. To prevent this from occurring, a vasoconstrictor such as epinephrine is often coadministered with the local anesthetic to keep the anesthetic at its site of action. This property of epinephrine also serves to reduce local blood loss during minor surgical procedures. Another reason for the lower incidence of toxic effects with local anesthetics is that the doses of local anesthetics are, on average, much smaller than those of the general anesthetics. If for some reason significant amounts of the locally administered anesthetic are absorbed systemically, cardiovascular and respiratory function may be compromised. Symptomatic and supportive therapy is usually all that is needed to reverse the toxic effects stemming from systemic absorption of the drug until it is eventually metabolized by the body.

Interactions

Few clinically significant drug interactions occur with the local anesthetics. Some of the more important drug-drug interactions are seen with bupivacaine, chloroprocaine, and etidocaine. When given with enflurane, halothane, or epinephrine, these drugs can lead to dysrhythmias.

Dosages

For the recommended dosages of local anesthetic drugs, see the Dosages table on this page.

Box 11-3	Chemical Groups of Local Anesthetics

Ester Type
benzocaine
chloroprocaine
cocaine
procaine
proparacaine
propoxycaine
tetracaine

Amide Type
bupivacaine
dibucaine
etidocaine
lidocaine
mepivacaine
prilocaine

DOSAGES

Local Anesthetic Drug

Drug	Pharmacologic Class	Usual Dosage Range	Indications
▶lidocaine (Xylocaine)	Amide local anesthetic	0.5%, 1% solution: 5-300 mg	Percutaneous infiltration
		1% solution: 200-300 mg	Caudal obstetric analgesia, thoracic nerve block
		1% solution: 100 mg each side	Paracervical obstetric analgesia
		1% solution: 50-100 mg	Sympathetic lumbar nerve block
		1% solution: 30-50 mg	Paravertebral nerve block
		1% solution: 30 mg	Intercostal nerve block
		1% solution: 50 mg	Sympathetic cervical nerve block
		1.5% solution: 225-300 mg	Brachial nerve block, caudal surgical anesthesia
		2% solution: 20-100 mg	Dental procedures
		2% solution: 200-300 mg	Lumbar anesthesia

Drug Profiles

Besides lidocaine, profiled here, local anesthetics include bupivacaine, chloroprocaine, etidocaine, mepivacaine, prilocaine, procaine, propoxycaine, and tetracaine. As noted earlier, there are two major types of local anesthetics as determined by chemical structure: amides and esters. These designations refer to the type of linkage between the aromatic ring and the amino group of the drug, two of the structural components that make an anesthetic an anesthetic. Lidocaine belongs to the amide class of local anesthetics. Some patients may report that they have allergic or anaphylactic reactions to the "caines," as they may refer to lidocaine and the other amide drugs. In these situations, it may be wise to try a local anesthetic of the amide type.

▶ **lidocaine**

Lidocaine (Xylocaine) is one of the most commonly used local anesthetics. It is available in several strengths, both alone and in different concentrations with epinephrine, and is used for both infiltration and nerve block anesthesia. It is available as a 0.5%, 1%, 1.5%, 2%, and 4% parenteral injection and in a 0.5%, 1%, 1.5%, and 2% concentration in combination with epinephrine as a parenteral injection. The epinephrine reduces blood loss from minor surgical procedures because of its vasoconstrictive properties, and it also reduces systemic absorption of lidocaine for the same reason. Lidocaine is now also available as a 5% patch for relief of postherpetic neuralgia. Lidocaine is classified as a pregnancy category B drug and is contraindicated in those who have a hypersensitivity to it. Commonly recommended dosages are listed in the table on page 169.

NEUROMUSCULAR BLOCKING DRUGS

NMBAs prevent nerve transmission in certain muscles, leading to paralysis of the muscles. They are often used with anesthetics for surgical procedures. Use of NMBAs requires artificial mechanical ventilation, because these drugs paralyze respiratory and skeletal muscles. The patient is rendered unable to breathe on his or her own. The drugs do not cause sedation or relieve pain; therefore, the health care provider should assume that the paralyzed patient is in pain and anxious and should take steps to relieve such symptoms with analgesics and anxiolytics.

Snakes and plants played a large role in the identification of the chemical structure of substances that cause paralysis and discovery of the related receptor. The beginning steps in the identification of the receptor involved study of the seemingly irreversible inhibition of nerve transmission in muscles by toxins in the venoms of krait snake species (e.g., *Bungarus multicinctus*) and the venoms of certain varieties of cobra (e.g., *Naja naja* or king cobra). Once the receptor at which these venoms work was identified, pharmacologic drugs that mimic the venoms and produce paralysis were developed.

Curare, a nondepolarizing NMBA, has a long and romantic history. It has been used for centuries by natives of South America along the Amazon and Orinoco rivers and in other parts of that continent for killing wild animals for food. Animals shot with arrows soaked in this plant substance normally die from paralysis of respiratory muscles. *Curare* is actually a generic term for various South American arrow poisons. The most potent of all curare alkaloids are the toxiferines, obtained from *Strychnos toxifera*. The seeds of the trees and shrubs of the genus *Erythrina*, widely distributed in tropical and subtropical areas, also contain substances with curare-like activity.

NMBAs are traditionally classified as depolarizing or nondepolarizing drugs. Succinylcholine is now the only commonly used depolarizing NMBA. Nondepolarizing NMBAs prevent acetylcholine (ACh) from acting at neuromuscular junctions. Consequently, the nerve cell membrane is not depolarized, the muscle fibers are not stimulated, and skeletal muscle contraction does not occur. Nondepolarizing NMBAs are typically classified into three groups based on their duration of action: short-, intermediate-, and long-acting drugs.

Mechanism of Action and Drug Effects

The original prototypical depolarizing NMBA was d-tubocurarine, the active ingredient of curare. It is a naturally occurring plant alkaloid that causes skeletal muscle relaxation or paralysis. It is no longer available on the U.S. market, however, but has been replaced by newer synthetic drugs. Succinylcholine, a synthetic drug, works similarly to the neurotransmitter ACh. Initially succinylcholine combines with cholinergic receptors at the motor endplate of muscle nerves to produce depolarization and muscle contraction. Repolarization and further muscle contraction are then inhibited as long as an adequate concentration of drug remains at the receptor site. Succinylcholine is metabolized much more slowly than ACh. Because of this slower metabolism, succinylcholine subjects the motor endplate to ongoing depolarizing stimulation and thus repolarization cannot occur. As long as sufficient succinylcholine concentrations are present, the muscle is unable to contract and a flaccid muscle paralysis results. This muscle paralysis is sometimes preceded by muscle spasms, which may damage muscles. These muscle spasms are termed *muscle fasciculations* and are most pronounced in the muscle groups of the hands, feet, and face. Injury to muscle cells may cause postoperative muscle pain and release potassium into the circulation. Small doses of nondepolarizing NMBAs are sometimes administered with succinylcholine to minimize these muscle fasciculations. This reduces the muscle pain caused by depolarizing drugs such as succinylcholine. Nondepolarizing NMBAs prevent ACh from acting at neuromuscular junctions. They behave as antagonists, blocking ACh from binding to the postsynaptic receptors. Consequently, the nerve cell membrane is not depolarized, the muscle fibers are not stimulated, and skeletal muscle contraction does not occur.

If hyperkalemia develops, it is usually mild and insignificant. Rarely, cardiac dysrhythmias or even cardiac arrest has occurred. Succinylcholine is normally deactivated by plasma cholinesterase. This enzyme breaks down succinylcholine, freeing up the receptor site and allowing repolarization of the motor endplate. The duration of action of succinylcholine after a single intubating dose is about 5 to 9 minutes because of the rapid breakdown of the drug by this enzyme.

Anticholinesterase drugs such as neostigmine, pyridostigmine, and edrophonium are antidotes and are used to reverse muscle paralysis. They work by preventing the enzyme cholinesterase from breaking down ACh. This causes ACh to build up at the motor endplate, and it eventually displaces the nondepolarizing NMBA molecule, returning the nerve to its original state.

To summarize the drug effects of the NMBAs, the first sensation that is typically felt is muscle weakness. This is usually followed by a total flaccid paralysis. Small, rapidly moving muscles such as those of the fingers and eyes are typically the first to be paralyzed. The next are those of the limbs, neck, and trunk. Finally, the intercostal muscles and the diaphragm are paralyzed.

Respirations stop as a result; the patient can no longer breathe on his or her own. Recovery of muscular activity after discontinuation of anesthesia usually occurs in the reverse order to the initiation of paralysis during anesthesia induction, and thus the diaphragm is ordinarily the first to regain function. Before causing paralysis, depolarizing drugs such as succinylcholine often evoke transient muscular fasciculations. For this reason, when succinylcholine is administered, muscle soreness may occur when the patient wakes up from anesthesia. One general anesthetic drugs that helps alleviate this common but undesirable effect is the newer inhalational drug sevoflurane.

CNS effects are usually minimal because of the chemical structure of most of the nondepolarizing drugs. They are quaternary ammonium compounds and are not able to penetrate the blood-brain barrier. The effects on the cardiovascular system vary depending on the NMBA used and the individual patient. Increases and decreases in blood pressure and heart rate have been seen. Some NMBAs cause a release of histamine, which can result in bronchospasm, hypotension, and excessive bronchial and salivary secretion. The gastrointestinal tract is seldom affected by NMBAs. When it is affected, decreased tone and motility typically result, which can lead to constipation or even ileus.

Indications

The main therapeutic use of NMBAs is for maintaining controlled ventilation during surgical procedures. When respiratory muscles are paralyzed by an NMBA, mechanical ventilation is easier because the body's desire to control respirations is eliminated by the NMBA; this allows the ventilator to have total control of respirations.

Because NMBAs reduce muscular contractions, they are also helpful when the muscle tissue itself is part of the surgical site. Short-acting NMBAs are often used to facilitate intubation with an endotracheal tube. This is commonly done to facilitate a variety of diagnostic procedures such as laryngoscopy, bronchoscopy, and esophagoscopy. When used for this purpose, NMBAs are often combined with anxiolytics or anesthetics. Additional nonsurgical applications include reduction of laryngeal or general muscle spasms, reduction of spasticity from tetanus and neurologic diseases such as multiple sclerosis, and prevention of bone fractures during electroconvulsive therapy. These drugs are also used for the diagnosis of myasthenia gravis.

Contraindications

Contraindications to NMBAs include known drug allergy and also may include previous history of malignant hyperthermia, penetrating eye injuries, and narrow-angle glaucoma.

Adverse Effects

The key to limiting adverse effects with most NMBAs is to use only enough of the drug to block the neuromuscular receptors. If too much is used, the risk is increased that other ganglionic receptors will be affected. Blockade of these other ganglionic receptors leads to most of the undesirable effects of NMBAs. The effects of ganglionic blockade in various areas of the body are listed in Table 11-7.

Nondepolarizing NMBAs have relatively few adverse effects when used appropriately. Their cardiovascular effects include blockade of autonomic ganglia resulting in hypotension, blockade of muscarinic receptors resulting in tachycardia, and release of histamine resulting in hypotension. Use of the depolarizing drug succinylcholine has been associated with hypokalemia, dysrhythmias, fasciculations, muscle pain, myoglobinuria, and increased intraocular, intragastric, and intracranial pressure, as well as malignant hyperthermia. **Malignant hyperthermia** (MH) is an uncommon, genetically linked adverse metabolic reaction to general anesthesia that includes a rapid rise in body temperature, tachycardia, tachypnea, and muscular rigidity. Patients known to statistically be at greater risk for MH include children, adolescents, and such musculoskeletal abnormalities as hernias, strabismus, ptosis, scoliosis, and muscular dystrophy. MH is treated with cardiorespiratory supportive care as needed to stabilize heart and lung function (e.g., beta blockers to slow heart rate, supplemental oxygen to reduce respiratory intensity), as well as with the skeletal muscle relaxant dantrolene (see Chapter 12).

Toxicity and Management of Overdose

The primary concern when NMBAs are overdosed is prolonged paralysis requiring prolonged mechanical ventilation (see the Preventing Medication Errors box). Cardiovascular collapse may also be seen and is thought to be the result of histamine release. Multiple medical conditions can predispose an individual to toxicity. These conditions increase the sensitivity of the individual to NMBAs and prolong their effects. These predisposing conditions are listed in Box 11-4.

Table 11-7	Effects of Ganglionic Blockade by Neuromuscular Blocking Drugs	
Site	**Part of Nervous System Blocked**	**Physiologic Effect**
Arterioles	Sympathetic	Vasodilation and hypotension
Veins	Sympathetic	Dilation
Heart	Parasympathetic	Tachycardia
Gastrointestinal tract	Parasympathetic	Reduced tone and tract motility; constipation
Urinary bladder	Parasympathetic	Urinary retention
Salivary glands	Parasympathetic	Dry mouth

> ### PREVENTING MEDICATION ERRORS
> #### Neuromuscular Blocking Drugs
>
> Neuromuscular blocking drugs are considered high-alert drugs because improper use may lead to severe injury or death. The Institute for Safe Medication Practice has published several examples of patient death or injury as a result of medication errors involving neuromuscular blocking drugs. Because these drugs paralyze the respiratory muscles, incorrect administration without sufficient ventilator support has resulted in patient deaths. There have been medication errors due to "sound-alike" drug names as well (e.g., vancomycin and vecuronium). Most facilities have followed recommendations to restrict access to these drugs, provide warning labels and reminders, and increase staff awareness of the dangers of these drugs.
>
> For more information, visit www.ismp.org/Newsletters/acutecare/articles/20050922.asp. Accessed July 23, 2006.

Box 11-4 Conditions That Predispose Patients to Toxic Effects from Neuromuscular Blocking Drugs

Acidosis
Amyotrophic lateral sclerosis
Hypermagnesemia
Hypocalcemia
Hypokalemia
Hypothermia
Myasthenia gravis
Myasthenic syndrome
Neonatal status
Neurofibromatosis
Paraplegia
Poliomyelitis

Box 11-5 Conditions That Oppose the Effects of Neuromuscular Blocking Drugs

Cirrhosis with ascites
Clostridial infections
Hemiplegia
Hypercalcemia
Hyperkalemia
Peripheral nerve transection
Peripheral neuropathies
Thermal burns

Box 11-6 Drugs That Interact with Neuromuscular Blocking Drugs

Additive Effects

Aminoglycosides
Calcium channel blockers
clindamycin
cyclophosphamide
cyclosporine
dantrolene
furosemide
Inhalation anesthetics
Local anesthetics
magnesium
polymyxin
procainamide
quinidine
trimethaphan

Opposing Effects

carbamazepine
Corticosteroids
phenytoin

Some conditions make it more difficult for NMBAs to work and therefore require higher doses of NMBAs. Although these conditions do not result in toxicity or overdose, they are worthy of mention and are listed in Box 11-5.

Interactions

Many drugs can interact with NMBAs, which can lead to either synergistic or opposing effects. Some antibiotics, when given concomitantly with an NMBA, can have additive effects. The aminoglycoside antibiotics are a common example. They produce neuromuscular blockade by inhibiting ACh release from the preganglionic terminal. The tetracycline antibiotics can also produce neuromuscular blockade, possibly by chelation of calcium, and calcium channel blockers have also been shown to enhance neuromuscular blockade. Some of the more notable drugs that interact with NMBAs are listed in Box 11-6.

Dosages

For the recommended dosages of selected NMBAs, see the Dosages table on page 173.

Drug Profiles

NMBAs are one of the most commonly used classes of drugs in the operating room. They are given primarily with general anesthetics to facilitate endotracheal intubation and to relax skeletal muscles during surgery. In addition to their use in the operating room, NMBAs commonly are administered in the ICU to paralyze mechanically ventilated patients. As noted earlier, the two basic types of NMBAs are depolarizing and nondepolarizing drugs. The only depolarizing drug available is succinylcholine. Nondepolarizing drugs can be classified in a variety of ways but are typically categorized by their chemical structure or their duration of action. Table 11-8 lists some nondepolarizing drugs currently in use.

Depolarizing Neuromuscular Blocking Drugs

As mentioned previously, succinylcholine is the only drug in this subclass of NMBAs. Succinylcholine has a structure similar to that of the parasympathetic neurotransmitter ACh. It stimulates the same neurons as ACh and produces the same physiologic responses initially. Unlike ACh, succinylcholine is metabolized slowly. Because of this slower metabolism, succinylcholine subjects the motor endplate to ongoing depolarizing stimulation. Repolarization cannot occur. As long as sufficient succinylcholine concentrations are present, the muscle loses its ability to contract and flaccid muscle paralysis results. Because of its quick onset of action, succinylcholine is most commonly used to facilitate endotracheal intubation. It is seldom used over long periods because of the unwanted effects that develop with continuous infusion.

▶ **succinylcholine**

Succinylcholine (Anectine) is the only currently available depolarizing NMBA. It is an ultra–short-acting, depolarizing skeletal muscle relaxant for intravenous administration. Succinylcholine is used as an adjunct to general anesthesia, to facilitate tracheal intubation, and to provide skeletal muscle relaxation during surgery or mechanical ventilation. It is contraindicated in patients with personal or familial history of malignant hyperthermia, skeletal muscle myopathies, and known hypersensitivity to the drug. It is available as a 20 mg/mL 20-mL solution, a 500-mg sterile powder, and a 1000-mg sterile powder. Pregnancy category C. The recommended dosage is given in the table on page 173.

Pharmacokinetics

Half-Life	Onset	Peak	Duration
Seconds	Rapid, ≈1 min	Rapid	4-6 min

Nondepolarizing Neuromuscular Blocking Drugs

Nondepolarizing NMBAs are commonly used to facilitate endotracheal intubation, reduce muscle contraction in an area that needs surgery, and facilitate a variety of diagnostic procedures. They are often combined with anxiolytics or anesthetics. They may also be used to induce respiratory arrest in patients on mechanical ventilation.

pancuronium

Pancuronium (Pavulon) is a long-acting nondepolarizing NMBA. It is used as an adjunct to general anesthesia to facilitate tracheal intubation and to provide skeletal muscle relaxation during surgery or

DOSAGES

Selected Neuromuscular Blocking Drugs

Drug	Pharmacologic Class	Usual Dosage Range		Indications
pancuronium (Pavulon)	Nondepolarizing NMBA (long acting)	**Pediatric** IV: 0.02 mg/kg		Intubation
		Adult IV: 0.04-0.1 mg/kg Continuous infusion: 0.1 mg/kg/hr		Mechanical ventilation
▶succinylcholine (Anectine, Quelicin, others)	Depolarizing NMBA (short acting)	**Pediatric** IV: 1-2 mg/kg IM: 3-4 mg/kg		Intubation
		Adult IV: 0.3-1.1 mg/kg IM: 3-4 mg/kg		Mechanical ventilation
▶vecuronium (Norcuron)	Nondepolarizing NMBA (intermediate acting)	**Pediatric** IV: 0.08-0.1 mg/kg		Intubation
		Adult IV: 0.08-0.1 mg/kg Continuous infusion: 0.1 mg/kg/hr		Mechanical ventilation

NMBA, Neuromuscular blocking drug; *IV,* intravenous; *IM,* intramuscular.

Table 11-8   Classification of Neuromuscular Blocking Drugs

Drug	Type of Compound
Short-Acting Drug	
mivacurium (Mivacron)	Benzylisoquinolinium
Intermediate-Acting Drugs	
atracurium (Tracrium)	Benzylisoquinolinium
rocuronium (Zemuron)	Steroid
vecuronium (Norcuron)	Steroid
Long-Acting Drugs	
doxacurium (Nuromax)	Benzylisoquinolinium
pancuronium (Pavulon)	Steroid
tubocuraine (dTC)	Benzylisoquinolinium

mechanical ventilation. It is most commonly employed for long surgical procedures that require prolonged muscle paralysis. Use of pancuronium is contraindicated in patients with known hypersensitivity to the drug. It is available as 1 g/mL 10-mL vials and 2 mg/mL 2- and 5-mL ampules. Pregnancy category C. The recommended dosage is given in the table on this page.

Pharmacokinetics

Half-Life	Onset	Peak	Duration
80-120 min	3-5 min	Rapid	60-100 min

▶ vecuronium

Vecuronium (Norcuron) is an intermediate-acting nondepolarizing NMBA. It is used as an adjunct to general anesthesia to facilitate tracheal intubation and to provide skeletal muscle relaxation during surgery or mechanical ventilation and is one of the most commonly used NMBAs. Long-term use in the ICU setting has resulted in prolonged paralysis and consequent difficulty weaning from mechanical ventilation. This is believed to be due to an active metabolite, 3-desacetyl vecuronium, which tends to accumulate with prolonged use. Use of vecuronium is contraindicated in patients with known hypersensitivity to the drug. It is available as 1 mg/mL 10- and 20-mL vials and 1 mg/mL 10-mL syringes. Pregnancy category C. The recommended dosage is given in the table on this page.

Pharmacokinetics

Half-Life	Onset	Peak	Duration
65-75 min	2.5-3 min	3-5 min	25-40 min

MODERATE SEDATION

Many types of procedures, including diagnostic and minor operative procedures, do not require as great a depth of anesthesia as do more extensive surgeries. **Moderate sedation,** *conscious sedation,* and *procedural sedation* are terms that all mean the same thing: namely, an anesthesia that does not lead to loss of consciousness. This technique uses combinations of several drugs that may be classified differently. For example, one or more benzodiazepines may be used with one or several narcotic agonists or opioids. Drugs may be given by intravenous, intramuscular, or spinal routes. The net effect is a type of anesthesia that allows the patient to remain conscious, respond verbally to commands, relax, and maintain an open airway. Mild amnesia for the procedure may occur. All types of moderate sedation have a more rapid recovery time than general anesthesia as well as a better safety profile because of lower cardiopulmonary risks.

In pediatric patients moderate sedation may be accomplished using an oral syrup form of midazolam with or without concurrent use of injected medications such as opiates. This technique can be especially helpful for pediatric patients who must undergo uncomfortable procedures such as wound suturing or diagnostic procedures requiring reduced movement such as computed tomography and magnetic resonance imaging. See Life Span Considerations: The Pediatric Patient on page 174 for other considerations.

PHARMACOKINETIC BRIDGE to Nursing Practice

With moderate (conscious or procedural) sedation or anesthesia, it is always important to understand the pharmacokinetic properties of the drugs used. For example, the intravenous

Life Span Considerations: The Pediatric Patient

Moderate or Conscious Anesthesia

- The American Academy of Pediatrics recommends that moderate or conscious sedation (anesthesia) be used to reduce anxiety, pain, and fear in the pediatric patient. The use of moderate anesthesia in the pediatric patient allows a procedure to be performed restraint free in most situations while keeping the patient responsive.
- Pediatric dosing often conforms to the following guidelines:
  - Morphine—pediatric dosing may be at 0.05 to 0.1 mg/kg intravenously (IV) over a 2-minute period and is ideal for long procedures or cases in which pain is anticipated after the procedure.
  - Fentanyl—pediatric dosing may be 0.5 to 1 mcg/kg with increments over 3 minutes to a maximum of three doses. Too rapid an IV injection may result in chest rigidity, which may need to be treated with muscle relaxants and possibly mechanical ventilation. Fentanyl is used often for short procedures.
  - Fentanyl citrate—oral transmucosal forms are dosed at 10 to 15 mcg/kg/hr and are used in monitored hospital settings. They are administered by having the patient suck on a stick (as with a lollipop).
  - Hydromorphone—pediatric dosing is at 0.015 to 0.02 mg/kg.
  - Meperidine—pediatric dosing is at 0.5 to 1 mg/kg over 2 minutes.
- Discharge status of the pediatric patient depends on the type of drugs and drug combinations used. Discharge after conscious or moderate sedation is based mainly on whether the following criteria are met:
  - Patient is alert and oriented compared with the baseline neurologic assessment.
  - Protective swallowing and gag reflexes are intact.
  - Vital signs are stable and consistent with baseline values for at least 30 minutes after the last dosing. Different health care facilities set different criteria that must be met and documented (blood pressure and pulse rate within normal limits or within 20 points of baseline, temperature lower than 38.3° C[101° F]).
  - Oxygen saturation is at least 95% on room air 30 minutes after the last dose.
  - Pain rating is at baseline levels or less.
  - Ambulation is at baseline.
  - An adult is present to get the patient home and remain with the patient for at least two half-lives of the various drugs used for the anesthesia.
  - If a reversal drug was administered, there has been time for the drug to be excreted.

form of diazepam has an onset of action of 1 to 5 minutes, peak effect time of 15 minutes, duration of action of 15 to 60 minutes, and half-life of 20 to 70 hours. (Half-life is the time it takes for 50% of the drug to be excreted from the body.) Therefore, if diazepam is used for sedation or anesthesia, the drug could be present in the body and cause effects for up to 70 hours. In the care of patients receiving drugs for anesthesia (whether for conscious or moderate anesthesia, or general or local anesthesia), these drug profile properties help the nurse to predict the drugs' onset of action, peak effect, and duration of action.

◆ NURSING PROCESS

◆ ASSESSMENT

Associated with each drug used in general and local anesthesia are some broad as well as very specific assessment parameters. First, for general anesthesia, once assessment for any drug or food allergies has been performed, the next group of major parameters to be assessed is the ABCs (*a*irway, *b*reathing, and *c*irculation). Assessment should also include a thorough survey of the patient's physical and mental status before, during, and after the administration of the various drugs used for general anesthesia. The nurse's responsibility is to assess and document previous reactions, both positive or negative (adverse), to general anesthetics and related drugs, so that the appropriate health care professionals, such as the anesthesiologist, nurse anesthetist, registered nurse, physician, and any other health care professional involved in the patient's care, can be notified.

For general anesthesia, it is important to identify and document any problems or areas of concern in the patient's profile. A patient's profile includes subjective and objective data. One very important area in the profile is drug use, including prescription drugs, over-the-counter drugs, herbals, supplements, and social and illegal drugs. Unusual and/or adverse reactions to any previously used drugs should be noted. Another important area to consider is the use of alcohol and nicotine. Excessive use of alcohol or illicit substances can alter the patient's response to general anesthesia. Also, if the patient has a history of alcohol abuse, withdrawal symptoms may occur during recovery from surgery. The patient's history of smoking is very important because nicotine has an adverse effect on the cilia in the respiratory system. The cilia become paralyzed and unable to perform the function of clearing foreign bodies from the airways assessment, weight, height, electrocardiogram, and chest radiograph (ordered by the physician or anesthesia personnel).

Other objective data includes physical assessment, weight, height, electrocardiogram, chest x-ray (as ordered, and laboratory tests, including hemoglobin, hematocrit, complete blood count, blood urea nitrogen level, creatinine level, alkaline phosphate level, prothrombin time, partial thromboplastin time, and platelet count. Results of tests for serum electrolytes (such as potassium, sodium, chloride, phosphorus, magnesium, and calcium), urinalysis with specific gravity, and a pregnancy test (indicated if a female patient is of childbearing age) should be assessed and findings documented. Results of these laboratory studies are important in establishing baseline organ function prior to the use of any form of anesthetic or related drugs.

Neurologic assessment should include motor assessments with bilateral and upper extremity versus lower extremity comparisons of strength, reflexes, grasp, and ability to move on command. Sensory assessment includes the same anatomical areas with comparison of response to various types of stimuli such as sharp, dull, soft, and cold versus warm. Swallowing ability and gag reflexes are also important to assess and document for baseline status and comparison. In addition, the patient's level of consciousness, alertness, and orientation to person, place, and time should be assessed. These motor, sensory, and cognitive parameters, when within normal limits, indicate an intact neurologic system. Other baseline parameters include the patient's intake and output as well as oxygen saturation levels.

One very significant reaction to assess for patients receiving general anesthesia is that of malignant hyperthermia. This is a rapid progression of hyperthermia that may be fatal if not promptly recognized and aggressively treated. It is an inherited condition, so questions about related signs and symptoms in the family and patient medical history would be important. These signs and symptoms include tachycardia, tachypnea, muscle rigidity, cyanosis, irregular heartbeat, fever, mottling of the skin, diaphoresis (profuse sweating), and an unstable blood pressure. Astute and careful monitoring for the slightest change in vital signs and the parameters listed previously and for the occurrence of any abnormality associated with the anesthesia is crucial to patient safety. Regardless of the degree of altered sensorium, there is a need for constant and intense assessment. Whether the assessment occurs during the preanesthesia, intraanesthesia, or postanesthesia period, the nurse should remember that no matter how intense and critical the situation, use of the basic ABCs will always be the starting point for prioritizing and organizing patient care. Other areas of assessment include drug interactions, cautions, and contraindications (see previous discussion in the pharmacology section).

Intravenously administered anesthetic drugs are usually combined with various sedatives-hypnotics, antianxiety drugs, opioid and nonopioid analgesics, antiemetics, and anticholinergics. These drugs are used to decrease some of the undesirable aftereffects of inhaled anesthetics. With any form of adjuvant drug (a drug given at the same time) use, the patient should be assessed for any problems in liver, renal, or cardiac functioning, because of the risk for complications or adverse events. Generally speaking, the use of general anesthetics (either intravenous or inhaled) carries a greater potential for more systemic, adverse effects in the patient related to overall CNS depression that affects all body systems.

With the use of conscious sedation, as with any anesthesia technique, assessment for cautions, contraindications, and drug interactions is important. Cautions and contraindications are similar to those for all other types of anesthesia, as are drug interactions. Because moderate sedation is often used in pediatric patients, there should be close assessment of organ function and diseases or conditions that could lead to excessive levels of the drug in the child's body. Even with the use of local anesthesia there are concerns about complications. Just because an anesthetic is local does not mean that adverse reactions will not occur—they do occur and may be rather severe. Adverse reactions to or complications with local anesthesia and intraspinal anesthesia include the following: reduced respiratory function and altered breathing patterns, hypotension, tachycardia, decreased respiratory rate, diminished sensation, and decreased motor responses. "Spinal headaches" may also be associated with intraspinal anesthesia and occur because of the leakage of cerebrospinal fluid from the insertion site. This type of headache is often severe and occurs when the patient stands or ambulates once the initial bedrest has ended. An assessment of blood pressure and other vital parameters, including respiratory

function, provides important baseline data, and a history of any previous headaches is important information for the patient profile.

Local-topical anesthetics used for either infiltration or nerve block anesthesia may be combined with other medications such as vasoconstrictors (e.g., epinephrine, phenylephrine, norepinephrine). The vasoconstrictors are used to help confine the local anesthetic to the injected area, prevent systemic absorption, and reduce bleeding. Systemic absorption of the vasoconstrictors results in hypertensive episodes that may be life-threatening, especially in patients who are at high risk (e.g., those with underlying arterial disease). When local-topical anesthetics such as lidocaine are used (e.g., when lacerations are sutured), the patient must be assessed for any preexisting illnesses and allergies. Blood pressure, pulse rate, respiration rate, and temperature also must be assessed and documented. In addition, information about any illnesses or conditions as well as a list of prescription medications, herbal products, supplements, and over-the-counter medications taken should be obtained and recorded. There is always concern about possible drug interactions or adverse effects that may be exacerbated by the use of the anesthetic and/or other drugs that are combined with the topical-local anesthetic drug. One example is the use of topical lidocaine with epinephrine. If this topical-local anesthetic combination gains access to the systemic circulation, the epinephrine may lead to hypertension, creating an even greater risk for hypertensive emergency than if plain lidocaine (without epinephrine) was used. Such a crisis would be at higher risk of occurring if the patient has hypertension or is taking medications, herbals, or supplements that elevate blood pressure.

For patients about to undergo anesthesia with NMBAs, a complete head-to-toe assessment should be performed and a thorough medical and medication history taken. The specific drug being used and whether it is depolarizing or nondepolarizing will guide nursing assessment and practices because of the NMBAs' action on the patient's neuromuscular functioning. All cautions, contraindications, and drug interactions must also be assessed (see previous discussion). Another concern with the use of NMBAs is that they are associated with an increase in intraocular pressure and intracranial pressure. Therefore, these anesthetic drugs should not be used at all or should be used with extreme caution (close monitoring of these pressures) in patients with glaucoma or closed head injuries. Patients receiving NMBAs should also receive a thorough respiratory assessment because of the impact of these drugs on the respiratory system, including a paralyzing effect on the muscles used for breathing. In fact, some of the NMBAs are often used to induce paralysis of respiratory muscles in patients requiring mechanical ventilation. Paralysis of respiratory muscles is necessary so that patients will relax and not fight the machine and work against the breaths the machine delivers. If an NMBA is indicated for other uses, it is critical to make sure that mechanical ventilation is available because of the potential for respiratory arrest.

Also indicated with the use of NMBAs is careful assessment of serum electrolyte levels, specifically potassium and magnesium levels. Imbalances in these electrolytes may lead to increased action of the NMBA with exacerbation of the drug's actions and adverse effects. Allergic reactions to NMBAs are most commonly characterized by rash, fever, respiratory distress, and pruritus. Drug interactions with herbal products are outlined in the Herbal Therapies and Dietary Supplements box on this page.

Once any type of anesthesia is discontinued, patient assessment continues with further notation of the patient's ABCs, vital signs, and other critical parameters (e.g., pulse oximetry, neurological assessment, urinary output). The nurse's responsibility is to provide continual assessment and care.

◆ NURSING DIAGNOSES

- Impaired gas exchange related to the anesthetic's CNS depressant effects with altered respiratory rate and effort (decreased rate, decreased depth)
- Decreased cardiac output related to the systemic effects of anesthesia
- Risk for injury related to the impact of anesthesia on the CNS (i.e., decreased sensorium)
- Anxiety related to the use of anesthesia and the possibility of surgery
- Deficient knowledge related to lack of information about anesthesia

◆ PLANNING

Goals

- Patient states the adverse effects of general or local anesthesia, including decreased sensorium.
- Patient states the potential complications of anesthesia involving the cardiac system.
- Patient experiences minimal or no respiratory complications related to anesthesia.
- Patient describes what to expect during recovery from anesthesia.
- Patient complies with postanesthesia care to help decrease the chance of complications.
- Patient follows instructions regarding preanesthesia and postanesthesia care.
- Patient verbalizes anxiety, fears, and concerns regarding anesthesia.

- Patient verbalizes purpose of and adverse effects and complications of anesthesia.

Outcome Criteria

- Patient experiences minimal to no adverse effects from anesthesia, such as myocardial depression, during and after anesthesia.
- Patient remains free of complications such as injury, falls, cardiac and respiratory depression, and hepatotoxicity during the preanesthesia, intraanesthesia, and postanesthesia periods.
- Patient experiences minimal anxiety or fear as a result of specific interventions and education.
- Patient is compliant with all interventions and treatments such as turning, coughing, and deep breathing once the anesthesia has been terminated.

◆ IMPLEMENTATION

Regardless of the type of anesthesia used, one of the most important nursing considerations during the preanesthesia, intraanesthesia, and postanesthesia periods is close and frequent observation of all body systems, with specific attention to the ABCs of nursing care (vital signs) and arterial oxygen saturation by pulse oximetry (SpO_2). These observations and interventions should be performed as frequently as needed depending on the patient's status and in keeping with the standard of care for anesthesia. Sudden elevation in the patient's body temperature (e.g., higher than 40° C [104° F]) while the patient is receiving general anesthesia may indicate malignant hyperthermia, and immediate intervention is needed to protect the patient from injury and possible death. Other nursing interventions include monitoring all body systems, implementing safety measures, and carrying out the physician's orders.

Oxygen is often administered after a patient has received general anesthesia to compensate for the respiratory depression that occurred during surgery as well as to elevate oxygen levels. Because oxygen is a drug, a doctor's order is needed for its administration. Continuous monitoring of SpO_2 is usually performed. In addition, hypotension and orthostatic hypotension are possible problems after anesthesia, so postural blood pressure measurements (supine and standing) are needed. Should the patient require pain management once the anesthesia has been terminated, the nurse must remember that the anesthetic and any adjuvant drugs used continue to have an effect on the patient. Therefore, administration of sedatives-hypnotics, narcotics, nonnarcotic analgesics, and other CNS depressants for pain relief should be done cautiously and only with close monitoring of vital signs. If the patient has received other medications (such as narcotics or CNS depressants) in a recovery area, dosages of drugs used in the postanesthesia period and on the general nursing unit may be decreased by one half or one fourth as ordered. This reduction will help to prevent any further CNS depression. For those patients receiving anesthetics that are quick acting and whose effects are reversed quickly, dosages of analgesics may not need to be altered.

For intravenous anesthesia, all resuscitative equipment—as well as a drug antidote—are usually readily available in case of cardiorespiratory distress or arrest. Neurologic indicators (e.g., reflexes, response to commands, level of consciousness), electrocardiogram, pulse oximetry readings, and vital signs are some of the parameters that need to be monitored frequently. Additional nursing interventions with anesthesia include the following: status of breath sounds should be assessed by auscultation (hypoventilation may be a complication of general anesthesia) and neurologic changes and status (no matter how small) and any change in sensations, such as noted with nerve blocks (local anesthesia), should be documented and reported. If changes occur in body parts distal to the site of local anesthesia or in locations where restraints were placed, the body part should be assessed for temperature, color, and presence or absence of pulses and the findings should be documented and reported to the physician. Improper positioning during surgery may lead to the injury of arteries and nerves and should be reported immediately.

Patients undergoing moderate sedation as the method of anesthesia should receive education about the technique. As noted earlier, recovery from this type of anesthesia is more rapid and the safety profile better than with general anesthesia, which has inherent cardiorespiratory risks. As with general anesthesia, the nurse should monitor the ABCs, vital signs, pulse oximetry readings, patient's level of consciousness. See Box 11-7 for more information on conscious sedation.

With regard to the use of topical or local anesthetics (e.g., lidocaine with or without epinephrine), solutions that are not clear and appear cloudy or discolored should not be used. Some anesthesiologists mix the solution with sodium bicarbonate to minimize local pain during infiltration, but this also causes a more rapid onset of action and a longer duration of sensory analgesia. If an anesthetic ointment or cream is used, the nurse should thoroughly cleanse and dry the area to be anesthetized before application of the drug.

If a topical or local anesthetic is being used in the nose or throat, the nurse must remember that it may cause paralysis and/or numbness of the structures of the upper respiratory tract, which can lead to aspiration. Exact amounts of the drug should be used, and it should be administered only at the prescribed times. Local anesthetics are not to be swallowed unless the physician has so instructed. Should this occur, the nurse must closely observe the patient, check his or her gag reflex, and expect to withhold food or drink until the patient's sensation and/or gag reflex has returned.

A patient who receives an NMBA should be monitored closely during and after anesthesia or initiation of mechanical ventilation. Vital signs and other parameters should be constantly monitored, with measurement of blood pressure, pulse, respirations (rate, depth, pattern, quality), SpO_2, and hand grasp strength (for neuromotor assessment). Intake and output are also monitored. Recovery from NMBAs is manifested by a decrease in paralysis of the face, diaphragm, legs, arms, and remainder of the body. The health care provider must reassure the patient of his or her condition as the patient begins to recover, because the patient may become frightened if communication is difficult during the recovery process.

Once anesthesia and procedures are completed and the patient is to be discharged or transferred, some general areas of patient teaching must be completed. One major focus is sharing information regarding health care resources available to the patient at home, should assistance be necessary. Home health care is often required and ordered by the physician, and if it is not ordered, there may be a need for additional resources for assistance at home. Education about home health care resources and assistance-in-living programs should be guided by

---

Box 11-7 Moderate or Conscious Sedation: What to Expect

What questions should the patient or caregiver ask about the technique of moderate or conscious sedation?
- Who will be providing this type of anesthesia?
- Who will be monitoring me or my loved one?
- Will there be constant monitoring of blood pressure, pulse rate, respiratory rate, and temperature?
- Will there be emergency equipment in the room, in case of need?
- Are the personnel qualified to administer these drugs? To administer advanced cardiac life support?
- What do I need to know about care at home? Will I need help? Can I drive after having the procedure?

What are the adverse effects of moderate or conscious sedation?
- Brief periods of amnesia (loss of memory)
- Headache
- Hangover
- Nausea and vomiting

What should be expected immediately following the procedure?
- Frequent monitoring
- Written postoperative instructions and care
- No driving, if the patient is driving age, for at least 24 hours after undergoing moderate sedation
- A follow-up contact by phone to check on the patient

Who can administer the conscious sedation?
- Moderate or conscious sedation is safe when administered by qualified providers. Certified registered nurse anesthetists, anesthesiologists, other physicians, dentists, and oral surgeons are qualified to administer conscious sedation.

Which procedures generally require moderate sedation?
- Breast biopsy
- Vasectomy
- Minor foot surgery
- Minor bone fracture repair
- Plastic or reconstructive surgery
- Dental prosthetic or reconstructive surgery
- Endoscopy (such as diagnostic studies and treatment of stomach, colon, and bladder cancer)

What are the overall benefits of this type of anesthesia?
- It is a safe and effective option for patients undergoing minor surgeries or diagnostic procedures.
- It allows patients to recover quickly and resume normal activities in a shorter period of time.

Data from American Association of Nurse Anesthetists: Conscious sedation: what patients should expect, 2005. Available at www.aana.com. For more information, see www.aana.com/patients/conscious.asp.

---

the findings of an at-home nursing assessment and the needs identified. Assistance with activities of daily living and/or assistance with health care–related procedures or interventions may be required. Some examples of health care procedures for which help might be needed are wound care, dressing changes, surgical site care, drawing of samples for laboratory studies, intravenous infusions, and administration of various medications through the intravenous, intramuscular, or subcutaneous route. Pain management may also need to be addressed (Chapter 10) with thorough teaching for the patient and those involved in care at home. Simple instructions provided using age-appropriate teaching strategies are always important (Chapter 6). Sharing of information about community resources is also important, especially for those who may need transportation, assistance with meals and housekeeping during the patient's recovery, and possibly rehabilitation at home. Some of these community resources may be agencies that are supported by city or state social service programs, Meals on Wheels, senior citizen support groups, and church-sponsored support resources. Many of these resources are free or have income-based fees. Teaching tips important for patients receiving general or local anesthesia are given in the Patient Teaching Tips.

◆ EVALUATION

The therapeutic effects of any general or local anesthetic include loss of sensation during a procedure (such as loss of sensation in the eye during corneal surgery) and loss of consciousness and re-flexes (such as insensitivity to pain during abdominal or other major procedures). The patient who has received general anesthesia should be constantly monitored for the occurrence of adverse effects of the anesthesia. These effects include myocardial depression, convulsions, respiratory depression, allergic rhinitis, and decreased renal or liver function. Patients who have received a local anesthetic also need to be constantly monitored for the occurrence of adverse effects (mostly stemming from the systemic absorption of the specific drug). These effects include bradycardia, myocardial depression, hypotension, and dysrhythmias. As mentioned earlier in this chapter, significant overdoses of local anesthetic drugs or direct injection into a blood vessel may result in cardiovascular collapse or cardiac or respiratory depression.

Patient Teaching Tips

General Anesthesia

- Inform the patient that it is important to know whether any medications the patient is taking may need to be discontinued and/or tapered before the anesthesia administration.
- Educate the patient about the route of administration and specific anesthetic being used. Include information about the action, use, adverse effects, and special precautions associated with the specific anesthetic used after the anesthesia has been discontinued.
- Encourage the patient and family members to openly discuss any fears or anxieties about anesthesia and related procedures or surgery.
- Instruct the patient about the postanesthesia process, especially if there is a need to turn, cough, and deep breathe (which helps to prevent atelectasis and pneumonia).
- Encourage ambulation with assistance as needed. This helps increase circulation and improve ventilation to the alveoli of the lungs; consequently, circulation to the legs will be improved (helps to prevent stasis of blood and possible blood clot formation in the leg veins).
- Encourage the patient to request pain medication if needed before pain becomes severe. Inform the patient that even though anesthesia has been administered, the patient may experience discomfort or pain from the procedure or surgery, even though anesthesia was used.
- Encourage the patient to rate his or her pain on a scale of 0 to 10, with 0 being no pain and 10 being the worst possible pain.
- Explain the rationale for any other treatments or procedures related to the anesthesia (such as epidural catheter placement; delivery of oxygen; administration of a gas; use of various tubes, catheters, or intravenous lines).

- Inform the patient that frequent measurement of vital signs and pulse oximetry monitoring are a standard of care and do not necessarily mean that a problem or complication exists.
- For a patient with diminished sensorium, ensuring that the bed side rails are up and that a call button is at the bedside is critical to patient safety. (Note that bed alarms are now generally used instead of side rails, but they may not always be available.) This information should be shared with the patient, family, or caregiver.
- Make sure that patients receiving NMBAs for mechanical ventilation know that although they may not be able to move (due to the paralyzing effects of the NMBA), they will still be able to hear.

Local Anesthesia

- Make sure the patient understands how local anesthetics work, what the adverse effects are, and why the specific local drug was selected.
- Inform a patient receiving local (spinal) anesthesia about the need for frequent assessments, measurement of vital signs, and system assessments during and after the procedure to monitor for and assess any complications.
- Share with the patient the fact that even though the anesthesia is local, there are still concerns regarding the procedure and adverse effects.

Miscellaneous

- Wound care instructions should be emphasized with return demonstrations from the patient or caregiver.

NCLEX Examination Review Questions

1. A patient is in the hospital for removal of a lymph node from his arm under local anesthesia. The physician has requested "lidocaine *with* epinephrine." Which of the following statements is the most accurate rationale for adding epinephrine?
   a. It helps calm the patient before the procedure.
   b. It helps minimize the risk of an allergic reaction.
   c. It enhances the effect of the local lidocaine.
   d. It helps to reduce local bleeding.
2. Which of the following patients is more prone to complications from general anesthesia?
   a. A 79-year-old female who is about to have her gallbladder removed
   b. A 49-year-old male athlete who quit heavy smoking 12 years ago
   c. A 30-year-old female who is in perfect health but has never had anesthesia
   d. A 50-year-old female scheduled for outpatient laser surgery for vision correction
3. Which of the following may occur in a patient who has been under general anesthesia for 3 to 4 hours for abdominal-thoracic surgery?
   a. Decreased urine output from use of vasopressors as anesthetics
   b. Increased cardiac output related to the effects of general anesthesia
   c. Risk for injury (fall) related to decreased sensorium for 2 to 4 days postoperatively
   d. Decreased gaseous exchange due to the CNS depressant effect of general anesthesia
4. Which of the following should be the nurse's main concern about a patient recovering from general anesthesia during the immediately postoperative period?
   a. Airway
   b. Pupillary reflexes
   c. Return of sensations
   d. Level of consciousness
5. A patient is recovering from surgery during which he received an NMBA. As he wakes up during recovery, he looks as if he is panicking and yet is unable to speak. Which of the following should be the nurse's reaction?
   a. Call the anesthesia department for reintubation because of an impaired airway
   b. Reassure the patient that he is recovering and that the medication is still wearing off
   c. Readminister the NMBA to help the patient calm down
   d. Increase oxygen administration and monitor oxygenation

1. d, 2. a, 3. d, 4. a, 5. b.

Critical Thinking Activities

A 53-year-old woman is scheduled to have a colonoscopy this morning, and she is very anxious. The nurse anesthetist has explained the conscious sedation that is planned, but the patient says after the anesthetist leaves the room, "I'm so afraid of feeling it during the test. Why don't they just put me to sleep?"

1. How does conscious sedation differ from general anesthesia?
2. How do you answer her question?
3. What is important to assess before this procedure is performed?

For answers, see http://evolve.elsevier.com/Lilley.

Central Nervous System Depressants and Muscle Relaxants

Objectives

When you reach the end of this chapter, you should be able to do the following:

1. Describe the impact of CNS depressants on all body systems.
2. Differentiate between the following terms: sedative-hypnotic drugs, barbiturates, benzodiazepines, muscle relaxants, and non-benzodiazepine drugs.
3. Identify the specific drugs within each category of CNS depressants.
4. Contrast the mechanism of action, indications, adverse effects, toxic effects, cautions, contraindications, dosage forms, routes of administration, and drug interactions of barbiturates, benzodiazepines, muscle relaxants, non-benzodiazepines, and miscellaneous sedative-hypnotic drugs.
5. Discuss the nursing process as it relates to the nursing care of a patient receiving any CNS depressants.
6. Discuss nonpharmacologic approaches to the treatment of sleep disorders.

e-Learning Activities

Companion CD
- NCLEX Review Questions: see questions 72-78
- Animations
- Audio Glossary
- Category Catchers
- Medication Errors Checklists
- IV Therapy Checklists

evolve Website (http://evolve.elsevier.com/Lilley)
- Nursing Care Plans • Frequently Asked Questions • Content Updates • WebLinks • Supplemental Resources • Elsevier ePharmacology Update • Medication Administration Animations

Drug Profiles

▶ baclofen, p. 189
▶ cyclobenzaprine, p. 189
dantrolene, p. 189
estazolam, p. 186
flurazepam, p. 187
pentobarbital, p. 184
phenobarbital, p. 184

quazepam, p. 187
secobarbital, p. 184
▶ temazepam, p. 187
triazolam, p. 187
▶ zaleplon, p. 188
▶ zolpidem, p. 188

▶ Key drug.

Glossary

Anxiolytic A medication that relieves anxiety. (p. 185)

Barbiturates A class of drugs that are chemical derivatives of barbituric acid. They can induce sedation and sleep. (p. 181)

Benzodiazepines A chemical category of drugs most frequently prescribed as sedative-hypnotic and anxiolytic drugs. (p. 185)

Gamma-aminobutyric acid (GABA) An inhibitory neurotransmitter found in the brain. (p. 181)

Hypnotics Drugs that, when given at low to moderate dosages, calm or soothe the central nervous system (CNS) without inducing sleep but when given at high dosages may cause sleep. (p. 181)

Non–rapid eye movement (non-REM) sleep One of the stages of the sleep cycle. It characteristically has four stages and precedes REM sleep. Most of a normal sleep cycle consists of non-REM sleep. (p. 181)

Rapid eye movement (REM) sleep One of the stages of the sleep cycle. Some of the characteristics of REM sleep are rapid movement of the eyes, vivid dreams, and irregular breathing. (p. 181)

REM interference A drug-induced reduction of REM sleep time. (p. 181)

REM rebound Excessive REM sleep following discontinuation of a sleep-altering drug. (p. 181)

Sedatives Drugs that have an inhibitory effect on the CNS to the degree that they reduce nervousness, excitability, and irritability without causing sleep. (p. 181)

Sedatives-hypnotics Drugs that can act in the body either as sedatives or as hypnotics. (p. 181)

Sleep A transient, reversible, and periodic state of rest in which there is a decrease in physical activity and consciousness. (p. 181)

Sleep architecture The structure of the various elements involved in the sleep cycle, including normal and abnormal patterns of sleep. (p. 181)

Tachyphylaxis The rapid appearance of a progressive decrease in response to a drug after repetitive administration of the drug. (p. 190)

Therapeutic index The ratio between the toxic and therapeutic concentrations of a drug. If the index is low, the difference between the therapeutic and toxic drug concentrations is small, and use of the drug is more hazardous. (p. 181)

Drugs that have a calming effect or that depress the central nervous system (CNS) are referred to as *sedatives* and *hypnotics*. A drug is classified as either a sedative or a hypnotic drug depending on the degree to which it inhibits the transmission of nerve impulses to the CNS. **Sedatives** reduce nervousness, excitability, and irritability without causing sleep, but a sedative can become a hypnotic if it is given in large enough doses. **Hypnotics** cause sleep. They have a much more potent effect on the CNS than do sedatives. Many drugs can act in the body as either a sedative or a hypnotic, and for this reason are called *sedatives-hypnotics*. Listed in Table 12-1 are some points of interest relating to sedatives-hypnotics.

Sedatives-hypnotics can be classified chemically into three main groups: barbiturates, benzodiazepines, and miscellaneous drugs. Before the sedative-hypnotic drugs are discussed in depth, it is important that the physiology of normal sleep be understood because of the significant effects these drugs can have on sleep patterns.

SLEEP

Sleep is defined as a transient, reversible, and periodic state of rest in which there is a decrease in physical activity and consciousness. Normal sleep is cyclic and repetitive, and a person's responses to stimuli are markedly reduced during sleep. During waking hours the body is bombarded with stimuli that provoke the senses of sight, hearing, touch, smell, and taste. These stimuli elicit voluntary and involuntary movements or functions. During sleep a person is no longer aware of the sensory stimuli within his or her immediate environment.

Sleep research involves study of the patterns of sleep, or what is sometimes referred to as **sleep architecture.** The architecture of sleep consists of two basic elements that occur cyclically: **rapid eye movement (REM) sleep** and **non–rapid eye movement (non-REM) sleep.** The normal cyclic progression of the stages of sleep is summarized in Table 12-2. Various sedative-hypnotic drugs affect

different stages of the normal sleep pattern. If usage is prolonged, emotional and psychologic changes can occur. An appreciation of this fact will help prevent the inappropriate use of long-term sleeping drugs. For example, prolonged sedative-hypnotic use may reduce the cumulative amount of REM sleep; this is known as **REM interference.** This can result in daytime fatigue since REM sleep provides a certain component of the "restfulness" of sleep. Upon discontinuing a sedative-hypnotic drug, **REM rebound** can occur where the patient has an abnormally large amount of REM sleep, often leading to frequent and vivid dreams. Abuse of sedative-hypnotic drugs is common and discussed in Chapter 8.

BARBITURATES

Barbiturates were first introduced into clinical use in 1903 and were the standard drugs for treating insomnia and producing sedation. Chemically they are derivatives of barbituric acid. Although almost 50 different barbiturates are approved for clinical use in the United States, only a handful are in common clinical use today. This is due in part to the favorable safety profile and proven efficacy of the class of drugs commonly referred to as *benzodiazepines*. Barbiturates can produce many unwanted adverse effects. They are habit forming and have a low **therapeutic index** (i.e., there is only a narrow dosage range within which the drug is effective, and above that range it is rapidly toxic). Barbiturates can be classified into four groups based on their onset and duration of action. Table 12-3 lists the drugs in each category and summarizes their pharmacokinetic characteristics.

Mechanism of Action and Drug Effects

Barbiturates are CNS depressants that act primarily on the brainstem in an area called the *reticular formation*. Their sedative and hypnotic effects are dose related, and they act by reducing the nerve impulses traveling to the area of the brain called the *cerebral cortex*. Their ability to inhibit nerve impulse transmission is in part due to their ability to potentiate the action of an inhibitory amino acid known as **gamma-aminobutyric acid (GABA),** which is found in high concentrations in the CNS. Barbiturates are capable of raising the convulsive or seizure threshold and are

---

Table 12-1	**Sedative-Hypnotic Drugs: Points of Interest**
Drug	**Point**
butabarbital	Effects last about 6-8 hr; use cautiously in elderly patients; keep tablets in an airtight container.
estazolam	Give with food to minimize GI upset; always make sure patients have swallowed medication.
flurazepam	Causes less REM rebound than the other benzodiazepines; use cautiously in elderly patients; give 15-30 min before bedtime.
pentobarbital	Short acting; can be given PO, by rectal suppository, or IM; IM injection given deep in large muscle mass; as with any of these drugs, patients should avoid caffeine intake for 4 hr before or after the time of dosing because of the decreased effectiveness that results.
phenobarbital	Long acting (up to 16 hr); in the body longer and thus can react with other medications such as alcohol and other CNS depressants; because of long duration, use cautiously in elderly patients with decreased liver and renal function.
quazepam	Give 15-30 min before bedtime; hangover common in elderly patients.
secobarbital	Same as for pentobarbital; given PO; as with any sedative-hypnotic drug, do not mix with alcohol.
temazepam	Induces sleep within 20-40 min; give 20-30 min before bedtime.
triazolam	Short-term use only; try other medications in this category, as ordered by a physician; use cautiously in elderly patients— causes confusion, so protect patient from injury.

CNS, Central nervous system; *GI,* gastrointestinal; *IM,* intramuscular(ly); *PO,* orally; *REM,* rapid eye movement.

Table 12-2 Stages of Sleep

Stage	Characteristics	Average Percentage of Time in Stage (for Young Adult)
Non-REM Sleep		
1	Dozing or feelings of drifting off to sleep; person can be easily awakened; insomniacs have longer stage 1 periods than normal.	2%-5%
2	Relaxation, but person can easily be awakened; person has occasional REMs and also slight eye movements.	50%
3	Deep sleep; difficult to wake person; respiratory rates, pulse, and blood pressure may decrease.	5%
4	Very difficult to wake person; person may be very groggy if awakened; dreaming occurs, especially about daily events; sleepwalking or bedwetting may occur.	10%-15%
REM Sleep		
	REMs occur; vivid dreams occur; breathing may be irregular.	25%-33%

Modified from McKenry LM, Salerno E: *Mosby's pharmacology in nursing—revised and updated,* ed 21, St Louis, 2003, Mosby.
REM, Rapid eye movement.

Table 12-3 Barbiturates: Onset and Duration

Category	Pharmacokinetics		Barbiturates
	Onset	Duration	
Ultrashort	IV: less than 15 min	IV: less than 2 hr	methohexital, thiamylal, thiopental
Short	PO: 15-20 min	PO: 2-4 hr	pentobarbital, secobarbital
Intermediate	PO: 20-30 min	PO: 2-4 hr	butabarbital
Long	PO: 30-60 min	PO: 6-8 hr	phenobarbital, mephobarbital

IV, Intravenous; *PO,* oral.

therefore also effective in treating status epilepticus and tetanus- or drug-induced convulsions. In addition, selected barbiturates are used as prophylaxis for epileptic seizures.

At low dosages, barbiturates act as sedatives. Increasing the dosage produces a hypnotic effect but also decreases the respira-

tory rate. At normal dosages they have little effect on the circulation. Barbiturates as a class are notorious enzyme inducers. They stimulate the action of enzymes in the liver that are responsible for the metabolism or breakdown of many drugs. By stimulating the action of these enzymes, they cause many drugs to be metabolized more quickly, which usually shortens their duration of action. Other drugs that are enzyme inducers are warfarin, theophylline, and phenytoin.

Indications

All barbiturates have the same sedative-hypnotic effects but differ in their potency, onset, and duration of action. They are used as hypnotics, sedatives, and anticonvulsants and also for anesthesia during surgical procedures. The various categories of barbiturates are used for the following therapeutic purposes:

Ultrashort acting: Anesthesia for short surgical procedures, anesthesia induction, control of convulsions, narcoanalysis, and reduction in intracranial pressure in neurosurgical patients

Short acting: Sedative-hypnotic and control of convulsive conditions

Intermediate acting: Sedative-hypnotic and control of convulsive conditions

Long acting: Sedative-hypnotic, epileptic seizure prophylaxis, and treatment of neonatal hyperbilirubinemia

Contraindications

Contraindications to barbiturate use include known drug allergy, pregnancy, significant respiratory difficulties, and severe liver disease.

Adverse Effects

The main adverse effects of barbiturates affect the CNS and include drowsiness, lethargy, dizziness, hangover (prolongation of drowsiness, lethargy, and dizziness), and paradoxical restlessness or excitement. Their chronic effects on normal sleep architecture can be detrimental. Sleep research has shown that adequate rest is obtained from the sleep process only when there are proper

Table 12-4 Barbiturates: Adverse Effects

Body System	Adverse Effects
Cardiovascular	Vasodilation and hypotension, especially if given too rapidly
Gastrointestinal	Nausea, vomiting, diarrhea, constipation
Hematologic	Agranulocytosis, thrombocytopenia, megaloblastic anemia
Nervous	Drowsiness; lethargy; vertigo; headache; mental depression; myalgic, neuralgic, or arthralgic pain
Respiratory	Respiratory depression, apnea, laryngospasm, bronchospasm, coughing
Other	Hypersensitivity reactions: urticaria, angioedema, rash, fever, serum sickness, Stevens-Johnson syndrome

amounts of REM sleep, which is sometimes referred to as *dreaming sleep*. Barbiturates deprive people of REM sleep, which can result in agitation and an inability to deal with normal stress. When the barbiturate is stopped and REM sleep once again takes place, a rebound phenomenon can occur. During this rebound the proportion of REM sleep is increased, the patient's dream time constitutes a larger percentage of total sleep, and the dreams are often nightmares. The adverse effects of barbiturates and the body systems affected are listed in Table 12-4. Barbiturates, as is the case with most sedative drugs, are also associated with an increased incidence of falls when used in the elderly. If they are recommended at all, the usual dose is reduced by half whenever possible.

Toxicity and Management of Overdose

Overdose frequently results in respiratory depression leading to respiratory arrest. Often this is done therapeutically to induce anesthesia. In this situation, however, the patient is ventilated mechanically and respiration is controlled or assisted mechanically. Another situation in which intentional overdoses are given for therapeutic reasons is the management of uncontrollable seizures. Patients in such a seizure state are sometimes put into what is called a *phenobarbital coma*. Because of the inhibitory effects of barbiturates on nerve transmission in the brain (possibly GABA mediated), the uncontrollable seizures can be stopped until appropriate serum levels of anticonvulsant drugs are reached.

An overdose of barbiturates produces CNS depression ranging from sleep to profound coma and death. Respiratory depression progresses to Cheyne-Stokes respirations, hypoventilation, and cyanosis. Affected patients often have cold, clammy skin or are hypothermic, and later they can exhibit fever, areflexia, tachycardia, and hypotension. Pupils are usually slightly constricted but may be dilated in cases of severe drug toxicity.

Treatment of an overdose is mainly symptomatic and supportive. The mainstays of therapy are maintenance of an adequate airway, assisted respiration, and oxygen administration if needed, along with fluid and pressor support as indicated. Multiple-dose (every 4 hours) nasogastric administration of activated charcoal is very effective in removing barbiturates from the stomach and the circulation. Barbiturates are highly metabolized by the liver, and they increase enzyme activity there. In an overdose, however,

the amount of barbiturate may overwhelm the liver's ability to metabolize it. This is the situation in which administration of activated charcoal may be helpful. Activated charcoal assists in pulling the drug from the circulation and eliminating it by means of the gastrointestinal (GI) tract. Some of the barbiturates (phenobarbital, aprobarbital, and mephobarbital) can be eliminated more quickly by the kidneys when the urine is alkalized. This keeps the drug in the urine and prevents it from being resorbed back into the circulation. Alkalization, along with forced diuresis, can hasten elimination of the barbiturate.

Interactions

The drug interactions possible with barbiturates can be intense and often dramatic. The risk encountered in the coadministration of barbiturates with alcohol, antihistamines, benzodiazepines, opioids, and tranquilizers is additive CNS depression. Most of the drug-drug interactions involving barbiturates are secondary to the effects of barbiturates on the hepatic enzyme system. As mentioned previously, barbiturates increase the activity of hepatic microsomal enzymes. This process is called *enzyme induction*. Induction of this enzyme system results in increased drug metabolism and breakdown. However, if two drugs are competing for the same enzyme system for metabolism, the result can be inhibited drug metabolism or breakdown. Examples are the administration of monoamine oxidase inhibitors (MAOIs), anticoagulants, glucocorticoids, tricyclic antidepressants, quinidine, and oral contraceptives with barbiturates. Coadministration of MAOIs and barbiturates can result in prolonged barbiturate effects. Coadministration of anticoagulants with barbiturates can result in decreased anticoagulation response and possible clot formation. Coadministration of barbiturates with oral contraceptives can result in accelerated metabolism of the contraceptive drug and possible unintended pregnancy. Women taking both types of medication concurrently should be advised to consider an additional method of contraception as a backup.

Laboratory Test Interactions

Barbiturates can also interact with body substances and affect the results of various laboratory tests. Barbiturates can cause an increase in the serum levels of bilirubin, glutamic-pyruvic transaminase (alanine aminotransferase [ALT]), glutamic-oxaloacetic transaminase (aspartate aminotransferase [AST]), and alkaline phosphatase.

Dosages

As previously mentioned, barbiturates can act as either sedatives or hypnotics depending on the dosage. Selected barbiturates and their recommended sedative and hypnotic dosages are listed in the Dosages table on page 184.

Drug Profiles

Barbiturates are available in a variety of dosage forms, including tablets, capsules, elixirs, injections, and suppositories. They are all rated as pregnancy category D drugs by the U.S. Food and Drug Administration (FDA). All barbiturates are considered prescription-only drugs because of the potential for misuse and the severe effects that result if they are not used appropriately. From a legal standpoint they are con-

DOSAGES

Selected Barbiturates

Drug	Onset and Duration	Usual Dosage Range	Indications
butabarbital (Buticaps, Butisol, Butalan)	Intermediate acting	**Pediatric**	
		PO: 2-6 mg/kg before surgery	Preop sedative
		Adult	
		PO: 15-30 mg tid-qid	Sedative
		50-100 mg before surgery	Preop sedative
		50-100 mg	Hypnotic
pentobarbital (Nembutal)	Short acting	**Pediatric**	
		IM/IV/PO: 2-6 mg/kg; rectal: 2 mo-1 yr, 30 mg; 1-4 yr, 30-60 mg; 5-12 yr, 60 mg; 12-14 yr, 60-120 mg HS	Anticonvulsant, preop sedative, sedative
		Adult	
		PO: 100-200 mg HS	Hypnotic
		IM: 150-200 mg; rectal: 120-200 mg HS; IV: 100 mg	Anticonvulsant, preop sedative, hypnotic
phenobarbital (Solfoton, Luminal)	Long acting	**Neonatal**	
		PO: 5-10 mg/kg/day	Treatment of hyperbilirubinemia
		Pediatric	
		PO: 6 mg/kg in 3 equally divided doses	Sedative
		IM/IV: 1-3 mg/kg	Preop sedative
		Adult	
		PO: 30-120 mg/day divided	Sedative
		100-320 mg HS	Hypnotic
		IM/IV: 100-200 mg 60-90 min before surgery	Preop sedative
secobarbital (Seconal)	Short acting	**Pediatric**	
		PO: 2-6 mg/kg	Preop sedative
		Adult	
		PO: 100 mg HS	Hypnotic
		200-300 mg 1-2 hr before surgery	Preop sedative

HS, At bedtime; *IM*, intramuscular; *IV*, intravenous; *PO*, oral; *preop*, preoperatively.

Table 12-5 Barbiturates: Controlled Substance Schedule

Schedule	Barbiturates
C-II	Pentobarbital, secobarbital
C-III	Butabarbital
C-IV	phenobarbital

sidered controlled substances. As discussed in Chapter 4, controlled substances are medications that the U.S. Drug Enforcement Administration has identified as drugs that have a high abuse potential. State laws are often more stringent than federal laws in terms of the way in which these drugs are dispensed; therefore, health care providers must be careful to comply with both federal and state laws. The controlled substance schedule classifications of selected barbiturates are listed in Table 12-5. Use of barbiturates is contraindicated in patients with known hypersensitivity reactions to them, latent porphyria, significant liver dysfunction, and known previous addiction.

pentobarbital

Formerly prescribed as a sedative-hypnotic for insomnia, pentobarbital is now principally used preoperatively to relieve anxiety and provide sedation. In addition, it is used occasionally to control status epilepticus or acute seizure episodes resulting from meningitis, poisons, eclampsia, alcohol withdrawal, tetanus, and chorea. Pentobarbital may also be used to treat withdrawal symptoms in patients who are physically dependent on barbiturates or nonbarbiturate hypnotics. Pregnancy category D. The sedative and hypnotic dosages are given in the Dosages table on this page.

Pharmacokinetics

Half-Life	Onset	Peak	Duration
PO: 35-50 hr	PO: 15-60 min	PO: 30-60 min	PO: 1-4 hr
IV: 35-50 hr	IV: Less than 1 min	IV: Less than 30 min	IV: 15 min

phenobarbital

Phenobarbital is the barbiturate most commonly prescribed, either alone or in combination with other drugs. It is considered the prototypical barbiturate and is classified as a long-acting drug. Phenobarbital is used for the prevention of generalized tonic clonic seizures and fever-induced convulsions. In addition, it has been useful in the treatment of hyperbilirubinemia in neonates. It has also been used for the treatment of Gilbert's syndrome. It is only rarely used today as a sedative-hypnotic drug. Pregnancy category D. See the table on this page for dosages.

Pharmacokinetics

Half-Life	Onset	Peak	Duration
PO: 53-118 hr	PO: 30 min	PO: 8-12 hr	PO: 10-12 hr
IV: 53-118 hr	IV: 5 min	IV: 30 min	IV: 4-10 hr

secobarbital

Secobarbital is used primarily as a hypnotic drug to induce sleep. It is now prescribed much less commonly than before because of the availability of the hypnotic benzodiazepines. It may be administered intravenously to control status epilepticus or acute seizures, similar to the way in which pentobarbital is used. It may also be given to maintain a steady state of unconsciousness during general, spinal, or regional anesthesia or to facilitate intubation procedures. Pregnancy category D. The common sedative and hypnotic dosages are given in the dosages table on page 184.

Pharmacokinetics

Half-Life	Onset	Peak	Duration
PO: 30 hr	PO: 15 min	PO: 2-4 hr	PO: 1-4 hr
IV: 30 hr	IV: 1-3 min	IV: Less than 30 min	IV: 15 min

BENZODIAZEPINES

Benzodiazepines are the most commonly prescribed sedative-hypnotic drugs and one of the most commonly prescribed classes of drugs. This is directly attributable to their favorable adverse effect profiles, efficacy, and safety. Even when a drug in this class is taken as the sole drug in an overdose (e.g., not with alcohol), it is relatively benign, causing little more than sedation. Benzodiazepines are classified as either anxiolytics or sedatives-hypnotics depending on their primary usage. An **anxiolytic** relieves anxiety. The benzodiazepines discussed in Chapter 15 are the ones that work primarily to produce sedation or sleep. There are five such benzodiazepines commonly used as sedative-hypnotic drugs. They are listed in Table 12-6 and can be further classified on the basis of their duration of action as either long acting or short acting.

Mechanism of Action and Drug Effects

As mentioned previously, the sedative and hypnotic action of benzodiazepines is related to their ability to depress activity in the CNS. The specific areas they affect in the CNS appear to be the hypothalamic, thalamic, and limbic systems of the brain. Recent research has indicated that there are specific receptors in the brain for benzodiazepines. These receptors are thought to be the same as those of the CNS inhibitory transmitter GABA. If they are not the same, then they are adjacent to the GABA receptors. Their depressant action on the CNS appears to be related to their ability to inhibit stimulation of the brain. They have many favorable characteristics compared with the barbiturates. They do not suppress REM sleep to the same extent as do barbiturates. They also do not induce hepatic microsomal enzyme activity and are

Table 12-6	**Sedative-Hypnotic Benzodiazepines**

Generic Name	Trade Name
Long Acting	
estazolam	ProSom
eszopiclone*	Lunesta
flurazepam	Dalmane
quazepam	Doral
Short Acting	
temazepam	Restoril
triazolam	Halcion
zaleplon*	Sonata
zolpidem*	Ambien

NOTE: The benzodiazepines discussed in Chapter 15 and those described here have similar pharmacologic properties. They all act as anxiolytics and sedatives-hypnotics. Different benzodiazepines are just more effective at one or the other pharmacologic effect.
*These drugs share many characteristics with the benzodiazepines but are classified as nonbenzodiazepine hypnotic drugs.

therefore safe to administer to patients who are taking medications metabolized by this enzyme system.

In terms of patient experience, benzodiazepines have a calming effect on the CNS. This causes the inhibition of hyperexcitable nerves in the CNS that might be responsible for initiating seizure activity. Similarly, this calming effect on the CNS makes benzodiazepines useful in controlling agitation and anxiety. It also reduces excessive sensory stimulation and induces sleep. In addition, benzodiazepines have been shown to induce skeletal muscle relaxation. Their receptors in the CNS are in the same area as those that play a role in alcohol addiction. Therefore, they are used in the treatment and prevention of the symptoms of alcohol withdrawal (see Chapter 15).

Indications

Benzodiazepines have a variety of therapeutic applications. They are most commonly used for sedation, sleep induction, skeletal muscle relaxation, and anxiety relief. They have also been used in the treatment of alcohol withdrawal, agitation, depression, and epilepsy. They are often combined with anesthetics, analgesics, and neuromuscular blocking drugs in what is called *balanced anesthesia* and also *moderate* or *"conscious" sedation.* (see Chapter 11). They are used in this setting mostly for their amnesiac properties, because most persons undergoing surgery would rather not remember the events of their procedure.

Contraindications

Contraindications to the use of benzodiazepines include known drug allergy, narrow-angle glaucoma, and pregnancy.

Adverse Effects

As a class, benzodiazepines have a relatively safe adverse effect profile. The adverse effects associated with their use are usually mild and primarily involve the CNS. The more commonly reported undesirable effects are headache, drowsiness, paradoxical excitement or nervousness, dizziness or vertigo, cognitive impairment, and lethargy. Benzodiazepines can create a significant fall hazard in frail elderly patients, however, and their use should be avoided when possible in this patient population. To help prevent adverse effects, the lowest effective dosages are recommended for all patients, especially the elderly. Because of the effect of the benzodiazepines on the normal sleep cycle, a hangover effect is sometimes reported. Other less common adverse effects are palpitations, dry mouth, nausea, vomiting, hypokinesia, and occasional nightmares.

Toxicity and Management of Overdose

An overdose of benzodiazepines may result in one or all of the following symptoms: somnolence, confusion, coma, and diminished reflexes. An overdose of just benzodiazepines rarely results in hypotension and respiratory depression. These are more commonly seen when benzodiazepines are taken with other CNS depressants such as alcohol or barbiturates. The same holds true for their lethal effects. In the absence of the concurrent ingestion of alcohol or other CNS depressants, benzodiazepine overdose rarely results in death.

The treatment of benzodiazepine intoxication is generally symptomatic and supportive. If ingestion is recent, decontamination of the GI system is indicated. As a rule of thumb, the administration

Table 12-7	Flumazenil Treatment Regimen	
Indication	**Recommended Regimen**	**Duration**
Reversal of conscious sedation or general anesthesia	Give 0.2 mg (2 mL) IV over 15 sec, then give 0.2 mg if consciousness does not occur; may be repeated at 60-sec intervals prn up to 4 additional times (maximum total dose, 1 mg)	1-4 hr
Management of suspected benzodiazepine overdose	Give 0.2 mg (2 mL) IV over 30 sec; wait 30 sec, then give 0.3 mg (3 mL) over 30 sec if consciousness does not occur; further doses of 0.5 mg (5 mL) can be given over 30 sec at intervals of 1 min up to a cumulative dose of 3 mg	1-4 hr

IMPORTANT NOTE: Flumazenil has a relatively short half-life and a duration of effect of 1-4 hr; therefore, if flumazenil is used to reverse the effects of a long-acting benzodiazepine, the dose of the reversal drug may wear off and the patient may become sedated again, requiring more flumazenil. *IV*, Intravenously.

Table 12-8	Benzodiazepines: Drug Interactions	
Drug	**Mechanism**	**Result**
cimetidine	Decreased benzodiazepine metabolism	Prolonged benzodiazepine action
CNS depressants	Additive effects	Increased CNS depression
MAOIs	Decreased metabolism	Increased benzodiazepine effects
Protease inhibitors	Decreased metabolism	Increased benzodiazepine effects

CNS, Central nervous system; *MAOI*, monoamine oxidase inhibitor.

of syrup of ipecac (an emetic drug used to induce vomiting in overdose) to produce gastric decontamination is contraindicated in patients who have ingested medications that cause sedation. The concern is that an unconscious patient induced to vomit could easily aspirate stomach contents. Therefore, gastric lavage is generally the best and most effective means of gastric decontamination. Activated charcoal and a saline cathartic may be administered after gastric lavage to remove any remaining drug. Hemodialysis is not useful in the treatment of benzodiazepine overdose. Flumazenil can be used to acutely reverse the sedative effects of benzodiazepines, although this is normally done only in cases of excessive overdose or sedation. Flumazenil antagonizes the action of benzodiazepines on the CNS by directly competing with benzodiazepines for binding at the benzodiazepine receptors in the CNS. It has a stronger affinity for the receptor than do the benzodiazepines, however, and knocks the benzodiazepine off the receptor, which reverses the sedative action of the benzodiazepine. The dosage regimens to be followed for the reversal of conscious sedation or general anesthesia induced by benzodiazepines and the management of suspected benzodiazepine overdose are summarized in Table 12-7.

Interactions

The potential drug interactions with the benzodiazepines are significant because of their intensity, particularly when they involve other CNS depressants (e.g., alcohol, analgesics). These drugs may result in further CNS depressant effects (including decreased blood pressure, respiratory rate, sedation, confusion, and diminished reflexes). Herbal interactions include kava kava and valerian, which may also lead to further CNS depression. Food-drug interactions include grapefruit or grapefruit juice, which alters drug absorption. Prior to

use of any drugs that are within the category of CNS depressants, it is always important to remember that when combined with other drugs affecting the CNS, there is a 90% chance of causing adverse drug reactions. The risks associated with the coadministration of these and some other drugs are described in Table 12-8.

Laboratory Test Interactions

No laboratory test interactions occur with the five benzodiazepines that are typically used as either sedatives or hypnotics.

Dosages

The benzodiazepines discussed in this chapter are those that are commonly used to treat insomnia. Therefore, the dosage recommendations given in the Dosages table on page 187 are those for achieving hypnotic effects. All drugs administered for the treatment of insomnia should be limited to short-term usage of 2 to 4 weeks or less. With long-term usage, rebound insomnia and severe withdrawal can develop. Elderly patients should also be started on lower dosages, because they generally experience a more pronounced effect from benzodiazepines.

Drug Profiles

Benzodiazepines are all prescription-only drugs, and they are designated as Schedule IV controlled substances. All five benzodiazepines discussed here have active metabolites that can accumulate during long-term use, especially in patients who have altered metabolic function (hepatic dysfunction) or altered excretion capabilities (renal dysfunction). There are several other benzodiazepines, but they are more commonly used to treat anxiety or agitation, to produce amnesia, and to relax skeletal muscles. These other benzodiazepines are discussed in detail in the appropriate chapters.

Zolpidem (Ambien), zaleplon (Sonata), and eszoplicone (Lunesta) share many characteristics with the benzodiazepines but are classified as nonbenzodiazepine hypnotic drugs. Zolpidem is a nonbenzodiazepine hypnotic of the imidazopyridine class, and zaleplon is a nonbenzodiazepine hypnotic of the pyrazolopyrimidine class. Eszoplicone is a newer, miscellaneous hypnotic drug (see Miscellaneous Drugs). The pharmacologic properties of these drugs are similar to those of the benzodiazepines in that they have sedative, anxiolytic, muscle relaxant, and anticonvulsive effects. They are indicated for the short-term (7- to 10-day) treatment of insomnia, are only available orally, and are designated as Schedule IV controlled substances.

estazolam

Estazolam (ProSom) is available in 1- and 2-mg tablets. The usual adult dosage is 1 to 2 mg at bedtime; the dosage for elderly patients is usually 0.5 mg at bedtime (see the Dosages table on p. 187). Pregnancy category X.

DOSAGES

Benzodiazepines: Selected Hypnotic Drugs

Drug	Onset and Duration Range	Usual Dosage Range	Indications
estazolam (ProSom)	Short acting	**Adult** PO: 1-2 mg HS **Elderly** PO: 0.5 mg HS	Hypnotic
flurazepam (Dalmane)	Long acting	**Adult** PO: 15-30 mg HS	Hypnotic
quazepam (Doral)	Long acting	**Adult** PO: 7.5 or 15 mg HS	Hypnotic
▶temazepam (Restoril)	Short acting	**Adult** PO: 15-30 mg HS **Elderly** PO: 7.5 mg HS	Hypnotic
triazolam, (Halcion)	Short acting	**Adult** PO: 0.25-0.5 mg HS **Elderly** PO: 0.125-0.25 mg HS	Hypnotic
▶zaleplon* (Sonata)	Short acting	**Adult** PO: 10 mg HS **Elderly** PO: 5 mg HS	Hypnotic
▶zolpidem* (Ambien)	Short acting	**Adult** PO: 10 mg HS **Elderly** PO: 5 mg HS	Hypnotic
eszoplicone* (Lunesta)	Long acting	**Adult:** PO: 2-5 mg HS **Elderly** PO: 1 mg HS	Hypnotic

HS, At bedtime; *PO,* oral.
*Nonbenzodiazepine drugs.

Pharmacokinetics

Half-Life	Onset	Peak	Duration
10-24 hr	20 min	2 hr	24 hr

flurazepam

Flurazepam (Dalmane) is available in 15- and 30-mg capsules. It is considered a long-acting hypnotic drug and is indicated for the short-term treatment of insomnia for periods of up to 4 weeks. Flurazepam has two active metabolites that account for its hypnotic effects. These active metabolites have also been shown to be responsible for inducing a hangover effect, causing lethargy or grogginess the morning after the medication has been taken. Pregnancy category X. The recommended dosages for adult and elderly patients are given in the table on this page.

Pharmacokinetics

Half-Life	Onset	Peak	Duration
50-100 hr	15-45 min	30-60 min	7-8 hr

quazepam

Quazepam (Doral) is available in 7.5- and 15-mg tablets. Quazepam is considered a long-acting hypnotic drug and is indicated for the short-term treatment of insomnia for periods of up to 4 weeks. Pregnancy category X. The recommended dosages for adult and elderly patients are given in the table on this page.

Pharmacokinetics

Half-Life	Onset	Peak	Duration
25-41 hr	30 min	2 hr	20 hr

▶ temazepam

Temazepam (Restoril) is available in 7.5-, 15-, and 30-mg capsules. Its use is contraindicated in patients who have narrow-angle glaucoma because it can exacerbate the glaucoma. It is indicated for the short-term treatment of insomnia. Pregnancy category X. The common dosages are given in the table on this page.

Pharmacokinetics

Half-Life	Onset	Peak	Duration
9.5-12.4 hr	30-60 min	2-3 hr	7-8 hr

triazolam

Triazolam (Halcion) is available in 0.125- and 0.25-mg tablets and is indicated for the short-term treatment of insomnia. The best approach with this drug is for the nurse to give the smallest effective dose for the shortest possible duration. Pregnancy category X. The common dosages are given in the table on this page.

Pharmacokinetics

Half-Life	Onset	Peak	Duration
2-5 hr	15-30 min	0.5-1.5 hr	6-7 hr

▶ *zaleplon*

Zaleplon (Sonata) is the newest short-acting nonbenzodiazepine hypnotic drug. However, its hypnotic effects do arise from chemical activity at the benzodiazepine-GABA receptor complex. It is indicated for the short-term treatment of insomnia and has been shown to be effective for up to 5 weeks. However, its use is ideally recommended for no more than 10 days to avoid dependency. It has no known contraindications except known allergy to the drug. A unique advantage of this drug stems from its very short half-life: patients whose sleep difficulties include early awakenings can dose themselves in the middle of the night as long as they take the drug at least 4 hours before they must arise. It is available in both 5- and 10-mg capsules. Pregnancy category C. Common dosages are given in the table on page 187.

Pharmacokinetics

Half-Life	Onset	Peak	Duration
1 hr	Rapid	1 hr	6-8 hr

▶ *zolpidem*

Zolpidem (Ambien) is a short-acting nonbenzodiazepine hypnotic drug. It is indicated for the short-term treatment of insomnia, and its use should be limited to 7 to 10 days of treatment. Zolpidem is currently contraindicated only in cases of known drug allergy. Zolpidem has a relatively short half-life compared with the benzodiazepines and no active metabolites. These two characteristics may account for the fact that less lethargy or grogginess is experienced in the morning after this medication has been taken than after taking the hypnotic benzodiazepines. It is available in 5- and 10-mg tablets. Pregnancy category B. The recommended dosage is given in the table on page 187.

Pharmacokinetics

Half-Life	Onset	Peak	Duration
1.4-4.5 hr	Unknown	1.6 hr	Unknown

MUSCLE RELAXANTS

A variety of conditions such as trauma, inflammation, anxiety, and pain can be associated with acute muscle spasms. Although there is no completely satisfactory form of therapy available for relief of skeletal muscle spasticity, muscle relaxants are capable of providing some relief. The muscle relaxants are a group of compounds that act predominantly within the CNS to relieve pain associated with skeletal muscle spasms. The majority of muscle relaxants are known as *central-acting skeletal muscle relaxants* because their site of action is the CNS. Central-acting skeletal muscle relaxants are similar in structures and action to other CNS depressants such as diazepam. It is believed that the muscle relaxant effects of these drugs are related to this CNS depressant activity. Only one of these compounds, dantrolene, acts directly on skeletal muscle. It belongs to a group of relaxants know as *direct-acting skeletal muscle relaxants*. It closely resembles GABA.

These drugs are most effective when they are used in conjunction with rest and physical therapy. When muscle relaxants are taken with alcohol, other CNS depressants, or opioid analgesics, enhanced CNS depressant effects are seen. In such cases, close monitoring and dosage reduction of one or both drugs should be considered.

Mechanism of Action and Drug Effects

As noted earlier, the majority of the muscle relaxants work within the CNS. Their beneficial effects are believed to come from their sedative effects rather than from direct muscle re-

laxation. Dantrolene has direct effects on skeletal muscle. All others have no direct effects on muscles, nerve conduction, or muscle-nerve junctions. One of the more effective drugs in this class, baclofen, is a derivative of GABA. It is believed to work by depressing nerve transmission in the spinal cord. The other drugs in this class are not derivatives of GABA but act by enhancing GABA's central inhibitory effects at the level of the spinal cord. These drugs are generally less effective than baclofen. Dantrolene acts directly on the excitation-contraction coupling of muscle fibers and not at the level of the CNS. It appears to exert its action by decreasing the amount of calcium released from storage sites in the sarcoplasmic reticulum.

As noted earlier, muscle relaxants have a depressant effect on the CNS. Their effects are the result of CNS depression in the brain primarily at the level of the brainstem, thalamus, and basal ganglia but also at the spinal cord. Dantrolene acts directly on skeletal muscles by decreasing the response of the muscle to stimuli. The effects of muscle relaxants are relaxation of striated muscles, mild weakness of skeletal muscles, decreased force of muscle contraction, and muscle stiffness. Other drug effects that may be experienced include generalized CNS depression manifested as sedation, somnolence, ataxia, and respiratory and cardiovascular depression.

Indications

Muscle relaxants are primarily used for the relief of painful musculoskeletal conditions such as muscle spasms. They are most effective when used in conjunction with physical therapy. They may also be used in the management of spasticity associated with severe chronic disorders such as multiple sclerosis and other types of cerebral lesions, cerebral palsy, and rheumatic disorders. Some relaxants are used to reduce choreiform movement in patients with Huntington's chorea, to reduce rigidity in patients with parkinsonian syndrome, or to relieve the pain associated with trigeminal neuralgia. Intravenous dantrolene is used for the management of the full-blown hypermetabolism of skeletal muscle that is characteristic of a malignant hyperthermia crisis. Another muscle relaxant, baclofen, has been shown to be effective in relieving hiccups.

Contraindications

The only usual contraindication to the use of muscle relaxants is known drug allergy, but contraindications for some drugs may also include severe renal impairment.

Adverse Effects

The primary adverse effects of muscle relaxants are an extension of their effects on the CNS and skeletal muscles. Euphoria, lightheadedness, dizziness, drowsiness, fatigue, and muscle weakness are often experienced early in treatment. These adverse effects are generally short lived, with patients growing tolerant to them over time. Less common adverse effects seen with the muscle relaxants include diarrhea, GI upset, headache, slurred speech, muscle stiffness, constipation, sexual difficulties in males, hypotension, tachycardia, and weight gain. Dantrolene has a strong potential to cause hepatotoxicity. However, this is rare, occurring in 0.1% to 0.2% of patients treated with the drug for more than 60 days.

Toxicity and Management of Overdose

The toxicities and consequences of an overdose of muscle relaxants primarily involve the CNS. There is no specific antidote or reversal drug for muscle relaxant overdoses. They are best treated with conservative supportive measures. More aggressive therapies are generally needed when muscle relaxants are taken along with other CNS depressant drugs as an overdose. Gastric lavage and close observation of the patient are recommended. An adequate airway should be maintained and means of artificial respiration should be readily available. Electrocardiographic monitoring should be instituted and large quantities of intravenous fluids should be administered to avoid crystalluria.

Interactions

When muscle relaxants are administered along with other depressant drugs such as alcohol and benzodiazepines, caution should be used to avoid overdosage. The combination of propoxyphene and orphenadrine has resulted in additive CNS effects. Mental confusion, anxiety, tremors, and additive hypoglycemic activity have been reported with this combination as well. A dosage reduction and/or discontinuance of one or both drugs is recommended.

Laboratory Test Interactions

A reducing substance in the urine of patients receiving metaxalone may produce false-positive results in glucose determinations using cupric sulfate (Benedict's solution, Clinitest, Fehling's solution) but does not interfere with glucose testing using glucose oxidase (Clinistix, Diastix, Tes-Tape). Although these types of tests are somewhat outdated, they are still used in some patient care settings.

Dosages

For an overview of dosages for the more commonly used muscle relaxants, see the Dosages table on this page.

Drug Profiles

Muscle relaxants are all prescription-only drugs and are all (except for one) centrally acting relaxants because of their site of action in the CNS. These include baclofen (Lioresal), carisoprodol (Rela, Soma), chlorphenesin (Maolate), chlorzoxazone (Paraflex), cyclobenzaprine (Flexeril), metaxalone (Skelaxin), methocarbamol (Robaxin, Mardaxin), and orphenadrine (Disipal, Norflex). Use of all muscle relaxants is contraindicated in patients who have shown a hypersensitivity reaction to them or have compromised pulmonary function, active hepatic disease, or impaired myocardial function.

▶ baclofen

Baclofen (Lioresal) is available in 10- and 20-mg tablets and in a 0.5- and a 2-mg/mL concentration for injection. The usual oral dosage is 5 mg 3 times daily for 3 days. The recommendation is then to increase the dose by 5 mg every 3 days until a maximum of 20 mg 3 times daily is reached, with titration to the desired response. When the drug is given via the intrathecal route, a compatible pump must be implanted. With this administration route a test dose should be administered initially to test for a positive response. The injection is diluted before infusion. Pregnancy category C.

Pharmacokinetics

Half-Life	Onset	Peak	Duration
2.5-4 hr	0.5-1 hr	2-3 hr	Longer than 8 hr

▶ cyclobenzaprine

Cyclobenzaprine (Flexeril) is available in a 10-mg dose. Cyclobenzaprine is a central-acting muscle relaxant that is structurally and pharmacologically related to the tricyclic antidepressants. The usual oral dosage is 10 mg 3 times daily for 1 week. Dosage can be increased to a maximum of 60 mg daily. Pregnancy category B.

Pharmacokinetics

Half-Life	Onset	Peak	Duration
1-3 days	1 hr	3-8 hr	12-24 hr

dantrolene

Dantrolene (Dantrium) is available in 25-, 50-, and 100-mg capsules and as a 20-mg parenteral injection. Dantrolene is a direct-acting muscle relaxant that is pharmacologically different from the central-

DOSAGES

Selected Muscle Relaxants

Drug	Pharmacologic Class	Usual Dosage Range	Indications
▶baclofen (Lioresal)	Central acting	**Adult** PO: 5 mg tid × 3 days, then 10 mg tid × 3 days, then 15 mg tid, then titrated to response Intrathecal: 120-1500 mcg/day	Spasticity
▶cyclobenzaprine (Flexeril)	Central acting	**Adult** PO: 10-20 mg tid	Spasticity
dantrolene (Dantrium)	Direct acting	**Pediatric** PO: 1 mg/kg/day given in divided doses bid-qid **Adult** PO: 25 mg/day; may increase to 25-100 mg bid-qid	Spasticity and malignant hyperthermia
		Pediatric and adult IV: 1 mg/kg, may repeat to total dose of 10 mg/kg	Malignant hyperthermia
metaxalone (Skelaxin)	Central acting	**Pediatric (older than 12 yr) and adult** PO: 400-800 mg tid-qid	Acute painful muscle spasticity
tizanidine (Zanaflex)	Central acting	**Adult** PO: 2-4 mg tid	Spasticity

IV, Intravenous; *PO,* oral.

acting relaxants in that it can work directly on the skeletal muscles. It can be administered orally to children at a dosage of 1 mg/kg/day in two to three divided doses or to an adult at a dosage of 25 mg/day. In adults, dantrolene dosage can be increased to 25 to 100 mg 2 to 4 times daily when given orally. Dantrolene is also indicated for the acute management of malignant hyperthermia. This serious condition can occur on its own or as a complication of general anesthesia. When dantrolene is given for malignant hyperthermia it is administered intravenously at a dosage of 1 mg/kg and may be repeated until a total dose of 10 mg/kg has been given. Pregnancy category C.

Pharmacokinetics

Half-Life	Onset	Peak	Duration
8 hr	0.5-1 hr	5 hr	12-24 hr

MISCELLANEOUS DRUGS

There are several other sedative-hypnotic medications that do not fall into the barbiturate or benzodiazepine drug classes. These drugs include chloral hydrate, glutethimide, methyprylon, ethchlorvynol, tizanidine, paraldehyde, and (most recently) eszoplicone. These are all prescription-only drugs. Of these six sedative-hypnotic drugs, chloral hydrate and tizanidine are the ones most commonly prescribed, because the other four are associated with severe adverse effects and are extremely toxic if taken inappropriately or in an overdose.

Chloral hydrate (Noctec) is one of the oldest nonbarbiturate, miscellaneous-category sedative-hypnotic drugs. It has the favorable characteristic of not suppressing REM sleep at the usual therapeutic doses, and the incidence of hangover effects associated with its use is low because of its relatively short duration of action. One potential disadvantage to its use is that tachyphylaxis can develop rather quickly. **Tachyphylaxis** is the rapid appearance of a progressive decrease in response to a pharmacologically or physiologically active substance after its repetitive administration. This makes chloral hydrate useful only for short-term therapy. High doses lead to dependence and cause GI tract irritation. The combination of alcohol and chloral hydrate leads to rapid loss of consciousness. This combination is commonly referred to as a "Mickey Finn."

Tizanidine (Zanaflex) is a short-acting, centrally active α-adrenergic receptor agonist similar to clonidine. Tizanidine is a muscle relaxant but is not chemically classified with the other major drug categories in this chapter. It has been shown to reduce spastic muscle tone and decrease the frequency of daytime muscle spasms and nighttime awakenings caused by spasms. It is indicated for increased muscle tone associated with spasticity. It has been used in Europe and Japan for over a decade but was approved relatively recently for use in the United States. It is most commonly used in patients with multiple sclerosis or spinal cord injury. The typical starting dosage is 4 mg at bedtime. It is then slowly titrated to a maintenance dosage of 4 mg 3 times daily. Patients are less likely to suffer from hypotension and bradycardia when it is slowly titrated.

Eszoplicone (Lunesta) is the newest prescription hypnotic to become available. It is the first such drug to be approved for long-term use in treatment of insomnia. The usual starting dose is 1 mg, with titration as needed to 2 or 3 mg nightly.

Nonprescription sleeping aids often contain antihistamines, and some may also contain analgesics such as aspirin or acet-aminophen. The most common antihistamines contained in over-the-counter sleeping aids are doxylamine, diphenhydramine, and pyrilamine. Besides having antihistaminic effects, these drugs are heavily sedating. They have a depressant effect on the CNS. Analgesics are sometimes added to offer some pain relief if pain is a component of the sleep disturbance or insomnia. As with other CNS depressants, such as barbiturates and benzodiazepines, patients should avoid the consumption of alcohol when taking these drugs. The combination may result in respiratory depression and death.

◆ NURSING PROCESS

◆ ASSESSMENT

Before administering any CNS depressant drug, whether a barbiturate, benzodiazepine, muscle relaxant, nonbenzodiazepine, or miscellaneous drug, the nurse needs to determine allergies and whether the patient has any conditions that would be contraindications or cautions to receiving the drug. The patient's mental status (mood, affect, level of consciousness, memory) should be assessed and documented, because a lack of sleep itself may lead to confusion, mood changes, and restlessness. A sleep diary or journal with a description of the patient's sleep habits, patterns, and any related problems may be available and would provide insight into a patient's insomnia. The nurse must also assess the patient's vital signs, including supine and erect blood pressures, respirations, and temperature, especially if the intravenous use of any of these drugs is planned. For example, if an intravenous dosage form of any of these drugs is administered, a rapid drop could occur in blood pressure and other vital parameters such as respiratory rate, so administering the drug per protocol is critical to patient safety. Also, the drug may need to be withheld if the blood pressure and other vital signs are below normal limits and are unable to sustain further decreases. In addition, a neurologic assessment should also be performed and documented before initiation of therapy.

Cautions, contraindications, and drug interactions for barbiturates were discussed earlier in the chapter. Other assessment data includes renal and liver function and lifespan considerations (e.g., because barbiturates rapidly cross the placenta and pass into breast milk; respiratory depression may be problematic in neonates during labor; withdrawal symptoms may appear in neonates born to women who have taken barbiturates during their last trimester). Barbiturates may produce paradoxical excitement in children and confusion and mental depression in the elderly, so baseline neurological assessment is needed.

Patients taking benzodiazepines and other chemically related drugs (benzodiazepine-like drugs) should be assessed for previous allergic reactions to these drugs. Cautious use with close monitoring of the patient's response to the drug and vital signs is indicated in patients who are anemic, suicidal, and have a history of alcohol or other substance abuse. Cautious use is also indicated in the elderly and the very young because of their increased sensitivity to these drugs as well as in those who are younger than the age of 18 years, are pregnant, or are lactating. In addition, before initiating drug therapy with the benzodiazepines and most other sedative-hypnotic drugs, the physician may order blood studies such as hematocrit, hemoglobin level, and red blood cell count. Tests of renal function (blood urea nitrogen or creatinine levels) or hepatic function (alkaline phosphatase) may be ordered to rule out any potential problems from organ dysfunction, such as a decreased excretion capability with renal dysfunction and decreased metabolic abilities with hepatic dysfunction. Life span assessment considerations regarding placental crossing and distribution of the drug into breast milk are similar to those for the barbiturates, and fetal abnormalities may occur if these drugs are used during the first trimester of pregnancy. Other assessment data related to lifespan include the fact that drug dosages may need to be decreased in children and the elderly to avoid ataxia and excessive sedation. Potential drug interactions have also been previously discussed and presented in Table 12-8, but it is significant to note that use of any other CNS depressant drug may lead to severe decreases of blood pressure, respiratory rate, reflexes, and level of consciousness.

For muscle relaxants, drug allergies should also be noted before use. A head-to-toe assessment, with focus on the neurologic system, should also be completed. Cautions, contraindications, and drug interactions were discussed previously. With the elderly, there is increased risk of CNS toxicity with possible hallucinations, confusion, and excessive sedation. Assessment associated with the use of miscellaneous drugs (e.g., chloral hydrate) includes taking a thorough health and medication history and examining the complete patient profile with associated laboratory studies. Cautions, contraindications, and drug interactions for miscellaneous drugs have been previously discussed.

With the non-benzodiazepines such as zaleplon, zolpidem tartrate, and eszopiclone, assessment should include a head-to-toe appraisal and a thorough health and medication history. Allergies to these drugs and to aspirin should be assessed and documented. If a patient has been allergic to aspirin, there is an associated risk of allergies to non-benzodiazepines. Other considerations include the need for assessment of any confusion and lightheadedness, especially in the elderly because of their increased sensitivity to these drugs.

◆ NURSING DIAGNOSES

- Impaired gas exchange related to the respiratory depression associated with CNS depressants
- Deficient knowledge related to inadequate information about the various CNS depressant drugs
- Disturbed sleep patterns related to the drug's interference with REM sleep
- Risk for injury and falls to self related to drug-related decreased sensorium
- Risk for injury to self related to possible drug overdose or adverse reactions related to drug-drug interactions (e.g., combined use of the drug with alcohol, tranquilizers, and/or analgesics)
- Risk for injury, addiction, related to physical or psychologic dependency on CNS drugs

◆ PLANNING
Goals

- Patient remains free of respiratory depression.
- Patient remains free of further sleep deprivation.
- Patient experiences little or no rebound insomnia.

- Patient remains free of self-injury and falls related to decreased sensorium.
- Patient complies with drug therapy and keeps follow-up appointments with the physician or other health care professional.
- Patient regains normal sleep patterns.
- Patient remains free of or experiences minimal adverse effects and toxic effects from sedative-hypnotic drugs, muscle relaxants, and other CNS depressants.
- Patient remains free of drug interaction effects.
- Patient experiences no problems with addiction.

Outcome Criteria

- Patient states the common adverse effects, toxic effects, and symptoms related to sedative-hypnotic drugs to be reported to the physician, such as drowsiness, confusion, and respiratory depression.
- Patient states ways to minimize self-injury and falls related to decreased sensorium, such as changing positions slowly.
- Patient states risk for REM interference from sedative-hypnotic drugs with associated sleep hangovers and uses non-pharmacologic measures as appropriate.
- Patient states the common adverse effects related to muscle relaxants such as euphoria, dizziness, drowsiness, and fatigue.
- Patient minimizes adverse effects and toxic effects by taking medications as prescribed.
- Patient states the common drug interactions with alcohol and other medications (e.g., tranquilizers and analgesics) that may be life threatening.
- Patient states the importance of taking measures to minimize problems with addiction, such as taking medication only as needed.
- Patient, family, or significant other states the need to contact physician about possible complications, such as respiratory depression.
- Patient demonstrates increased knowledge related to inadequate information about pharmacologic and non-pharmacologic treatment and regimen for sleeping disturbance.

◆ IMPLEMENTATION

For management of sleep disorders, the benzodiazepines and non-benzodiazepines are generally used, because the barbiturates have a greater addiction potential as well as more CNS depressant adverse effects. However, barbiturates may be indicated in specific situations. Short-acting barbiturates (e.g., secobarbital) should be given 15 to 30 minutes before bedtime, as should some of the intermediate-acting drugs (e.g., butabarbital). The longer-acting drugs such as phenobarbital have an onset of action of 60 minutes. Oral dosage forms are tolerated better when given with a light snack, crackers, or milk. Intramuscular injections should not be used unless absolutely necessary. With phenobarbital, the intramuscular route may be ordered, but the injection must be into the lateral aspect of the thigh and into an adequate muscle mass.

Intravenous use requires dilution with normal saline (NaCl) and other recommended solutions. Rates of administration are very important for safe use, and most of the drugs should not be administered any faster than 1 mg/kg/min with a maximum amount per minute. Guidelines for maximum amounts per minute are outlined in any authoritative drug source, such as a current drug handbook, or in the manufacturer's insert. Too rapid an infusion of a barbiturate may produce profound hypotension and marked respiratory depression. Should there be intravenous infiltration, the site may become red and tender, with tissue necrosis to follow. Some intravenous barbiturates have antidote protocols. With phenobarbital intravenous infiltration, 0.5% procaine solution should be injected into the affected area and moist heat applied. Protocol for management of intravenous infiltrations of a given drug should always be checked before intervening. Intravenous incompatibilities include amphotericin B, hydrocortisone, and hydromorphone, so these drugs should be given only after the intravenous line has been adequately flushed with NaCl. With intramuscular injection, the solution should be given deep into a large muscle mass to prevent tissue sloughing. However, this route should be avoided and used only when absolutely necessary. Administration of barbiturates also requires frequent CNS monitoring, with observation for level of consciousness, sedation, reflexes, and excessive drowsiness. Use of a bed alarm system or raising of side rails and assistance with ambulation are important for prevention of injury. If the patient is in the post-anesthesia care unit or other hospital setting, the nurse should monitor blood pressure, pulse, and respiratory rate. Abrupt withdrawal of barbiturates after prolonged therapy may produce adverse effects ranging from nightmares, hallucinations, and delirium to seizures. In addition, while the patient is taking barbiturates it is important to monitor the patient's red blood cell count, hemoglobin, and hematocrit because of the possible adverse effect of anemia.

Long-term use of barbiturates also requires monitoring of therapeutic blood levels of the drug. For example, the level of phenobarbital should be 10 to 30 mcg/mL. Patients with serum levels above 40 mcg/mL may experience toxicity. Toxicity and/or overdosage is manifested by cold clammy skin, respiratory rate less than 12 breaths/min, and severe CNS depression.

Patients taking benzodiazepines may become sedated and sleepy, so safety issues are important. If the patient is in the hospital setting, bed alarms should be used and/or side rails should be kept up (per hospital policy or physician's order), and assistance with ambulation should be provided. Safety at home should also be emphasized if any of the CNS depressant drugs are used. In addition, dependence may be a problem with the benzodiazepines, but not to the same degree as with the barbiturates. While taking these drugs, patients should avoid driving or participating in any activities that require mental alertness. These drugs should be taken on an empty stomach for faster onset; however, this often results in GI upset, so they can be taken with meals or a snack. Orally administered benzodiazepines have an onset of action of 30 minutes to 6 hours, depending on the drug (see the pharmacokinetics information in the drug profiles). These drugs should be given at the appropriate interval before bedtime to maximize the drug's effectiveness for sleep induction. In addition, it is crucial to patient compliance and safety to understand that drug tolerance may develop to many of the CNS depressant drugs. This means that the body develops physiologic tolerance to the drug so that larger dosages are required to produce the same therapeutic effect. Interrupting therapy helps to decrease such tolerance, not only with these drugs but with other drugs as well.

Most of the benzodiazepines (and other CNS depressants) actually interfere with REM sleep instead of aiding it. This is an important concept to understand, because REM sleep is the restful and nurturing part of the sleep cycle. With REM interference, REM rebound may occur, especially if the drug is taken long term and withdrawn abruptly. REM rebound is manifested by vivid dreams and nightmares. Of the benzodiazepines, REM interference is less problematic with flurazepam, quazepam, and estazolam, primarily because they produce fewer active metabolites. In addition, patients should be informed that REM interference and rebound may occur with just a 3- to 4-week regimen of drug therapy. To minimize REM interference, benzodiazepines and other drugs should be used only when nonpharmacologic methods fail and should be used with caution in all patients with sleep disorders. Other recommendations include use of these drugs for the specific period associated with each drug class (e.g., some are to be used for only short periods of time). Gradual weaning-off periods are recommended with benzodiazepines and all CNS depressants. Hangover effects are also associated with many of the CNS depressants but occur less frequently with benzodiazepines and non-benzodiazepines compared with barbiturates. The hangover effect is a residual drowsiness that results in impaired reaction times and occurs upon awakening. The intermediate- and long-acting hypnotics are often the culprits in this adverse effect.

Muscle relaxants have different indications than the barbiturates and benzodiazepines and are not indicated for insomnia as compared with other sedative-hypnotic drugs. Toxicities associated with these drugs are usually treated with support measures to airway, breathing, and circulation. Early identification of toxicity is critical to prompt treatment and to prevention of respiratory and other CNS depressant effects. Close monitoring of all vital parameters and level of consciousness is needed with use of these muscle relaxants, as well as assistance with ambulation and moving/changing positions to prevent syncope or dizziness. Purposeful and slow movements should be encouraged with these (and other) drugs. The greatest risk for hypotension is usually within 1 hour of dosing, so it is important for the patient to be more cautious with activity during this time frame.

The miscellaneous drug chloral hydrate should be given with fluids (e.g., 6 to 8 oz of water or juice). Capsule dosage forms should not be altered in any way and should be swallowed whole. Activities requiring mental alertness or driving a vehicle should be avoided while taking any of the miscellaneous drugs or the other CNS depressants discussed in this chapter. Gradual weaning off the drug is also recommended.

Non-benzodiazepines should be taken for the prescribed time and with attention to special instructions, such as the following: (1) For zaleplon, the drug should be taken as directed and right before bed due to its quick onset of action; very heavy and/or high-fat meals should *not* be taken within 2 hours of taking this drug because of interference with the drug's action. (2) For zolpidem, the drug should be given at bedtime and taken on an empty stomach with no crushing, chewing, or breaking of the oral dosage form. It is also important to emphasize that this drug may infrequently lead to temporary memory loss. To help avoid this adverse effect, it is recommended that patient not take a dose of the drug unless he or she has had a full night's sleep (e.g., at least 7 to 8 hours). As with any CNS depressant drug, tasks requiring mental alertness should be avoided until the patient's response to the drug is known. Tolerance and dependence are possible with prolonged use, and neither drug should be discontinued without gradual weaning.

HERBAL THERAPIES AND DIETARY SUPPLEMENTS
Kava (Piper methysticum)

Overview
Kava consists of the dried rhizomes of *Piper methysticum.* The drug contains kava pyrones (kawain). Extended continuous intake can cause a temporary yellow discoloration of the skin, hair, and nails.

Common Uses
Relief of anxiety, stress, restlessness; promotion of sleep

Adverse Effects
Skin discoloration, possible accommodative disturbances and pupillary enlargement, scaly skin (with long-term use)

Potential Drug Interactions
Alcohol, barbiturates, psychoactive drugs

Contraindications
Contraindicated in patients with Parkinson's disease, liver disease, or alcoholism; in those operating heavy machinery; and in pregnant and breast-feeding women

HERBAL THERAPIES AND DIETARY SUPPLEMENTS
Valerian (Valeriana officinalis)

Overview
Valerian root, consisting of fresh underground plant parts, contains essential oil with monoterpenes and sesquiterpenes (valerianic acids).

Common Uses
Relief of anxiety, restlessness, sleep disorders

Adverse Effects
Central nervous system (CNS) depression, hepatotoxicity, nausea, vomiting, anorexia, headache, restlessness, insomnia

Potential Drug Interactions
CNS depressants, monamine oxidase inhibitors, phenytoin, warfarin; may have enhanced relative and adverse effects when taken with other drugs (including other herbal products) that have known sedative properties (including alcohol)

Contraindications
Contraindicated in patients with cardiac disease or those operating heavy machinery

In summary, before giving any sedative hypnotic drug, it is always important to try non-pharmacologic measures to induce sleep. However, regardless of the drug given, safety and prevention of injury are most important considerations. In years past, the standard of care has always been to keep bed rails raised, and some facilities may still adhere to this safety measure. Most acute and long-term health care facilities, though, are using bed alarms that sound when the patient attempts to get out of bed. If one or both side rails need to be kept up for a given patient, then the reason why this is being implemented should be documented. The rationale for using a bed alarm instead of raising the side rails is to prevent injury in those patients who are demented, under the influence of any sort of mind- or consciousness-altering drug, or even just sleepy or groggy who try to climb or crawl out of bed. With the bed rails up, there is a greater potential for self-injury in such patients. (The use of bed alarms is mentioned throughout this text, but the rationale is explained only briefly from this chapter forward.) Documentation must be timely, clear, and concise and must reflect follow-up on the pa-

tient's response to the drug. It is also important for the nurse to document dose, route, time of administration, and safety measures taken.

♦ EVALUATION

Some of the criteria by which to confirm a patient's therapeutic response to a CNS depressant include the following: an increased ability to sleep at night, fewer awakenings, shorter sleep induction time, few adverse effects such as hangover effects, and an improved sense of well-being because of improved sleep. Therapeutic effects related to muscle relaxants include decreased spasticity, reduction of choreiform movements in Huntington's chorea, decreased rigidity in parkinsonian syndrome, and relief of pain from trigeminal neuralgia. The nurse must constantly watch for and document the occurrence of any of the adverse effects of benzodiazepines, barbiturates, and muscle relaxants. See the previous discussion on adverse effects for each type of drug. Toxic effects to evaluate for with the CNS depressants may range from severe CNS depression of all body systems to respiratory and circulatory collapse.

Patient Teaching Tips

- Encourage the patient to keep a journal of sleep habits and response to both drug and non-drug therapy (Box 12-1).
- Encourage the patient to always try non-pharmacologic measures first in an attempt to enhance sleep (see Box 12-1) because use of the CNS depressants often leads to interference with the REM stage of sleep, hangover effects, and/or tolerance.
- Inform the patient to always check with the physician or pharmacist before taking any over-the-counter medications because of the many drug interactions associated with CNS depressants and, more specifically, with sedative-hypnotic drugs.
- Make sure the patient knows to keep all medications out of the reach of children.
- Patients should be informed to take the medication only as prescribed. Instructions are usually given to the patient that if one dose does not work, the patient is not to double up on the dosage unless otherwise prescribed or directed.

- Patients should be fully informed of time constraints related to driving, operating heavy machinery/equipment, and participating in activities requiring mental alertness while taking these medications.
- Patients should be informed that they should never stop taking these medications abruptly to avoid possible withdrawal and/or rebound insomnia.
- Sedative-hypnotic drugs (used for sleep) are not intended for long-term use because of their adverse effects, interference with REM sleep, and addictive properties.
- Patients should be aware that hangover effects may occur with most of these drugs and that this is more problematic in the elderly.
- Educate the patient to avoid smoking in bed or when lounging.

Box 12-1 Sleep Diaries and Non-Pharmacologic Treatment of Sleep Disorders

Information for a Sleep Diary

- What time do you usually go to bed and wake up?
- How long and how well do you sleep?
- When were you awake during the night and for how long?
- How easy was it to go to sleep?
- How easy was it to wake up in the morning?
- How much caffeine or alcohol do you consume?
- What time did you last eat or drink (if after dinner)?
- Did you have any bedtime snacks?
- What emotions or stressors are present?
- What medications do you take daily?
- Do you smoke? How much and for how long?
- Do you consume alcohol? How much and for how long?
- Do you take any over-the-counter drugs? If so, what drug and for what reason? How much and for how long?
- Do you take any herbals? If so, which one? For what and for how long?

Nonpharmacologic Sleep Interventions

- Establish a set sleep pattern with a time to go to bed at night and a regular time to get up in the morning and stick to it. This will help to reset your internal clock.
- Sleep only as much as you need to feel refreshed and renewed. Too much sleep may lead to fragmented sleep patterns and shallow sleep.
- Keep bedroom temperatures moderate, if possible.
- Avoid caffeine-containing beverages and food within 6 hours of bedtime.
- Decrease exposure to loud noises.
- Avoid daytime napping.
- Avoid exercise late in the evening (i.e., not past 7 PM).
- Avoid alcohol in the evening. Rather than putting you to sleep, it actually results in fragmented sleep.
- Avoid tobacco at bedtime, because it disturbs sleep.
- Try to relax before bedtime with soft music, yoga, relaxation therapy, deep breathing, or light reading on a topic that is not intense or anxiety provoking.
- Drink a warm decaffeinated beverage, such as warm milk or chamomile tea, 30 minutes to 1 hour before bedtime.
- If you are still awake 20 minutes after going to bed, get up and engage in a relaxing activity (as noted previously) and go back to bed once you feel drowsy. Repeat as necessary.

Points to Remember

- Non-pharmacologic measures for sleep disorders should always be tried before resorting to treatment with medications.
- Nurses should understand the classification and pharmacokinetic properties of barbiturates. Short-acting barbiturates include pentobarbital sodium, secobarbital. Intermediate-acting barbiturates include amobarbital, aprobarbital, and butabarbital.
- The pharmacokinetics of each group of barbiturates lend specific characteristics to the drugs in that group. The nurse also needs to understand how these drugs are absorbed orally and used parenterally, as well as their onset, peak, and duration of action. In addition, the life-threatening potential of these drugs should never be minimized by the nurse or other health care provider administering the drug(s), because too rapid an infusion may precipitate respiratory or cardiac arrest.
- Nursing interventions for barbiturates include careful consideration of parenteral injection with complete knowledge about incompatibilities with other drugs in solution as well as dilutional fluid incompatibilities.
- Most sedative-hypnotic drugs suppress REM sleep and should only be used for the recommended period of time. This time frame varies according to the specific drug used.
- Muscle relaxants are often used for the treatment of muscle spasms, spasticity, and rigidity. They result in varying levels of decreased sensorium and CNS depression depending on the specific drug, dosage, and route of administration. Nurses need to understand that even though muscle relaxants are discussed in this chapter, they are not used as sedative-hypnotic drugs.

NCLEX Examination Review Questions

1. Which is an important nursing consideration regarding the administration of a benzodiazepine as a sedative-hypnotic drug?
   a. These drugs are intended for long-term management of insomnia.
   b. The drugs can be administered safely with other CNS depressants for insomnia.
   c. The drug should be used as a first choice for treatment of sleeplessness.
   d. The patient should be evaluated for the drowsiness that may occur the morning after a benzodiazepine is taken.
2. An older adult has been given a barbiturate for sleep induction, but the night nurse noted that the patient was awake most of the night, watching television and reading in bed. This type of reaction is known as
   a. an allergic reaction.
   b. a teratogenic reaction.
   c. a paradoxical reaction.
   d. an idiopathic reaction.
3. Which of the following interventions applies to the administration of a nonbenzodiazepine, such as zolpidem?
   a. These drugs are meant for long-term treatment of insomnia.
   b. Because of their rapid onset, they should be taken just before bedtime.

c. The patient should be cautioned about the high incidence of morning drowsiness that may occur after taking these drugs.
   d. These drugs are less likely to interact with alcohol.
4. The nurse should monitor the patient who is taking a muscle relaxant for which adverse effects?
   a. CNS depression
   b. Hypertension
   c. Peripheral edema
   d. Blurred vision
5. A patient on a cardiac medical-surgical unit is complaining of having difficulty sleeping. Which action should the nurse take first to address this problem?
   a. Administer a sedative-hypnotic drug if ordered
   b. Offer tea made with the herbal preparation valerian
   c. Encourage the patient to exercise by walking up and down the halls a few times if tolerated
   d. Provide an environment that is restful and reduce loud noises

1. d, 2. c, 3. b, 4. a, 5. d.

Critical Thinking Activities

1. Explain the difference between a drug that is a sedative and a drug that is a hypnotic.
2. One of your patients has been told to discontinue the use of flurazepam, which she has been taking for about 1 year. The health care provider gave no other instructions. As her home health nurse, does this cause you concern? Why or why not?
3. a. A patient has undergone conscious sedation with benzodiazepines for a brief diagnostic procedure. What drug can be given

to reverse the effects of the benzodiazepines? How is it administered?
   b. The patient woke up after the procedure, and vital signs have been stable. However, 3 hours after the procedure, the patient gradually becomes very sleepy. Is this a concern or is the patient just tired? What should the nurse expect to do at this time?

For answers, see http://evolve.elsevier.com/Lilley.

Antiepileptic Drugs

Objectives

When you reach the end of this chapter, you should be able to do the following:

1. Discuss the rationale for use of the various classes of antiepileptic drugs (AEDs) used in the management of the various forms of epilepsy.
2. Identify the various drugs within each of the following drug classes: iminostilbenes, benzodiazepines, barbiturates, hydantoins, and miscellaneous.
3. Identify the mechanisms of action, indications, cautions, contraindications, dosages, routes of administration, adverse effects, toxic effects, any related serum therapeutic levels and drug interactions for the various drugs within the different classifications of AEDs.
4. Develop a nursing care plan, including patient education, related to the nursing process for patients receiving antiepileptic drugs.

e-Learning Activities

Companion CD

- NCLEX Review Questions: see questions 79-89
- Animations
- Audio Glossary
- Category Catchers
- Medication Errors Checklists
- IV Therapy Checklists

Evolve Website (http://evolve.elsevier.com/Lilley)

• Nursing Care Plans • Frequently Asked Questions • Content Updates • WebLinks • Supplemental Resources • Elsevier ePharmacology Update • Medication Administration Animations

Drug Profiles

▶ carbamazepine, p. 204
▶ gabapentin, p. 205
  lamotrigine, p. 205
  levetiracetam, p. 205
  oxcarbazepine, p. 205
▶ phenobarbital, p. 200

▶ phenytoin, p. 204
  pregabalin, p. 205
  tiagabine, p. 205
  topiramate, p. 205
▶ valproic acid, p. 204
  zonisamide, p. 205

▶ Key drug.

Glossary

Anticonvulsant A substance or procedure that prevents or reduces the severity of epileptic or other convulsive seizures. (p. 197)

Antiepileptic drug A substance that prevents or reduces the severity of epilepsy and different types of epileptic seizures, not just convulsive seizures. (p. 197)

Autoinduction A metabolic process that occurs when a drug increases its own metabolism over time, leading to lower than expected drug concentrations. (p. 204)

Convulsion A type of seizure involving excessive stimulation of neurons in the brain and characterized by the spas-

modic contraction of voluntary muscles. (See also *seizure.*) (p. 197)

Epilepsy General term for any of a group of neurologic disorders characterized by recurrent episodes of convulsive seizures, sensory disturbances, abnormal behavior, loss of consciousness, or any combination of these. (p. 197)

International Classification of Seizures The most extensively used system for classifying seizures. Both the symptoms and characteristics of the various types of seizures are described. (p. 197)

Narrow therapeutic index (NTI) drugs Drugs that are characterized by a narrow difference between their therapeutic and toxic doses. (p. 199)

Primary or idiopathic epilepsy Epilepsy that develops without an apparent cause. More than 50% of cases of epilepsy are of unknown origin. (p. 197)

Secondary epilepsy Epilepsy that has a distinct cause (e.g., trauma). (p. 197)

Seizure Excessive stimulation of neurons in the brain leading to a sudden burst of abnormal neuron activity that results in temporary changes in brain function. (p. 197)

Status epilepticus A common seizure disorder characterized by generalized tonic-clonic convulsions that occur in succession. (p. 197)

Tonic-clonic seizure Formerly called grand mal seizure, this type of epilepsy is characterized by a series of generalized movements of tonic (stiffening) and clonic (rapid, synchronized jerking) muscular contraction. (p. 197)

Unclassified seizures Seizures that are not described by any of the seizure classifications. (p. 197)

EPILEPSY

A seizure disorder, or what is more commonly referred to as *epilepsy,* is not as specific a disease as, for example, cancer or diabetes. It is a broad syndrome of central nervous system (CNS) dysfunction that can manifest in many ways, from momentary sensory disturbances to convulsive seizures. Most likely, it involves the generation of excessive electrical discharges from nerves located in the area of the brain known as the *cerebral cortex.*

The terms **convulsion, seizure,** and **epilepsy** are often used interchangeably, but they do not have the same meaning. A seizure is a brief episode of abnormal electrical activity in the nerve cells of the brain. A convulsion is characterized by involuntary spasmodic contractions of any or all voluntary muscles throughout the body, including skeletal and facial muscles. Epilepsy is a chronic, recurrent pattern of seizures. These excessive electrical discharges can often be detected by an electroencephalogram (EEG), which is commonly obtained to help diagnose epilepsy. Other diagnostic aids that are helpful in the diagnosis of epilepsy are computerized tomography (CT) and magnetic resonance imaging (MRI). The information yielded by these diagnostic aids in conjunction with the common symptoms of the particular seizure disorder help establish the diagnosis. In particularly severe cases, patients may be observed in a hospital setting or sleep study laboratory with continuous EEG and video monitoring to determine detailed patterns of seizure activity in hopes of tailoring an effective treatment. Commonly reported symptoms are abnormal motor function, loss of consciousness, altered sensory awareness, and psychic changes.

The cause of more than 50% of the cases of epilepsy is unknown. That type of epilepsy for which a cause cannot be identified is called **primary or idiopathic epilepsy.** Other types of epilepsy have a distinct cause such as trauma, infection, cerebrovascular disorder, or other illness. These types of epilepsy are called **secondary epilepsy.** The chief causes of secondary epilepsy in children and infants are developmental defects, metabolic disease, or injury at birth. Acquired brain disorder is the major cause of secondary epilepsy in adults. Some examples are head injury, disease or infection of the brain and spinal cord, stroke, metabolic disorder, a primary or metastatic brain tumor, or some other recognizable neurologic disease. Interestingly, the elderly have the highest incidence of new-onset epilepsy than other age groups. Fortunately, seizures in the elderly are often well-controlled with drug therapy. The accurate diagnosis of a seizure disorder requires careful patient observation, a reliable patient history, and an EEG. Other diagnostic tests that are often used in revealing structural lesions of the CNS as the cause of the seizure disorder are CT and MRI (which are superior to the clinical examination), EEG, and routine skull radiographs. Of MRI and CT, MRI is more sensitive and is now preferred in the evaluation of a patient with seizures.

Seizures can be classified into distinct categories based on their characteristics. In traditional classifications, seizures were categorized as grand mal seizures **(tonic-clonic seizures),** petit mal seizures, Jacksonian epilepsy, and psychomotor attacks. Currently, the **International Classification of Seizures** involves a more systematic approach that divides seizures into two main types: partial and generalized. This system is more extensively used because it more adequately describes the symptoms and characteristics of the various types of seizures (Box 13-1). Under this newer nomenclature, two other classifications of seizures also exist: status epilepticus and unclassified. **Status epilepticus** seizures start out as either partial or generalized seizures and be-

---

Box 13-1   International Classification of Seizures

Partial Seizures
Description
Short alterations in consciousness, repetitive unusual movements (chewing or swallowing movements), psychologic changes, and confusion.

Simple Seizures
- No impaired consciousness
- Motor symptoms (most commonly face, arm, or leg)
- Hallucinations of sight, hearing, or taste along with somatosensory changes (tingling)
- Autonomic nervous system responses
- Personality changes

Complex Seizures
- Impaired consciousness
- Memory impairment
- Behavioral effects
- Purposeless behaviors
- Aura, chewing and swallowing movements, unreal feelings, bizarre behavior
- Tonic, clonic, or tonic-clonic seizures

Generalized Seizures
Description
Most often seen in children and commonly characterized by temporary lapses in consciousness lasting a few seconds. Staring off into space, daydreaming, and inattentive look are common symptoms. Patients may exhibit rhythmic movements of their eyes, head, or hands but do not convulse. May have several attacks per day.
- Both cerebral hemispheres involved
- Tonic, clonic, myoclonic, atonic, or tonic-clonic seizures and infantile spasms possible
- Brief loss of consciousness for a few seconds with no confusion
- Head drop or falling-down symptoms

---

come status epilepticus when there is no recovery between attacks. **Unclassified seizures** are those that do not clearly fit into any of the other categories. It should also be noted that seizure episodes can sometimes start off as partial and then become generalized. If the partial component is not noticed, the patient may be given drug therapy that is more suitable for generalized seizures and possibly not receive optimal treatment.

ANTIEPILEPTIC DRUGS

Antiepileptic drugs (or antiepileptics) are also called anticonvulsants. The term **antiepileptic drugs** (or AEDs) is a more appropriate term because many of these medications are indicated for the management of all types of epilepsy, not just with convulsions. **Anticonvulsants,** on the other hand, are medications that are used to prevent the seizures typically associated with epilepsy. In practice, however, there is significant overlap between these two terms, and both are often used interchangeably.

The combined goal of AED therapy is to control or prevent seizures while maintaining a reasonable quality of life. Approximately 70% of patients can expect to become seizure-free with modern drug therapy, and most will only take one AED. The remaining 30% of cases are more complicated, often requiring additional medications. Many AEDs have adverse effects, and balancing seizure control with adverse effects is often a difficult task. In most cases, the therapeutic goal is not to eliminate seizure activity but rather to maximally reduce the incidence of seizures while minimizing drug-induced toxicity. Many patients must take AEDs for their entire life. Treatment may eventually be stopped in some, but others will suffer repeated seizures if constant levels of AEDs are not maintained in their blood. In both children and adults, there is only a 40% chance of recurrence after the first partial or generalized seizure; therefore, many physicians choose not to initiate treatment after the first seizure. However, it is the consensus that AED therapy should be implemented in patients who have had two or more seizures.

There are several AEDs available. Sometimes, a combination of drugs must be used to control the disorder. Nonetheless, most seizure disorders can be controlled. To optimize drug selection for each patient, neurologists consider the efficacy of the drug for seizure types, adverse effect profile, likelihood of drug interactions, cost, ease of use, and availability of pediatric dosage forms. In addition, a number of AEDs are also used for other types of illnesses, including psychiatric disorders, migraine headaches, and neuropathic pain syndromes. Generally, single-drug therapy must fail before two-drug and then multiple-drug therapy is implemented. A patient should always be started on a single AED and the dosage slowly increased until the seizures are controlled or until clinical toxicity occurs. If the first AED does not work, the drug should be tapered slowly while a second AED is introduced. AEDs should never be stopped abruptly unless a severe adverse effect occurs. It is sometimes difficult to control a patient's seizures using a single AED, but monotherapy is likely to result in higher serum drug concentrations, fewer adverse effects, and better control.

Serum drug concentrations are useful guidelines in assessing the effectiveness of therapy. They should, however, be only guidelines. Maintaining serum drug levels within therapeutic ranges helps not only to control seizures but also to reduce adverse effects. There are established normal therapeutic ranges for many AEDs, but these are useful only as guidelines. Each patient should be monitored individually and the dosages adjusted based on the individual case. Many patients are maintained successfully below or above the usual therapeutic range. The goal should be to slowly titrate to the lowest effective serum drug level that controls the seizure disorder. This decreases the risk for medication-induced adverse effects and interactions. The serum concentrations of phenytoin, phenobarbital, carbamazepine, and primidone correlate better with seizure control and toxicity than do those of valproic acid, ethosuximide, and clonazepam. Emphasis should be placed primarily on the clinical symptoms and patient's history rather than on strict adherence to established drug concentration ranges.

There are six traditional classes of AEDs, and many new drugs have been marketed. These newer drugs were developed with the goal of eliminating many of the drug interactions and adverse effects associated with the older drugs. There is current debate in the literature as to whether patients benefit more from newer than older drugs. Prescribers must consider all pertinent nuances of both drugs used and the patient. It is reported that some newer AEDs may be less likely to cause undesirable drug interactions, compared to older drugs. This may especially bene-fit elderly patients, who are more likely to be on multiple medications and, therefore, more prone to drug interactions. Successful control of a seizure disorder hinges on selecting the appropriate drug class and drug dosage, the patient complying with the treatment regimen, and limiting toxicity.

The underlying cause of most cases of epilepsy is an excessive electrical discharge from abnormally functioning nerve cells (neurons) within the CNS. Therefore, the object of AED therapy is to prevent the generation and spread of these excessive discharges while simultaneously protecting surrounding normal cells.

Mechanism of Action and Drug Effects

Like many classes of drugs, the exact mechanism of action of the AEDs is not known with certainty. However, strong evidence shows that they alter the movement of sodium, potassium, calcium, and magnesium ions. The changes in the movement of these ions induced by AEDs result in stabilized and less responsive cell membranes. This ion theory may explain how AEDs decrease the excitability and responsiveness of brain neurons (nerve cells).

Theoretically, the primary pharmacologic effects of AEDs are threefold. First, they increase the threshold of activity in the area of the brain called the motor cortex. In other words, they make it more difficult for a nerve to be excited or they reduce the nerve's response to incoming electrical or chemical stimulation. Second, they act to depress or limit the spread of a seizure discharge from its origin. They do this by suppressing the transmission of impulses from one nerve to the next. Third, they can decrease the speed of nerve impulse conduction within a given neuron. AEDs may also have effects outside the neuron, indirectly affecting the area in the brain responsible for the problem by altering, for instance, the blood supply to that area. However, the overall effect is that AEDs stabilize neurons and keep them from becoming hyperexcited and generating excessive nerve impulses to adjacent neurons.

Indications

The major therapeutic indication for AEDs is the prevention or control of seizure activity. They are especially useful for maintenance therapy in patients with the chronic recurring type of seizures that are commonly associated with epilepsy. As evidenced by the wide range of seizure disorders listed in Box 13-1, epilepsy is a very diverse disorder. As a result, no one drug can control all types of epilepsy. Although our understanding of epilepsy is still growing, we have a good idea of the primary causes of many of the various seizure disorders. Each involves a distinct area of dysfunction and has certain characteristics that make particular drugs more effective than others in treating it. Therefore, particular drugs are indicated for the control of specific seizures. Some of the AEDs and the seizure disorders they are used to treat are listed in Table 13-1.

AEDs are chiefly used for the long-term maintenance treatment of epilepsy. However, AEDs are also useful for the acute treatment of convulsions and status epilepticus. Status epilepticus is a common seizure disorder that is a life-threatening emergency; it is characterized by generalized tonic-clonic convulsions that occur in succession. Affected patients typically do not regain consciousness between the many convulsions. Hypotension, hypoxia, and cardiac dysrhythmias complicate the disorder, and brain damage and death quickly ensue if prompt, appropriate therapy is not started. Therapy is typically diazepam (Valium), which is considered by many

Table 13-1 Antiepileptic Drugs of Choice

Simple	Complex	GTC	Absence	Myoclonic	Clonic	Tonic	Atonic
First Choice							
Carbamazepine	carbamazepine	carbamazepine	ethosuximide	valproic acid	valproic acid	valproic acid	valproic acid
Phenytoin	phenytoin	phenytoin	phenytoin				
Phenytoin	phenytoin	phenytoin	valproic acid				
Primidone	primidone	primidone					
Valproic Acid	valproic acid	valproic acid					
Second Choice							
Clonazepam	clonazepam	clonazepam	acetazolamide	clonazepam	clonazepam	clonazepam	clonazepam
Levetiracetam	zonisamide	zonisamide				topiramate	lamotrigine
	pregabalin	oxcarbazepine				zonisamide	levetiracetam
	tiagabine					oxcarbazepine	topiramate
Clorazepate	clorazepate	levetiraetam	clonazepam	lamotrigine	lamotrigine	clonazepam	
Lamotrigine	lamotrigine					lamotrigine	
						levetiracetam	
Topiramate	topiramate	lamotrigine		topiramate	topiramate	phenytoin	
Oxcarbaze-Pine	oxcarbazepine	topiramate					

GTC, Generalized tonic-clonic.

Table 13-2 Antiepileptic Drugs Used for Treatment of Status Epilepticus

Drug	Dose (mg/kg)	Onset	Duration	Half-Life	Adverse Effects
Diazepam	0.3-0.5 (<30 mg)	3-10 min	Minutes	35 hr	Apnea, hypotension, somnolence
Fosphenytoin	15-20 phenytoin equivalents (1.5 mg fosphenytoin =1 mg phenytoin)	15-30 min	12-24 hr	10-60 hr	Comparable to phenytoin (see below)
lorazepam*	0.05-0.1	1-20 min	Hours	15 hr	Apnea, hypotension, somnolence
Phenobarbital	15-20	10-30 min	4-10 hr	53-140 hr	Apnea, hypotension, somnolence
Phenytoin	15-20	5-30 min	12-24 hr	10-60 hr	Cardiac dysrhythmias, hypotension

*Off-label use (non–FDA-approved indication), but still sometimes used for this purpose.

to be the drug of choice. However, there are other drugs that are also useful for the treatment of status epilepticus. The drugs most commonly used are listed in Table 13-2.

Once status epilepticus is controlled, long-term drug therapy is begun with other drugs for the prevention of future seizures. Patients who undergo brain surgery or who have suffered severe head injuries may receive prophylactic AED therapy. These patients are at high risk for acquiring a seizure disorder, and often severe complications will arise if seizures are not controlled.

Contraindications

The only usual contraindication to AEDs is known drug allergy. Pregnancy is also a common contraindication, but the prescriber must consider the risks to mother and infant of untreated maternal epilepsy and the increased risks for seizure activity.

Adverse Effects

AEDs are plagued by many adverse effects, which often limit their usefulness. Drugs must be withdrawn from many patients because of some of these effects. In addition, although some medications are safer than others, AEDs do appear to be responsible for many birth defects in offspring of epileptic women. Each AED is associated with its own diverse set of adverse effects, which makes it difficult to categorize all of the classes of AEDs according to their common adverse effects. The various AEDs and their most common adverse effects are listed in Table 13-3.

Interactions

The drug interactions that can occur with the AEDs are many and varied, and these are summarized in Table 13-4. Significant drug interactions for selected drugs are also listed in Table 13-4.

Dosages

With certain AEDs, the safe and toxic levels are very close. Drugs that have a narrow difference between safe and toxic levels are called **narrow therapeutic index (NTI) drugs.** Table 13-5 lists the various AEDs that require monitoring of therapeutic plasma levels and their corresponding therapeutic levels. For an overview of dosages, see the Dosages table on p. 202.

It is important for the safe use of the various classes of drugs used in the management of seizure disorders for the nurse to understand the nursing process as it relates to each of these major classes. This discussion focuses on the different groups of the barbiturates, benzodiazepines, and hydantoins. Some of these AEDs, such as the barbiturates and benzodiazepines, are also discussed with the sedative-hypnotic drugs (Chapter 12).

Drug Profiles

All AEDs are prescription-only drugs. These drugs are associated with many characteristics that make it undesirable for patients to be taking them without the supervision of a qualified medical

Table 13-3   Adverse Effects of Selected Antiepileptic Drugs

Drug or Drug Class	Adverse Effects
Barbiturates	CNS: Drowsiness, dizziness, lethargy, paradoxical restlessness, excitement Gastrointestinal: Nausea, vomiting Other: Rash, Stevens-Johnson syndrome, urticaria
carbamazepine	Hematologic: Bone marrow suppression (aplastic anemia, agranulocytosis, thrombocytopenia) Integumentary: Exfoliative dermatitis, erythema multiforme, Stevens-Johnson syndrome Heart: Dysrhythmias, heart failure Other: Thrombophlebitis, vision and hearing disturbances, acute urinary retention, dyspnea, pneumonitis, pneumonia
divalproex (valproic acid)	Other: Pancreatitis, irregular menses, secondary amenorrhea, galactorrhea, rare breast enlargement, weight gain Hematologic: Thrombocytopenia
felbamate	Gastrointestinal: Anorexia, nausea, vomiting Other: Headache, intramenstrual bleeding, respiratory and urinary tract infections Pediatric: Fever, purpura, nervousness, somnolence
Hydantoins	Cardiovascular: Dysrhythmias, hypotension Integumentary: Exfoliative dermatitis, lupus erythematosus, Stevens-Johnson syndrome Hematologic: Bone marrow suppression (agranulocytosis, thrombocytopenia, megaloblastic anemia) Other: Neuropathies, gingival hyperplasia
topiramate	Hematologic: Purpura, leukopenia Integumentary: Dermatitis, rash, alopecia Other: Cognitive impairment, fatigue or somnolence, anorexia
tiagabine	Cognitive impairment, dizziness, somnolence, nausea, skin rash
zonisamide	Irritability, confusion, depression, cognitive impairment, anorexia, GI upset, diplopia
levetiracetam	Somnolence, headache, dizziness, asthenia, pharyngitis
lamotrigine	Headache, dizziness, somnolence, rash, nausea, rhinitis, pharyngitis, diplopia, fever
oxcarbazepine	Headache, dizziness, somnolence, NVD, fatigue, visual changes
gabapentin	Dizziness, somnolence, peripheral edema, NVD, visual changes
pregabalin	Dizziness, somnolence, dry mouth, edema, blurred vision, weight gain, difficulty concentrating

CNS, Central nervous system.

specialist. They are available in many oral, injectable, and rectal formulations. The U.S. Food and Drug Administration's (FDA's) pregnancy risk classification of AEDs is summarized in Table 13-6.

In most children and adults, epilepsy can be controlled with a first-line AED, such as carbamazepine, ethosuximide, phenobarbital, primidone, phenytoin, or valproic acid. For patients who do not respond to the first-line AEDs, there are a number of second-line AEDs that are used occasionally, such as the benzodiazepines, clonazepam and clorazepate; methsuximide; and acetazolamide. These are often used as first-line drugs for status epilepticus.

After valproic acid was introduced in 1978, no major new drugs for the treatment of epilepsy were introduced in the United States until the 1990s. Gabapentin, lamotrigine, and felbamate were all approved during this decade. Gabapentin and lamotrigine are primarily used as add-on drugs in adults who have partial seizures alone or with secondary generalized seizures. The FDA currently recommends that felbamate be given only to patients who have seizures that are refractory to treatment with all other medications and in whom risk-benefit considerations warrant its use. Reports of aplastic anemia and acute liver failure with this particular drug require that weekly or biweekly complete blood count (CBC) and liver function tests be performed.

AEDs that have more recently been approved are levetiracetam (Keppra), topiramate (Topamax), zonisamide (Zonegran), and pregabalin (Lyrica). These drugs fall under the miscellaneous category of AEDs and have greatly expanded the options currently available to patients with seizure disorders. Dosage, pregnancy category, and specific indication information appears in the corresponding table. The following general information applies to most AEDs as a group. If a given drug is to be replaced with another AED, the prescriber will often recommend gradual tapering off of the first drug and

gradual tapering up of the new one. For those drugs available in both tablet and suspension forms, switching from tablet to suspension will often result in more frequent, but smaller, doses for an equivalent total daily dose. Extended release forms are usually given in one to two divided daily doses. These dosage forms normally should not be crushed. In contrast, immediate-release tablets can usually be crushed, but neither of these rules are absolute. Check with a pharmacist when in doubt.

Barbiturates
> *phenobarbital*

Originally, two of the most commonly used AEDs were the barbiturates phenobarbital (Solfoton) and primidone (Mysoline). Primidone is metabolized in the liver to phenobarbital and phenylethylmalonamide, both of which have anticonvulsant properties. Phenobarbital has been used since 1912, principally for controlling tonic-clonic and partial seizures. Phenobarbital is still one of the first-line drugs for the management of status epilepticus and is an effective prophylactic drug for the control of febrile seizures. Although the use of phenobarbital for seizure emergencies is still common even in the more technically advanced societies, its use by the oral route for seizure prevention is much less so. However, in developing, third-world countries, oral phenobarbital is often the drug of choice for routine seizure prophylaxis because of its drastically lower cost compared to the newer AEDs more common in industrialized countries. By far, the most common adverse effect is sedation, but tolerance to this effect usually develops with continued therapy. In pediatric patients the most common adverse effects are irritability, hyperactivity, depression, sleep disorders, and cognitive abnormalities. Therapeutic effects are generally seen at serum drug levels of 15 to 40 mcg/mL. It interacts with many drugs because it is a major "inducer" of hepatic enzymes, causing more

Table 13-4 Drug Interactions of Selected Antiepileptic Drugs

Drug or Drug Class	Mechanism	Results
Carbamazepine		
Bone marrow depressants	Additive effect	Increased bone marrow toxicity
doxycycline, phenytoin, theophylline, Warfarin	Alters metabolism	Significant decrease in half-life
Grapefruit juice	Inhibits hepatic enzymes	Increased carbamazepine levels
divalproex (valproic acid)		
Barbiturates	Additive effect	Increased CNS depression
clonazepam	Not determined	May produce absence status
phenytoin	Not determined	May produce breakthrough seizures
tiagabine		
valproate	Not determined	Increased valproate levels
carbamazepine, phenytoin, phenobarbital.	Induction of hepatic enzymes	Reduced tiagabine levels
Hydantoins		
disulfiram, isoniazid, valproic acid	Inhibits hepatic enzymes	Increased hydantoin levels
Tricyclic antidepressants	Not determined	Possible seizures
Topiramate		
carbamazepine, phenytoin, valproic acid	Enzymatic induction	Reduced topiramate levels
metformin	Uncertain	Increased topiramate and metformin levels
Alcohol	Synergism	Increased CNS depression
Oral contraceptives, estrogens	Uncertain	Reduced OC/estrogen levels
digoxin	Uncertain	Reduced digoxin levels
zonisamide		
phenytoin, carbamazepine, phenobarbital	Enzymatic induction	Reduced zonisamide levels
levetiracetam		No major ones reported
lamotrigine		
acetaminophen, carbamazepine, oral contraceptives, progestins, oxcarbazepine, phenytoin	Uncertain	Reduced lamotrigine levels
valproic acid	Uncertain	Increased lamotrigine levels
oxcarbazepine		
phenytoin, phenobarbital	Uncertain	Reduced oxcarbazepine levels and increased phenytoin/phenobarbital levels
gabapentin		
Antacids		Reduced gabapentin absorption
cimetidine, hydrocodone, morphine		Increased gabapentin levels
pregabalin		None reported to date. Drug approved in 2005.

Table 13-5 Therapeutic Plasma Levels of NTI Antiepileptic Drugs

Antiepileptic Drug	Therapeutic Plasma Level (mcg/mL)
carbamazepine	3-14
clonazepam	0.02-0.08
divalproex	50-100
ethosuximide	40-100
phenobarbital	15-40
phenytoin	10-20
primidone	5-12
valproic acid	50-100

NTI, Narrow therapeutic index.

Table 13-6 Antiepileptic Drugs: FDA Pregnancy Risk Classification

Pregnancy Category	Anticonvulsant
C	acetazolamide, ethosuximide, gabapentin, lamotrigine, levetiracetam, oxcarbazepine, tiagabine, topiramate
D	Barbiturates (e.g., phenobarbital), carbamazepine, clonazepam, clorazepate, diazepam, divalproex, phenytoin, primidone, valproic acid, trimethadione (used only in refractory cases that do not respond to other drugs)

FDA, Food and Drug Administration.

rapid clearance of some drugs. Its major advantage is that it has the longest half-life of all the standard AEDs, which allows for once-a-day dosing. This can be a substantial advantage for patients who have a hard time remembering to take their medication or for those who have erratic schedules. A patient may take a dose 12 or even 24 hours too late and may still have therapeutic blood levels at that time. In addition, phenobarbital is the most inexpensive AED, cost-ing only pennies a day compared with several dollars a day for other AEDs.

Pharmacokinetics			
Half-Life	**Onset**	**Peak**	**Duration**
PO: 53-118 hr	PO: 20-60 min	PO: 8-12 hr	PO: 6-12 hr

DOSAGES

Selected Antiepileptic Drugs

Drug (Pregnancy Category)	Pharmacologic Class	Usual Dosage Range	Indications
▶carbamazepine (Tegretol, Tegretol XR) (D)	Iminostilbene	**Pediatric** PO: <9 yr, 10-20 mg/kg/day PO: 6-12 yr, 200-1000 mg/day **Pediatric/adult** PO: >12 yr, 400-2400 mg/day	Partial seizures with complex symptoms; tonic-clonic, mixed seizures; trigeminal—glossopharyngeal neuralgia
clonazepam (Klonopin) (D)	Benzodiazepine	**Pediatric** PO: ≤10 yr or 30 kg, 0.1-0.2 mg/kg/day divided tid **Adult** PO: 4-20 mg/day	Lennox-Gastaut; absence, akinetic, and myoclonic seizures
clorazepate dipotassium (Gen-XENE, Tranxene) (D)	Benzodiazepine	**Pediatric** PO: 9-12 yr, 15-60 mg/day **Adult/children** PO: >12 yr, 22-90 mg/day	Partial seizures
ethosuximide (Zarontin) (C)	Succinimide	**Pediatric** PO: 3-6 yr, 250 mg/day then adjust; >6 yr, 500 mg/day then adjust **Adult** PO: 500 mg/day then adjust	Absence seizures
fosphenytoin (Cerebyx) (D)	Hydantoin	**Pediatric** IV: 10-20 PE*/kg loading dose; may begin maintenance dosing 8-12 hr later using pediatric phenytoin dosing guidelines (see below) **Adult** IV: 10-20 PE*/kg loading dose; maintenance dose 4-6 mg/kg/day	Tonic-clonic seizures; psychomotor seizures, convulsions
▶gabapentin (Neurontin) (C)	Miscellaneous	**Pediatric** PO: 10-15 mg/kg/day divided tid, then adjust **Adult** PO: >18 yr, 900-1800 mg/day	Add-on therapy for partial seizures and neuropathic pain
lamotrigine (Lamictal) (C)	Miscellaneous	**Pediatric** PO: 2-12 yr, 5-15 mg/kg/day depending on other AEDs used **Adult** PO: 50-200 mg divided qd-bid	Partial seizures, Lennox-Gastaut syndrome
levetiracetam (Keppra) (C)	Miscellaneous	**Adult** PO: 500 mg bid-3000 mg/day Pediatric (per child neurologist)	Partial seizures
oxcarbazepine (Trileptal) (C)	Iminostilbene	**Pediatric** PO: 8-10 mg/kg/day divided bid; max 600 mg/day **Adult** 300-600 mg bid	Partial seizures
▶phenobarbital (Solfoton) (D)	Barbiturate	**Pediatric** PO: 3-5 mg/kg/day IM/IV: 10-20 mg/kg load, may repeat 5 mg/kg every 15-30 min until seizure is controlled or total dose of 40 mg/kg is reached **Adult** PO: 100-300 mg/day IM/IV: 200-800 mg followed by 120-240 mg dose every 20 min until seizure is controlled or a total dose of 1-2 g is reached **Pediatric** PO: 3-6 mg/kg/day	Partial, tonic-clonic seizures Convulsions Partial, tonic-clonic seizures Convulsions Prophylaxis for febrile convulsions Tonic-clonic; psychomotor seizures Convulsions

AED, Antiepileptic drug; *IM,* intramuscular; *IV,* intravenous; *PO,* oral.

*PE = phenytoin equivalent: 1.5 mg fosphenytoin to be given for each milligram of phenytoin desired. One PE = 1.5 mg fosphenytoin = 1 mg phenytoin.

DOSAGES

Selected Antiepileptic Drugs—cont'd

Drug (Pregnancy Category)	Pharmacologic Class	Usual Dosage Range	Indications
phenytoin (Dilantin) (D)	Hydantoin	**Pediatric** PO: 4-8 mg/kg/day IV: 15-20 mg/kg **Adult** PO: 300-600 mg/day IV: 15-20 mg/kg	Tonic-clonic; psychomotor seizures Convulsions
primidone (Mysoline) (D)	Barbiturate	**Pediatric** PO: <8 yr, 125-500 mg/tid Dosage for pediatric <8 yr is initially 50-125 mg at bedtime, slowly titrated up to 125-250 mg tid; >8 yr is initially 125-250 mg at bedtime, slowly titrated up to 250 mg; max 2 g/day **Adult/pediatric** PO: >8 yr, 250 mg 4-6 times/day; max 2 g/day	Partial seizures Tonic-clonic seizures Partial seizures
tiagabine (Gabitril) (C)	Miscellaneous	**Pediatric** PO: 12-18 yr, 4 mg qd-32 mg divided bid-qid **Adult** 4 mg qd-56 mg divided bid-qid	Partial seizures
topiramate (Topamax) (C)	Miscellaneous	**Pediatric** PO: 1-9 mg/kg/day **Adult** PO: 25-1600 mg/day	Multiple seizures
valproic acid (Depakene, Depakote) (D)	Miscellaneous	**Adult/pediatric** PO: 15-60 mg/kg/day divided bid-tid	Multiple seizures
zonisamide (Zonegram) (C)	Miscellaneous	**Pediatric** >16 yr, 100-400 mg/day **Adult** 100-400 mg/day	Partial seizures
pregabalin (Lyrica) (C)	Miscellaneous	**Adult** PO: 150-600 mg/day divided into 2 or 3 doses	Partial seizures

Life Span Considerations: The Pediatric Patient

AEDs

- Should a skin rash develop in a child or infant taking phenytoin, the drug should be discontinued immediately and the physician notified.
- Chewable dosage forms of AEDs should not be used for once-a-day administration, and IM injections of barbiturates or phenytoin should not be used in any patient.
- Family members, parents, significant others, or caregivers should be encouraged to keep a journal with a record of the signs and symptoms before, during, and after the seizure and before, during, and after the treatment with an AED.
- Wearing of a medical alert bracelet or necklace at all times should be encouraged with information about the diagnosis and medication therapy.
- Suspension forms of AEDs should always be shaken thoroughly before use, and graduated device or oral syringe used for more accurate dosing.
- Pediatric patients are more sensitive to barbiturates and may respond to lower than expected doses. They may also show more profound CNS depressive effects related to the AED or show depression, confusion, or excitement (a paradoxical reaction).
- Any excessive sedation, confusion, lethargy, hypotension, bradypnea, tachycardia, and/or decreased movement in pediatric patients taking any AED should be reported to the health care provider immediately.
- Carbamazepine is to be given with meals to reduce risk of GI distress. All suspension forms should be shaken well before use.
- Oral forms of valproic acid should not be given with milk because this may cause the drug to dissolve early and irritate mucosa. Do not give with carbonated beverages.

AED, Antiepileptic drug; *CNS,* central nervous system; *IM,* intramuscular.

Hydantoins

▸ *phenytoin*

Phenytoin (Dilantin) has been used as a first-line AED for many years. It is primarily indicated for the management of tonic-clonic and partial seizures. The most common adverse effects are lethargy, abnormal movements, mental confusion, and cognitive changes. Therapeutic drug levels are usually 10 to 20 mcg/mL. At toxic levels, phenytoin can cause nystagmus, ataxia, dysarthria, and encephalopathy. Long-term phenytoin therapy can cause gingival hyperplasia, acne, hirsutism, and hypertrophy of subcutaneous facial tissue resulting in an appearance known as "Dilantin facies." Scrupulous dental care can help prevent gingival hypertrophy. Another long-term consequence of phenytoin therapy is osteoporosis. Vitamin D therapy may be necessary to prevent this, particularly in women. Phenytoin can interact with other medications, for two main reasons. First, it is highly bound to plasma proteins and competes with other highly protein-bound medications for binding sites. Second, it induces hepatic microsomal enzymes, mainly the cytochrome P-450 system, thereby increasing the metabolism of other drugs and decreasing their levels.

Exaggerated phenytoin effects can be seen in patients with very low serum albumin concentrations. This scenario is most commonly seen in patients who are malnourished or have chronic renal failure. In these patients, it may be necessary to maintain phenytoin levels well below 20 mcg/mL. With lower levels of albumin in a patient's body, more free, unbound, pharmacologically active phenytoin will be present. Phenytoin has many advantages from the standpoint of long-term therapy. It is usually well tolerated, highly effective, and relatively inexpensive. It can also be given intravenously if needed. Phenytoin's long half-life allows it to be given only twice a day, and in some cases once a day. As stressed earlier, compliance with AED treatment is very important to seizure control. If a patient has to remember to take medication only once or twice a day, his or her compliance will be increased and, therefore, the likelihood of therapeutic drug levels being reached is increased, leading to better seizure control.

Parenteral phenytoin is adjusted chemically to a pH of 12 for reasons of drug stability. It is very irritating to veins when injected and should be given slowly (not exceeding 50 mg/min in adults), directly into a large vein through a large-gauge needle (or needleless system, preferably larger than 20 gauge) or intravenous (IV) catheter. Each injection should be followed by an injection of sterile saline through the same needle or intravenous catheter to avoid local venous irritation caused by the alkalinity of the solution. Continuous infusion should be avoided.

Soft-tissue irritation and inflammation has occurred at the site of injection with and without extravasation of intravenous phenytoin. Soft tissue irritation may vary from slight tenderness to extensive necrosis, sloughing, and in rare instances amputation. Improper administration, including subcutaneous (SC) or perivascular injection,

should be avoided to help prevent the possibility of these occurrences. Local irritation, inflammation, tenderness, necrosis, and sloughing have been reported with or without extravasation of intravenous phenytoin.

Fosphenytoin (Cerebyx) was developed in an attempt to overcome some of the physical shortcomings of phenytoin sodium. Fosphenytoin is a water-soluble, phosphorylated phenytoin derivative that can be given intramuscularly or intravenously without causing the burning on injection associated with phenytoin. Fosphenytoin is dosed in *phenytoin equivalents (PE)* as indicated in Table 13-7. The conversion factor is as follows: 1.5 mg of fosphenytoin is *equivalent* to 1 mg of phenytoin. Therefore, for a patient requiring a 100-mg injection dose of phenytoin, 150 mg would be the correct dose of fosphenytoin. Concentrations for IV dosages range from 1.5 mg to 25 mg PE/ml and at a rate of 150mg PE/min or less to avoid hypotension or cardiorespiratory depression. Should arrhythmias or hypotension occur, the infusion should be discontinued. Safety measures to be implemented post-infusion because of ataxia and dizziness, and vital signs should continue to be taken up to 2 hours post-infusion. Fosphenytoin (Cerebyx) should not be confused with Celebrex. IV; incompatabilities are numerous, so always check for in-syringe and in-solution incompatibilities (as is the case with any IV-administered drug). (see Table 13-7).

Pharmacokinetics

Half-Life	Onset	Peak	Duration
10-34 hr	2-24 hr	1.5-2.5 hr	6-12 hr

▸ *valproic acid*

Valproic acid (Depakene, Depakote, Depacon) is used primarily in the treatment of generalized seizures (absence, myoclonic, and tonic-clonic). It has also been shown to be effective for controlling partial seizures. The main adverse effects are drowsiness; nausea, vomiting, and other gastrointestinal disturbances; tremor; weight gain; and transient hair loss. The most serious adverse effects can be fatal: hepatotoxicity and pancreatitis. Valproic acid can interact with many medications. The main reasons for these interactions are protein binding and liver metabolism. It is highly bound to plasma proteins and competes with other highly protein-bound medications for binding sites. It also is highly metabolized by hepatic microsomal enzymes and competes for metabolism. This drug is available in both oral and injectable forms.

Pharmacokinetics

Half-Life	Onset	Peak	Duration
6-16 hr	15-30 min	1-4 hr	4-6 hr

Iminostilbenes

▸ *carbamazepine*

Carbamazepine (Tegretol) is the second most commonly prescribed AED in the United States, after phenytoin. It was marketed in the late 1960s for the treatment of epilepsy in adults after its efficacy and safety for the treatment of trigeminal neuralgia were proved. It was granted approval for use in pediatric patients in 1976. It is chemically related to the tricyclic antidepressants and is considered a first-line AED for the treatment of simple partial, complex partial, and generalized tonic-clonic seizures. It is contraindicated in patients with absence and myoclonic seizures and those who have shown a hypersensitivity reaction to it in the past. Carbamazepine is available as an oral suspension (100 mg/5 mL), a 200-mg tablet, and a 100-mg chewable tablet. There are also extended-release tablets available in 100, 200, and 400 mg. The typical therapeutic serum carbamazepine drug level is 4 to 12 mcg/mL, but as with all AEDs the therapeutic concentrations should be used only as a guideline. Carbamazepine is metabolized to carbamazepine epoxide, which has both anticonvulsant and toxic effects. Carbamazepine undergoes **autoinduction,** the process whereby a drug increases its own metabolism over time, leading to lower than expected drug concentrations. With carba-

Table 13-7	**Phenytoin Sodium Versus Fosphenytoin Sodium**	
	phenytoin sodium (Dilantin IV)	**fosphenytoin sodium (Cerebyx IM/IV)**
pH	12	8.6-9
Maximum infusion rate	50 mg/min	150 mg PE*/min
Admixtures	0.9% saline	0.9% saline or 5% dextrose

*150 mg fosphenytoin sodium =100 mg phenytoin sodium.
IM, Intramuscular; *IV,* intravenous; *PE,* phenytoin sodium equivalents.

mazepine, this process usually occurs within the first 2 months after the start of therapy.

Pharmacokinetics

Half-Life	Onset	Peak	Duration
14-16 hr	Slow	4-8 hr	12-24 hr

oxcarbazepine

Oxcarbazepine (Trileptal) is a keto analog of carbamazepine. Its precise mechanism of action is unknown, although it is known to block voltage-sensitive sodium channels, which aids in stabilizing excited neuronal membranes. It is indicated for partial seizures. In adults it may be used as either monotherapy or adjunct therapy with other AED(s). In children, it is only recommended as adjunct therapy.

Pharmacokinetics

Half-Life	Onset	Peak	Duration
2-9 hr	2-4 hr	2-3 days	Unknown

Miscellaneous Drugs
▶ gabapentin

Gabapentin (Neurontin) is an add-on drug for the treatment of partial seizures and partial seizures with secondary generalization in adults. It is also commonly used to treat neuropathic pain. The exact mechanism of action of gabapentin is unknown, although it is structurally related to the inhibitory neurotransmitter gamma-aminobutyric acid (GABA). Many believe that it works by increasing the synthesis and accumulation between neurons of GABA, hence, the drug name. It may also work by binding to an as yet undefined receptor site in the brain to produce anticonvulsant activity. Abrupt discontinuation of gabapentin can lead to withdrawal seizures. Its only usual contraindication is known drug allergy.

Pharmacokinetics

Half-Life	Onset	Peak	Duration
5-7 hr	Unknown	Unknown	Unknown

lamotrigine

Lamotrigine (Lamictal) is indicated for partial seizures in adults and for generalized seizures related to Lennox-Gastaut syndrome in both children and adult patients. It stabilizes neuronal cell membranes by blocking voltage-sensitive sodium channels, although its precise antiepileptic mechanism of action is unknown. It has no known contraindications other than drug allergy. Its pharmacokinetic parameters can vary widely when taken concurrently with other AEDs.

Pharmacokinetics

Half-Life	Onset	Peak	Duration
25-32 hr	Variable	1.7-2.2 hr	Unknown

levetiracetam

Levetiracetam (Keppra) is indicated as add-on therapy for partial seizures in adults. Its mechanism of action is unknown. However, it is generally well tolerated with the most common adverse effects being somnolence, asthenia, and dizziness. This drug has begun to be used successfully in children. Pediatric dosing information should be determined for each patient by a pediatric neurologist.

Pharmacokinetics

Half-Life	Onset	Peak	Duration
6-8 hr	Rapid	1 hr	Unknown

tiagabine

Tiagabine (Gabitril) is indicated as add-on therapy for partial seizures in adults and children 12 years of age and older. Its exact mechanism of action is unknown. Tiagabine exerts its beneficial ef-

fects by inhibiting the re-uptake of GABA from the neuronal synapses (spaces between neurons) in the brain. It has similar indications and adverse effects to topiramate. In February of 2005, the FDA issued a special warning regarding the use of tiagabine for "off-label" (non–FDA-approved) indications. Although tiagabine is effective in controlling epileptic seizures, there have been several case reports of *paradoxical* (opposite of what would intuitively be expected) seizures in non-epileptic patients who are treated with the drug for other indications. Most of these cases involved patients being treated for psychiatric disorders such as bipolar disorder. Of even greater concern is the fact that the seizure episodes in some of these cases progressed to status epilepticus. For these reasons, prescribers are currently advised to avoid off-label use of this drug. Again, the approved, *labeled* use is partial seizures in patients 12 years or older.

Pharmacokinetics

Half-Life	Onset	Peak	Duration
7-9 hr	Rapid	45 min	Unknown

topiramate

Topiramate is a structurally unique drug chemically related to fructose. Topiramate (Topamax) is indicated as add-on therapy for partial seizures in adults and children 2 years of age and older. Its exact mechanism of action is unknown. However, it is believed to work by blocking sodium channels in neurons, blocking glutamate activity, and enhancing GABA activity.

Pharmacokinetics

Half-Life	Onset	Peak	Duration
21 hr	Good; unaffected by food	2-4 hr	Unknown

zonisamide

Zonisamide (Zonegran) is a sulfonamide derivative indicated as add-on therapy for partial seizures in adults. Its exact mechanism of action is unknown. However, it is known to inhibit certain types of calcium currents in neuronal cell membranes. It does not have GABA activity. It is contraindicated in patients with known drug allergy to the drug itself or sulfonamide antibiotics ("sulfa drugs").

Pharmacokinetics

Half-Life	Onset	Peak	Duration
63 hr	Good	2-6 hr	Unknown

pregabalin

Pregabalin (Lyrica), like gabapentin, is structurally related to GABA, a major neurotransmitter that inhibits brain activity. However, the drug does not bind to GABA receptors, but rather to the alpha$_2$-delta receptor sites, which affect calcium channels in CNS tissues. This is believed to be related to its mechanism of action, although the full mechanism is still uncertain. The drug is indicated as add-on therapy for partial seizures in adult patients.

◆ NURSING PROCESS

◆ ASSESSMENT

When any of the AEDs are to be administered, the nurse should obtain a thorough health and medication history and physical assessment so that any possible allergies, drug interactions (see Table 13-4), and untoward reactions, concerns, contraindications, cautions to any of these medications can be known in advance. Review of the patient's history of seizure disorders is also important to assess and document, with emphasis on precipitating events, duration/frequency, and intensity of the seizure activity.

The nurse needs to also gather results from diagnostic studies and serum laboratory tests—especially those associated with cardiac, respiratory tract, renal, liver, hematologic, and CNS functioning.

Tiagabine, topiramate, and zonisamide are some of the more recent miscellaneous AEDs that have significant contraindications, cautions, and drug interactions that have been previously discussed in the pharmacology section of this chapter and discussed in Tables 13-3 and 13-4. In addition, assessment of mental status with attention to the patient's sensorium and level of consciousness before, during, and after drug therapy and/or seizure activity needs to be completed.

If barbiturates have been ordered, astute assessment of vital signs is especially important due to their central nervous system depression. Assess the room for safety measures (e.g., side rails up or use of a bed alarm system depending on facility policy), noise level (control of), and the presence of seizure precautions (keeping oxygen, suctioning equipment, and airway nearby, use of padded side rails, and IV access per facility policy). With barbiturates and phenytoins, assessing CBC levels and serum chemistry before initiating drug therapy and after the physician's order is also important with intervals of blood testing about every 2 weeks, should maintenance therapy continue.

Other assessment data include questioning the patient about possible "panic attacks," because high levels of anxiety or stress may precipitate seizure activity. Assess for autonomic nervous system responses to anxiety and "panic," such as cold, clammy hands; excessive sweating (diaphoresis); agitation; trembling of extremities; and complaints of "tension". Patients that are taking oral contraceptives with the drug topiramate should receive education about other means of contraception because of decreased effectiveness. It is also important to be aware of all *other uses* of AEDs, such as with valproic acid in manic episodes and migraine prevention, so that an appropriate assessment is done.

◆ NURSING DIAGNOSES
- Risk for injury related to decreased sensorium from drug-related CNS depression and adverse effects of AEDs
- Deficient knowledge related to lack of familiarity with and information concerning the use of AEDs
- Noncompliance (therapeutic regimen) related to patient's misuse of drugs or lack of understanding about the seizure disorder and its treatment

◆ PLANNING
Goals
- Patient experiences little or no adverse effects associated with noncompliance and/or with overtreatment or undertreatment.
- Patient can identify therapeutic effects of AEDs.
- Patient remains compliant with therapy and without major harm to self during AED treatment.

Outcome Criteria
- Patient will state the therapeutic drug effects and adverse effects of the AED (e.g., sedation, confusion, CNS depression).
- Patient (or family members) will state the importance of taking the medication exactly the way it has been prescribed, such as the same time every day.
- Patient will state the dangers associated with sudden withdrawal of the medication, such as rebound convulsions.
- Patient will maintain a protective environment at home and at work to minimize self-injury.

Implementation

Oral AEDs should be taken regularly at the same time every day at the recommended dose and with meals to diminish gastrointestinal upset. Oral suspensions should be shaken thoroughly and capsules should not be crushed, opened, or chewed—especially if extended or long release forms. Extended-release drugs are usually taken once a day, so be cautious with their use if more frequent dosing is ordered—always check and double check! If there are any questions about the medication order or the medication prescribed, the physician should be contacted immediately for clarification. It is best to give oral AEDs with water but not with juices, milk, or carbonated beverages. Topiramate and valproic acid, in particular, should be taken it their original oral dosage form but the "capsule" forms (not the delayed/extended release forms) may be opened and sprinkled in 1 teaspoon of soft food such as applesauce.

The following interventions are more drug or drug class-specific:
- Carbamazepine: This drug should *not* be given with grapefruit because of increased toxicity of the AED. If the drug is to be replaced with another AED, there should be a plan to decrease one drug prior to beginning low doses (at first) of the new AED. Serum therapeutic levels are presented in Table 13-5.
- Clonazepam: Tablets may be crushed as needed if they are regular release.
- Fosphenytoin: As a point of reference, 150 mg of this drug yields a 100 mg of phenytoin and the dose, concentration solution, and infusion rate of fosphenytoin would be expressed as a phenytoin equivalent (PE). Dilutional fluids include D5W or 0.9% NaCl, and rates of infusion should reflect manufacturer guidelines and are usually given at a rate of 150 mg PE/minute or less to avoid hypotension or cardiorespiratory depression. Should arrhythmias or hypotension occur, the infusion should be discontinued, patient vital signs monitored, and the physician contacted immediately. Safety measures (e.g., help with ambulation, moving slowly and purposefully) should be implemented with this drug (as with all other AEDs) and especially with IV infusions because of the adverse effects of ataxia and dizziness.
- For phenytoin, IV dosage forms should be given very cautiously, only with 0.9% NaCl (to avoid precipitation of the solution), given slowly/as ordered because of possible cardiovascular/respiratory collapse. CNS depression is always a concern; thus there is a need to frequently monitor the patient's vital signs. If existing IV lines are used that contain D5W or other solutions, the line should be flushed with NaCl before and after dosing to avoid precipitate formation. If infiltration of the IV site leads to subcutaneous tissue access, ischemia and sloughing may occur because of the high alkalinity of the drug (as with other AEDs) and hospital/facility policy as well as manufacturer guidelines should be reviewed for use of possible antidotes. If infiltration occurs, discontinue the solution but leave the needle in place until all orders from the physician have been received. Oral dosage forms that are sustained or extended release should never be opened, punctured, chewed, or broken/halved. Other regular forms of the drug may be crushed as needed. Gingival hyperplasia as an adverse effect requires that the patient receive frequent oral care on a daily basis, as well as frequent dental visits. CBC levels are often monitored very closely

within the first year of therapy (e.g., monthly for 1 year, then every 3 months).

- For barbiturates: Avoid abrupt withdrawal as with all AEDs and mix elixir dosage forms with fruit juice, milk, or water. Too rapid of infusion of IV dosage forms may lead to cardiovascular collapse and respiratory depression; therefore, vital signs and IV infusion rates should be frequently monitored.
- Valproic acid: Oral dosage forms are not to be given with carbonated beverages.

In addition to the above drug and drug class-related nursing interventions, it is also important to maintain patient safety, especially airway maintenance. Airway management is a major concern with seizure activity because muscles relax and the tongue may then fall back. The patient's airway may be maintained through the same technique used in airway management during CPR with the use of the chin lift or jaw thrust method. Provide rescue breathing if the patient is not breathing on their own at a rate of 1 breath every 5 seconds and if breathing on their own, just keep the airway open. Also important is maintaining seizure precautions according to hospital policy (e.g., making sure the patient is gently kept in bed or kept from falling, and maintaining quick access to oxygen and suctioning equipment). The dosage frequency of AEDs is important as well, so if such a medication is ordered to be taken, for example, every 6 hours, it should be given around the clock so that drug levels are maintained. See the Patient Teaching Tips for more information.

◆ EVALUATION

A therapeutic response to AEDs does not mean the patient has been cured of the seizures but only that seizure activity is decreased or absent. Any response to the medication should be documented in the nurses' notes. Because AEDs have other indications, such as chronic pain and migraines, the existing problem/condition/disorder should show improvement with minimal adverse effects. In addition, when monitoring and evaluating the effects of AEDs, the nurse needs to constantly assess the patient for mental status, mood and mood changes, sensorium, behavioral changes or changes in the level of consciousness, affect, eye problems or visual disorders, sore throat, and fever (blood dyscrasia is an adverse effect of the hydantoins). The occurrence of vomiting, diplopia, cardiovascular collapse, and Stevens-Johnson syndrome indicates toxicity of the bone marrow, and the physician should be contacted immediately and no further doses administered should these adverse and toxic effects occur. Therapeutic serum levels of the specific AED are ordered at baseline or at the start of therapy and frequently thereafter to monitor the amount of drug in the blood and to see if subsequent serum levels are subtherapeutic, therapeutic, or toxic. Subtherapeutic levels would mean that the drug may need to be increased in dosage amount by the physician or health care provider and toxic levels would require withholding or decreasing the dose—but only after a doctor's order! Specific AED blood levels are listed with each drug profile, as appropriate to the specific drug.

Patient Teaching Tips

- Patient should be aware of the sedating effects of drug therapy so that appropriate steps can be taken to ensure patient safety.
- Patient should be encouraged to avoid tasks requiring alertness to prevent harm to self until a steady state of the drug is achieved (takes 4-5 half-lives).
- Encourage patients to avoid alcohol and smoking while taking AEDs.
- Patients should be informed to not abruptly discontinue AEDs. Abrupt withdrawal may precipitate rebound seizure activity.
- Adverse effects that are most commonly associated with AEDs include drowsiness, but patients should be informed that this often decreases after several weeks of being on the drug.
- Patients should be informed that a reoccurrence of seizure activity is usually due to a lack of compliance.
- Patients should know that some AEDs cause photosensitivity (e.g., lamotrigine), so exposure to sunlight or tanning beds should be avoided. Patients should be instructed on use of sunscreen and protective clothing.

- Patients should be encouraged to avoid any form of stimulants (e.g., caffeine) because of higher risk for seizure activity.
- Patients taking topiramate should force fluids, unless contraindicated, to avoid renal calculi formation.
- It should be reemphasized to the patient that treatment of epilepsy is usually life-long and compliance is important to the effectiveness of therapy. Community and other appropriate resources (e.g., national and local support groups) should be discussed with the patient.
- The patient should be informed to contact the physician if any unusual reactions, such as glandular swelling, fever, sore throat, tarry stools, back pain, hematuria, easy bruising, lethargy, or mouth ulcers occur.
- Backup contraception is recommended with topiramate, and age-appropriate instructions should be thoroughly presented to the patient.

Points to Remember

- The terms for epilepsy (i.e., seizure and convulsion) have very different meanings and should not be used interchangeably:
  - *Epilepsy:* Disorder of the brain manifested as a chronic, recurrent pattern of seizures
  - *Seizure:* Abnormal electrical activity in the brain
  - *Convulsion:* A type of seizure (spasmodic contractions of involuntary muscles)
- Specific drugs are indicated for the different classifications of seizure disorders. The more common classifications are as follows:
  - *Partial:* Short alterations in consciousness, repetitive unusual movements, psychologic changes, and confusion
  - *Generalized:* Most common in childhood; temporary lapses in consciousness (seconds); rhythmic movement of eyes, head, or hands; does not convulse; and may have several a day
  - *Status epilepticus:* A common seizure disorder; a life-threatening emergency that is characterized by tonic-clonic convulsions and may result in brain damage and death if not treated immediately
- Nursing considerations include the following:
  - Nurse must distinguish between focal, primary, secondary, status, tonic-clonic, grand mal, and petit mal seizures and describe exactly what has occurred before, during, and after the seizure event.
  - Noncompliance is the most notable factor leading to treatment failure.
  - Therapeutic blood levels should be monitored at all times, and abrupt withdrawal of the AED avoided.
  - IV infusions of AEDs are very dangerous and should be managed cautiously and through adhering to hospital/facility policy or manufacturer guidelines.
  - Although there are many drug interactions, there are also many IV incompatibilities.

NCLEX Examination Review Questions

1. Which of the following reflects the most appropriate nursing action as related to IV phenytoin (Dilantin)?
   a. Give IV doses via rapid IV push.
   b. Administer in normal saline solutions.
   c. Administer in dextrose solutions.
   d. Ensure continuous infusion of drug.
2. The nurse is reviewing the current drugs taken by a patient who will be starting drug therapy with carbamazepine. Which of the following drugs may be a concern regarding interactions?
   a. Digoxin (Lanoxin)
   b. Acetaminophen (Tylenol)
   c. Diazepam (Valium)
   d. Warfarin (Coumadin)
3. Which of the following would the nurse expect to find in a patient with a phenytoin (Dilantin) level of 35 mcg/mL?
   a. Ataxia
   b. Hypertension
   c. Seizures
   d. No unusual response; this level is therapeutic.
4. Which of the following is most appropriate when administering an AED?
   a. Give on an empty stomach.
   b. May be stopped if seizure activity disappears.
   c. Take at the same time every day.
   d. Crush tablets if unable to swallow.
5. During assessment of a patient with a history of epilepsy, which question would be most important to pose to the patient about the disease and its treatment?
   a. "Do you have a family history of seizures?"
   b. "Do your seizures interfere with your appetite?"
   c. "Do you have severe migraines with the seizure?"
   d. "Do you experience any unusual sensations before the seizure occurs?"

1. b, 2. d, 3. a, 4. c, 5. d.

Critical Thinking Activities

1. Why is assessment of patients important in determining the most appropriate AED?
2. Why is it so important to be aware of concurrent medication administration, including over-the-counter drugs, with patients taking AEDs?
3. A 21-year-old patient has been brought to the emergency department in status epilepticus. She weighs 63 kg. The physician has decided to treat the woman as follows: intravenous diazepam (Valium) 0.3 mg/kg IV push; if no response, phenytoin (Dilantin), 15 mg/kg IV push.
   a. Calculate the dose for each of these drugs, and how they will be given.
   b. Specify what assessments are important when these drugs are given. How do you measure therapeutic response?

For answers, see http://evolve.elsevier.com/Lilley.

Antiparkinsonian Drugs

Objectives

When you reach the end of this chapter, you should be able to do the following:

1. Briefly discuss the pathophysiology related to Parkinson's disease (PD).
2. Identify the different classes of medications used as antiparkinsonian drugs, including first and second line of drugs used in therapy.
3. Discuss the mechanisms of action, dosages, indications, routes of administration, contraindications, cautions, adverse effects, and toxic effects associated with the use of antiparkinsonian drugs.
4. Develop a nursing care plan that includes all phases of the nursing process related to antiparkinsonian drugs.

e Learning Activities

Companion CD

- NCLEX Review Questions: see questions 90-95
- Animations
- Audio Glossary
- Category Catchers
- Medication Errors Checklists
- IV Therapy Checklists

Evolve Website (http://evolve.elsevier.com/Lilley)

• Nursing Care Plans • Frequently Asked Questions • Content Updates • WebLinks • Supplemental Resources • Elsevier ePharmacology Update • Medication Administration Animations

Drug Profiles

amantadine, p. 214
▶ benztropine mesylate, p. 217
bromocriptine p. 215
entacapone, p. 216
levodopa, p. 214

▶ levodopa-carbidopa, p. 214
▶ ropinirole, p. 215
▶ selegiline, p. 212

▶ Key drug.

Glossary

Akinesia   Reduction or lack of psychomotor activity of voluntary muscles. (p. 213)

Anticholinergic drugs   Drugs that block or impede the activity of the neurotransmitter acetylcholine (ACh) at cholinergic receptors in the brain. (p. 216)

Catechol ortho-methyltransferase (COMT) inhibitors   A class of indirect-acting dopaminergic drugs that work by inhibiting the enzyme COMT, which catalyzes the breakdown of dopamine. (p. 213)

Chorea   A condition characterized by involuntary, purposeless, rapid motions such as flexing and extending the fingers,

raising and lowering the shoulders, or grimacing. In some forms, the person is also irritable, emotionally unstable, weak, restless, and fretful. (p. 211)

Dopaminergic drugs   Drugs used to replace the deficiency of dopamine at dopamine receptors in the nerve endings, especially in the brain when treating Parkinson's disease (PD) (can be direct- or indirect-acting or replacement drugs). (p. 212)

Dyskinesia   An impaired ability to execute voluntary movements. (p. 211)

Dystonia   Impaired or distorted voluntary movement due to a disorder of muscle tone. The condition commonly involves the head, neck, and tongue and often occurs as an adverse effect of a medication. (p. 211)

Endogenous   Describes any substance produced by the body's own natural biochemistry (e.g., hormones, neurotransmitters). (p. 212)

Exogenous   Describes any substance produced outside of the body that may be taken into the body (e.g., a medication, food, or even an environmental toxin). (p. 212)

On-off phenomenon   A common experience of patients being medicated for Parkinson's disease in which they experience periods of greater symptomatic control ("on" time) alternating with periods of lesser symptomatic control ("off" time). (p. 214)

Parkinson's disease (PD)   A slowly progressive, degenerative neurologic disorder characterized by resting tremor, pill-rolling of the fingers, masklike facies, shuffling gait, forward flexion of the trunk, loss of postural reflexes, and muscle rigidity and weakness. (p. 210)

Presynaptic drugs   Drugs that exert their antiparkinsonian effects before the nerve synapse. (p. 213)

Wearing off phenomenon   A gradual worsening of Parkinsonian symptoms as a patient's medications begin to lose their effectiveness, despite maximal doses with a variety of medications. (p. 213)

PARKINSON'S DISEASE

Parkinson's disease (PD) is a chronic, progressive, degenerative disorder affecting the dopamine-producing neurons in the brain. Other chronic central nervous system (CNS) neuromuscular disorders include myasthenia gravis, dementia, and Alzheimer's disease. PD was initially recognized in 1817, at which time it was called "shaking palsy." James Parkinson first described the symptoms of both the early and advanced stages of the disease, along with the treatment options. It was not until the 1960s, however, that the underlying pathologic defect was discovered. It was then believed that Parkinson's disease was caused by a dopamine deficit in the area of the cerebral cortex called the *substantia nigra*, which is contained within another brain structure known as the *basal ganglia*. The substantia nigra and basal ganglia are parts of the brain that are included in the *extrapyramidal system*, which is involved in motor function, including posture, muscle tone, and smooth muscle activity.

It is now recognized that PD results from an imbalance in two neurotransmitters—dopamine (DA) and acetylcholine (ACh)—in the basal ganglia. This imbalance is caused by failure of the nerve terminals in the substantia nigra to produce the essential neurotransmitter dopamine. This neurotransmitter acts in the basal ganglia to control movements. Destruction of the substantia nigra leads to dopamine depletion. Dopamine is an inhibitory neurotransmitter, and ACh is an excitatory neurotransmitter in this area of the brain. A correct balance between these two neurotransmitters is needed for the proper regulation of posture, muscle tone, and voluntary movement. Patients who suffer from PD have an imbalance in these neurotransmitters, usually a deficiency of dopamine in the substantia nigra areas of the brain, as mentioned previously. This dopamine deficiency often leads to excessive ACh (cholinergic) activity due to the lack of a normal dopaminergic balancing effect. Figure 14-1 illustrates the difference in neurotransmitter concentrations in persons with normal balance and in patients with PD.

A significant advance in our understanding of the etiology and pathogenesis of PD came in 1983 when the potent neurotoxin 1-methyl-4-phenyl-1,2,3,6-tetrahydropyridine (MPTP) and its metabolic breakdown product 1-methyl-4-phenylpyridine (MPP) were discovered. This illegal substance has been produced in home laboratories and used for recreational purposes. MPTP and MPP selectively destroy the substantia nigra, the same area of the brain that is dysfunctional in PD. It has been shown that a parkinsonian syndrome that is almost identical to idiopathic PD develops in laboratory animals that are injected with this neurotoxin. Others theorize that PD is the result of an earlier head injury or of excess iron in the substantia nigra, which undergoes oxidation and causes the generation of toxic free radicals. In still another theory, it is thought that because dopamine levels naturally decrease with age, PD represents a premature aging of the *nigrostriatal cells* of the substantia nigra resulting from environmental or intrinsic biochemical factors, or both.

PD afflicts at least 1 million Americans. In most patients, the disease becomes apparent between 45 and 65 years of age, with a mean age of onset of 56 years. The number of patients with PD is expected to continue to increase as our elderly population grows. It occasionally occurs in younger people, especially after acute encephalitis or carbon monoxide or metallic poisoning. It

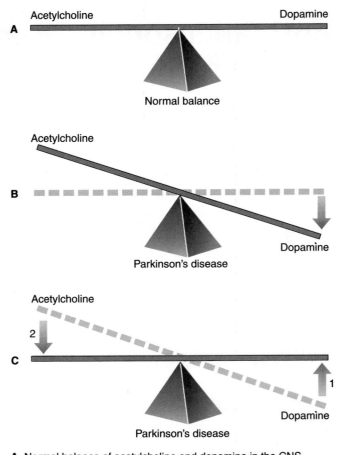

A, Normal balance of acetylcholine and dopamine in the CNS.
B, In Parkinson's disease, a decrease in dopamine results in an imbalance.
C, Drug therapy in Parkinson's disease is aimed at correcting the imbalance between acetylcholine and dopamine. This can be accomplished by either
  1. increasing the supply of dopamine or
  2. blocking or lowering acetylcholine levels.

FIGURE 14-1 The neurotransmitter abnormality of Parkinson's disease.

is usually idiopathic (of no known cause). Overall, there is a 2% chance of PD developing in a person during his or her lifetime. Males may be affected more often than females up to a ratio of 3 to 2. Family history does not seem to be a contributing factor. PD is also a prominent cause of disability because of the common accompanying motor complications.

There are no readily available laboratory tests that can detect or confirm PD. Results of computerized tomography (CT), magnetic resonance imaging (MRI), cerebrospinal fluid analysis, and electroencephalography are usually normal and of little diagnostic value. A positron emission tomography (PET) scan may offer some additional information. This new type of scanning involves intravenous (IV) injections of deoxyglucose with radioactive fluorine. The various shades of colors that show up indicate areas of abnormalities and assist in the diagnosis of neurologic disorders, including PD. CT, MRI, and PET may be useful tools for ruling out other possible diseases as causes of the symptoms. The diagnosis of PD is usually made on the basis of the classic symptoms and physical findings. The classic symptoms of PD are listed in Table 14-1.

Table 14-1   Classic Parkinsonian Symptom

Symptom	Description
Bradykinesia	Slowness of movement
Rigidity	"Cogwheel" rigidity, resistance to passive movement
Tremor	Pill rolling: tremor of the thumb against the forefinger, seen mostly at rest, is less severe during voluntary activity; starts usually on one side then progresses to the other; is the presenting sign in 70% of cases
Postural	Danger of falling, hesitation in gait as instability patient starts or stops walking

Table 14-2   Antiparkinsonian Drugs

Drug Category	Drugs
Anticholinergic drugs	benztropine, biperiden, procyclidine, trihexyphenidyl
Antihistamines (used for their anticholinergic effects)	diphenhydramine, orphenadrine
Dopamine receptor agonists (direct acting)	bromocriptine, levodopa, levodopa-carbidopa, pramipexole, ropinirole

Indirect-Acting Dopamine Receptor Agonists

MAO-B inhibitor	selegiline
COMT inhibitor	entacapone, tolcapone
Miscellaneous drugs	amantadine

COMT, Catechol O-methyltransferase; *MAO*, monoamine oxidase.

Unfortunately, PD is a progressive condition. With time, the number of surviving dopaminergic terminals that can take up exogenously administered levodopa and convert it into dopamine decrease. Rapid swings in the response to levodopa (known as the *on-off phenomenon*) also occur. The result is worsening PD when too little dopamine is present or dyskinesias when too much is present. **Dyskinesia** is the difficulty in performing voluntary movements that some patients with PD have. The two dyskinesias most commonly associated with antiparkinsonian therapy are **chorea** (irregular, spasmodic, involuntary movements of the limbs or facial muscles) and **dystonia** (abnormal muscle tone leading to impaired or abnormal movements). Symptoms of PD do not appear until approximately 80% of the dopamine store in the substantia nigra of the basal ganglia has been depleted. This means that by the time PD is diagnosed, only approximately 20% of the patient's original nigral dopaminergic terminals are functioning normally.

Nerve terminals can take up substances, store them, and release them for use when needed. It is this factor that forms the basis for antiparkinsonian treatment. As long as there are functioning nerve terminals that can take up dopamine, the symptoms of PD can be at least partially controlled. The blood-brain barrier does not allow exogenously supplied dopamine to enter the brain; however, it does allow levodopa, a naturally occurring dopamine precursor, to do so. After levodopa has been taken up by the dopaminergic terminal, it is converted into dopamine and then released as needed. Levodopa therapy can thus correct the neurotransmitter imbalance in patients with early PD who still have functioning nerve terminals.

The first step in the treatment of PD is a full explanation of the disease to the patient and his or her family members or significant others. Physical therapy, speech therapy, and occupational therapy are almost always needed when the patient is in the later stages of the disease. As previously discussed, drug therapy is aimed at increasing the levels of dopamine as long as there are functioning nerve terminals. It is also aimed at antagonizing or blocking the effects of ACh and slowing the progression of the disease. The drugs available for the treatment of PD and their respective categories are listed in Table 14-2.

SELECTIVE MONOAMINE OXIDASE INHIBITOR THERAPY

There are two subclasses of monoamine oxidase (MAO) in the body: MAO-A and MAO-B. As early as 1965, nonselective monoamine oxidase inhibitors (MAOIs), which inhibit both MAO-A and MAO-B, were being used to improve the therapeutic effect of levodopa in patients with PD. They were also among the first medications used to treat depression, but their use for this purpose has been widely supplanted by newer drug categories (as discussed in Chapter 15). However, a major adverse effect of these nonselective MAOIs has been that they interact with tyramine-containing foods (cheese, red wine, beer, and yogurt) because of their inhibitory activity against MAO-A. This has been called the "cheese effect," and one hazardous result can be severe hypertension. This has considerably restricted the therapeutic use of MAOIs. In 1974, selegiline, an amphetamine derivative, was introduced as an investigational treatment option for PD. As a selective MAO-B inhibitor, selegiline is much less likely to elicit the classic cheese effect at doses of 10 mg or less daily. In the years that followed, many investigational studies were conducted, and, in October 1989, selegiline received approval by the U.S. Food and Drug Administration (FDA) for use in conjunction with levodopa therapy in the treatment of PD. There was earlier speculation by researchers that selegiline, as well as possibly vitamins E (tocopherol) and C (ascorbic acid), might have antiparkinsonian effects due to "neuroprotective" activity at the neuronal (nerve cell) level. The results of some animal studies suggested this as a possibility. However, no human or animal studies to date have conclusively demonstrated this to be the case for any of these three substances.

Mechanism of Action and Drug Effects

MAOs are widely distributed throughout the body. The areas where concentrations are high are the liver, kidney, stomach, intestinal wall, and brain. As mentioned previously, there are two subclasses of MAOs: A and B. Most of MAO-B is in the CNS, primarily in the brain. The primary role of MAOs is the catabolism or breakdown of catecholamines, such as dopamine, norepinephrine, and epinephrine, as well as the breakdown of serotonin. Therefore, an MAO-B inhibitor such as selegiline causes an increase in the levels of dopaminergic stimulation in the CNS. This helps to counter the dopaminergic deficiency that arises from the PD pathology. Selegiline allows the dose of levodopa (see Dopaminergic Therapy in this chapter) to be decreased. Improvement in functional ability and decreased severity of symptoms are

Table 14-3	Selegiline: Adverse Effects
Body System	**Adverse Effects**
Cardiovascular	Hypotension, dysrhythmia, tachycardia, palpitations, angina, edema
Central nervous	Altered sensation, pain, dizziness, drowsiness, irritability, anxiety, extrapyramidal adverse effects, CNS depression and unresponsiveness, tremors, seizures
Gastrointestinal	Nausea, vomiting, constipation, diarrhea, anorexia
Respiratory	Asthma, shortness of breath, apnea

PREVENTING MEDICATION ERRORS

Look-Alike Drugs: Selegiline and Salagen

Be careful about look-alike drugs! Medication errors often occur when drug names are similar.

Selegiline is a MAOI that is used to treat Parkinson's disease. Salagen, an oral form of pilocarpine hydrochloride, is prescribed for relief of dry mouth symptoms, also known as xerostomia, in patients who have Sjögren's syndrome or who have received radiation therapy. To make it more confusing, both drugs are available in 5-mg tablets. Be sure to double-check the name and use of these drugs when receiving orders and instruct patients to check the drug names when getting these drugs filled at pharmacies.

For more information, visit www.ismp.org/newsletters/acutecare/articles/20050922_1.asp. Accessed July 23, 2006.

common after selegiline is added. However, only approximately 50% to 60% of patients show a positive response.

Indications

Selegiline is currently approved for use in combination with levodopa or levodopa-carbidopa. It is an adjunctive drug used when a patient's response to levodopa is fluctuating. Selegiline may also be somewhat beneficial as a prophylactic drug to delay patients' reduced responses to levodopa. Several studies have shown that selegiline-treated patients required levodopa therapy approximately 1.8 times later than control patients. One problem that patients with PD experience is that as their disease progresses it becomes more and more difficult to control it with levodopa. Ultimately, levodopa no longer controls the PD, and the patient is seriously debilitated. This generally occurs between 5 and 10 years after the start of levodopa therapy. Prophylactic selegiline use may delay the development of serious debilitating PD for 9 to 18 years. Because the average age of patients at the onset of PD is between 55 and 65 years, such a delay can prevent functional disability during the patient's life span, depending on the age at death.

Contraindications

Selegiline is normally contraindicated in cases of known drug allergy. Concurrent use of the opioid drug meperidine is contraindicated because of the likelihood of introducing a dangerous condition known as *serotonin syndrome* (see Chapter 15).

Adverse Effects

The most common adverse effects associated with selegiline use are mild and consist of nausea, lightheadedness, dizziness, abdominal pain, insomnia, confusion, and dry mouth. The adverse effects seen with selegiline use as they relate to the various body systems are listed in Table 14-3. Reactions seen when the dosage exceeds 10 mg/day include a hypertensive crisis (with the consumption of tyramine-containing food), memory loss, muscular twitches and jerks, and grinding of the teeth.

Interactions

The number of drugs with which selegiline interacts is relatively small, and the degree of interaction is dose dependent. At recommended doses of 10 mg/day, the drug maintains its selective MAO-B inhibition. However, at doses that exceed 10 mg/day, selegiline becomes a nonselective MAOI, contributing to the development of the cheese effect. Meperidine is contraindicated in

patients receiving nonselective MAOIs because this combination has been associated with the occurrence of fatal hypertensive episodes. It is suggested that meperidine, as well as other opioids, be avoided in patients taking more than 10 mg/day of selegiline. For the same reasons, combinations with other drugs, including dextroamphetamine, methylphenidate, dextromethorphan, sibutramine, and serotonin-selective reuptake inhibitors (SSRIs) (see Chapter 15) should also be avoided.

Dosage

For the recommended dosage of selegiline, see the table on page 215. Also see the Preventing Medication Errors box.

Drug Profiles

▶ *selegiline*

Selegiline (Eldepryl) is an MAO-B inhibitor used as an adjunctive drug along with levodopa to decrease the amount of levodopa needed.

Pharmacokinetics

Half-Life*	Onset	Peak	Duration
2 hr	1 hr	0.5-2 hr	1-3 days

*Selegiline has three active metabolites with long half-lives of 18 to 21 hours.

DOPAMINERGIC THERAPY

Because in PD little or no **endogenous** dopamine is produced, ACh is left as the predominant neurotransmitter in the brain, creating a state of imbalance. **Dopaminergic drugs** are used to provide **exogenous** replacement of the lost dopamine or enhance the function of the few neurons that are still producing their own dopamine. Dopaminergic drugs can be broken down into three categories based on their underlying mechanisms of action: those that release dopamine from remaining functional dopamine vesicles in presynaptic fibers of neurons or that inhibit dopamine-metabolizing enzymes (indirect acting), those that increase brain levels of dopamine by providing exogenous dopamine in tablet form (direct-acting/replacement), and dopaminergic agonists that act as dopamine substitutes and stimulate dopamine receptors directly in place of dopamine (direct-acting). The ultimate goal is to increase the levels of dopamine in the brain. By doing so and creating a balance with ACh, akinesias, the most detrimental complications of PD, can be reversed. **Akine-**

sias are symptoms such as a masklike facial expression and impaired postural reflexes. They eventually render the patient unable to care for himself or herself.

Mechanism of Action and Drug Effects

Levodopa and the combination product levodopa-carbidopa provide exogenous sources of dopamine that directly replace the deficient neurotransmitter dopamine in the substantia nigra. They are considered the cornerstone of the treatment of PD. Levodopa is the biologic precursor of dopamine required by the brain for dopamine synthesis. These drugs are also referred to as **presynaptic drugs** *or replacement drugs.* This is because they work presynaptically and attempt to increase brain levels of dopamine. Dopamine must be administered in this form because, as mentioned previously, exogenously administered dopamine cannot pass through the blood-brain barrier, whereas levodopa can. Once it does, it is converted directly into dopamine by the enzyme dopa-decarboxylase. Traditionally, very large doses of levodopa had to be administered to get enough dopamine to the brain because much of the levodopa administered was broken down outside the CNS by this same enzyme. These large doses resulted in high peripheral levels of dopamine and many unwanted adverse effects such as confusion, involuntary movements, gastrointestinal (GI) distress, and hypotension. Levodopa has even been known to cause dysrhythmias. These problems are avoided when levodopa is given with carbidopa, a peripheral decarboxylase inhibitor that does not cross the blood-brain barrier. Therefore, carbidopa prevents levodopa breakdown in the periphery. As a result, levodopa is allowed to reach and cross the blood-brain barrier, yet carbidopa does not cross this barrier. Once in the brain, the levodopa is then converted to dopamine, which can then exert its therapeutic antiparkinsonian effects by offsetting the dopamine ACh imbalance.

Originally developed and used for the prophylaxis and treatment of viral disorders, amantadine (Symmetrel) has proved to be a valuable adjunct to the traditional antiparkinsonian drugs. Amantadine appears to exert its antiparkinsonian effect by causing the release of dopamine and other catecholamines from their storage sites in the ends of nerve cells that are still intact and have not yet been destroyed by the disease process. Amantadine also blocks the reuptake of dopamine into the nerve endings, which allows more dopamine to accumulate both centrally and peripherally. Therefore, its dopaminergic effects are the result of its indirect actions on the nerve because amantadine does not directly stimulate dopamine receptors as do certain other types of PD drugs. Amantadine also has some anticholinergic properties. This may further help by controlling symptoms of dyskinesias.

Bromocriptine (Parlodel) and pergolide (Permax)* are dopaminergic agonists that directly stimulate the dopamine receptors. Chemically, bromocriptine is an ergot alkaloid similar to ergotamine in its chemical structure. Its antiparkinsonian effects are due to its ability to activate dopamine receptors and stimulate the production of more dopamine. This helps correct the imbalance between ACh and dopamine in the CNS. Pergolide, on the other hand, while also an ergot alkaloid, has no effect on dopamine synthesis or dopamine storage sites. It stimulates dopamine receptors in the substantia nigra of the brain, the area believed to be defective

in patients with PD. Bromocriptine is a D2 dopamine agonist, whereas pergolide stimulates D1-3 receptors. Another difference between these two postsynaptic drugs is that pergolide is 20 times more potent than bromocriptine and has a half-life that is 3 times longer than that of bromocriptine. Pramipexole (Mirapex) and ropinirole (Requip) are two new highly specific D2-3 dopamine agonists that were released in 1997. They are both nonergot drugs that are effective in early and late stages of PD.

Tolcapone (Tasmar) and entacapone (Comtan) are two drugs that belong to a totally new class of antiparkinsonian drugs, the **catechol ortho-methyltransferase (COMT) inhibitors.** COMT inhibitors help patients with PD by inhibiting COMT, the enzyme responsible for the breakdown of levodopa, the dopamine precursor. In this way, COMT inhibitors are also indirect-acting dopaminergic drugs. Tolcapone differs slightly from entacapone in that it may act both centrally and peripherally. Entacapone cannot cross the blood-brain barrier and therefore can act only peripherally. The main positive effect of these drugs is that they prolong the duration of levodopa benefit. Patients have less of a **wearing off phenomenon** and experience prolonged benefits. Along with amantadine, COMT inhibitors are also considered to be indirect-acting drugs and work as presynaptic drugs.

Indications

All three of these classes of dopaminergic drugs are used to treat various stages of Parkinson's disease, either alone or in combination with other drugs. Bromocriptine also inhibits the production of the hormone *prolactin,* which stimulates normal lactation. For this reason, it is used to treat women with excessive or undesired breast milk production *(galactorrhea)* and is also used for treatment of prolactin-secreting tumors.

Contraindications

Contraindications to dopaminergic drugs include known drug allergy, history of melanoma or any undiagnosed skin condition, and narrow-angle glaucoma. In addition, these drugs should also not be used until at least 14 days after MAOI therapy (except selegiline) is stopped.

Adverse Effects

There are many potential adverse effects associated with the dopaminergic drugs. The most common of these are listed in Table 14-4. Effects that may occur with any of these drugs include syncope, rhinorrhea, and abdominal pain. Unfortunately, postmarketing case reports of severe liver failure with tolcapone have led to strong recommendations against using this drug, unless the patient is significantly less responsive to other PD drugs and shows substantial benefit with tolcapone. Regular blood liver enzyme studies are necessary for patients taking this drug. At the time of this writing, tolcapone still remains on the U.S. market. To date, no similar pattern of adverse outcomes has been shown with the other available COMT inhibitor, entacapone, making it a better first choice for COMT inhibitor therapy for PD patients.

Interactions

The drug interactions involving dopaminergic drugs can cause significant adverse reactions, including a decrease in the efficacy of the dopaminergic drug, a hypertensive crisis, and reversal of the dopaminergic drug's effect. Hydantoins, when given with le-

---

*Peroglide was voluntarily removed from the market in March 2007.

Table 14-4 Dopaminergic Drugs: Adverse Effects

Body System	Adverse Effects
Amantadine	
Central nervous	Impaired concentration, dizziness, increased irritability, nervousness, blurred vision
Gastrointestinal	Anorexia, nausea, constipation, vomiting
Other	Purple-red skin spots; dryness of mouth, nose, and throat; increased weakness
Entacapone	
Central nervous	Involuntary movements (dyskinesias)
Gastrointestinal	Nausea, abdominal pain, diarrhea, decreased appetite
Other	Urine discoloration (brownish-orange)
Levodopa-Carbidopa	
Hematologic	Hemolytic anemia, agranulocytosis
Cardiovascular	Palpitations, orthostatic hypotension
Central nervous	Agitation; anxiety; psychotic and suicidal episodes; choreiform, dystonic, and other involuntary movements; headache and blurred vision
Ropinirole	
Cardiovascular	Syncope sometimes associated with bradycardia, symptomatic orthostatic hypotension
Central nervous	Hallucinations; somnolence; uncontrolled movement of body, face, tongue, arms, hands, and head
Gastrointestinal	Nausea

vodopa, increase the metabolism of levodopa, decreasing its effects. Haloperidol and phenothiazines, when given with levodopa, block dopamine receptors in the brain, resulting in decreased levodopa levels. Nonselective MAOIs taken concomitantly with dopaminergic drugs can result in inhibited metabolism, leading to a possible hypertensive crisis. Pyridoxine (vitamin B_6) promotes levodopa breakdown and may reverse levodopa effects. Carbidopa may help prevent this adverse outcome. The selective MAO-B inhibitor selegiline may be safely taken concurrently with COMT inhibitors.

Dosages

For the recommended dosages of the dopaminergic drugs, see the table on page 215.

Drug Profiles

levodopa

As described earlier, the treatment of PD centers around attempts to replace the dopamine deficiency. Dopamine does not cross the blood-brain barrier, whereas levodopa, a precursor of dopamine, does. However, levodopa is also converted into dopamine in the rest of the body outside the brain. This can cause many unwanted adverse effects, including cardiac dysrhythmias, hypotension, chorea, muscle cramps, and gastrointestinal distress.

Levodopa is contraindicated in patients who have shown a hypersensitivity reaction to it, those with narrow-angle glaucoma or a history of melanoma, and those concurrently taking MAOIs. Normally levodopa is taken orally, but the latest research literature describes

giving levodopa by intravenous or gastrointestinal infusion for the most severe PD cases. Time will tell whether or not this becomes conventional treatment.

Pharmacokinetics

Half-Life	Onset	Peak	Duration
1-3 hr	2-3 wk*	1-3 hr	<5 hr

*Therapeutic effect.

▶ levodopa-carbidopa

The peripheral decarboxylase inhibitor carbidopa does not cross the blood-brain barrier. However, it does prevent metabolism of levodopa to dopamine in the periphery (i.e., outside the CNS). This, in turn, limits peripheral dopamine-induced adverse effects, such as those described earlier. Instead, the levodopa can reach its site of action in the brain without being broken down. As a result, much lower daily doses of levodopa are needed. Levodopa-carbidopa (Sinemet, Sinemet CR) has become the cornerstone in the treatment of PD and is used much more commonly than levodopa alone. It also appears to limit the **on-off phenomenon** that some patients with PD experience. This phenomenon is seen in patients taking levodopa long term. Such patients may experience periods when they have good control ("on" time) and periods when they have bad control or breakthrough PD ("off" time). A variety of studies have shown that the controlled-release product, Sinemet CR (or generic), increases on time and decreases off time. When converting patients from conventional levodopa-carbidopa preparations, the dosage of Sinemet CR should include 10% to 30% more levodopa per day. The interval between dosages of Sinemet CR should be 4 to 8 hours during the waking day. Sinemet CR should not be crushed.

Levodopa-carbidopa is contraindicated in patients who have shown a hypersensitivity reaction to it, those with narrow-angle glaucoma or a history of melanoma, and those concurrently taking MAOIs.

Pharmacokinetics

Half-Life	Onset	Peak	Duration
1-3 hr	2-3 wk*	1-3 hr	<5 hr

*Therapeutic effect.

amantadine

Amantadine (Symmetrel) is believed to work in the CNS by eliciting the release of dopamine from nerve endings, causing higher concentrations of dopamine in the CNS. It is most effective in the earlier stages of PD when there are still significant numbers of nerves to act on and dopamine to be released. As the disease progresses, however, the population of functioning nerves diminishes, and so does amantadine's effect. Amantadine is usually effective for only 6 to 12 months. After amantadine fails to relieve the hypokinesia and rigidity, a dopamine agonist such as bromocriptine is usually tried next.

Amantadine is contraindicated in patients who have shown a hypersensitivity reaction to it, women who are lactating, and children younger than 1 year of age (amantadine is also an antiviral drug).

Pharmacokinetics

Half-Life	Onset	Peak	Duration
11-15 hr	48 hr	2-4 hr	6-12 wk

Dopamine Agonists

The traditional role of dopamine agonists (bromocriptine, pramipexole, ropinirole, and cabergoline) has been as adjunct to levodopa for management of motor fluctuations only. These drugs differ from levodopa in that they do not replace dopamine itself but still act by stimulation of dopaminergic receptors in the brain. The drugs have been evaluated as initial monotherapy and as combination therapy with low-dose levodopa in an attempt to delay levodopa therapy or reduce total exposure to the drug and associated motor complications. The newer drugs pramipexole, ropinirole, and cabergoline are more specific for the receptors associated with parkinsonian symp-

DOSAGES

Selegiline and Selected Dopaminergic Drugs

Drug (Pregnancy Category)	Pharmacologic Class	Usual Dosage Range	Indications
amantadine (Symmetrel) (C)	Indirect-acting dopamine agonist	**Adult** PO: 100-400 mg/day divided q12h	
bromocriptine (Parlodel) (D)	Direct-acting dopamine agonist	**Adult** PO: 2.5-90 mg/day	
entacapone (Comtan) (C)	Indirect-acting dopamine agonist	**Adult** PO: 200 mg with each dosage of levodopa, up to 8×/day	
levodopa (Larodopa) (C)	Direct-acting dopamine agonist/replacement	**Adult** PO: 500-8000 mg/day divided bid-qid	
▶levodopa-carbidopa (Sinemet) (C)	Direct-acting dopamine agonist/replacement	**Adult** PO: 10/100, 1 tab 3-8×/day; 25/100, 1 tab 3-6×/day; 25/250, 1 tab tid-qid CR: 1 tab bid; up to 2-8 tabs at 4- to 8-hr intervals	PD
pergolide (Permax) (B)*	Direct-acting dopamine agonist	**Adult** PO: Up to 5 mg/day in combination with levodopa-carbidopa	
pramipexole (Mirapex) (C)	Direct-acting dopamine agonist	**Adult** PO: 1.5-4.5 mg/day divided tid	
ropinirole (Requip) (C)	Direct-acting dopamine agonist	**Adult** PO: 0.25 mg tid slowly titrating to max dose of 24 mg/day	
▶selegiline (Eldepryl) (C)	Indirect-acting dopamine agonist/selective MAOI	**Adult** PO: 5 mg bid with breakfast and lunch in combination with levodopa-carbidopa, or 10 mg qam	
tolcapone (Tasmar) (C)	Indirect-acting dopamine agonist	**Adult** PO: 100-200 mg tid	

CR, Controlled release; *MAOI*, monoamine oxidase inhibitor; *PD*, Parkinson's disease.
*Pergolide was voluntarily removed from the market in March 2007.

toms, the D2 family (D2, D3, and D4). This in turn may have more specific antiparkinsonian effects with fewer adverse effects associated with generalized dopaminergic stimulation. These newer dopamine agonists have a promising role in the early treatment of PD. They appear to delay the start of levodopa therapy. Another benefit is that they have less ergot-like effects and dyskinesias. Bromocriptine is structurally similar to ergot derivatives and has some of their unwanted effects. These newer drugs have also shown efficacy in patients with advanced PD.

bromocriptine and pergolide*

Once amantadine becomes ineffective, a dopamine agonist such as pergolide (Permax) or bromocriptine (Parlodel) may be prescribed in its place. Bromocriptine differs from pergolide in that it only stimulates the dopamine 2 (D2) receptors and antagonizes or blocks the dopamine 1 (D1) receptors. Pergolide stimulates or acts as an agonist at both types of receptors. Eventually, levodopa-carbidopa is needed to control the patient's symptoms, but by using amantadine until it fails, and then a dopamine agonist until it fails, the need for levodopa therapy may be postponed for up to 3 years. These two drugs may also be given with levodopa-carbidopa so that lower doses of the levodopa are needed. This often results in prolonging the on periods, when PD is controlled, and decreasing the off periods, when PD is not controlled.

Bromocriptine is contraindicated in patients who have shown a hypersensitivity reaction to any of the ergot alkaloids, patients with severe ischemic disease, and those with severe peripheral vascular

disease. This is primarily because of bromocriptine's ability to stimulate dopamine receptors.

Pharmacokinetics (bromocriptine)

Half-Life	Onset	Peak	Duration
3-5 hr	0.5-1.5 hr	1-3 hr	4-8 hr

Pergolide is contraindicated in patients who have shown a hypersensitivity reaction to it or to other ergot alkaloids.

Pharmacokinetics (pergolide)

Half-Life	Onset	Peak	Duration
27 hr	15-30 min	1-3 hr	1-2 days

▶ ropinirole

Ropinirole (Requip) is a newer nonergot dopamine agonist indicated for monotherapy for PD and adjunctive therapy with levodopa. It is also approved by the FDA for moderate to severe primary restless legs syndrome. This is a nocturnal disorder characterized by excessive leg movements that disrupt sleep. It is highly selective for the D2 family of dopamine receptors. It is contraindicated in patients who have shown a hypersensitivity reaction to it.

Pharmacokinetics

Half-Life	Onset	Peak	Duration
3-5 hr	30 min	1-2 hr	6-10 hr

*Peroglide was voluntarily removed from the market in March 2007.

COMT Inhibitors

Inhibition of the enzyme in the body known as COMT is a new strategy for prolonging the duration of action of levodopa. As mentioned previously, this is a naturally occurring enzyme in the body that breaks down dopamine molecules. Two compounds were developed for this purpose: tolcapone (Tasmar) and entacapone (Comtan). Both drugs are reversible inhibitors of COMT. The major difference between them is that tolcapone has a longer duration of action. COMT inhibitors help patients with PD by inhibiting COMT, the enzyme responsible for the breakdown of levodopa. Tolcapone differs slightly from entacapone in that it may act centrally and peripherally. Entacapone cannot cross the blood-brain barrier and therefore can act only peripherally. The main positive effect of these drugs is that they prolong the duration of levodopa benefit. Patients have less wearing off and experience prolonged benefits. A "wearing-off" effect is what many Parkinson's patients experience as medications gradually begin to lose their effectiveness and disease symptoms worsen as a result. Along with amantadine, the COMT inhibitors are considered to be indirect-acting drugs and work as presynaptic drugs.

entacapone

Entacapone (Comtan) is a potent COMT inhibitor indicated for the adjunctive treatment of PD. The most recent safety information indicates that entacapone does not appear to be hepatotoxic. Hepatotoxicity was a problem with tolcapone, and no liver tests are required for patients taking entacapone. Entacapone is taken with levodopa and should be effective from the first dose. A patient with PD can feel the benefit of entacapone within a day or two. Entacapone is particularly effective in patients who are experiencing wearing off fluctuations. Entacapone, used with levodopa, can reduce the daily off time and increase the daily on time. The levodopa dose and dosing frequency can also be reduced in many cases. Entacapone is contraindicated in patients who have shown a hypersensitivity reaction to it. This drug is also now available in a combination tablet that contains various dosages of entacapone, carbidopa, and levodopa (Stalevo).

Pharmacokinetics

Half-Life	Onset	Peak	Duration
1.5-3.5 hr	1 hr	0.5-1.5 hr	6 hr

ANTICHOLINERGIC THERAPY

Anticholinergic drugs, or drugs that block the effects of ACh, are sometimes useful in treating the muscle tremors and muscle rigidity associated with PD. These two symptoms are caused by excessive cholinergic activity, which occurs due to lack of the normal dopamine balance. Anticholinergics do little, however, to relieve the bradykinesia (extremely slow movements) associated with PD. The rationale for the use of anticholinergics is to reduce excessive cholinergic activity in the brain. The first drugs in this category to be used were the belladonna alkaloids, atropine and scopolamine. However the anticholinergic adverse effects of dry mouth, urinary retention, and blurred vision can be excessive; therefore, new synthetic anticholinergics and antihistamines with better adverse effect profiles (e.g., benztropine and trihexyphenidyl) were developed.

Mechanism of Action and Drug Effects

All anticholinergics work in some way to block ACh (central cholinergic excitatory pathways). Because of the reduced number of dopamine-producing nerves associated with PD, the ACh-producing nerves are left unchecked, and ACh accumulates. This causes an overstimulation of the cholinergic excitatory pathways, resulting in muscle tremors and muscle rigidity. This is sometimes described as *cogwheel rigidity*. The muscle tremors are usually worse while the patient is at rest and consist of a pill-rolling movement and bobbing of the head. Anticholinergic drugs have either the opposite effect or oppose the effects of the neurotransmitter ACh, which is responsible for causing increased *s*alivation, *l*acrimation (tearing of the eyes), *u*rination, *d*iarrhea, increased *G*I motility, and possibly *e*mesis (vomiting). The acronym SLUDGE is often used to describe these cholinergic-induced effects. With these in mind, effects of anticholinergics would be the opposite of the SLUDGE symptoms—effects such as antisecretory effects (dry mouth or decreased salivation), urinary retention, decreased gastrointestinal motility (constipation), dilated pupils (mydriasis), and smooth muscle relaxation. These drugs readily cross the blood-brain barrier and, therefore, can get right to the site of the imbalance in the CNS—the substantia nigra. It is because of their ability to directly relax smooth muscles that the muscle rigidity and akinesia (lack of movement) are reduced.

Indications

Anticholinergic drugs are indicated as antidyskinetic drugs in PD. They are also used for the treatment of drug-induced extrapyramidal reactions such as those related to selected antipsychotic drugs.

Contraindications

Contraindications to anticholinergic drugs include known drug allergy, any type of GI or bladder outlet obstruction, cardiac disease, glaucoma, and myasthenia gravis.

Adverse Effects

The adverse effects associated with anticholinergic drug use are many, and the most common ones are listed in Table 14-5. They occur more commonly when the drugs are given in high doses. Anticholinergic-induced adverse effects are also more common in elderly patients. However, wise and judicious use of such drugs can lead to very effective treatment that is free of the unwanted adverse effects.

Interactions

The interactions that occur between anticholinergic drugs and other drugs and drug classes can be very damaging. Alcohol, CNS depressants, amantadine, phenothiazines, tricyclic antidepressants, and antihistamines can have an additive effect with anticholinergic drugs, resulting in enhanced CNS depressant effects. Antacids, when taken with anticholinergic drugs, alter gas-

Table 14-5	Anticholinergic Drugs: Adverse Effects

Body System	Adverse Effects
Central nervous	Drowsiness, confusion, disorientation, hallucinations
Gastrointestinal	Constipation, nausea, vomiting
Genitourinary	Urinary retention, pain on urination
Other	Blurred vision, dilated pupils (mydriasis), photophobia, dry skin

tric pH and reduce the absorption and decrease the therapeutic effects of anticholinergic drugs.

Dosages

For information on the dosages of benztropine and trihexyphenidyl in the treatment of PD, see the Dosages table on this page.

Drug Profiles

Anticholinergics are helpful in alleviating the muscle tremors and rigidity seen in patients with PD. They are not, however, as effective as the other drug classes used in the treatment of PD in correcting the underlying problem. They are very effective for the relief of only minimal symptoms and for the treatment of those patients who cannot tolerate or do not respond to dopamine replacement drugs such as levodopa or the dopaminergics such as amantadine and bromocriptine. Anticholinergics are also useful as adjuncts to these primary drugs. Treatment is usually started with small doses, which are gradually increased until the benefits or adverse effects appear. Some of the more commonly used drugs include trihexyphenidyl (Artane), diphenhydramine (Benadryl), and benztropine mesylate (Cogentin). Two of the drugs for this purpose are biperiden (Akineton) and procyclidine (Kemadrin). They must be used cautiously in older adults because significant adverse effects such as confusion, urinary retention, visual blurring, palpitations, and increased intraocular pressure can develop. The most commonly used drugs are the synthetic anticholinergics, which are associated with fewer of the adverse effects commonly seen with the belladonna alkaloid derivatives such as atropine and scopolamine.

▶ benztropine mesylate

Benztropine (Cogentin) is a synthetic anticholinergic drug that resembles both atropine and diphenhydramine (Benadryl) in its chemical structure. Biperiden (Akineton) and procyclidine (Kemadrin) are also synthetic anticholinergic drugs used in the treatment of PD. All have anticholinergic and antihistaminic properties and are primarily used as adjuncts in the treatment of all forms of PD. They are also useful in the treatment of phenothiazine-induced extrapyramidal reactions (see Chapter 15). Their use is contraindicated in cases of known drug allergy; in those who have narrow-angle glaucoma, myasthenia gravis, urinary retention, a history of peptic ulcer disease, megacolon, or prostate hypertrophy; and in children under 3 years of age.

Pharmacokinetics

Half-Life	Onset	Peak	Duration
4-8 hr	1 hr	2-4 hr	6-10 hr

◆ NURSING PROCESS

◆ ASSESSMENT

Antiparkinsonian drugs are used to treat Parkinson's disease to reduce the symptoms, as discussed in the earlier part of this chapter; however, some of the drugs have other indications that require additional assessment. For example, amantadine is used for Parkinson's but is also used to treat respiratory infections and control extrapyramidal reactions that occur as adverse effects to groups of drugs such as the phenothiazines. Bromocriptine, another antiparkinsonian drug, is also indicated to suppress milk "let-down" process for those new mothers who choose not to breast-feed.

After a patient is first confronted with the diagnosis of Parkinson's disease, the patient soon learns how the disease can affect every movement and alter activities of daily living (ADLs). This may be physiologically and emotionally stressful, and assessment of support systems and patient's status as a whole is needed throughout the period between diagnosis and treatment. In addition, it may take weeks before therapeutic improvement is seen. As soon as the disease process and associated diagnoses are understood, the patient becomes aware of the significance of drug therapy that is not without challenges. The nurse must begin with a thorough head-to-toe assessment with a medical and medication history. A nursing history should include questions about the following:

- Central nervous system: Have there been any changes or alterations in activities of daily living (ADLs), gait, balance, tremors, weakness, lethargy, and level of consciousness?
- Gastrointestinal (GI) and genitourinary (GU) systems: Have there been any changes in the patient's appetite? Changes in bowel or bladder patterns/habits?
- Psychological and emotional status: Any recent or past changes in mood, affect, depression, or any personality changes?
- Specific disease process: Have there been signs and symptoms of Parkinson's apparent in the patient such as masklike expression; speech problems; dysphagia; rigidity of arms, legs, and neck; tremors; insomnia; inability to perform daily activities; or the inability to maintain emotional stability?

DOSAGES

Selected Anticholinergic Drugs

Drug (Pregnancy Category)	Pharmacologic Class	Usual Dosage Range	Indications
▶ benztropine mesylate (Cogentin) (C)	Anticholinergic	**Adult** PO: 0.5-6 mg/day 1-4 mg bid	PD; drug-induced extrapyramidal symptoms
biperiden (Akineton) (C)		**Adult** PO: 2 mg 3-4×/day	
procyclidine (Kemadrin) (C)		**Adult** PO: 2.5 mg 3×/day	
trihexyphenidyl (Artane) (C)		**Adult** PO: 6-10 mg/day 5-15 mg/day	

PD, Parkinson's disease.

• Neurological system and motor control and movements: What is the usual state of muscle movement and state of voluntary versus involuntary motor control? Are muscle movements co-ordinated and smooth or uncoordinated and rigid or with tremors? (Note that these movements are of particular importance because of the tremors that occur with purposeful movements with Parkinson's disease.)

With dopaminergic drugs, such as levodopa, amantadine, levodopa-carbidopa, and ropinirole, a patient assessment should include vital signs, height, weight, medication and medical history, nursing history, nursing assessment, and a journal of presenting symptoms. All contraindications, cautions, and drug interactions should be noted. Motor skills, abilities and deficiencies, should also be assessed—specifically the presence of akinesia, tremors, staggering gait, rigidity, and drooling. Vital signs should be assessed, with attention to blood pressure because of the adverse effects of hypotension and risk for syncope. Assessment of urinary patterns is also important because of the possibility of urinary retention with several of the drugs. If ordered, make sure to assess for blood urea nitrogen (BUN) and creatinine as indicators of renal function and/or alkaline phosphatase levels as indicators for liver function. For lifespan considerations, it is also important to understand the gynecologic history of the patient and if they are pregnant and/or may be lactating, as some of the dopaminergics cross into the placenta and into breast milk and have unknown actions in the pediatric patient. Drug interactions related to the dopaminergics are presented in Table 14-4.

When anticholinergic drugs are prescribed, the nurse should assess the patient carefully to determine gross level of organ functioning (for those systems most affected by Parkinson's) such as with the gastrointestinal system, genitourinary system, cardiac systems, and visual stability. Assessment of these systems is important because of the fact that any preexisting cardiac irregularities, tachycardia, urinary retention, bladder difficulties or obstruction, myasthenia gravis, and/or acute narrow-angle glaucoma (mydriasis leads to an increase in intraocular pressure) may be worsened or exacerbated with the use of the anticholinergics. Mental status, occurrence of agitation, confusion, or psychotic-like behavior needs to be assessed for—especially in those 60 years of age or older—because they are at higher risk for these problems. Age is also a significant factor to consider because of the increased likelihood of adverse effects or toxicity. The elderly experience physiologic changes of most organ functions and thus the increased risk for adverse or untoward reactions to drugs. Cautions, contraindications, and drug interactions are discussed on page 216.

For the dopamine agonist drugs that are also antivirals (e.g., amantadine), baseline assessment of underlying viral or other infectious disease processes is important. In fact, if the drug is used for antiviral indications, therapy is usually not begun until a positive influenza test is obtained, but for use in patients with Parkinson's, the benefits of the drug may not be seen for several days after initiation of drug therapy. If used as a dopamine agonist for Parkinson's, it is always important to continue to monitor/assess the baseline functioning of the patient and degree of Parkinson-related symptoms with this group of drugs because of the possible decline in its effectiveness within 3 to 6 months of the initial therapy.

If a dopamine agonist/prolactin inhibitor is used, it is important to understand that this drug is also used for suppression of lactations; however, for those with Parkinson's, it is crucial to be aware of its action on the symptoms of the disease. If the drug is being used for other indications, such as hyperprolactinemia or infertility, an entirely different assessment is indicated (Chapter 33). Elderly patients require additional assessment of the central nervous system because of the adverse effects related to that system (such as headache, lightheadedness, and visual or auditory changes). Also, if the patient with Parkinson's is taking this medication long-term, assessment of the following adverse effects is crucial to patient safety: rhinorrhea, fainting (syncope), peptic ulcers, severe abdominal pain, and gastrointestinal hemorrhage. These should be reported to the patient's health care provider immediately.

The antiparkinsonian drugs classified as MAO type B inhibitors (e.g., selegiline HCl), are associated with many of the same assessment parameters, as discussed. In addition, cardiac status is important to know because of the problems with cardiac irregularities and hypotension. Assessment of dosing is also important because, as with other antiparkinsonian drugs, the lowest dose should be started initially with gradual increases over an approximately 3 to 4 week period. These drugs also require astute neurologic assessment because of the possibility of serious reactions such as CNS depression (see Table 14-3 and the previous text for more information on CNS-related adverse effects).

The COMT inhibitors (e.g., entacapone and/or tolcapone) also require assessment of baseline vital signs, especially because of the adverse effect of orthostatic hypotension and syncope, and these occur with more frequency than with the other antiparkinsonian drugs. Assessment of dosing time is also important because if "not" given 1 hour before or 2 hours after, the bioavailability of the drug is adversely effected. Serum transaminase levels should be assessed prior to and during drug therapy and if the patient's SGPT (ALT) is elevated even to the upper range of normal or higher, the drug will most likely be discontinued by the physician owing to the risk of onset of hepatic failure.

Life Span Considerations: The Elderly Patient
Antiparkinsonian Drugs

• Levodopa should be used cautiously, with close monitoring of elderly patients, especially if there is a history of cardiac, renal, hepatic, endocrine, pulmonary, ulcer, or psychiatric disease.
• The elderly patient taking levodopa is at an increased risk for experiencing adverse effects, especially confusion, loss of appetite, and orthostatic hypotension.
• Levodopa-carbidopa is often started at a low dose because of the increased sensitivity of the older patient to these medications and to salvage higher dosages for another point in time during treatment.
• Overheating is a problem in patients taking anticholinergics, and the elderly patient needs to be very careful and avoid excessive exercise during warm weather and excessive heat exposure.
• One of the main problems with the long-term use of levodopa is that its duration of effectiveness decreases over time; this is even more problematic for elderly patients. COMT inhibitors hold much promise for those elderly patients who are having the "wearing off" phenomenon; they help turn the "off" times into "on" times so that the drug begins to work throughout the entire day.

Elderly patients also suffer from a higher incidence of hallucinations as compared to the general population.

♦ NURSING DIAGNOSES

- Impaired physical mobility related to the disease process and adverse effects of the medications
- Disturbed body image related to changes in appearance and mobility due to the disease process
- Urinary retention related to the effects of the disease on the bladder with incomplete emptying
- Constipation related to the disease process with decreased peristalsis
- Risk for injury related to the physical limitations produced by the disease process
- Imbalanced nutrition, less than body requirements, related to pharmacotherapy and associated adverse effects
- Deficient knowledge related to lack of exposure to treatment regimen

♦ PLANNING

Goals

- Patient remains free of self-injury.
- Patient states the purpose of the specific medications prescribed for the disease.
- Patient states the adverse effects and toxic effects of medications.
- Patient regains as normal as possible bowel and bladder elimination patterns.
- Patient maintains adequate nutritional status.
- Patient remains as independent as possible.
- Patient is less anxious and fearful.
- Patient regains a positive self-concept.
- Patient remains compliant to therapy.

Outcome Criteria

- Patient (and significant others) states ways of preventing self-injury, such as the use of assistive devices.
- Patient states purposes, adverse effects, and toxic effects associated with the specific antiparkinson medications, such as emesis, nausea, instability, and palpitations.
- Patient states ways to prevent some of the adverse effects and toxic effects of antiparkinsonian medications such as frequent mouth care and increased fluids.
- Patient discusses ways to minimize problems associated with drug-induced alterations in bowel and bladder elimination patterns through changes in diet and fluid intake.
- Patient discusses measures to ensure an adequate nutritional status with possible antiemetic therapy.
- Patient begins to perform ADLs more independently.
- Patient openly verbalizes fears, anxieties, and changes in self-image with members of the health care team and supportive staff.

♦ IMPLEMENTATION

Nursing interventions associated with the various antiparkinsonian drugs will vary somewhat depending on the drug class but all will require close monitoring and comprehensive patient education. During the start of dopaminergic drug therapy, the patient should be assisted when walking because of the dizziness caused by these drugs. Oral doses should be given with food to help minimize gastrointestinal upset. It is also important for the nurse to remember that pyridoxine (vitamin B_6) in doses greater than 10 mg will reverse the effects of levodopa. Foods high in vitamin

B_6 should therefore also be avoided, and protein should be supplemented in the diet, but in divided amounts, with small, frequent meals, so that minimal protein is ingested during the actual dose of drug is taken. The patient should be encouraged to force fluids, unless contraindicated, drinking at least 2000 mL/day, as well as consume an adequate amount of food that is high in roughage and fiber. The doses of dopaminergics should be given as a single dose or in divided doses and may be given with or without food. Doses should be given several hours before bedtime to decrease the incidence of insomnia. Should edema, nausea, or vomiting occur, the patient should be encouraged to contact his or her health care provider immediately.

With the dopamine agonists, it is crucial to review (with the patient and family members) the concept of "drug holidays" with long-term use of levodopa. A drug holiday (usually a 10-day period) is sometimes used by physicians when drug therapy is not working. The patient is generally hospitalized so that when the drug is withdrawn and the patient is without drugs, he or she can be taken care of appropriately and have needs met. Depending on the severity of the disease process, a patient may be totally dependent on others for basic care and nutritional and elimination needs. A patient may even be immobilized by a contracted physical state and not able to turn in bed, thus requiring a controlled environment with around-the-clock medical and nursing care. The purpose for the drug holiday is to hopefully obtain more therapeutic effectiveness once the levodopa is "re-initiated," and the hope is also for the patient to respond to a lower dose of the drug. The newer COMT inhibitors have been shown to have more efficacy in patients with advanced forms of PD. After use of the various dosage forms of levodopa or levodopa/carbidopa, a COMT inhibitor may be added, having a quicker onset of therapeutic effects. With anticholinergic drugs, patients should take the medication as prescribed but after meals or at bedtime and avoid other medications without the consent or advice of a physician.

It is most important in the care of patients with PD to be aware of all other forms of therapies that may be beneficial, such as support groups, water aerobics, occupational and physical therapy, and use of community resources. Some community resources that may be helpful include community-wide recreation facilities, transportation services and assistance, Meals on Wheels, and alternative therapies, and consultation with an osteopathic physician or chiropractor may also be beneficial. Educational materials and emotional support resources should also be shared with the patient and family members because of the long-term and progressive nature of the disease process. Contacting research institutes about new treatment protocols may be a viable option for patients and family members along the continuum of the disease process, and information should be made available as appropriate. Patient education tips associated with the antiparkinsonian drugs are discussed below.

♦ EVALUATION

Monitoring the patient's response to any of the antiparkinsonian medications is crucial to documenting treatment success or failure. Therapeutic responses to the antiparkinsonian drugs include an improved sense of well-being; improved mental status; increased appetite; ability to perform ADLs, to concentrate, and to think clearly; and less intense parkinsonian manifestations, such as less tremor, shuffling of gait, muscle rigidity, and involuntary movements. In addition to monitoring for therapeutic responses, the nurse must also watch for the occurrence of adverse effects, such as confusion, anxiety, irritability, depression, paranoia, headache, weakness, lethargy, nausea, vomiting, anorexia, palpitations, postural hypotension, tachycardia, dry mouth, constipation, urinary retention, blurred vision, dark urine, difficulty swallowing, and nightmares.

Patients should immediately report to their physician any of the following signs and symptoms indicating possible overdose: excessive twitching, drooling, or eye spasms. Therapeutic effects of COMT inhibitors (such as entacapone) may be noticed within a few days, whereas other antiparkinsonian drugs may take weeks. Adverse effects to monitor for with COMT inhibitors include those mentioned previously but with fewer dyskinesias than with dopamine agonists.

Patient Teaching Tips

- Patients should take their medication as ordered. Around-the-clock dosing is usually the regimen in order to achieve steady blood levels, especially with the dopamine agonists.
- Patients should be instructed to avoid alcohol and to seek out advice about taking any other medications, over-the-counter drugs, or herbal medications.
- Patients should be encouraged to change positions slowly to avoid dizziness and possible syncope.
- Patients should be instructed to take sustained-release forms of the drug in their whole form and never crush or chew them.
- Patients should use alternative methods of contraception if taking oral contraceptives.
- With dopamine agonists or anticholinergic drugs, patients should be warned about the adverse effect of dry mouth. This may be managed with artificial saliva through drops or gum, frequent mouth care, forced fluids, and use of sugarless gum or hard candy.
- If a combination of levodopa/carbidopa is used, patients should be warned of a darkening in the color of sweat and urine, but with the emphasis that this change is harmless.
- Patients should be instructed to contact their health care providers should vision become blurred or mental alertness diminished, or if there is confusion and lethargy with any of the antiparkinsonian drugs.
- Patients should be informed about other adverse effects associated with antiparkinsonian drugs that should be reported should they occur; these include difficulty urinating, irregular pulse rate, and severe, uncontrolled movements of arms, legs, mouth, and tongue.
- Education about potential blood pressure problems should be emphasized, whether they are the adverse effect of postural hypotension or the occurrence of hypertensive crisis if a MAOI is taken mistakenly. MAOIs should not be used with these drugs, and, if needed, 2 weeks should pass between the time the MAOI is discontinued and the levodopa is initiated.
- It is important for the patient and family to understand that dopaminergics are often titrated to the patient's response. It may take 3 to 4 weeks before a therapeutic response is seen.
- Patients taking newer dopamine agonists (pramipexole and ropinirole) should be educated about the "sleep attacks" that may occur without warning.

- Patients should be encouraged to always use caution with any activity. Some of these drugs may be associated with lightheadedness.
- Because drugs like bromocriptine may cause constipation, measures to avoid this adverse effect need to be emphasized, including forcing fluids, increasing bulk/fiber in the diet, and using stool softeners as prescribed.
- Patients taking COMT inhibitors should be informed about how to minimize nausea and vomiting, such as taking the drug with food. Other instructions for COMT inihibitors should include information about the adverse effects of dizziness, drowsiness, and even nausea that may occur in the beginning of therapy but diminish as therapy continues.
- Patients taking COMT inhibitors should, with the initial onset of therapy, be encouraged to avoid tasks that require mental clarity or intact motor skills to avoid injury. COMT inhibitors may result in hallucinations within the first 2 weeks of therapy.
- Patients taking entacapone should be warned about the possiblility of the urine turning brownish-orange and that the therapeutic effects may take only a few days versus the few weeks associated with other antiparkinsonian drugs.
- A patient's health care provider should be contacted if he or she experiences any abnormal contractions of the head, neck, or trunk, as well as syncope, falls, itching, and/or jaundice.
- Educate patients about the goal of therapy, especially if entacapone is being used for helping the patient with the "wearing off" phenomena. This is a "waning" of the effects of a dose of levodopa before the scheduled time of the next dose, resulting in diminished motor ability and performance and the patient experiencing more "symptoms." If a COMT inhibitor is added to the levodopa or levodopa/carbidopa, the "wearing off" phenomenon is minimized and the therapeutic effects of the regimen are maximized. The patient can then expect the "off" time to go away and the drugs work through the whole day which (of course) is the goal in the treatment of patients with PD.
- Patients should be encouraged to never come off their medications abruptly and to contact a physician for further instructions should this occur.

Points to Remember

- The neurotransmitting abnormalities with PD include a chronic, progressive, degenerative disorder of dopamine-producing neurons in the brain, and patients with PD have elevated ACh levels and lowered dopamine levels.
- Signs and symptoms of PD include bradykinesia (slow movements), rigidity (cogwheel), tremor (pill-rolling), postural instability, dyskinesias (difficulty performing voluntary movements—two common ones: chorea and dystonias); chorea: irregular, spasmodic, involuntary movements of limbs or facial muscles; and dystonias: abnormal muscle tone in any tissue.
- Drug therapies for PD include the following mechanisms: dopamine agonism, MAO inhibition, anticholinergic effects, and COMT inhibition.
- COMT inhibitors are also associated with fewer "wearing off" effects and prolonged therapeutic benefits.
- Nursing care considerations include thorough patient care, including information on the various therapies involved and the variety of resources available in their community.

- Patient considerations include much family support along with options for care of the family member with PD. This is a long-term process and a chronic, debilitating disease. Patients and families should be given excellent patient care, including the "holistic" approach that we apply to all we do as nurses, and patient rights should be honored at all times.
- Patient care also requires much support and education about the disease process and the drugs indicated. The newer COMT inhibitors have a quicker onset of a few days compared with the several days required for onset by traditional drugs used for PD.
- Sleep attacks may occur with the newer dopamine agonists (pramipexole and ropinirole), and brownish-orange discoloration of the urine occurs with entacapone.

ACh, Anticholinergic; *COMT,* catechol ortho-methyltransferase; *MAO,* monoamine oxidase; *PD,* Parkinson's disease.

NCLEX Examination Review Questions

1. Which of the following should alert the nurse to a potential caution or contraindication with use of a dopaminergic drug for treatment of mild PD?
   a. Diarrhea
   b. Tremors
   c. Narrow angle glaucoma
   d. Unstable gait
2. A patient is taking entacapone as part of the therapy for Parkinson's disease. Which intervention is appropriate at this time?
   a. Notify the patient that this drug causes discoloration of the urine.
   b. Limit the patient's intake of tyramine-containing foods.
   c. Monitor liver studies as this drug can seriously affect liver function.
   d. Force fluids to prevent dehydration.
3. Patient teaching for antiparkinsonian drugs should include which statements?
   a. The drug should be stopped when tremors and weakness are relieved.
   b. If a dose is missed, take two doses to avoid significant decreases in blood levels.
   c. Notify the physician if the urine turns brownish-orange in color.

   d. Change positions slowly to prevent falling due to postural hypotension.
4. Which statement is true regarding new drug therapy for a patient who has PD and is not responding well to levodopa therapy:
   a. Adding haloperidol (Haldol) will reduce adverse effects of levodopa.
   b. Taking methyldopa (Aldomet) will increase available dopamine levels in the brain.
   c. Taking amantadine (Symmetrel) improves the effectiveness of levodopa.
   d. Adding carbidopa will prevent the peripheral destruction of levodopa and result in increased amounts in the brain.
5. Which statement should be included during patient teaching about the use of levodopa-carbidopa?
   a. There are very few drug interactions with levodopa-carbidopa.
   b. Therapeutic effects may take up to several weeks to a few months.
   c. Notify the physician immediately if darkening of urine or sweat occurs.
   d. Pyridoxine (vitamin B_6) helps protect the action of levodopa-carbidopa.

1. c, 2. a, 3. d, 4. d, 5. b.

Critical Thinking Activities

1. Mr. P. has been diagnosed with PD and is taking levodopa-carbidopa (Sinemet). He also has Alzheimer's disease and is taking tacrine (Cognex). What do you think about the use of these two medications together?
2. You discover that your client who has PD and is taking levodopa-carbidopa is also being given some of his wife's phenothiazine medication to make him "feel even better." Why is this combination unsafe and not rational?
3. Your patient has been placed on a dopaminergic for the management of PD. She also relates to you during the nursing history

   that she has a diet high in meats, poultry, and whole grain cereals, and takes a "megadose multivitamin" daily. What would be a concern you may have with this patient's diet and why?
4. How does levodopa help improve the function of the patient diagnosed with PD?
5. After long-term treatment, patients with PD are often placed on a "drug holiday." Explain the rationale for this approach to treatment.
6. Explain the physiology behind the "on-again/off-again" appearance of symptoms that occurs with long-term levodopa treatment.

For answers, see http://evolve.elsevier.com/Lilley.

Psychotherapeutic Drugs

Objectives

When you reach the end of this chapter, you should be able to do the following:

1. Identify the various psychotherapeutic drugs, such as antianxiety drugs, antidepressants, antimanic drugs, and antipsychotics.
2. Discuss the mechanisms of action, indications, therapeutic effects, adverse effects, toxic effects, drug interactions, contraindications, and cautions associated with the various psychotherapeutic drugs.
3. Develop a nursing care plan that includes all phases of the nursing process related to the administration of psychotherapeutic drugs.
4. Develop patient education guidelines for patients receiving psychotherapeutic drugs.

e-Learning Activities

Companion CD

- NCLEX Review Questions: see questions 96-108
- Animations
- Audio Glossary
- Category Catchers
- Medication Errors Checklists
- IV Therapy Checklists

evolve Website (http://evolve.elsevier.com/Lilley)

• Nursing Care Plans • Frequently Asked Questions • Content Updates • WebLinks • Supplemental Resources • Elsevier ePharmacology Update • Medication Administration Animations

Drug Profiles

▸ alprazolam, p. 227
▸ amitriptyline, p. 236
▸ bupropion, p. 234
  buspirone, p. 228
▸ chlordiazepoxide, p. 227
  clozapine, p. 242
▸ diazepam, p. 227
▸ fluoxetine, p. 234
  fluphenazine, p. 240
  haloperidol, p. 241
  hydroxyzine, p. 228

▸ lithium, p. 229
▸ lorazepam, p. 227
▸ mirtazapine, p. 234
▸ olanzapine, p. 242
  quetiapine, p. 242
▸ risperidone, p. 242
  trazodone, p. 233
  valproic acid, p. 229
  venlafaxine, p. 234
  ziprasidone, p. 242

▸ Key drug.

Glossary

Adjunct therapy Combination drug therapy used when a patient's condition does not respond adequately to a single drug (monotherapy), or used when a given combination of medications is known to have therapeutic benefits over a single drug. (See *monotherapy.*) (p. 231)

Affective disorders Emotional disorders that are characterized by changes in mood. (p. 224)

Agoraphobia Fear of leaving the familiar setting of home. (p. 224)

Akathisia Motor restlessness—a distressing experience of uncontrollable muscular movements that can occur as an adverse effect of many psychotropic medications. (p. 239)

Antihistamine Any substance capable of reducing the physiologic and pharmacologic effects of histamine, including a wide variety of drugs that block histamine receptors. (p. 225)

Antipsychotic Of or pertaining to a medication that counteracts or diminishes symptoms of psychosis. (See *psychosis.*) An older term for such medications is *neuroleptic.* (p. 237)

Anxiety The unpleasant state of mind in which real or imagined dangers are anticipated and/or exaggerated. (p. 224)

Anxiolytic Capable of reducing anxiety; usually said of a medication. (p. 225)

Benzodiazepine The most common group of psychotropic drugs currently prescribed to alleviate anxiety. (p. 225)

Biogenic amine hypothesis (BAH) Theory suggesting that depression and mania are due to alterations in neuronal and synaptic amine concentrations, primarily the catecholamines dopamine and norepinephrine, as well as the indolamines serotonin and histamine. (p. 230)

Bipolar disorder (BPD) A major psychologic disorder characterized by episodes of mania or hypomania, cycling with depression. (p. 224)

Black Box warning A special warning required by the U.S. Food and Drug Administration (FDA) in the commercial drug labeling for drugs that have shown a pattern of major adverse effects. (p. 231)

Depression An abnormal emotional state characterized by exaggerated feelings of sadness, melancholy, dejection, worthlessness, emptiness, and hopelessness that are inappropriate and out of proportion to reality. (p. 224)

Dopamine hypothesis Views dopamine dysregulation in certain parts of the brain as one of the primary contributing factors to the development of psychotic disorders (psychoses). (p. 238)

Dysregulation hypothesis   Views depression and affective disorders as not simply decreased or increased catecholamine and serotonin activity but as failures of the regulation of these systems. (p. 230)

Extrapyramidal symptoms   Refers to symptoms arising adjacent to the *pyrimidal* portions of the brain. Such symptoms involve various motion disorders similar to Parkinson's disease and are an adverse effect associated with use of various antipsychotic drugs. (p. 239)

Gamma-aminobutyric acid (GABA)   An inhibitory amino acid in the brain that functions to inhibit nerve transmission in the central nervous system (CNS). (p. 225)

Mania   A state characterized by an expansive emotional state; extreme excitement; excessive elation; hyperactivity; agitation; over-talkativeness; flight of ideas; increased psychomotor activity; fleeting attention; and sometimes violent, destructive, and self-destructive behavior. (p. 224)

Monoamine oxidase inhibitor (MAOI)   Any of a heterogeneous group of drugs used primarily in the treatment of depression. (p. 227)

Monotherapy   Pharmacologic therapy involving a single medication for a specific condition. (See *adjunct therapy*.) (p. 231)

Neuroleptic malignant syndrome   Refers to an uncommon but serious adverse effect associated with use of antipsychotic drugs and including such symptoms as fever, cardiovascular instability, and myoglobinemia (broken down muscle protein in the blood). (p. 239)

Neurotransmitter   Endogenous chemical in the body that serves to conduct nerve impulses between nerve cells (neurons). This type of neurotransmission occurs in both the CNS and the peripheral nervous system. However, the proposed mechanisms of both the pathology of and drug therapy for mental illness center around neurotransmitter function between neurons in various regions of the brain. (p. 225)

Permissive hypothesis   Implicates reduced concentrations of serotonin (5-HT) as the predisposing factor in individuals with affective disorders. (p. 230)

Psychosis   (Plural: psychoses) A type of serious mental illness that can take several different forms and is associated with being truly out of touch with reality, that is, unable to distinguish imaginary from real circumstances and events. Psychosis often results in significant disability. (p. 224)

Psychotherapeutics   Refers to the therapy of emotional and mental disorders. It may involve drug therapy (pharmacotherapy), a variety of counseling techniques, recreational therapy, and, in extreme cases, electroconvulsive therapy (ECT). (p. 223)

Psychotropic   Capable of affecting mental processes; usually said of a medication. (p. 223)

Selective serotonin reuptake inhibitor (SSRI)   Also called *serotonin selective* reuptake inhibitors. Any of a heterogenous group of newer medications used to treat depression and certain other mental illnesses. They work by selectively reducing postsynaptic reuptake of the neurotransmitter serotonin in the brain. (p. 231)

Serotonin syndrome   A collection of symptoms resulting from excessive activity of the neurotransmitter *serotonin* in the brain; may occur with any psychotropic drugs (e.g., anti-depressants or buspirone) that enhance brain serotonin activity (see Box 15-2). (p. 232)

Stigma   Widespread negative perceptions of and prejudice toward a specific group of people such as those with mental illness. (p. 224)

Tardive dyskinesia   A serious drug adverse effect involving disordered body movements and muscle tension that is associated with antipsychotic medications. (p. 239)

Tricyclic   A chemical class of antidepressant drugs that block reuptake of the amine neurotransmitters serotonin and norepinephrine. They are so named because their chemical structures include a distinctive three-ring segment. (p. 234)

The treatment of emotional and mental disorders is called **psychotherapeutics.** When a person's ability to cope with his or her environment to carry out the activities of daily living (ADLs) and to interact with others is seriously impaired, a **psychotropic** drug may be a treatment option. These drugs are among the most commonly prescribed drugs in the United States today. Because of the inherent subjectivity in the description and reporting of symptoms of mental illness, the effects of these drugs are less easily quantified than are many other types of medications. For example, it is usually not known with certainty how long a given psychotropic drug works in the body (duration of action). Thus, the effectiveness of psychotropic drug therapy is often measured by verbal reports from patients regarding the level of improvement (if any) in their social and occupational functioning. There are also several established tools that attempt to quantify patient response to psychotropic drug therapy, such as the Hamilton Depression Rating Scale (HAM-D). Of interest recently is the

---

CULTURAL IMPLICATIONS
Psychotherapeutic Drugs

Many racial and ethnic groups respond to drugs differently. For example, Asians have a lower activity of drug metabolism compared with whites as a result of various enzyme deficiencies. Asians often require lower doses of benzodiazepines and tricyclic antidepressants (TCAs) because they have lower levels of metabolizing enzymes (e.g., CYO2D6) and are, therefore, more sensitive to these drugs. β-blockers, specifically propranolol, are also problematic for Asians.

The commonly used antianxiety drug diazepam undergoes different metabolic pathways in the Chinese and Japanese population. These two groups are found to be poor "mephenytoin pathway" metabolizers. Approximately 20% of these individuals metabolize mephenytoin poorly, resulting in rapid drug accumulation. To prevent possible toxicity, lower doses are generally required. As related to nursing implications, nurses may need to watch these individuals more closely for sedation, overdosage, and other adverse reactions (to diazepam).

Researchers have also been identified genetic factors that help predict a response to antidepressants. A study of some 80 Mexican-Americans with depression found that depressed and highly anxious patients with certain variant genes had a 70% greater "reduction" in anxiety and a 30% greater "reduction" in depression in response to treatment with fluoxetine and desipramine than did other racial ethnic groups without the specific gene variation.

rapidly expanding area of study known as *pharmacogenomics* (Chapter 50). One objective of this field is to map genetic factors (genetic polymorphisms) that contribute to different patterns of activity of drug-metabolizing enzymes across different ethnic groups. To better understand the nature and goals of this treatment, the types and definitions of various mental disorders are presented first.

OVERVIEW OF MENTAL ILLNESS

Most people experience emotions such as anxiety, depression, and grief. They are normal human emotions. However, the effect of these emotions on a person's ability to engage in normal daily activities and to interact with others can vary considerably. The duration and intensity of these emotions can range from occasional depression or anxiety to a state of constant emotional distress that interferes with a person's ability to carry on normal ADLs.

There is often a lot of overlap among the symptoms of the many different psychiatric disorders, which can make it difficult to accurately diagnose a disorder. Complicating this issue further is the inherent subjectivity with which different patients experience their symptoms. Often a patient has ongoing symptoms that meet several criteria for several mental disorders. Such patients may be said to have a spectrum disorder. For example, research shows that more than half of chronically depressed adults also have a comorbid personality disorder, and one third have a comorbid anxiety disorder and/or a substance abuse disorder. Mentally ill people may also be more susceptible to various physical health problems than the general population. For example, obesity is significantly more common in patients with mental disorders. Because of the variety of economic, educational, and psychosocial issues that may preclude a mentally ill person from seeking psychiatric health care, many patients self-medicate with alcohol, tobacco, and illegal drugs. This generally worsens the problem.

Despite newer, more effective treatments for mental illness, a long-held societal **stigma** continues to be an obstacle for diagnosed patients. The National Alliance for the Mentally Ill (NAMI) is one major organization that advocates reducing this stigma. NAMI and its many state-level chapters recognize those with mental illness as *consumers* of mental health services. NAMI seeks to promote consumer well-being and autonomy through public education, research funding, and legislative advocacy.

Ideal mental health care usually involves many factors, including a carefully detailed patient interview (to help ensure accurate and complete diagnosis); carefully chosen and regularly monitored drug therapy (if indicated); and significant emotional support, which may range from formal psychotherapy to informal support groups, social and family support systems, and spiritual support systems that the patient values.

There are three main emotional and mental disorders: psychoses, affective disorders, and anxiety. A **psychosis** is a severe emotional disorder that often impairs mental function to the point of significant disability regarding ADLs. A hallmark of psychosis is a loss of contact with reality. Psychotic disorders primarily include schizophrenia and depressive and drug-induced psychoses.

Affective disorders, also called *mood disorders,* are characterized by changes in mood and range from **mania** (abnormally pronounced emotions) to **depression** (abnormally reduced emo-

tions). Some patients may exhibit both mania and depression, experiencing periodic swings in emotions, from extremely reduced emotions to very intense, hyperactive emotions. This is referred to as a **bipolar disorder (BPD).**

Depression is currently reported to have prevalence rates anywhere from 4.4% to 20%. Major depressive disorders (MDDs) are expected to become the second leading cause of disability by the year 2020. Common depressive symptoms include feelings of worthlessness, loss of interest or pleasure in most or all normal daily activities, frequent reduced energy level, drastic increase or decrease in appetite, insomnia or hypersomnia, and recurrent thoughts of death or suicide. In addition to being associated with often drastic reductions in quality of life and occupational and psychosocial functioning, depression is also associated with the occurrence of major sleep disturbances in up to 80% of patients with depression. Some sleep researchers report that a $1\frac{1}{2}$ hour loss of sleep on any given night may reduce alertness on the following day by 33%; therefore, insomnia associated with depression has even more far-reaching adverse effects on the patient. This loss in the patient's state of alertness may then be associated with accidents and even increased risk for suicide. Despite recent advances in pharmacotherapy for depression, it remains undertreated in many cases and, in fact, two current and significant epidemiologic studies have demonstrated that patients seeking treatment for depressive symptoms were not even offered antidepressant treatment in 52% to 75% of cases.

Anxiety is the unpleasant state of mind chiefly characterized by a sense of dread and fear. It may be based on actual anticipated or past experiences such as scheduled surgery or previous abuse. It may also stem from exaggerated responses to imaginary negative situations or to common everyday experiences that are only mildly disturbing to a mentally healthy person. Persistent anxiety is divided clinically into several distinct disorders that have been classified by the American Psychiatric Association. This classification is published in the fourth edition of the *Diagnostic and Statistical Manual for Mental Disorders* (DSM-IV). This reference delineates the demographic features and diagnostic criteria for the major psychiatric disorders and has categorized anxiety into the following six major disorders:

- Obsessive-compulsive disorder (OCD)
- Posttraumatic stress disorder (PTSD)
- Generalized anxiety disorder (GAD)
- Panic disorder
- Social phobia
- Simple phobia

Anxiety is a normal physiologic emotion, but the results of epidemiologic studies show that 2% to 6% of adults suffer from a GAD; 1% from a panic disorder; and 4% to 5% from **agoraphobia,** the fear of leaving the familiar setting of home. OCD was thought to be rare but is now observed to be twice as common as schizophrenia or panic disorder in the general population. Anxiety may occur as a result of a wide range of medical illnesses (e.g., cardiovascular or pulmonary disease, hypothyroidism, hyperthyroidism, pheochromocytoma, and hypoglycemia). Many of the anxiety disorders are situational. They arise because of a specific event and subside with time. The treatment of these disorders should be limited to psychotherapy, and possibly short-term drug therapy. However, when the anxiety disorder markedly affects a person's quality of life and relationships or interferes with the ability to function normally over a prolonged period (at least several months), longer-term pharmacotherapy in conjunction with psychotherapy is usually recommended.

The exact causes of mental disorders are not fully understood. Many theories have been advanced in an attempt to explain the causes and pathophysiology of mental dysfunction. In the biochemical imbalance concept, mental disorders are thought to arise as the result of abnormal levels of endogenous chemicals in the brain known as **neurotransmitters.** There is strong evidence indicating that the brain levels of catecholamines (especially dopamine and norepinephrine; Chapter 17) and indolamines (serotonin and histamine) play an important role in maintaining mental health. Other biochemicals that seem necessary for the maintenance of normal mental function are **gamma-aminobutyric acid (GABA);** the cholinergic neurotransmitter acetylcholine (Ach) (Chapter 19); and various inorganic ions such as sodium, potassium, and magnesium. Knowledge of these various etiologies, especially the biochemical imbalance theory, can aid in understanding psychotherapeutic drug action because many of the drugs used to treat psychoses, affective disorders, and anxiety block or stimulate the release of these endogenous neurotransmitters. It should be noted that most psychotropic drugs may have greater potency with elderly patients, especially frail elderly. For this reason, smaller starting doses and careful dosage titration are usually recommended for the elderly psychiatric patient, as is often the case with other medication classes.

ANTIANXIETY DRUGS

Medications are only one therapeutic option in people afflicted with the various anxiety disorders. Other therapeutic options include the nonpharmacologic treatment modalities of psychotherapy, exercise, and meditation. Although benzodiazepines are generally the first-line drug treatment for anxiety disorders, there are other classes of drugs that are also effective. The efficacy of certain classes of medications in the treatment of certain anxiety disorders and their superiority over other drug classes has been documented. These various drug classes are listed in Table 15-1 according to the anxiety disorders they effectively treat.

Mechanism of Action and Drug Effects

Of the several drug classes shown to be effective in the treatment of anxiety disorders, all reduce anxiety by reducing overactivity in the central nervous system (CNS). There are, however, differences among the various drug classes.

Benzodiazepines seem to exert their **anxiolytic** effects by depressing activity in the areas of the brain called the *brainstem* and the *limbic system.* Benzodiazepines are believed to accomplish this by increasing the action of GABA, an inhibitory neurotransmitter in the brain that functions to inhibit nerve transmission in the CNS. Benzodiazepines have specific receptor proteins (also known as *specific receptor binding sites*) in the same areas of the brain that govern the release of GABA. The binding of benzodiazepines with these sites/receptors produces anxiolytic effects, as well as the effects of sedation and muscle relaxation.

Antihistamines (Chapter 35) have also been used as anxiolytics because of their ability to depress the CNS by sedating the patient. The antihistamine most commonly used for the relief of anxiety is hydroxyzine. Its significant sedative effects are related to its antihistaminic properties. This can be advantageous for patients with comorbid insomnia such as that often associated with both depression and antidepressant therapy. However, sedative effects of any medication can also be hazardous, and patients should be warned to use caution when driving or operating dangerous machinery. There are two salt forms of hydroxyzine: hydroxyzine hydrochloride (Atarax) and hydroxyzine pamoate (Vistaril), both of which are effective anxiolytics. However, benzodiazepines, antidepressants, and buspirone (described later in this chapter) have emerged as the mainstays for treatment of ongoing anxiety disorders.

Miscellaneous anxiolytic drugs are the third class of anxiolytics and include the single drug buspirone (BuSpar). It has the advantage of being both nonsedating and non–habit-forming. It is described in more detail later in this chapter.

Besides their anxiolytic effects just mentioned, anti-anxiety drugs produce several other effects throughout the body, including sedative, hypnotic, appetite stimulating, analgesic, and anticonvulsant effects.

Indications

As stated earlier, both carbamates and barbiturates were used for many years to treat anxiety, but this is now unusual, since the introduction of newer drugs. Some antihistamines are used to treat anxiety because of their sedative adverse effects, but their primary pharmacologic effect is to block the actions of histamine released during exacerbations of allergic conditions.

Benzodiazepines are the largest and most commonly prescribed anxiolytic drug class because they offer several advantages over the other drug classes used to treat anxiety. At therapeutic doses, they have little effect on consciousness, they are

Table 15-1	**Various Anxiety Disorders: Drugs of Choice**				
Disorder	**TCAs**	**Benzodiazepines**	**MAOIs**	**Buspirone**	**SSRIs**
Panic disorder	+++	++++	+++	0	++++
Generalized anxiety disorder	+	++++	++	+++	
Obsessive-compulsive disorder	+++	+	+	0	++++
Posttraumatic stress disorder	+	+	+	+	
Simple phobia	0	+	0	0	
Social phobia	+	+	+	0	

MAOI, Monoamine oxidase inhibitor; *SSRI*, selective serotonin reuptake inhibitor; *TCA*, tricyclic and tetracyclic antidepressants; +, limited use and efficacy; ++, some use and efficacy; +++, frequent use, good efficacy; ++++, most frequent use, best efficacy; 0, no efficacy or use.

Table 15-2	Benzodiazepines: Approved Indications
Approved Indications	**Benzodiazepines**
Alcohol withdrawal	chlordiazepoxide, diazepam, lorazepam, oxazepam
Anxiety	alprazolam, chlordiazepoxide, clonazepam, clorazepate, diazepam, halazepam, lorazepam, oxazepam, prazepam
Depression (adjunct)	alprazolam, oxazepam
Muscle spasm	diazepam
Preoperative sedation	chlordiazepoxide, diazepam, lorazepam
Seizure disorders	clorazepate, diazepam

Table 15-3	Benzodiazepines: Common Adverse Effects
Body System	**Adverse Effects**
Central nervous	Drowsiness, sedation, loss of coordination, dizziness, blurred vision, headaches, paradoxical reactions (insomnia, increased excitability, hallucinations)
Cardiovascular	Hypotension
Hematologic	Blood dyscrasias, including anemia, leukopenia, thrombocytopenia
Gastrointestinal	Nausea, vomiting, constipation, dry mouth, abdominal cramping
Integumentary	Pruritus, skin rash

very safe from the standpoint of their adverse effect profile, and they do not interact with many other drugs. Six very commonly prescribed anxiolytic benzodiazepines are diazepam (Valium), lorazepam (Ativan), alprazolam (Xanax), clonazepam (Klonopin), chlordiazepoxide (Librium), and midazolam (Versed). In addition to treating anxiety these drugs are used for sedation, to produce muscle relaxation, to control seizures, as adjuvant drug therapy for depression, and to treat alcohol withdrawal. It should be noted that midazolam is only available in injectable form and is limited to use as a sedative and anesthetic during invasive medical or surgical procedures. One of its desirable qualities is that it reduces anxiety during and the patient's memory of painful medical procedures that do not require general anesthesia. This is known as *moderate sedation* (Chapter 11). It is also used to provide sedation and control acute anxiety and agitation in intensive care unit (ICU) patients when excessive movement might be harmful (e.g., spinal cord injury in a confused patient or a patient requiring mechanical ventilation). Benzodiazepines commonly used as sedative-hypnotics, as opposed to anxiolytics per se, are discussed with other CNS depressants and have slightly different therapeutic actions and pharmacokinetics from those of the benzodiazepines used to treat anxiety. Because of their wide range of effects, anxiolytic drugs are sometimes used for certain other indications in addition to anxiety, such as seizure disorders, insomnia, agitation, and pain control. The commonly used anxiolytic benzodiazepines and their approved indications are listed in Table 15-2.

Contraindications

Contraindications to anxiolytic drugs include known drug allergy, narrow-angle glaucoma, and pregnancy. A positive seizure history is a relative contraindication.

Adverse Effects

The most common undesirable effect of the anxiolytic drugs is an overexpression of their therapeutic effects. All of these classes of drugs decrease CNS activity, and many of the unwanted effects of these drugs are related directly to this action. Both antihistamines and benzodiazepines can cause hypotension. Benzodiazepines are by far more commonly used, and some of their other adverse effects of benzodiazepines are listed

in Table 15-3. Of particular note are *paradoxical* (opposite of what would normally be expected) reactions to the benzodiazepines and antihistamines, including hyperactivity and aggressive behavior. Although they are relatively uncommon, such reactions are more likely to occur in pediatric/adolescent as well as psychiatric patients. There are also case reports of increasing seizure frequency in epileptic patients receiving benzodiazepines. It should also be noted that all benzodiazepines are potentially habit-forming and addictive. Although they can provide significant symptom relief, they should be used judiciously and at the lowest effective dosages and frequencies needed for symptom control.

Toxicity and Management of Overdose

Overdose of antihistamines is usually not severe but may be associated with excessive sedation, hypotension, and seizures. There is no specific antidote, but in extreme cases a cholinergic drug (Chapter 19), such as physostigmine, may be used to treat anticholinergic adverse effects that are associated with antihistamines.

There is a potential for benzodiazepines to cause serious life-threatening toxicities, but when taken alone in normal doses in otherwise healthy patients, they are very safe, effective anxiolytics. When taken with other sedating medications or with alcohol, life-threatening respiratory depression or arrest can occur. This serious consequence can also occur in patients whose metabolism or elimination capabilities are impaired because of liver or kidney dysfunction. In such cases, benzodiazepines can accumulate and not be eliminated. This further accentuates their therapeutic and toxic actions. An overdose of benzodiazepines may result in one or any combination of the following symptoms: somnolence, confusion, coma, or respiratory depression. However, coma and respiratory depression are much less likely with benzodiazepines alone than with barbiturates or meprobamate.

The treatment for benzodiazepine intoxication is generally symptomatic and supportive. If ingestion is recent, decontamination of the gastrointestinal system is indicated. As a rule of thumb, gastric decontamination using syrup of ipecac (a drug used to in-

Box 15-1 Flumazenil Treatment Regimen

Recommended Regimen

0.2 mg (2 mL) of flumazenil intravenously over 15 seconds. If desired level of consciousness is not apparent after 45 additional seconds, readminister same dose every 60 seconds up to 4 additional times (total dose 1 mg).

Duration of Action

Usually 1 hour. If reversing the effects of a long-acting benzodiazepine, may need to readminister flumazenil as it wears off and the effects reappear (e.g., resedation).

duce vomiting in overdose) is contraindicated in patients who have ingested medications that cause sedation because of the risk for aspiration of the stomach contents and subsequent risk for aspiration pneumonia. Therefore, gastric lavage is generally the best and most effective means of gastric decontamination. Activated charcoal and a saline cathartic may be administered after gastric lavage to remove any remaining drug. Hemodialysis is usually not needed or useful in the treatment of benzodiazepine overdose but may be used in more extreme cases, especially those involving multiple types of drugs. A more likely treatment in such severe cases might also be the use of the benzodiazepine-specific antidote flumazenil (Romazicon). This drug is a benzodiazepine receptor blocker (antagonist) that is used to reverse the effects of benzodiazepines. Although it has been approved for benzodiazepine overdose, flumazenil has not been shown to reduce mortality or length of hospital stay. For this reason, its use for this indication is more limited. Instead, this drug is more commonly used to reverse benzodiazepine effects following procedures involving moderate sedation (described earlier and in Chapter 11). It opposes the actions of benzodiazepines by directly competing with benzodiazepines for binding at the benzodiazepine receptors in the CNS. It has a stronger affinity for these receptors and thus chemically forces the benzodiazepine drug molecules off the receptor, reversing their CNS depressant effects. The treatment regimen for the reversal of benzodiazepine overdose is summarized in Box 15-1.

Interactions

There are a few notable drug interactions that occur with the use of the anxiolytics, particularly benzodiazepines. As mentioned earlier, alcohol and CNS depressants, when coadministered with benzodiazepines, can result in additive CNS depression, and even death. Cimetidine, disulfiram, **monoamine oxidase inhibitors (MAOIs),** and tobacco all can decrease the metabolism of benzodiazepines and result in increased CNS depression.

Dosages

For the recommended dosages of selected antianxiety drugs, see the Dosages table on page 228.

Drug Profiles

Benzodiazepines

Benzodiazepines are contraindicated in patients who have shown a hypersensitivity reaction to them and in patients who have narrow-angle glaucoma. They are all Schedule IV drugs. Dosage and indication information appears in the corresponding table.

▸ alprazolam

Alprazolam (Xanax) is most commonly used as an anxiolytic and as an adjunct for the treatment of depression. The commonly recommended dosages are given in the table on page 228.

Pharmacokinetics

Half-Life	Onset	Peak	Duration
1 hr	1-2 hr	6-12 hr	

▸ chlordiazepoxide

Chlordiazepoxide (Librium) is used for many indications but is most commonly used for the treatment of alcohol withdrawal, for the relief of anxiety, and as a preoperative sedative drug.

When giving this drug intramuscularly (IM), it is recommended that nurses DO use only the diluent provided with the powdered drug ampule. However, this diluent should NOT be used when giving the drug intravenously (IV), because this diluent forms air bubbles during reconstitution. In this case, the appropriate diluent is sterile normal saline or sterile water for injection.

The commonly recommended dosages are given in the table on page 228.

Pharmacokinetics

Half-Life	Onset	Peak	Duration
9-34 hr	30-60 min	0.5-4 hr	12-24 hr

▸ diazepam

Diazepam (Valium) is one of the most commonly prescribed benzodiazepines. It is indicated for the relief of anxiety, alcohol withdrawal, and seizure disorders (e.g., status epilepticus); for sedation; and as an adjunct for the relief of skeletal muscle spasms. Diazepam has active metabolites that can accumulate in patients who have hepatic dysfunction because it is metabolized primarily in the liver. This can result in additive, cumulative effects that may be manifested as prolonged sedation, respiratory depression, or coma.

Pharmacokinetics

Half-Life	Onset	Peak	Duration
20-80 hr	30-60 min	1-2 hr	12-24 hr

▸ lorazepam

Lorazepam (Ativan) is a widely used benzodiazepine. It is currently approved for use in the management of anxiety disorders, for the short-term relief of acute anxiety, and as a preoperative medication to provide sedation and light anesthesia and to diminish patient recall (amnesia). It has also shown efficacy in the prevention and treatment of chemotherapy-related nausea and vomiting and the symptoms of acute alcohol withdrawal. Its injectable form requires refrigeration.

Pharmacokinetics

Half-Life	Onset	Peak	Duration
IV: 12-16 hr	IV: Rapid	IV: 15-20 min	IV: 4 hr
PO: 12-16 hr	PO: 15-45 min	PO: 2 hr	PO: 12-24 hr

Miscellaneous Drugs

There are several categories of drugs that can be used in the treatment of anxiety disorders. Although benzodiazepines are by far the most widely prescribed anxiolytics, often drugs in other categories may be prescribed because of certain advantages they offer. Some of the more commonly used drugs are described in this section. The efficacy of the carbamates in treating anxiety disorders, with meprobamate the prototype, has been shown. The antihistamine hydroxyzine and the nonbenzodiazepine anxiolytic buspirone are also very effective antianxiety drugs. Dosage and indication information appears in the corresponding table.

DOSAGES

Selected Antianxiety Drugs

Drug (Pregnancy Category)	Pharmacologic Class	Usual Dosage Range	Indications
▶alprazolam (Xanax) (D)	Benzodiazepine	**Adult** PO: 0.25-2 mg tid; do not exceed 6 mg/day	Anxiolytic
		Elderly PO: 0.25 mg bid-tid	Anxiolytic
buspirone (BuSpar) (B)	Miscellaneous	**Adult only** PO: 15-60 mg/day in 2-3 divided doses	Anxiolytic
▶chlordiazepoxide (Librium) (D)	Benzodiazepine	Pediatric PO:<6 yr, 5 mg bid-qid	Anxiolytic
		Adult PO: 5-25 mg tid-qid IM/IV: 50-100 mg, then 25 mg tid-qid for severe anxiety IM/IV: 50-100 mg q2-4h for alcoholism IM: 50-100 mg before surgery	Anxiolytic Anxiolytic, preop sedation
		Pediatric PO: >6 mo: 1.25 mg tid-qid	Anxiety, alcoholism, muscle spasm, convulsive disorders
hydroxyzine (Atarax, Vistaril) (C)	Antihistamine	**Pediatric** PO: 50 mg/day divided ≥6 yr: PO: 50-100 mg/day divided ≥6 yr: PO: 0.6 mg/kg ≥6 yr: IM: 1.1 mg/kg	Anxiolytic/pruritus Pre- and postop sedation Nausea/vomiting
		Adult PO: 50-100 mg qid IM: 50-100 mg q4-6h PO: 25 mg tid-qid PO: 50-100 mg IM: 25-100 mg	Anxiolytic Anxiolytic Pruritus Pre- and postpartum sedation Nausea/vomiting
▶lorazepam (Ativan) (D)	Benzodiazepine	**Adult** PO: 2-6 mg/day divided PO: 2-4 mg hs IM: 0.05 mg/kg to a max of 4 mg IV: 2-4 mg	Anxiolytic Preop sedation Preop sedation

hydroxyzine

Hydroxyzine is available in two different salt forms: hydrochloride salt (Atarax) and pamoate salt (Vistaril). Both forms are used to treat anxiety disorders. Hydroxyzine is an antihistamine that suppresses activity in the CNS, which makes it useful as both an anxiolytic and an antiemetic drug.

Pharmacokinetics

Half-Life	Onset	Peak	Duration
3-7 hr	15-30 min	15-30 min	4-6 hr

buspirone

Buspirone (BuSpar) is an anxiolytic drug that is distinctly different both chemically and pharmacologically from the benzodiazepines. Its precise mechanism of action is unknown, but it appears to have agonist activity at a subset of both serotonin and dopamine receptors. It is indicated for treatment of anxiety and is always taken on a scheduled (not prn) basis. Its only reported contraindication is drug allergy. The advantages of buspirone over benzodiazepines include its lack of the sedative properties and dependency potential of benzodiazepines. It also does not prevent or treat benzodiazepine withdrawal symptoms, and, therefore, although it may be used concurrently with benzodiazepines, it should be withdrawn gradually if it is to be discontinued. An additional advantage of buspirone is that it does not require dose adjustment for elderly patients because age has not been shown to affect the pharmacokinetics of the drug in the body. However, the drug is not currently approved for pediatric use. Potential drug interactions include a risk for serotonin syndrome (see Antidepressants in this chapter) when buspirone is used concurrently with any antidepressant with serotonergic activity, such as **selective serotonin reuptake inhibitors (SSRIs),** tricyclic antidepressants (TCAs), nefazodone, trazodone, and venlafaxine. Patients receiving both types of medications together should be monitored carefully. It is recommended that MAOIs not be used concurrently with buspirone due to a risk of hypertension. A washout period of at least 14 days after discontinuation of MAOI therapy should occur before starting buspirone.

Pharmacokinetics

Half-Life	Onset	Peak	Duration
2-3 hr	Up to 2-3 wk	40-60 min	Unknown

DRUGS USED TO TREAT AFFECTIVE DISORDERS

Several classes of drugs are used in the treatment of the affective disorders. The two main drug categories are antimanic drugs and antidepressant drugs.

ANTIMANIC DRUGS

Clinical evidence indicates that the catecholamines (dopamine and norepinephrine) play an important pathophysiologic role in the development of mania. Serotonin also appears to be involved. The original drugs currently available that can effectively alleviate the major symptoms of mania are the lithium salts. Lithium also continues to be shown effective in maintenance treatment of BPD. One theory on its effectiveness is that it is thought to potentiate serotonergic neurotransmission. A variety of medications may be used in conjunction with lithium to regulate mood or stabilize manic patients. Some of these adjunctive medications are benzodiazepines, carbamazepine, clozapine, dopamine receptor agonists, L-tryptophan, and calcium channel blockers (CCBs). More recently approved medications for acute manic episodes include the anticonvulsant valproic acid (Chapter 13) and the antipsychotic drug olanzapine (see the Atypical Antipsychotics section later in this chapter). Valproic acid is often a better choice than lithium in frail elderly patients because of the narrow therapeutic index, and closer monitoring requirements associated with lithium therapy. Lithium, valproic acid, and carbamazepine are also commonly referred to as "mood stabilizers" regarding their use in treating BPD.

Antidepressants are often needed as well to control the depressive side of bipolar disorder. A pharmacologic challenge is to choose antidepressants that are less likely to evoke manic responses secondary to the expected stimulating effects of the antidepressant medication. Several of the newer third-generation anticonvulsants (Chapter 13) have also recently become more firmly established in treating mania/hypomania, and to a lesser degree, depressive symptoms. These include lamotrigine, oxcarbazepine, and topiramate. Other recent studies have shown the atypical antipsychotic drugs risperidone, olanzapine, quetiapine, and ziprasidone to be effective for acute mania or hypomania.

Drug Profiles

▶ lithium

The antimanic effect of lithium is not fully understood. Results of studies indicate that lithium ions alter sodium ion transport in nerve cells, resulting in a shift in catecholamine metabolism. The therapeutic levels of lithium that are required are close to the toxic levels, but there is increasingly greater tolerance to these toxic levels during acute manic phases. For the management of acute mania, a lithium serum level of 1 to 1.5 mEq/L is usually required. Desirable long-term maintenance levels range between 0.6 and 1.2 mEq/L, and are best measured 8 to 12 hours (roughly the midpoint of the drug half-life) after the last dose, because the half-life usually ranges between 18 and 24 hours. Both sodium and lithium are monovalent positive ions—one can affect the other. Therefore, the patient's serum sodium levels should also be monitored. A sodium level that is kept in the normal range (135-145 mEq/L) helps to maintain therapeutic lithium levels.

Lithium carbonate (Eskalith, Lithane, and Lithobid) and lithium citrate (Cibalith-S) are the two currently available salts of lithium. There are no absolute contraindications to lithium therapy, and the adverse effects are dependent on the serum levels. Levels exceeding 1.5 to 2.5 mEq/L begin to produce toxicity, including gastrointestinal discomfort, tremor, confusion, somnolence, seizures, and possibly death. The most serious adverse effect is cardiac dysrhythmia. Other effects include drowsiness, slurred speech, epileptic-type seizures, choreoathetotic movements (involuntary wavelike movements of extremities), ataxia (generalized disturbance of muscular coordination), and hypotension. Long-term treatment may cause hypothyroidism.

The concurrent use of thiazides, angiotensin-converting enzyme (ACE) inhibitors, calcium channel blockers, and nonsteroidal antiinflammatory drugs can increase lithium toxicity.

Pharmacokinetics

Half-Life	Onset	Peak	Duration
18-24 hr	7-14 days*	0.5-2 hr	2-24 hr

*Therapeutic benefit for controlling mania.

valproic acid

The anticonvulsant valproic acid (Depakote, Depakene) has been used for seizure disorders for many years (Chapter 13). More recently, it has become one of the major drugs of choice for mania. Although lithium can be effective in both acute mania and for prevention of manic episodes, valproic acid is normally reserved for preventive drug therapy maintenance against manic episodes.

Pharmacokinetics

Half-Life	Onset	Peak	Duration
9-16 hr	1-3 days	1-4 hr	2-4 days

ANTIDEPRESSANT DRUGS

Antidepressants are the pharmacologic treatment of choice for major depressive disorders. Not only are they very effective in treating depression, they are also useful for treating other disor-

DOSAGES

Selected Antimanic Drugs

Drug (Pregnancy Category)	Pharmacologic Class	Usual Dosage Range	Indications
lithium carbonate (D)	Mood stabilizer	600-1200 mg/day	Mania, acute and prevention of
valproic acid (divalproex) (Depakote) (D)	Anticonvulsant, mood stabilizer	750-1500 mg/day	Mania, prevention of

ders, such as dysthymia, schizophrenia (as an adjunct), eating disorders, and personality disorders. Some of these drugs are also commonly used in the treatment of various medical conditions, including migraine headaches, chronic pain syndromes, and sleep disorders.

Many of the drugs currently used to treat affective disorders increase the levels of monoamine neurotransmitter concentrations in the CNS. Monoamine neurotransmitters include serotonin (also known as 5-hydroxytryptamine, or 5-HT), dopamine, and norepinephrine. This treatment is based on the belief that alterations in the levels of these types of neurotransmitters in the CNS are responsible for causing depression. One of the most widely held hypotheses advanced to explain depression in these terms is the **biogenic amine hypothesis (BAH).** Specifically, it postulates that depression results from a deficiency of neuronal and synaptic catecholamines (primarily norepinephrine) and mania from an excess of amines at the adrenergic receptor sites in the brain. This hypothesis is illustrated in Figure 15-1.

Another hypothesis advanced to explain the etiology of affective disorders is the **permissive hypothesis.** It implicates reduced concentrations of serotonin as the predisposing factor in patients with affective disorders. Depression results from decreases in both the serotonin and catecholamine levels, whereas mania results from increased catecholamine but decreased serotonin levels. The permissive hypothesis is illustrated in Figure 15-2.

A new leading theory attempting to explain the etiology of affective disorders is the **dysregulation hypothesis.** It is essentially a reformulation of the BAH. It views depression and affective disorders not simply in terms of decreased or increased catecholamine activity but as a failure of the regulation of these systems.

Recent research data indicate that early and aggressive antidepressant treatment increases the chances for full remission. The first 6 to 8 weeks of therapy constitute the acute phase. The primary goals during this time are to obtain a response to drug therapy and to improve the patient's symptoms. It is currently recommended that antidepressant drug therapy be maintained at the effective dose for an additional 8 to 14 months after remission of depressive symptoms. In choosing an antidepressant for a given patient, the patient's previous psychotropic drug response history (if any) should be considered. Information regarding any family history of depression with known drug responses may also be helpful. Therapeutic response is measured primarily by subjective patient feedback. In addition, there are a few measurement tools that attempt to quantify the patient response to drug therapy, such as the Hamilton Depression Rating Scale (HAM-D) and the Symptom Checklist-90 (SCL-90) anxiety factor score. A therapeutic nonresponse to antidepressant drug therapy is defined as failure to respond to adequate doses of at least 6 weeks of therapy. Twenty to thirty percent of patients who do not respond to the usual dose of a given antidepressant drug will respond to higher doses. Therefore, dose optimization, involving careful upward titration of medication dose for several weeks, is recommended before concluding that a given drug is ineffective for a particular patient. If it is decided that a switch to a different pharmacologic class of antidepressant is appropriate, research indicates that 40% to 60% of patients will respond to the second drug class attempted.

Nonresponse to at least two trials, including at least two different classes of antidepressants, is classified as *treatment-resistant depression (TRD).* Such cases can be treated by either switching to a different drug from the same or a different class or augmenting the initial drug therapy by adding a second drug. There is currently limited controlled research data regarding drug combination augmentation strategies, but more research is anticipated on this topic. In the meantime, clinicians rely on trial and error experience, their previous clinical experience in general, and considerations of specific patient factors (e.g., comorbid anxiety) when choosing combinations of psychiatric drug therapy. Antipsychotic drugs (discussed in detail later in this chapter) may also be used concurrently with antidepressants in treating some cases of TRD. This practice is currently well established for cases of MDD that also involve psychotic symptoms. Two issues currently under research include the use of antipsychotic

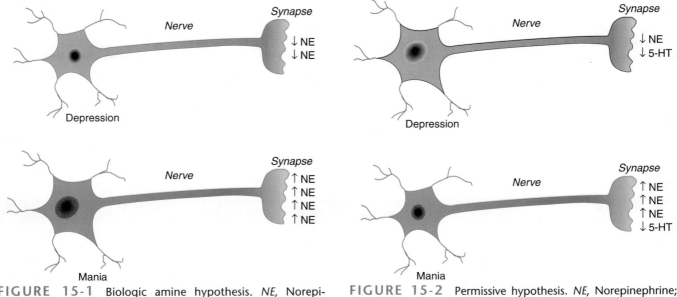

FIGURE 15-1 Biologic amine hypothesis. *NE,* Norepinephrine.

FIGURE 15-2 Permissive hypothesis. *NE,* Norepinephrine; *5-HT,* serotonin.

drugs as **monotherapy** for psychotic forms of MDD, and the potential use of antipsychotic drugs as **adjunct therapy** for non-psychotic TRD. The most severe cases of TRD may warrant a treatment attempt with electroconvulsive therapy (ECT). Current ECT techniques are greatly refined from similar treatments in past decades and are usually carried out in a postanesthesia care unit (PACU) or recovery room setting under general anesthesia. Seizure activity is induced in the anesthetized patient via externally applied electric shocks to the brain. It should be recognized that treatment failure in cases of depression may be due to a misdiagnosis or failure to treat comorbid mental illness (e.g., anxiety disorder, substance abuse) and/or comorbid nonpsychiatric illness (e.g., hypothyroidism). It may also be due to nonadherence to drug therapy, which is the cause in an estimated 20% of TRD cases. Thus, careful choice of drug therapy to minimize adverse effects may improve compliance with treatment and therapeutic outcome. It should also be recognized that one reason for treatment failure may be the discouragement associated with depression itself. This alone may cause patients to give up prematurely on their drug therapy, especially because antidepressants often take several weeks to reach their full effect. Effective psychotherapy and support groups can help encourage patients to be consistent with prescribed psychotropic drug therapy.

The drug categories most commonly used in the treatment of affective disorders are the SSRIs and the second- and third-generation antidepressants. Less commonly used are what are considered to be, although not formally classified as, the first-generation antidepressants. These include the TCAs and MAOIs. As of 2005, the FDA has issued special Black Box warnings regarding the use of all classes of antidepressants in both adult and pediatric patient populations. It should be kept in mind that most patients do not experience severe adverse effects with these medications, and many patients experience significant relief from depressive symptoms while on these medications. However, a meta-analysis combining data from 24 small studies of child and adolescent subjects indicated a higher risk for suicide in up to 4% of patients receiving these medications, compared with 2% receiving placebo. Later in the same year, the agency expressed similar concerns regarding adult patients. As a result, current recommendations for all patients receiving antidepressants include regular monitoring for signs of worsening depressive symptoms, especially when starting or changing the dose of medication. Patients should be evaluated by their health care provider immediately if they report, or others observe, signs of worsening depression or other emotional instability.

SELECTIVE SEROTONIN REUPTAKE INHIBITORS AND SECOND- AND THIRD-GENERATION ANTIDEPRESSANTS

These three drug classes can be described together as newer-generation antidepressants (NGAs) and are generally considered superior to TCAs and MAOIs in terms of their adverse-effect profiles. Because of this, they largely replaced TCAs and MAOIs as first-line drug therapy for depression in the 1980s following the introduction of the first SSRI, fluoxetine. The SSRIs include fluoxetine (Prozac), paroxetine (Paxil), sertraline (Zoloft), fluvoxamine (Luvox), citalopram (Celexa), and escitalopram (Lexapro). Escitalopram is one of the two stereoiso-

mers that make up citalopram. This chemical property gives it greater receptor specificity and therefore reduces the likelihood of adverse effects. Second-generation antidepressants include trazodone (Desyrel) and bupropion (Wellbutrin). Third-generation antidepressants include venlafaxine (Effexor), nefazodone (generic only), and mirtazapine (Remeron). Mirtazapine, a third-generation drug, along with the much less commonly used second-generation drug maprotiline, are also known as *tetracyclic drugs* because of the four connected rings that form the basis of their chemical structure; thus the tetracyclic drugs actually span more than one "generation" of antidepressants. In contrast, the TCAs are all solely first-generation drugs. For this reason, the terms *second-* and *third*-generation are more precise and less ambiguous when speaking of the tetracyclic antidepressants. Because maprotiline is rarely used, only mirtazapine is discussed in detail in this chapter.

These newer antidepressants offer several attractive advantages over the traditional TCAs and MAOIs. They are associated with significantly fewer and less severe systemic adverse effects, especially those to which older adults have little tolerance—anticholinergic and cardiovascular adverse effects. They are very safe and have very few drug-drug or drug-food interactions. However, it does take approximately the same amount of time for them to reach maximum clinical effectiveness as it does the TCAs and MAOIs, typically 4 to 6 weeks.

SSRIs were developed to slow or inhibit the reuptake of serotonin into presynaptic terminals (nerve endings) and thus to increase the levels of serotonin for neurotransmission at the postsynaptic nerve endings. Sertraline is the most selective of the three drugs in inhibiting serotonin as opposed to norepinephrine reuptake, and fluoxetine is the least selective. Fluoxetine is the only one that has an active metabolite. Fluoxetine, along with its active metabolite, has an elimination half-life of 2 to 4 days as opposed to a 1-day half-life for sertraline and paroxetine. A newer antidepressant in its own unique category is reboxetine (Vestra). It is a norepinephrine-selective reuptake inhibitor (NSRI). Currently, it is not yet widely used in the United States. A still newer drug, more closely related to the SSRIs, is duloxetine (Cymbalta). Approved by the FDA in 2002, this drug works as a strong inhibitor of both serotonin and norepinephrine and a weaker reuptake inhibitor of dopamine.

Mechanism of Action and Drug Effects

The inhibition of serotonin reuptake seems to be the primary clinically significant mechanism of action for the SSRIs, although SSRIs may also have weak effects on norepinephrine and dopamine reuptake. Second- and third-generation drugs are less selective and have activity at brain serotonin as well as norepinephrine and/or dopamine receptors. They are also referred to as *multimodal* or *multireceptor* drugs and have greater receptor specificity and a generally improved adverse effect profile when compared with first-generation drugs. The second- and third-generation drugs have chemical structures that differ from the SSRIs, and there is significant overlap between the pharmacologic activities of these two generations of medications. Nefazodone and trazodone are both primarily serotonin-reuptake inhibitors but also have a smaller inhibitory effect on norepinephrine reuptake. Mirtazapine has both noradrenergic (norepinephrine) and serotonergic (serotonin) effects but works by promoting presynaptic release of these two neurotransmitters and does not inhibit either their pre- or postsynaptic reuptake. The antidepressant activities of bupropion and venlafaxine are believed to affect all three major neurotransmitters: serotonin, norepinephrine, and, to a lesser degree, dopamine. The latest research is starting to suggest that these newer-generation multireceptor drugs may offer significant improvement outcomes in depression treatment over even the highly acclaimed SSRI drugs. Larger clinical studies are anticipated with these newer drugs, either alone or in combination with SSRI therapy.

The increase in serotonin, norepinephrine, or dopamine reuptake causes increased concentrations of these various neurotransmitters at nerve endings in the CNS, resulting in numerous functional changes associated with enhanced amine neurotransmission. This increased neurotransmitter concentration in the CNS also seems to lead to a decrease in REM sleep. In addition, it has a potentiating effect when given with opioid analgesics in that the increased serotonin concentration at nerve endings appears to work synergistically with the opioid analgesic in relieving pain.

Although all NGAs are associated with varying degrees of weight gain or loss, SSRIs are more commonly associated with anorectic activity and weight loss. This appetite-inhibiting action may result from the blocking of serotonin reuptake and the attendant increase in the serotonin concentration at the nerve endings. For this reason, SSRIs are sometimes used to treat eating disorders, such as bulimia nervosa, that involve compulsive overeating. Patients should be educated that antidepressant drugs commonly require several weeks before full therapeutic effects are realized. This requires some patience and faithful dosing on the part of patients.

Indications

All three classes of NGAs have been used to treat many affective disorders. Depression, BPD, obesity, eating disorders, OCD, panic attacks or disorders, social anxiety disorder, PTSD, premenstrual dysphoric disorder, and the neurologic disorder myoclonus are only some of the many disorders that this highly effective drug class can be used to treat. This list is expanding with continued research on these drugs. These newer antidepressant classes have also shown some beneficial effects in the treatment of various substance abuse problems such as alcohol dependence.

Contraindications

Contraindications to NGA use include known drug allergy, use sooner than 14 days after stopping MAOI therapy, and therapy with certain antipsychotic drugs such as thioridazine or mesoridazine. Additionally, a significant cardiac or seizure history may also be a contraindication due to relatively uncommon, but reported, cardiac effects and alterations in seizure threshold (see later). Bupropion is also contraindicated in cases of eating disorder and also seizure disorder because it can lower the seizure threshold.

Adverse Effects

NGAs offer an advantage over TCAs and MAOIs in that their adverse effect profiles are generally much safer. However, some adverse effects can be bothersome enough to cause patients to discontinue their antidepressant drug therapy. Up to two thirds of all depressed patients may discontinue therapy due to drug adverse effects. Some of the most common and bothersome adverse effects include insomnia, weight gain, and sexual dysfunction. Less commonly reported cardiac effects include chest pain, palpita-

tions, and QT-prolongation (on EKG). NGAs may also lower the seizure threshold in susceptible patients (i.e., those with previous seizure history). Bupropion, nefazodone, and mirtazapine are all associated with a reduced incidence of sexual adverse effects, and may serve as effective substitute or adjuvant (second) drugs. The sexual dysfunction primarily involves male impotence in terms of erectile dysfunction. Other drug alternatives to treat this condition (e.g., Viagra) are discussed in the chapter pertaining to men's health (see Chapter 34). One potentially hazardous adverse effect of any drug or combination of drugs that have serotoninergic activity is known as **serotonin syndrome**. The symptoms of this condition are listed in Box 15-2. Fortunately it is usually self-limiting on discontinuation of the causal drugs. The various adverse effects that can occur in patients taking second-generation antidepressants are listed in Table 15-4.

Interactions

NGAs are highly bound to plasma proteins such as albumin. When given with other drugs that are also highly bound to protein (warfarin and phenytoin), both compete for binding sites on the surface of albumin. This results in a more free, unbound drug and, therefore, a greater, more pronounced drug effect.

NGAs also have the capacity to inhibit cytochrome P-450. The cytochrome P-450 system is an enzyme system in the liver that is responsible for the metabolism of several drugs. Inhibition of this enzyme system results in higher levels of drugs because they accumulate rather than break down to their inactive metabolites. This also prolongs the action of drugs metabolized by the cytochrome P-450 system. The SSRIs fluoxetine and paroxetine seem to be more potent inhibitors of this enzyme system than sertraline. There is still controversy over whether the cytochrome P-450 system is inhibited. Many studies have shown that this event is minimal or even nonexistent. The most common and significant drug interactions are listed in Table 15-5.

To prevent the potentially fatal pharmacodynamic interactions that can occur between NGAs and MAOIs, a 2- to 5-week washout period is recommended between uses of the two classes of medications. NGAs that have a longer half-life, such as fluoxetine, require the longer washout period.

Box 15-2	Common Symptoms of Serotonin Syndrome

Delirium, agitation, tachycardia, sweating, myoclonus (muscle spasms), hyperreflexia, shivering, coarse tremors, and extensor plantar muscle responses (sole of foot). More severe cases may involve hyperthermia, seizures, rhabdomyolysis, renal failure, cardiac dysrhythmias, and disseminated intravascular coagulation.

Table 15-4	Newer Generation Antidepressants: Adverse Effects

Body System	Adverse Effects
Central nervous	Headache, dizziness, tremor, nervousness, insomnia, fatigue
Gastrointestinal	Nausea, diarrhea, constipation, dry mouth, weight loss/gain
Other	Sweating, sexual dysfunction

Table 15-5 Newer Generation Antidepressants: Drug Interactions

Drug	Mechanism	Result
carbamazepine	Decreases carbamazepine metabolism	Increased carbamazepine levels, carbamazepine toxicity, ocular changes, vertigo, tremor
MAOIs	Enhances serotonin activity	Hyperthermia, diaphoresis, shivering, tremor, seizures, ataxia, autonomic instability
TCAs	Increases TCA toxicity	Sedation, decreased energy, lightheadedness, dry mouth, constipation, elevated TCA levels
warfarin	Possible displacement of warfarin by NGAs from protein-binding sites	Increased warfarin effects

MAOI, Monoamine oxidase inhibitor; *NGA,* newer-generation antidepressant; *TCA,* tricyclic and tetracyclic antidepressants.

DOSAGES

Selected NGAs

Drug, Year Approved by FDA (Pregnancy Category)	Pharmacologic Class	Usual Dosage Range*	FDA-Approved Indications
trazodone (Desyrel), 1982 (C)	Second generation	PO: 25-600 mg/day, with larger doses divided	Depression, adjunct for insomnia
▶bupropion (Wellbutrin, Zyban, Wellbutrin SR), 1985; reintroduced 1989 (B)	Second generation	PO: 200-400 mg/day, divided	Depression (Wellbutrin), smoking cessation (Zyban)
▶fluoxetine (Prozac, Sarafem), 1987 (B)	SSRI	PO, SR: 150-450 mg/day, divided bid-tid PO: 10-80 mg/day, qd or bid	Depression, OCD, bulimia nervosa, premenstrual dysphoric disorder
sertraline (Zoloft), 1991 (B)	SSRI	PO: 25-200 mg/day, taken qd	Depression, OCD, panic disorder, PTSD
paroxetine (Paxil), 1992 (B)	SSRI	PO: 10-50 mg/day, taken qd	Depression, OCD, panic disorder, social anxiety disorder, GAD
venlafaxine (Effexor), 1993 (C)	Third generation	PO: 75-375 mg/day, divided bid	Depression; GAD (XR form)
fluvoxamine (Luvox), 1994 (C)	SSRI	50-300 mg/day, with larger doses divided bid	OCD
nefazodone (generic only), 1994 (C)	Third generation	200-600 mg/day, divided bid	Depression
▶mirtazapine (Remeron), 1996 (C)	Third generation	15-45 mg/day qhs	Depression
citalopram (Celexa), 1998 (C)	SSRI	20-40 mg/day taken qd—qAM or qPM	Depression
escitalopram (Lexapro), 2002 (C)	SSRI	10-20 mg/day	Depression, generalized anxiety disorder
duloxetine (Cymbalta), 2002 (C)	SNRI	30-60 mg/day	Depression, pain from diabetic neuropathy

*All dosages reflect usual adult dosage ranges. Pediatric doses may be more variable and should be specified by a pediatric practitioner.
FDA, Food and Drug Administration; *GAD,* generalized anxiety disorder; *NGA,* newer-generation antidepressant; *OCD,* obsessive—compulsive disorder; *PTSD,* posttraumatic stress disorder; *SSRI,* selective serotonin reuptake inhibitor.

Drug Profiles

The 1980s and 1990s were decades of much development in psychotropic pharmacotherapy. Several new classes of antidepressants alone were introduced during this period. TCAs and MAOIs may be thought of as first-generation antidepressants. Two drugs introduced in the 1980s, now classified as second-generation antidepressants, are trazodone and bupropion. Both are still commonly used. The six currently available SSRIs were introduced during the 1980s and 1990s. In chronologic order, they are fluoxetine, sertraline, paroxetine, fluvoxamine, citalopram, and escitalopram. The 1990s saw the introduction of another major class of antidepressants: the third-generation antidepressants. These are venlafaxine, nefazodone, and mirtazapine. All three of these newer drugs have proved to be valuable new antidepressants. They are highly effective as antidepressants and are associated with very few serious adverse effects, especially when compared with first-generation antidepressants. They are now considered first-line drugs in the treatment of depression, including for patients with concurrent symptoms of anxiety, patients with depression with suicidal ideations, and patients unable to tolerate adverse reactions to other drugs. One notable hazard of the first-generation drugs, especially the TCAs, is their tendency to cause fatal cardiac dysrhythmias following overdose. Because depressed patients are generally at greater risk for suicide attempts, the newer generations of antidepressant drugs usually provide a safer drug choice. Dosage and indication information for selected NGAs appears in the corresponding table.

trazodone

Trazodone (Desyrel) was marketed in the United States in 1982. It was the first of the second- generation antidepressants that could selectively inhibit serotonin reuptake but that negligibly affected norepinephrine reuptake. This allowed for one advantage of trazodone over TCAs in terms of its minimal adverse effect on the cardiovascular system. It is, however, very sedating. This can be severe and can impair cognitive function in older adults. However, the sedating effect of trazodone is often advantageous in helping depressed patients, who commonly have comorbid anxiety and/or insomnia, obtain effective sleep. Trazodone also has rarely been associated with transient nonsexual priapism. This is reportedly the result of α-adrenergic blockade. The use of trazodone is contraindicated in patients who have shown a hypersensitivity reaction to it.

Pharmacokinetics

Half-Life	Onset	Peak	Duration
6-9 hr	1-2 wk*	2-4 wk*	Weeks*

*Therapeutic effects.

▶ *bupropion*

Bupropion (Wellbutrin, Wellbutrin SR, Zyban), a second-generation antidepressant, was originally approved by the FDA in 1985 but was withdrawn by the manufacturer because of its apparently high potential for inducing seizures in nondepressed patients being treated for bulimia. Subsequent investigations revealed that the overall estimated frequency of seizures was approximately 0.4%, and the drug was reintroduced in 1989. Bupropion is a unique antidepressant in terms of both its structure and mechanism of action. It has relatively weak, but measurable, effects on brain serotonin activity, with little to no activity on MAO. Its strongest therapeutic effects appear to be primarily dopaminergic and noradrenergic in nature.

Bupropion is available in both immediate-release (for multiple daily dosing) and sustained-release (for single or double daily dosing) dosage forms. Bupropion is sometimes added as a second antidepressant for male patients experiencing sexual adverse effects (e.g., erectile dysfunction) secondary to SSRI therapy. The mechanism for this is unclear, but the drug is often effective in this situation. A new sustained-release form of bupropion, Zyban, has recently been approved as first-line therapy as an aid in smoking cessation treatment. Zyban is an innovative new treatment because it is the first nicotine-free prescription medicine used to treat nicotine dependence. Its exact mechanism of action in treating nicotine dependence is unknown, but it is believed to be related to the drug's ability to modulate dopamine and norepinephrine levels in the brain. Both of these neurotransmitters are believed to play an important role in maintaining nicotine addiction.

Bupropion is contraindicated in patients who have shown a hypersensitivity reaction to it, those with a seizure disorder (bupropion can lower the seizure threshold) or who currently or in the past have suffered from anorexia nervosa or bulimia, and those currently on MAOI treatment.

Pharmacokinetics

Half-Life	Onset	Peak	Duration
10-14 hr	Up to 4 wk*	3 hr	Weeks to months

*Therapeutic effects.

▶ *fluoxetine*

Fluoxetine (Prozac) was the first SSRI marketed for the treatment of depression. It was approved by the FDA in December of 1987. Since that time, it has become the number one prescribed antidepressant in the United States and one of the most commonly prescribed of all drugs. It is contraindicated in patients who have shown a hypersensitivity reaction to it and in those taking MAOIs.

Pharmacokinetics

Half-Life	Onset	Peak	Duration
1-3 days	1-4 wk*	6-8 hr	2-4 wk

*Therapeutic effects.

venlafaxine

Venlafaxine (Effexor, Effexor XR), a third-generation antidepressant, was approved in 1993. It is unique in that it is chemically unrelated to all other available antidepressants and that it has a trimodal mechanism

of action on the activity of three major brain neurotransmitters. Specifically, it has potent inhibitory effects on both serotonin and norepinephrine reuptake and weaker, although still significant, inhibitory effects on dopamine reuptake. Given this multi-neurotransmitter activity, it is not surprising that venlafaxine, along with many other newer antidepressants, is often associated with activating adverse effects such as nervousness and insomnia. However, patients often report rapid improvement in depressive symptoms. The drug is available in both immediate-release (for multiple daily dosing) and sustained release (for single or double daily dosing) dosage forms. Venlafaxine does have significant metabolic effects on various cytochrome P-450 enzyme systems and is contraindicated in cases of drug allergy and in combination with MAOIs. Concurrent use with other serotonergic drugs carries the risk for serotonin syndrome and is generally not recommended.

Pharmacokinetics

Half-Life	Onset	Peak	Duration
3-11 hr	1-7 days	1-2 hr	Unknown

▶ *mirtazapine*

Mirtazapine (Remeron), the newest of the third-generation antidepressants, was approved by the FDA in 1996. It is unique in that it promotes the presynaptic release in the brain of both serotonin and norepinephrine due to its antagonist activity in the presynaptic α2-adrenergic receptors (see Chapter 17) but does not inhibit the reuptake of either of these neurotransmitters. It is strongly associated with sedation in more than 50% of patients due to its histamine (H1) receptor activity and, therefore, is usually dosed once daily at bedtime. However, it has demonstrated significant improvement of symptoms in depressed patients, including frail elderly patients in the nursing home setting. Furthermore, although clearance of the drug may be somewhat reduced in elderly patients, no dosage adjustment is currently recommended. Mirtazapine is also sometimes helpful (mechanism unknown) in reducing the sexual adverse effects in male patients receiving SSRI therapy. Mirtazapine is contraindicated in cases of drug allergy and concurrent use of MAOIs.

Pharmacokinetics

Half-Life	Onset	Peak	Duration
20-40 hr	1-3 wk	2 hr	Unknown

TRICYCLIC ANTIDEPRESSANTS

Among the original, first-generation antidepressants, TCAs have largely been superseded as first-line antidepressant drug therapy following the introduction of the SSRIs in the 1980s, beginning with fluoxetine (Prozac). At this point TCAs are generally considered second-line drug therapy for patients who fail NGAs or as adjunct therapy with NGAs.

Mechanism of Action and Drug Effects

TCAs are believed to work by correcting the imbalance in the neurotransmitter concentrations of serotonin and norepinephrine at the nerve endings in the CNS (the biogenic amine hypothesis). This is accomplished by blocking the reuptake of the neurotransmitters and thus causing these neurotransmitters to accumulate at the nerve endings. Some also believe that these drugs may help regulate malfunctioning nerves (the dysregulation hypothesis). TCAs have several advantageous therapeutic effects, but their use is also associated with many adverse effects. Both the advantageous and adverse effects can be explained by the functions of the various receptors that these drugs affect. As previously mentioned, the therapeutic effects of TCAs result from their ability to inhibit the reuptake of norepinephrine and serotonin at the nerve

Table 15-6	**Tricyclic Antidepressants: Therapeutic and Undesirable Drug Effects by Receptor Site**
Blockade of	**Drug Effect***
Adrenergic receptors	Orthostatic hypotension, anti-antihypertensive effects
Dopaminergic receptors	Extrapyramidal and endocrine adverse effects
Histaminergic receptors	Sedation, weight gain
Muscarinic receptors	Dry mouth, constipation, blurred vision, tachycardia, urinary retention, confusion
Norepinephrine reuptake	*Antidepressant,* tremors, tachycardia, additive pressor effects with sympathomimetic drugs
Serotonergic receptors	*Alleviation of rhinitis,* hypotension
Serotonin reuptake	*Antidepressant,* nausea, headache, anxiety, sexual dysfunction

*Italicized effects are the therapeutic ones.

Table 15-7	**Tricyclic Antidepressants: Adverse Effects**
Body System	**Adverse Effects**
Cardiovascular	Tremors, tachycardia, orthostatic hypotension, dysrhythmias
Central nervous	Anxiety, confusion, extrapyramidal effects, sedation
Gastrointestinal	Nausea, constipation, dry mouth
Hematologic	Pancytopenia
Other	Blurred vision, urinary retention, weight gain, impotence

endings, but they also block muscarinic, histaminergic, adrenergic, dopaminergic, and serotonergic receptors. This nonselective antagonism of multiple receptor types contributes to their adverse effects. The therapeutic and undesirable effects as they relate to the receptors affected are presented in Table 15-6.

Indications

TCAs are used to treat depression. They have been available for more than 40 years. Overall, they have demonstrated a remarkable efficacy, and their adverse-effect profiles are well established. They are also considerably less expensive than most of the newer drugs, with many of them available in generic formulations. Some of the TCAs have additional specific indications besides depression. For example, imipramine is used as an adjunct in the treatment of childhood enuresis (bedwetting), and clomipramine is useful in the treatment of OCD. Besides their beneficial antidepressant effects, TCAs are useful as adjunctive analgesics in the treatment of various chronic pain syndromes, especially neuropathic pain (e.g., trigeminal neuralgia).

Contraindications

Contraindications for TCAs include known drug allergy, use sooner than 14 days after stopping MAOI therapy, and pregnancy. They are also not recommended in patients with any acute or chronic cardiac problems or seizure history. It is this effect that usually results in death when these medications are overdosed by a suicidal patient.

Adverse Effects

The most common undesirable effects of TCAs are due to their effects on various receptors, mostly the muscarinic receptors. Blockade of these receptors by TCAs results in many undesirable anticholinergic adverse effects, the most common being sedation, impotence, and orthostatic hypotension. These drugs may also cause disturbances in cardiac conduction and alter the seizure threshold. Elderly patients have a tendency to suffer more from dizziness, postural hypotension, constipation, delayed micturition, edema, and muscle tremors. The various undesirable effects as they relate to body systems are listed in Table 15-7.

Toxicity and Management of Overdose

TCA overdoses are notoriously lethal. It is estimated that 70% to 80% of patients who die of TCA overdose do so before reaching the hospital. The primary organ systems affected are the CNS and cardiovascular system, and death usually results from either seizures or dysrhythmias.

There is no specific antidote for TCA poisoning. Management efforts are aimed at decreasing drug absorption through the administration of multiple doses of activated charcoal. Administration of an alkaline drug such as sodium bicarbonate speeds up elimination of the TCA by alkalinizing the urine to a pH of greater than 7.55. CNS damage may also be minimized through the administration of diazepam, and cardiovascular events may be minimized by giving antidysrhythmics to control cardiac dysrhythmias. Other care includes basic life support in an intensive care setting to maintain vital organ functions. These processes must continue until enough of the TCA is eliminated to permit restoration of normal organ function.

Interactions

When taken with TCAs, adrenergics may result in increased sympathetic stimulation. Anticholinergics and phenothiazines taken with TCAs may result in increased anticholinergic effects. CNS depressants when taken with TCAs will have additive CNS depressant effects. MAOIs when taken with TCAs may result in increased therapeutic and toxic effects, including hyperpyretic crisis (excessive fever). TCAs can inhibit the metabolism of warfarin, resulting in increased anticoagulation effects.

Dosages

For the recommended dosages for selected TCA drugs, see the dosages table below.

DOSAGES

Selected Tricyclic Antidepressants

Drug (Pregnancy Category)	Usual Dosage Range	Indications
▶ amitriptyline (Elavil, Endep) (C)	**Adult** PO: 15-300 mg/day divided **Elderly** PO: 100-150 mg/day divided	Depression

Box 15-3 Cyclic Antidepressant Categories

Tertiary Amine TCAs
amitriptyline
doxepin
imipramine
trimipramine

Secondary Amine TCAs
amoxapine
desipramine
nortriptyline
protriptyline

Tetracyclic Antidepressants
maprotiline
mirtazapine

TCA, Tricyclic antidepressant.

Drug Profiles

TCAs are effective drugs in the treatment of various affective disorders, but they are also associated with serious adverse effects. Therefore, patients taking them need to be monitored closely. For this reason, all antidepressants are available only with a prescription, with the exception of some herbal products such as St. John's wort (see the Herbal Therapies box on this page). Many drugs in this class are rated as pregnancy category D drugs, making their use by pregnant women relatively more hazardous than most of the NGAs. There are many drugs in the TCA drug class, including the tertiary-amine and secondary-amine TCAs. The secondary-amine TCAs have a stronger noradrenergic (norepinephrine) receptor effect and may have a structural advantage over the tertiary-amine TCAs in augmenting drug therapy with SSRIs in TRD. Box 15-3 lists the various cyclic antidepressants according to their respective categories. Dosage and indication information appears in the corresponding table.

▶ *amitriptyline*
Amitriptyline (Elavil) is one of the oldest and most widely used of all the TCAs. It is the prototypical tertiary-amine TCA and is also used in the treatment of various pain disorders such as trigeminal neuralgia. It has very potent anticholinergic properties, which can lead to many adverse effects such as dry mouth, constipation, blurred vision, urinary retention, and dysrhythmias.

There are two combination products that contain amitriptyline: Limbitrol, which also contains chlordiazepoxide, and Etrafon or Triavil, which also contains perphenazine.

Pharmacokinetics

Half-Life	Onset	Peak	Duration
10-50 hr	7-21 days*	2-12 hr	6-12 hr

*Therapeutic antidepressant effect.

MONOAMINE OXIDASE INHIBITORS

MAOIs, along with TCAs, represent the first generation of antidepressant drug therapy. Although MAOIs are potent drugs, they are now considered to be second- or third-line drugs for the treatment of depression that is not responsive to other pharmacologic therapies, such as the SSRIs or TCAs. As mentioned previously, such cases are known as TRD. A serious disadvantage to MAOI use is their potential to cause a hypertensive crisis when taken with a substance containing tyramine, which is found in many common foods and beverages (see Table 15-9). Another chemical with a similar name is tyrosine. This is an amino acid that is a biochemical precursor of dopamine and is not to be confused

Table 15-8 MAOIs: Adverse Effects

Body System	Adverse Effects
Cardiovascular	Orthostatic hypotension, tachycardia, palpitations, other arrhythmias, edema
Central nervous	Dizziness, drowsiness, restlessness, insomnia, headache, ataxia, hallucinations, seizures, tremors, confusion
Gastrointestinal	Anorexia, abdominal cramps, nausea, dry mouth,
Other	Blurred vision, impotence, skin rashes, impotence, respiratory depression

MAOI, Monoamine oxidase inhibitor.

with tyramine, which comes from exogenous food and beverage sources. The adverse effects of MAOIs are listed in Table 15-8.

Two available MAOI antidepressants, phenelzine (Nardil) and tranylcypromine (Parnate), are nonselective inhibitors of both types A and B MAO. Both types of MAO are widely distributed throughout the body, including the brain. MAO-A preferentially metabolizes serotonin, norepinephrine, and tyramine. MAO-B preferentially metabolizes dopamine. By inhibiting the MAO enzyme system in the CNS of patients suffering from depression, amines such as dopamine, serotonin, and norepinephrine are not broken down, and, therefore, higher levels occur. This in turn alleviates the symptoms of depression. However, higher levels of tyramine can also result in the hazardous drug-food interactions associated with MAOIs. This interaction is described in the following section on MAOI toxicity. There is also an MAO type B selective inhibitor called selegiline (Eldepryl) (see Chapter 14). This medication is used primarily for treating Parkinson's disease. It should be noted that MAOIs, as with other antidepressants, might take 1 to 4 weeks or more to reach their full therapeutic effects. However, patients vary widely in the timing of their responsiveness. Furthermore, a variety of over-the-counter drugs (especially for cough/cold) can interact with MAOIs to cause adverse cardiovascular effects. The patient taking MAOIs should always read labels and/or consult the pharmacist when using any such products. Dosage information for selected MAOIs appears in the table on this page.

Toxicity and Management of Overdose

Clinical symptoms of MAOI overdose generally do not appear until about 12 hours after ingestion. The primary signs and symptoms are cardiovascular and neurologic in nature. The most seri- ous cardiovascular effects are tachycardia and circulatory collapse, and the neurologic symptoms of major concern are seizures and coma. Hyperthermia and miosis are also generally present in overdose. The recommended treatment is aimed at eliminating the ingested toxin and protecting the organs at greatest risk for damage—the brain and heart. Recommended treatments are gastric lavage, urine acidification to a pH of 5, and hemodialysis. MAOIs are one of the few drug classes that are capable of interacting with food, leading to a severe reaction. In this case, food containing the amino acid tyramine is the primary culprit, and a hypertensive crisis is the reaction. It is essential for both the patient and the nurse to know the various foods and drinks that should be avoided; these are listed in Table 15-9. Treatment of hypertensive crisis resulting from consumption of tyramine-containing foods or beverages may require intravenous administration of hypotensive drugs along with careful monitoring in an intensive care setting.

Interactions

A wide variety of drug interactions can occur with MAOIs. Sympathomimetic drugs can also interact with the MAOIs and together cause a hypertensive crisis. MAOIs can markedly potentiate the effects of meperidine, and, therefore, concurrent use is contraindicated. In addition, concurrent use of MAOIs with SSRIs carries the risk for serotonin syndrome. A washout period of at least 2 weeks after discontinuation of sertraline, paroxetine, or citalopram should occur before initiation of MAOI therapy. A 5-week washout period is necessary if switching to MAOIs from fluoxetine.

Dosages

For recommended dosage and indication information for selected MAOI drugs, see the table on this page.

Table 15-9	Food and Drink to Avoid When Taking MAOIs
Food/Drink	**Examples**
High Tyramine Content—Not Permitted	
Aged mature cheeses	Cheddar, blue, Swiss
Smoked/pickled meats	Herring, sausage, corned beef, smoked fish or poultry, salami, pepperoni
Aged/fermented meats	Chicken or beef liver pate, game fish, or poultry
Yeast extracts	Brewer's yeast
Red wines	Chianti, burgundy, sherry, vermouth
Italian broad beans	Fava beans
Moderate Tyramine Content—Limited Amounts Allowed	
Meat extracts	Bouillon, consommé
Pasteurized light and pale beer	
Ripe avocado	
Low Tyramine Content—Permissible	
Distilled spirits	Vodka, gin, rye, scotch (in moderation)
American and mozzarella	Cottage cheese, cream cheese
Chocolate and caffeinated beverages	
Fruit	Figs, bananas, raisins, grapes, pineapple, oranges
Soy sauce	
Yogurt, sour cream	

MAOI, Monoamine oxidase inhibitor.

DOSAGES

Selected MAOIs

Drug (Pregnancy Category)	Usual Dosage Range	Indications
phenelzine (Nardil) (C)	PO: Initial dose 45-90 mg/day divided tid, followed by dose reduction to minimal effective dose after therapeutic effect achieved	Depression, panic disorders
tranylcypromine (Parnate) (C)	20-60 mg/day divided bid	Depression

MAOI, Monoamine oxidase inhibitor.

ANTIPSYCHOTIC DRUGS

Antipsychotic drugs are used to treat serious mental illness such as depressive and drug-induced psychoses, schizophrenia, and autism. Antipsychotics are also used to treat extreme mania (as an adjunct to lithium), BPD, certain movement disorders (e.g., Tourette's syndrome), and certain other medical conditions (e.g., nausea, intractable hiccups). Antipsychotics have also been referred to as tranquilizers or *neuroleptics* because they produce a state of tranquillity and work on abnormally functioning nerves. However, these are both older terms that are now less commonly used.

Constituting about two thirds of all antipsychotics, phenothiazines are the largest group of antipsychotic drugs. Like many other drugs, phenothiazines were discovered by chance, in this case during research for new antihistamines. In 1951, chlorpromazine was the first phenothiazine to be discovered in this way. Phenothiazines are associated with a high incidence of anticholinergic adverse effects because they are so closely related to antihistamines. Therefore, since the early 1950s, researchers have been working on developing phenothiazines with few adverse effects. Although phenothiazines can provide much relief to the mentally ill patient, they can also cause many undesirable adverse effects.

Phenothiazines can be divided into three groups based on structural differences: aliphatic, piperidine, and piperazine. Besides the phenothiazine antipsychotics, there are four other categories of drugs that are commonly used to treat mental illness: thioxanthenes, butyrophenones, dihydroindolones, and dibenzoxazepines. Many of the therapeutic and toxic effects of the antipsychotics are the consequence of their chemical structures.

There is very little difference between traditional antipsychotics in their mechanisms of action; therefore, selection of an antipsychotic is based primarily on the least undesirable drug adverse effect and the patient's type of psychosis. Of the currently available antipsychotic drugs, no single drug stands out as either more or less effective in the treatment of the symptoms of psychosis. It should also be stressed that antipsychotic drug therapy does not provide a cure for mental illness but is only a way of chemically controlling the symptoms of the illness. These drugs represent a significant advance in our treatment of mental illnesses, as borne out by the fact that the early treatment of mental illnesses (before the 1950s) consisted of such extreme measures as isolation, physical restraint, shock therapy, and even lobotomy.

Over the past 6 or 7 years, a new class of antipsychotic medications has evolved. They are referred to as atypical antipsychotics (AAPs) or second-generation antipsychotics, and they differ from first-generation drugs in both their mechanisms of action and their adverse effect profiles. Some of these newer AAPs include clozapine (Clozaril), risperidone (Risperdal), olanzapine (Zyprexa), quetiapine (Seroquel), ziprasidone (Geodon), and, most recently, aripiprazole (Abilify). Newer antipsychotics gaining approval and showing great promise include sertindole and zotepine.

Mechanism of Action and Drug Effects

One thing that all antipsychotics have in common is some degree of blockage of dopamine receptors in the brain, thus decreasing the dopamine concentration in the CNS. Specifically, the older phenothiazines block the receptors to which dopamine normally binds postsynaptically in certain areas of the CNS, such as the limbic system and the basal ganglia. These are the areas associated with emotions, cognitive function, and motor function. This results in a tranquilizing effect in psychotic patients. Both the therapeutic and toxic effects of these drugs are the direct result of the dopamine blockade in these areas.

The newer AAPs mentioned previously block specific dopamine receptors called dopamine 2 (D_2) receptors, as well as specific serotonin receptors in the brain called serotonin 2 (5-HT2) receptors. The different mechanisms of action of the AAPs are responsible for their improved efficacy and improved safety profiles.

Antipsychotics have many effects throughout the body. Besides blocking the dopamine receptors in the CNS, they also block alpha receptors, which can result in hypotension and other cardiovascular effects. Many of the adverse effects of these drugs stem from their ability to block histamine receptors (anticholinergic effects). They also block serotonin receptors. This, in combination with their ability to block dopamine receptors in the chemoreceptor trigger zone and peripherally and with their ability to inhibit neurotransmission in the vagus nerve in the gastrointestinal tract, accounts for the ability of certain antipsychotics to function as antiemetics. Additional blocking of dopamine receptors in the brainstem reticular system also allows AAPs to have antianxiety effects.

All antipsychotics show some efficacy for the *positive* symptoms of schizophrenia, and, over time, the improvement may even increase. These so-called positive symptoms include hallucinations, delusions, and conceptual disorganization. Unfortunately, first-generation antipsychotics are much less effective for negative symptoms. Negative symptoms are apathy, social withdrawal, blunted affect, poverty of speech, and catatonia. It is these negative symptoms that account for most of the social and vocational disability caused by schizophrenia. Fortunately, newer generation antipsychotic drugs often have improved efficacy against the negative symptoms. Another drawback to first-generation antipsychotics is that they all cause extrapyramidal symptoms (EPS), including rigidity, tremor, bradykinesia (slow movement), and bradyphrenia (slow thought). To summarize, first-generation antipsychotics such as haloperidol are effective for controlling symptoms, but not all symptoms, not in all patients, and not without serious adverse effects. However, there is recent debate in the literature regarding the level of overall improvement between older and newer antipsychotic drugs.

Indications

As previously mentioned, the major therapeutic effect of antipsychotic drugs is the result of blockade of dopamine receptors in certain areas of the CNS. These are the areas where regulation of dopamine activity tends to be dysfunctional in psychotic patients. The extent to which such antidopaminergic drug therapy has been shown to control psychotic symptoms is one of the major factors supporting the **dopamine hypothesis** regarding the origins of the various psychotic disorders. Note that this type of drug therapy is in direct contrast to that for PD treatment, where dopaminergic activity needs to be enhanced instead of reduced. The various areas within the CNS where antipsychotics have a major effect are listed in Table 15-10.

Table 15-10 Major Dopamine Systems in the Brain

DA System	DA-Related Function	Effects of DA-Receptor Blockade
Hypothalamic-pituitary	Regulates prolactin secretion, temperature, appetite, emesis	Increased prolactin levels resulting in galactorrhea, amenorrhea, and decreased libido; loss of temperature regulation, increased appetite, and antiemetic effects
Mesocortical	Regulates behavior	Therapeutic antipsychotic effects
Mesolimbic	Regulates stereotypical and other behaviors	Therapeutic antipsychotic effects
Nigrostriatal	Mediates function of the extrapyramidal motor system (EPS movement)	Reversible: Dystonia, pseudoparkinsonism, akathisia Irreversible: TD (must catch early to reverse!)

DA, Dopamine; *EPS,* extrapyramidal symptoms; *TD,* tardive dyskinesia.

Contraindications

Contraindications to the use of antipsychotic drugs include known drug allergy; comatose state; and possibly significant CNS depression, brain damage, liver or kidney disease, blood dyscrasias, and uncontrolled epilepsy.

Adverse Effects

The adverse effects of the individual antipsychotic drugs are many and are important to remember. The goal is to choose a drug with the least bothersome adverse effect profile for a given patient. Individual patients may vary widely in their response to, and tolerance of, a given medication. These individual variances are usually not predictable, and often the medications that best help a given patient are discovered through a trial and error process. The common adverse effects caused by blockade of the dopamine, muscarinic (synonymous with cholinergic), histamine, and α-adrenergic receptors are listed in Table 15-11. These undesirable effects can also be classified according to the body system affected. Severe hematologic effects may include agranulocytosis (lack of *granulocytes* in the blood) and hemolytic anemia. Integumentary effects may include exfoliative dermatitis. CNS effects include drowsiness, **neuroleptic malignant syndrome** (NMS), **extrapyramidal symptoms** (EPS), and **tardive dyskinesia** (TD). NMS is a potentially life-threatening adverse effect that may include high fever, unstable blood pressure (BP), and myoglobinemia. EPS involve involuntary motor symptoms similar to those associated with Parkinson's disease (see Chapter 14). This drug-induced state is known as *pseudoparkinsonism* and includes such symptoms as **akathisia** (distressing motor restlessness) and acute dystonia (painful muscle spasms). Two anticholinergic medications, benztropine (Cogentin) and trihexyphenidyl (Artane) are commonly used to treat these symptoms. These drugs were introduced in Chapter 14 on Parkinson's disease. Tardive is a word that means "late-appearing." TD involves involuntary contractions of oral and facial muscles (e.g.,

involuntary tongue-thrusting) and choreoathetosis (wavelike movements of extremities) that usually appear only after continuous long-term antipsychotic therapy. Ocular adverse effects include blurred vision, corneal lens changes, epithelial keratopathy, and pigmentary retinopathy. Cardiovascular effects include postural hypotension. Additionally, electrocardiogram (ECG) changes, notably prolonged QT interval, are associated to varying degrees with all classes of antipsychotic drugs. Baseline and periodic ECGs, as well as serum potassium and magnesium levels, can help determine if a patient is at risk for such effects or diagnose newly acquired cardiac dysrhythmias. In such cases, another drug choice may still control symptoms without causing cardiac effects. The older first-generation drugs such as phenothiazines and haloperidol can also augment prolactin release, which can result in swelling of the breasts and milk secretion in women taking these drugs. Gynecomastia (breast tissue enlargement) can also be a distressing adverse effect in male patients.

The common adverse effects caused by antipsychotic drugs are listed in Table 15-12.

Low-potency antipsychotic drugs generally have a low incidence of EPS and a high incidence of sedation, anticholinergic adverse effects, and cardiovascular adverse effects. The opposite is true for high-potency antipsychotic drugs. They have a high incidence of EPS and a low incidence of sedation, anticholinergic adverse effects, and cardiovascular adverse effects.

Interactions

Major drug interactions include the following. Antacids and *tannic acids* (also known as *tannins;* e.g., in tea, grapes, wine) can decrease antipsychotic absorption when taken with these drugs. Antihypertensives may have additive hypotensive effects and CNS depressants may have additive CNS-depressant effects when taken with antipsychotics. With regard to clozapine in particular, grapefruit juice can enhance its effects (by reducing its metabolism) and nicotine can reduce its effects (by speeding its metabolism).

Table 15-11 Antipsychotics: Receptor-Related Adverse Effects

Receptor	Adverse Effects	Drug Category
α-adrenergic	Postural hypotension, lightheadedness, reflex tachycardia	Low-potency drugs
Dopamine	Extrapyramidal movement disorders, dystonia, parkinsonism, akathisia, TD	High-potency drugs
Endocrine	Prolactin secretion (galactorrhea, gynecomastia), menstrual changes, sexual dysfunction	Low-potency drugs
Histamine	Sedation, drowsiness, hypotension, weight gain	Low-potency drugs
Muscarinic (cholinergic)	Blurred vision, worsening of narrow-angle glaucoma, dry mouth, tachycardia, constipation, urinary retention, decreased sweating	Low-potency drugs

TD, Tardive dyskinesia.

Table 15-12 Antipsychotics: Adverse Effects

Body System	Adverse Effects
Cardiovascular	Orthostatic hypotension, syncope, dizziness, ECG changes, conduction abnormalities
Central nervous	Sedation, delirium, neuroleptic malignant syndrome
Gastrointestinal	Dry mouth, constipation, paralytic ileus, hepatotoxicity, weight gain
Genitourinary	Urinary hesitancy, urinary retention, impaired erection, priapism, ejaculatory problems
Hematologic	Leukopenia and agranulocytosis
Integumentary	Photosensitivity, hyperpigmentation, rash, pruritus
Metabolic and endocrine	Galactorrhea, irregular menses, amenorrhea, amenorrhea, decreased libido, increased appetite, polydipsia, impaired temperature regulation

Dosages

For recommended dosage and indication information for selected antipsychotic drugs, see the tables below and on page 240.

The first-generation antipsychotic drugs are currently still available on the U.S. market. However, their use in common clinical practice has been largely supplanted by the second-generation or "atypical" antipsychotic drugs, which generally have better adverse-effect profiles. All antipsychotics are prescription-only medications that are indicated for the treatment of various psychotic disorders. No single drug stands out as being either more or less effective in the treatment of the symptoms of psychosis. Some of the factors that should be considered before selecting an antipsychotic are the patient's history of response to a drug and the possible adverse-effect profile. Patients should be started with a low dose and titrated to the lowest effective dose, balancing between symptom relief and adverse effects, if any. Dosage and indication information appears in the corresponding table. Selected drugs are profiled in more detail below.

Table 15-13 lists compatible and incompatible liquids for dosing the liquid dosage forms of both older and newer generations of selected antipsychotic drugs.

Phenothiazines
fluphenazine

Fluphenazine (Prolixin) is available in three different salt forms, which give it varying degrees of antipsychotic potency. The decanoate and enanthate salt forms have the longest durations of action, and the hydrochloride salt form is fairly short in duration. Fluphenazine has the greatest potency of all the phenothiazines: 1 mg of the drug has the antipsychotic potency of 200 mg of chlorphenazine. It is primarily used to treat psychotic disorders and schizophrenia. It is considered to be a high-potency antipsychotic and is therefore associ-

DOSAGES

Selected First-Generation Antipsychotic Drugs

Drug (Pregnancy Category)	Pharmacologic Class	Usual Dosage Range	Indications
chlorpromazine (Thorazine) (C)	Alipatic phenothiazine	**Adult** PO, IM: 25-500 mg/day with larger doses divided; IM is usually for acute care only **Pediatric** PO, IM, IV: 0.5-1 mg/kg/dose q6-8 hr	Psychotic disorders, mania
fluphenazine (Prolixin) (C)	Piperidine phenothiazine	**Adult only** PO: 0.5-20 mg/day with larger doses divided tid-qid IM: 1.25-10 mg/day with larger doses divided tid-qid	Psychotic disorders
haloperidol (Haldol) (C)	Butyrophenone phenylbutylpiperidine	**Adult** PO, IM: 0.5-5 mg bid-tid Pediatric PO: 25-50 mcg/kd/day IM (acute care only): 2-5 mg up to q1h prn	
loxapine (Loxitane) (C)	Dibenzoxazepine dipenzepine	**Adult only** PO: 10 mg bid up to 250 mg/day divided bid-qid IM: 12.5-50 mg q4-6h	
molindone (Moban) (C)	Dihydroindolone	**Adult only:** PO: 50-225 mg/day divided tid-qid	
thiothixene (Navane) (C)	Thioxanthenes	**Adult** 2 mg tid to 60 mg/day divided tid	

Table 15-13 Compatibility of Selected Liquid Antipsychotic Dosage Forms with Beverages for Dosing Purposes*

Drug	Compatible with	Not Compatible with
risperidone	Water, coffee, orange juice, low-fat milk	Cola, tea
thioridazine	Water, fruit juice, carbonated, drinks, milk, (or pudding)	None listed
fluphenazine	Water, saline, homogenized milk, carbonated orange beverage, pineapple, apricot, prune, orange, tomato, and grapefruit juice	Beverages containing caffeine, tannics (e.g., tea), or pectinates (e.g., apple juice)
perphenazine	Water, saline, 7-Up, homogenized milk, carbonated orange beverages, pineapple, apricot, prune, orange, V-8, tomato, and grapefruit juice	Beverages containing caffeine, tannics (e.g., tea), or pectinates (e.g., apple juice)
haloperidol	Water, juice	None listed

*When in doubt, the nurse should consult the manufacturer's package insert and/or pharmacist for information about a specific drug product.

ated with a high incidence of EPS; however, the associated incidence of sedative, anticholinergic, and cardiovascular effects is low. It is contraindicated in patients who have shown a hypersensitivity reaction to phenothiazines and in those suffering from circulatory collapse, liver dysfunction, blood dyscrasias, comatose state, bone marrow depression, or alcohol or barbiturate withdrawal.

Pharmacokinetics

Half-Life	Onset	Peak	Duration
PO: 15-16 hr*	PO (HCl): 1 hr	PO (HCl): 1.5-2 hr	PO (HCl): 6-8 hr
IM: Up to 2 wk†	IM (HCl): 1 hr	IM (HCl): 1.5-2 hr	IM (HCl): 6-8 hr
	IM (enanthate): 24-72 hr	IM (enanthate): 1.5-2 hr	IM (enanthate): 1-3 wk
	IM (decanoate): 24-72 hr	IM (decanoate): Unknown	IM (decanoate): ≥4 wk
		IM (decanoate): Unknown	

*Following single dose.
†Following multiple intramuscular injections.

Butyrophenones
haloperidol

Haloperidol (Haldol) is structurally different from the thioxanthenes and the phenothiazines, but has similar antipsychotic properties. It is a high-potency neuroleptic drug that has a favorable cardiovascular, anticholinergic, and sedative adverse effect profile but can often cause EPS. Haloperidol is available in three salt forms: base, decanoate, and lactate. Haloperidol decanoate has an extremely long duration of effect. It is used primarily for the long-term treatment of psychosis and is especially useful in patients who are noncompliant with their drug treatment. It is contraindicated in patients who have shown a hypersensitivity reaction to it, those in a comatose state, those taking large amounts of CNS depressants, and those with PD.

Pharmacokinetics

Half-Life	Onset	Peak	Duration
PO/IM: 13-35 hr	PO: 2 hr	PO: 2-6 hr	PO: 8-12 hr
	IM (lactate): 20-30 min	IM (lactate): 30-45 min	IM (lactate): 4-8 hr
	IM (decanoate): 3-9 days	IM (decanoate): Unknown	IM (decanoate): 1 mo

Atypical Antipsychotics

Between 1975 and 1990 there was not a single new antipsychotic drug approved in the United States. Then, in 1990 came the approval of clozapine (Clozaril), the first of the atypical antipsychotics (AAPs). Clozapine was followed in 1995 by risperidone (Risperdal), in 1996 by olanzapine (Zyprexa), in 1997 by quetiapine (Seroquel), in 2001 by ziprasidone (Geodon), and in 2002 by aripiprazole (Abilify). The term *atypical antipsychotics* refers to the following advantageous properties of these drugs: reduced effect on prolactin levels compared with older drugs and improvement in the negative symptoms associated with schizophrenia. Although they are still fairly new compared with their first-generation counterparts, they also show a lower risk for NMS, EPS, and TD. These new drugs—plus several more in clinical trials—are revolutionizing the treatment of psychosis and schizophrenia. For these reasons, AAPs are also referred to and recognized as second-generation antipsychotic drugs. All five of the currently available AAPs have several pharmacologic properties in common. Antagonist activity at the dopamine D_1 receptor is believed to be the mechanism of antimanic activity. Serotonergic (serotonin agonist) activity at various serotonin (5-HT) receptor subtypes and α2-adrenergic (agonist) activity are both associated with antidepressant activity. α1-adrenergic receptor antagonist activity is associated with orthostatic effects, and histamine H_1 receptor antagonist activity is associated with both sedative and appetite stimulating effects. This last effect accounts for a common adverse effect of weight gain that is associated to various degrees with AAP drugs. This can cause or worsen obesity and even bring about diabetes. Clozapine and olanzapine are associated with the most weight gain, risperidone and quetiapine with less, and ziprasidone is considered weight neutral. Sedative effects may diminish over time and can actually be helpful for patients with insomnia. Although these five drugs all have similar pharmacologic properties, they vary in the degree of affinity that each may have for the various types of receptors. These subtle pharmacologic differences, along with often unknown and unpredictable physiologic patient differences, help to explain why some patients respond better (or not) to one medication versus another.

In April of 2005, the FDA issued a special Public Health Advisory concerning the use of atypical antipsychotic drugs in elderly patients for "off-label" (non–FDA-approved) uses. These medications are currently FDA-approved for schizophrenia and mania. In practice, however, they are also commonly used to control agitative behavioral symptoms in elderly patients with dementia, including dementia related to Alzheimer's disease. A meta-analysis combining the data of 17 smaller placebo-controlled studies found that elderly patients given AAPs for this reason were up to 1.7 times more likely to die during treatment. This FDA announcement serves to remind prescribers that AAPs are not officially indicated for dementia-related behavioral symptoms. The agency also recommends that patients so treated have their treatment plans re-evaluated by their health care provider.

Dosage and indication information appears in the corresponding table. Also, Table 15-13 lists compatible and incompatible liquids for dosing the liquid dosage forms of both older and newer generations of selected antipsychotic drugs.

DOSAGES

Selected Atypical Antipsychotic Drugs

Drug, Year Approved (Pregnancy Category)	Pharmacologic Class	Usual Dosage Range*	Indications
clozapine (Clozaril), 1989 (B)	Dibenzodiazepine dibenzepin	25-900 mg/day with larger doses divided tid	Psychotic disorders
risperidone (Risperdal), 1993 (C)	Benzisoxazole	PO: 1-8 mg/day qd-bid IM depot form (Risperdal Consta): 25-50 mg IM every two weeks	Psychotic disorders
olanzapine (Zyprexa), 1996 (C)	Thienobenzodiazepine dibenzepin	5-20 mg/day qd	Schizophrenia, bipolar mania
quetiapine (Seroquel), 1997 (C)	Dibenzothiazepine dibenzepin	25-800 mg/day with larger doses divided bid-tid	Schizophrenia
ziprasidone (Geodon), 2001 (C)	Dihydroindolone	20-80 mg bid	Schizophrenia
aripiprazole (Abilify, 2002) (C)	Quinolinone	10-30 mg once daily	Schizophrenia, bipolar mania

*All dosages reflect usual adult dosage ranges. Pediatric doses may be more variable and should be specified by a pediatric practitioner.

clozapine

Clozapine (Clozaril) is a unique antipsychotic drug. It is similar to loxapine in its chemical structure in that it is a piperazine-substituted tricyclic antipsychotic; however, pharmacologically it is different from all other currently available antipsychotics in terms of its mechanism of action. It also more selectively blocks the dopaminergic receptors in the mesolimbic system. Other antipsychotic drugs block dopamine receptors in an area of the brain called the neostriatum, but blockade in this area of the brain is believed to give rise to the unwanted EPS. Because clozapine has very weak dopamine-blocking abilities in this area, it is associated with minor or no EPS. In fact, although newer AAPs may be better tolerated and are not associated with the hematologic adverse effects associated with clozapine, clozapine is currently the AAP with the lowest reported incidence of such effects. This often makes clozapine the drug of choice for psychotic disorders in patients with comorbid PD because it will not worsen motor symptoms.

Clozapine has been extremely useful for the treatment of patients who have failed treatment with other antipsychotic drugs, especially those with schizophrenia. Patients taking clozapine must be monitored very closely for the development of agranulocytosis, a dangerous lack of white blood cell (WBC) production that is drug-induced. The risk for the development of agranulocytosis as the result of clozapine therapy is 1% to 2% after the first year; this compares with a risk of 0.1% to 1% for phenothiazines. For this reason, patients beginning clozapine therapy require weekly monitoring of WBC count for the first 6 months of therapy. The drug should be withheld if the count falls below $3000/mm^3$ until it rises above this value. It is also recommended that weekly WBC counts are evaluated for 4 weeks after discontinuation of the drug. Its use is contraindicated in patients who have shown a hypersensitivity reaction to it and in those with myeloproliferative disorders, severe granulocytopenia, CNS depression, or narrow-angle glaucoma or those who are in a comatose state.

Pharmacokinetics

Half-Life	Onset	Peak	Duration
6 hr	1-6 hr	Weeks	4-12 hr

▶ risperidone

Risperidone (Risperdal) was the second atypical antipsychotic to receive FDA approval. It is even more active than clozapine at the serotonin (5-HT 2A and 2C) receptors. It also has high affinity for α1- and α2-adrenergic receptors and histamine H1 receptors. It has lower affinity for the serotonin 5-HT 1A, 1C, and 1D receptors and the dopamine D1 receptor. It is effective for refractory schizophrenia, including negative symptoms, and causes minimal EPS at therapeutic dosages (1 to 6 mg/day). It also is not associated with the hematologic hazards and need for frequent WBC count monitoring that is necessary with clozapine. However, it can cause mild-to-moderate elevation of serum prolactin levels. The use of risperidone is contraindicated in patients who have shown a hypersensitivity reaction to it. It is available in both oral and a long-acting injectable form.

Pharmacokinetics

Half-Life	Onset	Peak	Duration
20-30 hr	1-2 wk*	Unknown	7 days

*Therapeutic effects.

▶ olanzapine

Olanzapine (Zyprexa) is the third of the AAPs to receive FDA approval. It interacts with dopamine D1-4 and serotonin 5-HT2A and 2C receptors. Like clozapine, it also has blocking action on a variety of other receptors, such as other serotonin receptors, α1-adrenergic receptors, and histamine receptors. Olanzapine is a thienobenzodiazepine derivative. It was designated 1S (new molecular entity) by the FDA and approved without advisory committee review to speed its availability for schizophrenic patients. Many previously disabled patients have experienced dramatic improvement in their level of day-to-day functioning. Olanzapine has only minor effects on the hepatic cytochrome P-450 enzyme systems, greatly reducing the likelihood of significant drug interactions. It also lacks the requirement for frequent monitoring of WBC count that is necessary with clozapine. However, it is associated with both weight gain and sedation. Its only absolute contraindication is drug allergy.

Pharmacokinetics

Half-Life	Onset	Peak	Duration
21-54 hr	>1 wk	6 hr	Unknown

quetiapine

A fourth AAP is quetiapine (Seroquel). Quetiapine is a dibenzothiazepine antipsychotic similar in structure to clozapine but seems to be much safer, especially from a hematologic standpoint. Quetiapine has affinity for dopamine D2 and D1 receptors; serotonin 5-HT1A, 2A, and 2C receptors; muscarinic (cholinergic) M1 receptors; histamine H1 receptors; and α1- and α2-adrenergic receptors. It also has minor effects on hepatic cytochrome P-450 enzyme systems, thus reducing the likelihood of serious drug interactions. The drug also blocks histamine and α-adrenergic receptors. This medication can cause ocular cataracts, and patients should have eye examinations every 6 months.

Pharmacokinetics

Half-Life	Onset	Peak	Duration
6 hr	2 days	1-2 hr	Unknown

ziprasidone

Ziprasidone (Geodon) is the fifth and newest of the atypical antipsychotics, approved in 2001. It is chemically classified as a benzothiazolylpiperazine. Its pharmacologic activity is comparable to that of quetiapine. It has antagonist activity at several serotonin-receptor subtypes, including 5-HT2A/2C, 5-HT1D, 5-HT7, and the D2 dopamine receptors. It has agonist activity at the 5-HT1A serotonin receptors. It has also been shown to cause what is considered to be a mild ECG change—slight prolongation of the QT interval. It is recommended that ziprasidone be taken with food to enhance its absorption. However, grapefruit and grapefruit juice have been shown to increase its blood concentration, and it is recommended that both be avoided while taking this drug.

Pharmacokinetics

Half-Life	Onset	Peak	Duration
7 hr	2-3 days	6-8 hr	Unknown

Antipsychotic Drugs Summary

All of these drugs have a place in the treatment of schizophrenia. The lack of traditional neurologic adverse effects is a tremendous benefit of the newer-generation atypical drugs. This encourages the early use of antipsychotics when therapy is the most beneficial. Physicians have been very reluctant in the past to prescribe drugs early in therapy. With the evolution of the AAPs, early therapy is not only possible but safe and relatively well tolerated.

◆ NURSING PROCESS

◆ ASSESSMENT

Both physical and emotional status of patients taking psychotherapeutic drugs need to be thoroughly assessed before, during, and after initiation of therapy. The potential for drug interactions, drug toxicity, drug overdosage, and other adverse effects associated with these drugs is great, and, thus, the need for an ongoing assessment. Constant assessment for any suicidal ideations or tendencies is important because patients may have covert, as well as overt, cues or thoughts. The potential for suicide with psychotherapeutic drugs with or without the combination or other drugs or alcohol should always be considered a risk. Many of the patients needing these medications are so mentally distressed that their physical needs go unmet, resulting in a complexity of other problems such as insomnia, poor health status, and weight loss or gain. Baseline blood pressure, pulse rate, body temperature, and body weight should be assessed and documented before, during, and after drug therapy. Postural (supine then standing) blood pressure readings are particularly important due to the adverse effect of postural hypotension associated with psychotherapeutics. The more potent, older drugs, such as MAOIs and TCAs, may lead to a significant drop in blood pressure and warrant even more astute assessment.

The patient's neurologic functioning should be assessed, including level of consciousness, mental alertness and level of motor and cognitive functioning. The Mini-Mental Status Examination (MMSE) is one tool that may be used to assess the cognitive impairment found with so many mental illnesses and is simple, cost efficient, and can be completed in about 20 minutes by the nurse/clinician. The MMSE is usually found in most nursing-assessment textbooks as well as psychiatric–mental health nursing textbooks. It includes an assessment with scoring of points in four major areas: level of orientation, attention and calculation ability, recall testing, and language skills. Other assessment tools include the six-item Blessed Orientation-Memory-Concentration Test; Clock Drawing Tasks and Functional Activities Questionnaire (for those with dementia) as well as Alzheimer's Disease Assessment Scale, the Mattis Dementia Rating Scale; the Severe Impairment Battery and the Hamilton Rating Scale (HAM-D). The HAM-D was previously discussed in this chapter. To complete the neurologic system assessment, assessment of baseline levels of motor responses/reflexes, presence of any tremors, agitation, as well as cold, clammy hands, sweating, and pallor (indicative of autonomic responses) should be performed and documented.

It is also important to assess laboratory studies performed, which are usually ordered before, during, and after psychotropic drug therapy. It is especially important in those who are in long-term therapy to prevent or identify early any possible complications and toxicity. Laboratory tests may include, but are not limited to, serum therapeutic levels/ranges of the specific drug—if appropriate, a complete blood cell count (CBC), erythrocyte sedimentation rate (ESR), serum electrolytes, glucose levels, blood urea nitrogen (BUN), liver function studies, serum vitamin B_{12}, and thyroid studies. If the patient is experiencing forms of dementia, other types of testing may be needed, such as genetic studies, computed tomography (CT) scan, or magnetic resonance imaging (MRI).

With psychotherapeutic drugs, the nurse should always assess the patient's mouth to make sure the patient has swallowed the entire oral dosage. This helps to prevent "hoarding" or "cheeking" of medications, a form of noncompliance that may lead to drug toxicity or overdose. If the assessment shows that this is a potential risk, use of liquid dosage forms, when available, may minimize such problems. Appetite, sleeping patterns, addictive

behaviors, elimination difficulties, hypersensitivity, and other complaints also need to be assessed and documented. Assessment of motor responses, such as trembling and agitation, as well as assessment of autonomic responses (cold, clammy hands, sweating and pallor) is also important to establishing baseline information.

Antianxiety Drugs

Antianxiety drugs are associated with many contraindications, cautions, and drug interactions, and specific pediatric and elderly concerns are presented in the boxes on p. 244. The elderly patient needs to be closely assessed and observed for oversedation and profound CNS depression for the duration of therapy. The elderly are often more sensitive to drugs, and, therefore, there is constant concern for their safety. It is also critical for nurses to document these assessment findings and make safety a top priority in all phases of the nursing process. Specific serum studies that may be ordered include CBC, lactate dehydrogenase (LDH), creatinine, alkaline phosphatase, and BUN. In addition, BP readings are important because of drug-related postural hypotension as an adverse effect. Pulse rate and temperature should also be assessed.

Eye problems may occur with benzodiazepines; therefore, baseline visual testing should be determined with a basic Snellen chart examination or by the appropriate health care provider—for example, an ophthalmologist or optometrist. Allergic reactions to some of these medications, such as clonazepam, are characterized by a red, raised rash. A significant reduction in bone marrow functioning may occur with possible blood dyscrasias, fever, sore throat, bruising, and jaundice. These "at risk" patients for complications would need even closer assessment. In addition, patients who are obese may become toxic within a shorter period of time as compared to those who are not obese. This occurs because several antianxiety drugs are lipid soluble and because most obese patients have a higher percentage of lipids, the lipid-soluble drug would have greater affinity for these tissues and stay in the body longer than anticipated, with a resultant prolonged half-life (and increased toxicity in obese patients).

Some benzodiazepines—as well as most drug groups—are associated with medication errors that are "sound alike/look alike" in nature. Assessing the drug order for the right drug is important because of this potential error that could occur and the negative consequences to the patient. Sound-alike benzodiazepine drugs that could be confused with other medications include the following:

- Clonazepam, Klonopin, and clonidine
- Diazepam and Ditropan
- Lorazepam and alprazolam
- Midazolam or Versed and VePesid or Vistaril

Other important assessment-related parameters for some of the specific benzodiazepines include the following:

(1) Lorazepam should be given cautiously (under very close supervision) if the patient is suicidal because its use is associated with suicide attempts. (2) Alprazolam should be administered only after assessment of mental status, anxiety, mood, sensorium, sleep patterns, and dizziness. (3) Chlordiazepoxide has significant assessment parameters such as monitoring for any blood dyscrasias (altered blood counts) or evidence of ataxia. (4) Clonazepam is commonly associated with blood dyscrasias; therefore, blood

Lifespan Considerations: The Pediatric Patient

Psychotherapeutic Drugs

- Pediatric patients are more likely to experience adverse effects from psychotropic drugs, especially EPS reactions. Close monitoring is needed.
- The incidence of Reye's syndrome and other adverse reactions is greater in pediatric patients taking psychotropic drugs who have had chickenpox, CNS infections, measles, acute illnesses, or dehydration.
- Lithium may lead to decreased bone density or bone formation in children; therefore, children receiving it should be closely monitored for signs and symptoms of lithium toxicity and bone disorders.
- TCAs are generally not prescribed for patients younger than 12 years of age. However, some antidepressants are used in children with enuresis, attention deficit disorders, and major depressive disorders and may be associated with adverse reactions such as changes in the ECG, nervousness, sleep disorder, fatigue, elevated BP, and gastrointestinal upset.
- Pediatric patients are generally more sensitive to the effects of most drugs, and this group of drugs is no exception. Be aware of the toxicity risk, which can be fatal. Should confusion, lethargy, visual disturbances, insomnia, tremors, palpitations, constipation, or eye pain occur, report this to the physician immediately.

BP, Blood pressure; *CNS,* central nervous system; *ECG,* electrocardiogram; *EPS,* extrapyramidal symptoms; *GI,* gastrointestinal; *TCA,* tricyclic antidepressants.

Lifespan Considerations: The Elderly Patient

Psychotherapeutic Drugs

- Elderly patients have higher serum levels of psychotherapeutic drugs because of changes in the drug distribution and metabolism processes, less serum albumin, decreased lean body mass, less water in tissues, and increased body fat. Because of these changes, elderly patients generally require lower doses of antipsychotic and antidepressant drugs.
- Orthostatic hypotension, anticholinergic adverse effects, sedation, and EPS are more common in elderly patients taking psychotherapeutic drugs.
- Careful evaluation and documentation of baseline parameters, including neurologic findings, are important to the safe use of these drugs.
- Increased anxiety is often associated with the use of TCAs.
- Patients with a history of cardiac disease may be at a greater risk for experiencing dysrhythmias, tachycardia, stroke, myocardial infarction, or heart failure.
- Lithium is more toxic in elderly patients and lower doses are often necessary. Close monitoring is important to its safe use in this age group. CNS toxicity, lithium-induced goiter, and hypothyroidism are more common in the elderly patient.

CNS, Central nervous system; *EPS,* extrapyramidal symptoms; *TCA,* tricyclic antidepressant.

studies, such as red blood cell (RBC) count, hematocrit (Hct), hemoglobin (Hgb), and reticulocytes should be performed every week for the first 4 weeks and then monthly.

Antimanic Drugs

Before administering antimanic drugs, such as lithium, a neurologic assessment, blood pressure, pulse, intake and output, hydration status, dietary intake, skin tone, and presence of edema are important to assess and document. Baseline levels of consciousness, gait and mobility levels, and assessment of neuromotor functioning are also important to assess because poor coordination, tremors, and weakness may be symptoms of toxicity to antimanic drugs. Laboratory studies often include measurement of the sodium, albumin, and uric acid. Specific gravity and a urinalysis may also be ordered. Serum levels of sodium are important to assess due to the fact that hyponatremia and hypovolemia place the patient at risk for lithium toxicity. In addition, serum lithium levels need to be assessed once drug therapy is initiated and usually every 3 to 4 days, especially during the initial phase of therapy. Generally speaking, with lithium it is best to have the levels done 8 to 12 hours after the dose of drug (therapeutic levels: 0.6-1.2 mEq/L with toxic levels above 1.5 mEq/L).

Antidepressants

There are many cautions, contraindications, and drug interactions to assess before giving antidepressants. Constant assessment for any suicidal ideations or tendencies is important because patients may have covert, as well as overt, suicidal "cues" or thoughts. The potential for suicide with psychotherapeutic drugs with or without the combination or other drugs or alcohol should always be considered a risk, whether with an antidepressant or other drug group. Many of the patients needing these medications are so mentally distressed that their physical needs go unmet, resulting in a complexity of other problems, such as insomnia, poor health status, and weight loss or gain. Baseline blood pressure, pulse rate, body temperature, and body weight should be assessed and documented before, during, and after drug therapy. Postural (supine then standing) blood pressure readings are important due to the adverse effect of postural hypotension. The more potent, older drugs, such as MAOIs and TCAs, may lead to a significant drop in blood pressure and warrant even more astute assessment.

With the SSRIs, serotonin syndrome may occur, especially when combining two or more such drugs. Any of the following drugs may also lead to hazardous adverse effects such as SSRIs, MAOIs, tryptophan, and herbal products, such as ginseng and St. John's wort. See Box 15-2 for common symptoms of serotonin syndrome.

Because the newer antidepressants are associated with fewer and less potent adverse effects, only a few MAOIs are used today in psychiatric mental health settings. Patients receiving MAOIs who have a history of suicide attempts or suicidal ideations, have seizure disorders, hyperactivity, diabetes, or psychosis need to be closely monitored. Suicidal thoughts/attempts are important to consider because "hoarding" these drugs may then be used by the patient to carry out suicide. These patients should be under the care of a health care professional (such as a psychiatrist, physician, or nurse practitioner) so that they may be closely monitored for destructive behaviors. MAOIs are known for their potentiation of hypertensive crisis when used with SSRIs, meperidine, and TCAs; this information is reemphasized here because of the risk of complications to the patient should this hypertensive event occur. Assess for dietary intake of tyramine if the patient is taking an MAOI (see the foods high in tyramine in Table 15-9).

Other parameters to assess with the MAO inhibitors include BP readings and postural BPs. These are important for the nurse to obtain because of the MAOI adverse effect of postural hypotension and subsequent risk of dizziness and even fainting. If the patient is hospitalized, it is recommended that the nurse assess supine and standing or sitting BPs at least with each shift or more frequent if needed. The nurse should wait 1 to 2 minutes after taking a supine BP before taking standing or sitting BP and pulse rate, and laboratory values such as those indicative of hepatic functioning (ALT, AST, bilirubin) as well as CBCs are needed to rule out contraindications or cautions.

Contraindications to the use of TCAs are numerous and have been previously discussed. In addition, it is crucial to understand that the elderly patient should be given these drugs only if absolutely necessary and only with careful monitoring. The elderly patient's blood pressure, pulse, CBC, weight, hepatic and renal studies should also be assessed. The extrapyramidal adverse effects are often worse in the elderly (e.g. worsening of tremors, inability to carry out ADLs). This syndrome may lead to progressive deterioration of motor activities, so baseline motor abilities are important to assess and document. It is important to reemphasize the drug interaction between TCAs and MAOIs. A hyperpyretic crisis may occur if TCAs are used with MAOIs and clonidine or with patients exhibiting high fever, convulsions, or a hypertensive crisis.

With second-generation antidepressants, cautious use in the elderly and cardiac patient is important. Bupropion may be preferred over other antidepressants because it has fewer anticholinergic, antiadrenergic, and cardiotoxic effects. However, the therapeutic effect of bupropion may not be reached for up to 4 weeks (as with many antidepressants); therefore, it is critical for the nurse to assess the patient for suicidal tendencies and support systems to ensure patient safety. Many of the antidepressants take weeks to have full therapeutic effect, and, therefore, close monitoring and observation of the patient are important until the drug begins to work. Due to the risk for seizures associated with second-generation antidepressants, an assessment should help to identify those patients with a history of seizures so that another medication may be used. Third-generation antidepressants have

several advantages over the older classes of antidepressants, but still have contraindications, cautions, and drug interactions. One important area to re-emphasize includes the fact that the elderly patient with decreased renal functioning should not take these drugs if at all possible. Concurrent use of third-generation antidepressants with any of the serotonergic (SSRIs) drugs carries the risk for serotonin syndrome and is to be avoided.

Antipsychotics

The antipsychotics require careful assessment of all body systems. Different antipsychotics are associated with different adverse effects—for example, olanzapine may cause an increase in total cholesterol, and the phenothiazines are associated with EPS and a high incidence of anticholinergic effects. Therefore, assessment of cardiovascular, cerebrovascular, neurologic, gastrointestinal, genitourinary, renal, hepatic, and hematologic functioning is important to safe and efficacious drug therapy. If there are significant diseases of one or several organ systems, the response to a drug may be more adverse and even dose-limiting—thus, the need for such close and astute assessment of the patient prior to and during drug therapy. Weight gain may occur, and, therefore, if the patient is experiencing adverse health conditions because of the adverse effect, another drug may need to be ordered. Changes in sex drive, oversedation, suicidal ideations, orthostatic changes in blood pressure, and insomnia related to some of these drugs—should they occur—need to be assessed thoroughly and reported as appropriate for the option of another drug. The common "anticholinergic" adverse effects of the phenothiazines (e.g., dry mouth, urinary hesitancy, constipation) and the EPS may be too bothersome for some patients and lead to the use of other drugs (as ordered by the physician!) for long-term treatment. All in all, it is the nurse with careful and astute assessment skills who is needed for the most effective and quality therapeutic regimen for each patient in need of psychotherapeutic drug therapy—and for each drug therapeutic regimen.

Haloperidol is similar to other high-potency antipsychotics because its sedating effects are low but the incidence of EPS is high. Assessment of baseline motor, sensory, and neurologic functioning is, therefore, very important to patient safety. With some of the antipsychotic drugs, patients may experience adverse effects of tremors and muscle twitching from the drug's blockade of dopamine receptors (dopamine generally has an "inhibitory" effect on specific motor movements in the musculoskeletal system). These "extrapyramidal" movements are manifested as parkinsonism-like and are very irritating and uncomfortable for the person experiencing them. Therefore, it would be important to know if there are underlying motor movement disturbances so that the best drug for the situation may be ordered. It is important with patients who have significant CNS disorders/symptoms and/or are taking medications that impact the CNS that antipsychotic drugs, like haloperidol be used only with extreme caution and with close monitoring.

Atypical antipsychotics (AAPs), such as quetiapine or clozapine, have many contraindications, cautions and drug interactions with newer drugs in this group showing great promise, as previously discussed. A thorough mental status examination should be performed and documented in the nurse's notes before initiation of these and other antipsychotic drugs. An assessment of musculoskeletal functioning and monitoring for any EPS reaction is also important as well as the need for assessment of the following laboratory studies: bilirubin and other liver function studies, renal studies, CBC, and urinalysis. BP readings, with postural BP readings, and standing, should be assessed and documented, with a drop of 20 mm Hg or more reported to the physician immediately. In addition, the health care provider may order reduced doses to avoid toxicity in the elderly. These drugs are also associated with a high degree of sedation and should be used very cautiously in elderly and other patients who are at risk for personal injury or harm or have limited motor and sensory capabilities. With risperidone use in elderly patients, it is important to assess for any unusual adverse effects, such as excessive sedation and sleepiness, that may lead to significant problems (e.g., safety concerns, falls, self injury) in the patient; another drug may be indicated. Patients taking non-phenothiazine antipsychotics or miscellaneous drugs require careful monitoring of BP as well as assessment for hepatic or cardiac disease due to drug-related drops in BP and tachycardia.

Antipsychotic drugs, in general, interact with many medications, herbals, and over-the-counter drugs and should be re-emphasized because of the nature of the reactions. These drugs include oral contraceptives, MAOIs, TCAs, SSRIs, erythromycin, quinolone antibiotics, the antibiotic ciprofloxacin (Cipro), nicotine, alcohol, antihistamines (e.g., diphenhydramine), antiepileptics, and narcotics. In addition, the antipsychotics may also interact with foods grilled over charcoal. Antipsychotic drugs are potent drugs that deserve close monitoring and attention to detail and, therefore, it is crucial for the nurse to update their knowledge about these drugs so that they can be proactive in the care of patients needing these medications.

In summary, all health care professionals who prescribe or administer psychotherapeutic drugs must remain current, competent, and very cautious about how they administer and monitor the use of these drugs. Safety is a major concern for any patient, and the concern is even greater when the drug being administered has significant adverse effects, contraindications, cautions, and drug interactions. The nurse must always take the time to assess the patient thoroughly before administering any psychotherapeutic drug and continue to assess the needs of the patient on an ongoing basis while using all resources to be sure the patient has all of their needs met.

◆ NURSING DIAGNOSES

- Risk for injury related to disease state and possible adverse effects of medications
- Disturbed thought processes related to neurochemical imbalance or cognitive processing problems
- Impaired social interaction related to various inadequacies felt by patient due to illnesses or isolation from others
- Imbalanced nutrition, less than body requirements, related to consequences of illness and/or its treatment
- Disturbed sleep patterns related to the illness or related drug therapy
- Situational low self-esteem related to illness/disease process, adverse effects of medication including sexual dysfunction
- Constipation related to adverse effects of psychotherapeutic drugs
- Urinary retention related to adverse effects of psychotherapeutic drugs

- Deficient knowledge related to lack of information about the specific psychotherapeutic drugs and their adverse effects
- Sexual dysfunction related to possible adverse effect of psychotherapeutic drugs

◆ PLANNING

Goals

- Patient does not sustain injury while on medication.
- Patient experiences no further deterioration in thought processes.
- Patient exhibits improved nutritional status.
- Patient regains normal sleep patterns.
- Patient exhibits (overtly and covertly) a more positive self-image.
- Patient remains free of any alterations in urinary elimination patterns.
- Patient remains free of altered bowel elimination patterns.
- Patient remains compliant with therapy.
- Patient is free of complications associated with the drug and with food and drug interactions.
- Patient is free of problems with sexual function.

Outcome Criteria

- Patient is free from falls, dizziness, and fainting attributable to adverse effects.
- Patient demonstrates improved or no deterioration in thought processes and is less hostile, withdrawn, and delusional once medication has reached steady state.
- Patient demonstrates more open and appropriate behavior and communication with health care team and significant others.
- Patient shows healthy nutrition habits with appropriate weight gain and a diet that includes foods from the U.S. Department of Agriculture (USDA) "MyPyramid" food guide (www.mypyramid.gov).
- Patient reports improved sleep patterns and feeling more rested.
- Patient openly discusses feelings of poor self-image and self-concept with staff.
- Patient reports any problems with urinary retention and identifies measures to reduce its occurrence
- Patient reports any difficulty with constipation if not manageable by fluids and dietary changes.
- Patient states the importance of taking medications exactly as prescribed at the same time every day and without omissions.
- Patient states the importance of appointments with the physician or other health care providers to follow improvement and monitor therapy.
- Patient states the common adverse effects of the medication and those adverse effects (e.g., confusion and changes in level of consciousness) to be reported to the physician.
- Patient lists those medications and foods to be avoided while taking any psychotherapeutic medication.
- Patient reports any problems with sexual function.

◆ IMPLEMENTATION

Regardless of the psychotherapeutic drug prescribed, several general nursing actions are important for safe administration. First and foremost is a firm but patient attitude combined with therapeutic communication. Simple explanations about the drug, action, and the length of time before therapeutic effects can be expected should be given after reading levels and an effective means of teaching/learning established. Once a thorough psychosocial and holistic approach has been implemented, vital signs should be monitored during therapy, especially in the elderly and in patients with a history of hypertension and cardiac disease. Any of these drugs should be taken exactly as prescribed and at the same time every day without failure. If omission occurs, the physician should be contacted immediately. Abrupt withdrawal of medication should be avoided due to the negative consequences to the patient and his or her mental status. Soliciting help from family members or other support systems should occur so that there are options for assistance with drug administration.

Antianxiety Drugs

Specific nursing interventions and patient education related to antianxiety drugs include the following: (1) Frequent checks of vital signs (e.g., BP) should be done, owing to adverse effects of orthostatic hypotension. (2) Wearing of elastic compression stockings is encouraged and changing positions slowly if orthostatic hypotension is problematic. (3) Encourage verbalizing of all disturbing thoughts (e.g., suicidal ideations, because these drugs and other psychotherapeutics should be dispensed only in small amounts to help minimize the risk for suicide attempt). (4) Intravenous routes of administration of these drugs should be only as prescribed, given over the recommended time with the proper diluent, and at a rate indicated by the manufacturer and as ordered by the physician, (5) Always administer intramuscular dosage forms in a large muscle mass and only as ordered or indicated. See the Patient Teaching Tips for more information.

Antimanic Drugs

The antimanic drug lithium is used mainly for patients who are in a manic state, and crucial to its safe use is that patient is adequately hydrated and in a state of electrolyte balance. Lithium may become toxic if excretion is decreased or if there is dehydration and/or hyponatremia present. See the Patient Teaching Tips for more information.

Antidepressants

Antidepressants must be administered carefully and exactly as ordered. It is important (with antidepressants as well as other psychotherapeutic drugs) to emphasize the fact that it may take several weeks before therapeutic effects are evident. The nurse must make sure that patients understand this and continue to take the medication as prescribed—even if they feel their condition is not improving. Careful monitoring of the patient, being readily available, and providing supportive care during this time is critical to the therapeutic approach. The time lapse before therapeutic effects are seen may put the patient at the highest risk for self-harm and/or suicide. Other nursing considerations include the following. (1) Most of these drugs are better tolerated if taken with food and at least 4 to 6 ounces of fluid. (2) Encourage assistance with ambulation and other activities if this is the first time on antidepressants or if the patient is elderly or weakened, to prevent falls and subsequent injury. (3) Postural hypotension, as an adverse effect, may also lead to dizziness or falls, and, therefore, caution with regular activities is recommended. (4) If the patient is receiving an SSRI, remember these are somewhat safer antidepressants, but they still need to be taken as prescribed. (5) Counsel the patient about potential sexual dysfunction if re-

lated to the particular medication. If sexual dysfunction occurs, explain that there are options, such as waiting to see if the adverse effect resolves, reducing the current dose of the drug (the health care professional—not the patient!), use of a "drug holiday," by the physician, where the patient is monitored closely—sometimes in a hospital setting—while the drug is discontinued and reinitiated, or open discussion about other medications or treatment options, if the adverse effect continues or worsens. See the Patient Teaching Tips for more information.

Specific nursing interventions for MAOIs and TCAs are as follows: (1) Remember that MAOIs are very potent antidepressants and are reserved for patients who do not respond to TCAs or other modes of therapy. (2) Adverse effects to report to their physician include orthostatic hypotension, dysrhythmias, ataxia, hallucinations, seizures, tremors, dry mouth, and impotence. (3) Encourage the patient to report this medication to all health care providers. (4) If an MAOI or TCA is prescribed and the patient requires some sort of surgical procedure, the drug will most likely need to be weaned carefully by the physician several weeks prior to the procedure due to known interactions with anesthesia. (5) With TCAs, it is important to know that blurred vision, excessive drowsiness or sleepiness, urinary retention, or constipation need to be reported to the physician immediately. (6) With some of the second- and third-generation antidepressants, it is important to inform patients that it may take up to 6 weeks for therapeutic effects and that tolerance to sedation will occur. (7) Bupropion and venlafaxine come in sustained-release forms and, therefore, have a convenient once- or twice-a-day dosing, and bupropion and mirtazapine may be used as antidotes for SSRI-induced sexual dysfunction.

Antipsychotics

Patients need to be aware that all antipsychotic drugs have to be taken exactly as prescribed to be effective. Different levels of paranoia or delusions may lead to suspicion and thus a mistrust of the nurse/physician and their treatment so that maintaining the level of trust through a therapeutic relationship is a vital link to compliance. Compliance is a key issue with psychotic illnesses because these patients are at higher risk for not taking medications and may not even follow-up or seek further medical advice. This is of major concern because the serum drug levels, such as haloperidol, need to be within a therapeutic range for the patient to feel better and be functional. If serum drug levels of haloperidol are less than 4 ng/mL, the patient may show symptoms of the mental disorder, whereas levels greater than 22 ng/mL may result in toxicity. Therefore, selection of an antipsychotic, its dosage, route of administration, risk for toxicity and/or suicidal potential as well as patient education and therapeutic support are all important factors to successful therapy. Because most antipsychotic drugs are quite potent, the nurse must be sure that oral dosage forms have actually been swallowed and not "tucked" in the side of the mouth or under the tongue to be discarded at a later time or taken with other dosages with a potentially "lethal" outcome. Oral forms of the antipsychotics are generally well absorbed and will cause less gastrointestinal upset if taken with food or a full glass of water, and use of hard candy or gum may help to relieve dry mouth. With any of the dosage forms, perspiration may be increased; therefore, patients should be warned about engaging in excessive activity or being exposed to hot or humid climates.

Excessive sweating could lead to dehydration and then drug toxicity.

Haloperidol may not necessarily be the best drug to use because of the risk for under- or over-medicating; other antipsychotics may be preferred. However, nurses need to understand that the older, more traditional drugs, such as chlorpromazine, are highly protein-bound and, as such, have many drug interactions and even more adverse effects that are often severe in nature, such as anticholinergic effects. Anticholinergic adrenal effects include photophobia, dry mouth, mydriasis with increased intraocular pressure, sedation, constipation, and urinary retention. Antiadrenergic effects include hypotension, as well as the increased risk for dysrhythmias, decreased cardiac output, and tachycardia. Other significant characteristics of the more traditional antipsychotics include EPS (occur in up 90% of the patients), dystonias, tardive dyskinesias, and neuroleptic malignant syndromes (occur in 50% of the patients). Sore throat, malaise, fever, and bleeding, due to drug-induced blood dyscrasias, should be reported to the physician immediately. In addition, the development of psychotherapeutic drugs is ever-growing, and currently there are a variety of atypical or newer drugs—such as clozapine, risperidone, olanzapine, and quetiapine—that may be preferred in treatment because of the minimal risk for tardive dyskinesia (TD), lower incidence of EPS, and an increase in cognition. Remaining current in practice is important!

With the newer antipsychotic drug, quetiapine, the nurse should assist patients with ambulation until they have been stabilized on the medication. Patients should be taught to change positions slowly to avoid fainting caused by postural hypotension. Increasing fluids may help decrease constipation, and sips of water, candy, and gum may help with dry mouth. Some of the other atypical antipsychotic drugs have the characteristics of fewer EPS, increased cognition, and reduction of TD and, therefore, may be used more commonly. The newer drugs, whether AAPs (dibenzodiazepine [clozapine], benzisoxazole [risperidone], thienobenzodiazepine [olanzapine], dibenzothiazepine [quetiapine], benzisothiazolyl [ziprasidone]) or other atypical drugs, such as sertindole and zotepine, may be the ones that are used more commonly. It is important for the nurse to remember that although these drugs have different qualities and fewer of the most serious adverse effects, there are still adverse effects and concerns associated with their use. These newer drugs do appear to be more efficient for those individuals who are treatment resistant or who are exhibiting many adverse effects. However, lethal blood dyscrasias, EPS, anticholinergic, antiadrenergic, and antihistamine adverse effects may occur with the use of clozapine, limiting its use.

Once therapy has been initiated, it is important for the nurse and other health care members involved in the patient's care to monitor drug therapy closely, including serum drug levels during follow-up visits. If the patient is suspected of being noncompliant, and serum drug levels are subtherapeutic, it is important to have the patient reevaluated by the prescribing physician and a possible switch to a parenteral dosage form. The parenteral dosage form is usually a depot (longer-releasing preparation) intramuscular injection that remains in the serum for up to one month, which may increase compliance and have a better therapeutic outcome. Antipsychotic drugs that are available for injection include chlorpromazine, chlorprothix-ene, fluphenazine, haloperidol, loxapine, mesoridazine, perphenazine, thiothixene, and trifluoperazine.

Patient education (see Patient Teaching Tips) and compliance are keys to successful treatment. Often it is the mental disorder itself that causes patient noncompliance. Patients must be taught that overdosages can occur when these drugs are mixed with alcohol and other CNS depressants, leading to respiratory and/or cardiovascular collapse, which are often fatal. But even in the best of circumstances, a lapse in therapy is possible and should always be considered. Keeping communication open with the patient and/or family/caregiver is important to developing trust and a sense of empathy. Although patient education may have been thorough, it is always best to emphasize that the patient can call the physician or clinic/"hotline" 24 hours a day. Phone numbers should be updated and shared frequently with the patient, and professional counseling should be available as needed with a mental health care provider (psychiatrist or nurse practitioner) and/or a licensed clinical worker so that the patient's progress is consistently monitored. Group therapy and support groups are also available for the patient and significant others.

◆ EVALUATION

Both the therapeutic effects of psychotropic medications and the patient's progress within the treatment regimen must be monitored at all times during and even after therapy. Mental alertness, cognition, affect, mood, ability to carry out ADLs, appetite, and sleep patterns are all areas that need to be closely monitored and documented. In addition to drug therapy, the patient must continue with other forms of therapy, with the goal of acquiring more effective coping skills. Along with psychotherapy, relaxation therapy, stress reduction and other positive lifestyle changes may be needed to help with the holistic treatment of the patient. Before evaluation of the specific psychotherapeutic drugs is discussed, it is important to mention that blood levels are often drawn with these drugs so that therapeutic levels are maintained and toxic levels and/or undermanagement are prevented.

The therapeutic effects of antianxiety drugs are evidenced by improved mental alertness, cognition, and mood; fewer anxiety and panic attacks; improved sleep patterns and appetite; more interest in self and others; less tension and irritability; and fewer feelings of fear, impending doom, and stress. Adverse effects to watch for in patients taking antianxiety drugs include hypotension, lethargy, fatigue, drowsiness, confusion, constipation, dry mouth, blood dyscrasias, lightheadedness, and insomnia. Adverse reactions to antidepressants in general consist of drowsiness, dry mouth, constipation, dizziness, postural hypotension, sedation, blood dyscrasias, and tremors. Overdose is evidenced by irritability, agitation, CNS irritability, seizures, and then progression to CNS depression with respiratory or cardiac depression.

Lithium's therapeutic effects are characterized by less mania and a "stabilizing" of the patient's mood. It is usually during the manic phase that lithium is better tolerated by the patient. Therapeutic levels of lithium range from 0.6 to 1.2 mEq/L and should be determined frequently, every few days initially and then at least every few months while the patient is on the drug. The nurse should also monitor the patient's mood, affect, and emotional stability. Adverse reactions to lithium include dysrhythmias, hypotension, sedation, slurred speech, slowed motor abilities, and weight gain. Gastrointestinal symptoms such as diarrhea and vomiting, drowsiness, weakness, and unsteady gait are indicative of overdose. The physician should be consulted immediately if these occur. Patients taking clozapine should exhibit improvement in their schizophrenic state. When evaluating for adverse effects such as development of agranulocytosis, it is important for the nurse to remember that it is associated with minor to no EPS.

As antidepressants, SSRIs may take up to 8 weeks to reach a full therapeutic effect. They are also associated with the therapeutic effects of improved depression/mental status; improved ability to carry out ADLs; less insomnia; and improved mood disorder without an overproduction of the adverse effects of weight gain, sedation, headache, insomnia, gastrointestinal upset and complaints, dizziness, agitation, and sexual dysfunction. Be sure to monitor for symptoms of serotonin syndrome. Other therapeutic effects of the SSRIs and other antidepressants are improved sleep patterns and nutrition, increased feelings of self esteem, decreased feelings of hopelessness, and an increased interest in self and appearance. MAOIs and TCAs may take up to 4 weeks for full therapeutic effects. Adverse effects include sedation, dry mouth, constipation, postural hypotension, blurred vision, seizures, and tremors. Toxic reactions may be manifested by confusion or hypotension and possibly by respiratory or cardiac distress.

The therapeutic effects of haloperidol, another antipsychotic drug, are similar to those of the other drugs, but the nurse should monitor his or her patient for adverse reactions that are particular to haloperidol. These include sedation; ticlike trembling movements of the hands, face, neck, and head; hypotension; and dry mouth. Overdose is manifested by severe sedation, hypotension, respiratory depression, and coma. It takes approximately 3 weeks for the therapeutic effects of haloperidol to appear, but it is still important for the nurse to watch the patient for possible dyskinesia and trembling during this early period. Should these occur, the nurse should consult the physician immediately to discuss possible actions. The therapeutic effects of other antipsychotic drugs (e.g., phenothiazines, nonphenothiazines, and quetiapine; AAPs) should include improvement in mood and affect and alleviation of the psychotic symptoms and episodes. Emotional instability, hallucinations, paranoia, delusions, garbled speech, and inability to cope should begin to abate once the patient has been on the medication for several weeks. It is critical that the nurse carefully monitors a patient's potential to injure himself or herself or others during the delay between the start of therapy and symptomatic improvement. It is also important that the nurse watches the patient for the development of adverse reactions to phenothiazines. These include dizziness and syncope stemming from orthostatic hypotension, tachycardia, confusion, drowsiness, insomnia, hyperglycemia, blood dyscrasias, and dry mouth. Overdose is manifested by excessive CNS depression, severe hypotension, and EPS, such as dyskinesias and tremors. These symptoms should be reported immediately to the physician. Other adverse effects to monitor with the AAPs include the anticholinergic-, antiadrenergic-, antihistaminic-, and prolactin-related adverse effects, as well as the risk for extrapyramidal adverse effects.

Patient Teaching Tips

Antianxiety Drugs

- Encourage patients to change positions slowly, especially from a sitting or reclining position, to avoid dizziness or fainting, and also to avoid operating heavy machinery or driving until the adverse effects of sedation or drowsiness have resolved.
- Patients need to know that tolerance often develops to the sedating properties of benzodiazepines, so drowsiness should improve over time.
- Patients should be informed to avoid OTC drugs and herbals without seeking advice from their health care provider.
- Inform patients that any psychotherapeutic drug (and *all* medications) should be kept out of the reach of children.
- Patients should avoid use of alcohol and other CNS depressants while taking these medications.
- Encourage patients to wear an ID bracelet/necklace with showing diagnosis and any drugs they are taking.
- Encourage patients to always keep a list of medications on their person at all times.
- Inform patient to take medications exactly as ordered and never go off the medications suddenly.
- Patients should report a lack of improvement or any fears, anxiety, or feelings of despair.

Antimanic Drugs

- Instruct the patient to take lithium at the same time every day and also how to handle missed doses. (If in doubt, encourage patients to contact their health care provider immediately.)
- Inform patients that adverse effects of lithium (e.g., fine hand tremors, increased thirst and urination, nausea, diarrhea, anorexia) are usually transient, but that they should report any excessive adverse effects.
- Patients should know to report the following adverse effects: extreme hand tremors, sedation, muscle weakness, vomiting, and vertigo.
- Adequate hydration should be emphasized, with up to 8 to 10 glasses of water daily (if not contraindicated).
- Patients need to be informed and reminded of follow-up visits with their health care provider so that serum drug levels and fluid and electrolyte status can be monitored to help decrease toxicity and maximize therapeutic effects.

Antidepressant Drugs

- Encourage an increase in dietary fiber and fluids to help minimize constipation.
- Measures to help with dry mouth should be shared with the patient, such as use of saliva substitutes, chewing gum, and allowing hard candy to dissolve. Diet forms of candy and gum are available.
- Should sedation and drowsiness continue past 2 to 3 weeks, a patient should know to contact the physician.
- Encourage patients to openly discuss any concerns about their medication and adverse effects such as gastrointestinal upset, sexual dysfunction, and weight gain.

- For patients taking these medications, they should be aware to not abruptly stop them. SSRIs require a tapering period of up to 1 to 2 months. Discontinuation syndrome may occur without a tapering period; this includes symptoms of dizziness, diarrhea, movement disorders, insomnia, irritability, visual disturbance, lethargy, anorexia, and lowered mood.
- Patient should know about all drug interactions, such as the strong interaction between SSRIs and MAOIs, St. John's wort (an herbal product), and/or tryptophan (a serotonin precursor found in foods). This interaction may pose a risk for the occurrence of serotonin syndrome.
- Encourage patients to seek out medical advice about self-treating a cold or flu due to possible drug interactions.

MAOIs and TCAs

- Encourage patients to contact their health care provider if they experience the following signs and symptoms of overdosage/toxicity: increased pulse rate, seizure activity, or changes in breathing, memory, alertness, and restlessness.
- Make sure the patient is aware that it takes approximately 1 to 4 weeks for the therapeutic effects of a MAOI to be seen; therefore, medication should be continued as prescribed.
- If taking a MAOI, emphasize to the patient to avoid OTC cold/flu products as well as foods high in tyramine (aged cheese, wine, beer, avocados, bananas, canned meats, yogurt, soy sauce, packaged soups, and sour cream). The concern for combining MAOIs and tyramine is that this interaction leads to serious elevations in blood pressure, heart palpitations/racing heart beat, neck stiffness, nausea and/or vomiting and severe headache. Should these problems occur, the patient must seek out medical care immediately due to possible CVA or stroke from hypertensive crisis.
- If patients are taking TCAs, they should be encouraged to report any blurred vision, excessive drowsiness or sleepiness, urinary retention, or constipation to their health care provider.
- With all medications, emphasize the importance of wearing a medic alert necklace/bracelet with a list of diagnoses and current drugs.

Haloperidol

- Emphasize the importance of avoiding hot baths, saunas, or hot climates due to risk of further drop in BP especially upon standing (postural hypotension). Injury to self may occur due to dizziness or fainting.
- Encourage patients to never stop medication abruptly because of the high risk for inducing a withdrawal psychosis.
- Patients should be advised to avoid sun exposure and, if outdoors, apply sunscreen liberally as per instructions and wear protective clothing.
- Patients should report immediately any sore throat, malaise, fever, and bleeding to their health care provider.

Points to Remember

- Psychosis is a major emotional disorder that impairs mental function. A person suffering from psychosis cannot participate in everyday life and shows the hallmark symptom of loss of contact with reality.
- Affective disorders are emotional disorders characterized by changes in mood and range from mania (abnormally elevated emotions) to depression (abnormally reduced emotions), and anxiety, a normal physiologic emotion, may be a healthy reaction but becomes pathologic when it becomes "life altering."
- Situational anxiety arises with specific life events, and nursing assessment is key to identifying "at risk" patients.
- Benzodiazepines remain the drug of choice for treatment of anxiety, are most often prescribed, are considered to be fairly safe, and do not interact with many other drugs.
- Nurses need to be aware that the SSRIs are often prescribed because of their superiority to TCAs and MAOIs in terms of adverse effect and safety profiles.

- Nurses need to understand terms used in everyday treatment regimens for mental health disorders. In the past, antipsychotics were called *tranquilizers* because they produce a state of tranquility. *Neuroleptics* are thus named because they work on abnormally functioning nerves. *Antipsychotics* and neuroleptics are terms that are used to refer to the drugs commonly used to treat serious mental illnesses. They are used to treat BPD, psychoses, schizophrenia, and autism.
- Nursing considerations related to psychotherapeutic drugs include astute assessment of medication and drug history and medical history.
- Nursing actions focus on adequate use of the nursing process with all types of psychotherapeutic medications and informing patients that their medications must be taken exactly as prescribed and that they need to avoid alcohol and other CNS depressants (as well as many other medications) to maintain patient safety. Frequent blood studies are needed to monitor therapeutic levels of the drugs.

NCLEX Examination Review Questions

1. While caring for a patient with alcohol withdrawal, the nurse knows which medication is most likely to be ordered as treatment for this condition?
   a. Lithium (Eskalith)
   b. Chlordiazepoxide (Librium)
   c. Alprazolam (Xanax)
   d. Bupropion (Wellbutrin)
2. Patient teaching for a patient receiving an MAOI would include instructing the patient to avoid which food product?
   a. Grapefruit juice
   b. Milk
   c. Shrimp
   d. Swiss cheese
3. After 4 weeks of treatment for depression, the nurse calls the patient to schedule a follow-up visit. Which finding should the nurse know to look for during the conversation with the patient?
   a. Weakness
   b. Hallucinations

   c. Suicidal ideations
   d. Difficulty with urination
4. The nurse is caring for a patient who has been taking clozapine (Clozaril) for 2 months. Which lab test should be monitored while the patient is on this medication?
   a. Platelet count
   b. Decreased WBC count
   c. Liver function studies
   d. Renal function studies
5. Which drug, when administered with lithium, increases the risk for toxicity?
   a. Thiazides
   b. Levofloxacin
   c. Calcium citrate
   d. Beta blockers

1. b, 2. d, 3. c, 4. b, 5. a.

Critical Thinking Activities

1. A 49-year-old patient comes in with a history of depression. He tells you that he used to be treated for it by a doctor in another country, but he "ran out of pills" a few weeks ago and did not know how to get a refill. He could not remember the name of the pill, but said it was for "depression." After a psychiatric evaluation, he is given a 2-week prescription for fluoxetine (Prozac). A few days later, his wife calls to describe "a terrible reaction" that he is having. She says that he is shaking, shivering, has a fever, and is somewhat confused and upset. She thinks he has a bad infection. What do you think has happened, and why?
2. Mrs. B. has inadvertently been given too much lorazepam and is experiencing respiratory arrest. You have identified that the use of the benzodiazepine reversal drug flumazenil is indicated. The dose called for is 0.2 mg delivered over 15 seconds, then another 0.2 mg if consciousness does not occur after 45 seconds, then

at 60-second intervals as needed up to a total dose of 1 mg. Flumazenil (Romazicon) is available as a 0.1-mg/mL vial. What dose should you draw up into the needle to deliver 0.2 mg each time?
3. A 51-year-old patient arrives at the doctor's office for his annual physical. As the intake nurse, you do a brief assessment and take a short drug history. You note that he states that he has started taking St. John's wort for depression and wants to know what the doctor thinks. You document this in the chart and research this information because you are not very familiar with herbal products. What is St. John's wort? Is it safe for patients to use for depressive symptoms? What information is important to remember about this herbal? What information is really crucial to share with patients in the future if they state that they are taking this supplement?

For answers, see http://evolve.elsevier.com/Lilley.

Central Nervous System Stimulants and Related Drugs

Objectives

When you reach the end of this chapter, you should be able to do the following:

1. Define the following terms: *analeptic, anorexiant, hyperactivity, attention deficit hyperactivity disorder, obesity,* and *migraine headache.*
2. Identify the various central nervous system (CNS) stimulants and their indications, contraindications, cautions, and drug interactions.
3. Discuss the therapeutic effects and adverse effects associated with the use of CNS stimulants.
4. Briefly describe the mechanisms of action, dosage forms, routes of administration, adverse effects, toxic effects, cautions, contraindications, and drug interactions associated with the various CNS stimulants.
5. Develop a nursing care plan encompassing all phases of the nursing process for a patient taking a CNS stimulant drug.

e-Learning Activities

Companion CD

- NCLEX Review Questions: see questions 109-114
- Animations
- Audio Glossary
- Category Catchers
- Medication Errors Checklists
- IV Therapy Checklists

evolve Website (http://evolve.elsevier.com/Lilley)

• Nursing Care Plans • Frequently Asked Questions • Content Updates • WebLinks • Supplemental Resources • Elsevier ePharmacology Update • Medication Administration Animations

Drug Profiles

▶ amphetamines, p. 254
atomoxetine, p. 255
▶ caffeine, p. 261
doxapram, p. 261
▶ methylphenidate, p. 255
modafinil, p. 255

orlistat, p. 259
▶ phentermine, p. 259
▶ sibutramine, p. 259
sodium oxybate, p. 255
▶ sumatriptan, p. 260

▶ Key drug.

Glossary

Amphetamines Central nervous system (CNS) stimulants that produce mood elevation or euphoria, increase mental alertness and capacity to work, decrease fatigue and drowsiness, and prolong wakefulness. (p. 254)

Analeptics CNS stimulants that have generalized effects on the brainstem and spinal cord, which in turn produce an increase in responsiveness to external stimuli and stimulates respiration. (p. 260)

Anorexiants Drugs used to control or suppress appetite. These also stimulate the CNS. (p. 257)

Attention deficit hyperactivity disorder (ADHD) Syndrome affecting children, adolescents, and adults that involves difficulty in maintaining concentration on a given task and/or hyperactive behavior. The term *attention deficit disorder (ADD)* has been absorbed under this broader term. (p. 253)

Cataplexy A condition characterized by abrupt attacks of muscular weakness and hypotonia triggered by an emotional stimulus such as joy, laughter, anger, fear, or surprise. It is often associated with narcolepsy. (p. 253)

CNS stimulants Drugs that stimulate specific areas of the brain or spinal cord. (p. 252)

Migraine A common type of recurring painful headache characterized by a *pulsatile* or throbbing quality, incapacitating pain, and photophobia. (p. 259)

Narcolepsy Syndrome characterized by sudden sleep attacks, cataplexy, sleep paralysis, and visual or auditory hallucinations at the onset of sleep. (p. 253)

Serotonin receptor agonists A new class of CNS stimulants used to treat migraine headaches; they work by stimulating 5-HT$_1$ receptors in the brain and are sometimes referred to as *selective serotonin receptor agonists* or *triptans*. (p. 259)

Sympathomimetic drugs CNS stimulants such as noradrenergic drugs (and, to a lesser degree, dopaminergic drugs) whose actions resemble or mimic those of the sympathetic nervous system. (p. 253)

CENTRAL NERVOUS SYSTEM STIMULANTS

Central nervous system (CNS) activity is regulated by a checks-and-balances system that consists of both excitatory and inhibitory neurotransmitters and their corresponding receptors in the brain and spinal cord tissues. CNS stimulation can result from either excessive stimulation of excitatory neurons or blockade of inhibitory neurons. **CNS stimulants** are a broad class of drugs that stimulate specific areas of the brain or spinal cord. However, most CNS stimulant drugs act by stimulating the excitatory neurons in the brain. They generally act by enhancing the activity in the brain of one or more of the excitatory neurotransmitters: dopamine (dopaminergic drugs), norepinephrine (noradrenergic drugs), and serotonin (serotonergic drugs). Dopamine is a metabolic precursor of norepinephrine, which is also a neurotransmitter within the sympathetic nervous system (SNS). The actions of noradrenergic drugs often resemble or mimic the actions of the SNS. For this reason, noradrenergic drugs (and, to a lesser degree, dopaminergic drugs

as well) are also called **sympathomimetic drugs.** Other sympathomimetic drugs are discussed further in Chapter 17.

There are three ways to classify CNS stimulant drugs. The first is on the basis of chemical structural similarities. Major chemical classes of CNS stimulants include amphetamines, serotonin agonists, sympathomimetics, and xanthines (Table 16-1). Second, these drugs can be classified according to their site of therapeutic action in the CNS (Table 16-2). Finally, they can be categorized according to five major therapeutic usage categories for CNS stimulant drugs (Table 16-3). These include anti–attention deficit, antinarcoleptic, anorexiant, antimigraine, and analeptic drugs. Anorexiants are drugs used to control obesity by suppression of appetite. Analeptics are drugs used by clinicians for specific CNS stimulation in certain clinical situations. Some therapeutic overlap exists among these drug categories.

Table 16-1	Structurally Related CNS Stimulants
Chemical Category	**CNS Stimulants and Related Drugs**
Amphetamines and related stimulants	dextroamphetamine, methamphetamine, benzphetamine, methylphenidate, dexmethylphenidate, pemoline, mazindol
Serotonin agonists	almotriptan, eletriptan, frovatriptan, naratriptan, rizatriptan, sumatriptan, zolmitriptan
Sympathomimetics	phentermine, phenidimetrazine
Xanthines	caffeine, theophylline, aminophylline
Miscellaneous	modafinil, sodium oxybate (CNS depressant), sibutramine (anorexiant), orlistat (lipase inhibitor), doxapram (analeptic)

CNS, Central nervous system.

Table 16-2	CNS Stimulants: Site of Action
Primary Site of Action	**CNS Stimulants**
Cerebrovascular system	Serotonin agonists
Cerebral cortex	Amphetamines, phenidates, pemoline, mazindol, modafinil
Hypothalamic and limbic regions	Anorexiants
Medulla and brainstem	Analeptics

CNS, Central nervous system.

Table 16-3	CNS Stimulants and Related Drugs: Therapeutic Categories
Category	**Drugs**
Anti-ADHD	dextroamphetamine, methamphetamine, methylphenidate, atomoxetine (norepinephrine reuptake inhibitor)
Antinarcoleptic	dextroamphetamine, methamphetamine, methylphenidate, mazindol, modafinil, sodium oxybate (CNS depressant)
Antimigraine (serotonin agonists)	almotriptan, eletriptan, frovatriptan, naratriptan, rizatriptan, sumatriptan, zolmitriptan
Anorexiant	methamphetamine, phentermine, phendimetrazine, diethylpropion, benzphetamine, sibutramine, orlistat (lipase inhibitor)
Analeptic	caffeine, doxapram, aminophylline, theophylline, modafinil (antinarcoleptic)

ADHD, Attention deficit hyperactivity disorder; *CNS,* central nervous system.

OVERVIEW OF PATHOPHYSIOLOGY

ATTENTION DEFICIT HYPERACTIVITY DISORDER

Attention deficit hyperactivity disorder (ADHD), formerly known as attention deficit disorder (ADD), is the most common psychiatric disorder in children; affecting 3% to 5% of school-aged children. Boys are affected from two to nine times as often as girls, although the disorder may be underdiagnosed in girls. Primary symptoms of ADHD center around a developmentally inappropriate ability to maintain attention span and/or the presence of hyperactivity and impulsivity. The disorder may involve predominantly attention deficit, predominantly hyperactivity or impulsivity, or a combination of both. It usually begins before 7 years of age (as early as age 3) and is officially diagnosable when symptoms last at least 6 months and occur in at least two different settings, according to the *Diagnostic and Statistical Manual of Mental Disorders.* Children with this disorder often outgrow it, but adult ADHD does occur. Drug therapy for both is essentially the same. Although there is some social controversy regarding possible overdiagnosis of, and overmedication for, this disorder, studies in twins indicate a degree of genetic predisposition and familial heritability. The disorder is commonly associated with other forms of mental illness, including depression, bipolar disorder, anxiety, and learning difficulties.

NARCOLEPSY

Narcolepsy is an incurable neurologic condition in which patients unexpectedly fall asleep in the middle of normal daily activities. These "sleep attacks" are reported to cause car accidents or near-misses in 70% or more of patients. Another major symptom of the disease is dysfunctional rapid eye movement sleep. **Cataplexy** is an associated symptom in at least 70% of narcolepsy cases. It involves sudden loss of voluntary (skeletal) muscle control with the exception of respiratory and ocular muscles. The condition is often associated with strong emotions (joy, laughter, anger, etc.), and commonly the knees buckle and the individual falls to the floor while still awake. Men and women are equally affected, with approximately 100,000 cases in the United States. Some genetic markers have been identified. Roughly half of patients with narcolepsy experience migraine headaches as well.

DRUGS FOR ATTENTION DEFICIT HYPERACTIVITY DISORDER AND NARCOLEPSY

CNS stimulants are the first-line drugs of choice for both ADHD and narcolepsy. Although there has been some public controversy regarding their use, these drugs have led to a 65% to 75% improvement in symptoms in treated patients compared with a placebo. In general, CNS stimulants elevate mood, produce a sense of increased energy and alertness, decrease appetite, and enhance task performance impaired by fatigue or boredom. Two of the oldest known stimulants are cocaine and amphetamine, which are prototypical drugs for this class. Cocaine is a natural alkaloid that was first extracted from the plant *Erythroxylon coca* in the mid-nineteenth century but had been used by natives of the Andes for its stimulant effects for centuries before. Caffeine, contained in coffee and tea, is another plant-derived CNS stimulant. Amphetamine sulfate was first synthesized in the late 1800s. It was subsequently used to treat narcolepsy and then to prolong the alertness of soldiers during World War II. Later variants of the drug, which are still used clinically, include dextroamphetamine sulfate, methamphetamine, and benzphetamine. The drugs currently used to treat both ADHD and narcolepsy include **amphetamines** as well as nonamphetamine stimulants. Methylphenidate, a synthetic amphetamine derivative, was first introduced for the treatment of hyperactivity in children in 1958.

Mechanism of Action and Drug Effects

Amphetamines stimulate areas of the brain associated with mental alertness, such as the cerebral cortex and the thalamus. The pharmacologic actions of amphetamines and sympathomimetic CNS stimulants are similar to the actions of the SNS in that the CNS and respiratory system are the primary body systems affected. CNS effects include mood elevation or euphoria, increased mental alertness and capacity for work, decreased fatigue and drowsiness, and prolonged wakefulness. The respiratory effects most commonly seen are relaxation of bronchial smooth muscle, increased respiration, and dilation of pulmonary arteries. CNS stimulants are potent drugs with a strong potential for tolerance and psychologic dependence. They are therefore classified as Schedule II drugs under the Controlled Substance Act. These drugs include amphetamine sulfate, its d-isomer dextroamphetamine sulfate (Dexedrine), methamphetamine hydrochloride (Desoxyn), benzphetamine (Didrex), and mixed amphetamine salts (Adderal), which includes various salts of both amphetamine and dextroamphetamine. Another stimulant, methylphenidate (Ritalin, Concerta), is structurally and functionally similar to amphetamine. Its d-isomer is the drug dexmethylphenidate (Focalin). The phenidates are also Schedule II drugs. Specialists sometimes recommend periodic "drug holidays" (e.g., one day per week) without medication to mitigate the addictive tendencies of these drugs.

The amphetamines and phenidates increase the effects of both norepinephrine and dopamine in CNS synapses by increasing their release and blocking their reuptake. As a result, both neurotransmitters are in contact with their receptors longer, which lengthens their duration of action. Nonamphetamine stimulants include mazindol, pemoline, and modafinil. Mazindol and pemoline work in a manner similar to the amphetamines and phenidates. Modafinil is also classified as an analeptic. It promotes wakefulness like the amphetamines and phenidates. It lacks sympathomimetic properties, however, and appears to work primarily by reducing γ-aminobutyric acid (GABA)–mediated neurotransmission in the brain. GABA is the principle inhibitory neurotransmitter in the brain. A newer nonstimulant drug, atomoxetine, is also being used to treat ADHD. It works by selective inhibition of norepinephrine reuptake.

Indications

The various amphetamines, methylphenidate, and pemoline are currently used to treat ADHD and narcolepsy. Dexmethylphenidate is currently indicated for ADHD alone. As noted earlier, the newer nonstimulant drug atomoxetine is also now used to treat ADHD. Amphetamine sulfate was also used to treat obesity in the early to mid twentieth century. However, the only amphetamines currently approved for this indication are benzphetamine and methamphetamine (see Anorexiants). The nonamphetamine stimulants mazindol and modafinil are indicated for narcolepsy, and mazindol is used to treat obesity as well.

Contraindications

Contraindications to the use of amphetamine and nonamphetamine stimulants include known drug allergy, marked anxiety or agitation, glaucoma, Tourette's syndrome, other tic disorders, and therapy with any monoamine oxidase inhibitor (MAOI) within the preceding 14 days. Pemoline is contraindicated in cases of known liver disease, and this drug is now less commonly used because of case reports of associated liver failure. Contraindications specific to atomoxetine include drug allergy, glaucoma, and recent MAOI use as mentioned previously.

Adverse Effects

Both amphetamine and nonamphetamine stimulants have a wide range of adverse effects that most often arise when these drugs are administered at dosages higher than the therapeutic dosages. These drugs tend to "speed up" body systems. For example, effects on the cardiovascular system include increased heart rate and blood pressure. Other adverse effects include, angina, anxiety, insomnia, headache, tremor, blurred vision, increased metabolic rate (beneficial in treatment of obesity), gastrointestinal (GI) distress, and dry mouth.

Interactions

The drug interactions associated with CNS stimulants vary greatly from class to class. Table 16-4 summarizes some of the more common interactions for all drug classes in this chapter.

Drug Profiles

Amphetamines and Related Stimulants

As noted earlier, the principal drugs used to treat ADHD and narcolepsy are the amphetamine and nonamphetamine stimulants. Dosages and other information appears in the Dosages table on page 256.

▶ *amphetamines*

The various amphetamine salts are the prototypical CNS stimulants used to treat ADHD and narcolepsy. Amphetamine is available in prescription form only for oral use, both as single-component dextroamphetamine sulfate and as a mixture of dextroamphetamine sulfate, dextroamphetamine saccharate, amphetamine sulfate, and amphetamine aspartate.

Table 16-4 CNS Stimulants: Common Drug Interactions

Drug	Mechanism	Result
Amphetamines and Other Stimulants		
β-blockers	Increased α-adrenergic effects	Hypertension, bradycardia, dysrhythmias, heart block
CNS stimulants	Additive toxicities	Cardiovascular adverse effects, nervousness, insomnia, convulsions
Digoxin	Additive toxicity	Increased risk of dysrhythmias
MAOIs	Increased release of catecholamines	Headaches, dysrhythmias, severe hypertension
TCAs	Additive toxicities	Cardiovascular adverse effects (dysrhythmias, tachycardia, hypertension)
Anorexiants and Analeptics		
CNS stimulants	Additive toxicities	Nervousness, irritability, insomnia, dysrhythmias, seizures
MAOIs	Increased release of catecholamines	Headach es, dysrhythmias, severe hypertension
Quinolones	Interference with metabolism	Reduced clearance of caffeine and prolongation of caffeine's effects
Serotonergic drugs	Additive toxicity	Cardiovascular adverse effects, nervousness, insomnia, convulsions
Serotonin Agonists		
Ergot alkaloids, SSRIs, MAOIs	Additive toxicity	Cardiovascular adverse effects, nervousness, insomnia, convulsions.

CNS, Central nervous system; *MAOIs,* monoamine oxidase inhibitors; *SSRIs,* selective serotonin reuptake inhibitors; *TCAs,* tricyclic antidepressants.

Pharmacokinetics (dextroamphetamine)

Half-Life	Onset	Peak	Duration
PO: 7-14 hr*	PO: 30-60 min	PO: Less than 2 hr	PO: 10 hr

*pH less than 6.6.

▶ methylphenidate

Methylphenidate (Ritalin, Concerta) is also a major drug of choice for the treatment of ADHD and narcolepsy and is the most widely prescribed drug for treatment of ADHD. As noted earlier, there is some controversy regarding its use, especially among apprehensive parents. However, with proper diagnosis of the disorder, proper dosing of the drug, and regular medical monitoring, many children can achieve significant improvement in school performance and social skills. Psychosocial problems within a child's family should be ruled out or addressed if they are contributing to the child's problems, regardless of whether the medication is prescribed.

Pharmacokinetics (Immediate Release)

Half-Life	Onset	Peak	Duration
PO: 1-3 hr	PO: 30-60 min	PO: 1-3 hr	PO: 4-6 hr

atomoxetine

Atomoxetine (Strattera) is the newest medication approved for treating ADHD in children older than 6 years of age and in adults. It was approved by the Food and Drug Administration (FDA) in 2002. This medication is not a controlled substance because it lacks addictive properties, unlike amphetamines and phenidates. For this reason, it has rapidly gained popularity as a therapeutic option for treating ADHD and has been used to treat over 2 million patients to date. In September of 2005, however, the FDA did issue a warning describing cases of suicidal thinking and behavior in small numbers of adolescent patients receiving this medication, similar to its previous warnings regarding adolescent use of antidepressant medications (Chapter 15). Atomoxetine currently remains on the market, but prescribers are advised to work with parents in providing prudent monitoring of any young patients taking this medication and to promptly reevaluate patients showing any behavioral symptoms of concern.

Pharmacokinetics

Half-Life	Onset	Peak	Duration
PO: 5-24 hr	PO: 60 min	PO: 1-2 hr	PO: 24-120 hr

modafinil

Modafinil (Provigil) is indicated for improvement of wakefulness in patients with excessive daytime sleepiness associated with narcolepsy. It has less abuse potential than amphetamines and methylphenidate and is a Schedule IV drug.

Pharmacokinetics

Half-Life	Onset	Peak	Duration
PO: 8-15 hr	PO: 1-2 mo*	PO: 2-4 hr	PO: Unknown

*Therapeutic effects.

Miscellaneous Narcolepsy Drugs
sodium oxybate

Sodium oxybate (Xyrem) is the sodium salt of γ-hydroxybutyrate, one of the notorious "date rape" drugs. It is currently one of only two drugs approved by the FDA for the treatment of cataplexy. (The other is viloxazine (Catatrol), an antidepressant that blocks norepinephrine reuptake.) As noted earlier, cataplexy is a condition characterized by acute attacks of muscle weakness and is often associated with narcolepsy. Distribution of this drug is carefully controlled due to its abuse potential. Prescribers who wish to use this medication for this restricted population of patients must contact the Xyrem Success Program at 1-866-XYREM-88 (1-866-997-3688). Sodium oxybate is considered an orphan drug and is currently legally available only through such restricted dispensing programs. It is classified as a Schedule III controlled substance for this limited medical use and is technically a CNS depressant rather than a stimulant. This drug is contraindicated in cases of sleep apnea, substance abuse, or concurrent use of hypnotic drugs.

Pharmacokinetics

Half-Life	Onset	Peak	Duration
PO: 30-60 min	PO: 30 min	PO: 30-75 min	PO: 1-5 hr

OBESITY

According to the National Institutes of Health and the Centers for Disease Control and Prevention, roughly 30.5% of Americans are *obese* and nearly two thirds (64.5%) are *overweight*. This translates into more than 60 million obese adults, with a higher incidence of obesity among women and minorities. Obesity was formerly defined as being 20% or more above one's ideal body weight based on population statistics for height, body frame, and gender. More recent data are based on a measurement known as the body mass index (BMI), defined as weight in kilograms divided by height in meters squared (= weight [kg]/[height in meters]^2). *Overweight* is now defined as a BMI of 25 to 29.9, whereas *obesity* is now defined as a BMI of 30 or higher. At any

DOSAGES

Selected CNS Stimulants and Related Drugs

Drug	Pharmacologic Class (Pregnancy Category)	Usual Dosage Range	Indications
almotriptan (Axert)	Serotonin receptor agonist (C)	**Adult only** PO: 6.25-12.5 mg × 1 dose; may repeat in 2 hr to a max of 12.5 mg/24 hr	Acute migraine with or without aura
▶amphetamine (Adderall)	CNS stimulant (C)	**Pediatric 3-5 yr** PO: 2.5 mg/day, increased weekly until desired effect **Pediatric 6 yr and older** PO: 5 mg once or twice daily, increased weekly until desired effect to a daily max of 40 mg	ADHD, narcolepsy
atomoxetine (Strattera)	Selective norepinephrine reuptake inhibitor (C)	**Pediatric (less than 70 kg)** PO: 0.5-1.2 mg/kg/day divided once or twice daily . **Adult (70 kg or more)** PO: 40-100 mg/day divided once or twice daily	ADHD
▶caffeine (No-Doz Maximum Strength, Vivarin)	Xanthine cerebral stimulant (B)	**Adult** PO: 5-10 mg tid 0.5-1 hr ac IM/IV: 500-1000 mg caffeine citrate or sodium benzoate **Premature infants** IV (caffeine citrate only): 20 mg/kg load followed by 5 mg/kg once daily	Need for mental alertness Respiratory depression (not commonly used in adults) Neonatal apnea, bronchopulmonary dysplasia
doxapram (Dopram)	Respiratory stimulant (analeptic) (B)	**Adult** PO: 100-200 mg q3-4h **Adult and pediatric older than 12 yr** 0.5-1 mg/kg IV as a single injection not to exceed 1.5 mg/kg, or infusion of 5 mg/min until desired effect, then reduced to 1-3 mg/min 1-2 mg IV given twice at 5-min intervals then repeated at 1-2 hr intervals prn Infusion of 1-2 mg/min for up to 2 hr	Postanesthetic respiratory depression Drug-induced respiratory depression COPD-associated hypercapnia
eletriptan (Relpax)	Serotonin receptor agonist (C)	**Adult only** PO: 20-40 mg × 1 dose; may repeat in 2 hr for a max of 80 mg/24 hr	Acute migraine with or without aura
frovatriptan (Frova)	Serotonin receptor agonist (C)	**Adult only** PO: 2.5 mg × 1 dose; may repeat at no less than 2-hr intervals up to max of 7.5 mg/24 hr	Acute migraine with or without aura
methylphenidate, extended-release (Concerta)	CNS stimulant (C)	**Pediatric and adult** 18-54 mg/day in a single dose	ADHD, narcolepsy
▶methylphenidate (Ritalin)	CNS stimulant (C)	**Pediatric 6 yr or older** PO: 5 mg bid before breakfast and lunch and increased weekly until desired effect to max of 60 mg/day **Adult** PO: 20-60 mg/day divided bid-tid 30-45 min ac	ADHD, narcolepsy
methylphenidate, extended release (Ritalin-SR)	CNS stimulant (C)	**Pediatric and adult** 20-60 mg/day in a single dose	ADHD, narcolepsy
modafinil (Provigil)	CNS stimulant (C)	**Adult** PO: 200 mg/day, up to 400 mg/day	Narcolepsy
naratriptan (Amerge)	Serotonin agonist (C)	**Adult** PO: 1-2.5 mg at onset of headache; may repeat × 1 after 4 hr, up to 5 mg/day	Acute migraine with or without aura
orlistat (Xenical)	Lipase inhibitor (B)	**Adult** PO: 120 mg tid with each meal containing fat	Obesity
rizatriptan (Maxalt, Maxalt-MLT)	Serotonin agonist (C)	**Adult** PO: 5-10 mg at onset of headache; may repeat × 1 after 2 hr, up to 30 mg/day	Acute migraine with or without aura

DOSAGES

Selected CNS Stimulants and Related Drugs—cont'd

Drug	Pharmacologic Class (Pregnancy Category)	Usual Dosage Range	Indications
▶sibutramine (Meridia)	CNS stimulant (anorexiant) (C)	**Adult** PO: 10 mg/day, up to max of 15 mg/day	Obesity
sodium oxybate (Xyrem)	CNS depressant (B)	**Adult only** PO: 2.25 g bid; may titrate upward by 1.5 g to a maximum of 9 g/day	Cataplexy (associated with narcolepsy)
▶sumatriptan (Imitrex)	Serotonin agonist (C)	**Adult** PO: 25, 50, or 100 mg, can repeat after 2 hr (max 40 mg/day) SC: 6 mg, can repeat in 1 hr (max 2 injections/day) Nasal spray: 5 or 20 mg, can repeat after 2 hr (max 40 mg/day)	Acute migraine with or without aura
zolmitriptan (Zomig, Zomig-ZMT)	Serotonin agonist (C)	**Adult** PO: ½-1 tablet (1.25 to 2.5 mg) at onset of headache (note that orally disintegrating tablets may not be broken in half) Nasal spray: 1 spray (5 mg) in one nostril at onset of headache Oral and nasal: may repeat × 1 after 2 hr, up to 10 mg/day	Acute migraine with or without aura

ADHD, Attention deficit hyperactivity disorder; *CNS,* central nervous system.

---

given time, one third of women and one quarter of men are trying to lose weight. Moreover, the incidence of obesity in young people aged 6 to 19 years has more than tripled since 1980. Obesity increases the risk for hypertension, dyslipidemia, coronary artery disease, stroke, type 2 diabetes mellitus, gallbladder disease, gout, osteoarthritis, sleep apnea, and certain types of cancer, including breast and colon cancer. An estimated 70% of diabetes risk in the United States can be attributed to excess weight. Some 300,000 deaths each year are linked to obesity, which makes it the second leading cause of preventable deaths in the United States. The related health care costs alone are currently estimated at more than $90 billion. Yet many people who attempt weight loss do so for cosmetic reasons, not for health reasons. Obese people are often stigmatized, at times even by the health care professionals treating them.

ANOREXIANTS

By definition, an *anorexiant* is any substance that suppresses appetite. Anorexiants are CNS stimulant drugs used to promote weight loss in obesity. These drugs include phentermine (Ionamin), benzphetamine (Didrex), methamphetamine (Desoxyn), phendimetrazine (Bontril), diethylpropion (Tenuate), and sibutramine (Meridia). As noted earlier, benzphetamine and methamphetamine are the only amphetamines currently approved for treating obesity. Orlistat (Xenical) is a related nonstimulant drug.

Mechanism of Action and Drug Effects

Anorexiants are CNS stimulants that are believed to work by suppressing appetite control centers in the brain. Some evidence suggests that they also increase the body's basal metabolic rate, including mobilization of adipose tissue stores and enhanced cellular glucose uptake, as well as reduce dietary fat absorption.

There are some minor differences between these drugs in terms of their individual actions. Phentermine, phendimetrazine, diethylpropion, methamphetamine, and benzphetamine resemble amphetamine sulfate in their chemical structures and CNS effects. These drugs are classified as both anorexiants and adrenergic (sympathomimetic) drugs. However, all appear to suppress appetite centers in the CNS through dopamine- and norepinephrine-mediated pathways. Sibutramine, the newest anorexiant, enhances dopamine, norepinephrine, and serotonin activity in the brain by inhibiting neuronal reuptake of these neurotransmitters. Its dopamine activity is weaker than its norepinephrine and serotonin activity. This kind of serotonergic activity is associated with enhanced feelings of satiety. All of these medications

EVIDENCE-BASED PRACTICE

An Applied Evidence-Based Review of the Diagnosis and Treatment of Obesity in Adults

Review

Because obesity is an epidemic in the United States and leads to substantial morbidity and mortality, a review was conducted to identify effective strategies for managing obesity and to provide a rationale for its diagnosis and treatment. This applied evidence-based review of research presents information about the diagnostic test characteristics of exact body mass index (BMI) and, for the appropriate and relevant treatment methods identified, reports the number of patients who need to be treated to achieve one positive outcome event. The review integrated support of recommendations from the following scientific bodies that are known for their work on adult obesity: The National Heart, Lung, and Blood Institute; The World Health Organization; The Canadian Task Force on Preventative Health Care; and The U.S. Preventative Task Force. Data were obtained from pertinent studies identified using MEDLINE, the Database of Abstracts of Reviews of Effectiveness, and the Cochrane Database of Systematic Reviews.

Type of Evidence

This was an applied evidence-based review of methods for diagnosing and treating adults with obesity. Various data in the following areas were summarized: evidence of increased health risk associated with obesity, evidence that reducing weight decreases disease risk, and evidence that reducing weight increases disease risk (e.g., increased risk of hip fracture). The review was based on a compilation and synthesis of the data, focusing on the role of primary care health care providers in the diagnosis and treatment of adult obese patients.

Results of Study

The various means of diagnosing obesity in adulthood were identified through the use of BMI rather than the gender-, height-, and age-specific tables used in the past. BMI (weight in kilograms divided by height in meters squared) is easily calculated and seen as a reliable measure for overweight/obese adults. Evidence on treatment modalities was also reviewed and presented. Data on the effectiveness of various interventions were reviewed. The weight loss interventions identified as being effective included diet, exercise, behavioral strategies, limited use of pharmacologic treatments in combination with strategies that change lifestyle, and surgery for selected morbidly obese patients. Because this chapter concerns central nervous system stimulants, it is relevant to mention that *serotonin-norepinephrine reuptake inhibitors* (e.g., sibutramine) *and gastrointestinal lipase inhibitors* (e.g., orlistat) were the specific drugs mentioned in this re-view. Surgical interventions discussed in the review were gastric bypass and gastroplasty.

Link of Evidence to Nursing Practice

This review emphasized the importance of using an applied evidence-based approach to investigating obesity management in adults. Diagnosis and treatment were the focus of the review, and excellent criteria were identified for the health care provider to use in everyday practice. Some of the key points relevant for clinicians to use when treating obese patients are as follows:

- Obesity should be managed as a chronic and relapsing disease.
- BMI should be used as a tool to diagnose obesity in patients and to guide decisions about treatment.
- A reduction of 10% of total body weight (identified as a "modest" reduction) yields results in improving and preventing hypertension, diabetes, and hyperlipidemia.
- Diet combined with exercise proved to be the most effective treatment method; sibutramine should be used with caution pending review by the Food and Drug Administration.
- Patients should be counseled to set a goal of a 10% decrease in total body weight.
- Patients should be counseled to exercise to increase energy expenditure rather than to attain aerobic fitness.
- Referral to a behavioral program to reinforce the health care provider's counseling should be considered.
- Being an advocate for social policies that promote health, good nutrition, and increased physical activity is important.

This review summarized various therapies and lifestyle changes for treating obesity. The importance of viewing obesity management as a lifelong process and applying a "chronic disease care" model that incorporates collaborative approaches to care was emphasized. Effective methods of diagnosis and treatment of adult obesity were identified. Although the review concentrated on the actions of the primary care provider during the clinical encounter, this was identified as a reactive approach; a more proactive strategy on the part of health care providers is critical to successful therapy. Major changes must occur in the health care of adults and children (because habits start early!) to put in place the necessary social policies and good nutrition and exercise habits that are needed to attack this problem. Nurses continue to play an important role in patient care and in the education of the community regarding all types of health care concerns, including the morbidity and mortality associated with obesity.

Based on Orzano JA, Scott JG: Diagnosis and treatment of obesity in adults: an applied evidence-based review, *J Am Board Fam Pract* 17(5):359-369, 2004. Available at www.medscape.com/viewarticle/489073_print.

also are believed to work in part by raising the patient's metabolic rate as another consequence of their activities in the brain.

Another relatively new drug is orlistat, which differs from the others in that it is not a CNS stimulant per se but works by irreversibly inhibiting the enzyme lipase. This results in absorption of decreased amounts of dietary fat from the intestinal tract and increased fat excretion in the feces.

Indications

Anorexiants are used for the treatment of obesity. However, their effects are often minimal without accompanying behavioral modifications involving diet and exercise. More specifically, these drugs are often used in obese patients with a body mass index (BMI) of 30 or more, or in patients with a BMI of 27 who are also hypertensive or have high cholesterol or diabetes.

Contraindications

Contraindications to anorexiants include drug allergy, any severe cardiovascular disease, uncontrolled hypertension, hyperthyroidism, glaucoma, mental agitation, history of drug abuse, eating disorders (e.g., anorexia, bulimia), and use of MAOIs (Chapter 15) within the previous 14 days. In addition, sibutramine should not be used concurrently with other serotonergic drugs, including selective serotonin reuptake inhibitors (Chapter 15), meperidine, lithium, or dihydroergotamine. Orlistat is contraindicated in cases of chronic malabsorption syndrome or cholestasis.

Adverse Effects

With the exception of diethylpropion, anorexiants may raise blood pressure and cause heart palpitations and even dysrhythmias at higher dosages. Ironically, at therapeutic dosages, they may actually reflexively slow the heart rate. Diethylpropion, however, has little cardiovascular activity. These drugs may also cause anxiety, agitation, dizziness, and headache. In addition to these effects, with sibutramine use there have been case reports of mania, intestinal obstruction, cardiac arrest, and stroke, among several other serious consequences. However, it should be recognized that obese patients commonly have multiple risk factors for such adverse events even when this drug is not taken. The most common adverse effects of orlistat include headache, upper respiratory tract infection (mechanism uncertain), and GI distress, including fecal incontinence.

Interactions

See Table 16-4.

Drug Profiles

Anorexiants

As noted earlier, amphetamine salts generally are no longer used for treatment of obesity because of their high abuse potential. The current major prescription anorexiants include phentermine and sibutramine. Several others have been mentioned earlier but are not as commonly prescribed. A newer nonstimulant drug also included here is the lipase inhibitor orlistat. All three of these medications offer generally improved safety and adverse effect profiles compared with the potent and highly addictive amphetamines.

▶ phentermine

Phentermine (Ionamin) is a sympathomimetic anorexiant that is structurally related to amphetamines but with much lower abuse potential. It is classified as a Schedule IV drug. This drug is not to be confused with several other drugs that were recalled by the FDA in the late 1990s (fenfluramine dexfenfluramine [Phen-Fen]) and 2000 (phenylpropanolamine) because of case reports of various adverse cardiovascular and/or pulmonary effects.

▶ sibutramine

Sibutramine (Meridia) is one of the newest anorexiants and is classified as a Schedule IV controlled substance. Sibutramine works by inhibiting the reuptake primarily of norepinephrine and serotonin (and to a lesser extent, dopamine), which results in reduced appetite.

Pharmacokinetics

Half-Life	Onset	Peak	Duration
PO: 14-16 hr	PO: 8 wk	PO: 6 mo*	PO: 12 mo*

*Therapeutic effects.

orlistat

Orlistat (Xenical), one of the newer anorexiants, is unrelated to other drugs in its category. As noted earlier, it works by binding to gastric and pancreatic enzymes called *lipases*. Blocking these enzymes reduces fat absorption by roughly 30%. Restricting dietary intake of fat to less than 30% of total calories can help reduce some of the GI adverse effects, which include oily spotting, flatulence, and fecal incontinence in 20% to 40% of patients. Decreases in serum concentrations of vitamins A, D, and E and β-carotene are seen as a result of the blocking of fat absorption. Supplementation with fat-soluble vitamins corrects this deficiency.

Pharmacokinetics

Half-Life	Onset	Peak	Duration
PO: 1-2 hr	PO: 3 mo*	PO: 6-8 hr	PO: Unknown

*Therapeutic effects.

MIGRAINE

A **migraine** is a common type of recurring headache, usually lasting from 4 to 72 hours. Typical features include a pulsatile quality with pain that worsens with each pulse. The pain is most commonly unilateral but may occur bilaterally on both sides of the head. Associated symptoms include nausea, vomiting, *photophobia* (avoidance of light), and *phonophobia* (avoidance of sounds). In addition, a minority of migraines are accompanied by an *aura,* which is a predictive set of altered visual or other senses (formerly termed "classic migraine"). However, the majority of migraines are without an aura (formerly termed "common migraine"). Migraines affect about 12% of the U.S. population, with a reported incidence in females roughly three times that in males. These headaches can occur at any age, but migraines commonly begin after age 10 and peak between the mid-twenties and early forties. They often fade after middle age. Familial inheritance of migraine is also well recognized. Precipitating factors include stress, emotionality, hypoglycemia, menses, estrogens (including oral contraceptives), exercise, alcohol, caffeine, cocaine, nitroglycerin, aspartame, and the food additive monosodium glutamate (MSG). Interestingly, over 50% of patients with narcolepsy report nocturnal migraines. Previously, migraines were thought to be caused by compensatory vasodilation when brain circulation was compromised for some unknown reason. According to this "vascular hypothesis," the enhanced intracranial circulation causes headache pain by displacing tissues within the cranial cavity. A more recent theory can be termed the "neurovascular hypothesis." It focuses on both neural structures of the trigeminal nerve itself as well as the vascular structures associated with this nerve, which affect intracranial circulation. This theory is supported by positron emission tomographic scans of the brain during a migraine attack. These neural structures are believed to have unpredictable episodes of inflammatory dysfunction that results in pain. This inflammatory process, like such processes in general, also causes increased blood flow to the affected area. It is driven by inflammatory mediator proteins such as the neuropeptides (nerve proteins) *substance P, calcitonin gene–related peptide,* and *neurokinin A,* all of which are potent vasodilators. In particular, falling brain and body serotonin levels are believed to be one major culprit, and this is reflected in the design of antimigraine drugs. During migraine, platelets release serotonin into the circulation where much of it is lost to body metabolism. Two drug classes work against migraine symptoms by enhancing serotonergic transmission in the brain: the ergot alkaloids (Chapter 17) and serotonergic agonists or *triptans*. These include sumatriptan, almotriptan, eletriptan, naratriptan, rizatriptan, zolmitriptan, and frovatriptan.

ANTIMIGRAINE DRUGS (SEROTONIN AGONISTS)

Serotonin receptor agonists, first introduced in the 1990s, have revolutionized the treatment of migraine headache. Like the ergot alkaloids mentioned in Chapter 17, these drugs work by stimulating serotonin receptors in the brain.

Mechanism of Action and Drug Effects

The chemical name for serotonin is 5-hydroxytryptamine or 5-HT. Physiologists have further identified two 5-HT receptor subtypes on which these drugs have their greatest effect: 5-HT_{1B} and 5-HT_{1D}. Triptans stimulate these receptors in cerebral arteries, causing vasoconstriction and normally reducing or eliminating headache symptoms. They also reduce the production of inflammatory neuropeptides. This is known as *abortive* drug therapy because it treats a headache that has already started.

Indications

Antimigraine drugs, also referred to as selective serotonin receptor agonists (SSRAs) are indicated for abortive therapy of an acute migraine headache. Although they may be taken during aura symptoms in patients who have auras with their headaches, these drugs are not indicated for *preventive* migraine therapy. Preventive therapy is indicated if migraine attacks occur one or more days per week. A variety of drugs are used for preventive therapy; most of them are discussed in more detail in other chapters. These include analgesics (e.g., acetaminophen, aspirin, ibuprofen), tricyclic antidepressants (Chapter 15), monoamine oxidase inhibitors (Chapter 15), β-blockers (Chapter 18), calcium channel blockers (Chapters 22 and 24), anticonvulsants (see Chapter 13), antiemetics (see Chapter 53), sedatives (Chapter 12), and the serotonergic drug cyproheptadine (Chapter 35). The newer serotonin-selective reuptake inhibitor antidepressants (see Chapter 15) have not proved effective, and in fact headache is a common adverse effect of this drug class. Among the most commonly used products is a tablet or capsule containing fixed combinations of either acetaminophen or aspirin plus the barbiturate butalbital plus the analeptic caffeine. In addition to potentiating the effects of the analgesics, caffeine can also enhance intestinal absorption of the ergot alkaloids (Chapter 17) and has a vasoconstricting effect, which can reduce cerebral blood flow to ease headache pain. Caffeine also has a diuretic effect, which may ultimately also reduce cerebral blood flow due to reduced vascular volume secondary to enhanced urinary output. In many cases, preventive drug therapy is also sufficient for abortive therapy. When it is not, triptans are now the most commonly prescribed drug class, followed by the ergot alkaloids.

Contraindications

Contraindications to triptans include drug allergy and the presence of serious cardiovascular disease, because of the vasoconstrictive potential of these medications.

Adverse Effects

As noted earlier, triptans have potential vasoconstrictor effects, including effects on the coronary circulation. Injectable dosage forms may cause local irritation at the site of injection. Other adverse effects include feelings of tingling, flushing (skin warmth and redness), and a congested feeling in the head or chest.

Interactions

See Table 16-4.

Drug Profiles

Serotonin Agonists

The serotonin agonists are a new class of CNS stimulants used to treat migraine headache. They can produce relief from moderate to severe migraines within 2 hours in 70% to 80% of patients. They work by stimulating 5-HT$_1$ receptors in the brain and are sometimes referred to as SSRAs or triptans. They are available in a variety of formulations, including oral tablets, sublingual tablets, subcutaneous

self-injections, and nasal sprays. A common effect of migraines is nausea and vomiting. Orally administered medications are therefore not tolerated by some patients. Nonoral (including sublingual) forms are advantageous for this reason. They also often have a more rapid onset of action, producing relief in some patients in 10 to 15 minutes, compared with 1 to 2 hours for tablets. Dosage and other information appears in the table on page 256.

▶ sumatriptan

Sumatriptan (Imitrex) was the original prototype drug for this class. As noted earlier, there are now seven triptans. Slight pharmacokinetic differences exist between some of these products, but their effects are comparable overall.

Pharmacokinetics

Half-Life	Onset	Peak	Duration
PO: 2.5 hr	PO: 0.5-1 hr	PO: 2.5 hr	PO: 4 hr

ANALEPTIC-RESPONSIVE RESPIRATORY DEPRESSION SYNDROMES

Analeptic drugs are now generally used much less frequently than they were in the earlier days of general anesthesia. This is because of advances in intensive respiratory care, including mechanical ventilation and improved anesthetic techniques, as well as the availability of newer medications with less toxicity. Nonetheless, there are several respiratory syndromes for which these medications are sometimes still used. Neonatal apnea, or periodic cessation of breathing in newborn babies, is a common condition seen in neonatal intensive care units. It is especially frequent among premature infants, whose pulmonary structures have not completed their gestational development due to preterm birth. Infants undergoing prolonged mechanical ventilation, especially at high pressures, often develop a chronic lung disease known as bronchopulmonary dysplasia. Postanesthetic respiratory depression occurs when a patient's spontaneous respiratory drive does not resume adequately and in a timely manner after general anesthesia. Respiratory depression may also be secondary to abuse of some drugs. Hypercapnia, or elevated blood levels of carbon dioxide, is often associated with later stages of chronic obstructive pulmonary disease (COPD). Analeptic drugs such as theophylline, aminophylline, caffeine, and doxapram may be used to treat one or more of these conditions.

ANALEPTICS

Analeptics include doxapram and the methylxanthines aminophylline, theophylline, and caffeine.

Mechanism of Action and Drug Effects

Analeptics work by stimulating areas of the CNS that control respiration, mainly the medulla and spinal cord. Methylxanthine analeptics (caffeine, aminophylline, and theophylline) also inhibit the enzyme *phosphodiesterase*. This enzyme breaks down a substance called *cyclic adenosine monophosphate* (cAMP). When these drugs block this enzyme, cAMP accumulates. This results in relaxation of smooth muscle in the respiratory tract, dilation of pulmonary arterioles, and stimulation of the CNS in general. Aminophylline is a *prodrug* (a drug formulated for greater solubility to facilitate administration) that is *hydrolyzed* (reacts with water molecules) to theophylline in the body; theophylline is metabolized to caffeine. Caffeine has an inherently stronger affinity for CNS stimulation; hence its popularity in coffee, tea, and soft drinks. As noted previously, it also helps to potentiate the effects of analgesics used for migraine and has a diuretic effect. The stimulant effects of caffeine are attributed to its antagonism (blocking) of adenosine receptors in the brain. Adenosine is associated with sleep promotion. The mechanism of action of doxapram is similar to that of the three methylxanthines, but it has a greater stimulant effect in the area of the brain that senses carbon dioxide content. When the carbon dioxide content of the blood is high, the respiratory center in the brain is stimulated to induce deeper and faster breathing in an attempt to exchange more carbon dioxide for inhaled oxygen.

Indications

Currently listed indications for analeptics include neonatal apnea, bronchopulmonary dysplasia, hypercapnia associated with COPD, postanesthetic respiratory depression, and respiratory depression secondary to drugs of abuse (e.g., opioids, alcohol, or barbiturates). However, these latter two conditions especially are now more commonly treated with specific reversal antidote drugs and/or mechanical ventilation until the overdosed drug wears off. In newborns, administration of caffeine is associated with less tachycardia, CNS stimulation, and feeding intolerance than administration of theophylline or aminophylline. The latter are also used for neonatal bradycardia as well as for asthma in older children and adults. Aminophylline is also sometimes given intravenously to treat anaphylaxis (Chapter 36).

Contraindications

Contraindications to the use of analeptics include drug allergy, peptic ulcer disease (especially for caffeine), and serious cardiovascular conditions. Concurrent use of other phosphodiesterase-inhibiting drugs such as sildenafil and similar drugs is also not recommended.

Doxapram use is contraindicated in newborns because of the benzyl alcohol contained in the injectable formulation of the drug. Its use is also contraindicated in patients with epilepsy or other convulsive disorders, those who have shown a hypersensitivity reaction to it, those showing evidence of head injury, those suffering from cardiovascular impairment or severe hypertension, and patients who have had a stroke.

Adverse Effects

At higher dosages, analeptics stimulate the vagal, vasomotor, and respiratory centers of the medulla in the brainstem, as well as skeletal muscles. Vagal effects include stimulation of gastric secretions, diarrhea, and reflex tachycardia. Vasomotor effects include flushing (warmth, redness) and sweating of the skin. Respiratory effects include elevated respiratory rate (which is normally desired). Skeletal muscle effects include muscular tension and tremors. Neurological effects include reduced deep-tendon reflexes.

Interactions

See Table 16-4.

Drug Profiles

Analeptic drugs include doxapram and the methylxanthines aminophylline, theophylline, and caffeine. The profiles for aminophylline and theophylline can be found in Part Six of this book on respiratory system drugs. The antinarcoleptic drug modafinil was discussed in the narcolepsy section of this chapter. Dosage and other information appears in the table on page 256.

▶ *caffeine*

Caffeine (No-Doz) is a CNS stimulant that can be found in over-the-counter (OTC) drugs and combination prescription drugs. It is also contained in many beverages and foods. Just a few of the many foods and drugs that contain caffeine are listed in Table 16-5. Caffeine use is contraindicated in patients with a known hypersensitivity to it and should be used with caution in patients who have a history of peptic ulcers or cardiac dysrhythmias or who have recently suffered a myocardial infarction. Caffeine is available in oral and injectable dosage forms.

Caffeine citrate is recommended for neonatal apnea, including that not responsive to other methylxanthines such as theophylline, because of the longer half-life of caffeine. The alternative caffeine product, caffeine sodium benzoate, is recommended for respiratory depression in adults only, because it is associated with *gasping syndrome* in infants and may also displace bilirubin into the blood from albumin binding sites in the circulation. This, in turn, could cause or worsen hyperbilirubinemia, a common condition in high-risk infants.

Pharmacokinetics

Half-Life	Onset	Peak	Duration
PO: 3-4 hr	PO: 15-45 min	PO: 50-75 min	PO: Less than 6 hr

doxapram

Doxapram (Dopram) is another analeptic that is commonly used in conjunction with supportive measures in cases of respiratory depression that involve anesthetics or drugs of abuse and in COPD-associated hypercapnia. In addition to vital signs and heart rhythm, deep-tendon reflexes are another monitoring parameter for prevention of overdosage of this drug.

Table 16-5 Caffeine-Containing Beverages and Drugs

Medication or Beverage	Amount of Caffeine
Nonprescription Medications	
Analgesics	
Anacin	32 mg/tab
Excedrin, Excedrin Aspirin-Free, Excedrin Migraine	65 mg/tab
Stimulants	
No-Doz Maximum Strength	100 mg/tab
Vivarin	200 mg/tab
Prescription Medications (for Migraines)	
Fioricet, Fiorinal	40 mg/tab
Esgic	40 mg/tab
Cafergot	10 mg/suppository
Beverages	
Coffee (brewed)	80-150 mg/5-oz cup
Coffee (instant)	80-150 mg/5-oz cup
Coffee (decaffeinated)	2-4 mg/5-oz cup
Tea (brewed)	30-75 mg/5-oz cup
Soft drinks	35-60 mg/12-oz cup
Cocoa	5-40 mg/5-oz cup

Pharmacokinetics

Half-Life	Onset	Peak	Duration
IV: 2-4 hr*	IV: Less than 30 sec	IV: Less than 2 min	IV: 5-12 min

*Metabolites: 4-8 hr.

◆ NURSING PROCESS

◆ ASSESSMENT

CNS stimulants are used for a variety of conditions and disorders. They have addictive potential, and a thorough medical history, physical assessment, and medication history must be obtained before their use. The CNS stimulants used for their *anorexiant* effect (see discussion in pharmacology section) include drugs that stimulate the release of catecholamines, and at higher dosages they suppress appetite, stimulate the respiratory center, and decrease drug-induced CNS depression (however, seizures may be a consequence of CNS stimulation). Other uses include an improvement in attentiveness and wakefulness. When the patient is about to receive these medications for weight loss, baseline weight and height measurements are needed, as is as documentation of vital signs with specific attention to pulse rate and blood pressure. The vital parameters of pulse rate and blood pressure are critical because of the adverse effects. A nursing history should include questions about lifestyle, exercise, nutritional habits, patterns, and knowledge, family history, self-esteem, stress levels, and mental status, and information related to contraindications, cautions, and drug interactions (see Table 16-4). It is important for the nurse to understand that cardiovascular and cerebrovascular diseases may be exacerbated to life-threatening levels with these drugs. In addition, psychoses may worsen, drug dependence may be exacerbated, and diabetics may need tighter insulin control or a decrease in insulin dosage (mainly because of concurrent dietary changes). Nutritional assessments should be documented, and attention should be given to the levels of fat-soluble vitamins because their reduction by the medication. The nurse should assess for and document underlying addictive behaviors, hypertension, and other disease states because of the higher risk of exacerbation with this drug. However, orlistat, the nonstimulant anorexiant (see the pharmacology section), is associated with a lower incidence of systemic adverse effects.

With drugs used for the management of *ADHD*, very cautious and continuous assessment is required. This should include measurement of vital signs and baseline weight and height as well as evaluation of the child's baseline growth and development and complete blood counts as needed. Usual sleep habits and patterns should be noted so that efforts can be made to prevent any sleep disturbances that may occur with these drugs. In addition, it is important to have baseline documentation of difficulties with cognition, attention, and mood so that successful treatment or need for change in therapy is identifiable. Typical behavior and attention span and history of social problems or problems in school are also important to assess and document before and during therapy. Parental support is important to the success of treatment, so a home assessment is usually performed by supporting organizations such as a public or private school or social services agency. Attention to daily dietary intake before drug therapy is initiated is important because of drug-related weight loss. It is crucial that the pediatric patient not experience too rapid or too much weight loss. Very important to the use of these drugs (as with all CNS stimulants) is a thorough cardiac assessment with attention to heart sounds, any history of chest pain or palpitations, and baseline pulse rate and rhythm and blood pressure. Before administering CNS stimulants, the nurse must carefully gather data from the patient's history that may raise concern regarding potential contraindications, cautions, and drug interactions (see previous discussion). The nurse should also assess for the use of any herbal preparations, OTC products, and beverages that may contain ginseng or caffeine (see Selected Herbal Compounds Used for Nervous System Stimulation).

An *analeptic* such as doxapram is used as a central respiratory stimulant; therefore, it is most likely be used in a hospital setting, specifically in intensive care units or postanesthesia units. The same concerns for contraindications, cautions, and drug interactions exist for this drug as for all CNS stimulants, but even closer attention must be paid to vital signs, especially heart rate and rhythm and blood pressure, to prevent complications. As with any CNS stimulant, it is also important to perform a thorough

---

HERBAL THERAPIES AND DIETARY SUPPLEMENTS

Selected Herbal Compounds Used for Nervous System Stimulation*

Common Name(s)	Uses	Possible Drug Interactions (Avoid Concurrent Use)
Ginkgo biloba, ginkgo	To enhance mental alertness; to improve memory or dementia	Warfarin, aspirin
Ginseng	To enhance impaired mental function and concentration	Drugs for diabetes that lower blood sugar (e.g., insulin, oral hypoglycemic drugs), monoamine oxidase inhibitors
Guarana	Nervous system stimulation, appetite suppression	Adenosine, disulfiram, quinolones, oral contraceptives, β-blockers, iron, lithium, phenylephrine (e.g., nasal spray), cimetidine, theophylline, tobacco

Data from Fetrow CW, Avila JR: *The complete guide to herbal remedies,* Springhouse, Pa, 2000, Springhouse.

*The information in this box does not imply author or publisher endorsement of these products. Although individual consumers often experience satisfying results with various herbal products, there is frequently little, if any, rigorously controlled research to demonstrate their efficacy at treating particular conditions. Patients should always be advised to communicate regularly with their health care practitioners about all medications used, including herbal remedies, to decrease the likelihood of possibly hazardous drug interactions.

Note also that sale of the herbal central nervous system stimulant known as ephedra or ma huang was officially banned by the Food and Drug Administration, effective April 2004, following its link to cases of myocardial infarction and stroke.

neurologic assessment with attention to any history of seizures because of the risk of exacerbation of seizures. With the use of doxapram, in particular, deep tendon reflexes should be noted before and during use of the drug.

The serotonin agonists, commonly used in the treatment of *migraines,* are not without adverse reactions, contraindications, cautions, and drug interactions, as previously discussed. Assessment should include measuring blood pressure, pulse rate and rhythm, and heart sounds, and taking a thorough cardiac history. Because an elevation in blood pressure may occur, even though it is usually only a slight elevation, these drugs should not be used in patients with uncontrolled hypertension. These drugs are not usually prescribed for patients with coronary artery disease unless a thorough cardiac evaluation has been performed and their use is approved. It is important to reemphasize the significant drug interactions with MAOIs (serotonin agonists should not be administered within 2 weeks of MAOI use), and serotonin agonists should not be taken within 24 hours of use of ergotamine-containing products or even dihydroergotamine or methysergide. Other triptans should not be taken within 24 hours of taking sumatriptan. In addition, the patient may also take OTC or other prescribed analgesics that contain caffeine, aspirin, and/or other nonsteroidal antiinflammatory drugs, so there should be assessment of allergy to the components as well as documentation of any problems with bleeding, GI upset, or ulcers prior to use of these adjunctive therapies.

✦ NURSING DIAGNOSES

- Anxiety related to the drug's adverse effect of CNS stimulation
- Decreased cardiac output related to the adverse effects of palpitations and tachycardia
- Deficient knowledge related to lack of information about the specific drug regimen
- Disturbed thought processes related to the CNS effects of the drug
- Disturbed sleep pattern (decreased sleep) related to drug effects
- Imbalanced nutrition, more than body requirements, due to presence of obesity
- Imbalanced nutrition, less than body requirements, related to adverse effects of the medication
- Pain related to migraine headaches
- Pain related to adverse effects of the drug such as headache and dry mouth
- Situational low self-esteem related to the impact of obesity, decreased sexual performance, and other adverse effects of the CNS stimulation

✦ PLANNING

Goals

- Patient appears less anxious or experiences no anxiety from the medication.
- Patient is free of cardiac symptoms and associated complications of drug therapy.
- Patient remains open to education about related drug and nondrug therapeutic regimens.
- Patient regains or maintains near normal body weight and BMI during therapy.
- Patient continues to undergo close to normal growth and development while taking medications.
- Patient experiences minimal sleep deprivation.

- Patient maintains positive self-esteem.
- Patient remains compliant with drug therapy and free from complications of treatment.

Outcome Criteria

- Patient communicates anxiety, anger, and feelings regarding self-image and self-esteem openly and as needed.
- Patient maintains appropriate weight loss without too rapid losses or gains throughout treatment (if a pediatric patient, normal growth and development patterns are continued with weight and height falling within normal limits on growth chart) while taking CNS stimulants.
- Patient shows improved sensorium and level of consciousness with increased attention span and cognition.
- Patient experiences more restful sleep using nonpharmacologic measures.
- Patient's vital signs, especially blood pressure and pulse, remain within normal limits.
- Patient states symptoms (e.g., palpitations, chest pain) to report to the physician immediately.
- Patient reports a decrease in headaches.
- Patient reports that medication is taken as ordered and consistently over the time of the therapeutic protocol.

✦ IMPLEMENTATION

Because *anorexiants* are generally used for a short period of time, it is very important to emphasize to the patient and all members of the patient's support system that a suitable diet, appropriate independent and/or supervised exercise program, and behavioral modifications are necessary to support a favorable result and to help the patient cease overeating and experience healthy weight loss. Medications are usually taken first thing in the morning, as ordered, to minimize interference with sleep, and they should not be taken within 4 to 6 hours of sleep. If the patient has been taking these drugs for a prolonged period of time, there should be a period of weaning upon discontinuation to avoid withdrawal symptoms and to avoid any chance of a rebound increase in appetite. Weight should be assessed weekly or as ordered, and often keeping a food diary helps with 24-hour recall of all intake. Caffeine should be avoided, including all caffeine-containing beverages and foods such as coffee, tea, sodas, and chocolate. Other products that contain caffeine include OTC analgesics such as Excedrin, OTC menstrual-symptom related compunds such as Midol, prescription analgesics such as ergotamine with caffeine, butalbital with aspirin and caffeine, and prescription drugs with an opioid such as butalbital with aspirin, caffeine, and codeine. Online resources and information are available at www.cspinet.org/nah/caffeine/caffeinecorner.htm. Dry mouth may be managed with frequent mouth care and the use of sugar-free gum or hard candy. Ice chips may help as well.

Other nursing considerations include emphasis on a holistic approach to treatment of obesity, including the possible use of hypnosis, biofeedback, and guided imagery as ordered. Keeping a journal to record responses to the drug therapy at home, play, and school is important for charting the effectiveness of the drug for any patient. Counseling is generally a part of the treatment, with the family involved in goal setting for the treatment regimen. The patient should be encouraged to keep follow-up visits with his or her physician. Supplementation with fat-soluble vitamins may be indicated. It is important also to watch for "tolerance" to the anorexiant.

With drugs used for ADHD, some pediatric patients may respond better to certain dosage forms such as immediate release, and dosing should be individualized and based on the patient's needs at different times during their school day (e.g., a noon dose for music lessons later in the afternoon). Scheduling of these medications and close communication with the family and patient is very important to successful treatment. It is also important to time medications, as ordered, for periods in which symptom control is most needed and sleep not altered. Generally speaking, once-a-day dosing is used with extended-release or long-acting preparations. Adequate and proper dosing will be manifested by good control in behavior and improvement during school time, and, if extended-release dosage forms work well, then the pediatric patient will not have to take the medication at school. Many times a stigma is associated with taking medications at school, and this may be prevented with long-acting preparations or other scheduling. To help decrease the occurrence of insomnia, the last daily dose should be taken 4 to 6 hours before bedtime. During therapy, the patient will also be monitored for continued physical growth with specific attention to weight. The physician may order times for "medication-free" weekends, holidays, or vacations, and the drug may also be discontinued periodically so that the need for the medication can be reassessed.

Doxapram may be administered intravenously (see the Dosages table on p. 256) but at different dosages depending on the purpose. Doxapram infusions should be given with use of an intravenous pump and with close monitoring. Because the patient's sensorium is generally diminished in this situation, placing the patient in Sims' or semi-Fowler's position is necessary to prevent aspiration. If adverse effects occur, the infusion should be discontinued immediately and the physician notified (see the pharmacology discussion).

SSRAs come in a variety of dosage forms. Rizatriptan comes in a disintegrating tablet or wafer that dissolves on the tongue, which leads to rapid absorption even if the patient is experiencing nausea and vomiting; it also comes in oral tablets. Use of the nasal spray or self-injectable forms of the serotonin agonists is desirable, especially in patients experiencing the nausea and vomiting that may occur with migraine headaches. Patient instructions about administration technique are very important. Self-injectable forms and nasal sprays also have the benefit of an onset of action of 10 to 15 minutes compared with 1 to 2 hours with tablet forms. Administration of a test dose for all dosage forms is usually recommended. See Patient Teaching Tips for more information.

◆ EVALUATION

Therapeutic responses to drugs used in the management of hyperkinesia include decreased hyperactivity, increased attention span and concentration, and improved behavior. The therapeutic response to drugs used for the management of narcolepsy is the ability to remain awake. Anorexiants should cause the patient's appetite to decrease and weight loss to occur. The nurse needs to monitor the patient for the development of adverse effects to these medications; these include changes in mental status, sensorium, mood, affect, and sleep patterns; physical dependency; irritability; and withdrawal symptoms such as headache, nausea, and vomiting.

Therapeutic effects of anorexiants include appetite control and weight loss for the treatment of obesity. Adverse effects of sibutramine include dry mouth, headache, insomnia, and constipation. It is important to monitor for adverse effects of these drugs, including worsening of headache, dry mouth, insomnia, tachycardia, cardiac irregularities, hypertension, and possible seizures due to excess CNS stimulation. Therapeutic effects of orlistat—another anorexiant but one that is a lipase inhibitor instead of a CNS stimulant—include appetite control in obesity. Adverse effects caused mainly by the drug's action of inhibiting lipase include flatulence with an oily discharge, spotting, and fecal urgency. The patient also needs to be closely evaluated for decreases in levels of fat-soluble vitamins (A, D, E, and K), because levels of these vitamins are affected by the decrease in absorption of fats. Therapeutic responses to modafinil include a decrease in sleepiness associated with narcolepsy. Adverse effects for which to monitor with modafinil include headache, nausea, nervousness, and anxiety.

Therapeutic responses to the serotonin agonists include an improvement in the frequency, duration, and severity of migraine headaches with improved daily functioning and performance because of the decrease in headaches. Adverse effects for which to monitor include pain at the injection site (temporary), flushing, chest tightness or pressure, weakness, sedation, dizziness, sweating, increase in blood pressure and pulse rate, and bad taste with the nasal spray formulation, which may precipitate nausea.

Patient Teaching Tips

CNS Stimulants in General

- Serotonin agonists should be taken at the exact time and frequency as ordered.
- Medications should be taken exactly as prescribed without skipping, omitting, or adding doses.
- Alcohol, OTC cold products, cough syrups that may contain alcohol, nicotine, and caffeine, should be avoided.
- The patient should keep a log of daily activities and record how the drug is working and any adverse effects.
- Sudden withdrawal of medications should be avoided.

Anorexiants

- The patient must be sure to follow all physician instructions regarding medications, diet, and exercise.
- Some of the medications may impair alertness and ability to think. The patient should be very cautious in engaging in such activities until these impairments are gone.
- The unpleasant taste of the medicine and/or dry mouth may be minimized by use of mouth rinses, ice chips, sugarless chewing gum, and/or hard candies.

Drugs Used to Treat ADHD

- Medication should be taken on an empty stomach 30 to 45 minutes before eating for maximal effects.
- The patient should keep scheduled appointments so that the physician can document progress.
- If the doctor thinks use of the medication should be discontinued, a weaning process with careful supervision is usually used.
- Extended-release or long-acting preparations should not be crushed, chewed, or broken, and they should be taken as directed.
- Dosage should not be increased or decreased because this may lead to complications. If the patient has any questions or concerns, the parents, caregiver, or physician should be contacted.

Antimigraine Drugs

- Foods containing tyramine should be avoided, because tyramine is known to precipitate severe headaches. Tyramine-containing foods include beer, wine, aged cheese, food additives, preservatives, artificial sweeteners, chocolate, and caffeine.
- Before using a nasal spray form of an antimigraine drug, the patient should gently blow the nose to clear the nasal passages. With head upright, the patient should close one nostril and insert the nozzle into the open nostril. While a breath is taken through the nose, the spray should be released. The nozzle should be removed, and the patient should gently breathe in through the nose and out through the mouth for 10 to 20 seconds. Some distaste may be experienced.
- The patient should avoid doing things that require alertness and rapid skilled movements while experiencing migraines and/or taking medications until the patient is feeling back to normal.
- The patient should keep a journal of all headaches, precipitators, and relievers, and should rate each headache on a scale of 0 to 10, where 0 is no pain and 10 is the worst pain ever. The patient should be sure to record other symptoms such as photophobia, nausea, and vomiting as well as their frequency and duration.
- When taking SSRAs, the patient should contact the physician immediately if he or she experiences palpitations, chest pain, and/or pain or weakness in the extremities.
- Injectable forms of sumatriptan should be given subcutaneously and as ordered. The patient should practice administering injections (without the medication) with the nurse at the doctor's office so that proper technique is used and comfort level achieved.
- Autoinjectors with prefilled syringes may be used. The syringe should be discarded after use.
- No more than two injections of sumatriptan should be administered during a 24-hour period and at least 1 hour should be allowed between injections.
- With injections of sumatriptan, the patient should contact a physician or emergency services immediately if he or she experiences swelling around the eyes, pain or tightness in the chest or throat, wheezing, and/or heart throbbing.
- Helpful online resources include www.ahsnet.org, www.stress.org, www.mbmi.org, www.aan.com, and www.achenet.org.

Points to Remember

- CNS stimulants are drugs that stimulate the brain or spinal cord (e.g., cocaine and caffeine).
- Actions of these stimulants mimic those of the SNS neurotransmitters norepinephrine, dopamine, and serotonin.
- Sympathomimetic drugs mimic the action of the sympathetic division of the autonomic nervous system.
- Included in the family of CNS stimulants are the amphetamines, analeptics, and anorexiants, with therapeutic uses for ADHD, narcolepsy, and appetite control.
- Because the analeptics stimulate respiration, they may be used to treat respiratory paralysis caused by overdose of opioids, alcohol, barbiturates, and general anesthetic drugs.
- Anorexiants control or suppress appetite. They may also be used to stimulate the CNS and work by suppressing appetite control centers in the brain.
- Contraindications to the use of anorexiants, as well as any CNS stimulant, include hypersensitivity, seizure activity, convulsive disorders, and liver dysfunction.
- The serotonin agonists are a newer class of CNS stimulants generally used to treat migraine headaches. They are to be avoided by patients who have coronary heart disease.

- Amphetamines elevate mood or produce euphoria, increase mental alertness and capacity for work, decrease fatigue and drowsiness, and prolong wakefulness.
- The analeptics have generalized effects on the brainstem and spinal cord, increase responsiveness to external stimuli, and stimulate respiration.
- Nursing considerations for children who take methylphenidate and other related drugs include recording baseline height and weight before initiating drug therapy and continuing to plot height and weight in a journal during therapy.
- Journaling is helpful in evaluating the effects of all drugs used to treat ADHD or migraines as well as in obesity treatment.
- Therapeutic responses to drugs used in the treatment of hyperkinesia include decreased hyperactivity, increased attention span and concentration, and improved behavior patterns.
- Adverse effects for which to monitor in individuals taking CNS stimulants include changes in mental status or sensorium, mood, affect, and sleep patterns; physical dependency; and irritability.
- Serotonin agonists may be administered subcutaneously, as a nasal spray, and as oral tablets. Any chest pain or tightness, tremors, vomiting, or worsening symptoms should be reported to the physician immediately.

NCLEX Examination Review Questions

1. A patient with narcolepsy will begin treatment with a CNS stimulant. Which of the following adverse effects is this patient likely to encounter?
   a. Bradycardia
   b. Nervousness
   c. Mental clouding
   d. Drowsiness at night
2. At a weight management clinic, a patient who was given a prescription for orlistat (Xenical) calls the clinic hotline because of a "terrible adverse effect." The nurse suspects that the patient is referring to:
   a. Nausea
   b. Sexual dysfunction
   c. Urinary incontinence
   d. Fecal incontinence
3. Patients receiving anorexiants are most likely being treated for which nursing diagnoses?
   a. Deficient fluid volume
   b. Disturbed sleep pattern
   c. Impaired memory
   d. Imbalanced nutrition, more than body requirements

4. A patient with a new prescription for sumatriptan (Imitrex) will need patient teaching on what topic before he self-administers this drug?
   a. Correct technique for subcutaneous injections
   b. Correct technique for intramuscular injections
   c. Proper placement of the transdermal patch
   d. The need to dissolve tablets under the tongue completely
5. Which statement is correct to make when reviewing atomoxetine (Strattera) therapy with the parents of an adolescent with ADHD?
   a. "Be sure to have your child blow his nose before administering the nasal spray."
   b. "This medication is used only when symptoms of ADHD are severe."
   c. "Be sure to contact the physician right away if you notice expression of suicidal thoughts."
   d. "If adverse effects become severe, stop the medication for 3 to 4 days."

1. b, 2. d, 3. d, 4. a, 5. c.

Critical Thinking Activities

1. The parents of a 10-year-old boy are concerned about the adverse effects of the medication their son is taking for ADHD. What will they need to monitor while he is taking medications for this condition?
2. A patient calls the headache clinic because she is unhappy about her medication. She says, "I've been taking zolmitriptan (Zomig)

to prevent headaches, but I am still having them." What does she need to know about the proper use of this drug?
3. Why would you, as a nurse, recommend or not recommend appetite suppressants for an adult who is obese?

For answers, see http://evolve.elsevier.com/Lilley.

Drugs Affecting the Autonomic Nervous System

STUDY SKILLS TIPS

- *PURR Application*
- *Study Groups*

PURR APPLICATION

Planning for the Part

The basic explanation provided for the PURR model in the Study Skills Tips for Part One demonstrates the application process as it relates to individual chapters. There is another application for the PURR model that can be very useful. This application encourages the learner to take a broader view of the assignment. In the case of this text, you have noticed that the chapters are grouped together into multiple chapter blocks called *parts*. Part organization is not some random process applied by the author to further complicate the subject. Part organization is a carefully considered process to put content together in a fashion that is logical and meaningful. Since the author has spent considerable time trying to link the chapters together in the most logical pattern, it is to your benefit as a student to learn to take advantage of the work already done for you.

Part Title

Begin the process of part planning by looking at the Part Three title, Drugs Affecting the Autonomic Nervous System. Then look at the part structure. There are four chapters contained in Part Three. All these chapters must be concerned with the autonomic nervous system. Even before you have read any chapter, you are beginning to look for the links that will establish a relationship, not only for the ideas in individual chapters but also the broader links that connect the four chapters in this part with each other and with the ideas that have come in earlier parts and will follow in later parts.

There is a clear example here of the way in which parts relate to one another. Look back at Part Two, Drugs Affecting the Central Nervous System. Clearly that part deals with some aspect of the nervous system, as does this part. One learning objective you should establish for yourself is determining the relationship between these two parts. You must be able to define and explain *central nervous system* and *autonomic nervous system*. However, defining these and just moving on limits the learning you can achieve. Ask yourself some additional questions that will help you establish a connection between these parts. "What are the differences in functions of the central and the autonomic nervous systems? Are there pharmacologic drugs that have application in both the central and autonomic nervous systems?" The principle is to keep stressing the links that must exist throughout all the parts and chapters you are studying. The normal study pattern that most students apply is one that focuses on the individual chapters, but it is essential that the broader scope of chapter and part be maintained.

Part Chapters

After considering the part title and looking for relationships between the new part and the previous parts, the next step in applying the Plan step of PURR s to spend a few minutes studying the chapter titles and looking for the relationships that must exist. Part Three has four chapters, and there is a clear pattern in these chapters. Chapters 17 and 18 both contain the term *adrenergic*. Clearly the two chapters are dealing with the same broad topic. However, Chapter 17 covers adrenergic drugs and Chapter 18 covers adrenergic-blocking drugs. Apply questioning strategies at this point. "What does adrenergic mean? What is an adrenergic drug?" These two questions are essential in mastering the content of Chapter 17 and should be questions that you ask yourself almost without thinking.

However, the next step is one that can greatly enhance your understanding when you start to read the material. This is a step that is easily overlooked. Notice that Chapter 17 deals with drugs and Chapter 18 deals with blocking drugs. There must be a difference between a *drug* and a *blocking drug*. Focus now with a few questions that will keep you aware that the content in Chapter 17 has a direct relationship to the content in Chapter 18. "What is the difference between a drug and a blocking drug? When is the pharmacologic application of a drug appropriate? Under what conditions should a blocking drug be chosen?" Then ask a question to help maintain the focus on the concept of the entire part. "What aspects of the autonomic nervous system are related to the adrenergic drugs and blocking drugs?"

Chapters 19 and 20

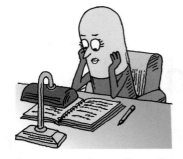

Once you begin to focus on the relationship of chapters within a part, certain things will begin to become apparent. Chapters 19 and 20 also cover drugs and blocking drugs. These two chapters develop the concept as related to cholinergics rather than adrenergics. However, the same questions you used as a focus for Chapters 17 and 18 can be recycled in setting up the study of Chapters 19 and 20. Simply replace the term *adrenergic* with *cholinergic* and you are ready to begin reading these two chapters with a clear personal learning objective.

Active Questioning

This is the key concept to master in working through the process for planning your learning for an entire part rather than for single chapters. The idea is to view the part as a whole rather than seeing only the content of individual chapters. The preceding discussion has provided a number of sample questions to help you begin the process. These questions should not be seen as the only questions you should ask, but rather as samples to help you develop a questioning process.

Keep in mind that you may or may not ask questions that are useful and appropriate when you are using only the chapter titles as the question stimulus. Some of the questions will prove to be very useful when reading the chapter. On the other hand, some of the initial questions you generate may have little or no application as you read and understand the content of an individual chapter. Do not worry about the quality of your questions when planning on the part level. Questions can (and sometimes

should) be revised or discarded when the details of the chapter become clearer. The important point is that you begin the part with some questions to help you focus your own reading and learning. Also, you will find that the more you apply active questioning as a part of your learning strategy, the better your questions will become.

Study Groups

A significant part of the PURR approach to learning is active questioning and rehearsing. When we engage others in this process, we have access to their ideas and understanding. We must also think through our own thoughts and make them clear to others. The best way to learn is to teach others.

Study groups are particularly helpful when anticipating test questions. With several minds working, you increase your odds of being correct. In nursing, your textbook learning is of no value until you learn to apply the knowledge and skills you are learning. Study groups provide a discussion venue to stimulate thinking about the nursing process. The critical thinking activities at the end of each chapter can serve as a basis for small group discussions. Study group members can share lecture notes, which is of value when you need to be absent or if you have an instructor who talks too fast. Relating with a study group keeps us alert while we are studying. It is hard to fall asleep or daydream when you are in the middle of a discussion. There are many advantages to working with a study group; however you must be careful when selecting the people to be in your group. Consider these four guidelines when establishing your study group:

1. Choose students who have **similar abilities and motivation** as you do. Socializing and gossiping can eat up valuable study time. Non-committed and underprepared classmates can be a drain.
2. Look for students who have a **common time to meet.**
3. Select classmates who have learning styles **different** from yours. They might understand the reading material or lecture material better than you. They may be able to draw a diagram that will help your learning.
4. Find students that have good communication skills; that is, people who know how to listen, ask good questions, and explain concepts.

Study groups are not for everyone; however they may be an alternative for you if you are having difficulty staying focused during your personal study time.

Adrenergic Drugs

Objectives

When you reach the end of this chapter, you should be able to do the following:

1. Briefly discuss the sympathetic nervous system in relation to drug therapy—specifically, the effects of adrenergic stimulation or sympathomimetic effects.
2. List the various drugs classified as adrenergic agonists or sympathomimetics.
3. Discuss the mechanisms of action, therapeutic effects, indications, adverse and toxic effects, cautions, contraindications, interactions, and available antidotes to overdosage for the various adrenergic agonists.
4. Discuss the nursing process as it relates to the administration of adrenergic drugs, including development of a nursing care plan for patients and caregivers.

e-Learning Activities

Companion CD
- NCLEX Review Questions: see questions 115-122
- Animations
- Audio Glossary
- Category Catchers
- Medication Errors Checklists
- IV Therapy Checklists

evolve Website (http://evolve.elsevier.com/Lilley)
• Nursing Care Plans • Frequently Asked Questions • Content Updates • WebLinks • Supplemental Resources • Elsevier ePharmacology Update • Medication Administration Animations

Drug Profiles

▶ albuterol sulfate, p. 275
▶ dobutamine, p. 277
▶ dopamine, p. 277
▶ epinephrine, pp. 276, 278
 fenoldopam, p. 278
 midodrine, p. 278

▶ norepinephrine, p. 278
 phenylephrine, p. 278
▶ pseudoephedrine, p. 276
▶ salmeterol, p. 276
 tetrahydrozoline, p. 276

▶ Key drug.

Glossary

α-adrenergic receptors A class of adrenergic receptors that are further subdivided into α_1- and α_2-adrenergic receptors, occur on the surface of postsynaptic effector cells, and are differentiated by their anatomic location in the tissues, muscles, and organs regulated by specific autonomic nerve fibers. (p. 270)

Adrenergic receptors Receptor sites for the sympathetic neurotransmitters norepinephrine and epinephrine. (p. 270)

Adrenergics Drugs that stimulate the sympathetic nervous system. They are also referred to as adrenergic agonists or

sympathomimetics because they mimic the effects of the sympathetic neurotransmitters norepinephrine and epinephrine. (p. 270)

Autonomic functions Bodily functions that are involuntary and result from physiologic activity of the autonomic nervous system. The functions often occur in pairs of opposing actions between the sympathetic and parasympathetic divisions of the autonomic nervous system. (p. 270)

Autonomic nervous system (ANS) A branch of the peripheral nervous system that controls autonomic bodily functions. It consists of the sympathetic nervous system and the parasympathetic nervous system. (p. 270)

β-adrenergic receptors Receptors located on postsynaptic effector cells of tissues, muscles, and organs stimulated by specific autonomic nerve fibers. β_1-adrenergic receptors are located primarily in the heart, whereas β_2-adrenergic receptors are located in the smooth muscle of the bronchioles and arterioles and in visceral organs. (p. 270)

Catecholamines Substances that can produce a sympathomimetic response. They are either endogenous catecholamines (such as epinephrine, norepinephrine, and dopamine) or synthetic catecholamine drugs (such as dobutamine). (p. 270)

Dopaminergic receptor A third type of adrenergic receptor (in addition to α-adrenergic and β-adrenergic receptors) located in various tissues and organs and activated by the binding of the neurotransmitter dopamine, which occurs in both endogenous and synthetic (drug) forms. (p. 270)

Mydriasis Pupillary dilation, whether natural (physiologic) or drug induced. (p. 273)

Ophthalmics Topically applied eye medications. (p. 273)

Positive chronotropic effect An increase in heart rate. (p. 273)

Positive dromotropic effect An increase in the conduction of cardiac electrical impulses through the atrioventricular node, which results in the transfer of nerve action potentials from the atria to the ventricles. This ultimately leads to a systolic heartbeat (ventricular contractions). (p. 273)

Positive inotropic effect An increase in the force of contraction of the heart muscle (myocardium). (p. 273)

Synaptic cleft The space either between two adjacent nerve cell membranes or between a nerve cell membrane and an effector organ cell membrane. (p. 271)

Adrenergics are a large group of both exogenous (synthetic) and endogenous (naturally occurring) substances. They have a wide variety of therapeutic uses depending on their site of action and their effect on receptors. Adrenergics stimulate the sympathetic nervous system (SNS) and are also called *adrenergic agonists.* They are also known as *sympathomimetics,* because they mimic the effects of the SNS neurotransmitters norepinephrine, epinephrine, and dopamine, which are chemically classified as **catecholamines.** In considering the adrenergic class of medications, it is helpful to understand how the SNS operates in relation to the rest of the nervous system.

SYMPATHETIC NERVOUS SYSTEM

Figure 17-1 depicts the divisions of the nervous system and shows the relationship of the SNS to the entire nervous system. The SNS is the counterpart of the parasympathetic nervous system (PSNS); together they make up the **autonomic nervous system (ANS).** They provide a checks-and-balances system for maintaining the normal homeostasis of the **autonomic functions** of the human body.

Throughout the body there are receptor sites for the catecholamines norepinephrine and epinephrine. These are referred to as **adrenergic receptors,** and these are the sites at which adrenergic

drugs bind and produce their effects. Adrenergic receptors are located in many anatomic sites, and many physiologic responses are produced when they are stimulated or blocked. Adrenergic receptors are further divided into **α-adrenergic receptors** and **β-adrenergic receptors,** depending on the specific physiologic responses caused by their stimulation. Both types of adrenergic receptors have subtypes, designated 1 and 2, which provide a further means of checks and balances that control stimulation and blockade, constriction and dilation, and the increased and decreased production of various substances.

The α_1- and α_2-adrenergic receptors are differentiated by their location relative to nerves. The α_1-adrenergic receptors are located on postsynaptic effector cells (the tissue, muscle, or organ that the nerve stimulates). The α_2-adrenergic receptors are located on the presynaptic nerve terminals. They control the release of neurotransmitters. The predominant α-adrenergic agonist response is vasoconstriction and central nervous system (CNS) stimulation.

The β-adrenergic receptors are all located on postsynaptic effector cells. The β_1-adrenergic receptors are primarily located in the heart; the β_2-adrenergic receptors are located in the smooth muscle of the bronchioles, arterioles, and visceral organs. A β-adrenergic agonist response results in bronchial, gastrointestinal (GI), and uterine smooth muscle relaxation; glycogenolysis; and cardiac stimulation. Table 17-1 contains a more detailed listing of the adrenergic receptors and the responses elicited when they are stimulated by a neurotransmitter or a drug that acts like a neurotransmitter (Figure 17-2).

Another type of adrenergic receptor is the **dopaminergic receptor.** When stimulated by dopamine, these receptors cause the

Table 17-1	**Adrenergic Receptor Responses to Stimulation**	
Location	**Receptor**	**Response**
Cardiovascular		
Blood vessels	α_1	Constriction
	β_2	Dilation
Cardiac muscle	β_1	Increased contractility
Atrioventricular node	β_1	Increased heart rate
Sinoatrial node	β_1	Increased heart rate
Endocrine		
Pancreas	β_1	Decreased insulin release
Liver	β_2	Glycogenolysis
Kidney	β_2	Increased renin secretion
Gastrointestinal		
Muscle	β_2	Decreased motility
Sphincters	α_1	Constriction
Genitourinary		
Bladder sphincter	α_1	Constriction
Penis	α_1	Ejaculation
Uterus	α_1	Contraction
	β_2	Relaxation
Respiratory		
Bronchial muscles	β_2	Dilation
Ocular		
Pupilary muscles of iris	α_1	Mydriasis

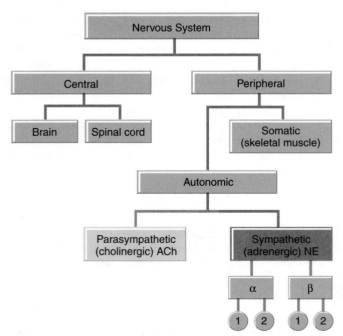

FIGURE 17-1 The sympathetic nervous system in relation to the entire nervous system. *ACh,* Acetylcholine; *NE,* norepinephrine.

vessels of the renal, mesenteric, coronary, and cerebral arteries to dilate, which increases blood flow to these tissues. Dopamine is the only substance that can stimulate these receptors.

Catecholamine neurotransmitter molecules are produced by the SNS and are stored in vesicles or granules located in the ends of nerves. Here the transmitter waits until the nerve is stimulated, then the vesicles move to the walls of nerve endings and release their contents into the space between the nerve ending and the effector organ, known as the **synaptic cleft.** The released contents of the vesicles (catecholamines) then have the opportunity to bind to the receptor sites located all along the effector organ. Once the neurotransmitter binds to the receptors, the effector organ responds. Depending on the function of the particular organ, this response involves smooth muscle contraction (e.g., skeletal muscles) or relaxation (e.g., GI and airway smooth muscles), an increased heart rate, the increased production of one or more substances (e.g., stress hormones), or constriction of a blood vessel. This process is halted by the action

of specific enzymes and by reuptake of the neurotransmitter molecules back into the nerve cell (neuron). Catecholamines are specifically metabolized by two enzymes, monoamine oxidase (MAO) and catechol ortho-methyltransferase (COMT). Each enzyme breaks down catecholamines but is responsible for doing it in a different area. MAO breaks down the catecholamines that are in the nerve ending, whereas COMT breaks down the catecholamines that are outside the nerve ending at the synaptic cleft. Neurotransmitter molecules may also be actively taken back up into the nerve ending by the action of various protein pumps within the cell membrane, a phenomenon known as *active transport*. This restores the catecholamine to the vesicle and provides another means of maintaining an adequate supply of the substance for future sympathetic nerve impulses. This process is illustrated in Figure 17-2. The sympathetic branch of the ANS is often described as having a "fight-or-flight" function because it allows the body to respond in a self-protective manner to dangerous situations.

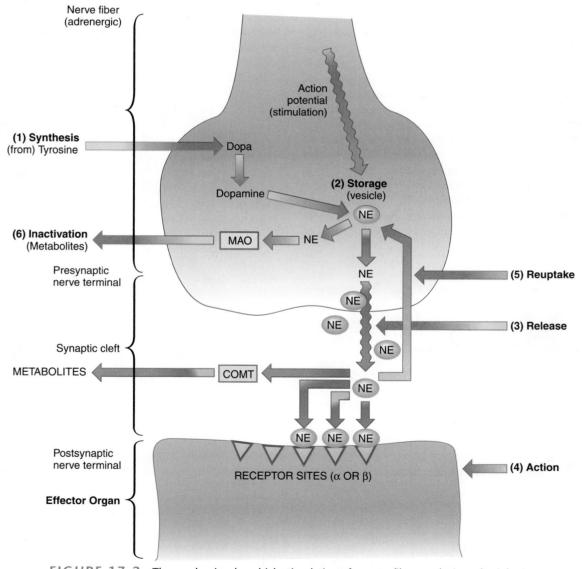

FIGURE 17-2   The mechanism by which stimulation of a nerve fiber results in a physiologic process; adrenergic drugs mimic this same process. *COMT,* Catechol ortho-methyltransferase; *MAO,* monoamine oxidase; *NE,* norepinephrine.

ADRENERGIC DRUGS

Drugs with effects that are similar to or mimic the effects of the SNS neurotransmitters norepinephrine, epinephrine, and dopamine are referred to as adrenergics. As mentioned previously, these neurotransmitters are known as *catecholamines*. This term also refers to adrenergic drugs that have a basic chemical structure similar to that of norepinephrine, epinephrine, or dopamine. Catecholamines produce a sympathomimetic response and are either endogenous substances such as epinephrine, norepinephrine, and dopamine or synthetic substances such as dobutamine, and phenylephrine.

Catecholamine drugs that are used therapeutically produce the same result as endogenous catecholamines. When epinephrine, dobutamine, or any of the adrenergic drugs is given, it bathes the area between the nerve and the effector cell (i.e., the synaptic cleft). Once there, the drug has the opportunity to induce a response. This can be accomplished in one of three ways: by direct stimulation, by indirect stimulation, or by a combination of the two.

A direct-acting sympathomimetic binds directly to the receptor and causes a physiologic response (Figure 17-3). Epinephrine is an example of such a drug. An indirect-acting sympathomimetic is an adrenergic drug that, when given, causes the release of the catecholamine from the storage sites *(vesicles)* in the nerve endings, which then binds to the receptors and causes a physiologic response (Figure 17-4). Amphetamine and other related anorexiants are examples of such drugs. A mixed-acting sympathomimetic both directly stimulates the receptor by binding to it and indirectly stimulates the receptor by causing the release of the neurotransmitter stored in vesicles at the nerve endings (Figure 17-5). Ephedrine is an example of a mixed-acting adrenergic drug.

There are also noncatecholamine adrenergic drugs such as phenylephrine, metaproterenol, and albuterol. These are structurally dissimilar to the endogenous catecholamines and generally have a longer duration of action than either the endogenous or synthetic catecholamines.

Catecholamines and noncatecholamines can act to varying degrees at different types of adrenergic receptors depending on the amount of drug administered. Examples of a few of the catecholamines and the dose-specific selectivity of these drugs for various adrenergic receptors are given in Table 17-2. Noncatecholamine drugs show comparable patterns of activity. Although adrenergics work primarily at postganglionic receptors (the receptors that immediately innervate the effector organ, gland, muscle, and so on), they may also work more centrally in the nervous system at the preganglionic sympathetic nerve trunks. The ability to do so depends on the potency of the specific drug and the dose used.

Although adrenergic drugs are classified most technically by their specific receptor activities, they may also be categorized in terms of their clinical effects. For example, phenylephrine is both an α_1-agonist and a vasopressive drug ("pressor"), whereas albuterol is both a β_2-agonist and a bronchodilator. Both classifications are suitable for most clinical purposes. However, it may sometimes be necessary to carefully choose an adrenergic drug with greater selectivity for a particular receptor type to avoid undesired clinical effects. In such a situation, detailed knowledge of the type and degree of receptor selectivity for different drugs may become more important.

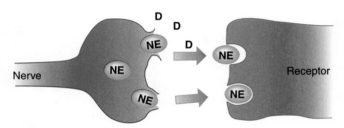

FIGURE 17-4 Mechanism of physiologic response to *indirect-acting* sympathomimetics. *D,* Drug; *NE,* norepinephrine.

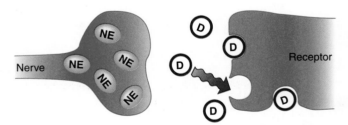

FIGURE 17-3 Mechanism of physiologic response to *direct-acting* sympathomimetics. *D,* Drug; *NE,* norepinephrine.

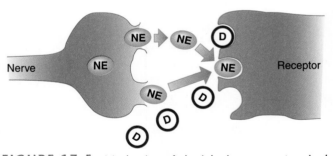

FIGURE 17-5 Mechanism of physiologic response to *mixed-acting* sympathomimetics. *D,* Drug; *NE,* norepinephrine.

Table 17-2 **Catecholamines and Their Dose-Response Relationship**		
Drug	**Dosage**	**Receptor**
dobutamine (Dobutrex)	Maintenance: 2-15 mcg/kg/min	$\beta_1 \gg \beta_2 > \alpha_1$
	High: 40 mcg/kg/min	
dopamine (Intropin)	Low: 0.5-2 mcg/kg/min	Dopaminergic
	Moderate: 2-4 or less than 10 mcg/kg/min	β_1
	High: 20-30 mcg/kg/min	α_1
epinephrine (Adrenalin)	Low: 1-4 mcg/min	$\beta_1 > \beta_2 \gg \alpha_1$
	High: 4-40 mcg/min	$\alpha_1 \geq \beta_1$

Mechanism of Action and Drug Effects

To fully understand the mechanism of action of adrenergics, one must have a working knowledge of normal adrenergic transmission, which takes place at the junction between the nerve (postganglionic sympathetic neuron) and the receptor site of the innervated organ or tissue (effector). The process of SNS stimulation is illustrated in Figure 17-2 and was discussed earlier in this chapter. When adrenergic drugs stimulate α_1-adrenergic receptor sites located on smooth muscles, vasoconstriction most commonly occurs. Many structures of the body are covered by smooth muscles with α_1-adrenergic receptors on them. The binding of adrenergic drugs to these α_1-adrenergic receptors on the smooth muscle of blood vessels, for instance, causes smooth muscle contraction that results in vasoconstriction. However, such drug binding can also cause the relaxation of GI smooth muscle, contraction of the uterus and bladder, male ejaculation, decreased insulin release, and contraction of the ciliary muscles of the eye, which causes the pupils to dilate (see Table 17-1). Stimulation of α_2-adrenergic receptors, on the other hand, actually tends to reverse sympathetic activity but is not of great significance either physiologically or pharmacologically.

There are β_1-adrenergic receptors on the myocardium and in the conduction system of the heart, including the sinoatrial node and the atrioventricular node. When these β_1-adrenergic receptors are stimulated by an adrenergic drug, three things result: (1) an increase in the force of contraction (**positive inotropic effect**), (2) an increase in heart rate (**positive chronotropic effect**), and (3) an increase in the conduction of cardiac electrical nerve impulses through the atrioventricular node (**positive dromotropic effect**). Activation of β_2-adrenergic receptors produces relaxation of the bronchi (bronchodilation) and uterus. Stimulation β_2-adrenergic receptors also causes increased glycogenolysis in the liver and an increase in renin secretion in the kidneys (see Table 17-1).

Indications

Adrenergics, or sympathomimetics, are employed in the treatment of a wide variety of illnesses and conditions. Their selectivity for either α- or β-adrenergic receptors and their affinity for certain tissues or organs determine the settings in which they are most commonly used. Some adrenergics are used as adjuncts to dietary changes in the short-term treatment of obesity. These drugs are discussed in greater detail in Chapter 16.

Respiratory Indications

Certain adrenergic drugs have an affinity for the adrenergic receptors located in the respiratory system and are classified as bronchodilators. They tend to preferentially stimulate the β_2-adrenergic receptors rather than the α-adrenergic receptors and cause bronchodilation. Of the two subtypes of β-adrenergic receptors, these adrenergic drugs are predominantly attracted more to the β_2-adrenergic receptors on the bronchial, uterine, and vascular smooth muscles than to the β_1-adrenergic receptors on the heart. These drugs are helpful in treating conditions such as asthma and bronchitis. Some common bronchodilators that are classified as predominantly β_2-selective adrenergic drugs include albuterol, bitolterol, ephedrine, epinephrine, formoterol, isoetharine, levalbuterol, metaproterenol, pirbuterol, salmeterol, and terbutaline. These drugs are discussed further in Chapter 36.

Indications for Topical Nasal Decongestants

The intranasal application of certain adrenergics can cause the constriction of dilated arterioles and a reduction in nasal blood flow, which thus decreases congestion. These adrenergic drugs work by stimulating α_1-adrenergic receptors and have little or no effect on β-adrenergic receptors. The nasal decongestants include epinephrine, ephedrine, naphazoline, oxymetazoline, phenylephrine, and tetrahydrozoline. They are discussed further in Chapter 35.

Ophthalmic Indications

In another topical application, some adrenergics are applied to the surface of the eye. These drugs are called **ophthalmics,** and they work in much the same way as nasal decongestants except that they affect the vasculature of the eye. When administered, they stimulate α-adrenergic receptors located on small arterioles in the eye and temporarily relieve conjunctival congestion by causing arteriolar vasoconstriction. The ophthalmic adrenergics include epinephrine, naphazoline, phenylephrine, and tetrahydrozoline.

Adrenergics can also be used to reduce intraocular pressure and dilate the pupils (**mydriasis),** properties that make them useful in the treatment of open-angle glaucoma. They accomplish these tasks by stimulating α- or β_2-adrenergic receptors, or both. The two adrenergics used for this purpose are epinephrine and dipivefrin. Ocular adrenergic drugs are discussed further in Chapter 58.

Cardiovascular Indications

The final group of adrenergics are sometimes referred to as *vasoactive sympathomimetics, vasoconstrictive drugs* (also known as vasopressive drugs, pressor drugs, or pressors), *inotropes,* or *cardioselective sympathomimetics* because they are used to support the cardiovascular system during cardiac failure or shock. These drugs have a variety of effects on the various α- and β-adrenergic receptors, and these effects can also be related to the specific dose of the adrenergic drug. Common vasoactive adrenergic drugs include dobutamine, dopamine, ephedrine, epinephrine, fenoldopam, metaraminol, methoxamine, norepinephrine, and phenylephrine.

Contraindications

The only usual contraindications to the use of adrenergic drugs are known drug allergy and severe hypertension.

Adverse Effects

Some of the most common unwanted CNS effects of the α-adrenergic drugs are headache, restlessness, excitement, insomnia, and euphoria. Possible cardiovascular adverse effects of the α-adrenergics include chest pain, vasoconstriction, hypertension, tachycardia, and palpitations or dysrhythmias. Effects on other body systems include anorexia, or loss of appetite; dry mouth; nausea; vomiting; and, rarely, taste changes.

The β-adrenergic drugs can adversely stimulate the CNS, causing mild tremors, headache, nervousness, and dizziness. These drugs can also have unwanted effects on the cardiovascular system, including increased heart rate (positive chronotropy), palpitations (dysrhythmias), and fluctuations in blood pressure. Other significant effects include sweating, nausea, vomiting, and

Life Span Considerations: The Elderly Patient
Use of β-Adrenergic Agonists

- Several physiologic changes occur in the cardiovascular system of the older individual. These changes include a decline in the efficiency and contractile ability of the heart muscle and a decrease in cardiac output and stroke volume. In most cases, the older adult adjusts to these changes without too much difficulty; however, if unusual demands are placed on this aging heart, problems and complications may arise. Unusual demands may occur with strenuous activities, excess stress, heat, and medication use. Therefore, when drugs are given that lead to changes in blood pressure, as with the β-adrenergics, the elderly patient may react negatively with either very high or very low blood pressure.
- Baroreceptors do not work as effectively in the elderly patient either. Reduced baroreceptor activity may lead to orthostatic hypotension even without medication adverse effects.
- Because of the possible presence of other medical conditions such as hypertension, peripheral vascular disease, and cardiovascular and/or cerebrovascular disease, the elderly patient must be monitored carefully before, during, and after administration of adrenergic drugs.
- An elderly patient, as well as a patient of any age, should immediately report the occurrence of any chest pain, palpitations, blurred vision, headache, seizures, or hallucinations to the physician or health care provider.
- Cautious use of OTC drugs, herbals, supplements, and other medications is recommended. This caution is due to polypharmacy, possible drug-drug interactions as well as the elderly person's increased sensitivity to many drugs and other products.
- Vital signs, especially blood pressure and pulse rate, should be monitored frequently and as needed when the patient is taking any of the adrenergic drugs because of their cardiovascular and cerebrovascular effects.
- The elderly often have decreased motor and cognitive functioning. Therefore, use of additional equipment and certain facilitating aids as well as provision of special instructions are needed to help ensure proper dosing of medications.

muscle cramps. See the Life Span Considerations box on this page for additional information.

Toxicity and Management of Overdose

The toxic effects of adrenergic drugs are mainly an extension of their common adverse effects (e.g., seizures from excessive CNS stimulation, hypotension or hypertension, dysrhythmias, palpitation, nervousness, dizziness, fatigue, malaise, insomnia, headache, tremor, dry mouth, and nausea). The two most life-threatening toxic effects involve the CNS and cardiovascular system. In the acute setting, seizures can be effectively managed with diazepam. Intracranial bleeding can also occur, often as the result of an extreme elevation in blood pressure. Such elevated blood pressure poses the risk of hemorrhage not only in the brain but elsewhere in the body as well. The best and most effective treatment in this situation is to lower the blood pressure using a rapid-acting sympatholytic drug (e.g., esmolol; Chapter 18). This can directly reverse the adrenergic-induced state.

Many adrenergic drugs are either synthetic analogues of the naturally occurring neurotransmitters (norepinephrine, epinephrine, and dopamine) or the actual endogenous adrenergic compounds. The majority of these compounds have very short half-

lives, and thus their effects are relatively short lived. Therefore, when these drugs are taken in overdose or signs and symptoms of toxicity develop, reversing the adverse effects takes a relatively short time. Stopping the drug should quickly cause the toxic symptoms to subside. The recommended treatment for overdose is often managing the symptoms and supporting the patient. If death occurs, it is usually the result of either respiratory failure or cardiac arrest. The treatment of overdose should be aimed at supporting these two body systems.

Interactions

The drug interactions that potentially can occur with adrenergic drugs are significant. Although many of the interactions result only in a diminished adrenergic effect because of direct antagonism at and competition for receptor sites, some reactions can be life threatening. The following are some of the more serious drug-drug interactions involving adrenergic drugs: When α- and β-adrenergic drugs are given with adrenergic antagonists (e.g., some classes of antihypertensive drugs), the drugs directly antagonize each other, which results in reduced therapeutic effects. Administration of adrenergics with anesthetic drugs or digoxin can cause increased risk of cardiac dysrhythmias. Tricyclic antidepressants, when given with adrenergics, can cause increased vasopressor effects, acute hypertensive crisis, and possibly respiratory depression. Administration of adrenergic drugs with MAO inhibitors can cause a possibly life-threatening hypertensive crisis. Antihistamines and thyroid preparations can also increase the effects of adrenergic drugs.

Laboratory Test Interactions

The α-adrenergic drugs can cause the serum levels of endogenous corticotropin (i.e., adrenocorticotropic hormone), corticosteroids, and glucose to be increased. Therefore, these laboratory test results should be interpreted with caution in patients receiving any of these medications.

Dosages

For the recommended dosages of various adrenergic drugs, see the Dosages tables on pages 276 and 277.

Drug Profiles

Adrenergics are used in the treatment of a variety of illnesses, and there are many indications for their use. Their selectivity for either α- or β-adrenergic receptors and their affinity for various tissues or organs define the settings in which they are most commonly used. Four frequently used therapeutic classes of adrenergic drugs are the bronchodilators (see Chapter 36), the ophthalmic drugs (see Chapter 58), nasal decongestants (see Chapter 35), and vasoactive drugs, which are emphasized in this chapter and in Chapter 23. It should be noted that receptor selectivity for the α_1, β_1, and β_2 receptor subtypes is *relative* (as opposed to *absolute*). Thus, there may be some overlap of drug effects between the different adrenergic classes of drugs, especially at higher dosages.

Bronchodilators

The bronchodilating adrenergic drugs act primarily to stimulate β_2-adrenergic receptors. They are very effective as antiasthmatic drugs and are used in the treatment of acute attacks because of their rapid onset of action and efficacy. Ephedrine and epinephrine also possess α-adrenergic activity. Although most of these drugs are prescription-only medications, a few are available over the counter (OTC).

DOSAGES

Selected Bronchodilators

Drug	Pharmacologic Class	Usual Dosage Range	Indications
albuterol (Proventil, Ventolin, others)	β-adrenergic agonist (β₂ predominant)	**Adult and pediatric older than 4 yr** MDI (inhalation aerosol): 1-2 puffs q4-6h **Pediatric 2-6 yr** PO syrup: 0.1-0.2 mg/kg tid, max 4 mg tid **Pediatric 6-14 yr** PO syrup: 2 mg tid-qid **Adult and pediatric older than 14 yr** PO syrup: 2-4 mg tid-qid **Adult and pediatric 12 yr and older** PO tabs: 2-4 mg tid-qid, max 32 mg/day **Pediatric 6-12 yr** PO tabs: 2 mg tid-qid, max 24 mg/day **Adult and pediatric 12 yr and older** Inhalation solution (via nebulizer device): 2.5 mg tid-qid diluted in 2.5 mL sterile NS **Pediatric 2-12 yr** Inhalation solution (via nebulizer device): Starting dose 0.1-0.15 mg/kg, max 2.5 mg tid-qid	
epinephrine (Primatene, Bronkaid, others)	Adrenergic agonist (α₁, β₁, β₂)	**Adult only** Inhaler: Dosage individualized starting at first symptoms of bronchospasm **Adult and pediatric 4 yr and older** Inhalation solution: 0.5 mL of racemic epinephrine diluted in 3 mL sterile water, up to q3h	
formoterol (Foradil)	β-adrenergic agonist (β₂ predominant)	**Adult and pediatric 5 yr and older** Inhalation capsule: 12 mcg q12h	Bronchodilation
isoetharine (Arm-a-Med)	β-adrenergic agonist (β₂ predominant)	**Adult only** Aerosol: 1-2 inhalations (340-680 mcg) q4h or more Solution: 0.25-0.5 mL of 1% solution diluted 1:3 with NS by oxygen aerosolization or IPPB; or 3-7 inhalations of undiluted 1% solution by hand nebulizer; consult package insert for percent solutions dosages	
	β-adrenergic agonist (β₂ predominant)	**Adult only** IV: 0.01 to 0.02 mg of diluted solution; repeated as needed to control bronchospasm occurring while under anesthesia	
levalbuterol (Xopenex)	β-adrenergic agonist (β₂ predominant)	**Adult and pediatric 12 yr and older** Inhalation solution: 0.63 mg tid-qid to 1.25 mg tid via nebulization	
salmeterol (Serevent)	β-adrenergic agonist (β₂ predominant)	**Adult and pediatric 12 yr and older** Inhalation aerosol: 2 inhalations q12h **Adult and pediatric 4 yr and older** Inhalation powder: 1 inhalation q12h	
terbutaline (Brethine, Brethaire, Bricanyl)	β-adrenergic agonist (β₂ predominant)	**Adult and pediatric 15 yr and older** PO tabs: 2.5 mg tid-qid up to 5 mg tid (q6h), max 15 mg/day **Pediatric 12-15 yr** PO tabs: 2.5 mg tid max Injection: 0.25 mg SC into lateral deltoid area; may repeat × 1 in 15-30 min, max 0.5 mg in 4 hr	

IPPB, Intermittent positive pressure breathing; *MDI*, metered-dose inhaler; *NS*, normal saline; *PO*, oral; *SC*, subcutaneous.

Activation of β₂-adrenergic receptors causes the bronchi to dilate. The selective β₂-adrenergics are the preferred bronchodilators because they produce fewer cardiac-related adverse effects (e.g., tachycardia) than the nonselective or β₁-selective β-adrenergic drugs. These drugs are available in oral, aerosol, and injection forms. Common dosages for selected bronchodilators appear in the table on this page.

▶ albuterol sulfate
Albuterol (Proventil, Ventolin, Volmax) is a selective β₂-adrenergic bronchodilator. Its use is contraindicated in patients with a known hypersensitivity to it. It can be administered orally and by inhalation.

It is available in a metered-dose inhaler and as 2- and 4-mg tablets, as well as extended-release tablets, oral syrup, inhalation solution, and inhalation capsules. Pregnancy category C. See the table on this page for the most common dosages.

Pharmacokinetics

Half-Life	Onset	Peak	Duration
PO: 4 hr	PO: 30 min	PO: 2.5 hr	PO: 6-8 hr
Inhaled: 4 hr	Inhaled: 5-15 min	Inhaled: 1-1.5 hr	Inhaled: 4-6 hr

▶ *epinephrine*

Epinephrine (Adrenalin) is a naturally occurring catecholamine produced by the adrenal medulla. It is a very potent mixed α- and β-adrenergic drug that produces vasoconstriction, increased blood pressure, cardiac stimulation, and dilation of the bronchioles. It is the drug of choice for the relief of acute asthma attacks and for the treatment of anaphylaxis. In addition, epinephrine is used to treat open-angle glaucoma, to restore cardiac rhythm in cardiac arrest, and to control bleeding in surgical procedures. It is also used as an ophthalmic drug and a nasal decongestant and is administered to prolong the activity of infiltrated local anesthetics. Its use is contraindicated in several conditions, including hypersensitivity, narrow-angle glaucoma, shock due to trauma, general anesthesia with halogenated drugs, coronary insufficiency, and labor. In addition, its administration with local anesthetics to the toes or fingers is not recommended, because distal circulation may be excessively decreased due to its vasoconstricting properties and the patient may be placed at risk for tissue necrosis (gangrene) and amputation. For those OTC products that contain epinephrine, such as Primatene Mist, cautious (if any) use is recommended because of the potential CNS stimulation and subsequent adverse effects, as well as the potential for drug dependency. Pregnancy category C. See the table on page 275 for selected dosage information.

Pharmacokinetics

Half-Life	Onset	Peak	Duration
SC: Variable (min)	SC: 5-10 min	SC: 20 min	SC: 4 hr
PO inhaled/IV: Variable (min)	PO inhaled/IV: 1 min	PO inhaled/IV: Less than 30 min	

▶ *salmeterol*

Salmeterol (Serevent) is a β$_2$-agonist indicated for long-term maintenance treatment of asthma, prevention of bronchospasm, and prevention of exercise-induced bronchospasm. It is not indicated for acute exacerbations of asthma or bronchospasms. Its use is contraindicated in patients with known hypersensitivity to salmeterol. It is available in a 25-mcg/dose aerosol inhaler and a 50-mcg/dose powder inhalation device. Pregnancy category C. Recommended dosages are given in the table on page 275. Salmeterol is also available in a combination product with fluticasone (Advair Diskus) (Chapter 36).

Pharmacokinetics

Half-Life	Onset	Peak	Duration
5.5 hr	10-20 min	3 hr	12 hr

Nasal Decongestants

The sympathomimetic drugs used as nasal decongestants consist of both α- and α–β-adrenergic drugs. The α-adrenergic activity of these drugs is responsible for causing vasoconstriction in the nasal mucosa. This produces shrinkage of the mucosa, which promotes easier nasal breathing and reduces nasal secretions. However, excessive use of nasal decongestants can lead to greater congestion because of a rebound phenomenon that occurs when use of the product is stopped. This rebound effect is not seen with the oral drugs. The decongestants are administered topically as nasal drops or sprays, which are instilled into each nostril. The ephedrine salts, phenylephrine hydrochloride, and pseudoephedrine can produce nasal decongestion when taken either as single therapy or in combination with other drugs, such as in allergy, cold, cough, and sinus relief preparations. Phenylephrine is usually administered via intranasal spray for this purpose, whereas pseudoephedrine is taken orally.

Relative contraindications to the use of the nasal decongestants are the same for all of these drugs and include hypersensitivity, diabetes, hypertension, thyroid disorders, and enlargement of the prostate gland. With routine use, adverse effects due to systemic absorption of nasally administered decongestants are usually minimal. However, all practitioners should be aware of the possibility of systemic adverse effects and educate patients accordingly if they are prescribed these drugs.

▶ *pseudoephedrine*

Pseudoephedrine (Sudafed, Afrin) is a natural plant alkaloid that is obtained from the ephedra plant. It is a stereoisomer of ephedrine and is a widely used oral decongestant. Actual ephedra products were banned by the FDA in 2004 due to severe adverse cardiovascular events. Pseudoephedrine is available in infant oral drops, oral solution, and tablet form. Some dosage forms are available OTC without prescription. Pregnancy category C. See the table on this page for recommended dosages.

Pharmacokinetics

Half-Life	Onset	Peak	Duration
Variable (min)	15-30 min	30-60 min	4-6 hr SR: 8-12 hr

SR, Sustained release.

Ophthalmic Decongestants

Ophthalmic decongestants are adrenergics that are applied topically to the eye. When instilled into the eye, they stimulate α-adrenergic receptors located on the small arterioles in the eye. This results in arteriolar vasoconstriction, which reduces conjunctival congestion and thus decreases redness in the eye. Although epinephrine, phenylephrine, and naphazoline are all used as ophthalmic decongestants, tetrahydrozoline is the drug most widely used.

tetrahydrozoline

Tetrahydrozoline (Murine, Visine) is applied topically to the eye to temporarily relieve congestion, itching, and minor irritation in patients with red and irritated eyes. It causes constriction of the blood

DOSAGES

Selected Nasal and Ophthalmic Decongestant Adrenergics

Drug	Pharmacologic Class	Usual Dosage Range	Indications
▶pseudoephedrine (Sudafed, Afrin, PediaCare Drops, others)	α–β-adrenergic	**Adult** PO tabs: 60 mg q4-6h, max 240 mg/day **Pediatric 6-12 yr** PO tabs: 30 mg q4-6h, max 120 mg/day **Pediatric 2-5 yr** PO tabs: 15 mg q4-6h, max 60 mg/day **Pediatric 1-2 yr** PO: 7 drops (0.2 mL)/kg q4-6h, max qid **Pediatric 3-12 mo** PO: 3 drops/kg q4-6h, max qid	Nasal decongestant
tetrahydrozoline (Tyzine, Tyzine Pediatric)	α-adrenergic	1-2 drops into eye(s) up to qid	Ophthalmic decongestant

PO, Oral

vessels of the eye and is sometimes also used during diagnostic eye procedures. It is the active ingredient in such OTC products as Visine, and Murine Plus eyedrops. Its use is contraindicated in patients with a hypersensitivity reaction to it and in those with narrow-angle glaucoma. Pregnancy category C. The recommended dosages are given in the table on page 276.

Pharmacokinetics

Half-Life	Onset	Peak	Duration
Variable (min)	Less than 3 min	Short (min)	4-8 hr

Vasoactive Adrenergics

Adrenergics that have primarily cardioselective effects are referred to as *vasoactive adrenergics*. They are used to support a failing heart or to treat shock. They may also be used to treat orthostatic hypotension. These drugs have a wide range of effects on α- and β-adrenergic receptors, depending on the dosage. The vasoactive adrenergics are very potent, quick-acting, injectable drugs. Although dosage recommendations are given in the table on this page, all of these drugs are titrated to the desired physiologic response. All of the vasoactive adrenergics (with the exception of midodrine) are rapid in onset, and their effects very quickly cease when administration is stopped. Therefore, careful titration and monitoring of vital signs and electrocardiogram (ECG) are required in patients receiving them.

▶ dobutamine

Dobutamine (Dobutrex) is a β_1-selective vasoactive adrenergic drug that is structurally similar to the naturally occurring catecholamine dopamine. Through stimulation of the β_1 receptors on heart muscle (myocardium), it increases cardiac output by increasing contractility (positive inotropy), which increases the stroke volume, especially in patients with heart failure. Dobutamine is available only as an intravenous injectable drug. Pregnancy category B. The recommended dosages are listed in the table on this page.

Pharmacokinetics

Half-Life	Onset	Peak	Duration
2-5 min	Less than 2 min	Less than 10 min	Less than 10 min

▶ dopamine

Dopamine (Intropin) is a naturally occurring catecholamine neurotransmitter in the SNS. It has potent dopaminergic and β_1- and α_1-adrenergic receptor activity, depending on the dosage. Dopamine, when used at low dosages, can dilate blood vessels in the brain, heart, kidneys, and mesentery, which increases blood flow to these areas (dopaminergic receptor activity). At higher infusion rates dopamine can improve cardiac contractility and output (β_1-adrenergic receptor activity). Use of the drug is contraindicated in patients who have a catecholamine-secreting tumor of the adrenal gland known as a *pheochromocytoma*. The drug is available only as an intravenous injectable drug. Pregnancy category C. The recommended vasoactive dosages are given in the table on this page.

Pharmacokinetics

Half-Life	Onset	Peak	Duration
Less than 2 min	2-5 min	Rapid	10 min

DOSAGES

Selected Vasoactive Adrenergics

Drug	Pharmacologic Class	Usual Dosage Range	Indications
▶dobutamine (Dobutrex)	β_1-adrenergic	**Pediatric** IV infusion: 2.5-15 mcg/kg/min **Adult** IV infusion: 2.5-40 mcg/kg/min	Cardiac decompensation
▶dopamine (Intropin)	β_1-adrenergic	**Adult and pediatric** IV infusion: 1-50 mcg/kg/min	Shock syndrome, cardiopulmonary arrest
▶epinephrine (Adrenalin)	α–β-adrenergic	**Pediatric** SC: 10 mcg/kg repeated q15min × 2 then q4h prn **Adult** SC: 0.1-0.5 mg repeated q10-15min if required **Neonatal** IV: 10-30 mcg/kg q3-5min if required **Pediatric** IV: 10 mcg/kg q3-5min if required **Adult** IV: 0.5-1 mg q3-5min if required	Anaphylaxis, cardiopulmonary arrest
fenoldopam (Corlopam)	D_1 agonist	**Adult only** IV: 0.1-1.6 mcg/kg/min for up to 48 hr	Hypertensive emergency in hospital setting
midodrine (ProAmatine)	α_1-adrenergic	**Adult only** PO: 10 mg tid (q3-4h when awake), max 40 mg/day	Orthostatic hypotension
▶norepinephrine (Levophed)	α–β-adrenergic	**Pediatric** IV infusion: 0.05-1 mcg/kg/min **Adult** IV infusion: 4-20 mcg/min	Hypotensive states
phenylephrine (Neo-Synephrine)	α-adrenergic	**Pediatric** (for hypotension during spinal anesthesia) SC/IM: 0.1 mg/kg/dose **Adult** IV infusion: 10 mg/250 or 500 mL IV solution, start at 100-180 mcg/min and titrate down to 40-60 mcg/min IM/SC: 2-5 mg IV: 0.1-0.5 mg	Hypotension, paroxysmal supraventricular tachycardia

IM, Intramuscular; *IV,* intravenous; *PO,* oral; *SC,* subcutaneous.

▶ *epinephrine*

Epinephrine (Adrenalin) is also an endogenous vasoactive catecholamine. It acts directly on both the α- and β-adrenergic receptors of tissues innervated by the SNS. It is used in emergency situations and is one of the primary vasoactive drugs used in many advanced cardiac life support protocols. The physiologic response it elicits is dose related. At low dosages it stimulates mostly β_1-adrenergic receptors, increasing the force of contraction and heart rate. It is also used to treat anaphylactic shock at these dosages because it has significant bronchodilatory effects via the β_2-adrenergic receptors in the lungs. At high dosages (e.g., intravenous drip), it stimulates mostly α-adrenergic receptors, causing vasoconstriction, which elevates the blood pressure. Pregnancy category C. The dosages recommended for the treatment of various disorders are given in the table on page 277.

Pharmacokinetics

Half-Life	Onset	Peak	Duration
Less than 5 min	Less than 2 min	Rapid	5-30 min

fenoldopam

Fenoldopam (Corlopam) is a peripheral dopamine 1 (D_1) agonist indicated for parenteral use in lowering blood pressure. Fenoldopam produces its blood pressure–lowering effects by inducing arteriolar vasodilation mainly through stimulation of D_1 receptors. It appears to be as effective as sodium nitroprusside for short-term treatment of severe hypertension and may have beneficial effects on renal function because it increases renal blood flow. It is available as a 10-mg/mL injection. Pregnancy category B. Recommended dosages are given in the table on page 277.

Pharmacokinetics

Half-Life	Onset	Peak	Duration
Longer than 5 min	5 min	20 min	10 min

midodrine

Midodrine (ProAmatine) is a prodrug converted to its active form, desglymidodrine, in the liver. It is this active metabolite that is responsible for the primary pharmacologic action of midodrine, which is α_1-adrenergic receptor stimulation. This α_1 stimulation causes constriction of both arterioles and veins, resulting in peripheral vasoconstriction. Midodrine is primarily indicated for the treatment of symptomatic orthostatic hypotension. Midodrine is available as 2.5- and 5-mg tablets. Pregnancy category C. Common dosages are given in the table on page 277.

Pharmacokinetics

Half-Life	Onset	Peak	Duration
Longer than 3-4 hr	45-90 min	1 hr	6-8 hr

▶ *norepinephrine*

Norepinephrine (Levophed) acts predominantly by directly stimulating α-adrenergic receptors, which leads to vasoconstriction. It also has some direct-stimulating β-adrenergic effects on the heart (β_1-adrenergic receptors) but none on the lung (β_2-adrenergic receptors). Norepinephrine is directly metabolized to dopamine and is used primarily in the treatment of hypotension and shock. Pregnancy category D. Common dosages are given in the table on page 277.

Pharmacokinetics

Half-Life	Onset	Peak	Duration
Less than 5 min	Immediate	1-2 min	1-2 min

phenylephrine

Phenylephrine (Neo-Synephrine) works almost exclusively on the α-adrenergic receptors. It is used primarily for short-term treatment to augment blood pressure in patients in shock, to control some dysrhythmias (supraventricular tachycardias), and to produce vasoconstriction in regional anesthesia. It is also administered topically as an ophthalmic drug and as a nasal decongestant. Common vasoactive dosages are listed in the table on page 277.

Pharmacokinetics

Half-Life	Onset	Peak	Duration
IV: Less than 5 min	IV: Immediate	IV: Rapid	IV: 15-20 min

◆ NURSING PROCESS

◆ ASSESSMENT

Adrenergic drugs have a variety of effects depending on the receptors they stimulate. Stimulation of the α-adrenergic receptors results in vasoconstriction of blood vessels. Stimulation of the β_1-adrenergic receptors produces cardiac stimulation, and β_2-adrenergic receptor stimulation results in bronchodilation. Because of these properties, especially the cardiac stimulation effects, use of adrenergic agonists requires careful patient assessment and monitoring to maximize therapeutic effects and minimize possible adverse effects.

A thorough patient assessment, including a health history and medication history with a listing of drug allergies, medications routinely used, and OTC drugs and herbals used, should be completed before any drug is administered. Other important assessment questions to pose include the following:

- Are there allergies to any medications, foods, topical products, environmental products, or other substance?
- Does the patient have asthma? If so, how frequent and severe are the attacks and what are factors that exacerbate the attacks and help them? Are there any other signs and symptoms besides bronchospasms, wheezing, or dyspnea (shortness of breath)? What previous treatments for asthma have been tried? Any successes or failures?
- Is there any history of transient ischemic attacks? Any history of cerebrovascular accident, stroke, hypertension, hypotension, cardiac irregularities, or other cardiovascular disease?

Assessment of renal and hepatic functioning is important before initiating treatment, especially in high-risk patients such as the elderly, because if the drugs cannot be excreted or metabolized properly then adverse effects and toxicity may occur. Assessment of cardiac functioning is also important because of the cardiac stimulation associated with these drugs. Adrenergic drugs may cause tachycardia, hypertension, myocardial infarction, or heart failure, so these drugs should be given cautiously or not at all in patients who are at risk for possible worsening of preexisting disease states or symptoms.

Baseline vital signs should be assessed (e.g., blood pressure, postural blood pressures, pulse rate, temperature, respiratory rate), with further specific attention given to peripheral pulses, skin color, and capillary refill (and with findings documented). Specific to the use of midodrine is the assessment of postural blood pressures and pulse rates (supine, sitting, and standing, as ordered) before and during drug administration. This should be done for short- and/or long-term use of this drug for the management of postural hypotension and accompanied with assessment of other problems such as dizziness, lightheadedness, and syncope. Assessment of the patient's symptoms and his or her perception of either disease progression or a decrease in symptoms is very important for effective and successful treatment.

With other adrenergic drugs, such as those used for broncho-dilating effects, the following parameters should be assessed more closely: respiratory status with breath sounds (normal and adventitious); respiratory rate, depth, and pattern; occurrence of difficulty in breathing; activity or exercise tolerance or intolerance; and pulse oximetry readings. Use of a peak flow respiratory meter and measurement of anterior-posterior diameter of the chest wall (increased in chronic lung disorders such as emphysema) may also be part of the assessment process. Physicians may order other respiratory function studies and measurement of arterial blood gas levels, as deemed necessary. Cautions, contraindications, life span considerations, and drug interactions should always be assessed prior to use of these and other drugs in this chapter (see the previous discussion on each drug and its related profile and dosage table). In addition, some of these drugs are used only for acute episodes of asthma, whereas other drugs are used year-round as preventative drugs. For example, the drug salmeterol is *not* used to treat acute attacks. In addition, the elderly may react to these drugs with increased sensitivity, which requires close assessment.

Epinephrine and similar drugs are used for their cardiac, bronchial, antiallergic, ophthalmic, and vasopressor effects. Assessment should focus on vital signs, breath sounds, arterial blood gas levels, and ECG findings. Liver and renal function test results also need to be assessed and documented. In addition, each system related to the specific action of the drug (e.g., respiratory system and bronchodilation) must also be assessed.

Overall, adrenergic drugs work in similar ways, but individual drugs may have some differences with regard to action, indications, and overall considerations. If the overall class of drugs and the way in which they work is known, however, then their related assessment parameters, cautions, contraindications, drug interactions, and life span–related considerations are easy to determine. If the drug is a pure adrenergic agonist, the net effect is stimulation of α-adrenergic receptors with vasoconstriction of blood vessels and subsequent elevation of blood pressure and heart rate. The nurse would then know to expect specific effects from the drug as well as to anticipate certain adverse effects. The drug may be used for the therapeutic effect of increased blood pressure, but an unwanted adverse effect could then be a hypertensive crisis. If the drug is a β-adrenergic agonist, it will stimulate both β_1 and β_2 receptors, which will lead to cardiac stimulation and bronchodilation. This β_1 action can also result in too much stimulation with severe tachycardia and possibly chest pain if coronary artery disease is present. Thus, by simply knowing the actions of a given drug, the nurse can draw conclusions about, anticipate, and be very alert to the drug's therapeutic action, adverse effects, cautions, contraindications, drug interactions, and toxicity.

◆ NURSING DIAGNOSES

- Decreased cardiac output related to cardiovascular adverse effects of these drugs
- Ineffective tissue perfusion related to intense vasoconstrictive reactions
- Acute pain related to adverse effects of tachycardia and palpitations
- Deficient knowledge regarding therapeutic regimen, adverse effects, drug interactions, and precautions related to the use of adrenergic drugs

- Risk for injury related to possible adverse effects (nervousness, vertigo, hypertension, or tremors) or to potential drug interactions
- Disturbed sleep patterns related to CNS stimulation caused by adrenergic drugs
- Noncompliance with drug therapy related to lack of information about the importance of taking the medication as ordered

◆ PLANNING

Goals

- Patient's symptoms improve because of the drug's therapeutic effects.
- Patient takes the drugs as ordered and follows directions explicitly.
- Patient remains compliant with the drug therapy regimen.
- Patient demonstrates adequate knowledge about the use of the specific medications.

Outcome Criteria

- Patient shows improvement in the disease process or condition for which the medication was given with subsequent decrease in the signs and symptoms of cardiac and/or respiratory problems.
- Patient states the importance of pharmacologic and nonpharmacologic treatment of the respiratory or other conditions that may be present, such as asthma.
- Patient states the importance of compliance with the drug regimen and adherence to the proper dosage of the medication to maximize therapeutic effects and minimize adverse effects.
- Patient experiences minimal adverse effects and complications, such as excessive CNS stimulation, insomnia, tachycardia, chest pain, and tremors.
- Patient states conditions and adverse effects associated with long-term at-home use that should be reported to the physician, such as chest pain, restlessness, and severe insomnia.
- Patient states the importance of scheduling and keeping follow-up appointments with the physician to monitor the effectiveness of drug therapy.

◆ IMPLEMENTATION

There are several nursing interventions that can maximize the therapeutic effects of adrenergic drugs and minimize their adverse effects. The nurse should always check the package inserts concerning dilutional solutions with parenteral dosage forms. For example, subcutaneous administration of the adrenergic agonist epinephrine to patients with asthma requires safe calculations and accurate dosing. A tuberculin syringe may be used with subcutaneous epinephrine may help with accuracy in both adult and pediatric patients.

When intravenous infusions of these drugs are administered for shock-related symptoms (hypotension), drugs such as dopamine will be used. Use of epinephrine and some of the other pure α-adrenergics results in vasoconstriction of the renal vessels and subsequent renal damage or shutdown. Therefore, when any of these drugs are given intravenously, the nurse must be sure to check and must be confident that the drug and dosage route are correct. For dopamine and similar drugs, the IV site should be checked frequently (e.g., every hour, as needed) for infiltration to be sure that the site remains intact and that the proper rate is being infused. Infiltration of an intravenous solution containing an adrenergic drug may lead to tissue necrosis from excessive vascular vasoconstriction around the IV site. Phentolamine is often used for the treatment of infiltration (Chapter 18). Also, with intravenous infusions the nurse must use only clear solutions and a proper dilutional solution and must always administer the drug with an IV infusion pump, with monitoring of the cardiac system. ECG monitoring may also be ordered. All of these drugs should be given per the manufacturer's directions and suggested infusion rates to avoid precipitating dangerously high blood pressure and pulse rate and subsequent complications.

When these drugs are to be administered by an inhaler or nebulizer, patient instruction about correct use, storage, and care of equipment should be complete, thorough, and age-appropriate. The patient also needs to know how to use a spacer correctly, because administration with this device is often ordered. Use of a spacer provides more effective delivery of inhaled doses of drug, but patient education must be thorough and easy to understand

(see Chapter 9 and the Patient Teaching Tips). With dosing of the adrenergics for bronchodilating effects, often two adrenergics are indicated, but because of different medications and actions, one inhaler may be for use in *acute* situations and the other may be for *long-term and/or preventative* use. This type of treatment regimen requires that the patient receive thorough, simple, and complete instructions and explanations about the method of delivery as well as the drugs used. This will help to minimize overdosage and risk of severe adverse effects such as hypertension, severe tachycardia, tremors, and CNS overstimulation.

The nurse must emphasize that these medications are to be used only as prescribed with regard to amount, timing, and spacing of doses. Because of their synergistic effects, when these medications (especially asthmatics) are used in combination with other types of bronchodilators, the patient must be very clear about what to do before, during, and after the dose is delivered. If the patient is taking an inhaled dosage form, he or she may also be taking an oral or parenteral form of the same or a similar drug. The reason for the use of more than one drug of the same drug class and the use of more than one route of administration is to achieve combined therapeutic effects. Patient education deserves extremely close attention with these regimens because of the need to prevent exacerbation of adverse effects, minimize drug interactions, and prevent severe vascular and cardiovascular adverse effects. Patients should immediately report any complaints of chest pain, palpitations, blurred vision, headache, seizures, or hallucinations.

Patients with chronic lung disease who are receiving adrenergic drugs should also avoid anything that may exacerbate their respiratory condition (e.g., food or other allergens, cigarette smoking) and implement measures that may help diminish the risk of respiratory infection. These measures may include avoiding those who are ill with colds and flu, avoiding crowded areas, remaining well nourished and rested, and maintaining fluid intake of up to 3000 mL/day to ensure adequate hydration (unless contraindicated). Keeping a journal of symptoms and any improvement or worsening in their condition while taking the medications may be very helpful.

Salmeterol is not to be used for relief of acute symptoms, and education about its dosing is important. The dosage of salmeterol is usually 2 puffs twice daily 12 hours apart for maintenance effects. For prevention of exercise-induced asthma, it is recommended that patients take 2 puffs $\frac{1}{2}$ to 1 hour before exercise and no additional doses for 12 hours. Always recheck these orders and directions. If another type of inhalant is used, such as a corticosteroid, the bronchodilator should be used first, with a 5-minute waiting period afterward before taking the second drug. All equipment should be rinsed, and the patient should be encouraged to rinse the mouth thoroughly after the use of any inhalant form of medication.

If ophthalmic forms of these drugs are used, the nurse must make sure that the medication has not expired and is also a clear solution. The eyedropper must not be allowed to touch the eye when the drug is applied to help prevent contamination of the remaining solution. With ophthalmic administration, drops and ointments should be applied into the conjunctival sac—not directly onto the eye itself.

Oral midodrine should be taken exactly as prescribed. This medication is usually ordered to be given with forcing of fluids

---

LEGAL AND ETHICAL PRINCIPLES

Infiltrating Intravenous (IV) Infusions

Nurses often encounter an infiltrating IV in the routine care of many of their patients. Every action taken is very important to the standard of care of the patient and in ensuring that the nurse has acted as any prudent nurse would. The assessment and action taken by the nurse can be important for the patient as in the case of *Macon-Bibb Hosp. Authority vs. Ross* (335 S.E. 2d 633-GA).

Situation

Ms. Ross was brought to the emergency department of the hospital with dyspnea, bradycardia, and a blood pressure (BP) of 250/150 mm Hg. She went into respiratory arrest at 2:55 PM; she was intubated with an endotracheal tube, and nitroprusside was administered intravenously to decrease her BP. Because of the rapid drop in BP, an IV administration of dopamine was started at 3:28 PM in her right wrist to increase her BP. When her BP was stable at 4:30 PM, she was transferred to the cardiac care unit. At midnight, a nurse noted that the intravenous catheter site had a "bruise bluish in color." The next notation was at 11:00 AM the following day, in which it was recorded that the patient's right arm was swollen and painful with a large blistered area around the intravenous catheter site. The same notation was made at 4:00 PM. It was not until 6:50 PM that a note indicated that a physician was informed of the infiltration. As a result of the extravasation of dopamine, the patient's lower right arm was permanently scarred. On a jury verdict, the court entered judgment for the patient. The hospital appealed.

The court of appeals affirmed the judgment of the lower court. It was noted that, although an infiltration may result from an improper technique, it may also be due to the size of the needle, the status of the patient's veins, or specific intolerance to an intravenous catheter. However, according to the expert nurse's testimony, supported by suitable references, dopamine should be infused into a "large vein," such as in the antecubital fossa, to minimize the risk for extravasation. In addition, dopamine should be monitored continuously for free flow. If extravasation of dopamine occurs, the recommended treatment of the site is infiltration with a saline solution of phentolamine (Regitine) within 12 hours.

The nurses were criticized for not being sufficiently knowledgeable regarding dopamine, which resulted in their failure to notify a physician of the patient's impaired tissue integrity.

From McKenry LM, Tessier E, Hogan M: *Mosby's pharmacology in nursing,* ed 22, St Louis, 2006, Mosby.

before the patient gets out of bed in the morning. Doses of the drug are also often front loaded in their dosing so that most of the doses occur in the morning when patients with orthostatic intolerance are usually more symptomatic. Patients should avoid taking this medication after 6 PM to prevent insomnia and possible supine hypertension.

◆ EVALUATION

Therapeutic effects of adrenergic drugs include the following. For vasoactive drugs, therapeutic effects include improved cardiac output (with increased urinary output), return to normal vital signs (e.g., blood pressure of 120/80 mm Hg or higher or gradual increases in blood pressure as indicated, pulse rate greater than 60 but less than 120 beats/min), improved skin color (pallor to pink) and temperature (cool to warm) in extremities, improved peripheral pulses, and increased level of consciousness. Therapeutic effects of drugs given for bronchial indications include a return to normal respiratory rate (more than 12 but fewer than 20 breaths/min), improved breath sounds throughout the lung

field with fewer adventitious (abnormal) sounds, increased air exchange in all areas of the lungs, decreased to no coughing, less dyspnea, improved partial pressure of oxygen and pulse oximeter readings, and tolerance of slowly increasing levels of activity. If the drugs are used for nasal congestion, the patient should report less congestion and improved ability to breathe. Therapeutic effects of midodrine include improved level of functioning and performance of the activities of daily living, fewer episodes of postural intolerance (dizziness, lightheadedness, and syncopal episodes), and more energy.

Evaluation for the occurrence of adverse effects with adrenergic drugs includes monitoring for stimulation of the systems that are affected, such as the cardiac system and the CNS. Adverse effects such as cardiac irregularities, hypertension, and tachycardia may occur. The nurse should be sure to monitor for chest pain as well. With the use of nasal decongestants, adverse effects of rebound nasal congestion, rhinitis, and nasal mucosal ulcerations are possible. See page 273 for additional information on adverse effects.

Patient Teaching Tips

- The patient should always take medications as prescribed; excessive dosing may cause CNS and cardiovascular stimulation, including tachycardia and palpitations.
- Be sure the patient is able to self-administer inhaled forms of medication. See Chapter 9 (p. 126) for instructions on using a metered-dose inhaler and a spacer. The patient should be sure to rinse the mouth thoroughly after taking inhaled preparations.
- The patient should report worsening of respiratory symptoms, dyspnea, distress, chest pain and/or cardiac palpitations to the health care provider immediately.
- The patient should not take any other medications (including OTC medications and herbal supplements) without the physician's approval.

- If adrenergic nasal decongestant sprays are used, the phenomenon of rebound nasal congestion may occur with overuse and can be prevented by taking the drug as prescribed.
- Should rebound nasal congestion occur, the patient should follow the instructions given by the physician or health care provider and use saline nasal spray for relief.
- The patient should rinse his or her mouth after each inhalation or use of a nebulizer.
- Mitodrine use requires careful dosing, as ordered and with use of a journal to record adverse effects, improvements in symptoms, or any worsening of symptoms.

Points to Remember

- Catecholamines are substances that produce a sympathomimetic response (stimulate the SNS). The naturally occurring or endogenous catecholamines include epinephrine, norepinephrine, and dopamine. An example of an exogenous catecholamine is dobutamine.
- Nursing considerations regarding the use of adrenergic agonist drugs to treat respiratory disorders include the following:
  - Patients should be taught to avoid respiratory irritants
  - Patients should be instructed to avoid contact with individuals who may have infections to help minimize situations that would exacerbate the original problem
  - Patients should be told to avoid OTCs or prescribed medications because of possible drug interactions with adrenergic agonists.

- With nasal preparations, rebound nasal congestion or ulcerations of the nasal mucosa may occur if drugs are overused; therefore, patients need to be educated to use these products only as directed.
- Midodrine use requires careful blood pressure monitoring, so education about supine blood pressures and journaling of measured blood pressure values is very important to the effective use of the drug.
- Inhaled forms of β-agonists are used for their bronchodilating action and must be taken only as prescribed with caution to avoid any overuse of the drug. Overdosage of these drugs may lead to severe cardiovascular, CNS, and cerebrovascular adverse effects and stimulation.

NCLEX Examination Review Question

1. The nurse caring for a patient who is receiving β-agonist drug therapy needs to be aware that these drugs cause:
   a. Increased cardiac contractility
   b. Decreased heart rate
   c. Bronchoconstriction
   d. Increased GI tract motility
2. During a teaching session for a patient who is receiving inhaled salmeterol, the nurse emphasizes that the drug is indicated for:
   a. Rescue treatment of acute bronchospasms
   b. Prevention of bronchospasm
   c. Reduction of airway inflammation
   d. Long-term treatment of sinus congestion
3. For a patient receiving a vasoactive drug such as intravenous dopamine, which of the following actions by the nurse is most appropriate?
   a. Monitor the gravity drip infusion closely and adjust as needed
   b. Assess the patient's cardiac function by checking the radial pulse
   c. Assess the intravenous site hourly to rule out infiltration
   d. Administer the drug by intravenous boluses according to the patient's blood pressure
4. A patient is receiving dobutamine for a worsening of heart failure. Vital signs yesterday were blood pressure, 150/88; pulse rate, 88 beats/min; respiration rate, 16 breaths/min. Vital signs now are blood pressure, 170/94; pulse rate, 110 beats/min; respiration rate, 20 breaths/min. The patient is now complaining of "chest tightness." Which statement is most appropriate regarding the patient's symptoms?
   a. The changes in vital signs are reflective of a therapeutic response to the drug.
   b. The patient most likely needs a dose of a β-agonist to elevate the heart rate and help with the heart failure.
   c. These changes reflect a need to switch to an oral form of dobutamine.
   d. The presence of chest pain and the changes in vital signs need to be evaluated immediately by the nurse and physician.
5. When a drug is characterized as having a negative chronotropic effect, the nurse knows to expect:
   a. Improved sinoatrial nodal firing
   b. Decreased heart rate
   c. Decreased ectopic beats
   d. Increased force of cardiac contractions

1. a, 2. b, 3. c, 4. d, 5. b.

Critical Thinking Activities

1. Why is it important to carefully assess elderly patients for the presence of medical conditions before administering any β-adrenergic agonist drugs?
2. Discuss the rationale for careful drug titration and monitoring of patients receiving vasoactive adrenergic drugs.
3. A patient has had an infiltration of a dopamine infusion. Describe what effects this may have on the patient and what can be done about it.

For answers, see http://evolve.elsevier.com/Lilley.

Adrenergic-Blocking Drugs

Objectives

When you reach the end of this chapter, you should be able to do the following:

1. Discuss the normal anatomy and physiology of the autonomic nervous system as it pertains to adrenergic-blocking drugs or sympatholytics.
2. List examples of specific drugs categorized as adrenergic antagonists or adrenergic blockers, including α- and β-blockers.
3. Discuss the mechanisms of action, therapeutic effects, indications, adverse and toxic effects, cautions, contraindications, dosages, and routes of administration for the various α-blockers, nonselective β-blockers, and β$_1$- and β$_2$-blockers.
4. Identify the antidotes used in the treatment of adrenergic-blocking drug overdosage.
5. Develop a nursing care plan that includes all phases of the nursing process related to the administration of adrenergic-blocking drugs

e-Learning Activities

Companion CD

- NCLEX Review Questions: see questions 123-133
- Animations
- Audio Glossary
- Category Catchers
- Medication Errors Checklists
- IV Therapy Checklists

evolve Website (http://evolve.elsevier.com/Lilley)

- Nursing Care Plans • Frequently Asked Questions • Content Updates • WebLinks • Supplemental Resources • Elsevier ePharmacology Update • Medication Administration Animations

Drug Profiles

Glossary

Agonists   Drugs with a specific receptor affinity that produce a "mimic" response. (p. 284)

Angina   Paroxysmal chest pain caused by myocardial ischemia. (p. 288)

Antagonists   Drugs that bind to adrenergic receptors and inhibit or block the action of neurotransmitters. (p. 284)

Cardioprotective   Term applied to β-blockers to inhibit stimulation of the heart by circulating catecholamines. (p. 288)

Cardioselective β-blockers   The β-blocking drugs that are selective for β$_1$-adrenergic receptors. Also called β$_1$-blocking drugs. (p. 287)

Dysrhythmias   Irregular heart rhythms; almost always called *arrhythmias* in clinical practice. (p. 288)

Extravasation   Leaking of fluid from the blood vessel into the surrounding tissues, as in the case of an infiltrated intravenous infusion. (p. 285)

Glycogenolysis   The production of glucose from glycogen in the liver, which is reduced by β-blockers. (p. 288)

Intrinsic sympathomimetic activity   Paradoxical action of some β-blocking drugs (e.g., acebutolol) that mimics the action of the sympathetic nervous system. (p. 288)

Lipophilicity   Chemical attraction of a substance (e.g., drug molecule) to lipid or fat molecules. (p. 288)

Nonselective β-blockers   The β-blocking drugs that block both β$_1$- and β$_2$-adrenergic receptors. (p. 287)

Orthostatic hypotension   Abnormally low blood pressure that occurs when a person assumes a standing position from a sitting or lying position. (p. 287)

Oxytocics   Drugs used to treat postpartum and postabortion bleeding caused by uterine relaxation and enlargement. They stimulate the smooth muscle of the uterus to contract. (p. 284)

Pheochromocytoma   A vascular adrenal gland tumor that is usually benign but secretes epinephrine and norepinephrine and thus often causes central nervous system stimulation and substantial blood pressure elevation. (p. 284)

Sympatholytics   Another name for adrenergic antagonists. (p. 284)

Vaughan Williams classification   System of classifying antidysrhythmic drugs. (p. 288)

The autonomic nervous system consists of the parasympathetic and sympathetic nervous systems. The class of drugs discussed in this chapter works primarily on the sympathetic nervous system

(SNS). As discussed in Chapter 17, the adrenergic agonist drugs stimulate the SNS. These drugs are called **agonists** because they bind to receptors and cause a response. The adrenergic blockers have the opposite effect and are therefore referred to as **antagonists.** They also bind to adrenergic receptors but in doing so inhibit or block stimulation by the SNS. They are also referred to as **sympatholytics** because they "lyse," or inhibit, SNS stimulation.

Throughout the body there are receptor sites for the endogenous sympathetic neurotransmitters norepinephrine and epinephrine. Such receptors are known as *adrenergic receptors,* and two basic types are found—α and β. There are subtypes of both the α- and β-adrenergic receptors, designated 1 and 2. The α_1- and α_2-adrenergic receptors are differentiated by their location on nerves. The α_1-adrenergic receptors are located on the tissue, muscle, or organ that the nerve is stimulating (postsynaptic effector cells). The α_2-adrenergic receptors are located on the actual nerves that stimulate the presynaptic effector cells. The β_1-adrenergic receptors are located primarily in the heart. The β_2-adrenergic receptors are located primarily on the smooth muscles of the bronchioles and blood vessels. It is at these various receptors that adrenergic blockers act, and these drugs are classified by the type of adrenergic receptor they block—α or β or, in a few cases, both. Hence, they are called *α-blockers, β-blockers,* or *α-β–blockers.*

α-BLOCKERS

The α-adrenergic–blocking drugs, or α-blockers, interrupt or block the stimulation of the SNS at the α-adrenergic receptor. Various physiologic responses occur when the stimulation of the α-adrenergic receptors is inhibited. Adrenergic blockade at the α-adrenergic receptors leads to vasodilation, decreased blood pressure, miosis or constriction of the pupil, and suppressed ejaculation. The ergot alkaloids dihydroergotamine mesylate, ergoloid mesylate, ergotamine tartrate, and ergonovine maleate are α-blockers that are used mainly for their vasoconstrictive properties. The α-blockers doxazosin, prazosin, and terazosin are used as antihypertensive drugs because they cause vasodilation. Both of these two groups of drugs block α-adrenergic receptors, but they have an affinity for different sites in the body and therefore the resulting effects differ. Other α-blockers are phenoxybenzamine, phentolamine, and tolazoline.

Mechanism of Action and Drug Effects

As mentioned earlier, α-blockers work by blocking or inhibiting the normal stimulation of the SNS. They do this either by direct competition with the SNS neurotransmitter norepinephrine or by a noncompetitive process. Most α-blockers are competitive in their actions. They have a higher affinity for the α-adrenergic receptor than does norepinephrine and can chemically displace norepinephrine molecules from the receptor. Once such a competitive α-blocker binds to the receptor, it causes the receptor to be less responsive. This blockade is reversible. Noncompetitive α-blockers work in a different fashion. They also bind to the α-adrenergic receptors, but this type of bond (a *covalent* bond) is irreversible. An example of an irreversible antagonist is phenoxybenzamine. Regardless of which way the blockade is accomplished, the result is a decreased response to stimulation of the SNS. Figure 18-1 illustrates these two mechanisms.

The α-blockers have many effects on the normal physiologic functions of the body. The effects of each drug can differ depending on the drug's selectivity for receptors in particular tissues or cells in the body. Ergot alkaloids, for example, can cause peripheral and cerebral vasoconstriction as well as the constriction of dilated arteries. Certain α-blockers can stimulate uterine contractions. Others can block α-adrenergic receptors on both vascular and nonvascular smooth muscle. The vascular smooth muscle receptors for which these α-blockers have an affinity are those in the bladder and its sphincters, the gastrointestinal tract and its sphincters, the prostate, and the ureters. The nonvascular smooth muscle receptors for which these drugs have an affinity are in the central nervous system (CNS), liver, and kidneys. Unlike ergot alkaloids, some α-blockers can induce arterial and venous dilation and thus decrease peripheral vascular resistance and blood pressure. Some α-blockers can also influence the concentration of certain neurotransmitters, causing a depletion of catecholamines such as norepinephrine and epinephrine. Others can directly block a neurotransmitter such as serotonin (5-hydroxytryptamine) or indirectly cause it to be depleted.

Indications

The α-blockers have many therapeutic effects, but these effects differ greatly depending on the particular drug. Ergot alkaloids constrict dilated arterioles in the brain that are often responsible for causing vascular headaches, such as migraines. The vasoconstriction that results from these drugs helps to relieve the symptoms associated with vascular migraines due to dilated arteries. Ergot alkaloids are also used as **oxytocics,** drugs given to control postpartum and postabortion bleeding caused by uterine relaxation and enlargement. These drugs increase the intensity of uterine contractions and induce local vasoconstriction.

The α-blockers such as doxazosin, prazosin, terazosin, and tamsulosin cause both arterial and venous dilation. This reduces peripheral vascular resistance and blood pressure. Thus, the first three drugs are used to treat hypertension. The α-adrenergic receptors are also present in the prostate and bladder. By blocking stimulation of α_1 receptors, these drugs reduce smooth muscle contraction of the bladder neck and the prostatic portion of the urethra. For this reason, α-blockers are given to patients with benign prostatic hyperplasia (BPH) to decrease resistance to urinary outflow. This reduces urinary obstruction and relieves some of the effects of BPH. Tamsulosin is used exclusively for treating BPH.

Other α-blockers can inhibit excitatory responses to adrenergic stimulation. These drugs noncompetitively block α-adrenergic receptors on smooth muscle and various exocrine glands. Because of this action, these α-blockers are very useful in controlling or preventing hypertension in patients who have a **pheochromocytoma,** a tumor that forms on the adrenal gland on top of the kidney and secretes norepinephrine, thus causing SNS stimulation. The α-blockers are also useful in the treatment of patients who have increased endogenous α-adrenergic agonist activity, which results in vasoconstriction. Three conditions in which this occurs are Raynaud's disease, acrocyanosis, and frostbite. Phenoxybenzamine is an α-blocker useful for the treatment of these syndromes.

Still other α-blockers are effective at antagonizing responses caused by injected catecholamines such as epineph-

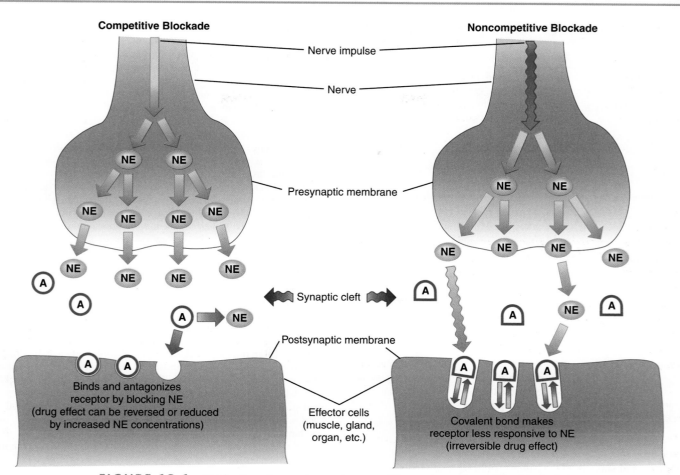

FIGURE 18-1 Mechanisms for α-adrenergic competitive and noncompetitive blockade by α-blockers. *A,* α-blocker; *NE,* norepinephrine.

---

rine and norepinephrine. These drugs cause peripheral vasodilation and decrease peripheral resistance by blocking catecholamine-stimulated vasoconstriction. They can also be used to treat pheochromocytomas. Because of their potent vasodilating properties and their fast onset of action, they are also used to prevent skin necrosis and sloughing after the **extravasation** of vasopressors such as norepinephrine or epinephrine. When these drugs extravasate, or leak out of the blood vessel into the surrounding tissue, they cause vasoconstriction and ultimately tissue death, or necrosis. If the vasoconstriction is not reversed quickly, the entire limb can be lost. Phentolamine, an α-blocker, can reverse this potent vasoconstriction and restore blood flow to the ischemic, vasoconstricted area.

Contraindications

Contraindications to the use of α-blocking drugs include known drug allergy and peripheral vascular disease and may include hepatic and renal disease, coronary artery disease, peptic ulcer, and sepsis.

Adverse Effects

The primary adverse effects of α-blockers are those related to their effects on the vasculature. The primary adverse effects of the α-blockers are listed by body system in Table 18-1.

Toxicity and Management of Overdose

In an acute overdose, the patient's stomach should be emptied immediately, either by inducing emesis by gastric lavage. After this, activated charcoal should be administered to bind to the drug and remove it from the stomach and the circulation. To hasten elimination of the drug bound to the activated charcoal, the

Table 18-1 α-Blockers: Adverse Effects

Body System	Adverse Effects
Cardiovascular	Palpitations, orthostatic hypotension, tachycardia, edema, dysrhythmias, chest pain
Central nervous	Dizziness, headache, drowsiness, anxiety, depression, vertigo, weakness, numbness, fatigue
Gastrointestinal	Nausea, vomiting, diarrhea, constipation, abdominal pain
Other	Incontinence, nosebleed, tinnitus, dry mouth, pharyngitis, rhinitis

Table 18-2 α-Blockers: Common Drug Interactions

Drug	Mechanism	Result
β-blockers		
Calcium channel blockers	Additive effects	Profound hypotension
Diuretics		
Protein-bound drugs	Competition for plasma protein-binding sites	Effects of increased free drug levels in plasma

first dose should be given with a cathartic such as sorbitol. Symptomatic and supportive measures should be instituted as needed. Blood pressure support with the administration of fluids, volume expanders, and vasopressor drugs and the administration of anticonvulsants such as diazepam for the control of seizures are examples of such measures.

Interactions

The most severe drug interactions with α-blockers are the ones that potentiate the effects of the α-blockers. The α-blockers as a whole are very highly protein bound and compete for binding sites with other drugs that are highly protein bound. Because of the limited sites for binding on proteins and the increased competition for these sites, more free α-blocker molecules circulate in the bloodstream. Drug that is not bound to protein is active, and thus the result is a more pronounced drug effect. Some of the common drugs that interact with α-blockers and the results of these interactions are listed in Table 18-2.

Dosages

For the recommended dosages of α-blockers, see the Dosages table on page 287.

Drug Profiles

The α-blockers are prescription-only drugs that are available in many dosage forms. The oral forms include tablets, capsules, solutions, and sublingual tablets. Parenteral formulations include intravenous, intramuscular, and subcutaneous injections. Some are also available as rectal suppositories. Most α-blockers are rated as pregnancy category C drugs by the U.S. Food and Drug Administration. Ergot alkaloids, however, are rated as pregnancy category X drugs.

ergotamine tartrate

Ergotamine (Ergostat) is an ergot alkaloid. All ergot alkaloids are obtained from a fungus called *Claviceps purpurea* that grows on rye. It causes vasoconstriction of dilated blood vessels in the brain and of the carotid arteries. These dilated arteries are responsible for causing vascular headaches such as migraines and cluster headaches. Ergotamine use is contraindicated in patients with peripheral vascular disease, coronary artery disease, sepsis, impaired hepatic or renal function, and severe hypertension, as well as in pregnant women. It is available as a sublingual 2-mg tablet, an aerosolized inhaler, and a rectal suppository that contains 2 mg of ergotamine and 100 mg of caffeine. Several combination drug preparations are also available in oral tablet form. These combinations vary; some of the other drugs combined with ergotamine in these preparations are belladonna alkaloids, phenobarbital, and caffeine. See the table on page 287 for dosing information for the 2-mg sublingual tablets and the aerosol preparation.

Pharmacokinetics

Half-Life	Onset	Peak	Duration
2 hr	30 min-2 hr	30 min-3 hr	24-48 hr

phenoxybenzamine hydrochloride

Phenoxybenzamine (Dibenzyline) is an α-blocker that reduces blood pressure by reducing peripheral vascular resistance. It is used to treat the hypertension caused by pheochromocytoma. Phenoxybenzamine is also useful in the treatment of vascular disorders such as frostbite, Raynaud's disease, and acrocyanosis, for which the underlying cause is increased α-adrenergic activity. Phenoxybenzamine directly blocks the α-adrenergic receptors and is therefore very useful in the treatment of these vasospastic disorders. Use of the drug is contraindicated in patients who have shown a hypersensitivity reaction to it or who have conditions in which hypotension is undesirable. It is available as a 10-mg oral capsule. The recommended dosage is given in the table on page 287.

Pharmacokinetics

Half-Life	Onset	Peak	Duration
24 hr	Less than 2 hr	4-6 hr	3-4 days

▶ phentolamine

Phentolamine (Regitine) is an α-blocker that reduces peripheral vascular resistance and is also used to treat hypertension. Like phenoxybenzamine, it is used to treat the high blood pressure caused by pheochromocytoma, but unlike that drug, it can also be used in the diagnosis of this catecholamine-secreting tumor. To help establish a diagnosis of pheochromocytoma using phentolamine, a single intravenous dose of the drug is given to the hypertensive patient who is suspected of having the tumor. If the blood pressure declines rapidly, it is highly likely that the patient has a pheochromocytoma. Phentolamine is available only as an intravenous preparation. This confers some advantages, however, because it can be used to treat the extravasation of vasoconstricting intravenous drugs such as norepinephrine, epinephrine, and dopamine, which when given intravenously can leak out of the vein, especially if the intravenous tube is not correctly positioned. If such a drug is allowed to extravasate into the surrounding tissue, the result is intense vasoconstriction, decreased blood flow, necrosis, and potential loss of the limb. When phentolamine is injected subcutaneously in a circular fashion around the extravasation site, it causes α-adrenergic receptor blockade and vasodilation, which in turn increases blood flow to the ischemic tissue and thus prevents permanent damage. Its use is contraindicated in patients who have shown a hypersensitivity to it, those who have experienced a myocardial infarction (MI), and those with coronary artery disease. The recommended dosages are given in the table on page 287.

Pharmacokinetics

Half-Life	Onset	Peak	Duration
19 min	Immediate	2 min	15-30 min

DOSAGES

Selected α-Adrenergic-Blocking Drugs

Drug	Pharmacologic Class	Usual Dosage Range	Indications
ergotamine tartrate (Ergostat)	α-blocker	**Adult only** SL tabs: 2 mg; repeat at ½-hr intervals; do not exceed 6 mg/day or 5 tabs/wk	Vascular headache
phenoxybenzamine hydrochloride (Dibenzyline)	α-blocker	**Adult only** PO: Initial dose of 10 mg bid; usual range 20-40 mg bid-tid	Hypertension
▶phentolamine (Regitine)	α-blocker	**Adult** IV: 5 mg 1-2 hr preop and 5 mg prn during surgery **Pediatric** IV: 1 mg 1-2 hr preop and 1 mg prn during surgery	Hypertension during surgery
		Adult IM/IV: 5 mg; repeat if necessary	Hypertensive episodes with pheochromocytoma
		Adult 5-10 mg diluted in 10 mL NS injected into extravasation site **Pediatric** 0.1-0.2 mg/kg into extravasation site	α-adrenergic drug extravasation
▶prazosin (Minipress)	α₁-blocker	**Adult only** PO: 1 mg bid-tid; maintenance range 6-15 mg/day divided bid-qid	Hypertension
tolazoline (Priscoline)	α-blocker	**Neonatal only** IV: 1-2 mg/kg via scalp vein, followed by 1-2 mg/kg/hr infusion	Neonatal pulmonary hypertension (persistent fetal circulation)

IM, Intramuscular; *IV,* intravenous; *NS,* normal saline; *PO,* oral; *preop,* preoperative; *SL,* sublingual.

▶ *prazosin*

Prazosin (Minipress) is an α_1-adrenergic–blocking drug primarily used to treat hypertension and to reduce urinary obstruction in men with BPH. Other drugs that are chemically and pharmacologically related to prazosin are doxazosin (Cardura), terazosin (Hytrin), and tamsulosin (Flomax). Its primary antihypertensive effects are related to its selective and competitive inhibition of α_1-adrenergic receptors. In men with BPH, prazosin relieves impaired urinary flow and urinary frequency by relaxing and dilating the vasculature and smooth muscle in the area surrounding the prostate. It also rather dramatically lowers blood pressure. A patient's ability to tolerate this drop in blood pressure must be taken into consideration when prescribing α-blockers for the treatment of BPH. Often when patients first start taking these drugs, they become very lightheaded and may even pass out when standing up after sitting or lying down. This is referred to as **orthostatic hypotension.** Although it is a fairly common problem specific to the α_1-blockers prazosin, doxazosin, terazosin, and tamsulosin, patients quickly acquire a tolerance to this effect, most after the first dose. Often patients taking their first dose are told to take it at bedtime and to be careful arising to circumvent this problem. Use of prazosin is contraindicated in patients who have shown hypersensitivity reactions to it. It is available for oral use in 1-, 2-, and 5-mg capsules and as a combination product with the diuretic polythiazide. The normally recommended dosages of prazosin are given in the table on this page.

Pharmacokinetics

Half-Life	Onset	Peak	Duration
2-3 hr	2 hr	1-3 hr	10 hr

tolazoline

Tolazoline (Priscoline) is an α-blocker that causes peripheral vasodilation and decreases peripheral resistance. It does this primarily through direct relaxation of vascular smooth muscle and the competitive blockade of α-adrenergic receptors. It is used primarily for the treatment of pulmonary hypertension in neonates when the hypertension causes the oxygen level in the neonate's bloodstream to decrease and the usual supportive measures are not able to compensate for this. Tolazoline use is contraindicated in patients who have had hypersensitivity reactions to it and in patients with known or suspected coronary artery disease. Its use is also contraindicated in patients who have suffered a stroke. It is available only as a parenteral (intravenous, intramuscular, or subcutaneous) injection. The normal dosages are given in the table on this page.

Pharmacokinetics

Half-Life	Onset	Peak	Duration
3-10 hr	Less than 30 min	30-60 min	3-4 hr

β-BLOCKERS

The β-adrenergic–blocking drugs (β-blockers) block SNS stimulation of the β-adrenergic receptors by competing with the endogenous catecholamines norepinephrine and epinephrine. The β-blockers can be either selective or nonselective, depending on the type of β-adrenergic receptors they antagonize or block. As mentioned earlier, β_1-adrenergic receptors are located primarily in the heart. The β-blockers selective for these receptors are sometimes called **cardioselective β-blockers,** or β_1-blocking drugs. Other β-blockers block both β_1- and β_2-adrenergic receptors, the latter of which are located primarily on the smooth muscles of the bronchioles and blood vessels. The β-blockers that block both types of β-adrenergic receptors are referred to as **nonselective β-blockers.** The drugs in the β-blocker class can be further categorized according to whether they do or do not have **intrinsic sympathomimetic activity.** Drugs with intrinsic sympathomimetic activity (acebutolol, penbutolol, pindolol) not only block β-adrenergic receptors but also partially stimulate them. This was initially believed to be an advantageous characteristic, but clinical experience has not borne this out. Some β-blockers also have α receptor–blocking activity, especially at higher dosages; examples of these drugs include carvedilol and labetalol. Box 18-1 lists the currently available β-blockers.

Mechanism of Action and Drug Effects

Because β-blockers compete with and block norepinephrine and epinephrine at the β-adrenergic receptors located throughout the body, the β-adrenergic receptor sites can no longer be stimulated by neurotransmitters and SNS stimulation is blocked. Although β-adrenergic receptors are located throughout the body, the most important ones in terms of these drugs are those located on the surface of the heart, the smooth muscle of the bronchi, and the smooth muscle of blood vessels. Cardioselective β_1-blockers block the β_1-adrenergic receptors on the surface of the heart. This reduces myocardial stimulation, which in turn reduces heart rate, slows conduction through the atrioventricular (AV) node, prolongs sinoatrial (SA) node recovery, and decreases myocardial oxygen demand by decreasing myocardial contractile force (contractility). Nonselective β-blockers also have this effect on the heart, but they block β_2-adrenergic receptors on the smooth muscle of the bronchioles and blood vessels as well.

Smooth muscle also surrounds the airways in the lungs called *bronchioles*. When β_2-adrenergic receptors in the bronchioles are blocked, the smooth muscle contracts, causing these airways to narrow. This may lead to shortness of breath. In addition, the smooth muscle that surrounds blood vessels controls the size of the blood vessels and can cause them to dilate or constrict depending on whether the α_1- or β_2-adrenergic receptors are stimulated. When β_2-SNS stimulation at these smooth muscles is blocked by a β-blocker, the muscles are then stimulated by unopposed SNS activity at the α_1-adrenergic receptors, which causes them to contract. This in turn increases peripheral vascular resistance. Furthermore, catecholamines promote **glycogenolysis,** the

---

Box 18-1 **Currently Available β-Blockers**
Nonselective β-Blockers
carteolol (Cartrol)
carvedilol (Coreg)
labetalol (Normodyne and Trandate)*
nadolol (Corgard)
penbutolol (Levatol)
pindolol (Visken)
propranolol (Inderal)
sotalol (Betapace)
timolol (Blocadren)
Cardioselective β-Blockers
acebutolol (Sectral)
atenolol (Tenormin)
betaxolol (Kerlone)
bisoprolol (Zebeta)
esmolol (Brevibloc)
metoprolol (Lopressor and Toprol XL)

*Blocks both α- and β-adrenergic receptors.

---

production of glucose from glycogen, and mobilize glucose in response to hypoglycemia. Nonselective β-blockers impair this process and also impede the secretion of insulin from the pancreas, which causes elevation of blood glucose level.

Finally, β-blockers can cause the release of free fatty acids from adipose tissue. This may result in moderately elevated blood levels of triglycerides and reduced levels of the "good cholesterol" known as high-density lipoproteins (HDLs).

Indications

The drug effects mentioned in the preceding section vary from β-blocker to β-blocker depending on the specific chemical characteristics of the drug. Some β-blockers are used primarily in the treatment of **angina,** or chest pain. These work by decreasing demand for myocardial energy and oxygen consumption, which helps shift the supply-and-demand ratio to the supply side and allows more oxygen to get to the heart muscle. This in turn helps relieve the pain in the heart muscle caused by the lack of oxygen.

Other β-blockers are considered **cardioprotective** because they inhibit stimulation of the myocardium by circulating catecholamines. Catecholamines are released during myocardial muscle damage such as that caused by an MI, or heart attack. When a β-blocker drug occupies myocardial β_1 receptors, circulating catecholamine molecules are prevented from binding to the receptors. Thus, the β-blockers protect the heart from being stimulated by these catecholamines, which would only further increase the heart rate and the contractile force and thereby increase myocardial oxygen demand. Because of this characteristic, β-blockers are commonly given to patients after they have suffered an MI to protect the heart from the stress caused by the compensatory release of catecholamines.

As mentioned previously, β-blockers also have a profound effect on the conduction system of the heart. The AV node normally receives impulse stimulation from the SA node and slows it down so that the ventricles have time to fill before they are stimulated to contract. Conduction in the SA node, which spontaneously depolarizes at the most frequent rate, is slowed by β-blockers, which results in a decreased heart rate. These drugs also slow conduction through the AV node. These effects of β-blockers on the conduction system of the heart make them useful drugs in the treatment of various types of irregular heart rhythms, called **dysrhythmias.** In the **Vaughan Williams classification** of antidysrhythmic drugs (Chapter 22), all β-blockers are categorized as class II drugs with the exception of sotalol, which has both class II and class III properties.

Their ability to reduce SNS stimulation of the heart, including reducing heart rate and the force of myocardial contraction (systole), renders β-blockers useful in treating hypertension. Traditionally β-blockers were thought to worsen heart failure. However, recent studies have shown benefit to the use of β-blockers. Certain β-blockers such as carvedilol and metoprolol have produced the best results to date. The form of heart failure that includes a diastolic dysfunction component responds especially favorably to β-blockers.

Because of their **lipophilicity** (attraction to lipid or fat), some β-blockers (e.g., propranolol) can easily gain entry into the CNS. These β-blockers are used to treat migraine headaches. In addition, the topical application of β-blockers to the eye has been very effective in treating ocular disorders such as glaucoma.

Contraindications

Contraindications to the use of β-blockers include known drug allergies and may include uncompensated heart failure, cardiogenic shock, heart block or bradycardia, pregnancy, severe pulmonary disease, and Raynaud's disease.

Adverse Effects

The adverse effects of β-blockers are primarily extensions of their pharmacologic activity. Most such effects are mild and diminish with time. Some of the most serious undesirable effects can be caused by acute withdrawal of the drug. For example, this may exacerbate the underlying angina the drug is being used to treat or it may precipitate an MI. The β-blockers may also mask the signs and symptoms of hypoglycemia. Adverse effects induced by β-blockers are listed by body system in Table 18-3.

Toxicity and Management of Overdose

After acute oral overdose of a β-blocker, the stomach should be emptied immediately, either by induction of emesis or by gastric lavage. Treatment consists primarily of symptomatic and supportive care. Atropine may be given intravenously for the management of bradycardia. If the bradycardia still persists, placement of a transvenous cardiac pacemaker should be considered. For the treatment of severe hypotension, vasopressors should be titrated until the desired blood pressure and heart rate are achieved. Intravenously administered diazepam may be useful for the treatment of seizures. Most β-blockers are dialyzable; therefore, hemodialysis may be useful in enhancing elimination in the event of severe overdose.

Interactions

Most of the drug interactions with β-blockers result from either the additive effects of coadministered medications with similar mechanisms of action or the antagonistic effects of various drugs.

Some of the common drugs that interact with β-blockers and the resulting effects are given in Table 18-4.

Dosages

For information on the recommended dosages for selected β-blockers, see the Dosages table on page 290.

Drug Profiles

The β-blockers are prescription-only drugs that are available in oral preparations as tablets and capsules and in parenteral forms for intermittent injection or continuous intravenous infusion. Topically administered forms are also available. Eyedrops containing a β-blocker are used in the treatment of glaucoma. Most β-blockers, except acebutolol and sotalol, are rated as pregnancy category C drugs. However, acebutolol is a category D drug, and sotalol is a category B drug.

acebutolol

Acebutolol (Sectral) is a cardioselective β₁-blocker used for the treatment of hypertension, ventricular and supraventricular dysrhythmias, and angina. It is also used in patients in the period immediately after an MI. It is commonly used alone as an antihypertensive drug or in combination with a diuretic for the additive antihypertensive effects. It is one of the few β-blockers that possesses intrinsic sympathomimetic activity. Its use is contraindicated in patients who have had a hypersensitivity reaction to it; in those with severe bradycardia, heart block greater than first degree, Raynaud's disease, or malignant hypertension; and in those in cardiogenic shock or cardiac failure. It is available for oral use in 200- and 400-mg capsules. Pregnancy category D. The commonly recommended dosages are given in the table on page 290.

Pharmacokinetics			
Half-Life	**Onset**	**Peak**	**Duration**
3-7 hr	1.5-3 hr	3-8 hr	10-24 hr

▶ atenolol

Atenolol (Tenormin) is a cardioselective β-blocker that is commonly used to prevent future MIs in patients who have had an MI. It is also used in the treatment of hypertension and angina. It is available as a 0.5-mg/mL injection for intravenous use and in 25-, 50-, and 100-mg tablets for oral use. Pregnancy category C. See the table on page 290 for the recommended dosages.

Pharmacokinetics			
Half-Life	**Onset**	**Peak**	**Duration**
IV: 6-7 hr	IV: Immediate	IV: Less than 5 min	IV: Less than 12 hr
PO: 6-7 hr	PO: 1 hr	PO: 2-4 hr	PO: 24 hr

carvedilol

Carvedilol (Coreg) is the newest β-blocker. It has many effects, including acting as a nonselective β-blocker, an α₁-blocker, a calcium channel blocker, and possibly as an antioxidant. It is used primarily in the treatment of heart failure but is also beneficial for hypertension and angina. It has been shown to slow the progression of heart failure

---

Table 18-3   β-Blockers: Common Adverse Effects

Body System	Adverse Effects
Cardiovascular	Atrioventricular block, bradycardia, heart failure, peripheral vascular insufficiency
Central nervous	Dizziness, mental depression, lethargy, hallucinations
Gastrointestinal	Nausea, vomiting, constipation, diarrhea, cramps, ischemic colitis
Hematologic	Agranulocytosis, thrombocytopenia
Other	Impotence, rash, alopecia, bronchospasms, dry mouth

Table 18-4   β-Blockers: Drug Interactions

Drug	Mechanism	Result
Antacids (aluminum hydroxide type)	Decrease absorption	Decreased β-blocker activity
Antimuscarinics, anticholinergics	Antagonism	Reduced β-blocker effects
Diuretics and cardiovascular drugs	Additive effect	Additive hypotensive effects
Neuromuscular blocking drugs	Additive effect	Prolonged neuromuscular blockade
Oral hypoglycemic drugs	Antagonism	Decreased hypoglycemic effects

DOSAGES

Selected β-Adrenergic-Blocking Drugs

Drug	Pharmacologic Class	Usual Dosage Range	Indications
acebutolol (Sectral)	β_1-blocker	**Adult** PO: 400-800 mg/day divided bid 600-1200 mg/day divided bid	Hypertension Premature ventricular beats
atenolol (Tenormin)	β_1-blocker	**Adult** PO: 50-100 mg/day daily or bid 50-200 mg/day divided daily or bid IV: 5 mg over 5 min; may repeat in 10 min	Hypertension Angina Acute MI
carvedilol (Coreg)	α-β-blocker	**Adult** PO: 3.125 mg bid; may double dose every 2 wk to highest tolerated dose, max 50 mg/day	Heart failure, angina, hypertension
esmolol (Brevibloc)	β_1-blocker	**Adult** IV: Bolus of 500 mcg/kg over 1 min, followed by 4 min at 50 mcg/kg/min and evaluate IV: 80 mg bolus over 30 min followed by 150 mcg/kg/min infusion	Supraventricular tachydysrhythmias Intraoperative/postoperative hypertension
labetalol (Normodyne, Trandate)	α_1-β-blocker	**Adult** PO: 200-800 mg/day divided bid IV: 20 mg with additional doses of 40-80 mg at 10-min intervals until desired effect or a total dose of 300 mg is injected; maintenance infusion of 2 mg/min initially and titrated to response	Hypertension Severe hypertension
metoprolol (Lopressor, Toprol XL)	β_1-blocker	**Adult** PO: 100-450 mg/day divided bid-tid IV/PO: 3 bolus injections of 5 mg at 2-min intervals followed in 15 min by 50 mg PO q6h for 48 hr; thereafter 100 mg PO bid	Hypertension, late MI Early MI
propranolol (Inderal)	β-blocker	**Adult** PO: 80-320 mg/day divided bid-qid 120-640 mg/day divided bid-tid 10-30 mg tid-qid 180-240 mg divided tid-qid 20-40 mg tid-qid 120-320 mg/day divided 160-240 mg/day divided 30-60 mg/day divided for 3 days before surgery with an α-blocker also IV: 1 mg slow IV push, may repeat every 5 min up to 5 mg	Angina Hypertension Dysrhythmias Post-MI Hypertrophic subaortic stenosis Essential tremor Migraine Pheochromocytoma surgery Serious dysrhythmias
sotalol (Betapace)	β-blocker	**Adult** PO: 160-320 mg/day divided	Life-threatening ventricular dysrhythmias

IV, Intravenous; *MI*, myocardial infarction; *PO*, oral.

and to decrease the frequency of hospitalization in patients with mild to moderate (class II or III) heart failure. Carvedilol is most commonly added to digoxin, furosemide, and angiotensin-converting enzyme (ACE) inhibitors when used to treat heart failure. Its use is contraindicated in patients with class IV decompensated heart failure, asthma, second- or third-degree AV block, cardiogenic shock, and severe bradycardia. It is available as 3.125-, 6.25-, 12.5-, and 25-mg tablets. Pregnancy category C. Recommended dosages are given in the table on this page.

Pharmacokinetics

Half-Life	Onset	Peak	Duration
IV: 6-8 hr	IV: 2-5 min	IV: 5-15 min	IV: 2-4 hr
PO: 7-10 hr	PO: 1-2 hr	PO: 1-2 hr	PO: Unknown

▶ esmolol

Esmolol (Brevibloc) is a very potent short-acting β_1-blocker. It is primarily used in acute situations to provide rapid, temporary control of the ventricular rate in patients with supraventricular tachydysrhythmias. Because of its very short half-life, it is given only as an intravenous infusion and is titrated to achieve the serum levels that control the patient's symptoms. It is available in 10- and 250-mg/mL concentrate for intravenous injection. Pregnancy category C. Recommended dosages are given in the table on this page.

Pharmacokinetics

Half-Life	Onset	Peak	Duration
9 min	Immediate	6 min	15-20 min

labetalol

Labetalol (Normodyne, Trandate) is unusual in that it can block both α- and β-adrenergic receptors. It is used in the treatment of severe hypertension and hypertensive emergencies to quickly lower the blood pressure before permanent damage is done. It is available both for parenteral use as a 5-mg/mL intravenous injection and for oral use as 100-, 200-, and 300-mg tablets. Pregnancy category C. The normal dosages are given in the table on this page.

Pharmacokinetics

Half-Life	Onset	Peak	Duration
IV: 6-8 hr	IV: 2-5 min	IV: 5-15 min	IV: 2-4 hr
PO: 6-8 hr	PO: 20-120 min	PO: 1-4 hr	PO: 8-24 hr

▶ metoprolol

Metoprolol is a β$_1$-blocker that has become a favorite of cardiologists for use in the post-MI patient. Recent studies of metoprolol have shown increased survival in patients given the drug after they have experienced an MI. It is available as a 1-mg/mL injection or as 50-, 100-, and 200-mg tablets (Lopressor) and 50-, 100-, and 200-mg extended-release tablets (Toprol-XL). It is also available in combination with the diuretic hydrochlorothiazide. Pregnancy category C. Commonly recommended dosages are given in the table on page 290.

Pharmacokinetics

Half-Life	Onset	Peak	Duration
IV: 3-4 hr	IV: Immediate	IV: 10 min	IV: 5-8 hr
PO: 3-7 hr	PO: 1 hr	PO: 2-4 hr	PO: 13-19 hr

▶ propranolol

Propranolol (Inderal) is the prototypical nonselective β$_1$- and β$_2$-blocking drug. It was one of the very first β-blockers to be used. The lengthy experience with it has revealed many uses for it. In addition to the indications mentioned for acebutolol, propranolol has been used for the treatment of tachydysrhythmias associated with cardiac glycoside intoxication and for the treatment of hypertrophic subaortic stenosis, pheochromocytoma, thyrotoxicosis, migraine headache, essential tremor, and many other conditions. The same contraindications that apply to the cardioselective β-blockers (cited in the discussion on acebutolol) hold for propranolol as well. In addition, its use is contraindicated in patients with bronchial asthma. It is available as a 1-mg/mL intravenous injection; as 60-, 80-, 120-, and 160-mg oral long-acting capsules; as 10-, 20-, 40-, 60-, 80-, and 90-mg tablets; and as 4-, 8-, and 80-mg/mL oral solutions. Pregnancy category C. The recommended dosages are given in the table on page 290.

Pharmacokinetics

Half-Life	Onset	Peak	Duration
3-5 hr	30 min	1-1.5 hr	6-8 hr

sotalol

Sotalol (Betapace) is a nonselective β-blocker that has very potent antidysrhythmic properties. It is commonly used for the management of difficult-to-treat dysrhythmias. Often these dysrhythmias are life-threatening ventricular dysrhythmias such as sustained ventricular tachycardia. It has properties characteristic of both a class II and a class III antidysrhythmic drug (Chapter 22), though many references list it as being one class or the other. Because it is a nonselective β-blocker, it causes some of the unwanted adverse effects typical of these drugs (e.g., hypotension). It is available in oral form in 80-, 160-, and 240-mg tablets. Pregnancy category B. Commonly recommended dosages are given in the table on page 290.

Pharmacokinetics

Half-Life	Onset	Peak	Duration
12 hr	Less than 1 hr	2.5-4 hr	8-12 hr

◆ NURSING PROCESS

◆ ASSESSMENT

Adrenergic-blocking drugs, or sympatholytics, produce a variety of effects on the patient, depending on the type of receptor blocked. Because of the clinical impact of these drugs, primarily on the cardiac and respiratory systems, their use requires careful assessment of the patient to minimize the adverse effects and maximize the therapeutic effects. Understanding the basic anatomy and physiology of adrenergic receptors and their subsequent actions if stimulated—or, in this case, blocked—is also critical in carrying out assessment and other aspects of the nursing process and drug therapy. If an adrenegic-blocking drug is nonselective, it blocks both α and β (β$_1$ and β$_2$) receptors and has blocking effects on blood vessels (α), heart rate (β$_1$), and bronchial smooth muscle (β$_2$). Therefore, if it is a nonselective drug, it will have the following actions:

- α-blocking, causing a block of the sympathetic stimulation of blood vessels (i.e., vasoconstriction); this will result in vasodilation and subsequent decrease in blood pressure.
- β$_1$-blocking, causing a block of the sympathetic effects on heart rate, contractility, and conduction with resulting bradycardia, negative inotropic effects (i.e., a decrease in contractility), and a decrease in conduction; this can help in treating several types of dysfunctional irregularities in heart rate.
- β$_2$-blocking, causing a block of the sympathetic effects on bronchial smooth muscle and of bronchodilating effects from smooth muscle relaxation; this will result in bronchoconstriction in the lungs.

However, if the drug is α, β$_1$, or β$_2$ blocking, the resulting effect will be related to the specific receptor or combination thereof. An understanding of these basic physiologic concepts helps the nurse to understand critical aspects of the administration of drugs that alter the function of the SNS (in this chapter, drugs that block sympathetic effects).

To begin a thorough assessment, the nurse should gather information about the patient's allergies and past and present medical conditions. Conducting a system overview and taking a thorough medication history should be part of this process. Some questions to pose to the patient include the following:

- Are you allergic to any medications or foods?
- Do you have a history of a chronic obstructive pulmonary disease such as emphysema, asthma, or chronic bronchitis?
- Do you have a history of hypotension, cardiac dysrhythmias, bradycardia, heart failure, or any other cardiovascular disease?

These questions are important, because α-blockers may precipitate hypotension, and β-blockers (β_1 and/or β_2) may precipitate bradycardia, hypotension, heart block, heart failure, bronchoconstriction, and/or increased airway resistance. Therefore, any preexisting condition that might be exacerbated by the use of these drugs may become a contraindication or caution. For example, with β_1-blocking drugs, the nurse needs to consider the types of conditions or diseases that would be exacerbated, such as preexisting bradycardia, decreased cardiac contractility, and decreased conduction. Another example is with β_2-blocking drugs, with consideration of conditions or diseases involving increased airway resistance because of the β_2-blocking effect of bronchoconstriction. Although previously discussed, it is critical to remember that these drug classes are used frequently, so adverse effects, cautions, contraindications, and drug interactions must be kept in mind. Patients should be asked whether they are taking any drugs that could possibly interact with the adrenergic-blocking drug that has been prescribed for them. These interacting drugs include α- and β-agonists (or stimulators). See Tables 18-1 and 18-3 for related adverse effects. See Tables 18-2 and 18-4 for drug interactions.

◆ NURSING DIAGNOSES

Nursing diagnoses related to the use of adrenergic antagonists, or sympatholytics, include, but are not limited to, the following:

- Ineffective tissue perfusion (cerebral and cardiovascular) related to the adverse effects of the disease of hypertension and the adverse effects of the drug (hypotension)
- Disturbed sensory perception related to the CNS adverse effects of the drug
- Risk for injury related to possible adverse effects of the adrenergic blockers (e.g., postural hypotension, numbness and tingling of the fingers and toes)
- Imbalanced nutrition, less than body requirements, due to nausea and vomiting related to the use of adrenergic blockers
- Deficient knowledge related to lack of information about the therapeutic regimen, adverse effects, drug interactions, and precautions to be taken

◆ PLANNING
Goals

- Patient maintains and regains adequate tissue perfusion.
- Patient's perception and CNS functioning remain intact.
- Patient is free of injury to self as the result of adverse effects of the medications.
- Patient takes medication exactly as prescribed and with minimal impact on nutrition.
- Patient experiences improvement in hypertension or relief of the symptoms for which the medication was prescribed.
- Patient remains compliant with the drug therapy regimen.
- Patient demonstrates an adequate knowledge concerning the use of the specific medications, their adverse effects, and the appropriate dosing routine to be followed at home.

Outcome Criteria

- Patient states that blood pressure readings are within the normal range and that adverse effects are minimal.
- Patient reports fewer symptoms of hypertension as well as more energy and clearer thinking without profound adverse effects.
- Patient is free of injury to self as the result of adverse effects of the medications.

EVIDENCE-BASED PRACTICE

β-Blockers

Review

The β-blockers are used to lower blood pressure and heart rate in patients with heart failure. A recent 5-year longitudinal study of more than 3000 patients was reported in *Lancet* (2003). The study compared clinical outcomes for treatment with carvedilol and metoprolol in patients with chronic heart failure.

Type of Evidence

The β-blockers carvedilol (Coreg) and metoprolol tartrate (Lopressor) were compared in a randomized, controlled trial known as the Carvedilol or Metoprolol European Trial (COMET).

Results of Study

The median survival time was 1.4 years longer in the group taking carvedilol than in the group taking metoprolol.

Link of Evidence to Nursing Practice

This study had a large sample size of 3000 participants and supports the use of β-blockers in the treatment of chronic heart failure. Chronic heart failure presents many challenges for nursing and for

the medical profession. Four types of drugs have commonly been used to treat heart failure: diuretics, angiotensin-converting enzyme inhibitors, β-blockers, and digitalis glycosides. Most patients with chronic heart failure receive some combination of these drugs. These drugs act to lower blood pressure, and their use in the treatment of chronic heart failure has been targeted at this effect. The lower the blood pressure is, the easier it is for blood to be ejected from the left ventricle to the rest of the body. Because the β-blockers lower blood pressure and heart rate, the results found for carvedilol and metoprolol continue to hold promise for patients who have this chronic, debilitating disease. Nurses must look to nursing research to further their knowledge and understanding of diseases as well as related pharmacologic and nonpharmacologic interventions and other treatment regimens. Research findings like these can improve patient care and lead to sound, evidence-based nursing practice.

Based on Poole-Wilson PA et al: Comparison of carvedilol and metoprolol on clinical outcomes in patients with chronic heart failure in the Carvedilol or Metoprolol European Trial (COMET): randomised controlled trial, *Lancet* 362(9377):7-13, 2003; Riggs JM: New therapies for heart failure, *RN* 67(3):29-33, 2004.

- Patient states the importance of both the pharmacologic and nonpharmacologic treatment of hypertension or other indication for the drug therapy.
- Patient states reasons for complying with the medication therapy without risking nutritional status.
- Patient reports effective blood pressure lowering or treatment with adrenergic blocker without risks and complications such as syncope, dizziness, and hypotension.
- Patient demonstrates the correct method of self-measurement of blood pressure using a digital cuff device or using community resources.
- Patient states the conditions that may occur of which the physician should be informed immediately, such as palpitations, chest pain, insomnia, and excessive agitation.
- Patient keeps all follow-up appointments with the physician to maintain safe therapy.
- Patient follows instructions to avoid sudden withdrawal of hypertensive drugs to prevent rebound hypertensive crises and experiences minimal complications.

◆ IMPLEMENTATION

Several nursing interventions can maximize the therapeutic effects of adrenergic-blocking drugs and minimize their adverse effects. Thorough patient education is required to ensure good compliance (see the Patient Teaching Tips). Patients taking α-blockers should be encouraged to change positions slowly to prevent or minimize postural hypotension. When α- and/or β-blockers are used, apical pulse rate (taken for 1 full minute) and both supine and standing blood pressures should be measured as ordered. Should there be any problems with dizziness, fainting, or lightheadedness, or should blood pressure be lower than 100 mm Hg systolic or pulse rate lower than 60 beats/min, the health care provider should be contacted.

In addition, daily weights measurements are important to monitor the progress of therapy and monitor for the adverse effect of edema. A good rule of thumb is that if the patient has an increase of 2 lb or more over a 24-hour period or 5 lb or more within 1 week, the health care provider should be contacted. Other symptoms to be reported include muscle weakness, shortness of breath, and collection of fluid in the lower extremities as noted by difficulty in putting on shoes or socks. The nurse should make sure that the patient is weaned off these medications slowly if indicated because of the rebound hypertension or chest pain that rapid withdrawal can precipitate. The nurse should remember basic anatomy and physiology; as mentioned previously, this will always help guide nursing actions and considerations related to these drugs.

With any of the adrenergic drugs, the patient's feedback, daily journal-keeping, and compliance to therapy is critical to successful treatment and prevention of adverse effects. In addition, patient education with attention to dietary intake of potassium, fluid intake, daily weights, recording of blood pressure and/or pulse rates before taking doses, reporting of adverse effects (e.g., postural hypotension and bradycardia), and edema or fluid collection is crucial to patient safety and effective therapy. See the Patient Teaching Tips for more information.

◆ EVALUATION

Therapeutic effects for which to monitor in patients receiving adrenergic-blocking drugs include, but are not limited to, the following:

- Decrease in blood pressure, pulse rate, and palpitations in patients with these specific problems before drug therapy
- Alleviation of the symptoms of the disorder for which the drug was indicated
- Return to normal blood pressure and pulse with lowering of the blood pressure toward 120/80 mm Hg and the pulse toward normal (60 beats/min) in patients with diagnosed hypertension
- Decrease in chest pain in patients with angina

Patients must also be monitored for the occurrence of the adverse effects of these medications, which include bradycardia, depression, fatigue, and hypotension, among others. See Tables 18-1 and 18-3 for other potential adverse effects.

Patient Teaching Tips

- Educate patients about the therapeutic effects and adverse effects of their drug therapy.
- Encourage patients to always have printed information about their medical conditions and medications on their persons at all times. Emphasize the importance of always wearing a medical alert bracelet or necklace that identifies the specific medical diagnosis and list of all medications (e.g., prescription, over-the-counter drugs, herbals, supplements). Patients should know to update their information frequently with their health care provider, and the changes should be dated. This list could also have a place for the patient to record blood pressures by date and time so that, with each visit to the physician, the medication list and blood pressure values are readily available.
- Inform patients that they should take medications exactly as prescribed and never stop the drugs abruptly (which can result in rebound hypertension); they should instead contact their health care providers.
- While taking adrenergic-blocking drugs, patients should be encouraged to avoid caffeine and other CNS stimulants to prevent excessive irritability of the cardiac and central nervous systems.
- Alcohol ingestion should be avoided because it will lead to vasodilation and a higher risk of hypotension and postural hypotension.

- Patients should contact the physician or health care provider if they experience palpitations, chest pain, confusion, weight gain, dyspnea, nausea, or vomiting. Other problems to report include swelling in the feet and ankles, shortness of breath, excessive fatigue, dizziness, and syncope.
- Patients who are prescribed β-blockers must always take the medication exactly as prescribed, no more and no less, and never try to catch up their dosing if they have missed more than one dose; in such cases, they should contact the health care provider for further instructions.
- Patients should be informed to change positions slowly to avoid dizziness and/or syncope. Exercise, exposure to heat in the environment or in a sauna, time in a tanning bed (due to greater vasodilation and a greater drop in blood pressure), and alcohol may lead to further vasodilation and subsequent syncope.
- Patients should report constipation or the development of any urinary hesitancy or bladder distention (discomfort over the symphysis pubis) to the health care provider for further instructions. Prevention of constipation through diet and fluids should be encouraged.
- Encourage the patient to immediately report any of the following to their health care provider: confusion, depression, hallucinations, nightmares, palpitations, and dizziness.

Points to Remember

- Adrenergic-blocking drugs block the stimulation of the α- and β_1- or β_2-adrenergic receptors, with a net result of blocking the effects of either norepinephrine or epinephrine on the receptor. This blocking action leads to a variety of physiologic responses depending on which receptors are blocked. Knowing how these receptors work allows the nurse to understand and predict the expected therapeutic effects of the drugs as well as the expected adverse effects.
- With α-blockers the predominant response is vasodilation. This is due to blocking of the α-adrenergic effect of vasoconstriction, which results in blood vessel relaxation.
- Vasodilation of blood vessels with the α-blockers results in a drop in blood pressure and a reduction in urinary obstruction that may lead to increased urinary flow rates. These are effects for which to monitor in patients taking α-blockers.
- β-blockers inhibit the stimulation of β-adrenergic receptors by blocking the effects of the SNS neurotransmitters norepinephrine, epinephrine, and dopamine. Stimulation of β_1 receptors leads to an increase in heart rate, conduction, and contractility. Stimulation of β_2 receptors results in bronchial smooth muscle relaxation or bronchodilation. Blocking of β_1 receptors therefore results in a *decrease* in heart rate, conduction, and contractility.

- Blocking of β_2 receptors leads to a *decrease* in bronchial smooth muscle relaxation, or bronchoconstriction.
- β-blockers are classified as either selective or nonselective. Selective β-blockers are also called *cardioselective* β-blockers and block only the β_1-adrenergic receptors in the heart that are located on the postsynaptic effector cells (i.e., the cells that nerves stimulate). The beneficial effects of the cardioselective β-blockers include decreased heart rate, reduced cardiac conduction, and decreased myocardial contractility with *no* bronchoconstriction. These drugs are a good choice for patients with hypertension who also have bronchospastic airway disease or other pulmonary lung disease.
- Nonselective β-blockers block both β_1- and β_2-adrenergic receptors and affect the heart and bronchial smooth muscle. These drugs are used to treat patients with hypertension who do not have a problem with bronchospasm or pulmonary airway disease.
- Nursing considerations for patients taking β-blockers include teaching patients that they should avoid sudden changes in position because of possible postural hypotension and instructing patients to report rapid weight gain or a decrease in heart rate below 60 beats/min.

NCLEX Examination Review Questions

1. When a patient has experienced infiltration of a peripheral infusion of dopamine, the nurse knows that injecting the α-blocker phentolamine (Regitine) will result in:
   a. Local vasoconstriction
   b. Local vasodilation
   c. Local analgesia
   d. Local hypotension

2. Which statement is most correct for a patient taking a β-blocker?
   a. The drug may be discontinued without any time constraints.
   b. Postural hypotension is not a problem with this drug.
   c. Weaning off the medication is necessary to prevent rebound hypertension.
   d. The patient should stop taking the medication at once if he or she gains 3 to 4 lb in a week.

3. The nurse providing teaching for a patient who has a new prescription for β₁-blockers will keep in mind that these drugs may result in:
   a. Tachycardia
   b. Tachypnea

   c. Bradycardia
   d. Bradypnea

4. A patient who has had a recent MI may be placed on which of the following drugs for its cardioprotective effects?
   a. metoprolol (Lopressor)
   b. esmolol (Brevibloc)
   c. prazosin (Minipress)
   d. phenoxybenzamine (Dibenzyline)

5. Before initiating therapy with a nonselective β-blocker, the nurse should assess the patient for the presence of:
   a. Hypertension
   b. Liver disease
   c. Pancreatitis
   d. Chronic bronchitis

1. b, 2. c, 3. c, 4. a, 5. d.

Critical Thinking Activities

1. Develop patient teaching plans for the use of one of the following medications:
   a. ergotamine tartrate (Ergostat)
   b. prazosin (Minipress)
   c. atenolol (Tenormin)

2. One of your patients, a 46-year-old mother of two adolescent children, is now taking propranolol (Inderal) for the control of tachycardia and hypertension. What instructions should you give her if she says, "Well, if it doesn't work after a month or two, I'll just quit taking it!"

3. A 69-year-old man is given a new prescription for prazosin (Minipress), 1 mg twice a day. The physician asks you to be sure to be "thorough in your teaching" about this drug. What points are important when discussing this drug therapy with your patient?

For answers, see http://evolve.elsevier.com/Lilley.

Cholinergic Drugs

Objectives

When you reach the end of this chapter, you should be able to do the following:

1. Briefly discuss the normal anatomy and physiology of the autonomic nervous system (ANS), including the events that occur during synaptic transmission in the parasympathetic division of the ANS.
2. Cite various examples of the cholinergic drugs, including newer drug therapy for treating Alzheimer's disease and dementia-related conditions.
3. Discuss the mechanisms of action, therapeutic effects, indications, adverse effects, dosage amounts, and routes of administration as well as any antidotes for the various cholinergic drugs.
4. Develop a nursing care plan that includes all phases of the nursing process related to the administration of cholinergic drugs.

e-Learning Activities

Companion CD
- NCLEX Review Questions: see questions 134-140
- Animations
- Audio Glossary
- Category Catchers
- Medication Errors Checklists
- IV Therapy Checklists

evolve Website (http://evolve.elsevier.com/Lilley)
- Nursing Care Plans • Frequently Asked Questions • Content Updates • WebLinks • Supplemental Resources • Elsevier ePharmacology Update • Medication Administration Animations

Drug Profiles

▶ bethanechol, p. 299	memantine, p. 302
cevimeline, p. 300	▶ physostigmine, p. 300
▶ donepezil, p. 301	▶ pyridostigmine, p. 300
galantamine, p. 301	rivastigmine, p. 302

▶ Key drug.

Glossary

Acetylcholine (ACh) Neurotransmitter responsible for transmission of nerve impulses to effector cells in the parasympathetic nervous system (PSNS). (p. 297)

Acetylcholinesterase (AChE) Enzyme responsible for the breakdown of ACh (also referred to simply as *cholinesterase*). (p. 298)

Alzheimer's disease A disease that is characterized by progressive mental deterioration manifested by loss of memory, ability to calculate, and visual-spatial orientation, as well as by confusion and disorientation. (p. 298)

Cholinergic drugs Drugs that stimulate the PSNS by mimicking ACh. (p. 298)

Direct-acting cholinergic agonists Cholinergic drugs that bind directly to cholinergic receptors to activate them. (p. 298)

Indirect-acting cholinergic agonists Cholinergic drugs that work indirectly by making more ACh available at the receptor site. (p. 298)

Irreversible cholinesterase inhibitors Drugs that form a permanent covalent bond with cholinesterase. (p. 298)

Miosis Contraction of the pupil. (p. 298)

Muscarinic receptors Effector-organ cholinergic receptors located postsynaptically in the smooth muscle, cardiac muscle, and glands supplied by parasympathetic fibers; so named because they can be stimulated by the alkaloid muscarine. (p. 297)

Nicotinic receptors Cholinergic receptors located in the *ganglia* (where presynaptic and postsynaptic nerve fibers meet) of both the PSNS and the sympathetic nervous system; so named because they can be stimulated by the alkaloid nicotine. (p. 297)

Parasympathomimetics Another name for cholinergic drugs that mimic the effects of ACh. (p. 298)

Reversible cholinesterase inhibitors Drugs that bind to cholinesterase for minutes to hours but do not form a permanent bond. (p. 298)

Cholinergics, cholinergic agonists, and *parasympathomimetics* are all terms that refer to the class of drugs which stimulate the parasympathetic nervous system (PSNS). For a better understanding of how these drugs work, it is helpful to know how the PSNS operates in relation to the rest of the nervous system.

PARASYMPATHETIC NERVOUS SYSTEM

The PSNS is the branch of the autonomic nervous system with nerve functions generally opposite those of the sympathetic nervous system (SNS) (Figure 19-1). The neurotransmitter responsible for the transmission of nerve impulses to effector cells in the PSNS is **acetylcholine (ACh).** A receptor that binds the ACh and mediates its actions is called a *cholinergic receptor.* There are two types of cholinergic receptor, as determined by their location and their action once stimulated. **Nicotinic re-** ceptors are located in the ganglia of both the PSNS and SNS. They are called *nicotinic* because they can also be stimulated by the alkaloid nicotine. The other cholinergic receptors are the **muscarinic receptors.** These receptors are located postsynaptically in the effector organs (i.e., smooth muscle, cardiac muscle, and glands) supplied by the parasympathetic fibers. They are called *muscarinic* because they are stimulated by the alkaloid muscarine, a substance isolated from mushrooms. Figure 19-2 shows how the nicotinic and muscarinic receptors are arranged in the PSNS.

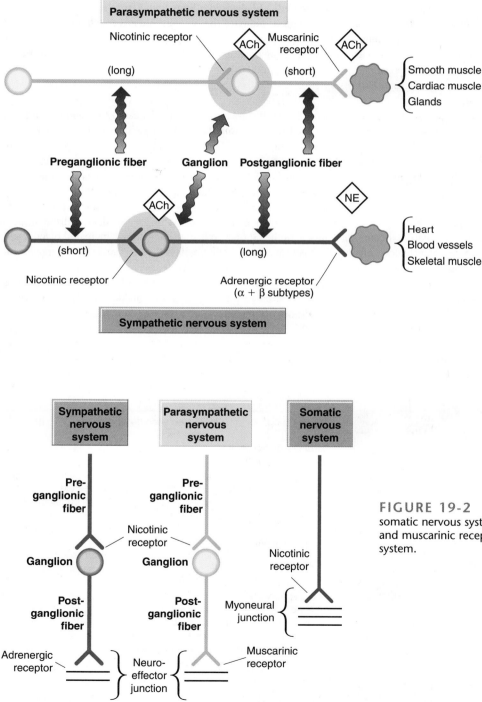

FIGURE 19-1   The parasympathetic and sympathetic nervous systems and their relationship to one another. *ACh,* Acetylcholine; *NE,* norepinephrine.

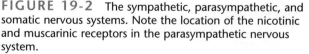

FIGURE 19-2   The sympathetic, parasympathetic, and somatic nervous systems. Note the location of the nicotinic and muscarinic receptors in the parasympathetic nervous system.

CHOLINERGIC DRUGS

Cholinergic drugs mimic the effects of ACh and are therefore sometimes referred to as **parasympathomimetics.** These drugs can stimulate cholinergic receptors either directly or indirectly. **Direct-acting cholinergic agonists** bind to cholinergic receptors and activate them. **Indirect-acting cholinergic agonists** act by stimulating postsynaptic nerve cell (neuronal) release of ACh at the receptor site, which allows the ACh to bind to and stimulate the receptor. They do this by inhibiting the action of **acetylcholinesterase (AChE),** the enzyme responsible for breaking down ACh, which is also referred to simply as *cholinesterase.* The indirect-acting cholinergic drugs bind to the cholinesterase in one of two ways: reversibly or irreversibly. **Reversible cholinesterase inhibitors** bind to cholinesterase for a period of minutes to hours; **irreversible cholinesterase inhibitors** bind to cholinesterase and form a permanent covalent bond. The body must then generate new enzymes to override the effects of the irreversible drugs. Box 19-1 lists the direct- and indirect-acting cholinergics.

These drugs are used to reduce intraocular pressure (IOP) in patients with glaucoma or in those undergoing ocular surgery (see Chapter 58), to treat various gastrointestinal (GI) and bladder disorders, to diagnose and treat myasthenia gravis, to treat **Alzheimer's disease,** and to treat excessively dry mouth (xerostomia) resulting from a disorder known as *Sjögren's syndrome.*

Mechanism of Action and Drug Effects

When ACh directly binds to its receptor, stimulation occurs. Once binding takes place on the membranes of effector cells (cells of the target tissues or organs), the permeability of the cells changes and calcium and sodium are permitted to flow into the cells. This depolarizes the cell membrane and stimulates the effector organ.

The effects of direct- and indirect-acting cholinergics are those that are generally seen when the PSNS is stimulated. There are many mnemonics to aid in remembering these effects. One is to think of the PSNS as the "rest-and-digest" system.

Cholinergic drugs stimulate the intestine and bladder, which results in increased gastric secretions, GI motility, and urinary frequency. They also stimulate the pupil to constrict, causing **miosis.** This helps decrease IOP. In addition, parasympathomimetic drugs cause increased salivation and sweating. Their cardiovascular effects include decreased heart rate and vasodilation. These drugs also cause the bronchi of the lungs to constrict and the airways to narrow.

ACh is also needed for normal brain function. It is in short supply in patients with Alzheimer's disease. At recommended dosages, cholinergics primarily affect the muscarinic receptors, but at high dosages the nicotinic receptors can also be stimulated. The desired effects come from muscarinic receptor stimulation; many of the undesirable adverse effects are due to nicotinic receptor stimulation. The various effects of the cholinergic drugs are listed in Table 19-1 according to the receptors stimulated.

Indications

Most of the direct-acting drugs (ACh, carbachol, and pilocarpine) are used topically to reduce IOP in patients with glaucoma or in those undergoing ocular surgery. They are poorly absorbed orally because they have large quaternary amines in their chemical structure. This limits their use mostly to topical application. One exception is the direct-acting cholinergic drug bethanechol, which can be administered orally or as a subcutaneous injection. It primarily affects the detrusor muscle of the urinary bladder and the smooth muscle of the GI tract. When given, it causes increased bladder and GI tract tone and motility, which thereby increases the movement of contents through these areas. It also causes the sphincters in the bladder and the GI tract to relax, which allows them to empty. It is therefore used to treat atony of the bladder and GI tract, which sometimes occurs after a surgical procedure.

Box 19-1 Cholinergic Drugs

Direct-Acting Drugs

bethanechol
carbachol
cevimeline
pilocarpine
succinylcholine

Indirect-Acting Drugs

ambenonium
demecarium
donepezil
echothiophate
edrophonium
galantamine
isoflurophate
methacholine
neostigmine
physostigmine
pyridostigmine
rivastigmine
tacrine

Table 19-1 Cholinergic Agonists: Drug Effects

Body Tissue	Response to Stimulation	
	Muscarinic	**Nicotinic**
Bronchi (lung)	Increased secretion, constriction	None
Cardiovascular		
Blood vessels	Dilation	Constriction
Heart rate	Slowed	Increased
Blood pressure	Decreased	Increased
Eye	Pupil constriction, decreased accommodation	Pupil constriction, decreased accommodation
Gastrointestinal		
Tone	Increased	Increased
Motility	Increased	Increased
Sphincters	Relaxed	None
Genitourinary		
Tone	Increased	Increased
Motility	Increased	Increased
Sphincter	Relaxed	Relaxed
Glandular secretions	Increased intestinal, lacrimal, salivary, and sweat gland secretion	—
Skeletal muscle	—	Increased contraction

Indirect-acting drugs work by increasing ACh concentrations at the receptor sites, stimulating the effector cells. They cause skeletal muscle contraction and are therefore used for the diagnosis and treatment of myasthenia gravis. Their ability to inhibit AChE also makes them useful for the reversal of neuromuscular blockade produced either by neuromuscular blocking drugs (NMBAs) or by anticholinergic poisoning. For this reason, the indirect-acting drug physostigmine is considered the antidote for anticholinergic poisoning as well as poisoning by irreversible cholinesterase inhibitors such as the organophosphates and carbonates, common classes of insecticides.

In the treatment of Alzheimer's disease, cholinergic drugs increase concentrations of ACh in the brain and thereby improve cholinergic function. The ability to increase ACh levels in the brain by inhibiting AChE and preventing the degradation of endogenously released ACh increases or maintains memory and learning capabilities. Fortunately, the last 2 decades have seen the introduction of four new medications that are specifically used to arrest or slow the progression of Alzheimer's disease. All are indirect-acting anticholinergic drugs, which means that they are inhibitors of the enzyme AChE. Although their therapeutic efficacy is often limited, these drugs can sometimes enhance a patient's mental status enough to make a noticeable, if temporary, improvement in the quality of life for patients as well as caregivers and family members. The most commonly used of these medications at this time is donepezil, but it should be kept in mind that patient response to these drugs, as with most other drug classes, is highly variable. For this reason, a failure to respond to maximally titrated dosages of one of these drugs should not necessarily rule out an attempt at therapy with another. Dosage information for all of these drugs appears in the Dosages table on page 301.

Contraindications

Contraindications to the use of cholinergic drugs include known drug allergy, GI or genitourinary (GU) tract obstruction (which may require surgical correction), bradycardia, defects in cardiac impulse conduction, hyperthyroidism, epilepsy, hypotension, chronic obstructive pulmonary disease, and Parkinson's disease.

Adverse Effects

The primary adverse effects of cholinergic drugs are the consequence of overstimulation of the PSNS. They are extensions of the cholinergic reactions that affect many body functions. The major effects are listed by body system in Table 19-2.

Table 19-2   Cholinergic Drugs: Adverse Effects

Body System	Adverse Effects
Cardiovascular	Bradycardia, hypotension, conduction abnormalities (atrioventricular block and cardiac arrest)
Central nervous	Headache, dizziness, convulsions
Gastrointestinal	Abdominal cramps, increased secretions, nausea, vomiting
Respiratory	Increased bronchial secretions, bronchospasms
Other	Lacrimation, sweating, salivation, loss of ocular accommodation, miosis

Interactions

The potential drug interactions that can occur with the cholinergics are significant because of their severity. Anticholinergics (such as atropine), antihistamines, and sympathomimetics may antagonize cholinergic drugs and lead to a decreased response to them. Other cholinergic drugs may have additive effects.

Toxicity and Management of Overdose

There is very little systemic absorption of the topically administered drugs and therefore little systemic toxicity. When administered locally in the eye, they can cause temporary ocular changes such as transient blurring and dimming of vision, which can be bothersome to the patient. Systemic toxicity with topically applied cholinergics is seen most commonly when longer-acting drugs are given repeatedly over a long period. This can result in overstimulation of the PSNS and all the attendant responses. Treatment is generally symptomatic and supportive, and the administration of a reversal drug (e.g., atropine) is rarely required.

The likelihood of toxicity is greater for cholinergics that are given orally or intravenously. The most severe consequence of an overdose of a cholinergic drug is a cholinergic crisis. The symptoms of such a reaction may include circulatory collapse, hypotension, bloody diarrhea, shock, and cardiac arrest. Early signs include abdominal cramps, salivation, flushing of the skin, nausea, and vomiting. Transient syncope, transient complete heart block, dyspnea, and orthostatic hypotension may also occur. These can be reversed promptly by the administration of atropine, a cholinergic antagonist. Severe cardiovascular reactions or bronchoconstriction may be alleviated by epinephrine, an adrenergic agonist. One way of remembering the effects of cholinergic poisoning is to use the acronym *SLUDGE,* which stands for salivation, lacrimation, urinary incontinence, diarrhea, GI cramps, and emesis.

Dosages

For the recommended dosages of the cholinergic drugs, see the Dosages table on page 301.

Drug Profiles

As noted earlier, of the direct-acting cholinergic drugs, bethanechol is the only drug that is administered orally. A drug formulation of acetylcholine itself and the drug carbachol are two cholinergics applied topically to the eye for the treatment of glaucoma or for the reduction of IOP during ocular surgery. They are discussed in greater detail in Chapter 58, as are the indirect-acting ocular cholinergics echothiophate, demecarium, and isoflurophate, which are used primarily for the treatment of eye disorders or for surgical purposes. The cholinergics are available in oral form as tablets and syrups, in topical form as eyedrops, and parenterally as intravenous and subcutaneous injections. All cholinergics are prescription-only drugs.

▶ bethanechol

Bethanechol (Urecholine) is a direct-acting cholinergic agonist that stimulates the cholinergic receptors located on the smooth muscle of the bladder. This stimulation results in increased bladder tone, increased motility, and relaxation of the sphincter of the bladder. It is used in the treatment of acute postoperative and postpartum nonobstructive urinary retention and for the management of urinary retention associated with neurogenic atony of the bladder. It has also been used to prevent and treat the adverse effects of other classes of drugs, such as bladder dysfunction induced by phenothiazine and

Review

The use of Razadyne (galantamine) to treat mild to moderate Alzheimer's disease was investigated in this particular study and found to produce improved cognitive functioning relative to a placebo after 6 months of therapy. This well-designed study examined the "safety, tolerability, and efficacy" of treatment with Razadyne, using either the non–extended-release or extended-release ER dosage forms. The study compared cognition and daily living skills of a group of individuals taking Razadyne against a group of patients receiving a placebo.

Type of Evidence

Results came from a well-developed research study conducted over a 6-month period and involved 965 patients. A randomized, double-blind, parallel-group, placebo-controlled, flexible-dose study compared the safety, tolerability, and efficacy of drug therapy in patients who were randomly assigned to receive at least one dose of placebo, Razadyne, or Razadyne ER. Score on the Alzheimer's Disease Cooperative Study Activities of Daily Living inventory was used as a secondary outcome measure. Primary outcome measures included scores on the Alzheimer's Disease Assessment Scale—Cognitive Subscale and the Clinician's Interview-Based Impression of Change with Caregiver Input tool. Observed case analysis at 2, 3, and 6 months was reported.

Results of Study

Results over the 6-month period showed that most patients treated with Razadyne ER experienced "significant improvement in cognition" compared with those receiving the placebo. Results of data from the group receiving Razadyne were not shown. However, at 6 months, most patients treated with Razadyne ER also showed no significant decline from baseline in the performance of the activities of daily living (ADLs) and had significantly better ADL scores than those taking the placebo. It is important to remember that this study involved patients diagnosed with mild to moderate Alzheimer's disease. Treatment with Razadyne ER helped to preserve cognitive and related functioning in these patients in home and community settings (see www.razadyne.com/active/janus/en_US/images/raz/cht_results_adls.jpg*MERGEFORMATINET). This study also found the following to be adverse effects of Razadyne ER: nausea, vomiting, diarrhea, loss of appetite, and weight loss.

Link of Evidence to Nursing Practice

The patients treated with Razadyne ER showed improvement in cognitive functioning. Drug-related adverse events were identified as well. By consulting the findings of drug research and specific clinical trials, nurses remain current and well informed about new and cutting-edge treatments for a variety of diseases, including Alzheimer's disease. The nurse can apply the findings of this study regarding improved cognition and possible adverse effects to the nursing process for individual patients taking the drug to treat Alzheimer's disease. One way to link this evidence to nursing practice is in patient education about the most frequent adverse effects of Razadyne ER use, such as nausea, vomiting, diarrhea, loss of appetite, and weight loss.

Based on Ortho-McNeil Pharmaceutical: Dear healthcare professional, March 31, 2005 (letter). Available at www.WebMD.com; more information available at www.ortho-mcneilneurologics.com.

---

tricyclic antidepressants. In addition, it is used in the treatment of postoperative GI atony and gastric retention, chronic refractory heartburn, and familial dysautonomia, as well as in diagnostic testing for infantile cystic fibrosis. Intramuscular and intravenous use are contraindicated. Its use is also contraindicated in patients with hyperthyroidism, peptic ulcer, active bronchial asthma, cardiac disease or coronary artery disease, epilepsy, and parkinsonism. It should also be avoided in patients with conditions in which the strength or integrity of the GI tract or bladder wall is questionable or with conditions in which increased muscular activity could prove harmful, such as known or suspected mechanical obstruction. Bethanechol is available in both oral and parenteral formulations. Pregnancy category C. Commonly recommended dosages are given in the table on page 301.

Pharmacokinetics

Half-Life	Onset	Peak	Duration
Variable	30-90 min	Less than 30 min	1-6 hr

cevimeline

Cevimeline (Evoxac) is a direct-acting cholinergic drug and is the newest medication in this class. It is used to stimulate salivation in patients with the disorder known as Sjögren's syndrome, which causes xerostomia (dry mouth). Its use is contraindicated in patients with any condition in which pupillary miosis might be undesirable, such as narrow-angle glaucoma or iritis, and also with uncontrolled asthma. Pregnancy category C. Dosage information appears in the Dosages table on page 301.

Pharmacokinetics

Half-Life	Onset	Peak	Duration
5 hr	Unknown	1-2 hr	Unknown

▶ physostigmine

Physostigmine (Antilirium) is a synthetic quaternary ammonium compound that is very similar in structure to other drugs in this class, including edrophonium, pyridostigmine (see later), neostigmine, and ambenonium. It is an indirect-acting cholinergic drug that works to increase ACh by inhibiting the enzyme that breaks it down. It has been shown to improve muscle strength and is therefore used in the symptomatic treatment of myasthenia gravis. Neostigmine, pyridostigmine, and ambenonium are the standard drugs used for symptomatic treatment of myasthenia gravis. Edrophonium, another indirect-acting cholinergic drug, is commonly used to diagnose this disorder. It is also useful for reversing the effects of nondepolarizing NMBAs after surgery. It may also be used in the treatment of severe tricyclic antidepressant overdoses. Its use is contraindicated in patients who have shown a hypersensitivity or severe cholinergic reaction to it. It should be used with caution in patients with epilepsy, bronchial asthma, bradycardia, recent coronary artery occlusion, hyperthyroidism, cardiac dysrhythmias, or peptic ulcer. It is available parenterally as an intravenous injection (1 mg/mL) and topically as an ophthalmic solution and ointment. Pregnancy category C. Recommended dosages are given in the table on page 301.

Pharmacokinetics

Half-Life	Onset	Peak	Duration
15-40 min	Less than 5 min	5 min	30-60 min

▶ pyridostigmine

Pyridostigmine (Mestinon) is also a synthetic quaternary ammonium compound and is very similar structurally to edrophonium, neostigmine, and ambenonium. It is an indirect-acting cholinergic drug and is used in the symptomatic treatment of myasthenia gravis. It is also useful for reversing the effects of nondepolarizing NMDAs after surgery. Its use is contraindicated in patients who have shown a hypersensitivity

DOSAGES

Selected Cholinergic Agonist Drugs

Drug	Pharmacologic Class	Usual Dosage Range	Indications
▶bethanechol (Urecholine)	Direct-acting muscarinic	**Adult** PO: 10-50 mg bid-qid (usually start with 5-10 mg, repeating hourly until urination, max 50 mg/cycle)	Postoperative and postpartum functional urinary retention
cevimeline (Evoxac)	Direct-acting muscarinic	**Adult** PO: 30 mg tid	Xerostomia (dry mouth) resulting from Sjögren's syndrome
memantine (Namenda)	NMDA-receptor antagonist	**Adult only** PO: Initial dose is 5 mg/day; may titrate by 5 mg/wk up to max daily dose of 20 mg	Alzheimer's dementia
▶physostigmine (Antilirium)	Anticholinesterase (indirect acting)	**Pediatric** IM/IV: 0.01-0.03 mg/kg repeated at 5-10 min intervals until desired effect or dose of 2 mg reached **Adult** IM/IV: 0.5-2 mg repeated q20min if needed	Myasthenia gravis, reversal of anticholinergic drug effects and TCA overdose
▶pyridostigmine (Mestinon)	Anticholinesterase (indirect acting)	**Pediatric** PO: 7 mg/kg/day divided into 5-6 doses IM/IV: 0.05-0.15 mg/kg/dose **Adult** PO: 60-1500 mg/day divided to provide max therapeutic effect SR tabs: 180-540 mg daily or bid IV: 10-20 mg with suitable anticholinergic	Myasthenia gravis Myasthenia gravis Reversal of nondepolarizing NMBAs

Currently Available Cholinergic Agonist Drugs Specifically for Treating Alzheimer's Disease (in Chronologic Order of Introduction to U.S. Market)

Drug, Year Introduced	Pharmacologic Class	Usual Dosage Range	Indications
tacrine (Cognex), 1993	Anticholinesterase (indirect acting)	**Adult** PO: 40-160 mg divided qid	
▶donepezil (Aricept), 1996	Anticholinesterase (indirect acting)	**Adult** PO: 5-10 mg/day as a single dose	Alzheimer's disease
rivastigmine (Exelon), 2000	Anticholinesterase (indirect acting)	**Adult** PO: 3-12 mg divided bid	
galantamine (Razadyne*), 2001	Anticholinesterase (indirect acting)	**Adult** PO: 16-32 mg divided bid	

IM, Intramuscular; *IV*, intravenous; *NMBA*, neuromuscular blocking drug; *PO*, oral; *SR*, sustained-release; *TCA*, tricyclic antidepressant.
*Reminyl was renamed Razadyne in 2005 to help avoid confusion with the diabetes drug Amaryl (glimepiride).

or severe cholinergic reaction to it. It should be used with caution in patients with epilepsy, bronchial asthma, bradycardia, recent coronary artery occlusion, hyperthyroidism, cardiac dysrhythmias, or peptic ulcer. It is available in oral form as a regular and extended-release tablet and as a solution. It is also available as a parenteral preparation. Pregnancy category C. Recommended dosages are given in the table on this page.

Pharmacokinetics

Half-Life	Onset	Peak	Duration
PO: Variable	PO: 30-45 min	PO: 2-5 min	PO: Less than 30 min
IV: Variable	IV: Less than 5 min	IV: 3-6 hr	IV: 2-4 hr

Cholinergic Agonists Used Specifically for Alzheimer's Disease

▶ donepezil

Donepezil (Aricept) is an indirect-acting anticholinesterase drug that works centrally in the brain to increase levels of ACh by blocking its breakdown. It is used in the treatment of mild to moderate Alzheimer's

disease. Drugs with anticholinergic properties should be avoided in patients taking donepezil because they may counteract the effects of donepezil.

Donepezil offers many advantages over tacrine (Cognex), the first drug in this class of indirect-acting anticholinesterase drugs. Donepezil is dosed only once a day compared with four times a day for tacrine. It is more specific for AChE in the central nervous system (CNS), which decreases the incidence of the drug interactions currently seen with tacrine. Donepezil is available for oral use. Pregnancy category C. Recommended dosages are given in the table on this page.

Pharmacokinetics

Half-Life	Onset	Peak	Duration
72-80 hr	3 wk*	3-4 hr	2 wk*

*Therapeutic effects.

galantamine

Galantamine (Razadyne) is an indirect-acting cholinergic drug. Its mechanism of action is inhibition of the enzyme AChE. It is indicated for the treatment of patients with mild to moderate dementia associated with Alzheimer's disease. Its only known contraindication is drug allergy. Reduced dosages are recommended for patients with moderate renal or hepatic impairment. This drug is *not* recommended for patients with severe renal or hepatic impairment. Adverse effects include nausea, vomiting, dizziness, anorexia (loss of appetite), and syncope. This drug, along with others in its class, has been shown in some cases to alter cardiac conduction in patients with and without prior cardiovascular disease. Therefore, all patients treated with galantamine, as well as other cholinergic drugs, should be considered at risk for cardiac conduction effects. Galantamine is available for oral use. Pregnancy category B. The recommended dosage is given in the table on page 301.

Pharmacokinetics

Half-Life	Onset	Peak	Duration
4-10 hr	Variable*	1 hr	Unknown*

*Onset and duration of drug action for this and other cholinergic drugs used to treat Alzheimer's dementia are difficult to quantify because both may vary significantly among patients. The practitioner should judge the therapeutic effect of these medications according to the degree of change in the patient's mental status.

rivastigmine

Rivastigmine (Exelon) is an indirect-acting cholinergic drug. Its mechanism of action is inhibition of the enzyme AChE. It is indicated for the treatment of patients with mild to moderate dementia associated with Alzheimer's disease. Its only known contraindication is drug allergy to rivastigmine or other carbamate compounds. One therapeutic advantage of rivastigmine compared with some similar drugs used to treat Alzheimer's dementia is that dosage adjustments are not needed or recommended for patients with renal or hepatic impairment. However, the lowest effective dosage should be used. Common adverse effects include dizziness, headache, nausea, vomiting, diarrhea, and anorexia. Rivastigmine is available in oral form. Pregnancy category B. The recommended dosage is given in the table on page 301.

Pharmacokinetics

Half-Life	Onset	Peak	Duration
1.5 hr	Variable*	1 hr	Unknown*

*Onset and duration of drug action for this and other cholinergic drugs used for Alzheimer's dementia are difficult to quantify because both may vary significantly among patients. The practitioner should judge the therapeutic effect of these medications according to the degree of change in the patient's mental status.

Miscellaneous Alzheimer's Disease Medications
memantine

In 2003, the Food and Drug Administration (FDA) approved a new medication for the treatment of Alzheimer's disease. Memantine (Namenda) is classified as an N-methyl D-aspartate (NMDA) receptor antagonist due to its inhibitory activity at the NMDA receptors in the CNS. Stimulation of these receptors is believed to be part of the Alzheimer's disease process. Memantine blocks this stimulation and thereby helps to reduce or arrest the patient's degenerative cognitive symptoms. As with all other currently available medications for this debilitating illness, the effects of this drug are likely to be temporary but may still afford some improvement in quality of life and general functioning for some patients. Its only current contraindication is known drug allergy. No pregnancy category is currently listed. The recommended dosage is given in the table on page 301.

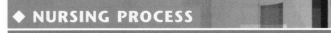

◆ NURSING PROCESS

◆ ASSESSMENT

Cholinergic drugs, or parasympathomimetics, produce a variety of effects stemming from their ability to stimulate the PSNS and mimic the action of ACh. These effects include the following:

- Decrease in heart rate
- Increase in GI and GU tone through increased contractility of the smooth muscle
- Increase in the contractility and tone of bronchial smooth muscle
- Increased respiratory secretions
- Miosis (pupillary constriction)

For patients taking cholinergic drugs, a thorough head-to-toe physical assessment, nursing history, and medication history should be taken before the drugs are given. Information about patient allergies and past and present medical conditions needs to be assessed and documented prior to administration of the cholinergic drugs. Cautions, contraindications, and drug interactions also need to be identified and documented (see the previous discussion).

Before a drug for Alzheimer's disease is used, the patient must be assessed for allergies to it, to other drugs, or to any piperidine derivative. Because galantamine and other related drugs may cause cardiac conduction problems in patients with and without prior cardiac problems, it is important to assess heart sounds, any cardiac problems (e.g., chest pain, irregularities), blood pressure, and pulse rate before and during therapy. Before initiation of drug therapy with donepezil, the nurse should assess and document the patient's: vital signs, GI and GU history and status, mental status, mood, affect, changes in mental behavior, depression, and level of consciousness or suicidal tendencies. Once the patient has begun taking the medication, it is critical for the nurse to continue to assess the patient's response to the drug, especially if there is no improvement within a 6-week period. At this point, the health care provider may find it necessary to adjust the dosage. The nurse should assess for use of herbals. Ginkgo may be used by some health care providers for organic brain syndrome (see the Herbal Therapies and Dietary Supplements box on this page). The patient must be assessed for possible medical contraindications and cautions, just as with prescription drugs. See the individual discussions earlier for information regarding other contraindications and drug interactions.

HERBAL THERAPIES AND DIETARY SUPPLEMENTS
Ginkgo (Ginkgo biloba)

Overview
The dried leaf of the ginkgo plant contains flavonoids, terpenoids, and organic acids that help ginkgo preparations exert their positive effects as an antioxidant and inhibitor of platelet aggregation.

Common Uses
Organic brain syndrome, peripheral arterial occlusive disease, vertigo, tinnitus

Adverse Effects
Stomach or intestinal upset, headache, bleeding, allergic skin reaction

Potential Drug Interactions
Aspirin, nonsteroidal antiinflammatory drugs, warfarin, heparin, anticonvulsants, ticlopidine, clopidogrel, dipyridamole, tricyclic antidepressants

Contraindications
None

◆ NURSING DIAGNOSES

- Acute pain related to the adverse effects of abdominal cramping caused by drug therapy
- Deficient knowledge of the therapeutic regimen, adverse effects, drug interactions, and precautions for cholinergic drugs
- Risk for injury related to the possible adverse effects of cholinergic drugs (bradycardia and hypotension)
- Decreased cardiac output related to the cardiovascular adverse effects of dysrhythmias, hypotension, and bradycardia
- Disturbed sensory perception related to the adverse CNS effects of cholinergic drugs

◆ PLANNING

Goals

- Patient receives or takes medications as prescribed.
- Patient experiences relief of the symptoms for which the medication was prescribed.
- Patient remains compliant with the drug therapy regimen.
- Patient demonstrates adequate knowledge concerning the use of the specific medication, its adverse effects, and the appropriate dosing at home.
- Patient remains free of self-injury resulting from the adverse effects of the medication.

Outcome Criteria

- Patient states the importance of both the pharmacologic and nonpharmacologic treatment of the GI or GU tract disorder or glaucoma in achieving good health.
- Patient states reasons for compliance with the medication therapy and the risks associated with noncompliance as well as the complications associated with overuse of the medication, such as bronchospasm, increased abdominal cramping, and decreased pulse and blood pressure.
- Patient states conditions under which to contact the physician, such as the occurrence of wheezing, bradycardia, and/or increased abdominal pain.
- Patient states the importance of scheduling and keeping follow-up appointments with the physician related to the management of the disorder for which medication has been prescribed.

◆ IMPLEMENTATION

Several nursing interventions can be implemented to maximize the therapeutic effects of cholinergic drugs and minimize their adverse effects. The nurse should be sure that patients who have undergone surgery ambulate as early as possible after the procedure (as ordered) to help minimize or prevent gastric and urinary retention and maximize the effects of these medications. For drugs used to treat myasthenia gravis, the oral medication should be given about 30 minutes before meals to allow for onset of action and therapeutic effects (e.g., decreased dysphagia). The packaging inserts should always be checked for instructions concerning dilutional drugs and the route of administration (e.g., bethanechol is administered orally or subcutaneously). Atropine is the antidote to cholinergic overdose; therefore, this medication should be available as necessary and per facility protocol and used only if ordered.

None of the drugs listed in this chapter is used as a "cure" for Alzheimer's disease, because there is no cure. The nurse should be honest with the patient, family, significant others, and caregivers about the fact that any of these drugs is given only for symptomatic improvement and not for cure. Of course, the nurse must always adhere to the American Nurses Association's Code of Ethics, maintain a high level of professionalism, and respect patients' rights when developing care plans. Any sharing of information with the patient, family, significant others, and caregivers must be done with the approval of the physician, with good intent, in compliance with any research protocol, and/or with the goal of being a patient advocate. When beginning any of these medications, the patient will most likely need continued assistance and help with activities of daily living and ambulation (because the medication may increase dizziness and cause gait imbalances at the initiation of treatment). The patient, family members, and/or caregivers also need to understand the importance of taking the medication exactly as ordered. In addition, the patient and anyone involved in the patient's daily care should be instructed about how the medication should be taken (such as the importance of taking the drug with food to decrease GI upset); should be informed of any possible interactions, concerns, or potential for harm; and should be told the importance of *not* withdrawing the medication abruptly. The patient must be weaned off all drugs over a period of time designated by the physician because of the potential for serious complications if weaning does not occur.

Most of the cholinergic agonists have dose-limiting adverse effects that include severe GI disturbances (nausea and vomiting). Also, blood pressure readings and corresponding pulse rates should be taken and recorded before, during, and after initiation of therapy. Dizziness with therapy is not unusual and may be an indication of the need for more assistance with care and ambulation. Ataxia may also indicate the need for further assessment and intervention by the nurse and health care provider. In addition, keeping a journal of these parameters as well as information about the patient's mental status, cognition, and ability to perform activities of daily living would be helpful to all involved in the patient's care.

Dosages may be changed by the physician after about 6 weeks if no response to the medication occurs. For patient safety, when galantamine and some of the other newer drugs are used, the nurse must take blood pressure and pulse and have electrocardiogram baseline studies available as ordered. The patient should be encouraged to report to the health care provider any new cardiac distress such as new chest discomfort or palpitations. Cevimeline, used to treat xerostomia (dry mouth), must be taken as ordered for maximal therapeutic effects.

In summary, because most of the cholinergic drugs are in the group of medications used to treat patients diagnosed with Alzheimer's disease, it is important that the individuals who comprise the support systems for these patients know some of the questions to which it would be helpful to get answers once a loved one is diagnosed with the disease. These questions include the following:

- What should we expect for our loved one? What will happen to the person emotionally and physically?
- What treatments are available and what drugs are deemed safe? What are the common adverse effects of drug therapy? How can adverse effects be minimized?
- What about diet, fluids, and exercise for our loved one?
- Are there herbals or any sort of supplements or over-the-counter drugs that would help with the disease or should they be avoided in the treatment of the disease?
- What will we need to do for long-term care or other living situations for our loved one?

- What are the expected costs for this person's care now and in the future? What are the costs of drug therapy? Other costs?
- What kind of help can we all receive emotionally? What about emotional support for our loved one?
- How can this disease affect intimate relationships?
- What type of attorney should we seek out? What about durable power of attorney and living wills? Other types of wills? Are these needed right away if we don't have these legal documents already?
- How do we all go on with our lives when our loved one is changing so drastically?
- Will life ever be normal again?
- What about research and clinical trials for treatment regimens? Should we pursue other treatments or do nothing new? What about drugs that are not FDA approved?
- How long will this process take? Just what can we expect over time?

◆ EVALUATION

The following are some therapeutic effects for which to monitor in patients receiving cholinergic drugs: In patients with myasthenia gravis, the signs and symptoms of the disease should be decreased but may not be completely alleviated. In patients suffering a decrease in GI peristalsis postoperatively, there should be an increase in bowel sounds, the passage of flatus, and the occurrence of bowel movements that indicate increased GI peristalsis. In patients who have a hypotonic bladder with urinary retention, micturition (voiding) should occur within about 60 minutes of the administration of bethanechol.

The nurse must also be alert to the occurrence of the adverse effects of these medications, including increased respiratory secretions, bronchospasms, nausea, vomiting, diarrhea, hypotension, bradycardia, and conduction abnormalities. For other adverse effects, see Table 19-2.

Therapeutic effects of most of the drugs used to manage Alzheimer's disease–related dementia or cognitive impairment may not occur for up to 6 weeks but include an improvement of the symptoms of the disease. Varying degrees of improvement in mood and a decrease in confusion usually occur. Adverse effects include nausea, vomiting, dizziness, and others. (See individual drug profiles for specific information.) Cardiac conductive disorders and hepatic problems are the associated adverse effects with galantamine.

Therapeutic effects of cevimeline include an improvement in moisture level in the mouth. Adverse effects are similar to those of the other cholinergic agonists.

Patient Teaching Tips

- Encourage participation of family, significant others, and/or caregivers in the care of patients with Alzheimer's disease.
- Encourage patients to take medications exactly as ordered and with meals to minimize GI upset. They should never double up on medication, if a dose has been omitted.
- Encourage patients to maintain consistent time spacing of doses of medication to optimize therapeutic effects and minimize adverse effects and toxicity.
- Patients (along with family, significant others, or caregivers) should be encouraged to call the physician or other health care provider if there is any increased muscle weakness, abdominal cramps, diarrhea, dizziness, ataxia, and/or difficulty breathing.
- Patients should be informed that if they are taking the medication for the treatment of myasthenia gravis, signs and symptoms associated with the disease should begin to decrease and so there should be fewer problems with ptosis (eyelid drooping) and diplopia (double vision), less difficulty swallowing and chewing, and an improvement in muscle weakness.
- If the medication is being taken for myasthenia gravis, patients should take it 30 minutes before meals so that the drug begins to work before the patient chews and swallows. This will help with strengthening muscles for chewing/eating.
- Educate patients that if they are taking a sustained-released or extended-release dosage form it should be taken as is and *not* crushed, chewed, or broken in any way.
- Patients should always wear or have on their person an identification bracelet or necklace with a medical diagnoses, list of medications, and any special requirements regarding emergency treatment and allergies.

Points to Remember

- *Cholinergics, cholinergic agonists,* and *parasympathomimetics* are all appropriate terms for the class of drugs that stimulate the PSNS (the branch of the autonomic nervous system that opposes the SNS).
- The primary neurotransmitter of the PSNS is ACh. There are two types of cholinergic receptors: nicotinic and muscarinic.
- Nicotinic receptors are located on preganglionic nerve fibers in the PSNS, SNS, and adrenal medulla. Muscarinic receptors are located on postsynaptic cells in muscles and glands (*not* on the nerves).
- Nursing considerations for the administration of cholinergic drugs include giving the drug as directed and monitoring the patient carefully for the occurrence of bradycardia, hypotension, headache, dizziness, respiratory depression, or bronchospasms. If these occur in a patient taking cholinergics, the health care provider must be contacted immediately.
- Nursing considerations for the administration of drugs used to treat Alzheimer's include the following: (1) It may take about 6 weeks for a therapeutic response to occur. (2) Cardiac screening (measurement of blood pressure, postural blood pressures, electrocardiogram) and neurologic screening is very important before the initiation of drug therapy. (3) Any new or different cardiac adverse effects, such as new chest discomfort or palpitations, should be reported to the physician or health care provider immediately.
- Patients taking cholinergics should always be encouraged to change positions slowly to avoid dizziness and fainting resulting from postural hypotension.

NCLEX Examination Review Questions

1. A patient is taking the direct-acting cholinergic drug bethanechol (Urecholine) before meals. After 3 days, he calls his health care provider's office and complains of occasional nausea and vomiting. Which of the following instructions is appropriate?
   a. "Continue to take it on an empty stomach to minimize GI upset."
   b. "If this continues, you can skip a dose and try it again tomorrow."
   c. "If these symptoms continue, take the doses in the evening."
   d. "Take this medication with meals to reduce GI upset."

2. The family of a patient who has recently been diagnosed with Alzheimer's disease is asking about the new drug prescribed to treat this disease. The patient's wife says, "I'm so excited that there are drugs that can cure this disease! I can't wait for him to start it." Which of the following replies from the nurse is appropriate?
   a. "The sooner he starts the medicine, the sooner it can have this effect."
   b. "These effects won't be seen for a few months."
   c. "These drugs do not cure Alzheimer's disease. Let's talk about what the physician said to expect with this drug therapy."
   d. "His response to this drug therapy will depend on how far along he is in the disease process."

3. When giving intravenous cholinergic drugs, the nurse must watch for symptoms of a cholinergic crisis. Which of the following is a symptom of this reaction?
   a. Peripheral tingling
   b. Hypotension
   c. Hypertension
   d. Tinnitus

4. A patient took an accidental overdose of a cholinergic drug while at home. He goes to the emergency department with severe abdominal cramping and bloody diarrhea. The nurse expects that which drug will be used to treat this patient?
   a. Atropine
   b. Physostigmine
   c. Lidocaine
   d. Protamine sulfate

5. A patient with myasthenia gravis has received a prescription for pyridostigmine (Mestinon). Which teaching point is appropriate for this patient?
   a. The drug is taken once in the mornings for maximum effect.
   b. The drug should be taken 30 minutes before eating meals.
   c. The drug should be taken 30 minutes after eating meals.
   d. This drug can be given without regard to meals.

1. d, 2. c, 3. b, 4. a, 5. b.

Critical Thinking Activities

1. Compare the uses for direct- and indirect-acting parasympathomimetics and the assessment of the patients who may take these drugs.
2. Describe the symptoms of cholinergic poisoning, or cholinergic crisis, and discuss its treatment.
3. An elderly neighbor wants to take Ginkgo (Ginkgo biloba) because he is worried about "losing it." He lives alone since being widowed last year and does not have any family members in the area. Review the drug box on Herbal Therapies and Dietary Supplements in this chapter and other sources, if desired. What would you say to him?

For answers, see http://evolve.elsevier.com/Lilley.

Cholinergic-Blocking Drugs

Objectives

When you reach the end of this chapter, you should be able to do the following:

1. Describe the function of cholinergic receptors with contrast of stimulation versus blocking of these receptors.
2. List the drugs that are cholinergic blockers.
3. Discuss the mechanisms of action, therapeutic effects, indications, adverse and toxic effects, dosages, routes of administration, contraindications, cautions, and drug interactions of the various cholinergic-blocking drugs.
4. Develop a nursing care plan that includes all phases of the nursing process related to the administration of cholinergic-blocking drugs.

e-Learning Activities

Companion CD

- NCLEX Review Questions: see questions 141-147
- Animations
- Audio Glossary
- Category Catchers
- Medication Errors Checklists
- IV Therapy Checklists

evolve Website (http://evolve.elsevier.com/Lilley)

- Nursing Care Plans • Frequently Asked Questions • Content Updates • WebLinks • Supplemental Resources • Elsevier ePharmacology Update • Medication Administration Animations

Drug Profiles

▶ atropine, p. 310
▶ benztropine mesylate (Chapter 14), p. 217
▶ dicyclomine, p. 310

glycopyrrolate, p. 310
scopolamine, p. 310
▶ tolterodine, p. 310

▶ Key drug.

Glossary

Anticholinergics Another name for cholinergic-blocking drugs. (p. 306)

Cholinergic-blocking drugs Drugs that block the action of acetylcholine (ACh) and substances similar to ACh at receptor sites in the synapse. Such drugs in effect block the action of the cholinergic nerves that transmit impulses through the release of ACh at their synapses. (p. 306)

Competitive antagonists Drugs or other substances that are antagonists or that resemble an endogenous human substance (metabolite) and interfere with its function in the body, usually by competing for its receptor sites or enzymes. Also called *antimetabolites*. (p. 306)

Mydriasis Dilation of the pupil of the eye caused by contraction of the dilator muscle of the iris. (p. 307)

CHOLINERGIC-BLOCKING DRUGS

Cholinergic blockers, anticholinergics, parasympatholytics, and *antimuscarinic drugs* are all terms that refer to the class of drugs that block or inhibit the actions of acetylcholine (ACh) in the parasympathetic nervous system (PSNS). **Cholinergic-blocking drugs** block the action of the neurotransmitter ACh at the muscarinic receptors in the PSNS. ACh released from a stimulated nerve fiber is then unable to bind to the receptor site and fails to produce a cholinergic effect. This is why the cholinergic blockers are also referred to as **anticholinergics.** Blocking the parasympathetic nerves allows the sympathetic (adrenergic) nervous system (SNS) to dominate. Because of this, cholinergic blockers have many of the same effects as the adrenergics. Figure 20-1 illustrates the site of action of the cholinergic blockers in the PSNS.

Cholinergic blockers have many important therapeutic uses and are one of the oldest groups of therapeutic drugs. Originally they were derived from various plant sources, but today these naturally occurring substances are only part of a larger group of cholinergic blockers that also include both synthetic and semisynthetic drugs. Box 20-1 lists the currently available cholinergic blockers grouped according to their chemical class.

Mechanism of Action and Drug Effects

Cholinergic blockers are largely **competitive antagonists.** They compete with ACh for binding at the muscarinic receptors of the PSNS. Once they have bound to the receptor, they inhibit nerve transmission at these receptors. This generally occurs at the neuroeffector junction of smooth muscle, cardiac muscle, and glands. Cholinergic blockers have little effect at the nicotinic receptors, although at high doses they can have partial blocking effects.

The major sites of action of the anticholinergics are the heart, respiratory tract, gastrointestinal (GI) tract, urinary bladder, eye, and exocrine glands. In general the anticholinergics have effects opposite those of the cholinergics at these sites of action. The blockade of ACh by cholinergic blockers causes the pupils to dilate and increases intraocular pressure. This can occur because the ciliary muscles and the sphincter muscle of the iris are innervated by cholinergic nerve fibers. Cholinergic blockers can there-

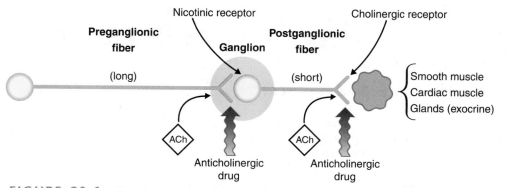

FIGURE 20-1   Site of action of cholinergic blockers in the parasympathetic nervous system. *ACh,* Acetylcholine.

Box 20-1	Cholinergic Blockers Grouped According to Chemical Class

Natural Drugs
atropine
belladonna
hyoscyamine
scopolamine

Synthetic and Semisynthetic Drugs
benztropine (see Chapter 14)
clidinium
dicyclomine
glycopyrrolate
homatropine
ipratropium
isopropamide
mepenzolate
methantheline
methscopolamine
oxybutynin
propantheline
solifenacin
tolterodine
trihexyphenidyl (Chapter 14)

Table 20-1	Cholinergic Blockers: Drug Effects
Body System	**Cholinergic-Blocking Effects**
Cardiovascular	Small doses: decrease heart rate
	Large doses: increase heart rate
Central nervous	Small doses: decrease muscle rigidity and tremors
	Large doses: cause drowsiness, disorientation, hallucinations
Eye	Dilate pupils (mydriasis), decrease accommodation by paralyzing ciliary muscles (cycloplegia)
Gastrointestinal	Relax smooth muscle tone of gastrointestinal tract, decrease intestinal and gastric secretions, decrease motility and peristalsis
Genitourinary	Relax detrusor muscle of bladder, increase constriction of internal sphincter; these two effects may result in urinary retention
Glandular	Decrease bronchial secretions, salivation, sweating
Respiratory	Decrease bronchial secretions, dilate bronchial airways

fore keep the sphincter muscle of the iris from contracting and allow unopposed radial muscle stimulation. The result is dilation of the pupil (**mydriasis**) and paralysis of the ocular lens (cycloplegia). This can be detrimental to patients with glaucoma, however, because it results in increased intraocular pressure.

In the GI tract, cholinergic blockers cause a decrease in GI motility, GI secretions, and salivation. In the cardiovascular system these drugs cause an increase in heart rate. In the genitourinary (GU) system, anticholinergics lead to decreased bladder contraction, which can result in urinary retention. In the skin they reduce sweating, and in the respiratory system they dry mucous membranes and cause bronchial dilation. These and other effects are listed by body system in Table 20-1. Many of these cholinergic-blocking drugs are available in a variety of forms, including intravenous, intramuscular, oral, and subcutaneous preparations.

Indications

At the level of the central nervous system (CNS), cholinergic blockers have the therapeutic effect of decreasing muscle rigidity and diminishing tremors. This is of benefit in the treatment of both Parkinson's disease (Chapter 14) and drug-induced extrapyramidal reactions. The therapeutic cardiovascular effects of anticholinergics are related to their cholinergic-blocking effects on the heart's conduction system. At low dosages the anticholinergics may actually slow the heart rate through their effects on the cardiac center in the portion of the brain called the *medulla.* At high dosages, cholinergic blockers block the inhibitory vagal (i.e., parasympathetic or cholinergic) effects on the pacemaker cells of the sinoatrial and atrioventricular nodes, which leads to acceleration of the heart rate due to unopposed sympathetic activity. Atropine is primarily used to treat cardiovascular disorders, such as in the diagnosis of sinus node dysfunction, the treatment of patients with symptomatic second-degree atrioventricular block, and provision of advanced life support in the treatment of sinus bradycardia that is accompanied by hemodynamic compromise.

As previously mentioned, when the cholinergic stimulation of the PSNS is blocked by cholinergic blockers, the SNS effects go unopposed. In the respiratory tract this results in decreased secretions from the nose, mouth, pharynx, and bronchi. It also causes relaxation of the smooth muscles in the bronchi and bronchioles, which results in decreased airway resistance and bronchodilation. Because of this, the cholinergic blockers have proved beneficial in treating exercise-induced bronchospasms, chronic bronchitis, asthma, and chronic obstructive pulmonary disease.

Gastric secretions and the smooth muscles responsible for producing gastric motility are both controlled by the PSNS, which is primarily under the control of muscarinic receptors. Cholinergic blockers antagonize these receptors, causing decreased secretions, relaxation of smooth muscle, and decreased GI motility and peristalsis. For these reasons cholinergic blockers are commonly used in the treatment of irritable bowel disease and GI hypersecretory states.

The effects that anticholinergics have on the bladder have made them useful in the treatment of such GU tract disorders as reflex neurogenic bladder and incontinence. They relax the detrusor muscles of the bladder and increase constriction of the internal sphincter. The ability of cholinergic blockers to decrease glandular secretions also makes them potentially useful drugs for reducing gastric and pancreatic secretions in patients with acute pancreatitis. They are also used preoperatively to reduce salivary secretions, which aids in intubation and other procedures (e.g., endoscopy) involving the oral cavity.

Contraindications

Contraindications to the use of anticholinergic drugs include known drug allergy, narrow-angle glaucoma, acute asthma or other respiratory distress, myasthenia gravis, acute cardiovascular instability (some exceptions were listed previously), and GI or GU tract obstruction or other acute GI or GU illness.

Adverse Effects

Many body systems are affected adversely by cholinergic blockers because of the site of action of these drugs. The muscarinic receptors are located in a variety of tissues, organs, and glands throughout the body. Therefore, blockade of these receptors by the anticholinergics produces a wide range of effects, some desirable, as described in the previous section, and some not so desirable, depending on the clinical situation. The various adverse effects of cholinergic blockers are listed by body system in Table 20-2.

Other factors contributing to the wide variety of possible adverse effects of cholinergic blockers are the relative affinity of the muscarinic receptors for specific drugs and the drug dosage. Certain patient populations are also more susceptible to the effects of these drugs. These groups include infants, older adults, fair-skinned children with Down syndrome, and children with spastic paralysis or brain damage.

Interactions

The potential drug interactions that can occur with cholinergic blockers are significant and often involve additive or synergistic drug effects. Knowledge of the broad categories of drugs that should not be coadministered with cholinergic blockers can help prevent potentially serious consequences. Additive cholinergic effects can be seen when antihistamines, phenothiazines, tricyclic antidepressants, and monoamine oxidase inhibitors are given with cholinergic blockers. Isopropamide can also alter the results of thyroid function tests.

Table 20-2	Cholinergic Blockers: Adverse Effects
Body System	**Adverse Effects**
Cardiovascular	Increased heart rate, dysrhythmias
Central nervous	Central nervous system excitation, restlessness, irritability, disorientation, hallucinations, delirium
Eye	Dilated pupils, decreased visual accommodation, increased intraocular pressure
Gastrointestinal	Decreased salivation, gastric secretions, motility
Genitourinary	Urinary retention
Glandular	Decreased sweating
Respiratory	Decreased bronchial secretions

Toxicity and Management of Overdose

The dosage of cholinergic blockers is particularly important because there is a very small difference between therapeutic and toxic dosages. Drugs with this characteristic are commonly referred to as having a *narrow therapeutic index*. The treatment of cholinergic blocker overdose consists of symptomatic and supportive therapy. The patient should be hospitalized, and close, continuous monitoring, including continuous electrocardiographic monitoring, should be initiated. The stomach should be emptied by whichever means is most appropriate, through induction of emesis with syrup of ipecac if the patient is awake and not having convulsions or through lavage if this is not the case. Activated charcoal has proven very effective in removing drug from the GI tract that has not already been absorbed. Ipecac is still available but used much less routinely than in the past.

Fluid therapy and other standard measures used for the treatment of shock should be instituted as needed. Delirium, hallucinations, coma, and cardiac dysrhythmias respond favorably to physostigmine treatment. Its routine use as an antidote for cholinergic blocker overdose is controversial, however. It has the potential to produce severe adverse effects such as seizures and cardiac asystole and should therefore be reserved for the treatment of patients who show extreme delirium or agitation or who could inflict injury on themselves.

Dosages

For the recommended dosages of selected cholinergic blockers, see the Dosages table on page 309.

Drug Profiles

All cholinergic blockers are prescription-only drugs. They are available in many dosage formulations: oral, topical, and injectable. Most of the cholinergic blockers are classified as pregnancy category C drugs; dicyclomine and mepenzolate are classified as pregnancy category B drugs.

Among the oldest and best known naturally occurring cholinergic blockers are the belladonna alkaloids. It is the belladonna alkaloid contained in the anticholinergic drugs that is responsible for their therapeutic effects. Of these, atropine is the prototypical drug. It has been in use for hundreds of years and continues to be widely administered because of its effectiveness. Besides atropine, scopolamine and hyoscyamine are the other major naturally occurring drugs. These drugs come from a variety of plants in the potato family (Solanaceae). Some examples

DOSAGES

Selected Cholinergic Antagonist (Anticholinergic) Drugs

Drug	Pharmacologic Class	Usual Dosage Range	Indications
▶atropine		**Pediatric** 0.01-0.02 mg/kg/dose preop and/or q4-6h 0.02 mg/kg, max 0.5 mg 0.05 mg/kg initial dose, repeat q10-30min prn **Adult** IM: 1 mg IV: 0.5-1 mg IV: 1-3 mg/dose, repeat prn until signs of atropine intoxication appear (e.g., tachycardia)	Preop control of secretions, therapeutic anticholinergic effect Treatment of bradycardia Anticholinesterase effect for organophosphate or carbamate poisoning (e.g., insecticides) Hypotonic radiography Treatment of bradycardia, CPR Anticholinesterase effect for organophosphate or carbamate poisoning (e.g., insecticides)
▶dicyclomine (Bentyl)		**Pediatric** PO: 5-10 mg tid-qid **Adult** PO: 80-160 mg/day divided qid	Treatment of irritable bowel syndrome
glycopyrrolate (Robinul)	Anticholinergic	**Pediatric** PO: 40-100 mcg/kg/dose tid-qid IM/IV: 4-10 mcg/kg/dose q3-4h, max 0.2 mg/dose or 0.8 mg/day IV (intraop): 4 mcg/kg, max 0.1 mg; may repeat q2-3min prn **Adult and pediatric 12 yr and older** PO: 1-2 mg bid-tid IM/IV: 0.1-0.2 mg tid-qid IM: 4.4 mcg/kg 30-60 min preop IV (intraop): 0.1 mg, may repeat q2-3min prn **Adult and pediatric** 0.2 mg for each 1 mg of neostigmine or 5 mg of pyridostigmine	Control of secretions Intraop control of secretions Treatment of peptic ulcer Preop control of secretions Intraop control of secretions Reversal of neuromuscular blockade
oxybutynin (Ditropan, Ditropan XL)		**Pediatric 1-5 yr** PO: 0.2 mg/kg/dose bid-qid **Adult and pediatric older than 5 yr** PO: 5 mg bid-qid **Adult only** PO ER tab: 5-30 mg/day in single or divided doses	Antispasmodic for neurogenic bladder (e.g., following spinal cord injury), overactive bladder
scopolamine (Transderm-Scop)		**Pediatric** 6 mcg/kg/dose, max 0.3 mg/dose; may repeat q6-8h **Adult** IM/IV/SC: 0.3-0.65 mg Transdermal patch: 1.5 mg patch behind ear q3days (delivers approx 1 mg scopolamine over 3 days); apply at least 4 hr before transportation	Preop control of secretions Preop control of secretions Motion sickness prevention
solifenacin (Vesicare)		**Adult** PO: 5-10 mg qd	Treatment of overactive bladder
▶tolterodine (Detrol, Detrol XL)		**Adult only** PO: 1-2 mg bid PO ER cap: 2-4 mg qd	Treatment of overactive bladder

CPR, Cardiopulmonary resuscitation; *ER,* extended-release; *IM,* intramuscular; *intraop,* intraoperative; *IV,* intravenous; *PO,* oral; *preop,* preoperative; *SC,* subcutaneous.

are *Atropa belladonna* (deadly nightshade), *Hyoscyamus niger* (henbane), and *Datura stramonium* (jimson weed or thorn apple).

Of the semisynthetic and synthetic cholinergic blockers, many are therapeutically useful drugs. These drugs are used in the treatment of a variety of illnesses and conditions ranging from irritable bowel syndrome to the symptoms of the common cold and are also administered preoperatively to dry up secretions. They are the synthetic counterparts of the plant-derived belladonna alkaloids and are generally more specific in binding predominantly with muscarinic receptors. They may also be associated with fewer adverse effects.

▶ atropine

Atropine is a naturally occurring antimuscarinic. It may be prepared synthetically but is usually obtained by extraction from various members of the Solanaceae family of plants (which includes deadly nightshade and jimson weed, as noted earlier). In general, atropine is more potent than scopolamine in its cholinergic-blocking effects on the heart and in its effects on the smooth muscles of the bronchi and intestines. Atropine is effective in the treatment of many of the conditions listed in the Indications section. It is also used preoperatively to reduce salivation and GI secretions, as is glycopyrrolate. Its use is contraindicated in patients with angle-closure glaucoma, adhesions between the iris and lens, certain types of asthma (not cholinergic associated), advanced hepatic and renal dysfunction, hiatal hernia associated with reflux esophagitis, intestinal atony, obstructive GI or GU conditions, and severe ulcerative colitis. It is available as a parenteral injection in several concentrations, as a 0.4-mg tablet, and in combination with phenobarbital as a oral solution, as well as in various ophthalmic preparations (Chapter 58). Pregnancy category C. The recommended dosages are given in the table on page 309.

Pharmacokinetics

Half-Life	Onset	Peak	Duration
IV: 2.5 hr	IV: Immediate	IV: 2-4 min	IV: 4-6 hr

▶ benztropine mesylate

For a discussion of benztropine (Cogentin), see page 217 in Chapter 14.

▶ dicyclomine

Dicyclomine (Bentyl) is a synthetic antispasmodic cholinergic blocker primarily used in the treatment of functional disturbances of GI motility such as irritable bowel syndrome. It has also been used alone and in combination with phenobarbital for the treatment of colic and enterocolitis in infants. It is most commonly administered in oral form as either a 10- or 20-mg capsule or tablet. It is also available as an orally administered syrup at a strength of 10 mg/5 mL. As a parenteral preparation, it is available as a 10-mg/mL intramuscular injection. Intravenous administration is not recommended. Use of the drug is contraindicated in patients who have a known hypersensitivity to anticholinergics and in those with narrow-angle glaucoma, GI tract obstruction, myasthenia gravis, paralytic ileus, GI atony, or toxic megacolon. Pregnancy category B. The recommended dosages can be found in the table on page 309.

Pharmacokinetics

Half-Life	Onset	Peak	Duration
9-10 hr	1-2 hr	1-1.5 hr	3-4 hr

glycopyrrolate

Glycopyrrolate (Robinul) is a synthetic antimuscarinic drug that blocks receptor sites in the autonomic nervous system that control the production of secretions and the concentration of free acids in the stomach. It is most commonly used as an adjunct in the treatment of peptic ulcer disease and as a preoperative medication to reduce salivation and excessive secretions in the respiratory and GI tracts. Its use is contraindicated in patients who are hypersensitive to it and in those with narrow-angle glaucoma, myasthenia gravis, GI or GU tract obstruction, tachycardia, myocardial ischemia, hepatic disease, ulcerative colitis, and toxic megacolon. It also should not be given to children younger than 3 years of age. Glycopyrrolate is available in oral form as 1- and 2-mg tablets and in parenteral form as a 0.2-mg/mL

intramuscular or intravenous injection. Pregnancy category B. The normal recommended dosages are given in the table on page 309.

Pharmacokinetics

Half-Life	Onset	Peak	Duration
IV: Variable	IV: 1 min	IV: 10-15 min	IV: 4 hr
PO: Variable	PO: Less than 45 min	PO: 1 hr	PO: 6 hr

scopolamine

Scopolamine (Transderm-Scōp) is another naturally occurring cholinergic blocker and one of the principal belladonna alkaloids. It appears to be the most potent antimuscarinic for the prevention of motion sickness. It seems to accomplish this by correcting the imbalance between ACh and norepinephrine in the higher centers in the brain, particularly in the vomiting center, that is responsible for the symptoms of motion sickness. Ipratropium, a derivative of scopolamine, has potent therapeutic effects on the lungs and is discussed in Chapters 35 and 36. Scopolamine is available in several different delivery systems that make it very useful for various indications. For the prevention of motion sickness it is available in a convenient transdermal delivery system, a patch that can be applied just behind the ear 4 to 5 hours before travel. It is also available in several parenteral formulations for injection by various routes: intravenous, intramuscular, and subcutaneous. The transdermal patch Transderm-Scōp is now available by prescription. Scopolamine is also available as a topical preparation for ocular indications and in oral form as a 0.4-mg tablet. The contraindications that apply to atropine apply to scopolamine as well. Pregnancy category C. The recommended dosages for various indications can be found in the table on page 309.

Pharmacokinetics

Half-Life	Onset	Peak	Duration
IV: Variable	IV: 30-60 min	IV: 30-45 min	IV: 4 hr
Patch: Variable	Patch: 4-5 hr	Patch: 6 hr	Patch: 72 hr

▶ tolterodine

Tolterodine (Detrol) is a relatively new muscarinic receptor blocker now being widely promoted for treatment of urinary frequency, urgency, and urge incontinence caused by bladder (detrusor) overactivity. Another, much older drug that is commonly used to treat these conditions is oxybutynin, which is one of the most commonly prescribed. Other drugs also used include propantheline, hyoscyamine, flavoxate, and the tricyclic antidepressant imipramine. The newest drug for this purpose is solifenacin (Vesicare). These drugs are less commonly used than tolterodine because of their antimuscarinic adverse effects, particularly dry mouth. Tolterodine appears to be associated with a much lower incidence of dry mouth, in part because of its pharmacologic specificity for the bladder as opposed to the salivary glands.

Tolterodine should not be used in patients with narrow-angle glaucoma or urinary retention. Patients with markedly decreased hepatic function or poor metabolizers taking drugs that inhibit cytochrome P-450 enzyme 3A4 (CYP3A4), such as erythromycin or ketoconazole, should start with 1 mg twice a day instead of the normal recommended dose of 2 mg twice a day. Tolterodine is available as 1- and 2-mg tablets. Pregnancy category C. Recommended dosages are given in the table on page 309.

Pharmacokinetics

Half-Life	Onset	Peak	Duration
2-4 hr	1 hr	1-2 hr	5 hr

◆ NURSING PROCESS

◆ ASSESSMENT

Anticholinergic drugs (parasympatholytics or cholinergic antagonists or blockers) produce a number of effects that result from the blocking of cholinergic receptors. Because of the variety of effects at different body sites (e.g., smooth muscle relaxation, decreased glandular secretion, mydriasis) the nurse must take a complete medical and medication history and perform a thorough head-to-toe assessment to help identify these contraindications or cautions to the use of the drugs. Drug interactions should also be noted. The head-to-toe assessment also helps in documenting baseline findings and providing data for evaluating drug effectiveness. Cautions, contraindications and drug interactions have been presented in the pharmacology section. Life span considerations for the elderly include increased susceptibility to the adverse effects of confusion, delirium, constipation, blurred vision and tachycardia; thus, the elderly require more careful assessment and monitoring.

◆ NURSING DIAGNOSES

- Ineffective tissue perfusion (cardiopulmonary) related to drug-induced tachycardia
- Risk for injury related to possible excessive CNS stimulation and adverse effects resulting in tremors, confusion, sedation, and amnesia
- Constipation related to adverse effects of anticholinergic (cholinergic-blocking) drugs
- Impaired gas exchange related to thickened respiratory secretions from adverse effects of the drug
- Urinary retention related to loss of bladder tone from adverse effects of cholinergic-blocking drugs
- Risk for injury related to decreased sweating and loss of normal heat-regulating mechanisms (especially in elderly patients and in those who engage in excessive exercise or who are in high environmental temperatures) and possible heat stroke due to effects of the drug on the temperature-regulating mechanisms
- Risk for falls related to changes in vision caused by the mydriatic (pupil dilating) effects of the medication
- Deficient knowledge related to lack of information about the therapeutic regimen, adverse effects, drug interactions, and precautions for the use of anticholinergic drugs

◆ PLANNING

Goals

- Patient self-administers medication as prescribed.
- Patient experiences relief of symptoms for which the medication was prescribed.
- Patient remains compliant with the drug therapy regimen.
- Patient demonstrates adequate knowledge about the use of the specific medication, adverse effects, and appropriate dosing at home.
- Patient is free of injury to self resulting from adverse effects from the medication.

Outcome Criteria

- Patient states the rationale for the use of cholinergic blockers in preoperative preparation, such as decreasing the risk of complications associated with anesthesia.
- Patient states the importance of compliance with the medication regimen, such as avoiding complications of Parkinson's disease.
- Patient states the importance of taking the medication as prescribed and not suddenly withdrawing the medication because of the risk of increasing adverse effects.
- Patient states those conditions of which the physician should be notified immediately if they occur (e.g., palpitations, dysrhythmias, chest pain).

- Patient keeps follow-up appointments with the physician to avoid unnecessary adverse effects of complications of treatment or noncompliance with the drug regimen.

◆ IMPLEMENTATION

A preventive focus for nursing care is important to the effective use of cholinergic-blocking drugs, especially with regard to patient teaching about how to decrease the need for these medications. There are several nursing interventions that may also maximize the therapeutic effects of anticholinergics and minimize the adverse effects, such as giving the drug on time and per the physician's order. For example, solifenacin (Vesicare) should be taken exactly as directed, and patients should be encouraged to contact their health care provider if symptoms do not improve. See the Patient Teaching Tips for more information.

Because drugs such as atropine and glycopyrrolate are compatible with some of the commonly used preoperative medications such as meperidine and morphine, they may be used in combination with these drugs and mixed in the same syringe for parenteral, preanesthetic medication. Whenever several medications are mixed together in one syringe, doses must al-

---

Life Span Considerations: The Elderly Patient
Overactive Bladder

- Overactive bladder affects the lives of 1 out of every 11 American adults, and the incidence increases with age.
- Some questions to pose to the elderly patient regarding this condition include the following:
  - Do you suddenly have the sudden and strong urge to urinate?
  - Do you urinate more than eight times within a 24-hour period?
  - Do you have to get up more than two times during the night to urinate?
  - Do you have "wetting" accidents?
  - Are these "wetting" accidents related to the uncontrollable urge to urinate?
- If the patient answers yes to some of these questions, the patient should be encouraged to contact his or her primary health care provider. A referral to a urologist may or may not be necessary.
- Various treatments are available nationwide in the United States. Some of these drug treatments have been presented, but another drug (released in January of 2005) is a different option for men and women experiencing the symptoms of overactive bladder. Solifenacin succinate (Vesicare) is taken once daily and treats all of the major symptoms of overactive bladder, including urgency, frequency, and urge-related incontinence.
- Solifenacin succinate was found to reduce the number of incontinence episodes over 12 weeks in studies of the drug involving more than 3000 patients with overactive bladder symptoms; 5- to 10-mg dosing of the drug produced improvement in all of the major symptoms. Use of this drug is contraindicated in patients with glaucoma, certain gastrointestinal or genitourinary tract problems, severe constipation, and/or urinary retention. Adverse effects include dry mouth, constipation, and blurred vision. If a patient experiences severe abdominal pain or is constipated for 3 or more days, the patient should contact his or her health care provider immediately.

Modified from http://myWebMD.com/content/tools/1/quiz/_overactive_bladder.htm, www.vesicare.com, www.yamanouchi.com, and www.gsk.com.

ways be calculated very carefully and compatibilities always double-checked! When an anticholinergic ophthalmic solution is given, the nurse must always check the concentration of medication and apply light pressure (i.e., for 15 to 30 seconds) with a tissue to the inner canthus of the eye. This helps to minimize the possibility of systemic absorption of the drug. Atropine may be combined with other cholinergic-blocking drugs (e.g., hyoscyamine) for treatment of lower urinary tract discomfort. This combination decreases GU spasms and GU hypermotility.

When a cholinergic-blocking drug is used to treat urinary tract disorders or dysfunction, the patient needs to be aware of the importance of taking the drug exactly as ordered, which may be as often as four times a day depending on the drug. In addition, in patients with altered renal or liver function, the dose or frequency of dosing of oxybutynin may need to be decreased because of the potential for toxicity. If anticholinergic drugs are taken at the same time as a CYP3A4 inhibitors (e.g., erythromycin), the possibility of complications exists. Oxybutynin should be taken as directed with fluids 1 hour before or 2 hours after meals if tolerated. Tolterodine should be taken as directed and with food. Also associated with the cholinergic-blocking drugs are the adverse effects of constipation and inability to sweat or perspire. See the Patient Teaching Tips for more information on these specific drugs.

◆ EVALUATION

Monitoring goals and outcome criteria should be a starting place for effective evaluation of therapy with these medications. In particular, therapeutic effects of cholinergic-blocking drugs include the following:

- For Parkinson's disease, patients experience improved ability to carry out the activities of daily living and fewer problems with tremors, salivation, and drooling.
- For relief of GI symptoms such as hyperacidity, patients report improved comfort and a decrease in symptoms of abdominal pain, nausea, vomiting, and heartburn.
- For urologic problems, patients show an improvement in urinary patterns with less hypermotility and increased time between voiding.
- In preoperative situations, patients experience fewer bronchospasms with induction of anesthesia and fewer problems with secretions because the cholinergic-blockers (anticholinergic drugs) dry out secretions, making them more viscous.

The nurse must also monitor the patient for the occurrence of adverse effects such as constipation, tachycardia, tremors, confusion, hallucinations, CNS depression (which occurs with large dosages of atropine), sedation, urinary retention, hot and dry skin, and fever. Toxicity of these drugs includes possible CNS depression with confusion and hallucinations and cardiovascular stimulation with severe tachycardia and palpitations.

Patient Teaching Tips

- Encourage patients to take the drug exactly as prescribed and to take the exact amount to prevent overdosage. Overdosage may cause life-threatening problems, especially in the cardiovascular and central nervous systems.
- Educate patients to practice regular oral hygiene with brushing of teeth twice daily; dental flossing; and minimizing the adverse effect of dry mouth through forcing fluids (if not contraindicated), using artificial saliva drops/gum, and sucking on sugar free hard candy as needed. Regularly scheduled dental visits should be encouraged because of the association between dry mouth and dental caries or gum disease.
- Encourage patients to exercise care when first taking the medications and to be very cautious when engaging in activities such as driving a car or operating machinery because of the blurred vision that commonly occurs with these medications.
- Inform patients of the adverse effect of increased sensitivity to light. Wearing dark/tinted glasses or sunglasses is encouraged.
- Patients should be encouraged to consult a health care provider before taking any other medications, including prescription drugs, OTC medications, herbals, and supplements.

- If the patient is elderly or is taking higher dosages of these medications, the risk of experiencing heat stroke or hyperthermia is increased because of the drug's interference with the normal heat-regulating mechanisms. Educate the elderly on how to prevent these problems (e.g., stay in a cool or shaded environment if outside in warm temperatures, wear protective clothing and hats/caps, take fluids regularly, avoid excessive heat and strenuous exercise in warm environments, avoid saunas or hot tubs). In addition, fans, air conditioners, and adequate ventilation may help to prevent overheating.
- Encourage patients to contact the health care provider if they experience any urinary hesitancy and/or retention, constipation, palpitations, tremors, confusion, sedation, amnesia, excessive dry mouth (especially if the patient has a chronic lung infection or other chronic lung disease), or fever.
- Educate patients that anticholinergic related constipation may be managed with increased bulk and fiber by dietary intake or the use of OTC fiber-containing supplements (as ordered) and fluids.
- Patients should report unresolved constipation, palpitations, alterations in gait, excessive dizziness, or difficulty in urinating.

Points to Remember

- *Cholinergic blockers, anticholinergics, parasympatholytics,* and *antimuscarinics* are all terms that refer to the drugs that block or inhibit the actions of acetylcholine (ACh) in the PSNS.
- The use of these cholinergic blockers allows the SNS to dominate. They are classified chemically as natural, semisynthetic, and synthetic anticholinergics. Anticholinergics may be competitive antagonists (blockers) and compete with ACh at the musca-

rinic receptors. In high dosages they result in partial blocking actions at nicotinic receptors. Anticholinergics bind to and block ACh at muscarinic receptors located on the cells stimulated by the parasympathetic nerve.
- The nurse should assess for possible contraindications such as benign prostatic hypertrophy, glaucoma, tachycardia, myocardial infarction, heart failure, and hiatal hernia.

NCLEX Examination Review Questions

1. Elderly patients taking anticholinergics should be reminded to
   a. avoid exposure to high temperatures.
   b. limit liquid intake to avoid fluid overload.
   c. begin an exercise program to avoid adverse effects.
   d. stop the medication if excessive mouth dryness occurs.
2. Contraindications to the use of anticholinergics include:
   a. Chronic bronchitis
   b. Peptic ulcer disease
   c. Irritable bowel syndrome
   d. Benign prostatic hypertrophy
3. Adverse effects associated with the use of cholinergic blockers include:
   a. Diaphoresis
   b. Dry mouth
   c. Diarrhea
   d. Urinary frequency
4. The nurse administering a cholinergic-blocking drug would expect to see which of the following effects in the patient?
   a. Miosis
   b. Increased muscle rigidity
   c. Increased bronchial secretions
   d. Decreased GI motility and peristalsis
5. During the assessment of a patient about to receive a cholinergic-blocking drug, the nurse should determine whether the patient is taking any drugs that may potentially interact with the anticholinergic, including:
   a. Narcotics, such as morphine sulfate
   b. Antibiotics, such as penicillin
   c. Tricyclic antidepressants, such as amitriptyline
   d. Anticonvulsants, such as phenobarbital

1. a, 2. d, 3. b, 4. d, 5. c.

Critical Thinking Activities

1. You are getting ready to administer preoperative medications to a 75-year-old woman undergoing minor surgery. She has a history of smoking, heart failure, and narrow-angle glaucoma. Why do you *not* administer the atropine preoperatively to this patient, as ordered? Also, what is your rationale for contacting the physician about this drug interaction and your subsequent action?
2. You are caring for a patient who has just experienced a cardiac arrest while in the intensive care unit. The patient is in second-degree heart block, has sinus bradycardia with a heart rate of 30 beats/min, and has lost consciousness. You expect that the cholinergic blocker _____ will be given to _____ the heart rate. *(Choose two responses.)*
   a. Dicyclomine
   b. Tolterodine
   c. Atropine
   d. Increase
   e. Decrease
3. You are on a deep-sea fishing trip with friends. One of the participants shows you the patch she is wearing because she gets "terribly seasick." She tells you that she has never used this patch before but that her friends recommended that she try it. After 3 hours, though, you notice that she is very restless and irritable. What drug do you think is contained in this patch? Are these expected adverse effects or a worse problem? Explain.
4. In preparation for emergency surgery, the order was to give 0.5 mg of atropine to your patient intravenously. The vial concentration is 1 mg/mL. In the haste of this emergency situation, 5 mL of the atropine solution is given. How many milligrams of atropine were given to your patient? What effects can you expect to see? What treatment will you expect to be ordered for this problem?
5. What are the advantages of the synthetic derivatives over the natural belladonna alkaloids?

For answers, see http://evolve.elsevier.com/Lilley.

Drugs Affecting the Cardiovascular and Renal Systems

STUDY SKILLS TIPS

- *Linking Learning*
- *Text Notation*

LINKING LEARNING

The Part Three Study Skills Tips stressed the importance of planning for the part as a whole. With that in mind, what is the focus of Part Four? The part title is Drugs Affecting the Cardiovascular and Renal Systems. What is the first question you think you should ask about this part? I would begin by asking, "What are the cardiovascular and renal systems?" This is a very obvious question and might seem to be so basic that it need not be asked, but the next eight chapters will all develop around this part title. Asking the obvious question is sometimes exactly the thing that should be done to get started.

Chapter Structure

Just as there is a structure to each part in the text, which is constant from one part to the next, there is also a structure in the chapters. This structure is a repeating model that was created by the authors in an attempt to organize the material and present it in the clearest way possible. The chapter structure is a valuable learning asset for those who make use of it.

Chapter Objectives

Each chapter begins with a set of objectives. These are established by the authors and serve to tell you what they expect you will know and be able to do when you have completed the chapter. It is sometimes tempting to ignore the objectives and get right on with the task of reading the chapter. Do not give in to that temptation. Read the objectives and spend some time thinking about what they reveal about the content of the chapter.

Example Based on Chapter 21 Objectives

Objective 1: Differentiate between the following terms: *inotropic, chronotropic,* and *dromotropic.*

What can you learn from this objective? First, there is the vocabulary. This objective makes it clear that you have some terms to learn. This means that you may want to have some blank note cards available to start setting up vocabulary cards for this chapter. In fact, you should write each of the terms in objective 1 on a separate card and be ready to complete the card as the terms are introduced and explained in the chapter.

The next thing that stands out in this first objective is that the three terms contain a common element: *tropic.* This should bring active questioning into play. What does the suffix *tropic* mean? Asking this question now is a way of noting that these three terms do have some common meaning. Also it serves to provide an immediate focus for personal learning when you begin to read the chapter.

Objective 2: Briefly discuss the effect of cardiac glycosides and positive inotropic drugs on the failing and/or diseased heart.

From this comes the potential for a new question relating to the first objective. What do *inotropic, chronotropic,* and *dromotropic* have to do with the heart? Just as it is essential to see the relationship between parts and chapters, it is also essential to see relationships within the chapters. These first two objectives should cause you to consider those relationships and make your own learning much more active.

Chapter Headings

The next chapter structure to consider in this process is the chapter headings. Chapter 21 has the major sections Heart Failure and Cardiac Dysrhythmias, Cardiac Glycosides, Phosphodiesterase Inhibitors, Miscella-neous Heart Failure Drug, and Nursing Process. What is the importance of this heading structure? It tells you that the authors will focus on the pharmacologic aspects first 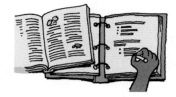 and then explain how this relates to nursing. This does not tell the learner a great deal about what to anticipate in terms of chapter content, but it does make clear a structure that is consistent in most of the chapters in this text.

Cardiac Glycosides are broken down into subsections in this chapter. Spend several minutes considering the organization of these subsections. The first subtopic to be treated is Mechanism of Action and Drug Effects. What is meant by mechanism of action? How do cardiac glycosides act? On what do they act? It does not matter that you cannot answer these questions at this point. What is important is that you ask them as a means of fostering an active and participatory learning attitude when you begin to read the chapter. Think, question, anticipate, and then read. This sequence will enhance your learning.

Continue this process of looking at the subtopics and thinking ahead to what will be explained in the chapter. These subsections are the same in every chapter, and this thinking process should become automatic very quickly.

Glossary

The next chapter structure is one that I have already stressed in previous Study Skills Tips, and it is one that is essential to learning. The glossary is a mini-dictionary for each chapter. Words that have not been introduced earlier in the text and that are central to the content of this chapter are presented here. The listing is in alphabetical order, which means that the glossary terms will not necessarily occur in the same order in the body of the chapter.

As you read the terms as presented in the glossary, be aware of the nature of the definition. A glossary definition is specific and brief. It is a very useful place to begin to learn the new terms in the chapter, but the definition presented may not be enough for full understanding. You will find that full understanding will come after reading the chapter and encountering the term within the fuller context of sentences and paragraphs of text that explain not only the term but how it applies in the particular situation.

Glossary and Text Relationship

The term *inotropic drug* is defined in the Chapter 21 glossary. As I read it, I understand that inotropic has to do with force or energy of muscle contractions. The glossary states that a positive inotropic drug is a drug that increases myocardial contractility. Some of this information is clear, and some of it is still somewhat hazy. It should become clearer when connected with the chapter text. The first paragraph of the chapter introduces inotropic drugs: "Drugs that increase the force of myocardial contraction are called positive **inotropic drugs,** and such drugs have a beneficial role in the treatment of failing heart muscle."

With this sentence I find I have a much clearer understanding of what is meant by *inotropic drugs,* and I have the added benefit of knowing that there are positive inotropic drugs. This is what must happen to fully master the content-specific vocabulary. You must see the core definition as presented in the glossary, but you must also read to determine how that core definition is expanded and exemplified in the body of the text.

When preparing vocabulary cards, it is not a good idea to simply copy the definition from the glossary and assume that definition will serve your purpose. Wait to fill out the card until after you encounter the same term in the body of the chapter, and then pick and choose the information from the glossary and the body that will provide you with the clearest understanding of the term. Also, when placing information on vocabulary cards, it is always useful to include a chapter number and page numbers so that you can locate the source of your definition quickly should you find it necessary later.

These chapter structures can provide you with a clear picture of what you are expected to learn and the organizational pattern in which the material will be presented. Being aware of the structures and making use of them in this way will improve your concentration when you begin to read the chapter for understanding and memory. The time spent working with chapter structure is not wasted and does not sig- 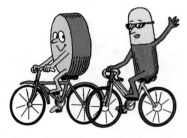 nificantly increase the study time of the chapter. In fact, the time you spend working with the objectives, headings, and glossary will generally save time when you are doing intensive reading and study.

TEXT NOTATION

Highlighting or underlining text materials is a tool that can be very helpful when rehearsing and reviewing materials after the study reading. The problem, as discussed in the *Study Guide,* is that it is often difficult to limit the quantity of material that is marked. Although a good general guideline is to try to limit yourself to marking no more than 20% to 25% of the total material, this guideline applies to large blocks of material. However, some paragraphs contain essential information and must be marked extensively, while other paragraphs may need only one or two sentences marked. In this Study Skills Tips section, the object is to look at how the author's structure and language can help you to select what should be marked.

Text Notation Application

Reproduced here are two paragraphs from Chapter 26 with my model underlining completed, followed by a discussion of the reasons for which I made the choices. You should not view the model underlining as a "perfect" example. The decision as to what to mark is very much an individual choice based on a number of factors, including prior experience with the subject matter and awareness of personal learning objectives and needs. These model paragraphs with accompanying discussion are intended to provide you with a basic model to adapt to your own learning style and needs.

Chapter 26, Paragraphs One and Two

Fluid and electrolyte management is one of the cornerstones of patient care. Most disease processes, tissue injuries, and surgical procedures greatly influence the physiologic status of fluids and electrolytes in the body. A prerequisite to the understanding of fluid and electrolyte management is knowledge of the extent and composition of the various body fluid compartments.

Approximately 60% of the adult human body is water. This is referred to as the *total body water* (TBW), and it is distributed to the three main compartments in the following proportions: **intracellular fluid (ICF), 67%; interstitial fluid (ISF), 25%; and plasma volume (PV), 8%.** This distribution is illustrated in Figure 26-1. The actual volume of fluid that would normally be in each compartment in an average 70-kg man with a TBW content of 60% of his TBW is shown in Table 26-1.

Discussion

The first thing you should notice is that the underlining I have done exceeds the 20% to 25% guideline. These are the first paragraphs in the chapter. First paragraphs are usually introductions to the topic and may vary a great deal in the quantity of important information. This chapter, in my view, contains a number of key points that must be considered. Because the content seems important, I have chosen to underline more.

Sentence one was chosen because of the word *cornerstones.* This word suggests that fluid management is extremely important in patient care and I must be sure to keep that focus throughout the chapter. Paying careful attention to the author's word choices plays a major role in selecting materials for text notation.

Paying attention to language led me to the third sentence, which begins, "A prerequisite to the understanding…" That phrase should immediately capture your attention. The phrase says that there is something that must be understood before anything else that follows will make complete sense. The phrase should also serve as an instant cue to generate a question for reading. "What is the prerequisite to understanding fluid and electrolyte management?" This question is answered directly by the sentence containing the phrase. The phrase serves as a language cue that there is something important. This in turn suggests that you probably will want to underline or highlight some information. The question helps you select what should be marked. Everything you do at this point serves as a guide to help you establish clear learning objectives and makes the process of selecting the best information for marking easier to accomplish.

The next segment was chosen because it stands out from the body of the paragraph. *Total body water* is italicized. This is a print convention used as a means of putting emphasis on something that the author believes to be of special importance. The decision to underline words and phrases that are already emphasized is a personal one. You may feel that, since the author has already marked it, you have no need to add your own marks. I find that my own marking, even of italicized or bold print material, serves as a double reminder of the importance of the information. This is an excellent example of what I mean when I say that text notation is highly personal. Whether you choose to add your own marking or not there is one aspect of this phrase that is essential. *Total body water* is part of the vocabulary of fluids and

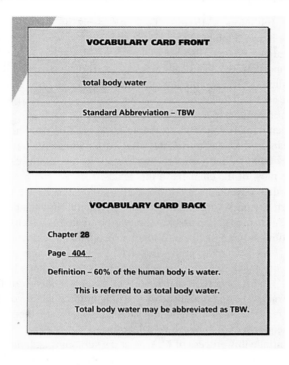

electrolytes. That means it is time to add to your vocabulary cards.

This term served as a lead-in to the next key point that I have marked. The next sentence is, "TBW is distributed to the three main compartments." Whenever you see a phrase with a number and a word such as *main,* you should be aware that this is potentially important material. This phrase should generate a new question that will aid in your selection of material to mark. "What are the three main compartments?" You see immediately that the rest of this sentence answers that question, and therefore identifies what needs to be marked. This marking also identifies three additional vocabulary items to be added to your cards for this chapter. As you set up your cards, be careful. One fluid is *intra-,* and the second is *inter-.* It would be easy to confuse the two, but they have very different meanings.

Chapter 26, Paragraph Three

The terms used to identify the various spaces within which the TBW is distributed can be quite confusing, and there are two basic approaches to distinguishing among the locations of the fluid. The TBW can be described as being in or out of the blood vessels, or vasculature. If this terminology is used, the term **intravascular fluid (IVF)** describes fluid inside the blood vessels and the term **extravascular fluid (EVF)** describes the fluid outside the blood vessels. Examples of EVF include lymph and cerebrospinal fluid. As you learn these concepts, recall the difference between the prefixes *intra-* (inside), *inter-* (between), and *extra-* (outside). The term **plasma** is used to describe the fluid that flows through the blood vessels that is intravascular. **Serum** is a closely related term (see glossary). ISF is the fluid that is in the space between cells, tissues, and organs. Both plasma and ISF make up extracellular volume. Both ISF and ICF make up extravascular volume. These terms are often confused and misused. Table 26-1 lists these definitions for further clarity and understanding.

Discussion

The language conventions and the print conventions (**bold**) are the same that I used to help in the previous paragraph. This paragraph also makes a point about the possibility of confusing and/ or misusing the terms introduced. Being told that there is confusing material suggests that it is crucial that you be able to identify, define, and explain each of the terms used, and that it will take some careful thought to do so. There is one additional point in this paragraph that is important. The last sentence points you to a table, Table 26-1. There are many tables in this text. Always remember that tables are often used in an effort to simplify complex material and to clarify the relationships between the items presented in the table. In these opening paragraphs, with the repeated reference to the confusing nature of the descriptions, Table 26-1 will almost certainly be important to your learning.

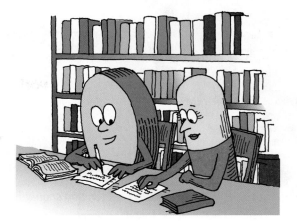

Positive Inotropic Drugs

Objectives

When you reach the end of this chapter, you should be able to do the following:

1. Differentiate between the following terms: *inotropic, chronotropic,* and *dromotropic.*
2. Briefly discuss the effect of cardiac glycosides and other positive inotropic drugs on the failing and/or diseased heart.
3. Compare the mechanisms of action, pharmacokinetics, indications, dosages, dosage forms, routes of administration, cautions, contraindications, adverse effects, and toxicity of the cardiac glycosides and other positive inotropics.
4. Briefly discuss rapid versus slow digitalization, including associated nursing considerations.
5. Identify significant drug, laboratory test, and food interactions associated with cardiac glycosides and other positive inotropic drugs.
6. Develop a nursing care plan that includes all phases of the nursing process for patients undergoing treatment with cardiac glycosides or other positive inotropics.

e-Learning Activities

Companion CD
- NCLEX Review Questions: see questions 148-158
- Animations
- Audio Glossary
- Category Catchers
- Medication Errors Checklists
- IV Therapy Checklists

evolve Website (http://evolve.elsevier.com/Lilley)
• Nursing Care Plans • Frequently Asked Questions • Content Updates • WebLinks • Supplemental Resources • Elsevier ePharmacology Update • Medication Administration Animations

Drug Profiles

▶ digoxin, p. 322   milrinone, p. 325
  digoxin immune Fab, p. 324

▶ Key drug.

Glossary

Atrial fibrillation   A common cardiac dysrhythmia involving atrial contractions that are so rapid that they prevent full repolarization of myocardial fibers between heartbeats. (p. 319)

Automaticity   A property of specialized excitable tissue that allows self-activation through the spontaneous development of an action potential, as in the pacemaker cells of the heart. (p. 320)

Cardiac glycosides   Glycosides (carbohydrates that yields a sugar and a nonsugar upon hydrolysis) that are derived from the plant species *Digitalis purpurea* and are used in the treatment of heart disease. (p. 319)

Chronotropic drugs   Drugs that influence the rate of the heartbeat. Positive chronotropic drugs increase the heart rate, whereas negative chronotropic drugs decrease it. (p. 319)

Dromotropic drugs   Drugs that influence the conduction of electrical impulses. Positive dromotropic drugs enhance the conduction of electrical impulses in the heart. (p. 319)

Ejection fraction   The proportion of blood that is ejected during each ventricular contraction compared with the total ventricular filling volume. It is an index of left ventricular function; the normal fraction is 65% (0.65). (p. 319)

Heart failure   An abnormal condition in which cardiac pumping is impaired as a result of myocardial infarction, ischemic heart disease, or cardiomyopathy. Failure of the ventricle to eject blood efficiently results in volume overload, chamber dilation, and elevated intracardiac pressure. The retrograde transmission of increased hydrostatic pressure from the left ventricle leads to pulmonary congestion; elevated right ventricular pressure leads to systemic venous congestion and peripheral edema. (p. 319)

Inotropic drugs   Drugs that influence the force or energy of muscular contractions, particularly contraction of the heart muscle. Positive inotropic drugs increase myocardial contractility. (p. 319)

Left ventricular end-diastolic volume   The total amount of blood in the ventricle immediately before it contracts, or the preload. Ventricular diastole begins with the onset of the second heart sound and ends with the onset of first heart sound. (p. 319)

Refractory period   The period during which a pulse generator (e.g., the sinoatrial node of the heart) is unresponsive to an input signal of specified amplitude and during which it is impossible for the myocardium to respond. This is the period during which the cardiac cell is readjusting its sodium and potassium levels and cannot be depolarized again. (p. 320)

Therapeutic index   The range of drug levels in the blood that is considered beneficial as opposed to toxic or ineffective. (p. 321)

Drugs that increase the force of myocardial contraction are called positive **inotropic drugs,** and such drugs have a beneficial role in the treatment of failing heart muscle. Drugs that increase the rate at which the heart beats are called positive **chronotropic drugs.** Drugs may also affect how quickly electrical impulses travel through the conduction system of the heart (the sinoatrial [SA] node, atrioventricular [AV] node, bundle of His, and Purkinje fibers). Drugs that accelerate conduction are referred to as positive **dromotropic drugs.** This chapter focuses on two of the main classes of positive inotropic drugs: **cardiac glycosides** and phosphodiesterase inhibitors.

Estimates are that close to 2 million office visits and 1.5 million hospital visits a year are necessitated by exacerbations of **heart failure.** The findings of one of the largest and most frequently cited studies involving patients with heart failure, the Framingham study, show that the 5-year survival rate in patients with heart failure is approximately 50%. Therefore, any drug that can lengthen survival in affected patients or help the failing heart perform its essential duties would be extremely valuable. The cardiac glycosides are a prime example. Data questioning their use were recently released, however. Digoxin therapy as a first-line treatment for heart failure did not improve mortality rates. Angiotensin-converting enzyme (ACE) inhibitors and diuretics were recommended as the mainstays; nevertheless, digoxin may still offer benefit in some patients.

HEART FAILURE AND CARDIAC DYSRHYTHMIAS

Heart failure is a pathologic state in which the heart is unable to pump blood in sufficient amounts from the ventricles (i.e., cardiac output is insufficient) to meet the body's metabolic needs. The signs and symptoms typically associated with this insufficiency constitute the syndrome of heart failure. This syndrome can be limited to the left ventricle (producing pulmonary edema and symptoms of dyspnea or cough) or to the right ventricle (producing symptoms such as pedal edema, jugular venous distention, ascites, and hepatic congestion), or it may affect both ventricles.

In patients with heart failure, the overworked, failing heart cannot meet the demands placed on it and blood is not ejected efficiently from the ventricles. This occurs because the **ejection fraction** (the amount of blood ejected with each contraction) compared with the total amount of blood in the ventricle just before contraction (**left ventricular end-diastolic volume**) is decreased. (Normally the ejection fraction is approximately 65% [0.65] of the total volume in the ventricle.) As more blood accumulates in the right and left ventricles, more pressure builds up in the blood vessels leading to the heart. The retrograde transmission of this increased hydrostatic pressure from the left ventricle leads to pulmonary congestion, whereas elevated right ventricular pressure causes systemic venous congestion and peripheral edema.

Because the heart cannot then meet the increased demands placed on it, the blood supply to certain organs is reduced. The organs most dependent on blood supply, the brain and heart, are the last to be deprived of blood. As an organ that is relatively less dependent on blood supply, the kidney has its blood supply shunted away. Therefore, the filtration of fluids and removal of waste products is impaired. When these fluids and waste products accumulate, the patient experiences such symptoms as pulmonary edema, shortness of breath, and peripheral edema resulting from kidney failure.

The physical defects producing heart failure are of two types: (1) a cardiac defect (myocardial deficiency such as myocardial infarction or valve insufficiency), which leads to inadequate cardiac contractility and ventricular filling, and (2) a defect outside the heart (e.g., systemic defects such as coronary artery disease, pulmonary hypertension, or diabetes), which results in an overload on an otherwise normal heart. Either or both of these defects may be present in a given patient. Common causes of myocardial deficiency and systemic defects are listed in Box 21-1.

A dysfunctional heart rhythm is technically termed a *cardiac dysrhythmia.* In practice, however, the term *arrhythmia* is also used, even though it literally means "no rhythm," or absence of heartbeat. In patients with supraventricular dysrhythmias, **atrial fibrillation,** or atrial flutter, the top aspects of the heart (the atria) may be contracting several hundred times a minute. Not only are the atria contracting too frequently, but several areas in the atria besides the SA node are then acting as the pacemaker of the heart. Normally the AV node controls how slowly or quickly impulses arrive in the ventricles, and it also has the ability to receive all of these depolarizations and allow only a certain number to pass through to the ventricles. This keeps the patient from going into ventricular fibrillation, which is fatal. It also gives the ventricles time to fill with blood, which is essential for normal perfusion. During atrial fibrillation or flutter, however, patients may show symptoms such as heart failure.

Box 21-1   Myocardial Deficiency and Increased Workload: Common Causes

Myocardial Deficiency
Inadequate Contractility
Myocardial infarction
Coronary artery disease
Cardiomyopathy
Infection
Inadequate Filling
Atrial fibrillation
Infection
Tamponade
Ischemia

Increased Workload
Pressure Overload
Hypertension
Outflow obstruction
Volume Overload
Hypervolemia
Congenital abnormalities
Anemia
Thyroid disease

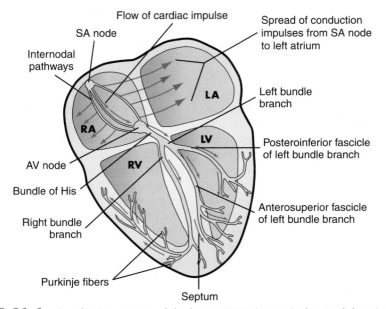

FIGURE 21-1 Conduction system of the heart. *AV,* Atrioventricular; *LA,* left atrium; *LV,* left ventricle; *RA,* right atrium; *RV,* right ventricle; *SA,* sinoatrial. *(Modified from Kinney M et al: Comprehensive cardiac care, ed 8, St Louis, 1996, Mosby; Lewis SM, Heitkemper MM, Dirksen SR: Medical-surgical nursing: assessment and management of clinical problems, ed 6, St Louis, 2004, Mosby.)*

All cells in the heart can depolarize spontaneously, a property called **automaticity.** The **refractory period** is the time when the cardiac cells are readjusting their sodium and potassium levels following depolarization. During this time the cardiac cells cannot depolarize again. It is the sodium-potassium adenosine triphosphatase (ATPase) pump that is responsible for the movement of potassium ions in and sodium ions out of the cardiac cells after they have depolarized, an action potential has been generated, and the electrical impulse has been promulgated through the myocardium. In patients with supraventricular tachydysrhythmias such as atrial fibrillation or flutter, the AV node may be circumvented and a greater number of electrical impulses than usual may arrive in the ventricle before the refractory period is over. This can potentially cause ventricular tachydysrhythmias (e.g., ventricular tachycardia or fibrillation), which are potentially more serious than the supraventricular tachydysrhythmias mentioned earlier. Figure 21-1 illustrates the conduction system of the heart. (The cardiac conduction system and the abnormalities responsible for causing dysrhythmias are described in greater detail in Chapter 22.)

CARDIAC GLYCOSIDES

Cardiac glycosides are one of the oldest and most effective groups of cardiac drugs. Not only do they have beneficial effects in the failing heart but they also help control the ventricular response to atrial fibrillation or flutter. They were originally obtained from either the *Digitalis purpurea* or *Digitalis lanata* plant, both commonly referred to as *foxglove.* For this reason, cardiac glycosides are sometimes referred to as *digitalis glycosides.* Cardiac glycosides have now been the mainstay of therapy for heart failure for more than 200 years, and they continue to be one of the most commonly used positive inotropic drugs. Digoxin is the most frequently prescribed cardiac glycoside and the only one currently available in the United States. Another drug with a similar-sounding name, *digitoxin,* is no longer on the U.S. market. The widespread and enduring popularity of digitalis is the result of many years of clinical use. Critically ill patients can often be restored to near-normal states within hours after initiating digoxin therapy, a process known as *digitalization.* It should be noted, however, that the emphasis in this chapter regarding heart failure focuses on systolic dysfunction or inadequate ventricular contractions *(systole)* during the pumping of the heart. Less common but still important is diastolic dysfunction, or inadequate ventricular filling during ventricular relaxation *(diastole).* This condition is most commonly associated with left ventricular hypertrophy secondary to chronic hypertension. However, it may also result from cardiomyopathy (e.g., virus induced), pericardial disease, and diabetes. Unlike with systolic heart failure, inotropic drugs (including digoxin) and vasodilators (Chapter 24) may not be the drugs of choice for diastolic dysfunction. Diuretic drugs (Chapter 25), on the other hand, are often used as part of therapy for both conditions.

Mechanism of Action and Drug Effects

The primary beneficial effect of a cardiac glycoside (e.g., digoxin) is thought to be an increase in myocardial contractility. This occurs secondarily to the inhibition of the sodium-potassium ATPase pump. When the action of this enzyme complex is inhibited, the cellular sodium concentration and subsequently the calcium concentration increase. The overall result is enhanced myocardial contraction. Digoxin also augments vagal (cholinergic or parasympathetic) tone, which results in increased diastolic filling between heartbeats secondary to reduced heart rate. This further enhances cardiac efficiency and output.

Cardiac glycosides also change the electrical conduction properties of the heart, and this markedly affects the conduction system and cardiac automaticity. Cardiac glycosides decrease the velocity (rate) of electrical conduction and prolong the refractory period in the conduction system. The particular area of the conduction system where this occurs is between the atria and the ventricles (SA node to AV node). The cardiac cells remain in a state of depolarization longer and are unable to start another electrical impulse, which also reduces heart rate and improves cardiac efficiency.

Digoxin produces the following dramatic inotropic, chronotropic, dromotropic, and other cardiac effects:

- A positive inotropic effect resulting in an increase in the force and velocity of myocardial contraction without a corresponding increase in oxygen consumption
- A negative chronotropic effect producing a reduced heart rate
- A negative dromotropic effect that decreases automaticity at the SA node, decreases AV nodal conduction, reduces conductivity at the bundle of His, and prolongs the atrial and ventricular refractory periods
- An increase in stroke volume
- A reduction in heart size during diastole
- A decrease in venous blood pressure and vein engorgement
- An increase in coronary circulation
- Promotion of diuresis as a result of improved blood circulation
- Palliation of exertional and paroxysmal nocturnal dyspnea, cough, and cyanosis

Indications

Cardiac glycosides are primarily used in the treatment of heart failure and supraventricular dysrhythmias. In heart failure the therapeutic effects of digoxin are secondary to its ability to increase the force of contraction—its positive inotropic action. This has many therapeutic benefits. Increasing the force of contraction increases the volume of blood ejected as a percentage of the left ventricular end-diastolic volume or preload (i.e., the ejection fraction). Because more blood is ejected with each contraction of the heart, less blood remains in the ventricle and thus less pressure builds up. With this, the symptoms of pulmonary edema, pulmonary hypertension, and right-sided ventricular failure subside, and tissue perfusion improves.

Another benefit of this positive inotropic action is that it promotes diuresis by ensuring that adequate blood is supplied to the kidneys. As a result, fluids are more completely filtered and waste products removed, which relieves shortness of breath and pulmonary edema.

Cardiac glycosides are also effective in the treatment of supraventricular dysrhythmias such as atrial fibrillation and atrial flutter because of their negative chronotropic and negative dromotropic actions. Automaticity, conduction velocity, and the refractory period are all affected. Digoxin can slow the depolarization of the SA node and other areas of the atria that may be acting as pacemakers. Thus, the cardiac glycosides such as digoxin directly slow conduction through the AV node (decreasing the ventricular rate) and increase the vagal action on the heart. In addition, the cardiac glycosides lengthen the refractory period, which allows the correct levels of sodium and potassium ions to be reached before depolarization.

Contraindications

Contraindications to the use of cardiac glycosides include known drug allergy and may include second- or third-degree heart block, atrial fibrillation (also an indication, so this is a clinical

judgment call), ventricular tachycardia or fibrillation, heart failure resulting from diastolic dysfunction, and subaortic stenosis (obstruction in the left ventricle below the aortic valve). However, these drugs may be used to treat some of these conditions, if recommended by a competent cardiologist, depending on the given clinical situation.

Adverse Effects

The adverse effects associated with cardiac glycoside use can be very serious. The primary cardiac glycoside in use today is digoxin, and close monitoring of the patient's clinical response to it and observation for the possible development of toxic symptoms is essential. Digoxin has a narrow **therapeutic index;** that is, the range of blood drug levels that is considered therapeutic is small. Monitoring of digoxin levels after the drug reaches steady state is necessary only if there is suspicion of toxicity, noncompliance, or deteriorating renal function. Low potassium levels can increase the potential for toxicity, known specifically for this drug as *digitoxicity*. Therefore, frequent serum electrolyte level checks are also important. Estimates are that as many as 20% of patients taking digoxin exhibit symptoms of toxicity. The common undesirable effects associated with cardiac glycoside use are listed in Table 21-1.

Toxicity and Management of Overdose

The treatment strategies for digoxin toxicity depend on the severity of the symptoms. These strategies can range from simply withholding the next dose to instituting more aggressive therapies. The steps usually taken in the management of cardiac glycoside toxicity are listed in Table 21-2.

Table 21-1	Cardiac Glycosides: Common Adverse Effects
Body System	**Adverse Effects**
Cardiovascular	Any type of dysrhythmia, including bradycardia or tachycardia
Central nervous	Headache, fatigue, malaise, confusion, convulsions
Eye	Colored vision (i.e., green, yellow, or purple), halo vision, or flickering lights
Gastrointestinal	Anorexia, nausea, vomiting, diarrhea

Table 21-2	Digoxin Toxicity: Step-by-Step Management
Step	**Actions**
1	Discontinue administration of drug.
2	Begin continuous electrocardiographic monitoring for cardiac dysrhythmias; administer any appropriate antidysrhythmic drugs as ordered.
3	Determine serum digoxin and electrolyte levels.
4	Administer potassium supplements for hypokalemia if indicated, as ordered.
5	Institute supportive therapy for gastrointestinal symptoms (nausea, vomiting, or diarrhea).
6	Administer digoxin antidote (i.e., digoxin immune Fab) if indicated, as ordered.

Life Span Considerations: The Pediatric Patient
Heart Failure and Cardiac Glycosides

The cause, symptoms, treatment, and prognosis of heart failure in children vary depending on age. In infants, the cause of heart failure is generally holes in the heart or other structural problems. In older children, the structure of the heart may be normal but the heart muscle may be weakened. Symptoms of heart failure differ depending on age and become worse with age because the heart must keep up with increased oxygen demands and energy demands.

- Symptoms may include poor growth, difficulty in feeding, and tachypnea; in older children, inability to tolerate exercise and other activities, the need to rest more often, and dyspnea with minimal exertion occur more frequently.
- Treatment is generally age and cause specific. For septal defects, surgery or medication may be indicated. For more complex problems, surgery may be needed within the first few weeks of life.
- Medications used include furosemide (a loop diuretic), angiotensin-converting enzyme inhibitors, β-blockers, and sometimes digoxin to help with heart pumping efficiency.
- Digoxin should be given on a regular time schedule 1 hour before or 2 hours after feeding. Dosing of the drug must be accompanied by close monitoring and individualized nursing care.
- Correct calculation of dosages is very important to safe and cautious nursing care. A one-decimal-point placement error will result in a tenfold dosage error, which could be fatal.
- All medication calculations should be double-checked by a second registered nurse or by a pharmacist or physician because of the narrow margin for error. Toxicity is manifested in children by nausea, vomiting, bradycardia, anorexia, and dysrhythmias.
- The physician should be notified immediately should the following symptoms indicative of heart failure develop: increased fatigue, sudden weight gain (2 lb or more in 24 hours), or respiratory distress.

Based on www.cincinnatichildrens.org/health/heart-encyclopedia/signs/chf.htm.

When significant toxicity develops as a result of cardiac glycoside therapy, the administration of digoxin immune Fab may be indicated. Digoxin immune Fab is an antibody that recognizes digoxin as an antigen and forms an antigen-antibody complex with the drug, thus inactivating the free digoxin. Digoxin immune Fab therapy is not indicated for every patient who is showing signs of digoxin toxicity. The following are the clinical settings in which its use may be indicated:

- Hyperkalemia (serum potassium level over 5 mEq/L) in a patient with digitoxicity
- Life-threatening cardiac dysrhythmias, sustained ventricular tachycardia or fibrillation, and severe sinus bradycardia or heart block unresponsive to atropine treatment or cardiac pacing
- Life-threatening digoxin overdose: more than 10 mg digoxin in adults; more than 4 mg digoxin in children

Interactions

A number of significant drug interactions are possible with cardiac glycosides. The common ones are listed in Table 21-3. One food, bran in large amounts, may decrease the absorption of oral

digitalis drugs. The herbal supplement hawthorne can reduce the effectiveness of cardiac glycosides. Hawthorne is used for hypertension and angina. Other specific food interactions are mentioned in Table 21-3.

Dosages

For dosage information for the cardiac glycosides, see the Dosages table on page 323. Also see the Preventing Medication Errors box on this page.

Drug Profiles

Cardiac glycosides get their name from their chemical structures. Glycosides are complex, steroidlike structures linked to sugar molecules. Because the particular drugs derived from the digitalis plant have potent actions on the heart, they are referred to as *cardiac glycosides*. Digoxin is currently the only prescribed digitalis preparation. Digoxin is a prescription-only drug and is classified as Pregnancy Category C.

▸ *digoxin*

Digoxin (Lanoxin, Lanoxicaps) is effective for the treatment of both heart failure and atrial fibrillation and flutter. It may also be used clinically to improve myocardial contractility and thus reverse cardiogenic shock or other low cardiac output states. Digoxin use is contraindicated in patients who have shown a hypersensitivity to it and in those with ventricular tachycardia and fibrillation, heart disease associated with beriberi, or hypersensitive carotid sinus syndrome. Normal therapeutic drug levels of digoxin should be between 0.5 and 2 ng/mL. Levels higher than 2 ng/mL are typically desirable for the treatment of atrial fibrillation. Digoxin is available in oral and injectable forms. It comes in parenteral form as 100- and 250-mcg/mL intravenous injections. Because of digoxin's fairly long duration of action and half-life, a loading, or "digitalizing," dose is often given to bring serum levels of the drug up to a desirable therapeutic level more quickly. See the table on page 323 for the recommended digitalizing doses and the daily oral and intravenous adult and pediatric dosages.

Pharmacokinetics

Half-Life	Onset	Peak	Duration
33-44 hr	30-120 min	2-6 hr	2-4 days

Table 21-3 Cardiac Glycosides: Drug Interactions

Interacting Drug	Mechanism	Result
Antidysrhythmics calcium (parenteral) reserpine	Increase cardiac irritability	Increased digoxin toxicity
Sympathomimetics amphotericin B chlorthalidone Loop diuretics Laxatives Steroids (adrenal) Thiazide diuretics	Produce hypokalemia	Increased digoxin toxicity
Antacids Antidiarrheals cholestyramine colestipol sucralfate	Decrease oral absorption	Reduced therapeutic effect
Anticholinergics	Increase oral absorption	Increased therapeutic effect
Barbiturates	Induce enzyme	Reduced therapeutic effect
β-blockers	Block β_1 receptors in heart	Enhanced bradycardic effect of digoxin
Calcium channel blockers	Block calcium channels in myocardium	Enhanced bradycardic and negative inotropic effects of digoxin
quinidine verapamil amiodarone	Decrease clearance	Increased digoxin levels (2×); digoxin dose should be reduced 50%

Use of a digoxin preparation can also interfere with the results of several laboratory tests. It can cause the plasma levels of estrone to be raised and the levels of lactate dehydrogenase and testosterone to be lowered. It can also cause the erythrocyte sodium concentration to be increased and the erythrocyte potassium concentration to be reduced.

In addition to interacting with other drugs and with laboratory tests, digoxin can interact with certain foods. The consumption of excessive amounts of potassium-rich foods can decrease its therapeutic effect, whereas the consumption of excessive amounts of licorice can increase digoxin toxicity as the result of the hypokalemia produced.

DOSAGES

Drugs for Heart Failure

Drug	Pharmacologic Class	Usual Dosage Range	Indications

▶digoxin (Lanoxin, Lanoxicaps)	Digitalis cardiac glycoside	**Pediatric**
		Digitalizing dose
		IV: Premature: 0.015-0.025 mg/kg
		    Newborn: 0.020-0.030 mg/kg
		    1 mo-2 yr: 0.030-0.050 mg/kg
		    2-5 yr: 0.025-0.035 mg/kg
		    5-10 yr: 0.015-0.030 mg/kg
		    Older than 10 yr: 0.008-0.012 mg/kg
		PO: Premature: 0.020-0.030 mg/kg
		    Newborn: 0.025-0.035 mg/kg
		    1 mo-2 yr: 0.035-0.060 mg/kg
		    2-5 yr: 0.030-0.040 mg/kg
		    5-10 yr: 0.020-0.035 mg/kg
		    Older than 10 yr: 0.010-0.015 mg/kg
		Usual maintenance dose, 20%-35% of digitalizing dose
		Adult
		PO/IV: Usual digitalizing dose, 1-1.5 mg/day; usual maintenance dose, 0.125-0.5 mg/day
			Heart failure, supraventricular dysrhythmias

milrinone (Primacor)	Phosphodiesterase inhibitor	**Adult** IV loading dose: 50 mcg/kg IV continuous infusion dose: 0.375-0.75mcg/kg/min	Heart failure Heart failure
nesiritide (Natrecor)	Recombinant human type-B natriuretic peptide	**Adult only (pediatric use not yet established)** IV: Initial bolus of 2 mcg/kg, followed by continuous infusion of 0.01 mcg/kg/min	Acutely decompensated heart failure in patients with dyspnea at rest or with minimal activity

digoxin immune Fab Digoxin CD

Digoxin immune Fab (Digibind, DigiFab) is the antidote for severe digoxin overdose and is indicated for the reversal of such life-threatening cardiotoxic effects as severe bradycardia, advanced heart block, ventricular tachycardia or fibrillation, and severe hyperkalemia. It has a unique mechanism of action. As previously mentioned, it works by binding to free (unbound) digoxin, which reverses the drug's effects and symptoms of toxicity. Use of digoxin immune Fab is contraindicated in patients who have shown a hypersensitivity to it. It is available only in parenteral form as a 40-mg vial. Digoxin immune Fab is dosed either in milligrams or by the number of vials, depending on the dose calculation method or the reference chart used. It is commonly dosed based on the patient's serum digoxin level in conjunction with his or her weight. The recommended dosages vary according to the amount of cardiac glycoside ingested. Each milligram can neutralize up to 15 mg of digoxin. For recommended dosages the nurse should consult the manufacturer's latest dosage recommendations. It is important to bear in mind that after digoxin immune Fab is given, all subsequent measurements of serum digoxin level will be elevated for days to weeks because of the presence of both the free (unbound) digoxin (toxic digoxin) and the digoxin that has been bound by the digoxin immune Fab (nontoxic digoxin). Therefore, after its administration, the clinical signs and symptoms of digoxin toxicity, rather than the digoxin serum levels, should be the primary focus in monitoring for the effectiveness of reversal therapy.

Pharmacokinetics

Half-Life	Onset	Peak	Duration
14-20 hr	Immediate	Immediate	Days to weeks

PHOSPHODIESTERASE INHIBITORS

As the name implies, phosphodiesterase inhibitors (PDIs) are a group of inotropic drugs that work by inhibiting the action of an enzyme called *phosphodiesterase*. The inhibition of this enzyme results in two very beneficial effects in an individual with heart failure: a positive inotropic response and vasodilation. For this reason this class of drugs may also be referred to as *inodilators* (inotropics and dilators). These drugs were discovered in the search for positive inotropic drugs with a better therapeutic window than digoxin. There are presently only two U.S. drugs in this category: inamrinone and milrinone. Inamrinone was originally named *amrinone,* but its name was modified to prevent confusion with the antidysrhythmic drug *amiodarone* (Chapter 22). These inodilators share a similar pharmacologic action with methylxanthines such as theophylline. Both types of drug inhibit the action of phosphodiesterase, which results in an increase in intracellular cyclic adenosine monophosphate (cAMP). However, the inodilators are more specific for phosphodiesterase type III, which is especially common in the heart and vascular smooth muscles.

Mechanism of Action and Drug Effects

The mechanism of action of PDIs differs from that of other inotropic drugs such as cardiac glycosides and catecholamines. The beneficial effects of PDIs come from the intracellular increase in cAMP, the buildup of which the phosphodiesterase enzyme normally prevents. Inamrinone and milrinone, the two currently available PDIs, work by selectively inhibiting phosphodiesterase type III, which as noted earlier is found in high concentrations in the heart and vascular smooth muscle. Inhibition of phosphodiesterase results in the availability of more calcium for the heart to use in muscle contraction. It also results in dilation of systemic or pulmonary blood vessels, which in turn decreases the workload of the heart. The effects on heart muscle lead to an increase in the force of contraction (i.e., positive inotropic action). The effects on the smooth muscle that surrounds blood vessels result in relaxation of smooth muscle and therefore causes dilation of blood vessels. The increased calcium present in heart muscle is also taken back up into its storage sites in the sarcoplasmic reticulum at a much faster rate than normal. As a result, the heart muscle relaxes more than normal and is also more compliant. In summary, PDIs have positive inotropic and vasodilatory effects. They may also increase heart rate in some instances and therefore may also have positive chronotropic effects.

Indications

PDIs are primarily used for the short-term management of heart failure. In the treatment of heart failure the therapeutic benefits of the inodilators are due to their inotropic and vasodilatory effects. The inodilators have a 10 to 100 times greater affinity for smooth muscle surrounding blood vessels than they do for heart muscle. This suggests that the primary beneficial effects of inodilators come from their ability to dilate blood vessels. This causes a reduction in afterload, or the force against which the heart must pump to eject its volume of blood.

Traditionally, PDIs are given to patients who can be closely monitored and who have not responded adequately to digoxin, diuretics, and/or vasodilators. PDIs do not require a receptor-mediated action to increase contraction. In contrast, with other positive inotropic drugs, such as β-agonists (e.g., dobutamine, dopamine), stimulation of a receptor is required to increase contraction. The repetitive stimulation of these receptors can cause the body to become less sensitive to the drug over time. In patients with end-stage heart failure who require positive inotropic support, a continual dosage increase is often needed to maintain positive results. As the dosages of these drugs are increased, they produce more unwanted cardiac effects. Because PDIs do not stimulate receptors to increase the force of contraction, they do not have this unwanted problem. Many hospitals that treat large numbers of patients with heart failure now manage patients with end-stage heart failure using weekly 6-hour infusions of PDIs. This has been shown to increase the quality of life and decrease the number of readmissions to the hospital for exacerbations of heart failure.

Contraindications

Contraindications to the use of PDIs include known drug allergy and may include the presence of severe aortic or pulmonary valvular disease and heart failure resulting from diastolic dysfunction.

Adverse Effects

Although inamrinone and milrinone are both PDIs, they have very different adverse effect profiles. The adverse effect that is most worrisome with inamrinone is thrombocytopenia. Inamrinone-induced thrombocytopenia occurs at a rate of about 2.4% and is more frequent when high doses are given over long periods. The other adverse effects associated with inamrinone therapy include dysrhythmia (3%), nausea (1.7%), and hypotension (1.3%). With long-term use, elevations in liver enzyme levels may occur.

The primary adverse effect seen with milrinone therapy is dysrhythmia. Milrinone-induced dysrhythmias are mainly ventricular. Ventricular dysrhythmias occur in approximately 12% of patients treated with this drug. Some other adverse effects associated with milrinone therapy are hypotension (2.9%), angina (chest pain) (1.2%), hypokalemia (0.6%), tremor (0.4%), and thrombocytopenia (0.4%).

Toxicity and Management of Overdose

No specific antidote exists for an overdose of either inamrinone or milrinone. Hypotension secondary to vasodilation is the primary effect seen with excessive doses of both drugs. The recommendation is to reduce the dose or temporarily discontinue the PDI if excessive hypotension occurs. This should be done until the patient's condition is stabilized. Initiation of general measures for circulatory support is also recommended.

Interactions

Concurrent administration of diuretics (see Chapter 25) may cause significant hypovolemia and reduced cardiac filling pressure. The patient should be appropriately monitored in an intensive care setting to detect and respond to these problems. Also, additive inotropic effects may be seen with coadministration of digoxin. Furosemide must not be injected into intravenous lines of inamrinone or milrinone because it will precipitate immediately. Glucose-containing solutions should not be used when mixing inamrinone. Such solutions will cause an 11% to 13% loss in inamrinone's activity over 24 hours because of a slow chemical interaction.

Dosages

For dosage information for the PDIs, see the Dosages table on page 323.

Drug Profiles

milrinone

Milrinone (Primacor) is one of the two presently available PDIs. Inamrinone was the first of the two PDIs to be used clinically for the short-term treatment of heart failure. As noted earlier, milrinone and inamrinone are referred to as inodilators because they exert both a positive inotropic effect and a vasodilatory effect. Both of these drugs are contraindicated in patients who have shown a hypersensitivity to them. Milrinone is marketed only as an intravenous product and is available in a 5-mg (1-mg/mL) Carpuject sterile cartridge unit and a 100-mL (200 mg/mL) in 5% dextrose injection. It is classified as a pregnancy category C drug. Recommended dosages are given in the table on page 323.

Pharmacokinetics

Half-Life	Onset	Peak	Duration
2.3 hr	5-15 min	6-12 hr	8-10 hr

MISCELLANEOUS HEART FAILURE DRUGS

The newest class of medications for heart failure currently includes only one drug: nesiritide (Natrecor). This drug is classified as a synthetic recombinant version of human B-type natriuretic peptide, which is a synthetic hormone that has vasodilating effects on both arteries and veins. This vasodilation takes place in the heart itself and throughout the body. A related hormone that occurs naturally in the body is *atrial natriuretic peptide,* which affects *vascular permeability.* Vascular permeability is the ability of plasma to flow between blood vessels and their surrounding tissues, which serves as one way for the body to regulate blood pressure. The effects of nesiritide on vascular permeability remain to be studied. A "recombinant" drug is one manufactured using recombinant DNA technology. This method is described further in later chapters, including Chapter 39. At this time, nesiritide is generally used in the intensive care setting as a final effort to treat severe, life-threatening heart failure, often along with several other cardiostimulatory medications. The manufacturer recommends that nesiritide not be used as a first-line drug for this purpose. Its only current contraindication is drug allergy, although it is not recommended for use in patients with low cardiac filling pressures, as typically measured in the intensive care unit. The drug was approved by the Food and Drug Administration in 2001. Currently identified drug interactions include additive hypotensive effects with coadministration of ACE inhibitors (Chapter 24) and diuretics (Chapter 25). The drug is categorized as pregnancy category C. Recommended dosages are given in the table on page 323.

◆ NURSING PROCESS

◆ ASSESSMENT

Before a cardiac glycoside or other positive inotropic drug is administered, a thorough assessment of the patient is required so that the drug can be used in the safest manner possible. An assessment of the patient's past and present medical history, drug allergies, family medical history (especially if positive for cardiac, hypertensive, and renal diseases), and complete medication history may yield findings that either dictate very cautious use of the drug or even contraindicate its use (Table 21-4). Before the nurse initiates therapy with digoxin and/or another positive inotropic drug, a number of clinical parameters and other data need to be assessed. These include the following:
- Blood pressure
- Pulse rate—both apical and radial for 1 full minute
- Peripheral pulse location and grading
- Capillary refill
- Presence of edema
- Heart sounds
- Breath sounds
- Weight
- Intake and output amounts
- Serum laboratory values such as potassium, sodium, magnesium, and calcium
- Electrocardiogram
- Renal function laboratory test results (blood urea nitrogen and creatinine levels)
- Liver function test results (levels of aspartate aminotransferase, alanine aminotransferase, creatine phosphokinase, lactate dehydrogenase, and alkaline phosphatase)
- Medication history and profile regarding prescription drugs, over-the-counter drugs, herbals, and nutritional supplements;

Table 21-4 Conditions Predisposing to Digitalis Toxicity

Condition/Disease	Significance
Use of cardiac pacemaker	A patient with this device may exhibit digitalis toxicity at lower doses than usual.
Hepatic dysfunction	Hepatic elimination of digitoxin is decreased, which necessitates a reduction in dosage.
Hypokalemia	The patient's risk of serious dysrhythmias is increased and the patient is more susceptible to digitalis toxicity.
Hypercalcemia	The patient is at higher risk of suffering sinus bradycardia, dysrhythmias, and heart block.
Atrioventricular block	Heart block may worsen with increasing levels or digitalis.
Dysrhythmias	Dysrhythmias may occur that did not exist before digitalis use and thus could be related to digitalis toxicity.
Hypothyroid, respiratory, or renal disease	Patients with these disorders require lower dosages because they cause delayed renal drug excretion.
Advanced age	Because of decreased renal function and the resultant diminished drug excretion along with decreased body mass in this patient population, a lower dose than usual is needed to prevent toxicity. The practice of polypharmacy may also lead to toxicity.
Ventricular fibrillation	Ventricular rate may actually increase with digitalis use.

for example, herbal products (e.g., Siberian ginseng) may increase digitalis drug levels; consuming large amounts of bran with digoxin will decrease the drug's absorption

- Dietary habits and a recall of meals and snacks for the previous 24 hours
- Inquiries about the intake of moderate to large amounts of bran and/or taking bran at the same time as the digitalis drug (which decreases the drug's absorption)
- Smoking history
- Alcohol intake

Other assessment data includes thorough monitoring of electrolytes because of the narrow therapeutic range with digoxin. With a narrow therapeutic range, there is but a small difference between a therapeutic serum level of digoxin and a toxic level. Because low levels of certain electrolytes (e.g., hypokalemia) may precipitate this drug's toxicity, close assessment is critical to preventing complications and further problems. Other laboratory tests serum calcium, magnesium, and sodium levels before and during drug therapy. In addition, the occurrence of edema (weight gain of 2 lb or more over a 24-hour period or 5 lb or more in 1 week) needs to be reported to the health care provider. The following systems should also be included: (1) neurological assessment, with notation of headache, depression, weakness, changes in level of consciousness, alertness/orientation vs. confusion, presence of restlessness, fatigue, lethargy, or occurrence of nightmares, (2) gastrointestinal assessment, with attention to changes in appetite, diarrhea vs. constipation, nausea, and vomiting, (3) cardiac assessment, with documentation of any irregularities, pulse rate of less than 60 beats/min or more than 100 beats/min, abnormal heart sounds, and abnormal ECG findings (if ordered), and (4) vision/sensory assessment, with notation of any changes such as green-yellow halos surrounding the peripheral field of vision. Also assess for complaints of anorexia, nausea, and vomiting, which indicate cardiac glycoside toxicity. See Table 21-1 for more information related to adverse effects. Cautions, contraindications, and drug interactions should also be assessed (see Tables 21-1, 21-2, and 21-3).

In summary, a head-to-toe physical assessment with thorough medical and medication history taking will help to prevent adverse and toxic reactions or at least help identify them early in the therapy. These drugs, although very helpful in management of heart failure, are not without concerns for toxicity. It is also important to assess support systems at home, because safe and effective therapy depends on close observation, monitoring of parameters such as daily weight, attention to complaints by the patient, and evaluation of how the patient is feeling and doing.

◆ NURSING DIAGNOSES
- Ineffective tissue perfusion, cardiopulmonary, related to the pathophysiologic influence of heart failure
- Deficient knowledge related to the first-time use of a cardiac glycoside or positive inotropic drug and subsequent lack of information on heart failure and its treatment
- Risk for injury related to limited information on the pathologic impact of heart failure and the potential adverse effects of drug therapy
- Imbalanced nutrition, less than body requirements, related to gastrointestinal adverse effects related to digoxin toxicity
- Noncompliance with therapy regimen related to lack of information about the drug's effects and adverse effects

◆ PLANNING
Goals
- Patient exhibits improved cardiac output once therapy is initiated.
- Patient states use, action, adverse effects, and toxic effects of therapy.
- Patient is free from injury related to medication therapy.
- Patient's appetite is improved or he or she is free of anorexia while taking positive inotropic drugs.

In planning for the administration of these preparations, the nurse must check the dosage and always double-check calculations as well as to double-check the patient's laboratory values. Administration of parenteral dosage forms needs preplanning so that all necessary equipment is gathered before giving the drug.

Outcome Criteria
- Patient has improved to strong peripheral pulses; increased endurance for activity; decreased fatigue; and pink, warm extremities.
- Patient has increased urinary output resulting from therapeutic effects of the drug.
- Patient has improved heart and lung sounds with decreased dysrhythmias and crackles.

- Patient loses appropriate weight and has less edema from the therapeutic effects of the drug (increased urinary output due to increased cardiac output).
- Patient's skin and mucous membranes (color and temperature) are improved to pink and warm.
- Patient maintains appetite while on therapy and reports anorexia, nausea, or vomiting immediately to the physician.
- Patient is free of toxicity as evidenced by absence of bradycardia and complaints of anorexia, nausea, or vomiting.
- Patient demonstrates proper technique for measuring radial pulse for 1 full minute before taking medication.
- Patient is able to cite drug-related problems to report to the physician, such as palpitations, dysrhythmias, chest pain, and pulse rate lower than 60 beats/min or greater than 100 beats/min.

◆ IMPLEMENTATION

Before administering any dose of a cardiac glycoside, all electrolyte and drug levels should be checked to be sure they are within normal limits. The nurse should *always* count the patient's apical pulse rate (auscultate the apical heart rate—found at the point of maximal impulse located at the fifth left midclavicular intercostal space—for *1 full minute*). If the pulse rate is 60 beats/min or less or more than 120 beats/min, then the dose is generally withheld and the physician notified immediately of the problem. Withholding of the dose is usually indicated; however, health care facilities and health care providers have their own protocols that apply to individual patients. In addition, the physician should be contacted if the patient experiences any of the following signs and symptoms (which may indicate digitalis toxicity): anorexia, nausea, vomiting, diarrhea, or visual disturbances such as blurred vision or the perception of green or yellow halos around objects. Remember that most institutions and/or nursing units follow some protocol or policy with regard to digitalis and its administration.

Other nursing interventions include checking the dosage form and prescribed amounts and the physician's order carefully to make sure that the correct drug dosage has been dispensed (e.g., 0.125 or 0.25 mg). Oral digoxin may be administered with meals but not with foods high in fiber (bran), because the fiber will bind to the digitalis and lead to altered absorption and bioavailability of the drug. If the medication is to be given intravenously, the following interventions are critical to patient safety: infuse undiluted intravenous forms at around 0.25 mg/min or over longer than a 5-minute period, or as per hospital protocol. The administration of intramuscular forms of cardiac glycosides is extremely painful and is not indicated or recommended because tissue necrosis and erratic absorption are often the outcome. Digoxin is incompatible with many other medications in solution or syringe, and compatibility must be double-checked before parenteral administration.

The nursing interventions for patients undergoing digitalization must be considered separately. Although not commonly used in contemporary practice, digitalization may still be performed in some areas of practice for the management of heart failure. Rapid digitalization (to achieve faster onset of action) is generally reserved for patients with heart failure and in acute distress. Such patients are hospitalized because digitalis toxicities can appear quickly in this setting and are directly correlated with the high drug concentrations used. Should the patient undergoing rapid digitalization exhibit any of the manifestations of toxicity, the physician should be contacted immediately. These patients should be observed constantly and serum drug and potassium levels measured frequently.

Slow digitalization is generally performed on an outpatient basis in patients with heart failure who are not in acute distress. In this situation, it takes longer for toxic effects to appear (depending on the specific drug's half-life) than with rapid digitalization. The main advantages of slow digitalization are that it can be performed on an outpatient basis, oral dosage forms can be used, and it is safer than rapid digitalization. The disadvantages are that it takes longer for the therapeutic effects to occur and the symptoms of toxicity are more gradual in onset and therefore more insidious.

Should toxicity occur and digoxin rise to a life-threatening level, the antidote, digoxin immune Fab, should be administered as ordered. It is given parenterally over 30 minutes and in some scenarios given as an intravenous bolus (or IV push) (e.g., if cardiac arrest is imminent). All vials of the drug should be refrigerated. The drug, stable for 4 hours after being mixed, should be used immediately and, if not used within this time frame, be discarded. Compatible solutions for dilution should be checked prior to infusion of the antidote. Blood pressure, apical pulse rate/rhythm, electrocardiogram, and serum potassium levels must be closely monitored and documented. The nurse must always watch for changes from patient baseline assessment values in the following: muscle strength; tremor; muscle cramping; mental status; cardiac irregular rhythms (from hypokalemia); and confusion, thirst, and cold, clammy skin (from hyponatremia). If toxicity improves, these signs and symptoms will improve (from baseline).

With inamrinone, intravenous forms should not be mixed with dextrose, and the true color of intravenous inamrinone solution is clear yellow (the majority of solutions are clear). Intake and output, heart rate, blood pressure, daily weight, respiration rate, heart sounds, and breath sounds should be recorded. Any evidence of hypokalemia should be noted and reported to the physician immediately. When giving these drugs (e,g., digoxin, inamrinone, milrinone, digoxin immune Fab) parenterally, an infusion pump must be used unless the order is to give them IV push.

◆ EVALUATION

Monitoring patients after the administration of positive inotropic drugs is critical for identifying therapeutic effects and adverse effects. Because positive inotropic drugs increase the force of myocardial contractility (positive inotropic effect), alter electrophysiologic properties (decrease rate, negative chronotropic effect), and decrease AV node conduction (negative dromotropic effect), the therapeutic effects include the following:

- Increased urinary output
- Decreased edema
- Decreased shortness of breath, dyspnea, and crackles
- Decreased fatigue
- Resolution of paroxysmal nocturnal dyspnea
- Improved peripheral pulses, skin color, and temperature

While the nurse is monitoring for therapeutic effects, it is essential (because of the low therapeutic index of digitalis preparations) for the nurse to assess the patient for the development of toxic effects described earlier. Monitoring laboratory values such as serum creatinine, potassium, calcium, sodium, and chloride levels, as well as watching the serum levels of digoxin (0.5 to 2 ng/mL), is important to ensure safe and efficacious treatment.

For patients receiving inamrinone, all vital signs and hemodynamic parameters (cardiac output, central venous pressure) must be constantly evaluated. Therapeutic effects of milrinone include an improvement in cardiac function with a corresponding improvement in the patient's heart failure. Adverse effects for which to monitor include hypotension, dysrhythmias, headache, ventricular fibrillation, chest pain, and hypokalemia. Patients taking milrinone should be evaluated for significant hypotension, and the drug should be discontinued or the infusion rate decreased per the physician's orders should this occur.

Patient Teaching Tips

- Patients should be instructed to take the radial pulse before each dose of digoxin. For elderly or physically or mentally challenged patients, it is important that home health care personnel supervise the medication regimen or that a hospital-based or cardiologist-managed heart failure clinic supervise therapy. This is important because these individuals are at risk for interactions with other medications, adverse effects, and toxicity.
- Patients should keep a journal at home in which they record the following: date, time of dose, amount of medication taken, dietary intake, weight, any unusual adverse effects or changes in condition, pulse rate, and any other miscellaneous comments.
- Patients should be encouraged to contact the physician or health care provider if they have any unusual complaints, if the pulse rate is below 60 beats/min or is erratic, if the pulse rate is 100 bpm or greater or if they are experiencing anorexia, nausea, or vomiting.
- Encourage the patient to report any of the following: palpitations or a feeling that the heart is racing, a change in heart rate, dizziness, fainting or blackout spells, and weight gain (2 lb or more in 24 hours or 5 lb or more in 1 week).
- Any changes in visual acuity should also be reported to the health care provider or home health care nurse immediately.
- Inform the patient to wear a medical alert bracelet or necklace or otherwise make sure their medical and medication history and information is on their person at all times. Make sure all information is updated frequently or with each visit to the physician.
- Encourage the patient to weigh daily, at the same time each day and with the same amount of clothing on because weight is an important indicator of fluid volume overload or exacerbation of heart failure. Be emphatic about the importance of compliance to medications, reducing the stress on the heart, rest and relaxation, watching weights daily, and keeping follow-up appointments with their physician, heart failure clinic, nurse practitioner, or other health care provider.
- Digoxin is usually taken once a day, and patients should be encouraged to take it at the same time every morning. If a dose is missed, the patient may take the omitted dose if no more than 12 hours have passed from the time the drug was to have been taken.
- If more than 12 hours have passed, the patient should know to *not* skip that dose, *not* double up on the next digoxin dose, and to contact the health care provider immediately for further instructions.
- Patients should *never* abruptly stop their digoxin (or other positive inotropics) because this could precipitate more cardiac problems and complications.
- Patients should be encouraged to consume foods high in potassium, especially if they are also taking a potassium-depleting diuretic. Encourage them to report any weakness, fatigue, or lethargy immediately to the health care provider.
- Encourage patients to report any worsening of dizziness or dyspnea or the occurrence of any unusual problems.
- Patients should avoid using antacids or eating ice cream, milk products, yogurt, or cheese for 2 hours before or after taking medication to avoid interference with the drug.

Points to Remember

- *Inotropic* drugs affect the force of myocardial contraction; positive inotropics (e.g., digoxin) increase the force of contractions and negative inotropics (e.g., β-blockers, calcium channel blockers) decrease myocardial contractility.
- *Chronotropic* drugs affect the rate at which the heart beats (beats/min); positive chronotropic drugs (e.g., epinephrine, atropine) increase the heart rate and negative chronotropic drugs decrease the heart rate.
- *Dromotropic* drugs affect the conduction of electrical impulses through the heart; positive dromotropic drugs increase the speed of electrical impulses through the heart, whereas negative drugs have the opposite effect.
- Nurses need to be aware of some important physiologic concepts such as ejection fraction. A patient's ejection fraction reflects the contractility of the heart and is about 65% (0.65) in a normal heart. This value decreases as heart failure progresses; therefore, patients with heart failure have low ejection fractions because their hearts are failing to pump effectively.
- Nurses need to be informed regarding contraindications to the use of digoxin, which include the following: a history of allergy to the digitalis medications, ventricular tachycardia and fibrillations, and AV block.
- Patients need to be aware of conditions that predispose to digitalis toxicity, including hypokalemia, hypercalcemia, hypothyroid states, renal dysfunction, and advanced age.
- Patients should be educated to measure pulse rate, and daily weight with daily journaling. Nurses should always take an apical pulse for 1 full minute when digoxin is administered, and patients should be instructed on taking radial pulses when at home.
- Patients should be encouraged to notify the health care provider immediately at the first signs of anorexia, nausea, or vomiting, or the occurrence of bradycardia with a pulse rate below 60 beats/min if the patient is taking digoxin.
- Nurses must be aware that hypotension, dysrhythmias, and thrombocytopenia are major adverse effects of inamrinone and milrinone use.

NCLEX Examination Review Questions

1. When teaching the patient about the signs and symptoms of cardiac glycoside toxicity, the nurse should alert the patient to watch for:
   a. Visual changes such as photophobia
   b. Flickering lights or halos around lights
   c. Dizziness when standing up
   d. Increased urine output
2. During assessment of a patient who is receiving digoxin, which finding would indicate an increased possibility of toxicity?
   a. Apical pulse rate of 62 beats/min
   b. Digoxin level of 1.5 ng/mL
   c. Serum potassium level of 2.0 mEq/L
   d. Serum potassium level of 4.8 mEq/L
3. When monitoring a patient who is receiving an intravenous infusion of inamrinone, the nurse will look for which adverse effect?
   a. Thrombocytopenia
   b. Proteinuria
   c. Anemia
   d. Decreased blood urea nitrogen and creatinine levels
4. When a patient is experiencing digitalis toxicity, in which of the following situations would it be appropriate to treat with digoxin immune Fab (Digibind)?
   a. Hypokalemia (serum potassium level lower than 3.5 mEq/L)
   b. Hyperkalemia (serum potassium level higher than 5 mEq/L)
   c. Apical heart rate of 60 beats/min
   d. Supraventricular dysrhythmias
5. Before beginning oral digoxin therapy, the nurse would note that which of the following drugs would cause a decrease in the absorption of the digoxin if the two are taken together?
   a. Loop diuretics
   b. Antidepressants
   c. Potassium
   d. Antidiarrheals

1. b, 2. c, 3. a, 4. b, 5. d.

Critical Thinking Activities

1. A nurse administered 125 mg of digoxin instead of 0.125 mg of digoxin intravenously. The patient has developed a severe heart block dysrhythmia, and the slow heart rate has not responded to administration of atropine and other measures. The patient will be receiving digoxin immune Fab. Explain how this medication works in this situation. How could this situation have been prevented?
2. Your patient, a 78-year-old man, has a potassium level of 3.0 mEq/L. He states that he has been nauseous and without an appetite and has experienced some diarrhea. He has been taking digoxin for the past few weeks for the treatment of recently diagnosed heart failure. Discuss the implication of hypokalemia in a patient who is taking digoxin and any negative consequences.
3. Explain why an older patient with hypothyroid disease is at increased risk for digitalis toxicity.

For answers, see http://evolve.elsevier.com/Lilley.

Objectives

Objectives

When you reach the end of this chapter, you should be able to do the following:

1. Describe the anatomy and physiology of a normal heart, including conduction, rate, and rhythm, and compare them with those of a heart with abnormal conduction and/or rhythm.
2. Define the term *dysrhythmia* and explain its causes and consequences for the patient.
3. Identify the most commonly encountered dysrhythmias.
4. Compare the various dysrhythmias with regard to their basic characteristics, the impact on the structures of the heart, and related symptoms.
5. Contrast the various classes of antidysrhythmic drugs, citing prototypes in each class and describing their mechanisms of action, indications, routes of administration, dosing, any related drug protocols, adverse effects, cautions, contraindications, drug interactions, and any toxic reactions.
6. Develop a nursing care plan that includes all phases of the nursing process for patients receiving each class of antidysrhythmics.

e-Learning Activities

Companion CD

- NCLEX Review Questions: see questions 159-169
- Animations
- Audio Glossary
- Category Catchers
- Medication Errors Checklists
- IV Therapy Checklists

evolve Website (http://evolve.elsevier.com/Lilley)

• Nursing Care Plans • Frequently Asked Questions • Content Updates • WebLinks • Supplemental Resources • Elsevier ePharmacology Update • Medication Administration Animations

Drug Profiles

adenosine, p. 348
▶ amiodarone, p. 347
▶ atenolol, p. 346
▶ diltiazem, p. 348
esmolol, p. 346
flecainide, p. 346
ibutilide, p. 347
▶ lidocaine, p. 343

▶ metoprolol, p. 346
mexiletine, p. 345
procainamide, p. 341
propafenone, p. 346
▶ propranolol, p. 346
quinidine, p. 342
▶ sotalol, p. 347
▶ verapamil, p. 348

▶ Key drug.

Glossary

Action potential Electrical activity consisting of a self-propagating series of polarizations and depolarizations that travel across the cell membrane of a nerve fiber during the transmission of a nerve impulse and across the cell membranes of a muscle cell during contraction or other activity of the cell. (p. 331)

Action potential duration (APD) For a cell membrane, the interval beginning with baseline (resting) membrane potential followed by depolarization and ending with repolarization to baseline membrane potential. (p. 333)

Arrhythmia Technically "no rhythm," meaning absence of heart beat rhythm (i.e., no heart beat at all). More commonly used in clinical practice to refer to any variation from the normal rhythm of the heartbeat. A synonymous term is *dysrhythmia*, which is the primary term used in this chapter and book. (p. 331)

Cardiac Arrhythmia Suppression Trial (CAST) The name of the major research study conducted by the National Heart, Lung, and Blood Institute to investigate the possibility of eliminating sudden cardiac death in patients with asymptomatic, non–life-threatening ectopy that has arisen after a myocardial infarction. (p. 346)

Depolarization The movement of positive and negative ions on either side of a cell membrane across the membrane in a direction that tends to bring the net charge to zero. (p. 332)

Dysrhythmia Any disturbance or abnormality in the rhythm of the heartbeat. (p. 331)

Effective refractory period (ERP) The period after the firing of an impulse during which a cell may respond to a stimulus but the response will not be passed along or continued as another impulse. (p. 333)

Internodal pathways (Bachmann's bundle) Special pathways in the atria that carry electrical impulses spontaneously generated by the sinoatrial node. These impulses cause the heart to beat. (p. 333)

Relative refractory period (RRP) The time after generation of an action potential during which a nerve fiber will show a (reduced) response only to a strong stimulus. (p. 333)

Resting membrane potential (RMP)   The transmembrane voltage that exists when the cell membranes of heart muscle (or other muscle or nerve cells) are at rest. (p. 331)

Sodium-potassium adenosine triphosphatase (ATPase) pump   A mechanism for transporting sodium and potassium ions across the cell membrane against an opposing concentration gradient. Energy for this transport is obtained from the hydrolysis of adenosine triphosphate (ATP) by means of the enzyme ATPase. (p. 331)

Sudden cardiac death   Unexpected, fatal cardiac arrest. (p. 346)

Threshold potential (TP)   The critical state of electrical tension required for spontaneous depolarization of a cell membrane. (p. 333)

Vaughan Williams classification   The system most commonly used to classify antidysrhythmic drugs. (p. 000; see also Table 22-3, p. 338)

DYSRHYTHMIAS AND NORMAL CARDIAC ELECTROPHYSIOLOGY

A **dysrhythmia** is any deviation from the normal rhythm of the heart. The term **arrhythmia** (literally "no rhythm") implies asystole, or no heartbeat at all. Thus, the more accurate term for an irregular heart rhythm is *dysrhythmia,* because a patient who has no cardiac rhythm is in asystole, or dead. Dysrhythmias can develop in association with many conditions. Some of the more common ones arise after a myocardial infarction (MI) or cardiac surgery or as the result of coronary artery disease. These dysrhythmias are usually serious and may require treatment with an antidysrhythmic drug or nonpharmacologic therapies (discussed later in this chapter), although not all require medical treatment. A cardiologist is usually consulted to make the judgment.

Disturbances in cardiac rhythm are the result of abnormally functioning cardiac cells. Therefore, an understanding of the pathologic mechanism responsible for dysrhythmias first requires review of the electrical properties of these cells. Figure 21-1 on page 320 illustrates the overall anatomy of the conduction system of the heart. Figure 22-1 illustrates some of the

properties of this system from the standpoint of a single cardiac cell. Inside a resting cardiac cell there exists a net negative charge relative to the outside of the cell. This difference in the electronegative charge exists in all types of cardiac cells and is referred to as the **resting membrane potential (RMP).** The RMP results from an uneven distribution of ions (e.g., sodium, potassium, and calcium) across the cell membrane. This is known as *polarization.* Each ion moves primarily through its own specific *channel,* which is a specialized protein molecule that sits across the cell membrane. These proteins work continuously to restore the specific intracellular and extracellular concentrations of each ion. At RMP, the ionic concentration *gradient* (distribution) for the different ions is such that potassium ions are more highly concentrated intracellularly, whereas sodium and calcium ions are both more highly concentrated extracellularly. For this reason, potassium is generally thought of as an intracellular ion, whereas sodium and calcium are generally thought of as extracellular ions. Negatively charged intracellular and extracellular ions such as chloride (Cl^-) and bicarbonate (HCO_3^-) also contribute to this uneven distribution of ions, which is known as a *polarized* state. This polarized distribution of ions is maintained by the **sodium-potassium adenosine triphosphatase (ATPase) pump,** an energy-requiring ionic pump. The energy that drives this pump comes from molecules of *adenosine triphosphate (ATP),* which are a major source of energy in cellular metabolism. Cardiac cells become excited when there is a change in this baseline distribution of ions across their membranes (RMP) that leads to the propagation of an electrical impulse. This change is known as an **action potential.** Action potentials normally occur in a continuous and regular manner in the cells of the cardiac conduction system, such as the *sinoatrial node, atrioventricular node,* and *His-Purkinje system.* This is because all of these tissues have the property of spontaneous electrical excitability known as *automaticity.* This excited state creates *action potentials,* which in turn generate electrical impulses that travel through the myocardium ultimately to create the heartbeat via contraction of cardiac muscle fibers. An action potential has five phases. *Phase 0* is also called the *upstroke* because it appears as an upward line on the graph of an action potential, as shown in Figure 22-2, *A* and *B.* Both of these figures graphically illustrate the cycle of electrical

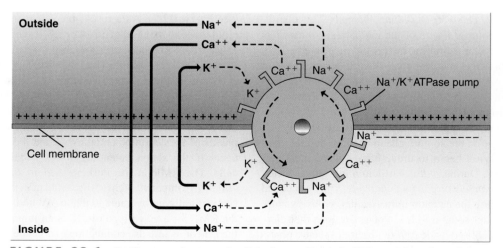

FIGURE 22-1   Resting membrane potential of a cardiac cell. *ATPase,* Adenosine triphosphatase.

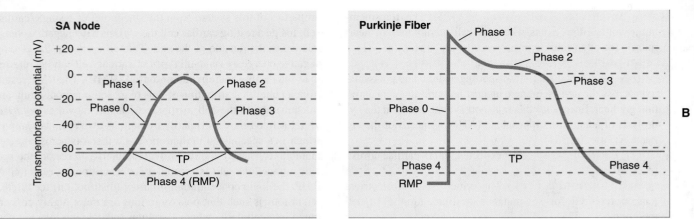

A   **B**

FIGURE 22-2 Action potentials. *RMP*, Resting membrane potential; *SA*, sinoatrial; *TP*, threshold potential.

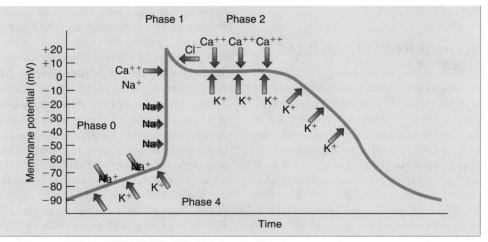

FIGURE 22-3 Purkinje fiber action potential.

changes that create an action potential. Note the variation in the shape of the curve of the graph depending on the relative conduction speed of the specific tissue involved (SA node vs. Purkinje fiber). A faster rate of conduction corresponds to a steeper slope on the graph. During phase 0, the resting cardiac cell membrane suddenly becomes highly permeable to sodium ions, which rush from outside of the cell membrane to inside *(influx)* through what are known as the *fast channels* or *sodium channels.* This disruption of the earlier *polarized* state of the membrane is known as **depolarization.** Depolarization can be thought of as a temporary equalization of positive and negative charges across the cell membrane. This releases spurts of electrochemical energy that drive the resulting electrical impulses through adjacent cells. *Phase 1* of the action potential begins a rapid process of *repolarization* that continues through *phases 2* and *3* to *phase 4,* which is the RMP. In phase 1, the sodium channels close and the concentrations of each ion begin to move back toward their ion-specific RMP levels. During *phase 2,* calcium ion influx occurs through the *slow channels* or *calcium channels.* They are called slow channels because the calcium influx occurs *relatively* more slowly than the earlier sodium influx. Potassium ions then flow from inside of the cell to outside *(efflux)* through specific potassium channels to offset the elevated positive charge caused by the influx of sodium and calcium ions. In the case of the Purkinje fi-

bers, this causes a partial plateau (flattening on the graph) during which the overall membrane potential changes only slightly, as seen in Figure 22-2, *B.* In *phase 3,* the ionic flow patterns of phases 0 to 2 are changed by the sodium-potassium ATPase pump (or, more simply, the *sodium pump*), which reestablishes the baseline polarized state by restoring both intracellular and extracellular concentrations of sodium, potassium, and calcium (see Figure 22-1). As a result, the cell membrane is ultimately repolarized to its baseline level or RMP *(phase 4).* Note that this entire process occurs over roughly 400 *milliseconds*—that is, four hundred thousandths (less than half) of *1* second.

However, there is some variation in this time period between different parts of the conduction system. As an example, Figure 22-3 illustrates the pattern of movement of sodium, potassium, and calcium ions into and out of a Purkinje cell during the four phases of the action potential. Note that there are several differences in the action potentials of SA nodal cells and Purkinje cells. The RMP in the Purkinje cell is approximately –80 to –90 mV, compared with –50 to –60 mV in the SA nodal cell (which is also comparable to that in AV nodal cells). The level of the RMP for a given type of cell is an important determinant of the *rate* of its impulse conduction to other cells. The less negative (i.e., the closer to zero) RMP at the onset of phase 0 of the action potential, the slower the upstroke *velocity* of phase 0. The *slope* of phase 0 is directly related to the impulse velocity. An upstroke with a steeper slope indicates faster conduction velocity. Thus, in the Purkinje cells, electrical conduction is relatively fast, and therefore electrical impulses are conducted quickly. These cells are referred to as *fast-response cells,* or *fast-channel cells,* and Purkinje fibers can therefore be thought of as fast-channel tissue. Many antidysrhythmic drugs affect the RMP and sodium channels, which in turn influences the rate of impulse conduction.

In contrast to Purkinje fibers, the cells of the SA node, because they have RMPs of −50 to −60 mV (i.e., less negative and closer to zero than those of Purkinje cells), have a slower upstroke velocity, or a slower phase 0. This is illustrated in Figure 22-2, *A* as an upstroke curve that is less steep, which indicates a relatively slower rate of electrical conduction in these cells.

Again, AV nodal cells are comparable to SA nodal cells in this regard. This slower upstroke in the SA and AV nodes is primarily dependent on the entry of calcium ions through the *slow channels* or *calcium channels* mentioned previously in the discussion of phase 3 in both nodal and Purkinje cells. This means that nodal action potentials are affected by calcium influx as early as phase 0, an effect that is less pronounced in the Purkinje action potentials, where calcium influx is more predominantly a phase 3 phenomenon. The nodes are therefore called *slow-channel tissue,* and conduction in these cells is slower than that in other parts of the conduction system. Drugs that affect calcium ion movement into or out of these cells (e.g., calcium channel blockers) tend to have significant effects on the SA and AV nodal conduction rates.

The interval between phase 0 and phase 4 is called the **action potential duration (APD)** (Figure 22-4). The period between phase 0 and midway through phase 3 is called the *absolute* or **effective refractory period (ERP).** During the ERP the cardiac cell cannot be restimulated to depolarize and generate another action potential. During the remainder of phase 3 until the return to the RMP (phase 4), the cardiac cell *can* be depolarized again if it receives a powerful enough impulse (such as one induced by drug therapy or supplied by an electrical *pacemaker*). This period is referred to as the **relative refractory period (RRP).** If a cardiac cell receives a strong enough stimulus during the RRP, it will be when the cell is at a relatively less negative membrane potential (i.e., closer to zero than when at RMP), which will result in a slower upstroke (phase 0) and slower impulse conduction than if it were stimulated while at RMP. Figure 22-4 illustrates these various aspects of an action potential. Again, the actual shape of the action potential curve varies in different parts of the conduction system.

The RMP of certain cardiac cells gradually decreases (becomes less negative) over time in ongoing cycles, and this is probably secondary to small changes in the flux of sodium and potassium ions. Depolarization eventually occurs when a certain critical voltage is reached (**threshold potential [TP]**). This process of spontaneous depolarization is referred to as *automaticity,* or *pacemaker activity,* as mentioned earlier in this section. It is normal when it occurs in the SA node (see Figure 21-1). When spontaneous depolarizations occur elsewhere, however, dysrhythmias often result.

Although the SA node, AV node, and His-Purkinje cells all possess the property of automaticity, only the SA node is the natural pacemaker of the heart because it spontaneously depolarizes the most frequently. The SA node has an intrinsic rate of 60 to 100 depolarizations or beats per minute; that of the AV node is 40 to 60 beats/min; and that of the ventricular Purkinje fibers is 40 or fewer beats/min. The action potentials and other properties in different areas of the heart are compared in Table 22-1.

As the pacemaker of the heart, the SA node, which is located near the top of the right atrium, generates the electrical impulse that ultimately produces the heartbeat. First, however, this impulse travels through the atria via specialized pathways called the **internodal pathways (Bachmann's bundle).** This causes contraction of atrial myocardial fibers, which creates the first heart sound. Next, the impulse reaches the AV node, which is located near the bottom of the right atrium. The AV node slows this very fast moving electrical impulse just long enough to allow the ventricles to fill with the blood that the contracting atria are just squeezing into them. If the AV node did not slow the impulse in

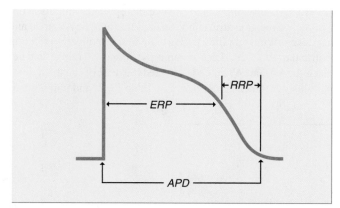

FIGURE 22-4 Aspects of an action potential. *APD,* Action potential duration; *ERP,* effective refractory period; *RRP,* relative refractory period.

Table 22-1	**Comparison of Action Potentials in Different Cardiac Tissue**			
Tissue	**Action Potential**	**Speed of Response**	**Threshold Potential (mV)**	**Conduction Velocity (m/sec)**
SA node	⋀	Slow	−60	Less than 0.05
Atrium	⋀	Fast	−90	1
AV node	⋀	Slow	−60	Less than 0.05
His-Purkinje system	⋀	Fast	−95	3
Ventricle	⋀	Fast	−90	1

AV, Atrioventricular; *SA,* sinoatrial.

this way, ventricular contraction would overlap that of the atria, which would result in a smaller volume of ejected ventricular blood and reduced cardiac output.

Next, the AV nodal cells generate an electrical impulse that passes into the *bundle of His* (or *His bundle*), a band of cardiac muscle fibers located between the right and left ventricles in what is called the *ventricular septum* (wall between the ventricles). The bundle of His distributes the impulse into both ventricles via the *right* and *left bundle branches*. Each branch terminates in the *Purkinje fibers* that are located in the myocardium of the ventricles. The stimulation of the Purkinje fibers causes ventricular contraction and ejection of blood from the ventricles. Blood from the right ventricle is pumped into the pulmonary circulation, whereas blood from the left ventricle is pumped into the systemic circulation to supply the rest of the body. The His bundle and Purkinje fibers are so named for the medical scientists who first identified them. Together, they are often referred to in the literature as the His-Purkinje system. Any abnormality in cardiac automaticity or impulse conduction often results in some type of dysrhythmia.

Electrocardiography

The electrophysiologic cardiac events described in detail earlier correspond more simply to the tracings of an electrocardiogram, abbreviated as ECG or EKG. EKG is still used more commonly in the United States, but it originates from a German spelling. Figure 22-5 illustrates the basic elements of a normal ECG tracing. The *P wave* corresponds to spontaneous impulse generation in the SA node followed immediately by depolarization of atrial myocardial fibers and their muscular contraction. This normally determines the heart rate and is affected by the balance between sympathetic and parasympathetic nervous system tone, the intrinsic automaticity of the SA nodal tissue, the mechanical stretch of atrial fibers due to incoming blood volume, and cardiac drugs. The *QRS complex* (or *QRS interval*) corresponds to depolarization and contraction of ventricular fibers. The *J point* marks the start of the *ST segment,* which corresponds to the beginning of ventricular repolarization. The *T wave* corresponds to completion of the

repolarization of these ventricular fibers. As an analogy, depolarization can be thought of as discharge or contraction of cardiac muscle fibers, whereas repolarization can be thought of as a relaxation of just-contracted muscle fibers to prepare for the next contraction (heartbeat). Note that the repolarization of the atrial fibers is obscured on the ECG tracing by the QRS complex and thus has no corresponding deflection in the tracing. The *U wave* is not always present, and its physiologic basis is uncertain. When it does occur, it is believed to arise from repolarization of Purkinje fibers or delayed repolarization of the ventricular cells that are among the last to depolarize earlier in the cycle of the heartbeat. The PR and QT intervals and the ST segment are parts of the ECG tracing that are often altered in recognizable ways by disease or by the adverse effects of certain types of drug therapy or drug interactions, as discussed in later sections of this chapter.

Common Dysrhythmias

A variety of cardiac dysrhythmias are recognized. Some are easier to treat than others using drug therapy and/or interventional cardiology procedures such as pacemakers, catheter ablation, cardioversion, and implantable cardioverters-defibrillators. These nonpharmacologic techniques are described in a later section of this chapter. Dysrhythmias are subdivided into several broad categories depending on their anatomical site of origin in the heart. *Supraventricular dysrhythmias* originate above the ventricles in the SA or AV node or atrial myocardium. *Ventricular dysrhythmias* originate below the AV node in the His-Purkinje system or ventricular myocardium. Dysrhythmias that originate outside the conduction system (i.e., in atrial or ventricular cells) are known as *ectopic,* and their specific points of origin are called *ectopic foci* (*foci* is the plural of the Latin word *focus*). *Conduction blocks* are dysrhythmias that involve disruption of impulse conduction between the atria and ventricles through the AV node and may also originate in the His-Purkinje system, directly affecting ventricular function. Less commonly, impulse conduction between the SA and AV node is affected. Several of the most common dysrhythmias are described in Table 22-2, and correspond-

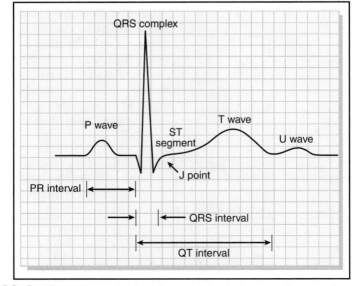

FIGURE 22-5 The waves and intervals of a normal electrocardiogram. (From Goldberger AL: *Clinical electrocardiography: a simplified approach,* ed 6, St Louis, 1999, Mosby.)

Table 22-2   Common Dysrhythmias

Dysrhythmia	Description	ECG Tracing
Supraventricular Dysrhythmias		
Atrial fibrillation (AF)	Rapid, ineffective atrial contractions	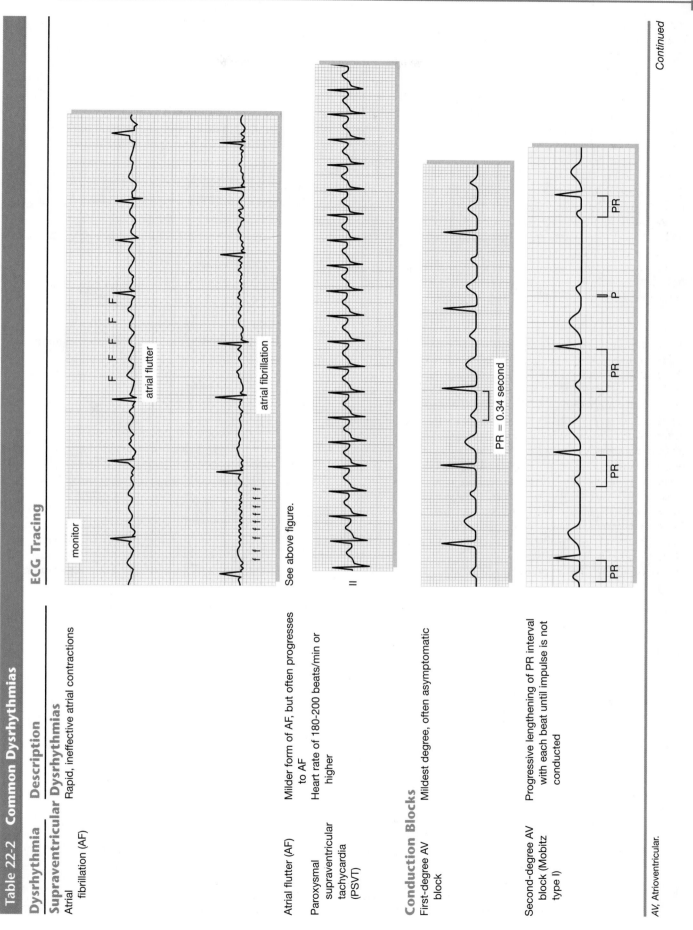
Atrial flutter (AF)	Milder form of AF, but often progresses to AF	
Paroxysmal supraventricular tachycardia (PSVT)	Heart rate of 180-200 beats/min or higher	See above figure.
Conduction Blocks		
First-degree AV block	Mildest degree, often asymptomatic	
Second-degree AV block (Mobitz type I)	Progressive lengthening of PR interval with each beat until impulse is not conducted	

AV, Atrioventricular.

Continued

Table 22-2 Common Dysrhythmias—cont'd

Dysrhythmia	Description	ECG Tracing
Second-degree AV block (Mobitz type II)	Similar to Mobitz type I, but more consistent in terms of number of failed impulses per unit of time	
Third-degree AV block (complete heart block)	No SA nodal impulses reach ventricles (but heartbeat often still occurs from ventricles' own automaticity—i.e., ectopic ventricular beats).	

Ventricular Dysrhythmias

Dysrhythmia	Description	ECG Tracing
Premature ventricular contractions (PVCs)	Contractions generated by impulses arising from ectopic foci within ventricular myocardium	
Nonsustained ventricular tachycardia (NSVT)	Relatively brief period (20 sec or less) in which ventricles contract rapidly on their own as well as in response to AV impulses	

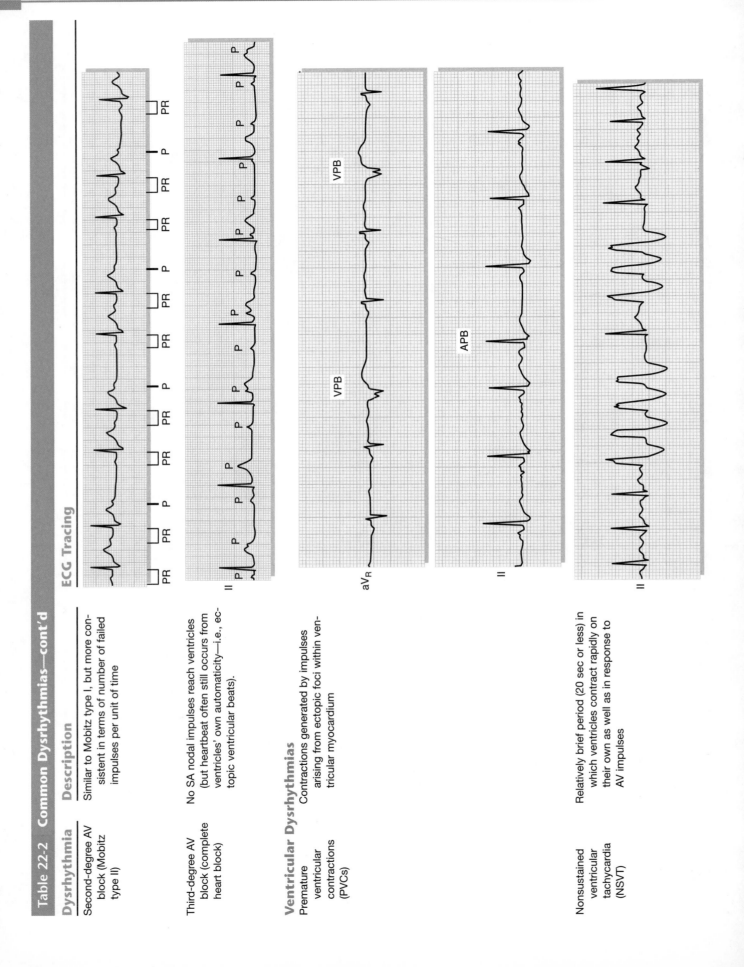

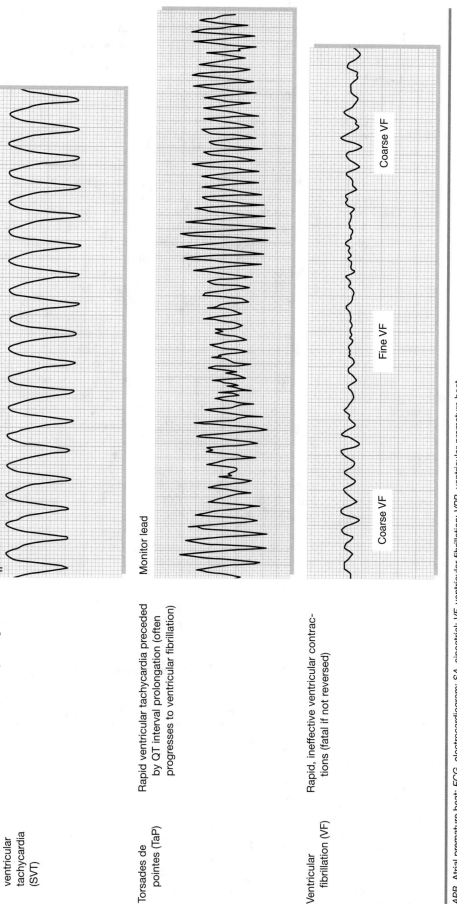

Sustained
ventricular
tachycardia
(SVT)

Same as above but more prolonged

Torsades de
pointes (TaP)

Rapid ventricular tachycardia preceded
by QT interval prolongation (often
progresses to ventricular fibrillation)

Monitor lead

Ventricular
fibrillation (VF)

Rapid, ineffective ventricular contractions (fatal if not reversed)

Coarse VF

Fine VF

Coarse VF

APB, Atrial premature beat; *ECG,* electrocardiogram; *SA,* sinoatrial; *VF,* ventricular fibrillation; *VPB,* ventricular premature beat.

ing ECG tracings are provided. They are also described further in the following text.

Among the supraventricular dysrhythmias, *atrial fibrillation* is a particularly common condition. It is characterized by rapid atrial contractions that only incompletely pump blood into the ventricles. Atrial fibrillation is notable in that it predisposes the patient to stroke. This is due to the fact that the blood tends to stagnate in the incompletely emptied atria and is therefore more likely to clot. If such blood clots manage to make their way into the left ventricle, they may be embolized to the brain and cause a stroke. Although there would theoretically be a similar risk for pulmonary embolism, this seems to be less of a clinical concern with atrial fibrillation than the risk of stroke. Patients with ongoing atrial fibrillation are often given anticoagulant therapy with warfarin to reduce the likelihood of stroke. *AV nodal reentrant tachycardia (AVNRT)* is a conduction disorder that often gives rise to a dysrhythmia known as *paroxysmal supraventricular tachycardia (PSVT)*. (The word *paroxysmal* means "sudden.") AVNRT occurs when electrical impulse transmission from the AV node into the His-Purkinje system of the ventricles is disrupted. As a result, some of the impulses circle backward *(retrograde impulses)* and reenter the atrial tissues to produce a tachycardic response. In Wolff-Parkinson-White (WPW) syndrome, ectopic impulses that begin near the AV node actually bypass the AV node and reach the His-Purkinje system before the normal AV-generated impulses. This is one cause of ventricular tachycardia, although it is technically supraventricular in origin. Varying degrees of *AV block* (often called *heart block*) involve varying levels of disrupted conduction of impulses from the AV node and His-Purkinje system to the ventricles. Although first-degree AV block is often asymptomatic, third-degree block or *complete heart block* often requires use of a cardiac pacemaker to ensure adequate ventricular function. There can also be blocks within the His-Purkinje system of the ventricles known as *bundle branch blocks. Premature ventricular contractions (PVCs)* occur when impulses originate from ectopic foci within the ventricles (His-Purkinje system). PVCs probably occur periodically in many people; they become problematic when they occur frequently enough to compromise systolic blood volume. *Ventricular tachycardia* refers to a rapid heartbeat from impulses originating in the ventricles. It can be nonsustained (brief) or sustained, requiring definitive treatment. Worsening ventricular tachycardia can deteriorate into *torsades de pointes*, an intermediate dysrhythmia that often further deteriorates into *ventricular fibrilla-*

tion. Ventricular fibrillation is fatal if not reversed, which most often requires electrical defibrillation. Interestingly, torsades de pointes often responds preferentially to intravenous magnesium sulfate.

ANTIDYSRHYTHMIC DRUGS

Numerous drugs are available to treat dysrhythmias. These drugs are categorized according to where and how they affect cardiac cells. Although other classifications are described in the literature, the most commonly used system for this purpose is still the **Vaughan Williams classification.** This system is based on the electrophysiologic effect of particular drugs on the action potential. This approach identifies four major classes of drugs: I (including Ia, Ib, and Ic), II , III, and IV. The various drugs in these four classes are listed in Table 22-3. The drug moricizine is somewhat unique in that it is classified simply as a class I drug, with properties of Ia, Ib, and Ic drugs. However, some references list it as class Ic. There is currently a gradual trend away from the use of class Ia drugs. The formerly available class Ic drug encainide was removed from the market after research indicated that the risk of fatal cardiac dysrhythmias associated with this drug overshadowed its dysrhythmia suppression effects. For similar reasons the other two class Ic drugs, flecainide and propafenone, are generally used in patients intolerant of other drugs. Nonetheless, several class I drugs of all types remain available in the United States as therapeutic options and so are included in this discussion. The class III drugs have emerged as among the most widely used antidysrhythmics at this time. The class IV drugs (calcium channel blockers) have limited usefulness in treating tachydysrhythmias (dysrhythmias involving tachycardia), unlike most of the other classes. The role of class II drugs (β-blockers) continues to grow in the field of cardiology, including in dysrhythmia management. Digoxin, the cardiac glycoside discussed in Chapter 21, still has a place in dysrhythmia management, especially in the prevention of dangerous ventricular tachydysrhythmias secondary to atrial fibrillation.

Mechanism of Action and Drug Effects

Antidysrhythmic drugs work by correcting, to varying degrees and by various mechanisms, abnormal cardiac electrophysiologic function. As membrane-stabilizing drugs, class I drugs exert their actions on the sodium (fast) channels. However, as already noted, there are some slight differences in the actions of the drugs in this

---

Table 22-3 Vaughan Williams Classification of Antidysrhythmic Drugs

Functional Class	Drugs
Class I: Membrane-stabilizing drugs; fast sodium channel blockers	moricizine
Ia: ↑ blockade of sodium channel, delay repolarization, ↑ APD	quinidine, disopyramide, procainamide
Ib: ↑ blockade of sodium channel, accelerate repolarization, ± APD	lidocaine, mexiletine, phenytoin
Ic: ↑ ↑ ↑ blockade of sodium channel, ± repolarization; also suppress reentry	flecainide, propafenone
Class II: β-blocking drugs	All β-blockers
Class III: Drugs whose principal effect on cardiac tissue is to ↑ APD	amiodarone, sotalol,* ibutilide, dofetilide
Class IV: Calcium channel blockers	verapamil, diltiazem
Other: Antidysrhythmic drugs that have the properties of several classes and therefore cannot be placed in one particular class	digoxin, adenosine

↑, Increase; ↓, decrease; ±, increase or decrease; *APD,* action potential duration.
*Sotalol also has Class II properties.

class, so that they are divided into three additional subclasses, with the previously noted exception of moricizine. These subclasses are Class Ia, Ib, and Ic drugs, and they depend on the magnitude of the effects of each drug on phase 0, the APD, and the ERP. Class Ia drugs (quinidine, procainamide, and disopyramide) block the sodium channels; more specifically, they delay repolarization and increase the APD. Class Ib drugs (mexiletine, phenytoin, and lidocaine) also block the sodium channels, but unlike class Ia drugs, they accelerate repolarization and decrease the APD. Phenytoin (Dilantin) is more commonly used as an anticonvulsant (Chapter 13) than as an antidysrhythmic drug. Tocainide, another drug in this class, has fallen out of use. Class Ic drugs (flecainide, propafenone) have a more pronounced effect on the blockade of sodium channels but have little effect on repolarization or the APD.

Class II drugs are the β-adrenergic blockers (β-blockers), and they are also commonly used as antianginal drugs (Chapter 23) and as antihypertensives (Chapters 18 and 24). They work by reducing or blocking sympathetic nervous system stimulation to the heart and, as a result, the transmission of impulses in the heart's conduction system. This results in depression of phase 4

depolarization. These drugs mostly affect slower-conducting cardiac tissues.

Class III drugs (amiodarone, sotalol, ibutilide, and dofetilide) increase the APD by prolonging repolarization in phase 3. They affect fast tissue and are most commonly used to manage dysrhythmias that are difficult to treat. Sotalol actually has properties of both Class II and Class III and is often listed as a member of one or the other class, depending on the specific reference used.

Class IV drugs are the calcium channel blockers, which, like β-blockers, are also used as both antianginal drugs (Chapter 23) and antihypertensives (Chapter 24). As their name implies, they work specifically by inhibiting the calcium channels, reducing the influx of calcium ions during action potentials. This results in depression of phase 4 depolarization. Diltiazem and verapamil are the calcium channel blockers most commonly used to treat cardiac dysrhythmias.

The mechanisms of action of the major classes of antidysrhythmics are summarized in Table 22-4. The effects of the various classes of drugs are presented in Box 22-1.

Table 22-4   Antidysrhythmic Drugs: Mechanisms of Action

	Vaughan Williams Class			
	I	**II**	**III**	**IV**
Action	Blocks sodium channels, affects phase 0	Decreases spontaneous depolarization, affects phase 4	Prolongs APD	Blocks slow calcium channels
Tissue	Fast	Slow	Fast	Slow
Effect on action potential	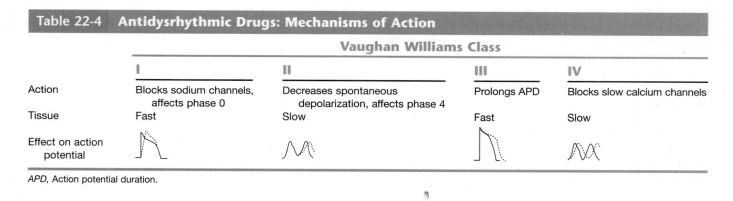			

APD, Action potential duration.

Box 22-1   Effects of Antidysrhythmic Drugs

Class I (moricizine)
- Prolong AV nodal conduction velocity
- Prolong bundle of His and Purkinje cell conduction velocity
- Prolong the PR and QRS complex intervals of the ECG
- Eliminate or reduces ectopic foci stimulation
- Have minimal effect on the SA node and automaticity

Class Ia (disopyramide, procainamide, quinidine)
- Depress myocardial excitability
- Prolong the ERP
- Eliminate or reduce ectopic foci stimulation
- Decrease inotropic effect
- Have anticholinergic (vagolytic) activity

Class Ib (lidocaine, mexiletine, phenytoin)
- Decrease myocardial excitability in the ventricles
- Eliminate or reduce ectopic foci stimulation in the ventricles
- Have minimal effect on the SA node and automaticity
- Have minimal effect on the AV node and conduction
- Have minimal anticholinergic (vagolytic) activity

Class Ic (flecainide, propafenone)
- Produce dose-related depression of cardiac conduction, especially in the bundle of His–Purkinje system

- Have minimal effect on atrial conduction
- Eliminate or reduce ectopic foci stimulation in the ventricles
- Have minimal anticholinergic (vagolytic) activity
- Flecainide use now reserved for the most serious dysrhythmias

Class II (β-blockers [e.g., atenolol, esmolol, metoprolol])
- Block β-adrenergic cardiac stimulation
- Reduce SA nodal activity
- Eliminate or reduce atrial ectopic foci stimulation
- Reduce ventricular contraction rate
- Reduce cardiac output and blood pressure

Class III (amiodarone, sotalol*, ibutilide, dofetilide)
- Prolong the ERP
- Prolong the myocardial action potential
- Block both α- and β-adrenergic cardiac stimulation

Class IV (diltiazem, verapamil)
- Prolong AV nodal ERP
- Reduce AV nodal conduction
- Reduce rapid ventricular conduction caused by atrial flutter

AV, Atrioventricular; *ECG*, electrocardiogram; *ERP*, effective refractory period; *SA*, sinoatrial.
*Sotalol also has Class II properties.

Indications

Antidysrhythmic drugs are effective in treating a variety of cardiac dysrhythmias. The antidysrhythmic drugs and the most common indications for their use are listed in Table 22-5.

Contraindications

Contraindications to the use of antidysrhythmic drugs include known drug allergy to a specific product and may include second- or third-degree AV block, bundle branch block, cardiogenic shock, sick sinus syndrome, and any other major ECG changes depending on the clinical judgment of a cardiologist. The reason for these concerns is that all antidysrhythmic drugs are potentially dysrhythmogenic themselves and can therefore worsen existing dysrhythmias. The risk of such an effect is greater in patients with structural heart damage (e.g., after MI). In particular, with AV block and bundle branch block, there is a danger of drug-induced ventricular failure if a given drug should further compromise already existing AV conduction delays. The safe prescribing of antidysrhythmic drugs is an area that requires especially strong clinical expertise and careful judgment on a case-by-case basis.

Adverse Effects

Adverse effects common to most antidysrhythmics include hypersensitivity reactions, nausea, vomiting, and diarrhea. Other common effects include dizziness, headache, and blurred vision. In addition, many antidysrhythmics are themselves capable of producing new dysrhythmias (*prodysrhythmic effect*). In addition, as with any drug class, there are also cases of unpredictable or *idiosyncratic* adverse effects that are not related to drug concentration in the body. The belief is that such effects will eventually be explained by genetic variations. Table 22-6 summarizes the most commonly reported adverse effects by specific drug. Effects that pertain specifically to the ECG tracing are summarized in Table 22-7.

Toxicity and Management of Overdose

The main toxic effects of the antidysrhythmics involve the heart, circulation, and central nervous system (CNS). Specific antidotes are not available, and the management of an overdose involves maintaining adequate circulation and respiration using general support measures and providing any required symptomatic treatment (Table 22-8).

Interactions

Antidysrhythmics can interact with many different categories of drugs. The most serious drug interactions are the ones that can result in dysrhythmias, hypotension or hypertension, respiratory distress, or any excessive therapeutic or toxic drug effects. Drug interactions occur when the presence of one drug strengthens or weakens the pharmacologic effects of another. This is most commonly seen when the first drug affects the activity of the enzymes that metabolize the second drug, either speeding or slowing its elimination. One particular interaction common to many antidysrhythmics is the potentiation of anticoagulant activity with warfarin (Coumadin). Because many patients receiving antidysrhythmic therapy also need warfarin, prothrombin time and international normalized ratio should be monitored appropriately and necessary adjustments made to the warfarin dosage. Other common interactions are summarized in Table 22-9. To explain the mechanism for each interaction is beyond the scope of this text. Readers needing more detailed information are encouraged to consult other appropriate references.

Table 22-5	Antidysrhythmic Drugs: Indication
Drug Class	**Indications**
Class Ia disopyramide procainamide quinidine	Atrial fibrillation, premature atrial contractions, premature ventricular contractions, ventricular tachycardia, Wolff-Parkinson-White syndrome
Class Ib lidocaine mexiletine phenytoin	Ventricular dysrhythmias only (premature ventricular contractions, ventricular tachycardia, ventricular fibrillation) Atrial and ventricular tachydysrhythmias caused by digitalis toxicity; long QT syndrome
Class Ic flecainide propafenone	Severe ventricular tachycardia and supraventricular tachycardia dysrhythmias, atrial fibrillation and flutter, Wolff-Parkinson-White syndrome
Class I moricizine	Symptomatic ventricular and life-threatening dysrhythmias
Class II β-blockers atenolol esmolol metoprolol propranolol	Both supraventricular and ventricular dysrhythmias (act as general myocardial depressants)
Class III amiodarone dofetilide ibutilide sotalol*	Life-threatening ventricular tachycardia or fibrillation Atrial fibrillation or flutter resistant to other drug therapy Same as amiodarone
Class IV CCBs diltiazem verapamil	Paroxysmal supraventricular tachycardia; rate control for atrial fibrillation and flutter

CCBs, Calcium channel blockers.
*Sotalol also has Class II properties.

Drug Profiles

Because the four classes of antidysrhythmics produce a variety of effects on the action potential of the cardiac cell, they exert a major influence on cardiac electrophysiologic function. The diversity of therapeutic effects and the attendant adverse effects pose a special challenge to the nurse, who is responsible for ensuring the safe and efficacious use of these drugs. Because the aspects of the nursing process that relate to the administration of these drugs differs for each of the four classes of drug, each group is discussed separately. Dosage and other information appears in the Dosages table on page 344.

Class Ia Drugs

Class Ia drugs are considered membrane-stabilizing drugs because they possess local anesthetic properties. They stabilize the membrane and have depressant effects on phase 0 of the action potential. These drugs include procainamide, quinidine, and disopyramide.

Table 22-6   Common Adverse Effects of Various Antidysrhythmic Drugs

Drug	Adverse Effects
amiodarone, diltiazem, disopyramide, dofetilide, flecainide, ibutilide, lidocaine, mexiletine, propafenone, quinidine (note that almost any drug can cause GI adverse effects)	Gastrointestinal effects, including one or more of the following (specific adverse effects may vary with drug): nausea, vomiting, diarrhea, abdominal pain, anorexia, constipation, weight gain, flatulence, bloating, taste disturbance
amiodarone, digoxin, disopyramide, dofetilide, flecainide, ibutilide, lidocaine, mexiletine, moricizine, phenytoin, procainamide, propafenone, quinidine	Central nervous system effects, including one or more of the following (specific adverse effects may vary with drug): tinnitus, hearing loss, visual disturbances, confusion, delirium, psychosis, giddiness, hallucinations, depression, dizziness, paresthesias, stupor, coma, seizures, fatigue, headache, tremor, anxiety, gait disturbance, somnolence (sleepiness), insomnia
quinidine (especially when taken with anticoagulants)	Bleeding
amiodarone, β-blockers, quinidine (secondary to antibodies to drug-platelet complexes)	Thrombocytopenia or other coagulation abnormalities
β-blockers, procainamide	Agranulocytosis
procainamide (especially in slow acetylators) and quinidine	Drug-induced lupuslike syndrome (idiosyncratic): arthralgia, fever, pleuropericarditis, hepatomegaly, positive result on antinuclear antibody test
β-blockers, disopyramide, flecainide, mexiletine, procainamide, propafenone	Muscular pain or weakness
procainamide	Raynaud's disease (idiopathic peripheral vascular compromise)
adenosine, β-blockers, flecainide, mexiletine	Chest pressure or pain
amiodarone, dofetilide, flecainide, ibutilide, moricizine, phenytoin, propafenone, sotalol, verapamil	Prodysrhythmic effects (see also Table 22-7)
lidocaine, procainamide	Elevated defibrillatory threshold
Lidocaine	Arterial spasms
amiodarone, phenytoin	Venous irritation, thrombophlebitis
amiodarone, β-blockers, moricizine	Heart failure
amiodarone, β-blockers, disopyramide, procainamide, verapamil	Hypotension
amiodarone, diltiazem	Edema
adenosine, amiodarone	Flushing
adenosine, amiodarone, β-blockers, disopyramide, flecainide, lidocaine, mexiletine, moricizine	Dyspnea
Amiodarone	Pulmonary toxicity (hypersensitivity pneumonitis, pulmonary fibrosis)
Quinidine	Fever
β-blockers, disopyramide, flecainide, lidocaine, mexiletine, procainamide, propafenone, quinidine	Rash, pruritus (itching)
β-blockers	Urticaria and other more serious dermatologic reactions (e.g., Stevens Johnson syndrome, toxic epidermal necrolysis)
amiodarone	Photosensitivity
amiodarone	Skin discoloration (blue-gray skin)
quinidine	Hemolytic anemia
disopyramide	Hypokalemia
β-blockers	Hyperkalemia
β-blockers, disopyramide	Elevated cholesterol, triglyceride levels
β-blockers	Hypoglycemia
β-blockers	Hyperglycemia
amiodarone	Hypothyroidism
amiodarone	Hyperthyroidism
amiodarone	Liver enzyme elevations or hepatitis
amiodarone, moricizine	Decreased libido

procainamide

The electrophysiologic effect of procainamide (Pronestyl, Procanbid, Procan SR) is similar to that of quinidine, but it differs from quinidine in that its indirect effect (anticholinergic action) is weaker. Procainamide is useful in the management of atrial and ventricular tachydysrhythmias. It is reported to be more effective in the treatment of ventricular disturbances, especially in suppressing premature ventricular contractions and preventing the recurrence of ventricular tachycardia. The intravenous form of procainamide is generally preferred over the intravenous form of quinidine. Procainamide is chemically related to the local anesthetic procaine. Significant adverse effects of the drug include ventricular dysrhythmias and blood disorders. It can cause a lupus erythematosus–like syndrome, which occurs in about 30% of patients on long-term therapy. It can also cause gastrointestinal effects such as nausea, vomiting, and diarrhea, but these are less intense than those produced by quinidine. Other adverse effects include fever, leukopenia, maculopapular rash, urticaria, pruritus, flushing, and torsades de pointes resulting from prolongation of the QT interval.

Use of procainamide is contraindicated in patients who have shown hypersensitivity reactions to it and in those with complete heart block, lupus erythematosus, and second- or third-degree heart block. It is available in both oral and injectable form.

Table 22-7   Common Electrocardiographic Effects of Various Antidysrhythmic Drugs

Drug	Effect
digoxin, verapamil	Asystole
amiodarone, β-blockers, digoxin, diltiazem, lidocaine, phenytoin, propafenone, verapamil	Bradycardia
amiodarone, β-blockers, disopyramide, lidocaine, quinidine, verapamil	SA nodal disturbance or depression
adenosine, propafenone	Atrial fibrillation
Digoxin	Supraventricular (atrial) tachycardia
amiodarone, β-blockers, diltiazem, disopyramide, lidocaine, propafenone, quinidine, verapamil	AV nodal disturbance or block
disopyramide, dofetilide, ibutilide, procainamide, propafenone, quinidine	Prolonged QRS or QT interval
amiodarone, β-blockers, lidocaine, propafenone	His-Purkinje block (bundle branch block)
amiodarone, digoxin, disopyramide, dofetilide, ibutilide, lidocaine, procainamide, propafenone, quinidine, sotalol	Ventricular tachycardia (with lidocaine, often occurs in association with supraventricular tachycardia; with sotalol, often occurs secondary to torsades de pointes)
disopyramide, dofetilide, ibutilide, quinidine, procainamide, sotalol	Torsades de pointes
mexiletine, propafenone	Premature ventricular contractions

Table 22-8   Selected Antidysrhythmic Drugs: Management of Overdose

Drug	Toxic Effect	Management
acebutolol	Bradycardia	1-3 mg IV atropine divided
	Bronchospasm	β₂-adrenergic or theophylline
	Cardiac failure	Digitalization
	Hypotension	Vasopressor
		Glucagon
adenosine	Usually self-limiting due to a very short half-life	Competitive antagonists caffeine or theophylline
amiodarone	Bradycardia	β-adrenergic drug
	Hypotension	Positive inotropic drug or vasopressor
digoxin	Decreased clearance due to drug interactions with other antidysrhythmic drugs (e.g., quinidine, verapamil, amiodarone)	See Chapter 21 for more information
disopyramide	Loss of consciousness, cardiac and respiratory arrest	Neostigmine for anticholinergic effects, emesis induction, activated charcoal, and hemodialysis
esmolol	Same as for acebutolol	Same as for acebutolol
flecainide	Reduced heart rate	Dopamine or dobutamine; acidify very alkaline urine
lidocaine	Convulsions	Diazepam or thiopental
mexiletine	Bradycardia, hypotension	Atropine; acidify urine to promote excretion
moricizine	Hypotension, heart failure, myocardial infarction	Gastric evacuation and advanced life support measures
phenytoin	Circulatory and respiratory arrest, convulsions	Life support measures when required
procainamide	Cardiac depression	IV pressor drugs and supportive measures
	Convulsions	Diazepam and mechanically assisted respiration
propafenone	Same as for acebutolol	Same as for acebutolol
propranolol	Cardiac dysrhythmias	Sodium lactate (reduces toxicity except in alkalosis); lidocaine
quinidine	Same as for acebutolol	Same as for acebutolol
sotalol	Convulsions	Diazepam or short-acting barbiturate
verapamil	Cardiac failure	Dopamine or dobutamine
	Conduction problems	Cardiac pacing
	Hypotension	Vasopressors, 10% calcium chloride solution

IV, Intravenous.

Pharmacokinetics

Half-Life	Onset	Peak	Duration
IV/IM: 3 hr	IV/IM: 10-30 min	IV/IM: 10-60 min	IV/IM: 3 hr
PO: 3 hr	PO: 0.5-1 hr	PO: 1-2 hr	PO: 3 hr (8 hr for extended-release dosage form)

quinidine

Quinidine (Quinidex, Cardioquin, Quinaglute, Dura-Tab) has both a direct action on the electrical activity of the heart and an indirect (anticholinergic) effect. Its anticholinergic action results in inhibition of the parasympathetic nervous system and allows sympathetic nervous system (SNS) activity to go unopposed. This accelerates the rate of electrical impulse formation and conduction. Significant adverse effects of the drug include cardiac asystole and ventricular ectopic beats. Like other cinchona alkaloids and the salicylates, quinidine can cause

Table 22-9   Common Drug Interactions for Selected Antidysrhythmic Drugs

Antidysrhythmic Drug	Interacting Drugs	Effects
quinidine	Other antidysrhythmics, antacids, cimetidine, verapamil, anticholinergics, digoxin, anticoagulants, β-blockers, tricyclic antidepressants	Enhanced quinidine activity*
quinidine	Barbiturates, cholinergics, rifampin, disopyramide, phenytoin, nifedipine	Reduced quinidine activity
procainamide	Other antidysrhythmics, anticholinergics, quinidine, cimetidine, ranitidine, quinolone antibiotics, antipsychotics, trimethoprim	Enhanced procainamide activity
disopyramide	Other antidysrhythmics, digoxin (possibly beneficial) macrolide antibiotics, quinolone antibiotics, antipsychotics	Enhanced disopyramide activity
disopyramide	phenytoin, rifampin,	Reduced disopyramide activity
lidocaine	Other antidysrhythmics, cimetidine	Enhanced lidocaine activity
flecainide	Other antidysrhythmics	Enhanced flecainide activity
propafenone	Other antidysrhythmics, cimetidine, quinidine, serotonin-selective reuptake inhibitors (SSRIs) (e.g., fluoxetine)	Enhanced propafenone activity
propafenone	rifampin	Reduced propafenone activity
propafenone	cyclosporine, digoxin, theophylline	Possible toxicity of these drugs
β-blockers	Other antidysrhythmics, cimetidine, clonidine, epinephrine, ergot alkaloids, oral contraceptives, diphenhydramine, haloperidol, hydralazine, hydroxychloroquine, loop diuretics	Enhanced β-blocker activity
β-blockers	Antacids, cholestyramine, ampicillin, rifampin, nonsteroidal antiinflammatory drugs (e.g., ibuprofen), phenothiazines (e.g., promethazine, quinolone antibiotics, salicylates, thyroid hormones	Reduced β-blocker activity
β-blockers	haloperidol, benzodiazepines, ergot alkaloids, gabapentin	Possible toxicity of these drugs
β-blockers	Sulfonylureas	Reduced hypoglycemic effect of these drugs
amiodarone	Other antidysrhythmics, cimetidine, quinolone antibiotics, SSRIs, ritonavir	Enhanced amiodarone activity
amiodarone	phenytoin, cholestyramine, rifampin	Reduced amiodarone activity
amiodarone	cyclosporine, digoxin, fentanyl, phenytoin, methotrexate, theophylline	Possible toxicity of these drugs
dofetilide, ibutilide	Other antidysrhythmics, cimetidine, amiloride, ketoconazole, trimethoprim-sulfamethoxazole, metformin, megestrol, prochlorperazine, triamterene, verapamil	Enhanced dofetilide or ibutilide activity
dofetilide, ibutilide	Potassium-wasting diuretics (i.e., thiazides, loop diuretics)	Hypokalemia, hypomagnesemia
calcium channel blockers (verapamil or diltiazem)	Other antidysrhythmics, cimetidine, ranitidine	Enhanced calcium channel blocker activity
calcium channel blockers (verapamil or diltiazem)	phenytoin, rifampin	Reduced calcium channel blocker activity
calcium channel blockers (verapamil or diltiazem)	Anesthetics, doxorubicin, benzodiazepines, buspirone, carbamazepine, digoxin, statins, steroids, tacrolimus, sirolimus, theophylline, vincristine	Possible toxicity of these drugs

*Note that enhanced activity of any antidysrhythmic drug may reach the level of drug toxicity, including potentially fatal cardiac dysrhythmias.

cinchonism. Symptoms of mild cinchonism include tinnitus, loss of hearing, slight blurring of vision, and GI upset. Contraindications to the use of the drug include hypersensitivity to it, thrombocytopenic purpura resulting from previous therapy, AV block, intraventricular conduction defects, and abnormal rhythms (prodysrhythmic effects such as torsades de pointes). Quinidine is available in both oral and parenteral (injectable) forms and in three different salt forms. The oral preparations include sulfate and gluconate salts.

Pharmacokinetics

Half-Life	Onset	Peak	Duration
PO: 6-7 hr	PO: 1-3 hr	PO: 0.5-6 hr	PO: 6-8 hr* (12 hr for sustained-release dosage form)

Class Ib Drugs

Class Ib drugs share many characteristics with class Ia drugs but are grouped together because they act preferentially on ischemic myocardial tissue. They have little effect on conduction velocity in normal tissue. Class Ib drugs have a weak depressive effect on phase 0 depolarization, the APD, and the ERP. They include lidocaine, mexiletine, and phenytoin.

▶ lidocaine

Lidocaine (Xylocaine) is the prototypical Ib drug. It is one of the most effective drugs for the treatment of ventricular dysrhythmias, but it can only be administered intravenously because it has an extensive first-pass effect (i.e., when it is taken orally, the liver metabolizes most of it to inactive metabolites). Because of its extensive hepatic metabolism, dosage reduction by 50% is recommended for patients in frank liver failure or cirrhosis. Dosage reductions may also be necessary in patients with renal impairment because of extensive excretion of the drug and its metabolites by the kidney.

Lidocaine exerts its effects on the conduction system of the heart by making it difficult for the ventricles to develop a dysrhythmia, an action known as *raising the ventricular fibrillation threshold*. It does this by decreasing the sensitivity of the cardiac cell membrane to

DOSAGES

Selected Antidysrhythmic Drugs

Drug Name (Pregnancy Category)	Pharmacologic Class	Usual Dosage Range	Indications
adenosine (Adenocard) (C)	Unclassified antidysrhythmic	**Adult** IV: 6-mg bolus over 1-2 sec; second rapid bolus of 12 mg as needed, which may be repeated a second time as needed	Supraventricular tachycardia, absence of normal sinus rhythm
▸amiodarone (Cordarone) (D)	Class III antidysrhythmic	**Adult** IV: 150 mg over 10 min, then 60 mg/hr for 6 hr, then 30 mg/hr as maintenance dose PO: 800-1600 mg/day for 1-3 wk, reduced to 600-800 mg/day for 5 wk; usual maintenance dose 400 mg/day PO: 200-400 mg/day	Ventricular dysrhythmias Atrial dysrhythmias
▸atenolol (Tenormin) (D)	β₁-blocker (class II antidysrhythmic)	**Adult** IV: 5 mg over 5 min followed by 5 mg over 10 min followed by 50 mg PO 10 min after last IV injection and another 50 mg PO 12 hr later, then 100 mg/day PO for a further 6-9 days PO (maintenance): 12.5 to 100 mg once daily	Acute MI
▸diltiazem (Cardizem)	Calcium channel blocker	**Adult** IV: Bolus dose 0.25 mg/kg over 2 min, second dose 0.35 mg/kg over 2 min after 15 min as needed, then 5-10 mg/hr or higher by continuous infusion	Supraventricular dysrhythmias
disopyramide (Norpace, Norpace CR)	Class Ia antidysrhythmic	**Adult** PO: 150 mg q6h; CR: 300 mg q12h with daily range of 400-800 mg divided	Ventricular dysrhythmias
esmolol (Brevibloc) (D)	β₁-blocker (class II antidysrhythmic)	**Adult** IV: Bolus dose of 500 mcg/kg/min followed by 4 min of 50 mcg/kg/min and evaluate	Supraventricular tachydysrhythmias
flecainide (Tambocor) (C)	Class Ic antidysrhythmic	**Adult** PO: 50 mg q12h, can be increased by 50 mg bid q4d until desired effect with daily max of 300 mg for PSVT 100 mg q12h with increment of 50 mg bid q4d as needed; usual dose 150 mg q12h with daily max of 400 mg	Paroxysmal supraventricular tachycardia–paroxysmal atrial flutter or fibrillation Sustained ventricular tachycardia
ibutilide (Corvert) (C)	Class III antidysrhythmic	**Adult** IV: 1-mg infusion over 10 min (if less than 60 kg, then 0.1 mL/kg)	Atrial fibrillation or flutter
▸lidocaine (Xylocaine) (B)	Class Ib antidysrhythmic	**Pediatric** IV: Suggested bolus dose, 1 mg/kg; usual maintenance infusion rate, 20-50 mcg/kg/min **Adult** IV: Bolus dose 50-100 mg; may be repeated in 5 min; do not exceed 200-300 mg over 1 hr; usual maintenance infusion rate 1-4 mg/min	Ventricular dysrhythmias Ventricular dysrhythmias
▸metoprolol (Lopressor) (D)	β₁-blocker	**Adult** IV/PO: 3 bolus injections of 5 mg at 2-min intervals followed by 50 mg PO q6h for 48 hr, thereafter 10 mg bid PO: 12.5-100 mg bid	Early MI Late MI
mexiletine (Mexitil) (C)	Class Ib antidysrhythmic	**Adult** PO: 200-300 mg q8h	Ventricular dysrhythmias
procainamide (Pronestyl, Pronestyl-SR, Procan SR, Procanbid) (C)	Class Ia antidysrhythmic	**Adult** PO: 250-500 mg q3-6h; SR: 0.5-1 g q6h; or Procanbid: 0.5-1 g q12h (alternate PO dose) IM: 0.5-1 g q4-8h until oral therapy possible IV: 100-200 mg q5min up to 1000 mg with a maintenance infusion of 1-4 mg/min	Atrial dysrhythmias, ventricular dysrhythmias Dysrhythmias during surgery Need for rapid dysrhythmia control

CR, Controlled (or continuous) release; *IV,* intravenous; *MI,* myocardial infarction; *PO,* oral; *PSVT,* paroxysmal supraventricular tachycardia.

DOSAGES

Selected Antidysrhythmic Drugs—cont'd

Drug Name (Pregnancy Category)	Pharmacologic Class	Usual Dosage Range	Indications
propafenone (Rythmol) (C)	Class Ic antidysrhythmic	**Adult** PO: Start with 150 mg q8h and increase q3-4d; usual range, 450-900 mg/day divided	Ventricular dysrhythmias
▸ propranolol (Inderal) (D)	β-blocker (class II antidysrhythmic)	**Adult** IV: 1-3 mg; if needed, repeated in 2 min and additional doses as needed q4h or longer; switch to PO as soon as possible PO: 10-30 mg q6-8h PO: 80-320 mg/day divided bid-qid	Serious dysrhythmias Angina
quinidine (Quinidex [sulfate], Cardioquin [polygalacturonate], Quinaglute, Dura-Tab [gluconate]) (C)	Class Ia antidysrhythmic	**Adult** *Gluconate* PO: 324-972 mg q8-12h IM: 600 mg followed by 400 mg q2-6h or more if needed IV: 200-750 mg infused at up to 10 mg/min *Sulfate* PO: 200-mg load; 100-600 mg q4-6h 200-300 mg tid-qid	Atrial dysrhythmias Ventricular dysrhythmias Ventricular dysrhythmias Atrial dysrhythmias Atrial fibrillation Atrial dysrhythmias
▸ sotalol (Betapace) (B)	Class II antidysrhythmic	**Adult** PO: 160-320 mg/day divided into 2-3 doses	Life-threatening dysrhythmias
▸ verapamil (Calan, Isoptin, Verelan) (C)	Calcium channel blocker (class IV antidysrhythmic)	**Pediatric** IV: 1 yr or younger: 0.1-0.2 mg/kg bolus over 2 min; repeat dose after 30 min IV: 1-15 yr: 0.1-0.3 mg/kg bolus over 2 min; do not exceed 5-mg dose; repeat dose not exceeding 10 mg may be given after 30 min **Adult** PO: Start with 80 mg tid-qid; daily range 240-480 mg IV: 2.5-5 mg bolus over 2 min; repeat dose of 5-10 mg may be given after 30 min	Supraventricular tachydysrhythmias

IM, Intramuscular; *SR,* sustained release.

impulses and decreasing the cell's ability to depolarize on its own (decreasing automaticity). Many of these effects are accomplished by blockade of fast sodium channels.

Lidocaine is the drug of choice for treating the acute ventricular dysrhythmias associated with MI. Significant adverse effects include CNS toxicities such as twitching, convulsions, and confusion; respiratory depression or arrest; and the cardiovascular effects of hypotension, bradycardia, and dysrhythmias. Use of the drug is contraindicated in patients who are hypersensitive to it, who have severe SA or AV intraventricular block, or who have Stokes-Adams or Wolff-Parkinson-White syndrome. Lidocaine is available only in parenteral form for intramuscular or intravenous administration. Intramuscular administration is recommended only in extenuating circumstances, such as when the patient is symptomatic and no intravenous or ECG equipment is available.

Pharmacokinetics

Half-Life	Onset	Peak	Duration
IV/IM: 8 min, 1-2 hr (terminal)	IV/IM: 2-15 min	IV/IM: 5-10 min	IV/IM: 20 min-1.5 hr

mexiletine

Mexiletine (Mexitil) is structurally and pharmacologically similar to lidocaine, and its effects on the conduction system of the heart are also very similar. A response to parenteral lidocaine does not predict

a response to mexiletine. Mexiletine effectively suppresses PVCs in patients experiencing an acute MI, chronic coronary artery disease, or digitalis toxicity and in those undergoing cardiac surgery. It has proved particularly useful when taken in combination with selected class Ia or Ic drugs or with β-blockers.

The most frequent adverse effects are nausea, vomiting, dizziness, and tremor. These reactions are usually not serious, however, and are dose related and minimized by taking the drug with food or an antacid. Contraindications to its use include hypersensitivity, cardiogenic shock, and second- or third-degree AV block. This drug is available only for oral use.

Pharmacokinetics

Half-Life	Onset	Peak	Duration
PO: 12 hr	PO: 0.5-2 hr	PO: 2-3 hr	PO: Unknown

Class Ic Drugs

Class Ic drugs (flecainide, propafenone) have a more pronounced effect on sodium channel blockade than class Ia and Ib drugs but have little effect on repolarization or the APD. These drugs significantly slow conduction in the atria, AV node, and ventricles. Because of their marked effect on conduction, these drugs strongly suppress PVCs, reducing or eliminating them in a large number of patients.

flecainide

Flecainide (Tambocor) is a chemical analogue of procainamide. A large, multicenter, double-blind, placebo-controlled study called the **Cardiac Arrhythmia Suppression Trial (CAST)** was conducted by the National Heart, Lung, and Blood Institute to determine whether the incidence of **sudden cardiac death** could be reduced in post-MI patients with asymptomatic non–life-threatening ectopy through the use of flecainide. The findings showed that the excessive mortality and nonfatal cardiac arrest rates in patients treated with this drug were actually comparable to or higher than those seen in patients who received the placebo. Because of these findings, the U.S. Food and Drug Administration (FDA) required that the labeling of flecainide be revised to indicate that its use should be limited to the treatment of documented life-threatening ventricular dysrhythmias such as sustained ventricular tachycardia. Treatment with this drug should be initiated in the hospital. This drug is not indicated for the management of less severe dysrhythmias such as nonsustained ventricular tachycardia or frequent PVCs.

Although flecainide is better tolerated than quinidine or procainamide and is more effective than mexiletine, it is also more prodysrhythmic. It is this prodysrhythmic potential that limits its use to the management of life-threatening dysrhythmias. Flecainide has a negative inotropic effect and depresses left ventricular function. Less serious but more common noncardiac adverse effects include dizziness, visual disturbances, and dyspnea. Contraindications to its use include hypersensitivity, cardiogenic shock, second- or third-degree AV block, and non–life-threatening dysrhythmias. It is available only for oral use.

Pharmacokinetics

Half-Life	Onset	Peak	Duration
Unknown	3 hr	Unknown	12-27 hr

propafenone

Propafenone (Rythmol) is similar in action to flecainide. It reduces the fast inward sodium current in Purkinje fibers and to a lesser extent in myocardial fibers. Unlike other class I drugs, propafenone has mild β-blocking effects. This may contribute to its overall effects on the conduction system. It is also believed to have calcium channel blocking effects, which may contribute to its mild negative inotropic effects.

Until recently, propafenone's use was limited to the treatment of documented life-threatening ventricular dysrhythmias such as sustained ventricular tachycardia. Recent findings suggest that at low dosages it has benefit in the treatment of atrial fibrillation as well. Treatment should also be started while the patient is in the hospital. Unlike flecainide, however, propafenone can be given to patients with depressed left ventricular function. It may be a better antidysrhythmic drug than disopyramide, procainamide, and quinidine in these patients. However, it should be used with caution in patients with heart failure, because it has some β-blocking properties and dose-dependent negative inotropic effects.

Propafenone is generally well tolerated. The most commonly reported adverse reaction is dizziness. Patients may also complain of a metallic taste, constipation, and headache, along with nausea and vomiting. These GI adverse effects may be reduced by taking propafenone with food. Propafenone use is contraindicated in patients with a known hypersensitivity to it and in those with bradycardia, bronchial asthma, significant hypotension, uncontrolled heart failure, cardiogenic shock, a various conduction disorders. It is available only for oral use.

Pharmacokinetics

Half-Life	Onset	Peak	Duration
2-10 hr	Unknown	3-5 hr	Unknown

Class II Drugs

Class II antidysrhythmics are also known as *β-blockers*. These drugs work by reducing or blocking SNS stimulation to the heart and the heart's conduction system. By doing this, β-blockers prevent catecholamine-mediated actions on the heart. This is known as a *cardioprotective* quality of beta-blockers. The resulting cardiovascular effects include a reduced heart rate, delayed AV node conduction, reduced myocardial contractility, and decreased myocardial automaticity. The pharmacologically induced effects of the β-blockers are especially beneficial after an MI because of the many catecholamines released at this time, which make the heart hyperirritable and predisposed to many types of dysrhythmias. The β-blockers offer protection from these potentially very dangerous complications. Several studies have demonstrated a significant reduction (on the average of 25%) in the incidence of sudden cardiac death after MI in patients treated with β-blockers on an ongoing basis.

Although there are several β-blockers, only a handful are commonly used as antidysrhythmic drugs. The only ones that are currently approved by the FDA for this purpose are acebutolol, esmolol, propranolol, and sotalol (which has class II and III properties). Selected drugs are described here. The class II drugs are classified as pregnancy category C drugs except acebutolol, pindolol, and sotalol, which are all category B drugs.

▶ atenolol

Atenolol (Tenormin) is a cardioselective β-blocker, which means that it preferentially blocks the β$_1$-adrenergic receptors that are located primarily in the heart. Noncardioselective β-blockers block not only the β$_1$-adrenergic receptors in the heart but also the β$_2$-adrenergic receptors in the lungs and therefore could exacerbate preexisting asthma or chronic obstructive pulmonary disease. In addition to having class II antidysrhythmic properties, atenolol is useful in the treatment of hypertension and angina. Its use is contraindicated in patients with severe bradycardia, second- or third-degree heart block, heart failure, cardiogenic shock, or a known hypersensitivity to it. This drug is available in both oral and injectable forms.

Pharmacokinetics

Half-Life	Onset	Peak	Duration
6-7 hr	1 hr	2-4 hr	24 hr

esmolol

Esmolol (Brevibloc) is a short-acting β-blocker with pharmacologic and electrophysiologic effects on the heart's conduction system similar to those of atenolol. Esmolol is also a cardioselective β-blocker that primarily and preferentially blocks the β$_1$-adrenergic receptors in the heart. It is used in the acute treatment of supraventricular tachydysrhythmias or dysrhythmias that originate above the ventricles and are fast instead of slow. It is also used to control hypertension and tachydysrhythmias that develop after an acute MI. Use of esmolol is contraindicated in patients with a known hypersensitivity to it or those with severe bradycardia, second- or third-degree heart block, heart failure, cardiogenic shock, or severe asthma. It is available only in injectable form.

Pharmacokinetics

Half-Life	Onset	Peak	Duration
IV: 9 min	IV: Very rapid	IV: Rapid	IV: Short

▶ metoprolol

Metoprolol (Lopressor, Toprol-XL) is another cardioselective β-blocker commonly given after an MI to reduce the risk of sudden cardiac death. It is also used in the treatment of hypertension and angina. The contraindications to metoprolol use are the same as those for the use of both atenolol and esmolol. It is available in both oral and injectable forms.

Pharmacokinetics

Half-Life	Onset	Peak	Duration
3-7 hr	1 hr	2-4 hr	13-19 hr

▶ propranolol

Propranolol (Inderal) was one of the first β-blockers introduced into clinical practice, which occurred in 1967. It was then primarily used in the treatment of dysrhythmias. Propranolol is a nonspecific β-blocker that blocks both β$_1$- and β$_2$-adrenergic receptors in the heart and lungs. Its primary effect on the conduction system of the heart is the blockade of cardiac β$_1$-adrenergic receptors, which prevents catecholamine-mediated stimulation of the heart. The resulting cardiovascular effects are a reduced heart rate, delayed AV node conduction, reduced myocardial contractility, and decreased myocardial automaticity. Propranolol is also believed to have membrane-stabilizing properties that may play a small role in its overall antidysrhythmic effect.

Because propranolol is the oldest of this class of drugs, there are now many indications for its use. Hypertension, angina, supraventricular dysrhythmias, ventricular tachycardia, the tachydysrhythmias associated with cardiac glycoside toxicity, hypertrophic subaortic stenosis, pheochromocytoma, thyrotoxicosis, migraines, post-MI, and essential tremor are just some of its uses. The contraindications to propranolol use are the same as those for atenolol. It is available in both oral and parenteral dosage forms.

Pharmacokinetics

Half-Life	Onset	Peak	Duration
IV: 3-5 hr	IV: 2 min	IV: 15 min	IV: 3-6 hr
PO: 3-5 hr	PO: 30 min	PO: 1-1.5 hr	PO: 6-8 hr

▶ sotalol

Sotalol (Betapace) is another nonselective β-blocker that is used to treat dysrhythmias. It is unique in that it possesses antidysrhythmic properties similar to those of the class III drugs (such as amiodarone) while simultaneously exerting β-blocker or class II effects on the conduction system of the heart. In addition, sotalol has prodysrhythmic properties similar to those of the class Ic drugs. This means that while patients are taking sotalol, it can cause serious dysrhythmias such as torsades de pointes or a new ventricular tachycardia or fibrillation. For this reason, sotalol is usually reserved for the treatment of documented life-threatening ventricular dysrhythmias such as sustained ventricular tachycardia.

Contraindications to sotalol use include hypersensitivity to it, bronchial asthma, cardiogenic shock, and sinus bradycardia. Sotalol is available only in oral form.

Pharmacokinetics

Half-Life	Onset	Peak	Duration
PO: 12 hr	PO: 1-2 hr	PO: 2-4 hr	PO: 12-24 hr

Class III Drugs

Class III drugs consist of amiodarone, sotalol (which also has class II properties), ibutilide, and dofetilide. Amiodarone controls dysrhythmias by inhibiting repolarization and markedly prolonging refractoriness and the APD. Ibutilide and dofetilide are both indicated for conversion of atrial fibrillation or flutter to a normal sinus rhythm. Amiodarone is indicated for the management of life-threatening ventricular tachycardia or ventricular fibrillation that is resistant to other drug therapy. This drug has also been very effective in the treatment of sustained ventricular tachycardias. Amiodarone has recently been used more frequently to treat atrial dysrhythmias as well.

▶ amiodarone

Amiodarone (Cordarone, Pacerone) markedly prolongs the APD and the ERP in all cardiac tissues. Besides exerting these dramatic effects, it is also known to block both the α- and β-adrenergic receptors of the SNS. Clinically it is one of the most effective antidysrhythmic drugs for controlling supraventricular and ventricular dysrhythmias. It is indicated for the management of sustained ventricular tachycardia, ventricular fibrillation, and nonsustained ventricular tachycardia. It is reported to be effective in 40% to 60% of all patients with ventricular tachycardia. Recently it has shown promise in the management of atrial dysrhythmias that are difficult to treat.

Amiodarone has many unwanted adverse effects, and these can be attributed to its chemical properties. Amiodarone is very lipophilic, or

Table 22-10	Recommendations for Oral Dosage after IV Infusion of Amiodarone

Duration of Amiodarone IV Infusion	Initial Daily Dose of Oral Amiodarone
Less than 1 wk	800-1600 mg
1-3 wk	600-800 mg
More than 3 wk	400 mg

IV, Intravenous.

fat loving. Therefore, it can penetrate and concentrate in the adipose tissue of any organ in the body, where it may cause unwanted effects. It also has iodine in its chemical structure. One organ that sequesters iodine from the diet is the thyroid gland. As a result, amiodarone can cause either hypothyroidism or hyperthyroidism. Adverse reactions occur in approximately 75% of patients treated with this drug, but the incidence is higher and the severity greater with higher dosages (those exceeding 400 mg/day) and prolonged therapy. The most common adverse effect is corneal microdeposits, which may cause visual halos, photophobia, and dry eyes. This occurs in virtually all adults who take the drug for longer than 6 months.

The most serious adverse effect is pulmonary toxicity, which is fatal in about 10% of patients and involves a clinical syndrome of progressive dyspnea and cough accompanied by damage to the alveoli. The result can be pulmonary fibrosis. Another serious complication of amiodarone therapy is that it not only may treat the dysrhythmias but also may provoke them.

Amiodarone has an exceptionally long half-life, approaching many days. As a result, the therapeutic as well as any adverse effects of amiodarone may linger long after the drug has been discontinued. In fact, it may take as long as 2 to 3 months after the drug has been stopped for some adverse effects to subside. For all these reasons, although it is very effective, amiodarone is typically considered a drug of last resort. Therapy is usually started in the hospital and is closely monitored until the patient's serum levels are within a therapeutic range.

Use of amiodarone is contraindicated in patients who have a known hypersensitivity to it and in those with severe sinus bradycardia or second- or third-degree heart block. For cases in which it is indicated to maintain the patient on long-term oral amiodarone therapy after intravenous amiodarone administration is discontinued, recommended conversions are available (Table 22-10). This drug is marketed in both oral and injectable forms.

Pharmacokinetics

Half-Life	Onset	Peak	Duration
PO: 15-100 days	PO: 1-3 wk	PO: 2-10 hr	PO: 10-150 days

▶ ibutilide

Ibutilide (Corvert) is a class III antidysrhythmic drug. Dofetilide (Tikosyn) is a similar drug with similar indications. Unlike the other two drugs in the class III group of antidysrhythmics, ibutilide is indicated for atrial dysrhythmias. Atrial fibrillation and atrial flutter cause irregular contractions of the heart and can lead to serious conditions such as decreased cardiac output, heart failure, low blood pressure, and stroke. Although other pharmacologic therapies are used to treat atrial fibrillation and flutter, ibutilide and dofetilide are the only drugs available for rapid conversion of these two conditions to normal sinus rhythm. The only other treatment that can produce rapid conversion is electrical cardioversion. Although it is effective, electrical cardioversion carries the risk, expense, and inconvenience of both the procedure itself and the anesthesia it requires.

Ibutilide is dosed based on patient weight. Use of ibutilide is contraindicated in patients who have previously demonstrated hypersensitivity to it. As with other antidysrhythmic drugs, ibutilide should be used with caution, because it can itself produce dysrhythmias, most significantly ventricular tachycardia and torsades de pointes. Class Ia antidysrhythmic drugs (e.g., disopyramide, quinidine, and procainamide) and other class III drugs (e.g., amiodarone and sotalol) should not be administered concomitantly with ibutilide, nor should they be given within 4 hours after infusion of ibutilide because of their potential to prolong refractoriness. Ibutilide is available only in injectable form.

Pharmacokinetics

Half-Life	Onset	Peak	Duration
6 hr	10 min	30 min	4 hr

Class IV Drugs

Class IV antidysrhythmic drugs are calcium channel blockers. Although more than nine such drugs are currently available, only a few are commonly used as antidysrhythmics. Besides being effective antidysrhythmics, calcium channel blockers are useful in the treatment of hypertension (Chapter 24) and angina. Verapamil and diltiazem are the two calcium channel blockers most commonly used for the following:

- Treating dysrhythmias, specifically those that arise above the ventricles (PSVT)
- Controlling the ventricular response to atrial fibrillation and flutter by slowing conduction and prolonging refractoriness of the AV node (i.e., preventing the ventricles from beating as fast as the atria)

These drugs block the slow inward flow of calcium ions into the slow (calcium) channels in cardiac conduction tissue. The conduction effects of these drugs are limited to the atria and the AV node, where conduction is prolonged and the tissues are made more refractory to stimulation. These drugs have little effect on the ventricular tissues.

▸ diltiazem

Diltiazem (Cardizem) is primarily indicated for the temporary control of a rapid ventricular response in a patient with atrial fibrillation or flutter and PSVT. Its use is contraindicated in patients with hypersensitivity, acute MI, pulmonary congestion, Wolff-Parkinson-White syndrome, severe hypotension, cardiogenic shock, sick sinus syndrome, or second- or third-degree AV block. Diltiazem is available in both oral and parenteral forms.

Pharmacokinetics

Half-Life	Onset	Peak	Duration
PO: 3.5-9 hr	PO: 0.5-1 hr	PO: 2-3 hr	PO: 4-8 hr
			PO: 12 hr*

*For extended-release product.

▸ verapamil

Verapamil (Calan, Isoptin, Verelan) has actions similar to those of diltiazem in that it also inhibits calcium ion influx across the slow calcium channels in cardiac conduction tissue. This results in dramatic effects on the AV node. Verapamil is used to prevent and convert recurrent PSVT and to control ventricular response in atrial flutter or fibrillation. It can also temporarily control a rapid ventricular response to these frequent atrial stimulations, usually decreasing the heart rate by at least 20%. Verapamil is not only used for the management of various dysrhythmias, but it is also used to treat angina, hypertension, and hypertrophic cardiomyopathy. The contraindications that apply to diltiazem apply to verapamil as well (Chapter 23). It is also available in both oral and parenteral forms.

Pharmacokinetics

Half-Life	Onset	Peak	Duration
PO: 2.8-7.4 hr	PO: 30 min	PO: 1-2 hr	PO: 6-8 hr
IV: 2-5 hr	IV: 1-2 min	IV: 3-5 min	IV: 10-60 min

Unclassified Antidysrhythmics
adenosine

Adenosine (Adenocard) is an unclassified antidysrhythmic drug. It is a naturally occurring nucleoside that slows the electrical conduction time through the AV node and is indicated for the conversion of PSVT to sinus rhythm. It is particularly useful when the PSVT has failed to respond to verapamil or when the patient has coexisting conditions such as heart failure, hypotension, or left ventricular dysfunction that limit the use of verapamil. Its use is contraindicated in patients with second- or third-degree heart block, sick sinus syndrome, atrial flutter or fibrillation, or ventricular tachycardia, as well as in those with a known hypersensitivity to it. It has an extremely short half-life of less than 10 seconds. For this reason, it is administered only intravenously and only as a fast intravenous push. It commonly causes asystole for a period of seconds. All other adverse effects are minimal because of its very short duration of action. Adenosine is available only in parenteral form.

Pharmacokinetics

Half-Life	Onset	Peak	Duration
Less than 10 sec	1 min	Immediate	1-2 min

PHARMACOKINETIC BRIDGE to Nursing Practice

A study of long-term oral amiodarone therapy for the treatment of dysrhythmias provides a different perspective on pharmacokinetics. To aid in evaluating the complex pharmacokinetic properties of amiodarone and developing an optimal dosing schedule for the drug in long-term oral drug therapy, serum concentrations of the drug and its metabolite, desethylamiodarone, were monitored in 345 Japanese patients receiving amiodarone. Serum concentrations of the drug and its metabolite were determined by a test called *chromatography*. In 245 participants who took fixed maintenance dosages of the drug for 6 months, there were small variations in the ratio of serum level of the actual drug and the serum level of its metabolite. (Review metabolism and related concepts in Chapter 2.) Other pharmacokinetic properties of amiodarone included an average clearance that was found to be slightly higher in women than in men, even though there was no difference between men and women with regard to age, dosage, or duration of action of the dose. Japanese patients had little variation in pharmacokinetics. From this study, one can see how important it is to fully understand basic pharmacokinetic principles (e.g., dosing, clearance, drug metabolism, serum concentrations) and their value as a very critical component of drug therapy and the nursing process. It is also important to note that culture, gender, age, and racial/ethnic group have an impact on the way each person responds to a drug and how each drug may vary in its action.

◆ NURSING PROCESS

◆ ASSESSMENT

Before administering any antidysrhythmic to a patient, the nurse must perform a thorough physical assessment and nursing assessment and obtain a complete medical history. Contraindications, cautions, and drug interactions for all of the antidysrhythmic drugs have been presented in the pharmacology section of the chapter as well as in various tables in the text. Other focuses of assessment include a baseline ECG with interpretation of the results and vital signs with attention to heart rate, rhythm, and character. Heart sounds and blood pressure, including postural blood pressures, should also be noted. Other signs and symptoms for which to assess include apical-radial pulse deficits, jugular vein distention, edema, prolonged capillary refill (longer than 5 seconds), decreased urinary output, activity intolerance, chest pain or pressure, dyspnea, syncope or dizziness, fatigue, nausea, changes in alertness, anxiety, and abnormal serum electrolyte levels. Renal and hepatic function studies are usually ordered to determine if dosages need to be adjusted due to age and altered excretion or metabolism of drugs. Altering of dosages is necessary in these situations to help prevent excessive accumulation and toxicity.

Blood counts should be assessed for the occurrence of problems with clotting (e.g., thrombocytopenia). There should be documentation of baseline neurological functioning and identification of any neuromuscular deficits, such as muscle weakness. These problems may be exacerbated by some of the antidysrhythmics (e.g., amiodarone, procainamide). Other assessment concerns associated with antidysrhythmics include close inspection of the skin for bruising and bleeding, as well as notation of bleeding gums, black tarry stools, hematuria, or hematemesis. All cautions, contraindications, and drug interactions should be assessed prior to use of these drugs, as well as other classes of antidysrhythmics (see previous discussion). One very important drug interaction to reemphasize is that of grapefruit juice, which inhibits metabolism by cytochrome P-450 3A4 hepatic enzymes (Chapter 2). This interaction with quinidine leads to increased blood levels and further risk of cinchonism (see Table 22-9). Use of lidocaine requires assessment of the central nervous and cardiovascular systems, with attention to heart rate and blood pressure. Further assessment of respiratory, thyroid, hepatic, and/or hypertensive conditions is needed with use of amiodarone. Use of this drug with fentanyl (an opioid) and St. John's wort (an herbal) should be avoided because of subsequent hypotension and bradycardia.

◆ NURSING DIAGNOSES

- Decreased cardiac output related to the pathology of the dysrhythmia
- Ineffective tissue perfusion related to the physiologic impact of dysrhythmias
- Risk for injury to self related to the drug adverse effects of hypotension, dizziness
- Deficient knowledge related to lack of experience with medication therapy
- Impaired gas exchange (decreased) related to adverse reaction to the medications
- Disturbed body image related to changes in lifestyle and sexual functioning caused by the disease process as well as by the adverse effects of medications
- Noncompliance with the medication regimen due to unpleasant adverse effects and lack of knowledge

◆ PLANNING

Goals

- Patient is free of injury to self during duration of drug therapy.
- Patient demonstrates adequate knowledge about drug therapy and related instruction.
- Patient regains normal respiratory patterns and experiences minimal respiratory-related adverse effects during drug therapy.

EVIDENCE-BASED PRACTICE

Antidysrhythmics and the Elderly Patient

Review

A review article presented a thorough examination of various research studies and clinical trials investigating the management of dysrhythmics in elderly patients. As noted in the article, the most interesting and recent application of pacemaker implantation has been for cardiac resynchronization in patients with advanced heart failure. Chronic heart failure is increasing in prevalence, with about 5 million individuals affected. Because elderly patients are more susceptible to atrial fibrillation, life-threatening ventricular dysrhythmias, and symptomatic bradycardia, it is very important for the clinician to be able to identify abnormal rhythms and initiate appropriate therapies to help prevent stroke and improve quality of life and survival. Data are reviewed in this article, but it is the summary of the various treatment modalities that is noteworthy.

Type of Evidence

This article provided a review of clinical trials and management of irregularities in heart rate in the elderly. It also presented a review of various treatment regimens.

Results of Study

Elderly patients are at increased risk for both atrial and ventricular irregularities even though they may be clinically healthy, and irregularity occurrence increases the risk of other problems in these patients. This study discussed the options of a new generation of oral anticoagulants and percutaneously implanted devices that may soon play a more expanded role in the management of atrial fibril-lation. Large clinical trial data have shown that the use of automatic implanted (AICDs) to treat ventricular tachydysrhythmias improves the survival of these patients in the appropriate setting. Biventricular pacing is also a treatment modality with an identifiable role in reducing morbidity in patients with heart failure. Other studies and trials evaluating the role of various treatment modalities in the management of cardiac irregularities in the elderly were also reviewed in this article. The treatment methods examined have provided elderly patients with the possibility of improved quality of life, decreased morbidity, and longer survival.

Link of Evidence to Nursing Practice

Elderly patients are subject to a variety of insults to their physiologic and psychologic status, and even if they are in normal health for their age, the risk for abnormal cardiac conditions and rhythms is high. The studies reviewed in this article provide evidence of improved quality of life and reduced morbidity and mortality with the use of these treatment modalities. It is important for the nurse to be aware of reliable, valid clinical trial data such as those examined in the article so that the nurse can support the patient and family throughout implementation of new treatment plans, including use of antidysrhythmics, anticoagulants, implanted pacemakers, cardioverters/defibrillators, and biventricular pacing. Research findings, such as the trial data reviewed in this article, may continue to improve patient care and lead to sound, evidence-based medical and nursing practice.

Based on Hanna IR et al: Approaching cardiac arrhythmias in the elderly patient, *MedGenMed* 7(4):24, 2005.

- Patient regains normal or near-normal cardiac output and tissue perfusion.
- Patient has improved tolerance to activity and improved general sense of well-being.
- Patient is free of complications associated with drug therapy.
- Patient maintains intact self-esteem and body image during drug therapy.
- Patient demonstrates adequate knowledge of drug therapy and its adverse effects.

Outcome Criteria
- Patient's symptoms of dysrhythmia, such as shortness of breath and chest pain, are decreased or alleviated by drug and/or nondrug therapy.
- Patient has normal breathing patterns (rate and rhythm) and no shortness of breath, cough, or chest pain.
- Patient exhibits signs and symptoms of improved cardiac output and tissue perfusion as evidenced by regular apical and radial pulses, vital signs within normal limits, and a decrease in weight, edema, crackles, and shortness of breath, attributable to compliance with therapy.
- Patient states the common adverse effects of the medication being taken, such as constipation, dry mouth, and dizziness.
- Patient experiences increase in energy and stamina and is able to carry out activities of daily living without symptoms.
- Patient states the importance of complying with the medication regimen and of scheduling and attending follow-up visits with the physician or health care provider.
- Patient openly discusses feelings of inadequacy and low self-esteem, fears, and negative feelings about self.

◆ IMPLEMENTATION

When being given class I antidysrhythmics, patients should continue to have their pulse rates (and other vital signs) monitored; if pulse rate is lower than 60 beats/min, the physician should be notified. Initially, the ECG and vital signs must be monitored closely because of possible prolongation of the QT interval by more than 50%. The end result may be the occurrence of a variety of conduction disturbances. Oral dosage forms should be taken as ordered and with food and fluids to help minimize GI upset. Intravenous dosing of any of the antidysrhythmic classes of drugs should be through use of an infusion pump. The various quinidine salts have ingredients that are specific to the given drugs and so the forms are not interchangeable. Any chest pain, hypotension, GI distress, dizziness or syncope, blurred vision, change in respiratory status, or edema should be reported to the physician immediately. Weight gain of 2 lb or more in 24 hours or 5 lb or more in 1 week should also be reported. Hypersensitivity to some of these drugs may occur 3 to 20 days into the therapy and is manifested by fever. Vials of lidocaine are usually identified as for cardiac or *not* for cardiac use. This is important to remember in reading the vial's label. Lidocaine solutions need to be used with extreme caution, and the nurse should be aware that the plain solution is used in various cardiac situations. Lidocaine is also used as an anesthetic, and the different concentrations of the drug are crucial to remember, as are their corresponding indications. It is important to remember that lidocaine comes in a solution with epinephrine, a potent vasoconstrictor. This combined solution comes in handy with suturing or repairing of wounds/lacerations to help

anesthetize (from the lidocaine) the area while also helping to control bleeding of the area (epinephrine vasoconstricts and decreases bleeding). The solution with epinephrine must *never* be used intravenously and *never* used except as a topical anesthetic with vasoconstrictor properties. Careful reading of a label is very important when using lidocaine or any of these drugs.

Parenteral solutions are usually stable for 24 hours. If the patient is also taking β-blockers, be sure to report any shortness of breath, edema, or skin rash. If the parenteral solution of any of these drugs appears discolored, it should be discarded and not used. With amiodarone, GI upset occurs during administration of loading doses and may be prevented by taking oral doses with food. Provision of a high-fiber diet with forcing fluids is also recommended to minimize constipation. If anorexia occurs, specific dietary changes should be made to improve appetite. See Patient Teaching Tips for more information.

◆ EVALUATION

The monitoring of patients receiving all classes of antidysrhythmics is important to confirm the therapeutic effects as well as identify the adverse and toxic effects.

- *Class I:* Therapeutic effects include improved cardiac output; decreased chest discomfort; decreased fatigue; improved vital signs, skin color, and urinary output; and conversion of irregularities to normal rhythm. Adverse effects include bradycardia, dizziness, headache, cinchonism, chest pain, heart failure, and peripheral edema. Toxic effects range from cardiac failure and bradycardia to CNS-related effects such as confusion or convulsions.
- *Class II:* Therapeutic effects include improved cardiac output; decreased chest discomfort; decreased fatigue; regular pulse rate or improvement in irregularities; and improved vital signs, skin color, and urinary output. Adverse effects include bradycardia, dizziness, headache, and peripheral edema. Toxic effects consist of cardiac failure, bradycardia, bronchospasms, hypotension, and conduction problems.
- *Class III:* Therapeutic effects include improved cardiac output; greater regularity in rhythm; decreased chest discomfort; decreased fatigue; and improved vital signs, skin color, and urinary output. Adverse effects include peripheral neuropathies, extrapyramidal symptoms, headache, fatigue, lethargy, bradycardia, hypotension, dysrhythmias, microdeposits on the cornea with visual disturbances, hypothyroidism or hyperthyroidism, nausea, vomiting, constipation, hepatic dysfunction with abnormal liver enzyme activity, electrolyte imbalances, photosensitivity, blue-gray skin color changes, severe pulmonary changes with development of pneumonitis, alveolitis at high dosages, pulmonary fibrosis, and pulmonary muscle weakness. The patient's thyroid function should be monitored carefully during therapy, so that abnormal function can be identified before any further adverse effects appear. Toxic effects include hypotension or hypertension and bradycardia.
- *Class IV:* Therapeutic effects include improved cardiac output, decreased chest discomfort, decreased fatigue, and improved vital signs, skin color, and urinary output. Adverse effects include bradycardia, heart failure, hypotension, AV conduction disorders, ventricular asystole, peripheral edema, and constipation. Toxic effects include hypotension, bradycardia, heart failure, and conduction disorders.

Patient Teaching Tips

- The patient should be warned not to crush or chew any of the oral sustained-release preparations. If portions of a tablet or capsule are noted in the patient's stool, he or she should know it is from the wax matrix of the drug dosage form. This means the drug matrix has not been absorbed and the physician should be contacted.
- If the use of an oral preparation is associated with GI distress, inform the patient to take the drug with food.
- Encourage the patient that if they need to use an antacid, it should be taken either 2 hours before or after the drug.
- Inform the patient that a well-balanced diet without an excess of alkaline ash foods, which include citrus fruits, vegetables, and milk, is recommended and that fluid intake should be increased up to 3 L/day (unless contraindicated).
- Encourage patients to limit and/or avoid the intake of caffeine (see Chapter 16 for a listing of foods and beverages containing caffeine).
- Medications should be taken exactly as prescribed without doubling up or omitting doses. If the patient forgets a dose or is ill and cannot take a dose, he or she should know to contact the health care provider for further instructions.
- Provide instructions to patients on how to take their pulse and blood pressure or to use community resources such as the local fire station or stopping by the physician's office just for a pulse and blood pressure check.
- Inform patients that a daily or weekly journal of symptoms, adverse effects, daily weights, a rating of how they feel, activity tolerance, blood pressure, and pulse rates will help with therapy. Also encourage them to weigh the same time every day and while wearing the same amount of clothing.
- Instruct the patient to call the physician immediately if there is a weight gain of 2 lb or more in 24 hours or 5 lb or more in 1 week.
- The patient should be cautioned to change positions slowly because postural hypotension can be an adverse effect of these drugs. Moving too quickly may lead to dizziness, syncope, and subsequent injury or falls.
- At the beginning of therapy or with any dosage increase, encourage the patient to avoid driving and other hazardous activities until sedating adverse effects are resolved.
- Instruct the patient on ways to manage dry mouth, such as use of sugarless gum or candy, eating ice chips, or rinsing the mouth frequently with water. Frequent dental visits are also encouraged.
- The patient should be cautioned to avoid exertion, hot weather, and saunas or hot tubs because of the possibility of fainting due to further blood vessel dilation from the heat and a subsequent drop in blood pressure (combined with adverse effects of hypotension with some of these drugs).
- Make sure the patient fully understands the need for carrying medical identification at all times, including an identification bracelet that lists disorders, medications, and allergies.
- Instruct patients that they should not abruptly discontinue their medication and should continue taking it as prescribed. They should be cautioned that sudden withdrawal of medication or stopping it on their own may be life threatening or lead to severe complications.
- Patients should know to report any dizziness, shortness of breath, or chest pain to their physician.
- With amiodarone, photosensitivity is an adverse effect, so the patient should avoid sun exposure and should wear sun-protective clothing and dark glasses when going outside. Sunscreens are ineffective because they do not block ultraviolet B light. Barrier sun blocks such as zinc or titanium chloride are needed.
- With amiodarone, the patient should be instructed on the need to report any blue-gray discoloration of the skin (often after 1 year, and especially on the face, neck, and arms) immediately to the health care provider. The patients should also report any jaundice, fever, numbness or tingling of extremities, blurred vision, or increased sensitivity to light.

Points to Remember

- The SA node, AV node, and bundle of His–Purkinje cells are all areas in which there is automaticity (cells can depolarize spontaneously). The SA node is the pacemaker because it can spontaneously depolarize easier and faster than the other areas.
- Any disturbance or abnormality in the normal pattern of the heartbeat and pulse rate is termed a *dysrhythmia.*
- Antidysrhythmic drugs are used to correct dysrhythmias; however, they may also cause dysrhythmias and for this reason are said to be *prodysrhythmic.* The Vaughan Williams classification is the system most commonly used to categorize antidysrhythmic drugs. It classifies groups of drugs according to where and how they affect cardiac cells and according to their mechanisms of action, as follows:
  - *Class I:* membrane-stabilizing drugs (examples are class Ia, quinidine; class Ib, lidocaine; class Ic, flecainide)
  - *Class II:* β-adrenergic blockers that depress phase 4 depolarization (e.g., propranolol)
  - *Class III:* drugs that prolong repolarization in phase 3 (e.g., amiodarone)
  - *Class IV:* calcium channel blockers that depress phase 4 depolarization (e.g., verapamil)
- Nursing actions for the various antidysrhythmics include astute nursing assessment and close monitoring of heart rate, blood pressure, heart rhythms, general well-being, skin color, temperature, and heart and breath sounds.
- The therapeutic responses to antidysrhythmics include a decrease in blood pressure in hypertensive patients, a decrease in edema, and restoration of a regular pulse rate or a pulse rate without major irregularities or with improved regularity compared to the irregularity that existed before therapy.
- Patient education about the dosage schedule and the adverse effects the patient should report to the physician is important for safe and effective therapy.

NCLEX Examination Review Questions

1. A patient with a rapid, irregular heart rhythm is being treated in the emergency department with adenosine. During administration of this drug, the nurse should be prepared to monitor the patient for which effect?
   a. Nausea and vomiting
   b. Transitory asystole
   c. Muscle tetany
   d. Hypertension

2. When assessing a patient who has been taking amiodarone for 6 months, which adverse reaction might the nurse identify?
   a. Glycosuria
   b. Dysphagia
   c. Photophobia
   d. Urticaria

3. The nurse is assessing a patient who has been taking quinidine and asks about adverse effects. Adverse effects associated with the use of this drug include which of the following?
   a. Muscle pain
   b. Tinnitus

   c. Chest pain
   d. Excessive thirst

4. A patient calls the family practice office to report that he has seen his pills in his stools when he has a bowel movement. What should be the nurse's response?
   a. "The pills are not being digested properly. You should be taking them on an empty stomach."
   b. "The pills are not being digested properly. You should be taking them with food."
   c. "What you are seeing is the waxy matrix that contained the medication, but the drug has been absorbed."
   d. "This indicates that you are not tolerating this medication and will need to switch to a different form."

5. Which condition would be a caution for the use of a class I antidysrhythmic?
   a. Tachycardia
   b. Hypertension
   c. Ventricular dysrhythmias
   d. Renal dysfunction

1. b, 2. c, 3. b, 4. c, 5. d.

Critical Thinking Activities

1. What special nursing considerations are important when administering adenosine to a patient who is experiencing PSVT that has not responded to treatment with calcium channel blockers?

2. Mrs. L. is about to be discharged home and will be taking quinidine for the treatment of ventricular ectopy. What instructions are important for her to understand before her discharge?

3. Many precautions are associated with the use of amiodarone (Cordarone). Discuss problems about which you would warn a patient taking this drug, especially in the summer in hot climates. What serious adverse effect may occur?

For answers, see http://evolve.elsevier.com/Lilley.

Antianginal Drugs

Glossary

Angina pectoris   Chest pain occurring when the heart's supply of blood carrying oxygen and energy-rich nutrients is insufficient to meet the demands of the heart. (p. 353)

Atherosclerosis   A common form of arteriosclerosis involving deposits of fatty, cholesterol-containing material *(plaques)* within arterial walls. (p. 353)

Chronic stable angina   Chest pain that has as its primary cause atherosclerosis, which results in a long-term but relatively stable level of obstruction in one or more coronary arteries. (p. 354)

Coronary arteries   Arteries that deliver oxygen to the heart muscle. (p. 353)

Coronary artery disease (CAD)   Any one of the abnormal conditions that can affect the arteries of the heart and produce various pathologic effects, especially a reduced supply of oxygen and nutrients to the myocardium. (p. 354)

Ischemia   Poor blood supply to an organ. (p. 353)

Ischemic heart disease   Poor blood supply to the heart via the coronary arteries. (p. 353)

Myocardial infarction (MI)   Gross necrosis of the myocardium following interruption of blood supply; it is almost always caused by atherosclerosis of the coronary arteries and is commonly called *heart attack.* (p. 354)

Reflex tachycardia   A rapid heartbeat caused by a variety of autonomic nervous system effects, such as blood pressure changes, fever, or emotional stress. (p. 355)

Unstable angina   Early stage of progressive coronary artery disease. (p. 354)

Vasospastic angina   Ischemia-induced myocardial chest pain caused by spasms of the coronary arteries. (p. 354)

ANGINA AND CORONARY ARTERY DISEASE

The heart is a very efficient organ, but it is very demanding in an aerobic sense because it requires a large supply of oxygen to meet the incredible demands placed on it. Pumping blood to all the tissues and organs of the body is a difficult job. The heart's much-needed oxygen supply is delivered to the heart muscle by means of the **coronary arteries.** When the heart's supply of blood carrying oxygen and energy-rich nutrients is insufficient to meet the demands of the heart, the heart muscle (or myocardium) aches. This is called **angina pectoris,** or chest pain. Poor blood supply to an organ is referred to as **ischemia.** When the organ involved is the heart, the condition is called **ischemic heart disease.**

Ischemic heart disease is the number one killer in the United States today, and the primary cause is a disease of the coronary arteries known as **atherosclerosis** (fatty plaque deposits in the arterial walls). When atherosclerotic plaques project from the walls into the lumens of these vessels, the vessels become narrow. The supply of oxygen and energy-rich nutrients needed for the heart to meet the demands placed on it is then decreased. This disorder is called **coronary artery disease (CAD).** An acute result of CAD and of ischemic heart disease is **myocardial infarction (MI),** or heart attack. It occurs when blood flow through the coronary arteries to the myocardium is completely blocked so that part of the heart muscle cannot receive any of the blood-borne nutrients (especially oxygen) necessary for normal function. If this process is not reversed immediately, that area of the heart will die and become *necrotic* (dead or nonfunctioning). Damage to a large enough area of the myocardium can be disabling or fatal.

The rate at which the heart pumps and the strength of each heartbeat (contractility) also influence oxygen demands on this organ. There are many substances and situations that can increase heart rate and contractility and thus increase oxygen demand. These include caffeine, exercise, and stress. These substances or situations result in stimulation of the sympathetic nervous system, which leads to increased heart rate and contractility. In an already overburdened heart, such as one in a patient with CAD, this can worsen the balance between myocardial oxygen supply and demand and result in angina. Some drugs that are used to treat angina are aimed at correcting the imbalance between myocardial oxygen supply and demand by decreasing heart rate and contractility. The β-blockers and the calcium channel blockers (CCBs) are two examples.

The pain of angina is a result of the following process: Under ischemic conditions when the myocardium is deprived of oxygen, the heart shifts to anaerobic metabolism to meet its energy needs. One of the byproducts of anaerobic metabolism is lactic acid. The accumulation of lactic acid and other metabolic byproducts causes the pain receptors surrounding the heart to be stimulated, which produces the heart pain known as *angina.* It is the same pathophysiologic mechanism responsible for causing the soreness in skeletal muscles after vigorous exercise.

There are three classic types of chest pain, or angina pectoris. **Chronic stable angina** has atherosclerosis as its primary cause. *Classic angina* and *effort angina* are other names for it. Chronic stable angina can be triggered by exertion or other stress (e.g., cold, emotions). The nicotine in tobacco as well as alcohol, coffee, and other drugs that stimulate the sympathetic nervous system can also exacerbate it. The pain of chronic stable angina is commonly intense but subsides within 15 minutes of either rest or appropriate antianginal drug therapy. **Unstable angina** is usually the early stage of progressive CAD. It often culminates in MI in subsequent years. For this reason, unstable angina is also called *preinfarction angina.* Another term for this type of angina is *crescendo angina,* because the pain increases in severity, as does the frequency of attacks. In the later stages, pain may even occur while the patient is at rest. **Vasospastic angina** results from spasms of the layer of smooth muscle that surrounds atherosclerotic coronary arteries. In contrast to chronic stable angina, this type of pain often happens at rest and without any precipitating cause. It does seem to follow a regular pattern, however, usually occurring at the same time of day. This type of angina is also called *Prinzmetal's angina* or *variant angina.* Dysrhythmias and electrocardiogram (ECG) changes often accompany these different types of anginal attacks.

ANTIANGINAL DRUGS

The three main classes of drugs used to treat angina pectoris are the nitrates and nitrites, the β-blockers, and the CCBs. Their various therapeutic effects are summarized and compared in Table 23-1. There are three main therapeutic objectives of antianginal drug therapy. It must (1) minimize the frequency of attacks and decrease the duration and intensity of the anginal pain; (2) improve the patient's functional capacity with as few adverse effects as possible; and (3) prevent or delay the worst possible outcome, MI. The overall goal of antianginal drug therapy is to increase blood flow to ischemic myocardium, decrease myocardial oxygen demand, or both. Figure 23-1 illustrates how drug therapy works to alleviate angina. Evidence exists to suggest that drug therapy may be at least as effective as angioplasty in treating this condition.

Table 23-1	**Antianginal Drugs: Therapeutic Effects**				
Therapeutic Effect	**Nitrates**	**β-Blockers***	**Amlodipine**	**Verapamil**	**Diltiazem**
Supply					
Blood flow	↑↑	↑	↑↑↑	↑↑↑	↑↑↑
Duration of diastole	0	↑↑↑	0/↑	↑↑↑	↑↑
Demand					
Preload†	↓↓	↑	↓/0	0	0/↓
Afterload	↓	0/↓	↓↓↓	↓↓	↓↓
Contractility	0	↓↓↓	↓	↓↓↓	↓↓
Heart rate	0/↑	↓↓↓	0/↓	↓↓	↓↓

↑, Increase; ↓, decrease; *0*, little or no effect.
*In particular, those that are cardioselective and do not have intrinsic sympathomimetic activity.
†*Preload* is pressure in the heart caused by blood volume. The nitrates effectively move part of this blood out of the heart and into blood vessels, thereby decreasing preload or filling pressure.

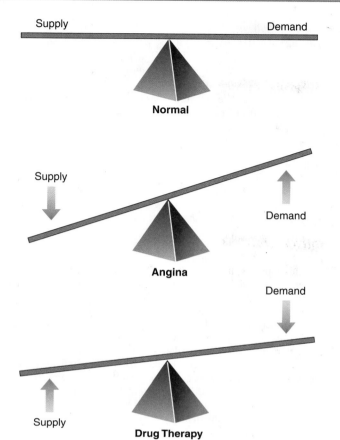

FIGURE 23-1 Benefit of drug therapy for angina through increasing oxygen supply and decreasing oxygen demands.

NITRATES AND NITRITES

Nitrates have long been the mainstay of both the prophylaxis and treatment for angina and other cardiac problems. This class of antianginal drugs was first discovered by Sir Thomas Lauder Brunton in England, who noted that amyl nitrite was just as effective as venesection (venipuncture with drainage of blood volume) in the management of angina. A few years later a chemically related substance, glyceryl trinitrate (nitroglycerin), was successfully isolated and used for this purpose. Today there are several chemical derivatives of these early precursors, all of which are organic nitrate esters. They are available in a wide variety of preparations, including sublingual, chewable, and oral tablets; capsules; ointments; patches; a translingual spray; and intravenous solutions. The following are the rapid- and long-acting nitrates available for clinical use:

- amyl nitrite (rapid acting)
- nitroglycerin (both rapid and long acting)
- isosorbide dinitrate (both rapid and long acting)
- isosorbide mononitrate (primarily long acting)

Mechanism of Action and Drug Effects

Medicinal nitrates and nitrites, more commonly referred to as simply *nitrates,* dilate all blood vessels. They predominantly affect venous vascular beds; however, they also have a dose-dependent arterial vasodilator effect. These vasodilatory effects are the result of relaxation of the smooth muscle cells that are part of the wall structure of veins and arteries. Particularly nota-

ble, however, is the potent dilating effect of nitrates on the coronary arteries, both large and small. This causes redistribution of blood and therefore oxygen to previously ischemic myocardial tissue and reduction of anginal symptoms. By causing venous dilation, the nitrates reduce venous return and, in turn, reduce the *left ventricular end-diastolic volume* (or *preload*), which results in a lower left ventricular pressure. Left ventricular systolic wall tension is thus reduced, as is myocardial oxygen demand. These and other nitrate drug effects are summarized in Table 23-1.

Coronary arteries that are diseased and that have been narrowed by atherosclerosis can still be dilated as long as there remains smooth muscle surrounding the coronary artery and the atherosclerotic plaque does not completely obstruct the arterial lumen. Exercise-induced spasms of atherosclerotic coronary arteries can also be reversed or even prevented by administration of nitrates, which encourages healthy physical activity in patients.

Indications

The nitrates are used for stable, unstable, and vasospastic (Prinzmetal's) angina. Long-acting dosage forms are used more for *prevention* of anginal episodes. Rapid-acting dosage forms, most often sublingual nitroglycerin tablets, or an intravenous drip in the hospital setting, are used to treat acute anginal attacks.

Contraindications

Contraindications to the use of nitrates include known drug allergy, as well as severe anemia, closed-angle glaucoma, hypotension, and severe head injury. This is because the vasodilatory effects of nitrates can worsen these latter conditions. In anemia, a drug-induced hypotensive episode can further compromise already reduced tissue oxygenation.

Adverse Effects

Nitrates are well tolerated, and most adverse effects are usually transient and involve the cardiovascular system. The most common undesirable effect is headache, which generally diminishes in intensity and frequency soon after the start of therapy. Other cardiovascular effects include tachycardia and postural hypotension. If nitrate-induced vasodilation occurs too rapidly, the cardiovascular system overcompensates and increases the heart rate, a condition referred to as **reflex tachycardia.** This may occur when significant vasodilation occurs that involves the systemic veins. When this happens, there is a large shift in blood volume toward the systemic venous circulation and away from the heart. Baroreceptors (blood pressure receptors) in the heart then falsely sense that there has been a dramatic loss of blood volume. At this point, the heart begins beating more rapidly to move the apparently smaller volume of blood more quickly throughout the body, especially toward the vital organs (including the heart itself). However, the same baroreceptors soon sense that there has not been a loss of blood volume but that the volume of blood missing in the heart is now in the periphery (e.g., venous system), and the heart rate slows back to normal.

Methemoglobinemia is an extremely rare adverse effect and usually occurs in patients with an inherited genetic propensity for the condition. Topical nitrate dosage forms can produce various types of contact dermatitis (skin inflammation), but these are actually reactions to the dosage delivery system and not to the nitroglycerin contained within.

Tolerance to the antianginal effects of nitrates can occur surprisingly quickly in some patients, especially those taking long-acting formulations or taking nitrates around the clock. In addition, cross-tolerance can arise when a patient receives more than one nitrate dosage form. To prevent this, a regular nitrate-free period is arranged to allow certain enzymatic pathways to replenish themselves. A common regimen with transdermal patches is to remove them at night for 8 hours and apply a new patch in the morning. This has been shown to prevent tolerance to the beneficial effects of nitrates.

Interactions

Nitrate antianginal drugs can produce additive hypotensive effects when taken in combination with alcohol, β-blockers, CCBs, phenothiazines, and erectile-dysfunction drugs such as sildenafil (Viagra).

Dosages

The organic nitrates are available in an array of forms and doses. See the Dosages table on this page for more information.

Drug Profiles

▶ isosorbide dinitrate

Isosorbide dinitrate (Isordil, Sorbitrate, Dilatrate-SR) is an organic nitrate and therefore a powerful explosive. It exerts the same effects as the other nitrates. When isosorbide dinitrate is metabolized in the liver, it is broken down into two active metabolites, both of which have the same therapeutic actions as isosorbide dinitrate itself. This drug is available in rapid-acting sublingual tablets, immediate-release tablets, and long-acting oral dosage forms.

Pharmacokinetics

Half-Life	Onset	Peak	Duration
Variable	1 hr	Unknown	4-6 hr

▶ isosorbide mononitrate

Isosorbide mononitrate (Imdur, Monoket, Ismo) is one of the two active metabolites of isosorbide dinitrate, but it has no active metabolites. Because of these qualities, it produces a more consistent, steady therapeutic response, with less variation in response within the same patient and between patients. It is available in both immediate- and sustained-release oral dosage forms.

Pharmacokinetics

Half-Life	Onset	Peak	Duration
5 hr	15-30 min	0.5-1 hr	5-12 hr

▶ nitroglycerin

Nitroglycerin is the prototypical nitrate and is made by many pharmaceutical companies; therefore, it goes by many different trade names (e.g., Nitro-Bid, Nitrostat). It has traditionally been the most important drug used in the symptomatic treatment of ischemic heart conditions such as angina. When given orally, nitroglycerin goes to the liver to be metabolized before it can become active in the body. During this process, a very large amount of the nitroglycerin is removed from the circulation. This is called a *large first-pass effect* (Chapter 2). For this reason, nitroglycerin is administered by many other routes to bypass the first-pass effect. It also is available in many formulations and has proved useful for the treatment of a variety of cardiovascular conditions. Tablets administered by the sublingual and buccal routes are used for the treatment of chest pain or angina of acute onset and for the prevention of angina when patients find themselves in situations likely to provoke an attack. Use of these routes is advantageous for ameliorating these acute conditions because the area under the tongue and inside the cheek is highly vascular. This means

DOSAGES

Selected Antianginal Nitrate Coronary Vasodilators

Drug (Pregnancy Category)	Pharmacologic Class	Usual Dosage Range	Indications
▶ isosorbide dinitrate (Isordil, Sorbitrate, Dilatrate-SR) (C)		**Adult** Chewable/SL: 2.5-10 mg q4-6h prn PO: 5-30 mg bid-tid and 40-80 mg q8-12h for SR formulations	
▶ isosorbide mononitrate (Imdur, Monoket, Ismo) (C)		**Adult** PO: 20 mg bid given 7 hr apart and 60-120 mg daily for SR formulations	
▶ nitroglycerin (Nitro-Bid, Nitrostat, Nitrol, others) (C)	Antianginal nitrate coronary vasodilator	**Adult** IV (continuous infusion): 5-20 mcg/min Ointment, 2%: 1-2 in ribbon q8h, up to 4-5 in ribbon q4h PO: 2.5-6.5 mg bid-tid during the day Spray: 0.4-0.8 mg onto or under the tongue prn Buccal: 1 mg q3-5h prn, place tablet between lip and gum Patch: 0.1 to 0.8 mg/hr applied once daily	Angina

IV, Intravenous; *PO,* oral; *SL,* sublingual; *SR,* sustained-release.

that the nitroglycerin is absorbed quickly and directly into the bloodstream, and hence its therapeutic effects occur rapidly.

Nitroglycerin also comes as a metered-dose aerosol that is sprayed under the tongue. Nitroglycerin is available in an intravenous form that is used for blood pressure control in hypertensive patients perioperatively; for the treatment of ischemic pain, heart failure, and pulmonary edema associated with acute MI; and in hypertensive emergency situations. Oral and topical dosage formulations are used for the long-term prophylactic management of angina pectoris. Topical formulations offer the same advantages as the sublingual and buccal formulations in that they also bypass the liver and the first-pass effect. They also allow for the continuous slow delivery of nitroglycerin, so that a steady dose of nitroglycerin is supplied to the patient. See the Preventing Medication Errors box.

Pharmacokinetics

Half-Life	Onset	Peak	Duration
SL: 1-4 min	SL: 2-3 min	SL: Unknown	SL: 0.5-1 hr

β-BLOCKERS

The β-adrenergic blockers, more commonly referred to as β-blockers, have become the mainstay in the treatment of several cardiovascular diseases. These include angina, MI, dysrhythmias (Chapter 22), and hypertension (Chapter 24). Most available β-blockers demonstrate antianginal efficacy, although not all have been approved for this use. Those β-blockers approved as antianginal drugs are atenolol, metoprolol, nadolol, and propranolol.

Mechanism of Action and Drug Effects

The primary drug effects of the β-blockers are related to the cardiovascular system. As discussed in previous chapters, the predominant β-adrenergic receptors in the heart are the β_1 receptors, located in the heart's conduction system and throughout the myocardium. The β-adrenergic receptors are normally stimulated by the binding of the neurotransmitters epinephrine and norepinephrine. These catecholamines are released in greater quantities during times of exercise or other stress to stimulate the heart muscle

to contract more strongly. At the normal heart rate of 60 to 80 beats/min, the heart spends 60% to 70% of its time in diastole. As the heart rate increases during stress or exercise, the heart spends more and more time in systole and less and less time in diastole. The physiologic consequence is that the coronary arteries receive increasingly less blood, and eventually the myocardium becomes ischemic. In an ischemic heart, the increased oxygen demand from increasing contractility (systole) also leads to increasing degrees of ischemia and chest pain. The physiologic act of systole requires energy in the form of adenosine triphosphate and oxygen. Therefore, any decrease in the energy demands on the heart is beneficial for alleviating conditions such as angina, in which the supply of these vital substances is already deficient because of the ischemia. When β receptors are blocked by β-blockers, the rate at which the pacemaker (sinoatrial node) fires decreases, and the time it takes for the node to recover increases. The β-blockers also slow conduction through the atrioventricular node and reduce myocardial contractility (negative inotropic effect). Both of these effects serve to slow the heart rate (negative chronotropic effect). These effects reduce myocardial oxygen demand, which aids in the treatment of angina by reducing the workload of the heart. Slowing the heart rate is also beneficial in patients with ischemic heart disease because the coronary arteries have more diastolic time to fill with oxygen- and nutrient-rich blood and deliver these substances to the myocardial tissues.

The β-blockers also have many therapeutic effects after an MI. After a patient has suffered an MI, there is a high level of circulating catecholamines (norepinephrine and epinephrine), the release of which has been triggered by the stress of the myocardial damage resulting from the infarction. These catecholamines will produce harmful consequences if their actions go unopposed. They essentially irritate the heart. They cause the heart rate to increase, which leads to a further imbalance in the supply and demand ratio, and they irritate the conduction system of the heart, which can result in dysrhythmias that can be fatal. The β-blockers block all of these harmful effects, and their use has been shown to improve the chances for survival in such patients. Unless strongly contraindicated, they should be given to all patients in the acute stages after an MI.

The β-blockers also suppress the activity of the hormone *renin*, which is the first step in the renin-aldosterone-angiotensin system. Renin is a potent vasoconstrictor released by the kidneys when they sense that they are not being adequately perfused. When β-blockers inhibit the release of renin, the blood vessels to and in the kidney dilate, which reduces blood pressure (Chapter 24).

Indications

The β-blockers are most effective in the treatment of typical *exertional* angina (i.e., that caused by exercise). This is because the usual physiologic increase in the heart rate and systolic blood pressure that occurs during exercise or stress is blunted, which thereby decreases the myocardial oxygen demand. It should be kept in mind that for an individual (often elderly) with significant angina, "exercise" may simply be carrying out the activities of daily living (ADLs) (bathing, dressing, cooking, housekeeping, etc.), which can become a major stressor for such patients. The β-blockers are also approved for the treatment of MI, hypertension (Chapter 24), cardiac dysrhythmias (Chapter 22), and

B1 = heart B2 = pulmonary

essential tremor. Some non–U.S. Food and Drug Administration (FDA)-approved but common uses include treatment of migraine headache and, in low dosages, even treatment of the tachycardia associated with stage fright.

Contraindications

There are a number of contraindications to the use of β-blockers, including systolic heart failure and serious conduction disturbances, because of the effects of β receptor blockade on heart rate and myocardial contractility. They should also be used with caution in patients with bronchial asthma, because any level of blockade of β_2 receptors can promote bronchoconstriction through unopposed parasympathetic (vagal) tone (see Adverse Effects). These contraindications are relative rather than absolute and depend on patient-specific risks and expected benefits of this drug therapy. Other relative contraindications include diabetes mellitus (due to masking of hypoglycemia-induced tachycardia), reduced mental alertness, and peripheral vascular disease (the drug may further compromise cerebral or peripheral blood flow).

Adverse Effects

The adverse effects of β-blockers result from the ability of the drug to block β-adrenergic receptors (β_1 and β_2) in various areas of the body. Therefore, blocking of β_1 receptors may lead to a decrease in heart rate, cardiac output, and cardiac contractility, whereas blocking of β_2 receptors may result in bronchoconstriction and increased airway resistance in patients with asthma or chronic obstructive pulmonary disease. β-blockers may lead to cardiac rhythm problems, decreased SA and AV nodal conduction, a decrease in systolic and diastolic blood pressures, and possible peripheral receptor blockade and/or decreased renin release from the kidneys. β-blockers are associated with masking tachycardia associated with hypoglycaemia. Fatigue, insomnia, and weakness may be related to negative effects on the cardiac and central nervous system. The β-blockers can also cause both hypoglycemia and hyperglycemia, which is of particular concern in diabetic patients. Other common β-blocker–related adverse effects are listed in Table 23-2.

Interactions

There are many important drug interactions that involve the β-blockers. The more common and important of these are listed in Table 23-3.

Dosages

For information on the dosages of selected β-blockers, see the Dosages table on this page.

Table 23-2 β-Blockers: Adverse Effects	
Body System	**Adverse Effects**
Cardiovascular	Bradycardia, hypotension, second- or third-degree heart block, heart failure
Central nervous	Dizziness, fatigue, mental depression, lethargy, drowsiness, unusual dreams
Metabolic	Altered glucose and lipid metabolism
Other	Wheezing, dyspnea, impotence

Drug Profiles

As pointed out earlier, b-blockers are the mainstay in the treatment of a wide range of cardiovascular diseases, mainly hypertension, angina, and the acute stages of MI. The three most commonly used

Table 23-3 β-Blockers: Common Drug Interactions		
Interacting Drug	**Mechanism**	**Result**
Anticholinergics, cimetidine	Antagonistic effects	Decreased level of β-blocker
	Decreased metabolism	Increased levels and pharmacodynamic effects of propranolol and metoprolol
Diuretics and antihypertensives	Additive effects	Hypotension
phenothiazine	Additive hypotensive effects	Hypotension and cardiac arrest
Phosphodiesterase type 5 inhibitors (e.g., sildenafil [Viagra])	Additive hypotensive effects	Potentially life-threatening hypotension
insulin and oral antidiabetic drugs	Additive hypoglycemic effects	Hypoglycemia; possibly requiring dosage adjustment of β-blocker or antidiabetic drugs

DOSAGES

Selected β-Adrenergic–Blocking Drugs			
Drug (Pregnancy Category)	**Pharmacologic Class**	**Usual Dosage Range**	**Indications**
▶atenolol (Tenormin) (C)		**Adult** PO: 50-200 mg/day as a single dose IV: 1.25-5 mg every 6 to 12 hr	
▶metoprolol (Lopressor, Toprol XL) (C)	β_1-blocker	**Adult** PO: 100-400 mg/day in 2 divided doses IV: 5 mg every 2 min × 3 doses, then PO therapy as indicated	Angina

IV, Intravenous; *PO,* oral.

β-blockers are carvedilol, metoprolol, and atenolol. Carvedilol is not indicated for angina per se, but it is instead indicated for congestive heart failure, essential hypertension, and left ventricular dysfunction. As noted previously, atenolol, metoprolol, nadolol, and propranolol all are indicated for angina. The drug profile for carvedilol appears in Chapter 18 on page 289.

▶ *atenolol*

Atenolol (Tenormin) is a cardioselective β₁-adrenergic receptor blocker and is indicated for the prophylactic treatment of angina pectoris. Use of atenolol after MI has been shown to decrease mortality. It is available in a parenteral form, which is an advantage because often during and immediately after an MI, blood flow to the gastrointestinal tract is poor and patients may be intubated, which rules out enteral administration of a drug. It is available in oral and injectable forms.

Pharmacokinetics

Half-Life	Onset	Peak	Duration
6-7 hr	1 hr	2-4 hr	24 hr

▶ *metoprolol*

Metoprolol (Lopressor) is also a cardioselective β₁-adrenergic receptor blocker that is used for the prophylactic treatment of angina and has many of the same characteristics as atenolol. It has shown similar efficacy in reducing mortality in the patients after MI and in treating angina. It is available in both oral (immediate release and long acting) and parenteral (injectable) forms.

Pharmacokinetics

Half-Life	Onset	Peak	Duration
3-7 hr	1 hr	2-4 hr	13-19 hr

CALCIUM CHANNEL BLOCKERS

The three chemical classes of calcium channel blockers are phenylalkylamines, benzothiazepines, and dihydropyridines, commonly represented by verapamil, diltiazem, and amlodipine, respectively (Table 23-4). Although they all block calcium channels, their chemical structures and therefore their mechanisms of action differ slightly. More than nine CCBs are available today, with more on the way. Those that are used for the treatment of

Table 23-4	**Classification of Calcium Channel Blockers**	
Generic Name	**Trade Name**	**Available Routes**
Benzothiazepines		
diltiazem	Cardizem, Dilacor, Tiazac, others	PO/IV
Dihydropyridines		
amlodipine	Norvasc	PO
bepridil	Vascor	PO
felodipine	Plendil	PO
isradipine	DynaCirc	PO
nicardipine	Cardene	PO/IV
nifedipine	Adalat, Procardia	PO
nimodipine	Nimotop	PO
Phenylalkylamines		
verapamil	Calan, Isoptin, Verelan	PO/IV

IV, Intravenous; *PO*, oral.

chronic stable angina are amlodipine, diltiazem, nicardipine, nifedipine, verapamil, and bepridil.

Mechanism of Action and Drug Effects

Calcium plays an important role in the excitation-contraction coupling process that occurs in the heart and vascular smooth muscle cells, as well as in skeletal muscle. Preventing calcium from entering into this process therefore prevents muscle contraction and promotes relaxation instead. Relaxation of the smooth muscles that surround the coronary arteries causes them to dilate. This increases blood flow to the ischemic heart, which in turn increases the oxygen supply and helps shift the supply and demand ratio back to normal. This dilation also occurs in the arteries throughout the body, which results in a decrease in the force (systemic vascular resistance) against which the heart must exert itself when delivering blood to the body (afterload). Decreasing the afterload reduces the workload of the heart and therefore reduces myocardial oxygen demand. This is the primary beneficial antianginal effect of the dihydropyridine CCBs such as amlodipine and nifedipine, but these drugs have a smaller negative inotropic effect than do verapamil and diltiazem.

Other cardiovascular effects of the CCBs include depression of the automaticity of and conduction through the sinoatrial and atrioventricular nodes because of their effects on the calcium channels (slow channels) within these tissues. For this reason, they are useful in treating cardiac dysrhythmias (Chapter 22). Finally, the CCBs reduce myocardial contractility and peripheral and coronary artery tone. Verapamil and diltiazem also decrease heart rate. Their strongest antianginal properties are secondary to their effects on myocardial contractility and the smooth muscle tone of peripheral and coronary arteries.

Indications

The therapeutic benefits of the CCBs are numerous. Because of their very acceptable adverse effect and safety profiles, they are considered first-line drugs for the treatment of such conditions as angina, hypertension, and supraventricular tachycardia. The CCBs are often particularly effective for the treatment of coronary artery spasms (vasospastic or Prinzmetal's angina). However, they may not be as effective as are β-blockers in blunting exercise-induced elevations in heart rate and blood pressure. The CCBs are also used for the short-term management of atrial fibrillation and flutter (Chapter 22), migraine headaches (Chapter 16), and Raynaud's disease (a type of peripheral vascular disease). Interestingly, the dihydropyridine CCB nimodipine is indicated solely for cerebral artery spasms associated with aneurysm rupture.

Contraindications

Contraindications to the use of CCBs include known drug allergy, acute MI, second- or third-degree atrioventricular block (unless the patient has a pacemaker), and hypotension.

Adverse Effects

The adverse effects of the CCBs are very limited and primarily relate to overexpression of their therapeutic effects. The most common of the CCB-related adverse effects are listed in Table 23-5.

Interactions

The drug interactions that can occur with CCBs vary with the particular drug, although there are not actually many such interactions. One of particular note because of its beneficial effect is the interaction that occurs between cyclosporin and diltiazem. Because diltiazem interferes with the metabolism and elimination of cyclosporin (and thus cyclosporin is not broken down as quickly), smaller doses of cyclosporin are needed. This is advantageous, because one of cyclosporin's most common and devastating effects is that it can destroy the kidney and cause renal failure. A particular food interaction of note is the fact that grapefruit juice can reduce the metabolism of calcium channel blockers. Other important drug interactions that involve CCBs are listed in Table 23-6.

Dosages

For information on the dosages of selected CCBs, see the Dosages table on this page.

Table 23-5	Calcium Channel Blockers: Adverse Effects
Body System	**Adverse Effects**
Cardiovascular	Hypotension, palpitations, tachycardia or bradycardia, heart failure
Gastrointestinal	Constipation, nausea
Other	Dermatitis, dyspnea, rash, flushing, peripheral edema, wheezing

Table 23-6	Calcium Channel Blockers: Common Drug Interactions	
Interacting Drug	**Mechanism**	**Result**
β-blockers	Additive effects	Bradycardia and atrioventricular block
digoxin	Interference with elimination	Possible increased digoxin levels
H$_2$ blockers	Decreased clearance	Elevated levels of calcium channel blockers

Drug Profiles

▶ diltiazem

Diltiazem (Cardizem, Dilacor, Tiazac) is the only benzothiazepine CCB. It has a particular affinity for the cardiac conduction system and is very effective for the oral treatment of angina pectoris resulting from coronary insufficiency and hypertension. It is one of the few CCBs that are also available in parenteral form, for which it is used for the treatment of atrial fibrillation and flutter along with paroxysmal supraventricular tachycardia. Verapamil is another CCB with similar indications. Two sustained-delivery formulations of Cardizem are available, which can be confused with each other. There is Cardizem SR, which is taken twice a day, and Cardizem CD, which is taken once a day. In addition to other brands of these two dosage forms, the drug is also available in several strengths of immediate-release capsule as well as intravenous form.

Pharmacokinetics

Half-Life	Onset	Peak	Duration
3.5-9 hr	30 min	2-3 hr	Up to 24 hr*

*With extended-release dosage forms.

amlodipine

Amlodipine (Norvasc) is currently the most popular CCB of the dihydropyridine subclass. It is indicated for both angina and hypertension and is available only for oral use.

Pharmacokinetics

Half-Life	Onset	Peak	Duration
30-50 hr	30-50 min	6-12 hr	24 hr

MISCELLANEOUS ANTIANGINAL DRUGS

Drug Profiles

ranolazine

Ranolazine (Ranexa) is the newest available antianginal drug, approved by the FDA in 2006 for chronic angina. Its mechanism of action is unknown, but it has antianginal and antiischemic effects that do not involve reductions in heart rate or blood pressure, unlike other

DOSAGES

Selected Calcium Channel–Blocking Drugs

Drug (Pregnancy Category)	Pharmacologic Class	Usual Dosage Range	Indications
▶diltiazem (Cardizem, Dilacor, Tiazac) (C)		**Adult** PO: Initial dose 30 mg qid ac and hs; range of 180-360 mg divided in 3-4 doses, or 1 daily for CD (extended-release) capsule; dosages of 480 mg/day may be needed	
amlodipine (Norvasc) (C)	Calcium channel blocker	**Adult** PO: 5-10 mg daily	Angina
verapamil (Calan, Covera-HS, Isoptin, Verelan) (C)		**Adult** PO: Initial dose 80-120 mg tid; range 240-480 mg/day divided; do not exceed 480 mg/day PO HS (extended release): 180 mg daily hs; max 480 mg/day	

PO, Oral.

antianginal drugs. Ranolazine is known to prolong the QT interval of the ECG. For this reason, this drug is reserved for patients who have failed to benefit from other antianginal drug therapy. In fact, ranolazine is contraindicated in patients with preexisting QT prolongation or hepatic impairment, in those on other QT-prolonging drugs (see Chapter 22 for examples), and in patients on moderately potent CYP3A inhibitors such as diltiazem. Other significant drug interactions include ketoconazole, and verapamil, both of which can raise ranolazine levels. Ranolazine can also raise digoxin levels enough to require adjustments in digoxin dose. The usual dose of ranolazine is 500 mg orally twice daily, which may be advanced to 1000 mg orally twice daily based on clinical symptoms. The drug is available only for oral use.

SUMMARY OF ANTIANGINAL PHARMACOLOGY

In patients with CAD, the clinical symptoms result from a lack or inadequate delivery of blood carrying oxygen and nutrients to the heart, which results in ischemic heart disease. Antianginal drugs such as nitrates, nitrites, β-blockers, and CCBs are used to reduce ischemia by increasing the delivery of oxygen- and nutrient-rich blood to cardiac tissues or by reducing oxygen consumption by the coronary vessels. Either of these mechanisms can reduce ischemia and lead to a decrease in anginal pain. Nitrates and nitrites work mainly by decreasing venous return to the heart (preload) and decreasing systemic vascular resistance (afterload). The CCBs decrease calcium influx into the smooth muscle, causing vascular relaxation. This either reverses or prevents the spasms of coronary vessels that cause the anginal pain associated with Prinzmetal's or chronic angina. The β-blockers help by slowing the heart rate and decreasing contractility, thereby decreasing oxygen demands. Although these groups of drugs have similar clinical effects, the nursing process required for each is somewhat specific because of the characteristics and effects of the drugs and the indications for and contraindications to their use.

PHARMACOKINETIC BRIDGE to Nursing Practice

Not only are the pharmacokinetic properties of nitrates very interesting, but their specific properties are critical to safe and accurate nursing care. Moreover, the patient's understanding of nitrate pharmacokinetics is also important because the level of the patient's knowledge may strongly influence compliance with the drug regimen and effectiveness of treatment for angina. The pharmacokinetics differ for the various dosage forms of nitroglycerin and are as follows:

Intravenous infusion: onset within 1-2 minutes (fastest of all dosage forms), peak time not applicable, duration of action 3-5 minutes; *sublingual tablet:* onset of action 2-3 minutes, peak action unknown, duration of action 0.5-1 hour; *transmucosal tablet:* onset 2-5 minutes, peak within 4-10 minutes, and duration of 3-5 hours; *extended-release tablet:* onset in 20-45 minutes, peak action varies, and duration of action between 3-8 hours; *topical ointment:* onset 15-60 minutes, peak within ½ to 2 hours, and duration of 3-8 hours; *transdermal patch:* onset 30-60 minutes, peak 1-3 hours, and duration of action 8-12 hours.

If the goal of treatment is to abort or treat a sudden attack of angina, then *rapid* onset of action is needed, so the clinical decision (by the physician) would be to prescribe either intravenous infusion, sublingual tablet (and/or lingual spray, which has a similar onset time), or transmucosal tablet. These dosage forms have pharmacokinetics that allow quick access of the drug to the bloodstream and lead to more rapid vasodilation. This provides more oxygenated blood to the myocardium and aborts acute attacks. If symptoms persist, more drastic medical management would be indicated. The quick-onset nitroglycerin dosage forms may also be used by the patient before engaging in activities known to provoke angina, such as increased physical activity, sexual intercourse, or other forms of physical exertion. If the purpose of treatment is maintenance therapy, the nitrate form must have other pharmacokinetic properties, such as a longer onset of action (because stopping an attack is not needed in this situation) and, more importantly, a longer duration of action to provide protection against angina. Use of ointments, transdermal patches, or extended-release preparations would be appropriate in such cases. If there is an acute episode of angina while on maintenance therapy, rapid onset of action would be indicated (as ordered). It is easy to see that thorough knowledge about a drug and its pharmacokinetics will allow the nurse to make safe and sound decisions about drug therapy for patients with angina.

◆ NURSING PROCESS

◆ ASSESSMENT

Before giving antianginal drugs, a health and medication history (e.g., listing of all prescription drugs, over-the-counter products, herbals, vitamins, and supplements) should be completed and documented. Weight, height, and vital signs, with attention to supine, sitting, and standing blood pressures, should also be noted. A systolic blood pressure reading of less than 90 mm Hg should be reported to the physician before a dose of any of these drugs are given. Apical pulse rates are preferred with drugs impacting blood pressure or heart rate and should be taken for 1 full minute with attention to rhythm and character. If the pulse rate is 60 beats/min or below, the physician should be contacted for further instructions. The nurse should also assess for any contraindications, cautions, and drug interactions (see the previous discussion in the pharmacology section). The patient's chest pain should also be thoroughly assessed, with documentation about onset, type, character (e.g., sharp, dull, piercing, squeezing, radiating), intensity, location, duration, precipitating factors (e.g., physical exertion, exercise, eating, stress, sexual intercourse), alleviating factors, and presence of nausea or vomiting. The physician may order an ECG, and the results should be reported/documented. The significant drug interaction with sildenafil, tadalafil, and/or vardenafil (used for erectile dysfunction) and nitrates is important to emphasize because of worsening of hypotensive responses, paradoxical bradycardia, and increased angina with risk of cardiac or cerebrovascular complications (from decreased perfusion). Elderly patients often have difficulty with blood pressure control due to normal age-related periods of hypotension, and use of antianginals may lead to worsening of hypotensive responses, paradoxical bradycardia, and increased angina. If patients are taking nitrates on a long-term basis, it is important to assess continued therapeutic responses because of the development of tolerance to the drug's effects. The physician should be notified if the patient begins to have more angina, and another antianginal or vasodilating drug may be ordered.

Concerns arise with the use of nonselective β-blockers or β₂ blockers in patients with bronchospastic disease because of the drug-related effects of bronchoconstriction and increased airway resistance. Therefore, if asthma or other respiratory problems are present, β-blockers would not be used. In addition, there are also concerns about the use of β-blockers in patients with hyperthyroidism, impaired renal or liver function, peripheral vascular disease, or diabetes. Hypoglycemia may occur in patients with previously controlled diabetes and nonselective β-blockers may also exacerbate preexisting heart failure. Assessment for edema is important because of drug-related edema. Weight gain of 2 lb or more over 24 hours or 5 lb or more in 1 week should be reported.

◆ NURSING DIAGNOSES

- Decreased cardiac output related to the pathology of CAD
- Ineffective tissue perfusion related to the physiologic impact of CAD
- Risk for injury to self related to the drug adverse effects of hypotension with subsequent dizziness and/or syncope
- Acute pain related to the pathologic impact of tissue ischemia on the heart
- Impaired physical mobility related to the impact of cellular ischemia
- Deficient knowledge related to first-time use of these drugs and a new diagnosis

◆ PLANNING

Goals

- Patient experiences fewer episodes of chest pain because of appropriate use of antianginal medication.
- Patient is able to perform ADLs and increase mobility with greater comfort, less chest pain, and increased stamina and energy.
- Patient tolerates moderate, supervised exercise while taking antianginals.
- Patient remains free of injury while on drug therapy.
- Patient states the rationale for medication therapy as well as adverse effects to report.

Outcome Criteria

- Patient states that there are more frequent periods of comfort while carrying out ADLs, engaging in supervised exercise, and performing moderate activity without reoccurring angina and without major adverse effects on follow-up with physician.
- Patient states measures to decrease risk of injury, such as changing positions slowly, keeping legs moving when in a still position, increasing fluid intake with medication regimen, and removing rugs or carpets that can cause tripping or slipping.
- Patient states symptoms that should be reported to the physician, such as syncope, excessive dizziness, severe headache, or increase in episodes of chest pain and/or its severity.

◆ IMPLEMENTATION

It is crucial for the nurse to always review and/or record the patient's vital signs and description of chest pain for the duration of therapy. Various dosage forms and routes of administration are used with the following nursing considerations: (1) *For*

any dosage form: The drug should always be administered while the patient is seated to avoid falls or injury from drug-induced hypotension. This may last for up to 30 minutes after dosing of the drug. When giving nitrates, the patient's chest pain should be monitored, rating of the pain on a scale of 1 to 10, before, during, and after therapy. The patient's response to drug therapy should be monitored through assessment of the patient's blood pressure, pulse rate, and presence of headache, dizziness, and/or lightheadedness. With the patient in a supine position, an appropriate dose of a nitrate should produce a clinical response of a fall in blood pressure of about 10 mm Hg and/or a rise in heart rate of 10 beats/min. Should the patient's systolic blood pressure fall to less than 90 mm Hg and/or pulse rate to less than 60 beats/min, the physician should be contacted. (2) *For oral dosage forms:* These should be taken as ordered before meals and with 6 oz of water. Extended-release preparations should not be crushed, chewed, or altered in any way. Acetaminophen may be given if there is a drug-related headache. (3) *For sublingual or buccal forms:* Tablets are to placed under the tongue (sublingual) or between the inner cheek mucosa and gum (buccal) as directed and *not* swallowed until the drug is completely dissolved. Remember that nitrates should be kept in its original packaging or container (e.g., sublingual or buccal tablets come in a small amber-colored glass container with a metal lid). Avoid exposure to light, plastic, cotton filler, and moisture. (4) *For ointment:* The proper dosing paper supplied by the drug company should be used to apply a thin layer on clean, dry, hairless skin of the upper arms or body. Areas below the knees and elbows should be avoided. The ointment should not be applied with the fingers unless using a gloved finger to avoid contact with the skin and subsequent absorption. A tongue depressor may also be used, but in most situations the ointment may be squeezed directly from the tube onto the proper dosing paper. Once the ointment is in place, it should *not* be rubbed into the skin, and the area should be covered with an occlusive dressing if not provided (e.g., plastic wrap). Application sites should be rotated, and all residue from the previous dose of ointment (and/or transdermal patch) should be gently removed with soap and water and the area patted dry. (5) *For transdermal forms:* The patch should be applied to a clean, residue-free, hairless area, and sites should be rotated. If cardioversion or use of an automated electrical defibrillator is required, the patch should be removed to avoid burning of the skin and damage to the defibrillator paddles. Be sure to locate and remove the old patch and any residual drug. (6) *For intravenous forms:* Intravenous dosing is for use in emergency situations only and in settings with close automatic monitoring of the blood pressure and pulse and constant ECG monitoring. Intravenous administration of nitrates may lead to sudden and severe hypotension, cardiovascular collapse, and shock. Always check for incompatibilities, use the proper diluent, and give intravenous solutions only through an infusion pump and as ordered. Intravenous dosage forms are available as ready-to-use injectable doses and are administered using *specific nonpolyvinylchloride* (non-PVC) plastic intravenous bags and tubing. The non-PVC infusion kits are used to avoid absorption or uptake of the nitrate by the intravenous tubing and bag. This prevents decomposition of the nitrate (with breakdown) into cyanide when the drug is exposed to light. Intravenous forms of nitroglycerin are stable for about 96 hours after preparation. If parenteral solutions are not clear and are discolored the solution should be discarded.

With isosorbide, tablets are best taken on an empty stomach; however, if the patient complains of headache or gastrointestinal upset, the medicine should be taken with meals. Oral tablets of isosorbide can be crushed; however, the sublingual and extended-release forms should *not* be crushed or chewed. In addition, if a "chewable" form is to be given, it should *not* be crushed, even though it is chewable. As with sublingual nitroglycerin, the patient should not swallow the medication until it is completely dissolved. If dizziness or lightheadedness occurs, assist and encourage the patient to change positions slowly. The nurse should monitor the patient's blood pressure, including orthostatic blood pressures, as well as anginal episodes with documentation of their severity and frequency.

CCBs should be given as ordered, and patients should take them as ordered without sudden or abrupt withdrawal. Weight should be measured daily (see the discussion of β-blockers), and the patient should be constantly monitored for edema and shortness of breath. The patient should be instructed to move and change positions slowly and with caution to prevent syncope. Constipation can be prevented. Should the patient experience cardiac irregularities, pronounced dizziness, nausea, or dyspnea, the physician should be contacted immediately. Intravenous administration of either CCBs or β-blockers requires use of an infusion pump and careful monitoring. See Patient Teaching Tips for more information.

β-blockers should be given as ordered and taken with or without food and without abrupt withdrawal. The patient's weight should be assessed every day at the same time, and if there is a gain of 2 lb or more in 24 hours or 5 lb or more in 1 week, the physician should be contacted immediately. With the use of these drugs, measures should be taken to reduce the incidence of orthostatic hypotension, such as having the patient dangle the legs before standing. Any dizziness, lightheadedness, mental depression, confusion, rash, or unusual bleeding or bruising should be reported to the physician. The patient should be informed that alcohol, saunas, hot tubs, hot showers, and hot weather or a hot environment will exacerbate vasodilation and increase the occurrence of orthostatic hypotension and a raise the risk for dizziness, syncope, and falls (as with all antianginals). With β-blockers, constipation may be a problem, which can be prevented by a high-fiber diet and increased water intake. Should the patient report that parts of any sustained-release forms of medication are appearing in the stool, the medication is possibly moving too rapidly through the gastrointestinal tract and the patient may need to be switched to another dosage form. The patient should be taught to monitor blood pressure correctly and to keep a journal in which the patient records all blood pressure readings, weights, and response to the medication regimen. Also, it should be remembered that the therapeutic effects of the β-blockers may take up to 1 to 2 weeks to appear. See the Patient Teaching Tips for more information on antianginals.

♦ EVALUATION

Patients taking antianginals must be monitored carefully for the occurrence of an allergic reaction, which may be manifested by dyspnea, swelling of the face, or hives. Evaluation of therapeutic effects includes a look at how goals and outcomes have been met, such as appropriate decrease in blood pressure, increase in cardiac output and tissue perfusion with decrease in angina, and a gradual increase in activity and performance of ADLs without exacerbation of anginal episodes. In addition, the patient must be monitored for adverse reactions such as headache, lightheadedness, dizziness, and decreased blood pressure, which may indicate the need to decrease the dosage. If the patient is receiving intravenous nitroglycerin, the nurse should evaluate for the development of pedal edema, abnormal skin turgor, nausea, vomiting, crackles, dyspnea, and orthopnea. If the patient experiences blurred vision, dry mouth, excessive drop in blood pressure and pulse rate, excessive facial or neck flushing, and/or worsening of angina, the physician should be notified immediately.

Patient Teaching Tips

Nitroglycerin

- The patient should be instructed that keeping a journal is a very good way of documenting how the patient feels, including how many anginal episodes occur, what happens, the character and intensity of the pain, frequency, and precipitating and relieving factors. Encourage the patient to also make notes about how the medication is tolerated.
- If patients are taking capsules or extended-release dosage forms, encourage them to not chew, crush, or alter the dosage form.
- *Aerosol and sublingual forms:* Encourage the patient taking *aerosol* dosage forms, to not shake the canister before lingual spraying and to avoid inhaling or swallowing the lingual aerosol until the drug is dispersed. With *sublingual* forms, inform the patient to take the medication at the first sign of chest pain and repeat every 5 minutes for up to a total of 3 doses. If after the third dose the patient is still having chest pain, instruct to immediately call 911! The sublingual dose should be placed under the tongue and the patient should avoid swallowing until the tablet is dissolved, with no eating or drinking until the drug has completely dissolved.
- Educate the patient about the best place to keep the medication away from moisture, light, heat, and cotton filler and to keep the medication in its original packaging (e.g., nitroglycerin in amber-colored glass container). Inform the patient to expect burning or stinging once the medication is placed under the tongue; if it does not burn, then the drug may have lost its potency and a new prescription must be obtained.
- It is important to emphasize that the medication is only potent for 3 to 6 months. Remind the patient to always have a fresh supply of the drug on hand, to plan ahead if traveling and (no matter the dosage form) to be seated or lie down when taking the medication to avoid falls secondary to a drop in blood pressure.
- Transmucosal tablets should be placed under the upper lip in the buccal pouch, which is located between the cheek and gum. The patient should be cautioned to avoid chewing or swallowing transmucosal dosage forms.

Continued

Patient Teaching Tips—cont'd

- With *all forms of nitrates*, educate patients about adverse effects such as flushing of the face, dizziness, fainting, brief throbbing headache, increase in heart rate, and lightheadedness. Inform them that headaches associated with nitrates last approximately 20 mintues (with sublingual forms) and may be easily managed with acetaminophen. If headaches are bothersome with the dosing of oral forms, the drug should be taken with meals, and patients should contact their physician if adverse effects continue. Educate patients that blurred vision, dry mouth, or severe headaches may indicate drug overdose and require immediate medical attention.
- Educate patients that while taking antianginals, they should avoid alcohol, hot environmental temperatures, saunas, hot tubs, and excessive exertion because these will lead to worsening of vasodilation with hypotension, possible fainting, or other cardiac events.
- If the physician prescribes it, educate the patient to take the nitroglycerin *before* stressful activities or events such as emotional situations, consumption of large meals, smoking, or sudden increase in activity (e.g., sexual intercourse). The patient should be instructed to follow the physician's directions very closely.
- With *ointment forms,* the patient should be told to use the appropriate dosage paper for application of ointment and not to use the fingers to apply the medicine. The medication can be pressed evenly directly from the tube onto the paper and to its dosing line. The patient should squeeze a thin line of ointment onto the paper and follow instructions regarding its application and the use of an occlusive dressing.
- With *transdermal nitrate* use, educate patients to apply the patch at the same time each day and to be sure to have only one patch in place at a time, with all residue cleansed off the skin before a new patch (or ointment) is applied. Educate about avoiding skinfolds, hairy areas, and any area distal to the knees or elbows. Other instructions are as follows: A patch should never be placed on irritated or open skin. If the transdermal patch becomes loose, the patient should take it off, gently remove the residue with soap and water, *pat* the area dry, and place another patch in another area. Rotation of sites is helpful in prevention of irritation with this form and with ointments. Sometimes the physician may order the patient to remove the patch for 8 hours at a specified time to prevent tolerance to the drug, because resistance does develop over time. Provide clear instructions about this type of regimen.

Isosorbide Dinitrate or Isosorbide Mononitrate

- Educate the patient about basic differences in oral nitrates (e.g., mononitrate form is well absorbed after oral dosing; dinitrate form is poorly absorbed, but its metabolite, isosorbide mononitrate, is active and well absorbed). It is important that the patient understand how these drugs work and know that the two drugs are *not interchangeable.*
- Educate the patient to take the medication exactly as prescribed and while lying down to avoid injury from sudden drop in blood pressure with subsequent dizziness, lightheadedness, and fainting.
- If the patient is taking isosorbide dinitrate, dosing may be scheduled for three times a day with a 12-hour drug-free interval, such as dosing at 0700, 1300, and 1900. The 12-hour drug-free interval will help prevent tolerance.
- The patient should be educated about how not to alter the dosage form; for example, no oral dosage form should be crushed. Oral tablet forms, as with all oral medications, should be taken with at least 6 to 8 oz of water.
- The patient should be instructed to keep a journal of episodes of angina along with blood pressure and pulse readings.
- Educate patients that while taking these drugs, they should always move cautiously and slowly, change positions gradually, and move their legs about or dangle them while sitting for a few moments before standing to help prevent dizziness and fainting.
- Educate patients that brands of these drugs should never be changed from one to the other and to avoid alcohol, heat, and saunas (see the previous tips for Nitroglycerin).

✳ Points to Remember

- Angina pectoris (chest pain) occurs because of a mismatch between the oxygen supply and oxygen demand, with either too high a demand for oxygen or too little oxygen delivery.
- The heart is a very aerobic (oxygen-requiring) muscle, and when it does not receive enough oxygen, pain (angina) occurs. When the coronary arteries that deliver oxygen to the heart muscle become blocked, a heart attack (MI) occurs.
- CAD is an abnormal condition of the arteries (blood vessels) that deliver oxygen to the heart muscle. These arteries may become narrowed, which results in reduced flow of oxygen and nutrients to the myocardium.
- Nitrates, CCBs, and β-blockers may be used to treat the symptoms of angina.
- Nitroglycerin is the prototypical nitrate. Nitrates dilate constricted coronary arteries, helping to increase the supply of oxygen and nutrients to the heart muscle. Nitrates also dilate all other blood vessels, which leads to the following effects: venous dilation results in a decrease in blood return to the heart (decreased preload), whereas arterial dilation results in a decrease of peripheral resistance (decreased afterload—that is, the pressure or force against which the left ventricle must pump). Isosorbide dinitrates were the first group of oral drugs used to treat angina; isosorbide mononitrates are new and improved nitrates used for angina therapy. Nitroglycerin is the main intravenous nitrate used to treat angina and hypertensive crisis.
- The β-blockers are also used to relieve angina and do so by decreasing the heart rate, which helps reduce the workload of the heart and decreases the oxygen demand of the heart.
- Nursing considerations for the use of all antianginals include the following:
  - Dosage forms for nitrates include conventional tablets, sublingual and buccal tablets, controlled-release and sustained release capsules, transdermal patch, topical ointment, and intravenous injection. Specific nursing interventions are associated with each dosage form. Hypotension is the most common adverse effect for all dosage forms. Extended-release tablets or transdermal patches are generally used for long-term angina prophylaxis, whereas lingual sprays and sublingual tablets are used for acute treatment.

Points to Remember—cont'd

- Quick-onset nitrates should be used to treat acute anginal attacks.
- CCBs and β-blockers may be associated with the adverse effects of postural hypotension, dizziness, headache, and edema.
- The nonselective β-blockers may exacerbate congestive heart failure, respiratory bronchospastic problems, and hypoglycemia.

- If the patient's pulse rate is 60 beats/min or lower, the physician should be contacted for further instructions.
- The patient should be sure to keep a fresh supply of sublingual nitroglycerin because the drug is only stable for 3 to 6 months.

NCLEX Examination Review Questions

1. A patient has a new prescription for transdermal nitroglycerin patches. The nurse teaches the patient that these patches are most appropriately used for which of the following?
   a. To relieve exertional angina
   b. To prevent palpitations
   c. To prevent the occurrence of angina
   d. To reduce the severity of anginal episodes
2. A nurse with adequate knowledge about the administration of intravenous nitroglycerin will recognize that which of the following statements is correct?
   a. The intravenous form is given by bolus injection.
   b. Because the intravenous forms are short-lived, the dosing must be every 2 hours.
   c. Intravenous nitroglycerin must be protected from exposure to light through use of special tubing.
   d. Intravenous nitroglycerin can be given via gravity drip infusions.
3. Which statement by the patient reflects the need for additional patient education about the CCB diltiazem (Cardizem)?
   a. "I can take this drug to stop acute anginal attacks."
   b. "I understand that food and antacids alter the absorption of this oral drug."
   c. "When the long-acting forms are taken, the drug cannot be crushed."
   d. "This drug may cause my blood pressure to drop, so I should be careful when getting up."

4. While assessing a patient with angina who is to start β-blocker therapy, the nurse is aware that the presence of which condition may be a problem if these drugs are used?
   a. Hypertension
   b. Essential tremors
   c. Exertional angina
   d. Asthma
5. A 68-year-old man has been taking the nitrate isosorbide dinitrate for 2 years for angina. He recently has been experiencing erectile dysfunction and wants a prescription for sildenafil (Viagra). Which response would the nurse most likely hear from the prescriber?
   a. "He will have to be switched to isosorbide mononitrate if he wants to take sildenafil."
   b. "Taking sildenafil with the nitrate may result in severe hypotension, so a contraindication exists."
   c. "I'll write a prescription, but if he uses it, he needs to stop taking the isosorbide for one dose."
   d. "These drugs are compatible with each other, and so I'll write a prescription."

1. c, 2. c, 3. a, 4. d, 5. b.

Critical Thinking Activities

1. Mr. J. is a 45-year-old man with stable angina who has recently been prescribed sublingual nitroglycerin tablets for the relief of his anginal attacks. He asks you how many milligrams of nitroglycerin are in his tablets. All the bottle says is "¹⁄₁₅₀ gr tablets." How many milligrams of nitroglycerin are in Mr. J.'s ¹⁄₁₅₀ gr tablets?
2. Mrs. A. had been shoveling snow all morning. As you work on the snow in your yard, you see her suddenly sit down in her driveway.

When you go over to check on her, she says that she took a nitroglycerin pill at the first sign of chest pain, just like the doctor told her to. The chest pain is gone at this time. What, if anything, should she have done differently?
3. Your patient has been switched from sublingual nitroglycerin to a transdermal form. What instructions do you need to give him regarding the difference in his therapeutic regimen?

For answers, see http://evolve.elsevier.com/Lilley.

Antihypertensive Drugs

Objectives

When you reach the end of this chapter, you should be able to do the following:

1. Briefly discuss the normal anatomy and physiology of the autonomic nervous system, including the events that take place within the sympathetic and parasympathetic divisions and how they relate to long-term and short-term control of blood pressure.
2. Define hypertension, with comparison of primary and secondary hypertension and their related manifestations.
3. Describe the protocol for treating hypertension as detailed in the *Seventh Report of the Joint National Committee on Prevention, Detection, Evaluation, and Treatment of High Blood Pressure* (JNC-7), including the rationale for its use.
4. List the criterion pressure values (in millimeters of mercury) for the new hypertension categories of normal pressure, prehypertension, hypertension stage 1, and hypertension stage 2 as defined in JNC-7.
5. Using the most recent guidelines, compare the various drugs used in the pharmacologic management of hypertension with regard to mechanism of action, specific indications, adverse effects, toxic effects, cautions, contraindications, dosages, and routes of administration.
6. Discuss the rationale for the nonpharmacologic management of hypertension.
7. Develop a nursing care plan that includes all phases of the nursing process for patients receiving antihypertensive drugs.

e-Learning Activities

Companion CD

- NCLEX Review Questions: see questions 190-204
- Animations
- Audio Glossary
- Category Catchers
- Medication Errors Checklists
- IV Therapy Checklists

evolve Website (http://evolve.elsevier.com/Lilley)

• Nursing Care Plans • Frequently Asked Questions • Content Updates • WebLinks • Supplemental Resources • Elsevier ePharmacology Update • Medication Administration Animations

Drug Profiles

bosentan, p. 380
▶ captopril, p. 377
carvedilol, p. 374
▶ clonidine, p. 373
enalapril, p. 377
eplerenone, p. 380

▶ hydralazine hydrochloride, p. 379
▶ losartan, p. 378
prazosin, p. 374
sodium nitroprusside, p. 380
treprostinil, p. 380

▶ Key drug.

Glossary

α₁-Blockers Drugs that primarily cause arterial and venous dilation through their action on peripheral sympathetic neurons. (p. 371)

Antihypertensive drugs Medications used to treat hypertension. (p. 367)

Cardiac output The amount of blood ejected from the left ventricle, measured in liters per minute. (p. 369)

Centrally acting adrenergic drugs Drugs that modify the function of the sympathetic nervous system in the brain by stimulating α_2 receptors, which has a reverse sympathetic effect that causes decreased blood pressure. (p. 371)

Essential hypertension Elevated systemic arterial pressure for which no cause can be found and which is often the only significant clinical finding; also called *primary* or *idiopathic hypertension.* (p. 379)

Ganglionic blocking drugs Drugs that prevent nerves from responding to the action of acetylcholine by occupying the receptor sites for acetylcholine (i.e., nicotinic receptors) on sympathetic and parasympathetic nerve endings. (p. 367)

Hypertension A common, often asymptomatic disorder in which blood pressure persistently exceeds 140/90 mm Hg. (p. 367)

Nicotinic receptor The receptor and site of action for acetylcholine in both the parasympathetic and sympathetic nervous systems. Nicotinic receptors are located at the junction of the preganglionic and postganglionic neurons of both of these systems. (p. 370)

Orthostatic hypotension A common adverse effect of adrenergic drugs involving a sudden drop in blood pressure when a person changes position, especially when rising from a seated or horizontal position. (p. 373)

Prodrug A drug that is inactive in its administered form and must be biotransformed in the liver to its active form. (p. 374)

Secondary hypertension   High blood pressure associated with a primary disease such as renal, pulmonary, endocrine, or vascular disease. (p. 368)

Significant advances have been made in the detection, evaluation, and treatment of high blood pressure, or **hypertension.** Over the past 40 years the development of new antihypertensive medications has had an enormous impact on the quality of life of affected persons by reducing the incidence of the various complications associated with hypertension and decreasing the adverse effects associated with these medications. Drug therapy for hypertension first became available in the early 1950s with the introduction of **ganglionic blocking drugs.** However, unpleasant adverse effects and inconsistent therapeutic effects were common problems with these **antihypertensive drugs.** Then in 1953 the vasodilator hydralazine was introduced. and in 1958 the thiazide diuretics became available. These drugs offered important advantages over the previous antihypertensive drug therapies. In addition, with the discovery of these newer drugs came a better understanding of the disease process itself.

Since that time, several additional drug categories have emerged, including loop diuretics (also called potassium-wasting diuretics), potassium-sparing diuretics, β-blockers (β receptor antagonists), angiotensin-converting enzyme (ACE) inhibitors, α_1-antagononists, α_2-agonists, angiotensin II receptor blockers (ARBs), calcium channel blockers (CCBs), and vasodilators. Although some of the medications mentioned in this chapter represent older classes of drugs, all are current therapeutic options listed in the treatment guidelines for hypertension published by the National Heart, Lung, and Blood Institute in May 2003. For this reason these selected older drugs are discussed in this chapter along with the newer drug classes.

HYPERTENSION

As many as 50 million people in the United States have some form of hypertension, which makes it the most common disease in the population of the Western hemisphere. Not only does hypertension affect a large portion of our society, but it has many severe consequences if left untreated. Hypertension is a major risk factor for coronary artery disease, cardiovascular disease, and death resulting from cardiovascular causes. It is the most important risk factor for stroke and heart failure, and it is also a major risk factor for renal failure and peripheral vascular disease.

The diagnosis and treatment of hypertension have varied considerably over the years, which has resulted in a great deal of misunderstanding. The *Seventh Report of the Joint National Committee on Prevention, Detection, Evaluation, and Treatment of High Blood Pressure (JNC-7)* was released in May 2003 (Box 24-1). This report provides the latest treatment guidelines for hypertension, which have been assembled by two large expert panels based on a review of the latest clinical research publications on the disease. As with previous such reports, the development of *JNC-7* was sponsored by the National Heart, Lung, and Blood Institute of the National Institutes of Health (NIH), the major

---

Box 24-1   New Hypertension Guidelines—The *Seventh Report*

The *Seventh Report of the Joint National Committee on the Detection, Evaluation, and Treatment of High Blood Pressure (JNC-7)* (May 2003) introduced further changes to the previous recommendations regarding identification and treatment of hypertension. It continued to emphasize an individualized approach to therapy, rather than the traditional stepped-care approach, as a means of addressing specific patient characteristics and needs and identifying pharmacologic alternatives. Health care providers were encouraged to consider quality of life, culture, ethnicity, use of concurrent therapies, demographic concerns, and presence of concomitant diseases in planning drug therapy for hypertension. These latest recommendations have been published and are available through the National Institutes of Health (NIH Publication No. 03-5231). Some of the major points in *JNC-7* can be summarized as follows:

- Normal blood pressure readings are considered to be a systolic blood pressure (SBP) of less than 120 mm Hg and a diastolic blood pressure (DBP) of less than 80 mm Hg. An SBP of 120 to 139 mm Hg or a DBP of 80 to 89 mm Hg is no longer considered to be "normal" or "high normal" but is identified as prehypertensive and requires lifestyle modifications to prevent cardiovascular disease and subsequent complications. Stage 1 hypertension is defined as an SBP of 140 to 159 mm Hg or a DBP of 80 to 89 mm Hg. Stage 2 hypertension is an SBP of more than 160 mm Hg or a DBP of more than 100 mm Hg.
- Blood pressure measurement techniques include the following:
  - In-office measurement should include two readings taken 5 minutes apart with the patient sitting in a chair and with elevated blood pressure confirmed in the other arm.

- Ambulatory blood pressure readings are indicated for patients who have elevated blood pressure in the presence of a physician or health care provider ("white coat" hypertension).
- Patient self-checks provide information on response to therapy and may help to improve adherence to the treatment regimen. (NOTE: This applies to adults age 18 years or older).
- A diagnostic workup for hypertension should include assessment for risk factors, comorbidities, causes of hypertension, and target organ damage; history taking and physical examination; recording of an electrocardiogram; and laboratory tests, including urinalysis, lipid panels, hematocrit, and other related studies.
- The patient should be evaluated for major risk factors for cardiovascular disease such as hypertension, obesity, lipid disorders, diabetes, cigarette smoking, physical inactivity, altered renal function, and age older than 55 years for men and 65 years for women.
- The patient should also be assessed for identifiable causes of hypertension, including sleep apnea, drug-induced hypertension, renovascular disease, and Cushing's syndrome.

The key message of *JNC-7* is that high DBP is no longer considered to be more dangerous than high SBP. This altered view reflects the results of many research studies as well as the year 2000 warning of the National Heart, Lung, and Blood Institute that elevated SBP is strongly associated with heart failure, stroke, and renal failure.

Modified from *Monthly prescribing reference* 21(10), October 2005. Available at www.prescribingref.com; Van Vlaanderen E: New hypertension guidelines, *Clin Advisor* 7:13-16, 2003.

governmental health research entity of the United States. The efforts of the Joint National Committee are intended to educate both health care professionals and the general public about the dangers of the disease and the importance of its treatment.

One of the major changes that appeared in the earlier *Sixth Report of the Joint National Committee on Prevention, Detection, Evaluation, and Treatment of High Blood Pressure (JNC-6)* in 1997 was a new classification system for blood pressure because of the realization that the previously applied term *mild hypertension* did not adequately reflect the serious nature of this condition. This became evident when it was found that although the vast majority of the 50 million Americans with hypertension have so-called mild hypertension, most of the morbidity and mortality actually occurs in this group. In addition, whereas pre–*JNC-6* reports had recommended a stepped-care pharmacologic approach to treating the illness, many practitioners believed that this approach no longer adequately reflected the current range of pharmacologic alternatives or furnished the type of care dictated by the current level of scientific understanding of the disorder. In *JNC-6* individualized therapy was proposed as a more appropriate treatment strategy than stepped care because it allowed specific patient circumstances to be addressed and pharmacologic alternatives to be considered. This individualized approach continues to be emphasized in *JNC-7*, with the recognition that some patients may require two or more medications, even as initial therapy, depending on their individual cardiovascular risk factors such as obesity, diabetes, and family history. Health care providers are therefore encouraged to adopt an individualized approach to the planning of drug therapy that takes into consideration the demographic concerns for the given patient, the presence of concomitant diseases, the use of concurrent therapies, and the patient's quality of life.

The classification scheme used to categorize individual cases of hypertension has been simplified to the following four stages based on blood pressure measurements: normal, prehypertension, stage 1 hypertension, and stage 2 hypertension. This revised classification scheme is presented in detail in Table 24-1.

Hypertension can also be defined by its cause. When the specific cause of hypertension is unknown, it may be called *essential, idiopathic,* or *primary hypertension.* About 90% of the cases of hypertension are of this type. **Secondary hypertension** makes up the other 10%. Secondary hypertension is most commonly the result of another disease such as pheochromocytoma (adrenal tumor), preeclampsia of pregnancy (a pregnancy complication involving acute hypertension, among other symptoms), or renal artery disease. It may also result from the use of certain medications. If the cause of secondary hypertension can be eliminated, blood pressure usually returns to normal.

EVIDENCE-BASED PRACTICE
Effects of Exercise on Blood Pressure in Those 55 Years of Age and Older

Review
The Senior Hypertension and Physical Exercise (SHAPE) study examined the effects of exercise on blood pressure in men and women 55 years of age or older with a diagnosis of mild hypertension. Those who participated in a 6-month exercise program showed greater reductions in diastolic (but not systolic) blood pressure than did subjects who did not exercise.

Type of Evidence
The participants were between 55 and 75 years of age, had systolic blood pressures (SBP) of 130 to 159 mm Hg or diastolic blood pressures (DBP) of 85 to 89 mm Hg, and were not taking any antihypertensive drugs. Fifty-three control subjects were asked to follow the standard recommendations for physical activity contained in the National Institute of Aging guidelines for exercise. They were also given dietary advice based on the American Heart Association Step 1 diet. In addition to receiving the same standard advice regarding diet and activity, the experimental group followed an exercise regimen based on the American College of Sports Medicine guidelines and participated in three supervised exercise sessions per week that included both resistance and aerobic training. Fifty-one individuals completed the exercise program between 1999 and 2003. The nonexercise group was not a true control group because these subjects may have made unreported lifestyle changes in response to the diet and exercise advice they received. SHAPE investigators were based at the Johns Hopkins School of Medicine and the National Institute on Aging.

Results of Study
The study reported significant mean decreases in SBP and DBP of 5.3 and 3.7 mm Hg, respectively, in the exercise group and 4.5 and 1.5 mm Hg, respectively, in the control group. The mean decrease in DBP was significantly greater in the exercisers than in the control group, but the difference in SBP in the two groups was not statistically significant. There was no difference between men and women in blood pressure reductions. The investigators pointed out that the main reason the decrease in SBP in the exercise group was smaller than anticipated was that increased arterial stiffness contributes to systolic hypertension in older patients. This age-related change may not be amenable to modification by exercise.

Link of Evidence to Nursing Practice
For older patients with hypertension, exercise has always been considered to be a lifestyle change that may help to decrease both SBP and DBP. Although this study did not find a larger decrease in blood pressure in the group that participated in the exercise program, as had been anticipated, other benefits were noted in this group: improvement in aerobic ability and fitness, increased strength, increase in lean body mass, and decrease in overall and abdominal obesity. Improved body composition accounted for 8% of the reduction in SBP and 17% of the reduction in DBP among the exercisers. This study may be helpful in establishing the importance of exercise training as a means of improving cardiovascular health in older men and women, as suggested by the SHAPE investigators. More research is needed to demonstrate the benefits of lifestyle changes for individuals in all age groups so that patients with hypertension can be educated regarding the importance of nonpharmacologic and pharmacologic treatment regimens for management of hypertension.

Based on Stewart KJ et al: Effect of exercise on blood pressure in older persons: a randomized controlled trial, *Arch Intern Med* 165:756-762, 2005.

Table 24-1   Classification and Management of Blood Pressure

BP Classification	SBP* (mm Hg)	DBP* (mm Hg)	Lifestyle Modification	Initial Drug Therapy	
				Without Compelling Indications†	With Compelling Indications†
Normal	Less than 120	and less than 80	Encourage		
Prehypertension	120-139	or 80-89	Yes	No antihypertensive drug indicated	Drug(s) for compelling indications‡
Stage 1 hypertension	140-159	or 90-99	Yes	Thiazide-type diuretics for most; may consider ACE inhibitor, ARB, BB, CCB, or combination	Drug(s) for compelling indications; other antihypertensive drugs (diuretics, ACE inhibitors, ARBs, BBs, CCBs) prn
Stage 2 hypertension	160 or higher	or 100 or higher	Yes	Two-drug combination for most§ (usually thiazide-type diuretic and ACE inhibitor, ARB, BB, or CCB).	

From U.S. Department of Health and Human Services: *Seventh report of the Joint National Committee on Prevention, Detection, Evaluation, and Treatment of High Blood Pressure (JNC-7),* Washington, DC, 2003, National Institutes of Health.
ACE, Angiotensin-converting enzyme; *ARB,* angiotensin II receptor blocker; *BB,* β-adrenergic blocker; *BP,* blood pressure; *CCB,* calcium channel blocker; *DBP,* diastolic blood pressure; *SBP,* systolic blood pressure.
*Treatment determined by highest BP category.
†Compelling indications include heart failure, previous myocardial infarction, high cardiovascular risk, diabetes mellitus, chronic kidney disease, and previous stroke.
‡Treat patients with chronic kidney disease or diabetes to BP goal of less than 130/80 mm Hg.
§Initial combined therapy should be used cautiously in those at risk for orthostatic hypotension.

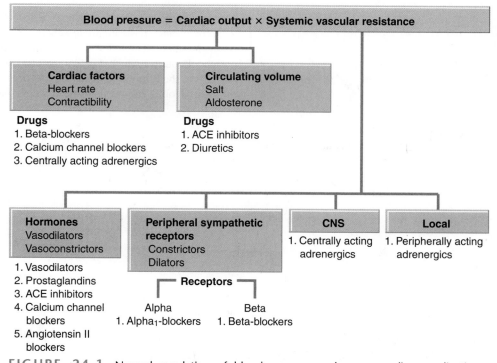

FIGURE 24-1   Normal regulation of blood pressure and corresponding medications. *ACE,* Angiotensin-converting enzyme; *CNS,* central nervous system.

Blood pressure is determined by the product of **cardiac output** and systemic vascular resistance (SVR). Cardiac output is the amount of blood that is ejected from the left ventricle and is measured in liters per minute. Normal cardiac output is 4 to 8 L/min. SVR is the force (resistance) the left ventricle has to overcome to eject its volume of blood. Numerous factors interact to regulate these two major variables and keep the blood pressure within normal limits. These are illustrated in Figure 24-1. These are the same factors that can cause high blood pressure and are the targets of action of many of the antihypertensive drugs.

ANTIHYPERTENSIVE DRUGS

As previously mentioned, the drug therapy for hypertension should be individualized to accommodate or complement the specific needs or concerns of the given patient. Important considerations in planning drug therapy are whether the patient has concomitant medical problems and what the impact of drug therapy on the patient's quality of life will be. For example, one very common adverse effect of almost any antihypertensive drug is

---

> ## Box 24-2 Categories and Subcategories of Antihypertensive Drugs
>
> ### Adrenergic Drugs
> - Centrally and peripherally acting adrenergic neuron blockers
> - Centrally acting α_2 receptor agonists
> - Peripherally acting α_1 receptor blockers
> - Peripherally acting β receptor blockers (β-blockers)
>   - Cardioselective (β_1 receptor blockers)
>   - Nonselective (β_1 and β_2 receptor blockers)
> - Peripherally acting dual α_1 and β receptor blockers
>
> ### Angiotensin-Converting Enzyme Inhibitors
>
> ### Angiotensin II Receptor Blockers
>
> ### Calcium Channel Blockers
> - Benzothiazepines
> - Dihydropyridines
> - Phenylalkylamines
>
> ### Diuretics
> - Loop diuretics
> - Potassium-sparing diuretics
> - Thiazides and thiazide-like diuretics
>
> ### Vasodilators
> Act directly on vascular smooth muscle cells, *not* through α or β receptors.

---

sexual dysfunction in male patients, which is the most common reason for noncompliance with drug therapy. Demographic factors, cultural implications, the ease of medication administration (e.g., a once-a-day dosing schedule or transdermal administration), and cost are other important considerations.

There are essentially seven main categories of pharmacologic drugs: diuretics, adrenergic drugs, vasodilators, ACE inhibitors, ARBs, CCBs, and vasodilators. Because all antihypertensive drugs (with the exception of diuretics) have some vasodilatory action, those in last category are also called *direct vasodilators* to differentiate them. Drugs in these classes may be used either alone or in combination. The various categories and subcategories of antihypertensive drugs are listed in Box 24-2. The diuretics are discussed in detail in Chapter 25 and therefore are not covered here.

REVIEW OF AUTONOMIC NEUROTRANSMISSION

The stimulation of the two divisions of the autonomic nervous system (ANS), the parasympathetic (PSNS) and sympathetic (SNS) nervous systems, is controlled by the neurotransmitters acetylcholine (ACh) and norepinephrine. The receptors for both divisions of the ANS are located throughout the body in a variety of tissues. ANS physiology is reviewed in greater detail in the introductory sections of Chapters 17 through 20. The preganglionic receptor for ACh in both the SNS and PSNS is the **nicotinic receptor.** It gets its name from the fact that it was the administration of the ganglionic stimulant *nicotine* that first revealed its existence. In both systems this receptor is located between the preganglionic and postganglionic fibers. The receptor located between the postganglionic fiber and the effector cells (i.e., the postganglionic receptor) is called the *muscarinic or cholinergic receptor* in the PSNS and the *adrenergic or noradrenergic receptor* (i.e., α or β receptor) in the SNS. Physiologic activity at

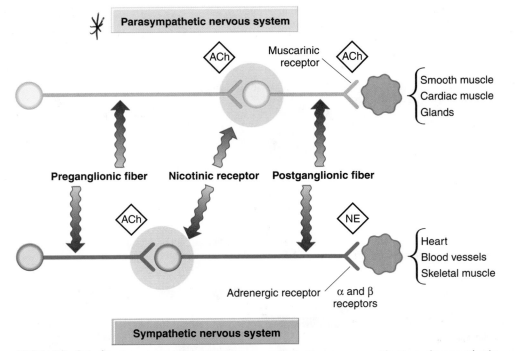

FIGURE 24-2 Location of the nicotinic receptors in the parasympathetic and sympathetic nervous systems. *ACh,* Acetylcholine; *NE,* norepinephrine.

The following are some important generalizations about demographics and the drugs used to treat hypertension:

- β-Blockers and angiotensin-converting enzyme (ACE) inhibitors have been found to be more effective in lowering blood pressure in whites than in African Americans.
- Calcium channel blockers and diuretics have been shown to be more effective in African American patients than in white patients.
- Captopril, used as monotherapy, to treat hypertension has been found to elicit a lesser response in African American patients, who are considered to be low-renin hypertensives, than in the general treatment population.
- Losartan used as monotherapy for hypertension has been found to be less effective in African American patients than in other racial groups because African American patients are low-renin hypertensives.

These findings are important to remember in the care of patients, whether they are in an inpatient setting, are being seen by a physician or a nurse practitioner, or are being screened by a nurse in the community. The significance of these cultural-ethnic factors is that they allow a better understanding of the dynamics of pharmacologic treatment in hypertensive patients of different ethnic groups and also underscore the importance of a thorough nursing assessment that includes attention to cultural influences. They also allow an appreciation of individual responses to drug therapy and aid in achieving more successful treatment of the disease. These responses are often considered by health care providers in selecting first-line therapy.

Results of many studies have supported a difference between African Americans and whites in response to antihypertensive drugs; however, conflicting findings in this area should be mentioned for balance. Although researchers have reported that, on average, African Americans and whites differ slightly in their responses to antihypertensive drugs, a metaanalysis published in the March 2004 issue of *Hypertension* found that the majority of African Americans and whites in the studies analyzed had similar responses to some of the more commonly used antihypertensives such as diuretics, β-blockers, calcium channel blockers, and ACE inhibitors. In this analysis, which pooled data on the use of common antihypertensives in some 9300 whites and 2900 African Americans, 81% to 95% of African Americans and whites were found to experience similar changes in blood pressure in response to each of the four groups of commonly used drugs. This analysis concluded that race, as examined in this context, had little value in predicting response to these drugs and that the responses of the two groups were overlapping. The reason to mention this research is that clinical decisions may be more efficient and of greater therapeutic value if drug treatment is based on considerations relevant to the given individual, such as indications and medical history, rather than being based solely on race. In summary, it is important for nurses to fully understand all the cultural and multifactor influences on pharmacologic therapies so that the nursing process can be implemented thoroughly and effectively.

Based on Rakel RE, Bope ET: *Conn's current therapy 2004,* Philadelphia, 2004, Saunders; Sehgal A: Overlap between whites and blacks in response to antihypertensive drugs, *Hypertension* 43:566-572, 2004.

muscarinic receptors is stimulated by ACh and cholinergic agonist drugs (Chapter 19) and is inhibited by cholinergic antagonists (anticholinergic drugs; Chapter 20). Similarly, physiologic activity at adrenergic receptors is stimulated by norepinephrine and epinephrine and adrenergic agonist drugs (Chapter 17) and inhibited by antiadrenergic drugs (adrenergic blockers, i.e., α or β receptor blockers; Chapter 18). Figure 24-2 shows how these various receptors are arranged in both the PSNS and SNS and indicates their corresponding neurotransmitters.

ADRENERGIC DRUGS

Adrenergic drugs are a large group of antihypertensive drugs, as shown in Box 24-2. The β-blockers and combined α-β–blockers were described in detail in Chapter 18. The adrenergic drugs discussed here exert their antihypertensive action at different sites.

Mechanism of Action and Drug Effects

Five specific drug subcategories are included in the adrenergic antihypertensive drugs as indicated in Box 24-2. Each of these subcategories of drugs can be described as having central action (in the brain) or peripheral action (at the heart and blood vessels). These drugs include the adrenergic neuron blockers (central and peripheral), the α_2 receptor agonists (central), the α_1 receptor blockers (peripheral), the β receptor blockers (peripheral), and the combination α_1 and β receptor blockers (peripheral).

The centrally acting α_2-adrenergic drugs clonidine, guanfacine, and methyldopa all act by modifying the function of the SNS. Because SNS stimulation leads to an increased heart rate and force of contraction, the constriction of blood vessels, and the release of renin from the kidney, the result is hypertension. The **centrally acting adrenergic drugs** work by stimulating the α_2-adrenergic receptors in the brain. The α_2-adrenergic receptors are unique in that receptor stimulation actually reduces sympathetic outflow, in this case from the central nervous system (CNS). The resulting lack of norepinephrine production reduces blood pressure. This stimulation of the α_2-adrenergic receptors also affects the kidneys, reducing the activity of renin. Renin is the hormone and enzyme that converts the protein precursor angiotensinogen to the protein angiotensin I, the precursor of angiotensin II (AII), a potent vasoconstrictor that raises blood pressure.

In the periphery the **α_1-blockers** doxazosin, prazosin, and terazosin also modify the function of the SNS. However, they do so by blocking the α_1-adrenergic receptors, which, when stimulated by circulating norepinephrine, produce increased blood pressure. Thus, when these receptors are blocked, blood pressure is decreased. The drug effects of the α_1-blockers are primarily related to their ability to dilate arteries and veins, which reduces peripheral vascular resistance and subsequently decreases blood pressure. This produces a marked decrease in the systemic and pulmonary venous pressures and an increase in cardiac output. The α_1-blockers also increase urinary flow rates and decrease outflow obstruction by preventing smooth muscle contractions in the bladder neck and urethra. This can be beneficial in cases of benign prostatic hypertrophy (BPH; see later).

The β-blockers also act in the periphery and include propranolol and atenolol as well as several other drugs. These drugs are discussed in more detail in Chapter 22 because they also have antidysrhythmic properties. Their antihypertensive effects are related to their reduction of the heart rate through β_1 receptor blockade. Furthermore, β-blockers also cause a reduction in the secretion of the hormone *renin* (see ACE inhibitors section), which in turn reduces both AII-mediated vasoconstriction and aldosterone-mediated volume expansion. Long-term use of β-blockers also reduces peripheral vascular resistance.

Two dual-action α_1 and β receptor blockers, which also act in the periphery at the heart and blood vessels, are currently available. These two drugs are labetalol and the newer medication carvedilol, which is growing in use. They have the dual antihypertensive effects of reduction in heart rate (β_1 receptor blockade) and vasodilation (α_1 receptor blockade). Figure 24-3 illustrates the site and mechanisms of action of the various antihypertensive drugs.

Indications

All of the drugs mentioned are used primarily for the treatment of hypertension, either alone or in combination with other antihypertensive drugs. Various forms of glaucoma may also respond to treatment by some of these drugs. Clonidine also has several unlabeled uses (not approved by the U.S. Food and Drug Administration [FDA] but still common), including prophylaxis against migraine headaches and the treatment of severe dysmenorrhea or menopausal flushing. It is also useful in the management of withdrawal symptoms in persons with opioid, nicotine, or alcohol dependency. The α_1-blockers doxazosin, prazosin, and terazosin have been used to relieve the symptoms associated with BPH. They have also proved effective in the management of severe

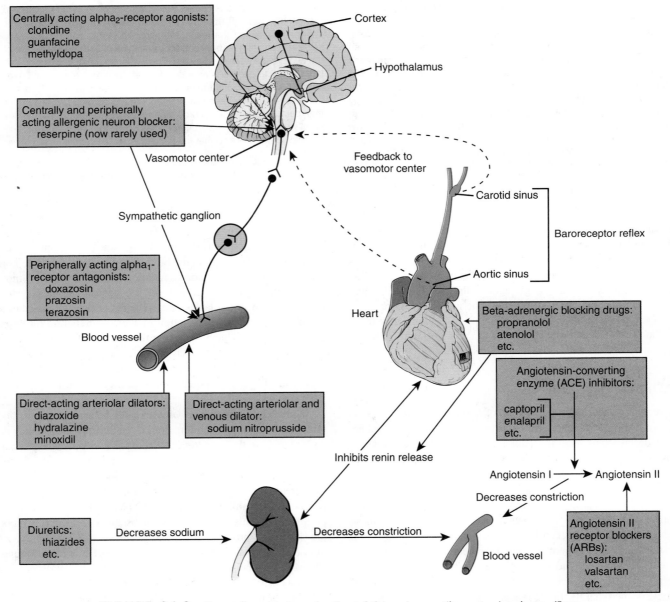

FIGURE 24-3 Site and mechanism of action of the various antihypertensive drugs. *(From U.S. Department of Health and Human Services: The seventh report of the Joint National Committee on Detection, Evaluation, and Treatment of High Blood Pressure (JNC-7), Washington, DC, 2003, National Institutes of Health. In Lewis SM, Heitkemper MM, Dirksen SR: Medical-surgical nursing: assessment and management of clinical problems, ed 6, St Louis, 2003, Mosby.)*

heart failure when used with cardiac glycosides (Chapter 21) and diuretics (Chapter 25).

Contraindications

Contraindications to the use of the adrenergic antihypertensive drugs include known drug allergy and may also include acute heart failure, concurrent use of monoamine oxidase inhibitors (Chapter 15), severe mental depression, peptic ulcer, colitis, and severe liver or kidney disease. Asthma may also be a contraindication to the use of any noncardioselective β-blocker (e.g., carvedilol). As mentioned in Chapter 21, the use of vasodilating drugs may also be contraindicated in cases of heart failure that is secondary to diastolic dysfunction.

Adverse Effects

Like all drug classes, adrenergic drugs can cause adverse effects. The most common adverse effects of these drugs are bradycardia with reflex tachycardia, postural and postexercise hypotension, dry mouth, drowsiness, sedation, dizziness, edema, constipation, and sexual dysfunction (e.g., impotence). Other effects include headaches, sleep disturbances, nausea, rash, peripheral pooling of blood, and cardiac disturbances such as palpitations. There is also a high incidence of **orthostatic hypotension** (a sudden drop in blood pressure during changes in position) in patients taking these drugs. This can even lead to a situation known as *first-dose syncope*, in which the hypotensive effect is severe enough to cause the patient to lose consciousness with even the first dose of medication. In addition, the abrupt discontinuation of the centrally acting α₂ receptor agonists can result in rebound hypertension. This may also be true for other antihypertensive drug classes, however. Nonselective drugs are also more commonly associated with bronchoconstriction (due to unrestrained parasympathetic tone) as well as metabolic inhibition of glycogenolysis in the liver, which can lead to hypoglycemia. However, hyperglycemic episodes are also among the adverse effects reported for this drug class. Any change in the dosing regimen for cardiovascular medications should be undertaken gradually and with appropriate patient monitoring and follow-up. Although the same is also true for most other classes of medications, abrupt dosage

changes of cardiovascular medications, either up or down, can be especially hazardous for the patient. Some of these drugs can also cause disruptions in blood count as well as in serum electrolyte levels and renal function. Periodic monitoring of white blood cell count, serum potassium and sodium levels, and urinary protein levels is recommended.

Interactions

Adrenergic drugs interact primarily with CNS depressants such as alcohol, benzodiazepines, and opioids. The additive effects of these combinations of drugs increase CNS depression. Terazosin can produce a reduced hematocrit reading. Other drug interactions that can occur with selected adrenergic drugs are summarized in Table 24-2. This list is merely representative and is not exhaustive. The nurse should always keep a drug information handbook available to check in cases in which a specific drug interaction is suspected.

Dosages

For information on the dosages of selected adrenergic antihypertensive drugs, see the Dosages table on page 374.

Drug Profiles

α₂-Adrenergic Receptor Stimulators (Agonists)

Of the three available α₂ receptor agonists—clonidine, guanfacine, and methyldopa—clonidine is by far the most commonly used and the prototypical drug for this class. Methyldopa is also used in the treatment of hypertension and is the drug of choice for treating hypertension in pregnancy. However, these drugs are not typically prescribed as first-line antihypertensive drugs because their use is associated with a high incidence of unwanted adverse effects such as orthostatic hypotension, fatigue, and dizziness. They may be used as adjunct drugs in the treatment of hypertension after other drugs have failed or may be used in conjunction with other antihypertensives such as diuretics.

▶ clonidine

Clonidine (Catapres) is used primarily for its ability to decrease blood pressure. As previously noted, clonidine is also useful in the management of opioid withdrawal. It has a better safety profile than the other centrally acting adrenergics and has the advantage of being available in several dosage formulations, including both topical and

Table 24-2 Adrenergic Drugs: Drug Interactions

Drug	Interacts with	Mechanism	Result
clonidine	Opioids, sedatives, hypnotics, anesthetics, alcohol	Additive	Increased CNS depression
	TCAs, MAOIs, appetite suppressants, amphetamines	Opposing actions	Decreased hypotensive effects
	Diuretics, nitrates, other antihypertensive drugs	Additive	Increased hypotensive effects
	β-blockers	Additive	May potentiate bradycardia and increase the rebound hypertension in clonidine withdrawal
guanfacine	Diuretics, other antihypertensive drugs	Additive	Increased hypotensive effects
	TCAs, ephedrine	Opposing effects	Decreased hypotensive effect
prazosin	Diuretics, other hypotensive drugs	Additive	Increased hypotension
	indomethacin	Opposing effects	Decreased hypotensive effect
	verapamil	Increased serum prazosin levels	Increased hypotension

CNS, Central nervous system; MAOIs, monoamine oxidase inhibitors; TCAs, tricyclic antidepressants.

DOSAGES

Selected Antihypertensive Drugs: Adrenergic Agonist and Antagonists

Drug (Pregnancy Category)	Pharmacologic Class	Usual Dosage Range	Indications
carvedilol (Coreg) (C)	Peripherally acting α_1, β_1, and β_2 receptor antagonist (blocker)	PO: 3.125-25 mg bid	Hypertension (also used in heart failure)
▶clonidine (Catapres, Catapres-TTS) (C)	Centrally acting α_2 receptor agonist	PO: Initial dose 0.1 mg daily-bid; may titrate up to a maximum of 2.4 mg/day, divided bid-qid. Transdermal patch: 0.1, 0.2, or 0.3 mg/24 hr, applied weekly	Hypertension (may have other unlabeled uses including treatment of psychiatric, cardiovascular, and gastrointestinal problems)
prazosin (Minipress) (C)	Peripherally acting α_1 receptor antagonist	PO: Initial dose 1 mg bid-tid; may titrate up to maximum of 20 mg/day, divided bid-qid	Hypertension

PO, Oral.

oral preparations. Clonidine should not be discontinued abruptly because this will lead to severe rebound hypertension. Its use is contraindicated in patients who have shown hypersensitivity reactions to it. See the table on this page for recommended dosages.

Pharmacokinetics

Half-Life	Onset	Peak	Duration
6-20 hr	30-60 min	3-5 hr	8 hr

α_1-Blockers

The α_1-blockers are doxazosin (Cardura), prazosin (Minipress), tamsulosin (Flomax), and terazosin (Hytrin). They are the newest of the adrenergics and have the best safety and efficacy profiles, but they are not free of adverse effects. Their use is contraindicated in patients who have shown a hypersensitivity to them. They are classified as pregnancy category C drugs. They are available only as oral preparations. Tamsulosin is not used to control blood pressure but is indicated solely for symptomatic control of BPH. This use is described further in Chapter 34.

prazosin

Prazosin (Minipress) is the oldest of the α_1-blockers and the prototype for this drug class. It reduces both peripheral vascular resistance and blood pressure by dilating both arterial and venous blood vessels. It has been shown to be beneficial in the treatment of hypertension, the relief of the symptoms of obstructive BPH, and as an adjunct to cardiac glycosides and diuretics in the treatment of severe heart failure. Recommended dosages are given in the table on this page.

Pharmacokinetics

Half-Life	Onset	Peak	Duration
2-3 hr	2 hr	1-3 hr	10 hr

Dual-Action α_1 and β Receptor Blockers
carvedilol

Carvedilol (Coreg), was approved by the FDA in 1995. At the present time its use in the ambulatory care setting is growing, and it seems to be well tolerated by most patients. In addition to hypertension, it is also indicated for mild to moderate heart failure in conjunction with digoxin, diuretics, and ACE inhibitors. Its contraindications include known drug allergy, cardiogenic shock, severe bradycardia or heart failure, bronchospastic conditions such as asthma, and various cardiac problems involving the conduction system. Dosage information appears in the table on this page.

Pharmacokinetics

Half-Life	Onset	Peak	Duration
IV: 6-8 hr	IV: 2-5 hr	IV: 5-15 min	IV: 2-4 hr
PO: 7-10 hr	PO: 1-2 hr	PO: 1-2 hr	PO: Unknown

ANGIOTENSIN-CONVERTING ENZYME INHIBITORS

The ACE inhibitors are a large group of antihypertensive drugs. There are currently 10 ACE inhibitors available for clinical use, in addition to various combination drug products in which a thiazide diuretic or a CCB is combined with an ACE inhibitor. The available ACE inhibitors are captopril (Capoten), benazepril (Lotensin), enalapril (Vasotec), fosinopril (Menopril), lisinopril (Prinivil, Zestril), moexipril (Univasc), perindopril (Aceon), quinapril (Accupril), ramipril (Altace), and trandolapril (Mavik). These drugs are very safe and efficacious and are often used as the first-line drugs in the treatment of both heart failure and hypertension. Some of the distinguishing characteristics of the various drugs that make up this large class of antihypertensives are summarized in Table 24-3. The ACE inhibitors as a class are very similar and differ in only a few of their chemical properties, but there are some significant differences among them in their clinical properties. Knowing these differences can help the practitioner select the proper drug for a particular patient.

Captopril has the shortest half-life and therefore must be dosed more frequently than any of the other ACE inhibitors. This may be an important drawback to its use in a patient who has a history of being noncompliant with his or her medication therapy. On the other hand, it may be best to start with a drug that has a short half-life in a patient who is still very critically ill and may not tolerate medications well, so that if problems arise they will be short lived. Both captopril and enalapril can be dosed multiple times a day.

Captopril and lisinopril are the only two ACE inhibitors that are not prodrugs. A **prodrug** is a drug that is inactive in its administered form and must be biotransformed in the liver to its active form to be effective. This characteristic of captopril and lisinopril is an important advantage in treating a patient with liver dysfunction; because all of the other ACE inhibitors are prodrugs, their transformation to active form in such patients is hindered.

Enalapril is the only ACE inhibitor that is available in a parenteral preparation. All other drugs are available only in oral formulations. All of the newer ACE inhibitors, such as benazepril, fosinopril, lisinopril, quinapril, and ramipril, have long half-lives and long durations of action, which allows them to be given only once a day. This is particularly beneficial for a patient who is

Table 24-3   ACE Inhibitors: Distinguishing Characteristics

Generic Name	Trade Name	Combination with Hydrochlorothiazide	Dosing Schedule	Route	Prodrug
benazepril	Lotensin	Lotensin HCT	Once a day	PO	Yes
captopril	Capoten	Capozide 25/15 and 25/25, Capozide 50/15 and 50/25	Multiple	PO	No
enalapril	Vasotec	Vaseretic	Multiple	PO/IV	Yes
fosinopril	Monopril	None		PO	Yes
lisinopril	Prinivil	Prinzide 12.5 and 25		PO	No
	Zestril	Zestoretic 12.5 and 25	Once a day	PO	No
moexipril	Univasc	None		PO	Yes
					Yes
perindopril	Aceon	None	Once to twice daily	PO	Yes
quinapril	Accupril	None		PO	
ramipril	Altace	None		PO	
trandolapril	Mavik	None	Once a day	PO	Yes

ACE, Angiotensin-converting enzyme; IV, Intravenous; PO, oral.

taking many other medications and may have difficulty keeping track of the various dosing schedules for each. A once-a-day medication regimen promotes better patient compliance.

All ACE inhibitors have detrimental effects on the unborn fetus and neonate. They are classified as pregnancy category C drugs for women in their first trimester and as pregnancy category D drugs for women in their second or third trimester. ACE inhibitors should be used by pregnant women only if there are no safer alternatives. Fetal and neonatal morbidity and mortality have been reported to have occurred in at least 50 cases in which women received ACE inhibitors during their pregnancies.

Many of the ACE inhibitors are combined with either a diuretic or a CCB. The advantage of such combination products is convenience. Often an individual with hypertension or heart failure must take many medications, including an ACE inhibitor, to control high blood pressure. Combination products are beneficial because they lead to greater patient compliance and decrease number of medications that must be taken. Examples of new combination ACE inhibitor–CCB products are benazepril and amlodipine (Lotrel); enalapril and diltiazem (Teczem); and trandolapril and verapamil (Tarka).

Mechanism of Action and Drug Effects

As is often the case with pharmaceutical innovations, the development of the ACE inhibitors was spurred by the discovery of an animal substance found to have beneficial effects in humans. This particular substance was the venom of a South American viper, which was found to inhibit kininase activity. Kininase is an enzyme that normally breaks down bradykinin, a potent vasodilator in the human body.

The ACE inhibitors have several beneficial cardiovascular effects. As their name implies, they inhibit angiotensin-converting enzyme, which is responsible for converting AI (formed through the action of renin) to AII. AII is a potent vasoconstrictor and induces aldosterone secretion by the adrenal glands. Aldosterone stimulates sodium and water resorption, which can raise blood pressure. Together, these processes are referred to as the renin-angiotensin-aldosterone system.

The primary effects of the ACE inhibitors are cardiovascular and renal. Their cardiovascular effects are due to their ability to reduce blood pressure by decreasing SVR. They do this by pre-venting the breakdown of the vasodilating substance bradykinin, and also substance P (another potent vasodilator), and preventing the formation of AII. These combined effects decrease afterload, or the resistance against which the left ventricle must pump to eject its volume of blood during contraction. The ACE inhibitors are beneficial in the treatment of heart failure because they prevent sodium and water resorption by inhibiting aldosterone secretion. This causes diuresis, which decreases blood volume and return to the heart. This in turn decreases preload, or the left ventricular end-diastolic volume, and the work required of the heart.

Indications

The therapeutic effects of the ACE inhibitors are related to their potent cardiovascular effects. They are excellent antihypertensives and adjunctive drugs for the treatment of heart failure. They may be used alone or in combination with other drugs such as diuretics in the treatment of hypertension or heart failure.

The beneficial hemodynamic effects of the ACE inhibitors have been studied extensively. Because of their ability to decrease SVR (a measure of afterload) and preload, ACE inhibitors can stop the progression of left ventricular hypertrophy, which is sometimes seen after a myocardial infarction (MI). This pathologic process is known as *ventricular remodeling*. The ability of ACE inhibitors to prevent it is termed a *cardioprotective effect*. ACE inhibitors have been shown to decrease morbidity and mortality rates in patients with heart failure. They should be considered the drugs of choice for hypertensive patients with heart failure. ACE inhibitors have also have been shown to have a protective effect on the kidneys, because they reduce glomerular filtration pressure. This is one reason that they are among the cardiovascular drugs of choice for diabetic patients. The various therapeutic effects of the ACE inhibitors are listed in Table 24-4, which lists the body substances on which ACE inhibitors act and the resulting beneficial hemodynamic effects.

Contraindications

Contraindications to the use of ACE inhibitors include known drug allergy, especially a previous reaction of angioedema (laryngeal swelling) to an ACE inhibitor. Patients with a baseline potassium level of 5 mEq/L or higher may not be suitable candidates for ACE inhibitor therapy because these drugs can promote hyperkalemia

Table 24-4 ACE Inhibitors: Therapeutic Effects

Body Substance	Effect in Body	ACE Inhibitor Action	Resulting Hemodynamic Effect
Aldosterone	Causes sodium and water retention	Prevents its secretion	Diuresis = ↓ plasma volume = ↓ filling pressures or ↓ preload
Angiotensin II	Potent vasoconstrictor	Prevents its formation	↓ SVR = ↓ afterload
Bradykinin	Potent vasodilator	Prevents its breakdown	↓ SVR = ↓ afterload

↓, Decreased; *ACE*, angiotensin converting enzyme; *SVR*, systemic vascular resistance.

DOSAGES

Selected Antihypertensive Drugs: ACE Inhibitors and Angiotensin II Receptor Blockers

Drug (Pregnancy Category)	Pharmacologic Class	Usual Dosage Range	Indications
▶captopril (Capoten, Capozide*) (C, first trimester; D, second and third trimesters)		**Adult** PO: 25-150 mg bid-tid PO: Usual dosage 1-2 tabs/day or more based on the ratio of the two drugs*	Hypertension, heart failure Hypertension
enalapril (Vasotec, Vaseretic*) (C, first trimester; D, second and third trimesters)	ACE inhibitor	**Adult** PO: 10-40 mg/day as a single dose or in 2 equal doses PO: 20-50 mg/day as a single dose with digoxin and diuretic IV: 1.25 mg q6h over a 5-min period PO: Usual dose 1-2 tabs/day	Hypertension Heart failure Hypertension
▶losartan (Cozaar) (C, first trimester; D, second and third trimesters) valsartan (Diovan) (C, first trimester; D, second and third trimesters)	Angiotensin II receptor blocker	**Adult** PO: 25-100 mg in 1-2 doses **Adult** PO: 80-320 mg in a single dose	Hypertension, heart failure

ACE, Angiotensin-converting enzyme; *IV*, intravenous; *PO*, oral.
*Fixed-combination tablet with hydrochlorothiazide.

(see later). All ACE inhibitors are contraindicated in lactating women, children, and patients with bilateral renal artery stenosis.

Adverse Effects

Major CNS effects of the ACE inhibitors include fatigue, dizziness, mood changes, and headaches. A characteristic dry, nonproductive cough is reversible with discontinuation of the therapy. A first-dose hypotensive effect can cause a significant decline in blood pressure. Other adverse effects include loss of taste, proteinuria, hyperkalemia, rash, pruritus, anemia, neutropenia, thrombocytosis, and agranulocytosis. In patients with severe heart failure whose renal function may depend on the activity of the renin-angiotensin-aldosterone system, treatment with ACE inhibitors may cause acute renal failure. ACE inhibitors tend to promote potassium resorption in the kidney, although they also promote sodium excretion due to their reduction of aldosterone secretion. For this reason, serum potassium levels should be monitored regularly. This is especially true when there is concurrent therapy with potassium-sparing diuretics, although many patients tolerate both types of drug therapy with no major problems. One rare, but potentially fatal, adverse effect is *angioedema*. This is a strong vascular reaction involving inflammation of submucosal tissues, which can progress to anaphylaxis.

Toxicity and Management of Overdose

The most pronounced symptom of an overdose of an ACE inhibitor is hypotension. Treatment is symptomatic and supportive and includes the administration of intravenous fluids to expand the blood volume. Hemodialysis is effective for the removal of captopril and lisinopril.

Interactions

Nonsteroidal antiinflammatory drugs can reduce the antihypertensive effect of ACE inhibitors. Concurrent use of ACE inhibitors and other antihypertensives or diuretics can have hypotensive effects. Giving lithium and ACE inhibitors together can result in lithium toxicity. Potassium supplements and potassium-sparing diuretics, when administered with ACE inhibitors, may result in hyperkalemia. As noted earlier, monitoring of serum potassium levels becomes especially important in these cases. Acetone may be falsely detected in the urine of patients taking captopril.

Dosages

For information on the dosages for selected ACE inhibitors, see the Dosages table on this page.

Drug Profiles

▶ captopril

Captopril (Capoten) was the first ACE inhibitor to become available and is considered the prototypical drug for the class. Several large multicenter studies have shown its clinical efficacy in minimizing or preventing the left ventricular dilation and dysfunction (also called *ventricular remodeling*) that can arise in the acute period after an MI and thereby improving the patient's chances of survival. It can also reduce the risk of heart failure in these patients and thus the need for subsequent hospitalizations for the treatment of heart failure. Because it has the shortest half-life of all of the currently available ACE inhibitors, captopril is an excellent drug to give to hospitalized patients who are in a fragile condition but need afterload and preload reduction. This reduction will decrease the workload of a failing heart. A very-long-acting drug may reduce the hemodynamic parameters too much and have lingering effects for which it may be difficult to compensate acutely. Recommended dosages are given in the table on page 376.

Pharmacokinetics

Half-Life	Onset	Peak	Duration
Less than 2 hr	15 min	1-2 hr	2-6 hr

enalapril

Enalapril (Vasotec, Vaseretic) is the only currently marketed ACE inhibitor that is available in both oral and parenteral preparations. The parenteral formulation (enalaprilat) is an active drug. It offers the hemodynamic benefit of inhibiting ACE activity in an acutely ill patient who cannot tolerate oral medications. Although its half-life is slightly longer than that of captopril, it may in some instances still have to be given twice a day. The oral form of enalapril differs from captopril in that it is a prodrug, and the patient must have a functioning liver for the drug to be converted into its active form. Like captopril, it has been shown in many large studies to improve a patient's chances of survival after an MI and to reduce the incidence of heart failure and the need for subsequent hospitalizations for the treatment of heart failure in these patients. Recommended dosages are given in the table on page 376.

Pharmacokinetics

Half-Life	Onset	Peak	Duration
PO: Less than 2 hr	PO: 1 hr	PO: 4-6 hr	PO: 12-24 hr

ANGIOTENSIN II RECEPTOR BLOCKERS

ARBs are one of the newest classes of antihypertensives. Losartan (Cozaar), eprosartan (Teveten), valsartan (Diovan), irbesartan (Avapro), candesartan (Atacand), olmesartan (Benicar), and telmisartan (Micardis) are all ARBs.

Mechanism of Action and Drug Effects

ARBs block the binding of AII to type 1 AII receptors. ACE inhibitors such as enalapril block conversion of AI to AII, but AII also may be formed by other enzymes that are not blocked by ACE inhibitors. For comparison, recall that ACE inhibitors block the breakdown of bradykinins and substance P, which accumulate and may cause adverse effects such as cough but might also contribute to the drugs' antihypertensive and cardiac and nephroprotective effects. Bradykinins are potent vasodilators and help to reduce blood pressure by dilating arteries and decreasing SVR.

In contrast to ACE inhibitors, ARBs affect primarily vascular smooth muscle and the adrenal gland. By selectively blocking the binding of AII to the type 1 AII receptors in these tissues, ARBs block vasoconstriction and the secretion of aldosterone. AII receptors have been found in other tissues throughout the body, but the effects of ARB blocking of these receptors is unknown.

Clinically, ACE inhibitors and ARBs appear to be equally effective for the treatment of hypertension. Both are well tolerated, but ARBs do not cause cough. There is evidence that ARBs are better tolerated and have lower mortality (after MI) than ACE inhibitors. It is not yet clear whether ARBs are as effective as ACE inhibitors in treating heart failure (cardioprotective effects); or in protecting the kidneys, as in diabetes. Both types of drugs are contraindicated for use in the second or third trimester of pregnancy. Whether one or more of these drugs, particularly the newer drugs, could prove to have unique adverse effects with long-term use is unknown.

Indications

The therapeutic effects of ARBs are related to their potent vasodilating properties. They are excellent antihypertensives and adjunctive drugs for the treatment of heart failure. They may be used alone or in combination with other drugs such as diuretics in the treatment of hypertension or heart failure. The beneficial hemodynamic effect of ARBs is their ability to decrease SVR (a measure of afterload). Their use is rapidly growing, and more and more studies are verifying their beneficial effects. Currently these drugs are used primarily in patients who have been intolerant of ACE inhibitors.

Contraindications

The only usual contraindications to the use of ARBs are known drug allergy, pregnancy, and lactation. ARBs such as losartan should be used very cautiously in elderly patients and in patients with renal dysfunction because of increased sensitivity to its effects and risk for more adverse effects in these patients. As with other antihypertensives, blood pressure and apical pulse rate should be assessed before and during drug therapy.

Adverse Effects

The most common adverse effects of ARBs are upper respiratory infections and headache. Occasionally dizziness, inability to sleep, diarrhea, dyspnea, heartburn, nasal congestion, back pain, and fatigue can occur. Rarely, anxiety, muscle pain, sinusitis, cough, and insomnia can also occur. Hyperkalemia is also much less likely to occur as compared with the ACE inhibitors.

Toxicity and Management of Overdose

Overdose may manifest as hypotension and tachycardia; bradycardia occurs less often. Treatment is symptomatic and supportive and includes the administration of intravenous fluids to expand the blood volume.

Interactions

ARBs can interact with cimetidine, phenobarbital, and rifampin. The drugs that interact with ARBs, the mechanism responsible, and the result of the interaction are summarized in Table 24-5. In addition, as is the case with ACE inhibitors, ARBs can promote hyperkalemia, especially when taken concurrently with potassium supplements (although this occurs much less frequently than with ACE inhibitors). However, patients' individual chemistry varies widely, and so monitoring of the serum potassium level

Table 24-5	Angiotensin II Receptor Blockers (ARBs): Drug Interactions	
Drug	**Mechanism**	**Result**
cimetidine	Competes for metabolism	Increased ARB effect
lithium	Inhibits lithium elimination	Increased lithium concentrations
phenobarbital, rifampin	Increase metabolism	Decreased ARB effect

is necessary for each patient. Potassium supplements may still be indicated for those patients with a tendency toward hypokalemia (whether acute or chronic).

Dosages

For information on the dosages for selected ARBs, see the table on page 376.

Drug Profile

▸ **losartan**

Losartan (Cozaar, Hyzaar) therapy has been shown to be beneficial in patients with hypertension and heart failure. More and more studies are showing the beneficial effects of ARBs, including losartan, in the treatment of heart failure. These studies indicate that ARBs are better tolerated and produce a marginally lower mortality rate (after MI) than treatment with ACE inhibitors.

The use of losartan is contraindicated in patients who are hypersensitive to any component of this product. It should be used with caution in patients with renal or hepatic dysfunction and in patients with renal artery stenosis. Breast-feeding women should not take losartan, because it can cause serious adverse effects on the nursing infant. Recommended dosages are given in the table on page 376.

Pharmacokinetics

Half-Life	Onset	Peak	Duration
6-9 hr	Unknown	3-4 hr	24 hr

CALCIUM CHANNEL BLOCKERS

CCBs have been discussed in some detail in the two previous chapters on antidysrhythmic drugs (Chapter 22) and antianginal drugs (Chapter 23). As a class of medications, they are used for several indications and have many beneficial effects and relatively few adverse effects. CCBs are primarily used for the treatment of hypertension and angina. Their effectiveness in treating hypertension is related to their ability to cause smooth muscle relaxation by blocking the binding of calcium to its receptors, which thereby preventing contraction. Because of their effectiveness and safety, they have been added to the list of first-line drugs for the treatment of hypertension. CCBs are used for many other indications as well. They are effective antidysrhythmics and they can prevent the cerebral artery spasms that can occur after a subarachnoid hemorrhage (nimodipine). They are also sometimes used in the treatment of Raynaud's disease and migraine headache.

DIURETICS

The diuretics are a highly effective class of antihypertensive drugs. They are listed as the current first-line antihypertensives in the *JNC-7* guidelines for the treatment of hypertension. They may be used as monotherapy (single-drug therapy) or in combination with drugs of other antihypertensive classes. Their primary therapeutic effect is decreasing the plasma and extracellular fluid volumes, which results in decreased preload. This leads to a decrease in cardiac output and total peripheral resistance, all of which decrease the workload of the heart. This large group of antihypertensives is discussed in detail in Chapter 25. The thiazide diuretics (e.g., hydrochlorothiazide) are the most commonly used diuretics for hypertension.

VASODILATORS

Vasodilators act directly on arteriolar and/or venous smooth muscle to cause relaxation. They do not work through adrenergic receptors. Some vasodilators (intravenous diazoxide and sodium nitroprusside) are particularly useful in the management of hypertensive emergencies when the blood pressure is severely, or even only moderately, elevated. However, there is a threat of end-organ damage, particularly in the brain, heart, or eyes.

Mechanism of Action and Drug Effects

The particular mechanism of action of the direct-acting vasodilators that makes them useful as antihypertensive drugs is their ability to directly elicit peripheral vasodilation. This results in a reduction in SVR. In general, the most notable effect of the vasodilators is their hypotensive effect. However, in recent years minoxidil (in its topical form) has also received increasing attention because of its effectiveness in restoring hair growth. This is described further in Chapter 57. Oral diazoxide has also proved to have significant antihypoglycemic effects. Diazoxide, hydralazine, and minoxidil work primarily through arteriolar vasodilation, whereas nitroprusside has both arteriolar and venous effects.

Indications

All of the vasodilators can be used to treat hypertension, either alone or in combination with other antihypertensives. Diazoxide is also an antihypoglycemic when administered orally. Sodium nitroprusside and intravenous diazoxide are reserved for the management of hypertensive emergencies. Minoxidil in its topical form is used to restore hair growth.

Contraindications

Contraindications include known drug allergy and may also include hypotension, cerebral edema, head injury, acute MI, and coronary artery disease.

As mentioned in Chapter 21, vasodilating drugs may also be contraindicated in cases of heart failure that is secondary to diastolic dysfunction.

Adverse Effects

Undesirable effects of diazoxide include dizziness, headache, orthostatic hypotension, dysrhythmias, sodium and water retention, nausea, vomiting, acute pancreatitis (rare), and hyperglycemia in diabetic patients. The adverse effects of hydralazine include dizziness, headache, anxiety, tachycardia, edema, nasal congestion, dyspnea, anorexia, nausea, vomiting, diarrhea, anemia, agranulocytosis, hepatitis, peripheral neuritis, systemic lupus erythematosus (SLE), and rash. Minoxidil adverse effects include T-wave electrocardiographic changes, pericardial effusion or tamponade, angina, breast tenderness, rash, and thrombocytopenia. Sodium nitroprusside effects include bradycardia, decreased platelet aggregation, rash, hypothyroidism, hypotension, methemoglobinemia, and, rarely, cyanide toxicity. Cyanide ions are a byproduct of nitroprusside metabolism. However, most drug dosages do not produce a large enough number of these ions to cause any serious effects.

Toxicity and Management of Overdose

The main symptom of diazoxide overdose or toxicity is hypotension, which can usually be controlled by placing the patient's bed in the Trendelenburg position. Sympathomimetics such as dopamine or norepinephrine may also be required. Hydralazine toxicity or overdose produces hypotension, tachycardia, headache, and generalized skin flushing. Treatment is supportive and symptomatic and includes the administration of intravenous fluids, digitalization if needed, and the administration of β-blockers for the control of tachycardia.

Minoxidil overdose or toxicity can precipitate excessive hypotension. Treatment is supportive and symptomatic and includes the administration of intravenous fluids. Norepinephrine and epinephrine should not be used to reverse the hypotension because of the possibility of causing excessive cardiac stimulation.

The main symptom of sodium nitroprusside overdose or toxicity is excessive hypotension. This drug is normally administered only to patients receiving intensive care. Under these conditions the infusion rate is usually carefully titrated to immediately visible results on a cardiovascular monitor that provides constant measurements of blood pressure from centrally placed venous or arterial catheters. For this reason excessive hypotension is usually avoidable. When it does occur, discontinuation of the infusion has an immediate effect because the drug is metabolized very rapidly (half-life of 10 minutes). Treatment for the hypotension is supportive and symptomatic; if necessary, pressor drugs can be infused to quickly raise blood pressure. The chemical structure of nitroprusside does contain cyanide groups, which are released upon its metabolism in the body and can theoretically result in cyanide toxicity, although this author has never observed or heard of such a case in his many years of hospital experience. Should this unlikely event occur, treatment can be administered using a standard cyanide antidote kit that includes sodium nitrite and sodium thiosulfate for injection and amyl nitrite for inhalation. However, the usual release of cyanide ions that accompanies therapy with this drug rarely, if ever, reaches sufficient concentration to paralyze respirations, as can be the case with occupational or wartime exposure to cyanide.

Interactions

Although the incidence of drug interactions with the direct-acting vasodilators (especially sodium nitroprusside) is low, as a class of drugs they are associated with a variety of drug interactions. These are summarized in Table 24-6.

Dosages

For dosage information for selected vasodilator drugs, see the Dosages table on page 380.

Table 24-6 Direct-Acting Vasodilators: Drug Interactions

Drug	Mechanism	Result
Diazoxide		
Antihypertensives/ thiazides	Additive effects	Increased hypotensive and hyperglycemic effects
hydralazine	Additive effects	Increased hypotensive effect
Oral anticoagulants	Protein storage displacement	Increased anticoagulant effect
Sulfonylureas	Hyperglycemic effect	Decreased hypoglycemic effect of sulfonylureas
Hydralazine		
Adrenergics	Antagonism	Decreased hypotensive effect
Antihypertensives	Additive effects	Increased hypotensive effect
Monoamine oxidase inhibitors	Alteration of biotransformation	Increased hypotensive effect
Minoxidil		
Antihypertensives/ thiazides	Additive effects	Increased hypotensive effect
guanethidine	Additive effects	Significant hypotensive effect
Sodium Nitroprusside		
Ganglionic blocking drugs	Additive effects	Increased hypotensive effect

Drug Profiles

▶ *hydralazine hydrochloride*

Hydralazine (Apresoline) is less commonly used now than when it first became available, but it is still effective for selected patients. It can be taken orally to treat routine cases of **essential hypertension** and it is also available in injectable form for hypertensive emergencies. However, its currently listed contraindications, in addition to drug allergy, include coronary artery disease and mitral valve dysfunction, such as that related to childhood rheumatic fever. A new combination drug product tablet includes both 37.5 mg of hydralazine and 20 mg of the antianginal drug isosorbide dinitrate (Chapter 23). This drug combination is known as BiDil, and it is specifically indicated as an adjunct for treatment of heart failure in self-identified black patients. This drug combination has been shown to improve patient survival and prolong time to hospitalization for heart failure in black patient populations. See the table on page 380 for dosage information.

Pharmacokinetics

Half-Life	Onset	Peak	Duration
IV: 1-2 hr	IV: 5-20 min	IV: 30-45 min	IV: 2-4 hr
PO: 3-7 hr	PO: 20-30 min	PO: 1-2 hr	PO: 6-12 hr

DOSAGES

Selected Antihypertensive Drugs: Vasodilators

Drug (Pregnancy Category)	Pharmacologic Class	Usual Dosage Range	Indications
diazoxide (Hyperstat) (C)		**Pediatric and adult** IV: 1-3 mg/kg repeated at 5-15 min intervals; maintenance doses can be given at 4-24 hr intervals if required (max of 150 mg/dose)	Acute hypertension
▶hydralazine hydrochloride (Apresoline) (C)		**Pediatric** PO: 0.75-7.5 mg/kg/day to a max of 200 mg/day **Adult** PO: 10 mg qid for 2-4 days, followed by 25 mg qid for balance of week; second and subsequent weeks 50 mg qid, then adjust to lowest effective dose for maintenance IV: 20-40 mg prn	
	Direct-acting peripheral vasodilator		Hypertension
minoxidil (Loniten) (C)		**Pediatric younger than 12 yr** PO: 0.25-1 mg/kg/day usually as a single dose; do not exceed 50 mg/day **Pediatric older than 12 yr and adult** PO: 10-40 mg/day as a single dose or divided; do not exceed 100 mg/day	
sodium nitroprusside (Nipride, Nitropress) (C)		**Pediatric and adult** IV: 0.3-10 mcg/kg/min	

IV, Intravenous; *PO,* oral.

sodium nitroprusside

Sodium nitroprusside (Nitropress), like diazoxide, is normally used in the intensive care setting for severe hypertensive emergencies and is titrated to effect by intravenous infusion. Its use is contraindicated in patients with a known hypersensitivity to it and in those with the compensatory hypertension associated with coarctation or arteriovenous shunt, congenital Leber's optic atrophy, or tobacco amblyopia (both of which may predispose the patient to cyanide toxicity), severe heart failure, and known inadequate cerebral perfusion (especially during neurosurgical procedures). Because of the risk for cyanide toxicity at maximal dosages (up to 10 mcg/kg/min) for extended periods, its use at such dosages is limited to no longer than 10 minutes. See the table on this page for dosage information.

Pharmacokinetics

Half-Life	Onset	Peak	Duration
2 min	Less than 2 min	2-5 min	1-10 min

MISCELLANEOUS ANTIHYPERTENSIVE DRUGS

Drug Profiles

Three newer medications exemplify some of the most recent antihypertensive drugs to be made available in the United States. These include eplerenone, bosentan, and treprostinil. All three of these drugs are currently indicated for adult use only.

eplerenone

Eplerenone (Inspra) is currently the only drug in a new class of antihypertensive drugs. It reduces blood pressure by blocking the actions of the hormone aldosterone at its corresponding receptors in the kidney, heart, blood vessels, and brain. Eplerenone is indicated for both routine treatment of hypertension and for post-MI heart failure. Its use is contraindicated in patients with known drug allergy, elevated serum potassium levels (higher than 5.5 mEq/L), or severe renal impairment and those using a medication that inhibits the action of the cytochrome P-450 enzyme CYP3A4. Many commonly used medications inhibit the action of this enzyme, including several antibiotic, antifungal, and antiviral drugs. Practitioners are advised to review the known drug interactions of all of their patient's concurrent used drugs before administering this medication. Recommended dosages are given in the Dosages table on page 381.

bosentan

Bosentan (Tracleer) is also currently the single drug in a new drug class and works by blocking the receptors of the hormone endothelin. Normally this hormone acts to stimulate the narrowing of blood vessels by binding to endothelin receptors (ET_A and ET_B) in the endothelial (innermost) lining of blood vessels and in vascular smooth muscle. Bosentan reduces blood pressure by blocking this action. However, currently its use is specifically indicated only for pulmonary artery hypertension in patients with moderate to severe heart failure. Its use is contraindicated in patients with known drug allergy, pregnancy, or significant liver impairment, and in patients receiving concurrent drug therapy with cyclosporine or glyburide. Recommended dosages are given in the table on page 381.

treprostinil

Treprostinil (Remodulin) lowers blood pressure through a combined mechanism of action by dilating both pulmonary and systemic blood vessels and by inhibiting platelet aggregation. Like

DOSAGES

Miscellaneous Antihypertensive Drugs

Drug (Pregnancy Category)	Pharmacologic Class	Usual Dosage Range	Indications
bosentan (Tracleer) (X)	Endothelin receptor antagonist	**Adult only** PO: Initial dose of 62.5 mg bid × 4 wk, then increase as tolerated to maintenance dose of 125 mg bid	Pulmonary artery hypertension in patients with moderate to severe heart failure
eplerenone (Inspra) (B)	Aldosterone receptor antagonist	**Adult only** PO: Initial dose of 25 mg once daily × 4 wk, then increase as tolerated to maintenance dose of 50 mg daily	Hypertension and to improve post-MI survival in patients with stable heart failure
treprostinil (Remodulin) (B)	Vasodilator and platelet aggregation inhibitor	**Adult only** Continuous subcutaneous infusion: 0.625-2.5 ng/kg/min	Pulmonary artery hypertension in severe heart failure

MI, Myocardial infarction; *PO,* oral.

LABORATORY VALUES RELATED TO DRUG THERAPY

Sodium Nitroprusside

Laboratory Test	Normal Ranges	Rationale for Assessment
Serum methemoglobin and serum cyanide	Normally there are no values with appropriate drug levels of sodium nitroprusside	Use of sodium nitroprusside may be associated with sequestion of hemoglobin (Hgb) as methemoglobin. The appearance of this clinically significant adverse effect of methemoglobinemia is rare (>10%). Patients receiving this drug at the maximum rate of 10 mcg/kg/min would take 16 or more hours to reach a total accumulated dose of 10 mg/kg, so serum laboratory testing is used to measure the amount of methemglobin. Significant clinical signs of this adverse effect include impaired oxygen delivery despite adequate cardiac output. When the sequestion is diagnosed, the treatment of choice is 1 to 2 mg/kg of methylene blue given intravenously over several minutes to allow binding of the metabolic byproduct of cyanide to methemoglobin as cyanmethemoglobin, but this should only be given as ordered and with extreme caution. In addition, sodium nitroprusside may lead to toxic reactions, even with doses that are within recommended dosage ranges; toxic reactions are evident by extreme hypotension, cyanide toxicity, or thiocyanate toxicity. Cyanide level assays are performed to detect if cyanide levels are in body fluids, but this is a difficult test to interpret and so not the most reliable method of monitoring. Other laboratory tests that may prove to be helpful in diagnosing cyanide toxicity include alterations of acid-base balance and venous oxygen concentrations. Actual cyanide levels in the blood may lag behind peak cyanide levels by an hour or more. Signs of thiocyanate toxicity include ringing of the ears (tinnitus), miosis, and hyperreflexia as well as methemoglobinemia.

bosentan, treprostinil is indicated specifically for pulmonary artery hypertension in patients with moderate to severe heart failure. Its only current contraindication is known drug allergy. It is also unique to date in being the only drug diluted to the nanogram level for administration. Recommended dosages are given in the table on this page.

◆ NURSING PROCESS

As mentioned earlier, a variety of drugs are used to treat hypertension. Although much of the nursing process related to their use is similar for all these drugs, there are some considerations very specific to the use of each particular drug class. Therefore, both general and specific information on these drugs and drug groups is presented.

It is also important for the nurse to understand that the guidelines published in May of 2003 regarding hypertension evaluation, classification, diagnosis, risk factors, identifiable causes, and blood pressure measurement techniques (NIH Publication No. 03-5231) apply to adults aged 18 years and older. One of the major differences in this newest report is the creation of a "prehypertension" category of hypertension defined as a systolic blood pressure of 120 to 139 mm Hg and/or diastolic blood pressure of 80 to 89 mm Hg. These guidelines were developed and implemented to encourage the management, both pharmacologic and nonpharmacologic, of hypertension early in the disease process instead of later when multiple organ damage may be present.

◆ ASSESSMENT

Before administering any antihypertensive drug to a patient, the nurse should obtain a thorough health history and perform a head-to-toe physical assessment, which are crucial for ensuring safe drug therapy. Parameters to measure and document include blood pressure, pulse rate, respirations, and pulse oximetry readings. Results of laboratory tests—especially those indicative of fluid and electrolyte imbalances, heart function and heart tissue damage, renal function, and liver function—should be monitored. These laboratory tests may include the following: (1) Serum sodium, potassium, chloride, magnesium, and calcium, (2) serum levels of troponin, which is usually elevated within 4 to 6 hours after onset of a heart attack begins and may be reliable up to 14 days after a heart attack, (3) renal function studies, including blood urea nitrogen and serum and urinary creatinine, and (4) hepatic function studies, including serum transaminase alanine aminotransferase (formerly called serum glutamic pyruvic transaminase) and aspartate aminotransferase.

Because hypertension may lead to cardiac, vascular, renal, hepatic, and retinal damage, assessment to determine how much organ damage has occurred is necessary. Laboratory tests will most likely be complimented with more sophisticated scans and imaging studies. Noninvasive ophtalmoscopic examination of the eye structures (e.g., optic nerve, optic disk, vasculature) by a professionally trained health care practitioner (e.g., nurse practitioner, physician assistant, physician, ophthalmologist, optometrist) allows easy visualization of the structures impacted by hypertension. If hypertensive retinopathy is present, the exam will reveal narrowing of blood vessels in the eye, oozing of fluid from these blood vessels, spots on the retina, swelling of the macula and optic nerve, and/or bleeding in the back of the eye. These problems may be prevented by controlling the blood pressure or treating hypertension with appropriate follow-up once it is diagnosed.

The nurse must also assess for conditions, factors, or variables that may be underlying causes for a patient's hypertension, such as the following:

- Addison's disease
- Coarctation of the aorta
- Coronary heart disease
- Culture and race/ethnicity
- Cushing's disease
- Family history of hypertension
- Nicotine use
- Obesity
- Peripheral vascular disease
- Pheochromocytoma
- Renal artery stenosis
- Renal or liver insufficiency
- Stressful lifestyle

Many of these factors demand very cautious use of antihypertensive drugs. Cautions and contraindications have been discussed, and it is also important to emphasize that the elderly and those with chronic illnesses are of special concern. These patients are at high risk for further compromise of their physical condition if they suffer from uncontrolled/untreated hypertension or the adverse effects of antihypertensives (e.g., fluid loss, dehydration, electrolyte imbalances, hypotension). For complete drug interactions associated with antihypertensives, see the pharmacology section in this chapter.

Use of *α-adrenergic agonists* demands close assessment of the patient's blood pressure, pulse rate, and weight before and during treatment because of their strong vasodilating properties

and hypotensive adverse effects. These drugs may also be associated with fluid retention and edema, so assessment of heart and breath sounds, monitoring of intake and output, and assessment for dependent and peripheral edema is necessary. The α-adrenergic drugs should always be used cautiously because of associated hypotensive-induced dizziness and syncope and should be used especially cautiously in the elderly or other patients with preexisiting dizziness and syncope. First-dose syncope generally occurs within 30 to 90 minutes of taking this drug and is often preceded by an increase in heart rate (120 to 160 beats/min). Careful assessment of blood pressures (supine and standing) and corresponding pulse rates is required before each dose of the drug and 30 to 60 minutes after the drug is given, especially for the first dose or two of the medication. Blood pressures and pulse rates (supine and standing) should always be assessed with any of the antihypertensive drugs, as should cautions, contraindications, and drug interactions. *Centrally acting α-blockers* require assessment of white blood cell counts, serum potassium and sodium, and protein in the urine. The route of administration for the given drug order should also be noted because of different concerns related to a specific route (e.g., assessment of skin sites for readiness for transdermal application [e.g., with clonidine]).

β-blockers and their mechanisms of action are important to remember prior to giving these drugs to a patient because of the risk for complications in certain patient populations. If a drug is a nonselective β-blocker, it blocks both β_1 and β_2 receptors and will block both cardiac and respiratory effects, whereas if a drug is only a β_1-blocking drug, the cardiac system will be affected (pulse rate and blood pressure will decrease) but there will be no β_2 effects, thus limiting any concern for respiratory problems (e.g., bronchoconstriction). Therefore, if a patient needs a β-blocker but has a restrictive airway problem, nonselective β-blockers should not be used in order to avoid bronchoconstriction. A β_1-specific blocker would be used to avoid a negative impact on the lungs. However, if there is no history of respiratory illnesses or concerns, these drugs may be very effective as antihypertensives. In addition, for patients with congestive heart failure, it is important to understand that β-blockers also have a negative inotropic effect on the heart (decrease contractility); their use would lead to worsening of heart failure, thus creating the need for a completely different type of antihypertensive.

With use of β-blockers, assessment should include measurement of blood pressure and apical pulse rate immediately before each dose; if the systolic blood pressure is less than 90 mm Hg or the pulse rate is less than 60 beats/min, the physician should be notified because of the risk of adverse effects (e.g., hypotension, bradycardia). The drug would usually be withheld as ordered or per protocol. These blood pressure and pulse rate parameters are also applicable with use of other antihypertensives. Breath sounds and heart sounds should also be assessed before and during drug therapy.

Use of *ACE inhibitors* require assessment of blood pressure, apical pulse rate, and respiratory status (because of the adverse effect of a dry, hacking, chronic cough). With regard to blood pressure, it is important to take blood pressure immediately before initial and subsequent doses of the drug so that extreme fluctuations may be identified early. Serum potassium, sodium, and chloride levels should also be assessed. Baseline cardiac functioning will most likely be ordered prior to initiation of therapy. Proteinuria is simple to assess through use of the dipstick method on the patient's first voided urine sample of the morning. Due to adverse effects of neutropenia and other blood disorders, a complete blood count should be performed before and during therapy, as ordered. *ARBs* should be used very cautiously in elderly patients and in patients with renal dysfunction because of increased sensitivity to the drug's effects and risk for more adverse effects.

Vasodilators require baseline neurologic assessment with noting of level of consciousness and cognitive ability. Extreme caution with the elderly is needed because they are more sensitive to the drug's effect on lowering of blood pressure and subsequently more problems with hypotension, dizziness, and syncope. See Chapters 22, 23, and 25 for further discussion on other antihypertensives.

In summary, many assessment parameters are similar for the various groups of antihypertensives. The difference in the level of assessment depends on the drug's impact on blood pressure as well as the individual's response to the medication and any preexisting illness or condition. Other aspects to be assessed in any patient receiving these drugs, as well as most other drugs, include the patient's cultural background, racial/ethnic group, reading level, learning needs, developmental and cognitive status, financial status, mental health status, support systems, and overall physical health. Always encourage patients to learn how to assess and monitor themselves and their individual responses to drug therapy.

✦ NURSING DIAGNOSES

- Deficient knowledge related to new prescribed drug regimen and lack of familiarity with medications and lifestyle changes
- Noncompliance with drug therapy related to lack of familiarity with or acceptance of the disease process
- Sexual dysfunction related to adverse effects of some antihypertensive drugs
- Risk for injury (e.g., possible falls) related to adverse effects of the antihypertensive drug such as dizziness, orthostatic hypotension, and syncope
- Acute pain related to headache as an adverse effect of drug therapy
- Ineffective tissue perfusion (renal, cardiac, cerebral) related to the impact of the disease process or possible severe hypotensive adverse effects of drug therapy
- Excess fluid volume related to adverse effects of edema
- Imbalanced nutrition, less than body requirements, related to the drug's adverse effects (e.g., impaired taste or loss of appetite)
- Constipation related to adverse effects of antihypertensive drugs
- Risk for injury (e.g., possible falls) related to possible CNS adverse effects such as paresthesia, sedation, tremors, weakness, and seizures
- Risk for injury to mucous membranes related to the adverse effects of the medication and decreased saliva (dry mouth)
- Disturbed body image related to the adverse effects of antihypertensives (e.g., impotence, sexual dysfunction, weight gain, fatigue)

✦ PLANNING

Nursing goals for antihypertensive therapy should focus on educating the patient and his or her family on the need for adequate management to prevent end-organ damage. These goals include making sure the patient understands the nature of the disease, its symptoms and treatment, and the importance of complying with the treatment regimen. The patient must also come to terms with the diagnosis as well as with the fact that there is no cure for the disease and treatment will be lifelong. The influence of chronic illness and the importance of nonpharmacologic therapy, stress reduction, and follow-up care must also be emphasized. The nurse needs to plan for ongoing assessment of blood pressure, weight, diet, exercise, smoking habits, alcohol intake, compliance with therapy, and sexual function in the patient receiving therapy for hypertension.

Goals

- Patient takes the drug exactly as prescribed.
- Patient experiences relief of symptoms for which the medication was prescribed (e.g., a decrease in blood pressure).
- Patient demonstrates adequate knowledge about the use of the specific medication, its adverse effects, and the appropriate dosing at home.
- Patient is free of self-injury resulting from adverse effects of drug therapy.
- Patient states the rationale and importance of antihypertensive therapy.
- Patient describes measures to implement to decrease the impact of the adverse effects of antihypertensive therapy.
- Patient reports any change in sexual patterns and function, bowel pattern changes, or activity intolerance.
- Patient remains compliant with the therapy regimen.

Outcome Criteria

- Patient states the risks and complications of potent antihypertensive drugs, such as tremors, decreased sweating, tachycardia, and hypotension.

CASE STUDY
Hypertension

Hypertension was diagnosed in Gina S. when she was 33 years old. Both her mother and sister have hypertension, and both were also in their thirties when it was diagnosed. Gina's most current blood pressure reading is 150/96 mm Hg, and for this reason the nurse practitioner has recommended that she see her primary care provider. After examining her, the physician prescribes atenolol (Tenormin) and relaxation therapy. After 14 days of this therapy, Gina's blood pressure is 145/86 mm Hg. Stress reduction has been the biggest obstacle in her treatment, because she is a lawyer with a prominent law firm and has found that her blood pressure is consistently elevated (160/100 mm Hg) whenever she measures it at work.

- What should Gina know about the expected therapeutic effects and adverse effects of atenolol?
- Discuss the differences between a drug such as atenolol and the drug propranolol (Inderal).
- What lifestyle changes would you, as her nurse, recommend that she make and, even more important, what information would you give her to help her change her lifestyle and more effectively reduce the stress in her life?

For answers, see http://evolve.elsevier.com/Lilley.

- Patient states conditions to report to the physician, such as syncope or chest pain.
- Patient states the importance of lifelong compliance with drug therapy for hypertension to decrease end-organ damage and complications.
- Patient follows instructions to change position slowly, monitor blood pressure, keep follow-up appointments with the physician, and keep a journal to help monitor the effects of therapy.
- Patient communicates openly with nurses and other members of the health care team regarding the disease, its treatment, and any concerns related to changes in body image.
- Patient reports to the physician immediately any pitting edema of the feet, hands, or sacral area or a weight gain of 2 lb or more within 24 hours or 5 lb or more in 1 week.
- Patient maintains normal nutritional status through adherence to a prescribed diet high in fiber and fluids and avoidance of alcohol.

◆ IMPLEMENTATION

Nursing interventions generally may help patients achieve stable blood pressure while minimizing adverse effects. Many patients have problems complying with treatment because the disease itself is silent or without symptoms. Because of this, patients are unaware of their blood pressure or think that if they don't feel bad then there is nothing wrong with them, which poses many problems for treatment. Also, the antihypertensives are associated with multiple adverse effects that may impact patients' self-concept and/or sexual integrity. Often these adverse effects lead patients to abruptly stop taking the medication. It is important to inform patients that any abrupt withdrawal is a serious concern because of the risk of developing "rebound hypertension." Rebound hypertension is characterized by a sudden and very high elevation of blood pressure. This places the patient at risk for a cerebrovascular accident or other cerebral or cardiac adverse event. It is important to understand that with *all* antihypertensives there is a risk of rebound hypertension, and prevention of this through patient education is critical to patient safety. Other interventions related to each major group of drugs are discussed subsequently. See the Patient Teaching Tips for more information.

Patients taking *α-adrenergic agonists,* such as methyldopa, will need to monitor their blood pressure and pulse rate at home or have these taken for them by a family member who has received instructions or by local fire department or rescue or emergency medical personnel. The blood pressure machines found in grocery stores do not provide as accurate readings as the aforementioned sources. These drugs are also associated with severe hypotension and first-dose syncope. To avoid injury, be sure patients are supine with the first dose of this drug. More than likely, these drugs will be prescribed to be given at bedtime to allow the patient to sleep through the drug's first-dose syncope. It may take 4 to 6 weeks for the drug to achieve its full therapeutic effects, so education about delayed onset of action and bedtime dosing is important in an attempt to avoid injury. There is the need to also continue to monitor the patient for dizziness, syncope, edema, and other adverse effects (e.g., shortness of breath, exacerbation of preexisting cardiac disorders). Diuretics may be ordered as adjunctive therapy to minimize the adverse effects of edema, but they may lead to more dizziness and electrolyte problems. *Centrally acting α-blockers* require the same type of nursing interventions as other α-blockers; however, as their name indicates, the mechanism of action of these drugs is central, so adverse effects are often more pronounced (e.g., hypotension, sedation, bradycardia, edema). See the Patient Teaching Tips for more information.

The *β-blockers* are either nonselective (block both β_1 and β_2 receptors; e.g., propranolol) or cardioselective (block mainly β_1 receptors; e.g., atenolol). With any β-blocker, careful compliance with the drug regimen is critical to patient safety. Patients taking β-blockers may experience an exacerbation of respiratory diseases such as asthma, bronchospasm, and chronic obstructive pulmonary disease (increased bronchoconstriction due to β_2 blocking) or an exacerbation of heart failure because of the drug's negative inotropic effects (decreased contractility due to β_1 blocking). Proper instructions about reporting adverse effects and for taking blood pressure and pulse rates must be clear and concise. In addition, if a β_1-blocker causes shortness of breath, it is most likely due to edema and/or exacerbation of congestive heart failure. Any dizziness, depression, confusion, or unusual bleeding or bruising should also be reported to the health care provider immediately. See the Patient Teaching Tips for more information.

ACE inhibitors must also be taken exactly as prescribed. If angioedema occurs, the physician should be contacted immediately. Should the drug need to be discontinued, weaning is recommended (as with all antihypertensives) to avoid rebound hypertension. Serum sodium and potassium levels should be monitored during therapy. Serum potassium levels increase as an adverse effect with these drugs and may lead to hyperkalemia with more complications. Urine samples may be checked for proteinuria and, because anorexia may also be a side effect, dietary and fluid intake should be monitored closely. Impaired taste may occur as an adverse effect and last up to 2 to 3 months after the drug has been discontinued. It is also important to educate the patient about the fact that it takes several weeks to see the full therapeutic effects and that potassium supplements should not be used with these drugs (due to the adverse effect of hyperkalemia).

ARBs must also be taken exactly as prescribed. They are often tolerated best with meals as with many antihypertensives. The dosage should not be changed nor the medication discontinued unless prescribed by the physician. With ARBs, if the patient has hypovolemia or hepatic dysfunction the dosage may need to be reduced. A diuretic such as hydrochlorothiazide may be ordered in combination with an ARB for patients who have hypertension with left ventricular hypertrophy. Losartan is also an option for patients at risk for stroke and for those who are hypertensive and have left ventricular hypertrophy. Most importantly, with ARBs, any unusual shortness of breath, dyspnea, weight gain, chest pain, or palpitations should be reported to the health care provider immediately.

Some nursing considerations for *vasodilators* are similar to those for other antihypertensives; however, their impact on blood pressure may be more drastic depending on the specific drug and dosage. Hydralazine given by injection may result in reduced blood pressure within 10 to 80 minutes after administration and requires very close monitoring of the patient. With hydralazine, SLE may be an adverse effect if the patient is taking more than 200 mg orally per day. If signs and symptoms of SLE occur, the drug should be discontinued, the physician should be contacted immediately, and the patient should be closely monitored. Electrocardiographic changes, cardiovascular inadequacies, and hypotension may have pronounced effects on the patient's cardiac status, and therefore the drug should *never* to be given without adequate monitoring and frequent assessment. Pyridoxine may help to diminish the adverse effect of peripheral neuritis.

Sodium nitroprusside must always be diluted per manufacturer's guidelines. Because this drug is a potent vasodilator, there may be extreme decreases in the patient's blood pressure. Close monitoring is therefore important for preventing further complications. Severe drops in blood pressure may lead to irreversible ischemic injuries and even death. The nurse must remember that sodium nitroprusside should never be infused at the maximum dose rate for more than 10 minutes. If this drug does not control a patient's blood pressure after 10 minutes, it will most likely be ordered to be discontinued. To help prevent complications of cyanide and thiocyanate toxicity, the nurse should (1) dilute the medication properly and avoid use of any solution that has turned blue, green, or red, (2) infuse only using a volumetric infusion pump, not through ordinary intravenous sets, (3) continuously monitor blood pressure during the infusion (often by invasive measures), and (4) when more than 500 mcg/kg of sodium nitroprusside is administered at a rate faster than 2 mcg/kg/min, be aware that this may result in production of cyanide at a more rapid rate than the patient can eliminate unaided. (See the Laboratory Values Related to Drug Therapy box on p. 381 for more information.)

CCBs and related nursing interventions are discussed only briefly here because these drugs are covered in other chapters. Drugs like enalapril and verapamil are to be taken exactly as prescribed with the warning to the patient not to puncture, open, or crush the extended-release or sustained-release tablets and capsules. The nurse must be aware that CCBs are negative inotropic drugs (used to decrease cardiac contractility), because this action may induce more signs of heart failure if these drugs are given with drugs that are used to increase cardiac contractility, such as digitalis glycosides. Monitoring of blood pressure and pulse rate before and during therapy will aid in prevention or early detection of any problems related to the negative inotropic effects (decreased contractility), negative chronotropic effects (decreased heart rate), and negative dromotropic effects (decreased conduction).

The nurse must remember always to base nursing interventions on a thorough assessment and plan of care that also includes consideration of the patient's cultural-ethnic group. This is particularly important with antihypertensives, because research studies have documented differences in responses to antihypertensives among different racial and ethnic groups. Some ethnic groups respond less favorably to certain drugs as than to others.

As with any disease, patients must be treated with respect and with an appreciation for a holistic approach to health care in which all physical, psychosocial, and spiritual needs are taken into consideration (see Cultural Implications box earlier in this chapter). In summary, some educational information to be conveyed to the patient has been mentioned for particular groups of drugs or specific drugs. The nurse must remember that patient education is of critical importance and plays an important part in ensuring compliance with the drug regimen and in decreasing the incidence of problems related to these medications.

◆ EVALUATION

Because patients with hypertension are at high risk for cardiovascular injury, it is critical for them to comply with both their pharmacologic and nonpharmacologic treatment regimens. Monitoring patients for the adverse effects (e.g., orthostatic hypotension, dizziness, fatigue) and toxic effects of the various types of antihypertensive drugs helps the nurse to identify potentially life-threatening complications. The most important aspect of the evaluation process is collecting data and monitoring patients for evidence of controlled blood pressure. Blood pressure should be maintained at less than 130/90 mm Hg. If compelling indications, such as diabetes mellitus or kidney disease, are present, then the blood pressure goal is lower than 130/80. Blood pressure should be monitored at periodic intervals, and patient education about self-monitoring is very important to the safe use of these drugs. In addition, the physician needs to examine the fundus of the patient's eyes, because this is a more reliable indicator of the long-term effectiveness of treatment than blood pressure readings. The patient must constantly be monitored for the development of end-organ damage and for specific problems that the medication can cause. Male patients receiving antihypertensives should be counseled and constantly monitored for any sexual dysfunction. This is important, because the patient may experience the dysfunction, and if the patient is not expecting it, he may not report the problem and decide to stop taking the medication abruptly, which places the patient at high risk for rebound hypertension and possible stroke or other complications. Communication is critical in these situations. Follow-up visits to the physician are important for monitoring these and other adverse effects and checking patient compliance. Therapeutic effects of antihypertensives in general include an improvement in blood pressure and in the disease process. Patients should report a return to a normal baseline level of blood pressure with improved energy levels and improved signs and symptoms of hypertension, such as less edema, improved breath sounds, no abnormal heart sounds, capillary refill in less than 5 seconds, and less shortness of breath (dyspnea). Adverse effects for which to monitor include all of the specific side effects discussed in the pharmacology section of the chapter as well as those described for each group of drugs earlier in the Nursing Process section.

Patient Teaching Tips

Antihypertensives in General

- Educate patients to take medications exactly as prescribed by the physician, to never double or omit doses, and to contact their physician if these instructions are not followed.
- The patient should be informed about the fact that successful therapy requires compliance to medications as well as any dietary restrictions (e.g., decreasing fatty foods or those high in cholesterol).
- The patient should always monitor stress levels and use biofeedback, imagery, and/or relaxation techniques or massage, as needed. Exercise, if approved by the physician, may also help in the management of hypertension and serves to relieve stress and is usually inclusive of supervised, prescribed exercise.
- The patient should avoid smoking and excessive alcohol intake as well as excessive exercise, hot climates, saunas, hot tubs, and hot environments. Heat may precipitate vasodilation and lead to worsening of hypotension with risk of fainting and injury to self.
- Frequent laboratory tests may be needed for the duration of therapy, so importance of follow-up appointments must be emphasized to patients.
- Educate the patient about keeping medications out of the reach of children, and if a transdermal patch is used, being sure it is intact and in place. There have been cases in which a patch that was placed on an adult and then dropped off has accidentally ended up on a crawling infant who picked up the fallen patch on the skin.
- Encourage the patient to always wear a medical alert bracelet or necklace and carry a medical identification card specifying the patient's diagnosis, noting allergies, and listing all medications taken (e.g., prescribed drugs, over-the-counter [OTC] medications, herbals, vitamins, and supplements). The same information should be kept in a visible location in the patient's car as well as in the patient's home on the refrigerator for emergency medical personnel.
- The patient should weigh daily at the same time every day and with the same amount of clothing, as well as record the weight in his or her journal.
- Blood pressure should be recorded, including postural blood pressures. The patient should be sure he or she feels comfortable in taking his or her own blood pressure and pulse rate. The patient should practice as needed and should never hesitate to ask for assistance.
- The patient should inform all health care providers (e.g., dentist, surgeon) that he or she is taking an antihypertensive drug.
- The patient should be sure to move purposefully and cautiously and to change positions slowly because of the possible adverse effect of postural hypotension and associated risk for dizziness, lightheadedness, and possible fainting and falls.
- The patient should be informed to always keep an adequate supply of hypertensive medications on hand, especially while traveling.
- Scheduling of periodic eye examinations (e.g., every 6 months) should be emphasized because of the need to evaluate treatment effectiveness and the impact of hypertension on the vasculature of the eyes.
- With successful therapy, the patient's condition will improve; however, the patient should be cautioned not to stop taking the medication just because he or she is feeling better. Lifelong therapy is usually required.
- Encourage patients to use saliva substitutes, sugar-free hard candy, or frequent fluids for management of dry mouth.

- Share with the patient measures to help with constipation, such as forcing fluids, increasing fiber and roughage, and contacting the physician if there is no relief of this adverse effect. Use of OTC drugs, herbals, or a prescription drug may be indicated.
- Sexual dysfunction may occur with antihypertensives, so encourage the patient to be open with reporting and discussion of any problems or concerns. Emphasize to the patient that should this adverse effect occur, there are options to help alleviate the problem, such as combination therapy that allows lower dosages of drugs to be used, as well as use of other types of antihypertensives. The patient should always report any problems to the physician, because solutions are usually available.
- Patients should know to never abruptly stop taking the medication for any reason, including sexual problems, because of the risk of severe hypertensive rebound. Avoiding abrupt withdrawal of *any* of the antihypertensives is critical to patient safety.
- The patient should be aware that antihypertensives may lead to depression, so any change in emotional status should be reported to the health care provider.

α-Adrenergic Agonists

- Educate the patient about avoiding alcohol and heat due to exacerbation of vasodilation and subsequent worsening of hypotension, leading to dizziness and possible fainting (syncope). This is appropriate for any of the antihypertensives.
- The patient should be careful at first with activities such as driving or activities requiring alertness. The patient may have to postpone driving and other activities until the drowsiness subsides.
- The patient should report any jaundice, unexplained fever, or flu-like symptoms to the physician immediately.
- Taking daily weights is recommended each morning before breakfast, at the same time and wearing the same amount of clothing each day. Information should be recorded in a daily journal along with blood pressure readings. The patient should be instructed to report an increase in weight by 2 lbs or more over a 24-hour period or 5 lbs or more in 1 week.
- Because centrally acting blockers may also affect the patient's sexual functioning (e.g., causing impotence or decreased libido), patients should be informed of these possible adverse effects and to contact their health care provider if problematic for them. Other treatment options may be indicated.
- Inform patients to apply the transdermal patch dosage form of clonidine to nonhairy areas of the skin as ordered and to rotate sites.

β-Blockers

- The patient should be cautioned to move and change positions slowly to avoid possible dizziness, fainting, and falls and should be instructed to report a pulse rate of less than 60 beats/min, any peripheral numbness, dizziness, weight gain (see earlier), or systolic blood pressure of 90 mm Hg or lower to the physician.
- Prolonged sitting or standing and excessive physical exercise may also lead to exacerbation of hypotensive effects, so encourage the patient to avoid these activities or counteract them with healthier alternatives such as pumping the feet up and down while sitting.

Points to Remember

- All antihypertensives in some way affect cardiac output and/or SVR.
  - Cardiac output is the amount of blood ejected from the left ventricle measured in liters per minute.
  - SVR is the force the left ventricle must overcome to eject its end-diastolic volume.
- The major groups of antihypertensives are diuretics (see Chapter 25), α-blockers, centrally active α-blockers, β-blockers, ACE inhibitors, vasodilators, CCBs, and ARBs.
- ACE inhibitors work by blocking a critical enzyme system responsible for the production of angiotensin II (a potent vasoconstrictor). They prevent (1) vasoconstriction caused by angiotensin II, (2) aldosterone secretion and therefore sodium and water resorption, and (3) the breakdown of bradykinin (a potent vasodilator) by angiotensin II.
- ARBs work by blocking the binding of angiotensin at the receptors; the end result is a decrease in blood pressure.
- CCBs may be used to treat angina, dysrhythmias, and hypertension and help to reduce blood pressure by causing smooth muscle relaxation and dilation of blood vessels. If calcium is not present, then the smooth muscle of the blood vessels cannot contract.
- Aspects of the nursing process related to the use of antihypertensives include the following:
  - A thorough nursing assessment should include finding out whether the patient has any underlying causes of hypertension, such as renal or liver dysfunction, a stressful lifestyle, Cushing's disease, Addison's disease, renal artery stenosis, peripheral vascular disease, or pheochromocytoma.
- The nurse should always assess for the presence of contraindications, cautions, and potential drug interactions before administering any of the antihypertensive drugs. Contraindications include a history of MI or chronic renal disease. Cautious use is recommended in patients with renal insufficiency and glaucoma. Drugs that interact with antihypertensive drugs include other antihypertensive drugs, anesthetics, and diuretics.
- Patients should be managed by both pharmacologic and nonpharmacologic means. They should be encouraged to consume a diet low in fat, make any other necessary modifications in their diet (such as a possible decrease in the intake of sodium, and increase in fiber intake), engage in regular supervised exercise, and reduce the amount of stress in their lives.
- Therapeutic effects include fewer hypertension-related symptoms such as chest pain and severe headaches, and decreased blood pressure readings.
- Adverse effects for which to constantly monitor include tachycardia, confusion, CNS depression, and constipation.

NCLEX Examination Review Questions

1. Which of the following adverse effects is of most concern for the older adult patient taking antihypertensive drugs?
   - a. Dry mouth
   - b. Hypotension
   - c. Restlessness
   - d. Constipation
2. When giving antihypertensive drugs, the nurse must consider giving the first dose at bedtime for which of the following classes of drugs?
   - a. α-Blockers such as prazosin (Minipress)
   - b. Diuretics such as furosemide (Lasix)
   - c. ACE inhibitors such as captopril (Capoten)
   - d. Vasodilators such as hydralazine (Apresoline)
3. A 56-year-old man started antihypertensive drug therapy 3 months earlier and is in the office for a follow-up visit. While the nurse is taking his blood pressure, he informs the nurse that he has had some problems with sexual intercourse. Which of the following would be the most appropriate response by the nurse?
   - a. "Not to worry. Tolerance will develop."
   - b. "The physician can work with you on changing the dose and/or drugs."
   - c. "Sexual dysfunction happens with this therapy, and you must learn to accept it."
   - d. "This is an unusual occurrence, but it is important to stay on your medications."
4. When a patient is being taught about the potential adverse effects of an ACE inhibitor, which of the following should be mentioned as possibly occurring when this drug is taken to treat hypertension?
   - a. Hypokalemia
   - b. Nausea
   - c. Dry, nonproductive cough
   - d. Sedation
5. A patient has a new prescription for an adrenergic drug. During a review of the patient's list of current medications, which would cause concern about a possible interaction with this new prescription?
   - a. A benzodiazepine taken as needed for allergies
   - b. A multivitamin with iron taken daily
   - c. An oral anticoagulant taken daily
   - d. A nonsteroidal antiinflammatory drug taken as needed for joint pain

1. b, 2. a, 3. b, 4. c, 5. a.

Critical Thinking Activities

1. Primary hypertension has been diagnosed in a 53-year-old woman, and the β-blocker carvedilol has been prescribed. Before initiating therapy, what past medical conditions should the nurse inquire about during the nursing assessment?
2. A 78-year-old woman has been admitted to the emergency department for the treatment of a possible acute MI and has another diagnosis of acute hypertensive crisis. One of the physician's orders is to start a sodium nitroprusside infusion. What is the purpose of using sodium nitroprusside?
3. A 63-year-old African American man has a new diagnosis of stage 2 hypertension. He has been treated for type 2 diabetes for 2 years but admits that he does not follow his diet as he should. His urinalysis shows traces of protein, but his retinal examination shows no defects. What drug therapy would you expect to see ordered for this patient? What is the treatment goal for this patient? Explain.

For answers, see http://evolve.elsevier.com/Lilley.

Diuretic Drugs

Objectives

When you reach the end of this chapter, you should be able to do the following:

1. Describe the normal anatomy and physiology of the renal system.
2. Briefly discuss the impact of the renal system on blood pressure regulation.
3. Describe how diuretics work in the renal system.
4. Distinguish among the different classes of diuretics with regard to mechanisms of action, indications, dosages, routes of administration, adverse effects, toxicity, cautions, contraindications, and drug interactions.
5. Develop a nursing care plan that includes all phases of the nursing process for patients receiving diuretics.

e-Learning Activities

Companion CD
- NCLEX Review Questions: see questions 205-220
- Animations
- Audio Glossary
- Category Catchers
- Medication Errors Checklists
- IV Therapy Checklists

evolve Website (http://evolve.elsevier.com/Lilley)
• Nursing Care Plans • Frequently Asked Questions • Content Updates • WebLinks • Supplemental Resources • Elsevier ePharmacology Update • Medication Administration Animations

Drug Profiles

acetazolamide, p. 391
amiloride, p. 395
▶ furosemide, p. 392
▶ hydrochlorothiazide, p. 397

▶ mannitol, p. 394
metolazone, p. 397
▶ spironolactone, p. 395
triamterene, p. 395

▶ Key drug.

Glossary

Afferent arterioles The small blood vessels approaching the glomerulus (proximal part of nephron). (p. 389)

Aldosterone A mineralocorticoid steroid hormone produced by the adrenal cortex that mediates the actions of the renal tubule in the regulation of sodium and potassium balance in the blood. (p. 389)

Ascites An abnormal intraperitoneal accumulation of fluid (defined as a volume of 500 mL or greater) containing large amounts of protein and electrolytes. (p. 392)

Collecting duct The most distal part of the nephron between the distal convoluted tubule and the ureters, which lead to the urinary bladder. (p. 389)

Distal convoluted tubule The part of the nephron immediately distal to the ascending loop of Henle and proximal to the collecting duct. (p. 389)

Diuretics Drugs or other substances that tend to promote the formation and excretion of urine. (p. 389)

Efferent arterioles The small blood vessels exiting the glomerulus. At this point blood has completed its filtration in the glomerulus. (p. 389)

Filtrate The material that passes through a filter. In the case of the kidney, the filter is the glomerulus and the filtrate is the extracted material from the blood (normally liquid) that ultimately becomes urine. (p. 389)

Glomerular capsule The open, rounded, and most proximal part of the proximal convoluted tubule that surrounds the glomerulus and receives the filtrate from the blood. (p. 389)

Glomerular filtration rate (GFR) The volume of ultrafiltrate extracted per unit of time from the plasma flowing through the glomeruli of the kidney. (p. 389)

Glomerulus The cluster of kidney capillaries that marks the beginning of the nephron and is immediately proximal to the proximal convoluted tubule. (p. 389)

Loop of Henle The part of the nephron between the proximal and distal convoluted tubules. (p. 389)

Nephron The microscopic functional filtration unit of the kidney, consisting of (in anatomical order from proximal to distal) the glomerulus, proximal convoluted tubule, loop of Henle, distal convoluted tubule, and collecting duct, which empties urine into the ureters. There are approximately 1 million nephrons in each kidney. (p. 389)

Open-angle glaucoma A condition in which pressure is elevated in the eye because of obstruction of the outflow of aqueous humor but access to the trabecular meshwork remains open. (p. 391)

Proximal convoluted (twisted) tubule The part of the nephron that is immediately distal to the glomerulus and proximal to the loop of Henle. (p. 389)

Ultrafiltration   Filtration at a *microscopic* level; the term is often used to describe the filtration function of the kidneys, with the filtrate referred to more specifically as *ultrafiltrate.* (p. 389)

The drugs that accelerate the rate of urine formation are termed **diuretics,** and they accomplish this through a variety of mechanisms. The result is the removal of sodium and water from the body.

Diuretics were discovered by accident when it was noticed that a mercury-based antibiotic had a very potent diuretic effect. Thus began the early developmental stages of diuretic drugs. All the major classes of diuretic drugs in use today were developed between 1950 and 1970, and they remain among the most commonly prescribed drugs in the world. The Seventh Joint National Committee on the Detection, Evaluation, and Treatment of Hypertension recently reaffirmed the role of diuretics, especially the thiazides, as the first-line drugs in the treatment of hypertension. The hypotensive activity of diuretics is due to many different mechanisms. They cause direct arteriolar dilation, which decreases peripheral vascular resistance. They also reduce extracellular fluid volume, plasma volume, and cardiac output, which may account for the decrease in blood pressure. They have long been the mainstay of therapy not only for hypertension but also for heart failure. Two of their advantages are their relatively low cost and their favorable safety profile compared with many other drug classes. The main problem with their use is the metabolic adverse effects that can result from excessive fluid and electrolyte loss. These effects are usually dose related and are therefore controllable with dosage *titration* (careful adjustment).

This chapter reviews the essential properties and actions of the following important classes of diuretic drugs: carbonic anhydrase inhibitors, loop diuretics, osmotic diuretics, potassium-sparing diuretics, and thiazide and thiazide-like diuretics. Before these drug classes are discussed in detail, however, it is important to quickly review kidney function, because all diuretics work primarily in the kidneys.

OVERVIEW OF RENAL PHYSIOLOGY

The kidney plays a very important role in the day-to-day functioning of the body. It filters out toxic waste products from the blood while simultaneously conserving essential substances. This delicate balance between elimination of toxins and retention of essential chemicals is maintained by the **nephron.** The nephron is the main structural unit of the kidney, and each kidney contains approximately 1 million of them. It is in the nephron where diuretic drugs exert their effect. The initial filtering of the blood takes place in the **glomerulus,** a cluster of capillaries surrounded by the **glomerular capsule.** The rate at which this filtering occurs is referred to as the **glomerular filtration rate (GFR),** and it is used as a gauge of how well the kidneys are functioning as filters. Normally about 180 L of blood are filtered through the nephrons every day. The GFR, which can also be thought of as the rate at which blood flows into and out of the

glomerulus, is regulated by the small blood vessels approaching the glomerulus (**afferent arterioles**) and the small blood vessels exiting the glomerulus (**efferent arterioles).** A mnemonic (memory aid) for remembering which arteriole is which is "A for *approach* and *afferent*" and "E for *exit* and *efferent*." Alterations in blood flow such as those that occur in a patient in shock can therefore have a dramatic effect on kidney (renal) function. In situations of low blood flow, the kidney receives less blood, and therefore less diuretic gets to its site of action. For this reason diuretics may have diminished effects, although they are often used to restore or enhance renal blood flow and glomerular filtration in such situations. This is especially true of the loop diuretics.

The **proximal convoluted (twisted) tubule** or, more simply, *proximal tubule,* anatomically follows the glomerulus and resorbs 60% to 70% of the sodium and water from the filtered fluid (*ultrafiltrate,* resulting from the process of **ultrafiltration**) back into the bloodstream. Blood vessels surround the nephrons and allow substances to be directly resorbed from or secreted into the bloodstream. This process is one of active transport that requires energy in the form of adenosine triphosphate molecules. The active transport of sodium and potassium ions back into the blood causes the passive resorption of chloride and water. The chloride ions (Cl^-) and water passively follows the sodium ions (Na^+) and, to a lesser extent, potassium ions (K^+) by osmosis. Another 20% to 25% of sodium is resorbed back into the bloodstream in the ascending **loop of Henle.** Here it is the chloride that is actively resorbed, and the sodium passively follows it.

The remaining 5% to 10% of sodium resorption takes place in the **distal convoluted tubule,** often called simply the *distal tubule,* which anatomically follows the ascending loop of Henle. In the distal tubule, sodium is actively filtered in exchange for potassium or hydrogen ions, a process regulated by the hormone **aldosterone.** The **collecting duct** is the final common pathway for the **filtrate** that started in the glomerulus. It is here that antidiuretic hormone acts to increase the absorption of water back into the bloodstream, thereby preventing it from being lost in the urine. The entire nephron, along with the sites of action of the different classes of diuretics, is shown in Figure 25-1.

DIURETIC DRUGS

The various diuretics are classified according to their sites of action within the nephron, their chemical structure, and their diuretic potency. The sites of action of the various diuretics are determined by the way in which they affect the various solute (electrolyte) and water transport systems located along the nephron (see Figure 25-1). The commonly used classes of drugs and the individual drugs in these classes are listed in Table 25-1. The most potent diuretics are the loop diuretics, followed by mannitol, metolazone (a thiazide-like diuretic), the thiazides, and the potassium-sparing diuretics. The potency of these diuretics is a function of where they work in the nephron to inhibit sodium and water resorption. The more sodium and water they inhibit from resorption, the greater the amount of diuresis and therefore the greater the potency.

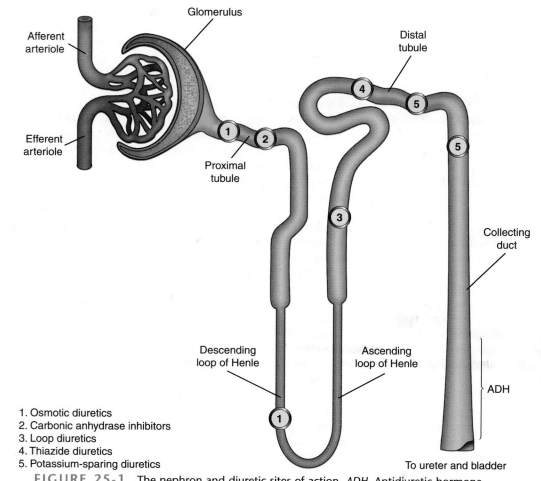

1. Osmotic diuretics
2. Carbonic anhydrase inhibitors
3. Loop diuretics
4. Thiazide diuretics
5. Potassium-sparing diuretics

FIGURE 25-1 The nephron and diuretic sites of action. *ADH,* Antidiuretic hormone.

Table 25-1 Classification of Diuretics

Class	Drugs
Carbonic anhydrase inhibitors	acetazolamide, dichlorphenamide, methazolamide
Loop diuretics	bumetanide, ethacrynic acid, furosemide, torsemide
Osmotic diuretics	mannitol
Potassium-sparing diuretics	amiloride, spironolactone, triamterene
Thiazide and thiazide-like diuretics	bendroflumethiazide, benzthiazide, chlorthalidone, chlorothiazide, hydrochlorothiazide, hydroflumethiazide, indapamide, methyclothiazide, metolazone, polythiazide, trichlormethiazide

CARBONIC ANHYDRASE INHIBITORS

Carbonic anhydrase inhibitors (CAIs) are chemical derivatives of sulfonamide antibiotics. As their name implies, CAIs inhibit the activity of the enzyme carbonic anhydrase, which is found in the kidneys, eyes, and other parts of the body. The site of action of the CAIs is the location of the carbonic anhydrase enzyme system along the nephron, primarily in the proximal tubule. For instance, acetazolamide acts principally in the proximal tubule, which as previously described is directly distal to the glomerulus.

Mechanism of Action and Drug Effects

As previously noted, the carbonic anhydrase system in the kidney is located just distal to the glomerulus in the proximal tubules, where roughly two thirds of all sodium and water is resorbed into the blood. Here a specific active transport system operates that exchanges sodium for hydrogen ions. For sodium and thus water to be resorbed back into the blood, hydrogen must be exchanged for it. Without hydrogen, this cannot occur, and the sodium and water will be eliminated with the urine. Carbonic anhydrase helps to make the hydrogen ions available for this exchange. When its actions are inhibited by a CAI such as acetazolamide, little sodium and water can be resorbed into the blood and they are eliminated with the urine. The CAIs reduce the formation of hydrogen (H^+) and bicarbonate (HCO_3^-) ions from carbon dioxide and water by the noncompetitive, reversible inhibition of carbonic anhydrase activity. This results in a reduction in the availability of these ions, mainly hydrogen, for use by active electrolyte transport systems.

The reduction in the formation of bicarbonate and hydrogen ions by CAIs can have many effects on other parts of the body.

The metabolic acidosis induced by CAIs is beneficial in the prevention of certain seizure conditions. In addition, both the respiratory and metabolic acidosis induced by CAIs may increase oxygenation during hypoxia by increasing ventilation, cerebral blood flow, and the dissociation of oxygen from oxyhemoglobin, all of which is usually beneficial to the patient. An undesirable effect of CAIs is that they elevate the blood glucose level and cause glycosuria in diabetic patients. This may be due in part to CAI-enhanced potassium loss through the urine.

Indications

The therapeutic applications of CAIs are wide and varied. They are commonly used in the treatment of glaucoma, edema, epilepsy, and high-altitude sickness.

CAIs are used principally as adjunct drugs in the long-term management of **open-angle glaucoma** that cannot be controlled by topical miotic drugs or epinephrine derivatives alone. Administration of these drugs together can increase the outflow of aqueous humor, the obstruction of which is responsible for the glaucoma. They are also used short term in conjunction with miotics to lower intraocular pressure in preparation for ocular surgery in patients with acute ocular disorders or narrow-angle glaucoma and as an adjunct in the treatment of secondary glaucoma.

CAIs, particularly acetazolamide, are used to manage the edema secondary to heart failure that has become resistant to other diuretics. However, as a class, CAIs are much less potent diuretics than loop diuretics or thiazides, and the metabolic acidosis they induce diminishes their diuretic effect in 2 to 4 days.

Acetazolamide may be a useful adjunct to other anticonvulsants in the prophylactic management of various forms of epilepsy. Tolerance to the anticonvulsant effects of CAIs develops quickly, however, and they may be ineffective for prolonged therapy. Acetazolamide is also effective in both the prevention and treatment of the symptoms of high-altitude sickness. These symptoms include headache, nausea, shortness of breath, dizziness, drowsiness, and fatigue.

Contraindications

Contraindications to the use of CAIs include known drug allergy and may include hyponatremia, hypokalemia, severe renal or hepatic dysfunction, adrenal gland insufficiency, and cirrhosis.

Adverse Effects

The more common undesirable effects of CAIs are metabolic abnormalities such as acidosis and hypokalemia. These drugs may also cause drowsiness, anorexia, paresthesias, hematuria, urticaria, photosensitivity, and melena (blood in the stool).

Interactions

Significant drug interactions that occur with CAIs include an increase in digitalis toxicity when CAIs and digitalis are given together, stemming from the hypokalemia that CAIs may induce. The concomitant use of CAIs and corticosteroids may also cause hypokalemia, and their use with oral hypoglycemic drugs and quinidine may induce greater activity or toxicity of the latter drugs.

Dosages

For information on the dosages of acetazolamide, see the following drug profile.

Drug Profiles

Although there are three CAIs (see Table 25-1), by far the most widely prescribed is acetazolamide, and thus it is the only CAI profiled here.

acetazolamide

Use of acetazolamide (Diamox) is contraindicated in patients who have shown a hypersensitivity to it and to sulfonamides, as well as in those with significant liver or kidney dysfunction, low serum potassium or sodium levels, acidosis, or adrenal gland failure. Acetazolamide is available in both oral and parenteral forms. A recommended dosage for pediatric patients is oral administration of 5 mg/kg/day. A common oral dosage for adults is 250 to 375 mg/day given on alternate days. Pregnancy category C.

Pharmacokinetics

Half-Life	Onset	Peak	Duration
PO: 10-15 hr	PO: 1 hr	PO: 2-4 hr	PO: 8-12 hr

LOOP DIURETICS

Loop diuretics (bumetanide, ethacrynic acid, furosemide, and torsemide) are very potent diuretics. Bumetanide, furosemide, and torsemide are chemically related to the sulfonamides antibiotics.

Mechanism of Action and Drug Effects

Loop diuretics have renal, cardiovascular, and metabolic effects. Their renal effects are their major mechanism of action. These drugs act primarily along the thick ascending limb of the loop of Henle, blocking chloride and, secondarily, sodium resorption. They are also believed to activate renal prostaglandins, which results in dilation of the blood vessels of the kidneys, the lungs, and the rest of the body (i.e., reduction in renal, pulmonary, and systemic vascular resistance). The beneficial hemodynamic effects of loop diuretics are a reduction in both the preload and central venous pressures, which are the filling pressures of the ventricles. These actions make them very useful in the treatment of the edema associated with heart failure, hepatic cirrhosis, and renal disease.

Loop diuretics are particularly useful when rapid diuresis is needed, because of their rapid onset of action. In addition, the diuretic effect lasts at least 2 hours. A distinct advantage they have over thiazide diuretics is that their diuretic action continues even when creatinine clearance decreases below 25 mL/min. This means that even when the function of the kidney diminishes, loop diuretics can still work. Because of their potent diuretic effect and the duration of this effect, loop diuretics are often effective when given in a single daily dose. This allows the renal tubule time to partially compensate for the potassium depletion and other electrolyte derangements that often accompany around-the-clock diuretic therapy. Despite this, the major adverse effect of loop diuretics is electrolyte disturbances. Prolonged administration of high dosages can also result in hearing loss stemming from ototoxicity, although this is rare.

Summary of Major Drug Effects of Loop Diuretics

As previously noted, loop diuretics produce a potent diuresis and subsequent loss of fluid. The resulting decreased fluid volume leads to a decreased return of blood to the heart, or de-

creased filling pressures. This has the following cardiovascular effects:
- Reduces blood pressure
- Reduces pulmonary vascular resistance
- Reduces systemic vascular resistance
- Reduces central venous pressure
- Reduces left ventricular end-diastolic pressure

The metabolic effects of the loop diuretics are secondary to the electrolyte losses resulting from the potent diuresis. Major electrolyte losses include loss of sodium and potassium and, to a lesser extent, calcium. Changes in the plasma levels of insulin, glucagon, and growth hormone have also been observed in association with loop diuretic therapy.

Indications

Loop diuretics are used to manage the edema associated with heart failure and hepatic or renal disease, to control hypertension, and to increase the renal excretion of calcium in patients with hypercalcemia. As with certain other classes of diuretics, they may also be indicated in cases of heart failure resulting from diastolic dysfunction.

Contraindications

Contraindications to the use of loop diuretics include known drug allergy and may include allergy to sulfonamide antibiotics, hepatic coma, or severe electrolyte loss.

Table 25-2	Loop Diuretics: Common Adverse Effects
Body System	**Adverse Effects**
Central nervous	Dizziness, headache, tinnitus, blurred vision
Gastrointestinal	Nausea, vomiting, diarrhea
Hematologic	Agranulocytosis, thrombocytopenia, neutropenia
Metabolic	Hypokalemia, hyperglycemia, hyperuricemia

Table 25-3	Loop Diuretics: Common Drug Interactions	
Interacting Drug	**Mechanism**	**Results**
Aminoglycosides capreomycin chloroquine vancomycin	Additive effect	Increased neurotoxicity, especially ototoxicity
Corticosteroids digoxin	Hypokalemia	Additive hypokalemia Increased digoxin toxicity
lithium	Decrease in renal excretion	Increased lithium toxicity
NSAIDs	Inhibition of renal prostaglandins	Decreased diuretic activity
Sulfonylureas	Decrease in glucose tolerance	Hyperglycemia

NSAIDs, Nonsteroidal antiinflammatory drugs.

Adverse Effects

Common undesirable effects of the loop diuretics are listed in Table 25-2. Other less common effects associated with bumetanide therapy include muscle cramps, dry mouth, arthritic pain, and encephalopathy. These are more likely to occur in patients with preexisting liver disease, which may require selection of a different drug. Ethacrynic acid may cause neutropenia and, rarely, episodes of Henoch-Schönlein purpura. Furosemide can produce erythema multiforme, exfoliative dermatitis, photosensitivity, and in rare cases aplastic anemia. Torsemide may rarely cause thrombocytopenia, agranulocytosis, leukopenia, and neutropenia. It may also cause a severe skin disorder called *Stevens-Johnson syndrome.*

Toxicity and Management of Overdose

Electrolyte loss and dehydration, which can result in circulatory failure, are the main toxic effects of loop diuretics that require attention. Treatment involves electrolyte and fluid replacement.

Interactions

Loop diuretics exhibit both neurotoxic and nephrotoxic properties, and they produce additive effects when given in combination with drugs that have similar toxicities. The drug interactions are summarized in Table 25-3.

Loop diuretics also affect certain laboratory results. They cause increases in the serum levels of uric acid, glucose, alanine aminotransferase, and aspartate aminotransferase. Their combined use with a thiazide (especially metolazone) results in the blockade of sodium and water resorption at multiple sites in the nephron, a property referred to as *sequential nephron blockade,* which increases their effects. The reduction in vascular resistance induced by loop diuretics may be impeded when these drugs are taken concurrently with nonsteroidal antiinflammatory drugs (NSAIDs) because these two drug classes have opposite effects on prostaglandin activity.

Dosages

For the recommended dosages of loop diuretics, see the Dosages table on page 393.

Drug Profiles

The currently available loop diuretics are bumetanide, ethacrynic acid, furosemide, and torsemide. As a class they are very potent diuretics, but this potency varies for the different drugs. The equipotent doses of these various drugs are as follows:

Pharmacokinetics			
bumetanide	**ethacrynic acid**	**furosemide**	**torsemide**
1 mg	50 mg	40 mg	10 mg

▶ furosemide

Furosemide (Lasix) is by far the most commonly used loop diuretic in clinical practice and the prototypical drug in this class. Structurally it is related to the sulfonamide antibiotics (Chapter 37). It has all the therapeutic and adverse characteristics of the loop diuretics mentioned earlier. It is primarily used in the management of pulmonary edema and the edema associated with heart failure, liver disease, nephrotic syndrome, and **ascites** (the accumulation of fluid in the peritoneal area). It has also been used in the treatment of hypertension, usually that caused by heart failure.

Furosemide use is contraindicated in patients who have shown a hypersensitivity to sulfonamides; in infants and lactating women;

DOSAGES

Selected Loop Diuretics and Osmotic Diuretics

Drug	Pharmacologic Class	Usual Dosage Range	Indications
bumetanide (Bumex)	Loop diuretic	**Adult** PO: 0.5-2 mg/day as a single dose IM/IV: 0.5-1 mg; may be repeated at intervals of 2-3 hr but do not exceed a total dose of 10 mg/day	Edema
ethacrynic acid (Edecrin)		**Pediatric** IV: 1 mg/kg/dose; max 3 mg/kg/day PO: Initial dose 25 mg/day; max 3 mg/kg/day **Adult** IV: 0.5-1 mg/kg; max 200 mg/day	
furosemide (Lasix)		**Pediatric** IM/IV: 1 mg/kg/dose; do not exceed 6 mg/kg/day PO: 2 mg/kg as a single dose; do not exceed 6 mg/kg/day **Adult** IM/IV: 20-40 mg/dose; max 600 mg/day; administer high-dose IV therapy as a controlled infusion at a rate of 4 mg/mL or less PO: 20-80 mg/day as a single dose	Heart failure, hypertension, renal failure, pulmonary edema, cirrhosis
mannitol (Resectisol, Osmitrol)	Osmotic diuretic	**Adult** IV infusion: 50-200 g/day, 1.5-2 g/kg over 30-60 min Suggested loading dose of 25 g, followed by an infusion rate to produce a urine flow of at least 100 mL/hr	Renal failure, abnormally high intraocular or intracranial pressure Drug intoxication (to induce diuresis)
torsemide (Demadex)	Loop diuretic	**Adult** PO/IV: 20-200 mg once daily	Edema

IM, Intramuscular; *IV*, intravenous; *PO*, oral.

and in patients suffering from anuria, hypovolemia, and electrolyte depletion. It is available in oral form as a 40 mg/5 mL and a 10 mg/mL solution. It is also available as 20-, 40-, and 80-mg tablets. In parenteral form it is available as a 10 mg/mL injection. Pregnancy category C. Recommended dosages are given in the Dosages table on this page.

Pharmacokinetics

Half-Life	Onset	Peak	Duration
1-2 hr	1 hr	1-2 hr	6-8 hr

OSMOTIC DIURETICS

The osmotic diuretics include mannitol, urea, organic acids, and glucose. Mannitol, a nonabsorbable solute, is the most commonly used of these drugs.

Mechanism of Action and Drug Effects

Mannitol works along the entire nephron. Its major site of action, however, is the proximal tubule and descending limb of the loop of Henle. Because it is nonabsorbable, it produces osmotic pressure in the glomerular filtrate, which in turn pulls fluid, primarily water, into the renal tubules from the surrounding tissues. This process also inhibits the tubular resorption of water and solutes, which produces a rapid diuresis. Ultimately this reduces cellular edema and increases urine production, causing diuresis. However, it produces only a slight loss of electrolytes, especially sodium. Therefore, mannitol is not indicated for patients with peripheral edema because it does not promote sufficient sodium excretion.

Mannitol may induce vasodilation and in doing so increase both glomerular filtration and renal plasma flow. This makes it an excellent drug for preventing kidney damage during acute renal failure. It is also often used to reduce intracranial pressure and cerebral edema resulting from head trauma. In addition, mannitol treatment may be tried when elevated intraocular pressure is unresponsive to other drug therapies.

Indications

Mannitol is the osmotic diuretic of choice. It is commonly used in the treatment of patients in the early, oliguric phase of acute renal failure. For it to be effective in this setting, however, enough renal blood flow and glomerular filtration must still remain to enable the drug to reach the renal tubules. Increased renal blood flow resulting from the dilation of blood vessels supplying blood to the kidneys is another therapeutic benefit of mannitol therapy in such patients. It can also be used to promote the excretion of toxic substances, reduce intracranial pressure, and treat cerebral edema. In addition, it can be used as a genitourinary irrigant in the preparation of patients for transurethral surgical procedures and as supportive treatment in patients with edema induced by other conditions.

Contraindications

Contraindications to the use of mannitol normally include known drug allergy, severe renal disease, pulmonary edema (loop diuretics are used instead), and active intracranial bleeding.

Adverse Effects

The significant undesirable effects of mannitol include convulsions, thrombophlebitis, and pulmonary congestion. Other less significant effects are headaches, chest pains, tachycardia, blurred vision, chills, and fever.

Interactions

There are no drugs that interact significantly with mannitol.

Dosages

For the recommended dosages of mannitol, see the Dosages table on page 393.

Drug Profiles

▶ *mannitol*

Mannitol (Osmitrol) is the prototypical osmotic diuretic. Its use is contraindicated in patients with a hypersensitivity to it as well as in those suffering from anuria, severe dehydration, pulmonary congestion, or cerebral hemorrhage. Treatment should be terminated if severe cardiac or renal impairment develops after the initiation of therapy. It is available only in parenteral form as 5%, 10%, 15%, 20%, and 25% solutions for intravenous injection. Mannitol may crystallize when exposed to low temperatures. This is more likely to occur when concentrations exceed 15%. Because of this, mannitol should always be administered intravenously through a filter, and vials of the drug are often stored in a warmer in the pharmacy. Pregnancy category C. Recommended dosages are given in the Dosages table on page 393.

Pharmacokinetics

Half-Life	Onset	Peak	Duration
1.5 hr	0.5-1 hr	0.25-2 hr	6-8 hr

POTASSIUM-SPARING DIURETICS

The currently available potassium-sparing diuretics are amiloride, spironolactone, and triamterene. These diuretics are also referred to as aldosterone-inhibiting diuretics because they block the aldosterone receptors. In fact, spironolactone is a competitive antagonist of aldosterone and for this reason causes sodium and water to be excreted and potassium to be retained. It is the most commonly used of the three drugs.

Mechanism of Action and Drug Effects

These drugs work in the collecting ducts and distal convoluted tubules, where they interfere with sodium-potassium exchange. As noted earlier, spironolactone competitively binds to aldoste-

rone receptors and therefore blocks the resorption of sodium and water that is induced by aldosterone secretion. These receptors are found primarily in the distal tubule. Amiloride and triamterene do not bind to aldosterone receptors. However, they inhibit both aldosterone-induced and basal sodium reabsorption, working in both the distal tubule and collecting ducts. They are often prescribed for children with heart failure, because pediatric cardiac problems are frequently accompanied by an excess secretion of aldosterone, and the loop and thiazide diuretics are often ineffective in their management.

Because around 3% of the total filtered urine volume reaches the collecting ducts, the potassium-sparing diuretics are relatively weak compared with the thiazide and loop diuretics. When diuresis is needed, they are generally used as adjuncts to thiazide treatment. This combination is beneficial in two respects. First, the drugs have synergistic diuretic effects; second, the two drugs counteract the adverse metabolic effects of each other. The thiazide diuretics cause potassium, magnesium, and chloride to be lost in the urine, and the potassium-sparing diuretics counteract this by elevating the potassium and chloride levels.

Life Span Considerations: The Pediatric Patient
Diuretics

- Pediatric dosages of diuretic medications should be calculated carefully, regardless of whether the patient is in the hospital or in the home setting. Weight should be measured daily at the same time every day and should be recorded so that therapeutic and/or adverse effects of diuretics can be assessed. Because pediatric patients are at greater risk for adverse effects and toxicity, they need closer and more cautious daily assessment to avoid excess fluid volume and electrolyte loss, hypotension, and shock.
- The half-life of furosemide is increased in neonates, so the interval between doses may need to be lengthened, as ordered by the physician.
- The oral forms of diuretics may be taken with food or milk and should be taken early in the day and at the same time every day.
- Lengthy exposure to either heat or sun should be avoided because it may precipitate heat stroke, exhaustion, and fluid volume loss in pediatric patients taking diuretics.
- Thiazide diuretics cross the placenta and pass through to the fetus, and small amounts are distributed in breast milk; thus, breast-feeding is not advised for mothers who are taking these drugs. For children, oral solutions of thiazide diuretics are available.
- Laboratory tests that may be altered by diuretics include increased serum levels of calcium, bilirubin, creatinine, glucose, and uric acid. Adverse effects, including potassium depletion and loss of volume, may be worse in pediatric patients because of age and increased sensitivity to these drugs.
- Loop diuretics may also interfere with laboratory findings in pediatric patients. Blood urea nitrogen, uric acid, and serum glucose levels may be increased, whereas calcium, chloride, magnesium, potassium, and sodium levels may be decreased.

Indications

The therapeutic applications of the potassium-sparing diuretics vary depending on the particular drug. Spironolactone and triamterene are used to treat hyperaldosteronism and hypertension and to reverse the potassium loss caused by the potassium-wasting (e.g., loop, thiazide) diuretics. One common feature of various types of heart failure is a hyperactive renin-angiotensin-aldosterone system. Research has identified this hyperactivity as a causative factor in permanent ventricular myocardial wall damage, known as *remodeling,* following myocardial infarction. Various clinical drug trials are increasingly demonstrating a cardioprotective benefit of spironolactone, owing to its aldosterone-inhibiting activity, in preventing this remodeling process. The uses for amiloride are similar to those for spironolactone and triamterene, but amiloride is less effective in the long term. It may be more effective than spironolactone or triamterene in the treatment of metabolic alkalosis, however. It is primarily used in the management of heart failure. As with certain other classes of diuretics, potassium-sparing diuretics may also be indicated in cases of heart failure due to diastolic dysfunction.

Contraindications

Contraindications to the use of potassium-sparing diuretics include known drug allergy, hyperkalemia (i.e., serum potassium level exceeding 5.5 mEq/L), and severe renal failure or anuria. Triamterene use may also be contraindicated in cases of severe hepatic failure.

Adverse Effects

Potassium-sparing diuretics have several common undesirable effects, which are listed in Table 25-4. There are also some significant adverse effects that are specific to individual drugs. Spironolactone can cause gynecomastia, amenorrhea, irregular menses, and postmenopausal bleeding. Triamterene may reduce folic acid levels and cause the formation of kidney stones and urinary casts. It may also precipitate megaloblastic anemia. Hyperkalemia may occur when potassium-sparing diuretics are used in combination with each other and/or with other potassium-sparing drugs such as angiotensin-converting enzyme (ACE) inhibitors (Chapter 24, as well as the Interactions section, which follows). However, adverse effects from triamterene use are rare.

Interactions

The concomitant use of potassium-sparing diuretics and lithium, ACE inhibitors, or potassium supplements can result in significant drug interactions. The administration of ACE inhibitors or potassium supplements in combination with potassium-sparing diuretics can result in hyperkalemia. When lithium and potassium-sparing diuretics are given together, lithium toxicity can result. NSAIDs can inhibit renal prostaglandins, decreasing

blood flow to the kidneys and therefore decreasing the delivery of diuretic drugs to this site of action. This in turn can lead to a diminished diuretic response.

Dosages

For the recommended dosages of potassium-sparing diuretics, see the Dosages table on page 396.

Drug Profiles

amiloride

Amiloride (Midamor) is generally used in combination with a thiazide or loop diuretic in the treatment of heart failure. Hyperkalemia may occur in as many as 10% of the patients who take amiloride alone. It should be used with caution in patients suffering from renal impairment or diabetes mellitus and in elderly patients. It has only weak antihypertensive properties. Amiloride is available only in oral form. It is also available in combination with hydrochlorothiazide. Pregnancy category B. Recommended dosages are given in the dosages table on page 396.

Pharmacokinetics

Half-Life	Onset	Peak	Duration
6-9 hr	2 hr	6-10 hr	24 hr

spironolactone

Structurally, spironolactone (Aldactone) is a synthetic steroid that blocks aldosterone receptors. It is used in high dosages for the treatment of ascites, a condition commonly associated with cirrhosis of the liver. The serum potassium level should be monitored frequently in patients who have impaired renal function or who are currently taking potassium supplements, because hyperkalemia is a common complication of spironolactone therapy. It is the potassium-sparing diuretic most commonly prescribed for children who have heart failure, because pediatric heart failure often causes excess aldosterone to be secreted, which in turn causes increased sodium and water resorption. Recently spironolactone has been shown to reduce morbidity and mortality in patients with severe heart failure when added to standard therapy. This is believed to be due primarily to its reduction of ventricular remodeling after myocardial infarction. Of the three commonly used potassium-sparing diuretics, spironolactone has the greatest antihypertensive activity. It is available only in oral form. It also is available in combination with hydrochlorothiazide. Pregnancy category D. Recommended dosages are given in the Dosages table on page 396.

Pharmacokinetics

Half-Life	Onset	Peak	Duration
13-24 hr	1-3 days	2-3 days	2-3 days

triamterene

As previously mentioned, the pharmacologic properties of triamterene (Dyrenium) are similar to those of amiloride. Like amiloride, triamterene acts directly on the distal renal tubule of the nephron to depress the resorption of sodium and the excretion of potassium and hydrogen, processes otherwise stimulated at that site by aldosterone. It has little or no antihypertensive effect. Triamterene is available only in oral form as 50- and 100-mg capsules. It also is available in combination with hydrochlorothiazide. Pregnancy category D. Recommended dosages are given in the Dosages table on page 396.

Pharmacokinetics

Half-Life	Onset	Peak	Duration
2-3 hr	2-4 hr	6-8 hr	12-16 hr

Table 25-4	Potassium-Sparing Diuretics: Common Adverse Effects
Body System	**Adverse Effects**
Central nervous	Dizziness, headache
Gastrointestinal	Cramps, nausea, vomiting, diarrhea
Other	Urinary frequency, weakness, hyperkalemia

DOSAGES

Selected Potassium-Sparing Diuretic Drugs

Drug	Pharmacologic Class	Usual Dosage Range	Indications
amiloride (Midamor)		**Adult** PO: 5-20 mg/day	Edema, heart failure (as an adjunct to kaliuretic diuretics)
▶spironolactone (Aldactone)	Potassium-sparing diuretics	**Pediatric** PO: 3.3 mg/kg/day in single or divided doses **Adult** PO: 25-200 mg/day	Edema, hypertension, heart failure, ascites
triamterene (Dyrenium)		**Adult** PO: 100 mg bid; do not exceed 300 mg/day	

PO, Oral.

THIAZIDES AND THIAZIDE-LIKE DIURETICS

Thiazide and thiazide-like diuretics are generally considered equivalent in their effects. Thiazide diuretics, like several of the loop diuretics, are chemical derivatives (benzothiadiazines) of sulfonamide antibiotics. Chlorthalidone is distinguished by its prolonged half-life of up to 72 hours. Metolazone may be more effective than other drugs in this class in the treatment of patients with renal dysfunction. Hydrochlorothiazide is undoubtedly the most commonly prescribed and the least expensive of the generic preparations. The thiazide diuretics include bendroflumethiazide, chlorothiazide, methyclothiazide, and trichlormethiazide. The thiazide-like diuretics are very similar in action to the thiazides and include chlorthalidone, indapamide, and metolazone. Of all of the drugs just mentioned, hydrochlorothiazide and metolazone are by far the most commonly prescribed in practice, although the others currently remain on the U.S. market.

Mechanism of Action and Drug Effects

Thiazides are used as adjunct drugs in the management of heart failure, hepatic cirrhosis, and edema of various origins. The primary site of action of thiazides and thiazide-like diuretics is the distal convoluted tubule, where they inhibit the resorption of sodium, potassium, and chloride. This results in osmotic water loss. Thiazides also cause direct relaxation of the arterioles (small blood vessels), which reduces peripheral vascular resistance (afterload). Decreased preload (filling pressures) and decreased afterload (the force the ventricles must overcome to eject the volume of blood they contain) are the beneficial hemodynamic effects. This makes them very effective for the treatment of both heart failure and hypertension.

As renal function decreases, the efficacy of thiazides diminishes, probably because delivery of the drug to the site of activity is impaired. Thiazides generally should not be used if creatinine clearance is less than 30 to 50 mL/min. Normal creatinine clearance is 125 mL/min. The only exception is metolazone, which remains effective to a creatinine clearance of 10 mL/min. The major adverse effects of the drugs stem from the electrolyte disturbances they produce. They are noted for precipitating hypokalemia and hypercalcemia, as well as metabolic disturbances such as hyperlipidemia, hyperglycemia, and hyperuricemia.

Indications

The thiazide and thiazide-like diuretics are used in the treatment of edematous states, idiopathic hypercalciuria, and diabetes insipidus, in addition to hypertension. Any of these drugs can be used either as monotherapy or in combination with other drugs. This group of diuretics may also be useful as adjunct drugs in the treatment of edema related to heart failure, hepatic cirrhosis, and corticosteroid or estrogen therapy. As with certain other classes of diuretics, they may also be indicated in cases of heart failure due to diastolic dysfunction.

Contraindications

Contraindications to the use of thiazides and thiazide-like diuretics include known drug allergy, hepatic coma (metolazone), anuria, and severe renal failure.

Adverse Effects

As previously mentioned, major adverse effects of the thiazide and thiazide-like diuretics relate to the electrolyte and metabolic disturbances they cause. These are mainly reduced potassium levels and elevated levels of calcium, lipids, glucose, and uric acid. Other effects, such as gastrointestinal disturbances, skin rashes, photosensitivity, thrombocytopenia, pancreatitis, and cholecystitis, are less common. Dizziness and vertigo are common adverse effects of metolazone therapy and are attributed to sudden shifts in the plasma volume brought about by the drug. Headache, impotence, and decreased libido are other important adverse effects of these drugs. Many of these adverse effects are dose related and are seen at higher doses, especially those above 25 mg. The more common adverse effects of the thiazide and thiazide-like diuretics are listed in Table 25-5.

Table 25-5   Thiazide and Thiazide-Like Diuretics: Potential Adverse Effects

Body System	Adverse Effects
Central nervous	Dizziness, headache, blurred vision, paresthesia, decreased libido
Gastrointestinal	Anorexia, nausea, vomiting, diarrhea, pancreatitis, cholecystitis
Genitourinary	Impotence
Hematologic	Jaundice, leukopenia, purpura, agranulocytosis, aplastic anemia, thrombocytopenia
Integumentary	Urticaria, photosensitivity
Metabolic	Hypokalemia, glycosuria, hyperglycemia, hyperuricemia, hypochloremic alkalosis

Table 25-6   Thiazide and Thiazide-Like Diuretics: Common Drug Interactions

Interacting Drug	Mechanism	Results
Corticosteroids	Additive effect	Hypokalemia
diazoxide	Additive effect	Hyperkalemia
digoxin	Hypokalemia	Increased digoxin toxicity
lithium	Decreased clearance	Increased lithium toxicity
NSAIDs	Inhibition of renal prostaglandins	Decreased diuretic activity
Oral hypoglycemics	Antagonism	Reduced therapeutic hypoglycemic effect

NSAIDs, Nonsteroidal antiinflammatory drugs.

DOSAGES

Thiazide and Selected Thiazide-Like Diuretic Drugs

Drug	Pharmacologic Class	Usual Dosage Range	Indications
▶ hydrochlorothiazide (Esidrix, HydroDIURIL)	Thiazide diuretic	**Pediatric** PO: Less than 6 mo, 3.3 mg/kg/day; 6 mo-2 yr, 12.5-37.5 mg/day in 2 doses; 2-12 yr, 37.5-100 mg/day in 2 doses **Adult** PO: 25-200 mg/day, usually divided PO: 25-100 mg/day **Elderly** 12.5-25 mg/day	Edema, heart failure (as an adjunct to kaliuretic diuretics)
metolazone (Mykrox, Diulo, Zaroxolyn)	Thiazide-like diuretic	**Adult** PO: 2.5-20 mg/day	

PO, Oral.

Toxicity and Management of Overdose

An overdose of these drugs can lead to an electrolyte imbalance resulting from hypokalemia. Symptoms include anorexia, nausea, lethargy, muscle weakness, mental confusion, and hypotension. Treatment involves electrolyte replacement.

Interactions

Thiazides and related drugs interact with corticosteroids, diazoxide, digitalis, and oral hypoglycemics. The mechanisms and results of these interactions are summarized in Table 25-6. Excessive consumption of licorice can lead to an additive hypokalemia in patients taking these drugs.

Dosages

For information on the dosages for thiazides and thiazide-like diuretics, see the Dosages table on this page.

Drug Profiles

▶ hydrochlorothiazide

Hydrochlorothiazide (Esidrix, HydroDIURIL), which is considered the prototypical thiazide diuretic, is a very commonly prescribed and inexpensive thiazide diuretic. It is also a very safe and effective diuretic. Hydrochlorothiazide is used in combination with many other drugs: methyldopa, propranolol, spironolactone, triamterene, hydralazine, ACE inhibitors, β-blockers, and labetalol. Dosages exceeding 50 mg/day rarely produce additional clinical results and may only increase drug toxicity. This property is known as a *ceiling effect.*

Hydrochlorothiazide use is contraindicated in patients with a known hypersensitivity to thiazides or sulfonamides and in those suffering from anuria, renal decompensation, or hypomagnesemia. It is available only in oral form. Pregnancy category B. Recommended dosages are given in the Dosages table on this page.

Pharmacokinetics

Half-Life	Onset	Peak	Duration
5.6-14.8 hr	2 hr	4 hr	6-12 hr

metolazone

Metolazone (Mykrox, Zaroxolyn) is a thiazide-like diuretic that appears to be more potent than the thiazide diuretics. This greater potency is most visible in patients with renal dysfunction. One striking advantage of metolazone is that, as noted earlier, it remains effective to a creatinine clearance as low as 10 mL/min. It may also be given in combination with loop diuretics to produce potent diuresis in patients with severe symptoms of heart failure. Metolazone use is contraindicated in patients with a known hypersensitivity to thiazides or sulfonamides, in those with anuria, and in pregnant or lactating women. It is available only in oral form. Pregnancy category B. Recommended dosages are given in the Dosages table on this page.

Pharmacokinetics

Half-Life	Onset	Peak	Duration
6-20 hr	1 hr	1-2 hr	Up to 24 hr

◆ NURSING PROCESS

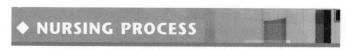

◆ ASSESSMENT

Before giving a patient any type of diuretic, the nurse should obtain a complete patient history, including medication history and nursing history. A thorough physical assessment should be completed and all findings documented. Because fluid volume levels and electrolyte concentrations are affected by diuretics, the patient's baseline fluid volume status (as indicated by vital signs, weight, and intake and output measurements) should be assessed and documented. Postural blood pressures (BPs) (e.g., lying, sitting, standing) should be assessed before and during drug therapy because of diuretic-induced fluid volume loss. This volume loss may lead to postural hypotension or a drop in blood pressure (e.g., of 20 mm Hg or more) upon standing. Skin turgor, status of moisture levels of mucous membranes, and capillary refill are also important to assess with diuretic therapy.

Serum potassium, sodium, chloride, magnesium, calcium, uric acid, and creatinine levels should also be measured and documented as ordered. Other laboratory studies may include arterial blood gases and blood pH. Cautious use of diuretics, with close monitoring of fluid volume status, electrolyte levels, and vital signs, is recommended in patients with the following disorders or conditions: hypokalemia, hypovolemia, renal disease, liver disease, lupus erythematosus, diabetes, chronic obstructive pulmonary disease, and gout. Loop diuretics are more potent than thiazides, combination products, and/or potassium-sparing diuretics, so these drugs may pose more problems for patients of any age. Patients with altered renal or liver functioning may also react more sensitively to diuretics and subsequent fluid volume loss. Cautions, contraindications, and drug interactions associated with all of the various diuretics have been previously discussed. Potassium-sparing diuretics may lead to hyperkalemia, and the patient's blood levels of potassium need to be closely monitored. In addition, a significant concern exists with loop diuretics that is important for nursing assessment; the concern is that they adversely react with other medications that are ototoxic or nephrotoxic (e.g., sulfonamide antibiotics).

◆ NURSING DIAGNOSES
- Decreased cardiac output related to adverse effects of diuretics
- Deficient fluid volume related to drug effects of diuretics
- Risk for injury related to postural hypotension and dizziness
- Deficient knowledge related to lack of experience with newly prescribed diuretic therapy
- Acute pain related to occurrence of headache from adverse effects of diuretics
- Noncompliance with the treatment regimen related to lack of information about the adverse effects of the medications

◆ PLANNING
Goals
- Patient regains fluid and electrolyte balance.
- Patient remains free of the complications associated with diuretic use.
- Patient remains free of injury to self while taking diuretics.
- Patient remains compliant with the therapy regimen.

Outcome Criteria
- Patient maintains normal levels of electrolytes (sodium, potassium, and chloride) while taking diuretics.
- Patient continues to show or regains normal cardiac output while on diuretic therapy as evidenced by vital signs, adequate intake, and output within normal limits (pulse less than 100 and higher than 60 beats/min; blood pressure 120/80; urine output less than or equal to 30 mL/hr).
- Patient's skin is pliable and without edema or dryness.

- Patient rises slowly and changes positions slowly and cautiously while receiving diuretics.
- Patient states the importance of and rationale for follow-up visits with the physician, such as monitoring for adverse effects, dehydration, and fluid and electrolyte imbalances.
- Patient reports dizziness, fainting, palpitations, tingling, confusion, or disorientation to the physician immediately.

◆ IMPLEMENTATION
Blood pressure, pulse rate, intake and output, and daily weights should continue to be measured and recorded during diuretic therapy. Changes from the initial assessment data (see earlier) that would alert the nurse to possible problems with the drug therapy include complaints of weakness, fatigue, tremor, muscle cramping, changes in mental status, and cold clammy skin. Diuretic therapy may also precipitate cardiac irregularities, and so heart rate and rhythm are important parameters to continue to watch and document. Fluid loss may lead to constipation, thus requiring measures to prevent this through dietary changes or use of naturally occurring bulk formers (e.g., Metamucil-type drugs). Diuretics should always be given exactly as directed but with consideration of the patient's age and related needs. Dosing and timing of the drugs are often very important to enhance therapeutic effects and minimize adverse effects. Because diuretics taken late in the afternoon or evening may lead to nocturia, the patient may experience sleep deficit, so these medications should be scheduled for morning dosing. Safety concerns exist with nocturia, especially with the elderly, because getting up in the middle of the night with possible confusion and dizziness may create the potential for falls and injury.

Loop diuretics (if taken at high doses as ordered) may put patients at greater risk for volume and electrolyte depletion (e.g., hypokalemia, hyponatremia, dehydration). Monitoring of therapy should include frequent BP and pulse rate, hydration status,

---

CASE STUDY

Diuretic Therapy

Primary hypertension has been diagnosed in Ms. G., a 47-year-old woman. Blood pressure readings have been ranging between 158 and 172 mm Hg systolic and 94 and 110 mm Hg diastolic. Average blood pressure over the past month has been 156/96 mm Hg. There is a strong family history of hypertension. Ms. G. is a single parent of two adolescents. She is also trying to keep up with her responsibilities as a full-time assistant professor of education at a local urban university and works more than 40 hours a week. There is no evidence of renal insufficiency or cardiac damage at this time, nor is there evidence of retinopathy or other signs and symptoms of end-organ disease. No other problems are reported. Ms. G. is started on 50 mg of hydrochlorothiazide daily with a small dose of the β-blocker atenolol.

- Discuss the antihypertensive effects of hydrochlorothiazide.
- What sort of information must you share with this patient to increase compliance and decrease adverse effects? What should she be educated about concerning her disease process and the impact of compliance with the drug therapy regimen?
- What should be included in her daily regimen (e.g., exercise, diet, journaling)?
- What other nonpharmacologic measures should you tell the patient about that can help her control her blood pressure?

For answers, see http://evolve.elsevier.com/Lilley.

Life Span Considerations: The Elderly Patient

Diuretic Therapy

- Measurements of the patient's height, weight, intake and output, blood pressure, pulse rate, respiratory rate, temperature; assessment of breath and heart sounds and edematous areas; and monitoring of serum sodium, potassium, and chloride levels should occur before and during diuretic drug therapy, so that adverse effects and/or complications can be minimized or identified early.

- It should be emphasized to the elderly patient that diuretics should be taken at the same time every day. They are generally ordered to be taken in the morning to help prevent nocturia (voiding at night), which can result in lack of sleep. More importantly, nocturia can lead to injury if the individual needs to get out of bed to void, becomes dizzy and/or confused, and falls. A bedside commode may be used to decrease the risk of injury.

- If the elderly patient is living alone and has minimal or no assistance with the medication regimen, visits from a home health or other health care professional may help ensure safety, efficacy, and compliance not only in taking the medication but also in following all aspects of the therapeutic regimen.

- Caution should be exercised in the administration of diuretics to the elderly because they are more sensitive to the therapeutic effects of these drugs (often reacting to smaller dosages of medi-cation than are required by other patients) and are more sensitive to the adverse effects of diuretics such as dehydration, electrolyte loss, dizziness, and syncope.

- Patients should be encouraged to change positions slowly because of the risk of orthostatic hypotension and subsequent falls and injury. Daily weights, blood pressures, and overall well-being should be recorded daily.

- Carrying a card outlining medical history, blood pressure readings, names and telephone numbers for contact persons, and list of medications is important to ensure safety and minimize complications. The card should be formatted so that it can fit in a wallet, with a copy placed in the kitchen on the refrigerator door or in another visible location so that it will be easily available to emergency personnel. Copies of the card should be given to the caregiver(s), family members, significant others, physicians, dentist, and relevant health care personnel. The card should be updated at regular intervals by the patient or another adult or by a physician involved in the patient's care. Such a card can be made easily using standard card stock or an index card. It can be placed in a wallet sleeve or can even be laminated and information entered using an erasable pen or pencil. The following sample shows the headings and content for such a card:

1. Name: _____
2. Age: _____   3. Blood type: _____   4. Drug/food allergies: _____
5. Medical history (circle all that apply and write in any not listed):

Anemia	Depression	Nerve problems
Asthma	Diabetes	Pacemaker or defibrillator device
Bleeding problems	Difficulty swallowing	Recent weight gain
Blood clots	Heart problems	Recent weight loss
Breathing problems	High blood pressure	Stroke
Cancer	Low blood pressure	Thyroid problems

   Others: _____

6. Current medications:
   Prescription drugs
      Name of drug: _____
      Dose amount: _____
      Frequency of doses: _____
      Condition for which drug is taken: _____
   Over-the-counter drugs
      Name of drug: _____
      Dose amount: _____
      Frequency of doses: _____
      Condition for which drug is taken: _____
   Herbals, vitamins, and other preparations
      Name of drug: _____
      Dose amount: _____
      Frequency of doses: _____
      Condition for which substance is taken: _____

7. Surgery (list all):
   Date: _____ Type and purpose: _____
   Any complications: _____
8. Prosthetics used: _____
9. Dental problems or concerns: _____
10. Wear glasses _____ Use hearing aid(s) _____ Need help with mobility _____
11. Other important information that should be known in case of emergency: _____
12. Contact names and telephone numbers: _____

capillary refill, and daily weights. Acute hypotensive episodes may also occur with higher doses of loop diuretics and precipitate syncope and falls, so safety measures should be implemented. Most oral diuretics should be taken with food to help minimize gastric upset. If giving intravenous dosage forms, it is crucial to check for diluents as well as drug incompatibilities. Rates of infusion should be confirmed and an infusion pump used. With potassium-sparing diuretics, potassium is reabsorbed and not excreted (as previously discussed), so hyperkalemia, rather than hypokalemia, may become problematic. Signs and symptoms of hyperkalemia include nausea, vomiting, diarrhea, and abdominal cramping (Chapter 26) and should be reported immediately. See the Patient Teaching Tips for more information.

◆ EVALUATION

The therapeutic effects of diuretics include the resolution of or reduction in edema, fluid volume overload, heart failure, or hypertension or a return to normal intraocular pressures (if used for that purpose). The patient must also be monitored for the occurrence of adverse reactions to the diuretics, such as metabolic alkalosis (arterial blood gas values should be monitored), drowsiness, lethargy, hypokalemia, tachycardia, hypotension, leg cramps, restlessness, and a decrease in mental alertness. With potassium-sparing diuretics, hyperkalemia may be the adverse effect for which to monitor with the therapeutic regimen. All goals and outcome criteria should be used in the evaluation process.

Patient Teaching Tips

- Patients taking diuretics need to be informed about the following: (1) They should maintain proper nutritional intake and fluid volume status with attention to eating potassium-rich foods, except when contraindicated or when taking potassium-sparing diuretics. (2) Foods high in potassium include bananas, oranges, dates, raisins, plums, fresh vegetables, potatoes (white and sweet), meat, fish, apricots, whole grain cereals, and legumes. (3) Potassium supplementation may be recommended by a physician when a patient's potassium level is below 3 mEq/L (Chapter 26). (4) Frequent laboratory tests may be indicated at the beginning of therapy and during the use of diuretics. (5) Patients need to change positions slowly and to rise slowly after sitting or lying to prevent dizziness and possible fainting (syncope). (6) Forcing fluids may be needed, if not contraindicated, to maintain adequate hydration. (7) Patients should report any unusual adverse effects or problems to their health care provider immediately. (8) Keeping a daily journal with notation of weight, how the patient feels each day, and any other important information relative to their diagnosis and medical treatment is important. (9) Prevent constipation with an increase in fiber, bulk, roughage, and fluids if not contraindicated.

- Patients should be educated about the signs and symptoms of hypokalemia, such as weakness, leg cramps, and other cramping. In addition, encourage patients to avoid hot climates, excessive sweating, fever, and the use of saunas or hot tubs. Heat raises core body temperature and cause further loss of potassium and sodium through sweat. It is also known that should the patient experience excessive sweating, vomiting, or other fluid loss, hypovolemia may be exacerbated.
- If the patient is taking a diuretic along with a digitalis preparation, the patient, family members, and anyone involved in the patient's care should be educated about how to monitor pulse rate. Emphasize the warning signs and symptoms of digitalis toxicity, such as anorexia, nausea, vomiting, and bradycardia (a pulse rate of less than 60 beats/min).
- For patients with diabetes mellitus who are also taking thiazide and/or loop diuretics, educate them about close monitoring of blood glucose levels. These diuretics may cause elevation of blood glucose.

Points to Remember

- The five main types of diuretics are CAIs and loop, osmotic, potassium-sparing, and thiazide and thiazide-like diuretics.
- The loop, potassium-sparing, and thiazide and thiazide-like diuretics are the most commonly used. The nurse must remember that the loop diuretics are more potent than the thiazides, combination diuretics, and potassium-sparing diuretics. The three most commonly prescribed loop diuretics are furosemide, bumetanide, and torsemide.
- Thiazide diuretics are the most commonly used diuretics and are the least expensive because several generic preparations are available. Hydrochlorothiazide is considered the prototypical thiazide diuretic and is used as adjunctive therapy to manage hepatic cirrhosis, edema, and heart failure. Related adverse metabolic effects for which the nurse needs to monitor include hypokalemia, hypercalcemia, hyperlipidemia, hyperglycemia, and hyperuricemia.
- Adverse effects for which the nurse should monitor in patients taking loop and/or thiazide diuretics include metabolic alkalosis,

drowsiness, lethargy, hypokalemia, tachycardia, hypotension, leg cramps, restlessness, and decreased mental alertness. When potassium-sparing diuretics are used, hyperkalemia with nausea, vomiting, and diarrhea may occur.
- Nurses must have a thorough knowledge of renal anatomy and physiology and how it relates to the action of the various diuretics; for example, if a loop diuretic is given, its site of action is the loop of Henle and it causes the excretion of sodium, potassium, and chloride into the urine.
- Methods for monitoring excess and deficit fluid volume states include assessment of skin and mucous membranes, blood pressure, pulse rate, intake and output, and daily weights.
- The nurse should always be concerned about the more vulnerable patient populations, such as the elderly, those with a chronic illness, and patients with altered renal or liver function.

NCLEX Examination Review Questions

1. The nurse is reviewing the medications that have been ordered for a patient for whom a loop diuretic has been newly prescribed. The loop diuretic may have a possible interaction with which of the following?
   a. vitamin C
   b. warfarin
   c. penicillins
   d. NSAIDs

2. When monitoring laboratory test results for patients receiving loop and thiazide diuretics, the nurse knows to look for which of the following?
   a. Decreased serum levels of potassium
   b. Increased serum levels of potassium
   c. Decreased serum glucose levels
   d. Increased serum levels of sodium

3. When the nurse is checking the laboratory data for a patient taking spironolactone (Aldactone), which result would be a potential concern?
   a. Serum sodium level of 140 mEq/L
   b. Serum potassium level of 3.6 mEq/L
   c. Serum potassium level of 5.8 mEq/L
   d. Serum magnesium level of 2.0 mg/dL

4. Which of the following statements should be included in patient education for an 81-year-old woman with heart failure who is taking daily doses of spironolactone (Aldactone)?
   a. "Be sure to eat foods that are high in potassium."
   b. "Avoid foods that are high in potassium."
   c. "Change positions slowly, because this drug causes severe hypertension-induced syncope."
   d. "A weight gain of 2 to 3 lb in 24 hours is normal."

5. A patient with diabetes has a new prescription for a thiazide diuretic. Which statement should the nurse include when teaching the patient about the thiazide drug?
   a. "You should take the thiazide at night to avoid interactions with the diabetes medicine."
   b. "There is nothing for you to be concerned about when you are taking the thiazide."
   c. "Monitor your blood glucose closely, because the thiazide may cause the levels to decrease."
   d. "Monitor your blood glucose closely, because the thiazide may cause the levels to increase."

1. d, 2. a, 3. c, 4. b, 5. d.

Critical Thinking Activities

1. Mr. G. is a 64-year-old man who has been admitted to the coronary care unit because he is experiencing heart failure. He has been given 80 mg of furosemide every 6 hours, but has experienced no relief of his pulmonary and peripheral edema. The physician would like to change his diuretic to bumetanide. What is the equivalent daily dose of bumetanide?

2. What type of teaching would be appropriate for a patient who is beginning treatment with a potassium-sparing diuretic?

3. Describe the antihypertensive effects of loop diuretics in the treatment of hypertension.

For answers, see http://evolve.elsevier.com/Lilley.

Fluids and Electrolytes

Objectives

When you reach the end of this chapter, you should be able to do the following:

1. Identify the various fluid and electrolyte solutions commonly used in the management of fluid and electrolyte disorders.
2. Discuss the mechanisms of action, indications, dosages, routes of administration, contraindications, cautions, adverse effects, toxicity, and drug interactions of various fluid and electrolyte solutions.
3. Compare the various solutions used to expand and/or decrease a patient's fluid volume and electrolytes with consideration of how they work, why they are used, and specific antidotes to any toxic effects.
4. Develop a nursing care plan that includes all phases of the nursing process for patients receiving fluid and electrolyte solutions.

e-Learning Activities

Companion CD

- NCLEX Review Questions: see questions 221-225
- Animations
- Audio Glossary
- Category Catchers
- Medication Errors Checklists
- IV Therapy Checklists

evolve Website (http://evolve.elsevier.com/Lilley)

• Nursing Care Plans • Frequently Asked Questions • Content Updates • WebLinks • Supplemental Resources • Elsevier ePharmacology Update • Medication Administration Animations

Drug Profiles

albumin, p. 407
dextran, p. 407
sodium chloride, pp. 406, 411

sodium polystyrene sulfonate, p. 410

Glossary

Blood The fluid that circulates through the heart, arteries, capillaries, and veins, carrying nutriment and oxygen to the body cells. Consists of *plasma*, its liquid component, plus three major solid components in the form of *erythrocytes* (red blood cells or RBCs), *leukocytes* (white blood cells or WBCs), and *platelets*. (p. 403)

Colloid A state of matter in which large molecules or aggregates of molecules that do not precipitate and that measure between 1 and 100 nm are dispersed in another medium. (p. 406)

Colloid oncotic pressure (COP) The osmotic pressure exerted by a colloid in solution, such as that produced when the concentration of protein in the plasma on one side of a

blood vessel cell wall membrane is higher than that in the neighboring *interstitial fluid* (ISF). (p. 403)

Crystalloids A substance in a solution that diffuses through a semipermeable membrane. (p. 404)

Dehydration Excessive loss of water from the body tissues. It is accompanied by an imbalance in the essential electrolyte concentrations, particularly sodium, potassium, and chloride. (p. 403)

Edema The abnormal accumulation of fluid in interstitial spaces. (p. 403)

Extracellular fluid (ECF) That portion of the body fluid comprising the ISF and blood plasma. The adult body contains about 11.2 L of ISF, constituting about 16% of the body weight, and about 2.8 L of plasma, constituting about 4% of the body weight. (p. 403)

Extravascular fluid (EVF) Fluids in the body that are outside the blood vessels. (p. 403)

Gradient A difference in the concentration of a substance on two sides of a permeable barrier. (p. 404)

Hydrostatic pressure (HP) The pressure exerted by a liquid. (p. 403)

Hyperkalemia Abnormally high potassium concentration in the blood; most often due to defective renal excretion but can also be due to excessive dietary potassium. (p. 408)

Hypernatremia Abnormally high sodium concentration in the blood; may be due to defective renal excretion, but more commonly due to excessive dietary sodium or from aggressive therapy. (p. 410)

Hypokalemia A condition in which there is an inadequate amount of potassium, the major intracellular cation, in the bloodstream. (p. 408)

Hyponatremia A condition in which there is an inadequate amount of sodium, the major extracellular cation, in the bloodstream, caused either by inadequate excretion of water or by excessive water intake. (p. 410)

Interstitial fluid (ISF) ECF that fills in the spaces between most of the cells of the body. Note also: an *interstice* is defined as a small space within a tissue. (p. 403)

Intracellular fluid (ICF) Fluid located within cell membranes throughout most of the body. It contains dissolved solutes that are essential to maintaining electrolyte balance and healthy metabolism. (p. 403)

Intravascular fluid (IVF) The fluid inside blood vessels. (p. 403)

Isotonic Having the same concentration of a solute as another solution, hence exerting the same osmotic pressure as that solution, such as an isotonic saline solution that contains an amount of salt equal to that found in the intracellular and ECF. (p. 403)

Osmotic pressure The pressure exerted on a semipermeable membrane separating a solution from a solvent; the membrane being impermeable to the solutes in the solution and permeable only to the solvent. (p. 403)

Plasma The watery, straw-colored fluid component of lymph and blood in which the leukocytes, erythrocytes, and platelets are suspended. (p. 403)

Serum The clear, cell-free portion of the blood from which fibrinogen has also been separated during the clotting process, as typically carried out with a laboratory sample. (p. 403)

Fluid and electrolyte management is one of the cornerstones of patient care. Most disease processes, tissue injuries, and surgical procedures greatly influence the physiologic status of fluids and electrolytes in the body. A prerequisite to the understanding of fluid and electrolyte management is knowledge of the extent and composition of the various body fluid compartments.

PHYSIOLOGY OF FLUID BALANCE

Approximately 60% of the adult human body is water. This is referred to as the *total body water* (TBW), and it is distributed to the three main compartments in the following proportions: **intracellular fluid (ICF)**, 67%; **interstitial fluid (ISF)**, 25%; and **plasma volume (PV)**, 8%. This distribution is illustrated in Figure 26-1. The actual volume of fluid that would normally be in each compartment in an average 70-kg man with a TBW content of 60% of his TBW is shown in Table 26-1.

The terms used to identify the various spaces within which the TBW is distributed can be quite confusing, and there are two basic approaches to distinguishing among the locations of the fluid.

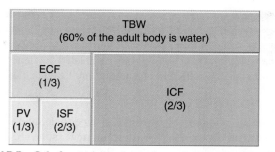

FIGURE 26-1 Distribution of total body water (TBW). *ECF,* Extracellular fluid; *ICF,* intracellular fluid; *ISF,* interstitial fluid; *PV,* plasma volume.

The TBW can be described as being in or out of the **blood** vessels, or vasculature. If this terminology is used, the term **intravascular fluid (IVF)** describes fluid inside the blood vessels and the term **extravascular fluid (EVF)** describes the fluid outside the blood vessels. Examples of EVF include lymph and cerebrospinal fluid. As you learn these concepts, recall the difference between the prefixes *intra-* (inside), *inter-* (between), and *extra-* (outside). The term **plasma** is used to describe the fluid that flows through the blood vessels that is intravascular. **Serum** is a closely related term (see glossary). ISF is the fluid that is in the space between cells, tissues, and organs. Both plasma and ISF make up extracellular volume. Both ISF and ICF make up extravascular volume. These terms are often confused and misused. Table 26-1 lists these definitions for further clarity and understanding.

What, then, keeps fluid inside the blood vessels? All the fluid outside the cells, the **extracellular fluid (ECF),** which consists of both the plasma and the ISF, has about the same concentration of electrolytes. However, there is one big difference between the plasma and the ISF. The plasma has a protein concentration four times greater than that of the ISF. It consists primarily of albumin but also includes globulin and fibrinogen, The reason for this higher intravascular concentration of protein is that these solutes (proteins) have a molecular weight that exceeds 69,000 daltons, and this makes them too large to pass through the walls of the blood vessels. Because of the difference in concentration of plasma proteins, fluid flows from the area of low protein concentration in the interstitial compartment to the area of high concentration inside the blood vessel to try to create an **isotonic** environment on either side of the blood vessel wall. (*Isotonic* means an equal concentration of solutes across a membrane.) The protein in the blood vessels, therefore, exerts a constant **osmotic pressure** that prevents the leakage of too much plasma through the capillaries into the tissues. Because proteins suspended in plasma constitute a *colloidal* state, this particular pressure is called **colloid oncotic pressure (COP),** and normally it is 24 mm Hg. The opposing pressure, that exerted by the ISF, is called **hydrostatic pressure (HP),** and normally it is 17 mm Hg, which, of course, is less than the COP. The phenomenon of COP is illustrated in Figure 26-2.

This regulation of the volume and composition of body water is essential for life because it is the medium in which all metabolic reactions occur. The body maintains the volume and composition remarkably constant by maintaining a balance between intake and excretion. The amount of water gained each day is kept roughly equal to the amount of water lost. When, for some reason, the body cannot maintain this equilibrium, therapy with various agents becomes necessary. If the amount of water gained exceeds the amount of water lost, a water excess or overhydration occurs. Such fluid excesses often accumulate in interstitial spaces, such as in the pericardial sac, intrapleural space, peritoneal cavity, joint capsules, and lower extremities. This is referred to as **edema.** If the quantity of water lost exceeds that gained, a water deficit, or **dehydration,** occurs. Death often occurs when 20% to 25% of the TBW is lost.

Dehydration leads to a disturbance in the balance between the amount of fluid in the extracellular compartment and that in the intracellular compartment. Sodium is the principle extracellular electrolyte, and plays a primary role in maintaining water concentration in the body due to its highly osmotic chemistry. In the initial stages of dehydration, water is lost first from the extracel-

Table 26-1   Fluid Location: Descriptive Terms and Actual Volumes

Name	Location	Actual Volumes (in a 70-kg Man with a TBW Content of 60% of his Total Body Weight)
If the Point of Reference Is the Cells, These Terms Are Used		
Intracellular fluid (ICF)	Inside of cells	28,000 mL
Extracellular fluid (ECF)	Outside of cells	14,000 mL (composed of both intravascular plasma and ISF)
If the Point of Reference Is the Blood Vessels, These Terms Are Used		
Intravascular fluid or plasma volume (PV)	In blood vessels	3500 mL
Extravascular fluid (EVF)	Out of blood vessels	38,500 mL
If the Point of Reference Is the Tissues, These Terms Are Used		
Interstitial fluid (ISF)	In the spaces between cells, tissues, and organs but not in the plasma or the cells	10,500 mL

ISF, Interstitial fluid; *TBW,* total body water.

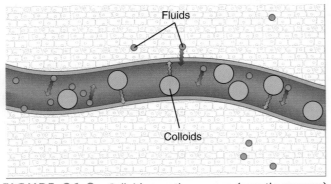

Fluids

Colloids

FIGURE 26-2   Colloid osmotic pressure (oncotic pressure). As shown, the colloids inside the blood vessel are too large to pass through the vessel wall. The resulting oncotic pressure exerted by the colloids draws fluid from the surrounding tissues and other extravascular spaces into the blood vessels and also keeps fluid inside the blood vessel.

Table 26-2   Types of Dehydration

Type of Dehydration	Characteristics
Hypertonic	Caused when water loss is greater than sodium loss, resulting in a concentration of solutes outside the cells and causing the fluid inside the cells to move to the extracellular space, thus dehydrating the cells. Example: Elevated temperature resulting in perspiration.
Hypotonic	Caused when sodium loss is greater than water loss, resulting in higher concentrations of solute inside the cells, thus pulling fluid from outside the cells (plasma and interstitial spaces) into the cells. Examples: Renal insufficiency and inadequate aldosterone secretion.
Isotonic	Caused by a loss of sodium and water from the body, resulting in a decrease in the volume of extracellular fluid. Examples: Diarrhea and vomiting.

Table 26-3   Conditions Leading to Fluid Loss or Dehydration and Associated Corresponding Symptoms*

Condition	Associated Symptoms
Bleeding	Tachycardia and hypotension
Bowel obstruction	Reduced perspiration and mucous secretions
Diarrhea	Reduced urine output (oliguria)
Fever	Dry skin and mucous membranes
Vomiting	Reduced lacrimal (tears) and salivary secretions

*There may be overlap involving more than one of the symptoms depending on the patient's specific condition.

lular compartments. The nature of further fluid losses, COP changes, or both depends on the type of clinical dehydration (Table 26-2). Clinical conditions that can result in dehydration and fluid loss, as well as the symptoms of dehydration and fluid loss, are listed in Table 26-3.

When fluid that has been lost must be replaced, there are three categories of agents that can be used to accomplish this: crystalloids, colloids, and blood products. The clinical situation dictates which category of agents is most appropriate.

CRYSTALLOIDS

Crystalloids are fluids given by intravenous (IV) injection that supply water and sodium to maintain the osmotic **gradient** between the extravascular and intravascular compartments. Their plasma volume-expanding capacity is related to their sodium concentration. The different crystalloids are listed in Table 26-4.

Mechanism of Action and Drug Effects

Because crystalloids work by osmosis, hypertonic saline (3% sodium chloride) is more efficient than normal saline (NS) (0.9% sodium chloride) for expanding the PV.

Crystalloid solutions contain fluids and electrolytes that are normally found in the body. They do not contain proteins (col-

Table 26-4 Crystalloids

| Product | Composition (mEq/L) | | | | | | Volume (mL) | Cost* |
	Na	Cl	K	Ca	Mg	Lactate		
NS	154	154	0	0	0	0	1000	1
Hypertonic saline	513	513	0	0	0	0	500	1
Lactated Ringer's	130	109	4	3	0	28	1000	2.5×
D₅W	0	0	1	0	0	0	1000	2×
Plasma-Lyte	140	103	10	5	3	8	1000	5×

*Relative cost; example: D_5W is two times the cost of hypertonic saline.
Ca, Calcium; Cl, chloride; D_5W, 5% dextrose in water; K, potassium; Mg, magnesium; Na, sodium; NS, normal saline.

loids), which are necessary to maintain the COP and prevent water from leaving the plasma compartment. In fact, the administration of large quantities of crystalloid solutions for fluid resuscitation decreases the COP, owing to a dilutional effect. Compared with the distribution of colloids, crystalloids are also distributed faster into the interstitial and intracellular compartments, which makes them better for treating dehydration than for expanding the PV alone, such as in hypovolemic shock. That is to say, crystalloids cannot expand the PV on a longer-term basis, nor can colloids, and even in the short term, much larger fluid volumes are required.

Indications

Crystalloid solutions are most commonly used as maintenance fluids. They are used to compensate for insensible fluid losses, to replace fluids when there are body-fluid deficits, and to manage specific fluid and electrolyte disturbances. Crystalloids also promote urinary flow. They are much less expensive than colloids and blood products. In addition, there is no risk for viral transmission or anaphylaxis and no alteration in the coagulation profile associated with their use, unlike blood products. The choice whether to use a crystalloid or colloid depends on the severity of the condition. Following are the common indications for either crystalloid or colloid replacement therapy:
- Acute liver failure
- Acute nephrosis
- Adult respiratory distress syndrome
- Burns
- Cardiopulmonary bypass
- Hypoproteinemia
- Reduction of the risk for deep vein thrombosis (DVT)
- Renal dialysis
- Shock

Contraindications

Contraindications to the use of crystalloids include known drug allergy to a specific product, hypervolemia, and may include severe electrolyte disturbance, depending on the type of crystalloid used.

Adverse Effects

Crystalloids are a very safe and effective means of replacing needed fluid. They do, however, have some unwanted effects. Because they contain no large particles, such as proteins, they do not stay within the blood vessels and can leak out of the plasma into the tissues and cells. This may result in edema anywhere in the body, due to osmo-

Table 26-5 Crystalloids and Colloids: Dosing Guidelines

| | Crystalloids and Colloids | | | |
	0.9% NS	3% NS	5% Colloid*	25% Colloid†
To Raise Plasma Volume by 1 L, Administer:	5-6 L	1.5-2 L	1 L	0.5 L
Fluid Compartment Distributed to:				
Plasma	25%	25%	100%	200%-300%
Interstitial space	75%	75%	0	Decreased fluid levels
Intracellular space	0	0	0	Decreased fluid levels

*Isooncotic solutions such as 5% albumin, dextran 70, and hetastarch.
†Hyperoncotic solutions such as 25% albumin.
NS, Normal saline.

sis from the crystalloid itself. Peripheral edema and pulmonary edema are two common examples. Crystalloids also dilute the proteins that are in the plasma, further reducing the COP. Because crystalloids cannot carry oxygen, their use may result in decreased oxygen tension due to a dilutional effect on erythrocyte concentration. Typically, large volumes (liters of fluid) are required for crystalloids to be effective. As a result, large or prolonged infusions may worsen acidosis or alkalosis, or adversely affect central nervous system (CNS) function, due to fluid overload. Another disadvantage of crystalloids is that their effects are relatively short-lived.

Interactions

Interactions with crystalloid solutions are rare because they are very similar if not identical to normal physiologic substances. Certain electrolytes contained in lactated Ringer's solution may be incompatible with other electrolytes, forming a chemical precipitate.

Dosages

For the recommended dosages of crystalloids, see Table 26-5.

Drug Profiles

The most commonly used crystalloid solutions are normal saline (NS or 0.9% sodium chloride) and lactated Ringer's solution. The available crystalloid solutions and their compositions are summarized in Table 26-4. Sodium chloride is also discussed briefly in the section on electrolytes and in the nursing process under electrolytes.

sodium chloride

Sodium chloride (salt, NaCl) is available in several concentrations, the most common being 0.9%. This is the physiologically normal concentration of sodium chloride, and for this reason it is referred to as *normal saline* (NS). Other concentrations are 0.45% ("half-normal"), 0.2% ("quarter-normal"), and 3% (hypertonic saline). These solutions have different indications, and they are used in different situations, depending on how urgently fluid volume restoration is needed and/or the extent of the sodium loss.

Sodium chloride is a physiologic electrolyte that is present throughout the body's water. For this reason, there are no hypersensitivity reactions to it. It is safe to administer it during any stage of pregnancy, but it is contraindicated in patients with hypernatremia and/or hyperchloremia. Hypertonic saline injections (3% and 5%) are contraindicated in the presence of increased, normal, or only slightly decreased serum electrolyte concentrations. Sodium chloride is also available as a 650-mg tablet and as 0.45%, 0.9%, 3%, and 5% solutions.

Pharmacokinetics

Plasma Volume	Colloid Oncotic	Duration of
Expansion 60-70 mL	Pressure 30 mm Hg	Expansion Few hours

*500 mL of NS will expand the plasma volume by 60 to 70 mL.

The dose of sodium chloride administered depends on the clinical situation. The volume of crystalloid or colloid needed to expand the plasma volume (PV) by 1 liter (1000 mL) is given in Table 26-5, and this can be used as a general guide to dosing.

COLLOIDS

Colloids are protein substances that increase the COP and effectively move fluid from the interstitial compartment to the plasma compartment by pulling the fluid into the blood vessels. Normally, this task is performed by the three blood proteins: albumin, globulin, and fibrinogen. However, for them to be effective, the total protein level must be in the range of 7.4 g/dL. If this level drops below 5.3 g/dL, the COP then drops below the HP and fluid shifts out of blood vessels into the tissues. When this happens, colloid replacement therapy is required to reverse this process by increasing the COP. The COP decreases with age and also with hypotension and malnutrition. The commonly used colloids are listed in Table 26-6.

Table 26-6 Commonly Used Colloids

Product	Composition (mEq/L)		Volume (mL)	Cost*
	Na	**Cl**		
Dextran 70†	154	154	500	1
Dextran 40†	154	154	500	2×
Hetastarch	154	154	500	5×
5% Albumin	145	145	500	10
25% Albumin	145	145	100	10

*Using the cost of dextran 70 as the means of comparison.
†Dextran is available in NaCl, which has 154 mEq/L of both Na and Cl. It is also available in 5% dextrose in water (D₅W), which contains no Na or Cl.
Cl, Chloride; *Na*, sodium.

Mechanism of Action and Drug Effects

The mechanism of action of colloids is related to their ability to increase the COP. As previously explained, because the colloids cannot pass into the extravascular space, there is ordinarily a higher concentration of colloid solutes (solid particles) inside the blood vessels (intravascular space) than outside the blood vessels. Fluid thus moves toward this hypertonic area, from the EV space, in an attempt to make it isotonic. Because colloids increase the blood volume, they are sometimes called *plasma expanders*. They also make up part of the total PV.

Colloids increase the COP and move fluid from outside the blood vessels to inside the blood vessels. They can maintain the COP for several hours. They are naturally occurring products and consist of proteins (albumin), carbohydrates (dextrans or starches), fats (lipid emulsion), and animal collagen (gelatin). Usually they contain a combination of both small and large particles. The small particles are eliminated quickly and promote diuresis and perfusion of the kidneys; the larger particles maintain the PV. Albumin is the one exception in that it contains particles that are all the same size.

Indications

Colloids are used to treat a wide variety of conditions (see list on p. 000). Clinically, colloids are superior to crystalloids in their ability to maintain the PV for a longer term. However, crystalloids are less expensive and are less likely to promote bleeding. On the other hand, crystalloids are more likely to cause edema because of the larger volumes needed to achieve the desired clinical effect, but they are still better than colloids for emergency short-term plasma volume expansion.

Contraindications

Contraindications to the use of colloids include known drug allergy to a specific product, hypervolemia, and may include severe electrolyte disturbance.

Adverse Effects

Colloids are relatively safe agents, although there are some disadvantages to their use. They have no oxygen-carrying ability and contain no clotting factors, unlike blood products. Because of this, they can alter the coagulation system through a dilutional effect, resulting in impaired coagulation and, possibly, bleeding. They may also dilute the plasma protein concentration, which, in turn, may impair the function of platelets. Rarely, dextran therapy causes anaphylaxis or renal failure.

Interactions

Because colloid solutions are so compatible with many drugs, they are sometimes used as the medium for delivering them. The anesthetic drug propofol (Diprivan) (Chapter 11) is such an example. It is delivered in a 10% lipid emulsion.

Dosages

For the recommended dosages of colloids, see Table 26-5.

Drug Profiles

The specific colloid used for replacement therapy varies from institution to institution. The three most commonly used are 5% albumin, dextran 40, and hetastarch. They are all very quick in onset and have a long duration of action. They are metabolized in the liver and excreted by the kidneys, with albumin the one exception. It is metabolized by the reticuloendothelial system and excreted by the kidneys and the intestines. Hetastarch is a synthetic colloid with properties similar to albumin and dextran.

albumin

Albumin (Albuminar, Albutein, Plasbumin) is a natural protein that is normally produced by the liver. It is responsible for generating approximately 70% of the COP. Human albumin is a sterile solution of serum albumin that is prepared from pooled blood, plasma serum, or placentas obtained from healthy human donors. It is pasteurized (heated at 60° C for 10 hours) to destroy any contaminants.

Albumin is contraindicated in patients with a known hypersensitivity to it and in those with heart failure, severe anemia, or renal insufficiency. Albumin is available only in parenteral form in concentrations of 5% and 25%. Pregnancy category C. See Table 26-5 for the dosing guidelines.

Pharmacokinetics

Half-Life	Onset	Peak	Duration
16 hr	<1 min	Unknown	<24 hr

dextran

Dextran (Gentran, LMD, Rheomacrodex) is a solution of glucose. It is available in two concentrations, dextran 40 and the more concentrated dextran 70 and dextran 75, and it has a molecular weight similar to that of albumin. Dextran 40 is the more commonly used of the two and is a low-molecular-weight polymer of glucose. It is a derivative of sugar that has actions similar to those of human albumin in that it expands the PV by drawing fluid from the interstitial space to the intravascular space.

Dextran is contraindicated in patients with hypersensitivity to it and in those with heart failure, renal insufficiency, and extreme dehydration. It is available only in parenteral form in either a 5% dextrose solution or a 0.9% sodium chloride solution. Pregnancy category C. See Table 26-5 for the dosing guidelines.

Pharmacokinetics

Half-Life	Onset	Peak	Duration
2-6 hr (D-40)	<5 min	Unknown	4-6 hr
12 hr (D-70)	1 hr	Unknown	12 hr

BLOOD PRODUCTS

Blood products can be thought of as biologic drugs. All of them can augment the PV. Red blood cell (RBC)-containing products can also improve tissue oxygenation, as well as augment PV. Blood products are also the most expensive and are less available than crystalloids and colloids because they are natural products and require human donors. The available blood products are listed in Table 26-7. They are most often indicated when a patient has 25% or more blood volume.

Mechanism of Action and Drug Effects

The mechanism of action of blood products is related to their ability to increase the COP, and hence, the PV. They do so in the same manner as colloids and crystalloids, by pulling fluid from the extravascular space to the intravascular space. Because of this they are also considered plasma expanders. Red blood cell (RBC) products also have the ability to carry oxygen. They can maintain the COP for several hours to days, and because they come from human donors, they have all the benefits (and hazards) that human blood products have. They

Table 26-7   Blood Products

Product	Dosage	Cost*
Cryoprecipitate	1 unit	1
FFP		1.7×
PRBCs		2.2×
PPF		1
Whole blood		3.33

*Using the cost of cryoprecipitate as the means of comparison.
FFP, Fresh frozen plasma; *PPF,* plasma protein fractions; *PRBC,* packed red blood cell.

Table 26-8   Blood Products: Indications

Blood Product	Indication
Cryoprecipitate and PPF	To manage acute bleeding (>50% blood loss slowly or 20% acutely)
FFP	To increase clotting factor levels in patients with a demonstrated deficiency
PRBCs	To increase oxygen-carrying capacity in patients with anemia, in patients with substantial hemoglobin deficits, and in patients who have lost up to 25% of their total blood volume
Whole blood	Same as for PRBCs, except that whole blood is more beneficial in cases of extreme (>25%) loss of blood volume since whole blood also contains plasma, the chief fluid volume of the blood; it also contains plasma proteins, the chief osmotic component, which help draw fluid back into blood vessels from surrounding tissues

FPP, Fresh frozen plasma; *PPF,* plasma protein fraction; *PRBCs,* packed red blood cells.

are administered when a person's body is deficient in these products.

Indications

Blood products are used to treat a wide variety of clinical conditions, and the blood product used depends on the specific indication. The available blood products and specific conditions they are used to treat are listed in Table 26-8.

Contraindications

There are no absolute contraindications to the use of blood products. However, because of the risk for transfer of infectious disease, although remote, their use should be based on careful clinical evaluation of the patient's condition.

Adverse Effects

Blood products can produce undesirable effects, some potentially serious. Because these products come from other humans, they can be incompatible with the recipient's immune system. These incompatibilities are tested for before the administration of the particular blood product by determining the respective blood types of the donor and recipient and by doing cross-matching

Table 26-9	**Suggested Guidelines for Blood Products: Management of Bleeding**
Amount of Blood Loss	**Fluid of Choice**
≤20% (slow loss)	Crystalloids
20%-50% (slow loss)	Nonprotein plasma expanders (dextran and hetastarch)
>50% (slow loss) or 20% (acutely)	Whole blood or PRBCs, and/or PPF and FFP
≥80% lost	As above, but for every 5 units of blood given, administer 1-2 units of FFP and 1-2 units of platelets to prevent the hemodilution of clotting factors and bleeding

FPP, Fresh frozen plasma; *PPF,* plasma protein fraction; *PRBCs,* packed red blood cells.

tests to screen for incompatibility between selected blood proteins. This helps reduce the likelihood of the recipient rejecting the blood products, which would, in turn, precipitate transfusion reactions and anaphylaxis. These products can also transmit pathogens from the donor to the recipient. Examples of such pathogens are hepatitis and HIV. Various preparation techniques are now used to reduce this risk for pathogen transmission, resulting in a drastic reduction in the incidence of such problems.

Interactions

As with crystalloids and colloids, blood products are very similar if not identical to normal physiologic substances; therefore, they interact with very few substances. Calcium and drugs such as aspirin, which normally affect coagulation, may interact with these substances when infused in the body in much the same way they interact with the body's own blood components.

Dosages

For the dosage guidelines pertaining to blood products, see Table 26-9.

Drug Profiles

Packed red blood cells (PRBCs) and fresh frozen plasma are among the most commonly used blood products. All of the blood products are derived from pooled human blood donors. Other less commonly used, but still important, blood products include whole blood, plasma protein fraction, cryoprecipitate, and platelets.

Packed Red Blood Cells

PRBCs are obtained by the centrifugation of whole blood and their separation from plasma and the other cellular elements. The advantage to PRBC use is that their oxygen-carrying capacity is better than that of the other blood products, and they are less likely to cause cardiac fluid overload. Their disadvantages include high cost, limited shelf life, fluctuating availability, and their ability to transmit viruses, cause allergic reactions, and bleeding abnormalities. The suggested guidelines are given in Table 26-9.

Fresh Frozen Plasma

Fresh frozen plasma (FFP) is obtained by centrifuging whole blood and thereby removing the cellular elements. The resulting plasma is then frozen at −18° C. FFP is not recommended for routine fluid re-

suscitation, but it may be used as an adjunct to massive blood transfusion in the treatment of patients with underlying coagulation disorders. The plasma-expanding capability of FFP is similar to that of dextran but slightly less than that of hetastarch. The disadvantage of FFP use is that it can transmit pathogens. The suggested guidelines are given in Table 26-9.

PHYSIOLOGY OF ELECTROLYTE BALANCE

As noted earlier in this chapter, the chemical composition of the fluid compartments varies from compartment to compartment. The principal electrolytes in the ECF are sodium cations (Na^+) and chloride anions (Cl^-); the major electrolyte of the ICF is the potassium cation (K^+). Other important electrolytes are calcium, magnesium, and phosphorus. These different chemical components are vital to the normal function of all body systems. They are controlled by the renin–angiotensin–aldosterone system (RAAS), antidiuretic hormone (ADH) system, and sympathetic nervous system (SNS). When these neuroendocrine systems are out of balance, adverse electrolyte imbalances commonly result.

POTASSIUM

Potassium is the most abundant cationic (positively charged) electrolyte inside cells (the intracellular space), where the normal concentration is approximately 150 mEq/L. Approximately 95% of the potassium in the body is intracellular. In contrast, the potassium content outside the cells in the plasma ranges from 3.5 to 5 mEq/L. These plasma levels are critical to normal body function.

Potassium is obtained from a variety of foods, the most common being fruit and juices, fish, vegetables, poultry, meats, and dairy products. It has been estimated that for normal body functions to be maintained, a person must consume 5 to 10 mEq of potassium per day. Fortunately, the average daily diet usually provides 35 to 100 mEq of potassium, which is well above the required daily amount. Excess dietary potassium is usually excreted by the kidneys in the urine. However, if the kidneys lose their ability to filter and secrete waste products, potassium can accumulate, leading to toxic levels, and these, in turn, can precipitate ventricular fibrillation and cardiac arrest. Hyperaldosteronism and potassium-sparing diuretics can alter normal potassium balance as well. **Hyperkalemia** is the term for an excessive serum potassium level, and it is defined as a serum potassium level exceeding 5.5 mEq/L. There are several causes of hyperkalemia. One, renal failure, was just mentioned. Others are as follows:

- Angiotensin-converting enzyme (ACE) inhibitors
- Burns
- Excessive loss from cells
- Infections
- Metabolic acidosis
- Potassium supplements
- Potassium-sparing diuretics
- Trauma

The opposite of hyperkalemia is **hypokalemia,** or a deficiency of potassium. This condition is more often the result of

Box 26-1   Symptoms of Hypokalemia

Early
Anorexia
Hypotension
Lethargy
Mental confusion
Muscle weakness
Nausea

Late
Cardiac dysrhythmias
Neuropathy
Paralytic ileus
Secondary alkalosis

excessive potassium loss than of poor dietary intake, however. As with hyperkalemia, there are multitudes of clinical conditions that can cause it. These include the following: *(causes)*

- Alkalosis
- An increased secretion of mineralocorticoids (hormones of the adrenal cortex)
- Burns*
- Corticosteroids
- Crash diets
- Diarrhea
- Hyperaldosteronism
- Ketoacidosis
- Large amounts of licorice
- Loop diuretics
- Malabsorption
- Prolonged laxative misuse
- Thiazide diuretics
- Thiazide-like diuretics
- Vomiting

Too little serum potassium can also greatly increase the toxicity associated with digitalis preparations, and this can precipitate serious ventricular dysrhythmias.

The early detection of hypokalemia is important in the prevention of the serious, life-threatening consequences of this metabolic disturbance if it goes undetected. The key to early detection is knowing its early symptoms, which are generally mild and can easily go undetected. Both the early (mild) symptoms and late (severe) symptoms of hypokalemia are listed in Box 26-1. The treatment of hypokalemia involves both identifying and treating the cause and restoring the serum potassium levels to normal (greater than 3.5 mEq/L). The consumption of potassium-rich foods can usually correct mild hypokalemia, but clinically significant hypokalemia requires the oral or parenteral administration of a potassium supplement, which usually contains potassium chloride.

Mechanism of Action and Drug Effects

The importance of potassium as the primarily intracellular electrolyte is highlighted by the enormous number of life-sustaining reactions and everyday physiologic functions that require it, functions that we take for granted and that would not be possible without it. Muscle contraction, the transmission of nerve im-

pulses, and the regulation of heartbeats (the pacemaker function of the heart) are just a few of these functions.

Potassium is also essential for the maintenance of acid–base balance, isotonicity, and the electrodynamic characteristics of the cell. It plays a role in many enzymatic reactions, and it is an essential component of gastric secretion, renal function, tissue synthesis, and carbohydrate metabolism.

Indications

Potassium replacement therapy is called for in the treatment or prevention of potassium depletion in patients whenever dietary measures prove inadequate. Potassium salts commonly used for this purpose include potassium chloride, potassium phosphate, and potassium acetate. The chloride is required to correct the hypochloremia (low chloride) that commonly accompanies potassium deficiency, and phosphate is used to correct hypophosphatemia. The acetate salt may be used to raise the blood pH in acidotic conditions.

Other therapeutic effects of potassium are related to its role in the contraction of muscles and the maintenance of the electrical characteristics of cells. Potassium salts may be used to stop irregular heartbeats (dysrhythmias) and to manage the tachyarrhythmias that can occur after cardiac surgery. Potassium may also be used to treat thallium poisoning and to help increase muscular strength in some patients with myasthenia gravis.

Contraindications

Contraindications to potassium replacement products include known allergy to a specific drug product, hyperkalemia from any cause, severe renal disease, acute dehydration, untreated Addison's disease, severe hemolytic disease, and conditions involving extensive tissue breakdown (e.g. multiple trauma, severe burns).

Adverse Effects

The adverse effects of oral potassium therapy are primarily limited to the gastrointestinal (GI) tract and occur with the oral administration of potassium preparations. These GI effects include diarrhea, nausea, and vomiting. More significant ones include GI bleeding and ulceration. The parenteral administration of potassium usually produces pain at the injection site. Cases of phlebitis have been associated with IV administration, and the excessive administration of potassium salts can lead to hyperkalemia and toxic effects.

Toxicity and Management of Overdose

The toxic effects of potassium are the result of hyperkalemia. Symptoms include muscle weakness, paresthesia, paralysis, cardiac rhythm irregularities that can result in ventricular fibrillation, and cardiac arrest. The treatment instituted depends on the degree of the hyperkalemia and ranges from regimens for reversing life-threatening problems to simple dietary restrictions. In the event of severe hyperkalemia, the intravenous administration of sodium bicarbonate, calcium gluconate or chloride, or dextrose solution with insulin is often required. These drugs correct severe hyperkalemia by causing a rapid intracellular shift of potassium ions, thus reducing the serum potassium concentration. Such interventions are often followed with orally or rectally administered sodium polystyrene sulfonate (e.g., Kayexalate) or hemodialysis to eliminate the extra potassium from the body. Less critical levels can be reduced with dietary restrictions.

*Burn patients can exhibit either hyperkalemia or hypokalemia.

Interactions

Concurrent use of potassium-sparing diuretics and ACE inhibitors can produce a hyperkalemic state. Concurrent use of diuretics, amphotericin B, and mineralosteroids can produce a hypokalemic state.

Dosages

Fluid and electrolyte therapy involves replacing any deficit losses and/or providing maintenance levels for specific patient requirements. Accordingly, specific dosage amounts of fluids or electrolytes depend on several clinical factors, including the following:

- Specific patient losses
- Efficacy of patient physiologic systems involved in fluid and electrolyte metabolism, especially adrenal, cardiovascular, and kidney functions
- Current drug therapy for pathologic conditions that complicate the amount and duration of replacement
- Selection of oral or parenteral replacement formulations

Suggested dosage guidelines with subsequent adjustments for potassium are 10 to 20 mEq administered orally several times a day or parenteral administration of 30 to 60 mEq every 24 hours.

Drug Profiles

Potassium supplements are administered to either prevent or treat potassium depletion. The acetate, bicarbonate, chloride, citrate, and gluconate salts of potassium are available for oral (PO) administration. The parenteral salt forms of potassium for intravenous administration are acetate, chloride, and phosphate.

The dosage of potassium supplements is usually expressed in milliequivalents of potassium and depends on the requirements of the individual patient. The different salt forms of potassium deliver varying milliequivalent amounts of potassium. These various salt forms and how many grams of each are needed to yield 40 mEq are given in Table 26-10.

Potassium is contraindicated in patients with severe renal disease, severe hemolytic disease, or Addison's disease and in those suffering from hyperkalemia, acute dehydration, or extensive tissue breakdown stemming from multiple traumas. Potassium is available in many different oral and intravenous formulations. It is available in oral form as a tablet and powder for solution, an extended-release capsule and tablet, and an elixir and solution. It is also available as an injection for intravenous use. Pregnancy category A.

Pharmacokinetics

Half-Life	Onset	Peak	Duration
IV: Variable	IV: Immediate	IV: Rapid	IV: Variable
PO: Variable	PO: <30 min	PO: 30 min	PO: Variable

Table 26-10   **Potassium: Various Salt Forms**

Salt Form	Amount (g) Needed to Yield 40 mEq of Potassium
Acetate	3.9
Chloride	3.0
Citrate	4.3
Dibasic phosphate	3.5
Gluconate	9.4
Monobasic phosphate	5.4

sodium polystyrene sulfonate (potassium exchange resin)

Sodium polystyrene sulfonate (Kayexalate, Kionex, SPS) is known as a *cation exchange resin* that is used to treat hyperkalemia. For this purpose it is usually administered orally via nasogastric tube or as an enema. It works in the intestine, where potassium ions from the body are exchanged for sodium ions in the resin. Although the drug effects in each case are unpredictable, approximately 1 mEq of potassium is lost from the body per gram of resin administered. It has no listed contraindications per se, but it can cause disturbances in electrolytes other than potassium, such as calcium and magnesium. For this reason, patients' electrolytes should be closely monitored during treatment with SPS. It is typically dosed in multiples of 15 to 30 g until desired effect on serum potassium. Onset of action varies from 2 to 12 hours, with the oral route generally faster than rectal administration. It is available in 15-g/60 mL suspensions and in a powder for reconstitution. Pregnancy category C.

SODIUM

Although sodium is discussed under colloids earlier in this chapter, it is also presented here in the electrolyte section because it is most commonly given for replenishing purposes. Sodium is the counterpart to potassium in that potassium is the principal cation (positively charged substance) inside cells, and sodium is the principal cation outside cells. The normal concentration of sodium outside cells is 135 to 145 mEq/L, and it is maintained through the dietary intake of sodium in the form of sodium chloride, which is obtained from salt; fish; meats; and other foods flavored, seasoned, or preserved with salt.

Hyponatremia is the condition of sodium loss or deficiency and occurs when the serum levels decrease below 135 mEq/L. It is manifested by lethargy, hypotension, stomach cramps, vomiting, diarrhea, and seizures. Some of the same conditions that cause hypokalemia can also cause hyponatremia, and these are listed on page 409. Other causes of hyponatremia are excessive perspiration, occurring during hot weather or physical work; prolonged diarrhea or vomiting, especially in young children; renal disorders; and adrenocortical impairment.

Hypernatremia is the condition of sodium excess and occurs when the serum levels of sodium exceed 145 mEq/L. Some of the symptoms are water retention (edema) and hypertension. The most common cause is poor renal excretion stemming from kidney malfunction. Inadequate water consumption and dehydration are other causes. Symptoms of hypernatremia include red, flushed skin; dry, sticky mucous membranes; increased thirst; temperature elevation; and decreased or absent urination.

Mechanism of Action and Drug Effects

As one of the body's electrolytes, sodium performs many physiologic roles necessary for the normal function of the body. It is the major cation in ECF and is principally involved in the control of water distribution, fluid and electrolyte balance, and osmotic pressure of body fluids. Sodium also participates along with both chloride and bicarbonate in the regulation of acid–base balance. Chloride, the major extracellular anion (negatively charged substance), closely complements the physiologic action of sodium. Sodium is also capable of causing diuresis.

Indications

Sodium is primarily administered in the treatment or prevention of sodium depletion when dietary measures have proved inadequate. Sodium chloride is the primary salt used for this purpose.

Mild hyponatremia is usually treated with the oral administration of sodium chloride tablets and/or fluid restriction. Pronounced sodium depletion is treated with NS or lactated Ringer's solution administered intravenously. These drugs are discussed earlier in this chapter.

Contraindications

The only usual contraindications to the use of sodium replacement products are known drug allergy to a specific product and hypernatremia.

Adverse Effects

The oral administration of sodium chloride can cause gastric upset consisting of nausea, vomiting, and cramps. Venous phlebitis can be a consequence of its parenteral administration.

Toxicity and Management of Overdose

Hypernatremia leads to hypertension, edema, thirst, tachycardia, weakness, convulsions, and possibly coma. Treatment consists of increased fluid intake and dietary restrictions. In more serious cases, diuretics may be required to enhance urinary sodium excretion. Intravenous administration of dextrose in water solution (e.g., D_5W, $D_{10}W$) may also be helpful, by both intravascular sodium dilution and enhanced urine volume output.

Interactions

Sodium is not known to interact significantly with any drugs.

Dosages

Fluid and electrolyte therapy involves replacing any deficit losses and/or providing maintenance levels for specific patient requirements. Accordingly, specific dosage amounts of fluids or electrolytes depend on several clinical factors, as follows:

- Specific patient losses
- Efficacy of patient physiologic systems involved in fluid and electrolyte metabolism, especially adrenal, cardiovascular, and kidney functions
- Current drug therapy for pathologic conditions that complicate the amount and duration of replacement
- Selection of oral or parenteral replacement formulations

Suggested dosage guidelines with subsequent adjustments for sodium chloride are 1 to 2 g administered orally several times a day or parenteral administration of 1 L of sodium chloride injection (NS).

Drug Profiles

sodium chloride

Sodium chloride is primarily used as a replacement electrolyte for either the prevention or treatment of sodium loss. It is also used as a diluent for the infusion of compatible drugs and in the assessment of kidney function after a fluid challenge. Sodium chloride is contraindicated in patients who are hypersensitive to it. It is available in many intravenous preparations and in oral form as a 650-mg tablet and as 1-g and 2.25-g tablets. Pregnancy category C.

Pharmacokinetics

Half-Life	Onset	Peak	Duration
Unknown	Immediate	Rapid	Variable

◆ NURSING PROCESS

◆ ASSESSMENT

For fluid replacement, patients' needs vary, and any medications or solutions ordered should be given exactly as ordered and without substitution. However, a physician's order should never be taken for just face value without confirming the order against authoritative resources, meaning that the nurse is responsible for making sure that whatever is given or done to the patient is accurate and safe and meets a standard of care. As a brief review, parenterally administered hydrating solutions (e.g., 5% dextrose in water [D_5W]) are used mainly for the prevention of dehydration. Isotonic solutions (e.g., 0.9% normal saline) are customarily used to augment extracellular volume in patients experiencing blood loss, severe vomiting, or any condition that leads to a chloride loss equal to or greater than the sodium loss. Isotonic normal saline (0.9% NS) is also used as diluting fluid for blood transfusions because D_5W results in hemolysis of red blood cells (in transfusions). Hypertonic solutions (3%) are used to treat hypotonic expansion, such as that resulting from water intoxication.

After all physician orders are verified and checked for accuracy and completeness (as with all drugs), there should be assessment of the medication/solution, the patient, and the intravenous site (if applicable). The nurse must also assess the following areas as related to intravenous infusions of fluids and/or electrolytes: solution to be infused, infusion equipment, infusion rate of solution/medication per minute, concentration of parenteral solution, related mathematical calculations, laboratory values (e.g., sodium, chloride, potassium), and parenteral compatibilities. More specific assessment of the patient who is to receive a parenteral replacement solution should focus on gathering information on the patient's medical history, including diseases of the gastrointestinal, renal, cardiac, and/or hepatic systems. A medication history should focus on a listing of prescription drugs, over-the-counter (OTC) medications, supplements, and herbals. A dietary history is also important and should include specific dietary habits and a dietary recall of the last 24 hours. Fluid volume and electrolyte status (through laboratory testing, urinary specific gravity, vital signs, and intake and output) should be assessed and documented. The skin and mucous membranes also reflect a patient's hydration status and would be important to assess, including skin turgor and/or rebound elasticity of skin over the top of the hand and other areas over the body. The findings would be documented as "immediate" turgor or "delayed" turgor. It would be appropriate to count the number of seconds that the patient's skin stays in the pinched-up position, with normal return being immediately or within 3 to 5 seconds.

Potassium is presented first in the discussion of electrolytes, and one important place to begin with assessment is knowing the normal range, which is 3.5 to 5 mEq/L. Levels below 3.5 mEq/L (hypokalemia) may result in a variety of problems such as cardiac irregularities and muscle weakness. Tartrazine sensitivity, mostly noted in patients with aspirin allergies, should be assessed carefully if a patient is taking potassium chloride because of a risk of cross-sensitivity. Potassium supplementation should be avoided or used with extreme caution in patients taking ACE inhibitors and with potassium sparing diuretics (such as spirono-

Calcium

Laboratory Test	Normal Ranges	Rationale for Assessment
Serum calcium	9-10.5 mg/dL or 4.65-5.28 mg/dL (ionized level)	Calcium supplementation may be deemed necessary whenever the level of calcium drops below normal ranges. In addition to reporting of normal levels of serum calcium is reporting of ionized calcium. Serum ionized calcium is the amount of calcium not bound to protein. Clinical signs and symptoms of hypocalcemia include abnormal neuromuscular contractions and tremors. There are other assessment tests for the presence of abnormal neuromuscular contractions. The two classic tests are the Chvostek's and Trousseau's signs. Chvostek's sign is elicited *gently* tapping the face at a point just anterior to the ear and below the zygomatic bone with the blunt end of a reflex hammer. A positive response for hypocalcemia includes twitching of the psilateral facial muscles and is suggestive of neuromuscular excitability secondary to hypocalcemia. Trousseau's sign is elicited by inflating a sphygmomanometer cuff (blood pressure cuff) for several minutes. A positive response includes muscular contraction with flexion of the wrist and metacarpophalangeal joints, hyperextension of the fingers, and flexion of the thumb on the palm. This muscle contraction is indicative of neuromuscular excitability secondary to hypocalcemia. These tests, in addition to serum calcium testing, may be helpful in confirming the presence of hypocalcemia.

Modified from Urbano FL: Signs of hypocalcemia: Chvostek's and Trousseau's signs, *Hosp Physician,* March 2000, p. 43.

lactone). These drugs are associated with adverse effects of hyperkalemia and, if given with potassium supplementation, could worsen hyperkalemia and possibly result in severe cardiac compromise and possible cardiac arrest. Oral potassium supplements are irritants and can be ulcerogenic. If a patient has a history of ulcers or GI bleeding, the supplementation should not be given orally and the physician should be contacted for further insructions.

Normal ranges of serum potassium often vary depending on the institution and/or physician. When it comes to identification and treatment of hyperkalemia, the normal range of potassium must be established. It is important to realize that potassium levels of 5.3 mEq/L may be identified as abnormally high, while other labs may identify 5.0 mEq/L as being abnormally high. High (and low) serum potassium levels should be reported. However, a serum level exceeding 5.5 mEq/L is considered by most sources as being toxic and dangerous to the patient and should be reported immediately to the physician. With close monitoring of patients, the dangerous effects of hyperkalemia will hopefully be prevented and/or identified early and treated appropriately to prevent potentially life-threatening complications (see previous discussion of hyperkalemia).

Vein access remains an issue with parenteral potassium supplementation because of irritation to the veins with infiltration or if the concentration has not been mixed thoroughly. Some important factors to consider for peripheral venous access include the following (for potassium, sodium, fluid, and any other sort of medication given per intravenous route): (1) Attempt use of distal veins first. (2) Know the purpose of using potassium and other electrolytes. (3) Set rate as ordered and recalculated for infusion. (4) Know the anticipated duration of therapy. (5) Assess overall condition of the veins. (6) Know restrictions imposed by the patient's history (e.g., affected arm of a patient with a mastectomy and lymph node dissection). For the postmastectomy and stroke patient, these situations may be associated with inadequate circulation and lead to edema and other complications.

Sodium is another electrolyte that is an ingredient in various intravenous replacement solutions. Hyponatremia, or serum sodium below 135 mEq/L, if not resolved with dietary and/or oral intake, may need to be treated with parenteral infusions. Venous access sites should be carefully chosen because of possible irritation of the vein and subsequent phlebitis. If there is overzealous replacement, hyponatremic states may lead to hypernatremia and fluid overload, edema, worsening of heart failure, dyspnea, and rales. Continual monitoring of vital signs, hydration status of skin and mucus membrane, and level of consciousness is important to safe replacement and prevention of further complications.

Hypernatremia also requires careful assessment. Identifying any precipitating events, medical concerns, and at-risk patient situations are important to finding early solutions for treatment. The at-risk population for hypernatremia include the elderly; those with renal and cardiovascular diseases, patients receiving sodium supplements, or with increased sodium intake, and those with decreased fluid intake. All electrolytes require assessment of cautions, contraindications, and drug interactions.

Albumin and other colloids are associated with cautions, contraindications, and drug interactions that need to be assessed. It is also important to assess the patient's hematocrit (Hct), hemoglobin (Hgb) levels, and serum protein levels. Monitoring of the patient's blood pressure, pulse rate, respiratory status, and intake and output amounts should be documented. Assessment for dyspnea or hypoxia should also be noted and reported prior to use of these drugs. Laboratory interference is seen with alkaline phosphatase, which is increased when albumin is given.

When giving blood or blood components, the nurse should obtain a thorough history regarding transfusions received the patient's response. Any history of adverse reactions to transfusions should be reported to the physician and the nature of these reactions documented. It is also important to assess the status of venous access areas as well as to check the patient's laboratory values (e.g., Hct, Hgb, white blood cells [WBCs], red blood cells [RBCs], platelets, and clotting factors). Baseline vital signs should be noted before infusing the blood/blood product. Even the general appearance of the patient, energy levels, ability to carry out activities of daily living,and color of extremities are important to note. During the infusion of blood components, be alert to the occurrence of fever and blood in the urine, which are both indicative of an adverse reaction.

In summary, safety and caution are top priorities in patients receiving any drug, including fluid and electrolyte replacements. Excess levels of fluid and electrolytes and deficits may pose tremendous risks to patients and, therefore, the nurse must assess thoroughly so that safety and caution are maintained. In addition, because so many patients receive therapies in the home setting, the nurse has even more accountability and responsibility for astute and thorough assessment before, during, and after therapy.

◆ NURSING DIAGNOSES
- Risk for falls related to fluid and electrolyte imbalances
- Risk for imbalanced fluid volume related to drug-induced fluid excess or deficits and electrolyte excesses or deficits
- Risk for injury related to complications of the transfusion or infusion of blood products, blood components, or related agents
- Deficient knowledge about treatment regimen related to lack of patient education about electrolyte disturbances and influence of treatment

◆ PLANNING
Goals
- Patient has minimal problems with volume overload related to the transfusion or infusion.
- Patient begins minimal exercise and shows increased tolerance daily.
- Patient participates in activities as he or she can tolerate them.
- Patient states measures to implement to minimize self-injury related to altered blood component levels or altered fluid and electrolyte levels.
- Patient states the rationale for treatment and the adverse effects of replacement agents.
- Patient states symptoms and problems to report to the physician.

Outcome Criteria
- Patient remains free of self-injury as the result of adverse reactions (dizziness, volume overload, hypersensitivity) to the transfusion or infusion or as the result of an allergic reaction.
- Patient regains the ability to engage in normal or near-normal exercise, showing increased tolerance daily as evidenced by walking small distances and increasing to regular supervised exercise.
- Patient participates in activities according to his or her ability to tolerate them without dyspnea or chest pain.
- Patient demonstrates a return to normal or near-normal values of blood components or fluid and electrolyte levels.
- Patient sees the physician for follow-up as ordered to monitor laboratory values pertinent to treatment.

◆ IMPLEMENTATION
Continued monitoring of the patient during fluid or electrolyte therapy is crucial to ensure safe and effective treatment. It is also important to continue monitoring so that adverse effects may be identified early and to help prevent complications of overzealous treatment and/or undertreatment. All serum electrolyte levels should not exceed normal ranges (see the pharmacology section).

With parenteral dosing, the nurse must monitor infusion rates as well as appearance of the fluid or solution (i.e., potassium and saline solutions are clear, whereas albumin is brown, clear, and viscous). The IV site must also be monitored frequently as per facility policy and nursing standards of care for evidence of infiltration (e.g., swelling, cool to the touch around IV site, no or decreased flow rate and no blood return from IV catheter) or thrombophlebitis (e.g., swelling, redness, heat and pain at site). Volume overload, drug toxicity, fever, infection, and emboli are other complications of IV therapy.

With the administration of any fluid or electrolyte solution, a steady and even flow rate must be maintained to prevent complications. Infusion rates must follow physician's orders and calculations must be re-checked for accuracy. The IV site, tubing, IV bag, fluids, and/or solutions as well as expiration dates should all be checked whether with infusion of replacement fluids or electrolytes. Always behave in a prudent, safe, and thorough manner when administering fluids and electrolyte solutions and remember that elderly and/or pediatric patients have their increased sensitivity to these solutions and fluids (as well as most medications). Patients at risk for deficits in volume, especially the elderly, should be informed of the impact of a hot, humid environment on physiologic functioning and of exacerbation by excess perspiration. Water is at the crux of every metabolic reaction that occurs within the body, and when there are deficits, physiologic reactions are negatively impacted and composition of fluids and electrolytes altered. For any age group, staying hydrated at all times is a preventative measure.

Oral preparations of potassium should be prescribed whenever possible, as opposed to parenteral dosage forms. The oral dosage forms should be prepared as per manufacturer inserts or per policy and standard of care. Generally, oral forms of potassium must not be taken with food to minimize gastric distress or irritation. Powder or effervescent forms should be prepared according to the package guidelines and mixed thoroughly with at least 4 to 6 oz of fluids prior to the actual taking of the medication. Enteric-coated and sustained-released forms may still result in gastric upset and lead to ulcer development (ulcerogenic). Although the risk for gastrointestinal adverse effects may be minimized with these dosage forms, the medicine should still be taken with food or a snack. The safest and most effective intervention includes frequent and close monitoring for complaints of nausea, vomiting, abdominal pain, or bleeding (such as blood in the stool and/or the occurrence of hematemesis or blood in vomitus). Should abnormalities be noted, continue to monitor vital signs and other parameters and report findings to the physician immediately. Serum levels of potassium should be monitored during therapy as well.

For the patient who is at risk for hypokalemia, educational materials and patient teaching should encourage certain foods high in potassium. The minimal daily requirement for potassium is between 40 and 50 mEq for adults and 2 to 3 mEq/kg of body weight for infants. Identification of foods containing potassium should be shared with the patient and include some of the following: two medium-sized bananas or an 8-oz glass of orange juice contains 45 mEq; 20 large dried apricots contain 40 mEq; and a level teaspoon of salt substitute (KCl) contains 60 mEq of potassium. Conversely, if the patient is already hyperkalemic, these are food items that should be avoided. See previous discussion concerning use of Kayexylate to treat hyperkalemia. See the Patient Teaching Tips for more information.

Potassium chloride is the salt customarily used for intravenous infusions. Potassium chloride comes with the concern and caution of avoiding overdosage due to the possibility of cardiac arrest. It is always important to remember that intravenous dosage forms of potassium MUST always be given in a DILUTED form. There is NO use or place for UNDILUTED potassium because undiluted potassium is associated with cardiac arrest. Therefore, parenteral forms of potassium should be diluted properly. Nowadays, most pharmacies "pre-mix" the infusion; however, it is still imperative to double check the concentration and amount of diluent. Never assume that whatever was pre-mixed is 100% correct because whatever the nurse administers is their responsibility. Diluted potassium should also be given only in situations where there is adequate urine output of at least 30 mL/hour. Manufacturer instructions and policy protocols generally recommend that intravenous solutions be given at concentrations less than 40 mEq/L of potassium and a rate not exceeding 20 mEq/hr. Another precautionary measure that must be followed is to avoid adding KCl to an already existing intravenous solution because the exact concentration would not be accurately calculated, thus risking complications, overdosage, or toxicity. Make sure that all IV fluids are labeled appropriately and documented, as with any medication. If there is need for very close monitoring of the IV fluid rate, an infusion pump may be used. There is *no* place for IV push or IV bolus potassium replacement!

Replacement of sodium carries the same concern for dosing and route of administration. With situations where the patient is only mildly depleted, an increase in oral intake of sodium should be tried. Food items high in sodium include catsup, mustard, cured meats, cheeses, potato chips, peanut butter, popcorn, and table salt. In some situations, salt tablets may be necessary. If the patient is given salt tablets, it is very important that he or she also takes plenty of fluids of up to 3000 mL/24 hr—unless contraindicated. If the sodium deficit requires intravenous replacement, venous access issues and drip rate are as important as with volume and potassium infusions (see previous discussion regarding intravenous infusion and intravenous sites).

The IV infusion of albumin and other colloids should always be done slowly and cautiously and with careful monitoring to prevent fluid overload and heart failure, especially in those patients who are at particular risk for heart failure. Fluid overload would be evidenced by shortness of breath, crackles in bases of lungs, decreased pulse oximeter readings, edema of dependent areas, and increase in weight (see the previous parameters). Serum hematocrit and hemoglobin values should also be determined in advance of therapy—as well as during and after—so that any dilutional factors could be determined. For example, if a patient has received albumin and other colloids too quickly, and hypervolemia results, the patient's hemoglobin and hematocrit may actually be decreased. This decrease would then be due to a dilutional factor from too much volume as related to concentra-tion of solutes. Clinically, the patient would appear to be anemic, but, in fact, the deficit would be attributed to the increase in volume. It is also important to remember that albumin is to be given at room temperature.

For infusion of blood, it is essential to always check the expiration date of blood and/or blood components to make sure that the blood is not outdated. Under NO circumstances should outdated blood be used! Policies at most hospitals and other health care agencies require that blood and blood products be double checked by another registered nurse BEFORE the blood is hung and infused. This is important in preventing a mix up of blood types. Blood types should always be a major concern because of the possible complications that can occur, some life threatening, if the wrong blood type is given or if the blood is given to the wrong person. The five "Rights" of drug administration remain critical in all that nurses do with medications, and administering blood is no exception.

When infusing blood and blood products, all vital signs and related parameters should be documented before, during, and after administration of a blood product, component (e.g., PPF, platelets, and FFP), or solution. The patient should then be assessed and the findings documented. Vital signs should also be checked and recorded. A transfusion reaction would most likely be noted by the occurrence of the following: apprehension, restlessness, flushed skin, increased pulse and respirations, dyspnea, rash, joint or lower back pain, swelling, fever and chills (a febrile reaction beginning 1 hour after the start of administration and possibly lasting up to 10 hours), nausea, weakness, and jaundice. These signs and symptoms should be reported to the physician immediately, and regardless of when the reaction occurs, the blood or product should be stopped and IV line kept patent with isotonic NS solution infusing at a low drip. Always follow the facility's protocol for transfusion reactions.

In summary, patients taking any type of fluid or electrolyte substance, colloid, or blood component should be encouraged to immediately report unusual adverse effects to their physician. Such complaints include chest pain, dizziness, weakness, and shortness of breath.

◆ EVALUATION

The therapeutic response to fluid, electrolyte, and blood or blood component therapy includes normalization of fluid volume and laboratory values, including RBCs, WBCs, Hgb, Hct, sodium, and potassium. In addition to these laboratory values, evaluation of the patient's cardiac, respiratory, musculoskeletal, and gastrointestinal functioning is also important. Energy levels and tolerance to activities of daily living should return to normal. There should be improved skin color, minimal to no dyspnea, chest pain, weakness, or fatigue. Blood volume that has been correctly treated will be evidenced by a return to normal of the laboratory values, improved vital signs, an increase in energy, and near-normal O_2 saturation levels. The therapeutic response to albumin therapy includes an elevation of blood pressure, decreased edema, and increased serum albumin levels. Monitoring for the adverse effects of any of these drugs and/or solutions should occur frequently and include monitoring for distended neck veins; shortness of breath; anxiety; insomnia; expiratory crackles; frothy, blood-tinged sputum; and cyanosis.

Patient Teaching Tips

- As needed, educate patients about the difference in signs and symptoms of hyponatremia and hypernatremia. Hyponatremia is manifested by lethargy, hypotension, stomach cramps, vomiting, diarrhea, and possibly seizures. Hypernatremia is manifested by red, flushed skin; dry, sticky mucous membranes; increased thirst; temperature elevation; and a decrease in or absence of urination.
- Make sure the patient knows to inform all of his or her health care professionals about all medications they are taking, including OTC drugs, herbals, supplements, and prescription drugs.
- Share information with the patient about how to take oral potassium chloride. Include directions about mixing any powdered or liquid solutions in at least 4 to 8 oz of cold water or juice, drinking the entire mixture slowly, and taking the dose with food.
- Encourage patients taking potassium supplements to inform their health care provider should they experience GI upset, abdominal pain, muscle cramps/weakness, fatigue, or irregular heartbeat. Share with the patient the many drug interactions, including antacids, diuretics, and digitalis drugs.
- A diet high in potassium such as bananas, oranges, leafy green vegetables, spinach, potatoes, lentils, fish, chicken, turkey, ham, beef, and milk.
- Sustained-release capsules and tablets must be swallowed whole and should not be crushed, chewed, or allowed to dissolve in the mouth. This would increase adverse effects. Do not crush, chew, or suck the pills because this may increase adverse effects.
- Encourage patients to report any difficulty in swallowing, painful swallowing, or feeling as if the capsule/tablet is stuck in their throat. Other serious adverse effects that need to be reported include vomiting of coffee ground–like material, stomach/abdominal pain, and swelling and black/tarry stools.
- Extended-release dosage forms should be taken in full. If difficulty swallowing occurs with the whole tablet, and if approved by their health care provider, encourage patients to break the tablet in half and take each half separately, drinking half a glass of water (4 oz) with each and taking the entire dose within a few minutes. Encourage the patient to not save a half for later. If the tablet must be dissolved as prescribed, the patient should know to allow 2 minutes for the tablet to dissolve in 4 oz of water, stir for 30 seconds, and then drink immediately. Adding 1 oz of water to the glass with swirling and then drinking the residual will allow adequate dosing. Water is recommended as the solution for mixing the extended dosage.
- Effervescent tablets should be dissolved as directed, with emphasis on at least 3 oz of cold water per tablet. Patients should be informed to take the dose as soon as fully dissolved, sipping the mixture over 5 to 10 minutes and taking the dose after food to minimize GI upset.
- Tell patients that salt substitutes contain potassium, so another alternative should be recommended if patients are hyperkalemic.
- Inform the patient to report any feelings of irritation (e.g., burning) at the IV site at any time.
- Salt tablets should be taken as prescribed, with caution, and with adequate fluid intake.

Points to Remember

- TBW is divided into intracellular (inside the cell) and extracellular (outside the cell) compartments. Fluid volume "outside" cells is either in the plasma (intravascular volume) or between the tissues, cells, or organs (ISF).
- Colloids are large protein particles that cannot leak out of the blood vessels. Because of their greater concentration inside blood vessels, fluid is pulled into the blood vessels. Examples of colloids include albumin, hetastarch, and dextran. Albumin must be administered with caution because of the high risk for hypervolemia and possibly heart failure. The nurse needs to monitor intake and output, weights, heart and breath sounds, as well as laboratory values appropriate to the situation and albumin.
- Blood products are also known as *oxygen-carrying resuscitation fluids*. They are the only class of fluids that are able to carry oxygen because they are the only fluids that contain hemoglobin. Patients should show improved energy and increasing tolerance for activities of daily living. The nurse should also be monitoring pulse oximeter readings.
- Dehydration may be hypotonic, resulting from the loss of salt; hypertonic, resulting from fever with perspiration; or isotonic, resulting from diarrhea or vomiting. Each form of dehydration is treated differently. The nurse should carefully assess intake and output as well as skin turgor assessment, urine specific gravity, and blood values of potassium, sodium, chloride, etc.
- Hypertonic solutions should be given slowly (less than 100 mL/hr) because of the risk for hypervolemia due to overzealous replacement.
- Symptoms of hypokalemia include lethargy, weakness, fatigue, respiratory difficulty, paralysis, and even possible paralytic ileus.

CAUTION: When replacing potassium via IV infusions, the nurse should never give undiluted potassium chloride because it can result in ventricular fibrillation and cardiac arrest due to hyperkalemia. Nursing units should only use diluted potassium (e.g., 1000 mL of IV fluids premixed by the manufacturer of the drug and IV fluids). The nurse should never exceed recommended IV dosages of potassium (e.g., usual dose per 1000 mL of IV fluids is 40 mEq).
- Treatment of hyperkalemia is with the use of Kayexylate. Adverse effects that the nurse needs to be aware of include the following: nausea, stomach pain, loss of appetite, constipation, or diarrhea may occur. If these effects persist or worsen, notify the physician immediately. Unlikely to occur but should be reported promptly are the following: swelling, muscle cramps, dizziness, mental, or mood changes. Very unlikely to occur but needed to be reported promptly includes the following: fast/slow/irregular pulse, muscle weakness, muscle spasm.
- Blood products may cause hemolysis of RBCs, and, therefore, adverse reactions such as fever, chills, and back pain should be watched for continually. Hematuria may occur if the hemolysis reaction is present. If noted, the nurse should notify the physician immediately, the IV infusion discontinued, and the nature of the reactions and all actions taken documented. Vital signs and frequent monitoring of the patient before, during, and after infusions are critical to patient safety. Blood products should be given only with NS 0.9% because D_5W will also cause hemolysis of the blood product.

NCLEX Examination Review Questions

1. While setting up a transfusion of packed red blood cells, the nurse remembers to follow which principle?
   a. The IV line should be flushed with NS before the blood is added to the infusion.
   b. The IV line should be flushed with dextrose before the blood is added to the infusion.
   c. Check the patient's vital signs after the infusion is completed.
   d. Flushed skin and fever are expected reactions to a blood transfusion.
2. When preparing an intravenous solution that contains potassium, the nurse knows that a contraindication to the potassium infusion would be:
   a. Diarrhea
   b. Serum potassium of 2.8 mEq/L
   c. Serum potassium of 5.6 mEq/L
   d. Dehydration
3. When assessing a patient who has an order for albumin administration, the nurse knows that a contraindication for albumin would be:
   a. Acute liver failure.
   b. Heart failure.
   c. Severe burns.
   d. Fluid-volume deficit.
4. The nurse is preparing an infusion for a patient who has deficient clotting due to hemophilia. Which type of infusion will this patient receive?
   a. Albumin 5%
   b. Packed RBCs
   c. Whole blood
   d. Fresh frozen plasma
5. While monitoring a patient who is receiving an infusion of 3% NS, the nurse should look for:
   a. Bradycardia
   b. Hypotension
   c. Decreased skin turgor
   d. Fluid overload

1. a, 2. c, 3. b, 4. d, 5. d.

Critical Thinking Activities

1. Compare the three types of dehydration. List an example of each type.
2. Discuss the importance of crystalloids and their therapeutic effectiveness. Provide examples of crystalloids and the conditions for which they would be ordered.
3. Compare the use of crystalloids with that of colloids.

For answers, see http://evolve.elsevier.com/Lilley.

Coagulation Modifier Drugs

Objectives

When you reach the end of this chapter, you should be able to do the following:

1. Discuss the mechanisms of action of coagulation modifiers such as anticoagulants, antiplatelet drugs, antifibrinolytics, and thrombolytics.
2. Compare the indications, cautions, contraindications, adverse effects, routes of administration, and dosages of the various coagulation modifiers.
3. Discuss the administration procedures for the various coagulation modifiers.
4. Identify drug interactions associated with the use of coagulation modifiers, specific observations related to their use, and any available antidotes.
5. Develop a nursing care plan that includes all phases of the nursing process for patients receiving anticoagulants, antiplatelet drugs, antifibrinolytics, and thrombolytics.

e-Learning Activities

Companion CD

- NCLEX Review Questions: see questions 226-242
- Animations
- Audio Glossary
- Category Catchers
- Medication Errors Checklists
- IV Therapy Checklists

evolve Website (http://evolve.elsevier.com/Lilley)

• Nursing Care Plans • Frequently Asked Questions • Content Updates • WebLinks • Supplemental Resources • Elsevier ePharmacology Update • Medication Administration Animations

Drug Profiles

▶ alteplase, p. 431
aminocaproic acid, p. 429
argatroban, p. 425
▶ aspirin, p. 427
▶ clopidogrel, p. 428
desmopressin, p. 429

▶ enoxaparin, p. 423
▶ eptifibatide p. 428
▶ heparin, p. 424
lepirudin, p. 425
▶ streptokinase, p. 431
▶ warfarin, p. 423

▶ Key drug.

Glossary

Anticoagulant   A substance that prevents or delays coagulation of the blood. (p. 419)

Antifibrinolytic drug   A drug that prevents the lysis of fibrin and in doing so promotes clot formation. (p. 421)

Antiplatelet drug   A substance that prevents platelet plugs from forming, which can be beneficial in defending the body against heart attacks and strokes. (p. 419)

Antithrombin III (AT-III)   A substance that inactivates ("turns off") three major activating factors of the clotting cascade activated II (thrombin), activated X, and activated IX. (p. 421)

Beta-hemolytic streptococci (group A)   The pyogenic streptococci of group A that cause hemolysis of red blood cells in blood agar in the laboratory setting. These organisms cause most of the acute streptococcal infections seen in human beings. (p. 430)

Clot   Insoluble solid elements of blood (cells, fibrin threads, etc.) that have chemically separated from the liquid (plasma) component of the blood. (p. 417)

Coagulation   The process of blood clotting. More specifically, the sequential process by which the multiple coagulation factors of the blood interact in the *coagulation cascade*, ultimately forming an insoluble fibrin clot. (p. 418)

Coagulation cascade   The series of steps beginning with the *intrinsic* or *extrinsic* pathways of coagulation and proceeding through the formation of a *fibrin clot*. (p. 419)

Deep vein thrombosis (DVT)   The formation of a thrombus in one of the deep veins of the body. The deep veins most commonly affected are the iliac and femoral veins. (p. 421)

Embolus   A blood clot *(thrombus)* that has been dislodged from the wall of a blood vessel and is traveling throughout the bloodstream. Emboli that lodge in critical blood vessels can result in ischemic injury to a vital organ (e.g., heart, lung, brain) and result in disability or death. (p. 418)

Enzyme   A protein molecule that catalyzes chemical reactions of other substances without being altered or destroyed in the process. (p. 422)

Fibrin   A stringy, insoluble protein produced by the action of thrombin on fibrinogen during the clotting process; a major component of blood *clots* or *thrombi* (see *thrombus*). (p. 419)

Fibrin-specificity   Property of newer thrombolytic drugs to activate plasminogen to plasmin only in the presence of established clots having fibrin threads versus systemic plasminogen activation throughout the body, which increased bleeding risk. The latter is associated with older thrombolytic drugs known as *thrombolytic enzymes.* (p. 430)

Fibrinogen   A plasma protein that is converted into fibrin by thrombin in the presence of calcium ions. (p. 426)

Fibrinolysis   The continual process of fibrin decomposition produced by the actions of the enzymatic protein *fibrinolysin.* It is the normal mechanism for removing small fibrin clots and is stimulated by anoxia, inflammatory reactions, and other kinds of stress. (p. 419)

Fibrinolytic system   An area of the circulatory system undergoing fibrinolysis. (p. 419)

Hemorrheologic drug   A drug that alters the function of platelets without compromising their blood-clotting properties. (p. 419)

Hemostasis   Arrest of bleeding, either by the physiologic properties of vasoconstriction and coagulation or by mechanical, surgical, or pharmacologic means. (p. 418)

Hemostatic drug   A procedure, device, or substance that arrests the flow of blood. (p. 421)

Plasmin   The enzymatic protein that breaks down fibrin into fibrin degradation products; is derived from plasminogen. (p. 419)

Plasminogen   A plasma protein that is converted to plasmin. (p. 419)

Pulmonary embolism   The blockage of a pulmonary artery by foreign matter such as fat, air, tumor, or a thrombus that usually arises from a peripheral vein. (p. 421)

Stroke   Occlusion of the blood vessels of the brain by an embolus, thrombus, or cerebrovascular hemorrhage, resulting in ischemia of the brain tissue. (p. 421)

Thromboembolic event   An event in which a blood vessel is blocked by an embolus carried in the bloodstream from the site of its formation. The tissue supplied by an obstructed artery may tingle and become cold, numb, cyanotic, and eventually necrotic (dead). (p. 421)

Thrombolytic drug   A drug that dissolves thrombi by functioning similarly to *tissue plasminogen activator.* (p. 421)

Thrombus   Technical term for a blood clot (plural: *thrombi*); an aggregation of platelets, fibrin, clotting factors, and the cellular elements of the blood that is attached to the interior wall of a vein or artery, sometimes occluding the vessel lumen. (p. 418)

Tissue plasminogen activator   A naturally occurring plasminogen activator secreted by vascular endothelial cells in the walls of blood vessels. Thrombolytic drugs are based on this blood component. (p. 419)

COAGULATION AND HEMOSTASIS

Hemostasis is a general term for any process that stops bleeding. This can be by mechanical means (e.g., compression to bleeding site) or even surgical means (e.g., surgical clamping or cauterization of a blood vessel). When hemostasis occurs due to physiologic clotting of blood, it is called **coagulation,** which is the process of blood-clot formation. The technical term for a blood clot is **thrombus,** and a thrombus that is not stationary but moves through blood vessels from its point of origin is called an **embolus.** Normal hemostasis involves the complex interaction of substances that promote clot formation and substances that either inhibit coagulation or dissolve the formed clot. Substances that promote coagulation

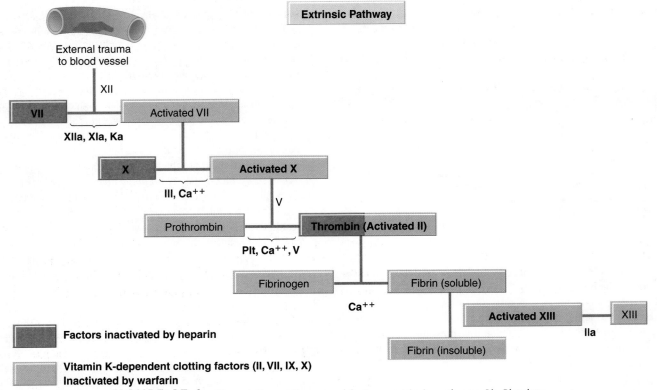

FIGURE 27-1   Coagulation pathway and factors: extrinsic pathway. *Plt,* Platelets.

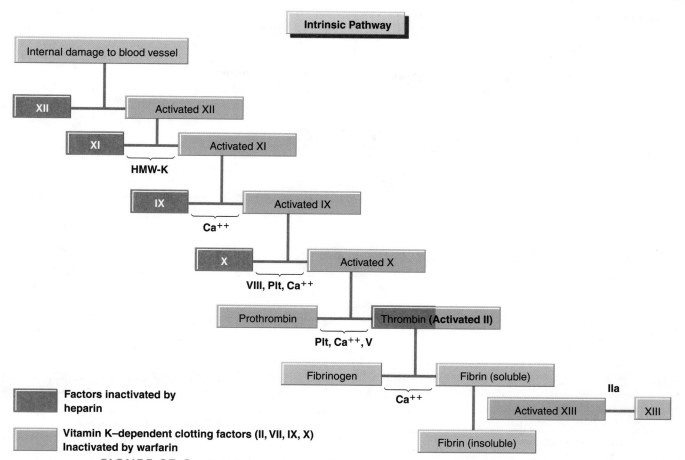

FIGURE 27-2 Coagulation pathway and factors: intrinsic pathway. *HMW-K,* High-molecular weight kininogen; *Plt,* platelets.

include *platelets, von Willebrand factor, activated clotting factors,* and *tissue thromboplastin.* Substances that inhibit coagulation include *prostacyclin, antithrombin III,* and *proteins C* and *S.* Additionally, **tissue plasminogen activator** is a natural substance that dissolves clots that are already formed.

The coagulation system is illustrated in Figures 27-1 and 27-2. It is called a *cascade* (or **coagulation cascade**) because each activated clotting factor serves as a catalyst that amplifies the next reaction. The result is a large concentration of a clot-forming substance called **fibrin.** The coagulation cascade is typically divided into the intrinsic and extrinsic pathways, and these pathways are activated by different types of injury. When blood vessels are damaged by penetration from the outside (e.g., knife or bullet wound), thromboplastin, a substance contained in the walls of blood vessels, is released. This initiates the *extrinsic pathway* by activating factors VII and X (see Figure 27-1). All of the components of this *intrinsic pathway* are present in the blood in their inactive forms (see Figure 27-2). This pathway is activated when factor XII comes in contact with exposed collagen on the *inside* of damaged blood vessels. Figures 27-1 and 27-2 illustrate the steps that occur in the extrinsic and intrinsic pathways, respectively, and the factors involved. They also illustrate the site of action of two commonly used anticoagulant drugs: warfarin and heparin.

Once a clot is formed, and fibrin is present, the **fibrinolytic system** is activated. This is the system that initiates the breakdown of clots and serves to balance the clotting process. **Fibri-**nolysis is the reversal of the clotting process. It is the mechanism by which formed thrombi are *lysed* (broken down) to prevent excessive clot formation and blood vessel blockage. It is the fibrin in the clot that binds to a circulating protein known as **plasminogen.** This converts plasminogen to **plasmin.** Plasmin is the enzymatic protein that eventually breaks down the fibrin thrombus into *fibrin degradation products.* This keeps the thrombus localized to prevent it from becoming an embolus that can travel to obstruct a major blood vessel in the lung, heart, or brain. Figure 27-3 illustrates the fibrinolytic system.

COAGULATION-MODIFYING DRUGS

The drugs discussed in this chapter aid the body in reversing or achieving hemostasis, and they can be broken down into several main categories based on their actions. **Anticoagulants** inhibit the action or formation of clotting factors and, therefore, prevent clots from forming. **Antiplatelet drugs** prevent platelet plugs from forming by inhibiting platelet aggregation, which can be beneficial in preventing heart attacks and strokes. Other drugs alter platelet function without preventing them from working. These are sometimes referred to as **hemorrheologic drugs.** Sometimes clots form and totally block a blood vessel. When this happens in one of the coronary arteries, a heart attack occurs, and the clot blocking the blood vessel must be lysed to prevent or

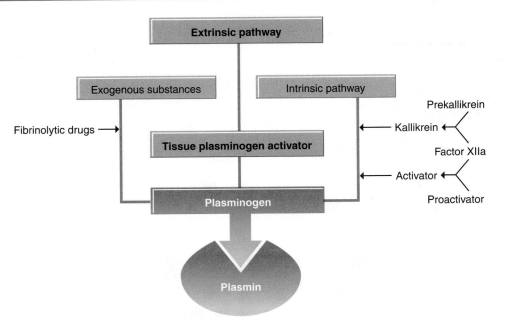

FIGURE 27-3 The fibrinolytic system.

Table 27-1 Coagulation Modifiers: Comparison of Drug Subclasses

Type of Coagulation Modifier and Mechanism of Action	Drug Class	Individual Drugs
Prevent Clot Formation *Anticoagulants*		
Inhibits clotting factors IIa (thrombin) and Xa	Heparins	unfractionated heparin ("heparin") and low molecular weight heparins (enoxaparin [Lovenox], dalteparin [Fragmin], tinzaparin [Innohep])
Inhibits vitamin K–dependent clotting factors II, VII, IX, and X	Coumarins	warfarin (Coumadin)
Inhibits clotting factors IIa and Xa	Glycosaminoglycans	danaparoid (Orgaran)
Inhibits thrombin (factor IIa)	Direct thrombin inhibitors	antithrombin III (human) (Thrombate), desirudin (Iprivask), lepirudin (Refludan), argatroban (Argatroban), bivalirudin (Angiomax)
Inhibits factor Xa	Selective factor Xa inhibitor	fondaparinux (Arixtra)
Antiplatelet Drugs		
Interfere with platelet function	Aggregation Inhibitors	cilostazol (Pletal), clopidogrel (Plavix)
	Aggregation Inhibitors/ Vasodilators	treprostinil (Remodulin)
	Glycoprotein IIb/IIIa Inhibitors	abciximab (ReoPro), eptifibitide (Integrilin), tirofiban (Aggrastat)
	Miscellaneous	anagrelide (Agrylin), dipyridamole (Persantine)
Promote Clot Formation *Antifibrinolytics*		
Prevent lysis of fibrin	Systemic hemostatics	aminocaproic acid (Amicar), tranexamic acid (Cyklokapron), aprotinin (Trasylol)
Reduce Blood Viscosity	Hemorrheologics	pentoxyfilline (Trental)
Lyse A Preformed Clot		
Thrombolytics	Thrombolytic enzymes	streptokinase (Streptase)
	Tissue plasminogen activators	alteplase (Activase, Cathflo Activase), reteplase (Retavase), tenecteplase (TNKase)
	Recombinant human activated Protein C	drotrecogin alfa (Xigris)
Reversal Drugs	Heparin antagonist	protamine sulfate
	Warfarin antagonist	vitamin K

minimize damage to the myocardial muscle. **Antifibrinolytic drugs,** also known as **hemostatic drugs,** have the opposite effect of these other classes of drugs; they actually *promote* blood coagulation and are helpful in the management of conditions in which excessive bleeding would be harmful.

The **thrombolytic drugs** lyse (break down) clots, or *thrombi,* that have already formed. This is a unique difference between thrombolytics and the anticoagulants, which can only prevent the formation of a clot. The various drugs in each category of coagulation modifiers are listed in Table 27-1. Understanding the individual coagulation modifiers and their mechanisms of action requires a basic working knowledge of the coagulation pathway and coagulation factors, which is provided in the next section.

ANTICOAGULANTS

Drugs that prevent the formation of a clot by inhibiting certain clotting factors are called anticoagulants. These drugs are only given prophylactically because they have no direct effect on a blood clot that has already formed or on ischemic tissue injured as the result of an inadequate blood supply caused by the clot. By decreasing blood coagulability, anticoagulants prevent intravascular thrombosis. Their uses vary from preventing clot formation to preventing the extension of an established clot, or a thrombus.

Once a clot forms on the wall of a blood vessel, it may dislodge and travel through the bloodstream. This is referred to as an **embolus.** If it lodges in a coronary artery, it causes a myocardial infarction (MI); if it obstructs a brain vessel, it causes a **stroke;** if it goes to the lungs, it is a **pulmonary embolism;** and if it goes to the veins in the legs, it is a **deep vein thrombosis (DVT).** Collectively, these complications are called **thromboembolic events** because they involve a thrombus becoming an embolus and causing an adverse cardiovascular "event." Anticoagulants can prevent all of these from occurring if used in the correct manner. There are both orally and parenterally administered anticoagulants, and each drug has a slightly different mechanism of action and indications. All of them have their own risks, mainly the risk for causing bleeding. The mechanisms of action of the anticoagulants vary depending on the drug. Drug classes of anticoagulants include older drugs such as unfractionated heparin and warfarin. But there are also several newer drug classes, including low molecular weight heparins (LMWHs), glycosaminoglycans, antithrombin drugs, and a selective factor Xa inhibitor. Dosages, indications, and other information appear in the corresponding dosage table.

Mechanism of Action and Drug Effects

Anticoagulants are also called *antithrombotic* drugs because they all work to prevent the formation of a clot or thrombus, a condition known as *thrombosis.* All anticoagulants work in the clotting cascade but do so at different points. As shown in Figures 27-1 and 27-2, heparin works by binding to a substance called **antithrombin III (AT-III),** which turns off three main activating factors: activated II (also called *thrombin*), activated X, and activated IX. (Factors XI and XII are also inactivated but do not play as important a role as the other three factors.) Of these, the thrombin is the most sensitive to the actions of heparin. AT-III is the major natural inhibitor of thrombin in the blood. The overall effect of heparin is that it turns off the coagulation pathway and prevents clots from forming. As previously noted, however, it cannot lyse a clot. The drug name "heparin" usually refers to *unfractionated* heparin, which is a relatively large molecule, and is derived from various animal sources. In contrast, LMWHs are synthetic and have a smaller molecular structure. These include enoxaparin (Lovenox), dalteparin (Fragmin), and tinzaparin (Innohep). All three work similarly to heparin. Heparin primarily binds to activated factors II, X, and IX. LMWHs differ from heparin in that they are much more specific for activated factor X (Xa) than for activated factor II (IIa = thrombin). This property confers upon LMWHs a much more predictable anticoagulant response. As a result, frequent laboratory monitoring of bleeding times such as activated partial thromboplastin times (aPTTs), which are imperative with unfractionated heparin, are not required with LMWHs.

Warfarin (Coumadin) also works by inhibiting vitamin K synthesis by bacteria in the gastrointestinal tract. This, in turn, inhibits production of clotting factors II, VII, IX, and X. These four factors are normally synthesized in the liver and are known as *vitamin K–dependent clotting factors.* As with heparin, the final effect is the prevention of clot formation. Figures 27-1 and 27-2 show where in the clotting cascade this occurs.

The *glycosaminoglycan* class currently includes one drug, danaparoid. This drug prevents fibrin formation by inhibiting clotting factors Xa (in conjunction with AT-III) and IIa (in conjunction with both AT-III and *heparin cofactor II [HC II]).* In contrast, fondaparinux (Arixtra) inhibits thrombosis by its molecular specificity against factor Xa alone. There are also currently five antithrombin drugs, which inhibit the thrombin molecules directly, one natural and four synthetic. The natural drug is human antithrombin III (Thrombate), which is isolated from the plasma of human donors. The four synthetic drugs include desirudin (Iprivask), lepirudin (Refludan), argatroban (Argatroban), and bivalirudin (Angiomax). All of these drugs work similarly to inhibit thrombus formation.

CASE STUDY

Heparin Therapy

In the past 2 years, Mr. L., a 56-year-old attorney, has suffered three episodes of DVT. All occurred without complications and all were treated successfully with anticoagulant therapy and bedrest. He now arrives at the urgent care center because of increased pain and swelling in his left calf that has lasted for the past 3 days. Initially he is given 5000 units of heparin. On admission to the hospital for anticoagulant therapy he is started on a continuous infusion of 25,000 units of heparin in 1000 mL of 0.9% sodium chloride.

- What nursing actions should be implemented to ensure the accuracy and safety of the continuous heparin infusion?
- What patient findings would indicate a therapeutic response to the heparin therapy?

Mr. L. suddenly complains of numbness and tingling in his lower extremities with accompanying changes in muscle strength and sensation 12 hr after the initiation and continuation of heparin therapy. What would be the most appropriate nursing actions to implement?

DVT, Deep vein thrombosis.
For answers, see http://evolve.elsevier.com/Lilley.

Indications

The ability of anticoagulants to prevent clot formation is of benefit in certain settings in which there is a high likelihood of clot formation. These include an MI; unstable angina; atrial fibrillation; indwelling devices such as mechanical heart valves; and conditions in which blood flow may be slowed and blood may pool, such as major orthopedic surgery. As previously mentioned, the ultimate consequence of a clot can be a stroke or a heart attack, a DVT, or a pulmonary embolism (PE); therefore, the prevention of these serious events is the ultimate benefit of these drugs. Warfarin is indicated for *prevention* of any of these events, whereas both unfractionated heparins and LMWHs are used for both prevention and treatment. LMWHs, especially enoxaparin, are also routinely used as anticoagulant "bridge" therapy in situations in which a patient must stop warfarin for surgery or other invasive medical procedures. The remainder of the antithrombotic drugs have similar but more restricted indications, which are listed in the corresponding dosage table.

Contraindications

Contraindications to the use of anticoagulants are generally very similar between the different drugs, and include known drug allergy to a specific product and usually include any acute bleeding process of high risk for such an occurrence, as well as thrombocytopenia. Some examples include leukemia or other major blood dyscrasias, pregnancy, gastrointestinal obstruction, serious inflammation (e.g., colitis), infection, and recent surgery or other invasive medical procedure. Warfarin is strongly contraindicated in pregnancy, whereas the other anticoagulants are rated in lower pregnancy categories (B or C).

Adverse Effects

Bleeding is the main complication of anticoagulation therapy, and the risk increases with increasing dosages. Such bleeding may be localized (e.g., hematoma at site of injection) or systemic. It also depends on the nature of the patient's underlying clinical disorder and is increased in patients also taking high doses of aspirin or other drugs that impair platelet function. One particularly notable adverse effect of heparin is *heparin-induced thrombocytopenia (HIT)*, which is also called *heparin-associated thrombocytopenia (HAT)*. This is an allergic reaction that is mediated by the production of immunoglobulin (Ig)G antibodies. The greatest risk to the patient with HIT is the paradoxical occurrence of thrombosis, something that heparin normally prevents or alleviates. The incidence of this disorder ranges from 5% to 15% of patients and is higher with *bovine* (cow-derived) versus *porcine* (pig-derived) heparins. As listed in the dosage table, the direct thrombin inhibitors lepirudin and argatroban are both specifically indicated for treating HIT. Other adverse effects are listed in Table 27-2.

Interactions

The drug interactions involving the oral anticoagulants are profound and complicated, and the drugs and the result of an interaction are given in Table 27-3. The main interaction mechanisms responsible for increasing anticoagulant activity include the following:

- **Enzyme** inhibition of biotransformation (metabolism)
- Displacement of the drug from inactive protein-binding sites

Table 27-2   Anticoagulants: Common Adverse Effects

Drug Subclass	Adverse Effects
Heparins	Bleeding, hematoma, nausea, anemia, thrombocytopenia, fever, edema
Glycosaminoglycans	Bleeding, insomnia, headache, dizziness, rash, pruritus, nausea, constipation, vomiting, fever, injection site pain, edema, joint pain, asthenia, anemia, urinary retention, or urinary tract infection
Direct thrombin inhibitors	Bleeding, dizziness, chest discomfort, nausea, constipation, chills, shortness of breath, fever, urticaria, heart and kidney failure (lepirudin, argatroban), cardiac arrhythmias (argatroban), hypotension (argatroban and bivalirudin)
Selective factor Xa inhibitors	Bleeding, hematoma, dizziness, confusion, rash, gastrointestinal distress, urinary tract infection, urinary retention, anemia

- Decrease in vitamin K absorption or synthesis by the bacterial flora of the large intestines
- Alteration in the platelet count or activity

Drugs that can increase the activity of heparin include aspirin, intravenous (IV) ethacrynic acid, and the oral anticoagulants. Antihistamines, digitalis, and the tetracyclines may partially antagonize the anticoagulant effects of heparin by inducing (promoting activity of) enzymes that metabolize heparin. The drugs that cause this are listed in Table 27-3. In terms of laboratory test interactions, heparin can alter the serum levels of lipids, glucose, thyroxine, aspartate aminotransferase (AST), alanine aminotransferase (ALT), and can also affect triiodothyronine (T_3) uptake.

Toxicity and Management of Overdose

Treatment of the toxic effects of anticoagulants is aimed at reversing the underlying cause. Although the toxic effects of heparin, LMWHs, and warfarin are hemorrhagic in nature, the management of each is different. Symptoms that may be attributed to toxicity or an overdose of anticoagulants are hematuria, melena (blood in stool), petechiae, ecchymoses, and gum or mucous membrane bleeding. In the event of either heparin or warfarin toxicity, the drug should be discontinued immediately. In the case of heparin, this alone may be enough to reverse the toxic effects because of its short half-life (1 to 2 hours). In severe cases or when large doses have been given intentionally (i.e., during cardiopulmonary bypass for heart surgery), IV injection of protamine sulfate is indicated. This drug is a specific heparin antidote and forms a complex with heparin, completely reversing its anticoagulant properties. This occurs in as few as 5 minutes. In general, 1 mg of protamine can reverse the effects of 100 units of heparin. Heparin comes from three different sources, and each source has a different anticoagulant potency. In theory, however,

Table 27-3 Anticoagulants: Drug Interactions

Drug	Mechanism	Result
Warfarin		
acetaminophen (high doses) amiodarone bumetanide furosemide	Displaces from inactive protein-binding sites	
aspirin/other NSAIDs Broad-spectrum antibiotics cephalosporin	Decreases platelet activity	Increased anticoagulant effect
Mineral oil Vitamin E	Interferes with vitamin K	
aminoglutethimide Barbiturates carbamazepine glutethimide rifampin	Enzyme inducer	Decreased anticoagulant effect
amiodarone cimetidine ciprofloxacin erythromycin ketoconazole metronidazole omeprazole Sulfonamides	Enzyme inhibitor	Increased anticoagulant effect
cholestyramine sucralfate	Impairs absorption of warfarin	Decreased anticoagulant effect
Heparin		
aspirin/other NSAIDs	Decrease platelet activity	
ethacrynic acid Oral anticoagulants Thrombolytics Cephalosporins Penicillins	Additive	Increased anticoagulant effect
Glycosaminoglycans, direct thrombin inhibitors, selective factor Xa inhibitors Any other anticoagulant, antiplatelet, or thrombolytic drugs	Additive	Increased bleeding risk

NSAID, Nonsteroidal antiinflammatory drug.

the protamine dosing should vary depending on the type of heparin given (1 mg of protamine for 90 units of heparin sodium from bovine lung tissue, 100 units of heparin calcium from porcine intestinal mucosa, and 115 units of heparin sodium from porcine intestinal mucosa). Protamine may also be used to reverse the effects of LMWHs. A 1-mg dose of protamine equal to that of the LMWH should be used (e.g., 1 mg protamine/1 mg enoxaparin). If the heparin overdose has resulted in a large blood loss, replacement with packed red blood cells (PRBCs) may be necessary.

In the event of warfarin toxicity or overdose, again the first step is to discontinue the warfarin. As with heparin, the toxicity associated with warfarin use is an extension of its therapeutic effects on the clotting cascade. However, because warfarin functionally inactivates the vitamin K–dependent clotting factors and because these clotting factors are synthesized in the liver, it may take 36 to 42 hours before the liver can resynthesize enough clotting factors to reverse the warfarin effects. IV injection of vitamin K (phytonadione) can hasten the return to normal coagulation. The dose and route of administration of the vitamin K depend on the clinical situation and its acuity (i.e., how quickly the warfarin-induced effects must be reversed). High doses of vitamin K (10 to 15 mg) given intravenously should reverse the anticoagulation within 6 hours. If the warfarin therapy needs to be resumed, warfarin resistance is likely to occur, because a large dose of vitamin K will maintain its warfarin reversal effects for up to 1 week. The use of lower doses of vitamin K, if clinically feasible, may minimize this effect. In acute situations in which bleeding is severe and the time it would take for the vitamin K to take effect is too great, it may be necessary to administer transfusions of human plasma or clotting factor concentrates.

With regard to the glycosaminoglycans (namely, danaparoid), protamine sulfate provides only partial neutralization of its anti-Xa activity, and there is no other known specific antidote. Transfuse with other blood products as clinically indicated. Transfusions may also be indicated for overdoses of antithrombin drugs and the selective factor Xa inhibitor fondaparinux, which also lack specific antidotes. These drugs may also be removed with hemodialysis.

Dosages

For dosage information on anticoagulants, see the Dosages table on page 424.

Drug Profiles

Of the anticoagulants, warfarin is available only for oral use. The rest are by IV and/or subcutaneous (SC) injection only. Intramuscular (IM) injection of these drugs is contraindicated due to their propensity to cause anticoagulation with large ecchymoses at the site of injection.

▶ warfarin

Warfarin sodium (Coumadin) is a pharmaceutical derivative of the natural plant anticoagulant known as *coumarin*. Warfarin is the most commonly prescribed oral (PO) anticoagulant and is only available for oral use, as noted earlier. Use of this drug requires careful monitoring of the prothrombin time/International Normalized Ratio (PT/INR), which is a standardized measure of the degree to which a patient's blood coagulability has been reduced by the drug. A normal INR (without warfarin) is 1.0, whereas a therapeutic INR (with warfarin) ranges from 2 to 3.5, depending on the indication for use of the drug (e.g., atrial fibrillation, thromboprevention, prosthetic heart valve). Elderly patients older than 65 years may have a lower INR threshold for bleeding complications and should be monitored accordingly.

Pharmacokinetics

Half-Life	Onset	Peak	Duration
0.5-3 days	12-24 hr	3-4 days	2-5 days

▶ enoxaparin

Enoxaparin (Lovenox) is the prototype LMWH, and is obtained by enzymatically cleaving large unfractionated heparin molecules into small fragments. These smaller fragments of heparin have a greater affinity for factor Xa than for factor IIa and have a higher degree of bioavailability and a longer elimination half-life than unfractionated heparin. Laboratory monitoring, as done for heparin, is not necessary with enoxaparin because of its high bioavailability and greater affinity for factor Xa. It is available only in injectable form. Other antico-

DOSAGES

Selected Anticoagulant Drugs

Drug (Pregnancy Category)	Pharmacologic Class	Usual Dosage Range	Indications
▶heparin (generic only) (C)	Natural anticoagulant	**Pediatric** IV: Initial 50 units/kg, then 12-25 units/kg/hr, increased by 2-4 units/kg/hr q6-8h prn **Adult** SC: 10,000-20,000 units followed by 8000-10,000 units tid IV: 10,000 units followed by 5000-10,000 units 4-6 ×/day IV infusion: 20,000-40,000 units/day ACT or aPTT determines maintenance dose	Thrombosis/embolism, coagulopathies (e.g., DIC), DVT, and PE prophylaxis, clotting prevention (e.g., open heart surgery, dialysis)
▶warfarin (X)	Coumarin anticoagulant	PT or INR determines maintenance dose, usually 2-10 mg/day	Thromboprevention and treatment in DVT, PE, atrial fibrillation, post-MI
▶enoxaparin (Lovenox) (B)	LMWH	**Adult** SC: 30-100 mg every 12 hours	Prevention and treatment of thromboembolic and ischemic processes in postoperative, unstable angina, and post-MI situations
dalteparin (Fragmin) (B)	LMWH	**Adult** SC: 2500-5000 units once daily.	
tinzaparin (Innohep) (B)	LMWH	**Adult** SC: 175 units/kg once daily	DVT prophylaxis only
antithrombin III (Human; Thrombate III) (B)	Human antithrombin	**Adult** IV: calculated by weight based on desired AT-III level	Hereditary AT-III deficiency in surgical, OB, or thrombosis settings
desirudin (Iprivask) (C)	Synthetic thrombin inhibitor	**Adult** SC: 15 mg every 12 hours	DVT prophylaxis in hip surgery
lepirudin (Refludan) (B)	Synthetic thrombin inhibitor	**Adult** IV: 0.4 mg/kg bolus, then 0.15 mg/kg continuous infusion × 2-10 days.	Thromboprevention in patients with HIT
argatroban (Argatroban) (B)	Synthetic thrombin inhibitor	**Adult** IV: 350 mcg/kg bolus then 25-30 mcg/kg/min until ACT in desired range.	Thromboprevention and treatment in HIT; and in PCI in patients at risk for HIT
bivalirudin (Angiomax) (B)	Synthetic thrombin inhibitor	**Adult** IV: 1 mg/kg bolus, then 2.5 mg/kg/hr (with aspirin, 325 mg daily)	Thromboprevention in unstable angina
fondaparinux (Arixtra) (B)	Selective Factor Xa inhibitor	**Adult** SC: 2.5 mg once daily	DVT prophylaxis in hip/knee surgery

agulants with comparable pharmacology and indications include danaparoid and fondaparinux.

Pharmacokinetics

Half-Life	Onset	Peak	Duration
4.5 hr	3-5 hr	4-5 hr	12 hr

▶ *heparin*

Heparin (generic only) is a natural mucopolysaccharide anticoagulant obtained from the lungs, intestinal mucosa, or other suitable tissues of primarily sheep, cows, and pigs. One brand name for some of the commonly used heparin products is Hep-Lock. However, this brand name refers only to small vials of aqueous heparin IV flush solutions used to maintain patency of heparin-lock IV insertion sites. This type of use for heparin is fundamentally different from the sys-

temic use of heparin for its anticoagulant cardiovascular effects as discussed in this chapter. Furthermore, heparin solutions used for such heparin lock flushes is usually in a lower concentration than heparin used for systemic cardiovascular purposes. In fact, some institutions routinely used normal saline (0.9% sodium chloride) as a flush for heparin lock intravenous ports and have moved away from using heparin flush solutions per se for this purpose.

Heparin is available in only in injectable form in multiple strengths ranging from 10 to 40,000 units per mL.

Pharmacokinetics

Half-Life	Onset	Peak	Duration
1-2 hr	SC: 20-60 min IV: Immediate	SC: 2-4 hr	Dose-dependent

lepirudin

Lepirudin (Refludan) is a recombinant, yeast-derived inhibitor of thrombin. It is used specifically for heparin-induced thrombocytopenia (HIT) and is only available for IV use. Like heparin, it is monitored using the aPTT. Argatroban is another drug in this class with the same indication. Other drugs in this class with more variable indications include human antithrombin III (for hereditary deficiency), desirudin (for DVT prophylaxis), and bivalirudin (for unstable angina).

Pharmacokinetics

Half-Life	Onset	Peak	Duration
1.3 hr	Not listed	Not listed	Dependent on length of infusion

argatroban

Argatroban, which has the same trade name, is a synthetic direct thrombin inhibitor that is derived from the amino acid L-arginine. It is indicated for both active HIT and for *percutaneous coronary intervention (PCI)* procedures in patients at risk for HIT (i.e., those with history). It is only given IV.

Pharmacokinetics

Half-Life	Onset	Peak	Duration
30-50 min	Immediate	1-3 hr	Dependent on length of infusion

PLATELET PHYSIOLOGY

Another class of coagulation modifiers that prevent clot formation is the antiplatelet drugs. The anticoagulants work in the clotting cascade. In contrast, antiplatelet drugs work to prevent the platelet *adhesion* to the site of blood vessel injury, which actually occurs before the clotting cascade. An understanding of the role of platelets in the clotting process is essential to understanding how antiplatelet drugs work.

Platelets normally flow through blood vessels without adhering to their surfaces. Blood vessels can be injured by a disruption of blood flow, trauma, or the rupture of plaque from a vessel wall. When such events occur, substances such as collagen and fibronectin, which are present in the walls of blood vessels, become exposed. Collagen is a potent stimulator of platelet adhesion, as is a prevalent component of the platelet membranes themselves, *glycoprotein IIb/IIIa* (GP IIb/IIIa). Once platelet adhesion occurs, stimulators (compounds such as adenosine diphosphate [ADP], thrombin, thromboxane A_2 [TXA_2], and prostaglandin H_2 are released from the activated platelets. These cause the platelets to *aggregate* (accumulate) at the site of injury. Once at the site of vessel injury, the platelets change shape and release *their* contents, which include ADP, serotonin, and platelet factor 4 (PF4). The hemostatic function of these substances is twofold. First, they function as platelet recruiters, attracting additional platelets to the site of injury; second, they are potent vasoconstrictors. Vasoconstriction limits blood flow to the damaged blood vessel to reduce blood loss.

A platelet plug that has formed at a site of vessel injury is not stable and can be dislodged. The clotting cascade is therefore stimulated to form a more permanent *fibrin* plug (blood clot). The role of platelets and their relationship to the clotting cascade are illustrated in Figure 27-4.

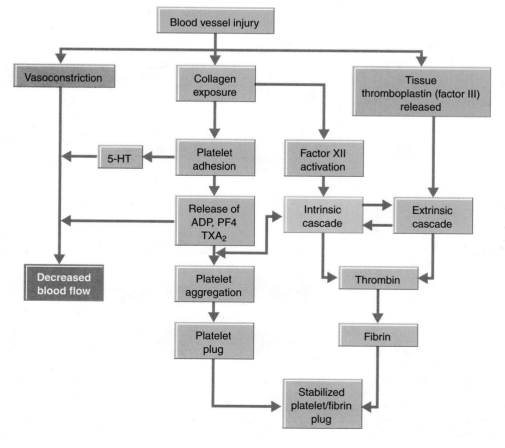

FIGURE 27-4 Relationship between platelets and clotting cascade. *ADP,* Adenosine diphosphate; *5-HT,* serotonin; *PF4,* platelet factor 4; *TXA_2,* thromboxane A_2.

ANTIPLATELET DRUGS

The mechanisms of action of the antiplatelet drugs vary depending on the drug. Aspirin, clopidogrel, dipyridamole, pentoxifylline, cilostazol, anagrelide, abciximab, tirofiban, and eptifibatide all affect the normal function of platelets. Dosage, indications, and other information appears in the designated table.

Mechanism of Action and Drug Effects

Many of the antiplatelet drugs affect the *cyclooxygenase* pathway, which is one of the common final enzymatic pathways in the complex *arachidonic acid* pathway that operates within platelets and on blood vessel walls. This pathway as it functions in both platelets and blood vessel walls is illustrated in Figure 27-5.

Aspirin is also widely used for its analgesic, antiinflammatory, and antipyretic (antifever) properties (Chapter 44). In terms of its anticoagulant effects, aspirin (acetylsalicylic acid) acetylates and inhibits cyclooxygenase in the platelet irreversibly such that the platelet cannot regenerate this enzyme. Therefore, the effects of aspirin last the life span of a platelet, or 7 days. This irreversible inhibition of cyclooxygenase in the platelet prevents the formation of TXA_2, a substance that causes blood vessels to constrict and platelets to aggregate. Thus, by preventing TXA_2 formation, aspirin prevents these actions, resulting in dilation of the blood vessels and prevention of platelets from aggregating or forming a clot. In addition, aspirin may also affect vitamin K–dependent clotting factors VII, IX, and X, by interfering with the action of vitamin K, in a manner similar to warfarin. Ironically, aspirin has the additional drawback of preventing the formation of *prostacyclin*, a beneficial *anti*coagulant substance that causes blood vessel dilation and inhibits platelet aggregation. However, this procoagulant effect of aspirin is not as pronounced as its anticoagulant effects.

Dipyridamole, another antiplatelet dug, also works to inhibit platelet aggregation by preventing the release of *adenosine diphosphate (ADP), platelet factor 4 (PF4)*, and TXA_2, all substances that stimulate platelets to aggregate or form a clot. Figure 27-4 shows how these substances accomplish this. Dipyridamole may also directly stimulate the release of prostacyclin and inhibit the formation of TXA_2 (see Figure 27-5).

Clopidogrel is a drug that belongs to one of the newest classes of antiplatelet drugs called the *ADP inhibitors*. Its use has largely superceded that of the original ADP inhibitor ticlopidine. Its mechanism of action is entirely different from that of aspirin in that it inhibits platelet aggregation by altering the platelet membrane so that it can no longer receive the signal to aggregate and form a clot. This signal is in the form of **fibrinogen** molecules, which attach to glycoprotein receptors (GP IIb/IIIa) on the surface of the platelet. Clopidogrel inhibits the activation of this receptor. Clopidogrel has been shown to be somewhat better than aspirin at reducing the number of heart attacks, strokes, and vascular deaths in at-risk patients.

Pentoxifylline, another antiplatelet drug, is a methylxanthine derivative with properties similar to those of other methylxanthines, such as caffeine and theophylline (Chapter 36). It was one of the earliest antiplatelet drugs, but is now much less

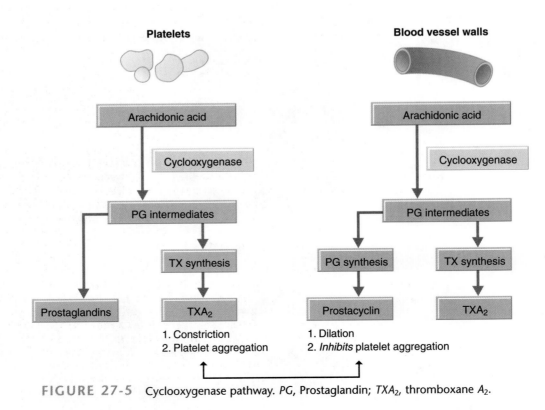

FIGURE 27-5 Cyclooxygenase pathway. *PG*, Prostaglandin; *TXA₂*, thromboxane *A₂*.

commonly used. It reduces the viscosity of blood by increasing the flexibility of red blood cells (RBCs) and reducing the aggregation of platelets. It is sometimes referred to as a *hemorrheologic drug,* or a drug that alters the fluid dynamics of the blood. The antiplatelet effects of pentoxifylline are attributed to its inhibition of ADP, serotonin, and PF4 (see Figure 27-4). Pentoxifylline also stimulates the synthesis and release of prostacyclin from blood vessels (see Figure 27-5). In addition, it may have effects on the fibrinolytic system by raising the plasma concentrations of tissue plasminogen activator (see Figure 27-3).

Cilostazol is another antiplatelet drug that works through inhibition of *type 3 phosphodiesterase* (PDE-3) in the platelets and primarily lower-extremity blood vessels. Its effects are to reduce platelet aggregation and promote vasodilation.

The newest available antiplatelet class of drugs is the GP IIb/IIIa inhibitors. They work by blocking the receptor protein by the same name that occurs in the platelet wall membranes. This protein plays a role in promoting the aggregation of platelets in preparation for fibrin clot formation. There are currently three available drugs in this class: tirofiban (Aggrastat), eptifibatide (Integrilin), and abciximab (ReoPro).

Indications

The therapeutic effects of the antiplatelet drugs depend on the particular drug. Aspirin has multiple therapeutic effects, but many of them vary depending on the dose. Aspirin is officially recommended for stroke prevention by the American Stroke Society in daily doses of 50 to 325 mg. Clopidogrel is also used for reducing the risk for fatal and nonfatal thrombotic stroke, and is used for prophylaxis against *transient ischemic attacks (TIAs)* as well for post-MI thromboprevention. Dipyridamole is used as an adjunct to warfarin in the prevention of postoperative thromboembolic complications. It is also used to decrease platelet aggregation in various other thromboembolic disorders. The GP IIb/IIIa inhibitors are used to treat acute unstable angina, MI, and during PCI, such as angioplasty. Their purpose is to prevent the formation of thrombi. This is known as *thromboprevention.* This treatment approach is based on the fact that *prevention* of thrombus formation is easier and less risky overall from a pharmacologic standpoint than is lysing a formed thrombus. Pentoxifylline is indicated for peripheral vascular disease, whereas cilostazol is indicated specifically for *intermittent claudication* (pain and cramping in the calf muscles associated with walking). It has been shown to be superior to pentoxifylline in improving exercise tolerance in elderly patients.

Contraindications

Contraindications to the use of antiplatelet drugs include known drug allergy to a specific product, thrombocytopenia, active bleeding, leukemia, traumatic injury, GI ulcer, vitamin K deficiency, and recent stroke.

Adverse Effects

The potential adverse effects of the various antiplatelet drugs can be serious, and they all pose a risk for inducing a serious bleeding episode. The most common adverse effects are listed in Table 27-4.

Table 27-4	Selected Antiplatelet Drugs: Adverse Effects
Body System	**Adverse Effects**
Aspirin	
Central nervous	Stimulation, drowsiness, dizziness, confusion, flushing
Gastrointestinal	Nausea, vomiting, gastrointestinal bleeding, diarrhea, heartburn
Hematologic	Thrombocytopenia, agranulocytosis, leukopenia, neutropenia, hemolytic anemia, bleeding
Clopidogrel	
Cardiovascular	Chest pain, hypertension, edema
Central nervous	Flulike symptoms, headache, dizziness, fatigue
Gastrointestinal	Abdominal pain, dyspepsia, diarrhea, nausea
Miscellaneous	Epistaxis and integumentary disorders, including rash and pruritis (itching)
GP IIb/IIIa Inhibitors	Bleeding, bradycardia, dizziness, edema, leg pain, pelvic pain, chills

Interactions

There are some potentially dangerous drug interactions that can occur with antiplatelet drugs. The concurrent use of dipyridamole, with aspirin, clopidogrel, and/or nonsteroidal antiinflammatory drugs (NSAIDs) produces additive antiplatelet activity and increased bleeding potential. There may also be allergic cross-reactivity between aspirin and NSAIDs. When aspirin is given with oral antidiabetic drugs, the patient can experience a loss of diabetic control. The combined use of steroids or NSAIDs with aspirin can increase the ulcerogenic effects of aspirin. The combined use of aspirin and heparin with GP IIb/IIIa inhibitors also further enhances antiplatelet activity and increases the likelihood of a serious bleeding episode. In spite of all of the above, it is not uncommon to see patients on daily maintenance doses of aspirin for thrombopreventive purposes. However, the most commonly used dose in this situation is the "baby aspirin" dose of 81 mg versus the standard adult dose of 325 mg.

Drug Profiles

Antiplatelet drugs are extremely useful in the management of thromboembolic disorders. Each has unique pharmacologic properties, and, therefore, they all are somewhat different from one another.

Dosages

For information on the dosages of selected antiplatelet drugs, see the Dosages table on page 428.

▶ aspirin

Aspirin is available in many combinations with other prescription and nonprescription drugs and goes by many product names. One unique contraindication for aspirin is its use in children and teenagers with flulike symptoms. This situation is associated with cases of Reye's syndrome, a rare, acute, and sometimes fatal condition involving hepatic and central nervous system (CNS) damage (Chapter 44). Aspirin is available in both oral and rectal forms.

DOSAGES

Selected Antiplatelet Drugs

Drug (Pregnancy Category)	Pharmacologic Class	Usual Dosage Range	Indications
▶aspirin (C/D)	Salicylate antiplatelet	**Adult** PO: 81-325 mg once daily PO: 325-1300 mg/day	MI prophylaxis TIA prophylaxis
▶clopidogrel (Plavix) (B)	ADP Inhibitor	**Adult** PO: 75 mg qd; 300-375 mg may be given as a one-time loading dose after coronary stent implantation	Reduction of atherosclerotic events; acute coronary syndrome without ST segment elevation
▶eptifibatide (Integrilin) (B)	GP IIb/IIIa inhibitor	IV: Single bolus followed by continuous infusion; specific doses are based on patient weight from 37 to >121 kg*	Unstable angina, MI, percutaneous coronary procedures
pentoxifylline (Trental) (C)	Antiplatelet/hemorrheologic	**Adult** PO: 400 mg tid with meals	Claudication associated with peripheral arterial disease
cilostazol (Pletal) (C)	Antiplatelet	**Adult** PO: 100 mg twice daily.	Intermittent claudication

*See table in package insert for specific dose.
ADP, Adenosine diphosphate; *GP,* glycoprotein; *MI,* myocardial infarction; *TIA,* transient ischemic attack.

Pharmacokinetics

Half-Life	Onset	Peak	Duration
2-3 hr	15-30 min	0.25-2 hr	4-6 hr

▶ clopidogrel

Clopidogrel (Plavix) is currently the most widely used ADP inhibitor on the market. It has superceded ticlopidine (Ticlid) due to its associated serious adverse reactions, including life-threatening neutropenia and agranulocytosis. It was initially believed that clopidogrel might be free from such adverse effects. However, there are some emerging case reports of clopidogrel-associated hematologic adverse effects of comparable severity. This drug is available only for oral use.

Pharmacokinetics

Half-Life	Onset	Peak	Duration
8 hr	1-2 hr*	1 hr*	7-10 days

*Onset and peak values can be reduced by giving a loading dose of 300-375 mg.

▶ eptifibatide

Eptifibatide (Integrilin) is a GP IIb/IIIa inhibitor, along with tirofiban (Aggrastat) and abciximab (ReoPro). They are usually administered in intensive care or cardiac catheterization lab settings where continuous cardiovascular monitoring is the norm. All are available only for IV use.

Pharmacokinetics

Half-Life	Onset	Peak	Duration
2-2.5 hr	1 hr	Unknown	4 hr

ANTIFIBRINOLYTIC DRUGS

The individual antifibrinolytic drugs have varying mechanisms of action, but all prevent the lysis of fibrin, the substance that helps make the platelet plug insoluble and anchors the clot to the damaged blood vessel (see Figures 27-1 and 27-2). The term *antifibrinolytic* refers to what these drugs do, which is to prevent the lysis of fibrin; in doing so, they actually *promote* clot formation. For this reason, they are also called *hemostatic* drugs. They have the opposite effects of anticoagulant and antiplatelet drugs, which *prevent* clot formation. There are three synthetic antifibrinolytics—aminocaproic acid, tranexamic acid, and desmopressin—and one natural antifibrinolytic drug—aprotinin. Dosages, indications, and other information appear in the designated table. There are also hemostatic drugs that are used *topically* (on the skin or tissue surface) in surgical settings to stop excessive bleeding. These include topical thrombin, microfibrillar collagen, absorbable gelatin, and oxidized cellulose.

Mechanism of Action and Drug Effects

Antifibrinolytics vary in several ways, depending on the particular drug. The various antifibrinolytic drugs and their proposed mechanisms of action are described in Table 27-5.

The drug effects of the antifibrinolytics are very specific and limited. They do not have many effects outside of their hematologic ones. Aminocaproic acid, tranexamic acid, and aprotinin prevent the breakdown of fibrin, which prevents the destruction of the formed platelet clot. Desmopressin causes a dose-dependent increase in the concentration of plasma factor VIII (von Willebrand factor), along with an increase in the plasma concentration of tissue plasminogen activator. The overall effect of this is increased platelet aggregation and clot formation. This drug is also an analog of antidiuretic hormone (ADH) and is discussed further in Chapter 29 (Pituitary Drugs).

Indications

Antifibrinolytics are useful in both the prevention and treatment of excessive bleeding resulting from systemic hyperfibrinolysis or surgical complications. They have also proved successful in arresting excessive oozing from surgical sites such as chest tubes, as well as in reducing the total blood loss and the duration of bleeding in the postoperative period.

Desmopressin may also be used in patients who have hemophilia A or type I von Willebrand's disease.

Contraindications

Contraindications to the use of antifibrinolytic drugs include known drug allergy to a specific product and disseminated intravascular coagulation (DIC), which could be worsened by these drugs.

Adverse Effects

The adverse effects of antifibrinolytic drugs occur uncommonly and are mild. However, there have been rare reports of these drugs causing thrombotic events, such as acute cerebrovascular thrombosis and acute MI. The common adverse effects of antifibrinolytics are listed in Table 27-6.

Interactions

The concurrent use of drugs such as estrogens or oral contraceptives with aminocaproic acid, tranexamic acid, and aprotinin may have an additive effect, resulting in increased coagulation. Few specific interactions have been reported for desmopressin, although it should be given cautiously in patients receiving lithium, large doses of epinephrine, demeclocycline, heparin, or alcohol, because these combinations may lead to a reduced antidiuretic response to the desmopressin. Drugs such as chlorpropamide and fludrocortisone may potentiate the antidiuretic response, leading to edema.

Dosages

For information on the dosages of aminocaproic acid and desmopressin, see the Dosages table on this page.

Table 27-5 Antifibrinolytics: Mechanisms of Action

Antifibrinolytic Drug	Mechanism of Action
Synthetic drugs: aminocaproic acid and tranexamic acid	Form a reversible complex with plasminogen and plasmin. By binding to the lysine-binding site of plasminogen, these drugs displace plasminogen from the surface of fibrin. This prevents plasmin from lysing the fibrin clot. Therefore, these drugs can only work if a clot has formed.
Natural drug: aprotinin	Inhibits the proteolytic enzymes trypsin, plasmin, and kallikrein, which lyse proteins that destroy fibrin clots. By inhibiting these enzymes, aprotinin prevents the degradation of the fibrin clot. It is also thought to inhibit the action of the complement system.
Other synthetic drug: desmopressin (DDAVP)	Works by increasing factor VII (von Willebrand factor), which anchors platelets to damaged vessels via the GP Ib platelet receptor. It appears that desmopressin acts as a general endothelial stimulant, stimulating factor VIII, prostaglandin I2, and plasminogen activator.

GP, Glycoprotein.

Drug Profiles

aminocaproic acid

Aminocaproic acid (Amicar) is a synthetic antifibrinolytic drug used to prevent and control the excessive bleeding that can result from surgery or overactivity of the fibrinolytic system. It is available in both oral and parenteral preparations.

Pharmacokinetics

Half-Life	Onset	Peak	Duration
2 hr	Unknown	1.2 hr	<3 hr*

*For intravenous formulation.

desmopressin

Desmopressin (DDAVP) is a synthetic polypeptide. It is structurally very similar to vasopressin, which is antidiuretic hormone (ADH), the natural human posterior pituitary hormone. Because of these physical characteristics, it is most often used to increase the resorption of water by the collecting ducts in the kidneys to prevent or

Table 27-6 Antifibrinolytics: Adverse Effects

Body System	Adverse Effects
Cardiovascular	Dysrhythmias, orthostatic hypotension, bradycardia
Central nervous	Headache, dizziness, fatigue, hallucinations, psychosis, convulsions
Gastrointestinal	Nausea, vomiting, abdominal cramps, diarrhea

DOSAGES

Selected Antifibrinolytic Drugs

Drug (Pregnancy Category)	Pharmacologic Class	Usual Dosage Range	Indications
aminocaproic acid (Amicar) (C)	Hemostatic	**Adult** IV infusion: 4-5 g during first hr, then 1-1.25 g at 1-hr intervals up to a daily max of 30 g	Excessive bleeding caused by systemic hyperfibrinolysis or urinary fibrinolysis
desmopressin (DDAVP) (B)	Synthetic posterior pituitary hormone	**Adult** IV: 0.3 mcg/kg infused over 15-30 min; preop use: drug is administered 30 min before surgery	Surgical and postop hemostasis and management of bleeding in patients with hemophilia A or type I von Willebrand's disease

control polydipsia, polyuria, and dehydration in patients with diabetes insipidus caused by a deficiency of endogenous posterior pituitary vasopressin or in patients with polyuria and polydipsia resulting from trauma or surgery in the pituitary region.

Desmopressin also causes a dose-dependent increase in plasma factor VIII (von Willebrand factor), along with an increase in tissue plasminogen activator, resulting in increased platelet aggregation and clot formation. Desmopressin is contraindicated in patients with a known hypersensitivity to it and in those with nephrogenic diabetes insipidus. It is available in both injectable and intranasal dosage forms. Desmopressin nasal spray is used for primary nocturnal enuresis.

Pharmacokinetics

Half-Life	Onset	Peak	Duration
<2 hr	15-30 min	1.1-2 hr	Unknown

THROMBOLYTIC DRUGS

Thrombolytics are coagulation modifiers that lyse thrombi in the blood vessels that supply the heart with blood, the coronary arteries. This reestablishes blood flow to the blood-starved heart muscle. If the blood flow is reestablished early, the heart muscle and left ventricular function can be saved. If blood flow is not reestablished early, the affected area of the heart muscle becomes ischemic, and eventually necrotic and nonfunctional.

Thrombolytic therapy made its debut in 1933 when a substance that would break down fibrin clots was isolated from a patient's blood. This substance was determined to be produced by a bacterium growing in the patient's blood. The bacterium was found to be **beta-hemolytic streptococci (group A),** and the substance was eventually called *streptokinase (SK).*

SK was first used in a patient in 1947 to dissolve a clotted hemothorax, but it was not until 1958 that the first patient with an acute MI received it. In 1960, a naturally occurring human plasminogen activator called *urokinase* became available, which was found to exert fibrinolytic effects on pulmonary emboli (clots in the lungs). However, the results of the early thrombolytic trials conducted during the 1960s and 1970s and made up of patients who had had an acute MI were not taken seriously by the medical community. It was not until the 1980s that DeWood and colleagues demonstrated that the underlying cause of acute MIs was a coronary artery occlusion. This marked the start of rapid growth in the use of thrombolytic drugs for the early treatment of acute MIs. Since that time, several new thrombolytics have become available for this and other clinical uses. *Tissue plasminogen activator* and *anisoylated plasminogen streptokinase activator complex (APSAC)* are two of these drugs. With the advent of these new thrombolytics came the results of several large landmark thrombolytic research studies. These studies showed that early thrombolytic therapy could bring about a 50% reduction in mortality, a reduction in the infarct size, an improvement in left ventricular function, and a reduction in the incidence and severity of congestive heart failure. These findings and developments, along with a better understanding of the pathogenesis of acute MIs, have led the way in the advancements made in the treatment of acute MIs. Currently available thrombolytic drug classes include thrombolytic enzymes (streptokinase [Streptase]), tissue plasminogen activators (anistreplase [Eminase], alteplase [t-PA, Activase], reteplase [Retavase],

and tenecteplase [TNKase]); and a recombinant human activated protein C (doctrecogin alfa [Xigris]). Dosages, indications, and other information appear in the designated table.

Mechanism of Action and Drug Effects

There is a fine balance between the formation and dissolution of a clot. As discussed previously, the coagulation system is responsible for forming clots, whereas the fibrinolytic system is responsible for dissolving clots. The natural fibrinolytic system within blood takes days to break down a clot (thrombus). This is of little value in the case of a clotted blood vessel supplying blood to the heart muscle. Necrosis of the myocardium would not be prevented by these natural means, but thrombolytic drug therapy activates the fibrinolytic system to break down the clot (thrombus) in the blood vessel quickly so that the delivery of blood to the heart muscle via the coronary arteries is quickly reestablished. This prevents myocardial tissue (heart muscle) and heart function from being destroyed. Thrombolytics accomplish this by activating the conversion of plasminogen to plasmin, which breaks down, or lyses, the thrombus (see Figure 27-3). Plasmin is a proteolytic enzyme, which means that it breaks down proteins. It is a relatively nonspecific serine protease that is capable of degrading such proteins as fibrin, fibrinogen, and other procoagulant proteins such as factors V, VIII, and XII. In other words, the substances that form clots are destroyed by plasmin. Essentially, thrombolytic drugs work by mimicking the body's own process of clot destruction. Although the individual thrombolytic drugs are somewhat diverse in their actions, they all have this common result.

Streptokinase (SK), the original thrombolytic enzyme, binds with plasminogen to form an SK-plasminogen complex, which then acts on other plasminogen molecules to form plasmin. The plasmin formed then lyses the clots. SK is not *clot specific.* Not only does it break down the thrombus in the coronary artery, but it also breaks down clots anywhere in the body. In other words, it activates fibrinolysis throughout the body. This can be helpful with clots in the leg, for example. The APSAC is an SK-plasminogen complex that has been chemically modified by acylation, allowing a prolonged half-life. In contrast to the newer thrombolytic drugs, the thrombolytic enzymes are not clot-specific, which increases the risk for bleeding complications. The newer thrombolytics have chemical specificity for fibrin threads **(fibrin-specificity)** and work primarily at the site of a clot. They still carry some bleeding risk, but much less than that of the thrombolytic enzymes.

Tissue plasminogen activator (t-PA) is a naturally occurring plasminogen activator secreted by vascular endothelial cells (the walls of blood vessels). However, the amount secreted naturally is not sufficient to dissolve a coronary thrombus quickly enough to restore circulation to the heart and save the heart muscle. t-PA is now made through recombinant DNA techniques and thus can be administered in quantities sufficient enough to dissolve a coronary thrombus quickly. Again, it is fibrin-specific (clot-specific), meaning that only the fibrin clot stimulates t-PA to convert plasminogen to plasmin. Therefore, it has as great a propensity to induce a systemic thrombolytic state, compared to the thrombolytic enzymes.

Indications

The purpose of all the thrombolytic drugs is to activate the conversion of plasminogen to plasmin, the enzyme that breaks down a thrombus. The presence of a thrombus that interferes significantly with normal blood flow on either the venous or the arterial side of the circulation is an indication for the use of thrombolytic therapy. An exception to this may be a thrombus that has formed in blood vessels that directly connects with the central nervous system (CNS). The indications for thrombolytic therapy include acute MI, arterial thrombosis, DVT, occlusion of shunts or catheters, PE, and acute ischemic stroke.

Contraindications

Contraindications to the use of thrombolytic drugs include known drug allergy to the specific product and any preservatives and concurrent use with other drugs that alter clotting.

Adverse Effects

The most common undesirable effect of thrombolytic therapy is internal, intracranial, and superficial bleeding. Other problems include hypersensitivity, anaphylactoid reactions, nausea, vomiting, and hypotension. These drugs can also induce cardiac dysrhythmias.

Toxicity and Management of Overdose

Acute toxicity primarily causes an extension of the adverse effects of the thrombolytic agent. Treatment is symptomatic and supportive as thrombolytic drugs have a relatively short half-life and no specific antidotes.

Interactions

The most common effect of drug interactions is an increased bleeding tendency resulting from the concurrent use of anticoagulant, antiplatelet, or other drugs that affect platelet function.

A laboratory test interaction that can occur with thrombolytic drugs is a reduction in the plasminogen and fibrinogen levels.

Dosages

For information on the dosages of SK and alteplase, see the Dosages table on this page.

Drug Profiles

All thrombolytic drugs exert their effects by activating plasminogen and converting it to plasmin, which is capable of digesting fibrin, a major component of clots.

▶ alteplase

Alteplase (Activase) is a naturally occurring t-PA secreted by vascular endothelial cells. The pharmaceutically available t-PA is made through recombinant DNA techniques, and modified mammalian hamster ovary cells produce the substance. It is clot (fibrin)-specific and, therefore, does not produce a systemic lytic state. In addition, because it is present in the human body in a natural state, its administration for therapeutic use does not induce an antigen–antibody reaction. Therefore, it can be readministered immediately in the event of reinfarction. t-PA has a very short half-life of 5 minutes. It is believed to open the clogged artery faster, but its action is short-lived. Therefore, it is given concomitantly with heparin to prevent reocclusion of the infarcted blood vessel. Alteplase is also available only in parenteral form. There is also a smaller dosage form known as Cathflo Activase that is used to flush clogged IV or arterial lines.

Pharmacokinetics

Half-Life	Onset	Peak	Duration
5 min	Unknown	Varies with dose	Unknown

▶ streptokinase

SK (Streptase) is the oldest thrombolytic drug, the one produced from β-hemolytic streptococci. It binds with plasminogen, and this SK–plasminogen complex then acts on other plasminogen molecules to form plasmin. As mentioned previously, SK is not clot specific. Because it is made from a nonhuman source, it is antigenic and may provoke allergic reactions. This happens because the body's immune

DOSAGES

Selected Thrombolytic Drugs

Drug (Pregnancy Category)	Pharmacologic Class	Usual Dosage Range	Indications
▶ alteplase (Activase) (C)	Tissue plasminogen activator	**Adult** IV: 100 mg over 90 min given as a 15-mg IV bolus, then 50 mg over 30 min, then 35 mg over 60 min	Acute MI
		IV: 100 mg over 2 hr or 30-50 mg over 1.5-2 hr via pulmonary artery	PE
		IV: 0.9 mg/kg (total dose not to exceed 90 mg) given as an IV bolus over 1 min, given within 3 hr of onset of symptoms	Acute ischemic stroke
▶ streptokinase (Streptase, Kabikinase) (C)	Thrombolytic enzyme	**Adult** IV: 1.5 million IU infused over 60 min or intracoronary infusion initiated with a bolus of 20,000 IU followed by 2000 IU/min for 1 hr	Acute MI
		IV: Loading dose of 250,000 IU over 30 min followed by a maintenance infusion of 100,000 IU/hr for 24-72 hr	DVT, arterial thrombosis and embolism, PE
		IV: 250,000 IU into each occluded limb of the cannula over 25-35 min and clamped for 2 hr followed by aspiration of the infusion cannula with saline and reconnection of the cannula	Arteriovenous cannula occlusion

DVT, Deep vein thrombosis; *MI,* myocardial infarction; *PE,* pulmonary embolism.

system recognizes it as a foreign substance (an antigen) and launches an antibody against it, resulting in an antigen–antibody reaction. These antibodies develop approximately 5 days after SK therapy and persist for 6 months to 1 year. It is recommended that patients not be retreated with SK or APSAC during this period. Hypotension secondary to vasodilation occurs in approximately 10% to 15% of patients given SK. SK is contraindicated in patients with a known hypersensitivity to it, in patients who have recently undergone surgery, and those with active internal bleeding, aneurysm, uncontrolled hypotension, intracranial or intraspinal neoplasm, and trauma. It is available only in parenteral form.

Pharmacokinetics

Half-Life	Onset	Peak	Duration
18 min, then 83 min	1 hr	Varies with dose	24-36 hr

◆ NURSING PROCESS

A variety of conditions warrant the use of coagulation modifiers ranging from the clotting of a PIC line, a central venous catheter, clot prevention in coronary artery bypass grafting, major vessel injury, and thrombophlebitis to venous and/or arterial thromboembolism. The drugs that are used to treat these different conditions are varied in their mechanisms of action and have general as well as very specific nursing process–related issues.

◆ ASSESSMENT

The nursing process related to these drugs will be discussed by drug class with specific drugs mentioned, as deemed appropriate. Nursing assessment associated with *all coagulation modifying* drugs should begin with a thorough nursing history, medication history, and brief physical assessment, including the following: medical history, family history, dietary habits, changes in body weight over time, ADLs, exercise habits, employment activities, success with previous medication/treatment regimens, blood pressure, pulse rate, respirations, body weight, and height. Laboratory tests usually ordered include baseline complete blood counts, hemoglobin, hematocrit, lipoprotein fractionation, triglyceride and cholesterol levels as well as various clotting studies. The appropriate serum laboratory tests that should be performed for baseline and maintenance levels are presented in the Laboratory Values Related to Drug Therapy box.

LABORATORY VALUES RELATED TO DRUG THERAPY

Anticoagulants

Laboratory Test	Normal Ranges	Rationale for Assessment
Partial thromboplastin time (PTT)	Normal control values are between 21 and 35 seconds, with therapeutic ranges aimed at 1.5 to 2.5 times the normal control value. Some laboratory testing centers use values between 2 to 2.5 times the normal control value.	This blood test detects defects in the intrinsic thromboplastin system and is used to monitor anticoagulant/ heparin therapy. If patient values are more than 2.5 times the control value, the patient may be receiving too much anticoagulant and the dosage will need adjustment by the physician. If patient values are less than 1.5, then the patient may not be receiving enough anticoagulant and is at risk for clotting.
aPTT (activated partial thromboplastin time)	With heparin therapy, aPTT values should fall between 1.5 to 2.5 times the control or baseline value. Normal control values are 25 to 35 seconds, so therapeutic values should then be approximately between 45 and 70 seconds.	Therapeutic levels of aPTT indicate decreased levels of clotting factors and subsequent clotting activity. aPTT is a more sensitive part of PTT and often replaces it. It is used to see if there are deficiencies in the patient's intrinsic coagulation pathway and monitor heparin therapy. aPTT is sensitive to changes in blood clotting factors, except for factor VII. Therefore, it is used to reflect normal blood coagulation. With continuous IV infusions of heparin, aPTT levels can be drawn at any time, but with intermittent infusions the aPTT should be drawn approximately 1 hour before a dose of heparin is scheduled to be given.
Prothrombin time (PT)	The normal control PT value ranges from 11 to 13 seconds, with therapeutic levels of anticoagulation aimed at 1.5 times the control or about 18 seconds.	Prothrombin is a vitamin-K dependent protein, a major component of the clotting process. It reflects the activity of clotting and is used to monitor effectiveness of warfarin therapy. PT values vary with each laboratory center and are based on the specifics of the testing procedure.
International normalized ratio (INR)	Target levels of INR range from 2 to 3 or average 2.5. For individuals taking warfarin for treatment of recurring systemic clots or emboli or having mechanical heart valves, the goal of INR may be 2.5 to 3.5, with a middle value of 3.	This is a routine test to evaluate coagulation while patients are on warfarin. When the therapy is initiated, the INR and PT should be done daily until a "stable" daily dose is reached or when a dose maintains the PT and INR within therapeutic ranges and does not cause bleeding. INR results actually reflect a dose of warfarin given 36 to 72 hours prior to the actual testing. Advantages of INR testing include the fact that there is more consistency among laboratories and a more consistent warfarin dosage. Some laboratories will report both INR and PT together.

Assessment of the skin/areas identified as potential SC injection sites for heparin and LWMHs is very important to safe administration techniques. For these specific drugs, *avoid* any area within 2 inches of the umbilicus as well as open wounds, scars, open/abraded areas, incisions, drainage tubes, stomas, or areas of bruising/oozing because these sites would then be at higher risk for further tissue trauma with injection of anticoagulant. Of course, the area being referenced is the subcutaneous fatty area across the lower abdomen and between the iliac crests.

There should be a thorough assessment of the following "at risk" factors as related to the patient's clotting disorder: immobility, history of limited activity or prolonged bedrest (e.g., generally for more than 5 days), dehydration, obesity, smoking, congestive heart failure, mitral or aortic stenosis, coronary heart disease with documented athero/arteriosclerosis, peripheral vascular disease, pelvic, gynecologic/genitourinary, abdominal, orthopedic or vascular major surgeries, history of thrombophlebitis, deep vein thrombosis, thromboembolism including pulmonary embolism, myocardial infarct, atrial fibrillation, edema of the periphery, trauma to the lower extremities, use of oral contraceptives, current extended airline travel time. If the patient has a positive history of clotting disorders and/or thromboembolism, be sure to assess and document the following: (1) For thrombophlebitis of the leg: presenting signs and symptoms such as calf edema, pain/warmth/redness directly over the vessel (more indicative of a superficial clot), increased diameter measurement of the calf of the affected leg, pain in the calf with dorsiflexion (often called Homan's sign; however, this is a very controversial method of assessment) or pain upon gentle compression of the calf muscle against the tibial bone. (2) For pulmonary embolism: chest pain, cough, dyspnea, tachypnea, drop in O_2 saturation (by oximetry or blood gasses), hemoptysis, tachycardia, drop in blood pressure, and possible shock.

With use of the *parenteral anticoagulant* heparin, assessment of the patient is very to quality nursing care and should include allergies, contraindications, cautions, and drug interactions. It is also important to assess conditions that pose an at risk situation for a patient, such as severe hypertension, ulcer disease, ulcerative colitis, aneurysms, malignant hypertension, alcoholism, and head injuries. An important caution for heparin's use is with pregnancy or lactation; however, should there be a need for an anticoagulant in pregnancy, heparin is the drug of choice, not warfarin. Other information is presented in Table 27-1. It is crucial to patient safety that nurses remember that heparin is NOT interchangeable unit for unit with another class of anticoagulants, *the low weight molecular heparins (LWMHs).* It is important to know that heparin sodium contains benzyl alcohol, and, therefore, allergy to this additional component needs to be assessed. The nurse should also note if the herbal products ginkgo and ginseng are being used because they may affect blood coagulation. Although their use leads to fewer adverse reactions in some patients, LWMHs are still associated with the contraindications, cautions, and drug interactions previously discussed. The same parameters discussed earlier with heparin would also be appropriate with the LWMHs. In addition, LWMHs contain sulfites and benzyl alcohol, and allergies to these substances should be assessed. It is important to note again that the LWMHs differ from standard heparin and also differ amongst themselves, so they are not interchangeable. Indications for LWMHs may include outpatient anticoagulant therapy, which is a trend for the use of these drugs because they are given subcutaneously, and they require less frequent/close monitoring—as compared to heparin. Clotting studies should also be assessed prior to therapy.

Warfarin and its related contraindications, cautions, and drug interactions have been previously discussed in this chapter. All of the previously mentioned parameters and laboratory studies are applicable to warfarin. Because of the drug's action, warfarin should be withdrawn—as ordered—prior to dental procedures or in the event of any evidence of tissue necrosis, gangrene, diarrhea, intestinal flora imbalances, and steatorrhea; thus, there is a need for close assessment. Important to emphasize with this drug is the fact that warfarin is indicated for prophylaxis/long-term treatment of a variety of thromboembolic disorders (see the Pharmacaology section for specifics) and requires constant and astute assessment of the patient and clotting activities or lack thereof. Most health care providers use standard protocols of warfarin to assist in the dosing of the drug based on INR values. The most common starting dose for warfarin is 5 mg daily. However, the dose can range from 1 to 10 mg, and occasionally even higher (e.g., 12 mg) depending on individual patient response. In most situations, dosage for adults is between 1 and 5 mg orally every day. In addition, warfarin's pharmacokinetics are important to assess and understand because it takes about 3 days for the drug to reach a steady state. Patients on heparin may receive warfarin prior to discontinuation of heparin for anticoagulation.

With *antiplatelet* drugs, a thorough nursing history, medication history, and physical assessment should be performed. Possible drug interactions, cautions, and contraindications have been discussed, but close assessment of any bleeding is most important to patient safety. Because aspirin, NSAIDs, and other antiplatelets alter bleeding times, these drugs should be withheld for 5 to 7 days prior to surgical procedures. Specific guidelines are generally given by the physician to avoid the concurrent use of other anticoagulants, antiplatelets, and fibrinolytics. With aspirin and its related ototoxicity, it is important to not give drugs that have the same adverse effect (e.g., ototoxicity) such as with aminoglycosides (e.g., vancomycin). Baseline cardiovascular assessment is needed with documentation of general history, history of chest pain, complete blood count, hemoglobin/hematocrit, platelet counts, PT, and INR values. This would provide values against which therapy values can be compared. Along with the above parameters, if platelet counts are at or fall below 80,000 cells/mm³, the physician should be notified, and antiplatelet therapy will most likely not be initiated (or will be discontinued). In addition, it is important to patient safety to reemphasize the fact that aspirin is not to be used in children and teenagers, any patient with any bleeding disorder, children with flu-like symptoms, pregnant or lactating women, or patients with a vitamin K deficiency or peptic ulcer disease. These are situations in which there would be major consequences if used; for example, there is a high risk for Reye's syndrome with aspirin use in children and teenagers, teratogenic effects, or ulcers, or bleeding tendencies. In addition, it is always important to know how each of the drugs works in the body so that there is a sound knowledge base for critical thinking-based decision—for example, call the physician and not administer two antiplatelets at the same time or give a thrombolytic with heparin, warfarin, aspirin, or NSAIDs. This type of critical drug information is very important to making sure that the patient receives the safest and most appropriate care during all phases of the nursing process.

The *glycoprotein IIb/IIIa inhibitors*—for example, eptifibatide (Integrilin), tirofiban (Aggrastat), and abciximab (ReoPro)—are associated with the same baseline assessment information (e.g., vital signs, medical history, history of chest pain/cardiac disease, complete blood cell counts, hemoglobin, hematocrit, renal function tests, platelet counts). Prior to and during therapy, should platelet counts fall below 90,000/mm^3 or be at that level to begin with, the physician should be contacted for further orders. *Antifibrinolytics* require the same astute assessment of baseline parameters and laboratory testing; however, there are additional concerns for patients with altered cardiac, renal, or hepatic functioning. These are situations in which the physician may need to decrease the dosage of medication. Serum potassium levels should be noted prior to therapy because of drug-induced hyperkalemia.

Thrombolytics also require similar assessment parameters, baseline complete blood cell counts, and clotting studies. There is always major concern and various contraindications for the use of alteplase (Activase, t-PA) and other thrombolytics (e.g., active internal bleeding, history of stroke, cerebral neoplasms, arteriovenous malformation, aneurysms, known bleeding disorders, severe uncontrolled hypertension, intracranial or intraspinal surgery or trauma within, for example, the past 2 months. Assessment of any arterial puncture, venous cut-down sites, PICC line sites, and central infusion ports/sites should be constantly assessed for bleeding. Intramuscular injections may pose problems with bleeding, and, therefore, other dosage forms may be indicated. As with any drugs that alter clotting and platelet activity, the thrombolytics are associated with risk for bleeding from wounds or the gastrointestinal, genitourinary, or respiratory tracts, so any drainage, urine, stool, emesis, sputum, and secretions should be assessed for presence of blood.

◆ NURSING DIAGNOSES

- Ineffective tissue perfusion related to the clotting disorder or thrombus formation
- Impaired physical mobility related to tissue injury or decreased tissue perfusion from coagulation disorders
- Risk for injury related to possible adverse reactions to any of the drugs that alter blood clotting
- Deficient knowledge related to medication treatment regimen due to lack of information
- Acute pain related to symptoms of underlying clotting disorder or ischemia
- Deficient knowledge related to new medication regimen and need for altered lifestyle
- Activity intolerance related to underlying clotting disorder or ischemia

◆ PLANNING
Goals

- Patient experiences increased comfort and relief of pain.
- Patient exhibits improved blood flow as the result of the therapeutic effects of the anticoagulants.
- Patient remains free from injury stemming from either the disease or the medication being taken.
- Patient is compliant with the lifestyle changes required and with the medication therapy.

- Patient demonstrates adequate knowledge regarding medication therapy and its potential adverse effects.

Outcome Criteria

- Patient experiences relief of symptoms such as decreased pain, swelling, and edema once tissue perfusion is regained as the result of medication therapy.
- Patient shows improved circulation with warm extremities or strong pedal pulses or experiences a return to his or her pre-disease state of tissue perfusion.
- Patient is free of bruising, bleeding problems, or any other adverse reaction to the medication.
- Patient states the rationale for the use of the medication regimen, such as decreased clotting or clot formation.
- Patient states the nature of and rationale for the lifestyle changes needed, such as improved diet, exercise, and no smoking.
- Patient states the adverse effects, how to monitor for complications of the anticoagulants, the importance of coming in for follow-up appointments with the physician and of frequent laboratory studies, and when to contact the physician to prevent complications such as hemorrhage.

◆ IMPLEMENTATION

Vital signs, heart sounds, peripheral pulses, and neurologic checks are routinely monitored in all patients during and immediately after anticoagulant therapy. The various laboratory values to be monitored are presented in the Laboratory Values Related to Drug Therapy box on page 432. If there is any change in pulse rate or rhythm, BP, or level of consciousness and/or occurrence of unexplained restlessness, contact the physician immediately, as it may indicate bleeding or hemorrhage.

Knowledge of the proper techniques of administration is crucial for safe and effective use of any clotting-altering drug (Box 27-1). The anticoagulant is given by subcutaneous or intravenous routes but *not* intramuscularly. Inadvertent intramuscular injection can be easily avoided if the nurse uses only subcutaneous syringes that are usually made available in prefilled syringes that include a ½-inch (1.5-cm), 25- to 28-gauge needle. No major harm would result from a subcutaneous dose being inadvertently administered given intravenously. If rapid anticoagulation is needed, the physician generally orders IV heparin, either by continuous or intermittent infusion. During continuous intravenous infusion or subcutaneous injection, monitoring of daily clotting studies may be ordered. The effects are reversed with the intravenous administration of protamine sulfate. With subcutaneous heparin, several doses of protamine sulfate may be needed to reverse the anticoagulant effect because of the variable rates of absorption of this dosage form. See Box 27-1 for the procedure for the intermittent or continuous intravenous administration of heparin.

LMWHs are given by subcutaneous injection in the abdominal area using the same techniques used with heparin, with a few differences. Prefilled syringes of LMWHs are available for inpatient use and for at-home treatment. Solutions may be clear to pale yellow in color. Usual length of therapy is approximately 5 to 10 days, and it is important to constantly be aware of any bleeding problems while the patient is taking this and other clot-altering drugs. CBCs, platelet counts, and stool for occult blood are all tests that will most likely be done during therapy for "monitoring" purposes. Tests for occult blood in the stool can be

Box 27-1   Anticoagulation Therapy and Related Nursing Considerations

Subcutaneous Heparin Injections

- After thoroughly checking the physician's order, assess the patient for the existence of any allergies, contraindications, cautions, or drug interactions.
- Wash hands thoroughly. Prefilled syringes are available for convenience as well as accurate technique/dosing and should be used whenever possible. As a point of reference, the prefilled syringe comes with a tuberculin syringe to draw up the exact dose of heparin. For a 25- to 28-gauge needle, the length of the needle is ½ to ⅝ of an inch. In situations when the medication is not available in a prefilled or premeasured syringe, a tuberculin syringe is used because it is the correct gauge and needle length. See Chapter 9 for more information on technique and on the process of medication administration.
- See Chapter 9 for specific information about the technique for giving heparin or LWMH injections and for a review on safe medication administration.
- Check injection site for bleeding or bruising and document any pertinent information. Technique is important with subcutaneous injections of heparin (Chapter 9), and the nurse should *not* massage or rub the site before or after the injection. *Do not aspirate* before injecting to avoid/prevent the occurrence of hematoma formation.
- Make sure the patient is comfortable, then remove your gloves and wash your hands. Document your intervention and any other pertinent data.

Intravenous Heparin Administration

- Always double-check the specific physician's order for dosage, rate of infusion, and time and route before beginning therapy and always practice the Five Rights of Medication Administration to prevent overdosing or erroneous dosing. Make sure the proper diluent is used and the compatibility of solutions or other drugs is checked before beginning the infusion.
- For the continuous IV administration of heparin, an IV pump must be used to ensure a precise rate of infusion.
- Continuous dosing is preferred over intermittent dosing because continuous dosing helps with blood levels of the drug and because intermittent IV dosing is associated with a higher risks for bleeding abnormalities.
- The use of continuous IV infusions generally begins with a loading dose and is followed by a maintenance dose. Be aware that

dosage adjustments are made exactly as ordered. The patient's aPTT level and/or other related clotting studies are used as parameters for dosing of heparin or LWMHs.
- For intermittent infusions, a heparin lock was used in the past. Heparin locks are now referred to as *intermittent infusion locks* or *saline locks* (because the locks are flushed with isotonic saline and not heparin).
- Intermittent infusions of heparin are usually ordered to be given every 4 to 6 hours because of heparin's short half-life. Intermittent infusions and all other types of IV infusions include use of needle-less systems!
- Regardless of the type of IV infusion (e.g., intermittent or continuous IV infusion), it is crucial to check the site to determine whether infiltration has occurred so that hematoma formation may be prevented. If infiltration is suspected, the lock should be removed and replaced in a new site before the next scheduled infusion. Document your actions in the nurse's notes.
- Therapeutic dosage of heparin is guided by aPTT with a targeted level of 1.5 to 2.5 times the control/normal. aPTTs are drawn within 24 hours of beginning therapy, 24 to 48 hours after therapy starts and 1 to 2 times weekly for about 3 to 4 weeks on an average. With long-term therapy, aPTTs are monitored 1 to 2 times per month.

Oral Anticoagulant Administration

- It is important to recheck the physician's orders and the patient's medication and medical history before administering the drug. Always check to make sure the patient has no known hypersensitivity to the drug.
- Scored tablets may be crushed and may be given with or without regard to food.
- There are many more drugs that can interact with oral anticoagulants than with heparin, especially those that are highly protein bound (such as the ones listed in Table 27-3). Always check the patient's medication list before initiating therapy with warfarin.
- Dosages of warfarin are calculated based upon INR blood values. INRs are also used to monitor the effectiveness of therapy. Remember, however, dosing is highly individualized!
- Oral anticoagulants should be administered at the same time every day to maintain steady blood levels.
- Document the dose, time of administration, and any other pertinent facts.

aPTT, Activated partial thromboplastin times; *INR,* international normalized ratio; *NS,* normal saline.

---

done simply if the occult stool test paper with its developer is available. It simply helps to identify hidden blood in the stool, which may occur as an adverse effect with LWMHs, as well as any clotting-altering drugs.

When the *oral anticoagulant,* warfarin, is prescribed, therapy is often initiated while the patient is still on heparin. This overlapping is done purposefully so that when the heparin is eventually discontinued, the blood levels of warfarin have been allowed for, and therapeutic anticoagulation levels are achieved. The full therapeutic effect of warfarin does not occur until 4 to 5 days after the first dose. The patient who has been on heparin for anticoagulation and is switched to warfarin must have this overlap of activity so that prevention of clotting is continuous. Monitoring the various clotting studies is still of utmost priority, as is watching for any clotting or bleeding problems. The administration procedures for warfarin are outlined in Box 27-1. For conversion from heparin to an oral anticoagulant such as warfarin, the dose

of the oral drug should be the usual initial amount with PT-INR levels used to help the physician determine the next appropriate dosage of warfarin. Once there is continuous therapeutic anticoagulation coverage, and warfarin is on board, the heparin or LWMH may then be discontinued without tapering. Should uncontrolled bleeding occur with any of these medications, the nurse must take action to control bleeding as well as institute emergency measures to stabilize the patient's condition, and the physician should be contacted immediately.

Of benefit with the use of anticoagulants is the use of antidotes. The antidote to hemorrhage or uncontrolled bleeding resulting from heparin or LMWH therapy is protamine sulfate. This antidote is given intravenously and may be given in an undiluted form over a 10-minute time frame and *not to exceed* 5 mg/minute or 50 mg in any 10 minute period. The benchmark dose is based on the fact that 1 mg of protamine sulfate neutralizes 90 to 115 units of heparin. It is important to note that too-rapid infusion may lead to acute hypotensive episodes, bradycardia, dyspnea, and transient feelings of warmth and flushing. aPTT ranges and hematocrit levels are generally used at this point to monitor bleeding, clotting, and risk for bleeding. Be sure to always watch the patient, especially for any changes in blood pressure and pulse rate. The antidote to oral anticoagulant (warfarin sodium) therapy is vitamin K, which is preferably given via the SC route, although oral, IV, and IM dosage forms are available. This drug may lead to rare occurrences of severe reactions such as dyspnea, dizziness, rapid/weak pulse, chest pain, and hypotension that may progress to shock and cardiac arrest. Continual monitoring of the patient's vital signs, cardiac parameters, and bleeding times/clotting studies continue to be very important.

The patient being treated with *antiplatelets* (or any clot-altering drug) should be constantly monitored for signs and symptoms of bleeding during and after their use: epistaxis, hematuria, hematemesis, easy/excessive bruising, blood in the stools, and bleeding gums. If there are invasive procedures or use of injections, appropriate pressure should be applied to bleeding sites, and all areas of venous/arterial catheter insertion should be closely watched for bleeding. Extended release dosage forms should be taken in their entire dosage form and without chewing or crushing. Enteric coated aspirin is recommended to be taken with 6 to 8 oz of water and with food to help decrease gastrointestinal upset. To avoid irritation to the esophagus, make sure the patient knows to remain upright and not lie down for up to 30 minutes after the dose of aspirin. If the aspirin has a strong, vinegar-like odor, discard the drug. With clopidogrel therapy, interventions are similar to that of aspirin. The patient should report any of the following: aches in the joints, back pain, dizziness, severe headache, dyspepsia, flu-like signs and symptoms, and epigastric pain. These drugs are often discontinued, as ordered, for 7 days prior to surgery. However, some surgical procedures (e.g., cardiovascular surgery) may warrant the patient to remain in an anticoagulated state intra-operatively. Oral forms of dipyridamole are recommended to be taken on an empty stomach; however, if not tolerated, it may be taken with food. If nausea occurs, cola, unsalted crackers, or dry toast may help to alleviate this adverse effect. In addition, it may take up to 2 to 3 months of continuous therapy for the drug to reach therapeutic levels. Encourage patients to change positions slowly and to take their time going from lying to sitting to standing due to the adverse effect of dizziness and postural hypotension with antiplatelets and all other drugs in this chapter.

Nursing considerations associated with the *glycoprotein (GP) IIb/IIIa inhibitors*, such as abciximab, eptifibatide, and tirofiban, include some similar, and yet, different, nursing actions. Close monitoring of all vital signs, electrocardiogram (ECG) readings, peripheral pulses, heart sounds, skin color, and temperature are all important parts of nursing care during and after the use of these drugs. Because these drugs are used in combination with heparin to treat individuals suspected of having acute coronary syndrome or with percutaneous transluminal coronary angioplasty (PTCA), there is always concern for the stability of the patient as well as a high risk for serious bleeding and/or extension of an acute myocardial infarct. The patient in this situation is at risk for other medical complications, and this may be intensified by the drug. Avoidance of further invasive procedures,

while the patient is on this type drug, is important to help prevent risks for bleeding. If invasive procedures are demanded it will be crucial to constantly monitor for bleeding and observe all vital parameters before, during, and after the procedure. Intravenous tirofiban should be protected from light, and any unused solutions should be discarded 24 hours after an infusion has been started. No other drugs should be used with this drug/infusion except for heparin, which may be given through the same IV line. Abciximab, in particular, can be given by bolus or by continuous infusions with infusion rates monitored closely (PTCA). In particular, manufacturer guidelines identify the need for sterile, nonpyrogenic, low protein–binding 0.2- or 0.22-micron filter, and while the vascular shield is in position, the patient should remain on complete bed rest with head of bed elevated at 30 degrees. The affected extremity should be maintained in a straight position with constant monitoring of peripheral pulses, color, and temperature of distal extremities. Once the sheath is removed, application of pressure to the femoral artery is required for at least 30 minutes, either by manual or mechanical pressure. A pressure dressing should be applied once bleeding has stopped. The site should be closely monitored for any oozing or bleeding.

If there is serious bleeding, the glycoprotein IIb/IIIa receptor inhibitor and heparin (the usual protocol for PTCA) should be discontinued immediately, the patient should be monitored closely, and the physician should be notified immediately for emergency treatment. Always move and handle these patients with caution, and avoid unnecessary trauma/injury due to risk for hematoma formation or bleeding. DO NOT take blood pressures in the lower extremities but keep a close and constant watch on the patient's blood pressure (for hypotension), pulse rate (for tachycardia), as well as for any complaints of abdominal/back pain, severe headache, and any other signs and symptoms of hemorrhage. When removing adhesive or sticky tape, always be careful to not tear or rip the skin, which would lead to tissue trauma and further risk for bleeding. aPTT levels should be monitored post-procedure, and there should be very close monitoring for bleeding with attention to IM injection sites, arterial or venous puncture sites, and bleeding from nasogastric tubes and/or urinary catheters. These procedures should be avoided, if at all possible, during or immediately after the angioplasty.

With *antifibrinolytics*, it is important to have an understanding of the rationale for the use of these drugs, such as to stop bleeding from overdosages of thrombolytic drugs or to control bleeding during cardiac surgery. Aminocaproic and tranexamic acid are usually given IV until bleeding is controlled. These drugs require very close patient monitoring, and if there is any change in motor strength or level of consciousness, the physician should be notified. Nurses have to apply the knowledge of certain adverse effects of drugs (like these) so that nursing care may be focused on prevention of complications, maintenance of safety, and a return to a healthier state. Because of drug-induced skeletal myopathies, creatine kinase and other liver function studies should be monitored. It is also important to monitor heart rate and blood pressure with attention to quality/strength of peripheral pulses. For the patient with hemophilia, tranexamic acid may be used to help decrease bleeding from dental extractions. Close monitoring of these patients for any oral bleeding would be important with post-dental care at home.

Nursing considerations related to *thrombolytics* are very similar to those for drugs previously discussed in this chapter. Specifically, their IV administration should be prepared per manufacturer guidelines and per protocol. Invasive procedures should be avoided during the use of these drugs as well as simultaneous use of anticoagulants or antiplatelets. IV infusion sites should be monitored frequently for bleeding, redness, and pain. Intramuscular injections of other drugs are contraindicated to prevent tissue damage/bleeding. Any bleeding from gums or mucous membranes or the occurrence of epistaxis and increased pulse (greater than 100 beats/min) should be reported to the physician immediately, and all vital signs should be monitored frequently. Other nursing considerations include monitoring for hypotension, restlessness, and a decrease in Hgb and Hct, which should be reported to the physician immediately. Patients should be instructed to report pink, red, or cloudy urine; black, tarry stools or frank red blood in the stools; abdominal or chest pain; dizziness; or severe headache. Reconstitution for intravenous dosing should be done with NaCl or D_5W. Solutions should be rolled gently and not shaken to maintain a stable solution. Continual monitoring of INR, aPTT, platelets, and fibrinogen levels should occur and within 2 to 3 hours after the use of thrombolytics. The patient's fibrinogen level may be measured to check for actual fibrinolysis. With the breakdown of fibrin (or fibrinolysis), INR or aPTT levels will increase, or be prolonged. Should bleeding occur, the physician will most likely discontinue the drug and replace fibrinogen with infusions of whole blood plasma or with cryoprecipitate. The above-mentioned antifibrinolytics (e.g., aminocaproic acid/tranexamic acid), may also be given.

Patient teaching tips for several of the clot-altering drugs are listed in the box on page 438.

◆ EVALUATION

Monitoring for the therapeutic and adverse effects of clotting-altering drugs is crucial for their safe use. Because these drugs are used for a variety of purposes, therapeutic responses vary. Some of the therapeutic effects include decreased chest pain and a decrease in dizziness, as well as other neurologic symptoms. Adverse effects may include drops in blood pressure, headache, hematoma formation, irritation and pain at the injection site, hemorrhage, thrombocytopenia, shortness of breath, chills, and fever. Early signs of drug overdose for any of the clotting-altering drugs include bleeding of the gums while brushing teeth, unexplained nosebleeds or bruising, and heavier-than-usual menstrual bleeding. Abdominal pain, back pain, bloody or tarry stools, bloody urine, constipation, blood in the sputum, severe or continuous headaches, and the vomiting of frank red blood or a coffee ground substance (old blood) are all possible indications of internal bleeding. The adverse effects of aspirin use include gastrointestinal upset or bleeding, heartburn, headache, hepatitis, thrombocytopenia, agranulocytosis, leukopenia, neutropenia, hemolytic anemia, prolonged PT, tinnitus, hearing loss, rapid pulse, wheezing, hypoglycemia, hyponatremia, and hypokalemia. Adverse effects of antiplatelets include postural hypotension, headache, weakness, syncope, gastrointestinal upset, rash, flushing of the face, and dizziness. It is necessary to continually monitor liver, renal, and clotting function in patients on long-term aspirin and other anti-clotting therapy. Therapeutic effects of clopidogrel—and like drugs—include a decrease in the occurrence of clotting events such as transient ischemic attacks (TIAs) and strokes. Adverse effects for which to monitor with these drugs include increased bleeding tendencies, flulike symptoms, headache, fatigue, chest pain, and epistaxis. Therapeutic levels of anticoagulants and other clotting-altering drugs are also monitored by laboratory tests such as aPTT, PT, and INR, are presented in the Laboratory Values Related to Drug Therapy box on page 432. Remember, however, that aPTT levels are used with heparin, PT, and INR with warfarin. Once the level of the particular drug stabilizes, and maintenance therapy is ongoing, the clotting studies may be drawn at 1- to 4-week intervals, depending on the specific drug, patients' responses, and their overall physical condition. Should a heparin or LWMH overdose occur, the antidote is protamine sulfate whereas vitamin K, or phytonadione, is the antidote to oral anticoagulant overdose (see Nursing Considerations).

The continuous monitoring of the patient for the signs and symptoms of internal or external bleeding is crucial during both the initiation and maintenance of therapy. Therapeutic effects of antifibrinolytics include the arrest of oozing of blood from a surgical site or a decrease in blood loss. Therapeutic levels of anticoagulants and other clotting-altering drugs are also monitored by laboratory tests. The standard tests for determining the effects of heparin therapy include aPTT with a therapeutic value of 1.5 to 2.5 times the control value. INR and PT values are used to monitor warfarin therapy and are discussed in the Laboratory Values Related to Drug Therapy box on page 432. In case of the need for reversal of the anticoagulation effects, there are antidotes available—for example, heparin with an antidote of protamine sulfate and warfarin with the antidote of vitamin K (see Implementation).

Because of the complexity and life-threatening nature of the conditions for which these drugs are used, the nurse must continually monitor and re-evaluate the patient's response to the treatment, document responses accordingly, and always keep goals and outcome criteria within the plan of care to serve as a benchmark. From the evaluation phase, the patient will hopefully emerge with full therapeutic effects and minimal adverse and/or toxic effects as related to drug therapy.

Patient Teaching Tips

- Educate patients that these drugs are given for specific purposes (e.g., prevention of serious complications related to clotting, such as with strokes, heart attacks, heart valve replacements, mini strokes [TIAs or transient ischemic attacks], deep vein thrombosis in the legs). It is important to understand that a healthy lifestyle is an important part of therapy and will most likely include eating the right foods, weight reduction if needed, smoking cessation, controlling blood pressure, and stress reduction.

- Inform patients that medications must be taken exactly as prescribed because too little may lead to a clot and too much may lead to bleeding. Regular follow-up appointments are an important part of patient care, with frequent blood tests to monitor therapeutic effects versus adverse effects of the medication. The results of the blood tests will assist health care providers to determine proper dosage.

- Encourage patients to inform all their health care providers, including dentists, about their medications.

- Encourage patients to carry an identification card on their person and/or wear a medical alert necklace or bracelet that states the medical diagnosis and drugs being taken. Including the physician's name and phone number and any allergies is also recommended.

- Home heparin therapy may require that patients receive injections for a period of time. It is the LWMHs that are usually used in these situations. Patients need to understand that if they are switched to warfarin (Coumadin) from heparin, there may be an overlap of taking the warfarin and heparin for approximately 3 to 5 days to allow therapeutic levels of the oral warfarin to occur before discontinuing heparin. This process may occur in the hospital or at home. Enoxaparin (LWMH) is usually given for up to 3 months. Complete and thorough instructions and return demonstrations are an important part of patient education (Chapter 9).

- Emphasize the importance for patients to report any unusual bleeding from anywhere on their body, onset of a severe headache, blurred vision, vomiting up blood, dizziness, fainting, fever, muscular or limb weakness, rash, nose bleeds, or any excessive vaginal or menstrual bleeding.

- Educate patients about applying direct pressure for 3 to 5 minutes or longer as needed for any superficial bleeding.

- Educate patients to keep a journal on how they are feeling daily as well as how they are tolerating their medication. They should also include any adverse effects or problems.

- To help prevent clot formation in the arteries, the physician may prescribe other interventions to help reduce risk factors for cardiovascular disease, such as a low-fat, low-cholesterol diet; medication to lower cholesterol if deemed necessary; weight reduction if ordered; controlling blood pressure if hypertensive; avoiding smoking; managinge stress; and regular exercise.

- Educate the patient on how to help prevent clot formation in their leg veins. If prone to blood clots in the legs or deep vein thrombosis, there are measures to help minimize situations that may make the blood slow or sluggish, such as to avoid wearing tight fitting clothing, minimize periods of sitting for prolonged periods of time, not cross legs at the knees, avoid tight-fitting socks, avoid periods of prolonged bedrest, make sure to stop and walk around every 1 to 2 hours when on long trips, stay well hydrated, and do leg/foot exercises.

- With any of the anticoagulants (oral and/or heparin/LWMHs) or clot-altering drugs, encourage patients to avoid brushing their teeth with a hard-bristled toothbrush, shaving with a straight razor, and/or avoid engaging in any activity that would increase the risk for tissue injury. They should understand why they need to be very careful when shaving, trimming their nails, gardening, and/or participating in rough or contact sports, and they should take every precaution to protect self from injury.

- Patients should be educated that while on anticoagulants they should avoid eating large amounts of foods high in vitamin K, such as broccoli, brussels sprouts, collard greens, kale, lettuce, mustard greens, and tomatoes. These foods will interact with the drug and decrease its effectiveness.

- Capsicum pepper, feverfew, garlic, ginger, ginkgo, and ginseng are some herbals that have potential interactions, especially to warfarin, and patients should receive a list of commonly encountered drug interactions. Make sure patients know to report any of the following to their physician immediately: decrease in urine output; constant ringing in the ears; swelling of the feet, ankles, or legs; dark urine; clay-colored stools; abdominal pain; rash (discontinue use if rash occurs); and blurred vision or the perception of halos around objects.

- Educate patients to never make up for any missed doses and to not double-up on doses. If in doubt of what to do, they should contact their physician for further instructions.

- If patients are taking aspirin or aspirin products, they should be taken with at least 8 oz of water and/or with food to help minimize stomach upset. Taking oral warfarin with food may help decrease GI upset.

- Educate patients that use of any of these medications requires that containers should be kept out of the reach of children and medications be kept in a container with a childproof top/lid. All equipment/syringes/needles should be kept out of reach of children or other individuals.

Points to Remember

- Coagulation modifiers work by the following: (1) preventing clot formation, (2) promoting clot formation, (3) lysing a preformed clot, or (4) reversing the action of anticoagulants.
- Anticoagulants, antiplatelet drugs, antifibrinolytics, thrombolytics, and reversal drugs are all examples of coagulation modifiers.
- The coagulation system is as follows: Clot formation takes place concurrently as clot destruction; clot destruction is governed by the fibrinolytic system; clot formation is accomplished by the coagulation pathway, of which there is an extrinsic and an intrinsic pathway.
- Warfarin prevents clot formation by inhibiting vitamin K–dependent clotting factors (II, VII, IX, and X) and is used prophylactically to prevent clots from forming; It cannot lyse preformed clots.
- The degree of anticoagulation (for any of the medications) is monitored by the PT.
- Heparin prevents clot formation by binding to antithrombin III and by doing so turns off certain activating factors. The overall effect is to turn off the coagulation pathway and prevent clots from forming. Heparin does not lyse (break down) a clot. Nurses should remember that heparin is given IV or subcutaneously.
- Antiplatelet drugs prevent clot formation by preventing platelet involvement in clot formation. All of these drugs affect normal platelet function and should be given to patients only after thorough assessment of the patient with a medical history and medication profile.
- Antifibrinolytics prevent lysis of fibrin, thus promoting clot formation, and have the opposite effects of anticoagulants.
- Thrombolytics are able to break down or lyse preformed clots in blood vessels that supply the heart with blood. Examples of drugs include SK and APSAC. SK is derived from group A β-hemolytic streptococci and converts plasminogen to plasmin, which breaks down thrombi. Therapeutic effects that the nurse should monitor for include improved tissue perfusion, decreased chest pain, and prevention of further myocardial damage. Adverse effects include nausea, vomiting, hypotension, and bleeding.
- The therapeutic effects of most coagulation modifier drugs include improved circulation, tissue perfusion, decreased pain, and prevention of further tissue damage. Before using any of these drugs, it is important for the nurse to perform a thorough physical assessment and record findings, as well as monitor any pertinent laboratory values such as INR, aPTT, and PT.
- Nursing care is very individualized depending on the patient, thorough assessment data, existing medical conditions, and the specific drug. It is the nurse's responsibility to know everything about the patient and the drug for safe administration and for quality nursing care.

NCLEX Examination Review Questions

1. The nurse is monitoring a patient who is receiving antithrombolytic therapy in the emergency room because of a possible myocardial infarction. Which of the following adverse effects would be the highest concern at this time?
   a. Dizziness
   b. BP 130/98 mm Hg
   c. Slight bloody oozing from the IV-insertion site
   d. Irregular heart rhythm
2. A patient is receiving instructions for warfarin therapy, and asks the nurse about what medications she can take for headaches. The nurse should tell her to avoid which type of medication?
   a. Opioids
   b. Acetaminophen (Tylenol)
   c. NSAIDs
   d. There are no restrictions while on warfarin.
3. The nurse is teaching a patient about self-administration of the LMWH enoxaparin (Lovenox). Which statement should be included in this teaching session?
   a. "We will need to teach a family member how to give this drug in your arm."
   b. "This drug is given in the folds of your abdomen, but at least 2 inches away from your navel."
   c. "This drug needs to be taken at the same time every day with a full glass of water."
   d. "Be sure to massage the injection site thoroughly after giving the drug."
4. A patient is receiving warfarin (Coumadin) therapy as part of the treatment for a pulmonary embolism. The nurse monitors the results of which laboratory test to check the drug's effectiveness?
   a. PT-INR levels
   b. aPTT levels
   c. Vitamin K levels
   d. Platelet counts
5. A patient has received a double dose of heparin during surgery, and is bleeding through his incision site. While the surgeons are working to stop the bleeding at the incision site, the nurse will prepare to do which action at this time?
   a. Prepare to give intravenous vitamin K as an antidote.
   b. Prepare to give intravenous protamine sulfate as an antidote.
   c. Call the blood bank for an immediate platelet transfusion.
   d. Obtain an order for packed RBCs.

1. d, 2. c, 3. b, 4. a, 5. b.

Critical Thinking Activities

1. Mrs. F.W., age 63, has had hip replacement surgery, and will be receiving enoxaparin (Lovenox) 30 mg SC every 12 hours. Explain the rationale behind this medication order.
2. If a patient decides to take garlic tablets to reduce his cholesterol level, is there a concern if he is taking warfarin? Explain.
3. Explain the rationale for a patient to receive warfarin and heparin together.

For answers, see http://evolve.elsevier.com/Lilley.

CHAPTER 28

Antilipemic Drugs

Objectives

When you reach the end of this chapter, you should be able to do the following:

1. Explain the pathology of primary and secondary hyperlipidemia, including causes and risk factors.
2. Discuss the different types of lipoproteins and their role in cardiovascular diseases and in hyperlipidemia.
3. List the various drug classes with specific drugs that are used to treat hyperlipidemia.
4. Compare the various drugs used to treat hyperlipidemia, including the rationale for treatment, indications, mechanisms of action, dosages, routes of administration, adverse effects, toxicity, cautions, contraindications, and associated drug interactions.
5. Develop a nursing care plan that includes all phases of the nursing process for the patient receiving an antilipemic drug.

e-Learning Activities

Companion CD

- NCLEX Review Questions: see questions 243-257
- Animations
- Audio Glossary
- Category Catchers
- Medication Errors Checklists
- IV Therapy Checklists

evolve Website (http://evolve.elsevier.com/Lilley)

• Nursing Care Plans • Frequently Asked Questions • Content Updates • WebLinks • Supplemental Resources • Elsevier ePharmacology Update • Medication Administration Animations

Drug Profiles

▶ atorvastatin, p. 447
▶ cholestyramine, p. 448
ezetimibe, p. 450

gemfibrozil, p. 450
▶ niacin, pp. 448, 449

▶ Key drug.

Glossary

Antilipemic A drug that reduces lipid levels. (p. 440)

Apolipoprotein The protein component of a lipoprotein. (p. 441)

Cholesterol A fat-soluble crystalline steroid alcohol found in animal fats and oils and egg yolk and widely distributed in the body, especially in the bile, blood, brain tissue, liver, kidneys, adrenal glands, and myelin sheaths of nerve fibers. (p. 440)

Chylomicrons Minute droplets of lipoproteins; the forms in which dietary fats are absorbed from the small intestine. Chylomicrons consist of about 90% triglycerides and small amounts of cholesterol, phospholipids, and proteins. (p. 441)

Exogenous lipids Lipids originating outside the body or an organ (e.g., dietary fats) or produced as the result of external causes, such as a disease caused by a bacterial or viral agent foreign to the body. (p. 441)

Foam cells The characteristic initial lesion of atherosclerosis, also known as the *fatty streak.* (p. 442)

HMG–CoA reductase inhibitors A class of cholesterol-lowering drugs that work by inhibiting the rate-limiting step in cholesterol synthesis; also commonly referred to as *statins* (see *statins*). (p. 445)

Hypercholesterolemia A condition in which greater-than-normal amounts of cholesterol are present in the blood. High levels of cholesterol and other lipids may lead to the development of atherosclerosis and serious illnesses such as coronary heart disease. (p. 441)

Lipoprotein Conjugated protein in which lipids form an integral part of the molecule. Lipoproteins are synthesized primarily in the liver; contain varying amounts of triglycerides, cholesterol, phospholipids, and protein; and are classified according to their composition and density. (p. 441)

Statins A class of cholesterol-lowering drugs that are more formally known as *HMG–CoA reductase inhibitors.* (p. 444)

Triglycerides A compound consisting of a fatty acid (oleic, palmitic, or stearic) and a type of alcohol known as *glycerol.* Triglycerides make up most animal and vegetable fats and are the principal lipids in the blood, where they circulate bound to a protein, forming high- and low-density lipoproteins (HDLs and LDLs). (p. 440)

An understanding of **antilipemic** drugs begins with an understanding of how **cholesterol** and **triglycerides** are transported and used in the human body and how lipoproteins, apolipoproteins, receptors, and enzyme systems are involved in these processes. Also essential is an understanding of the basic mechanisms underlying lipid abnormalities and the link between hyperlipidemia and coronary heart disease (CHD). Armed with this knowledge, the clinician can develop and implement a rational approach to treatment using both nonpharmacologic and pharmacologic interventions. Some patients also use dietary supplements for control of hyperlipidemia (see the Herbal Therapies and Dietary Supplements boxes on p. 441).

Garlic (allium sativum)

Overview
Garlic obtains its pharmacologic effects from the active ingredient allinin.

Common Uses
Antispasmodic, antiseptic, antibacterial and antiviral, antihypertensive, antiplatelet, lipid-lowering activity

Adverse Effects
Dermatitis, vomiting, diarrhea, anorexia, flatulence, antiplatelet activity

Potential Drug Interactions
May inhibit iodine uptake, warfarin, diazepam, protease inhibitors

Contraindications
Contraindicated in patients about to undergo surgery within 2 weeks and in patients with HIV or diabetes.
   Follow manufacturer directions on bottle or box for use of specific preparations.

Flax

Overview
Flax is a flowering annual found in the Europe, Canada, and the United States. Both the seed and the oil of the plant are used medicinally.

Common Uses
Atherosclerosis, hypercholesterolemia, hypertriglyceridemia; as well as gastrointestinal distress (esp., constipation), menopausal symptoms, and bladder inflammation, among various other uses.

Adverse Effects
Diarrhea, allergic reactions.

Potential Drug Interactions
Antidiabetic drugs: Theoretically can potentiate hypoglycemic effects.
Anticoagulant drugs: Theoretically can potentiate anticoagulant effects by reducing platelet aggregation and prolonging bleeding time.

Contraindications
Pregnancy (need more info), bowel obstruction; use with caution in diabetes and cardiovascular disease.
   Follow manufacturer directions on bottle or box for use of specific preparations.

LIPIDS AND LIPID ABNORMALITIES

PRIMARY FORMS OF LIPIDS

Triglycerides and cholesterol are the two primary forms of lipids in the blood. Triglycerides function as an energy source and are stored in adipose (fat) tissue. Cholesterol is primarily used to make steroid hormones, cell membranes, and bile acids. Triglycerides and cholesterol are both water-insoluble fats that must be bound to specialized lipid-carrying proteins called **apolipoproteins.** This combination of triglycerides and cholesterol with an apolipoprotein is referred to as a **lipoprotein.** Lipoproteins transport lipids via the

Table 28-1   Lipoprotein Classification

Lipid Content	Lipoprotein Classification	Protein Content
Most	Chylomicron	Least
	VLDL	
↓	LDL	↑
	IDL	
Least	HDL	Most

HDL, High-density lipoprotein; *IDL,* intermediate-density lipoprotein; *LDL,* low-density lipoprotein; *VLDL,* very-low-density lipoprotein.

blood. They are made up of a lipid core of triglycerides or cholesterol esters, or both, which is surrounded by a thin layer of phospholipids, apolipoproteins, and cholesterol. There are various types of lipoproteins, and they are classified according to their density and the type of apolipoproteins they contain. These various types of lipoproteins and their classifications are listed in Table 28-1.

CHOLESTEROL HOMEOSTASIS

There is a complex array of biochemical factors and reactions that are all part of physiologic (normal) cholesterol homeostasis. Figure 28-1 summarizes the major concepts that are described. Fats are taken into the body through the diet and are broken down in the small intestine to form triglycerides. These triglycerides are in turn incorporated into **chylomicrons** in the cells of the intestinal wall, which are then absorbed into the lymphatic system. The primary purpose of chylomicrons is to transport lipids obtained from dietary sources (**exogenous lipids**) from the intestines to the liver to be used to make steroid hormones, lipid structural components for peripheral body cells, and bile acids.

The liver is the major organ where lipid metabolism occurs. The liver produces very-low-density lipoprotein (VLDL) from both endogenous and exogenous sources. The major role of VLDL is the transport of endogenous lipids to peripheral cells. Once VLDL is circulating, it is enzymatically cleaved by lipoprotein lipase and loses triglycerides. This creates intermediate-density lipoprotein (IDL), which is soon also cleaved by lipoprotein lipase, creating low-density lipoprotein (LDL). Cholesterol is almost all that is left in LDL after this process. Any tissues that require LDL, such as endocrine cells, possess LDL receptors. LDL and about half of IDL are reabsorbed from the circulation into the liver by means of LDL receptors on the liver.

HDL is produced in the liver and intestines and is also formed when chylomicrons are broken down. Lipids that are not used by peripheral cells are transferred as cholesterol esters to HDL. HDL then transfers the cholesterol esters to IDL to be returned to the liver. HDL is responsible for the "recycling" of cholesterol. HDL is sometimes referred to as the good lipid (or "good cholesterol") because it is believed to be cardioprotective.

If the liver has an excess amount of cholesterol, the number of LDL receptors on the liver decreases, resulting in an accumulation of LDL in the blood. One explanation for **hypercholesterolemia** (cholesterol in the blood), therefore, is this downregulation (reduced production) of hepatic LDL receptors. A major function of the liver is to manufacture cholesterol, a process that requires acetyl coenzyme A (CoA) reductase. Inhibition of this enzyme thus results in decreased cholesterol production by the liver.

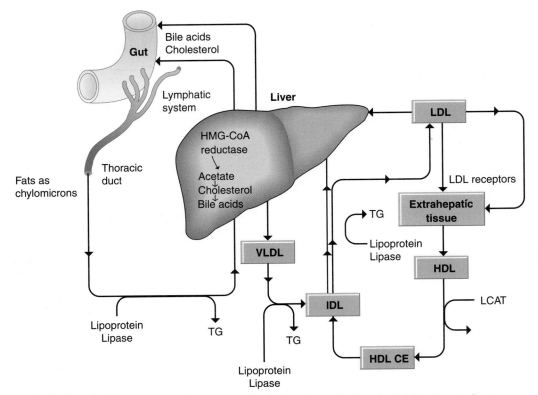

FIGURE 28-1 Cholesterol homeostasis. *CE,* Cholesterol ester; *HDL,* high-density lipoprotein; *HMG-CoA,* hydroxymethylglutaryl-coenzyme A; *IDL,* intermediate-density lipoprotein; *LCAT,* lecithin cholesterol acetyltransferase; *LDL,* low-density lipoprotein; *TG,* triglyceride; *VLDL,* very-low-density lipoprotein.

ATHEROSCLEROTIC PLAQUE FORMATION

Fundamental to the study of hyperlipidemia is an understanding of the processes by which lipids and lipoproteins participate in the formation of atherosclerotic plaque, and subsequently the development of CHD. When the serum cholesterol levels are elevated, circulating monocytes adhere to the smooth endothelial surface of the coronary vasculature. These monocytes burrow into the next layer of the blood vessel (subendothelial tissue) and change into macrophage cells, which then take up cholesterol from circulating lipoproteins until they become filled with fat. Soon they become what are known as **foam cells,** the characteristic precursor lesion of atherosclerosis, also known as the *fatty streak.* Once this process is established, it is usually present throughout the coronary and systemic circulation.

LINK BETWEEN CHOLESTEROL AND CORONARY HEART DISEASE

Numerous epidemiologic trials have shown that as blood cholesterol levels increase in the members of a population, the incidence of death and disability related to CHD also increases. The risk for CHD in patients with cholesterol levels of 300 mg/dL is three to four times greater than that in patients with levels less than 200 mg/dL. The absolute incidence of CHD in premenopausal women and women on estrogen replacement therapy is approximately 25% less than that of men.

This is thought to be secondary to the effects of estrogen because the risk for CHD climbs considerably in postmenopausal women. There has been emerging controversy, however, regarding this longstanding belief because two recent estrogen replacement therapy (ERT) trials did not demonstrate prevention of cardiovascular events in women receiving ERT. Other experimental studies that looked for any benefits of low-dose estrogen therapy in *male* patients also did not demonstrate significant cardioprotective efficacy.

Statistics show that half of all Americans, both male and female, will die of a heart attack. Thus the thrust of treatment is two-pronged: primary prevention of cardiac events in patients with risk factors and secondary prevention of subsequent cardiac events in individuals who have previously suffered a cardiac event (e.g., myocardial infarction [MI]). The benefits of primary prevention as it refers to cholesterol reduction have been illustrated in a variety of recent trials. Some of the larger and more recent trials are the Lipid Research Clinics (LRC) Coronary Primary Prevention Trial, the Helsinki Heart Study, and the West of Scotland Coronary Prevention Study (WOS). The LRC trial used the drug cholestyramine, the Helsinki study used the drug gemfibrozil, and the WOS used the hydroxymethylglutaryl (HMG)–CoA reductase inhibitor pravastatin. These studies help reinforce the belief that in patients with known risk factors for CHD, drug therapy with an antilipemic drug can reduce the occurrence of CHD. First-time heart attack and death caused by heart disease can be reduced with drug therapy.

EVIDENCE-BASED PRACTICE

Statins and Stroke Reduction in Patients With and Without Coronary Heart Disease

Review

The purpose of this study was to look at management of lipid levels as an important component of stroke prevention. This meta-analysis of randomized clinical trials focused on determining the effects of lipid-lowering interventions (statins, fibrates, resins, n-3 fatty acids, and diet) for the prevention of nonfatal and fatal strokes. Data sources include Medline, EMBASE/Excerpta Medica, Pascal, and Index Medicus in the article posted in volume 8 of *EBN Journal*, July 2005 issue.

Type of Evidence and Type of Research

A meta-analysis of randomized clinical trials with a 0.5- to 6.1-year follow-up were used to study the topic of statins and reduction of strokes. This analysis was conducted with the goal of comparing dietary or pharmaceutical lipid-lowering interventions with those in a placebo or "usual" diet group, who had follow-up in the past 6 months and had data on nonfatal and fatal strokes and total mortality. Sixty-five randomized, controlled trials were included with a pooled intervention group and a pooled control group.

Results of Study

Data found that statins reduced the risk of nonfatal and fatal stroke more than the group with controlled interventions in patients with and without coronary heart disease combined. Fibrates, resins, n-3 fatty acids, and dietary interventions were found to be no more effective than control interventions for reducing risk for nonfatal and fatal stroke. Several research studies were quoted within the commentary of this study, and it was

stated that the findings from Briel and colleagues show the importance of statin treatment in helping to reduce the incidence of stroke in patients with and without heart disease. It is thought that statins have a "pleiotropic" (meaning "multiple") effect—but not through lipoprotein changes but through other effects such as antiinflammatory and endothelial protection. Although the authors in this study (Briel M, et al.) did not confirm the benefits of non-"statin" lipid-lowering therapy, they also did not dismiss the merits of such treatments. The findings of a lack of treatment effects with the non-statins could be attributed to small "cohorts" and other variables.

Link of Evidence to Nursing Practice

This study emphasizes the importance of looking at different treatment options with certain individual variables with the use of statins in reducing nonfatal and fatal strokes in the above population. Although the significance and benefits of statins are known, many patients remain inadequately treated. Nurses play a major role here in the assessment and interventions for a cardiovascular (CV) patient as well as a significant role in the pharmacologic management of CV patients. Nurses continue to play an important part in patient and community education of the risk factors for stroke, including the presence of coronary artery disease and hyperlipidemia as well as education about compliance to all types of interventions and therapies, contemporary nursing practice, and the resultant pain management technique used by nurses.

Modified from Briel M et al: Effects of statins on stroke prevention in patients with and without coronary heart disease: a meta-analysis of randomized clinical trials, *Am J Med* 117:596-606, 2004; Briel M et al: Review: statins reduce non-fatal and fatal strokes in patients with and without coronary heart disease, *Evid Based Nurs* 8:86, 2005.

The benefits of secondary prevention as it refers to cholesterol reduction have been illustrated in a variety of recent trials as well. Some of the larger and more recent trials are the Cholesterol Lowering Atherosclerosis Study (CLAS), the Familial Atherosclerosis Treatment Study, and the Scandinavian Simvastatin Survival Study (4S trial). CLAS used the drugs colestipol and niacin, the Familial Atherosclerosis Treatment Study used the drugs niacin/colestipol and lovastatin/colestipol, and the 4S trial used the drug simvastatin. These secondary prevention trials showed that in patients with documented CHD, treatment with a cholesterol-lowering drug has many positive outcomes. Three of these are decreased coronary events, regression of coronary atherosclerotic lesions, and prolonged survival.

Measures taken early in a person's life to reduce and maintain cholesterol levels in a desirable range should have a dramatic effect in terms of preventing CHD and the death and disability it causes. These include lifestyle modifications related to diet, weight, and activity level. Diets lower in saturated fat and higher in fiber and plant chemicals known as sterols and stanols and possibly the substitution of soy-based proteins for animal proteins appear to promote healthier lipid profiles. These are among the latest dietary recommendations made in 2001 by the third National Cholesterol Education Program Adult Treatment Panel III (NCEP-ATP III) from the National Institutes of Health (NIH). The eating of fatty fish or dietary supplements containing omega-3 fatty acids appears to have

beneficial effects on triglyceride and HDL levels and is currently recommended by the American Heart Association (AHA). The AHA also strongly emphasizes the substantial therapeutic benefits of even modest weight reduction and exercise in both improvement of lipid profiles and reduction of the likelihood of heart disease.

HYPERLIPIDEMIAS AND TREATMENT GUIDELINES

The decision to prescribe hyperlipemic drugs as an adjunct to diet therapy in patients with an elevated cholesterol level should be based on the patient's clinical profile. This includes the patient's age, sex, menopausal status for women, family history, and response to dietary treatment, as well as the presence of risk factors (other than hyperlipidemia) for premature CHD and the cause, duration, and the phenotypic pattern of the patient's hyperlipidemia.

As mentioned earlier, a major source of guidance for antilipemic treatment at the disposal of health care professionals in the United States has been the National Cholesterol Education Program (NCEP), which has been developed in close cooperation with other major professional organizations such as the AHA. This program has two main thrusts, both aimed at reducing the total risk for CHD in the population of the United States. One is focused on the entire population and consists of general guidelines for the prevention of CHD. It emphasizes the appropriate dietary intake of total cholesterol and saturated fat, weight control, physical activity, and the control of other lifestyle risk factors. The other aspect is focused on the management of individual patients who are at increased risk for CHD. The original guidelines for the detection, evaluation, and treatment of high serum cholesterol levels in adults were published in 1988 and 2001. They were updated again in July of 2004. In these guidelines, the selection of diet and drug therapy options is determined by the presence of certain risk factors. The latest guidelines are the first to include CHD risk equivalents. These are other conditions, such as diabetes, that have been statistically calculated to equate one's 10-year risk for a major coronary event (e.g., MI) for those patients who do not currently have CHD. These risk factors and risk equivalents are listed in Box 28-1.

When the decision to institute drug therapy has been made, the choice of drug should then be determined by the specific lipid profile of the patient. There are five identified patterns or phenotypes of hyperlipidemia, and these are determined by the nature of the plasma (serum) concentrations of total cholesterol, triglyc-

erides, and lipoprotein fractions (HDL, LDL, IDL, VLDL). These various types of hyperlipidemias are listed in Table 28-2. The process of characterizing a patient's specific lipid profile in this way is referred to as *phenotyping*.

One of the basic tenets of the NCEP guidelines is that all reasonable nonpharmaceutical means of controlling the blood cholesterol level (e.g., diet, exercise) should be tried for at least 6 months and found to fail before drug therapy is considered. Because the drug therapy for hyperlipidemias entails a long-term commitment to the therapy, factors that should be considered before the initiation of therapy are the type and magnitude of dyslipidemia, the age and lifestyle of the patient, the relative indications and contraindications of different drugs and drug categories for a given patient, potential drug interactions, adverse effects, and the overall cost of therapy. The 2004 updated NCEP guidelines recommend that all patients with LDL cholesterol levels exceeding 190 mg/dL and those with LDL cholesterol levels between 160 and 190 mg/dL who have CHD or two or more risk factors for heart disease be considered for drug therapy after an adequate trial of dietary and other nondrug therapies has proved ineffective. The treatment decisions that should be made based on the LDL cholesterol levels are listed in Table 28-3. The updated guidelines even recommend optional use of drug therapy to reduce LDL to less than 70 mg/dL, in "very high risk" patients, and less than 100 in moderately high-risk patients. "Very high-risk" patients include those with active cardiovascular disease with other major risk factors such as diabetes, continued smoking, or *metabolic syndrome.* Metabolic syndrome is a set of risk factors associated with obesity, including hypertriglyceridemia and low HDL. "Moderately high risk" patients include those without cardiovascular disease but have two or more risk factors.

Box 28-2 lists the current symptoms described for patients with metabolic syndrome.

There are currently four established classes of drugs used to treat dyslipidemia: HMG–CoA reductase inhibitors (**statins),** bile acid sequestrants, the B-vitamin niacin (vitamin B_3, also known as *nicotinic acid),* and the fibric acid derivatives (fibrates). In addition to all of these drugs, the newest drug, *ezetimibe (Zetia),* is a cholesterol absorption inhibitor. In many cases, patient outcomes are improved with various combinations of these drugs. One of the newest examples of this is the combination

---

Box 28-1 Coronary Heart Disease: Risk Factors

Positive Risk Factors
- Age:
  - Male: ≥45 years
  - Female: ≥55 years or women with premature menopause not on estrogen replacement therapy
- Family history:
  - History of premature CHD (e.g., MI or sudden death before 55 years of age in father or other male first-degree relative, or before 65 years of age in mother or other female first-degree relative)
  - Current cigarette smoker
  - Hypertension: >140/90 mm Hg, or on antihypertensive medication
  - Low HDL cholesterol level: <35 mg/dL
  - Diabetes mellitus

Negative Risk Factors
- High HDL cholesterol: ≥60 mg/dL—if the HDL cholesterol is ≥60 mg/dL, subtract one risk factor

CHD, Coronary heart disease; *HDL,* high-density lipoprotein; *MI,* myocardial infarction.

Table 28-2 Types of Hyperlipidemias

		Lipid Composition	
Phenotype	**Lipoprotein Elevated**	**Cholesterol (mg/dL)**	**Triglyceride**
I	Chylomicrons	>300	>3000
IIa	LDL	>300	Normal ≅ 148
IIb	LDL, VLDL	>300	Normal ≅ 148
III	IDL	>400	>600 (1-3 × higher than cholesterol)
IV	VLDL	Normal or mildly elevated ≅ 250	>400
V	VLDL, chylomicrons	>300	>2000

IDL, Intermediate-density lipoprotein; *LDL,* low-density lipoprotein; *VLDL,* very-low-density lipoprotein.

Table 28-3	Treatment Decisions Based on LDL Cholesterol Level	
Patient Category	**Initiation Level**	**LDL Goal**
Dietary Therapy		
Without CHD and with <2 risk factors (low risk)	≥160 mg/dL (4.1 mmol/L)	<160 mg/dL (4.1 mmol/L)
Without CHD and with ≥2 risk factors (moderately high risk)	≥130 mg/dL (3.4 mmol/L)	<130 mg/dL (3.4 mmol/L)
With CHD (high or very high risk)	≥100 mg/dL (2.6 mmol/L)	<100 mg/dL (2.6 mmol/L)
Drug Therapy		
Without CHD and with <2 risk factors (low risk)	≥190 mg/dL (4.9 mmol/L)	<160 mg/dL (4.1 mmol/L)
Without CHD and with ≥2 risk factors (moderately high risk)	≥160 mg/dL (4.1 mmol/L)	<130 mg/dL (3.4 mmol/L)
With CHD (high or very high risk)	≥130 mg/dL (3.4 mmol/L)	<100 mg/dL (2.6 mmol/L)

CHD, Coronary heart disease; *LDL,* low-density lipoprotein.

Box 28-2 | Identifying Features of the Metabolic Syndrome

- Waist circumference greater than 40 inches in men or 30 inches in women
- Serum triglycerides of 150 mg/dL or more
- HDL cholesterol less than 40 mg/dL in men or less than 50 mg/dL in women
- Blood pressure at 130/85 or higher
- Fasting serum glucose more than 110 mg/dL

---

tablet Vytorin, which contains both the statin drug atorvastatin and ezetimibe.

HMG–CoA REDUCTASE INHIBITORS

The rate-limiting enzyme in cholesterol synthesis is known as HMG–CoA reductase. The class of medications that competitively inhibit this enzyme, the **HMG–CoA reductase inhibitors,** are the most potent of the drugs available for reducing plasma concentrations of LDL cholesterol. Lovastatin was the first drug in this class to be approved for use, and this occurred in 1987. Since that time, six other HMG–CoA reductase inhibitors have become available on the U.S. market: pravastatin, simvastatin, atorvastatin, cerivastatin, fluvastatin, and rosuvastatin. Because of the shared suffix of their generic names, these drugs are often collectively referred to as statins. The maximum extent to which these lipid levels are lowered may not occur until 6 to 8 weeks after the start of therapy. Few direct comparisons of the statins have been published. However, the authors of the published account of one such study concluded that the following doses of

drugs would yield the same reduction in the LDL cholesterol level: simvastatin, 10 mg; pravastatin, 20 mg; and lovastatin, 20 mg. This particular study did not assess fluvastatin or atorvastatin.

Mechanism of Action and Drug Effects

Statins lower the blood cholesterol level by decreasing the rate of cholesterol production. The liver requires HMG–CoA reductase to produce cholesterol. It is the rate-limiting enzyme in the reactions needed to make cholesterol. The statins inhibit this enzyme, thereby decreasing cholesterol production. When less cholesterol is produced, the liver increases the number of LDL receptors to augment the recycling of LDL from the circulation back into the liver, where it is needed for the synthesis of other needed substances such as steroids, bile acids, and cell membranes. Lovastatin and simvastatin are administered as inactive drugs or prodrugs that must be biotransformed into their active metabolites in the liver. In contrast, pravastatin is administered in its active form.

Indications

The statins are still recommended by the latest National Cholesterol Education Program-Adult Treatment Panel III (NCEP-ATP III) guidelines as first-line drug therapy for hypercholesterolemia (elevated LDL cholesterol, or LDL-C), the most common and dangerous form of dyslipidemia. More specifically, they are indicated for the treatment of type IIa and IIb hyperlipidemia and have been shown to reduce the plasma concentrations of LDL cholesterol by 30% to 40%. Their cholesterol-lowering properties are dose-dependent in that the larger the dose, the greater the cholesterol-lowering effects. A 10% to 30% decrease in the concentrations of plasma triglycerides has also been observed in patients receiving any of these drugs. Another very important therapeutic effect of the statins is an overall tendency for the HDL cholesterol level to increase by 2% to 15%, a known beneficial risk factor (i.e., a negative risk factor) against cardiovascular disease.

These drugs also appear to be equally effective in their ability to reduce LDL cholesterol concentrations. However, simvastatin and atorvastatin are more potent on a milligram basis. Atorvastatin appears to be more effective in lowering triglycerides than other HMG–CoA reductase inhibitors. Combined drug therapy with more than one class of antilipemic drugs may be necessary for desired results, and the statins are often combined with niacin or fibrates for this purpose, though this combination can increase the risk of adverse drug effects (see Adverse Effects).

Contraindications

Contraindications to the use of HMG–CoA reductase inhibitors (statins) include known drug allergy and pregnancy. Other contraindications may include liver disease or elevation of liver enzymes.

Adverse Effects

Generally speaking, however, the HMG–CoA reductase inhibitors available for clinical use have proved to be well-tolerated, with significant adverse effects being fairly uncommon. Mild,

Table 28-4   HMG—CoA Reductase Inhibitors: Potential Adverse Effects

Body System	Adverse Effects
Central nervous	Headache, dizziness, blurred vision, ophthalmoplegia, fatigue, nightmares, insomnia
Gastrointestinal	Constipation, cramps, diarrhea, nausea, changes in bowel function
Other	Myalgias, skin rashes

transient gastrointestinal disturbances, rash, and headache have been the most common problems. These and other less common adverse effects are listed in Table 28-4. Elevations in liver enzymes may also occur, and the patient should be monitored for excessive elevations, which may indicate the need for alternative drug therapy. Dose-dependent elevations in liver enzyme activity to values greater than three times the upper limit of normal have been noted in 0.4% to 1.9% of patients taking HMG—CoA reductase inhibitors. The serum creatine phosphokinase (CPK) concentrations may be increased by more than 10 times the normal level in patients receiving these drugs. Most of these patients have remained asymptomatic, however. In August of 2001, Bayer Corporation voluntarily recalled from the market its drug cerivastatin (Baycol) because of increasing numbers of serious adverse effects.

A less common but still clinically important adverse effect is myopathy (muscle pain), which may progress to a serious condition known as *rhabdomyolysis*. This is a condition involving the breakdown of muscle protein leading to myoglobinuria, which is the urinary elimination of the muscle protein myoglobin, the oxygen-carrying pigment of muscle tissue that is similar to a single subunit of hemoglobin (Hb). This abnormal urinary excretion of protein can place a severe strain on the kidneys, possibly leading to acute renal failure and even death. This myopathy is uncommon (less than 0.1%) during monotherapy for dyslipidemia with statins alone, but it appears to be dose-dependent and is more common in patients receiving a statin in combination with cyclosporine, niacin, gemfibrozil (a fibrate), or erythromycin. Patients receiving statin therapy should be advised to immediately report any unexplained muscular pain or discomfort to their health care providers. When recognized reasonably early, rhabdomyolysis is usually reversible with discontinuation of the statin drug. In June of 2004, the U.S. Food and Drug Administration (FDA) published a Public Health Advisory summarizing recent reports of myopathy and rhabdomyolysis cases associated with rosuvastatin (Crestor), one of the newer statin drugs. Zeneca Pharmaceuticals, the manufacturer of this drug, altered its labeling for the drug, listing risk factors for myopathy symptoms. These include age older than 65 years, hypothyroidism, renal insufficiency, and concurrent use of the immunosuppressant drug cyclosporine and the antihyperlipidemic drug gemfibrozil. The FDA also required Zeneca to make a 5-mg strength tablet available for those patients with significant risk factors

for drug toxicity, with a maximum recommended daily dose of 10 mg for these patients. In March of 2005, the FDA published a second Public Health Advisory regarding reports of both myopathy and renal failure associated with rosuvastatin as well as other statin drugs. Although these adverse effects are relatively uncommon, and although much benefit is often derived from their use, prescribers are advised to use minimal effective doses, with regular laboratory blood monitoring of liver and kidney function (every 3 to 6 months). Patients should also be educated regarding these serious, although uncommon, adverse drug effects, and instructed to immediately report signs of toxicity, including muscle soreness, changes in urine color, fever, malaise, nausea, or vomiting.

Toxicity and Management of Overdose
Very limited data are available on the nature of toxicity and overdose in patients taking HMG—CoA reductase inhibitors. Treatment, if needed, is supportive and based on presenting symptoms.

Interactions
HMG—CoA reductase inhibitors should be used cautiously in patients taking oral anticoagulants. In addition, the coadministration of these drugs with other classes of antilipemics, oral anticoagulants, oral antidiabetic drugs, erythromycin, gemfibrozil, insulin, niacin, and even grapefruit juice, has been observed to rarely lead to the development of rhabdomyolysis. Patients are advised to limit grapefruit juice to less than one quart daily, which is probably more than most people drink. The mechanism of this interaction is as follows: Components in grapefruit juice inactivate one of the *cytochrome P450* enzymes, specifically CYP3A4, in both the liver and intestines. This enzyme plays a key role in statin metabolism. The presence of grapefruit juice in the body may, therefore, result in sustained levels of unmetabolized statin drug, increasing the risk for major drug toxicity (e.g., rhabdomyolysis).

Laboratory Test Interactions
Laboratory interactions that can occur include increases in the aspartate aminotransferase (AST) levels and activated clotting time, thrombocytopenia, and transient eosinophilia.

Dosages
For dosage information on atorvastatin, see the following drug profile.

Drug Profiles

The HMG—CoA reductase inhibitors, or statins, are all potent inhibitors of the enzyme that catalyzes the rate-limiting step in the synthesis of cholesterol. There are currently five statins on the market in the United States: atorvastatin (Lipitor), fluvastatin (Lescol), lovastatin (Mevacor), pravastatin (Pravachol), and simvastatin (Zocor). There are some minor differences between drugs in this class of antilipemics; the most dramatic difference is that of potency. All five drugs are prescription-only drugs and are contraindicated in pregnant or lactating women and in those suffering from active liver dysfunction or with elevated serum transaminase levels of unknown cause. They are pregnancy category X drugs.

There is little evidence to recommend one drug over another, with the exception of fluvastatin, which may be somewhat less effective than the others.

▶ atorvastatin

Atorvastatin (Lipitor) has become the most commonly used drug in this class of cholesterol-lowering drugs. It is used primarily to lower total and LDL cholesterol as well as triglycerides. It is indicated for the treatment of type IIa and IIb hyperlipidemias. Atorvastatin has also been shown to raise good cholesterol, the HDL component. All statins are generally dosed once daily, usually with the evening meal or at bedtime. One particular advantage of atorvastatin is that it can be dosed at any time of day. However, bedtime dosing provides drug levels in a timeframe that correlates better with the natural *diurnal* (daytime) rhythm of cholesterol production in the body. The recommended dosage for atorvastatin is 10 to 80 mg daily. It is available only in tablet form in strengths of 10-, 20-, 40-, and 80-mg. Pregnancy category X.

Pharmacokinetics

Half-Life	Onset	Peak	Duration
14 hr	1-2 hr	2 wk*	Unknown

*Maximum therapeutic effect.

OTHER ANTILIPEMIC DRUGS

BILE ACID SEQUESTRANTS

Bile acid sequestrants, also called *bile acid–binding resins* and *ion-exchange resins,* include cholestyramine, colestipol, and colesevelam. The first two of these drugs have been used widely for more than 20 years and have been evaluated extensively in well-controlled clinical trials. They were actually the original prescription anticholesterol drugs. They have proven efficacy, but their powdered forms are somewhat messy to use. Colestipol is also available in tablet form. Colesevelam is a newer drug with a similar mechanism of action, but is only available in tablet form. These drugs are now considered second-line drugs in most cases in lieu of the more potent *statins.* However, they are still a suitable alternative in patients intolerant of the statins. Generally these drugs lower the plasma concentrations of LDL cholesterol by 15% to 30%. They also increase the HDL cholesterol level by 3% to 8% and increase hepatic triglyceride and VLDL production, which may result in a 10% to 50% increase in the triglyceride level.

Mechanism of Action and Drug Effects

Bile acid sequestrants bind bile, preventing the resorption of the bile acids from the small intestine. Instead, an insoluble bile acid-and-resin (drug) complex is excreted in the bowel movement. Bile acids are necessary for the absorption of cholesterol from the small intestine, yet are also synthesized from cholesterol by the liver. This is one natural way that the liver excretes cholesterol from the body. The more that bile acids are excreted in the feces, the more the liver converts cholesterol to bile acids. This reduces the level of cholesterol in the liver, and thus, the circulation as well. The liver then attempts to compensate for the loss of cholesterol by increasing the number of LDL receptors on its surface. Circulating LDL molecules bind to these receptors to be taken up into the liver, which also has the benefit of reducing circulating LDL in the blood stream.

Table 28-5	Bile Acid Sequestrants: Adverse Effects
Body System	**Adverse Effects**
Gastrointestinal	Constipation, heartburn, nausea, belching, bloating
Other	Bleeding, headache, tinnitus, burnt odor of urine

Indications

Bile acid sequestrants may be used as primary or adjunct drug therapy in the management of type II hyperlipoproteinemia. One common strategy is to use them along with statins for an additive drug effect in reducing LDL cholesterol. In addition, cholestyramine is used to relieve the pruritus associated with partial biliary obstruction. The newest drug in this class, colesevelam, may be better tolerated by higher risk patients who are intolerant of other antihyperlipemic therapy, including organ transplant recipients, and those with serious liver or kidney disease.

Contraindications

Contraindications to the use of bile acid sequestrants include known drug allergy and biliary or bowel obstruction.

Adverse Effects

The adverse effects of colestipol, cholestyramine, and colesevelam are similar; however, colesevelam is reported to have fewer gastrointestinal adverse effects and drug interactions. Constipation is a common problem and may be accompanied by heartburn, nausea, belching, and bloating. These adverse effects tend to disappear over time, however. Many patients require extra education and support to help them deal with the gastrointestinal effects and comply with the medication regimen. It is important that therapy is initiated with low doses and patients instructed to take the drugs with meals to reduce the adverse effects. Increasing the dietary fiber intake or taking a fiber supplement such as psyllium (Metamucil and others), as well as increasing fluid intake, may relieve constipation and bloating. These drugs may also cause mild increases in the triglyceride levels. The most common adverse effects of the bile acid sequestrants are listed in Table 28-5.

Toxicity and Management of Overdose

Because the bile acid sequestrants are not absorbed, an overdose could cause obstruction of the gastrointestinal tract. Therefore, treatment of an overdose involves restoring gut motility.

Interactions

The significant drug interactions associated with the use of bile acid sequestrants are limited to the absorption of concurrently administered drugs. All drugs should be taken at least

1 hour before or 4 to 6 hours after the administration of ion-exchange resins. In addition, high doses of a bile acid sequestrant will decrease the absorption of fat-soluble vitamins (A, D, E, and K).

Dosages

For dosage information on bile acid sequestrants, see the table on this page.

Drug Profiles

The bile acid sequestrants cholestyramine, colestipol, and colesevelam are indicated for the treatment of type IIa and IIb hyperlipidemia. They lower the cholesterol level, in particular the LDL cholesterol level, by increasing the destruction of LDL. However, their use may result in increases in the very low-density lipoprotein (VLDL) cholesterol level. Because of the high incidence of gastrointestinal adverse effects in patients taking these drugs, compliance with the prescribed dosage schedules is often poor. However, educating patients about the purpose and expected adverse effects of therapy can foster improved compliance. Patients must be warned not to take bile acid sequestrants concurrently with other drugs because the drug interactions can be very pronounced. Other drugs must be taken at other times of the day. This cannot be overemphasized.

cholestyramine

Cholestyramine (Questran, Questran Light) is a prescription-only drug that is contraindicated in patients with a known hypersensitivity to it and in those suffering from complete biliary obstruction. It may interfere with the distribution of the proper amounts of fat-soluble vitamins to the fetus or nursing infant of pregnant or nursing women taking the drug.

NIACIN

Niacin, or nicotinic acid, is not only a very unique lipid-lowering drug, it is also a vitamin. For its unique lipid-lowering properties to be realized, much larger doses of the drug are required than are commonly given when it is used as a vitamin. Niacin is a B vitamin, specifically vitamin B_3. It is an effective and inexpensive medication that exerts favorable effects on the plasma concentrations of all lipoproteins. Niacin is often given in combination with other antilipemic drugs to enhance the lipid-lowering effects.

Mechanism of Action and Drug Effects

Although the exact mechanism of action of niacin is unknown, the beneficial effects are believed to be related to its ability to inhibit lipolysis in adipose tissue, decrease esterification of triglycerides in the liver, and increase the activity of lipoprotein lipase. The drug effects of niacin are primarily limited to its ability to reduce the metabolism or catabolism of cholesterol and triglycerides. Niacin decreases the LDL levels moderately (10% to 20%), decreases the triglyceride levels (30% to 70%), and increases the HDL levels moderately (20% to 35%). Niacin is also a vitamin needed for many bodily processes. In large doses, it may produce vasodilation that is limited to the cutaneous vessels. This effect seems to be induced by prostaglandins. Niacin also causes the release of histamine, resulting in an increase in gastric motility and acid secretion. Niacin may also stimulate the fibrinolytic system to break down fibrin clots.

Indications

Niacin has been shown to be effective in lowering lipid levels. This includes triglyceride, total serum cholesterol, and LDL cholesterol levels. It also brings about an increase in the HDL cho-

DOSAGES

Selected Antilipemic Drugs

Drug (Pregnancy Category)	Pharmacologic Class	Usual Dosage Range	Indications
atorvastatin (Lipitor) (X)	HMG–CoA reductase inhibitor	**Adult** PO: 10-80 mg/day	
cholestyramine (Questran) (C)	Antilipemic ion-exchange resin	**Adult** PO: Powder, 9 g 1-6 ×/day	
colesevelam (WelChol) (B)	Antilipemic ion-exchange resin	**Adult** PO: (325-mg tablets) three tablets BID with meal or six tablets once daily with meal	
colestipol hydrochloride (Colestid) (C)	Antilipemic ion-exchange resin	**Adult** PO: Granules: 5-30 g/day once or in divided doses; tabs: 2-16 g/day	
ezetimibe (Zetia) (C)	Cholesterol absorption inhibitor	**Adult** PO: 10 mg 1× /day	Hyperlipidemia
fenofibrate (Tricor) (C)	Fibric acid derivative	**Adult** PO: 67 mg/day initial dose; max 201 mg/day	
gemfibrozil (Lopid) (C)	Fibric acid derivative	**Adult** PO: 600 mg bid 30 min ac in AM and PM	
simvastatin (Zocor) (X)	HMG–CoA reductase inhibitors	**Adult** PO: 10-80 mg/day	
niacin (nicotinic acid, vitamin B3) (A; C if dose exceeds RDA)	B vitamin	**Adult** PO: 1.5 to 6 gm/day in 2-4 divided doses.	

RDA, Recommended daily allowance.

Table 28-6	Nicotinic Acid: Potential Adverse Effects
Body System	**Adverse Effects**
Gastrointestinal	Abdominal discomfort; gastrointestinal distress
Integumentary	Cutaneous flushing, pruritus, hyperpigmentation
Other	Blurred vision, glucose intolerance, hyperuricemia, dry eyes (rare), hepatotoxicity

lesterol levels. Niacin may also lower the lipoprotein (a) level, except in patients with severe hypertriglyceridemia. It has been shown to be effective in the treatment of types IIa, IIb, III, IV, and V hyperlipidemias.

Niacin's effects on triglyceride levels begin to be noticed after 1 to 4 days of therapy, with the decrease in the levels ranging from 20% to 80%. The decline in the LDL levels is less, with the maximum decrease ranging from 10% to 15%. The maximum effects of niacin are seen after 3 to 5 weeks of continuous therapy.

Contraindications

Contraindications to the use of niacin include known drug allergy and may include liver disease, hypertension, peptic ulcer, and any active hemorrhagic process.

Adverse Effects

Niacin can cause flushing, pruritus, and gastrointestinal distress. Small doses of aspirin or nonsteroidal antiinflammatory drugs (NSAIDs) may be taken 30 minutes before niacin to minimize the cutaneous flushing. These undesirable effects can also be minimized by starting patients on a low initial dosage and increasing it gradually, and by having patients take the drug with meals. The most common adverse effects associated with niacin therapy are listed in Table 28-6.

Interactions

The major drug interactions associated with niacin are minimal. One interaction of note: when niacin is taken concomitantly with an HMG–CoA reductase inhibitor, the likelihood of myopathy development is greatly increased.

Dosages

For dosage information on niacin, see the following drug profile for this drug.

Drug Profiles

▶ niacin

Used alone or in combination with other lipid-lowering drugs, niacin (nicotinic acid, vitamin B_3) (Nicobid, Slo-Niacin) is a very effective, inexpensive medication that, as previously mentioned, has beneficial effects on LDL cholesterol, triglyceride, and HDL cholesterol levels. Drug therapy with niacin is usually initiated at a

small daily dose taken with or after meals to minimize the adverse effects previously discussed. Liver dysfunction has been observed in individuals taking sustained-release (SR) forms of niacin, not immediate-release (IR) forms. However, newer extended-release (ER) dosage forms, which dissolve more slowly than the IR forms but faster than the SR forms, appear to have even better adverse effect profiles, including less hepatotoxicity and flushing of the skin. Niacin is contraindicated in patients who have shown a hypersensitivity to it, in those with peptic ulcer, hepatic disease, hemorrhage, or severe hypotension, and in lactating women. It is also not recommended for patients with gout. Niacin is available over the counter (OTC) and by prescription.

Pharmacokinetics

Half-Life	Onset	Peak	Duration
45 min	Unknown	30-70 min	Unknown

FIBRIC ACID DERIVATIVES

Current fibric acid derivatives include gemfibrozil and fenofibrate. These drugs primarily affect the triglyceride levels but may also lower the total cholesterol and LDL cholesterol levels and raise the HDL cholesterol level. They are often collectively referred to as *fibrates*.

Mechanism of Action and Drug Effects

Fibric acid drugs are believed to work by activating lipoprotein lipase, an enzyme responsible for the breakdown of cholesterol. This enzyme usually cleaves off a triglyceride molecule from VLDL or LDL, leaving behind lipoproteins. Fibric acid derivatives can also suppress the release of free fatty acid from adipose tissue, inhibit the synthesis of triglycerides in the liver, and increase the secretion of cholesterol into bile. They have been shown to reduce triglyceride levels and serum VLDL and LDL concentrations. Independent of their lipid-lowering actions, fibric acid derivatives can also induce changes in blood coagulation. This involves a tendency for them to decrease platelet adhesiveness. They can also increase plasma fibrinolysis, the process that causes fibrin and, therefore, clots to be broken down.

Indications

The fibric acid derivatives gemfibrozil and fenofibrate all decrease the triglyceride levels and increase the HDL cholesterol level by as much as 25%. Both decrease the LDL concentrations in patients with type IIa and IIb hyperlipidemias but increase the LDL levels in patients with type IV and V hyperlipemias. They are indicated for the treatment of type III, IV, and V hyperlipidemias, and in some cases the type IIb form, although other classes of antilipemics are usually attempted first.

Contraindications

Contraindications to the use of fibrates include known drug allergy and may include severe liver or kidney disease, cirrhosis, or gallbladder disease.

Adverse Effects

As a class, the most common adverse effects of the fibric acid derivatives are abdominal discomfort, diarrhea, nausea, headache, blurred vision, increased risk for gallstones, and prolonged

Table 28-7 Fibric Acid Derivatives: Potential Adverse Effects

Body System	Adverse Effects
Gastrointestinal	Nausea, vomiting, diarrhea, gallstones, acute appendicitis
Genitourinary	Impotence, decreased urine output, hematuria, increased risk for urinary hematuria, increased risk for urinary tract infections and viral infections
Other	Drowsiness, dizziness, rash, pruritus, alopecia, eczema, vertigo, headache

prothrombin time. Liver function tests may also show increased enzyme levels. The more common adverse effects are listed in Table 28-7.

Toxicity and Management of Overdose

The management of fibrate overdose, which is uncommon, is supportive care based on presenting symptoms. Gastrointestinal decontamination or use of gastric lavage may be indicated for large overdoses.

Interactions

Gemfibrozil can also enhance the action of oral anticoagulants, thus also necessitating careful dose adjustments of these latter drugs. The risk for myositis, myalgias, and rhabdomyolysis is increased when either gemfibrozil or fenofibrate is given with a statin. Fenofibrate may also raise the blood level of ezetimibe, if taken concurrently.

Laboratory test interactions that can occur in patients taking gemfibrozil include a decrease in the hemoglobin (Hb) level, hematocrit (Hct) value, and white blood cell count. In addition, the AST, activated clotting time (ACT), lactate dehydrogenase, and bilirubin levels can be increased.

Dosages

For dosage information on gemfibrozil and fenofibrate, see the table on page 448.

Drug Profiles

Fibric Acid Derivatives (Fibrates)

The fibric acid derivatives gemfibrozil and fenofibrate are prescription-only drugs and are now the only two available drugs in this class. They are both pregnancy category C drugs and are contraindicated in patients with hypersensitivity, preexisting gallbladder disease, significant hepatic or renal dysfunction, and primary biliary cirrhosis. Both drugs decrease the triglyceride and increase the HDL levels by as much as 25%. They are good drugs for the treatment of mixed hyperlipidemias.

gemfibrozil

Gemfibrozil (Lopid) is a fibric acid derivative that decreases the synthesis of apolipoprotein B (Apo B) and lowers the VLDL level. It can also increase the HDL level. In addition, it is highly effective for lowering plasma triglyceride levels. In a very large trial, the Helsinki study, the triglyceride levels of the group receiving gemfibrozil were reduced by as much as 43% compared with the control group. The total cholesterol and LDL levels were

reduced by 11% and 10%, respectively, and the HDL level was increased by 10%. Gemfibrozil is indicated for the treatment of type IV and V hyperlipidemias, and, in some cases, the type IIb form. The specific dosing recommendations are given in the table on page 448.

Pharmacokinetics

Half-Life	Onset	Peak	Duration
1.3-1.5 hr	Unknown	1-2 hr	Unknown

Cholesterol Absorption Inhibitors

ezetimibe

Ezetimibe (Zetia) is currently the only cholesterol absorption inhibitor, approved by the FDA in 2002. Ezetimibe has a novel mechanism of action in that it selectively inhibits absorption in the small intestine of cholesterol and related sterols. The result is a reduction in several blood lipid parameters: total cholesterol, LDL cholesterol (LDL-C), Apo B, and triglycerides. However, serum levels of HDL cholesterol (HDL-C), the so-called "good cholesterol," have been shown to actually increase with the use of ezetimibe. These beneficial effects thus far appear to be further enhanced when ezetimibe is taken with a statin drug, rather than either type of drug taken alone, although ezetimibe may be used as monotherapy. In several small studies, ezetimibe was not shown to interact significantly with cimetidine, warfarin, digoxin, oral contraceptives, or antacids. However, fibric acid derivatives (fibrates) have been shown to significantly increase the serum levels of ezetimibe. It is not yet known whether this is harmful, but currently, concurrent use of ezetimibe and fibrates is not recommended. The use of ezetimibe with bile acid sequestrants has been shown thus far to reduce the serum level of ezetimibe by 55% and 80% in two small studies. Concurrent use of these two types of drugs is not yet contraindicated, but it should be recognized that the extent of LDL reduction normally promoted by ezetimibe is likely to be reduced with this drug combination. Ezetimibe is contraindicated in cases of demonstrated allergy to the drug or active liver disease or unexplained elevations in serum liver enzymes. It may be taken with or without food, and for patient convenience, may be dosed at the same time as a statin drug, if prescribed.

Pharmacokinetics

Half-Life	Onset	Peak	Duration
22 hr	Unknown	4-12 hr	Unknown

◆ NURSING PROCESS

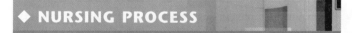

◆ ASSESSMENT

Before initiating antilipemic therapy in a patient, the nurse should obtain a thorough health and medication history, including any OTC drugs, herbals, and prescription drugs. Hypersensitivity to any of these drugs is also important to assess. It is important to assess the patient's dietary patterns; exercise program and frequency; weight; height; vital signs; and documentation over time, such as weeks of data—especially food intake. Also, use of tobacco, alcohol, and social drugs with information about frequency, amount, and duration of use should be documented. Some of the lipid disorders are hereditary and, as such, require a thorough assessment of the family history. Positive risk factors for CHD to assess for in patients include some of the following:

- Age (male 45 years old or older; female 55 years old or older)
- Smoking
- HDL levels 35 mg/dL or less

- Diabetes mellitus
- Family history of premature CHD

Cautions, contraindications, and drug interactions should be assessed prior to using any of the antilipemics. Serum lipid values and lipoprotein levels also need to be assessed and include the following normal ranges: (1) lipids—cholesterol levels 150 to 240 mg/dL, (2) triglycerides 40 to 190 mg/dL, and (3) lipoproteins—LDL 60 to 160 mg/dL and HDL 29 to 77 mg/dL. With use of cholestyramine, which contains aspartame, it is of particular interest to know if there is a history of phenylketonuria (PKU). Patients with PKU cannot properly process the amino acid phenylalanine, a component of protein. It is known that high levels of phenylalanine lead to behavioral, cognitive, and learning dysfunction as early as 3 weeks of age. Dietary restrictions must continue throughout the lifespan, with adult patients requiring monthly testing of phenylalanine. Because of the aspartame in cholestyramine, another class of an antilipemics would be indicated as ordered to prevent further complications from this disorder.

HMG–CoA reductase inhibitors (the statins) must not be used in patients younger than 10 years of age and other contraindications; cautions and drug interactions have been previously discussed in the pharmacology section of this chapter. The patient's intake of alcohol is also important to assess in regard to amounts and period of time that alcohol intake has occurred because of the potential of liver dysfunction associated with the majority of lipid-lowering drugs. These drugs could then more adversely affect the already damaged liver. Assessment of liver enzymes that are indicative of liver function should also be performed, including the following: AST (aspartate aminotransferase), CPK (creatine phosphokinase), and/or ALT (alanine aminotransferase). Lipid/lipoprotein levels also need to be assessed before, during, and after drug therapy with the statins as well as other antilipemic drugs. Myopathies and rhabdomyolysis should also be assessed for during and after drug therapy. Should blood levels of tranaminases increase and myopathy and/or rhabdomyolysis occur, the drug will most likely be discontinued by the physician. Also, with these drugs and others in this class, cultural influences need to be assessed, owing to the individual's belief on how to control diet and cholesterol levels. Cultural practices need to also be considered because of possible herbal and homeopathic therapies. Bile acid sequestrants, niacin, and fibric acid derivatives and their related contraindications, cautions, and drug interactions have been previously discussed, but always check for the numerous drug interactions.

◆ NURSING DIAGNOSES

- Imbalanced nutrition, more than body requirements, related to poor dietary habits of high fat intake
- Deficient knowledge related to a lack of knowledge about the disease and related complications
- Deficient knowledge related to a lack of understanding of drug therapy and need for lifestyle changes
- Impaired home maintenance related to lack of experience with lifestyle changes and unfamiliar medication therapy
- Imbalanced nutrition, less than body requirements, related to vitamin A, D, E, and K deficits from adverse effects of antilipemics

◆ PLANNING
Goals
- Patient remains compliant with both nonpharmacologic and pharmacologic therapy.
- Patient remains free of the complications associated with antilipemics due to appropriate use of the drug.
- Patient sees physician regularly and as indicated for the treatment of hyperlipidemia and to repeat laboratory studies until normal values return.
- Patient maintains homeostasis and nutritional well-being while taking the antilipemic drug.

Outcome Criteria
- Patient states the importance of pharmacologic and nonpharmacologic therapy to his or her overall health and safety, such as for decreasing the risk for CHD.
- Patient states the rationale of therapy as well as its adverse effects and expected therapeutic effects (i.e., decreasing lipid levels, gastrointestinal adverse effects, and therapeutic response of improved lipid profile).
- Patient states those conditions that may arise of which the physician should be notified, such as jaundice and abdominal pain.
- Patient states that cholesterol levels should return to a <200 mg/dL level within approximately 6 to 8 weeks.
- Patient states the importance of follow-up care with the physician to monitor for changes in liver function studies as well as the lipid levels.
- Patient states measures to adequately maintain levels of fat-soluble vitamins.

◆ IMPLEMENTATION

Patients who are taking antilipemics for a long period may have altered levels of the fat-soluble vitamins and may then require supplementation of vitamins A, D, and K. Antilipemics may also cause problems with the liver and biliary systems, and they may cause gastrointestinal tract problems such as constipation. Appropriate actions need to be taken to avoid or minimize constipation, such as increasing fiber and fluids. Monitoring blood studies per the health care provider's instructions often includes serum transaminases and other liver function studies.

With the HMG-CoA reductase inhibitors, monitoring serum levels of the aforementioned components is often done every 6 to 8 weeks for the first 6 months of statin therapy and then often every 3 to 6 months. If a lipid profile is ordered, emphasize to the patient that they should fast for 12 to 14 hours and that the following desired levels are hopefully achieved: cholesterol <200 mg/dL; triglycerides <150 mg/dL; LDL <130 mg/dL; and, HDL >60 mg/dL (these are the good lipids). Because severe cardiovascular diseases or cerebral vascular accidents (CVA; also known as a "stroke") are associated with cholesterol levels >240 mg/dL, LDLs >160 mg/dL, and HDLs <35 mg/dL, it is critical to maintenance of health and prevention of complications to continue with any prescribed nonpharmacologic and/or pharmacologic therapies (regardless of the specific antilipemic used). These drugs should never be discontinued abruptly.

Bile acid sequestrants often come in powder form and should be mixed thoroughly with fruit (e.g., crushed pineapple) or other food or fluids (at least 4 to 6 oz of fluid). The powder may not mix completely at first, but patients should be sure to mix the

LABORATORY VALUES RELATED TO DRUG THERAPY

Coronary Heart Disease

Laboratory Test	Normal Ranges	Rationale for Assessment
Lipid panel with serum cholesterol, triglycerides, and lipids	Serum cholesterol levels <200 mg/dL or <5.17 mmol/L Triglyceride levels <150 mg/dL Low-density lipoprotein (LDL) cholesterol level <100 mg/dL (<2.6 mmol/L) High-density lipoprotein (HDL) cholesterol level 60 mg/dL (1.56 mmol/L) or greater Very-low–density lipoprotein (VLDL) <130 mg/dL (<3.4 mmol/L)	A lipid panel is a serum test that measures lipids, fats, and fatty substances used as a source of energy in the body. Lipids include cholesterol, triglycerides, HDL, and LDL. When a lipid panel is ordered, the levels include all of the following: total cholesterol, triglycerides, HDL, LDL, very-low–density lipoproteins (VLDL), ratio of total cholesterol to HDL, and ratio of LDL to HDL. Lipid levels are important to health status and are indicators of health; if there are abnormalities (e.g., high cholesterol, triglycerides, HDL, VLDL and LDL levels), the individual is at increased risk for heart disease and stroke. Dietary and other lifestyle changes may be implemented to help decrease the bad cholesterol levels (LDL and VLDL) and elevate the good cholesterol levels (HDL). Medical treatment protocols may also be implemented to help prevent heart attack and strokes.

The values in this table are provided by the National Cholesterol Education Program (NCEP) of the National Institutes of Health (NIH).

dose as much as possible and then dilute any undissolved portion with additional fluid. The powder should be dissolved for at least 1 full minute without stirring. Stirring is not recommended with most powders because it causes them to clump. Powder and/or granule dosage forms are *never* to be taken in dry form. It is important that colestipol be taken 1 hour before or 4 to 6 hours after any other oral medication and/or meals because of the high risk for drug–drug or drug–food interactions. Cholestyramine should be taken just before meals or with meals and never given to a patient with PKU because it contains aspartame (see previous discussion). To prevent injuries from falls, patients should be encouraged to change positions slowly and to lie down should they get dizzy (from orthostatic changes).

With niacin, flushing of the face may occur, and the patient should be aware of this side effect. Postural hypotensive adverse effects demand that the patient change positions slowly and with caution, as well as lie down should further dizziness occur. To minimize the gastrointestinal upset, patients should take these medications with fluids or food. With niacin, aspirin and careful drug titrating after a doctor's order may help to minimize some of the adverse effects, including flushing of the skin and hyperuricemia.

◆ EVALUATION

Evaluation of goals and outcome criteria is the best place to begin when trying to evaluate the therapeutic versus adverse effects of these medications. In addition, cholesterol and triglyceride levels are used to monitor the patient's response to the medication regimen and specific levels are mentioned in the nursing assessment. While on antilipemics and integrated as a part of a change in lifestyle, patients remain on a low-fat, low-cholesterol diet. Patients receiving an antilipemic drug need to be monitored for therapeutic and adverse effects during their therapy. The therapeutic effects of both nonpharmacologic and pharmacologic measures are evidenced by a decrease in cholesterol and triglyceride levels to within normal levels (see previous serum laboratory values). Another commonly monitored marker, as a risk factor for atherosclerotic heart disease, is *C-reactive protein*. Any elevation of this protein is associated with greater risk for major ischemic heart disease (e.g., myocardial infarction). Nonpharmacologic measures include a low-fat, low-cholesterol diet; supervised, moderate exercise; weight loss; cessation of smoking and drinking; and relaxation therapy. If there is no response to pharmacologic therapy after about 3 months, the medication is generally withdrawn. Fenofibrate may be increased at 4- to 8-week intervals depending on the triglyceride levels. Adverse effects to monitor for include gastrointestinal upset, increased liver enzyme levels, hepatomegaly, myalgias, and other effects mentioned earlier in the chapter. Patients should be closely monitored for baseline renal/liver function and throughout the treatment regimen for the development of liver or renal dysfunction.

Patient Teaching Tips

- Encourage patients to notify their health care providers should there be any new or troublesome symptoms or if there is persistent gastrointestinal upset, constipation, gas, bloating, heartburn, nausea, vomiting, abnormal or unusual bleeding, and yellow discoloration of the skin. Other symptoms to report include muscle pain, decreased sex drive, impotence, and difficulty urinating.
- All medications—including antilipemics—must be kept out of the reach of children and protected with childproof lids/tops.
- Educate patients about the need for eating plentiful amounts of raw vegetables, fruit, and bran and at least 2000 mL of fluids a day to prevent the constipation that is commonly experienced with antilipemics.
- Patients should inform all health care providers about all medications they are taking, including OTC medications and herbal products.
- Inform patients to let all health care providers know about all medications they are taking, including antilipemics. These drugs are highly protein-bound, and, therefore, they are associated with many drug interactions, including drugs that a dentist may prescribe. In addition, these drugs may alter clotting if taken on a long-term basis, and, therefore, bleeding with dental work may occur.
- Educate patients about early signs of a peptic ulcer, including nausea and abdominal discomfort followed by abdominal pain and distention, and that these should be reported immediately to their physician.

- Inform patients to engage in moderate daily exercise as ordered by their physician and with supervision at first—especially if not used to exercising—and to change positions slowly due to possible dizziness and potential for falls.
- If a once-a-day dosage scheme is chosen, the medications should be taken with the evening meal.
- Encourage patients to store these medications away from heat and moisture to avoid alteration in the drug and its components.
- With the HMG-CoA reductase inhibitors or "statin" drugs, educate patients about the following measures: (1) Take the medication with at least 6 oz of water or with meals to help minimize gastric upset. (2) It may take several weeks before therapeutic results are seen, and frequent laboratory testing will occur at about every 3 to 6 months. (3) If taking one of the "statin" drugs, an ophthalmic examination is needed prior to and during therapy due to the problems reported with visual acuity. (4) Other side effects may include a decrease in libido, and if there are any severe muscle aches or pain, chest pain, or other unexplained pain, patients should contact their physician immediately.
- If patients are taking a bile acid sequestrant, make sure they contact their health care provider immediately should stools appear black and tarry.
- All patients should receive nutritional consultation and menu planning assistance related to a low-fat diet.
- Encourage patients to never abruptly discontinue their medication.

Points To Remember

- There are two primary forms of lipids: triglycerides and cholesterol.
- Triglycerides function as an energy source and are stored in adipose (fat) tissue.
- Cholesterol is primarily used to make steroid hormones, cell membranes, and bile acids.
- Lipids and lipoproteins participate in the formation of atherosclerotic plaque, which leads to CHD and nurses need to understand the pathology involved in this disease process so that proper/appropriate patient education may occur.
- Nurses need to understand that when plaque forms in the blood vessels that supply the heart with needed oxygen and nutrients, there will be eventual decrease in the lumen size of blood vessels and a reduction of oxygen and nutrients that can reach the heart.
- Antilipemic drugs are used to lower the high levels of lipids within the blood (triglycerides and cholesterol).
- The major classes of antilipemics are:
  - HMG–CoA reductase inhibitors
  - Bile acid sequestrants
  - Niacin
  - Fibric acid derivatives
  - Cholesterol absorption inhibitor (Zetia)

- The mechanisms of action vary with each class and each drug.
- Nurses need to thoroughly understand the effects of the HMG—CoA reductase inhibitors and that they lower blood cholesterol levels by decreasing the rate of cholesterol production and inhibit the enzyme necessary for the liver to produce cholesterol.
- While taking a nursing history, it is important for the nurse to assess the patient for any possible drug interactions and for a history of PKU (as related to use of cholestyramine).
- Fat-soluble vitamins may need to be prescribed for patients taking these medications long-term because the antilipemics have long-term effects on the liver's production of these vitamins.
- When using the powder or granule oral-based forms of these drugs, they must be mixed with noncarbonated liquids and *never* taken dry.
- Monitoring for adverse effects with the antilipemics includes monitoring liver and renal function studies.
- The statins have gained much attention for their adverse effects of muscle aches and pain due to breakdown of muscle tissue. Some patients suffer irreversible renal damage and severe pain and may have to switch dosages or drugs as ordered by their health care provider.

NCLEX Examination Review Questions

1. The nurse is administering a bile acid sequestrant drug, and implements which action to help to reduce adverse effects?
   a. Taking the medication with grapefruit juice.
   b. Taking a small dose of aspirin or a NSAID 30 minutes before the dose.
   c. Taking the medication dry without mixing it.
   d. Increasing dietary fiber intake.
2. When administering niacin, the nurse needs to monitor for which adverse effect?
   a. Cutaneous flushing
   b. Low back pain
   c. Headache
   d. Constipation
3. Which point is important to emphasize to a patient taking an antilipemic medication?
   a. Take on an empty stomach before meals.
   b. A low-fat diet is not necessary while on these medications.
   c. It is important to report muscle pain as soon as possible.
   d. Improved cholesterol levels should be evident within 2 weeks.
4. When assessing a patient before giving a new order for an antilipemic medication, which condition would be a potential contraindication?
   a. Diabetes insipidus
   b. Pulmonary fibrosis
   c. Elevated liver studies
   d. Hyperlipidemia
5. A patient currently taking a statin may have a higher risk of developing rhabdomyolysis when also taking which product?
   a. NSAIDs
   b. Gemfibrozil
   c. Orange juice
   d. Fat soluble vitamins

1. d; 2. a; 3. c. 4. c. 5. b.

Critical Thinking Activities

1. Flushing of the face and neck may occur with the administration of nicotinic acid. What would you suggest to a patient to help decrease these reactions and their unpleasantness?
2. Is the following statement true or false? Explain your answer. Antilipemics may be safely taken without concern of other medications, especially prescribed medications, and may be discontinued abruptly.
3. Your patient has just informed you that he was told that it was okay to take his colestipol powder without fluids. Are you concerned about this? Explain your answer.

For answers, see http://evolve.elsevier.com/Lilley.

Drugs Affecting the Endocrine System

STUDY SKILLS TIPS

- *Questioning Strategy*

QUESTIONING STRATEGY

One of the most important activities for learning is to become actively involved with the text. The best way to achieve this involvement is to develop the habit of asking questions. These questions can be generated using a number of different cues and structures that are part of the part and chapter structure. Some of what you anticipate as related material will not be correct, so you will adjust your expectations as you read the material. For now, focus on asking a lot of questions and making use of everything you know, which can help start the process of answering your questions.

Part Title

As you begin each new part, ask a question to focus your attention, seeking to learn what all the chapters in this part have in common. In Part Five, this question is: "What is the endocrine system?" This same question could be asked of Parts Two through Nine by simply replacing *endocrine* with the appropriate system for the specific part. Looking at the chapter titles in the part tells us that the endocrine system has to do with the pituitary drugs, thyroid and antithyroid drugs, antidiabetic and hypoglycemic drugs, adrenal drugs, women's health drugs, and men's health drugs. Although this answer is far too general to demonstrate any real understanding of the endocrine system, it is a beginning and helps keep you aware of what you need to learn from each chapter.

Chapter Titles

Chapter titles provide the first mechanism that can be used to generate questions. The first question to ask about each chapter is a very basic one, involving what the chapter is about. That question is also answered immediately. "What is Chapter 29 about?" It is about pituitary drugs.

The next question is equally obvious but also extremely important. The question to ask next is, "To what do pituitary (Chapter 29), thyroid and antithyroid (Chapter 30), antidiabetic (Chapter 31), adrenal (Chapter 32), women's health (Chapter 33), and

men's health (Chapter 34) refer?" Take the chapter title and state it as a question. What do you know about these subjects?

Chapter Objectives

To enhance your study, turn each chapter objective into one or more questions. Here are some possible questions using the objectives from Chapter 31.

Objective 1: Discuss the normal actions and functions of the pancreas and their regulation by a feedback system.

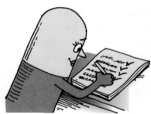

- What are the normal actions and functions of the pancreas?
- What is the feedback system for the pancreas?

Objective 2: Contrast type 1 and type 2 diabetes mellitus with regard to age of onset, signs and symptoms, pharmacologic and nonpharmacologic treatment, drug therapy, incidence, and etiology.

- What is type 1 diabetes mellitus?
- What is type 2 diabetes mellitus?
- How do types 1 and 2 diabetes mellitus differ in age of onset, signs and symptoms, treatment, drug therapy, incidence, and etiology?

Because the objectives tell you what the authors expect you to know at the end of the chapter, starting out with questions based on the objectives will improve your learning and probably save you time.

Chapter Headings

The same principle can be applied to each of the topic headings set out in the chapter. Continuing to use Chapter 31 as a model, here are some samples of questions that might be useful as preparation for reading.

Type 1 Diabetes Mellitus

- What is type 1 diabetes?
- What is mellitus?

As you start to process the chapter headings, you should also notice that they begin to answer some of the questions from the chapter objectives. This is a good time to begin setting up vocabulary cards.

Mechanism of Action and Drug Effects

- What is the mechanism of action of insulin?
- Is there more than one mechanism?
- What are the most important drug effects of insulin?
- Where do these effects take place?
- What is the evidence of these effects?

The idea is to focus on the major content of the chapter and establish a guide for learning as you read.

Print Conventions Within the Body of the Chapter

Print conventions are useful in this study skills strategy. The use of *italics,* **bold,** <u>underlining</u>, and multiple colors of ink are examples of print conventions. They are designed to catch your attention. Use them as a basis for questions.

In the first paragraph of Chapter 31, the first obvious print convention is the word **insulin**. It is printed in bold. If you let your eyes float down the page and do not read anything, this word stands out. It must be important.

- What is insulin?
- What is the relationship between insulin and type 1 diabetes mellitus?

There are more words on the first page of the chapter text that are in the same print style. Apply the same procedure to these terms. Also, notice that two of the terms, **glycogen** and **glycogenolysis,** must have some direct relationship because the second term contains the first term. The basic question in each case is, "What does the term mean?" However, there should be more to your questions than just the basics. *Glycogenolysis* seems to mean that there is some operation or activity taking place. Ask yourself the following:

- What happens in glycogenolysis?
- Where does glycogenolysis occur?
- When does glycogenolysis occur?
- How does it relate to type 1 diabetes mellitus?

Chapter Tables

Tables serve as a summary of information discussed in the chapter. You can learn a great deal from tables if you take the time.

Look at Table 31-1. The table summarizes characteristics of type 1 and type 2 diabetes. There are two obvious questions for each type.

- What is type 1 (and type 2) diabetes?
- What are its characteristics?

Use these questions to study Table 31-1 and you will find that all the information you need to respond to these questions is found here. It may be useful to make a first pass throughout the chapter focusing only on the tables before you begin to read. You will learn a great deal about some of the topics, and you will have established background information that will help you ask better questions and read with better understanding.

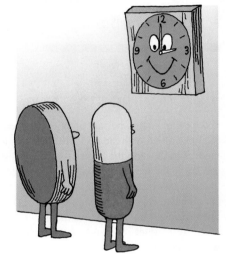

The time you spend asking questions makes the reading and learning go more quickly. Another benefit is that some of the questions you ask appear on tests. These questions will be easy for you to answer. This promotes test-taking confidence, and better test scores result in better grades. If you have not been using questioning strategy up to this point in your text, begin now. After you use the strategy for two or three chapters, you will find that the benefits far outweigh the time it takes.

Pituitary Drugs

CHAPTER 29

Objectives

When you reach the end of this chapter, you should be able to do the following:

1. Describe the normal function of the anterior and posterior segments of the pituitary gland and the impact of the pituitary gland on the human body.
2. Compare the various pituitary drugs as related to their indications, mechanisms of action, dosages, routes of administration, adverse effects, cautions, contraindications, and drug interactions.
3. Develop a nursing care plan that includes all phases of the nursing process for patients receiving pituitary drugs, such as corticotrophin, desmopressin, octreotide, somatropin, and vasopressin.

e-Learning Activities

Companion CD

- NCLEX Review Questions: see questions 258-264
- Animations
- Audio Glossary
- Category Catchers
- Medication Errors Checklists
- IV Therapy Checklists

evolve Website (http://evolve.elsevier.com/Lilley)

- Nursing Care Plans • Frequently Asked Questions • Content Updates • WebLinks • Supplemental Resources • Elsevier ePharmacology Update • Medication Administration Animations

Drug Profiles

▶ corticotropin, p. 460

▶ Key drug.

Glossary

Hypothalamus   The gland above and behind the pituitary gland and the **optic chiasm** from which both glands are suspended beneath the middle area of the bottom of the brain. It secretes the hormones vasopressin and oxytocin, which are stored in the posterior pituitary, and also secretes several hormone-releasing factors that stimulate the anterior pituitary to secrete a variety of hormones that control many body functions. (p. 457)

Negative feedback loop   In endocrinology, where the production of one hormone by its source gland is controlled by the levels of a second hormone, which is produced by a second gland after being stimulated by the hormone from the first gland. The source gland of the first hormone then reduces production of that hormone, until blood levels of the second hormone fall below a certain minimum level needed for specific hormonal effects, then the cycle begins again. (p. 458)

Neuroendocrine system   The system that regulates the reactions of the organism to both internal and external stimuli and involves the integrated activities of the endocrine glands and nervous system. (p. 457)

Optic chiasm   The part of the hypothalamus formed by the crossing of optic nerve fibers from the medial half of each retina. (p. 457)

Pituitary gland   An endocrine gland suspended beneath the brain that supplies numerous hormones that control many vital processes. (p. 458)

ENDOCRINE SYSTEM

The maintenance of physiologic stability is the main goal of the endocrine system, and it must accomplish this task despite constant changes in the internal and external environments. Every cell, and hence organ, in the body comes under its influence. The endocrine system communicates with the nearly 50 million target cells in the body using a chemical "language" called *hormones.* These are a large group of natural substances with chemical structures that are highly specific for causing physiologic effects in the cells of their target tissues. They are secreted into the bloodstream in response to the body's needs and travel through the blood to their site of action—the target cell.

For decades the pituitary gland was believed to be the master gland that regulated and controlled the other endocrine glands in this very diverse system. However, the discovery of strong evidence that the central nervous system (CNS), specifically the **hypothalamus**, controls the pituitary has caused this older belief to be discarded. The hypothalamus and pituitary are now viewed as functioning together as an integrated unit, with the primary direction coming from the hypothalamus. For this reason, the system is now commonly referred to as the **neuroendocrine system.** In fact, the endocrine system can be considered in much the same way as the CNS. Each is basically a system for signaling, and each operates in a stimulus-and-response manner. Together these two systems essentially govern all bodily functions.

The **pituitary gland** is made up of two distinct glands—the anterior pituitary (adenohypophysis) and posterior pituitary (neurohypophysis). They are individually linked to and communicate with the hypothalamus, and each gland secretes its own different set of hormones. These various hormones are listed in Box 29-1 and shown in Figure 29-1.

Hormones are either water or lipid soluble. The water-soluble hormones are protein-based substances such as the catecholamines norepinephrine and epinephrine. The receptors for these hormones are usually located on cell membranes. These hormones bind to their receptors on the cell surface, whereupon they either directly activate the cell to perform a function or cause a chemical signal to be sent by means of a "second messenger" inside the cell to generate an appropriate cellular response. The lipid-soluble hormones consist of the steroid and thyroid hormones. They are capable of crossing the plasma membrane through the process of simple diffusion and of binding with receptors within the cell nucleus, where they stimulate a specific cellular response.

The activity of the endocrine system is regulated by a system of surveillance and signaling usually dictated by the body's ongoing needs. Hormone secretion is commonly regulated by the **negative feedback loop.** This is best explained using a fictional ex-

ample: When gland X releases hormone X, this stimulates target cells to release hormone Y. When there is an excess of hormone Y, gland X "senses" this and inhibits its release of hormone X.

PITUITARY DRUGS

There are a variety of drugs that affect the pituitary gland. They are generally used for the following purposes: as replacement drug therapy to make up for a hormone deficiency; and as diagnostic aids to determine whether there is hypofunction or hyperfunction of a patient's hormonal functions. The currently identified anterior and posterior pituitary hormones and the drugs that mimic or antagonize their actions are listed in Table 29-1. Many of these hormones have been synthesized, and some of them have already been discussed in other chapters.

The anterior pituitary drugs discussed in this chapter include corticotropin, somatotropin, somatrem, and octreotide; the posterior pituitary drugs discussed in this chapter consist of vasopressin and desmopressin.

Mechanism of Action and Drug Effects

The mechanisms of action of the various pituitary drugs differ depending on the drug, but overall they either augment or antagonize the natural effects of the pituitary hormones. Exogenously administered corticotropin elicits all of the same pharmacologic responses as those elicited by the endogenous corticotropin (also known as *adrenocorticotropic hormone [ACTH]*). Regardless of whether it is exogenous or endogenous in origin, corticotropin travels to the adrenal cortex located just above the kidneys and stimulates the secretion of cortisol (the drug form of which is hydrocortisone [Solu-Cortef]). Cortisol has many antiinflammatory effects, including reduction of inflammatory leukocyte functions, edema, and scar tissue formation. Cortisol also promotes renal retention of sodium, which can result in edema and hypertension.

The drugs that mimic growth hormone (GH) are somatropin and somatrem. These drugs promote growth by stimulating vari-

---

Box 29-1   Hormones of the Anterior and Posterior Pituitary

Anterior Pituitary Adenohypophysis
- Adrenocorticotropic hormone (ACTH)
- Follicle-stimulating hormone (FSH)
- Growth hormone (GH)
- Luteinizing hormone (LH)
- Prolactin (PH)
- Thyroid-stimulating hormone (TSH)

Posterior Pituitary (Neurohypophysis)
- Antidiuretic hormone (ADH)
- Oxytocin

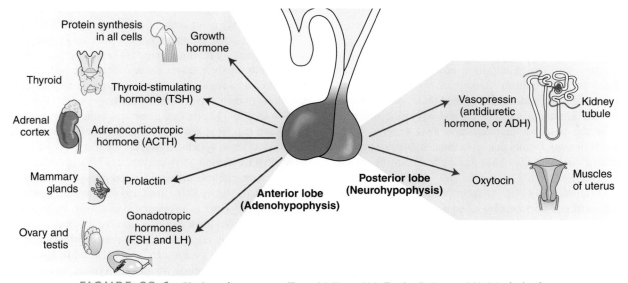

FIGURE 29-1   Pituitary hormones. *(From McKenry LM, Tessier E, Hogan MA:* Mosby's pharmacology in nursing, *ed 22, St Louis, 2006, Mosby.)*

Table 29-1   Anterior and Posterior Pituitary Hormones and Drugs

Hormone	Function/Mimicking Drug
Anterior Pituitary	
Adrenocorticotropic hormone	Targets adrenal gland; mediates adaptation to physical and emotional stress and starvation; redistributes body nutrients; promotes synthesis of adrenocortical hormone (glucocorticoids, mineralocorticoids, androgens); involved in skin pigmentation. *Corticotropin*: Diagnosis of adrenocortical insufficiency.
Follicle-stimulating hormone	Stimulates oogenesis and follicular growth in females and spermatogenesis in males. *Menotropins*: Same pharmacologic effects as FSH; many of the other gonadotropins also stimulate FSH (Chapter 33).
Growth hormone	Regulates anabolic processes related to growth and adaptation to stressors; promotes skeletal and muscle growth; increases protein synthesis; increases liver glycogenolysis; increases fat mobilization. *Somatropin, somatrem*: Human GH for hypopituitary dwarfism. *Octreotide*: A synthetic polypeptide structurally and pharmacologically similar to GH release-inhibiting factor; it inhibits GH.
Luteinizing hormone	Stimulates ovulation and estrogen release by ovaries in females; stimulates interstitial cells in males to promote spermatogenesis and testosterone secretion. *Gonadotropins*: Many of the drugs discussed in Chapter 33 stimulate LH.
Prolactin	Targets mammary glands; stimulates lactogenesis and breast growth. *Bromocriptine*: Inhibits action of PH and therefore inhibits lactogenesis (Chapter 14).
Thyroid-stimulating hormone	Stimulates secretion of thyroid hormones T_3 and T_4 by the thyroid. *Thyrotropin*: Increases the production and secretion of thyroid hormones (Chapter 30).
Posterior Pituitary	
Antidiuretic hormone	Increases water resorption in distal tubules and collecting duct of nephron; concentrates urine; causes potent vasoconstriction. *Vasopressin*: ADH; performs all the physiologic functions of ADH. *Desmopressin*: A synthetic vasopressin.
Oxytocin	Targets mammary glands; stimulates ejection of milk and contraction of uterine smooth muscle. *Pitocin*: Has all the physiologic actions of oxytocin (see Chapter 33).

ADH, Antidiuretic hormone; *FSH,* follicle-stimulating hormone; *GH,* growth hormone; *LH,* luteinizing hormone; *PH, prolactin; T_3,* triiodothyronine; *T_4,* thyroxine.

ous anabolic (tissue-building) processes, including nitrogen retention and increased cellular protein synthesis; liver glycogenolysis (to raise blood sugar levels); lipid mobilization from body fat stores; and retention of sodium, potassium, and phosphorus. Both drugs promote linear growth in children who lack normal amounts of the endogenous hormone.

A drug that antagonizes the effects of the natural GH is octreotide, and it does so by inhibiting GH release. It is a synthetic polypeptide that is structurally and pharmacologically similar to GH release–inhibiting factor, which is also called *somatostatin.* It also reduces plasma concentrations of vasoactive intestinal polypeptide (VIP), a protein secreted by a type of tumor known as *VIPoma* that causes profuse watery diarrhea.

The drugs that affect the posterior pituitary, such as vasopressin and desmopressin, mimic the actions of the naturally occurring antidiuretic hormone (ADH). They increase water resorption in the distal tubules and collecting ducts of the nephrons, and concentrate urine, reducing water excretion by up to 90%. Vasopressin is also a potent vasoconstrictor (hence, its name) in larger doses, and is, therefore, used in certain hypotensive emergencies. Desmopressin causes a dose-dependent increase in the plasma levels of factor VIII (antihemophilic factor), von Willebrand's factor (acts closely with factor VIII), and tissue plasminogen activator. These properties make it useful in certain blood disorders. The drug form of oxytocin mimics the endogenous hormone, promoting uterine contractions (Chapter 33).

Indications

Corticotropin is used in the diagnosis of, but not usually the treatment of, adrenocortical insufficiency. Upon diagnosis, the actual drug therapy generally involves replacement hormonal therapy using drug forms of the deficient corticosteroid hormones. These drugs are discussed in more detail in Chapter 32. Corticotropin is also used for the treatment of multiple sclerosis and corticotropin insufficiency caused by long-term corticosteroid use (e.g., prednisone therapy in asthma patients). Its antiinflammatory and immunosuppressant properties may also be useful in patients with normal adrenocortical function. Somatropin and somatrem are recombinantly make human GH. They are effective in stimulating skeletal growth in patients suffering from an inadequate secretion of normal endogenous GH, such as those with hypopituitary dwarfism. Octreotide is of benefit in alleviating certain symptoms of carcinoid tumors stemming from the secretion of VIP, including severe diarrhea and flushing and potentially life-threatening hypotension associated with a carcinoid crisis. Vasopressin and desmopressin are used to prevent or control polydipsia (excessive thirst), polyuria, and dehydration in patients with diabetes insipidus caused by a deficiency of endogenous ADH. Because of their vasoconstrictor properties, they are useful in the treatment of various types of bleeding, in particular gastrointestinal hemorrhage. Because of its effects on various blood-clotting factors, desmopressin is also useful in the treatment of hemophilia A and type I von Willebrand's disease. Vasopressin and desmopressin are also occasionally used after cranial surgery that may involve the pituitary gland.

Table 29-2 Corticotropin: Common Adverse Effects

Body System	Adverse Effects
Central nervous	Convulsions, dizziness, euphoria, insomnia, headache, depression, psychosis
Endocrine	Diabetes
Gastrointestinal	Nausea, vomiting, peptic ulcer perforation, pancreatitis
Genitourinary	Water and sodium retention, hypokalemia
Musculoskeletal	Hypocalcemia with possible pathologic bone fractures
Ocular	Cataracts
Other	Sweating, acne, hyperpigmentation, weakness, muscle atrophy, myalgia, arthralgia

Table 29-3 Desmopressin and Vasopressin: Common Adverse Effects

Body System	Adverse Effects
Cardiovascular	Increased blood pressure
Central nervous	Drowsiness, headache, lethargy, flushing
Gastrointestinal	Nausea, heartburn, cramps
Genitourinary	Uterine cramping
Other	Nasal irritation and congestion, tremor, sweating, vertigo

BP, Blood pressure.

Table 29-4 Growth Hormone Analogs: Common Adverse Effects

Body System	Adverse Effects
Central nervous	Headache
Endocrine	Hyperglycemia, ketosis, hypothyroidism
Genitourinary	Hypercalciuria
Other	Rash, urticaria, antibodies to GH, inflammation at injection site

GH, Growth hormone.

Contraindications

Contraindications for the use of pituitary drugs vary with each individual drug and are listed in each of the drug profiles included in this chapter. Because even small amounts of these drugs can initiate major physiologic changes, all of them should be used with special caution in patients with such acute or chronic illnesses such as migraine headaches, epilepsy, and asthma.

Adverse Effects

Most of the adverse effects of the pituitary drugs are specific to the individual drug. Those drugs possessing similar hormonal effects generally have similar adverse effects. The most common adverse effects of the pituitary drugs described here are listed in Tables 29-2 to 29-4.

Interactions

Selected interactions involving pituitary drugs are summarized in Table 29-5.

Dosages

For the recommended dosages of pituitary drugs, see the Dosages table on page 461.

Drug Profiles

▶ corticotropin

Corticotropin (Acthar) is contraindicated in patients who have shown a hypersensitivity to it; in those with scleroderma, osteoporosis, heart failure, peptic ulcer disease, hypertension, or primary adrenocortical insufficiency or hyperfunction; and in those who have undergone recent surgery. It is available in two parenteral forms, a regular form that may be given by intravenous (IV), intramuscular (IM), or subcutaneous (SC) injection, and a repository form, which may be given intramuscularly or subcutaneously, that has more prolonged effects. Pregnancy category C. Common dosages are listed in the table on page 461.

Pharmacokinetics

Half-Life	Onset	Peak	Duration
Unknown	Rapid	1 hr	3 days*

*For repository form.

Table 29-5 Selected Drug Interactions Involving Pituitary Drugs

Pituitary Drug	Interacting Drug	Potential Result
Corticotropin (ACTH)	Diuretics, amphotericin B	Enhanced urinary potassium loss
	Aspirin	Reduced salicylate levels and efficacy
	Barbiturates, hydantoins (e.g., phenytoin)	Reduced ACTH efficacy; reduced phenytoin efficacy
Desmopressin	Carbamazepine, chlorpropamide, clofibrate	Enhanced desmopressin effects
	Lithium, alcohol, demeclocycline, heparin	Reduced desmopressin effects
Octreotide	Cyclosporine	Case report of transplant rejection
	Vitamin B₁₂	Reduced vitamin B_{12} levels (monitor B_{12} levels with chronic therapy)
Somatropin and somatrem	Glucocorticoids	Reduction of growth effects
Vasopressin	Carbamazepine, fludrocortisone, tricyclic antidepressants	Enhanced antidiuretic effect
	Demeclocycline, norepinephrine, lithium, heparin, alcohol	Reduced antidiuretic effect

DOSAGES

Selected Pituitary Drugs

Drug	Pharmacologic Class	Usual Dosage Range	Indications
▸corticotropin (Acthar, ACTH; Repository IM dosage forms: H.P. Acthar Gel, ACTH-80)	Adrenal cortex stimulating hormone	**Adult*** IV: 10-25 units in 500 mL of D5W over 8 hr IM: 80-120 units/day×2-3 wk IM, SC repository injection: 40-80 units q24-72h	Diagnosis of adrenocortical insufficiency Exacerbation of multiple sclerosis
desmopressin (DDAVP, Stimate)	ADH, antihemophilic hormone	Adult and pediatric ≥6 yr Intranasal spray only: 0.1-0.4 mL (10-40 mcg) qhs **Adult** Intranasal: 0.1-0.4 mL divided qd-tid IV/SC: 0.5-1 mL divided bid Pediatric 3 mo-12 yr Intranasal spray: 0.05-0.3 mL divided qd-bid **Adult and pediatric** PO: Initial dose, both adult and pediatric, is 0.05 mg tab with careful titration upward as needed based on diurnal response **Adult and pediatric** IV infusion: 0.3 mcg/kg, diluted in 50 mL of NS (use 10 mL of saline diluent in patients weighing <10 kg) Intranasal spray: 1 spray per nostril (300 mcg total dose); use a single spray (150 mcg) in patients weighing <50 kg	Primary nocturnal enuresis Central cranial diabetes insipidus Hemophilia A and type 1 von Willebrand's disease
octreotide (Sandostatin, Sandostatin LAR Depot)	Somatostatin (GH inhibitor) analog	**Adult†** IV/SC: Initial dose of 50 mcg bid-tid; may titrate up to 500 mcg tid IV/SC: 100-750 mcg/day divided bid-qid Depot IM: 10-30 mg q4wk	Acromegaly Metastatic carcinoid tumors (to control flushing and diarrhea symptoms) VIPomas
somatrem (Protropin)	GH analog	IM/SC: Calculate a maximum weekly dose of up to 0.3 mg/kg and divide this dose into 6-7 daily injections	Growth failure
somatropin (Genotropin, Humatrope, Serostim, others)	GH analog	**Adult and pediatric** Dosages vary widely among the many products on the market; a typical dosage regimen is on the order of 0.16-0.24 mg/kg/wk divided into 6-7 daily IM or SC injections; consult product insert.	Growth failure; AIDS-related wasting syndrome (Serostim only)
vasopressin (Pitressin)	Natural or synthetic ADH	**Adult** IM/SC 5-10 units bid-qid Pediatric 2.5-10 units bid-qid	Diabetes insipidus; prevention or treatment of postoperative abdominal distension; dispersal of abdominal gas to improve imaging in abdominal x-ray studies

*Pediatric use is uncommon and should only occur following careful medical evaluation, preferably by a pediatric endocrinologist.
†Normally used only in adults.
ADH, Antidiuretic hormone; *D5W*, 5% dextrose in water; *GH*, growth hormone; *NS*, normal saline.

◆ NURSING PROCESS

◆ ASSESSMENT

Before administering any of the pituitary drugs, the nurse should perform a thorough nursing assessment, obtain a complete medication history, and document findings. Questions about hyper-sensitivity should be posed to the patient and documented. Baseline weight, blood pressure, serum glucose levels, cholesterol, and electrolytes should be assessed and documented.

Contraindications, cautions, and drug interactions for the use of pituitary drugs vary with each individual drug and are listed in each of the drug profiles included in this chapter and in Box 29-2. Small doses of these drugs may initiate major physiologic changes and, as

Box 29-2	**Pituitary Drugs: Assessment Data**

Assessment Parameters	Cautions and Drug Interactions	Contraindications
Corticotropin		
Baseline vital signs	**Cautions:**	Allergy
Electrolyte values	Pregnancy	Osteoporosis
Blood glucose levels	Lactation	Heart failure
Chest x-ray study	Liver disease	Ulcer disease
CBC, I&O, weight	Mental illness	Scleroderma
Cortisol levels	Myasthenia gravis	Fungal infections
Allergy to pork because of	Gout	Recent surgery
cross-sensitivity	Hypothyroidism	Adrenocortical hypo- and
	Latent tuberculosis	hyperfunction
	Clotting disorders	(primary)
	History of tuberculosis (possible reemergence of the disease)	No long-term therapy in
	Seizures	the pediatric patient
	Renal dysfunction	
	Drug Interactions:	
	Alcohol	
	Aspirin	
	Steroids	
	Diuretics	
	Amphotericin B (increases hypokalemia)	
	Oral hypoglycemics	
	Digoxin (increased risk for toxicity)	
	Hepatic enzyme inducers (may decrease drug's effect)	
	Hypocalcemia	
	Live virus vaccines (may lead to viral replication)	
	Insulin	
	Potassium supplements	
Desmopressin		
Vital signs with BP lying and	**Cautions:**	Allergy to drug or to
standing q4h	Depression or suicidal tendencies	TCAs
CBC: Leukocytes	Narrow-angle glaucoma	Glaucoma
Cardiac enzymes	Increased intraocular pressure	MI (recovery phase)
Weight every wk	Seizure disorder	BPH
ECG	Children <12 yr	Seizure disorder
	Chronic migraines	Children <12 yr
	Asthma	
	Drug Interactions:	
	Carbamazepine	
	Chlorpropamide	
	Clofibrate (result in additive effects of the desmopressin)	
	Lithium	
	Alcohol	
	Demeclocycline	
	Heparin (may result in decreased therapeutic effects of the desmopressin)	
Octreotide		
	Cautions:	Allergy
	Insulin-dependent diabetes	
	Chronic renal failure	
	Insulin, oral hypoglycemics, glucagons, and growth hormone (alters blood glucose)	

BP, Blood pressure; *BPH,* benign prostatic hypertrophy; *CBC,* complete blood count; *ECG,* electrocardiogram; *GH,* growth hormone; *I&O,* intake and output; *MI,* myocardial infarction; *TCA,* tricyclic antidepressant.

Box 29-2 Pituitary Drugs: Assessment Data—cont'd

Assessment Parameters	Cautions and Drug Interactions	Contraindications
Somatropin and Somatrem		
Thyroid function studies	**Cautions:**	Drug allergy
GH antibodies	Diabetes mellitus	Intracerebral lesions
	Hypothyroidism	Closed epiphyseal plates
	Pregnancy	
	Cancer	
	Drug interactions:	
	Glucocorticoids	
	Androgens	
	Thyroid hormones	
	Corticosteroids (impaired growth)	
Vasopressin		
Pulse and vital signs, especially	**Cautions:**	Allergy
with IM/IV dosage forms	Coronary artery disease	Chronic renal disease
Intake and output	Pregnancy	
Weight	Migraines	
Edema	Seizures	
	Asthma	
	Vascular disease	
	Renal and cardiac diseases	
	Nephritis	
	Drug interactions:	
	Carbamazepine	
	Clofibrate	
	Lithium	
	Epinephrine	
	Norepinephrine	
	Demeclocycline	
	Heparin	
	Alcohol	
	Chlorpropamide	
	Urea	
	Fludrocortisone	
	Ganglionic blocking drugs (e.g., mecamylamine)	
	Drugs for water loss (e.g., furosemide, mannitol, ethacrynic acid)	
	TCAs (e.g., amitriptyline, nortriptyline)	

IM, Intramuscular; *IV,* intravenous.

such, should be used with special caution in patients with acute or chronic illnesses such as migraine headache, epilepsy, asthma, and other chronic disease processes. Other growth hormones should be avoided when using other drugs that antagonize their effects.

◆ NURSING DIAGNOSES

- Disturbed body image related to specific disease processes or drug adverse effects and their influence on physical characteristics
- Excess fluid volume related to adverse effects of various pituitary drugs
- Fatigue related to the adverse effects associated with the various pituitary drugs
- Acute pain related to gastrointestinal adverse effects of the various pituitary drugs
- Deficient knowledge related to new treatment with various pituitary drugs

◆ PLANNING

Goals

- Patient maintains positive body image.
- Patient maintains normal fluid volume and electrolyte status while on various pituitary drugs.

- Patient returns to normal or pre-therapy levels of activity.
- Patient experiences little to no pain related to medication-induced gastrointestinal upset or epigastric distress.
- Patient remains compliant with medication therapy.
- Patient is without self-injury related to adverse effects of medications.

Outcome Criteria

- Patient openly verbalizes fears, anxieties, and concerns with health care professionals regarding body image changes related to disease process and medication therapy.
- Patient's sodium level is within normal limits while on medication therapy.
- Patient states ways to decrease edema caused by medication, such as dietary precautions.
- Patient experiences minimal gastrointestinal upset and gastric distress by taking medication with food or at mealtimes.
- Patient states measures to employ to diminish the risk for falls related to the musculoskeletal and neurologic (seizures) adverse effects of medication.
- Patient performs activities of daily living and other normal activity without difficulty.

- Patient states the importance of follow-up visits to the physician for monitoring of compliance, therapeutic effects, and adverse reactions.

◆ IMPLEMENTATION

Corticotropin is available in intramuscular, subcutaneous, and intravenous forms and in gel and repository forms. Gel forms should be at room temperature when administered, and intramuscular injections should be administered using a 21-gauge needle. Intravenous injections should be given over 2 minutes, or as designated in the packaging insert, and should be diluted with the recommended amounts of normal saline solution. This drug should never be stopped or doses changed without a physician's order. Patients on long-term therapy will need to be weaned off the drug with medical supervision. Dentists and other physicians involved in the patient's care should be aware of corticotropin therapy up to the previous 12 months. Patients receiving corticotropin should avoid vaccinations during drug therapy. Patients receiving corticotropin and corticotropin-like drugs should be encouraged to maintain adequate hydration of up to 2000 mL per day, unless this is contraindicated. Fluids should be low in sodium content, especially if the patient has cardiac disorders. In addition, doses should not be changed or stopped without a physician's order. It is also very important for the patient to be aware of adverse effects that need to be reported to their physician. These include muscle twitching (positive Trousseau's sign or Chvostek's signs) from possible hypocalcemia, muscle weakness, numbness, tingling and cramping (from hypokalemia), nausea, vomiting, electrocardiographic changes, and irritability. Emotional status, mood, and ability to sleep may be affected by this drug, and, therefore, these adverse effects or problems need to be monitored and documented throughout the entire treatment regimen.

Desmopressin should be administered per physician's orders because it may vary per indication (i.e., diabetes insipidus vs. other forms of pituitary dysfunction). Injection sites for somatropin should be rotated; injections are usually given subcutaneously (somatrem may be given intramuscularly as well). Vasopressin is administered intravenously, into the ventral gluteal muscle, or under the skin in the subcutaneous tissue but only as prescribed by the physician. To minimize adverse effects, drink one or two glasses of water when receiving this medication or as directed by a doctor. Always check the clarity of the parenteral solutions before using the medication. If there are visible particles or any fluid discoloration, the solution should not be used. Be alert to the adverse effects of nausea, diarrhea, pallor, abdominal pain, and flatus (gas). If these worsen or persist, the physician or health care provider should be notified immediately. Severe headache, sweating, chest pain, tremors, heart irregularities, unexplained weight gain, blood in the stool, black tarry stools, and/or seizure activity should be reported to the physician.

◆ EVALUATION

Once goals and outcome criteria have been evaluated, therapeutic responses to these drugs should be evaluated. For corticotropin, there should be less inflammation and improved symptoms as related to the indication. For desmopressin and vasopressin, there should be decreased or elimination of severe thirst and improved urinary output. For somatropin, there is an expectation for increased growth in patients in which it is indicated. For corticotropin and somatropin, expected adverse effects include dependent edema, moon face, pulmonary edema, infection, and mental status changes that include increased aggressive behavior and irritability. Somatropin may increase serum calcium levels. Desmopressin and vasopressin may cause similar adverse effects as corticotropin and somatropin but with additional adverse effects of hypertension, nausea, gastrointestinal upset, tremors, respiratory distress, and drowsiness. Allergic reactions to these drugs may include rash, urticaria, fever, and dyspnea. If these problems occur, the drug should be discontinued and the physician notified.

Patient Teaching Tips

- Patients should avoid alcohol while taking these medications.
- Patients should be encouraged to avoid abrupt discontinuation of these drugs because of the negative impact on pituitary hormones and the impact on blood levels of the various hormones.
- Patients should also be counseled that the medication does not lead to a cure but does help alleviate the symptoms of the disease.
- Routes and techniques of administration should be carefully discussed with the patient and anyone else involved in their care. With pediatric patients, demonstration of the technique of administration should be done with the family or caregiver before discharge and reevaluated with repeat demonstrations. Written instructions should always be used with patients of any age!
- Educate patients to keep a journal about the drug therapy and how the drugs are being tolerated.
- As with any medication or illness, a medical alert bracelet, necklace or card (in the wallet) should be kept on their person at all times.
- Patients should notify their physician if they experience fever, sore throat, joint pain, or muscular pain.

Points to Remember

- The pituitary gland is composed of two distinct glands: anterior and posterior. Each distinct gland has its own set of hormones: *anterior:* thyroid-stimulating hormone (TSH), GH, ACTH, prolactin (PH), follicle-stimulating hormone (FSH), luteinizing hormone (LH); *posterior:* ADH, oxytocin.
- Pituitary drugs are used to either mimic or antagonize the action of endogenous pituitary hormones.
- Drugs that mimic the action of endogenous pituitary hormones include corticotropin, somatropin, somatrem, vasopressin, and desmopressin. Drugs that antagonize the actions of endogenous pituitary hormones include octreotide, which suppresses or inhibits certain symptoms related to carcinoid tumors.

- Nursing assessment for those patients receiving corticotropin should include baseline vital signs, electrolyte values (sodium, potassium, chloride), blood glucose levels, chest x-ray studies, weight, and cortisol levels. Patients taking desmopressin should be assessed with documentation of vital signs, including both supine and standing blood pressure and pulse rates. Other assessment data should include complete blood count (CBC), cardiac and liver enzyme activity, electrocardiogram (ECG), and weight.
- Patients receiving somatropin should have thyroid function and growth hormone levels assessed and documented. Assessment should include vital signs, intake and output amounts, weight, and presence and status of edema.

NCLEX Examination Review Questions

1. During a teaching session for a patient who will be taking corticotropin, the nurse should include which statement?
   a. "Vaccinations should be avoided while on this medication."
   b. "Stop taking the medication if you experience adverse effects."
   c. "Restrict fluids to avoid fluid volume excess."
   d. "Be sure to increase your sodium and potassium intake while on this drug."
2. During an assessment of a patient who has been taking corticotropin for 4 weeks, the nurse recognizes which assessment finding as a possible indication of hypocalcemia?
   a. Joint pain
   b. Muscle twitching
   c. Decreased reflexes
   d. Visual disturbances
3. The nurse is reviewing the medication list for a patient who will be starting therapy with somatropin. Which drug would be a concern that would need to be addressed before the patient starts this new drug?
   a. NSAID therapy for arthritis
   b. Antidepressant therapy
   c. Penicillin
   d. Thyroid hormones

4. A patient who is about to be given corticotropin is also taking a diuretic, intravenous heparin, penicillin, and an opioid as needed for pain. The nurse should be watchful for what possible interaction?
   a. Hypokalemia due to an interaction with the diuretic
   b. Decreased anticoagulation due to an interaction with the heparin
   c. Decreased effectiveness of the penicillin
   d. Increased sedation if the opioid is given
5. When monitoring the therapeutic effects of intranasal desmopressin in a patient who has diabetes insipidus, which assessment would the nurse look for as an indication that the medication therapy is successful?
   a. Increased insulin levels
   b. Decreased diarrhea
   c. Improved nasal patency
   d. Decreased thirst

1. a, 2. b, 3. d, 4. a, 5. d.

Critical Thinking Activities

1. Vasopressin and desmopressin are structurally identical or similar to what endogenous hormone?
2. Discuss the purpose of octreotide therapy for a patient who has a cancerous tumor.

3. Your patient is excited that he is beginning therapy with pituitary drugs and is positive about a cure. What would be your most appropriate response and why?

For answers, see http://evolve.elsevier.com/Lilley.

Objectives

When you reach the end of this chapter, you should be able to do the following:

1. Briefly describe the normal anatomy and physiology of the thyroid gland.
2. Discuss the various functions of the thyroid gland and related hormones.
3. Describe the differences in the diseases resulting from the hyposecretion and hypersecretion of the thyroid gland.
4. Identify the various drugs used to treat the hyposecretion and hypersecretion states of the thyroid gland.
5. Discuss the mechanisms of action, indications, dosages, routes of administration, contraindications, cautions, drug interactions, and adverse effects related to the various drugs used to treat hypothyroidism and hyperthyroidism.
6. Develop a nursing care plan that includes all phases of the nursing process for patients receiving thyroid replacement as well as for patients receiving antithyroid drugs.

e-Learning Activities

Companion CD

- NCLEX Review Questions: see questions 265-271
- Animations
- Audio Glossary
- Category Catchers
- Medication Errors Checklists
- IV Therapy Checklists

evolve Website (http://evolve.elsevier.com/Lilley)

• Nursing Care Plans • Frequently Asked Questions • Content Updates • WebLinks • Supplemental Resources • Elsevier ePharmacology Update • Medication Administration Animations

Drug Profiles

▶ levothyroxine, p. 468 ▶ propylthiouracil, p. 469

▶ Key drug.

Glossary

Hyperthyroidism A condition characterized by excessive production of the thyroid hormones. Also called thyrotoxicosis. (p. 469)

Hypothyroidism A condition characterized by diminished production of the thyroid hormones. (p. 467)

Thyroid-stimulating hormone (TSH) An endogenous substance secreted by the pituitary gland that controls the release of thyroid gland hormones and is necessary for the growth and function of the thyroid gland (also called thyrotropin). As a drug preparation, TSH increases the uptake of radioactive iodine in the thyroid and the secretion of thyroxine by the thyroid gland. (p. 467)

Thyroxine (T$_4$) The principle thyroid hormone that influences the metabolic rate. (p. 466)

Triiodothyronine (T$_3$) A secondary thyroid hormone that also affects body metabolism. (p. 466)

THYROID FUNCTION

The thyroid gland lies across the larynx in front of the thyroid cartilage ("Adam's apple"). Its lobes extend laterally on both sides of the front of the neck. It is responsible for the secretion of three hormones essential for the proper regulation of metabolism: **thyroxine (T$_4$), triiodothyronine (T$_3$),** and calcitonin (Chapter 33). It is also close to and communicates with the parathyroid gland, which lies just above and behind it. The parathyroid gland consists of two pairs of bean-shaped glands. These glands are made up of encapsulated cells, which are responsible for maintaining adequate levels of calcium in the extracellular fluid, primarily by mobilizing calcium from bone.

T$_4$ and T$_3$ are produced in the thyroid gland through the iodination and coupling of the amino acid tyrosine. The iodide (I$^-$, the ionized form of iodine) needed for this process is acquired from the diet, and about 1 mg of iodide is needed per week. This iodide is sequestered by the thyroid gland, where it is absorbed from the blood and concentrated to 20 times its blood level. It is here that it is also converted to iodine (I2), which is combined with the tyrosine to make diiodotyrosine. The combination of two molecules of diiodotyrosine causes the formation of thyroxine, which therefore has four iodine molecules in its structure (T$_4$). Triiodothyronine is formed by the coupling of one molecule of diiodotyrosine with one molecule of monoiodotyrosine, thus it has three iodine molecules in its structure (T$_3$). The biologic potency of T$_3$ is about four times greater than that of T$_4$, but T$_4$ is present in much greater quantities. After the synthesis of these two thyroid hormones, they are stored in a complex with thyroglobulin (a protein that contains tyrosine and an amino acid) in the follicles in the thyroid gland called the *colloid*. When the thyroid gland is signaled to do so, the thyroglobulin–thyroid hormone complex is then enzymatically broken down to release T$_3$ and T$_4$ into the circulation. This entire process is triggered by **thyroid-stimulating hormone (TSH),** also called *thyrotropin.* Its release from the anterior pituitary is stimulated when the blood levels of T$_3$ and T$_4$ are low.

The thyroid hormones are involved in a wide variety of bodily processes. They regulate lipid and carbohydrate metabolism; are essential for normal growth and development; control the heat-regulating system (thermoregulatory center in the brain); and have various effects on the cardiovascular, endocrine, and neuromuscular systems. Therefore, hyperfunction or hypofunction of the thyroid gland can lead to a wide range of serious consequences.

HYPOTHYROIDISM

There are three types of **hypothyroidism.** Primary hypothyroidism stems from an abnormality in the thyroid gland itself and occurs when the thyroid gland is not able to perform one of its many functions, such as releasing the thyroid hormones from their storage sites, coupling iodine with tyrosine, trapping iodide, or converting iodide to iodine, or any combination of these defects. It is the most common of the three types of hypothyroidism. Secondary hypothyroidism begins at the level of the pituitary gland and results from reduced secretion of the TSH needed to trigger the release of the T$_3$ and T$_4$ stored in the thyroid gland. Tertiary hypothyroidism is caused by a reduced level of the thyrotropin-releasing hormone (TRH) from the hypothalamus. This, in turn, reduces TSH and thyroid hormone levels. Knowledge of the underlying cause of the hypothyroidism allows one to treat the cause and by so doing eliminate the deficiency.

Hypothyroidism can also be classified by when it occurs in life. Hyposecretion of thyroid hormone during youth may lead to cretinism. Cretinism is a condition characterized by low metabolic rate, retarded growth and sexual development, and possibly mental retardation. Hyposecretion of thyroid hormone as an adult may lead to myxedema. Myxedema is a condition characterized by decreased metabolic rate but also involves loss of mental and physical stamina, gain in weight, loss of hair, firm edema, and yellow dullness of the skin.

Some forms of hypothyroidism may result in the formation of a goiter, which is an enlargement of the thyroid gland resulting from its overstimulation by elevated levels of TSH. The TSH level is elevated because there is little or no thyroid hormone in the circulation.

THYROID AUGMENTATION DRUGS

All three types of hypothyroidism are amenable to thyroid hormone replacement using various thyroid preparations. These drugs can be either natural or synthetic in origin. The natural thyroid preparations are derived from the thyroids of animals such as cattle and hogs. There is currently only one such preparation available in the United States, which is called simply *thyroid* or *thyroid, desiccated.* Desiccation is the term for the drying process used to prepare this drug form, which basically consists of pulverized animal thyroid gland. All of the natural preparations are standardized according to their iodine content. The synthetic thyroid preparations are levothyroxine (T$_4$), liothyronine (T$_3$),

and liotrix, the latter drug containing a combination of T$_4$ and T$_3$ in a 4:1 ratio. The approximate clinically equivalent doses of the drugs are given in Table 30-1. This information is useful for guiding dosage adjustments when switching a patient from one thyroid hormone to another.

Mechanism of Action and Drug Effects

The thyroid drugs work in the same manner as the endogenous thyroid hormones, affecting many body systems. At the cellular level they work to induce changes in the metabolic rate, including protein, carbohydrate, and lipid metabolism; increase oxygen consumption, body temperature, blood volume, and overall cellular growth and differentiation. These drugs also stimulate the cardiovascular system, by increasing the number of myocardial beta-adrenergic receptors. This in turn, increases the sensitivity of the heart to catecholamines and ultimately increases cardiac output. Additionally, thyroid hormones increase renal blood flow and the glomerular filtration rate, which results in a diuretic effect.

Indications

The thyroid preparations are given to replace what the thyroid gland cannot itself produce to achieve normal thyroid levels (euthyroid). The various thyroid preparations are used in the treatment of all three forms of hypothyroidism, although levothyroxine is generally the preferred drug because its hormonal content is standardized and its effect is therefore predictable. The thyroid drugs can also be used for the diagnosis of suspected hyperthyroidism (as a TSH-suppression test) and in the prevention or treatment of various types of goiters. They are also used for replacement hormonal therapy in patients whose thyroid glands have been surgically removed or destroyed by radioactive iodine in the treatment of thyroid cancer or hyperthyroidism. Hypothyroidism should also be treated during pregnancy, with the dose of prescribed thyroid hormones adjusted every four weeks to maintain the TSH at the lower end of the normal range. Fetal growth may be retarded if maternal hypothroidism is untreated during pregnancy.

Contraindications

Contraindications to thyroid preparations include known drug allergy to a given drug product, recent myocardial infarction (MI), adrenal insufficiency, or hyperthyroidism.

Adverse Effects

The adverse effects of thyroid medications are usually the result of overdose. The most significant adverse effect is cardiac dysrhythmia with the risk for life-threatening or fatal irregu-

Table 30-1	Thyroid Drugs: Clinically Equivalent Doses
Thyroid Drug	**Approximate Equivalent Dose**
Natural Thyroid Preparation	
Thyroid	60-65 mg (1 gr)
Synthetic Thyroid Preparations	
Levothyroxine	≥100 mcg
Liothyronine	25 mcg
Liotrix	50 mcg/12.5 mcg

larities. Other more common undesirable effects are listed in Table 30-2.

Interactions

Thyroid drugs may enhance the activity of oral anticoagulants, which may need reduced doses. Thyroid preparations taken concurrently with digitalis glycosides may decrease serum digitalis levels. Cholestyramine binds to thyroid hormone in the gastrointestinal tract, possibly reducing the absorption of both drugs. Diabetic patients taking a thyroid drug may require increased doses of their hypoglycemic drugs. In addition, the use of thyroid preparations with epinephrine in patients with coronary disease may induce coronary insufficiency.

Dosages

For the recommended dosages of the thyroid drugs, see the dosages table below.

Table 30-2 Thyroid Drugs: Common Adverse Effects

Body System	Adverse Effects
Cardiovascular	Tachycardia, palpitations, angina, dysrhythmias, hypertension, cardiac arrest
Central nervous	Insomnia, tremors, headache, anxiety
Gastrointestinal	Nausea, diarrhea, increased or decreased appetite, cramps
Other	Menstrual irregularities, weight loss, sweating, heat intolerance, fever

Drug Profiles

As previously mentioned, there are several drugs that may be used for hypothyroidism. The most commonly used are the synthetic drugs, although some patients get better results with the animal-derived products. There are many factors that must be considered before the initiation of drug therapy with a thyroid drug. These include the desired ratio of T_3 to T_4, the cost, and the desired duration of effect. The thyroid hormone replacement drugs are classified as pregnancy category A drugs. They are all contraindicated in patients who have had a hypersensitivity reaction to them in the past and in those suffering from adrenal insufficiency, MI, or hyperthyroidism.

▸ *levothyroxine*

Levothyroxine (Levoxyl, Levothroid, Synthroid, others), or T_4, is the most commonly prescribed synthetic thyroid hormone, and is generally considered the drug of choice. One advantage it has over the natural thyroid preparations is that it is chemically pure, being 100% T_4 (thyroxine), making its drug effects more predictable than both natural thyroid products, which contain T_3 and T_4 in varying ratios (depending on the animal source), and synthetic T_3/T_4 combination drugs (e.g., liotrix). Its half-life is long enough that it only needs to be administered once a day. It is available in oral (PO) form and in parenteral form. Pregnancy category A. Liothyronine, liotrix, and desiccated thyroid ("thyroid") are other drug examples. Switching between different brands of levothyroxine during treatment can destabilize the course of treatment and should be minimized. Thyroid function tests should be monitored more carefully when switching is necessary due to drug supply or cost concerns such as the patient's insurance provider drug formulary requirements. Common dosages are given in the table on this page.

Pharmacokinetics

Half-Life	Onset	Peak*	Duration*
9-10 days	2 days	3-4 wk	1-3 wk

*Therapeutic effects.

DOSAGES

Selected Thyroid Drugs

Drug (Trade Names)	Pharmacologic Class	Usual Dosage Range	Indications
▸levothyroxine (Synthroid, Levoxyl, others)	Synthetic levothyroxine (thyroid hormone T_4)	**Adult** PO: 25-300 mcg/day (25-200 mcg/day most common) IM/IV: 50% of oral dose	Hypothyroidism
		IV: 200-500 mcg in a single dose; repeat next day 100-300 mcg if necessary	Myxedema coma
		Pediatric 0-12 yr PO: 25-150 mcg/day	Congenital hypothyroidism
liothyronine* (Cytomel, Triostat)	Synthetic liothyronine (thyroid hormone T_3)	**Adult only** PO: 25-100 mcg/day	Hypothyroidism
		IV: 25-50 mcg/dose	Myxedema coma
liotrix (Thyrolar)	Synthetic thyroid hormone T_3-T_4 combination	**Adult** PO: 15-120 mg/day†	Hypothyroidism
		Pediatric 0-12 yr 25-150 mcg/day‡	Congenital hypothyroidism
thyroid (Armour Thyroid, S-P-T, others)	Desiccated (dried) animal thyroid gland	**Adult** PO: 15-120 mg/day	Hypothyroidism
		Pediatric 0-12 yr 15-90 mg/day	Congenital hypothyroidism

*Liothyronine is synonymous with triiodothyronine (T_3).
†Dose is measured in milligrams of total thyroid activity. See table in drug profile.
‡Dose is measured in micrograms of levothyroxine (T_4) component only. See table in drug profile.

HYPERTHYROIDISM

The excessive secretion of thyroid hormones, or **hyperthyroidism,** may be caused by several different diseases and drugs. Some of the more common diseases are Graves' disease, which is the most common cause; Plummer's disease, which is also known as *toxic nodular disease* and is the least common cause; multinodular disease; and thyroid storm, which is usually induced by stress or infection.

Hyperthyroidism can affect multiple body systems, resulting in an overall increase in metabolism. Commonly reported symptoms are diarrhea, flushing, increased appetite, muscle weakness, fatigue, palpitations, irritability, nervousness, sleep disorders, heat intolerance, and altered menstrual flow.

ANTITHYROID DRUGS

The treatment of hyperthyroidism may be aimed at treating either the primary cause or the symptoms of the disease. Antithyroid drugs, iodides, ionic inhibitors, and radioactive isotopes of iodine are used to treat the underlying cause, and drugs such as β-blockers are used to treat the symptoms. The focus of the discussion here is on the antithyroid drugs called the *thioamide* derivatives, namely methimazole and propylthiouracil. Besides the thioamides, radioactive iodine may be used to treat hyperthyroidism. Radioactive iodine (^{131}I) works by destroying the thyroid gland, in a process known as *ablation.* It does this by emitting destructive beta rays once it is taken up into the follicles of the thyroid gland. It is a commonly used treatment for both hyperthyroidism and also thyroid cancer. Surgery is a nonpharmacologic means of treating hyperthyroidism and involves removal of part or all of the thyroid gland. It is usually a very effective way to treat hyperthyroidism, but lifelong hormone replacement therapy is normally required.

Mechanism of Action and Drug Effects

Methimazole and propylthiouracil act by inhibiting the incorporation of iodine molecules into the amino acid tyrosine, a process required to make both monoiodotyrosine and diiodotyrosine, the precursors of T_3 and T_4. By doing this, the formation of thyroid hormone is impeded. Propylthiouracil has the added ability to inhibit the conversion of T_4 to T_3 in the peripheral circulation. Neither drug can inactivate already existing thyroid hormone, however.

The drug effects of methimazole and propylthiouracil are primarily limited to the thyroid gland, their overall effect being a decrease in the thyroid hormone level. The administration of these medications to patients suffering from hyperthyroidism lowers the high levels of thyroid hormone, thereby normalizing the overall metabolic rate.

Indications

Antithyroid drugs are used to palliate hyperthyroidism and to prevent the surge in thyroid hormones that occurs after the surgical treatment of or during the radioactive iodine therapy for hyperthyroidism or thyroid cancer. In some types of hyperthyroidism, such as that seen in the Graves' disease, the long-term administration of these drugs (several years) may induce a spontaneous remission. Surgical resection of the thyroid *(thy-*

roidectomy) is often used in both patients who are intolerant of antithyroid drug therapy and pregnant women, in whom both antithyroid drugs and radioactive iodine therapy are usually contraindicated.

Contraindications

The only usual contraindications to the use of the two antithyroid drugs is known drug allergy. These drugs should be avoided in pregnancy whenever possible, and, in fact, both are rated pregnancy category D. However, they are sometimes used in the lowest effective dose to treat hyperthyroidism that is exacerbated by the metabolic demands of pregnancy.

Adverse Effects

The most damaging or serious adverse effects of the antithyroid medications are liver and bone marrow toxicity. These and the more common adverse effects of methimazole and propylthiouracil are listed in Table 30-3.

Interactions

Drug interactions that occur with antithyroid drugs include additive leukopenic effects when they are taken in conjunction with other bone marrow depressants and an increase in the activity of oral anticoagulants.

Dosages

See the Dosages table on page 470 for the recommended dosages of methimazole and propylthiouracil.

Drug Profiles

▸ **propylthiouracil**

Propylthiouracil (PTU) is the other thioamide antithyroid drug and is also rated as a pregnancy category D drug. The contraindications to its use are the same as those for methimazole. Approximately 2 weeks of therapy with propylthiouracil may be necessary before symptoms improve. It is available only in oral form as a 50-mg tablet. Methimazole is the only alternative drug in this class. Common dosages are given in the table on page 470.

Table 30-3   Antithyroid Drugs: Common Adverse Effects

Body System	Side/Adverse Effects
Central nervous	Drowsiness, headache, vertigo, fever, paresthesia
Gastrointestinal	Nausea, vomiting, diarrhea, jaundice, hepatitis, loss of taste
Genitourinary	Smoky colored urine, decreased urine output
Hematologic	Agranulocytosis, leukopenia, thrombocytopenia, hypothrombinemia, lymphadenopathy, bleeding
Integumentary	Rash, pruritus, hyperpigmentation
Musculoskeletal	Myalgia, arthralgia, nocturnal muscle cramps
Renal	Increased blood urea nitrogen and serum creatinine
Other	Enlarged thyroid, nephritis

BUN, Blood urea nitrogen.

DOSAGES

Selected Antithyroid Drugs

Drug	Pharmacologic Class	Usual Dosage Range	Indications
methimazole (Tapazole)	Antithyroid	**Adult** PO: 15-60 mg/day **Pediatric** PO: 0.2-0.4 mg/kg/day divided tid; max 30 mg/day	Hyperthyroidism
▶propylthiouracil* (generic only)	Antithyroid	**Adult** 300-900 mg/day **Pediatric 6-10 yr** PO: 50-150 mg/day **Pediatric >10 yr** PO: 150-300 mg/day	

*Often abbreviated PTU.

Pharmacokinetics

Half-Life	Onset	Peak*	Duration
1-2 hr	5 days	17 wk	2-4 hr

*Therapeutic effects.

PHARMACOKINETIC BRIDGE to Nursing Practice

Thyroid replacements possess very specific characteristics—as with many drugs—in regard to their pharmacokinetics. Nurses must understand the pharmacokinetics to critically think their way through a clinical situation with patients who are taking the specific drug. Understanding the specifics of what happens to the various drugs once they have been administered will allow the nurse to be more competent in decision-making with the patient and lead to a more quality, efficient, and knowledge-based nursing care plan.

For the drug levothyroxine (Synthroid, Levothroid, Levoxyl, Novothyrox), the pharmacokinetic characteristics include a half-life of 9 to 10 days, onset of action of 2 days, peak effects within 3 to 4 weeks, and a duration of action of 1 to 3 weeks and takes 4 to 5 days for the drug to be decreased in the body by 50% or to have it eliminated by this amount. Peak effects occur in up to 4 weeks, and the drug will stay in the serum for up to 3 weeks after it has been discontinued. Between the half-life characteristics, the risk for toxicity is of concern because of this prolonged half-life. Toxicity would be manifested by the following: weight loss, tachycardia, nervousness, tremors, hypertension, headache, insomnia, menstrual irregularities, and cardiac irregularities. Another important pharmacokinetic property is that the drug is more than 99% protein bound. A highly protein-bound drug acts like a "biological" sustained release drug and remains in the body longer and so is more likely to be in the serum to react with other drugs (therefore, more drug interactions with highly protein-bound drugs). In addition, the protein-binding characteristic may lead to toxicity due to the drug remaining in the blood for prolonged periods of time.

Knowing the pharmacokinetics of levothyroxine is critical to the safe and efficient administration of the drug. Therefore, based on the drug's pharmacokinetics, we know that the effects of levothyroxine are long-acting and pose more risks. In summary, before moving on to the nursing process, it is important to understand the significance of pharmacokinetics as it applies to this specific drug as a hormone replacement.

◆ NURSING PROCESS

◆ ASSESSMENT

Assessment of the patient taking thyroid supplements for hypothyroidism includes monitoring vital signs to compare to future vital signs. T_3 and T_4 levels should also be assessed before and during drug therapy. Thyroid stimulation hormone (TSH) levels will need to be assessed, as well. It is also important to take a medical history as well as a medication history to be aware of the prescription, nonprescription, and over-the-counter drugs as well any herbal and supplements. Cautions, contraindications, and drug interactions associated with the use of thyroid hormone have been previously discussed and should be assessed prior to the initiation of these drugs. A female's menses may be impacted by changes in hormone levels, so a baseline reproductive/gynecologic history is important. It is also important to remember that certain thyroid hormones may work faster than others (see the Pharmacokinetic Bridge to Nursing Practice section on this page). Lifespan considerations include the elderly because of their increased sensitivity to thyroid effects. Individualization of dosage is recommended because no two patients are ever identical in their response.

For antithyroid drugs, such as propylthiouracil and methimazole, it is important to first assess vital signs as well as signs and symptoms of thyroid crisis or what is often called "thyroid storm." These include tachycardia, cardiac irregularities, fever, heart failure, flushed skin, confusion, apathetic attitude, behavioral changes, possible hypotension, and vascular collapse. Baseline weight and intake/output measurements should also be assessed in patients receiving antithyroid and thyroid preparations. Assessing for thyroid storm also means assessing for potential causes, including thyroidectomy or abrupt withdrawal of antithyroid drugs. Other causes include excess thyroid replacement or failure to give antithyroid medications before thyroid surgery. Related cautions, contraindications, and drug interactions of antithyroid drugs must also be assessed prior to use.

Life Span Considerations: The Elderly Patient
Thyroid Hormones

- The elderly patient is much more sensitive to thyroid hormone replacement therapy (as they are more sensitive to most drugs). They are also more likely to suffer more adverse reactions to thyroid hormones than patients in any other age group.
- They have more consequences because their hepatic and renal functioning is decreased and the drug is highly protein bound.
- The nurse should ensure that the medication regimen in an elderly patient is highly individualized as ordered.
- If elderly patients begin to experience stumbling, falling, depression, incontinence, cold intolerance, and weight gain, they should contact their physician.
- With the elderly, it is also important to note that drug therapy should be initiated with caution and using very individualized dosages. If higher doses are necessary, increases should be with the doctor's guidance and gradually!

♦ **NURSING DIAGNOSES**
- Risk for injury related to the adverse effects of the medication
- Risk for infection related to the bone marrow depression caused by antithyroid medication
- Acute pain related to the adverse effects of the medication
- Decreased cardiac output related to adverse effects of the thyroid drugs
- Deficient knowledge related to lack of experience with self-administration of the medication

♦ **PLANNING**
Goals
- Patient remains free from injury as the result of the adverse effects of the medication.
- Patient is monitored closely (e.g., for thyroid levels) while taking the medication.
- Patient remains free of infection while receiving antithyroid medication.
- Patient maintains normal energy levels while on thyroid drugs.
- Patient experiences minimal adverse effects resulting from the medication.
- Patient demonstrates an understanding of the use of the thyroid drug and its adverse effects and the need for compliance by stating such information.

Outcome Criteria
- Patient states the measures to implement to decrease the likelihood of self-injury related to the drug's adverse effects, such as frequent laboratory checks and monitoring of vital signs.
- Patient states the importance of follow-up appointments with the physician for frequent blood studies and monitoring of therapeutic effects.
- Patient states ways to decrease the risk for infection while receiving an antithyroid medication, such as avoiding persons with infections, eating a proper diet, and getting adequate rest.
- Patient uses relaxation techniques to deal with the nervousness and irritability caused by the drugs or the diseases.

♦ **IMPLEMENTATION**

When administering thyroid drugs, it is important for the nurse to give the medication at the same time each day to maintain consistent blood levels of the drug. If possible, it is best to administer thyroid drugs taken once daily in the morning to decrease the likelihood of insomnia that may result from evening dosing. It is also very important to avoid interchanging brands due to problems with bioequivalence between different manufacturers. Thyroid hormones should be given before breakfast to prevent insomnia because if a thyroid hormone is taken too late in the day, the patient will experience increased energy. If needed, tablets may be crushed. If the patient is scheduled to undergo any radioactive isotope studies, the thyroid medication is usually discontinued about 4 weeks before the test, but only with a physician's order.

♦ **EVALUATION**

A therapeutic response to thyroid drugs is reflected by the disappearance of the symptoms of hypothyroidism, including depression, constipation, loss of appetite, weight gain, cold intolerance, syncope, and dry and brittle hair. Increased nervousness, irritability, mood changes, angina, and palpitations are adverse effects that need to be reported to the physician immediately. Clues that a patient is receiving inadequate doses include a return of the symptoms of hypothyroidism (see previous discussion).

A therapeutic response to antithyroid medications would be characterized by weight gain, decreased pulse, a return to a normal blood pressure, and decreased serum levels of T_4. Symptoms of overdose include cold intolerance, depression, and edema. The patient should be encouraged to report the development of any swelling, sore throat, lesions, or other signs of inflammation. Clues that a patient is not receiving adequate doses include tachycardia, insomnia, irritability, fever, and diarrhea.

Patient Teaching Tips

- Inform patients to never discontinue the drug abruptly and that drug therapy is life-long.
- Emphasize the importance of keeping follow-up visits because thyroid function tests are essential and needed to document therapeutic and/or adverse effects.
- Encourage patients not to interchange brands and to be sure that the pharmacy is refilling their medication with the correct brand.
- Emphasize the importance of reporting chest pain, weight loss, tremors, and insomnia.
- Inform parents and/or caregivers that children may suffer from hair loss at the beginning of therapy but also note that it is reversible.

- Children may experience increased aggressiveness during the first few months of therapy; parents should be educated about this possible behavioral change.
- Patients should be encouraged to keep a journal of daily energy levels and appetite during the initiation of drug therapy.
- Inform patients that it may take up to 3 weeks to see the full therapeutic effects of thyroid drugs.
- Antithyroid medications are better tolerated when taken with meals or a snack. These drugs should also be given at the same time every day to maintain consistent blood levels of the drug, and they should never be withdrawn abruptly.

Continued

Patient Teaching Tips—cont'd

- Encourage patients taking antithyroid (or thyroid) drugs that they should not take any over-the-counter (OTC) medications without physician approval.
- Encourage patients taking antithyroid medications to avoid eating foods high in iodine, such as soy, tofu, turnip, seafood, and some breads.

- Patients should avoid using iodized salt or decrease intake—as prescribed.
- Make sure the patient or caregiver is able to take pulse rate and record it.
- Illnesses, weight gain, cold intolerance, and depression should be reported to the physician immediately.

Points to Remember

- Thyroxine (T_4) and triiodothyronine (T_3) are the two hormones produced by the thyroid gland; thyroid hormone is made by iodination and coupling with the amino acid tyrosine.
- Thyroid replacement is generally done carefully by a health care provider with frequent monitoring of serum levels until there appears to have stabilization. Nurses must monitor and review laboratory values to be sure that serum levels are within normal limits to avoid possible toxicity.
- Hyperthyroidism is caused by excessive secretion of thyroid hormone from the thyroid gland and may be attributed to different diseases (Graves' disease, Plummer's disease, and multinodular

disease) or drugs. Important information about the patient's medical history should always be assessed and documented appropriately.
- Patients should report the occurrence of excitability, irritability, or anxiety to their health care provider because these symptoms may indicate levothyroxine toxicity.
- With antithyroid medications, the nurse should be aware of possible toxic reactions such as agranulocytosis, pancytopenia, and life-threatening hepatitis.

NCLEX Examination Review Questions

1. When monitoring the lab values of a patient who is taking antithyroid drugs, the nurse knows to watch for:
   a. Increased platelet counts.
   b. Decreased white blood cell counts.
   c. Decreased BUN.
   d. Increased blood glucose levels.
2. The pharmacy has called a patient to notify her that the current brand of thyroid replacement hormone is on back order. The patient calls the clinic to ask what to do. Which is the best response by the nurse?
   a. "Go ahead and take the other brand that the pharmacy has available for now."
   b. "You should stop the medication until your current brand is available."
   c. "You can split the thyroid pills that you have left so that they will last longer."
   d. "Let me ask your physician what should be done; we will need to watch how you do if you switch brands."
3. When assessing the older adult patient, the nurse keeps in mind that certain nonspecific symptoms may represent hypothyroidism in older patients, such as:
   a. Leukopenia, anemia.
   b. Loss of appetite, polyuria.

   c. Weight loss, dry cough.
   d. Cold intolerance, depression.
4. To help with the insomnia associated with thyroid hormone replacement therapy, the nurse should teach the patient to:
   a. Take half the dose at lunch time and the other half 2 hours later.
   b. Use a sedative to assist with falling asleep.
   c. Take the dose first thing in the morning.
   d. Reduce the dosage as needed if sleep is impaired.
5. When teaching a patient who has a new prescription for thyroid hormone, the nurse should instruct the patient to notify the physician if which adverse effect is noted?
   a. Palpitations
   b. Headache
   c. Anxiety
   d. Appetite changes

1. b, 2. d, 3. d, 4. c, 5. a.

Critical Thinking Activities

1. Your patient has been taking thyroid drugs for about 16 months and has recently noted palpitations and some heat intolerance. Should you be concerned about this or is this a fairly benign reaction to thyroid replacement? Explain your answer.
2. Explain "thyroid storm" and potential causes.
3. A 33-year-old man, a new admission from the medical surgical unit to the step-down ICU, underwent a thyroidectomy 2 days

ago. While reviewing the orders you note that the patient is to be started on his thyroid medication upon transfer to your unit. The written orders specify that 25 mcg of levothyroxine should be given once daily. However, the pharmacy has sent 25 mcg of liothyronine, another thyroid replacement product. Because the dose of each is the same, is it okay to administer the liothyronine? Explain your answer.

For answers, see http://evolve.elsevier.com/Lilley.

Antidiabetic Drugs

Objectives

When you reach the end of this chapter, you should be able to do the following:

1. Discuss the normal actions and functions of the pancreas.
2. Contrast type 1 and type 2 diabetes mellitus with regard to age of onset, signs and symptoms, pharmacologic and nonpharmacologic treatment, incidence, and etiology.
3. Discuss the various factors influencing blood glucose level in nondiabetic individuals and in patients with either type of diabetes mellitus.
4. Identify the various drugs used to manage type 1 and type 2 diabetes mellitus.
5. Discuss the mechanisms of action, indications, contraindications, cautions, drug interactions, and adverse effects associated with the various categories of insulin and the various oral hypoglycemic drugs.
6. Compare rapid-, short-, intermediate-, and long-acting insulins in regard to their onset of action, peak effects, duration of action, indications, adverse effects, cautions, contraindications, drug interactions, dosages, and routes.
7. Compare the signs and symptoms and related treatment of hypoglycemia and hyperglycemia.
8. Develop nursing care plans that include all phases of the nursing process for patients with type 1 or type 2 diabetes with a focus on medication regimens.

e-Learning Activities

Companion CD

- NCLEX Review Questions: see questions 272-287
- Animations
- Audio Glossary
- Category Catchers
- Medication Errors Checklists
- IV Therapy Checklists

evolve Website (http://evolve.elsevier.com/Lilley)

• Nursing Care Plans • Frequently Asked Questions • Content Updates • WebLinks • Supplemental Resources • Elsevier ePharmacology Update • Medication Administration Animations

Glossary

Diabetes mellitus A complex disorder of carbohydrate, fat, and protein metabolism resulting primarily from the lack of insulin secretion by the beta cells of the pancreas or from de-fects of the insulin receptors; it is commonly referred to simply as *diabetes*. There are two major types of diabetes: type 1 and type 2. (p. 474)

Diabetic ketoacidosis (DKA) Severe metabolic complication of uncontrolled diabetes which, if untreated, leads to diabetic coma and death. (p. 476)

Gestational diabetes Diabetes that develops during pregnancy. It may resolve after pregnancy but may also be a precursor of type 2 diabetes in later life. (p. 478)

Glucagon Hormone produced by the alpha cells in the islets of Langerhans that stimulates the conversion of glycogen to glucose in the liver. (p. 474)

Glucose One of the simple sugars that serves as a major source of energy. It is found in foods (e.g., fruits, refined sweets) and also is the final breakdown product of complex carbohydrate metabolism in the body; it is also commonly referred to as *dextrose*. (p. 474)

Glycogen A polysaccharide that is the major carbohydrate stored in animal cells. (p. 474)

Glycogenolysis The breakdown of glycogen to glucose. (p. 474)

Hemoglobin A1c (HbA1c) Hemoglobin molecules to which glucose molecules are bound; blood levels of hemoglobin A1c are used as a diagnostic measure of average daily blood glucose levels in the monitoring of diabetes; it is also called *glycosylated hemoglobin* or *glycated hemoglobin*. (p. 488)

Hyperglycemia A fasting blood glucose level of 126 mg/dL or higher or a nonfasting blood glucose level of 200 mg/dL or higher. (p. 474)

Hyperosmolar nonketotic syndrome (HNKS) A metabolic complication of uncontrolled diabetes, similar in severity to DKA but without ketosis and acidosis. (p. 476)

Hypoglycemia A blood glucose level of less that 50 mg/dL. (p. 488)

Impaired fasting glucose level A prediabetic state defined as a fasting glucose level of at least 110 mg/dL but lower than 126 mg/dL; it is sometimes called *prediabetes*. (p. 475)

Insulin A naturally occurring hormone secreted by the beta cells of the islets of Langerhans in the pancreas in response to increased levels of glucose in the blood. (p. 474)

Ketones Organic chemical compounds produced through the oxidation of secondary alcohols (e.g., fat molecules), including dietary carbohydrates. (p. 474)

Polydipsia Chronic excessive intake of water; it is a common symptom of diabetes. (p. 474)

Polyphagia Excessive eating; it is a common symptom of diabetes. (p. 474)

Polyuria Increased frequency or volume of urinary output; it is a common symptom of diabetes. (p. 474)

Type 1 diabetes mellitus Diabetes mellitus that is a genetically determined autoimmune disorder involving a complete or nearly complete lack of insulin production; it most commonly arises in children or adolescents. (p. 476)

Type 2 diabetes mellitus A type of diabetes mellitus that most commonly presents in middle age. The disease may be controlled by lifestyle modifications, oral drug therapy, and/or insulin, but patients are not necessarily dependent on insulin. (p. 476)

PANCREAS

The pancreas is a large, elongated organ that is located behind the stomach. It is both an exocrine gland (secreting digestive enzymes through the pancreatic duct) and an endocrine gland (secreting hormones directly into the bloodstream and not through a duct). The endocrine functions of the pancreas are the focus of this chapter. Two main hormones are produced by the pancreas: **insulin** and **glucagon.** Both hormones play an important role in the regulation of glucose homeostasis, specifically the use, mobilization, and storage of glucose by the body. **Glucose** is one of the primary sources of energy for the cells of the body. It is also the simplest form of carbohydrate (sugar) found in the body and is often referred to by the name of its D-ISOMER FORM, *dextrose.* There is a normal amount of glucose that circulates in the blood to meet requirements for quick energy. However, not all of the glucose consumed is needed. When the quantity of glucose in the blood is sufficient, the excess is stored as **glycogen** in the liver and, to a lesser extent, in skeletal muscle tissue, where it remains until the body needs it. Glucose is also stored in adipose tissue as triglyceride body fat.

When more circulating glucose is needed, glycogen—primarily that stored in the liver—is converted back to glucose through a process called **glycogenolysis.** The hormone responsible for initiating this process is glucagon. Glucagon has only minimal effects on muscle glycogen and adipose tissue triglyceride stores.

Glucagon is a protein hormone consisting of a single chain of amino acids (polypeptide chain). Its molecules are about half the size of those of insulin. Glucagon is released from the alpha cells of the islets of Langerhans in the pancreas. The beta cells of these same islets secrete insulin, a protein hormone composed of two amino acid chains (acidic A chain and basic B chain) joined by a disulfide linkage. There is a continuous homeostatic balance in the body between the actions of insulin and those of glucagon. This natural balance normally serves to maintain physiologically optimal blood glucose levels, which normally ranging between 70 and 100 mg/dL. Because of the critical role of the pancreas in producing and maintaining these two hormones, the drastic measure of *pancreatic transplant* is now sometimes undertaken to treat diabetes that has not been successfully controlled by other means. Another extreme treatment involves continuous insulin administration via a mechanized *insulin pump.*

Other substances that function as glucose regulators include cortisol, epinephrine, and growth hormone. These work synergistically with glucagon to counter the effects of insulin and cause increases in the blood glucose level. As mentioned, insulin serves several important metabolic functions in the body. It stimulates carbohydrate metabolism in skeletal and cardiac muscle and in adipose tissue by facilitating the transport of glucose into these cells. In the liver, insulin facilitates the phosphorylation of glucose to glucose-6-phosphate, which is then converted to glycogen for storage. By causing glucose to be stored in the liver as glycogen, insulin keeps the glomerular filtrate of the kidney free of glucose. Without insulin, the kidneys are unable to absorb the excess glucose in the glomerular filtrate and lose large amounts of glucose (a critical body nutrient and energy source), **ketones,** and other solutes into the urine. This loss of nutrient energy sources eventually leads to **polyphagia** (excessive appetite), weight loss, and malnutrition. The presence of these solutes in the distal renal tubules and collecting ducts also draws large volumes of water into the urine through *osmotic diuresis*, which leads to **polyuria** (excessive urination), dehydration, and **polydipsia** (excessive thirst). Polydipsia results from increased *serum osmolality* (i.e., relatively greater concentrations of solutes in the body caused by excess urinary water loss).

Insulin also has a direct effect on fat metabolism. It stimulates lipogenesis and inhibits lipolysis and the release of fatty acids from adipose cells. In addition, insulin stimulates protein synthesis and promotes the intracellular shift of potassium and magnesium, thereby decreasing elevated blood concentrations of these electrolytes. The actions of insulin are antagonized by the following body substances: somatropin (growth hormone), the adrenomedullary hormones epinephrine and norepinephrine, the adrenocortical hormones cortisol and aldosterone, thyroid hormones, and estrogens.

DIABETES MELLITUS

Hyperglycemia is a state involving excessive concentrations of glucose in the blood and results when the normal counterbalancing actions of glucagon and insulin fail to maintain normal glucose homeostasis (i.e., serum levels of 70 to 100 mg/dL). Complications in protein and fat metabolism (*dyslipidemia;* Chapter 28) are also involved. The current key diagnostic criterion for **diabetes mellitus** is hyperglycemia with a fasting plasma glucose level of more than 126 mg/dL. Diagnostic indicators are described in more detail in Box 31-1.

Diabetes mellitus, more commonly referred to simply as *diabetes,* is primarily a disorder of carbohydrate metabolism that in-

Box 31-2 Major Long-Term Consequences of Diabetes (Type 1 and Type 2)

Pathology	Possible Consequences
Macrovascular (Atherosclerotic Plaque)	
Coronary arteries	Myocardial infarction
Cerebral arteries	Stroke
Peripheral vessels	Peripheral vascular disease (e.g., neuropathies [see below], foot ulcers, possible amputations)
Microvascular (Capillary Damage)	
Retinopathy (retinal damage)	Partial or complete blindness
Neuropathy (autonomic and somatic nerve damage, due to both metabolic alterations and compromised circulation)	Autonomic nerve damage: For example, diabetic gastroparesis, bladder dysfunction, unawareness of hypoglycemia
	Somatic nerve damage: For example, diabetic foot ulcer and/or leg or foot amputation (resulting from undetected injuries due to loss of sensation and also from compromised circulation)
Nephropathy (kidney damage)	Proteinuria (microalbuminuria), chronic renal failure (may require dialysis or kidney transplantation)

Diabetes mellitus has been recognized since 1550 BC, when Egyptians wrote of a malady they called *honeyed urine.* The first step toward discerning the cause of diabetes mellitus occurred in 1788 when Thomas Cawley, an English physician, voiced his suspicion that the source of the illness lay in the pancreas. However, it took over a century to prove this, and it took even longer to discover the substance, insulin, that is secreted from the pancreas, the lack of which is responsible for causing the disease. It was known that this substance, whatever it was, was needed by those afflicted with the illness, but the substance could not be identified. Not until the early 1920s was insulin finally isolated. Its discovery is now considered one of the greatest triumphs of twentieth-century medicine, and its use in the treatment of diabetes mellitus has proved to be life saving for millions of people afflicted with the disease.

Diabetes mellitus is not actually a single disease, however, but a group of diseases. For this reason, it is often regarded as a syndrome rather than a disease. In some cases, diabetes is caused by a relative or absolute lack of insulin that is believed to result from the destruction of beta cells in the pancreas. As a result, insulin cannot be produced. Hyperglycemia can also be caused by defects in insulin receptors. The proteins that serve as insulin receptors normally occur in several tissues, including liver, muscle, and adipose tissue. These proteins customarily function in coordination with insulin molecules to remove glucose molecules from the blood. When these proteins become defective, they no longer respond normally to insulin molecules. The result is that glucose molecules remain in the blood, rather than being stored in the tissues. Two major types of diabetes mellitus are currently recognized and designated by the American Diabetes Association (ADA): type 1 and type 2. Type 1 diabetes was previously also called *insulin-dependent diabetes mellitus (IDDM)* or *juvenile-onset diabetes.* Type 2 diabetes was previously also called *non–insulin-dependent diabetes mellitus (NIDDM)* or *adult-onset diabetes.* The numerical designations for both conditions were adopted by the ADA as the preferred terms in 1995.

The previous designations were abandoned for several reasons. One reason is that many patients with type 2 diabetes *do* eventually become dependent on insulin therapy for control of their illness. A second reason is that the current epidemic of both child and adult obesity in the United States is increasing the incidence of type 2 diabetes in children and adolescents. This condition is now called *maturity-onset diabetes of youth (MODY)* and refers in general to hyperglycemia in persons younger than 25 years of age. Obesity is one of the major risk factors for the development of type 2 diabetes. Non-white ethnic groups including African, Asian, and Hispanic Americans and Native Americans are all at higher risk for the disease than are whites. The usual differences between type 1 and type 2 diabetes mellitus are listed in Table 31-1. Interestingly, approximately 10% of patients with type 2 diabetes have circulating antibodies that suggest an autoimmune origin for the disease. This condition is known as *latent autoimmune diabetes in adults (LADA)* and is basically a more slowly progressing form of type 1 diabetes. The most common signs and symptoms of any type of diabetes are elevated blood glucose level (higher than 126 mg/dL) or **impaired fasting glucose level** (110 mg/dL or higher but less than 126 mg/dL), and polyuria, polydipsia, polyphagia, glucosuria, weight loss, and fatigue.

volves either a deficiency of insulin, a tissue (e.g., muscle, liver) resistance to insulin, or both. Whatever the cause of the diabetes, the result is hyperglycemia. Uncontrolled hyperglycemia correlates strongly with serious long-term adverse health effects related to both *macroangiopathy* and *microangiopathy.* Macroangiopathy involves large vessel damage usually related to deposition of atherosclerotic plaque. This compromises both central and peripheral circulation. In contrast, microangiopathy involves damage to the capillary vessels, which impairs peripheral circulation. In addition, both autonomic and somatic nerve damage occur, caused primarily by the metabolic changes themselves and to a lesser degree by the compromised circulation. Box 31-2 lists common long-term complications of diabetes.

Table 31-1 Type 1 and Type 2 Diabetes: Characteristics		
Characteristic	**Type 1**	**Type 2**
Etiology	Autoimmune destruction of beta cells in the pancreas	Multifactorial genetic defects; strong association with obesity and insulin resistance resulting from a reduction in the number or activity of insulin receptors
Incidence	10% of cases	90% of cases
Onset	Juvenile onset, age younger than 20 yr	Previously maturity onset, age older than 40 yr; now increasingly seen in younger adults and even adolescents—attributed to obesity epidemic
Endogenous insulin	Little or none	Normal levels
Insulin receptors	Normal	Decreased or defective
Body weight	Usually nonobese	Obese (80% of cases)
Treatment	Insulin	Weight loss, diet and exercise, oral hypoglycemics if necessary; only about one third of all patients need insulin

Type 1 Diabetes Mellitus

Type 1 diabetes mellitus is characterized by a lack of insulin production or by the production of a defective insulin, which results in acute hyperglycemia. Affected patients require exogenous insulin to lower blood glucose level and prevent diabetic complications. It is believed that a genetically determined autoimmune reaction gradually destroys the insulin-producing beta cells of the pancreatic islets of Langerhans (Figure 31-1). The *preclinical* phase of beta cell destruction may be prolonged, possibly lasting several years. At some critical point, a rapid transition from preclinical to clinical type 1 diabetes occurs. This transition is believed to be triggered by a specific event such as an acute illness or major emotional stress. An unidentified viral infection is also strongly suspected as an environmental trigger. The stressor(s) trigger the release of the counterregulatory hormones cortisol and epinephrine. These hormones then mobilize glucagon to release glucose from the storage sites in the liver. This only further increases the already rising levels of glucose in the blood secondary to islet cell damage. At some point during this crisis cascade of events an autoimmune reaction may be initiated that destroys the insulin-producing beta cells of the pancreatic islets of Langerhans. The result is essentially a complete lack of endogenous insulin production by the pancreas, which necessitates chronic replacement insulin therapy. Fortunately, type 1 diabetes accounts for fewer than 10% of all diabetes cases. Historically, oral antidiabetic drugs (discussed later in this chapter) have not been effective in treating type 1 diabetes, although the matter is being investigated by a small number of researchers.

Acute Diabetic Complications: Diabetic Ketoacidosis and Hyperosmolar Nonketotic Syndrome

When blood glucose levels are high but no insulin is present to allow glucose to be used for energy production, the body may break down fatty acids for fuel, producing ketones as a metabolic byproduct. If this occurs to a sufficient degree, **diabetic ketoacidosis (DKA)** may result. DKA is a complex multisystem complication of uncontrolled diabetes. Without treatment, DKA will lead to coma and death. DKA is characterized by extreme hyperglycemia, the presence of ketones in the serum, acidosis, dehydration, and electrolyte imbalances. Approximately 25% to 30% of patients with newly diagnosed type 1 diabetes mellitus present with DKA. Another complication of comparable severity that is

also triggered by extreme hyperglycemia is **hyperosmolar nonketotic syndrome (HNKS).** The most common precipitator of DKA and HNKS is some type of physical or emotional stress. It was formerly believed that DKA occurred only in type 1 diabetes and HNKS occurred only in type 2 diabetes. However, it is now recognized that both disorders can occur with diabetes of either type, and this overlap is increasingly common with the rapidly decreasing age of type 2 diabetic patients.

Table 31-2 describes the subtle differences between these two acute diabetic complications. Treatment for either involves fluid and electrolyte replacement as well as intravenous insulin therapy (more common for DKA).

Type 2 Diabetes Mellitus

Type 2 diabetes mellitus, which was once thought to be a mild form of type 1 diabetes mellitus, is an important disorder that is often poorly treated. Of all the forms of diabetes mellitus it is by far the most common, accounting for at least 90% of all cases of diabetes mellitus and affecting as much as 20% of the population over 70 years of age. Over 17 million people in the United States have this disease. In part because this form of diabetes does not always require insulin therapy, there are many common and dangerous misconceptions regarding type 2 diabetes mellitus: that it is a mild diabetes; that it is easy to treat; and that tight metabolic control is unnecessary because these patients, who are mostly older adults, will die before diabetic complications develop. The clinical realities of this disease demonstrate otherwise, however.

Type 2 diabetes mellitus is caused by both insulin resistance and insulin deficiency, but there is not an absolute lack of insulin as in type 1 diabetes. As previously noted, one of the normal roles of insulin is to facilitate the uptake of circulating glucose molecules into tissues to be used as energy. In type 2 diabetes all of the main target tissues of insulin (muscle, liver, and adipose tissue) are hyporesponsive (resistant) to the effects of the hormone. Not only is the absolute number of insulin receptors in these tissues reduced, but their individual sensitivity and responsiveness to insulin is decreased as well. Therefore, it is possible for a patient with type 2 diabetes mellitus to have normal or even elevated levels of insulin yet still have high blood glucose levels. Another reason for this paradoxical situation is that the altered insulin receptor dynamics also cause the liver to overproduce

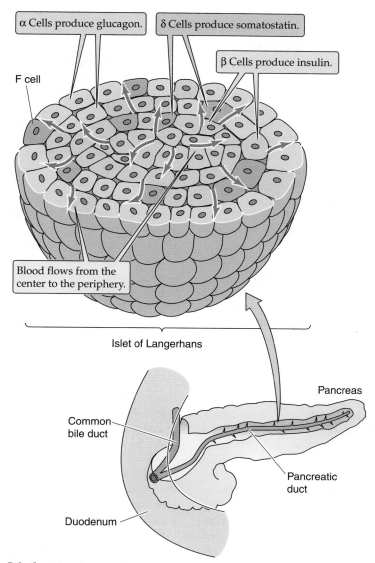

FIGURE 31-1   Islet of Langerhans. *(From Boron WF, Boulapaep EL:* Medical physiology, *Phila-delphia, 2003, Saunders.)*

Table 31-2	**Comparison of Some Salient Features of Diabetic Ketoacidosis and Hyperosmolar Nonketotic Syndrome**

	Condition	
Feature	**Diabetic Ketoacidosis**	**Hyperosmolar Nonketotic Syndrome**
Age of patient	Usually younger than 40 yr	Usually older than 40 yr
Duration of symptoms	Usually less than 2 days	Usually longer than 5 days
Serum glucose level	Usually less than 800 mg/dl	Usually higher than 800 mg/dl
Serum Na level	More likely to be normal or low	More likely to be normal or high
Serum K level	High, normal, or low	High, normal, or low
Serum HCO_3 level	Low	Normal
Ketone bodies	At least 4+ in 1:1 dilution	Less than 2+ in 1:1 dilution
pH	Low	Normal
Serum osmolality	Usually less than 350 mOsm/kg	Usually more than 350 mOsm/kg
Cerebral edema	Often subclinical; occasionally clinical	Not evaluated if subclinical; rarely clinical
Prognosis	3% to 10% mortality	10% to 20% mortality
Subsequent course	Insulin therapy required in virtually all cases	Insulin therapy not required in many cases

From Harmel AP, Mathur R: *Davidson's diabetes mellitus: diagnosis and treatment,* ed 5, Philadelphia, 2004, Saunders.

glucose, which exacerbates the already present hyperglycemic condition. All of these processes also result in impaired postprandial (after a meal) glucose metabolism. This is another problematic feature of type 2 diabetes that contributes to the hazardous hyperglycemic state.

In addition to the reduction in the number and sensitivity of insulin receptors in type 2 diabetes, there is often reduced insulin secretion by the pancreas. This insulin deficiency results from a loss of the normal responsiveness of the beta cells in the pancreas to elevated blood glucose levels. When the beta cells do not recognize glucose, they do not secrete insulin, and the normal insulin-facilitated transport of glucose into cells of muscle, liver, and adipose tissue does not occur. This situation is analogous to the loss of responsiveness of insulin receptors to insulin described earlier. Both insulin resistance and insulin deficiency may induce or aggravate one another.

Type 2 diabetes is a multifaceted disorder. Although loss of blood glucose control is its primary hallmark, several other significant conditions are strongly associated with the disease. These include obesity, coronary heart disease, dyslipidemia, hypertension (Chapter 24), microalbuminuria (spilling of protein into the urine), and changes in the blood that increase the risk for thrombotic (blood clotting) events. For patients with type 2 diabetes, the ADA recommends the regular use of aspirin for prevention of coronary artery heart disease and antihyperlipidemic drug therapy (Chapter 28), when applicable, in addition to any necessary antidiabetic drug therapy. These comorbidities are strongly associated with the development of type 2 diabetes and are collectively referred to as *metabolic syndrome* (also known as *insulin-resistance syndrome* and *syndrome X*). Roughly 90% of patients with diabetes are obese at the time of initial diagnosis. Obesity serves only to worsen the insulin resistance, because adipose tissue is often the site of a large proportion of the body's defective insulin receptors. These precipitating factors of type 2 diabetes, and the disease itself, are highly inherited (hereditary). However, the current obesity epidemic, driven by both widespread lack of exercise and a high-fat, high-carbohydrate diet, is increasingly leading to this disease even in teenage patients.

Gestational Diabetes

Gestational diabetes is a type of hyperglycemia that develops during pregnancy. Relatively uncommon, it occurs in about 4% of pregnancies. The use of insulin is necessary to decrease the risk of birth defects. In most cases gestational diabetes subsides after delivery. However, as many as 30% of patients are estimated to develop type 2 diabetes within 10 to 15 years.

All pregnant women should have blood glucose screenings at regular prenatal visits. Women who develop gestational diabetes should be screened for lingering diabetes 6 to 8 weeks postpartum. They should also be advised of their increased risk for recurrent diabetes and of the importance of regular medical checkups. Finally, women who are known to be diabetic before pregnancy should ideally have detailed prepregnancy counseling (and therefore preferably a planned pregnancy) and prenatal care from a physician experienced in managing pregnancies in diabetic women. Specific drug therapy issues pertaining to gestational diabetes are discussed further in the section on insulinase.

Prevention and Screening

Both macrovascular and microvascular problems are now recognized at fasting plasma glucose (FPG) levels as low as 126 mg/dL, with "fasting" being defined loosely as an overnight fast (no food from midnight until after the blood sample is taken in the morning). Impaired fasting glucose level is defined as an FPG level higher than or equal to 110 mg/dL but less than 126 mg/dL. This condition often proves to be a precursor to diabetes and is therefore sometimes referred to as *prediabetes.* Another recognized prediabetic condition is *impaired glucose tolerance,* which is identified using an oral glucose challenge test (see Box 31-1). The ADA, the National Institute of Diabetes and Digestive and Kidney Disease, and the Centers for Disease Control and Prevention recommend that all adults 45 years of age and older be screened for elevated FPG levels every 3 years. Several preventive measures are also recommended. Reducing alcohol consumption is helpful because alcohol is broken down in the body to simple carbohydrates, which leads to increases in blood glucose level. Regular exercise also lowers blood glucose levels by increasing insulin receptor sensitivity, the loss of which is a primary problem in type 2 diabetes. Exercise also reduces body fat and tends to reduce high blood pressure.

Nonpharmacologic Treatment Interventions

Patients diagnosed with type 1 diabetes almost always require insulin therapy. However, the initial treatment of type 2 diabetes should consist of weight loss and lifestyle changes. In some cases, these interventions may be sufficient to arrest the disease and avoid the need for drug therapy. The benefits of weight loss, as noted earlier, are that it not only lowers the blood glucose and lipid levels of these patients, but it also reduces another common comorbidity, hypertension. Other recommended lifestyle changes include improved dietary habits (e.g., consumption of a diet higher in protein and lower in fat and carbohydrates), smoking cessation, reduced alcohol consumption, and regular physical exercise. Cigarette smoking doubles the risk of cardiovascular disease in diabetic patients, largely because of its effects on peripheral vascular circulation and respiratory function. In fact, smoking cessation would probably save far more lives than antihypertensive, antilipemic, and antidiabetic drug treatment together!

ANTIDIABETIC DRUGS

The two major classes of drugs used to treat diabetes mellitus are the insulins and the oral hypoglycemic drugs. These drugs are more broadly referred to as *antidiabetic drugs,* and they are aimed at producing a normoglycemic or euglycemic (normal blood glucose) state.

INSULINS

The primary treatment for type 1 diabetes mellitus is insulin therapy. Patients with type 2 diabetes are not generally prescribed insulin until other measures—namely, lifestyle changes and oral drug therapy—no longer provide adequate glycemic control. There are currently two main sources of insulin. It can be extracted from domesticated animals or synthesized in laboratories using recombinant deoxyribonucleic acid (DNA) technology. Insulin was originally isolated from cattle, but beef-derived insulin is no longer available on the U.S. market. Insulin isolated from pigs, known as *porcine insulin,* has a chemical structure that differs from human insulin by only one amino acid. Porcine insulin has also been supplanted by human-derived insulin products. The development of recombinant DNA technologies has led to widespread use of recombinant insulins that follow the natural chemical structure of the human insulin molecule. Recombinant insulin is produced by bacteria or yeast that have been altered to contain the genetic information necessary for them to reproduce an insulin that is exactly like human insulin. The pharmacokinetic properties of insulin (onset of action, peak effect, and duration of action) can also be altered by making various minor modifications to either the insulin molecule itself or the drug formulation (final product). This practice has led to the development of many different insulin preparations, including several combination insulin products that contain more than one type of insulin in the same solution. Chemical manipulation of insulin activity in this way helps to meet the often very individual time-oriented metabolic demands for insulin of diabetic patients. Table 31-3 compares the pharmacokinetic parameters of various commonly prescribed insulin products. Further modifications can be accomplished by mixing compatible insulin preparations in the syringe before ad-

ministration. The latest syringe compatibility data for currently available insulin products appear in Table 31-4. Patients should be thoroughly educated regarding how, when, and whether they should (or should not) mix different types of insulin. Some combinations are chemically incompatible and can result in undesirable alteration of glycemic effects.

Mechanism of Action and Drug Effects

Exogenously administered insulin functions as a substitute for the endogenous hormone. It serves to replace the insulin that is either not made at all or is made defectively in the body of a diabetic patient. The drug effects of exogenously administered insulin are many and involve many body systems. They are the same as those of normal endogenous insulin. That is, exogenously administered insulin restores the diabetic patient's ability to metabolize carbohydrates, fats, and proteins; to store glucose in the liver; and to convert glycogen to fat stores.

Indications

All insulin preparations can be used to treat both type 1 and type 2 diabetes, but each patient requires careful customization of the dosing regimen for optimal glycemic control. Additional therapeutic approaches such as lifestyle modifications (e.g., improved dietary and exercise habits) are also indicated and, for type 2 diabetes, oral drug therapy as well. The use of intensive insulin therapy and tight glucose control is described in Box 31-3.

Contraindications

Contraindications to the use of all insulin products include known drug allergy to the specific product. Insulin also should never be administered to an already hypoglycemic patient.

Adverse Effects

Hypoglycemia resulting from an insulin overdose can result in shock and possibly death. This is the most immediate and serious adverse effect of insulin. Other more common adverse effects of insulin therapy are listed in Table 31-5. The reader may notice that some of the effects listed (e.g., tachycardia, delirium, sweating) can be associated with *either* hypoglycemia or hyperglycemia. The *clinical* symptoms of these two conditions can overlap.

Table 31-3	Human Insulins and Analogues: Comparison of Pharmacokinetic Properties		
Insulin Preparation	**Onset of Action**	**Peak Action**	**Duration of Action**
lispro*/aspart*	5-15 min	1-2 hr	4-6 hr
human regular	30-60 min	2-4 hr	6-10 hr
human NPH/Lente	1-2 hr	4-8 hr	10-18 hr
Ultralente	2-4 hr	8-14 hr	18-24 hr
glargine*	1-2 hr	Flat	24 hr

From Colwell JA: *Diabetes: hot topics,* Philadelphia, 2003, Hanley & Belfus.
*Insulin analogue.

Table 31-4	Insulin Mixing Compatibilities

Type of Insulin	Compatible with
regular (Humulin R, Novolin R, Velosulin BR)	All insulins except glargine, Lente, Ultralente, and glulisine (see below)
regular	Lente or Ultralente*
regular or insulin glulisine (Apidra)	NPH only; may use mixture immediately or store for future use; draw up NPH after regular insulin or insulin glulisine
insulin lispro (Humalog), insulin aspart (NovoLog)	Regular, NPH, Lente, and Ultralente; inject mixture 15 min before meal†
insulin glargine (Lantus)	Must give alone due to low pH of diluent
NPH 70% and regular insulin 30% (Humulin 70/30, Novolin 70/30)	
NPH 50% and regular insulin 50% (Humulin 50/50)	
insulin lispro protamine suspension 75% and insulin lispro 25% (Humalog Mix 75/25)	Premixed; do not mix with other insulins

*These combinations are not normally recommended unless the patient has already achieved adequate control on this mixture. If so, the patient should standardize the length of time between mixing and injection because of chemical interactions that delay the onset of action of the regular insulin. For this reason this mixture must be used soon after preparation; it is not suitable for storage for future use.
†Normally used as alternatives to regular insulin and therefore not usually given with it.

The importance of tight glucose control in patients with type 1 and type 2 diabetes appears obvious. In fact, the value of patients' maintaining especially careful control of their blood glucose levels was demonstrated in three large research studies in the 1990s: the Diabetes Control and Complications Trial (DCCT; 1993) sponsored by the National Institutes of Health, the Kumamoto study in Japan (1995), and the United Kingdom Prospective Diabetes Study (UKPDS; 1998). The DCCT focused on type 1 patients only and demonstrated improved outcomes with intensive insulin therapy. Intensive therapy was defined as either three insulin injections daily or administration of a rapid-acting insulin (regular, lispro, or aspart) by continuous subcutaneous insulin infusion (CSII). External CSII pumps are now being used in clinical practice. They are normally preprogrammed to deliver a basal dose of insulin around the clock, with premeal boluses delivered via the pump as needed. The patient can adjust these bolus doses based on premeal blood glucose measurements. The Kumamoto study and UKPDS both focused on patients with type 2 diabetes and included the use of both insulin and oral antidiabetic drugs. All three studies showed that patients who optimize, or even merely improve, their blood glucose control have a reduced incidence of long-term complications associated with the disease. These complications include both microvascular effects (retinopathy, nephropathy, neuropathy) and macrovascular effects (myocardial infarction, stroke, and peripheral vascular disease). The reductions in microvascular and neuropathic complications were especially dramatic, whereas the reductions in macrovascular complications were observable but were not statistically significant. Nonetheless, such studies underscore the importance of helping each patient maintain the best possible glycemic control through an individualized treatment regimen.

Table 31-5 Insulin: Common Adverse Effects

Body System	Adverse Effects
Cardiovascular	Tachycardia, palpitations
Central nervous	Headache, lethargy, tremors, weakness, fatigue, delirium, sweating
Metabolic	Hypoglycemia
Other	Blurred vision, dry mouth, hunger, nausea, flushing, rash, urticaria, anaphylaxis

This underscores the need to teach patients and their caregivers to measure and track their blood glucose levels when any acute symptoms arise.

Interactions

Drug interactions that can occur with the insulins are significant. The β-blockers, chlorthalidone, corticosteroids, diazoxide, epinephrine, ethacrynic acid, furosemide, isoniazid (for tuberculosis), niacin, phenytoin, thiazides, sympathomimetic drugs, and thyroid hormones (both endogenous and exogenous) can all antagonize the hypoglycemic effects of insulin (which results in elevated blood glucose levels). Alcohol, anabolic steroids, sulfa drugs, angiotensin-converting enzyme (ACE) inhibitors, guanethidine, monoamine oxidase inhibitors (MAOIs), propranolol, and the salicylates can all increase insulin's hypoglycemic effects, which leads to lower blood glucose levels.

Dosages

See the Dosages table on page 481 for the recommended dosages of the various insulin drugs.

Drug Profiles

Insulins

The primary treatment for both type 1 diabetes and gestational diabetes is insulin therapy. There are currently four major classes of insulin, as determined by their pharmacokinetic properties: rapid acting, short acting, intermediate acting, and long acting (Table 31-6). As previously mentioned, insulin is usually only a therapy of last resort for type 2 diabetes. However, some clinicians elect to prescribe insulin earlier than previously for patients who achieve less than desirable glycemic control with oral drugs and/or experience adverse reactions to them. The insulin dosage regimen for all diabetic patients is highly individualized and may consist of one or more types of insulin administered at either fixed dosages or variable dosages in response to self-measurements of blood glucose level. Because porcine (pork-derived) insulin products have actions are derived from a different animal species, they are more likely to be allergenic. For this reason they are seldom used today in developed countries, except in the unusual case of a patient who is intolerant of other insulins or achieves better glycemic control with a porcine product. With insulins, color and appearance is important to understand for patient safety and for the prevention of adverse effects and complications. Several insulins appear as clear, colorless solutions. These include regular insulin, insulin lispro (Humalog), and insulin glargine (Lantus). Other insulins, such as NPH insulin (insulin isophane) are white opaque (cloudy) solutions. This issue is discussed further in the Implementation subsection under Nursing Process.

If an insulin is rapid or short acting, then the nurse knows to expect the insulin to be clear, whereas intermediate-acting insulin is cloudy. It should also be noted that all of the Lente insulin products have been largely replaced in clinical practice by other types of insulin, including lispro and glargine. The Lente insulin products are included here because they currently remain on the U.S. market and are still used occasionally. Comparative pharmacokinetic parameters for several commonly used insulin products appear in Table 31-3.

Two special patient populations for whom careful attention is required during insulin therapy are pediatric patients and pregnant women (Table 31-7). Insulin dosages for both are calculated by weight as they are for the general adult population. The usual dosage range is 0.5 to 1 units/kg/day as a total daily dose. However, the nurse must be aware of a few important differences regarding the use of some of the more unusual insulin products in pediatric populations. The rapid-acting insulin lispro is approved for use in children older than 3 years of age and is often used concurrently with oral sulfonylurea therapy (discussed later in the chapter). However, the combination lispro product Humalog 75/25 that contains 75% insulin lispro protamine (an intermediate-acting insulin) and 25% insulin lispro (a rapid-acting insulin) is *not* currently approved for use in children younger than 18 years of age. The other rapid-acting product, insulin aspart (NovoLog), also is *not* currently approved for pediatric use. Any insulin therapy that falls outside of standard dosing guidelines should generally be prescribed by a trained pediatric endocrinologist, who must provide careful monitoring of the patient. Children need age-appropriate education and supervision from health care professionals and parents, which includes a safe and gradual transfer of responsibility for self-management of their illness.

Pregnant women also require special care with regard to diabetes management. Gestational diabetes reportedly occurs in roughly 4% of pregnancies in the United States. Although most of these mothers will return to a normal glycemic state after pregnancy, they also have a 30% to 60% risk of developing diabetes again in later life. Although all currently available oral and injectable antidiabetic drugs are classified as pregnancy category B or C, oral medications are

DOSAGES

Human-Based Insulin Products

Drug (Pregnancy Category)	Pharmacologic Class	Usual Dosage Range	Indications
Rapid-Acting insulin aspart (NovoLog) (C) ▸insulin lispro (Humalog) (B) insulin glulisine (Apidra) (C)	Human recombinant rapid-acting insulin analogues	SC: 0.5-1 unit/kg/day; doses are highly individualized to desired glycemic control; rapid-acting insulins are best given 15 min before a meal All three may be given per sliding scale; may also be given via continuous subcutaneous infusion pump (but not IV)	
Short-Acting ▸regular insulin (Humulin R, Novolin R, Velosulin BR) (B)	Human recombinant short-acting insulin	SC only: Same dosage as insulin aspart and insulin lispro; SC doses of regular insulin are best given 30 to 60 min before a meal Regular insulin may also be given per sliding scale and is the only insulin that can be given IV as a continuous infusion	
Intermediate-Acting ▸insulin isophane suspension [NPH] (Humulin N, Novolin N) (B) insulin zinc suspension [Lente] (Lente Iletin II, Humulin L) (B)	Human recombinant intermediate-acting insulin analogues	SC only: Same dosage as insulin aspart, insulin lispro, and regular insulin	Diabetes mellitus type 1 and type 2
Long-Acting ▸insulin glargine (Lantus) (C) insulin zinc suspension, extended [Ultralente] (Humulin-U) (B)	Human recombinant long-acting insulin analogues	SC only: Same dosage as others but is approved only for once- or twice-daily dosage (basal dosing)	
Combination Insulin Products NPH 70% and regular insulin 30% (Humulin 70/30, Novolin 70/30) (B) NPH 50% and regular insulin 50% (Humulin 50/50) (B)	Human recombinant intermediate-acting and short-acting combination insulin products	SC only: Same dosage as others	
insulin lispro protamine suspension 75% and insulin lispro 25% (Humalog Mix 75/25) (B)	Human recombinant intermediate-acting and rapid-acting combination insulin product		

NOTE: Boldface type denotes insulin solutions that normally appear cloudy (opaque). The remaining insulin products should appear clear and colorless, and should not be used otherwise.

IV, Intravenous; *SC,* subcutaneous.

generally not recommended for pregnant patients because of a lack of firm safety data. In contrast, insulin use in pregnant women is much better studied and understood. For this reason, insulin therapy is the only currently recommended drug therapy for pregnant women with diabetes. Roughly 15% of women who develop gestational diabetes require insulin therapy during pregnancy. All insulin products are classified as pregnancy category B drugs except for the glargine and aspart products, which are pregnancy category C drugs. Insulins, both endogenous and exogenous, do not normally cross the placenta.

However, insulin is normally excreted into human milk. Because this is a natural process, nursing mothers may still receive insulin therapy. Nevertheless, it is currently unknown whether insulin glargine is excreted in breast milk, and so it should not be used in women while they are breast-feeding. Optimization of insulin therapy and diet is especially important for a nursing mother, because inadequate or excessive glycemic control may reduce milk production. Effective glycemic control during pregnancy is also essential, because infants born to women with gestational diabetes have a twofold to threefold greater risk of congenital anomalies. In addition, the incidence of stillbirth is directly related to the degree of maternal hyperglycemia. Weight reduction is generally *not* advised for these women because it can jeopardize fetal nutritional status.

Rapid-Acting Insulins
▶ insulin lispro and insulin aspart

There are currently three insulin products that are classified as rapid acting. These have the most rapid onset of action (roughly 15 minutes) but often also a shorter duration of action than other insulin categories. These products include insulin lispro, insulin aspart, and, most recently, insulin glulisine (Apidra). Their effects are most like those of the endogenous insulin produced by the pancreas in re-

sponse to a meal. After a meal, the glucose that is ingested stimulates the pancreas to secrete insulin. This insulin then chemically facilitates uptake of the excess glucose at hepatic insulin receptor sites for storage in the liver as glycogen. In people with diabetes mellitus, the insulin response to meals is deficient; therefore, a rapid-acting insulin product is often used within 15 minutes of mealtime. This corresponds to the time required for the onset of action of these products.

Insulin lispro was approved by the U.S. Food and Drug Administration (FDA) in 1996, becoming the first new insulin product to appear on the U.S. market in 14 years. Produced using recombinant DNA technology, both insulin lispro and insulin aspart are able to more closely mimic the body's natural rapid insulin output after consumption of a meal compared than did previous insulin products. For this reason both are usually dosed within 15 minutes of beginning a meal. Insulin glulisine was approved in 2005. Both insulin lispro and insulin glulisine are also approved for use in subcutaneous (not intravenous) continuous infusion pumps, which are now sometimes used in the most severely diabetic patients. However, the successful use of this device, as with diabetes treatment in general, requires a motivated and attentive patient.

Short-Acting Insulin
▶ regular insulin

Regular insulin (Humulin R, Novolin R, Velosulin BR) is currently the only insulin that is classified as a short-acting insulin. Some references still classify it as a rapid-acting insulin. However, the two other rapid-acting insulins, insulin lispro and insulin aspart, actually have a faster onset of action than regular insulin, as indicated earlier and in Table 31-3, hence the newer designation for regular insulin as published in January 2003 by the ADA. Regular insulin is the only insulin product that can be dosed via intravenous bolus, intravenous infusion, or even intramuscularly. These routes, especially the intravenous infusion route, are often used in cases of DKA or coma associated with uncontrolled type 1 diabetes.

Regular insulin solution was actually the first medicinal insulin product developed and was originally isolated from bovine (cow)

Table 31-6 Sources of Available Insulin Products

Activity Classification	Human Recombinant Insulins
Rapid Acting	
insulin lispro	Humalog
insulin aspart	NovoLog
Short Acting	
Regular	Humulin R, Novolin R, Velosulin BR
Intermediate Acting	
insulin isophane suspension (NPH)	Humulin N, Novolin N
insulin zinc suspension (Lente)	Humulin L, Novolin L
Long Acting	
insulin glargine	Lantus
insulin zinc suspension, extended (Ultralente)	Humulin U

Table 31-7 Considerations for the Use of Antidiabetic Drugs and Insulin

Drug	Pediatric Considerations	Pregnancy and Lactation Considerations	Elderly Considerations
glimepiride	Safety and efficacy not established	Not recommended in pregnancy; unknown if this drug crosses into breast milk	Hypoglycemia more difficult to identify in the elderly. Age-related renal dysfunction may increase sensitivity to the glucose-lowering action.
glipizide glyburide	Safety and efficacy not established	Crosses the placenta and is found in breast milk; not recommended for pregnant or lactating women	Age-related renal dysfunction may lead to toxic effects and hypoglycemic responses.
insulin	No age-related precautions in pediatric patients; use of insulin lispro contraindicated in children younger than 18 years of age	Drug of choice for treatment during pregnancy; not secreted into breast milk, but lactation may decrease actual insulin requirements	The elderly with altered visual, cognitive, or motor abilities may have difficulty maintaining safe compliance with the drug regimen.
metformin	Safety and efficacy not established	Distributed in breast milk in animals	Elderly patients may require dosage adjustment if renal dysfunction occurs.
repaglinide	Safety and efficacy not established	Unknown if this drug is distributed in breast milk	No age-related precautions, but the elderly are more prone to hypoglycemia.
rosiglitazone	Safety and efficacy not established	Unknown if this drug crosses the placenta or if it is distributed into the breast milk; not recommended for pregnant or lactating women	No age-related concerns.

and porcine (pig) sources. It is now primarily made from human insulin sources using recombinant DNA technology.

To clarify some of the differences between regular insulin and the newer rapid-acting drugs, both insulin lispro and insulin aspart are human insulin analogues. This means that they are insulin molecules with synthetic alterations to their chemical structures that alter their onset or duration of action. Both of these insulins have a faster onset of action and a shorter time to peak plasma level, but also a shorter duration of action, than does regular insulin. Table 31-3 outlines these differences in more detail.

Intermediate-Acting Insulins
▶ *insulin zinc suspension (Lente) and insulin isophane suspension (NPH)*
Currently available intermediate-acting insulin products include two basic types: (1) insulin zinc suspension (Lente insulin), and (2) insulin isophane suspension (also known as NPH insulin). NPH is an acronym for neutral protamine Hagedorn insulin, the original name of this type of insulin.

Lente insulin is an intermediate-acting insulin that contains zinc; 70% is long-acting insulin zinc (crystalline insulin suspension, or Ultralente) and 30% is a more rapid-acting amorphous (noncrystalline) insulin suspension. The result is a cloudy insulin suspension with a usual onset of action of about 1 to 2 hours. NPH insulin is a sterile suspension of zinc insulin crystals and protamine sulfate in buffered water for injection. It also appears as a cloudy or opaque suspension.

Because of their intermediate onset of action, the effects of these insulins are slower to occur and more prolonged than those of endogenous insulin.

Long-Acting Insulins
▶ *extended insulin zinc suspension (Ultralente) and glargine*
Two long-acting insulin products are now available: extended insulin zinc suspension (Humulin U Ultralente) and insulin glargine (Lantus). The duration of action of Ultralente was prolonged through the addition of even more zinc, specifically zinc chloride, than was added to create the intermediate-acting Lente insulin product. Ultralente, like the Lente and NPH insulins, appears as a white, opaque suspension. In contrast, insulin glargine is normally a clear colorless solution. It is a recombinant DNA–produced insulin analogue and is unique in that it provides a constant level of insulin in the body. This enhances its safety because its effects do not rise and fall as with other insulins. Therapy is often initiated with once-daily dosing, but the drug may be dosed every 12 hours, depending on the patient's glycemic response. Ultralente may sometimes be dosed more than once daily as well. Both of these long-acting insulin products have longer onsets and durations of action than endogenous (regular) insulin. Because they help provide a more prolonged, consistent blood glucose level, they are sometimes referred to as *basal* insulins.

Often for those being switched from twice-daily NPH to glargine, the initial daily glargine dose is reduced to 80% of the previous total NPH dose, with a range of 2 to 100 IU.

Fixed-Combination Insulins
Currently available fixed combination insulin products include Humulin 70/30, Humulin 50/50, Novolin 70/30, and Humalog Mix 75/25. Each of these products contains two different insulins, one faster-acting type and one slower-acting type, which work together in the body to optimize glycemic control. The numerical designations indicate the relative percentages of each of the two components in the product. Notice that in each case the numbers add to up 100 (percent). These products were developed to more closely simulate the varying levels of endogenous insulin that occur normally in nondiabetic people. To maintain constant blood glucose levels both after and between meals, insulin must be present. In most insulin regimens, patients take a combination of a rapid-acting insulin to deal with the surges in glucose that occur after meals and an intermediate or long-acting insulin for the period between meals when glucose

levels are lower. However, this requires the mixing and administration of different types of insulins. Fixed-combination products were developed in an attempt to simplify the dosing process. The percentage of faster- and slower-acting components in each of the available combination insulin products is specified in the table on page 481. The insulin lispro protamine component of Humalog Mix 75/25 is a modified insulin lispro molecule with a longer duration of action.

Sliding-Scale Insulin Dosing
An important method for dosing insulin is referred to as the *sliding-scale method*. In this method, subcutaneous doses of rapid-acting (regular) or short-acting (lispro or aspart) regular insulin are adjusted according to blood glucose test results. This method is typically used in treating hospitalized diabetic patients whose insulin requirements may vary drastically because of stress (e.g., infections, surgery, acute illness), inactivity, or variable caloric intake, including receipt of *total parenteral nutrition (TPN)*. Sliding-scale insulin administration may also be used in type 1 patients on intensive insulin therapy. When an individual is on a sliding-scale insulin regimen, blood glucose concentrations are determined several times a day (e.g., before meals and at bedtime for patients on normal meal schedules, or every 4 to 6 hours around the clock for patients on TPN or enteral tube feedings). This enables the patient to obtain fasting blood glucose values and values before meals. Subcutaneously administered regular insulin is then ordered in an amount that increases with the increase in blood glucose level.

Example:
- No insulin for a blood glucose value of less than 140 mg/dL
- 2 units for a blood glucose value of 141-199 mg/dL
- 4 units for a blood glucose value of 200 to 249 mg/dL
- 6 units for a blood glucose value of 250 to 299 mg/dL
- 8 units for a blood glucose value of 300 mg/dL or greater

ORAL ANTIDIABETIC DRUGS

As previously described, type 2 diabetes is usually a very complex illness. Effective treatment involves several elements, including lifestyle modifications (e.g., diet, exercise, smoking cessation), careful monitoring of blood glucose levels, and possibly therapy with one or more drugs. In addition, the treatment of associated comorbid conditions is a necessity that only serves to further complicate the entire process.

If normal blood glucose levels are not achieved after 2 to 3 months of lifestyle modifications, treatment with an oral antidiabetic drug is often prescribed. However, the patient should be clearly advised that the ability of any drug therapy to improve the health of any diabetic patient is aided by appropriate changes in diet and activity level. Such drug therapy may fail or become inadequate without an effort by the patient to make behavioral changes. Once-daily dosage forms of various oral drugs are increasingly popular, as is the case with insulins (e.g., glargine). As is the case with drug therapy in general, reduced frequency of dosing is associated with increased patient adherence to the drug regimen and improved therapeutic outcomes.

Mechanism of Action and Drug Effects
Sulfonylureas
The sulfonylureas are a group of oral antidiabetic drugs that are able to stimulate insulin secretion from the beta cells of the pancreas. This increased insulin then helps to transport the glucose out of the blood and into the tissues, cells, and organs in which it is needed. Because of these actions, the sulfonylureas may be broadly considered oral hypoglycemic drugs. These drugs have

many other beneficial effects besides their ability to stimulate insulin release from the pancreas. They may also enhance the actions of insulin in muscle, liver, and adipose tissue, which allows these tissues to take up and store glucose more easily as a later source of energy. They may also increase the availability of insulin by preventing the liver from breaking insulin down as fast as it ordinarily would (reduced hepatic clearance). In summary, the overall effect of the sulfonylureas is that they improve both insulin secretion and the sensitivity to insulin in tissues.

The sulfonylureas have been the backbone of oral pharmacologic therapy for type 2 diabetes mellitus for more than 30 years. Their primary beneficial effect in patients with type 2 diabetes mellitus is to stimulate insulin secretion from beta cells in the pancreas. This means that the patient must still have functioning beta cells. Thus these drugs work best during the early stages of the disease when there is preserved beta cell function. Selected sulfonylurea drugs and their comparative durations of action are listed in Table 31-8. Although the first-generation drugs listed are less commonly used now than before, they are still available and preferred by some patients and prescribers. The action of these drugs forces the extra glucose out of the blood (the site of its harmful effects) and into cells, tissues, and organs (in which it can be used as energy or stored as fuel). The sulfonylurea compounds also increase the sensitivity of the insulin receptor proteins in the cells of the muscles, liver, and fat to the effects of insulin.

Meglitinides

Repaglinide and nateglinide are currently the only two drugs in the meglitinide class. They are structurally different from the sulfonylureas but have a similar mechanism of action in that they also increase insulin secretion from the pancreas.

Biguanide

Late in 1994, metformin, a drug that had been used abroad since the 1950s, was approved for use in the United States. Metformin is currently the only drug classified as a *biguanide*. Like the sulfonylureas, it is now among the most commonly used oral drugs for treating type 2 diabetes. Metformin differs significantly from the sulfonylureas in that it does not increase insulin secretion from the pancreas and thus does not cause hypoglycemia. Metformin works by decreasing the production of glucose as well as increasing its uptake.

Metformin is believed to exert its beneficial effects in type 2 diabetes mellitus via three mechanisms: (1) it decreases glucose production by the liver; (2) it decreases intestinal absorption of glucose; and (3) it improves insulin receptor sensitivity in the liver, skeletal muscle, and adipose tissue. This results in increased peripheral glucose uptake and use and decreased hepatic production of triglycerides and cholesterol. Unlike sulfonylureas and insulins, metformin does not produce hypoglycemia. Metformin also affects the intestines by decreasing the absorption of glucose.

Thiazolidinediones

The third major drug category to emerge for the oral treatment of type 2 diabetes mellitus is the thiazolidinediones. The first drug in this class to be used in the United States was troglitazone (Rezulin). In 2000, it was removed from the market because of concerns about liver toxicity. However, two newer thiazolidinediones have taken its place: pioglitazone and rosiglitazone. They offer efficacy similar to that of troglitazone with less risk of toxicity. Thiazolidinediones are also referred to as *insulin-sensitizing drugs*, as well as *glitazones*. Thiazolidinediones work to decrease insulin resistance by enhancing the sensitivity of insulin receptors in such areas as the liver, skeletal muscle, and adipose tissue. These drugs are also known to directly stimulate peripheral glucose uptake and storage, as well as to inhibit glucose and triglyceride production in the liver.

Thiazolidinediones, also known as glitazones, work to decrease insulin resistance by enhancing the insulin sensitivity of insulin receptors in such areas as the liver, skeletal muscle, and adipose tissue. This results in enhanced glucose uptake and storage. Thiazolidinediones work at two of the primary sites in the body that are abnormal in patients with type 2 diabetes mellitus: the liver and the skeletal muscle. In the presence of endogenous or exogenous insulin, thiazolidinediones reduce gluconeogenesis, glucose output, and triglyceride synthesis in the liver. They increase glucose uptake and use in skeletal muscle, and they increase glucose uptake and decrease fatty acid output in adipose tissue. Thiazolidinediones have no known effect on insulin secretion.

α-Glucosidase Inhibitors

Less commonly used than the oral drug classes described previously are the α-glucosidase inhibitors acarbose and miglitol. The α-glucosidase inhibitors work by reversibly inhibiting the en-

Table 31-8	**Sulfonylurea Drugs: Qualitative Comparison of Pharmacokinetic Properties**			
Drug	**Potency**	**Onset of Action**	**Duration of Action**	**Active Metabolite?**
First Generation				
acetohexamide (generic only)	Low	Fast	Long	Yes
chlorpropamide (Diabinese)	Low	Fast	Very long	Yes
tolazamide (Tolinase)	Low	Slow	Long	Yes
tolbutamide (Orinase)	Low	Fast	Short	No
Second Generation				
glimepiride (Amaryl)	High	Intermediate	Long	Yes
glipizide (Glucotrol, Glucotrol XL)	High	Fast	Long	No
glyburide (DiaBeta, Micronase, Glynase PresTab)	High	Slow	Long	Yes

zyme α-*glucosidase.* This enzyme is found in the brush border (villi) of the small intestine and is responsible for the hydrolysis of oligosaccharides and disaccharides to glucose and other monosaccharides. When this enzyme is blocked, glucose absorption is delayed. The timing of administration of the α-glucosidase inhibitors is important. When an α-glucosidase inhibitor is taken with the first bite of a meal, excessive postprandial blood glucose elevation (a glucose "spike") can be prevented or reduced.

Indications

Sulfonylurea drugs are used to lower the blood glucose levels in patients when diet and lifestyle changes have failed to do so, although beta cell function must be preserved for the drugs to have this action. The biguanide metformin and the α-glucosidase inhibitors are indicated as monotherapy in patients with type 2 diabetes mellitus. They are used as an adjunct to dietary measures to lower blood glucose levels when hyperglycemia cannot be satisfactorily managed through diet alone. Metformin may be used concomitantly with a sulfonylurea when dietary measures and metformin or a sulfonylurea drug alone does not result in adequate glycemic control. The α-glucosidase inhibitors may be used in this way as well. The thiazolidinediones (or glitazones) are most commonly used alone or with a sulfonylurea, metformin, or insulin in patients with type 2 diabetes mellitus.

Contraindications

Contraindications to the use of all antidiabetic drugs generally include known drug allergy and active hypoglycemia. They may also include severe liver or kidney disease, depending on the required metabolic pathways of the drug in question. These oral drugs are generally not used during pregnancy; insulin therapy is preferred because it not only is safer for the fetus but also provides for the more careful glycemic control that is so critical during pregnancy.

Adverse Effects

Sulfonylureas

The most serious adverse effects of sulfonylureas involve the hematologic system and include agranulocytosis, hemolytic anemia, thrombocytopenia, and cholestatic jaundice. Effects on the gastrointestinal (GI) system include nausea, epigastric fullness, and heartburn. Erythema, photosensitivity, hypoglycemia, and morbilliform and maculopapular eruptions are other undesirable effects.

Meglitinides

The most commonly reported adverse effects of the meglitinides include headache, hypoglycemia, dizziness, weight gain, joint pain, and upper respiratory infection or flulike symptoms.

Biguanide

The biguanide metformin primarily affects the GI tract. The most common adverse effects of therapy with metformin are abdominal bloating, nausea, cramping, a feeling of fullness, and diarrhea. These effects are all usually self-limiting and transient, and can be lessened by starting with low dosages, titrating up slowly, and taking the medication with food. Less common adverse effects with metformin are a metallic taste and a reduction in vitamin B_{12} levels. Lactic acidosis is extremely rare with metformin

and is lethal in 50% of cases. Unlike sulfonylureas, metformin does not cause hypoglycemia.

Thiazolidinediones

Rosiglitazone and pioglitazone both may cause moderate weight gain, edema, and mild anemia, possibly as a result of fluid retention. The safety of thiazolidinedione use in pregnant women, in children, and in patients with heart failure has not been established. There is concern that hepatic toxicity may be an effect of the entire class of thiazolidinediones. Laboratory measurement of liver alanine aminotransferase (ALT) levels is recommended before treatment is begun to assess baseline liver function, and ALT levels should be measured periodically thereafter per clinical judgment. If the ALT level rises above 2.5 to 3 times the normal upper limit, ALT monitoring should be done more frequently and the drug should be discontinued if ALT levels do not return to normal values.

α-Glucosidase Inhibitors

The α-glucosidase inhibitors acarbose and miglitol also have adverse effects that primarily involve the GI tract. They can cause flatulence, diarrhea, and abdominal pain. At high dosages they may also elevate levels of hepatic enzymes (transaminases). Unlike sulfonylureas they do not cause hypoglycemia, hyperinsulinemia, or weight gain.

Interactions

Sulfonylureas

The potential drug interactions that can occur with sulfonylureas are significant. Their hypoglycemic effect is increased when they are taken concurrently with alcohol, anabolic steroids, β-blockers, chloramphenicol, guanethidine, MAOIs, oral anticoagulants, phenylbutazone, or sulfonamides. Herbal supplements that are reported to increase the likelihood of hypoglycemia when given with sulfonylureas include garlic and ginseng.

Drugs that are capable of reducing the hypoglycemic effect of sulfonylureas include adrenergics, corticosteroids, thiazides, and thyroid preparations. In addition, the drugs in some drug classes have sufficient chemical similarity to the sulfonylureas that *allergic cross-reactivity* may be seen. These drug classes include loop diuretics (e.g., furosemide) and sulfonamide antibiotics (e.g., sulfamethoxazole). Sulfonylureas may also interact with alcohol in a way similar to disulfiram (Antabuse), which is used to deter alcohol ingestion in individuals with chronic alcoholism. Such a *disulfiram-type reaction* includes acute discomforts such as vomiting and hypertensive episodes.

Meglitinides

The hypoglycemic effects of the meglitinides may be increased if they are given with drugs such as fluconazole, gemfibrozil, nonsteroidal antiinflammatory drugs, pioglitazone, sulfonamides. Reduced hypoglycemic effects have been reported with drugs such as phenobarbital, phenytoin, carbamazepine, nafcillin, and thiazide diuretics.

Biguanide

Metformin concentrations can be increased when the drug is given concomitantly with furosemide and nifedipine. When it is given with cationic drugs such as cimetidine or digoxin, competition for renal tubular secretion occurs, which results in increased metformin concentrations. In addition, the concurrent use of metformin with iodinated (iodine-containing) radiologic contrast media has been associated with both acute renal failure and lactic acidosis. For these reasons, metformin therapy should be discontinued at least 48 hours before the patient undergoes any radiologic study that requires such contrast media and should be withheld for at least 48 hours after the procedure. The integrity of the patient's renal function should also be confirmed via blood sampling after the procedure before the patient is allowed to resume metformin therapy.

Thiazolidinediones

Clinically important interactions between rosiglitazone and other drugs have not been reported. Levels of low-density lipoprotein and high-density lipoprotein cholesterol increase between 12% and 19% in individuals taking rosiglitazone, but triglyceride levels may actually decrease. Pioglitazone, on the other hand, is partly metabolized by cytochrome P-450 3A4 (CYP3A4). Serum concentrations of pioglitazone may be increased if the drug is taken concurrently with a CYP3A4 inhibitor such as ketoconazole. However, pioglitazone raises low-density lipoprotein cholesterol only slightly and lowers serum triglyceride concentrations.

α-Glucosidase Inhibitors

Other potential drug interactions include medications that can cause hyperglycemia as an adverse effect, including loop and other types of diuretics, corticosteroids, estrogens, phenothiazines, thyroid replacement hormones, antiepileptic drugs, the antilipemic drug niacin, sympathomimetics (often found in cold products that are OTC), digoxin, and intestinal adsorbents.

Dosages

For the recommended dosages of oral antidiabetic drugs, see the Dosages table on this page.

Drug Profiles

Sulfonylurea drugs are the oldest class of oral medications used for diabetes. There are two categories, or generations, of sulfonylurea drugs. The first-generation sulfonylureas are the older low-potency drugs acetohexamide, tolbutamide, chlorpropamide, and tolazamide. These are still available but are now used much less frequently than newer drugs. The second-generation sulfonylureas are the newer high-potency drugs glimepiride, glyburide, and glipizide.

The newer drug categories include the biguanides, α-glucosidase inhibitors, meglitinides, and thiazolidinediones. Currently the only biguanide used in the United States is metformin. Two α-glucosidase inhibitors, acarbose and miglitol, are presently available. The meglitinides include repaglinide and nateglinide. The newest class of drugs used to treat patients with type 2 diabetes mellitus is the thiazolidinediones. Pioglitazone and rosiglitazone both belong to this class and are currently the only thiazolidinediones available. Several combination drug products are also marketed, including rosiglitazone plus metformin (Avandamet), glyburide plus metformin (Glucovance), and glipizide plus metformin (Metaglip). Dosage information for selected drugs appears in the Dosages table on this page.

acarbose

acarbose (Precose) is one of the two currently available α-glucosidase inhibitors. The other drug in this drug category is miglitol (Glyset). As noted earlier, these drugs work by blunting the elevation of blood

DOSAGES

Selected Oral Antidiabetic Drugs

Drug (Pregnancy Category)	Pharmacologic Class	Usual Dosage Range	Indications
acarbose (Precose) (B)	α-glucosidase inhibitor	PO: 25-100 mg tid, taken with first bite of meal	
chlorpropamide (Diabinese) (C)	First-generation sulfonylurea	PO: 100-500 mg divided daily or bid (max daily dose 750 mg)	
glimepiride (Amaryl)	Second-generation sulfonylurea	PO: 1-8 mg daily	
▸glipizide (Glucotrol, Glucotrol XL) (C)	Second-generation sulfonylurea	PO: 5-40 mg daily (max single dose 15 mg)	
▸glyburide (DiaBeta, Micronase, Glynase PresTab) (C)	Second-generation sulfonylurea	PO: 1.25-20 mg/day divided daily or bid	
▸metformin (Glucophage, Glucophage XR) (B)	Biguanide	PO: 500 mg bid or 850 mg daily; max daily dose 2550 mg for adults and 2000 mg for pediatric patients aged 10-16 yr	Diabetes mellitus type 2
repaglinide (Prandin) (C)	Meglitinide	PO: 0.5-4 mg tid; best taken 15 min before a meal	
▸rosiglitazone (Avandia) (C)	Thiazolidinedione	PO: 2-8 mg divided daily or bid	

Combination Oral Drugs

Drug (Pregnancy Category)	Pharmacologic Class	Usual Dosage Range	Indications
glyburide/metformin (Glucovance) (C)	Combination sulfonylurea/ biguanide	PO: 1-2 tabs daily or bid	
rosiglitazone/metformin (Avandamet) (C)	Combination thiazolidinedione/ biguanide	PO: 1-2 tabs daily or bid	

glucose levels after a meal. To work optimally they should be taken with the first bite of each meal. They also may be taken concomitantly with sulfonylurea drugs or with metformin. Acarbose use is contraindicated in patients with a hypersensitivity to α-glucosidase inhibitors, DKA, cirrhosis, inflammatory bowel disease, colonic ulceration, partial intestinal obstruction, or chronic intestinal disease.

Pharmacokinetics

Half-Life	Onset	Peak	Duration
2-3 hr	1-1.5 hr	14-24 hr	9-15 hr

▶ glipizide

Glipizide (Glucotrol) is a second-generation sulfonylurea drug with a potency much greater than that of the first-generation drugs. For this reason the common doses of glipizide are 5 and 10 mg compared with 100 to 500 mg for the first-generation drugs. In contrast to another second-generation sulfonylurea, glyburide, glipizide has a very rapid onset and short duration of action, with no active metabolites. This confers many benefits. The rapid onset of action allows it to function much like the body normally does in response to meals when greater levels of insulin are required rapidly to deal with the increased glucose in the blood. When a patient with type 2 diabetes mellitus takes glipizide, it rapidly stimulates the pancreas to release insulin. This, in turn, facilitates the transport of excess glucose from the blood into the cells of the muscles, liver, and adipose tissues.

Its short duration of action compared with that of glyburide prevents long-term stimulation of the beta cells in the pancreas, which may otherwise cause the beta cells to become resistant to the effects of the sulfonylurea drugs. It may also cause them to make too much insulin and thereby induce hyperinsulinemia, which can cause the muscle, liver, and fat tissues to become resistant to the effects of insulin.

Glipizide use is contraindicated in cases of known drug allergy as well as in type 1 or brittle diabetes. Unlike most other oral antidiabetic drugs, it is not contraindicated in patients with severe renal failure. It works best if given 30 minutes before meals. This allows the timing of the insulin secretion induced by the glipizide to correspond to the elevation in the blood glucose level induced by the meal in much the same way as endogenous insulin levels are raised in a person without diabetes.

Pharmacokinetics

Half-Life	Onset	Peak	Duration
1-1.5 hr	1-3 hr	10-24 hr	1-1.5 hr

▶ glyburide

Glyburide (DiaBeta, Micronase, Glynase PresTab) is another second-generation sulfonylurea drug. It differs from the first-generation oral hypoglycemic drugs in its greater potency and from glipizide in its slower onset and longer duration of action and the fact that it has active metabolites. These differences can have significant consequences. Because of its relatively slow onset of action, glyburide is less desirable for the treatment of the short-term elevations in blood glucose levels that occur after meals. However, its longer duration of action makes it better for the long-term, constant stimulation of the pancreas, causing it to release a constant amount of insulin. This may be beneficial in controlling blood glucose levels during the night and/or throughout the day. It has the same contraindications as glipizide.

Pharmacokinetics

Half-Life*	Onset	Peak	Duration
2-4 hr	1-1.5 hr	4 hr	20-24 hr

*When assays have been performed to measure metabolite levels, the terminal elimination half-life has been found to average 10 hr.

glimepiride

Glimepiride (Amaryl) is the newest of the sulfonylurea drugs. It has properties comparable to those of glyburide and glipizide described previously, except that it has an onset of action that is intermediate between that of glipizide and glyburide, as indicated in Table 31-8.

Pharmacokinetics

Half-Life	Onset	Peak	Duration
5-9 hr	2-3 hr	2-3 hr	24 hr

▶ metformin

Metformin (Glucophage) is currently the only biguanide oral antidiabetic drug. It works primarily by inhibiting hepatic glucose production and increasing the sensitivity of peripheral tissue to insulin. Because its mechanism of action differs from that of sulfonylurea drugs, it may be given concomitantly with these drugs.

Metformin use is contraindicated in patients with a hypersensitivity to biguanides, hepatic or renal disease, alcoholism, or cardiopulmonary disease.

Pharmacokinetics

Half-Life	Onset	Peak	Duration
1.5-5 hr	Less than 1 hr	1-3 hr	24 hr

repaglinide

Repaglinide (Prandin) is one of two antidiabetic drugs classified as meglitinides, the other being nateglinide (Starlix). These drugs have a mechanism of action similar to that of the sulfonylureas in that they also stimulate the release of insulin from pancreatic beta cells. They are often especially helpful in the treatment of patients who have erratic eating habits, because the drug dose is skipped when a meal is missed. Contraindications include known drug allergy.

Pharmacokinetics

Half-Life	Onset	Peak	Duration
2-3 hr	15-60 min	1 hr	4-6 hr

▶ rosiglitazone

Rosiglitazone (Avandia) is classified as a glitazone or thiazolidinedione derivative. It is marketed for the treatment of patients with type 2 diabetes. Rosiglitazone and pioglitazone (Actos) are used alone or with a sulfonylurea, metformin, or insulin. Thiazolidinedione antidiabetic drugs work by decreasing insulin resistance. As noted earlier the safety of these drugs for use in pregnant women, children, and individuals with heart failure has not been established.

Pharmacokinetics

Half-Life	Onset	Peak	Duration
3-4 hr	Unknown	1 hr	Unknown

MISCELLANEOUS ANTIDIABETIC DRUGS

Amylin Mimetic

In 2005, the first amylin mimetic drug was approved by the FDA. It is known as pramlintide (Symlin; pregnancy category C) and works by mimicking the action of the natural hormone amylin. *Amylin* is a protein in the body that is stored with and secreted with insulin from the pancreas in response to food intake. It affects the postprandial blood levels of glucose in the following three ways.

1. It slows gastric emptying.
2. It suppresses glucagon secretion, which reduces hepatic glucose output.
3. It centrally modulates appetite and satiety (sense of having eaten enough).

The drug is indicated for use in patients with type 1 or type 2 diabetes receiving mealtime insulin who have failed to achieve optimal glucose control with insulin and/or oral antidiabetic drugs. Its use is contraindicated in patients with known drug allergy (including allergy to its *metacresol* component), gastroparesis or other impaired GI motility, hypoglycemia, or **hemoglobin A1c (HbA1c)** level of more than 9%; in patients who are poorly adherent with insulin therapy or self-monitoring of blood glucose level; and in pediatric patients. Adverse effects include self-limiting nausea, vomiting, and dizziness, especially in overdose. The drug itself does not cause hypoglycemia, but if the patient is taking any preprandial rapid- or short-acting insulin product, the insulin dose usually needs to be reduced by 50%. Pramlintide can delay the oral absorption of any drug and should be given at least 1 hour before any concentration-dependent oral medication (including oral contraceptives and antibiotics). It can also alter insulin pharmacokinetics in the body and should not be mixed with any insulin products. Recommended dosage ranges are from 15 to 60 mcg for type 1 diabetes and 60 to 120 mcg for type 2 diabetes, given before any major meal (defined as more than 250 kcal or more than 30 g of carbohydrates). The drug is given only by subcutaneous injection.

Incretin Mimetic

Also in 2005, the first *incretin mimetic,* exenatide, was approved. Exenatide (Byetta; pregnancy category C) works by mimicking the class of hormones known as *incretins,* which normally enhance glucose-driven insulin secretion from pancreatic beta cells. These hormones also suppress excessive glucagon secretion and delay gastric emptying. The result is reduction of both fasting and postprandial glucose concentrations in patients with type 2 diabetes. This drug is indicated only for patients with type 2 diabetes and is contraindicated in those with drug allergy or type 1 diabetes. Possible adverse effects include hypoglycemia, dizziness, and nausea. Like pramlintide (see earlier), this drug can delay absorption of other orally administered drugs because of its slowing of gastric emptying. In patients who also receive metformin, the metformin dose does not need to be changed, because metformin does not cause hypoglycemia. However, in patients taking sulfonylurea drugs the dose may need to be reduced if hypoglycemia appears on initiation of exenatide therapy. The usual starting dosage is 5 mcg within 1 hour of both the morning and evening meals. If needed, the dosage may be increased to 10 mcg twice daily before meals after 1 month on the 5-mcg dose.

In September of 2005, an advisory committee recommended to the FDA that it approve the drug Exubera, an inhaled insulin product. Exubera is expected to be marketed in September of 2006. Evidence suggests that it could eventually replace injected insulin for many diabetic patients.

HYPOGLYCEMIA

Hypoglycemia is an abnormally low blood glucose level (generally below 50 mg/dL). When the cause is organic and the effects are mild, treatment usually consists of dietary modifications, primarily a higher intake of protein and lower intake of carbohydrates, to prevent a rebound postprandial hypoglycemic effect. Hypoglycemia is also a common adverse effect of many antidiabetic drugs when their pharmacologic effects are greater than expected. Because the brain needs a constant amount of glucose to function, early symptoms of hypoglycemia include the central nervous system (CNS) manifestations of confusion, irritability, tremor, and sweating. Later symptoms include hypothermia and seizures. Without adequate restoration of normal blood and CNS glucose levels, coma and death will occur.

GLUCOSE-ELEVATING DRUGS

Oral forms of concentrated glucose are available for patients to use in the event of a hypoglycemic crisis. Dosage forms include rapidly dissolving buccal tablets and semisolid gel forms designed for oral use and rapid mucosal absorption. It should be pointed out that table sugar, which is sucrose, will not produce as rapid an effect as the glucose products intended for use by diabetic patients. This is because sucrose is a *disaccharide* (two-molecule) sugar that must first be digested in the body to yield glucose as a *monosaccharide* (one-molecule) by-product. In the hospital setting, intravenous glucose is an obvious option. Concentrations of up to 50% dextrose in water ($D_{50}W$) are most often used for this purpose. Although solutions with glucose concentrations of up to 70% are also available, these are usually used for TPN preparations rather than acute treatment of hypoglycemia.

In addition to oral and/or intravenous glucose, two other drugs are specifically used for the treatment of hypoglycemia. Glucagon, a natural hormone secreted by the pancreas, has also been synthesized in the laboratory and is now available as an injection to be given when a quick response to hypoglycemia is needed. Diazoxide is another drug that may be given to correct abnormally low blood glucose levels. It works by inhibiting the release of insulin from the pancreas and is most commonly given to patients with long-term illnesses that are causing hypoglycemia. An example of such an illness is a pancreatic cancer that causes the pancreas to oversecrete insulin, which results in too much insulin in the blood, or hyperinsulinemia. The oral form of diazoxide is used for these purposes. There is also an intravenous form that is used for the treatment of hypertensive emergencies (very high blood pressure) in intensive care unit settings.

PHARMACOKINETIC BRIDGE to Nursing Practice

Provision of insulin therapy by continuous subcutaneous insulin infusion (CSII) is becoming an option for selected patients with diabetes to minimize the risks and complications of the disease. Other treatment options used to achieve tight control are multiple daily injections of insulin (MDI), but the onset, peak and duration of action of the drug will depend on the specific insulin used. With CSII, normal serum glucose levels are maintained by the continuous delivery of basal insulin with food intake—primarily carbohydrate consumption—being covered by bolus doses of insulin. Insulin pumps (e.g., CSII) lead to a more rapid, consistent absorption of the drug, and hypoglycemia is reduced. Research has also shown that use of an insulin pump helps to decrease the occurrence of elevated pre-breakfast serum glucose levels, or what is often called the *dawn phenomenon* (referring to the dawn of the day). Because the insulin pump delivers insulin through the subcutaneous route and due to the infusion being a continuous one, fewer problems occur that were previously associated with once or twice daily injections. Patients using CSII achieve mean serum glucose and HbA1c levels that remain somewhat lower than those associated with MDI, thus creating less risk for hypoglycemia. Understanding new and different drugs (with their associated pharmacokinetic properties) allows the nurse to help patients achieve higher quality of life, minimize risks, and maximize wellness.

◆ NURSING PROCESS

◆ ASSESSMENT

Before administering any type of antidiabetic drug, the nurse must assess the patient's knowledge about the disease and recommended treatment(s). Head-to-toe physical assessment, medication history, and nursing assessment need to be completed and documented. A medication history should include a list of current medications, including over-the-counter (OTC) drugs, herbals, and supplements. Assessment of appropriate laboratory test results (e.g., fasting blood glucose level, HbA1c level) should include noting any abnormalities compared to baseline levels. The physician's order for insulin must also be assessed so that the correct route, type of insulin (e.g., clear [rapid- or short-acting] or cloudy [intermediate-acting or NPH]), and dosage are implemented correctly. With assessment, it is important to note that allergic reactions are less likely to occur with recombinant human insulins than with pork insulins because of the similarity with endogenous insulin. Contraindications, cautions, and drug interactions associated with the various forms of insulin have already been discussed and should be thoroughly assessed prior to giving any insulin. Oral antidiabetic drugs also require close assessment of contraindications, cautions, and drug interactions, with an additional concern for other drugs that have chemical-structural similarity with sulfonylureas (e.g., furosemide, sulfamethoxazole) because of the increased risk for cross sensitivity.

The nurse must also be aware that patients who are elderly and malnourished may react adversely to the biguanides. Contraindications, cautions, and drug interactions for this drug class have been previously discussed. Also important to remember is the interaction between metformin and the radiopaque dyes used for certain diagnostic purposes (e.g., CT scan with contrast). The interaction is associated with an increased risk for renal dysfunction. With thiazolidinediones, one important caution to emphasize in addition to those previously discussed is their use in patients with elevated ALT levels. Baseline ALT levels should therefore be measured before drug therapy is begun and periodically thereafter (e.g., every 3 months or as ordered).

Cultural factors must also be assessed in relation to compliance with a therapeutic regimen. Unstable serum glucose levels require immediate attention, so assessment of any signs and symptoms of hypoglycemia (e.g., acute onset of nervousness, sweating, lethargy, weakness, cold and clammy skin, change in sensorium) or symptoms of hyperglycemia (e.g., tachycardia, blood glucose levels that exceed 150 mg/dL, changes in respiration [Kussmaul's respiration]) should be completed. Assessment is even more critical for a diabetic patient who is also under stress, has an infection or is ill, is pregnant or lactating, or is experiencing trauma or any change in health status. With treatment, diabetics are at risk of hypoglycemia, with the potential danger of losing consciousness; thus there is a need for constant assessment of serum glucose levels and neurological status.

CASE STUDY
Diabetes Mellitus

B.G. is a 58-year-old male who was diagnosed with type 2 adult-onset diabetes mellitus 10 years ago. Although he has type 2 diabetes mellitus, he has needed to take insulin for the last 2 years. He has been recovering, without complications, from a laparoscopic cholecystectomy, but his blood glucose levels have shown some wide fluctuations over the past 24 hours. The physician has changed his insulin to lispro (Humalog) to see if it will provide better control of his blood glucose levels.

- What is the rationale for the use of oral antidiabetic drugs in a patient with type 2 diabetes? Why do some patients with type 2 diabetes have to begin taking insulin? What can be done to measure the control of the patient's diabetes, short term and long term?
- What are the pharmacokinetics of lispro?
- What special instructions, if any, should be given to B.G. about the lispro before he is discharged home from the hospital?

For answers, see http://evolve.elsevier.com/Lilley.

◆ NURSING DIAGNOSES

- Risk for injury related to neurologic deficits (e.g., neuropathies) associated with diabetes mellitus
- Risk for infection related to the pathologic impact of diabetes associated with altered immune system function
- Imbalanced nutrition, more than body requirements, leading to weight gain associated with diabetes
- Deficient knowledge related to lack of information about diabetes mellitus, its management, and prevention of disease-related complications
- Ineffective therapeutic regimen management related to lack of experience with a significant daily treatment regimen

◆ PLANNING
Goals

- Patient remains free from self-injury and complications of diabetes.
- Patient remains free of infection.
- Patient maintains adequate weight control and dietary habits in the overall management of diabetes.
- Patient states the effects of diabetes on body function.
- Patient remains compliant with the medical regimen and adheres to treatment protocols.
- Patient states the importance of adherence to medication regimens, lifestyle changes, dietary restrictions, and avoidance of high-risk behaviors.
- Patient states the action and adverse effects of insulin or the oral hypoglycemic drugs.

Outcome Criteria

- Patient performs self-assessment and foot care as directed and as needed to maintain healthy skin.
- Patient immediately reports elevated temperature, difficult-to-heal lesions or sores, and any unusual redness of any area of the skin to his or her health care provider.
- Patient observes the diet recommended by the ADA or other dietary advisor per the orders of the physician or nutritional consult.
- Patient eats a healthy diet, gets sufficient rest and relaxation, and notifies the physician should any unusual problems occur with changes in customary activity (e.g., nausea and vomiting).

- Patient keeps all scheduled appointments with health care providers to monitor therapeutic effectiveness and assess for complications of therapy.
- Patient takes medication as scheduled, monitors blood glucose levels, and watches for any signs and symptoms of hyperglycemia or hypoglycemia.

◆ IMPLEMENTATION

With any patient who is taking insulin or oral antidiabetic drugs, the nurse must always check serum glucose levels (and other related laboratory values) before giving the drug so that accurate baseline glucose levels are obtained and documented. An additional check of the medication order and the prepared dosage should be carried out with another registered nurse. Insulin should be rolled between the hands before the prescribed dosage is withdrawn to avoid air in the syringe and inaccurate dosage administration. Insulin may be stored at room temperature if it is to be used within 1 month; otherwise, it must be refrigerated. Refrigeration is also recommended in warm or hot climates or temperatures. If insulin is discolored or is expired, it should not be used. For information about the handling, mixing, storage, and administration of insulin see Box 31-4.

Insulin should be administered subcutaneously at a 90-degree angle unless the patient is emaciated, in which case it should be administered at a 45-degree angle. Only regular insulin may be administered intravenously, but use of this route is controversial because of absorption of the insulin into the intravenous bag and/or tubing. Only insulin syringes should be used and are easy to identify because they have orange caps and are calibrated in units (U) not milliliters (mL). The syringe has a pre-attached needle that is 29 gauge (and ½ inch in length). When mixing insulins (if ordered), the regular or rapid-acting insulin (unmodified and *clear*) should be withdrawn first, followed by withdrawal of the intermediate-acting or NPH (modified and cloudy), but only after the appropriate amount of air has been injected (which is equal to the prescribed number of units) into the vials. Air should be injected into the intermediate insulin vial, followed by injection of air into the regular or rapid-/short-acting insulin vial. This helps prevent contamination of the rapid-acting insulin by the intermediate-acting insulin (see Table 31-3 and Chapter 9). Some fixed combinations of insulin products come pre-mixed.

Understanding the action of the insulin and its related pharmacokinetics (e.g., onset, peak, duration) is critical to safe care and for patient education. For example, it is important to know that lispro insulin is more rapidly absorbed than regular insulin with an onset of action of 15 minutes and peak effect of 1 to 2 hours, so lispro must be given 15 minutes before meals as compared to 30 minutes before meals as with regular insulin. Lispro insulin mixted with NPH should be given immediately after the insulins are mixed and also 15 minutes before meals. The physician's orders should be also be checked for any dietary changes (e.g., possible increase in carbohydrates and decrease in fat intake to avoid postprandial hypoglycemia).

Box 31-4 Administration, Handling, and Storage of Insulin

Dosages, Storage, Handling, and Mixing

1. Individualize insulin dosages (e.g., use sliding scales as ordered) and monitor closely for adequate control of hypoglycemia and hyperglycemia.
2. Adjust dosages, as ordered, to achieve premeal and bedtime serum glucose levels of 90 to 130 mg/dL in adults.
3. Store insulin for current use at room temperature. Avoid extreme temperatures and exposure to sunlight because the insulin's protein structure will be permanently denatured. Extra vials not in use should be stored in the refrigerator. Vials being used in high environmental temperatures should also be stored in the refrigerator, but insulin should *never* be given cold. Never freeze insulin. To maintain drug stability, insulin should be stored for up to 1 month at room temperature and for up to 3 months in the refrigerator.
4. Discard unused vials if they have not been used for several weeks (or follow hospital policy). Do not use any insulin that does not have the proper clarity or color (e.g., clear for regular, cloudy for NPH).
5. Store prefilled insulin syringes in the refrigerator for up to 1 week. Store the syringe with the needle pointing upward to avoid clogging within the hub of the needle.

Administration

1. Administer insulin subcutaneously (Chapter 9), however, regular insulin may be given intravenously in special situations (e.g., drip in patient with diabetic ketoacidosis; in postoperative patients) if ordered.
2. Roll the drug vial gently between hands without shaking to avoid bubble formation in the vial, which may lead to inaccurate dosage withdrawal. Give mixed insulins within 5 minutes of mixing to avoid binding of the solution and subsequent altered activity of the drugs.
3. Administer insulin at the recommended times, but always with meals or meal trays ready. Give insulin lispro approximately 15 minutes before meals (it has a quicker onset of action) and only after monitoring the patient's fasting serum glucose level (as with all insulin administration). Give regular and rapid-acting insulin 30 minutes before a meal, and give NPH insulin 30 to 45 minutes before mealtime.
4. When giving regular and NPH insulin at the same time (if ordered), mix the two appropriately (see discussion of mixing insulins in the Implementation subsection under Nursing Process). This mixture is usually given at least 30 minutes before mealtime.
5. Administer insulin subcutaneously at a 90-degree angle in most cases. If the patient is emaciated, a 45-degree angle may be more effective. Insulin syringes should always be used (see previous discussion and Chapter 9).
6. Instruct patients taking insulin injections to rotate sites within the same general location for about 1 week before moving to a new location (e.g., all injections for a week in the upper right thigh before moving a little lower on the right thigh). This technique allows for better insulin absorption. Each injection site should be at least ½ to 1 inch away from the previous injection site. If this practice is followed, it will be approximately 6 weeks before the patient will have to rotate to a totally new area of the body. Note the following sites for subcutaneous insulin injections: thigh areas (front and back) and outer areas of the upper arm (middle third of the upper arm between the shoulder and the elbow).
7. Mix intranasal insulin forms with a surfactant according to package or pharmacist's instructions for safe administration and storage. Teach the patient that the surfactant may be irritating to the nares and to notify the health provider if this occurs.
8. Continuous subcutaneous insulin injections and/or multiple daily injections may be ordered for tight glucose control.

Regardless of whether pork or recombinant human insulin is used, understanding the peak, onset, and duration of action of the specific insulin will help the nurse determine when the food should be administered. The intermediate-acting insulins, such as NPH and the many combination products of regular and intermediate insulin, have onsets of action ranging from 30 minutes to 1 to 2 hours; therefore, this is the time interval with which the nurse must work to ensure that the patient eats (i.e., immediately before or at the time of onset of action). In the hospital setting, be sure that meal trays have arrived on the unit before giving insulin to avoid time lapses and subsequent hypoglycemic episodes. The nurse must also be sure that other forms of allowed foods are available to the patient in case meals are delayed and insulin has already been administered.

Patients may require dosing by a sliding-scale method, which includes subcutaneous regular insulin doses adjusted according to serum glucose test results. Sliding scale may be used for hospitalized diabetic patients experiencing drastic changes in serum glucose levels due to physical and/or emotional stress, infections, surgery, acute illness, inactivity, or variable caloric intake, as well as in patients needing intensive insulin therapy. When this insulin regimen is used, blood glucose levels are measured several times a day (e.g., every 4 hours, every 6 hours, or at specified times such as 7 AM, 11 AM, 4 PM, and midnight) to obtain fasting and/or pre-meal blood glucose values.

Oral antidiabetic drugs are usually given at least 30 minutes before meals. Some of the sulfonylureas are to be taken with breakfast, α-glucosidase inhibitors are always to be taken with the first bite of each main meal, and the thiazolidinediones are to be given once daily or in two divided doses. Exact timing of the dose should always be checked against the physician's order and with consideration of the drug's onset of action. With metformin (as with any antidiabetic drug or insulin) it is important for the nurse and/or patient to know what to do if symptoms of hypoglycemia occur—for example, the patient should take glucagon; eat glucose tablets or gel, corn syrup, or honey; drink fruit juice or a non-diet soft drink; or eat a small snack such as crackers or half a sandwich. If the patient receiving metformin is to undergo diagnostic studies with contrast dye, the physician will need to discontinue the drug prior to the procedure and restart it after the tests only after reevaluation of the patient's renal status. It is critical to the safe and efficient use of oral antidiabetics to be sure that food will be or is being tolerated before the dose is given. If the oral drug and/or insulin is taken and no meal is consumed or it is consumed at a later time than usual, hypoglycemia may be problematic and result in negative health consequences and even unconsciousness. Because rosiglitazone and pioglitazone may both cause moderate weight gain and edema, it is important to weigh the patient daily at the same time every day and with the same amount of clothing. Several combination drug products are also available, including rosiglitazone plus metformin, glyburide plus metformin, and glipizide plus metformin, which should be given exactly as prescribed.

In special situations (e.g., the patient is NPO and is taking either an oral antidiabetic drug or insulin), it is crucial for the nurse to follow the physician's orders regarding drug administration. If there are no written orders about this situation, make sure to contact the physician for further instructions. If a patient is on NPO status but is receiving an intravenous solution of dextrose, the physician may still order insulin, but this should always be clarified. The physician should also be contacted if a patient becomes ill and unable to take the usual dosage of an oral antidiabetic drug (or insulin). Patients should always wear a medical alert bracelet, necklace, or tag with the diagnosis, list of medications, and emergency contact information.

It is also very important that the nurse stay informed and up-to-date about the latest research on diabetes. For example, there is a strong correlation between diabetes and heart disease, and microvascular problems are recognized as occurring at FPG levels of 126 mg/dL. As noted earlier, the ADA, the National Institute of Diabetes and Digestive and Kidney Disease, and the Centers for Disease Control and Prevention recommend that all adults 45 years of age and older be tested for elevated FPG levels every 3 years. Lifestyle changes for patients with high FPG levels may include decreased alcohol consumption, regular exercise to help lower blood glucose levels by increasing insulin sensitivity, and periodic medical follow-up. See the Evidence-Based Practice box on page 492 for more information on specific nursing research related to diabetes and its application to nursing practice.

In summary, there are many nursing considerations related to drug therapy in patients with diabetes mellitus. Patient education is also very important and should begin the moment the patient has entered into the health care system or upon diagnosis. Instruction that is tailored to the patient's educational level and with use of appropriate teaching-learning concepts and teaching aids is important to patient compliance. In addition, the nurse should be sure that all resources are made available to patients (e.g., financial assistance, visual assistance, dietary plans, daily menus, ADA information, transportation assistance, and Meals on Wheels and other community resources). See the Patient Teaching Tips for more specific information.

◆ EVALUATION

It is important for the nurse to understand current therapeutic guidelines. The prevailing key diagnostic criterion for diabetes mellitus is hyperglycemia with an FPG of higher than 126 mg/dL; however, the therapeutic response to insulin and any of the oral antidiabetic drugs is a decrease in blood glucose to the level prescribed by the physician or to near-normal levels. Most often, fasting blood glucose levels (no <60 mg/dL or >110 mg/dL, or a level designated by the physician) are used to measure the degree of glycemic control. To get a picture of the patient's compliance with the therapy regimen for several months previously, the level of HbA1c is measured. This value reflects how well the patient has been doing with diet and drug therapy. Patients with diabetes need to be monitored frequently by health care providers (as well as at home) to make sure they are adhering to the therapy regimen as evidenced by normalization of blood test results. Monitor the patient for indications of hypoglycemia or hyperglycemia and insulin allergy. With insulin lispro, because the onset of action is more rapid than with regular insulin and the duration of action is shorter, it is crucial for the nurse and the patient to monitor blood glucose levels very closely until the dosage is regulated and blood glucose is at the level the physician desires. Should a patient be switched from one insulin or oral antidiabetic drug to another, glucose levels must be monitored very closely at home or by the health care professional. Always evaluate whether identified goals and outcome criteria are being met and plan nursing care accordingly.

Tight Insulin Control

Review

Research has confirmed that intensive insulin therapy, although it carries many challenges, can help some patients with diabetes reduce complications and experience a better quality of life. More than 20 million Americans, or about 7% of the population, have diabetes mellitus, and serious complications and organ damage can result from the pathologic process. Heart disease, kidney disease, vascular disease, blindness, and amputations are the most common of the severely debilitating and/or fatal complications. Diabetes remains the fifth leading cause of death in the United States. One possible regimen to minimize risks and/or major complications as well as allow a more normal lifestyle is intensive insulin therapy is to use continuous subcutaneous insulin infusions (CSII) via pump or by multiple daily injections (MDI). Research has shown that tight insulin control through intensive therapy may well be the way to reduce morbidity and mortality.

Type of Evidence

The Diabetes Control and Complications Trial (DCCT) studied intensive therapy as compared with conventional therapy in a population of 1441 teenagers and young adults with type 1 diabetes. Intensive therapy involved hospitalization for stabilization of the disease and patient education, frequent dosing of insulin guided by the results of at least four serum glucose tests a day, four daily insulin injections or use of insulin pump, monthly office visits, frequent telephone calls between the patients and nurse educators, dietary consultation and exercise. Follow-up investigations occurred 4 years later.

Results of Study

The study found a 39% to 76% reduction in the incidence of various complications associated with diabetes in those receiving intensive therapy. Specifically, the findings of the DCCT showed that lowering blood glucose levels reduced the risk of eye disease by 75%, of kidney disease by 50% and of nerve disease by 60%. DCCT participants were not expected to have many heart-related problems, because their average age was 27 years when the study was initiated; however, electrocardiography, blood pressure tests, and serum laboratory tests of lipid levels were performed for all participants to look for signs of cardiovascular disease. The study showed that the participants who received intensive therapy had significantly lower risks of developing hyperlipidemia and subsequent cardiovascular/coronary heart disease. The risks of intensive therapy identified in the DCCT included

hypoglycemia severe enough to require the assistance of another individual, and because of this risk, DCCT researchers did not recommend intensive therapy for patients younger than 13 years of age, patients with heart disease or advanced complications, older adults, or patients with a history of frequent severe hypoglycemia.

A follow-up investigation 4 years later (in 1997), the Epidemiology of Diabetes Interventions and Complications study, found that the original intensive therapy group continued to have a lower risk of eye, nerve, and kidney disease even though control had become less intensive. In 2003, some 6 years later, the patients still had reduced rates of nerve damage. Because of the long-term nature of the study and the moderately sized research sample, the results hold promise for the treatment of diabetics in those individuals willing to invest the required time, energy, and lifestyle changes.

Link of Evidence to Nursing Practice

The patients who are the best candidates for CSII are those who are diligent and committed to self-management of their diabetes, are willing to spend the time it takes to record serum glucose levels and insulin values in a journal four or more times a day, will make monthly or more frequent visits to their health care professionals, and are able to monitor carbohydrate intake closely. Individuals who have motor or cognitive impairments as well as those who are not committed to the intensive therapy may be unable to adhere to the strict regimen. The evidence strongly indicates the value of tight control of glucose levels in helping to reduce long-term complications associated with diabetes. Not all patients are willing to spend the time and effort required to achieve tight glucose control, and the regimen is very stressful; however, every patient has the right to be informed of this option and its associated benefits and risks. This study produced ground-breaking results and has made an impact on the care of diabetic patients today. Many of the 1441 participants have been involved in the research for more than 20 years. To obtain more information for patients, contact the American Diabetes Association at 1-800-342-2383. In practicing evidence-based nursing, nurses look at new treatment approaches and their potential for improving patient care, as with the new therapy examined in this study. Although the costs of intensive therapy are high, they are offset by the decrease in other medical expenses related to the complications of diabetes and by the improved quality of life.

Based on National Institute of Diabetes and Digestive and Kidney Diseases: National diabetes statistics, 2004. Available at http:/diabetes.niddk.nih.gov/dm/pubs/statistics/index.htm; Dow N: Tight insulin control: Making it work, *RN* 68(7):44-52, 2005; National Institute of Diabetes and Digestive and Kidney Diseases: Diabetes Control and Complications Trial (DCCT), 2001. Available at http://diabetes.niddk.nih.gov/dm/pubs/control; American Diabetes Association: Intensive diabetes control yields less nerve damage years later, 2004. Available at www.diabetes.org/for-media/2004-press-releases/neuropathy.jsp.

Patient Teaching Tips

Insulin Therapy

- Always encourage the use of medical alert jewelry or an alert card.
- Instruct the patient on drawing up insulin, storage, the equipment needed, mixing (if ordered), and the technique for insulin injections.
- Demonstrate how to draw up the prescribed dose of insulin, how to inject the drug properly, how to rotate insulin injection sites, and how to keep notes in a journal.
- How to monitor blood (serum) glucose levels at the prescribed intervals should be demonstrated and the specific glucometer machine's instructions emphasized. Thorough instructions about the importance of exercise, hygiene, foot care, the prescribed dietary plan, and weight control should also be given.
- Encourage the patient to avoid smoking and alcohol consumption, follow all dietary instructions, and never skip meals or skip insulin.

- Explain the difference between hypoglycemia and hyperglycemia (see previous discussion for specific signs and symptoms) and emphasize the treatment of each (e.g., having quick sources of glucose on hand, such as candy, sugar packets, OTC glucose tablets, sugar cubes, honey, corn syrup, orange juice, and non-diet soda beverages) for hypoglycemia and having more insulin on hand for hyperglycemia. Encourage possession of quick dosage forms of glucose at all times!
- Inform the patient about situations or conditions that lead to altered serum glucose (e.g., fever, illness, stress, increased activity or exercise, surgery, emotional distress). Encourage the patient to contact the health care professional if any of these occur.
- Educate about the importance of knowing pre-meal serum glucose levels prior to taking insulin, and that insulin is given in relation to meal times, specifically breakfast.

Patient Teaching Tips—cont'd

- Instructions should include storage of insulin at room temperature unless the patient is traveling or is in a very hot climate because heat will alter insulin.
- Emphasize the importance of having adequate supplies of insulin and equipment and making sure to store safely and away from children. If needed, magnifying glass attachments are available for syringes and vials.
- Review and demonstrate mixing of insulins (see Chapter 9 and previous discussion in this chapter) and rotation of sites.
- Inform the patient to notify the physician if the patient notes any yellow discoloration of the skin, dark urine, fever, sore throat, weakness, or unusual bleeding or easy bruising (with any antidiabetic drug regimen).
- Review ADA recommendations for fasting serum glucose level measurement. For adults, the ADA recommends maintaining preprandial glucose levels of 90 to 130 mg/dL, peak postprandial levels of 180 mg/dL, and a glycosylated hemoglobin (HbA1c) level below 7%.
- Emphasize the importance of HbA1c monitoring (e.g., at least two times a year for those with good glycemic control; quarterly for patients not at goal, having changed their therapy, or not being compliant with the therapy) (Table 31-9). These recommendations apply to those taking oral antidiabetic drugs as well.
- Review lifestyle modifications, including weight control, glucose level maintenance with diet and exercise and/or drug therapy. Type 2 diabetics will have a greater therapeutic response to diet and exercise and glucose level control as compared to type 1 diabetics. Follow ADA recommendations for fasting serum glucose level measurement. Educate patients about the importance of supervised exercise until condition stabilizes. A nutritional consult may be needed, with specific menu planning to help the patient with changes in intake (e.g., low-fat diet with 160 to 300 g of carbohydrates).

- Emphasize the importance of American Heart Association recommendations for diabetics (e.g., 30 minutes of exercise daily; for patients with any neurologic changes in the extremities due to diabetes, exercise will most likely include use of a treadmill, prolonged walking, swimming or aquatic aerobics, bicycling, rowing, chair exercises, arm exercises, and non–weight bearing exercises).
- Educate patients with any form of diabetes that lifelong treatment and control, with strict management of drug therapy and glucose monitoring, is critical to reducing complications.
- Emphasize strict foot care, beginning with assessment of feet and toes every day. Other actions to prevent infections of the foot and possible gangrene (from diabetes-induced decreased circulation) include the following: (1) Soaking feet daily or as ordered in lukewarm water, with adequate drying and application of moisturizing lotion afterwards, (2) checking feet and legs for color, temperature, edema, and the appearance of any open sores, reddened areas, and so on, (3) contacting the health care provider for further instructions if there is suspicion of any type of wound or alteration in skin intactness, (4) having frequent pedicures and trimming of nails by a podiatrist or a licensed, certified individual, and (5) reporting of any unusual changes in the skin and intactness of the feet or nails or nail beds. A thermometer may be needed to check water.
- Educate about not skipping meals or medications; if problems with either occur, patients should contact their health care provider.
- Some of the oral antidiabetic drugs cause sensitivity to light, and so patients should always wear protective eyewear and sunscreen and to avoid unprotected sun exposure (including exposure to tanning beds).
- Be sure to educate patients that some oral antidiabetic drugs interact negatively with alcohol and cause a disulfiram-type reaction characterized by acute illness with vomiting and hypertension.

Table 31-9   Diabetes Care: Correlation of Glycosylated Hemoglobin Levels with Mean Serum Glucose Levels

Hemoglobin A1c (%)	Mean Serum Glucose Levels (mg/dL)	Mean Serum Glucose Levels (mmol/L)
6	135	7.5
7	170	9.5
8	205	11.5
9	240	13.5
10	275	15.5
11	310	17.5
12	345	19.5

Source: American Diabetes Association.

Points to Remember

- Insulin normally facilitates removal of glucose from the blood and its storage as glycogen in the liver.
- Type 1 diabetes mellitus was formerly known as *insulin-dependent diabetes (IDDM)* or *juvenile-onset diabetes*. Little or no endogenous insulin is produced by individuals with type 1 diabetes. It is much less common than type 2 diabetes and affects only about 10% of all diabetic patients. Patients with type 1 diabetes usually are not obese. Type 2 diabetes mellitus is much more common than type 1 diabetes.

- The primary treatment for type 1 diabetes mellitus is insulin therapy. Patients with type 2 diabetes are not generally prescribed insulin until other measures—namely, lifestyle changes and oral drug therapy—no longer provide adequate glycemic control. There are currently two main sources of insulin. It can be extracted from domesticated animals or synthesized in laboratories using recombinant deoxyribonucleic acid (DNA) technology. Insulin was originally isolated from cattle, but beef-derived insulin is no longer available because of mad cow disease.

Continued

Points to Remember—cont'd

- For type 2 diabetics, effective treatment involves several elements, including lifestyle modifications (e.g., diet, exercise, smoking cessation), careful monitoring of blood glucose levels, and possibly therapy with one or more drugs. If normal blood glucose levels are not achieved after 2 to 3 months of lifestyle modifications, treatment with an oral antidiabetic drug is often prescribed.
- Complications associated with diabetes include retinopathy, neuropathy, nephropathy, hypertension, cardiovascular disease, and coronary artery disease.
- The nurse should always check for allergies to specific medications and to pork before giving insulin.
- Patients need to learn the signs and symptoms of hypoglycemia and hyperglycemia and the methods of treating them at home. They also need to know when to contact the physician.
- Review ADA recommendations for fasting serum glucose levels (e.g., maintenance of preprandial glucose levels of 90 to 130 mg/dL, peak postprandial levels of 180 mg/dL, and a glycosylated hemoglobin (HbA1c) level below 7%).

- Exact timing of the dose of insulin or oral antidiabetic drug should always be carefully checked against the physician's order and with consideration of the drug's pharmacokinetics, including onset of action, peak, and duration of action.
- Information on foot care and the prevention of infection should be part of the patient education given to individuals with diabetes.
- The techniques of CSII and MDI hold promise for patients by giving them tight control of serum glucose levels, which can help to decrease the complications of diabetes.
- The nurse must remember that oral antidiabetic drugs are *not* to be used in pregnant women.
- A quick form of glucose should be kept available for patients taking arcabose because of the hypoglycemic reactions associated with this type of insulin. The nurse should make sure that patients know to keep such forms of glucose accessible for management at home.

NCLEX Examination Review Questions

1. Which of the following is most appropriate regarding the nurse's administration of insulin lispro to a hospitalized patient?
   a. It should be given half an hour before a meal.
   b. It should given 15 minutes before the patient begins the meal.
   c. It should be given half an hour after the meal.
   d. The timing of the insulin injection does not matter with insulin lispro.
2. Which of the following statements would be appropriate to include in patient teaching regarding type 2 diabetes?
   a. "Insulin injections are never used with type 2 diabetes."
   b. "Because you are not taking insulin injections, it is not necessary to measure your blood glucose levels."
   c. "Alcohol should be avoided because it can cause your blood glucose to fall to lower than normal levels."
   d. "Patients with type 2 diabetes usually have better control over their diabetes than those with type 1 diabetes."
3. A therapeutic response to oral antidiabetic drugs would include which of the following?
   a. Fewer episodes of DKA
   b. Weight gain of 10 lb
   c. Hemoglobin A1c levels of 6%
   d. Glucose levels of 170 mg/dL

4. When teaching the patient about drugs that interact with insulin, the nurse should instruct the patient to avoid which of the following OTC products, unless otherwise instructed by the physician?
   a. Acetaminophen products
   b. Aspirin products
   c. Vitamin C
   d. Iron supplements
5. A patient with type 2 diabetes has a new prescription for repaglinide (Prandin). After a week, she calls the office to ask what to do because she keeps missing meals. "I work right through lunch sometimes, and I'm not sure if I should take it or not. What should I do?" What is the nurse's best response?
   a. "You should try not to skip meals, but if that happens, you should also skip that dose of Prandin."
   b. "We will probably need to change your prescription to insulin injections because you can't eat meals on a regular basis."
   c. "Go ahead and take the pill when you first remember that you missed it."
   d. "Take both pills with the next meal and try to eat a little extra to make up for what you missed at lunchtime."

1. b, 2. c, 3. c, 4. b, 5. a.

Critical Thinking Activities

1. Type 1 diabetes mellitus has recently been diagnosed in a 240-lb, 25-year-old woman. When she is admitted to your unit for additional testing and control of her diabetes, she is placed on a 1500-calorie diabetic diet and prescribed 30 units of NPH insulin to be given every day at 7:30 AM. At 4 PM on the first day of therapy she becomes diaphoretic, weak, and pale. What should you do, and how would you explain these symptoms to the patient?

2. Compare the action of metformin (Glucophage) with that of regular insulin, glyburide (DiaBeta), and acarbose (Precose). What other oral antidiabetic drug(s) have an action similar to that of metformin?
3. What actions would be necessary in the nursing care of a patient with type 1 diabetes mellitus who is on NPO status for surgery but has orders for the usual morning (before breakfast) dose of Humulin N insulin? Explain your answer.

For answers, see http://evolve.elsevier.com/Lilley.

Adrenal Drugs

Objectives

When you reach the end of this chapter, you should be able to do the following:

1. Discuss the normal anatomy, physiology, and related functions of the adrenal glands, including specific hormones released from the glands.
2. Briefly compare the hormones secreted by the adrenal medulla with those secreted by the adrenal cortex.
3. Contrast Cushing's syndrome and Addison's disease.
4. Compare the actions and functions of glucocorticoids and mineralocorticoids, including what they do, what diseases alter them, and how they are used in pharmacotherapy.
5. Contrast the mechanisms of action, indications, dosages, routes of administration, cautions, contraindications, drug interactions, and adverse effects for glucocorticoids, mineralocorticoids, and antiadrenal drugs.
6. Develop a nursing care plan that includes all phases of the nursing process for patients taking adrenal and antiadrenal drugs.

e-Learning Activities

Companion CD

- NCLEX Review Questions: see questions 288-294
- Animations
- Audio Glossary
- Category Catchers
- Medication Errors Checklists
- IV Therapy Checklists

evolve Website (http://evolve.elsevier.com/Lilley)

- Nursing Care Plans • Frequently Asked Questions • Content Updates • WebLinks • Supplemental Resources • Elsevier ePharmacology Update • Medication Administration Animations

Drug Profiles

▶ aminoglutethimide, p. 500   ▶ prednisone, p. 500
▶ fludrocortisone, p. 499

▶ Key drug.

Glossary

Addison's disease Life-threatening condition caused by failure of adrenocortical function. (p. 496)

Adrenal cortex Outer portion of the adrenal gland. (p. 495)

Adrenal medulla Inner portion of the adrenal gland. (p. 495)

Aldosterone Mineralocorticoid hormone produced by the adrenal cortex that acts on the renal tubule to regulate sodium and potassium balance in the blood. (p. 496)

Cortex General anatomical term for the outer layers of a body organ or other structure. (p. 495)

Corticosteroids Any of the natural or synthetic adrenocortical hormones; that is, those produced by the cortex of the adrenal gland (adrenocorticosteroids). (p. 496)

Cushing's syndrome Metabolic disorder characterized by abnormally increased secretion of the adrenocortical steroids. (p. 496)

Epinephrine Endogenous hormone secreted into the bloodstream by the adrenal medulla; also a synthetic drug that is an adrenergic vasoconstrictor and also increases cardiac output. (p. 496)

Glucocorticoids A major group of corticosteroid hormones that regulate carbohydrate, protein, and lipid metabolism and inhibit the release of corticotropin. (p. 496)

Medulla General anatomical term for the most interior portions of an organ or structure. (p. 495)

Mineralocorticoids A major group of corticosteroid hormones that regulate electrolyte and water balance; in humans the primary mineralocorticoid is aldosterone. (p. 496)

Norepinephrine An adrenergic hormone, also secreted by the adrenal medulla, that increases blood pressure by causing vasoconstriction but does not appreciably affect cardiac output; it is the immediate metabolic precursor to epinephrine. (p. 496)

ADRENAL SYSTEM

The adrenal gland is an endocrine organ that sits on top of the kidney like a cap. It is composed of two distinct parts called the **adrenal cortex** and the **adrenal medulla** that both structurally and functionally are very different from one another. In general, the term **cortex** refers to the outer layers of various organs (e.g., cerebral cortex), while the term **medulla** refers to the most internal layers. The adrenal cortex comprises roughly 80% to 90% of the entire adrenal gland; the remainder is the medulla. The adrenal cortex is made up of regular endocrine tissue (hormone driven), and the adrenal medulla is made up of neurosecretory endocrine tissue (driven by both hormones and peripheral autonomic nerve impulses). Therefore, the adrenal gland actually functions as two different endocrine glands, each secreting different hormones.

The adrenal medulla secretes two important hormones, both of which are catecholamines. These are **epinephrine,** or adrenaline, which accounts for about 80% of the secretion, and **norepinephrine,** or noradrenaline, which accounts for the other 20%. (Both of these hormones are discussed in Chapter 17 and are not described further in this chapter in any detail.) Some characteristics of the adrenal cortex and the adrenal medulla and the various hormones secreted by each are presented in Table 32-1.

The hormones secreted by the adrenal cortex, which are the focus of this chapter, are broadly referred to as **corticosteroids** because they arise from the cortex and they are made from the steroid known as cholesterol. There are two types of corticosteroids—**glucocorticoids** and **mineralocorticoids.** These are secreted by two different layers, or zones, of the cortex. The zona glomerulosa, which is the outer layer, secretes the mineralocorticoids, and the zona fasciculata, which lies under the zona glomerulosa, secretes the glucocorticoids. A third, inner layer, the zona reticularis, secretes small amounts of sex hormones. All the hormones secreted

by the adrenal cortex are steroid hormones; that is, they have the steroid chemical structure (see Figure 33-2).

The mineralocorticoids get their name from the fact that they play an important role in regulating mineral salts (electrolytes) in the body. In humans the only physiologically important mineralocorticoid is **aldosterone.** Its primary role is to maintain normal levels of sodium in the blood (sodium homeostasis) by causing sodium to be resorbed from the urine back into the blood in exchange for potassium and hydrogen ions. In this way aldosterone not only regulates blood sodium levels but also influences the potassium levels in the blood and blood pH.

Overall, the corticosteroids are necessary for many vital bodily functions. Some of the more important ones are listed in Box 32-1. Without these hormones, life-threatening consequences may arise.

Adrenal corticosteroids are synthesized as needed; the body does not store them as it does other hormones. The body levels of these hormones are regulated by the hypothalamic-pituitary-adrenal (HPA) axis in much the same way that the levels of hormones secreted by the endocrine glands discussed in previous chapters (pancreas, thyroid, and pituitary) are regulated. As the name implies, this axis consists of a very organized system of communication between the adrenal gland, the pituitary gland, and the hypothalamus. As is the case for the other endocrine glands, it uses hormones as the messengers and a negative feedback mechanism as the controller and maintainer of the process. This feedback mechanism operates as follows: When the level of a particular corticosteroid is low, corticotropin-releasing hormone is released from the hypothalamus into the bloodstream and travels to the anterior pituitary, where it triggers the release of adrenocorticotropic hormone (ACTH; also called *corticotropin*). The ACTH is transported in the blood to the adrenal cortex, where it stimulates the production of the corticosteroids. Corticosteroids are then released into the bloodstream. When they reach peak levels, a signal (negative feedback) is sent to the hypothalamus, and the HPA axis is inhibited until the level of the corticosteroid again falls below physiologic threshold, whereupon the axis is stimulated once again.

The oversecretion (hypersecretion) of adrenocortical hormones can lead to a group of signs and symptoms called **Cushing's syndrome.** The hypersecretion of glucocorticoids results in the redistribution of body fat from the arms and legs to the face, shoulders, trunk, and abdomen, which leads to the characteristic "moon face." Such a glucocorticoid excess can be due to any one of several causes, including ACTH-dependent adrenocortical hyperplasia or tumor, ectopic ACTH-secreting tumor, or excessive administration of steroids. The hypersecretion of aldosterone, or primary aldosteronism, leads to increased retention of water and sodium, which causes muscle weakness due to the potassium loss.

The undersecretion (hyposecretion) of adrenocortical hormones causes a condition known as **Addison's disease.** It is associated with decreased blood sodium and glucose levels, increased potassium levels, dehydration, and weight loss. The combination of a mineralocorticoid (fludrocortisone) and a glucocorticoid (prednisone or some other suitable drug) is used for treatment.

ADRENAL DRUGS

All the naturally occurring corticosteroids are also available as exogenous drugs, and there are also higher-potency synthetic analogues. The adrenal glucocorticoids are an extremely large

---

Table 32-1   Adrenal Gland: Characteristics

Type of Tissue	Type of Hormone Secreted	Specific Drugs/ Hormones Secreted
Adrenal Cortex		
Endocrine	Glucocorticoids	adrenocorticotropic hormone, betamethasone, cortisone, dexamethasone, hydrocortisone, methylprednisolone, paramethasone, prednisolone, triamcinolone
	Mineralocorticoids	aldosterone, desoxycorticosterone, fludrocortisone
Adrenal Medulla		
Neuroendocrine	Catecholamines	epinephrine, norepinephrine

Box 32-1   Adrenal Cortex Hormones: Biologic Functions

Glucocorticoids
Antiinflammatory actions
Carbohydrate and protein metabolism
Fat metabolism
Maintenance of normal blood pressure
Stress effects

Mineralocorticoids
Blood pressure control
Maintenance of serum potassium levels
Maintenance of pH levels in the blood
Sodium and water resorption

group of steroids, and they are categorized in various ways. They can be classified by whether they are a natural or synthetic corticosteroid, by the method of administration (e.g., systemic, topical), by their salt and water retention potential (mineralocorticoid activity), by their duration of action (i.e., short, intermediate, or long acting), or by some combination of these methods. The only corticosteroid drug with exclusive mineralocorticoid activity is fludrocortisone. Its uses are much more specific than the glucocortocoids and are discussed in the designated drug profile for fludrocortisone. The currently available synthetic adrenal hormones and adrenal steroid inhibitors are listed in Table 32-2.

Mechanism of Action and Drug Effects

The action of the corticosteroids is related to their involvement in the synthesis of specific proteins. There are several steps to this process. Initially the steroid hormone binds to a receptor on the surface of a target cell to form a steroid-receptor complex, which is then transported through the cytoplasm to the nucleus of that target cell. Once inside the nucleus of the target cell, the complex stimulates the cell's deoxyribonucleic acid (DNA) to produce messenger ribonucleic acid (mRNA), which is then used as a template for the synthesis of a specific protein. It is these proteins that exert specific effects.

Most of the corticosteroids exert their effects by modifying enzyme activity; therefore, their role is more intermediary than direct. As previously mentioned, the naturally occurring mineralocorticoid aldosterone affects electrolyte and fluid balance by acting on the distal renal tubule to promote sodium resorption from the nephron into the blood, which pulls water and fluid along with it. In doing so it causes fluid and water retention, which leads to edema and hypertension. Aldosterone also promotes potassium and hydrogen excretion.

The glucocorticoid drugs hydrocortisone (called *cortisol* in its naturally occurring form) and cortisone have some mineralocorticoid activity and therefore have some of the same effects as aldosterone (i.e., fluid and water retention). Their other main effect is the inhibition of inflammatory and immune responses. Glucocorticoids primarily inhibit or help control the inflammatory response by stabilizing the cell membranes of inflammatory cells called *ly-sosomes,* decreasing the permeability of capillaries to the inflammatory cells, and decreasing the migration of white blood cells into already inflamed areas. They may lower fever by reducing the release of interleukin-1 from white blood cells. They also stimulate the *erythroid cells* that eventually become red blood cells. The glucocorticoids also promote the breakdown (catabolism) of protein, the production of glycogen in the liver (glycogenesis), and the redistribution of fat from peripheral to central areas of the body.

Indications

All of the systemically administered glucocorticoids have a similar clinical efficacy but differ in their potency and duration of action and in the extent to which they cause salt and water retention (Table 32-3). These drugs have broad indications, including the following:

- Adrenocortical deficiency
- Adrenogenital syndrome
- Bacterial meningitis (particularly in infants)
- Cerebral edema
- Collagen diseases (e.g., systemic lupus erythematosus)
- Dermatologic diseases (e.g., exfoliative dermatitis, pemphigus)
- Endocrine disorders (thyroiditis)
- Gastrointestinal (GI) diseases (e.g., ulcerative colitis, regional enteritis)
- Exacerbations of chronic respiratory illnesses such as asthma and chronic obstructive pulmonary disease
- Hematologic disorders (reduce bleeding tendencies)
- Ophthalmic disorders (e.g., nonpyogenic inflammations)
- Organ transplantation (decrease immune response to prevent organ rejection)
- leukemias and lymphomas (palliative management)
- Nephrotic syndrome (remission of proteinuria)
- Spinal cord injury

Glucocorticoids are also administered by inhalation for the control of steroid-responsive bronchospastic states. Nasally administered glucocorticoids are used to manage rhinitis and to prevent the recurrence of polyps after surgical removal (Chapter 36). The topical steroids are used in the management of inflammations in the eye, ear, and skin.

Table 32-2 **Available Synthetic Corticosteroids**		
Type of Hormone	**Method of Administration**	**Individual Drugs**
Adrenal steroid inhibitor	Systemic	aminoglutethimide, trilostane, mitotane, ketoconazole, metyrapone
Glucocorticoid	Topical	alclometasone dipropionate, amcinonide, betamethasone benzoate, betamethasone dipropionate, betamethasone valerate, clobetasol propionate, clocortolone pivalate desonide, desoximetasone, dexamethasone sodium phosphate, diflorasone diacetate, fluocinolone acetonide, fluocinonide, flurandrenolide, fluticasone propionate, halobetasol propionate, halcinonide, hydrocortisone acetate, hydrocortisone valerate, methylprednisolone acetate, mometasone furoate, triamcinolone
	Systemic	beclomethasone, cortisone, dexamethasone, hydrocortisone, methylprednisolone, prednisolone, prednisone, triamcinolone
	Inhaled	beclomethasone, dexamethasone, flunisolide, triamcinolone acetonide, fluticasone
	Nasal	beclomethasone dipropionate, dexamethasone sodium phosphate, flunisolide, triamcinolone acetonide
Mineralocorticoid	Systemic	fludrocortisone acetate

Table 32-3 Systemic Glucocorticoids: A Comparison

Drug	Origin	Duration of Action	Equivalent Dose (mg)*	Salt and Water Retention Potential
betamethasone	Synthetic	Long	0.75	Very low
cortisone	Natural	Short	25	High
dexamethasone	Synthetic	Long	0.75	Very low
hydrocortisone	Natural	Short	20	High
methylprednisolone	Synthetic	Intermediate	4	Low
prednisolone	Synthetic	Intermediate	5	Low
prednisone	Synthetic	Intermediate	5	Low
triamcinolone	Synthetic	Intermediate	4	Very low

*Drugs with higher potency require smaller milligram doses than those with lower potency. This column illustrates the approximate dose equivalency between different drugs that is expected to achieve a comparable therapeutic effect.

Contraindications

Contraindications to the administration of glucocorticoids include drug allergy; contraindications may include cataracts, glaucoma, peptic ulcer disease, psychiatric/mental health problems, and diabetes mellitus. The adrenal drugs may intensify these diseases. Glucocorticoids are often avoided, because of their immunosuppressant properties, in the presence of any serious infection, including septicemia, systemic fungal infections, and varicella. One exception to this rule is tuberculous meningitis, for which glucocorticoids may be used to prevent inflammatory central nervous system damage. Caution is emphasized in any patient with gastritis, reflux disease, ulcer disease, or diabetes, as well as with cardiac/renal and/or liver dysfunction.

Adverse Effects

The potent metabolic, physiologic, and pharmacologic effects of the corticosteroids can influence every body system, so that they can produce a wide variety of significant undesirable effects. The more common of these are summarized in Table 32-4.

Interactions

Systemically administered corticosteroids can interact with many drugs:

- Their use with non–potassium-sparing diuretics (e.g., thiazides, loop diuretics) can lead to severe hypocalcemia and hypokalemia.
- Their use with aspirin, other nonsteroidal antiinflammatory drugs (NSAIDs), and other ulcerogenic drugs produces additive GI effects.
- Their use with anticholinesterase drugs produces weakness in patients with myasthenia gravis.
- Their use with immunizing biologicals inhibits the immune response to the biological.
- Their use with antidiabetic drugs may reduce the hypoglycemic effects of the latter.

There are many other drugs that can interact with glucocorticoids; these include the following: thyroid hormones, antifungal drugs (such as fluconazole), barbiturates, hydantoins, oral anticoagulants, oral contraceptives, potassium-depleting diuretics, theophylline, and somatrem. Concerns about these specific drugs and interactions include the following: (1) antifungals decrease renal clearance of the adrenal drug, (2) barbiturates increase the metabolism of the prednisone and similar drugs, and (3) oral contra-

Table 32-4 Corticosteroids: Common Adverse Effects

Body System	Adverse Effects
Cardiovascular	Heart failure, cardiac edema, hypertension—all due to electrolyte imbalances (e.g., hypokalemia, hypernatremia)
Central nervous	Convulsions, headache, vertigo, mood swings, psychic impairment, nervousness, insomnia
Endocrine	Growth suppression, Cushing's syndrome, menstrual irregularities, carbohydrate intolerance, hyperglycemia, hypothalamic-pituitary-adrenal axis suppression
Gastrointestinal	Peptic ulcers with possible perforation, pancreatitis, ulcerative esophagitis, abdominal distension
Integumentary	Fragile skin, petechiae, ecchymosis, facial erythema, poor wound healing, hirsutism, urticaria
Musculoskeletal	Muscle weakness, loss of muscle mass, osteoporosis
Ocular	Increased intraocular pressure, glaucoma, exophthalmos, cataracts
Other	Weight gain

ceptives can increase the half-life of adrenal drugs. Various other drug interactions may be possible between adrenal drugs and over-the-counter (OTC) drugs and herbals. The nurse should educate the patient to read package labeling and consult with a pharmacist when in doubt.

Dosages

For information on the recommended dosages of adrenal drugs, see the Dosages table on page 499.

Drug Profiles

Corticosteroids

The systemic corticosteroids consist of 13 chemically different but pharmacologically similar hormones. They all exert varying degrees of glucocorticoid and mineralocorticoid effects. Their differences are due to slight changes in their chemical structures.

DOSAGES

Selected Antiadrenal and Corticosteroid Drugs

Drug	Pharmacologic Class	Usual Dosage Range	Indications
▶ aminoglutethimide (Cytadren)	Adrenal corticosteroid inhibitor (antiadrenal drug)	**Adult** PO: 250 mg q6h; titrate in increments of 250 mg to a max daily dose of 2000 mg	Cushing's syndrome
dexamethasone (Decadron, Hexadrol, Dexone, others)	Synthetic long-acting glucocorticoid	**Adult** PO/IV/IM: 0.75-9 mg/day divided bid-qid **Pediatric** PO/IV/IM: 0.5-2 mg/kg/day divided q6h	Wide variety of endocrine disorders (including adrenocortical insufficiency) and rheumatic, collagen, dermatologic, allergic, ophthalmic, respiratory, hematologic, neoplastic, GI, and nervous system disorders; edematous states
dexamethasone acetate (Dexasone LA, Dexone LA, others)	Synthetic long-acting repository glucocorticoid	**Adult only** IM: 8-16 mg q1-3wk Intralesional: 0.8-1.6 mg Intraarticular and soft tissue: 4-16 mg q1-3wk	Same as dexamethasone Inflammation Inflammation
▶ fludrocortisone (Florinef)	Synthetic mineralocorticoid	**Adult and pediatric (including infant)** PO: 0.05-0.2 mg q24h	Addison's disease; salt-losing adrenogenital syndrome
hydrocortisone (Cortef, Hydrocortone, others)	Natural short-acting glucocorticoid	**Adult** PO: 20-240 mg/day **Pediatric** PO: 2.5-10 mg/kg/day divided q6-8 hr	Adrenocortical insufficiency; many inflammatory conditions
hydrocortisone sodium succinate (Solu-Cortef, A-HydroCort)	Natural water-soluble, short-acting glucocorticoid	**Adult** IV/IM: 100-500 mg q2-6hr, depending on condition and patient response **Pediatric** IV/IM: 1.5 mg/kg/day divided daily-bid	Adrenocortical insufficiency
▶ prednisone (Orasone, Deltasone, Sterapred, Liquid Pred, others)	Synthetic intermediate-acting glucocorticoid	**Adult** PO: 5-60 mg/day Pediatric PO: 0.05-2 mg/kg/day divided daily-qid	Wide variety of endocrine disorders (including adrenocortical insufficiency) and rheumatic, collagen, dermatologic, allergic, ophthalmic, respiratory, hematologic, neoplastic, GI, and nervous system disorders; edematous states

GI, Gastrointestinal; *IM,* intramuscular; *IV,* intravenous; *PO,* oral.

Corticosteroid drugs can cross the placenta and produce fetal abnormalities. For this reason, they are classified as pregnancy category C drugs. They may also be secreted in breast milk and cause abnormalities in the nursing infant. Their use is contraindicated in patients who have exhibited hypersensitivity reactions to them in the past as well as in patients with fungal or bacterial infections. Short- or long-term use can lead to a condition known as *steroid psychosis.* In addition, the cessation of long-term treatment with these drugs requires a tapering of the daily dose, because the administration of the exogenous hormones causes the endogenous production of the hormones to stop. Tapering of daily doses allows the HPA axis the time to recover and to start stimulating the normal production of the endogenous hormones.

▶ **fludrocortisone**

Fludrocortisone (Florinef) is contraindicated in cases of systemic fungal infection. Adverse effects generally pertain to water retention and include congestive heart failure, hypertension, and elevated in-tracerebral pressure (e.g., leading to seizures). Other potential adverse effects involve several body systems and include skin rash, menstrual irregularities, peptic ulcer, hyperglycemia, hypokalemia, potassium loss, muscle pain and weakness, compression bone fractures, glaucoma, and thrombophlebitis, among others. Drug interactions include anabolic steroids (increased edema); barbiturates, hydantoins, rifamycins (increased fludrocortisone clearance), estrogens (reduced fludrocortisone clearance), amphotericin B and thiazide and loop diuretics (hypokalemia), anticoagulants (enhanced or reduced anticoagulant activity), antidiabetic drugs (reduced activity leading to hyperglycemia), digoxin (increased risk for arrhythmias due to fludrocortisone-induced hypokalemia), salicylates (reduced efficacy), and vaccines (increased risk of neurologic complications). Fortunately, adverse effects and serious drug interactions secondary to fludrocortisone therapy are uncommon due to the relatively small doses of the drug that are normally prescribed. This drug is available only in oral form as a 0.1-mg tablet. Pregnancy category C. Recommended dosages are given in the table on page 499.

Pharmacokinetics

Half-Life	Onset	Peak	Duration
PO: 18-36 hr	PO: 10-20 min	PO: 1.7 hr	PO: Unknown

▸ **prednisone**

Prednisone (Orasone, Meticorten, Deltasone, Sterapred) is one of the four intermediate-acting glucocorticoids; the others are methylprednisolone, prednisolone, and triamcinolone. These drugs have half-lives that are more than double those of the short-acting corticosteroids (2 to 5 hours), and therefore they have much longer durations of action. Prednisone is the preferred oral glucocorticoid for antiinflammatory or immunosuppressant purposes. Along with methylprednisolone and prednisolone, it is also used for exacerbations of chronic respiratory illnesses such as asthma and chronic bronchitis. This drug has only minimal mineralocorticoid properties and therefore alone is inadequate for the management of adrenocortical insufficiency (Addison's disease).

Prednisolone, a prednisone metabolite, is also the liquid drug form of prednisone. Prednisone itself comes in solid form. Pregnancy category C. Recommended dosages are given in the table on page 499.

Pharmacokinetics

Half-Life	Onset	Peak	Duration
18-36 hr	Unknown	1-2 hr	36 hr

Antiadrenals

Aminoglutethimide and metyrapone are adrenal steroid inhibitors. They obstruct the normal actions or function of the adrenal cortex by inhibiting the conversion of cholesterol into adrenal corticosteroids. Metyrapone is currently used only as a diagnostic drug to assess ACTH production by the hypothalamic-pituitary axis. Aminoglutethimide is indicated for the treatment of Cushing's syndrome, which results from an overproduction of corticosteroids by the adrenal gland. Use of antiadrenals is contraindicated in patients who have shown a previous hypersensitivity reaction to them. Their most common adverse effects are nausea, anorexia, dizziness, and skin rash.

▸ **aminoglutethimide**

Aminoglutethimide (Cytadren) is the most commonly used of the three antiadrenal drugs in the treatment of Cushing's syndrome, metastatic breast cancer, and adrenal cancer (Chapters 47 and 48). It is available only in oral form. Pregnancy category D. Recommended dosages are given in the table on page 499.

Pharmacokinetics

Half-Life	Onset	Peak	Duration
9 hr	Unknown	Unknown	Unknown

◆ NURSING PROCESS

◆ ASSESSMENT

Before administering any of the adrenal or antiadrenal drugs, the nurse should perform a thorough physical assessment to determine the patient's nutritional and hydration status, baseline weight, intake and output, vital signs (especially blood pressure ranges), skin condition, and immune status. Important baseline laboratory values include serum sodium, serum potassium, blood urea nitrogen, serum glucose, hemoglobin, and hematocrit. These serum tests are important because some

of the adverse effects that are expected with adrenal drugs. For instance, serum potassium levels usually decrease and blood glucose levels increase when a glucocorticoid such as prednisone is given. In addition, the patient's muscle strength and body stature should be assessed and documented. Hepatic functioning may also be assessed through liver enzyme testing. All of these parameters must be assessed and documented before, during, and after therapy so that baseline comparisons will be available to evaluate therapeutic effectiveness and/or adverse effects.

Specific contraindications, cautions, and drug interactions (including prescription drugs, OTC drugs, and herbals) associated with the adrenal and antiadrenal drugs should be assessed thoroughly and have been previously discussed. Assessment of variables associated with lifespan include concerns with use of these medications during pregnancy and lactation. Growth suppression may occur in children who are receiving long-term adrenal drug therapy (e.g., glucocorticoids) if the epiphyseal plates of the long bones have not closed, but there are often situations where benefits outweigh risks of the drug's adverse effects. Elderly patients are more prone to adrenal suppression with prolonged adrenal therapy and may require dosage alterations by the physician to minimize the impact of the drug on muscle mass, plasma volume, renal and hepatic function, blood pressure, and serum glucose and electrolyte levels. These drugs may exacerbate muscle weakness and fatigue as well as osteoporosis. In addition, because the adrenal drugs are associated with adverse effects of sodium retention, patients with edema and cardiac disease must be closely assessed for exacerbation of these conditions.

◆ NURSING DIAGNOSES

- Imbalanced nutrition, more than body requirements, related to increased appetite resulting from adrenal drug therapy
- Disturbed body image related to the physiologic effects of diseases of the adrenal gland on the body or the cushingoid appearance due to drug therapy (with prednisone)
- Excess fluid volume related to the fluid retention associated with glucocorticoid and mineralocorticoid use
- Risk for infection related to the antiinflammatory, immunosuppressive, metabolic, and dermatologic effects of long-term glucocorticoid therapy
- Impaired skin integrity related to the adverse effects of glucocorticoids
- Risk for injury related to adverse effects of adrenal drug therapy, such as changes in sensorium and confusion

◆ PLANNING

Goals

- Patient describes the healthy diet to follow during treatment.
- Patient experiences minimal body image disturbances.
- Patient exhibits minimal complications resulting from the fluid retention caused by mineralocorticoid therapy.
- Patient is free of infection during adrenal drug therapy.
- Patient's skin and mucous membranes remain intact during treatment.
- Patient maintains normal fluid and electrolyte levels.
- Patient remains free of changes in sensorium and possible confusion or dizziness from adrenal therapy.
- Patient states symptoms to report immediately to the physician should they occur.

Outcome Criteria

- Patient eats adequate food according to the food guide pyramid and maintains weight within the normal range with adequate menu planning.
- Patient openly verbalizes fears about body image disturbances to health care providers.
- Patient experiences minimal problems with fluid volume excess and does not gain more than 2 lb/wk.
- Patient notifies the physician if fever (over 100° F or 38° C) occurs.
- Patient performs frequent mouth and skin care to prevent infections and maintain intactness.
- Patient implements measures to minimize major electrolyte imbalances during adrenal drug therapy.
- Patient changes positions slowly and walks carefully to prevent injuries resulting from dizziness or syncope (from postural hypotension for which mineralocorticoids are taken).
- Patient identifies symptoms to report to the physician, such as a weight gain of more than 2 lb/24 hours or 5 lb or more/week, shortness of breath, edema, dizziness, and syncope.
- Patient experiences minimal problems when being weaned off of adrenal drugs such as prednisone.

♦ IMPLEMENTATION

The nurse must understand how the glucocorticoids work so that the patient can be given proper explanations and education reflecting these fundamental concepts in order to maximize therapeutic effects and minimize adverse effects. Points to remember when giving these drugs include the following: (1) Hormone production by the adrenal gland is influenced by time of day and follows a diurnal (daily or 24-hour) pattern with *peak* levels occurring early in the morning between 6 AM and 8 AM, a *decrease* during the day, and a *lower peak* in the late afternoon between 4 PM and 6 PM. (2) Cortisol levels increase in response to both emotional and physiologic stress. (3) Cortisol levels also increase when *endogenous* levels decrease due to a physiologic negative feedback system. (4) When *exogenous* glucocorticoids are given, *endogenous* levels decrease; for endogenous production to resume, exogenous levels must be decreased *gradually* so that hormone levels respond to the negative feedback system. (5) The best time to give exogenous glucocorticoids is early in the morning (6 AM to 9 AM), because this leads to the least amount of adrenal suppression.

Some of the systemic forms of adrenal drugs (e.g., prednisone) may be given by the oral, intramuscular, intravenous, or rectal route. All parenteral forms should be mixed as per manufacturer guidelines and intravenous dosages given over the recommended time frame. Intramuscular forms should always be administered into a large muscle mass such as the ventral gluteal site with rotation of sites (if giving frequent injections) to prevent tissue trauma and irritation.

Oral dosage forms should be given with milk, food, or nonsystemic antacids (such as Al^+, Ca^{2+}, or Mg^+), unless contraindicated, to minimize GI upset. Another option is for the physician to order an H_2-receptor antagonist or proton pump inhibitors to prevent ulcer formation (glucocorticoids are often ulcerogenic). Patients should be encouraged to avoid alcohol, aspirin, or NSAIDs to minimize gastric irritation and/or gastric bleeding. In long-term therapy, alternate-day dosing of glucocorticoids will help minimize the adrenal suppression. With oral and all other forms of glu-

cocorticoids that are given short and/or long term, abrupt withdrawal must be avoided. Abrupt withdrawal of adrenal drugs (e.g., prednisone) may lead to Addisonian crisis, which may be life-threatening. Signs and symptoms of Addison's disease or adrenal insufficiency include fatigue, nausea, vomiting, and hypotension.

Other adrenal drug dosage forms include intraarticular, intrabursal, intradermal, intralesional, and intrasynovial routes. Intraarticular injections should not be overused, and should a joint be injected with medication, the patient should rest that area for up to 48 hours after the injection. Topical dosage forms are also available and may be applied to the skin or eye or administered by inhalation as ordered. These drug dosage forms should be used as ordered and only according to the instructions in the package insert, which, for example, may specify the use of an occlusive dressing. The skin should be clean and dry before application of a topical drug. Gloves should be worn and the medication applied with either a sterile tongue depressor or a cotton-tipped applicator. Sterile technique should be used if the skin is not intact. Nasally administered glucocorticoids (e.g., beclomethasone) should be used exactly as ordered. Any written instructions that come with the product should be read and followed carefully. Patients should be instructed that before using the nasal spray, they should first clear the nasal passages and then use the spray per instructions. After the nasal passages are cleared, the container is placed gently inside the nasal passage and the medication is released at the same time that the patient breathes in through the nose.

Glucocorticoid inhalers should be used strictly as ordered and the negative consequences of overuse explained to the patient. Inhalers containing adrenal drugs (e.g., corticosteroids) may lead to oral mucosal/cavity and laryngeal/pharyngeal fungal (candidiasis) infections. After inhalers with these medications are used, the patient should always rinse the mouth with lukewarm water to help prevent fungal overgrowth and further complications. Hoarseness, fungal infections (candidiasis), throat irritation, and dry mouth are possible adverse effects associated with the use of inhaled corticosteroids and should be reported to the health care provider immediately. See Chapter 9 and Patient Teaching Tips for more information.

If a patient is receiving long-term maintenance glucocorticoid therapy and requires surgery, the nurse should be sure that the patient's medical records are reviewed carefully. In addition, all nursing documentation and notes should be reviewed. If the preoperative orders do not include the maintenance dosage, the nurse should contact the surgeon and/or other physician and ensure that they are aware of the situation and the possible need for a rapid-acting corticosteroid. After surgery, the dosage of steroid may well be increased, with a gradual decrease in dosage over several days until the patient returns to baseline. In addition, the nurse should keep in mind that healing may be decreased if the patient has been on long-term therapy.

In summary, because of their suppressed immune systems, patients taking corticosteroids should avoid contact with people with infections and should report any fever, increased weakness and lethargy, or sore throat. Monitoring nutritional status, weight, fluid volume, electrolyte status, skin turgor, and glucose levels during therapy is very important to ensure safe and effective therapy. Administration in one daily morning dose is recommended to minimize adrenal suppression. Physicians or health care providers should be notified if there is any weakness, joint pain, dyspnea, fever, dysrhythmias, depression, edema, or other unusual symptoms.

♦ **EVALUATION**

A therapeutic response to corticosteroids includes a resolution of the underlying manifestations of the disease, such as a decrease in inflammation, increased feeling of well-being, less pain and discomfort in the joints, decrease in lymphocytes, or other improvement in the condition for which the medication was ordered. Adverse effects include weight gain; increased blood pressure; pulse irregularities; sodium increase and potassium loss, mental status changes such as aggression, depression, or psychosis; electrolyte disturbances; elevated glucose levels; decreased healing; GI upset; and ulcer-related symptoms. The systemic drugs may cause potassium depletion, which is manifested by fatigue, nausea, vomiting, muscle weakness, and dysrhythmias. Cushing's syndrome is characterized by moon face, truncal obesity, increase in blood glucose and sodium levels and a loss of potassium, wasting of muscle mass, buffalo hump, and other features that have been thoroughly presented in this chapter. Cataract formation and osteoporosis may also occur. Addisonian crisis occurs with a rapid drop of cortisol level (e.g., abrupt withdrawal of medication) and is manifested by hypotension, weight loss, dehydration, and decreased blood glucose level. Therapeutic responses to aminoglutethimide include a decrease in the size of the tumor and a decrease in Cushing's syndrome. Adverse effects for which to monitor include jaundice, skin lesions, hypotension, headache, lethargy, weakness, GI upset, and hepatotoxicity.

Patient Teaching Tips

- The patient should be instructed on the importance of drug therapy, its method of administration, to follow exact instructions, and to never stop the medication abruptly. Encourage patients to contact the physician if there are situations that prevent proper dosing. If a once-a-day dose is missed, the patient should take the dose as soon as possible after remembering that the dose was missed. If the dose is *not* remembered until close to the time for the next dose, then the patient should skip the dose and resume the dosing on the next day without doubling up. Inform the patient of what to expect with long-term glucocorticoid therapy, including changes in body appearance with acne, buffalo hump, truncal obesity, moon face, thinning of the extremities, and cataract formation.
- Educate the patient about the importance of bone health and prevention of falls because long-term therapy may lead to osteoporosis. The physician may suggest a daily supplement of oral calcium and vitamin D.
- Inform the patient to report to the physician any signs and symptoms of acute adrenal insufficiency, such as anorexia, hypotension, hypoglycemia, weakness, nausea, psychologic changes, and restlessness. The patient should also report vomiting and diarrhea

or other acute illnesses. Other problems to report include weight gain, lower extremity edema, muscle weakness, and severe and/or continual headache.
- Fludrocortisone should be taken with food or milk to minimize GI upset. Weight gain 2 lb or more/24 hours or 5 lb or more/week with any adrenal drug should be reported to the physician as soon as possible.
- Abrupt withdrawal from adrenal drugs is not recommended because this may precipitate an adrenal crisis.
- Encourage use of a journal to document responses to treatment, blood pressure readings, daily weight measurements, and any adverse effects experienced.
- The patient should keep return appointments with the physician so that electrolyte levels can be monitored. Also, emphasize the importance of maintaining a low-sodium and high-potassium diet as ordered.
- Encourage the patient to wear a medical identification bracelet or necklace with the diagnosis and list of medications and allergies. A medical card with important relevant information should be on the person at all times and updated frequently.

Points to Remember

- The adrenal gland is an endocrine organ that is located on top of the kidneys and is composed of two distinct tissues: the adrenal cortex and the adrenal medulla. The adrenal medulla secretes two important hormones: epinephrine (80%) and norepinephrine (20%); the adrenal cortex secretes two classes of hormones known as *corticosteroids:* glucocorticoids and mineralocorticoids.
- The biologic functions of glucocorticoids include antiinflammatory actions; maintenance of normal blood pressure; carbohydrate, protein, and fat metabolism; and stress effects.
- The biologic functions of mineralocorticoids include sodium and water resorption, blood pressure control, and maintaining potassium levels and pH levels of the blood.
- Patients taking adrenal drugs may receive them by various routes, such as orally, intramuscularly, intravenously, intranasally, intraarticularly, and by inhalation; some are also administered by means of a rectal enema.

- Nurses should follow the manufacturer's guidelines for dilution and administration. Intramuscular forms of adrenal drugs should be administered deep into a large muscle, such as the ventral gluteal site. Steroid inhalers should be used as ordered and only after adequate patient education; patients should rinse the mouth after their use to avoid oral fungal infections (oral candidiasis) and oral-pharyngeal irritation.
- Adverse effects for which to monitor include weight gain, increase in blood pressure, pulse irregularities, mental status changes such as aggression or depression, electrolyte disturbances, elevated glucose levels, changes in nutritional status, decreased healing, GI tract upset, and ulcer-related symptoms.
- With once-a-day dosing of these drugs, adrenal suppression from corticosteroid therapy may be minimized if the dose is given between 6 AM and 9 AM, but it should only be given as ordered.

NCLEX Examination Review Questions

1. When monitoring for a therapeutic response to aminoglutethimide, the nurse will look for which of the following?
   a. Increase in Cushing's syndrome characteristics
   b. Decrease in Cushing's syndrome characteristics
   c. Increased lymphocyte levels
   d. Growth suppression
2. Which statement of the patient shows a poor understanding of the teaching about oral corticosteroid therapy that the patient has received?
   a. "I will report any fever or sore throat symptoms."
   b. "I will stay away from anyone who has a cold or infection."
   c. "I can stop this medication if I have severe adverse effects."
   d. "I should take this drug with food or milk."
3. During long-term corticosteroid therapy, the nurse should monitor the patient for Cushing's syndrome, which is manifested by which characteristic?
   a. Weight loss
   b. Truncal obesity

c. Muscle weakness
d. Thickened hair growth

4. When teaching a patient who has been prescribed a daily dose of prednisone, the nurse knows that the patient should be told to take the medication at which time of day to help reduce adrenal suppression?
   a. In the morning
   b. At lunchtime
   c. At dinnertime
   d. At bedtime
5. Which teaching is appropriate for a patient who is taking an inhaled glucocorticoid for asthma?
   a. "Exhale while pushing in on the canister of the inhaler."
   b. "Blow your nose after taking the medication."
   c. "Rinse the mouth thoroughly after taking the medication."
   d. "Do not rinse the mouth after taking the medication."

1. b, 2. c, 3. b, 4. a, 5. c.

Critical Thinking Activities

1. A 19-year-old man is admitted through the emergency department after a motorcycle accident. He is conscious upon admission, has stable vital signs, and has minimal cuts and abrasions on the left side of his body. You perform a thorough neurologic examination and find absence of sensation to light touch and pinprick and lower extremity paralysis. Reflexes are absent below the groin area. The physician orders high-dose intravenous methylprednisolone. What is the purpose of this medication and what should you, as the nurse, watch for while the patient is receiving this medication?

2. You are caring for a patient who is taking 100 mg of hydrocortisone orally. The physician decides that he is more familiar with prednisone and wants to change the patient's medication to the equivalent oral dose of prednisone. What will be the equivalent dose of prednisone?
3. Discuss how drug therapy benefits patients with Addison's disease.

For answers, see http://evolve.elsevier.com/Lilley.

Women's Health Drugs

Objectives

When you reach the end of this chapter, you should be able to do the following:

1. Discuss the normal anatomy and physiology of the female reproductive system.
2. Discuss the normal hormonally mediated feedback system and how it regulates the female reproductive system.
3. Describe the variety of disorders affecting women's health and the drugs used to treat these disorders.
4. Discuss the rationale for the various treatments involving estrogen, progesterone, uterine motility–altering drugs, alendronate, and other drugs related to women's health, with indications, adverse effects, cautions, contraindications, drug interactions, dosages, and routes of administration.
5. Develop a nursing care plan that includes all phases of the nursing process for patients receiving any of the drugs related to women's health (e.g., estrogens, progestins, uterine mobility–altering drugs, alendronate and related drugs).

e-Learning Activities

Companion CD

- NCLEX Review Questions: see questions 295-299
- Animations
- Audio Glossary
- Category Catchers
- Medication Errors Checklists
- IV Therapy Checklists

evolve Website (http://evolve.elsevier.com/Lilley)

- Nursing Care Plans • Frequently Asked Questions • Content Updates • WebLinks • Supplemental Resources • Elsevier ePharmacology Update • Medication Administration Animations

Drug Profiles

▶ alendronate, p. 514
calcitonin, p. 515
choriogonadotropin alfa, p. 516
clomiphene, p. 516
▶ dinoprostone, p. 517
▶ estrogen, p. 508
▶ medroxyprogesterone, p. 510
megestrol, p. 510

▶ menotropins, p. 516
▶ methylergonovine, p. 517
mifepristone, p. 517
▶ oxytocin, p. 517
raloxifene, p. 514
ritodrine, p. 519
terbutaline, p. 519

▶ Key drug.

Glossary

Chloasma Hyperpigmentation from the hormone melanin in the skin, involving brownish macules on the cheeks, forehead, lips, and/or neck; a common dermatologic adverse effect of female hormonal medications products (also called *melasma*). (p. 508)

Corpus luteum The structure that forms on the surface of the ovary after every ovulation and acts as a short-lived endocrine organ that secretes progesterone. (p. 505)

Endocrine glands Glands that secrete one or more hormones directly into the blood. (p. 505)

Estrogens The collective term for one of two major classes of female sex steroid hormones (the other is the *progestins*); of the estrogens, estradiol is responsible for most estrogenic physiologic activity. (p. 505)

Fallopian tubes The passages through which ova are carried from the ovary to the uterus. (p. 505)

Gonadotropin The hormone that stimulates the testes and ovaries. (p. 505)

Hormone replacement therapy (HRT) The term used to describe any replacement of natural body hormones with hormonal drug dosage forms. Most commonly, HRT refers to estrogen replacement therapy for treating symptoms associated with menopause-related estrogen deficiency. (p. 507)

Implantation The attachment to, penetration of, and embedding of the fertilized ovum in the lining of the uterine wall; it is one of the first stages of pregnancy. (Also called *nidation*, from the Latin word *nidus* meaning "nest".) (p. 505)

Menarche The first menses in a young woman's life and the beginning of cyclic menstrual function. (p. 505)

Menopause The cessation of menses that marks the end of a woman's childbearing capability. (p. 505)

Menses The normal flow of blood that occurs during menstruation. (p. 505)

Menstrual cycle The recurring cycle of changes in the endometrium in which the decidual layer is shed, regrows, proliferates, is maintained for several days, and is shed again at menstruation unless a pregnancy begins. (p. 505)

Nucleic acids Compounds involved in energy storage and release as well as in the determination and transmission of genetic characteristics. (p. 507)

Osteoporosis A condition characterized by the progressive loss of bone density and thinning of bone tissue; it is associated with increased risk of fractures. (p. 513)

Ova Female reproductive or germ cells (singular: ovum; also called *eggs*). (p. 505)

Ovarian follicles The location of egg production and ovulation in the ovary; the follicle is the precursor to the corpus luteum. (p. 505)

Ovaries The pair of female gonads located on each side of the lower abdomen beside the uterus. They store the *ova* (eggs) and release ova during the ovulation phase of the menstrual cycle. (p. 505)

Ovulation The rupture of the ovarian follicle, which results in the release of an unfertilized ovum into the peritoneal cavity, from which it normally enters the Fallopian tube. (p. 505)

Progestins The collective term for one of the two major classes of female hormones (the other is the *estrogens*); of the progestins, progesterone is responsible for most progestational physiologic activity. (p. 505)

Puberty The period of life when the ability to reproduce begins. (p. 505)

Uterus The hollow, pear-shaped female organ in which the fertilized ovum is implanted (see *implantation*) and the fetus develops. (p. 505)

Vagina The part of the female genitalia that forms a canal from its external orifice through its vestibule to the uterine cervix. (p. 505)

OVERVIEW OF FEMALE REPRODUCTIVE FUNCTIONS

The female reproductive system consists of the **ovaries, fallopian tubes, uterus, vagina,** and external structure known as the *vulva.* The development of these primary sex structures, initiation of their subsequent reproductive functions (starting at **puberty**), and their maintenance are controlled by pituitary **gonadotropin** hormones and the female sex steroid hormones—the **estrogens** and **progestins.** Pituitary gonadotropins include follicle-stimulating hormone (FSH) and luteinizing hormone (LH). Both play a primary role in hormonal communication between the pituitary gland (Chapter 29) and the ovaries in the continuous regulation of the **menstrual cycle** from month to month.

Estrogens are also responsible for stimulating the development of secondary female sex characteristics, including characteristic breast, skin, and bone development and distribution of body fat and hair. Progestins help create optimal conditions for pregnancy in the endometrium just after **ovulation** and also promote the start of **menses** in the absence of a fertilized ovum.

The ovaries (female gonads) are paired glands located on each side of the uterus. They function both as **endocrine glands** and as reproductive glands. As reproductive glands, they produce mature **ova** within **ovarian follicles,** which are then ovulated—that is, released into the space in the peritoneal cavity between the ovary and the fallopian tube. Fingerlike projections known as *fimbriae* lie adjacent to each ovary and serve to catch the released ovum and guide it into the fallopian tube. Once inside the fallopian tube the ovum is moved through its lumen to the uterus. This movement is accomplished through the muscular contractions of the tube walls and the actions of ciliated cells inside the lumen of the

tube, which "beat" in the direction of the uterus. Fertilization of the ovum, when it occurs, often takes place in the fallopian tube.

As endocrine glands, the ovaries are responsible for producing the two major classes of sex steroid hormones, estrogens and progestins. Chemically speaking, each of these two major classes includes several distinct hormones. However, only two of these hormones occur in significant amounts, and these two have the greatest physiologic activity. These are the estrogen estradiol and the progestin progesterone. Estradiol is the principle secretory product of the ovary and has several estrogenic effects. One of these effects is the regulation of gonadotropin (FSH and LH) secretion via negative feedback to the pituitary gland. Others include promotion of the development of women's secondary sex characteristics, monthly endometrial growth, thickening of the vaginal mucosa, thinning of the cervical mucus, and growth of the ductal system of the breasts. Progesterone is the principle secretory product of the **corpus luteum** and has progestational effects. These include promotion of tissue growth and secretory activity in the endometrium following the estrogen-driven *proliferative phase* of the menstrual cycle. This important secretory process is required for endometrial egg **implantation** and maintenance of pregnancy. Other progestational effects include induction of menstruation when fertilization has not occurred and, during pregnancy, inhibition of uterine contractions, increase in the viscosity of cervical mucus (which protects the fetus from external contamination), and growth of the alveolar glands of the breasts.

The uterus consists of three layers: the outer protective *perimetrium*, the muscular *myometrium*, and the inner mucosal layer known as the *endometrium*. The myometrium provides the powerful smooth muscle contractions needed for childbirth. The endometrium is the site of the following:

- Implantation of a fertilized ovum and subsequent development of the fetus
- Initiation of labor and birthing of the infant
- Menstruation

The vagina serves as a common passageway for birthing and menstrual flow. In addition, it is a receptacle for the penis during sexual intercourse and for the sperm after male ejaculation.

The menstrual cycle usually takes roughly 1 month to complete. Menstrual cycles begin during puberty with the first menses (**menarche**) and cease at **menopause,** which in most women occurs between 45 and 55 years of age. The hormonally controlled menstrual cycle consists of four distinct but interrelated phases that occur in overlapping sequence. Phase names correspond to activity in either the ovarian follicle or the endometrium (Table 33-1).

- **Phase 1:** The *menstruation phase,* which initiates the cycle and lasts from 5 to 7 days.
- **Phase 2:** The *follicular phase,* during which a mature ovum develops from an ovarian follicle. This phase is also called the

Table 33-1 Phases of the Menstrual Cycle

Phase	Ovarian Follicle Activity	Endometrium Activity
Phase 1	Menstruation	Menstruation
Phase 2	Follicular phase (preovulatory)	Proliferative phase
Phase 3	Ovulation	Ovulation
Phase 4	Luteal phase (postovulatory)	Secretory phase

proliferative or *preovulatory phase* and is characterized by rising estrogen secretion from the ovary and LH secretion from the pituitary gland. It terminates on or about day 14 of the cycle.

- **Phase 3:** The *ovulation phase* involves release of the unfertilized ovum from the ovary. This process occurs over a roughly 24- to 48-hour period starting at about day 14. Both estrogen and LH levels peak near this time.

- **Phase 4:** The final phase of the cycle is called the *luteal* or *postovulatory phase*. It is also known as the *secretory phase*. It occurs when the corpus luteum forms from the ruptured ovarian follicle. The corpus luteum is a mass of secretory cells on the surface of the ovary. Its primary function is to produce progesterone, which helps to optimize the endometrial mucosa for implantation of a fertilized ovum. The corpus luteum also serves as an initial source of the progesterone needed during early pregnancy. This function is later assumed by the developing placenta. If fertilization does not occur, the rising progesterone levels in the blood initiate the start of menstruation. The corpus luteum then degenerates and the menstrual cycle begins again on or about day 28.

Figure 33-1 illustrates the sequence of hormone secretions and related events that take place during the menstrual cycle.

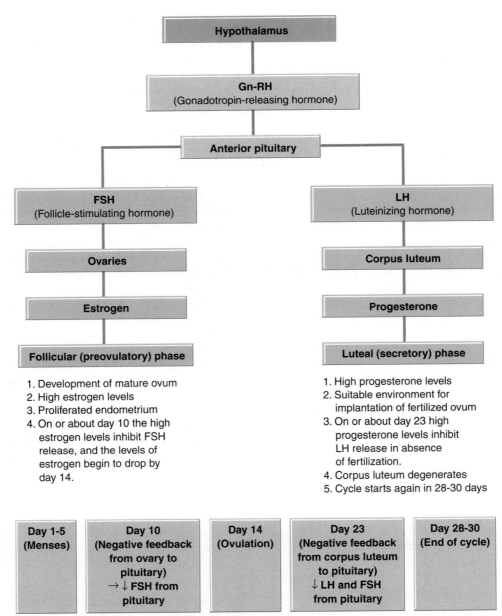

FIGURE 33-1 Hormonal activity during the monthly menstrual cycle. Gonadotropin-releasing hormone (Gn-RH) from the hypothalamus stimulates the pituitary gland, causing it to secrete follicle-stimulating hormone (FSH) early in the cycle (coinciding with the menses) and later luteinizing hormone (LH). FSH stimulates the ovaries to produce estrogen (primarily estradiol). Later in the cycle the combined surges in the levels of estrogen, Gn-RH, FSH, and LH stimulate ovulation. The corpus luteum then secretes estrogen and progesterone, providing negative feedback to the hypothalamus and pituitary gland to reduce Gn-RH, FSH, and LH secretions. If the ovum (egg) is not fertilized by a spermatozoon, levels of estrogen and progesterone then fall to their monthly lows, Gn-RH and FSH rise again, and the onset of menses begins a new cycle.

FEMALE SEX HORMONES

ESTROGENS

There are three major endogenous estrogens: estradiol, estrone, and estriol. All are synthesized from cholesterol in the ovarian follicles and have the basic chemical structure of a steroid, known as the steroid nucleus (Figure 33-2). For this reason they are sometimes referred to as steroid hormones. Estradiol is the principal and most active of the three and represents the end product of estrogen synthesis.

The exogenous estrogenic drugs, those used as drug therapy, were developed because most of the endogenous estrogens are inactive when taken orally. These synthetic drugs fall into two categories, steroidal and nonsteroidal, as follows:

Steroidal:
- Conjugated estrogens (Premarin)
- Synthetic conjugated estrogens (Cenestin)
- Esterified estrogens (Estratab, Menest)
- Estradiol transdermal (Estraderm, FemPatch, Climara, Vivelle, Menostar others)
- Estradiol cypionate (depGynogen, Depo-Estradiol Cypionate, DepoGen)
- Estradiol valerate (Delestrogen, Gynogen L.A. 20, Valergen)
- Ethinyl estradiol (Estinyl)
- Estradiol vaginal dosage forms (Vagifem, Estring, Estrace Vaginal Cream, others)
- Estrone (Estrone Aqueous, Kestrone 5)
- Estropipate (Ogen, Ortho-Est)

Nonsteroidal:
- Chlorotrianisene (TACE)
- Dienestrol (DVA)
- Diethylstilbestrol
- Diethylstilbestrol diphosphate (Stilphostrol)

The most popular estrogen product in use today is an estrogen mixture known as conjugated estrogens. It contains a combination of natural estrogen compounds equivalent to the average estrogen composition of the urine of pregnant mares, hence its brand name of Premarin. There is now a nonanimal source for this conjugated estrogen mixture. A product called Cenestin is composed of various conjugated estrogens obtained from soy and yam plants. This product was developed in response to consumer demand from women who wanted an alternative to an animal-derived product. Some women obtain other natural estrogen products from naturopathic prescribers and prefer these to standard prescription drugs such as Premarin. Patients report varying degrees of satisfaction with the numerous products available, and it can take both time and patience to find the best choice for a given individual. Ethinyl estradiol is one of the more potent estrogens and is most commonly found in oral contraceptive drugs.

Nonsteroidal estrogen products are no longer available in the United States because major adverse effects occurred when one of them, diethylstilbestrol (DES), was used in obstetrics. Box 33-1 describes this important episode in medical history.

Mechanism of Action and Drug Effects

The binding of estrogen to estrogen receptors stimulates the synthesis of **nucleic acids** (deoxyribonucleic acid [DNA] and ribonucleic acid [RNA]) and proteins, which are the building blocks for all living tissue. Estrogens are also required at puberty for the development and maintenance of the female reproductive system and the development of female secondary sex characteristics, a process known as *feminization.*

Estrogens produce their effects in estrogen-responsive tissues, which have a large number of estrogen receptors. These tissues include the female genital organs, the breasts, the pituitary gland, and the hypothalamus. At the time of puberty the production of estrogen increases greatly. This causes initiation of the menses, breast development, redistribution of body fat, softening of the skin, and other feminizing changes. Estrogens play a role in the shaping of body contours and development of the skeleton. For instance, long bones are usually inhibited from growing, with the result that females are usually shorter than males.

Indications

Estrogens are used in the treatment or prevention of a variety of disorders that primarily result from estrogen deficiency. These conditions are listed in Box 33-2. **Hormone replacement therapy (HRT)** to counter such estrogen deficiency is most commonly known for its benefits in treating menopausal symptoms (e.g., hot flashes).

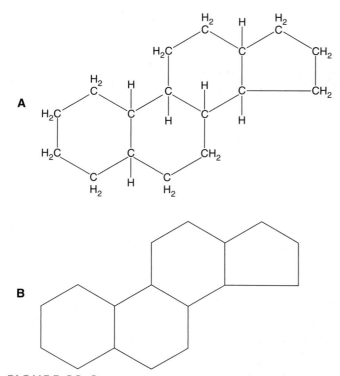

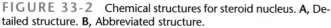

FIGURE 33-2   Chemical structures for steroid nucleus. **A,** Detailed structure. **B,** Abbreviated structure.

Box 33-1 Diethylstilbestrol

Between 1940 and 1971, an estimated 6 million mothers and their fetuses were exposed to diethylstilbestrol (DES). The drug was used to prevent reproductive problems such as miscarriage, premature delivery, intrauterine fetal death, and toxemia. This use resulted in significant complications of the reproductive system in both female and male offspring. Two large groups have been established to monitor these complications: the Registry for Research on Hormonal Transplacental Carcinogenesis and the National Cooperative Diethylstilbestrol Adenosis (DESAD) Project.

Contraindications

Contraindications for estrogen administration include known drug allergy, any estrogen-dependent cancer, undiagnosed abnormal vaginal bleeding, pregnancy, and active thromboembolic disorder (e.g., stroke, thrombophlebitis) or a history of such a disorder.

Box 33-2 Indications for Estrogen Therapy

- Atrophic vaginitis (shrinkage of the vagina and/or urethra)
- Hypogonadism
- Oral contraception (in combination with a progestin)
- Ovarian failure or castration
- Uterine bleeding
- Breast or prostate cancer (palliative treatment of advanced inoperable cases)
- Kraurosis vulvae (atrophy and shrinkage of the skin of the vulva)
- Osteoporosis treatment and prophylaxis
- Prevention of postpartum lactation
- Dysmenorrhea (painful or difficult menstruation)
- Vasomotor symptoms of menopause (e.g., hot flashes)

Table 33-2 Estrogens: Common Adverse Effects

Body System	Adverse Effects
Cardiovascular	Hypertension, thrombophlebitis, edema
Gastrointestinal	Nausea, vomiting, diarrhea, constipation, abdominal pain
Genitourinary	Amenorrhea, breakthrough uterine bleeding, enlarged uterine fibromyomas
Dermatologic	Chloasma (facial skin discoloration; also called melasma) hirsutism, alopecia
Other	Tender breasts, fluid retention, decreased carbohydrate tolerance, headaches

Adverse Effects

The most serious adverse effects of the estrogens are thromboembolic events. Very infrequently these drugs cause erythema multiforme, a rare skin disorder characterized by acute eruptions of macules, papules, or subdermal vesicles with a multiform appearance on the hands and forearms. It can be recurrent or may run a severe course and terminate fatally in Stevens-Johnson syndrome, one of the most severe dermatologic drug reactions. The most common undesirable effect of estrogen use is nausea. More commonly, photosensitivity may occur with estrogen therapy. However, one common dermatologic effect of note is known as **chloasma.** This may be distressing to the patient in terms of her body image. It consists of brownish, macular spots that often occur on the forehead, cheeks, lips, and neck. This and other adverse effects are listed in Table 33-2.

Interactions

Estrogens can decrease the activity of the oral anticoagulants, and the concurrent administration of rifampin and St. John's wort can decrease their estrogenic effect. Their use with tricyclic antidepressants (TCAs) may promote TCA toxicity. Smoking should be avoided during estrogen therapy, because this, too, can diminish the estrogenic effect and add to the risk for thrombosis.

Dosages

See the Dosages table on this page for the recommended dosages of some of the many available estrogen products.

Drug Profiles

▶ *estrogen*

Estrogen is indicated for the treatment of many clinical conditions, primarily those resulting from estrogen deficiency (see Box 33-2). Many of these conditions occur around menopause, when the endogenous estradiol level is declining. Any estrogen capable of binding to the estro-

---

DOSAGES

Selected Estrogenic Drugs

Drug (Pregnancy Category)	Pharmacologic Class	Usual Dosage Range	Indications
▶conjugated estrogens (Cenestin, Premarin) (X) and esterified estrogens (Estratab, Menest) (X)	Estrogenic hormone mixture	PO: 0.3-1.25 mg/day PO: 0.625-1.25 mg/day PO: 10 mg tid × 3 mo PO: 1.25 mg/day cyclically, 3 wk on, 1 wk off PO: 0.3-0.625 mg/day cyclically PO: 1.25-2.5 mg tid PO: 1.25 mg q4h × 24 hr, then 1.25 mg daily × 7-10 days	Atrophic vaginitis, kraurosis vulvae Vasomotor symptoms of menopause Breast cancer (palliative; male and female) Female castration, ovarian failure Female hypogonadism Prostate cancer Abnormal uterine bleeding
estradiol (Estrace) (X)	Estrogenic hormone	1-2 mg daily PO: 10 mg tid × 3 mo PO: 0.5 mg daily cyclically	Vasomotor symptoms of menopause, female castration, ovarian failure Breast cancer, prostate cancer Osteoporosis prophylaxis
estradiol transdermal (Estraderm, FemPatch, Vivelle, Climara, Menostar) (X)	Estrogenic hormone	Transdermal patch: 1 patch applied once or twice weekly to lower abdomen (not breast) ranging from 0.025 to 0.1 mg (instructions may vary by product)	Vasomotor symptoms of menopause

PO, Oral.

gen receptors in target organs can alleviate menopausal symptoms. As a general rule, the smallest dosage of estrogen that relieves the symptoms or prevents the condition is used. Although many women receive estrogen or estrogen-progestin therapy for many months or years, some clinicians (and patients) may prefer that the patient be weaned from such therapy in light of the known adverse effects.

Two recent studies performed as part of the Women's Health Initiative (WHI), a large research program sponsored by the National Institutes of Health (NIH), demonstrated the possible detrimental effects of estrogen and estrogen-progestin therapy. Both studies attempted to determine the value of HRT, if any, in preventing diseases and conditions commonly affecting older women, including breast cancer, heart disease, stroke, and hip fracture. The WHI was launched in 1991 under the direction of the National Heart, Lung, and Blood Institute (NHLBI). In one of the WHI studies of HRT, research subjects who took a certain estrogen-progestin combination product were found to have an increased risk of breast cancer, heart disease, stroke, and blood clots, although their risk of hip fractures and colon cancer was reduced. These preliminary results were so alarming that this study of combined estrogen-progestin therapy was discontinued in 2002. A part of the WHI investigation focusing on cognitive function, the WHI Memory Study, also identified adverse cognitive effects in women receiving combination estrogen-progestin therapy. These patients showed an increased risk of developing dementia and demonstrated reduced performance on tests of cognitive function. A second HRT study was begun in which women who had undergone hysterectomy received estrogen alone without progestin. In March 2004, however, these participants were advised to stop taking their assigned medication because the estrogen-only therapy appeared to be associated with an increased risk

of stroke. The data also indicated that estrogen therapy had no effect on the rates of coronary heart disease or breast cancer but was associated with a reduced rate of hip fracture. Given these results, the view of the NHLBI is that the increased risk of stroke does not justify the use of preventive estrogen therapy in healthy women, especially since no beneficial effect on heart disease (risk reduction) was demonstrated.

Follow-up of the WHI study subjects is scheduled to continue until 2010. At this time, the NHLBI recommends that estrogens *not* be used for the prevention of cardiovascular disease. However, HRT, given in the lowest effective dosages and for the shortest possible duration of treatment, is still recommended for alleviation of menopausal symptoms, based on the needs of each patient. Also recommended is the use of topical hormonal products if treatment is required only for vulvovaginal atrophy. In addition, although estrogen therapy is still endorsed for prevention of postmenopausal osteoporosis, the recommendation is that they be considered only for those women judged to be at especially high risk for osteoporosis and that nonestrogen osteoporosis medications also be strongly considered as an alternative or supplementary therapy.

The principal pharmacologic effects of all estrogens are similar because there are only slight differences in their chemical structures. These differences yield drugs of different potencies, which in turn makes them useful for a variety of indications. They also allow the drugs to be given by different routes of administration and at often highly customized dosages.

Many fixed estrogen-progestin combination products have emerged over the years. Their use is commonly referred to as *continuous combined hormone replacement therapy*. The rationale for the development of these drugs is that the use of estrogen therapy alone has been associated with an increased risk of endometrial hyperplasia, a possible precursor of endometrial cancer. The addition of continuously administered progestin to an estrogen regimen reduces the incidence of endometrial hyperplasia associated with unopposed estrogen therapy. Examples of these fixed combinations are conjugated estrogens with medroxyprogesterone, norethindrone acetate with ethinyl estradiol, and estradiol with norethindrone.

PROGESTINS

Available progestational medications, or progestins, include both natural and synthetic drugs. Progesterone is the most active natural progestational hormone and is the primary progestin component in most drug formulations. It is produced by the corpus luteum after each ovulation and during pregnancy by the placenta. In addition, there are two other major natural progestins. The first is 17-hydroxyprogesterone, an inactive metabolite of progesterone. The second is pregnenolone, a chemical precursor to all steroid hormones that is synthesized from cholesterol in the ovary as was described for the estrogens. Because orally administered progesterone is relatively inactive and parenterally administered progesterone causes local reactions and pain, chemical derivatives were developed that are effective orally and also more potent. Their actions are also more specific and of longer duration. The following are some of the most commonly used progestins:

- Hydroxyprogesterone (Hylutin)
- Medroxyprogesterone (Amen, Cycrin, Provera, Depo-Provera)
- Megestrol (Megace)
- Norethindrone acetate (Aygestin)
- Norgestrel (Ovrette, Ovral)
- Progesterone (Prometrium, Crinone)

Mechanism of Action and Drug Effects

All of the progestin products produce the same physiologic responses as those produced by progesterone itself. These responses include induction of secretory changes in the endometrium, including diminished endometrial tissue proliferation; an increase in the basal body temperature; thickening of the vaginal mucosa; relaxation of uterine smooth muscle; stimulation of mammary alveolar tissue growth; feedback inhibition (negative feedback) of the release of pituitary gonadotropins (FSH and LH); and alterations in menstrual blood flow, especially in the presence of estrogen.

Indications

Progestins are useful in the treatment of functional uterine bleeding caused by a hormonal imbalance, fibroids, or uterine cancer; in the treatment of primary and secondary amenorrhea; in the adjunctive and palliative treatment of some cancers and endometriosis; and alone or in combination with estrogens, in the prevention of conception. They may also be helpful in preventing a threatened miscarriage and alleviating the symptoms of premenstrual syndrome. Specifically, medroxyprogesterone, hydroxyprogesterone, and progesterone have all been used to treat hormone imbalance, primary or secondary amenorrhea, and functional bleeding of the uterus, although medroxyprogesterone is the one most commonly used. Norethindrone and norgestrel may be used to treat female hormone imbalance and endometriosis but are more commonly used alone or in combination with estrogens as contraceptives. Megestrol is commonly used as adjunct therapy in the treatment of breast and endometrial cancers. When estrogen replacement therapy is initiated after menopause, progestins are often included to decrease the endometrial proliferation that can be caused by unopposed estrogen. Formulations of progesterone itself are also used to treat female infertility (see Dosages table on page 511).

Contraindications

Contraindications for progestin use are similar to those for estrogens, as listed earlier.

Adverse Effects

The most serious undesirable effects of progestin use include liver dysfunction, commonly manifested as cholestatic jaundice; thrombophlebitis; and thromboembolic disorders such as pulmonary embolism. The more common adverse effects are listed in Table 33-3.

Interactions

There are reports of possible decreases in glucose tolerance when progestins are taken with antidiabetic drugs, and the dosage of the antidiabetic drug may need to be adjusted. The concurrent use of medroxyprogesterone or norethindrone and aminoglutethimide or rifampin induces increased metabolism of the progestin.

Table 33-3	Progestins: Common Adverse Effects
Body System	**Adverse Effects**
Gastrointestinal	Nausea, vomiting
Genitourinary	Amenorrhea, spotting, changes in menstrual flow, changes in cervical erosion and secretions
Other	Edema, weight gain or loss, allergic rash, pyrexia, somnolence or insomnia, depression

Dosages

For recommended dosages of the progestins, see the Dosages table on page 511.

Drug Profiles

▶ medroxyprogesterone

Medroxyprogesterone (Amen, Cycrin, Provera, Depo-Provera) inhibits the secretion of pituitary gonadotropins, which prevents follicular maturation and ovulation, stimulates the growth of mammary tissue, and has an antineoplastic action against endometrial cancer. Medroxyprogesterone is used to treat uterine bleeding, secondary amenorrhea, endometrial cancer, and renal cancer and is also used as a contraceptive. Its most common use is to prevent endometrial cancer caused by estrogen replacement therapy. It is also sometimes used as adjunct therapy in certain types of cancer (see Chapter 48). Medroxyprogesterone is available in both oral and parenteral preparations.

Pharmacokinetics

Half-Life	Onset	Peak	Duration
14.5 hr	Unknown	IM: 2-7 hr	IM: 3 mo

megestrol

Megestrol (Megace) is a synthetic progestin that differs structurally from progesterone only in the addition of a methyl group on the steroid nucleus and a double bond. Although megestrol shares the actions of the progestins, it is primarily used in the palliative management of recurrent, inoperable, or metastatic endometrial or breast cancer. It has also been used in the management of anorexia, cachexia, or unexplained substantial weight loss in patients with acquired immunodeficiency syndrome (AIDS). In addition, it may be used to stimulate appetite and promote weight gain in patients with cancer. It is available only for oral use.

Pharmacokinetics

Half-Life	Onset	Peak	Duration
34 hr	6-8 wk	Unknown	4-10 mo

CONTRACEPTIVE DRUGS

Contraceptive drugs are medications used to prevent pregnancy. Contraceptive devices are nondrug methods of pregnancy prevention such as intrauterine devices (IUDs), male and female condoms, cervical diaphragms, and so forth. Patients must be informed, for their own safety, of the fact that contraceptive drug therapy serves only to prevent pregnancy and does not protect them from sexually transmitted diseases, including human immunodeficiency virus (HIV) infection/AIDS. This even includes spermicidal drugs such as the over-the-counter (OTC) foams for intravaginal use. These products most often contain the spermicide nonoxynol-9, which does kill sperm cells to prevent pregnancy but does not necessarily kill microbes capable of causing sexually transmitted diseases, including HIV infection.

Aside from sexual abstinence, oral contraceptives are the most effective form of birth control currently available. Estrogen-progestin combinations, often referred to as "the pill," are oral contraceptives that contain both estrogenic and progestational steroids. The most common estrogenic component is ethinyl estradiol, a semisynthetic steroidal estrogen. The most common progestin component is norethindrone.

The currently available oral contraceptives may be *biphasic*, *triphasic*, or *monophasic*, in terms of the doses taken at different

DOSAGES

Selected Progestational Drugs

Drug (Pregnancy Category)	Pharmacologic Class	Usual Dosage Range	Indications
▸medroxyprogesterone acetate (Provera, others) (X)		PO: 2.5-10 mg/day for set number of days or cyclically (smaller doses may be given on a continuous daily basis)	Amenorrhea, uterine bleeding
		PO: 2.5-10 mg/day on last 10-13 days of each month to accompany estrogen dosing	Vasomotor symptoms of menopause
megestrol (Megace) (X)	Progestin	PO: 400-1000 mg/wk	Metastatic endometrial or renal cancer
		400-800 mg/day	Severe weight loss in male and female patients with HIV/AIDS
		PO: 40 mg bid-qid	Uterine bleeding
		PO: 40-800 mg/day in divided doses	Breast or endometrial cancer
progesterone (Prometrium, Progestasert, Crinone)* (D)		Intravaginal gel: 90 mg/day for up to 12 wk	Progesterone deficiency in infertility
		IM: 5-10 mg daily × 6-8 days	Amenorrhea or functional uterine bleeding
		PO: 400 mg qpm†	Secondary amenorrhea

AIDS, Acquired immunodeficiency syndrome; *HIV,* human immunodeficiency virus (infection); *IM,* intramuscular; *PO,* oral.
*These products are sometimes used to promote and/or maintain pregnancy as part of an assisted reproductive technology regimen.
†Formulation contains peanut oil and is contraindicated in patients with a peanut allergy.

times of the menstrual cycle. The biphasic drugs contain a fixed estrogen dose but a low progestin dose for the first 10 days and a higher dose for the rest of the cycle and are available in 21- or 28-day dosage packages. The triphasic oral contraceptives contain three different estrogen-progestin dose ratios that are administered sequentially during the cycle and are provided in 21- or 28-day dosage packages. The triphasic products most closely duplicate the normal hormonal levels of the female cycle. These contraceptives also come in *monophasic* forms, in which the estrogen and progestin doses are the same throughout the cycle. There are also oral contraceptives that are progestin-only drugs. The monophasic and triphasic oral contraceptives are the most numerous on the market and the most widely prescribed. Some patients (e.g., those with menstrual irregularities) may require special assistance in selecting drug products with their prescribers. Three other important contraceptive medications are a long-acting injectable form of medroxyprogesterone, a transdermal contraceptive patch, and, most recently, an intravaginal contraceptive ring.

Mechanism of Action and Drug Effects

Contraceptive drugs prevent ovulation by inhibiting the release of gonadotropins and by increasing uterine mucous viscosity, which results in (1) decreased sperm movement and fertilization of the ovum, and (2) possible inhibition of implantation (nidation) of a fertilized egg (zygote) into the endometrial lining.

Oral contraceptives have many of the same hormonal effects as those normally produced by endogenous estrogens and progesterone. The contraceptive effect results mainly from the suppression of the hypothalamic-pituitary system that they induce, which in turn prevents ovulation. Other incidental benefits to their use are that they improve menstrual cycle regularity and decrease blood loss during menstruation. A decreased incidence

of functional ovarian cysts and ectopic pregnancies has also been associated with their use.

Indications

Oral contraceptive drugs are primarily used to prevent pregnancy. In addition, they are used to treat endometriosis and hypermenorrhea and to produce cyclic withdrawal bleeding in patients with amenorrhea. Occasionally combination oral contraceptives are used to provide postcoital emergency contraception. Emergency contraception pills are not effective if the woman is already pregnant (i.e., egg implantation has occurred). They should therefore be taken within 72 hours of unprotected intercourse with a follow-up dose 12 hours after the first dose. They are intended to prevent pregnancy after known or suspected contraceptive failure or unprotected intercourse. Preven and Alesse are two ethinyl estradiol-levonorgestrel combination products that are commonly used for this indication. One new oral contraceptive of note is Seasonale, which includes both estrogen and progestin components. It is sold in packages containing 3 months worth of medication, including 1 week's worth of nonhormonal tablets. This is because Seasonale reduces a woman's menstrual cycles to once every 3 months.

Contraindications

Contraindications to the use of oral contraceptives include known drug allergy to a specific product, pregnancy, and known high risk for or history of thromboembolic events such as myocardial infarction, venous thrombosis, pulmonary embolism, or stroke.

Adverse Effects

Common adverse effects associated with the use of oral contraceptives are listed in Table 33-4. These effects include hypertension, thromboembolism, alterations in carbohydrate and lipid metabolism, increases in serum hormone concentrations, and alterations in serum metal and plasma protein levels. It is the estrogen component that appears to be the source of most of these metabolic effects.

Interactions

Several drugs and drug classes that can potentially reduce the effectiveness of oral contraceptives, which can possibly result in an unintended pregnancy. These include the following:

- Antibiotics
- Barbiturates

Table 33-4	Oral Contraceptives: Common Adverse Effects	
Body System	**Adverse Effects**
Cardiovascular	Hypotension, thrombophlebitis, edema, thromboembolism, pulmonary embolism, myocardial infarction
Central nervous	Dizziness, headache, migraines, depression, stroke
Gastrointestinal	Nausea, vomiting, diarrhea, anorexia, pancreatitis, cramps, constipation, increased appetite, increased weight, cholestatic jaundice
Genitourinary	Amenorrhea, cervical erosion, breakthrough bleeding, dysmenorrhea, breast changes

- griseofulvin
- isoniazid
- rifampin

The effectiveness of other drugs may be reduced when they are taken with oral contraceptives. These include the following:

- Anticonvulsants
- β-blockers
- guanethidine
- Hypnotics
- Hypoglycemic drugs
- Oral anticoagulants
- theophylline
- TCAs
- Vitamins

Dosages

For the recommended dosages of oral contraceptives, see the Dosages table on this page.

Drug Profiles

Contraceptive Drugs

The Dosages table on this page provides selected examples of the many contraceptive drugs available. All work in similar fashion to prevent pregnancy. If they are used during pregnancy, however, they can cause termination of pregnancy, and for this reason they are clas-

DOSAGES

Selected Contraceptive Drugs

Drug (Pregnancy Category)	Pharmacologic Class	Usual Dosage Range	Indications
Oral Contraceptives			
norethindrone and ethinyl estradiol (Ortho-Novum, Necon, Jenest, others) (X)	Biphasic: fixed estrogen–variable progestin 21- or 28-day products	For the most reliable contraceptive action, the patient should take all preparations according to instructions from prescriber or patient information product insert, at intervals not to exceed 24 hr	Prevention of pregnancy
norethindrone and ethinyl estradiol (Loestrin, Modicon, Necon, others) (X)	Monophasic: fixed estrogen-progestin combinations; 21- or 28-day products; 28-day products contain 7 inert tabs		
norethindrone and ethinyl estradiol (Ortho-Novum 7/7/7, Estrostep, Tri-Norinyl, others) (X)	Triphasic: 3 or 4 monthly phases of variable estrogen and progestin combinations; 21- or 28-day products; 28-day products contain 7 inert tabs		
Injectable Contraceptives (Depot)			
▶medroxyprogesterone (Depo-Provera) (X)	Progestin-only injectable contraceptive	IM: 150 mg q3mo	Prevention of pregnancy
Transdermal Contraceptives			
norelgestromin and ethinyl estradiol (X)	Fixed-combination estrogen-progestin transdermal contraceptive	Transdermal patch: 1 patch applied weekly × 3 wk each month, scheduled around menses in wk 4	Prevention of pregnancy
Intravaginal Contraceptives			
etonogestrel–ethinyl estradiol vaginal ring (NuvaRing) (X)	Fixed-combination estrogen-progestin intravaginal contraceptive	1 ring inserted into vagina by patient and left in place for 3 wk, followed by 1-wk removal; new ring is then inserted 1 wk later	Prevention of pregnancy

IM, Intramuscular.

sified as pregnancy category X drugs by the Food and Drug Administration (FDA). Drugs that are *intended* for termination of pregnancy are known as *abortifacients* and are discussed later in this chapter.

CURRENT DRUG THERAPY FOR OSTEOPOROSIS

Approximately 23 million women in the United States are currently affected by **osteoporosis** or low bone mass with increased risk of fracture. Nearly 40% of U.S. women over 50 years of age will develop an osteoporotic fracture, and the annual costs to society equal nearly $11 billion. Risk factors for postmenopausal osteoporosis include white or Asian descent, slender body build, early estrogen deficiency, smoking, alcohol consumption, low-calcium diet, sedentary lifestyle, and family history of osteoporosis. Although osteoporosis is primarily a disorder that affects women, up to 20% of persons with this condition are men.

Until recently, supplementation with calcium and vitamin D was strongly recommended for all women and men considered at risk for osteoporosis (e.g., those with a family history of the disorder). These supplements were thought to play a major role in the prevention of this common bone disorder. The recommended calcium intake usually ranged from 1000 to 1500 mg daily depending on age, frame, and hormone status. However, in February 2006, the NHLBI announced the results of the calcium–vitamin D trial of the WHI, which followed patients for 7 years to examine the preventive effects of calcium and vitamin D supplementation. The conclusion was that such supplements led to a more modest than expected reduction in hip and other fractures, had no preventive effects with regard to colon polyps or cancer as previously believed, and increased the risk of kidney stones. Again, this particular study focused exclusively on female patients. The current recommendation is that women, especially those over age 60, should *consider,* in discussions with their health providers, taking calcium and vitamin D supplements for bone health. No new recommendations were issued regarding the use of other medications that enhance body calcium levels such as calcitonin or teriparatide, the use of any other osteoporosis medications, or the use of these medications in male patients.

Three major drug classes are currently the mainstays of treatment of existing osteoporosis: the bisphosphonates, the selective estrogen receptor modulators (SERMs), and the hormone calcitonin. Currently available bisphosphonates used for osteoporosis prevention and treatment include alendronate, ibandronate, and risedronate. Currently raloxifene (Evista) and tamoxifen (Nolvadex) are the available SERMs. Tamoxifen is primarily used in oncology settings and is discussed further in Chapter 48. Raloxifene has primarily been investigated for use in the prevention of osteoporosis, although many studies suggest that it may be beneficial in the treatment of osteoporosis as well. A drug form of the hormone calcitonin is also commonly used.

Mechanism of Action and Drug Effects

Bisphosphonates

The bisphosphonates work by inhibiting osteoclast-mediated bone resorption, which in turn indirectly enhances bone mineral density. *Osteoclasts* are bone cells that break down bone, causing calcium to be reabsorbed into the circulation; this resorption eventually leads to osteoporosis if not controlled or countered by adequate new bone formation. These drugs have become the primary drugs of choice for this condition because their use is backed by the strongest clinical evidence to date indicating reversal of lost bone mass and reduction of fracture risk.

Selective Estrogen Receptor Modulators

Raloxifene helps prevent osteoporosis by stimulating estrogen receptors on bone and increasing bone density in a manner similar to the estrogens themselves.

Calcitonin

Like the natural thyroid hormone, calcitonin directly inhibits osteoclastic bone resorption.

Teriparatide

In contrast to the other therapies described thus far, which inhibit bone resorption, teriparatide is the first and currently the only drug available that acts by stimulating bone formation. It is a derivative of parathyroid hormone and works to treat osteoporosis by modulating the body's metabolism of calcium and phosphorus in a manner similar to natural parathyroid hormone.

Indications

Raloxifene is primarily used for the prevention of postmenopausal osteoporosis. The bisphosphonates and calcitonin are used in both the prevention and treatment of osteoporosis. Teriparatide is used primarily for the subset of osteoporosis patients at highest risk of fracture (e.g., those with prior fracture).

Contraindications

Bisphosphonates

Contraindications to bisphosphonate use include drug allergy, hypocalcemia, esophageal dysfunction, and the inability to sit or stand upright for at least 30 minutes after taking the medication.

Selective Estrogen Receptor Modulators

The use of SERMs is contraindicated in women with a known allergy to these drugs, in women who are or may become pregnant, and in women with a venous thromboembolic disorder, including deep vein thrombosis, pulmonary embolism, and retinal vein thrombosis, or with a history of such a disorder.

CASE STUDY

Osteoporosis

T.L. is a relatively healthy 73-year-old female with newly diagnosed postmenopausal osteoporosis. She has been prescribed treatment with alendronate (Fosamax) 10 mg orally every day. Approximately 5 days after initiating treatment, T.L. experiences dysphagia and odynophagia. She is scheduled for an endoscopy in the morning to rule out ulcerative esophagitis.

- What is alendronate and what are the indications for its use?
- How could the adverse reaction to this medication have been prevented?
- What drugs show significant interactions with alendronate?

For answers, see http://evolve.elsevier.com/Lilley.

Calcitonin

Contraindications to calcitonin use include drug allergy or allergy to salmon (the drug is salmon derived).

Teriparatide

Contraindications to the use of teriparatide include drug allergy.

Adverse Effects

The primary adverse effects of SERMs are hot flashes and leg cramps. Like estrogens they can increase the risk of venous thromboembolism and they are teratogenic. Leukopenia may also occur and predispose the patient to various infections. Post-menopausal women taking raloxifene were no more likely to develop breast, uterine, or ovarian cancer than women taking a placebo. The most common adverse effects of bisphosphonates include headache, gastrointestinal (GI) upset, and joint pain. However, the bisphosphonates are usually well tolerated. There is a risk of esophageal burns with these medications if they become lodged in the esophagus before reaching the stomach. For this reason the patient should take these medications with a full glass of water and remain sitting upright or standing for at least 30 minutes. Common adverse effects of calcitonin include flushing of the face, nausea, diarrhea and reduced appetite. Common adverse effects of teriparatide include chest pain, dizziness, hypercalcemia, nausea, and arthralgia.

Interactions

Cholestyramine and ampicillin decrease the absorption of raloxifene, and raloxifene can decrease the effects of warfarin. Calcium supplements and antacids can interfere with the absorption of the bisphosphonates, and therefore these drugs should be spaced 1 to 2 hours apart to avoid this interaction. Calcium supplements, although often needed by patients with osteoporosis, are also more likely to cause hypercalcemia in patients receiving calcitonin. In addition, there have been case reports of teriparatide-associated hypercalcemia that has been implicated in digitalis toxicity.

Dosages

For the recommended dosages of osteoporosis drugs, see the Dosages table on this page.

Drug Profiles

▸ alendronate

Alendronate (Fosamax) is an oral bisphosphonate and the first nonestrogen-nonhormonal option for preventing bone loss. This drug works by inhibiting and/or reversing osteoclast-mediated born resorption. Recall that *osteoclasts* are the bone cells that cause breakdown or *resorption* of bone tissue as part of their normal physiology. However, unchecked osteoclastic activity often leads to osteoporosis if not managed, so this drug class represents a major breakthrough in the treatment of osteoporosis. It is indicated for the prevention and treatment of osteoporosis in men and in postmenopausal women. It is also indicated for the treatment of glucocorticoid-induced osteoporosis in men and for the treatment of Paget's disease in women.

Data show that alendronate therapy may reduce the risk of hip fracture by 51%, of spinal fracture by 47%, and of wrist fracture by 48%. Precautions should be taken in patients with dysphagia, esophagitis, esophageal ulcer, or gastric ulcer, because the drug can be very irritating. Case reports of esophageal erosions have been published. It is recommended that alendronate be taken with an 8-oz glass of water immediately upon arising in the morning and that the patient not lie down for at least 30 minutes after taking it. When patients whose condition has been stabilized on alendronate are hospitalized and cannot comply with these recommendations, the medication is often withheld. Alendronate has an extremely long terminal half-life, and going several days without taking a dose will do little to reduce the therapeutic efficacy of the drug.

Both alendronate and a similar drug, risedronate, are available only in tablet form for daily or weekly oral use. In 2005, the FDA also approved another bisphosphonate, ibandronate, which is dosed orally once per month.

Pharmacokinetics

Half-Life	Onset*	Peak*	Duration*
Longer than 10 yr due to storage of drug in bone tissue	3 wk	Unknown	Unknown

*Therapeutic effect.

raloxifene

Raloxifene (Evista) is a SERM. It is used primarily for the prevention of postmenopausal osteoporosis. Interestingly, raloxifene has positive effects on cholesterol level, but it is not normally used specifically for this purpose. It may not be the best choice for women near menopause, because use of the drug is associated with the adverse effect of hot flashes. It is available only for oral use.

DOSAGES

Selected Drugs Used Specifically for Osteoporosis

Drug (Pregnancy Category)	Pharmacologic Class	Usual Dosage Range	Indications
▸ alendronate (Fosamax) (C)	Bisphosphonate	PO: 5 mg/day or 35 mg/wk PO: 10 mg/day or 70 mg/wk	Osteoporosis prevention and treatment
ibandronate (Boniva) (C)	Bisphosphonate	PO: 2.5 mg/day or 150 mg/mo IV: 3 mg IV push q3 mo (by health professional)	Osteoporosis prevention and treatment
calcitonin, salmon (Calcimar, Miacalcin, others) (C)	Calcitonin hormonal substitute derived from salmon	IM/SC: 100 units/day Nasal spray: 200 units (1 spray)/day	Osteoporosis prevention
raloxifene (Evista) (X)	Selective estrogen receptor modulator	PO: 60 mg/day	Osteoporosis treatment
teriparatide (Forteo) (C)	Parathyroid hormone derivative	SC: 20 mcg once/day in thigh or abdomen	Osteoporosis prevention and treatment

IM, Intramuscular; *PO,* oral; *SC,* subcutaneous.

Pharmacokinetics

Half-Life	Onset	Peak	Duration
27 hr	Unknown	Unknown	Unknown

calcitonin

Calcitonin, in its drug forms, is derived from salmon (fish) sources. Although it is available in both injectable form and nasal spray, the nasal spray (Miacalcin) is now more commonly used.

Pharmacokinetics (Nasal Spray)

Half-Life	Onset	Peak	Duration
43 min	Unknown	30-40 min	Unknown

DRUG THERAPY RELATED TO PREGNANCY, LABOR, DELIVERY, AND THE POSTPARTUM PERIOD

FERTILITY DRUGS

Infertility in women generally results from absence of ovulation (anovulation), which is normally due to various imbalances in female reproductive hormones. Such imbalances can occur at the level of the hypothalamus, the pituitary gland, the ovary, or any combination of these. Supplements of estrogens or progestins may be used to fortify the blood levels of these hormones when ovarian output is inadequate. The use of drug forms of these hormones was described earlier in this chapter.

Hormone deficiencies at the hypothalamic and pituitary levels are often treated with gonadotropin ovarian stimulants. These drugs stimulate increased secretion of gonadotropin-releasing hormone (Gn-RH) from the hypothalamus, which then results in increased secretion of FSH and LH from the pituitary gland. These hormones, in turn, stimulate the development of ovarian follicles and ovulation. They also stimulate ovarian secretion of the estrogens and progestins that are part of the normal ovulatory cycle. Proper selection and dosage adjustment of fertility drugs often requires the expertise of a fertility specialist. The various medical techniques used in the treatment of infertility, including drug therapy, are now collectively referred to as *assisted reproductive technology.* One particularly common specific technique is *in vitro fertilization,* which a woman's ovum is fertilized with her partner's sperm in a laboratory and the fertilized ovum is then medically implanted into the woman's uterus. Infants born through the use of this technique are commonly referred to as "test tube babies." The success of such fertilization techniques may be further aided with the use of medications such as those described earlier. Representative examples of ovulation stimulants include the drugs clomiphene, menotropins, and choriogonadotropin alfa.

Mechanism of Action and Drug Effects

Clomiphene is a nonsteroidal ovulation stimulant that works by blocking estrogen receptors in the uterus and brain. This results in a false signal of low estrogen levels to the brain. The hypothalamus and pituitary gland then increase their production of Gn-RH (from the hypothalamus) and FSH and LH (from the pituitary), which stimulates the maturation of ovarian follicles. Ideally this leads to ovulation and increases the likelihood of conception in a previously infertile woman.

Menotropins is the drug name for a standardized mixture of FSH and LH that is derived from the urine of postmenopausal women. The FSH component stimulates the development of ovarian follicles, which leads to ovulation. The LH component stimulates the development of the corpus luteum, which supplies female sex hormones (estrogens and progestins) during the first trimester of pregnancy. Choriogonadotropin alfa is a recombinant form (i.e., developed with recombinant DNA technology) of the hormone human chorionic gonadotropin (hCG). This hormone is naturally produced by the placenta during pregnancy and can be isolated from the urine of pregnant women. It is an analogue of LH and can provide a substitute for the natural LH surge that promotes ovulation. It does this by binding to LH receptors in the ovary and stimulating the rupture of mature ovarian follicles and the subsequent development of the corpus luteum. Human chorionic gonadotropin also maintains the viability of the corpus luteum during early pregnancy. This is critical, because the corpus luteum provides the supply of estrogens and progestins necessary to support the first trimester of pregnancy until the placenta assumes this role. Choriogonadotropin alfa is often given in a carefully timed fashion after FSH-active therapy such as menotropins or clomiphene therapy, when patient monitoring indicates sufficient maturation of ovarian follicles.

Indications

These drugs are used primarily for the promotion of ovulation in anovulatory female patients. They may also be used to promote spermatogenesis in infertile men. As was mentioned in the Progestins section, progesterone formulations are also used to treat female infertility.

Contraindications

Contraindications to the use of the ovarian stimulants include known drug allergy to a specific product and may also include primary ovarian failure, uncontrolled thyroid or adrenal dysfunction, liver disease, pituitary tumor, abnormal uterine bleeding, ovarian enlargement of uncertain cause, sex hormone–dependent tumors, and pregnancy.

Adverse Effects

The most common adverse effects of the ovulation stimulants are listed in Table 33-5.

Table 33-5	Fertility Drugs: Most Common Adverse Effects
Body System	**Adverse Effects**
Cardiovascular	Tachycardia, phlebitis, deep vein thrombosis, hypovolemia
Central nervous	Dizziness, headache, flushing, depression, restlessness, anxiety, nervousness, fatigue
Gastrointestinal	Nausea, bloating, constipation, abdominal pain, vomiting, anorexia
Other	Urticaria, ovarian hyperstimulation, multiple pregnancies, blurred vision, diplopia, photophobia, breast pain, fever

DOSAGES

Selected Fertility Drugs

Drug (Pregnancy Category)	Pharmacologic Class	Usual Dosage Range	Indications
choriogonadotropin alfa (Ovidrel) (X)	Ovulation stimulant, recombinant	SC: 250 mcg given 1 day after last dose of follicle stimulant (e.g., menotropins)	Female infertility
clomiphene (Clomid, Milophene, Serophene) (X)	Ovulation stimulant	PO: 50-100 mg daily × 5 days; repeatable cycle depending on response	Female infertility in selected patients
▶ menotropins (Pergonal, Repronex) (X)	Gonadotropins (FSH-LH) ovulation stimulant	IM: 1 ampule daily × 9-12 days, followed by chorionic gonadotropin	Female infertility, male infertility

FSH, Follicle-stimulating hormone; *IM,* intramuscular; *LH,* luteinizing hormone; *PO,* oral; *SC,* subcutaneous.

Interactions

Few drugs interact with fertility drugs. The most notable are the TCAs, the butyrophenones (e.g., haloperidol), the phenothiazines (e.g., promethazine), and the antihypertensive drugs methyldopa and reserpine. When any of these drugs is taken with the fertility drugs, prolactin concentrations may be increased, which may impair fertility.

Dosages

For recommended dosages of the fertility drugs, see the Dosages table on this page.

Drug Profiles

choriogonadotropin alfa

Choriogonadotropin alfa (Ovidrel) is a synthetic recombinant analogue of natural hCG and its effects are similar to those of this hormone. These effects include the rupture of mature ovarian follicles (and ovulation) and maintenance of the corpus luteum. Natural forms of hCG, isolated from the urine of pregnant women, are also still marketed. Choriogonadotropin alfa is currently available only in injectable form.

Pharmacokinetics

Half-Life	Onset	Peak	Duration
5.6 hr	2 hr	6 hr	36 hr

clomiphene

Clomiphene (Clomid, Milophene, Serophene) is primarily used to stimulate the production of pituitary gonadotropins, which in turn induces the maturation of the ovarian follicle and eventually ovulation. It is currently available only for oral use.

Pharmacokinetics

Half-Life	Onset	Peak	Duration
5 days	4-12 days	Unknown	1 mo

▶ menotropins

Menotropins (Pergonal) is a purified preparation of the gonadotropins FSH and LH that is extracted from the urine of postmenopausal women. Other available medications with similar composition and functions include urofollitropin, follitropin alfa, and follitropin beta. Menotropins is available only in injectable form.

Pharmacokinetics

Half-Life	Onset	Peak	Duration
Unknown	Unknown	Unknown	Unknown

LABOR, DELIVERY, AND POSTPARTUM DRUGS: UTERINE-ACTIVE MEDICATIONS

A variety of medications are used to alter the dynamics of uterine contractions either to promote or to prevent the start or progression of labor. In the immediately postpartal period, medications may also be used to promote rapid shrinkage of the uterus to reduce the risk of postpartum hemorrhage.

Uterine Stimulants

Four types of drugs are used to stimulate uterine contractions: ergot derivatives, prostaglandins, the progesterone antagonist mifepristone (RU-486), and the hormone oxytocin. These drugs all act on the uterus, a highly muscular organ that has a complex network of smooth muscle fibers and a large blood supply. These drugs are often collectively referred to as *oxytocics,* after the naturally occurring hormone oxytocin, whose action they mimic. The uterus undergoes several changes during normal gestation and childbirth that at different times make it either resistant or susceptible to various hormones and drugs. Oxytocin is one of the two hormones secreted by the posterior lobe of the pituitary gland. The other is vasopressin, which is also known as antidiuretic hormone.

Mechanism of Action and Drug Effects

The uterus of a woman who is not pregnant is relatively insensitive to oxytocin, but during pregnancy the uterus becomes more sensitive to this hormone and is most sensitive at term (the end of gestation).

During childbirth, oxytocin stimulates uterine contraction, and during lactation it promotes the movement of milk from the mammary glands to the nipples. Another class of oxytocic drugs is the prostaglandins, natural hormones involved in regulating the network of smooth muscle fibers of the uterus. This network is known as the *myometrium.* The prostaglandins cause very potent contractions of the myometrium and may also play a role in the natural induction of labor. When the prostaglandin concentrations increase during the final few weeks of pregnancy, mild myometrial contractions, commonly known as Braxton Hicks contractions, are stimulated. The third major class of oxytocic drugs is the ergot alkaloids, which are also potent simulators of uterine muscle. These drugs increase the force and frequency of uterine contractions. One of the most politically charged prescription drug approvals ever made by the FDA was approval of the progesterone antagonist mifepristone (Mifeprex), also known as the "abortion pill." This drug also stimulates uterine contractions and is used to induce elective termination of pregnancy.

Indications

Oxytocin is available in a synthetic injectable form (e.g., Pitocin). This drug is used to induce labor at or near full-term gestation and to enhance labor when uterine contractions are weak and ineffective. Oxytocic drugs are also used to prevent or control uterine bleeding after delivery, to induce completion of an incomplete abortion (including miscarriages), and to promote milk ejection during lactation.

The prostaglandins may be used therapeutically to induce labor by softening the cervix (cervical ripening) and enhancing uterine muscle tone. They may also be used to stimulate the myometrium to induce abortion during the second trimester when the uterus is resistant to oxytocin. Examples of these drugs are dinoprostone and misoprostol.

Ergot alkaloids are used after delivery of the infant and placenta to prevent postpartum uterine atony (lack of muscle tone) and hemorrhage.

Mifepristone is used to induce abortion and is often given with the synthetic prostaglandin drug misoprostol for this purpose.

Contraindications

Contraindications to the use of labor-inducing uterine stimulants include known drug allergy to a specific product and may include pelvic inflammatory disease, cervical stenosis, uterine fibrosis, high-risk intrauterine fetal positions before delivery, placenta previa, hypertonic uterus, uterine prolapse, or any condition in which vaginal delivery is contraindicated (e.g., increased bleeding risk). Contraindications to the use of abortifacients include known drug allergy as well as the presence of an IUD, ectopic pregnancy, concurrent anticoagulant therapy or bleeding disorder, inadequate access to emergency health care, or the inability to understand or comply with follow-up instructions.

Adverse Effects

The most common undesirable effects of oxytocic drugs are listed in Table 33-6.

Interactions

Few clinically significant drug interactions occur with the oxytocic drugs. The most common and important of these involve sympathomimetic drugs. Combining drugs that produce vasoconstriction, such as sympathomimetics, with the oxytocic drugs can result in severe hypertension.

Table 33-6	Oxytocic Drugs: Most Common Adverse Effects
Body System	**Adverse Effects**
Cardiovascular	Hypotension or hypertension, chest pain
Central nervous	Headache, dizziness, fainting
Gastrointestinal	Nausea, vomiting, diarrhea
Genitourinary	Vaginitis, vaginal pain, cramping
Other	Leg cramps, joint swelling, chills, fever, weakness, blurred vision

Dosages

For the recommended dosages of selected oxytocic drugs, see the Dosages table on this page.

Drug Profiles

▶ dinoprostone

Dinoprostone (Prostin E_2, Cervidil, Prepidil) is a synthetic derivative of the naturally occurring hormone prostaglandin E_2. It is used for the termination of pregnancy from the twelfth through the twentieth gestational weeks, for evacuation of the uterine contents in the management of missed abortion or intrauterine fetal death up to 28 weeks of gestational age, for the management of nonmetastatic gestational trophoblastic disease, and for ripening of an unfavorable cervix in pregnant women at or near term when there is a medical or obstetric need for labor induction. It is available only for vaginal use in various dosage forms.

Pharmacokinetics

Half-Life	Onset	Peak	Duration
Gel: N/A	Gel: Rapid	Gel: 30-45 min	Gel: Unavailable
Suppository: N/A	Suppository: 10 min	Suppository: Unavailable	Suppository: 2-3 hr

N/A, Not applicable.

▶ methylergonovine

The ergot alkaloid methylergonovine (Methergine) is used primarily in the immediately postpartal period to enhance myometrial tone and reduce the likelihood of postpartum uterine hemorrhage. Its use is contraindicated in patients with a known hypersensitivity to ergot medications and in those with pelvic inflammatory disease. It also should not be used for augmentation of labor, before delivery of the placenta, or during a spontaneous abortion. Methylergonovine is available in both oral and injectable forms.

Pharmacokinetics

Half-Life	Onset	Peak	Duration
PO: Less than 2 hr	PO: 5-15 min	PO: 30 min	PO: 3 hr
IM: N/A	IM: Less than 5 min	IM: Not listed	IM: Not listed

N/A, Not applicable.

mifepristone

Mifepristone (Mifeprex, RU-486) is a synthetic steroid compound that functions as a progesterone receptor antagonist. This action promotes uterine contractions and evacuation of uterine contents. The drug is primarily used for elective termination of pregnancy and is normally followed by a dose of the synthetic steroid misoprostol. Mifepristone is currently available only for oral use. In July of 2005, the FDA reported the occurrence of four deaths following abortions induced by mifepristone. These four deaths were attributed to sepsis from *Clostridium sordellii*, an anaerobic bacterial species. As of March of 2006, the FDA had reported two additional deaths associated with the use of this drug but did not list specific causes. In all six cases, it is uncertain whether the use of mifepristone played a direct role in the deaths. However, the agency has warned health providers and their patients to be aware of these cases and of each patient's risk factors for sepsis when considering the use of this drug for termination of pregnancy.

Pharmacokinetics

Half-Life	Onset	Peak	Duration
18 hr	Unknown	90 min	Unknown

▶ oxytocin

The drug oxytocin (Pitocin, Syntocinon) is the synthetic form of the endogenous hormone oxytocin and has all of its pharmacologic properties.

DOSAGES

Selected Uterine Stimulants

Drug (Pregnancy Category)*	Pharmacologic Class	Usual Dosage Range	Indications
▶dinoprostone (Prostin E₂, Prepidil, Cervidil) (X)	Prostaglandin E₂ abortifacient and cervical ripening drug	Vaginal suppository (Prostin E₂): 1 suppository (20 mg) into vagina at 3-5 hr intervals until uterine evacuation	Termination of pregnancy; uterine evacuation in cases of miscarriage or benign hydatidiform mole
		Cervical gel (Prepidil): 0.5 mg into cervical canal at 6-hr dosing intervals (max 1.5 mg/24 hr)	Cervical ripening for induction of labor
		Vaginal suppository (Cervidil): 10 mg into posterior vaginal fornix (space behind cervix) × 1 dose	Cervical ripening for induction of labor
▶methylergonovine (Methergine) (X)	Oxytocic ergot alkaloid	IM/IV: 0.2 mg after delivery of placenta, repeatable at 2-4 hr intervals	Postpartum uterine atony and hemorrhage
		PO: 0.2 mg tid-qid for up to 7 days postpartum	
▶oxytocin (Pitocin, Syntocinon) (X)	Oxytocic hypothalamic hormone	IV infusion: 1-20 milliunits/min, titrated to effect	Labor induction
		IV infusion: 10-40 units in 1 L of D₅LR titrated to effect	Postpartum uterine atony and hemorrhage
		IM: 10 units in a single dose after delivery of placenta	
mifepristone (RU-486, Mifeprex) (X)	Progesterone antagonist abortifacient	PO: 600 mg in a single dose on day 1, followed by 400 mcg of the prostaglandin drug misoprostol on day 3 (see misoprostol)	Termination of pregnancy
misoprostol (Cytotec) (X)	Prostaglandin	PO: 400 mcg in a single dose on day 3 following administration of mifepristone on day 1 (see mifepristone)	Termination of pregnancy

D₅LR, Dextrose 5% in lactated Ringer's solution; *IM*, intramuscular; *IV*, intravenous; *PO*, oral.
*Use of these medications is contraindicated in pregnancy (pregnancy category X) unless needed for the indications listed.

Pharmacokinetics

Half-Life	Onset	Peak	Duration
IV: 3-5 min	IV: Immediate	IV: Immediate	IV: 1 hr
IM: 3-5 min	IM: Less than 5 min	IM: Immediate	IM: 2-3 hr

Uterine Relaxants

When contractions of the uterus begin before term, it may be desirable to stop labor, because premature birth increases the risk of neonatal death. Postponing delivery by relaxing the uterine smooth muscles and helping prevent contractions and the induction of labor increases the likelihood of the infant's survival. However, this measure is generally employed only after the twentieth week of gestation, because spontaneous labor occurring before the twentieth week is commonly associated with a nonviable fetus and thus is usually not interrupted. Only uterine contractions occurring between about 20 and 37 weeks of gestation are considered premature labor.

The nonpharmacologic treatment of premature labor includes bed rest, sedation, and hydration. Drugs given to inhibit labor and maintain the pregnancy are called *tocolytics*. Two commonly used tocolytic drugs are ritodrine and terbutaline. Terbutaline and ritodrine are both classified as β-adrenergic drugs (see Chapter 17) and work by directly relaxing uterine smooth muscle. However, it should be noted that this use of terbutaline is "off-label," meaning that the drug is not officially approved by the FDA for this purpose. Concentrated solutions of the electrolyte magnesium sulfate are also used intravenously for this purpose. This section focuses on terbutaline and ritodrine.

Mechanism of Action and Drug Effects

One common characteristic of tocolytics is that they relax uterine smooth muscle and stop the uterus from contracting. As previously mentioned, terbutaline and ritodrine work by directly relaxing uterine smooth muscle. They do so by stimulating β-adrenergic receptors located on the bronchial tree, peripheral vasculature, and uterine smooth muscles. These are believed to be primarily β₂-adrenergic receptors. The β₁-adrenergic receptors are located in the heart and are not stimulated by terbutaline or ritodrine except at high dosages.

The drug effects of terbutaline and ritodrine are related to their β-adrenergic effects. When the bronchial β-adrenergic receptors are stimulated by these β-agonists, the bronchi dilate and airway resistance decreases. When the β-adrenergic receptors of the peripheral vasculature are stimulated by these β-agonists, the blood vessels dilate and blood pressure decreases. Finally, when the β-adrenergic receptors located on the uterine smooth muscle are stimulated by the β-agonists terbutaline and ritodrine, the uterine smooth muscle relaxes and premature contractions are thus halted.

Indications

Both terbutaline and ritodrine are used to inhibit uterine contractions in preterm labor. As noted earlier, both drugs are adrenergic agonists. Terbutaline was originally used as a bronchodilator in the symptomatic treatment of bronchial asthma and reversible bronchospasm (Chapter 36).

Contraindications

Contraindications to the use of ritodrine and terbutaline include known drug allergy, cardiac dysrhythmia, pheochromocytoma (an adrenal tumor), pregnancy before the twentieth week of gestation, eclampsia, hypertension, thyrotoxicosis, antepartum hemorrhage, intrauterine fetal death, maternal cardiac disease, pulmonary hypertension, and uncontrolled diabetes.

Adverse Effects

The most common adverse effects of terbutaline and ritodrine are listed in Table 33-7.

Toxicity and Management of Overdose

The toxicity stemming from an overdose of tocolytics and its management are similar to those for the other adrenergic drugs and are discussed in Chapter 17. For example, β-blockers may be used for terbutaline overdose.

Interactions

Few drugs interact with uterine relaxants. The most notable are sympathomimetic drugs and β-blockers. Sympathomimetic drugs may have additive cardiovascular effects when given with uterine relaxants, and β-blockers may have antagonistic effects when combined with uterine relaxants.

Dosages

For the recommended dosages of ritodrine and terbutaline, see the Dosages table on this page.

Drug Profiles

ritodrine

Ritodrine (Yutopar) is indicated for the prevention of preterm labor. It is available only in injectable form.

Pharmacokinetics

Half-Life	Onset	Peak	Duration
IM/IV: 2-3 hr	IM/IV: Less than 15 min	IM/IV: 20-40 min	IM/IV: Unknown
PO: 2 hr	PO: Less than 1 hr	PO: 30-60 min	PO: Unknown

terbutaline

Terbutaline (Brethine) is indicated for the prevention of preterm labor; it may also be used as a bronchodilator in the symptomatic treatment of asthma. It should be noted that the preterm labor indication is actually "unlabeled," meaning that it is not actually FDA-approved for this use; the original indication for terbutaline was for respiratory problems. However, clinical obstetrical practice has demonstrated the utility of this drug for preterm labor. Terbutaline is available in both oral and injectable forms. The injectable form is most commonly used for obstetrical purposes.

Pharmacokinetics

Half-Life	Onset	Peak	Duration
PO: 20 hr	PO: 30-45 min	PO: 1-2 hr	PO: 6-8 hr
IV: 20 hr	IV: 5 min	IV: 30-60 min	IV: 1.5-4 hr

◆ NURSING PROCESS

✦ ASSESSMENT

In this section, estrogen and progesterone drugs are discussed first, and then medroxyprogesterone, megestrol, menotropins, the gonadotropins, and clomiphene are covered. Next information on uterine motility–altering drugs is provided, followed by a discussion of dinoprostone and, finally, consideration of the bisphosphonates and calcitonin. Before initiating therapy with any of the hormonal drugs (e.g., estrogens, progestins) or other women's health-related drugs, the patient's blood pressure, weight, blood

Table 33-7	Tocolytic Drugs: Most Common Adverse Effects
Body System	**Adverse Effects**
Cardiovascular	Palpitations, tachycardia, hypertension, dysrhythmias, altered maternal and fetal heart rate and blood pressure, chest pain
Central nervous	Tremors, anxiety, insomnia, headache, dizziness, nervousness
Gastrointestinal	Nausea, vomiting, anorexia, bloating, constipation, diarrhea
Metabolic	Hyperglycemia, hypokalemia
Other	Rash, dyspnea, hyperventilation, glycosuria, lactic acidosis

DOSAGES

Selected Uterine Relaxants

Drug (Pregnancy Category)	Pharmacologic Class	Usual Dosage Range	Indications
ritodrine (Yutopar) (B)	β₂-selective adrenergic agonist	IV infusion: 50-100 mcg/min titrated dose	Preterm labor
terbutaline (Brethine) (B)	β₂-selective adrenergic agonist	IV infusion: 2.5-30 mcg/min, titrated to effect PO: 2.5-10 mg q4-6h as long as needed and tolerated by patient	Preterm labor (unlabeled, non–FDA approved use)

FDA, Food and Drug Administration; *IV,* intravenous; *PO,* oral.

glucose levels, and results of liver and renal function tests should be documented. Drug allergies, contraindications, cautions, and drug interactions should also be assessed and documented. Patient assessment should also include a thorough medication history, medical history, and menstrual history as well as documentation of vital signs, weight, any underlying cardiac and malignant diseases, and hormonal levels—if appropriate. Assessment of emotional stability is also important because of therapy-related depression. Results of the patient's last physical exam, clinician performed breast exam and a gynecological exam should be noted, as well.

Estrogen-only hormones should be given only after the following disorders and conditions have been ruled out: abnormal uterine bleeding, thromboembolic disorders, pregnancy, incomplete long-bone growth, photosensitivity (a more common adverse effect with conjugated estrogens), estrogen receptor–positive breast cancer, personal history or family history of breast cancer, early menstruation, pregnancies late in life, endocrine disorders, renal and/or liver dysfunction, fluid retention disorders, and seizure activity. Assessment should also include questions about breast examination and breast self-examination practices and dates of when they had their last complete physical examination and Papanicolaou (Pap) smear. The nurse must also assess patients' baseline levels of knowledge about estrogens and use of hormones, whether for contraception or replacement therapy. The patient's readiness to learn, educational level, and degree of compliance with other medication regimens must also be assessed. The success of treatment with oral contraceptives, hormonal replacement medication and other therapies depends heavily on understanding instructions.

With oral contraceptive drugs (e.g., combination estrogen-progestin drugs), the patient should be assessed—in addition to the above—for cerebral and coronary vascular disease, jaundice, thromboembolic disorders and malignancies of the reproductive tract or abnormal vaginal bleeding. There should also be close monitoring of patients with the following: uncontrolled hypertension, migraine headaches, visual disturbances, hyperlipidemia, asthma, blood dyscrasias, diabetes mellitus, congestive heart failure, depression and seizures. The concern is for exacerbation of any of these problems/disorders and subsequent complications. Patients who smoke should also be closely monitored because of the increased risk of complications in smokers, especially those older than age 35 years. A smoking history should include documentation of number of packs per day and number of years the patient has smoked. When combination oral contraceptives are used in emergency situations for postcoital conception, the same contraindications, cautions, and drug interactions apply even if for one-time use.

With hormones that are progestin/progesterone only, much of the aforementioned information is applicable and although medroxyprogesterone and megestrol have similar actions, their indications are varied, e.g., amenorrhea and abnormal uterine bleeding for medroxyprogesterone, and palliative treatment of breast and endometrial cancers and promotion of increased appetite in patients with AIDS for megestrol. Assessment of the appropriate parameters related to these drugs and their actions should be noted, as well.

An understanding of menotropins is critical to patient safety and assessment of the patient's knowledge about the drug and its use is important. Human chorionic gonadotropin is usually administered only after laboratory tests have determined the sufficiency of follicular development. A complete physical assessment is needed with attention to the menstrual-reproductive history and cardiac, renal, and liver functioning. Abdominal assessment is important, and preexisting diseases and abdominal pain should be noted. This is needed because if the ovary is overstimulated, moderate ovarian enlargement with or without abdominal pain and/or distention may occur. If over-stimulation is severe, the patient may experience nausea, vomiting, diarrhea, oliguria, ascites, electrolyte disturbances, and thromboembolic events.

Use of clomiphene requires assessment of the patient's medical and medication history as well as a thorough review of the menstrual history. Medical history is critical, especially reproductive and uterine status, because use of the drug may result in multiple births. Family stability and economic status must be assessed because of the risk of multiple births to make sure that as healthy a home as possible exists for everyone concerned. Cardiac, liver, and renal status must also be assessed, as ordered.

Terbutaline has an unlabeled use of inhibiting premature labor and should be used only in women in premature labor who are in their twentieth to thirty-seventh week of gestation. Women with other complications of pregnancy or with seizures, hypertension, diabetes, asthma, diabetes, cardiac dysrhythmias, angina, or hypokalemia may receive this drug but only if they are monitored very closely and if the benefits outweigh the risks. Terbutaline's contraindications, cautions and drug interactions have been previously discussed, however, vital signs, with emphasis on maternal pulse rate and blood pressure and fetal heart rate and a baseline electrocardiogram should be assessed and results available prior to use of the drug. Remember that β-agonists or β-stimulants will decrease therapeutic effects of terbutaline. The environment should be assessed as well. The setting should be a quiet one but should provide for constant maternal and fetal monitoring and the safe administration of the drug. Ritodrine was the drug of choice in previous years but has been replaced with terbutaline. If ritodrine is ordered, it is important to assess the same parameters as listed above with terbutaline and it should not be given in women prior to the twentieth week of gestation.

Before administering uterine stimulants (e.g., oxytocin or prostaglandins), the nurse should measure and document the patient's blood pressure, pulse, and respiration. Fetal heart rate and contraction-related fetal heart rates should also be determined and recorded. Because oxytocin therapy is associated with vasopressive and antidiuretic effects, it is even more important than normally to know fluid volume status. The nurse should know that when these drugs are administered, maternal blood pressure will decrease initially but will then rise (sometimes by up to 30%), and cardiac output and stroke volume will subsequently increase. Assessment for complications associated with the use of these drugs should include measurement of all vital signs, monitoring of intake and output, and observation for signs and symptoms of water intoxication (e.g., headache, fatigue, nausea, anorexia, lethargy, disorientation, seizures or coma, tachycardia, hypotension, and muscular cramps and weakness), which may even be fatal if not appropriately identified. Fetal distress and uterine contractions for either hypertonic or hypotonic patterns should be assessed frequently and documented. For labor and delivery, the patient's cervix should be ready for induction or be rated at a Bishop score of 5 or higher. Constant monitoring of maternal blood pressure, pulse, contractions, and fluid status, as well as fetal heart rate, monitoring is needed. Oxytocin is *not* used during the first trimester except in some cases of spontaneous or induced abortion. The same considerations apply to the ergot alkaloids (e.g., methylergonovine), and the patient's vital signs and fetal heart rate should be assessed. A baseline neurologic assessment is important with attention to seizures. The nurse should continually assess for the signs of acute overdose, including nausea, vomiting, abdominal pain, numbness and tingling of the extremities, and hypertension. Contraindications, cautions, and drug interactions have been previously discussed as well as with the remaining women's health drugs.

The use of dinoprostone or other prostaglandin E_2 drugs is indicated in specific situations requiring termination of pregnancy. Questioning about the presence of fibroids, pelvic inflammatory disease, pelvic stenosis, respiratory disease, and recent or past pelvic surgery should be posed and documented. For bisphosphonates, such as alendronate, there are many contraindications, cautions, and drug interactions; however, assessment of the following is important to patient safety: occurrence of thromboembolisms, premenopausal state, deep-vein thrombosis, pulmonary embolism, concurrent estrogen therapy, anticipated immobility or bed rest (the drug should be discontinued 72 hours before the patient becomes immobile), aspiration risk, renal or liver dysfunction, high levels of calcium, the use of other drugs that are considered to be GI irritants, the presence of esophageal abnormalities, delayed esophageal emptying, and the inability to remain upright in either a sitting or standing position (remaining upright helps to prevent esophageal erosion and ulcers from reflux of the drug back into the esophagus). Drug interactions have been discussed earlier in the chapter, but the nurse should note that any drugs that are associated with GI distress or ulcers (e.g., aspirin, nonsteroidal antiinflammatory drugs) should be avoided. Other drugs in this category require similar assessment. Concerns about prolonged immobility should be addressed as well.

◆ NURSING DIAGNOSES

- Risk for infection related to possible drop in white blood cell count due to the effects of SERMs
- Disturbed body image related to the effects of abnormal hormonal levels, osteoporosis, or other female-related diseases or disorders
- Deficient knowledge related to lack of information on first-time drug therapy
- Acute pain related to a disorder of the female reproductive tract and related drug therapy
- Disturbed body image related to abnormal estrogen and/or progestin levels, problems with pregnancy, and/or bone loss disorders
- Anxiety related to various female disorders and possible complications of the associated therapy
- Ineffective sexuality patterns related to abnormal levels of estrogen
- Decisional conflict related to the risks versus benefits of postmenopausal estrogen replacement therapy

- Risk for injury to the mother related to the adverse effects of uterine mobility–altering drugs
- Risk for injury to the infant related to premature labor and/or the adverse effects of tocolytics.
- Excess fluid volume related to the adverse effect of retention associated with hormonal drugs and tocolytics

◆ PLANNING
Goals

- Patient is free of body image disturbances.
- Patient states the rationale for hormonal replacement, combination oral contraceptives, osteoporosis drugs, uterine relaxants, or fertility drugs.
- Patient states the adverse effects of specific medications.
- Patient states the importance of compliance with hormonal therapy and other recommended pharmacologic and nonpharmacologic measures for the treatment of premature labor, preeclampsia and/or fertility disorders.
- Patient openly states the need for improved sexual functioning and image before and during treatment.
- Patient verbalizes fears and concerns about the use of hormonal therapy.
- Patient verbalizes fears and concerns about pregnancy and its outcome.

Outcome Criteria

- Patient openly verbalizes concerns, fears, and anxieties about body image changes and the need for medication.
- Patient is compliant with the pharmacologic and nonpharmacologic therapy regimen and achieves successful management of osteoporosis, breast cancer, infertility, preeclampsia, or premature labor, or experiences effective birth control.
- Patient is free of complications and disturbing adverse effects associated with each group of drugs, such as chest pain, leg pain, blurred vision, thrombophlebitis, and leukopenia.
- Patient returns for regular follow-up visits with the physician to monitor the therapeutic and adverse effects of treatment.
- Patient engages in positive sexual patterns and habits while receiving hormonal therapy.
- Patient is free of complications associated with uterine mobility–altering drugs.

◆ IMPLEMENTATION

Both estrogens and progestins should be administered in the lowest dosages possible and the dosages titrated as needed, but only as ordered. Intramuscular doses should be given deep in large muscle masses and the injection sites rotated. Oral forms should be taken with food or milk to minimize GI upset. Progestin-only oral contraceptive pills are taken daily. It is important for the patient to take this oral contraceptive at the same time every day so that effective hormonal serum levels are maintained. Because use of the progestin-only pill leads to a higher incidence of ovulatory cycles, there is an associated increased rate of contraceptive failure. The nurse should remember that this type of pill is usually prescribed for those women who cannot tolerate estrogens or those for whom estrogens are contraindicated. Often it is more effective in women who are older than 35 years of age. Combination estrogen-progestin pills contain low doses of drug. The low-dose monophasic and multiphasic types are provided as 21 days of pills followed by 7 days of placebo treatment, and the patient needs to understand how this treatment regimen works. The nurse should emphasize to the patient that the reduction in the level of estrogen has been associated with a decrease in adverse effects and a decrease in the risk for liver tumors, hypertension, and cardiovascular changes; however, more breakthrough bleeding will occur.

Medroxyprogesterone should be given as ordered. Megestrol is given orally and the patient should know whether the drug is being given to improve appetite so that appropriate dietary measures can be implemented. Menotropins should be given as ordered and requires frequent monitoring for the duration of therapy. Nausea, vomiting, dizziness, shortness of breath, severe headache, blurred vision, or swelling of the feet should be reported. Gonadotropin hormones are usually given intramuscularly, and if they are given in conjunction with menotropins, the dose is usually ordered to be given 1 day after the last menotropin dose. Fertility drugs such as clomiphene are often self-administered. The provision of specific instructions regarding how to administer the drug at home and how to monitor drug effectiveness is very important to improve the success of treatment. Journal tracking of the medication regimen is helpful to those involved in the care of the infertile patient or couple. See Patient Teaching Tips for more information.

Terbutaline use requires close and frequent monitoring of maternal blood pressure, pulse, temperature, and respirations. Terbutaline is usually given by intravenous pump with titration upward to the prescribed dose. Lactated Ringer's solution, dextrose 5% in water, or 0.9% normal saline should be used as ordered to help prevent fluid overload. Oral dosage forms are used for maintenance and can be administered at home, generally for long-term therapy. The patient should be positioned in the left lateral recumbent position to minimize hypotension, increase renal blood flow, and increase blood flow to the fetus.

Frequent measurement of intake and output as well as maternal vital signs and fetal heart rate is critical to preventing complications of therapy. Breath sounds should be auscultated for crackles or rhonchi as needed to help monitor fluid status. The nurse should check for pedal edema and notify the physician immediately of any signs and symptoms of pulmonary edema or other signs of fluid overload. The rate of infusion or the dosage should be decreased, as ordered, if adverse effects such as tachycardia, hypotension, or nervousness develop. An antidote that may be prescribed for adverse reactions to terbutaline is the β-blocker propranolol. The nurse must also be aware that these preterm labor patients should be monitored frequently for any increase in the intensity, duration, or frequency of their contractions, as well as any palpitations, anxiety, shortness of breath, vomiting, dizziness, or tachycardia. In addition, any loss of fetal movement should be immediately reported to the physician. If the patient is also diabetic and/or is receiving potassium-sparing diuretics (e.g., spironolactone), the physician will most likely order frequent measurement of serum glucose and/or potassium levels. Oral forms of terbutaline (or ritodrine, if ordered) may be prescribed for home use while the patient is on bed rest to try to suppress premature onset of labor. The patient must be sure to keep all follow-up appointments.

Oxytocin should be administered only as ordered, and any instructions or protocols should be strictly followed. The cervix must be ripe (see earlier). Prostaglandin E₂ may be instilled vaginally to help accomplish this if the mother's cervix is not ripe or at a Bishop score of 5 or higher. Because oxytocin has vasopres-

sive and antidiuretic properties, the patient is at risk for hypertensive episodes as well as fluid retention, and constant monitoring of maternal blood pressure and pulse rate as well as fetal monitoring is required. Patients should report any of the following: strong contractions, edema, symptoms of water intoxication, palpitations, chest pain, and any changes in fetal movement. IV infusions (use of infusion pumps) of oxytocin should be with the proper dilutional fluid and rate. To minimize the adverse effects of the drug, intravenous piggyback dosing is often ordered so that the diluted oxytocin solution can be discontinued immediately if maternal and/or fetal decline occurs while an intravenous line with hydration is maintained. Doses are generally titrated as ordered and are based on the progress of labor and degree of fetal tolerance to the drug. Should the labor progress at 1 cm/hr, oxytocin may no longer be needed. The decision is made by the physician and on an individual basis. Generally speaking, with oxytocin therapy, if there are hypertensive responses or major changes in the maternal vital signs *or* if the fetal heart rate decreases *or* if fetal movement stops, the physician should be contacted immediately. Hyperstimulation may also occur. If contractions are more frequent than every 2 minutes and last longer than 1 minute later (and are accompanied by changes in other parameters), the infusion should be stopped and the physician contacted immediately. If this does occur, it is critical also to place the patient on the left side, maintain administration of intravenous fluids, and give oxygen as ordered, (generally via tight face mask at 10 to 12 L/min). If there is concern about overstimulation, discuss concerns with the physician and document actions thoroughly.

Dinoprostone is given by vaginal suppository to those who are 12 to 20 weeks pregnant and are seeking termination and/or to those patients in whom evacuation of the uterus is needed for the management of incomplete spontaneous abortion or intrauterine fetal death (up to 28 weeks). The drug should be given exactly as ordered, and the patient should be monitored closely.

The success of therapy with drugs such as alendronate depends on providing thorough patient teaching and ensuring that the patient understands all aspects of the drug regimen. With alendronate, the nurse must emphasize the need to take the medication upon rising in the morning with a full glass (6 to 8 oz) of water at least 30 minutes before the intake of any food, other fluids, or other medication. In addition, the nurse must emphasize that the patient should remain upright in either a standing or sitting position for approximately 30 minutes after taking the drug to help prevent esophageal erosion or irritation. The patient taking raloxifene should be informed that the drug needs to be discontinued 72 hours before and during prolonged immobility. Therapy may be resumed once the patient becomes fully ambulatory and as ordered. See the Patient Teaching Tips.

◆ EVALUATION

Therapeutic responses to the various drugs discussed in this chapter should be measured by evaluating whether goals and outcome criteria have been met. Many drugs have been discussed, often with several indications for use; thus, the therapeutic response would be the occurrence of the indicated therapeutic effect, and the nurse would then also monitor for the associated adverse effects and/or toxicity. Therapeutic effects of *estrogens* may range from prevention of pregnancy to a decrease in menopausal symptoms to reduction in the size of a tumor. Adverse effects of estrogens may include thromboembolism, edema, jaundice, abnormal vaginal bleeding, hyperglycemia, nausea, vomiting, increased appetite, and weight gain. Therapeutic responses to *progestins* include a decrease in abnormal uterine bleeding and the disappearance of menstrual disorders (e.g., amenorrhea). The adverse effects of progestins include edema, hypertension, cardiac symptoms, changes in mood and affect, and jaundice.

Therapeutic effects of *oxytocin* and other uterine stimulants include stimulation of labor and control of postpartum bleeding, whereas adverse effects may include drop in pulse rate, dysrhythmias, severe abdominal pain, and shock-like symptoms (e.g., decrease in BP, increase in pulse rate). These adverse effects may indicate a dangerous complication and medical emergency. The primary therapeutic effect of *terbutaline* is the absence of preterm labor with adverse maternal effects such as palpitations,

nausea, vomiting, headache, jitteriness, tremors, chest pain, and anxiety. Adverse neonatal effects include hypoglycemia, ileus, hypotension, and hypocalcemia.

The therapeutic effects of *fertility drugs* include successful fertilization with adverse reactions of hot flashes, abdominal discomfort, blurred vision, GI upset, nervousness, depression, weight gain, and hair loss. Multiple births and birth defects are other possible consequences of therapy. The therapeutic effects of *dinoprostone* include therapeutic termination of pregnancy with adverse effects of severe cramping and bleeding. Therapeutic effects of *alendronate* and related drugs include increased bone density and prevention or management of osteoporosis with adverse effects of leukopenia, decreased platelet levels, thrombophlebitis, hot flashes, and leg cramps.

Patient Teaching Tips

- Hormonal drugs are usually tolerated better if taken with food or milk to minimize GI upset.
- With use of oral contraceptives and any form of HRT with estrogens and/or progestins, encourage the patient to openly discuss concerns about the medications. The patient should be assured that although risks may be associated with HRT, the physician will weigh each case individually and make the decision in each situation based on the benefits versus risks, but with the ultimate decision from the patient.
- With estrogens and progestins, encourage the patient to report the following to the health care provider immediately: chest pain, leg pain, blurred vision, headache, neck stiffness, neck pain, loss of vision, numbness of extremities, severe headache, edema, yellow discoloration of the skin or sclera, clay-colored stools, and abnormal vaginal bleeding.
- Patients should be advised to report any weight gain of more than 5 lb in 1 week or 2 lb or more in a 24-hour period to the health care provider. The patient should also report any breakthrough bleeding, change in menstrual flow, and breast tenderness.
- Instruct the patient to take oral contraceptives exactly as ordered and to be compliant with follow-up annual examinations, including a pelvic examination, Pap smear, and practitioner-performed breast examination. The patient should be instructed on monthly breast self-examinations, with return demonstrations with emphasis on the ideal time to perform a breast self-examination (e.g., 7 to 10 days after the menses). Follow-up appointments and annual examinations by a health care provider must be emphasized!
- Patients should be instructed to avoid sunlight or be sure to apply sunscreen because of increased sensitivity to sunlight and tanning beds.
- If the patient is using progesterone-only intravaginal gel with other gels, the patient should be sure to insert the other gels at least 6 hours before or after the progesterone-based product.
- Progesterone-filled intrauterine inserts are placed in the uterine cavity by a physician, and their use should be accompanied with thorough education regarding their use for 1 year after insertion and then the need to have them replaced. Patients should report abnormal uterine bleeding, cramping, abdominal pain, and amenorrhea to the physician.
- The patient using an estrogen/progestin vaginal ring for contraception should be instructed on what to expect with its insertion, and that it is to be removed in 3 weeks and a new ring inserted after another 1 week. This contraceptive device requires thorough teaching and follow-up, including insertion and removal techniques and a return demonstration prior to the patient leaving

the physician's office. Inform patients that menstruation will follow in about 2 to 3 days after the ring is removed and to be sure to replace the used ring in its foil pouch, discard it in the trash, and not flush it down the commode.
- With emergency oral contraception, the patient should take the first dose of this drug as soon as possible after intercourse, because it is more effective when taken early, but it may be used up to 72 hours after the event. A second dose is taken 12 hours later. One product contains only progestin, and one is a combination of progestin and estrogen; the two are equally effective when prescribed appropriately.
- The patient should take the dose of oral contraceptives at the same time every day. If one dose is missed, the patient should take the dose as soon as it is remembered and use a backup form of contraception. More specific instructions should be provided in regard to the omission of more than one pill and/or 1 day and should be specific to the prescribed oral contraceptive drug. It is important for patient safety and compliance to provide patients with a phone number for answering questions about dosing, omissions, etc.
- Instruct the patient about the fact that oral contraceptives may prevent pregnancy, but sexual intercourse is only considered safe if combined with use of condoms to prevent sexually transmitted diseases.
- Inform the patient about the significant interactions between oral contraceptives and certain antibiotics (Chapters 37 and 38) and the need for backup contraception.
- Encourage patients to *always* inquire about this interaction when taking antibiotics and to use a backup form of contraception. St. John's wort may also diminish the effectiveness of the oral contraceptive, so provide additional information about drug interactions.
- Instruct patients taking bisphosphonates (e.g., alendronate) to take the drug exactly as prescribed and to take it at least 30 minutes before the first morning beverage, food, or other medication. It must be taken with at least 6 to 8 oz of water. Patients must understand the importance of remaining upright for at least 30 minutes after taking the medication to prevent esophageal and GI adverse effects. Esophageal irritation, dysphagia, severe heartburn, and retrosternal pain must be reported to the physician immediately to prevent severe reactions.
- Encourage patients to inquire about taking supplemental calcium and vitamin D if taking bisphosphonates and to inquire about the best timing of their dosing.
- Educate the patient about making lifestyle changes as recommended, such as engaging in weight-bearing exercise (e.g., walking), stopping smoking, and limiting or eliminating alcohol intake.

Points to Remember

- Three major estrogens are synthesized in the ovaries: estradiol (the principal estrogen), progestrone, and estradiol. Exogenous estrogens can be classified into two main groups: steroidal estrogens (e.g., conjugated estrogens, esterified estrogens, estradiol) and non- nonsteroidal estrogens (e.g., chlorotrianisene, dienestrol, diethylstilbestrol).
- Progestins have a variety of uses, including treatment of uterine bleeding and amenorrhea and adjunctive and palliative treatment of some cancers.
- Oral contraceptives containing a combination of estrogens and progestins are the most effective form of birth control currently available.
- Uterine stimulants (sometimes called *oxytocic drugs*) include ergot derivatives, prostaglandins, and oxytocin.
- Uterine relaxants (often called *tocolytic drugs*) are used to stop preterm labor and maintain pregnancy by halting uterine contractions. The most commonly used drug is terbutaline.

- A thorough nursing assessment is necessary to ensure the safe and effective use of female reproductive drugs. Information should be obtained on the patient's past medical problems, history of menses and problems with the menstrual cycle, medications taken (prescribed and OTC), number of pregnancies and miscarriages, last menstrual period, and any related surgical or medical treatments.
- The nurse is responsible for determining the response of the mother and fetus to drugs such as oxytocin through monitoring of the frequency of contractions, the progress of labor, and fetal tolerance. The dose should be titrated per the physician's order.
- Drugs that alter uterine motility are potentially very dangerous to the mother and the fetus. The nurse should watch the infusion carefully while closely monitoring the patients (mother and fetus). Intravenous infusions should be given only with intravenous pumps.

NCLEX Examination Review Questions

1. The nurse is assessing a patient who is to receive dinoprostone. Which of the following would be a contraindication to the use of this drug?
   a. Pregnancy at 15 weeks' gestation.
   b. Gastrointestinal upset or ulcer disease
   c. Ectopic pregnancy
   d. Incomplete abortion
2. When teaching a patient who is taking oral contraceptive therapy for the first time, the nurse relates that adverse effects may include which of the following?
   a. Dizziness
   b. Nausea and vomiting
   c. Tingling in the extremities
   d. Polyuria
3. Which of the following situations is an indication for an oxytocin (Pitocin) infusion?
   a. Termination of a pregnancy at 12 weeks
   b. Hypertonic uterus
   c. Cervical stenosis in a patient who is in labor
   d. Induction of labor at full term

4. After a patient has been taught about drug therapy with the SERM raloxifene, which statement from the patient reflects a good understanding of the instruction?
   a. "When I fly to Europe I will need to stop taking this drug at least 3 days before I travel."
   b. "I can continue this drug even when traveling as long as I take it with 8 oz of water each time."
   c. "After I take this drug I must sit upright for at least 30 minutes."
   d. "One advantage of this drug is that it will reduce my hot flashes."
5. A patient calls the clinic because she realized she missed one dose of an oral contraceptive. Which statement from the nurse is appropriate? *Select all that apply.*
   a. "Go ahead and take the missed dose now, along with today's dose."
   b. "Don't worry, you are still protected from pregnancy."
   c. "Please come in to the clinic for a reevaluation of your therapy."
   d. "Wait 7 days, then start a new pack of pills."
   e. "You will need to use a backup form of contraception until next cycle."

1. c, 2. b, 3. d, 4. a, 5. a, e.

Critical Thinking Activities

1. K.T. has spent 14 hours in labor with her first pregnancy and has made little progress. She is becoming exhausted, and the uterine contractions have decreased in strength. She is now receiving an oxytocin infusion. What will you monitor while she is receiving this drug?

2. Why are oxytocics such as oxytocin (Pitocin) and Ergotrate used to treat postpartum and postabortion bleeding caused by uterine relaxation and enlargement?
3. What is the primary mechanism by which oral contraceptives prevent pregnancy?

For answers, see http://evolve.elsevier.com/Lilley.

Men's Health Drugs

Objectives

When you reach the end of this chapter, you should be able to do the following:

1. Discuss the normal anatomy, physiology, and functions of the male reproductive system.
2. Compare the various men's health drugs, with discussion of their rationale for use, dosages, and dosage forms.
3. Describe the mechanisms of action, dosages, adverse effects, cautions, contraindications, drug interactions, and routes of administration for the various men's health drugs.
4. Develop a nursing care plan that includes all phases of the nursing process for patients receiving any of the men's health drugs for treatment of benign prostatic hypertrophy, sexual dysfunction, hormone deficiency, or prostate cancer.

e-Learning Activities

Companion CD

- NCLEX Review Questions: see questions 300-304
- Animations
- Audio Glossary
- Category Catchers
- Medication Errors Checklists
- IV Therapy Checklists

evolve Website (http://evolve.elsevier.com/Lilley)

- Nursing Care Plans • Frequently Asked Questions • Content Updates • WebLinks • Supplemental Resources • Elsevier ePharmacology Update • Medication Administration Animations

Drug Profiles

finasteride, p. 528
▶ sildenafil, p. 529
▶ testosterone, p. 530

▶ Key drug.

Glossary

Anabolic activity Any metabolic activity that promotes the building up of body tissues, such as the activity produced by testosterone that causes the development of bone and muscle tissue; also called *anabolism*. (p. 526)

Androgenic activity The activity produced by testosterone that causes the development and maintenance of the male reproductive system and male secondary sex characteristics. (p. 525)

Androgens Male sex hormones responsible for mediating the development and maintenance of male sex characteristics. Chief among these are testosterone and its various biochemical precursors. (p. 525)

Benign prostatic hypertrophy (BPH) Nonmalignant (noncancerous) enlargement of the prostate gland. (p. 526)

Catabolism The opposite of anabolic activity; any metabolic activity that results in the breakdown of body tissues; also called *catabolism*. Examples of conditions in which catabolism occurs are debilitating illnesses such as end-stage cancer and starvation. (p. 526)

Erythropoietic effect The effect of stimulating the production of red blood cells (erythropoiesis). (p. 526)

Prostate cancer A malignant tumor within the prostate gland. (p. 527)

Testosterone The main androgenic hormone. (p. 525)

MALE REPRODUCTIVE SYSTEM

The male reproductive system consists of several structures, of which the testes and seminiferous tubules are the most important to the discussion in this chapter because they produce the primary male hormones. The testes, a pair of oval glands located in the scrotal sac, are the male gonads. The testes produce male sex hormones. The seminiferous tubules, which are channels in the testes, are the site of spermatogenesis, which is the process by which mature sperm cells are produced.

Androgens are the group of male sex hormones (primarily testosterone) that mediate the normal development and maintenance of the primary male sex characteristics (normal male genital anatomy) as well as the secondary sex characteristics. Secondary male sex characteristics include advanced development of the prostate, seminal vesicles (two glands adjacent to the prostate), penis, and scrotum, as well as male hair distribution, laryngeal enlargement and thickening of the vocal cords; and male body musculature and fat distribution. Androgens must be secreted in adequate amounts for these characteristics to appear. Probably the most important androgen is **testosterone,** which is produced from clusters of interstitial cells located between the seminiferous tubules. Besides having **androgenic activity,** testosterone is also involved in the development of bone and muscle tissue; inhibition of protein **catabolism** (metabolic breakdown); and retention of nitrogen, phosphorus, potassium, and sodium. These functions contribute to its **anabolic activity.** The hormone initiates the synthesis of specific proteins needed for androgenic and anabolic activity by binding to chromatin (strands of deoxyribonucleic acid [DNA]) in the nuclei of interstitial cells. In addition, testosterone appears to have an **erythropoietic effect** in that it stimulates the production of red blood cells (Chapter 56).

ANDROGENS AND OTHER DRUGS PERTAINING TO MEN'S HEALTH

There are several synthetic derivatives of testosterone, and these were developed with the intention of improving the pharmacokinetic and pharmacodynamic characteristics of the naturally occurring hormone. One way that this was accomplished was by combining various esters with testosterone, which prolonged the duration of action of the hormone. For example, testosterone propionate is formulated as an oily solution and its hormonal effects last for 2 to 3 days; the effects of testosterone cypionate and testosterone enanthate in oil last even longer. The effects of testosterone cypionate and testosterone enanthate in oil last even longer; these drugs can be administered once every 2 to 4 weeks. Orally administered testosterone has very poor pharmacokinetic and pharmacodynamic characteristics because most of the dose is metabolized and destroyed by the liver before it can reach the circulation (first-pass effect). To circumvent this problem, researchers developed methyltestosterone and fluoxymesterone. Both are synthetic dosage forms (tablets or capsules) designed to be effective following oral administration. Methyltestosterone is also available in a buccal tablet, which is dissolved in the buccal cavity, the space in the mouth between the cheek and teeth, and in an injectable form. Newer transdermal dosage forms for testosterone, including skin patches and a gel, have provided another way to circumvent the first-pass effect that occurs with oral administration of this hormone.

There are other chemical derivatives of naturally occurring testosterone known as *anabolic steroids.* These are synthetic drugs that closely resemble the natural hormone but possess high anabolic activity. Currently four anabolic steroid drug products are commercially available. These include oxymetholone (Anadrol-50), stanozolol (Winstrol), oxandrolone (Oxandrin), and nandrolone (Deca-Durabolin). These drugs are not commonly used, but Food and Drug Administration (FDA)–approved indications include anemia, hereditary angioedema, and metastatic breast cancer. Unlabeled (non–FDA-approved) uses for oxandrolone include treatment of human immunodeficiency virus wasting syndrome (debilitation related to disease-induced nutritional malabsorption) and alcoholic hepatitis. Anabolic steroids have a great potential for misuse by athletes, especially body builders and weight lifters, because of their muscle-building properties. Improper use of these substances can have many serious consequences, such as sterility, cardiovascular diseases, and even liver cancer. For this reason anabolic steroids are currently classified as Schedule III controlled substances by the U.S. Drug Enforcement Administration. This classification implies that misuse of these drugs can lead to psychologic or physical dependence or both. Another synthetic androgen is danazol. Its labeled uses include treatment of endometriosis, hereditary angioedema, and fibrocystic breast disease in women.

Mechanism of Action and Drug Effects

The drug forms of the natural and synthetic androgens and the synthetic anabolic steroids have effects similar to those of the endogenous androgens. These include stimulation of the normal growth and development of the male sex organs (primary sex characteristics) and development and maintenance of the secondary sex characteristics. One reason for the growth-promoting effects of androgens is that they stimulate the synthesis of ribonucleic acid (RNA) at the cellular level, thereby promoting cellular growth and reproduction. They also retard the breakdown of amino acids. These properties contribute to an increased synthesis of body proteins, which aids in the formation and maintenance of muscle tissue. Another potent anabolic effect of androgens is the retention of nitrogen, also essential for protein synthesis. Nitrogen also promotes the storage in the body of inorganic phosphorus, sulfate, sodium, and potassium, all of which have important metabolic roles, including protein synthesis, nerve impulse conduction, and muscular contractions. All of these effects result in weight gain and an increase in muscular strength. Finally, androgens also stimulate the production of erythropoietin by the kidney, which leads to enhanced erythropoiesis (red blood cell synthesis). However, the administration of exogenous androgens causes the release of endogenous testosterone to be inhibited as a result of the feedback inhibition of pituitary luteinizing hormone. Large doses of exogenous androgens may also suppress sperm production as a result of the feedback inhibition of pituitary follicle-stimulating hormone, leading to infertility.

Androgen inhibitors are drugs that block the effects of naturally occurring (endogenous) androgens in the body. This is accomplished via inhibition of a specific enzyme, 5α-reductase. For this reason these drugs are also called 5α-reductase inhibitors. As previously mentioned, androgens maintain secondary sex characteristics, one of which is the growth and maintenance of the prostate. For unknown reasons, normal male physiology results in a common enlargement of the prostate known as **benign prostatic hypertrophy (BPH).** This process begins as early as 30 years old and is present in at least 85% of men by the age of 80 years. The most troubling symptom is usually varying degrees of obstructed urinary outflow. Although surgical treatment by *transurethral resection of the prostate* (TURP) is a common strategy, BPH is also often amenable to treatment with a 5α-reductase ("five-alpha-reductase") inhibitor. There are currently two such drugs, finasteride and dutasteride. Finasteride, the prototype drug for this class, works by inhibiting this enzyme that normally converts testosterone to 5α-dihydrotestosterone (DHT). DHT is actually a somewhat more potent type of testosterone and is the principal androgen responsible for stimulating prostatic growth, as well as other male primary and secondary sex characteristics. Finasteride can dramatically lower the prostatic DHT concentrations, which helps to ease the passage of urine made difficult by the enlarged prostate. Fortunately, finasteride does not cause antiandrogen adverse effects that might be expected such as loss of muscle strength, and fertility.

The drug effects of finasteride are limited primarily to the prostate, but this drug may also affect 5α-reductase–dependent processes elsewhere in the body, such as in the hair follicles, skin, and liver. For example, it has been noted that men taking finasteride experience increased hair growth. Therefore, finasteride is also indicated for the treatment of male-pattern baldness. Research has demonstrated that the pharmacologic inhibition of

5α-reductase prevents the thinning of hair caused by increased levels of DHT. Finasteride is indicated for the treatment of baldness only in men, not in women. This is true even though testosterone and DHT serve ironically to promote normal male hair growth (e.g., facial hair), as well as hair loss (baldness or *alopecia*) in both sexes. Finasteride can be teratogenic in pregnant women, but its use in women of any age (pregnant or not) is still not recommended by its manufacturer. However, another medication, minoxidil, can be used topically to treat baldness in both men and women. It is discussed in more detail in Chapter 57.

Another class of drugs that may be used to help alleviate the symptoms of obstruction due to BPH are the α_1-adrenergic blockers. These drugs are discussed in greater detail in Chapter 17. The α_1-adrenergic blockers that are most commonly used for symptomatic relief of obstruction secondary to BPH are terazosin (Hytrin), doxazosin (Cardura), and tamsulosin (Flomax). Tamsulosin appears to have a greater specificity for the α_1-receptors in the prostate and thus may cause less hypotension.

There are also two other classes of androgen inhibitors. The first includes the androgen receptor blockers flutamide, nilutamide, and bicalutamide. These drugs work by blocking the activity of androgen hormones at the level of the receptors in target tissues (e.g., prostate). For this reason these drugs are used in the treatment of **prostate cancer.** The second class is the gonadotropin-releasing hormone (Gn-RH) analogues, including leuprolide, goserelin, and triptorelin. These drugs work by inhibiting the secretion of pituitary gonadotropin, which eventually leads to a decrease in testosterone production. Both androgen receptor blockers and Gn-RH analogues are used most commonly to treat prostate cancer and are discussed in further detail in Chapter 48.

CULTURAL IMPLICATIONS

Men's Health Concerns and Screening

Prostate cancer is the leading cancer diagnosed among men in the United States, and black men in America have the highest rate of prostate cancer in the world. In fact, between the years of 1996 and 2000, the age-adjusted death rate from prostate cancer among black men in the United States was more than double that of non-Hispanic white men. The causes of these higher rates of prostate cancer in black men are largely unknown; however, higher mortality rates are associated with late detection.

Researchers have studied the impact of culture on health-seeking behaviors among many of the racial/ethnic groups (e.g., Asians, Native Americans, Latinos) in an attempt to gain greater understanding about the role of culture in health-related behaviors. However, despite the research, there is little known about the impact of culture and health-seeking behaviors among black men. A goal of *Healthy People 2010* is to eliminate disparities among racial/ethnic groups, and black men suffer a higher burden of disease as compared to other groups and have been labeled as *endangered species* because of health, social, political, and psychological issues. Thus, more studies need to focus on their culture and communication with health care providers and the subsequent impact on the black male's knowledge, health belief systems, and health practices as related to prostate cancer screening.

From Braithwaite RL: The health status of black men. In Braithwaite RL, Taylor SE, eds: *Health issues in the black community*, ed 2, San Francisco, 2001, Jossey-Bass Publishers; Woods DV et al: Culture, black men, and prostate cancer: What is reality? *Cancer Control,* Lee Moffitt Cancer Center and Research Institute, Inc., 2004. Available at www.medscape.com/viewarticle/497924.

Sildenafil is the first oral drug approved for the treatment of erectile dysfunction. Sildenafil works by inhibiting the action of the enzyme phosphodiesterase. This in turn allows the buildup in the penis of the chemical cyclic guanosine monophosphate, which causes relaxation of the smooth muscle in the corpora cavernosa (erectile tubes) of the penis and permits the inflow of blood. Nitric oxide is also released inside the corpora cavernosa during sexual stimulation and contributes to the erectile effect. Two drugs that are similar but have a longer duration of action are vardenafil (Levitra) and tadalafil (Cialis). A second type of drug used to treat erectile dysfunction is the prostaglandin alprostadil. This drug must be given by injecting it directly into the erectile tissue of the penis or pushing a suppository form of the drug into the urethra.

A list of all of the men's health drugs mentioned in the chapter appears in Box 34-1. More information on selected drugs can be found in the Drug profiles section. Antiandrogens and gonadotropin-releasing hormone analogs are discussed in the antineoplastic drug chapters (Chapters 47 and 48).

Indications

The primary use for androgens is as hormone replacement therapy. Indications for other types of drugs discussed in this chapter are listed in Table 34-1.

Box 34-1	Currently Available Men's Health Drugs

α_1-Adrenergic Blockers
doxazosin
tamsulosin
terazosin

Anabolic Steroids
nandrolone
oxandrolone
oxymetholone
stanozolol

Other Androgens
danazol
fluoxymesterone
methyltestosterone
testosterone

Antiandrogens
bicalutamide
flutamide
nilutamide

5α-Reductase Inhibitors
finasteride
dutasteride

Gonadotropin-Releasing Hormone Analogues
goserelin
leuprolide
triptorelin

Peripheral Vasodilator
minoxidil

Drugs for Erectile Dysfunction
sildenafil
tadalafil
vardenafil

Table 34-1 Men's Health Drugs: Indications

Drug	Indication
danazol	Endometriosis
	Fibrocystic breast disease
danazol and stanozolol	Hereditary angioedema
finasteride	Benign prostatic hypertrophy
	Male androgenetic alopecia
fluoxymesterone and methyltestosterone	Inoperable breast cancer
	Male hypogonadism
	Postpartum breast engorgement
methyltestosterone	Postpubertal cryptorchidism
minoxidil	Hypertension
	Female and male androgenetic alopecia
nandrolone	Metastatic breast cancer
oxymetholone	Various anemias
sildenafil, tadalafil, vardenafil	Erectile dysfunction
testosterone	Primary or secondary hypogonadism

Table 34-2 Mens' Health Drugs: Selected Adverse Effects

Drug Class	Adverse Effects
α_1-Adrenergic blockers	Tachycardia, hypotension, chest pain, syncope, depression, dizziness, drowsiness, asthenia, rash, pruritus, impotence, urinary frequency, upper body muscular pain, dyspnea, flu-like symptoms, visual changes, headache
Androgens (including anabolic steroids)	Headache, increased or reduced libido, anxiety, depression, acne, male pattern baldness, hirsuitism, nausea, abnormal liver function tests, hepatic neoplasms, priapism, polycythemia, elevated cholesterol, anaphylaxis (injection)
5α-Reductase inhibitors	Reduced libido, reduced semen volume, hypotension, dizziness, drowsiness
Peripheral vasodilator (topical minoxidil)	Topical route usually limited to localized dermatologic reactions, including erythema, dermatitis, eczema, pruritus; possible systemic reactions theoretically include edema, chest pain, hyper/hypotension, headache, dizziness, nausea, vomiting, diarrhea, sexual dysfunction, anemia, thrombocytopenia, and muscular pain
Drugs for erectile dysfunction	Dizziness, headache, dyspepsia, nasal congestion, muscular pain, chest pain, hyper/hypotension, rash, dermatitis, abnormal liver function tests, dry mouth, nausea, vomiting, diarrhea, gingivitis, priapism

Contraindications

Contraindications to the use of androgenic drugs include known androgen-responsive tumors. Use of sildenafil, vardenafil, and tadalafil is also contraindicated in men with major cardiovascular disorders, especially if they use nitrate medications such as nitroglycerin. Finasteride is contraindicated in women (especially pregnant women) and children.

Adverse Effects

Although they are rare, some of the most devastating effects of androgenic steroids occur in the liver, where they cause the formation of blood-filled cavities, a condition known as *peliosis of the liver.* This condition is a possible consequence of the long-term administration of androgenic anabolic steroids and can be life threatening. Other serious hepatic effects are hepatic neoplasms (liver cancer), cholestatic hepatitis, jaundice, and abnormal liver function. Fluid retention is another undesirable effect of androgens and may account for some of the weight gain seen in persons taking them. The serious adverse effects that can be caused by the androgens far outweigh the advantages to be gained from their use in those seeking improved athletic ability. Other less serious adverse effects of androgens are listed in Table 34-2.

Sildenafil, vardenafil, and tadalafil appear to have relatively favorable adverse effect profiles. In patients with preexisting cardiovascular disease, especially those taking nitrates (e.g., nitroglycerin, isosorbide mononitrate, dinitrate), these drugs can lower blood pressure substantially, potentially leading to more serious adverse events. Headache, flushing, and dyspepsia are the most common adverse effects reported. *Priapism* or abnormally prolonged penile erection is another relatively uncommon, but possible, adverse effect of both the erectile dysfunction drugs and the androgens. This condition is a medical emergency and warrants urgent medical attention. It is simply due to an excessive therapeutic drug response. As of this writing, the FDA is currently investigating unexplained case reports of visual losses in men using these drugs. At this time, all remain on the U.S. market and have not been recalled.

Finasteride has been reported to cause loss of libido, loss of erection, ejaculatory dysfunction, hypersensitivity reactions, gynecomastia, and severe myopathy. The drug has also caused a 50% decrease in prostate-specific antigen (PSA) concentrations. Pregnant women should not handle crushed or broken tablets on a regular basis because of the possibility of topical absorption, which can lead to teratogenic effects.

Interactions

All androgens, when used with oral anticoagulants, can significantly increase or decrease anticoagulant activity. They can also enhance the hypoglycemic effects of oral hypoglycemic (antidiabetic) drugs. Concurrent use with cyclosporine increases the risk of cyclosporine toxicity and is not recommended.

Dosages

For recommended dosages of the men's health drugs, see the Dosages table on page 529.

Drug Profiles

finasteride

Finasteride (Proscar, Propecia) use is contraindicated in patients who have shown a hypersensitivity to it and in pregnant women, and it is considered potentially dangerous for a pregnant woman even to handle crushed or broken tablets. The drug is currently available in two tablet forms of 1- and 5-mg strengths. The lower strength is indicated for androgenetic alopecia in men. The higher strength is indicated for BPH. A similar but newer drug, dutaste-

DOSAGES

Selected Men's Health Drugs

Drug	Pharmacologic Class	Usual Dosage Range	Indications
danazol (Danocrine)	Synthetic androgen	**Adult** PO: 200-800 mg/day divided bid and reduced to a dose that maintains amenorrhea, usually given over 3-9 mo 100-400 mg/day divided bid × 4-6 mo 200 mg bid-tid, reduced by 50% after a favorable response, given at 1-3 mo intervals	Endometriosis Fibrocystic breast disease Hereditary angioedema
finasteride (Propecia, Proscar)	5α-reductase inhibitor	**Adult** PO: 1 mg daily (Propecia) PO: 5 mg daily (Proscar)	Male androgenetic alopecia (baldness) (males only) BPH
vardenafil (Levitra)	Phosphodiesterase inhibitor	**Adult** PO: 2.5-20 mg 1 hr before intercourse; no more than once daily	Erectile dysfunction
fluoxymesterone (Halotestin)	Synthetic androgen	**Adult** PO: 10-40 mg/day divided daily-qid **Adult and adolescent** PO: 5-20 mg/day	Inoperable breast cancer (in women) Delayed puberty or hypogonadism (in males)
methyltestosterone (Methitest, Virilon, Android, others)	Synthetic androgen	**Adult** PO: 50-200 mg/day **Adult and adolescent** PO/IM: 10-50 mg/day	Inoperable breast cancer (in women) Delayed puberty or hypogonadism (in males)
▶sildenafil (Viagra)	Phosphodiesterase inhibitor	**Adult (males only)** PO: 25-100 mg 1 hr before intercourse, no more than once daily	Erectile dysfunction
dutasteride (Avodart)	5α-reductase inhibitor	**Adult** PO: 0.5 mg daily	BPH
▶testosterone cypionate (Depo-Testosterone)	Androgenic hormone	**Adult** IM: 200-400 mg q2-4wk **Adult and adolescent** IM: 50-400 mg q2-4wk	Inoperable breast cancer (in women) Delayed puberty or hypogonadism (in males)
testosterone, transdermal (Testoderm, Andro-derm, AndroGel)	Androgenic hormone	**Adult and adolescent** Testoderm patch (applied only to scrotal skin): 4-6 mg/day Androderm patch (applied to skin of back, abdomen, upper arms, or thighs): 2.5-5 mg/day AndroGel (applied to shoulders, arms, or abdominal skin): 5 g daily (delivers 50 mg of testosterone)	Male hypogonadism

BPH, Benign prostatic hypertrophy; *IM*, intramuscular; *PO*, oral.

ride, is also indicated for BPH and is currently available in 0.5-mg capsule form. Both drugs are contraindicated in women and children. Pregnancy category X (for both). Refer to the table on this page for dosage information.

Pharmacokinetics

Half-Life	Onset	Peak	Duration
4-15 hr*	3-12 mo†	8 hr‡	Unknown

*Varies with age.
†To reduce prostate size.
‡To lower 5α-dihydrotestosterone concentrations.

▶ *sildenafil*

Sildenafil (Viagra) is the first oral drug approved by the FDA for the treatment of erectile dysfunction. Another currently available drug for the treatment of erectile dysfunction is an injectable form of the prostaglandin alprostadil. Sildenafil potentiates the physiologic sexual response, causing penile erection after sexual arousal by relaxing smooth muscle and increasing blood flow into the penis.

Sildenafil use is contraindicated in patients with a known hypersensitivity to it. Sildenafil can potentiate the hypotensive effects of nitrates, and its administration to patients who are using organic nitrates in any form, either regularly or intermittently, is therefore contraindicated. Dosage information for sildenafil and vardenafil appears in the table on this page. Sildenafil use is contraindicated in patients with a known hypersensitivity to it. Sildenafil can potentiate the hypotensive effects of nitrates, and its administration to patients who are using organic nitrates in any form, either regularly or intermittently, is therefore contraindicated. Two newer drugs for erectile dysfunction include vardenafil and tadalafil.

Pharmacokinetics

Half-Life	Onset	Peak	Duration
4 hr	0.5-1 hr	1 hr	4 hr

▶ *testosterone*

Testosterone (Androderm, AndroGel, Delatestryl, Depo-Testosterone, Testoderm, Testopel) is a naturally occurring anabolic steroid. It is used for primary and secondary hypogonadism but may also be used to treat oligospermia in men and inoperable breast cancer in women, where its purpose is to counteract tumor-enhancing estrogen activity. When it is used as hormone replacement therapy, a transdermal product is desirable. There are presently two transdermal patch formulations. They attempt to mimic the normal circadian variation in testosterone concentration seen in young healthy men, in whom the maximum testosterone levels occur in the early morning hours and the minimum concentrations occur in the evening. Of the two available transdermal delivery systems, Testoderm is always applied to the scrotal skin, whereas Androderm is always applied to skin elsewhere on the body and never to the scrotal skin.

Testosterone use is contraindicated in patients with severe renal, cardiac, or hepatic disease, hypersensitivity, or genital bleeding, and in pregnant or lactating women. Testosterone is considered a Schedule III controlled substance under the Anabolic Steroids Control Act. It is available as intramuscular injections, transdermal gel, transdermal patches, and even implantable pellets. Pregnancy category X. Common dosages are listed in the table on page 529.

Pharmacokinetics

Half-Life	Onset	Peak	Duration
10-100 min	1-2 hr	2-4 hr	2 hr-4 wk depending on dosage form

PHARMACOKINETIC BRIDGE
to Nursing Practice

Drugs used to manage erectile dysfunction (e.g., sildenafil) essentially work in the same way as the body to assist the male patient in achieving an erection. The related pharmacokinetics must be understood so that the drug is given safely and effectively. Sildenafil is a rapidly absorbed drug with maximal plasma concentrations within 30 to 120 minutes after oral dosing and if taken on an empty stomach. Peak time is at an average of 60 minutes. If the drug is taken with a high-fat meal, absorption will be delayed, and it may take an additional 60 minutes for the drug to reach peak levels. This is yet another example of how specific drug pharmacokinetics can be affected by variables in a patient's everyday life and habits. Another pharmacokinetic property is that patients who are 65 years of age or older have reduced clearance of sildenafil and may experience increased plasma concentrations of free (or pharmacolgocially active) drug. This could possibly lead to drug accumulation and/or possible toxicity.

◆ NURSING PROCESS

✦ ASSESSMENT

Before any drug is given to a male patient for the treatment of benign or malignant diseases of the male reproductive tract, presenting symptoms should be thoroughly assessed and a complete history of past and present medical diseases or conditions should be obtained. In addition, assessment of the patient's urinary elimination patterns should be documented. The physician

Life Span Considerations: The Elderly Patient
Sildenafil: Use and Concerns

- Over 10 million men experience erectile dysfunction (ED). The incidence of ED increases as age increases. About 2% of affected men are in their forties and 23% are 65 years of age or older.
- Sildenafil (Viagra) is a prescription medication that is commonly ordered to treat ED, but it is not without concerns and cautions for the patient. This is especially true for elderly patients, who generally have other medical conditions (e.g., renal disorders, hypertension, diabetes) and are usually taking more than one other prescribed medication.
- Liver function declines with age; therefore, drugs may not be metabolized as effectively in older adults as they are in younger adults. In addition, sildenafil is highly protein bound, which causes it to stay in the body longer and thus create more drug interactions.
- A decreased dosage of sildenafil is generally indicated for patients over 65 years of age and for those with liver or renal impairment.
- Adverse effects to be concerned about in all patients, particularly older patients, include headache, flushing, urinary tract infection, diarrhea, rash, and dizziness.
- Sildenafil should be used cautiously in patients who have cardiac disease and angina, because these patients are at greater risk for complications, especially if they are taking nitrates for their cardiovascular disease.
- Discussing topics of a sexual nature may be comfortable for some patients but very anxiety producing for others. It is important for nurses to be aware of cultural and gender differences in how individuals perceive their own sexuality and how they generally deal with sexual performance issues.
- Nurses must be respectful of each individual's beliefs and feelings not only about his or her sexuality but also about other parts of the patient's whole self. This requires knowledge, sensitivity, and objectivity.

Based on information from Lacy CF et al: *Drug information handbook,* ed 11, Hudson, Ohio, 2003, Lexi-Comp.

usually performs a rectal examination for BPH or other pathology and documents findings, and will order a serum PSA test before initiating therapy. Special handling precautions should be followed for some of these drugs because of potential teratogenic effects (e.g., finasteride should not be handled by pregnant nurses or caregivers). The patient should also be assessed for liver impairment. For patients with prostate cancer, PSA levels should be assessed before therapy and as needed because levels should decrease with successful treatment.

Drugs for erectile dysfunction should be given only after a medical-physical examination, thorough nursing assessment, and medication history have been completed. Serum phosphorus levels also need to be documented. Bowel sounds and bowel patterns should be assessed with notation of any dysphagia or gastrointestinal motility disorders (which may occur with sildenafil). Contraindications, cautions, and drug interactions have been previously discussed and should be assessed prior to the use of this drug (and all drugs in this class).

With testosterone and related drugs, the patient should be assessed for diabetes and/or cardiac disease because of possible edema and subsequent added stress on the heart. Because androgenic anabolic steroids (e.g., testosterone) may increase weight, have a negative impact on bone growth, and elevate serum levels of potassium, chloride, nitrogen, phosphorus, and cholesterol, the nurse should assess for obesity, recent weight gain, bone disorders, and electrolyte imbalances before, during, and after therapy. Height, vital signs, and intake and output should be assessed and results of the following laboratory tests analyzed: renal function tests (blood urea nitrogen and creatinine levels), cardiac enzyme assay, liver function tests (lactate dehydrogenase, creatine phosphokinase, and bilirubin levels), and PSA levels. A history of male breast cancer, prostate cancer, and/or gynecomastia should also be ruled out prior to drug therapy.

◆ NURSING DIAGNOSES

- Disturbed body image related to sexual dysfunction and/or diseases of the male reproductive tract
- Fatigue related to the adverse effects of medications
- Excess fluid volume related to possible adverse effects (sodium retention)
- Impaired urinary elimination related to BPH
- Ineffective sexuality patterns related to the effects of treatment with testosterone and drugs used for erectile dysfunction
- Sexual dysfunction (male) related to inability to perform sexually due to erectile dysfunction
- Risk for injury related to the adverse effects of therapy with drugs used for erectile dysfunction
- Risk for situational low self-esteem related to sexual dysfunction secondary to medications and/or disease states
- Deficient knowledge related to misinterpretation of information about self-medication

◆ PLANNING

Goals

- Patient maintains positive body image.
- Patient maintains normal activity levels during drug therapy with testosterone.
- Patient maintains normal sodium and fluid volume levels during drug therapy.
- Patient attains near-normal urinary elimination patterns.
- Patient experiences minimal alterations in sexual integrity and function during testosterone therapy.
- Patient remains compliant with drug therapy regimen.
- Patient verbalizes feelings and concerns about actual or perceived changes in sexual patterns and functioning.

Outcome Criteria

- Patient verbalizes feelings, fears, and anxieties concerning potential for alteration in body image related to the disease process or the adverse effects of treatment with testosterone and related men's health drugs.
- Patient maintains healthy activity level during drug therapy and suffers minimal fatigue with gradual increase in activities of daily living.
- Patient states measures to be taken (such as dietary changes) to minimize edema related to sodium retention stemming from the use of large dosages of testosterone.
- Patient verbalizes feelings, anxieties, and fears of alteration in sexual patterns or functioning during drug therapy.
- Patient takes medications as prescribed and with appropriate follow-up.

◆ IMPLEMENTATION

Finasteride may be given orally without regard to meals but should be protected from exposure to light and heat. When used for treatment of the urinary symptoms of BPH, finasteride and

related drugs should be administered orally for approximately 6 months, at which time the condition should be reevaluated. Patients taking drugs for erectile dysfunction should be warned about potential adverse effects, such as flushing of the face, headache, nasal congestion, heartburn, diarrhea, urinary tract infections, blue-tinged vision, blurred vision and light sensitivity, and dizziness. There have been concerns in the media about heart-related deaths and this drug, so patient education is crucial to patient safety. Additionally, the patient has the right to accurate and appropriate education about risk factors and concerns about level of activity and physical exertion. See the Patient Teaching Tips for more information.

The therapeutic effects of testosterone are maximized when the drug is taken as ordered and at regular intervals so that steady levels are maintained. If the drug is being used for hypogonadism or induction of puberty, dosages may be managed differently, so that at the end of the growth spurt the patient is placed on maintenance dosages. Testoderm transdermal patches should be placed on clean, dry scrotal skin that has been shaved for optimal skin contact and should be replaced every 22 to 24 hours or as ordered. Androderm patches should be placed on clean, dry skin on the back, abdomen, upper arms, or thighs; the scrotum and bony areas (shoulder, hip) should be avoided. These patches are often ordered to be changed every 7 days. Because various types of transdermal patch are available, the nurse should be sure the patient understands which type of patch is to be used, where, and how it is to be applied and how. Buccal tablets should be placed between the cheek and gum and allowed to dissolve before swallowing. If the drug is given intramuscularly, the vial of medication should be mixed thoroughly by agitating it before withdrawing the prescribed amount of medication. See the Herbal Therapies and Dietary Supplements box for a description of saw palmetto, an herbal supplement that is often taken to relieve symptoms of enlarged prostate.

◆ EVALUATION

The therapeutic effects of drugs related to the male reproductive tract include improvement of the condition and/or signs and symptoms for which the patient is being treated, such as hypogonadism, sexual dysfunction, erectile dysfunction, and urinary elimination problems caused by BPH. The therapeutic effects of some drugs (e.g., finasteride) may not be seen for 6 to 12 months, so it is important for the nurse to observe and monitor the patient for the intended effects of the drugs.

In addition, the nurse should evaluate for the adverse effects of these medications (see the pharmacology section for specific adverse effects). Goals and outcome criteria should always be evaluated to see if the patient's needs have been met.

Patient Teaching Tips

- With finasteride, education about the drug's therapeutic effects as well as adverse effects should must occur at the patient's educational level. Adverse effects include impotence, decrease in the amount of ejaculate, and decreased libido; however, the nurse should emphasize that these adverse effects may be transient and that sexual functioning is not otherwise altered. There should be education about the fact that there are special handling precautions for female family members, significant others, or caregivers who are pregnant or of childbearing age. This includes *not* handling any broken or crushed tablets, which could result in exposure to the drug and the risk of teratogenic effects.
- With sildenafil, explain to the patient that it should be taken about 1 hour before sexual activity and that the patient should not be taking this medication if also taking nitrates.
- Inform patients that drug therapy for erectile dysfunction is not effective without sexual stimulation and arousal.
- With testosterone, the patient should be educated about the therapeutic as well as adverse effects with use of age-appropriate education strategies. Follow-up appointments should also be emphasized as being an important aspect of an effective therapy.
- Educate patients about the transdermal dosage form and how it should be discarded in a trash can once the drug has been unwrapped and applied, so that accidental application or ingestion by children (or anyone else) may be minimized.
- Inform patients taking buccal dosage forms of testosterone that there should not be any eating or drinking while the dosage form is in place.
- Educate the patient to report any of the following adverse effects in order to receive further instructions: for male patients, swelling of the extremities, jaundice, or prolonged painful erections; for female patients, hoarseness, deepening of the voice, menstrual irregularities, acne, or facial hair growth. Dosage amounts may be changed or the drug may be discontinued by the physician should these effects occur.
- Educate patients about avoiding abrupt withdrawal of testosterone.

Points to Remember

- The most commonly used drugs related to male health and the male reproductive tract are finasteride, sildenafil, and testosterone. The nurse needs to know how these drugs work and what their adverse effects, contraindications, cautions, and drug interactions are for their safe and effective use.
- Testosterone is responsible for the development and maintenance of the male reproductive system and secondary sex characteristics. Oral testosterone has very poor pharmacokinetic and pharmacodynamic characteristics, and therefore it is recommended that testosterone be administered via injection (parenteral route) or a transdermal patch.
- Methyltestosterone was developed to circumvent the problems associated with the oral administration of testosterone.
- Patients taking testosterone should be told to avoid abrupt withdrawal of the medication. Weaning off of the drug, if ordered, is generally done over several weeks.
- Finasteride is usually indicated to stop growth of the prostate in men with BPH and to treat men with androgenic alopecia.

- Finasteride may be given orally without regard to meals but should be protected from exposure to light and heat.
- Patients taking drugs for erectile dysfunction (e.g., sildenafil) should be warned about potential adverse effects, such as flushing of the face, headache, nasal congestion, heartburn, diarrhea, urinary tract infections, blue-tinged vision, blurred vision and light sensitivity, and dizziness.
- There are major concerns about heart-related deaths associated with nitrates and drugs used for erectile dysfunction. Patient education should focus on prevention of drug interactions and related adverse effects and complications.
- The therapeutic effects of drugs related to the male reproductive tract include improvement of the condition and/or signs and symptoms for which the patient is being treated, such as hypogonadism, sexual dysfunction, erectile dysfunction, and urinary elimination problems caused by BPH. It is important to note that the therapeutic effects of most of the drugs do not occur immediately and may take 6 to 12 months.

NCLEX Examination Review Questions

1. Which is important to monitor when a patient is taking finasteride (Proscar)?
   a. Complete blood count
   b. PSA levels
   c. Blood pressure
   d. Fluid retention
2. The nurse is performing an assessment of a patient who is asking for a prescription for sildenafil (Viagra). Which of the following findings would be a contraindication to its use?
   a. Age of 65 years
   b. History of hypertension
   c. Medication list that includes nitrates
   d. Medication list that includes saw palmetto
3. During a counseling session for a group of teenage athletes, the use of androgenic steroids is discussed. The nurse will explain that which of the following is a rare but devastating effect of androgenic steroid use?
   a. Peliosis of the liver
   b. Bradycardia
   c. Kidney failure
   d. Tachydysrhythmias
4. The nurse is teaching a patient about the possible adverse effects of erectile dysfunction drugs. If the patient experiences priapism, or an erection that lasts longer than 4 hours, he should know to do which of the following:
   a. Stay in bed until the erection ceases
   b. Apply an ice pack for 30 minutes
   c. Turn on his left side and rest
   d. Seek medical attention
5. A patient is asking about the use of saw palmetto for prostate health. The nurse tells him that drugs that interact with saw palmetto include which of the following?
   a. Acetaminophen (Tylenol)
   b. Nitrates
   c. Nonsteroidal antiinflammatory drugs
   d. Antihypertensive drugs

1. b, 2. c, 3. a, 4. d, 5. c.

Critical Thinking Activities

1. How do finasteride and methyltestosterone differ in their mechanisms of action?
2. Why might an androgen be prescribed for a patient suffering from anemia?
3. Develop a teaching plan addressing the risks of anabolic steroid use for an 18-year-old male football player and weight lifter.

For answers, see http://evolve.elsevier.com/Lilley.

PART 6

Drugs Affecting the Respiratory System

STUDY ON THE RUN, PURR

The basic approach in applying Study on the Run (SOTR) is to make use of small blocks of time that are otherwise nonproductive. Plan, Rehearse, and Review do not require that the entire chapter be covered in one study session. These steps produce their benefits by promoting repetition of learning.

Where Is the Time?

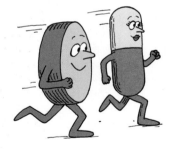

SOTR time is everywhere. In the course of a single day you might have an hour or more that can be used for SOTR actions. It is just a matter of becoming aware of little bits and pieces of your day that can ordinarily slip away without being productive. Small blocks of time are everywhere in your day; it just takes a little creativity on your part to become aware of them. Finishing an exam early, standing in the checkout line, waiting for the teakettle to boil, or even waiting for the washing machine to finish the last spin before you change loads can be time used for SOTR. Get creative and be flexible. Remember, every minute of time you use this way is a minute of time you will not have to find later.

SOTR and Plan

Remember the importance of questioning as an essential component in Plan. Look at the chapter objectives for Chapter 36. There are five objectives presented for this chapter. Work on the questions for as many of these objectives as can be accomplished in the time you have. If you complete questions for only two objectives, do not look upon it as failure to complete something. Instead, learn to view what you have done as that much less to do later. The time you spend now frees up that much more time during your large blocks of study time for intense study reading.

Will you forget the questions you generated in this session before you have the opportunity to read the chapter? If you make it a habit to ask questions as a continuing part of all study, you will find that you remember the focus questions very well. If you have trouble remembering your own questions, write the questions in the margins of the text. Gradually you will find that questioning becomes such an automatic procedure that you will be able to dispense with writing questions. You will remember them.

SOTR and Vocabulary

One of the most challenging aspects of a course like this is the almost overwhelming vocabulary load. If the new vocabulary load is not enough, there is also the need to keep reviewing previous parts and chapters because some term that was introduced three chapters ago has reappeared and you do not remember it clearly. Creating your own vocabulary cards is a perfect SOTR activity.

The basic card model is simple. The word, common form, prefix, or suffix appears on the card front. The back of the card may have just a little information (the minimum being a definition of what is on the front) or may contain considerable information. I recommend that you include part, chapter, and page number on the back so that you can locate the term quickly if the need arises. In addition, you may want to add a specific example from the text or of your own creation to help clarify the term. Put as much information on the back as you find useful.

Creating Vocabulary Cards with SOTR

Use the time between classes to create several personal vocabulary cards. Grab your text and your blank note cards. Open to the next chapter you will be studying. Flip over to the glossary pages. Write the first word from the glossary on the front of a blank note card. Flip the card over. Write the part and chapter numbers and the page number for the glossary on the card. Pick a standard location for this. Put these numbers in a top or bottom corner, but make sure you put them in the same corner every time. Eventually this becomes a habit and makes the preparation process faster. It also helps when you are making use of the cards because you will know exactly what information you put on the card and where you put it. Put this card aside and repeat the process with the next term in the glossary. In those few minutes before you go to class you can have completed the basic preparation for a full set of cards covering the 14 terms in the Chapter 36 glossary.

Notice that all I proposed was that you copy the term and the location information. I did not tell you to copy the definition in the glossary at this time. The term, used in the context of a sentence and a paragraph, may be much easier to understand. If, as you read the chapter, you feel that the glossary definition is also useful to have on this card, you can always flip back by using the location information you put on the card.

SOTR and Vocabulary Review

Your vocabulary cards are ideal for SOTR action. Carry a deck of cards with you at all times. Whenever you have even a minute or two, you can pull out a stack of cards from previous chapters or the current chapter. Use the oral ask-and-answer method discussed in the *Study Guide*. For instance, the first term in the glossary for Chapter 36 is *allergen*. Ask yourself aloud, "What is an allergen?" Then try to answer the question aloud. Answer: "An allergen is a substance that produces an allergic reaction." It is not necessary to recall the exact answer presented in the glossary and/or chapter. What is important is that you respond with a clear and meaningful answer. The answer given above is not exactly the same

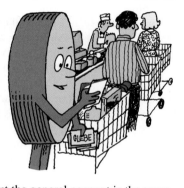

as that stated in the glossary, but the general concept is the same. Once you have stated your answer, turn the card over and check to make sure that you were correct. Each time you do this with a term, you are strengthening your long-term memory and will find that it takes less and less time to recall the terms you need.

Vocabulary cards can also be used with your study group. You may want to give oral quizzes to each other. This is one sure way to check that your answer is stated clearly.

SOTR and Chapter Review

It can be overwhelming if you think that review means rereading the material and that you therefore need large blocks of uninterrupted time. There is a much more efficient way to review, and it works well in short time blocks, which makes it a perfect technique for SOTR.

Look at the first page of Chapter 35. You should instantly see a number of visible structures that make it easy to review key terms and concepts without rereading the entire block of material. First, there is the chapter title: Antihistamines, Decongestants, Antitussives, and Expectorants. What are antihistamines? This is a question you would have generated when you were engaged in the Plan step of PURR. Now that you have read the chapter, repeat the question and answer it aloud. Answer aloud because you will hear what you say and will either know the material or need to mark it to come back and reread. Now ask a more complex question: "What is the role of antihistamines? What do they do?" Now try to answer these questions. If you can, then you do not need to reread to find out what antihistamines are. Next, looking at page 537, you will notice some things in **bold print.** Apply the same process. Using the boldface words and phrases as stimulus, ask questions and try to answer them to your own satisfaction. If you cannot develop a satisfactory answer, then you know that some rereading is needed. However, it is very focused. You are not trying to reread everything on the page, only the material right there that is associated with the term.

Looking further down the page you will see a list. Look at the previous sentence: "This explains why the release of excessive amounts of histamine can lead to anaphylaxis and severe allergic symptoms and may result in any or all of the following physiologic changes..." Ask questions. If you can answer, no reading is necessary. If you cannot answer, you know that the answers are found immediately after this sentence in the indented list. Use the structures in the chapter to accomplish focused review. Comprehension is improved, long-term memory is strengthened, and your test grades will reflect this.

The benefits of SOTR are enormous. There are no drawbacks. You are using time that otherwise would be "wasted," and this time now becomes productive study time. The more active you become in looking for SOTR opportunities, the more you will find. The more SOTR time you spend the better student you will become.

Antihistamines, Decongestants, Antitussives, and Expectorants

Objectives

When you reach the end of this chapter, you should be able to do the following:

1. Provide specific examples of the drugs categorized as antihistamines, decongestants, antitussives, and expectorants.
2. Discuss the mechanisms of action, indications, contraindications, cautions, drug interactions, adverse effects, dosages, and route of administration for antihistamines, decongestants, antitussives, and expectorants.
3. Develop a nursing care plan that includes all phases of the nursing process for patients taking any of the antihistamines, decongestants, antitussives, and/or expectorants.

e-Learning Activities

Companion CD

- NCLEX Review Questions: see questions 305-311
- Animations
- Audio Glossary
- Category Catchers
- Medication Errors Checklists
- IV Therapy Checklists

evolve Website (http://evolve.elsevier.com/Lilley)

- Nursing Care Plans • Frequently Asked Questions • Content Updates • WebLinks • Supplemental Resources • Elsevier ePharmacology Update • Medication Administration Animations

Drug Profiles

benzonatate, p. 545
codeine, p. 545
▶ dextromethorphan, p. 545
▶ diphenhydramine, p. 540

▶ guaifenesin, p. 546
▶ loratadine, p. 540
naphazoline, p. 543

▶ Key drug.

Glossary

Adrenergics (sympathomimetics) Drugs that stimulate the sympathetic nerve fibers of the autonomic nervous system that use epinephrine or epinephrine-like substances as neurotransmitters. (p. 541)

Antagonist Any drug that exerts an action opposite to that of another or competes for the same receptor sites. (p. 537)

Anticholinergics (parasympatholytics) Drugs that block the action of acetylcholine and similar substances at acetylcholine receptors, which results in inhibition of the transmission of parasympathetic nerve impulses. (p. 541)

Antigens Substances that, upon entering to the body, are capable of inducing specific immune responses and in turn reacting with the specific products of such responses, such as certain antibodies and specifically sensitized T lymphocytes.

Antigens can be soluble (e.g., a foreign protein) or particulate or insoluble (e.g., a bacterial cell). (p. 538)

Antihistamines Substances capable of reducing the physiologic and pharmacologic effects of histamine, including a wide variety of drugs that block histamine receptors. (p. 537)

Antitussive A drug that reduces coughing, often by inhibiting neural activity in the cough center of the central nervous system. (p. 544)

Corticosteroids Any of the hormones produced by the adrenal cortex, either in natural or synthetic drug form. They influence or control many key processes in the body, such as carbohydrate and protein metabolism, the maintenance of serum glucose levels, electrolyte and water balance, and the functions of the cardiovascular system, skeletal muscle, kidneys, and other organs. (p. 541)

Decongestants Drugs that reduce congestion or swelling, especially of the upper or lower respiratory tract. (p. 541)

Empiric therapy A method of treating disease based on observations and experience without an understanding of the precise cause of or mechanism responsible for the disorder or the way in which the therapeutic drug or procedure produces improvement or cure. (p. 537)

Expectorants Drugs that increase the flow of fluid in the respiratory tract, usually by reducing the viscosity of bronchial and tracheal secretions, and facilitate their removal by coughing and ciliary action. (p. 545)

Histamine antagonists Drugs that compete with histamine for binding sites on histamine receptors. (p. 537)

Influenza A highly contagious infection of the respiratory tract caused by a myxovirus and transmitted by airborne droplets. (p. 537)

Nonsedating antihistamines Newer medications that work peripherally to block the actions of histamine and therefore do not have the central nervous system effects of many of the older antihistamines; also called *second-generation antihistamines* or *peripherally acting antihistamines*. (p. 540)

Reflex stimulation   An irritation of the respiratory tract occurring in response to an irritation of the gastrointestinal tract. (p. 544)

Rhinovirus   Any of about 100 serologically distinct ribonucleic acid (RNA) viruses that cause about 40% of acute respiratory illnesses. (p. 537)

Sympathomimetic drugs   A class of drugs whose effects mimic those resulting from the stimulation of organs and structures by the sympathetic nervous system. They do this by occupying adrenergic receptor sites and acting as agonists or by increasing the release of norepinephrine at postganglionic nerve endings. (p. 543)

Upper respiratory tract infection (URI)   Any infectious disease of the upper respiratory tract, including the common cold, laryngitis, pharyngitis, rhinitis, sinusitis, and tonsillitis. (p. 537)

COLD MEDICATIONS

Most common colds result from a viral infection, most often infection with a **rhinovirus** or an **influenza** virus. These viruses normally invade the tissues (mucosa) of the upper respiratory tract (nose, pharynx, and larynx) to cause an **upper respiratory tract infection (URI).** The inflammatory response elicited by these invading viruses stimulates excessive mucus production. This fluid drips behind the nose, down the pharynx and into the esophagus and lower respiratory tract, which leads to symptoms

HERBAL THERAPIES AND DIETARY SUPPLEMENTS

Echinacea *(Echinacea)*

Overview

The three species of echinacea used medicinally are *Echinacea angustifolia*, *Echinacea pallida*, and *Echinacea purpurea*. Echinacea has been shown in clinical trials to reduce cold symptoms and recovery time when taken early in the illness. This is believed to be due to its immunostimulant effects. At this time there is no strong research evidence to warrant recommending the herb for urinary tract infections, wound healing, or prevention of colds; further study is needed to provide evidence of its therapeutic effects and indications.

Common Uses

Stimulation of immune system, antisepsis, treatment of viral infections and influenza-like respiratory infections, promotion of healing of wounds and chronic ulcerations

Adverse Effects

Dermatitis, upset stomach or vomiting, dizziness, headache, unpleasant taste

Potential Drug Interactions

Amiodarone, cyclosporine, phenytoin, methotrexate, ketoconazole, barbiturates; tolerance likely to develop if used for more than 8 weeks. Because some preparations have a high alcohol content, they may cause acetaldehyde syndrome in patients taking disulfiram (Antabuse) to prevent alcohol abuse (Chapter 8).

Contraindications

Contraindicated for patients with acquired immunodeficiency syndrome, tuberculosis, connective tissue diseases, multiple sclerosis

typical of a cold: sore throat, coughing, and upset stomach. The irritation of the nasal mucosa often triggers the sneeze reflex and also causes the release of several inflammatory and vasoactive substances, which results in the dilation of the small blood vessels in the nasal sinuses and leads to nasal congestion. The treatment of the common symptoms of URI involves the combined use of antihistamines, nasal decongestants, antitussives, and expectorants. Many are even available without prescription. However, these drugs can only relieve the symptoms of a URI. They can do nothing to eliminate the causative pathogen. Antiviral drugs are currently the only drugs that can do this, but treatment with these mediations is often hampered by the fact that the viral cause cannot be readily identified. Because of this, the treatment rendered can only be based what is believed to be the most likely cause, given the presenting clinical symptoms. Such treatment is called **empiric therapy.** Some patients seem to gain benefit from the use of herbal products and other supplements, such as vitamin C, in preventing the onset of cold signs and symptoms or at least in decreasing their severity. One herbal product commonly used for colds is echinacea (see Herbal Therapies and Dietary Supplements box on p. 537). The practitioner should recognize, however, that there is limited controlled research data regarding the efficacy of herbal products and also that some of them can have significant drug-drug or drug-disease interactions.

ANTIHISTAMINES

Histamine is a bodily substance that performs many functions. It is involved in nerve impulse transmission in the central nervous system (CNS), dilation of capillaries, contraction of smooth muscles, stimulation of gastric secretion, and acceleration of the heart rate. There are two types of cellular receptors for histamine. Histamine-1 (H_1) receptors mediate smooth muscle contraction and dilation of capillaries, and histamine-2 (H_2) receptors mediate the acceleration of the heart rate and gastric acid secretion. This explains why the release of excessive amounts of histamine can lead to anaphylaxis and severe allergic symptoms and may result in any or all of the following physiologic changes:

- Constriction of smooth muscle, especially in the stomach and lungs
- Increase in body secretions
- Vasodilation and increased capillary permeability, which results in the movement of fluid out of the blood vessels and into the tissues, causing a drop in blood pressure and edema

Antihistamines are drugs that directly compete with histamine for specific receptor sites. For this reason, they are also called **histamine antagonists.** Antihistamines that compete with histamine for the H_2 receptors are called H_2 **antagonists** or *H_2 blockers* and include such drugs as cimetidine, ranitidine, famotidine, and nizatidine. Because they act on the gastrointestinal (GI) system, they are discussed in detail in Part Nine, which deals with the drugs that affect this system. This chapter focuses on the H_1 antagonists (also called *H_1 blockers*); these are the drugs more commonly known by the name *antihistamines*. They are very useful drugs because approximately 10% to 20% of the general population is sensitive to various environmental allergens. Histamine is a major inflammatory mediator of many allergic disorders, such as allergic rhinitis (e.g., hay fever and mold, dust allergies), anaphylaxis, angioedema, drug fevers, insect bite reactions, and urticaria (itching).

H_1 antagonists include drugs such as diphenhydramine, chlorpheniramine, and fexofenadine. They are of greatest value in the treatment of nasal allergies, particularly seasonal hay fever. They are also given to relieve the symptoms of the common cold, such as sneezing and runny nose. In this regard they are palliative, not curative; that is, they can help alleviate the symptoms of a cold but can do nothing to destroy the virus causing it.

The clinical efficacy of the more than one dozen different antihistamines is very similar, although they have varying degrees of antihistaminic, anticholinergic, and sedating properties. The particular actions of, and hence the indications for, a particular antihistamine are determined by its specific chemical makeup. All antihistamines compete with histamine for the H_1 receptors in areas such as the smooth muscle surrounding blood vessels and bronchioles. They also affect the secretions of the lacrimal, salivary, and respiratory mucosal glands, which are the primary anticholinergic actions of antihistamines. Because of their antihistaminic properties, they are indicated for the treatment of allergies. These drugs also differ from each other in their potency and their adverse effects, especially in the degree of drowsiness they produce. The antihistaminic, anticholinergic, and sedative properties of some of the more commonly used antihistamines are summarized in Figure 35-1. These effects make them useful for the treatment of problems such as vertigo, motion sickness, insomnia, and cough. Several classes of antihistamines are listed in Table 35-1, along with their various anticholinergic and sedative effects.

Mechanism of Action and Drug Effects

During allergic reactions, histamine and other substances are released from mast cells, basophils, and other cells in response to **antigens** circulating in the blood. The histamine molecules then bind to and activate other cells in the nose, eyes, respiratory tract, GI tract, and skin, producing the characteristic allergic signs and symptoms. For example, in the respiratory tract histamine causes extravascular smooth muscle (e.g., in the bronchial tree) to contract, whereas antihistamines cause it to relax. Also, histamine causes pruritus by stimulating nerve endings. Antihistamines can prevent or alleviate this itching.

Circulating histamine molecules normally bind to histamine receptors on basophils and mast cells. This stimulates further release of histamine stored within these cells. Antihistamine drugs work by blocking the histamine receptors on the surfaces of basophils and mast cells, thereby preventing the release and actions of histamine stored within these cells. They do not push off histamine that is already bound to a cell surface receptor but compete with histamine for unoccupied receptors. Therefore, these drugs are most beneficial when given early in a histamine-mediated reaction, before all of the free histamine molecules bind to cell membrane receptors. The binding of H_1 blockers to these receptors prevents the adverse consequences of histamine binding: vasodilation; increased GI, respiratory, salivary, and lacrimal secretions; and increased capillary permeability with resultant edema. The various drug effects of antihistamines are listed in Table 35-2.

Indications

Antihistamines are most beneficial in the management of nasal allergies, seasonal or perennial allergic rhinitis (e.g., hay fever), and some of the typical symptoms of the common cold. They are also useful in the treatment of allergic reactions, motion sickness, Parkinson's disease (due to their anticholinergic effects), and vertigo. In addition, they are sometimes used as a sleep aid.

Contraindications

Use of antihistamines is generally contraindicated in cases of known drug allergy. They should also not be used as the sole drug therapy during acute asthmatic attacks. In such cases a rapidly acting bronchodilator such as albuterol, or in extreme cases epinephrine, is generally the most urgently needed medication. Other

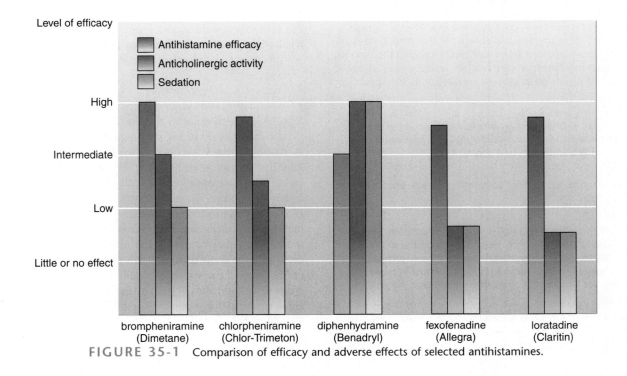

FIGURE 35-1 Comparison of efficacy and adverse effects of selected antihistamines.

Table 35-1 Effects of Various Antihistamines

Chemical Class	Anticholinergic Effects	Sedative Effects	Comments
Alkylamines			
brompheniramine	Moderate	Low	Cause less drowsiness and more CNS stimulation; suitable for daytime use
chlorpheniramine	Moderate	Low	
dexchlorpheniramine	Moderate	Low	
Ethanolamines			
clemastine	High	Moderate	Substantial anticholinergic effects; commonly cause sedation; at usual dosages, drowsiness occurs in about 50% of patients; diphenhydramine and dimenhydrinate also used as antiemetics
diphenhydramine	High	High	
dimenhydrinate	High	High	
Ethylenediamines			
pyrilamine	Low to none	Low	Weak sedative effects, but adverse GI effects are common
tripelennamine	Low to none	Moderate	
Phenothiazine			
promethazine	High	High	Drugs in this class are principally used as antipsychotics; some are useful as antihistamines, antipruritics, and antiemetics
Piperidines			
azatadine	Moderate	Moderate	Commonly used in the treatment of motion sickness; hydroxyzine is used as a tranquilizer, sedative, antipruritic, and antiemetic
cyproheptadine	Moderate	Low	
hydroxyzine	Moderate	Moderate	
phenindamine	Moderate	Low to none	
Miscellaneous			
fexofenadine	Low to none	Low to none	Very few adverse anticholinergic or sedative effects; almost exclusively antihistaminic effects; can be taken during the day because no sedative effects occur; in general they are longer acting and have fewer adverse effects than other classes
loratadine	Low to none	Low to none	

CNS, Central nervous system; *GI,* gastrointestinal.

Table 35-2 Antihistamines: Drug Effects

Body System	Histamine Effects	Antihistamine Effects
Cardiovascular (small blood vessels)	Dilates blood vessels, increases blood vessel permeability (allows substances to leak into tissues)	Reduces dilation of blood vessels and increased permeability
Immune (release of various substances commonly associated with allergic reactions)	Released from mast cells along with several other substances, which results in allergic reactions	Does not stabilize mast cells or prevent the release of histamine and other substances, but does bind to histamine receptors and prevent the actions of histamine
Smooth muscle (on exocrine glands)	Stimulates salivary, gastric, lacrimal, and bronchial secretions	Reduces salivary, gastric, lacrimal, and bronchial secretions

contraindications may include narrow-angle glaucoma, cardiac disease, kidney disease, hypertension, bronchial asthma, chronic obstructive pulmonary disease (COPD), peptic ulcer disease, seizure disorders, benign prostatic hypertrophy (BPH), and pregnancy. Fexofenadine is not recommended for patients under 6 years of age or those with renal impairment. Desloratadine is not recommended for pediatric patients. Loratadine is not recommended for patients under 2 years of age. Antihistamines should generally be used with caution in patients with impaired liver function or renal insufficiency, as well as with lactating mothers.

Adverse Effects

Drowsiness is usually the chief complaint of people who take antihistamines, but the sedative effects vary from class to class (see Table 35-1). Fortunately, sedative effects are much less common, although still possible, with the newer "nonsedating" drugs. The anticholinergic (drying) effects of antihistamines can cause adverse effects such as dry mouth, changes in vision, difficulty urinating, and constipation. Reported adverse effects and adverse effects of the antihistamines are listed in Table 35-3.

Table 35-3	Antihistamines: Reported Adverse Effects
Body System	**Adverse Effects**
Cardiovascular	Local anesthetic (quinidine-like) effect on the cardiac conduction system, which can result in dysrhythmias, arrest, hypotension, palpitations, syncope, dizziness, death (see Interactions section)
Central nervous	Sedation (mild drowsiness to deep sleep), dizziness, muscular weakness, paradoxical excitement, restlessness, insomnia, nervousness, seizures
Gastrointestinal	Anorexia, nausea, vomiting, diarrhea or constipation, hepatitis, jaundice
Other	Dryness of mouth, nose, and throat; urinary retention; impotence; vertigo; visual disturbances; blurred vision; tinnitus; headache; rarely agranulocytosis, hemolytic anemia, leukopenia, thrombocytopenia, pancytopenia

Interactions

When fexofenadine is given with erythromycin or ketoconazole, increased fexofenadine concentrations can result. Ketoconazole, cimetidine, and erythromycin may increase concentrations of loratadine. Alcohol, monoamine oxidase inhibitors (MAOIs), and CNS depressants may increase the CNS depressant effects of diphenhydramine and cetirizine. Concurrent use of anticholinergic drugs and MAOIs may also lead to more anticholinergic adverse effects such as dry mouth and constipation. Antihistamine effects may be potentiated excessively by interactions with apple, grapefruit and orange juice as well as St. John's wort. Rifampin reduces the absorption of fexofenadine. An allergist will usually recommend discontinuation of antihistamine drug therapy at least 4 days prior to allergy testing.

Dosages

For the recommended dosages for selected antihistamines, see the Dosages table on page 541.

Drug Profiles

Although some antihistamines are prescription drugs, most are available over the counter (OTC). Antihistamines are available in many dosage forms to be administered orally, intramuscularly, intravenously, or topically.

Nonsedating Antihistamines

A major advance in antihistamine therapy occurred with the development of the **nonsedating antihistamines** loratadine, cetirizine, and fexofenadine. These drugs were developed in part to eliminate many of the unwanted adverse effects (mainly sedation) of the older antihistamines. These drugs work peripherally to block the actions of histamine and therefore do not have the CNS effects that many older antihistamines do. For this reason these drugs are also called *peripherally acting antihistamines* because they tend not to cross the blood-brain barrier, unlike their traditional counterparts. Another advantage of these drugs over the older antihistamines is that they have longer durations of action, which allows some of them to be taken only once a day. This further increases compliance. These three drugs replace the two original nonsedating antihistamines terfenadine and astem-

izole, which were withdrawn from the U.S. market in the 1990s following several cases of fatal drug-induced cardiac dysrhythmias. Fexofenadine is actually the active metabolite of terfenadine but is not associated with such severe cardiac effects, nor are loratadine or cetirizine.

▶ loratadine

Loratadine (Claritin) is a nonsedating antihistamine. It needs to be taken only once a day. Structurally it is similar to cyproheptadine and azatadine, but unlike these drugs it cannot distribute into the CNS, which alleviates the sedative effects associated with traditional antihistamines. Loratadine is used to relieve the symptoms of seasonal allergic rhinitis (e.g., hay fever) as well as chronic urticaria. Loratadine has recently been converted to OTC status. However, a drug containing its primary active metabolite, desloratadine, has recently come on the U.S. market and is currently available by only by prescription (see drug profile).

Drug allergy is the only contraindication to the use of loratadine. The drug is available in oral form as a 10-mg tablet, as a 1-mg/mL syrup, as a 10-mg rapidly disintegrating tablet, and in a combination tablet with the decongestant pseudoephedrine. Pregnancy category B. See the table on page 541 for dosage information.

Pharmacokinetics

Half-Life	Onset	Peak	Duration
8.4-24 hr	1-3 hr	8-12 hr	24 hr

Traditional Antihistamines

The traditional antihistamines are the older drugs that work both peripherally and centrally. They also have anticholinergic effects, which in some cases make them more effective than nonsedating antihistamines. Some of these commonly used older drugs are diphenhydramine, brompheniramine, chlorpheniramine, dimenhydrinate, meclizine, and promethazine. These drugs are used either alone or in combination with other drugs in the symptomatic relief of many disorders ranging from insomnia to motion sickness. Many patients respond to and tolerate the older drugs quite well, and because many are generically available they are much less expensive. These drugs are available both OTC and by prescription.

▶ diphenhydramine

Diphenhydramine (Benadryl) is an older, traditional antihistamine that works both peripherally and centrally. It also has potent anticholinergic and sedative effects. In fact, it is still often used as a hypnotic drug because of its sedating effects. This use is not generally advised in elderly patients, however, because of the "hangover" effect and increased potential for falls. Diphenhydramine is one of the most commonly used antihistamines, in part because of its excellent safety profile and efficacy. It has the greatest range of therapeutic indications of any antihistamine available. It is used for the relief or prevention of histamine-mediated allergies and motion sickness, the treatment of Parkinson's disease (due to its anticholinergic effects), and the promotion of sleep. It is also used in conjunction with epinephrine in the management of anaphylaxis and in the treatment of acute dystonic reactions.

Diphenhydramine is classified as a pregnancy category B drug, and its use is contraindicated in patients with a known hypersensitivity to it, nursing mothers, neonates, and patients with lower respiratory tract symptoms. It is available in oral, parenteral, and topical preparations. In oral form, diphenhydramine is available as capsules, tablets, and liquid, as well as in several combination products that contain other cough and cold medications. In parenteral form, diphenhydramine is available as an injection. In topical form, diphenhydramine is available as a cream, gel, and spray. It also is available in combination with several other drugs that are commonly given topically, such as calamine, camphor, and zinc oxide. These combination preparations come in the form of aerosols, creams, gels, and lotions. The recommended dosages for the oral and injectable forms are given in the dosages table on page 541.

DOSAGES

Selected Antihistamines

Drug	Pharmacologic Class	Usual Dosage Range	Indications
Nonsedating Antihistamines			
cetirizine (Zyrtec)	H₁ antihistamine	**Adult and pediatric 6 yr and older** 5-10 mg once daily **Pediatric 2-5 yr** 2.5 mg once daily	Allergic rhinitis, chronic urticaria
desloratadine (Clarinex)	H₁ antihistamine	**Adult and pediatric 12 yr and older only** 5 mg once daily	Allergic rhinitis, chronic urticaria
fexofenadine (Allegra)	H₁ antihistamine	**Adult and pediatric 12 yr and older** 60 mg bid or 180 mg once daily **Pediatric 6-11 yr** 30 mg bid	Allergic rhinitis, chronic urticaria
▶loratadine (Claritin)	H₁ antihistamine	**Adult and pediatric 6 yr and older** 10 mg once daily **Pediatric 2-5 yr** 5 mg once daily	Allergic rhinitis, chronic urticaria
Traditional Antihistamines (More Commonly Associated with Sedation)			
chlorpheniramine (Chlor-Trimeton; less sedating)	H₁ antihistamine	**Pediatric 2-5 yr** 1 mg (¼ of a 4-mg tab) **Pediatric 6-12 yr** 2 mg q4-6h, max 12 mg/24 hr **Adult** Immediate-release tabs or syrup: 4 mg q4-6h, max 24 mg/24 hr **Adult and pediatric 12 yr and older** Timed-release tabs: 8 mg q8-12h or 12 mg q12h, max 24 mg/24 hr **Pediatric 6-12 yr** 8 mg once daily at bedtime or during the day	Allergic rhinitis
▶diphenhydramine (Benadryl; more sedating)	H₁ antihistamine	**Pediatric more than 10 kg** PO/IM/IV: 12.5-25 mg tid-qid **Adult and pediatric 12 yr and older** PO: 50 mg at bedtime **Adult only** PO/IM/IV: 25-50 mg tid-qid **Adult only** 25-50 mg tid-qid	Allergic disorders, nighttime insomnia, motion sickness Nighttime insomnia Allergic disorders, PD symptoms Motion sickness

IM, Intramuscular; *IV,* intravenous; *PD,* Parkinson's disease; *PO,* oral.

Pharmacokinetics

Half-Life	Onset	Peak	Duration
2-7 hr	15-30 min	1-2 hr	4 hr

DECONGESTANTS

Nasal congestion is due to excessive nasal secretions and inflamed and swollen nasal mucosa. The primary causes of nasal congestion are allergies and URIs, especially the common cold. There are three separate groups of nasal **decongestants: adrenergics (sympathomimetics),** which are the largest group; **anticholinergics (parasympatholytics),** which are somewhat less commonly used; and selected topical **corticosteroids** (intranasal steroids).

Nasal decongestants can be taken orally to produce a systemic effect, can be inhaled, or can be administered topically to the nose. Each method of administration has its advantages and disadvantages. Decongestants administered by the oral route include pseudoephedrine, which is available OTC. A commonly used nasal decongestant spray is phenylephrine, which is also OTC.

Drugs administered by the oral route produce prolonged decongestant effects, but the onset of action is more delayed and the effect less potent than those of decongestants applied topically. However, the clinical problem of rebound congestion associated

Goldenseal (*Hydrastis canadensis*)

Overview

Goldenseal is found in wooded areas from the northeastern to midwestern United States. It is the dried root of the plant that is most commonly used for its various biologically active alkaloids. These components have been shown to have antibacterial, antifungal, and antiprotozoal activity. The alkaloid berberine has both anticholinergic and antihistaminic activity.

Common Uses

Treatment of upper respiratory tract infections, allergies, nasal congestion, and numerous genitourinary, skin, ophthalmic, and otic conditions.

Adverse Effects

Gastrointestinal (GI) distress, emotional instability, mucosal ulceration (e.g., when used as a vaginal douche).

Potential Drug Interactions

Gastric acid suppressors (including antacids, histamine H_2 blockers [e.g., ranitidine], proton pump inhibitors [e.g., omeprazole]): theoretically reduced effectiveness due to acid-promoting effect of herb

Antihypertensives: theoretically reduced effectiveness due to vasoconstrictive activity of herb.

Contraindications

Acute or chronic GI disorders; pregnancy (has uterine stimulant properties); should be used with caution by those with cardiovascular disease

Data from Jellin J et al: *Natural medicines comprehensive database,* ed 6, Stockton, Calif, 2004, Therapeutic Research Faculty; Skidmore-Roth L: *Mosby's handbook of herbs and natural supplements,* ed 2, St Louis, 2004, Mosby.

with topically administered drugs is almost nonexistent with oral dosage forms. Rebound congestion occurs because of the very rapid absorption of drug through mucous membranes and delivery to adrenergic receptor within respiratory tissues, followed by a more rapid decline in therapeutic activity. This is in contrast to oral dosage forms, which provide a more gradual increase and decline in pharmacological activity due to the time required for GI absorption. Inhalation decongestants used orally include desoxyephedrine and propylhexedrine.

The topical administration of adrenergics into the nasal passages produces a potent decongestant effect with a prompt onset of action. However, sustained use of these drugs for several days can cause rebound congestion, which only exacerbates the condition. Decongestants suitable for nasal inhalation include the following:

- ephedrine (Pretz-D)
- naphazoline (Privine)
- oxymetazoline (Afrin)
- phenylephrine (Neo-Synephrine, Sinex)
- tetrahydrozoline (Tyzine Pediatric Drops)

Inhaled intranasal steroids and anticholinergic drugs are not generally associated with rebound congestion and are often used prophylactically to prevent nasal congestion in patients with chronic upper respiratory tract symptoms. Commonly used intranasal steroids include the following:

- beclomethasone dipropionate (Beconase, Vancenase)
- budesonide (Pulmicort Turbuhaler, Rhinocort, Rhinocort Turbuhaler)
- flunisolide (Nasalide)
- fluticasone (Flonase)
- triamcinolone (Nasacort)

The only commonly used intranasal anticholinergic drug at this time is ipratropium nasal spray (Atrovent).

Mechanism of Action and Drug Effects

Nasal decongestants are most commonly used for their ability to shrink engorged nasal mucous membranes and relieve nasal stuffiness. Adrenergic drugs (e.g., ephedrine, oxymetazoline) accomplish this by constricting the small arterioles that supply the structures of the upper respiratory tract, primarily the blood vessels surrounding the nasal sinuses. When these blood vessels are stimulated by α-adrenergic drugs, they constrict. Because sympathetic nervous system stimulation produces the same effect, these drugs are sometimes referred to as *sympathomimetics.* Once these blood vessels shrink, the nasal secretions in the swollen mucous membranes are better able to drain, either externally through the nostrils or internally through reabsorption into the bloodstream or lymphatic circulation.

Nasal steroids are aimed at the inflammatory response elicited by invading organisms (viruses and bacteria) or other antigens (e.g., allergens). The body responds to these antigens by producing inflammation in an effort to isolate or wall off the area and by attracting various cells of the immune system to consume and destroy the offending antigens. Steroids exert their antiinflammatory effect by causing these cells to be turned off or rendered unresponsive. It should be kept in mind, however, that the goal is *not* complete immunosuppression of the respiratory tract but rather the modulation of inflammatory symptoms to improve patient comfort and air exchange. The drug effects of intranasal steroids are discussed in more detail in Chapter 36.

Indications

Nasal decongestants reduce the nasal congestion associated with acute or chronic rhinitis, the common cold, sinusitis, and hay fever or other allergies. They may also be used to reduce swelling of the nasal passages and to facilitate visualization of the nasal and pharyngeal membranes before surgery or diagnostic procedures.

Contraindications

Contraindications to the use of decongestants include drug allergy and, in the case of adrenergic drugs, narrow-angle glaucoma, uncontrolled cardiovascular disease, hypertension, diabetes, hyperthyroidism, and prostatitis. Other contraindications may include situations in which the patient is unable to close his or her eyes (such as after a cerebrovascular accident [CVA]), as well as patients with a history of stroke or transient ischemic attacks, cerebral arteriosclerosis and long-standing asthma, CVA or transient ischemic attacks (TIAs), BPH, and diabetes.

Adverse Effects

Adrenergic drugs are usually well tolerated. Possible adverse effects of these drugs include nervousness, insomnia, palpitations, and tremor. The most common adverse effects of intranasal steroids are localized and include mucosal irritation and dryness.

Although a topically applied adrenergic nasal decongestant can be absorbed into the bloodstream, the amount is usually too small to cause systemic effects at normal dosages. Excessive dosages of these medications, however, are more likely to cause systemic effects elsewhere in the body. These may include cardiovascular effects such as hypertension and palpitations and CNS effects such as headache, nervousness, and dizziness. These systemic effects are the result of α-adrenergic stimulation of the heart, blood vessels, and CNS.

Interactions

There are few significant drug interactions with nasal decongestants. Systemic **sympathomimetic drugs** and sympathomimetic nasal decongestants are more likely to cause drug toxicity when given together. MAOIs may result in additive pressor effects (e.g., raising of the blood pressure) when given with sympathomimetic nasal decongestants. Other drug interactions include furazolidone, guanethidine, monoamine oxidase inhibitors, methyldopa, and urinary acidifiers and alkalinizers.

Dosages

For the recommended dosages of naphazoline, the only nasal decongestant profiled, see the Dosages table on this page.

Drug Profiles

Many of the decongestants are OTC drugs, but the more potent drugs that can cause serious adverse effects are available only by prescription. Use of adrenergic drugs is usually contraindicated in patients with diabetes, hypertension, cardiac disease, thyroid dysfunction, prostatitis, or a known hypersensitivity to these drugs. Although nasal steroids are relatively safe, their use is also contraindicated in some circumstances, including in patients with nasal mucosal infections (because of their ability to depress the body's immune response as part of their antiinflammatory effect) or known drug allergy.

Many inhaled corticosteroids (e.g., beclomethasone, dexamethasone, flunisolide) are discussed in greater detail in Chapter 36. The adrenergic drugs (e.g., naphazoline) are discussed in this chaper. Both of these drug categories are generally first-line drugs for the treatment of chronic nasal congestion.

naphazoline

Naphazoline (Privine) is chemically and pharmacologically very similar to the other sympathomimetic drugs oxymetazoline, tetrahydrozoline, and xylometazoline. When these drugs are administered intranasally they cause dilated arterioles to constrict, which reduces nasal blood flow and congestion. During a cold the blood vessels that

DOSAGES

Selected Decongestant, Expectorant, and Antitussive Drugs

Drug	Pharmacologic Class	Usual Dosage Range	Indications
benzonatate (Tessalon Perles)	Nonopioid antitussive	**Adult and pediatric older than 10 yr** 100-200 mg tid	
codeine (as part of a combination product such as Dimetane-DC, Tussar SF, Novahistine DH, Robitussin A-C, others)	Opioid antitussive	**Adult and pediatric older than 12 yr** 10-20 mg q4-6h, max 120 mg/24 hr **Pediatric 6-12 yr** 5-10 mg q4-6h, max 60 mg/24 hr **Pediatric 2-5 yr** 2.5-5 mg q4-6h, max 30 mg/24 hr	Cough suppression
dextromethorphan (as part of a combination product such as Vicks Formula 44, Robitussin-DM, others)	Nonopioid antitussive	**Adult and pediatric older than 12 yr** 10-30 mg q4-8h, max 120 mg/24 hr **Pediatric 6-12 yr** 5-10 mg q4h or 15 mg q6-8h, max 60 mg/24 hr **Pediatric 2-6 yr** 2.5-7.5 mg q4-8h, max 30 mg/24 hr	
guaifenesin [glyceryl guaiacolate] (Guiatuss, Humibid, Robitussin, others)	Expectorant	**Adult and pediatric 12 yr and older** 100-400 mg q4h, max 2400 mg/24 hr **Pediatric 6-12 yr** 100-200 mg q4h, max 1200 mg/24 hr **Pediatric 2-6 yr** 50-100 mg q4h, max 600 mg/24 hr	Relief of respiratory congestion, cough suppression
naphazoline (Privine)	α-Adrenergic vasoconstrictor	**Adult and pediatric 12 yr and older** 0.05%, 1 or 2 drops or sprays in each nostril q6h prn, usually for no more than 3-5 days	Relief of nasal congestion

surround the nasal sinus are usually dilated and engorged with plasma, white blood cells, mast cells, histamines, and many other blood components that are involved in fighting infections of the respiratory tract. This swelling, or dilation, blocks the nasal passages, which results in nasal congestion. Naphazoline and its chemically related cousins are classified as pregnancy category C drugs and have the same contraindications as the other nasal decongestants. Naphazoline for nasal administration is available as a 0.05% solution and is meant to be instilled into each nostril. Common dosages for this drug are given in the dosages table on page 543.

Pharmacokinetics

Half-Life	Onset	Peak	Duration
Unknown	5-10 min	Unknown	2-6 hr

ANTITUSSIVES

Coughing is a normal physiologic function and serves the purpose of removing potentially harmful foreign substances and excessive secretions from the respiratory tract. The cough reflex is stimulated when receptors in the bronchi, alveoli, and pleura (lining of the lungs) are stretched. This causes a signal to be sent to the cough center in the medulla of the brain, which in turn stimulates the cough. Although most of the time coughing is a beneficial response, there are times when it is not useful and may even be harmful (e.g., after a surgical procedure such as hernia repair or in cases of nonproductive or "dry" cough). In these situations it may enhance patient comfort and reduce respiratory distress to inhibit this otherwise normal response through the use of an **antitussive** drug. There are two main categories of antitussive drugs: opioid and nonopioid.

Although all opioid drugs have antitussive effects, only codeine and its semisynthetic derivative hydrocodone are used as antitussives. Both drugs are effective in suppressing the cough reflex, and if they are taken in the prescribed manner, their use should not lead to dependency. These two drugs are usually incorporated into various combination formulations with other respiratory drugs and are rarely used alone for the purpose of cough suppression.

Nonopioid antitussive drugs are less effective than opioid drugs and are available either alone or in combination with other drugs in an array of OTC cold and cough preparations. Dextromethorphan is the most widely used of these antitussive drugs and is a derivative of the synthetic opioid levorphanol. Benzonatate is another nonopioid drug.

Mechanism of Action and Drug Effects

The opioid antitussives codeine and hydrocodone suppress the cough reflex through direct action on the cough center in the CNS (medulla). Opioid antitussives also provide analgesia and have a drying effect on the mucosa of the respiratory tract, which increases the viscosity of respiratory secretions. This helps to reduce symptoms such as runny nose and postnasal drip. The nonopioid cough suppressant dextromethorphan works in the same way. Because it is not an opioid, however, it does not have analgesic properties, nor does it cause addiction or CNS depression. Another nonopioid antitussive is benzonatate. Its mechanism of action is entirely different from that of the other drugs. Benzonatate suppresses the cough reflex by anesthetizing (numbing)

the stretch receptor cells in the respiratory tract, which prevents **reflex stimulation** of the medullary cough center.

Indications

Although they have other properties, such as analgesic effects for the opioid drugs, antitussives are used primarily to stop the cough reflex when the cough is nonproductive and/or harmful.

Contraindications

The only absolute contraindication to the antitussives is drug allergy. Relative contraindications include opioid dependency (for opioid antitussives) and high risk for respiratory depression (e.g., in frail elderly patients). Patients with these conditions are often able to tolerate lower medication dosages and still experience some symptom relief.

Additional contraindications and cautions include the following: benzonatate: no known contraindications and cautious use in those with productive cough; codeine: see hydrocodone; dextromethorphan: contraindications of hyperthyroidism, advanced cardiac and vessel disease, hypertension, glaucoma and having taken MAOIs within the past 14 days; diphenydramine: see antihistamines; hydrocodone: contraindication with alcohol and extreme caution with CNS depression, anoxia, high serum levels of carbon dioxide (hypercapnia), and respiratory depression, and cautions of increased intracranial pressure, impaired renal function, and liver diseases, as well as BPH, Addison's disease, and COPD.

Adverse Effects

The following are the common adverse effects and adverse effects of selected antitussive drugs:

- *benzonatate:* dizziness, headache, sedation, nausea, constipation, pruritus, and nasal congestion
- *codeine:* sedation, nausea, vomiting, lightheadedness, and constipation
- *dextromethorphan:* dizziness, drowsiness, and nausea
- *diphenhydramine:* sedation, dry mouth, and other anticholinergic effects
- *hydrocodone:* sedation, nausea, vomiting, lightheadedness, and constipation

Interactions

Very few drug interactions occur with benzonatate, although some are associated with the use of opioid antitussives and dextromethorphan. Opioid antitussives (codeine and hydrocodone) may potentiate the effects of other opioids, general anesthetics, tranquilizers, sedatives and hypnotics, tricyclic antidepressants, MAOIs, alcohol, and other CNS depressants. Dextromethorphan may also potentiate the serotonergic effects of MAOIs, and thus concurrent administration is contraindicated.

Dosages

For the recommended dosages of selected antitussive drugs, see the Dosages table on page 543.

Drug Profiles

Antitussives come in many oral dosage forms and are available both with and without a prescription. Most of the narcotic antitussives are available only by prescription because of the associated abuse potential. Dextromethorphan is the most popular nonnarcotic antitussive available OTC.

benzonatate

Benzonatate (Tessalon Perles) is a nonopioid antitussive drug that, as mentioned earlier, is thought to work by anesthetizing or numbing the cough receptors. It is available only in oral form as a 100-mg capsule. Its use is contraindicated in patients with a known hypersensitivity to it. Pregnancy category C. Common dosages are listed in the Dosages table on page 543.

Pharmacokinetics

Half-Life	Onset	Peak	Duration
Unknown	15-20 min	Unknown	3-8 hr

codeine

Codeine (Dimetane-DC, Tussar SF, Novahistine DH, Robitussin A-C) is a very popular opioid antitussive drug. It is used in combination with many other respiratory medications to control coughs. Because it is an opioid it is potentially addictive and can depress respirations as part of its CNS depressant effects. For this reason codeine-containing cough suppressants are more tightly controlled substances. Although most states allow OTC purchase of at least one oral liquid combination product, the purchaser must usually be at least 18 years of age and be willing to sign a log book kept in the pharmacy. More commonly the patient has obtained a prescription for such products. These cough suppressants are available in many oral dosage forms: solutions, tablets, capsules, and suspensions. Their use is contraindicated in patients with a known hypersensitivity to opiates and in those who have respiratory depression, increased intracranial pressure, seizure disorders, or severe respiratory disorders. Pregnancy category C. Common dosages are listed in the table on page 543.

Pharmacokinetics

Half-Life	Onset	Peak	Duration
2.9 hr (plasma)	30-60 min	1-2 hr	4-6 hr

▶ dextromethorphan

Dextromethorphan (Vicks Formula 44, Robitussin-DM) is a nonopioid antitussive that is available alone or in combination with many other cough and cold preparations. It is widely used because it is safe and nonaddicting and does not cause respiratory or CNS depression. Its use is contraindicated in cases of drug allergy, asthma or emphysema, or persistent headache. Dextromethorphan is available as lozenges, solution, liquid-filled capsules, granules, tablets (chewable, extended release, and film coated), and extended-release suspension. Pregnancy category C. Common dosages are listed in the table on page 543.

Pharmacokinetics

Half-Life	Onset	Peak	Duration
Unknown	15-30 min	Unknown	3-6 hr

EXPECTORANTS

Expectorants aid in the expectoration (i.e., coughing up and spitting out) of excessive mucus that has accumulated in the respiratory tract by breaking down and thinning out the secretions. They are administered orally either as single drugs or in combination with other drugs to facilitate the flow of respiratory secretions by reducing the viscosity of tenacious secretions. The actual clinical effectiveness of expectorants is somewhat questionable, however. Placebo-controlled clinical evaluations have failed to strongly confirm that expectorants reduce the viscosity of sputum. Despite this, expectorants are popular drugs, are contained in most OTC cold and cough preparations, and provide symptom relief for many users. The most common expectorant in OTC products is guaifenesin (formerly known as glyceryl guaiacolate). Two other expectorants are less commonly used and are available only by prescription. These are iodinated glycerol and potassium iodide.

Mechanism of Action and Drug Effects

Expectorants have one of two different mechanisms of action, depending on the drug. The first is reflex stimulation, in which loosening and thinning of respiratory tract secretions occurs in response to an irritation of the GI tract produced by the drug. Guaifenesin is the only such drug currently available. The second mechanism of action is direct stimulation of the secretory glands in the respiratory tract. Iodine-containing products (iodinated glycerol and potassium iodide) are believed to work in this way.

Indications

Expectorants are used for the relief of productive cough commonly associated with the common cold, bronchitis, laryngitis, pharyngitis, pertussis, influenza, and measles. They may also be used for the suppression of coughs caused by chronic paranasal sinusitis. By loosening and thinning sputum and the bronchial secretions, they may also indirectly diminish the tendency to cough.

Contraindications

Contraindications include drug allergy and possibly hyperkalemia (for potassium-containing expectorants).

Adverse Effects

The adverse effects of expectorants are minimal. The most common adverse effects of the individual expectorants are listed in Table 35-4.

Interactions

The drug interactions most commonly associated with expectorant use occur with the iodinated products. These drugs may produce an additive or synergistic hypothyroid effect when used concurrently with lithium or antithyroid drugs. Their use with other potassium-containing drugs or potassium-sparing diuretics may lead to the development of hyperkalemia, which can result in cardiac dysrhythmias or cardiac arrest.

Dosages

The recommended dosages of guaifenesin, the only expectorant profiled, are given in the Dosages table on page 543.

Table 35-4	Expectorants: Reported Adverse Effects
Expectorant	**Adverse Effects**
guaifenesin	Nausea, vomiting, gastric irritation
iodinated glycerol	Gastrointestinal irritation, rash, enlarged thyroid gland
potassium iodide	Iodism, nausea, vomiting, taste perversion

Drug Profiles

▶ guaifenesin

Guaifenesin (Guiatuss, Humibid, Robitussin) is a very commonly used expectorant that is available in several different oral dosage forms: capsules, tablets, solutions, and granules. It is used in the symptomatic management of coughs of varying origin. It is beneficial in the treatment of productive coughs because it thins mucus in the respiratory tract that is difficult to cough up. There is little published pharmacokinetic data on guaifenesin, but its half-life is estimated to be approximately 1 hour. This short half-life helps to explain why it is usually dosed several times throughout the day. However, though this drug remains popular, there is some literature evidence to suggest that it has no greater therapeutic activity than water in terms of loosening respiratory tract secretions. Pregnancy category C. See the table on page 543 for the common dosages.

◆ NURSING PROCESS

◆ ASSESSMENT

When the patient is to be given drugs to treat symptoms related to the respiratory tract, the nurse should begin the assessment by gathering data about the condition and determining whether symptoms are caused by an allergic reaction. Obtaining the patient's medical history and medication profile, completing a thorough head-to-toe physical assessment, and taking a nursing history are critical to understanding possible causes, risks, or links to diseases or conditions such as allergy, a cold, or flu. For example, if an allergic reaction to a drug, food, or substance has occurred, the patient may be experiencing signs and symptoms such as hives, wheezing or bronchospasm, tachycardia, or hypotension, whereas if the cause is a cold or flu, the symptoms will be different and will be treated completely differently in most cases. The drug of choice is then selected based on the severity of the symptoms and their cause.

Before administering the traditional antihistamines such as diphenhydramine, chlorpheniramine, or brompheniramine, the nurse must ensure that the patient has no allergies to this group of medications, even though these drugs are used for allergic reactions. Contraindications, cautions, and drug interactions need to be assessed with this and all other drugs. Use of these antihistamines is of concern in patients who are experiencing an acute asthma attack and in those who have lower respiratory tract disease or are at risk for pneumonia. The rationale for not using these drugs in these situations is because antihistamines dry up secretions; if the patient cannot expectorate the secretions, the secretions may become viscous (thick), occlude airways, and lead to atelectasis or further infection or occlusion of the bronchioles. It is also important to know that these drugs may lead to paradoxical reactions in the elderly, with subsequent irritability as well as dizziness, confusion, sedation and hypotension.

Most nonsedating antihistamines (e.g., fexofenadine, loratadine, desloratadine, cetirizine) are not to be used in patients younger than 6 years of age. Allergies and other contraindications, cautions, and drug interactions should be assessed prior to use. It is important to remember with the traditional and nontraditional antihistamines that if allergy testing is to be performed, these medications should be discontinued at least 4 days before the testing, but only with a physician's order.

With antitussive therapy, assessment is tailored to the patient and the specific drug. Most of these drugs result in sedation, dizziness, and drowsiness, so assessment of the patient's safety is very important. A history of allergies, contraindications, cautions, and drug interactions should be completed and documented. Respiratory assessment (as with all of the drugs in this chapter) should include rate, rhythm and depth, as well as breath sounds, presence of cough, and description of cough and sputum if present. For individuals with chronic respiratory disease, the physician may order serum levels of carbon dioxide, PaO_2, and other blood gas information (e.g., blood pH).

Use of decongestants requires assessment of contraindications, cautions, and drug interactions. Because decongestants are available in oral, nasal drops/sprays, and eyedrop dosage forms, any condition that could affect the functional structures of the eye or nose may be a possible caution or contraindication. Decongestants may increase blood pressure and heart rate, so there should be assessment and documentation of the patient's blood pressure, pulse, and other vital parameters.

Inhaled intranasal steroids and anticholinergic drugs are not generally associated with rebound congestion but may be used prophylactically to prevent nasal congestion in patients with chronic upper respiratory tract symptoms. Contraindications, cautions, and drug interactions, as with all the drugs in this chapter, need to be thoroughly assessed prior to use. For patients who have a cough and need to bring up secretions more easily, expectorants are often recommended or prescribed. Assessment of cough and sputum, if present, should be noted in addition to all of the previously identified parameters.

◆ NURSING DIAGNOSES

- Impaired gas exchange related to the disorder, condition, or disease affecting the respiratory system and various respiratory-related signs and symptoms
- Deficient knowledge related to the effective use of cold medications and other related products due to lack of information and patient teaching
- Ineffective airway clearance related to diminished ability to cough and/or a suppressed cough reflex (with antitussives)
- Risk for injury or falls related to the sedating adverse effects of many of these related drugs
- Risk for injury related to sensory-perceptual alterations from drug-induced drowsiness and/or sedation

CASE STUDY
Decongestants

A 22-year-old college student has suffered with allergy symptoms since moving into his dormitory. When he calls the student health center, he is told to try an over-the-counter nasal decongestant. He tries this and is excited about the relief he experiences until 2 weeks later, when his symptoms return. He calls the student health center again, upset because his symptoms are now worse.

- What explanation do you have for the worsening symptoms?
- What patient education should he have received about this type of drug?
- What other over-the-counter drugs and nonpharmacologic measures could be suggested for this situation?

For answers, see http://evolve.elsevier.com/Lilley.

◆ PLANNING

Goals

- Patient states rationale for the use of antihistamine, expectorant, antitussive, or decongestant.
- Patient states the adverse effects of medication.
- Patient states the importance of compliance with the therapy regimen.
- Patient identifies symptoms to report to the physician.
- Patient states the importance of follow-up appointments with the physician.
- Patient indicates relief of symptoms with treatment.
- Patient regains near-normal or normal (baseline) respiratory patterns and function.
- Patient remains free of excessive drowsiness or sedation.

Outcome Criteria

- Patient remains compliant with the antihistamine, antitussive, decongestant, or expectorant medication regimen until symptoms are resolved or the physician orders discontinuation.
- Patient takes medications exactly as prescribed to avoid complications of therapy, achieve maximal effectiveness, and minimize adverse effects.
- Patient reports any of the following symptoms to the physician immediately: increase in cough, congestion, shortness of breath, chest pain, fever (a temperature above 100.4° F or 38° C), or any change in sputum production or color (i.e., if not clear or if a change from baseline).
- Patient identifies specific safety precautions to help prevent injury related to drug-induced CNS depressant adverse effects, such as moving purposefully and slowly, asking for assistance as needed, minimizing use of other CNS depressant drugs, and, if elderly or at high risk for injury, obtaining assistance with activities of daily living and with mobility.
- Patient reports resolution of symptoms and an improved health status, such as return of temperature to baseline, return of secretions or sputum to clear color and normal consistency, return to normal breathing rate and patterns, and clearing of breath sounds.

◆ IMPLEMENTATION

Patients taking traditional antihistamines (e.g., diphenhydramine) should take the medications as prescribed. Most of these medications, including the OTC antihistamines, are best tolerated when taken with meals. Although food may slightly decrease absorption of these drugs, it has the benefit of minimizing the GI upset these drugs may cause. Patients who experience dry mouth should be encouraged to chew or suck on candy (sugar-free if needed) or OTC throat, cough, or cold lozenges, or to chew gum, as well as to perform frequent mouth care to ease the dryness and related discomfort. Other OTC or prescribed cold or cough medications should not be taken with antihistamines unless they were previously approved or ordered by the physician because of the potential for serious drug inter-

actions. Dosage amounts and routes may vary depending on whether the patient is elderly, adult aged, or under the age of 12 years, so proper dosing and usage should be encouraged. Blood pressure and other vital signs should be monitored as needed. The elderly and children should be monitored for any paradoxical reactions, which are common with these drugs.

If patients are receiving any of the newer nonsedating antihistamines, the drugs should be taken very carefully and as directed. Reduced dosages may be needed for patients who are elderly or have decreased renal functioning. These newer H_1 receptor antagonist drugs do not cross the blood-brain barrier as readily as do older antihistamines and are therefore less likely to cause sedation. They are generally very well tolerated with minimal adverse effects.

With antitussives, chewable or lozenge forms of the drugs should be used exactly as ordered. Drowsiness or dizziness may occur with the use of antitussives; therefore, patients should be cautioned against driving a car or engaging in other activities that requires mental alertness until they feel back to normal. If the antitussive contains codeine, the CNS depressant effects of the narcotic opiate may further depress breathing and respiratory effort. Other antitussives, such as dextromethorphan, as well as the codeine-containing drugs should be given at evenly spaced intervals so that the drug reaches a steady state.

Patients taking decongestants, such as pseudoephedrine or phenylephrine, are generally using the drugs for nasal decongestion. These drugs come in oral dosage forms, including sustained-release and chewable forms. With the use of any of the drugs discussed in this chapter and the disorders or diseases for which they are being taken, it is also important to encourage fluid intake of up to 3000 mL a day, unless contraindicated. The fluid helps to liquefy secretions, assists in breaking up thick secretions, and makes it easier to cough up secretions.

Patient teaching tips for these drugs are presented on page 548.

◆ EVALUATION

A therapeutic response to drugs given to treat respiratory conditions, such as antihistamines, antitussives, decongestants, and expectorants, includes resolution of the symptoms for which the drugs were originally prescribed or taken. These symptoms may include cough; nasal, sinus, or chest congestion; nasal, salivary, and lacrimal gland hypersecretion; motion sickness; sneezing; watery, red, or itchy eyes; itchy nose; allergic rhinitis; and allergic symptoms. Some of the antihistamines, such as diphenhydramine, are also helpful as sleep aids, and a therapeutic response when taken for this purpose would be the successful induction of sleep. Adverse effects for which to monitor in patients using any of these drugs include excessively dry mouth, drowsiness, oversedation, dizziness (lightheadedness), paradoxical excitement, nervousness, dysrhythmias, palpitations, GI upset, urinary retention, fever, dyspnea, chest pain, headache, and insomnia, depending on the drug prescribed.

Patient Teaching Tips

- Educate patients about the possibility of tolerance to the sedating effects of traditional antihistamines. Patients should be informed to avoid activities that require alertness until tolerance to sedation occurs or until a patient accurately judges the fact that the drug has no impact on motor skills or responses to motor activities. Other areas to include in patient education include a list of drugs for the patient to avoid, including alcohol and CNS depressants.

- With traditional and nonsedating antihistamines, patients may require use of a humidifier to help liquefy sections, making expectoration of sputum easier. Fluids should be encouraged unless contraindicated.

- Patients with upper or lower respiratory symptoms or disease processes should know to avoid dry air, smoke-filled environments and allergens.

- Encourage the patient to *always* check possible drug interactions because of the many OTC and prescription drugs that could lead to adverse effects if taken concurrently.

- Educate the patient about taking the medication with food to help avoid GI upset.

- Inform the patient to report to the health care provider any difficulty breathing, palpitations, hallucinations, or tremors.

- Antitussives should be taken with caution, with the patient being fully aware of the fact that he or she should report fever, chest tightness, change in sputum from clear to colored, difficult or noisy breathing, activity intolerance, and weakness.

- Instruct the patient to use decongestants only as ordered and adhere to dose and frequency instructions. Emphasize the fact that frequent, long-term, or excessive use of decongestants (whether oral forms or nasal inhaled forms) may lead to rebound congestion in which the nasal passages become more congested as the effects of the drug wear off; when this occurs, the patient generally uses more of the drug, precipitating a vicious cycle with more congestion. Patients should be encouraged to report excessive dizziness, heart palpitations, weakness, sedation, and/or excessive irritability to the physician.

- Patients taking expectorants should avoid alcohol or use of products containing alcohol, and they should not use these medications for longer than 1 week. If cough or symptoms continue, they should know to contact their physician. Fluids should be encouraged (unless contraindicated) to help thin secretions for easier expectoration.

Points to Remember

- There are two types of histamine blockers: H_1 blockers and H_2 blockers. H_1 blockers are the drugs to which most people are referring when they use the term *antihistamine*. H_1 blockers prevent the harmful effects of histamine and are used to treat seasonal allergic rhinitis, anaphylaxis, reactions to insect bites, and so forth. H_2 blockers are used to treat gastric acid disorders, such as hyperacidity or ulcer disease.

- Patients should be educated thoroughly about the purposes of their medication, the expected adverse effects, and the drugs that possibly lead to negative interactions. Patients should be informed about the availability of newer, nonsedating antihistamines. Patients taking a nonsedating antihistamine—or *any* drug—should know to inform their physicians and other health care providers (e.g., dentists) that they are taking this medication. The nurse should be sure also to educate patients about measures to decrease the dry mouth associated with nonsedating antihistamines.

- Decongestants work by causing constriction of the engorged and swollen blood vessels in the sinuses, which decreases pressure and allows mucous membranes to drain. Nurses must under-

stand the action of these drugs and know other important information such as significant adverse effects, including cardiac and CNS stimulating effects that may result in palpitations, insomnia, restlessness, and nervousness.

- Nonopioid antitussive drugs may also cause sedation, drowsiness, or dizziness. Patients should not drive a car or engage in other activities that require mental alertness if these adverse effects occur. Codeine-containing antitussives may lead to CNS depression; they should be used cautiously and should not be mixed with anything containing alcohol.

- Any of the drugs presented in this chapter may interact with many OTC preparations, especially other OTC cold products; therefore, patients should always check the package insert to determine drug interactions.

- Decongestants and expectorants are recommended to treat cold symptoms, but patients should be encouraged to report to the physician a fever of over 100.4° F, cough, or other symptoms lasting longer than 4 days with decongestants or any other of the drugs presented in this chapter.

NCLEX Examination Review Question

1. When assessing a patient who is to receive a decongestant, the nurse will recognize that a potential contraindication to this drug is:
   a. Glaucoma
   b. Fever
   c. Ulcer disease
   d. Allergic rhinitis
2. When giving decongestants, the nurse must remember that these drugs have α-stimulating effects that may result in:
   a. Fever
   b. Bradycardia
   c. Hypertension
   d. CNS depression
3. The nurse is reviewing a patient's medication orders for prn (as necessary) medications that can be given to a patient who has pneumonia with a productive cough. Which drug should the nurse choose?
   a. An antitussive
   b. An expectorant
   c. An antihistamine
   d. A decongestant

4. An antitussive cough medication would be the best choice for which patient?
   a. A patient with a productive cough
   b. A patient with chronic paranasal sinusitis
   c. A patient who has had recent abdominal surgery
   d. A patient who has influenza
5. A patient is taking a decongestant to help reduce symptoms of a cold. The nurse should instruct the patient to observe for which possible symptom, which may indicate an adverse effect of this drug?
   a. Increased cough
   b. Dry mouth
   c. Slower heart rate
   d. Heart palpitations

1. a, 2. c, 3. b, 4. c, 5. d.

Critical Thinking Activities

1. Why should antihistamines be used with caution in asthmatic patients?
2. Discuss the problem of rebound congestion when nasal spray decongestants are used. Does this phenomenon also occur with oral decongestants? Explain your answer.

3. What additional nursing interventions would be helpful for an older patient without major medical problems who is taking guaifenesin?

For answers, see http://evolve.elsevier.com/Lilley.

Bronchodilators and Other Respiratory Drugs

Objectives

When you reach the end of this chapter, you should be able to do the following:

1. Describe the anatomy and physiology of the respiratory system.
2. Discuss the impact of respiratory drugs on various lower and upper respiratory tract diseases and conditions.
3. List the various classifications of drugs, with specific examples of each class.
4. Discuss the mechanisms of action, indications, contraindications, cautions, drug interactions, dosages, routes of administration, adverse effects, and toxic effects of the bronchodilators and other respiratory drugs.
5. Develop a nursing care plan that includes all phases of the nursing process for patients who use bronchodilators and other respiratory drugs.

e-Learning Activities

Companion CD

- NCLEX Review Questions: see questions 312-327
- Animations
- Audio Glossary
- Category Catchers
- Medication Errors Checklists
- IV Therapy Checklists

evolve Website (http://evolve.elsevier.com/Lilley)

- Nursing Care Plans • Frequently Asked Questions • Content Updates • WebLinks • Supplemental Resources • Elsevier ePharmacology Update • Medication Administration Animations

Drug Profiles

▶ albuterol, p. 554
fluticasone, p. 560
ipratropium, p. 555
methylprednisolone, p. 561
▶ montelukast, p. 558
▶ theophylline, p. 556

▶ Key drug.

Glossary

Allergen   Any substance that evokes an allergic response. (p. 551)

Allergic asthma   Bronchial asthma caused by hypersensitivity to an allergen or allergens. (p. 551)

Alveoli   Microscopic sacs in the lungs where oxygen is exchanged for carbon dioxide; also called *air sacs*. (p. 551)

Antibodies   Immunoglobulins produced by lymphocytes in response to bacteria, viruses, or other antigenic substances. (p. 551)

Antigen   A substance (usually a protein) that causes the formation of an antibody and reacts specifically with that antibody. (p. 551)

Asthma attack   The onset of wheezing together with difficulty breathing. (p. 551)

Bronchial asthma   General term for recurrent and reversible shortness of breath resulting from narrowing of the bronchi and bronchioles; it is often referred to simply as *asthma*. (p. 551)

Bronchodilators   Medications that improve airflow by relaxing bronchial smooth muscle cells (e.g., xanthines, adrenergic agonists). (p. 552)

Chronic bronchitis   Chronic inflammation of the bronchi. (p. 551)

Emphysema   A condition of the lungs characterized by enlargement of the air spaces distal to the bronchioles. (p. 551)

Immunoglobulins   Proteins belonging to any of five structurally and antigenically distinct classes of antibodies present in the serum and external secretions of the body; they play a major role in immune responses; *immunoglobulin* is often abbreviated *Ig*. (p. 551)

Lower respiratory tract (LRT)   The division of the respiratory system composed of organs located almost entirely within the chest. (p. 550)

Status asthmaticus   A prolonged asthma attack. (p. 551)

Upper respiratory tract (URT)   The division of the respiratory system composed of organs located outside the chest cavity (thorax). (p. 550)

The main function of the respiratory system is to deliver oxygen to, and remove carbon dioxide from, the cells of the body. To perform this deceptively simple task requires a very intricate system of tissues, muscles, and organs called the respiratory system. It consists of two divisions or tracts: the upper and lower respiratory tracts. The **upper respiratory tract (URT)** is composed of the structures that are located outside of the chest cavity or *thorax*. These are the nose, nasopharynx, oropharynx, laryngopharynx, and larynx. The **lower respiratory tract (LRT)** is located almost entirely within the thorax and is composed of the trachea, all segments of the bronchial tree, and the lungs. The URT and LRT have four main accessory structures that aid in their overall function. These are the oral cavity (mouth), the rib cage, the muscles of the rib cage (intercostal muscles), and the diaphragm. The URT and LRT together with the accessory structures make up the respiratory system, and the elements of this system are in constant communication with each other as they perform the vital function of respiration and the exchange of oxygen for carbon dioxide.

The air we breathe is a mixture of many gases. During inhalation, oxygen molecules from the air diffuse across the semipermeable membranes of the **alveoli,** where they are exchanged for carbon dioxide molecules, which are exhaled. The lungs also filter, warm, and humidify the air we breathe. The oxygen is then delivered to the cells by the blood vessels of the circulatory system. It is here that the respiratory system transfers the oxygen it has extracted from inhaled air to the hemoglobin protein molecules contained within red blood cells. It is also here that the cellular metabolic waste product carbon dioxide is collected from the tissues by the red blood cells. This waste is then transported back to the lungs via the circulatory system, where it diffuses back across the alveolar membranes and is then exhaled into the air. The respiratory system also plays a central role in speech, smell, and regulation of pH (acid-base balance).

DISEASES OF THE RESPIRATORY SYSTEM

Several diseases impair the function of the respiratory system. Those that affect the URT include colds, rhinitis, and hay fever. These conditions and the drugs used to treat them are discussed in Chapter 35. The major diseases that impair the function of the LRT include asthma, **emphysema,** and **chronic bronchitis.** The one feature these diseases have in common is that they all involve the obstruction of airflow through the airways. Chronic obstructive pulmonary disease (COPD) is the name applied collectively to emphysema and chronic bronchitis because the obstruction is relatively constant. Asthma that is persistent and present most of the time despite treatment is also considered a COPD. Cystic fibrosis and infant respiratory distress syndrome are other disorders that affect the LRT, but because the treatment for them places more emphasis on nonpharmacologic than on pharmacologic measures, they are not a focus of the discussion in this chapter.

ASTHMA

Bronchial asthma is defined as a recurrent and reversible shortness of breath and occurs when the airways of the lung (bronchi and bronchioles) become narrow as a result of bronchospasm, inflammation and edema of the bronchial mucosa, and the production of viscid (sticky) mucus. The alveolar ducts and alveoli distal to the bronchioles remain open, but the obstruction to the airflow in the airways prevents carbon dioxide from getting out of the air spaces and oxygen from getting into them. Wheezing and difficulty breathing are the symptoms. When an episode has a sudden and dramatic onset, it is referred to as an **asthma attack.** Most asthma attacks are short, and normal breathing is subsequently recovered. However, an asthma attack may be prolonged for several minutes to hours and may not respond to typical drug therapy. This is a condition known as **status asthmaticus** and often requires hospitalization. The onset of asthma occurs before 10 years of age in 50% of patients and before 40 years of age in about 80% of patients.

There are three categories of asthma: allergic, idiopathic, and mixed allergic-idiopathic asthma. Approximately 2% of the general population is affected by one of these three types. Allergic asthma accounts for approximately 30% to 35% of the cases of asthma, idiopathic asthma for about 35% to 50%, and the mixed form for the remaining cases.

Allergic asthma is caused by a hypersensitivity to an allergen or allergens in the environment. An **allergen** is any substance that elicits an allergic reaction. In patients with seasonal asthma the allergen is a substance such as pollen or mold, which is present only periodically (seasonally). The offending allergens in patients with nonseasonal asthma are substances such as dust, mold, and animal danders, which are present in the environment throughout the year. Cigarette smoke, from either smoking or exposure to secondhand smoke, is another common allergen. Examples of common food allergens include nuts, eggs, and corn. Exposure to the offending allergen in a patient with either type of allergic asthma causes an immediate allergic reaction in the form of an asthma attack. This attack is mediated by antibodies already present in the patient's body that chemically recognize the allergen to be a foreign substance, or **antigen.** These **antibodies** are specialized immune system proteins known as **immunoglobulins.** The antibody in asthma sufferers is usually immunoglobulin E (IgE), which is one of the five types of antibodies in the body (the others are IgG, IgA, IgM, and IgD). On exposure to the allergen, the patient's body responds by mounting an immediate and potent antigen-antibody reaction (*immune response*). This reaction occurs on the surfaces of cells such as *mast cells* that are rich in *histamines, leukotrienes,* and other substances involved in the immune response. These substances are collectively known as *inflammatory mediators,* and they are released from the mast cells as part of the immune response. This in turn, as described in the previous chapter, triggers the mucosal swelling and bronchoconstriction that are characteristic of an allergic asthma attack. The sequence of events that occurs in a patient with allergic asthma is shown in Box 36-1.

Box 36-1   Steps Involved in an Attack of Allergic Asthma

- The offending allergen provokes the production of hypersensitive antibodies (most commonly immunoglobulin E [IgE]) that are specific to the allergen. This immunologic response initiates patient sensitivity.
- The IgE antibodies are homocytotropic and collect on the surface of mast cells, thus sensitizing the patient to the allergen.
- Subsequent allergen contact provokes the antigen-antibody reaction on the surface of mast cells.
- Mast cell integrity is then violated, and these cells release chemical mediators stored in the cell. They also synthesize and then release other chemical mediators. These mediators include bradykinin, eosinophil chemotactic factor of anaphylaxis, histamine, prostaglandins, and slow-reacting substance of anaphylaxis (SRS-A).
- The released chemical mediators, especially histamine and SRS-A, trigger bronchial constriction and an asthma attack.

Box 36-2	Classifications of Drugs Used to Treat Asthma

Long-Term Control
Antileukotriene drugs
cromolyn
Inhaled steroids
ipratropium
Long-acting β₂-agonists
nedocromil
theophylline

Quick Relief
Intravenous systemic corticosteroids
Short-acting inhaled β₂-agonists

Table 36-1	Stepwise Therapy for the Management of Asthma

Step	Drug Classification
Step 1: Mild intermittent	Short-acting inhaled β₂-agonists prn
Step 2: Mild persistent	Cromolyn or nedocromil (particularly in children) and low-dose inhaled corticosteroids (preferred) plus short-acting inhaled β₂-agonists prn Theophylline and antileukotriene drugs considered second line
Step 3: Moderate persistent	Medium-dose inhaled corticosteroids Long-acting bronchodilator (salmeterol preferred) Short-acting inhaled β₂-agonists prn
Step 4: Severe persistent	High-dose inhaled corticosteroids Long-acting bronchodilators Systemic corticosteroids Short-acting inhaled β₂-agonists prn

The specific cause of idiopathic, or intrinsic, asthma is unknown. It is not mediated by IgE, and there is often no family history of allergies in affected patients. However, certain factors have been noted to precipitate asthma attacks in these patients, including respiratory infections, stress, cold weather, and strenuous work or exercise. As the name implies, mixed allergic-idiopathic asthma results from a combination of allergic and idiopathic factors. Patients with any type of asthma who know their suspected "triggers," whether an allergen, weather, or other factor, are advised to avoid these triggers as much as is feasible as part of managing their disease. When it is not feasible or advisable to avoid a certain trigger (e.g., exercise), patients should work with their health care providers to mitigate the response to these triggers through appropriate drug therapy (e.g., use of a bronchodilator inhaler before exercise or other strenuous activity).

The National Asthma Education and Prevention Panel (NAEPP) of the National Heart, Lung, and Blood Institute has maintained ongoing guidelines for the diagnosis and management of asthma since 1989. The current guideline revision was published in 2002. In general, these guidelines classify asthma medications as either for long-term symptom control or rapid symptom relief. The specific drugs in each classification are listed in Box 36-2. The guidelines advocate the use of a stepwise approach in the treatment of asthma. The particular steps and recommended drug classifications for treatment at each step are listed in Table 36-1.

CHRONIC BRONCHITIS

Chronic bronchitis is a continuous inflammation of the bronchi. The inflammation in the associated bronchioles (smaller bronchi) is responsible for most of the airflow obstruction. Chronic bronchitis involves the excessive secretion of mucus and certain pathologic changes in the bronchial structure. The disease can arise as a result of repeated episodes of acute bronchitis or in the context of chronic generalized diseases. It is usually precipitated by prolonged exposure to bronchial irritants. One of the most common is cigarette smoke. Some patients acquire the disease because of other predisposing factors such as viral or bacterial pulmonary infections during childhood. Others may have mild impairment of the ability to inactivate *proteolytic* (protein-destroying) enzymes, which then damage the airway mucosal tissues. Unknown genetic characteristics may be responsible as well.

EMPHYSEMA

Emphysema is a condition in which the air spaces enlarge as a result of the destruction of the alveolar walls. This appears to be caused by the effect of proteolytic enzymes released from leukocytes in response to alveolar inflammation. Because the alveolar walls are then partially destroyed, the surface area available for oxygen and carbon dioxide exchange is reduced, which impairs effective respiration. As with chronic bronchitis, smoking appears to be the primary irritant responsible for precipitating the underlying inflammation that leads to the development of emphysema. There is also an associated genetic deficiency in some people of the enzyme α_1-antitrypsin.

TREATMENT OF DISEASES OF THE LOWER RESPIRATORY TRACT

In the past the treatment of asthma and other COPDs focused primarily on the use of drugs that cause the airways to dilate. Now there is a greater understanding of the pathophysiology of asthma. The emphasis of research has shifted from the bronchoconstriction component of the disease to the inflammatory component. This is also reflected in the various medication classes used to treat COPDs, although bronchodilators still play an important role. A synopsis of the mechanisms of action of the various classes of antiasthmatic drugs is provided in Table 36-2.

BRONCHODILATORS

Bronchodilators are an important part of the pharmacotherapy for all COPDs. These drugs are able to relax bronchial smooth muscle bands to dilate the bronchi and bronchioles that are narrowed as a result of the disease process. There are three classes of such drugs: β-agonists, anticholinergics, and xanthine derivatives.

β-ADRENERGIC AGONISTS

The β-agonists are a large group of drugs that are commonly used during the acute phase of an asthmatic attack to quickly reduce airway constriction and restore airflow to normal. They are agonists or stimulators of the adrenergic receptors in the sympathetic nervous system. The β- and α-adrenergic receptors are discussed in Chapters 17 and 18. The β-agonists imitate the effects of norepinephrine on these receptors. For this reason they are also called sympathomimetic bronchodilators. Available asthma-related drugs in this class include albuterol (e.g., Ventolin), epinephrine, metaproterenol (Alupent), and ephedrine.

Mechanism of Action and Drug Effects

The β-agonists dilate airways by stimulating the β_2-adrenergic receptors located throughout the lungs.

There are three subtypes of these drugs, based on their selectivity for β_2 receptors:
1. Nonselective adrenergic drugs, which stimulate the α, β_1 (cardiac), and β_2 (respiratory) receptors. Example: epinephrine.
2. Nonselective β-adrenergic drugs, which stimulate both β_1 and β_2 receptors. Example: metaproterenol.
3. Selective β_2 drugs, which primarily stimulate the β_2 receptors. Example: albuterol.

These drugs can also be categorized according to their routes of administration as oral, injectable, or inhalational drugs. The various β-agonist bronchodilators are listed in Table 36-3.

The bronchioles are surrounded by smooth muscle. If this smooth muscle contracts, the airways are narrowed and the amount of oxygen and carbon dioxide exchanged is reduced. The action of β-agonist bronchodilators begins at the specific receptor stimulated and ends with the dilation of the airways, but many reactions must take place at the cellular level for this bronchodilation to occur. When a β_2-adrenergic receptor is stimulated by a β-agonist, adenylate cyclase, an enzyme needed to make cyclic adenosine monophosphate (cAMP), is activated. The increased

Table 36-2   Mechanisms of Antiasthmatic Drug Action

Antiasthmatic	Mechanism in Asthma Relief
Anticholinergics	Block cholinergic receptors, thus preventing the binding of cholinergic substances that cause constriction and increase secretions
Antileukotriene drugs	Modify or inhibit the activity of leukotrienes, which decreases arachidonic acid–induced inflammation and allergen-induced bronchoconstriction
β-Agonists and xanthine derivatives	Raise intracellular levels of cAMP, which in turn produces smooth muscle relaxation and dilates the constricted bronchi and bronchioles
Corticosteroids	Prevent the inflammation commonly provoked by the substances released from mast cells
Mast cell stabilizers (cromolyn and nedocromil)	Stabilize the cell membranes of the mast cells in which the antigen-antibody reactions take place, thereby preventing the release of substances such as histamine that cause constriction

cAMP, Cyclic adenosine monophosphate.

PREVENTING MEDICATION ERRORS

Oral Ingestion of Capsules for Inhalation Devices

Some inhalation products use capsules and a device that pierces the capsules to allow the powdered medication to be inhaled with a special inhaler. Two products, Foradil Aerolizer (formoterol fumarate inhalation powder) and Spiriva HandiHaler (tiotropium bromide inhalation powder) contain such capsules. Even though these capsules are packaged with inhaler devices, they closely resemble oral capsules. The FDA has received reports that the capsules have been taken orally by patients, resulting in potential adverse effects. If the capsules are swallowed instead of taken with the inhalation device, the medication's onset of action may be delayed, the efficacy is reduced, and as a result the patient receives inadequate drug delivery. The FDA has taken steps to work with the drug manufacturers to mark the packaging clearly. Nurses need to be certain to instruct patients on the proper use and correct route of administration for these inhaled drugs to prevent confusion with oral products.

From the FDA Safety Page: *Misadministration of capsules for inhalation.* (Tezky T, Holquist C), April 4, 2005. Available at www.drugtopics.com/drugtopics/article/articleDetail.jsp?id=153758. Accessed September 8, 2006.

Table 36-3   β-Agonist Bronchodilators

Drug	Type	Brand Names	Administration
albuterol	β_2	Proventil, Ventolin	PO, inhalation
bitolterol	β_2	Tornalate	Inhalation
ephedrine	α-β	None (various generic)	PO, IM, IV, SC
epinephrine	α-β	Adrenalin, Primatene, Bronkaid, Bronitin, Medihaler-Epi	SC, IM, inhalation
isoetharine	β_1-β_2	None (various generic)	Inhalation
metaproterenol	β_1-β_2	Alupent	PO, inhalation
levalbuterol	β_2	Xopenex	Inhalation
metaproterenol	β_1-β_2	Alupent, Metaprel	PO, inhalation
pirbuterol	β_2	Maxair	Inhalation
salmeterol	β_2	Serevent, Serevent Diskus	Inhalation
terbutaline	β_2	Brethine, Bricanyl	PO, SC, inhalation

IM, Intramuscular; *IV,* intravenous; *PO,* oral; *SC,* subcutaneous.

levels of cAMP made available by adenylate cyclase cause bronchial smooth muscles to relax, which results in bronchial dilation and increased airflow into and out of the lungs.

Nonselective adrenergic agonist drugs such as epinephrine also stimulate α-adrenergic receptors, causing constriction within the blood vessels. This vasoconstriction reduces the amount of edema or swelling in the mucous membranes and limits the quantity of secretions normally produced by these membranes. In addition, such drugs also stimulate β_1 receptors, which results in cardiovascular adverse effects such as an increase in heart rate, force of contraction, and blood pressure, as well as CNS effects such as nervousness and tremor.

Drugs such as albuterol that predominantly stimulate the β_2 receptors have more specific drug effects. By predominantly stimulating the β_2-adrenergic receptors of the bronchial and vascular smooth muscles, they cause bronchodilation and may also have a dilating effect on the peripheral vasculature, which results in a decrease in diastolic blood pressure. In addition, the β_2 agonists are thought to stimulate the sodium-potassium adenosine triphosphatase ion pump contained in cell membranes. This facilitates a temporary shift of potassium ions from the bloodstream into the cells, which results in a temporary decrease in serum potassium levels. For this reason, these drugs are also useful in treating patients with acute hyperkalemia. Finally, stimulation of β_2 receptors in uterine smooth muscle can cause beneficial uterine relaxation (see Indications).

Indications

The primary respiratory therapeutic effect of the β-agonists is the relief of bronchospasm related to bronchial asthma, bronchitis, and other pulmonary diseases. However, they are also used for beneficial therapeutic effects outside the respiratory system. Because some of these drugs have the ability to stimulate both β_1- and α-adrenergic receptors, they may be used to treat hypotension and shock. They can also stimulate a shift of potassium out of the blood and into cells. For this reason, as noted earlier, β_2-agonists can be used to treat hyperkalemia (e.g., that associated with renal failure).

The drugs terbutaline and ritodrine both have the added ability to stimulate the β_2 receptors on the uterus that control uterine contractions; they are used to produce uterine relaxation and prevent premature labor in pregnant women (Chapter 33). Although used less often than terbutaline, ritodrine is still available and is indicated solely for this purpose.

Contraindications

Contraindications include drug allergy, uncontrolled cardiac dysrhythmias, and high risk of stroke (because of the vasoconstrictive drug actions).

Adverse Effects

Mixed α-β–agonists produce the greatest array of undesirable effects. These include insomnia, restlessness, anorexia, cardiac stimulation, hyperglycemia, tremor, and vascular headache. The adverse effects of the nonselective β-agonists are limited to β-adrenergic effects, including cardiac stimulation, tremor, anginal pain, and vascular headache. The β_2 drugs can cause both hypertension and hypotension, vascular headaches, and tremor. Overdose management may include careful administration of a

β-blocker while the patient is under close observation. Because the half-life of most adrenergic agonists is often relatively short, however, the patient may just be observed while the body eliminates the medication.

Interactions

The use of a nonselective β-blocker with β-agonist bronchodilators antagonizes the bronchodilation. The use of β-agonists with monoamine oxidase inhibitors and other sympathomimetics is best avoided because of the enhanced risk for hypertension. Concurrent use with xanthines and digoxin increase the risk of cardiac toxicity and may also reduce digoxin serum levels. Hypokalemia and electrocardiographic changes are more likely to occur with concurrent use of diuretics. Patients with diabetes may require an adjustment in the dosage of their hypoglycemic drugs, especially patients receiving epinephrine, because of the increased blood glucose levels that can occur.

Dosages

For recommended dosages of selected β-agonists, see the Dosages table on page 555.

Drug Profiles

▶ albuterol

Albuterol (Proventil, Ventolin, Volmax) is one of six β_2-specific bronchodilating β-agonists. Other similar drugs include bitolterol (Tornalate), levalbuterol (Xopenex), pirbuterol (Maxair), salmeterol (Serevent Diskus), and terbutaline (Brethine). Although albuterol is the most commonly used drug in this class, salmeterol has a unique 12-hour duration of action, which makes it an attractive alternative. If albuterol is used too frequently, dose-related adverse effects may be seen, because albuterol loses its β_2-specific actions especially at larger dosages. As a consequence, the β_1 receptors are stimulated, which causes nausea, increased anxiety, palpitations, tremors, and an increased heart rate.

Albuterol is available for both oral and inhalational use. Inhalational dosage forms include metered-dose inhalers (MDIs) as well as solutions for inhalation. The levorotatory isomeric form of albuterol, levalbuterol, is strictly for inhalational use and is sometimes prescribed as an albuterol alternative for patients with certain risk factors (e.g., tachycardia, including tachycardia associated with albuterol treatment).

Pharmacokinetics

Half-Life	Onset	Peak	Duration
Inhaled: 3-4 hr	Inhaled: 0.5-2 hr	Inhaled: 2-3 hr	Inhaled: 3-4 hr

ANTICHOLINERGICS

Currently there are two anticholinergic drugs used in the treatment of COPD: ipratropium and tiotropium.

Mechanism of Action and Drug Effects

On the surface of the bronchial tree are receptors for acetylcholine (ACh), the neurotransmitter for the parasympathetic nervous system. When the parasympathetic nervous system releases ACh from its nerve endings, the neurotransmitter binds to the ACh receptors on the surface of the bronchial tree, which results in bronchial constriction and narrowing of the airways. Anticholin-

DOSAGES

Bronchodilators

Drug (Pregnancy Category)	Pharmacologic Class	Usual Dosage Range	Indications
▶ albuterol (Proventil, Proventil Repetabs, Ventolin, Volmax, others) (C)	β_2-agonist	**Pediatric 2-6 yr** PO: 0.1-0.2 mg/kg tid **Pediatric 7-11 yr** PO: 2 mg tid-qid **Adult and pediatric 12 yr and older** PO: 2-4 mg tid-qid Inhalation solution: 2.5 mg tid-qid **Adult and pediatric 4 yr and older** MDI: 2 puffs q4-6h Powder capsules: 200 mcg via inhalation q4-6h	Asthma, bronchospasm
epinephrine (Adrenalin, Primatene, Bronkaid) (C)	α-β-agonist	**Pediatric (all ages)** SC: 10 mcg/kg **Adult** SC/IM: 0.1-0.5 mg q15min-q4h IV: 0.1-0.25 mg Inhalation spray: 0.2 mg/inhalation prn	
ipratropium (Atrovent) (B)	Anticholinergic	**Adult and pediatric 12 yr and older** MDI: 2 puffs qid Nasal spray, 0.03%: 2 sprays bid-tid Nasal spray, 0.06%: 2 sprays tid-qid Inhalation solution: 500 mcg tid-qid	
metaproterenol (Alupent) (C)	β_1-β_2-agonist	**Pediatric** PO: <2 yr: 0.4 mg/kg/dose 3-4 x/day 2-6 yr: 1-2.6 mg/kg/day divided tid-qid 6-9 yr: 10 mg/dose 3-4 x/day >9 yr to adult: 20 mg 3-4 x/day **Children >12 yrs and adult** MDI: 1-2 puffs 4-6 ×/day Inhalation solution: Infant/child (to 11 yr): 0.01-0.02 mg/kg diluted in 2-3 mL normal saline q4-6 hr Children >12 yrs and adult 0.2-0.3 mL of full strength (5%) solution in 2-3 mL	

IM, Intramuscular; *IV,* intravenous; *MDI,* metered-dose inhaler; *PO,* oral; *SC,* subcutaneous.

ergic drugs block these ACh receptors to prevent bronchoconstriction. This indirectly causes airway dilation.

Indications

Because their actions are slow and prolonged, anticholinergics are used for prevention of the bronchospasm associated with chronic bronchitis or emphysema and not for the management of acute symptoms.

Contraindications

The only usual contraindication to the use of bronchial anticholinergic drugs is drug allergy, including allergy to atropine or to soy lecithin (found in some of the inhalational formulations), which may include allergy to peanut oils, peanuts, soybeans, and other legumes (beans).

Adverse Effects

The most commonly reported adverse effects of ipratropium and tiotropium therapy are related to the drug's anticholinergic effects and include dry mouth or throat, nasal congestion, heart palpitations, gastrointestinal (GI) distress, headache, coughing, and anxiety. It is classified as a pregnancy category B drug, and its use is contraindicated in patients with a known hypersensitivity to it or to atropine or any of its derivatives.

Drug Interactions

Possible additive toxicity may occur when anticholinergic bronchodilators are taken with other anticholinergic drugs.

Dosages

See the Dosages table on this page.

Drug Profiles

ipratropium

Ipratropium (Atrovent) is the oldest and most commonly used anticholinergic bronchodilator. It is pharmacologically very similar to atropine (Chapter 20). It is available both as a liquid aerosol for inhalation and as an MDI; both form are usually dosed twice daily. A newer but similar drug is tiotropium (Spiriva), which is formulated for once-daily dosing. Many patients also benefit from taking both a β_2-agonist and an anticholinergic drug, with the most popular combination being albuterol and ipratropium. Although many patients receive the two drugs separately, there are two available combination products containing both of these drugs: Combivent (an MDI) and DuoNeb (an inhalation solution).

Pharmacokinetics

Half-Life	Onset	Peak	Duration
1.6 hr	5-15 min	1-2 hr	4-5 hr

XANTHINE DERIVATIVES

The natural xanthines consist of the plant alkaloids caffeine, theobromine, and theophylline, but only theophylline and caffeine are currently used clinically. Synthetic xanthines include aminophylline, dyphylline, and oxtriphylline. Caffeine, which is actually a metabolite of theophylline, has other uses described later.

Mechanism of Action and Drug Effects

The mechanisms of action of the different xanthine drugs are similar. They all cause bronchodilation by increasing the levels of the energy-producing substance cAMP. They do this by competitively inhibiting phosphodiesterase, the enzyme responsible for breaking down cAMP. In patients with COPD, cAMP plays an integral role in the maintenance of open airways. Higher intracellular levels of cAMP contribute to smooth muscle relaxation and also inhibit IgE-induced release of the chemical mediators that drive allergic reactions (histamine, slow-reacting substance of anaphylaxis [SRS-A], and others).

Xanthine derivatives also have other beneficial drug effects besides those involving respiratory function. Theophylline is metabolized to caffeine in the body, whereas aminophylline is metabolized to theophylline. Theophylline and other xanthines also stimulate the CNS, but to a lesser degree than caffeine. This stimulation of the CNS has the beneficial effect of acting directly on the medullary respiratory center to enhance respiratory drive. In large doses, theophylline and its derivatives may stimulate the cardiovascular system, which results in both an increased force of contraction (positive inotropy) and an increased heart rate (positive chronotropy). The increased force of contraction raises cardiac output and hence blood flow to the kidneys. This, in combination with the ability of the xanthines to dilate blood vessels in and around the kidney, increases the glomerular filtration rate, producing a diuretic effect.

Indications

Xanthines are used to dilate the airways in patients with asthma, chronic bronchitis, or emphysema. They may be used in mild to moderate cases of acute asthma and as an adjunct drug in the management of COPD. However, xanthines are now deemphasized as treatment for milder asthma because of their greater potential for drug interactions and the greater interpatient variability in therapeutic drug levels in the blood. Because of their relatively slow onset of action, xanthines are more often used for the prevention of asthmatic symptoms than for the relief of acute asthma attacks. However, they are often preferred as adjunct bronchodilators for patients with chronic bronchitis or emphysema.

Caffeine is primarily used without prescription as a CNS stimulant, or analeptic (Chapter 16), to promote alertness (e.g., for long-duration driving or studying). It is also used as a cardiac stimulant in infants with bradycardia and to enhance respiratory drive in infants in neonatal intensive care units. It is not normally used clinically in adults for these purposes, although theoretically it would have similar effects.

Contraindications

Contraindications to therapy with xanthine derivatives include drug allergy, uncontrolled cardiac dysrhythmias, seizure disorders, hyperthyroidism, and peptic ulcers. Caffeine, which as noted earlier is a metabolite of theophylline, is known as a *secretagogue*. Such compounds stimulate gastric secretions; hence, the contraindication of peptic ulcer.

Adverse Effects

The common adverse effects of the xanthine derivatives include nausea, vomiting, and anorexia. In addition, gastroesophageal reflux has been observed to occur during sleep in patients taking these drugs. Cardiac adverse effects include sinus tachycardia, extrasystole, palpitations, and ventricular dysrhythmias. Transient increased urination and hyperglycemia are other possible adverse effects. Overdose and other toxicity of xanthine derivatives are usually treated by the administration of repeat doses of activated charcoal. Syrup of ipecac, while formerly used more regularly, is now rarely recommended by poison control centers for poisonings or overdoses of any kind.

Interactions

The use of xanthine derivatives with any of the following drugs causes the serum level of the xanthine derivative to be increased: allopurinol, cimetidine, macrolide antibiotics (e.g., erythromycin), quinolones (e.g., ciprofloxacin), influenza vaccine, rifampin, and oral contraceptives. Their use with sympathomimetics, or even caffeine, can produce additive cardiac and CNS stimulation. A reported herbal interaction is the tendency of St. John's wort (*Hypericum perforatum*) to enhance the rate of xanthine drug metabolism, presumably by enhancing the activity of the enzymes in the liver that normally metabolize the xanthine. Thus, higher dosages of theophylline and other xanthine derivatives may be needed in patients using this popular herbal preparation. Cigarette smoking has a similar effect because of the enzyme-inducing effect of nicotine. Food interactions include charcoal broiling, high protein, and low carbohydrate foods. These substances may reduce serum levels of xanthines through various metabolic mechanisms.

Dosages

For the recommended dosages of selected theophylline salts, see the Dosages table on page 557.

Drug Profiles

▸ *theophylline*

Theophylline (Bronkodyl, Elixophyllin, Slo-Bid, Theo-Dur, Theo-24, Quibron-T, Uniphyl) is the most commonly used xanthine derivative. It is available in oral, rectal, injectable (as aminophylline), and topical dosage forms. Besides theophylline, which occurs in various

DOSAGES

Theophylline Salts

Drug (Pregnancy Category)	Pharmacologic Class	Usual Dosage Range	Indication
aminophylline (multiple generic preparations) (C)	Xanthine-derived bronchodilator	**Pediatric 6 mo-16 yr** IV: 0.8-1.2 mg/kg/hr continuous infusion **Adult** IV: 0.1-0.7 mg/kg/hr continuous infusion	
▶theophylline (Bronkodyl, Elixophyllin, Theo-Dur, Uniphyl, others) (C)	Xanthine-derived bronchodilator	**Pediatric*** PO: 2-6 mg/kg **Adult*** PO: 400-600 mg/day in 1-4 divided doses	Asthma

IV, Intravenous; *PO,* oral.

*The dosage schedules and dosage forms used vary widely depending on age and clinical status.

Table 36-4   Available Theophylline Preparations

Dosage Form	Strengths
Oral	
Capsules	100 and 200 mg
Extended-release capsules	100, 125, 200, and 300 mg
Solution	27 and 50 mg/5 mL
Tablets	100, 125, 200, and 300 mg
Extended-release tablets	100, 200, 300, 400, 450, and 600 mg
Parenteral (as Aminophylline)*	
Injection	25 mg/mL
Rectal (as Aminophylline)*	
Suppository	250 and 500 mg

*Aminophylline (a theophylline prodrug) = 79% theophylline.

salt forms, the other xanthine bronchodilators used clinically for the treatment of bronchoconstriction are aminophylline, dyphylline, and oxtriphylline. All three of these are theophylline prodrugs that are metabolized to theophylline in the body. Aminophylline is the most commonly used of these prodrugs and is sometimes given intravenously to patients with status asthmaticus who have not responded to fast-acting β-agonists such as epinephrine. The numerous theophylline preparations are listed in Table 36-4.

The beneficial effects of theophylline can be maximized by maintaining levels in the blood within a certain target range. If these levels become too high, many unwanted adverse effects can occur. If the levels become too low, the patient receives little therapeutic benefit. Although the optimal level may vary from patient to patient, a common target therapeutic range for theophylline blood level is 10 to 20 mcg/mL. While most standard references indicate adverse effects are uncommon at therapeutic ranges below 20 mcg/mL, some practitioners advise maintaining the level between 5 and 15 mcg/mL. Laboratory monitoring of drug blood levels is common to ensure adequate dosage, especially in the hospital setting.

Pharmacokinetics

Half-Life	Onset	Peak	Duration
PO: 7-9 hr (highly variable)*	PO: Unknown	PO: 1-2 hr	PO: Varies with dosage form

*Depending on pulmonary, heart, and liver function; smoking history; and dosage form.

NONBRONCHODILATING RESPIRATORY DRUGS

Bronchodilators are just one type of drug used to treat asthma, chronic bronchitis, and emphysema; these drugs include beta-adrenergic agonists and xanthines. There are also other drugs that are effective in suppressing various underlying causes of some of these respiratory illnesses. These include antileukotriene drugs (montelukast, zafirlukast, and zileuton), and corticosteroids (beclomethasone, budesonide, dexamethasone, flunisolide, fluticasone, and triamcinolone). Another drug class known as *mast cell stabilizers* is now rarely used. However, these drugs are still listed in the NAEPP guidelines as *alternative* therapy and include cromolyn and nedocromil. As their class name implies, they work by stabilizing the cell membranes of mast cells to prevent the release of inflammatory mediators such as histamine.

ANTILEUKOTRIENE DRUGS

A newer class of asthma medications called *leukotriene receptor antagonists (LTRAs),* or antileukotriene drugs, is available. Antileukotriene drugs became the first new class of asthma medications to be introduced in the United States in more than 20 years when the first of these was made available in the 1990s.

Before the development of antileukotriene drugs, most asthma treatments focused on relaxing the contraction of bronchial muscles with bronchodilators. In the last decade, researchers have begun to understand how asthma symptoms are caused by the immune system at the cellular level. A chain reaction starts when a trigger allergen, such as cat hair or dust, initiates a series of chemical reactions in the body. Several substances are produced, including a family of molecules known as *leukotrienes (LTs)*. In people with asthma, LTs cause inflammation, bronchoconstriction, and mucus production. This in turn leads to coughing, wheezing, and shortness of breath. Antileukotriene drugs prevent LTs from attaching to receptors located on circulating immune cells (e.g., lymphocytes in the blood) as well as local immune cells within the lungs (e.g., alveolar macrophages). This alleviates asthma symptoms in the lungs by reducing inflammation.

Mechanism of Action and Drug Effects

Currently two subclasses of antileukotriene drugs are available. These subclasses differ in the mechanism by which they block the inflammatory process in asthma. The first subclass of antileukotriene drugs acts by an indirect mechanism and inhibits the enzyme 5-lipoxygenase, which is necessary for LT synthesis. Zileuton (Zyflo) is the only drug of this type currently available. The second subclass of antileukotriene drugs act more directly by binding to the D_4 leukotriene receptor subtype (LTD$_4$) in respiratory tract tissues and organs. These drugs include montelukast (Singulair) and zafirlukast (Accolate).

The drug effects of antileukotriene drugs are primarily limited to the lungs. Through their reduction of LT synthesis or action, they prevent smooth muscle contraction of the bronchial airways, decrease mucus secretion, and reduce vascular permeability (which reduces edema). Other anti-LT effects of these drugs include prevention of the mobilization and migration of such cells as neutrophils and lymphocytes into the lungs. This also serves to reduce airway inflammation.

Indications

The antileukotriene drugs montelukast, zafirlukast, and zileuton are used for the prophylaxis and long-term treatment of asthma in adults and children 12 years of age and older. Montelukast is the most widely used of these drugs and has also been approved for treatment of allergic rhinitis, a condition discussed in Chapter 35. These drugs are not meant for the management of acute asthmatic attacks. Improvement with their use is typically seen in about 1 week.

Contraindications

Drug allergy or other previous adverse drug reaction is the primary contraindication to the use of the antileukotriene drugs. Allergy to povidone, lactose, titanium dioxide, or cellulose derivatives is also important to note because these are inactive ingredients in these drugs.

Adverse Effects

The adverse effects of antileukotriene drugs differ depending on the specific drug. Zileuton and zafirlukast both can cause headaches. The most commonly reported adverse effects of zileuton, after headaches, are dyspepsia, nausea, dizziness, and insomnia.

The most common adverse effects of zafirlukast, after headaches, are nausea and diarrhea. Both drugs may also lead to liver dysfunction. For this reason, liver enzyme levels should be monitored regularly in patients taking these drugs, especially early in the course of therapy.

There have been some case reports of the occurrence of Churg-Strauss syndrome in patients receiving montelukast. This syndrome is characterized by systemic necrotizing vasculitis (destruction of blood vessels) and is often manifested by tender subcutaneous nodules, large skin plaques, and markedly elevated eosinophil count in the blood (eosinophilia). It is usually treated with systemic (intravenous or oral) corticosteroid therapy.

Interactions

Montelukast has fewer drug interactions than zafirlukast or zileuton. It does not interact with theophylline, warfarin, digoxin, prednisone, or either the estrogen or progestin components of combination oral contraceptives. Phenobarbital decreases montelukast concentrations. For information on the drugs that interact with zafirlukast and zileuton, see Table 36-5.

Dosages

For recommended dosages of selected antileukotriene drugs, see the Dosages table on page 559.

Drug Profiles

Antileukotriene drugs are a new class of asthma medications. As note earlier, the three antileukotriene drugs currently available are zileuton, zafirlukast, and montelukast. They are used primarily for oral prophylaxis and long-term treatment of asthma. These drugs are not recommended for treatment of acute asthma attacks.

▸ **montelukast**

Montelukast (Singulair) is the third drug to become available in the antileukotriene class. It belongs to the same subcategory of antileukotriene drugs as zafirlukast. Montelukast and zafirlukast work by blocking LTD$_4$ receptors to augment the inflammatory response. Montelukast offers the advantage of being U.S. Food and Drug Administration approved for use in children 2 years of age and older. It also has fewer adverse effects and drug interactions than zafirlukast. Use of montelukast is contraindicated in patients with a known hypersensitivity to it. It is available only for oral use. Pregnancy category B. Common dosages are given in the table on page 559.

Table 36-5	**Drug Interactions: Antileukotriene Drugs**	
Drug	**Mechanism**	**Result**
Montelukast (Singulair)		
phenobarbital, rifampin	Increased metabolism	Decreased montelukast levels
Zafirlukast (Accolate)		
aspirin	Decreased clearance	Increased zafirlukast levels
erythromycin	Decreased bioavailability	Decreased zafirlukast levels
tolbutamide, phenytoin, carbamazepine	Inhibited metabolism	Increased tolbutamide, phenytoin, and carbamazepine levels
warfarin	Decreased clearance	Increased warfarin levels
Zileuton (Zyflo)		
propranolol	Decreased clearance	Increased propranolol levels
theophylline	Decreased clearance	Increased theophylline levels
warfarin	Decreased clearance	Increased warfarin levels

DOSAGES

Selected Antileukotriene Drugs

Drug (Pregnancy Category)	Pharmacologic Class	Usual Dosage Range	Indications
▶montelukast (Singulair) (B)	Leukotriene receptor antagonist	**Pediatric 2-5 yr** PO: 4 mg daily in evening **Pediatric 6-14 yr** PO: 5 mg daily in evening **Adult and pediatric 15 yr and older** PO: 10 mg daily in evening	Asthma (prophylaxis and maintenance treatment)
zafirlukast (Accolate) (B)	Leukotriene receptor antagonist	**Adult and pediatric 12 yr and older** PO: 20 mg bid	
zileuton (Zyflo) (C)	Leukotriene synthesis inhibitor	**Adult and pediatric 12 yr and older** PO: 600 mg qid	

PO, Oral.

Pharmacokinetics			
Half-Life	**Onset**	**Peak**	**Duration**
2.7-5.5 hr	30 min	3-4 hr Chewable tablet: 2.5 hr	24 hr

CORTICOSTEROIDS

Corticosteroids, also known as *glucocorticoids,* are either naturally occurring or synthetic drugs used in the treatment of COPDs for their antiinflammatory effects. All have actions similar to those of the natural steroid hormone cortisol, which is chemically the same as the drug hydrocortisone. Synthetic steroids are now more commonly used in drug therapy. They can be given by inhalation, orally, or even intravenously in severe cases of asthma when the drug cannot get to the airways because of the obstruction. Corticosteroids administered by inhalation have an advantage over orally administered corticosteroids in that their action is limited to the topical site in the lungs. This generally prevents systemic effects. The chemical structures of the corticosteroids given by inhalation have also been slightly altered to limit their systemic absorption from the respiratory tract. The corticosteroids administered by inhalation include the following:

- beclomethasone dipropionate (Beclovent, Vanceril)
- budesonide (Pulmicort Turbuhaler)
- dexamethasone sodium phosphate (Decadron Phosphate Respihaler)
- flunisolide (Aerobid)
- fluticasone (Flonase, Cutivate, Flovent)
- triamcinolone acetonide (Azmacort)

The systemic use of corticosteroids was described in Chapter 32. The most commonly used systemic corticosteroids for respiratory illness include the following:

- prednisone (oral)
- methylprednisolone (intravenous or oral)

Mechanism of Action and Drug Effects

Although the exact mechanism of action of the corticosteroids has not been determined, it is conjectured that they have the dual effect of both reducing inflammation and enhancing the activity of β-agonists. The corticosteroids previously mentioned produce their antiinflammatory effects through a complex sequence of actions. The overall effect is to prevent various nonspecific inflammatory processes. These include the accumulation of inflammatory mediators as well as altered vascular permeability (which causes edema).

They essentially work by stabilizing the membranes of cells that normally release very harmful bronchoconstricting substances (e.g., histamine, SRS-A). These cells include *leukocytes,* which is another name for white blood cells (WBCs). There are five different types of WBC, each with its own specific characteristics. The five types of WBC, their role in the inflammatory process, and the way in which corticosteroids inhibit their normal action, combat inflammation, and produce bronchodilation are summarized in Table 36-6. In particular, inflammatory mediators are primarily released by *lymphocytes* in the circulation as well as by *mast cells* and *alveolar macrophages.* These latter two cell types are stationary (noncirculating) inflammatory cells that remain localized in the various tissues and organs of the respiratory tract.

Corticosteroids have also been shown to restore or increase the responsiveness of bronchial smooth muscle to β-adrenergic receptor stimulation, which results in more pronounced stimulation of the β_2 receptors by β-agonist drugs such as albuterol. It may take several weeks of continuous therapy before the full therapeutic effects of the corticosteroids are realized.

Indications

Inhaled corticosteroids are now used for the primary treatment of bronchospastic disorders to control the inflammatory responses that are believed to be the cause of these disorders. They are often used concurrently with bronchodilators, primarily β-adrenergic agonists. The systemic (versus inhaled) use of corticosteroids for a variety of illnesses was described in Chapter 32. In respiratory illnesses, systemic corticosteroids are generally used only for acute exacerbations. Their long-term use is avoided because of the associated long-term adverse effects (see later). The NAEPP recommends long-term use only in cases of truly disabling illness in which the benefits of the drug therapy arguably outweigh the adverse effects. When a more pronounced antiinflammatory effect is needed, however, as in an acute exacerbation of asthma

Table 36-6 White Blood Cells (Leukocytes)		
WBC Type*	**Role in Inflammation**	**Corticosteroid Effect**
Granulocytes		
Neutrophils (65%)	Contain powerful lysosomes (very small bodies that hold cellular digestive enzymes); release chemicals that destroy invading organisms and also attack other WBCs	Stabilize cell membranes so that inflammation-causing substances are not released
Eosinophils (2%-5%)	Function mainly in allergic reactions and protect against parasitic infections; ingest inflammatory chemicals and antigen-antibody complexes	Little if any effect
Basophils (0.5%-1%)	Contain histamine, an inflammation-causing substance, and heparin, an anticoagulant	Stabilize cell membranes so that histamine is not released
Agranulocytes		
Lymphocytes (25%)	Two types: T lymphocytes and B lymphocytes; T cells attack infecting microbial or cancerous cells; B cells produce antibodies against specific antigens	Decrease activity of the lymphocytes
Monocytes (3%-5%)	Produce macrophages, which can migrate out of the bloodstream to such places as mucous membranes, where they are capable of engulfing large bacteria or virus-infected cells	Inhibited macrophage accumulation in already inflamed areas, thus preventing more inflammation

*Value in parentheses is the percentage of all leukocytes represented by the given type.
WBC, White blood cell.

or other COPD, intravenous corticosteroids (e.g., methylprednisolone) are often used.

Contraindications

Drug allergy is the primary contraindication. It should also be emphasized that these drugs are not intended as sole therapy for acute asthma attacks. Inhaled corticosteroids are contraindicated in patients who are hypersensitive in response to glucocorticoids, in patients whose sputum tests positive for *Candida* organisms, and in patients with systemic fungal infection.

Adverse Effects

The main undesirable local effects of typical doses of inhaled corticosteroids in the respiratory system include pharyngeal irritation, coughing, dry mouth, and oral fungal infections. Most of the drug effects of inhaled corticosteroids are limited to their topical site of action in the lungs. Because of the chemical structure of these inhaled dosage forms, there is relatively little systemic absorption of the drugs when they are administered by inhalation at normal therapeutic doses. However, the degree of systemic absorption is more likely to be increased in patients who require higher inhaled doses. When there is significant systemic absorption, which is most likely with high-dose intravenous or oral administration, corticosteroids can affect any of the organ systems in the body. Some of these systemic drug effects include adrenocortical insufficiency, increased susceptibility to infection, fluid and electrolyte disturbances, endocrine effects, CNS effects (insomnia, nervousness, seizures), and dermatologic and connective tissue effects, including brittle skin, bone loss, and osteoporosis.

One important point to remember pertains to patients who are switched to inhaled corticosteroids after receiving systemic corticosteroids, especially at high dosages for an extended period. Patient deaths have been reported due to adrenal gland failure in such cases when the switch to inhaled corticosteroids is made quickly and the dosage of systemic corticosteroids is not reduced gradually. Preven-

tion of this occurrence requires careful clinical monitoring with slow tapering of drug dosages. The patient dependent on systemic corticosteroids may need up to 1 year of recovery time after discontinuation of systemic therapy. There is evidence that bone growth is suppressed in children and adolescents taking corticosteroids. This suppression is more apparent in children receiving larger systemic (versus inhaled) dosages over longer treatment durations. Growth should be tracked (e.g., with standardized charts) and medications should be reevaluated should growth suppression become evident. In some cases, supplemental growth hormone may be prescribed.

Interactions

Drug interactions are more likely to occur with systemic (versus inhaled) corticosteroids. These drugs may increase serum glucose levels, possibly requiring adjustments in dosages of antidiabetic drugs. Because of interactions related to metabolizing enzymes, they may also raise the blood levels of the immunosuppressants cyclosporine and tacrolimus. Likewise, the antifungal drug itraconazole may reduce clearance of the steroids, whereas phenytoin, phenobarbital, and rifampin, may enhance it. There is also greater risk for hypokalemia with concurrent use of potassium-depleting diuretics such as hydrochlorothiazide and furosemide.

Dosages

For recommended dosages of selected corticosteroids, see the Dosages table on page 561.

Drug Profiles

fluticasone

Fluticasone is administered intranasally (Flonase) (1 inhalation in each nostril daily) and by oral inhalation (Flovent) (usually 1 inhalation by mouth twice daily). Recently fluticasone became available in a combination formulation with the bronchodilator salmeterol (Advair Diskus).

DOSAGES

Selected Corticosteroids

Drug (Pregnancy Category)	Pharmacologic Class	Usual Dosage Range	Indications
budesonide (Pulmicort Turbuhaler, Pulmicort Respules, Rhinocort, Rhinocort Aqua) (C)	Synthetic glucocorticoid	**Adult and pediatric 6 yr and older** MDI: 1-2 puffs bid Nasal spray: 2 sprays in each nostril bid or 4 sprays in each nostril once daily **Pediatric 12 mo-8 yr** Inhalation solution: 0.5-1 mg daily-bid	Asthma (prophylaxis and maintenance treatment) Allergic rhinitis Asthma (prophylaxis and maintenance treatment)
fluticasone propionate (Flovent, Flovent Rotadisk, Flonase) (C)	Synthetic glucocorticoid	**Adult and pediatric 12 yr and older** Flovent MDI, 3 strengths available: 88-880 mcg bid **Pediatric 4-11 yr** Flovent Rotadisk inhalation powder, 3 strengths available: 50-100 mcg bid **Adult and pediatric 12 yr and older** Flovent Rotadisk inhalation powder, 3 strengths available: 100-1000 mcg bid	Asthma (prophylaxis and maintenance treatment); seasonal allergic rhinitis
prednisone (Deltasone, others) (C)	Synthetic glucocorticoid	Dose varies widely, depending on severity of disease; usual oral dose 1-100 mg daily, usually tapered down	Exacerbations of asthma or other COPD
methylprednisolone (Solu-Medrol injection, Medrol tablets) (C)	Synthetic glucocorticoid	Dose varies as above, but usually 40-125 mg IV, daily-tid, usually tapered down Oral taper: usually from 24 to 2 mg daily	Exacerbations of asthma or other COPD

COPD, Chronic obstructive pulmonary disease; *IV,* intravenous; *MDI,* metered-dose inhaler.

Pharmacokinetics

Half-Life	Onset	Peak	Duration
Inhaled: 3 hr	Inhaled: Unknown	Inhaled: Unknown	Inhaled: Up to 1 day

CASE STUDY

Chronic Obstructive Pulmonary Disease

Ms. B. is a 73-year-old woman who worked in the local traffic tunnel for about 25 years and has had chronic obstructive pulmonary disease (COPD) for 10 years, caused by exposure to environmental pollutants while on the job and by cigarette smoking. She is now retired and is frequently admitted to the hospital for treatment of her condition. She quit smoking about 8 years ago. She is now in the hospital for treatment of an acute exacerbation of her COPD and an upper respiratory tract infection. The physician has ordered the following: aminophylline intravenously per respiratory therapy protocol, intravenous continuous infusion at a rate of 0.8 mg/kg/hr; chest physiotherapy bid and prn; cephalothin antibiotic therapy, 1 g intravenously in 30 mL normal saline q8h; measurement of intake and output; daily weight measurement; assessment of vital signs with breath sounds q2h and prn until stable; and albuterol inhaler, 2 puffs q4h per respiratory therapy protocol.

- What nursing interventions would be most appropriate for helping this patient conserve energy while enhancing O_2 and CO_2 gas exchange?
- What is the rationale for using the continuous intravenous infusion of aminophylline?
- What are the reasons for prescribing the albuterol inhaler and the antibiotic? Be specific about the reasons for each.
- What would be the most important patient education guidelines to impart to Ms. B. concerning the use of an oral xanthine drug (theophylline) and the albuterol inhaler at home?

For answers, see http://evolve.elsevier.com/Lilley.

methylprednisolone

Methylprednisolone is a systemic corticosteroid available in both oral (Medrol) and injectable (Solu-Medrol) forms.

Pharmacokinetics

Half-Life	Onset	Peak	Duration
IV: 3-4 hr	IV: 1-2 hr	IV: Unknown	IV: 24-36 hr

◆ NURSING PROCESS

◆ ASSESSMENT

The net drug effect of β-agonists, xanthine derivatives, anticholinergics, leukotriene receptor antagonists (or antileukotrienes), and corticosteroids is improved airflow in airway passages and increased oxygen supply. Cautions, contraindications, and drug interactions (discussed previously) should be assessed before they are administered. In a thorough assessment of patients receiving any of the respiratory drugs, the patient's skin color, temperature, respiration rate (which should be more than 12 and less than 24 breaths/min), depth and rhythm, breath sounds, blood pressure, and pulse should be monitored as needed. The nurse should also determine if the patient is having problems with cough, dyspnea, orthopnea, or hypoxia, or has other signs or symptoms of respiratory distress. The patient should also be assessed for the presence of any of the following: sternal retractions, cyanosis, restlessness, activity intolerance, cardiac irregularities, palpitations, hypertension, tachycardia, or use of accessory muscles to breathe. The anterior-posterior diameter of the thorax should be determined, and pulse oximetry should be assessed to determine oxygen saturation levels. Assess for history of allergies and specific allergens (e.g., dust, pollen, mold, mildew, nuts or other foods). If a cough is present, its character, frequency, and presence of sputum should be noted. The color of sputum should also be noted. A complete medication history, noting prescription drugs, over-the-counter (OTC) drugs, herbal products, alternative therapies, use of nebulizers and/or humidifiers, use of a home air conditioner, and intactness of heating/air conditioning system should be documented. Note the characteristics of any respiratory symptoms (e.g., seasonally induced, exercise- or stress-induced) and if there is a family history of respiratory diseases. Identify any environmental exposures and precipitating/alleviating factors for any respiratory symptoms and/or disease processes. An excellent resource for asthma may be found online at http://asthma.com/asthma control test.html. Assessment of smoking habits should also be noted because of exacerbation of respiratory symptoms/problems and due to the interaction of nicotine with many respiratory drugs.

Cardiac status may be compromised due to respiratory distress; this is the reason for assessing blood pressure, pulse rate, heart sounds and ECG if ordered. The physician may order blood gases with attention to pH, oxygen, carbon dioxide levels, and serum bicarbonate levels. Assess the patient's nail beds for abnormalities (e.g., clubbing, cyanosis), and assess the area around the lips. Restlessness may be due to hypoxia, so this symptom should be further evaluated. If chest x-rays, scans, or MRIs have been ordered, be sure to review the findings. Along with a physical assessment comes the need for an emotional assessment because anxiety, stress, and fear may only further compromise the patient's respiratory status and oxygen levels. Be sure to note the

age of the patient because of increased sensitivity to drugs in elderly and pediatric patients.

The β-agonists and their cautions, contraindications, drug interactions, and general overview of respiratory assessment associated with these drugs have been discussed previously; however, it is important to emphasize that assessment of allergies to the fluorocarbon propellant (in inhaled dosage forms) should also be noted. Assess the patient's intake of caffeine (e.g., chocolate, tea, coffee, candy, and sodas) and the patient's use of OTC medications containing caffeine (e.g., appetite suppressants, pain relievers). The intake of caffeine is important to determine because caffeine has sympathomimetic effects and causes an increase in adverse effects that are similar to those associated with albuterol and other β-agonists (e.g., tachycardia, hypertension, headache, nervousness, tremors). Educational level and readiness to learn should also be assessed for preparation of patient education (e.g., instructions about the use of dosage forms such as MDIs).

Respiratory anticholinergic drugs and their cautions, contraindications, and drug interactions have been discussed previously. Assessments for patients taking these drugs should include those mentioned earlier as well as assessment for any history of benign prostatic hypertrophy (because of drug-induced urinary retention) or glaucoma (because of drug-induced increase in intraocular pressure). Patients with an allergy to soy lecithin, peanut oils, peanuts, soybeans, or other legumes have shown a higher risk of allergy to the anticholinergics, and this information should be assessed prior to using these drugs. Ipratropium and its aerosol forms have been associated with bronchospasms, so the patient should be assessed for preexisting problems with the use of MDIs.

Assessment with the use of xanthine derivatives (e.g., theophylline) should include identification of any contraindications, cautions, and drug interactions. Cardiovascular and CNS stimulation may occur with these drugs, thus requiring astute cardiac and neurological assessment. GI ulcers may occur with these drugs too, so assessment of bowel patterns and preexisting disease (e.g., ulcers) is also important. Results of renal and liver function tests should also be assessed if these are ordered. As with anticholinergics, xanthines may cause urinary retention, so baseline assessment of urinary patterns and/or benign prostatic hypertrophy is important. A dietary assessment should include questions about consumption of a low-carbohydrate, high-protein diet and intake of charcoal-broiled meat. These dietary practices may lead to increased theophylline elimination and possibly decreased therapeutic levels, whereas a high-carbohydrate, low-protein diet may decrease excretion of the drug and lead to theophylline toxicity. Effects of the xanthines may be increased by other xanthine-containing foods (e.g., those containing caffeine). Other concerns include prescription drugs and OTC drugs containing caffeine (e.g., some antimigraine drugs).

With corticosteroids, baseline assessment of vital signs, breath sounds, and heart sounds should occur. Age should be noted because corticosteroids are not recommended in pediatric patients in whom growth is still occurring. As with the other drugs in this chapter, awareness of basic information about these drugs, in particular their action, is very important to safe use and prevention of medication errors. For example, glucocorticoids are used for their antiinflammatory effects, β-agonists and xanthines for their bron-

---

Life Span Considerations: The Elderly Patient

Xanthine Derivatives

- Xanthine derivatives should be administered cautiously with careful monitoring in the elderly because sensitivity to these drugs is increased in this patient population due to decreased drug metabolism.
- The elderly should be assessed for signs and symptoms of xanthine toxicity, which include nausea, vomiting, restlessness, insomnia, irritability, and tremors. The nurse should be very cautious in assessing restlessness and concluding that it is drug related, because it may be caused by hypoxia secondary to respiratory difficulties and not by the medication.
- Elderly patients should be told never to chew or crush sustained-released dosage forms; to be careful of drug interactions, especially with other asthma-related drugs or bronchodilators; and to take the medication at the same time every day.
- The elderly should be advised never to omit or double up on doses. If a dose is missed, the patient should contact the physician or health care provider for further instructions.
- Monitoring of serum levels of the drug should be initiated to avoid possible toxicity and to make sure blood levels are therapeutic. Assistance with transportation and expenses may be needed and can be sought through various community resources.
- Lower dosages may be necessary initially in the elderly, not only because of their increased sensitivity to the drug but also because of the possibility of decreased in liver and renal functioning. Close monitoring for adverse effects and toxicity should be part of everyday therapy, and palpitations and increased blood pressure (from cardiovascular and central nervous system stimulation) should be noted and reported.

chodilating effects, and anticholinergics for their blockage of cholinergic receptors. Knowing what drugs do and why they are used helps to prevent or decrease medication errors and adverse effects. (See Chapter 32 for more information on these antiinflammatory/adrenal drugs.)

With antileukotrienes, it is important to assess for contraindications, cautions, and drug interactions. Liver functioning should be determined because of specific concerns about the use of these drugs in patients with altered hepatic function. As with other medications, the elderly are more sensitive to these drugs.

◆ NURSING DIAGNOSES

- Impaired gas exchange related to pathophysiologic changes caused by respiratory disease
- Fatigue related to the disease process
- Risk for injury related to bronchospasms of the disease and to the adverse effects of various respiratory medications
- Anxiety related to the "unknowns" associated with respiratory disease and to the adverse effects of drug therapy
- Disturbed sensory perception related to the CNS stimulation caused by bronchodilators
- Deficient knowledge related to unfamiliarity with the medication treatment regimen and the disease process
- Ineffective tissue perfusion related to the adverse effects of albuterol and other β-agonist drugs
- Noncompliance with the medication regimen related to undesirable adverse effects of drug therapy

◆ PLANNING

Goals

- Patient experiences minimal exacerbations of the disease while compliant with the medication regimen.
- Patient states the importance of rest to recovery.
- Patient is free of self-injury related to the disease or to the adverse effects of the medication.
- Patient remains compliant with the medication regimen and with the nonpharmacologic therapies.
- Patient follows up with health care providers as instructed by the physician.
- Patient does not increase or decrease the dosage or stop taking the medication without the approval of the physician.
- Patient's respiratory status improves because of compliance with the medication therapy.
- Patient's circulation remains intact and strong during therapy.

Outcome Criteria

- Patient briefly describes the disease process, its signs and symptoms, and the precipitating factors.
- Patient states measures to take to prevent self-injury resulting from the disease or the adverse effects of the medication, such as taking medications as prescribed.
- Patient is well rested, with plans to rest during periods of disease exacerbation.
- Patient states the expected adverse effects of the drug being taken, such as palpitations, nervousness, mood changes, and insomnia.
- Patient contacts the physician if increased dyspnea, shortness of breath, increased cough, or fever occurs.
- Patient states the importance of taking the medication as prescribed, the reasons for not increasing or decreasing the dosage of the drug, and the importance of not stopping the drug

therapy to prevent complications and exacerbations related to the disease or the adverse effects of medications.
- Patient states situations to report to the physician that are indicative of poor circulation, such as swelling of the feet, bluish discoloration to nail beds and/or lips, coolness of the extremities, and heart palpitations.

◆ IMPLEMENTATION

Nursing interventions that apply to patients with respiratory disease processes (e.g., COPD, asthma, other upper and lower respiratory tract disorders) include patient education and an emphasis on compliance and prevention, in addition to the specific actions related to the prescribed drug therapy. Measures to implement to prevent, relieve, or decrease the manifestations of the disease should be emphasized to the patient at all times, and the patient's awareness of specific precipitating and relieving factors should be increased. Bronchodilators and other respiratory drugs should be given exactly as prescribed and by the prescribed route (e.g., parenterally, orally, by intermittent positive pressure breathing, or by inhalation). The proper method for administering the inhaled forms of these drugs should be demonstrated to the patient, who should provide a return demonstration. The patient should also be strongly discouraged from taking more than the prescribed dose of the β-agonists, xanthines, and other respiratory drugs because of the excessive cardiac demands and cardiac and CNS stimulation (hypertension and tachycardia) that may occur. The use of MDIs requires coordination to inhale the medication correctly and to obtain approximately 10% of drug delivery to the lungs. One minute should be allowed between puffs, and the use of a spacer may be indicated to increase the amount of drug delivered. See the Legal and Ethical Principles box for information concerning the environmental hazards associated with MDIs. Dry powder inhalers are small, hand-held devices that deliver a specific amount of dry micronized power with each inhaled breath. Their use does not require the same coordination as do MDIs, they deliver about 20% of the drug to the lung, and they have no propellants and thus do not pose problems for the environment. One minute should also be allowed between each puff. A nebulizer dosage form delivers small amounts of misted droplets of the drug to the lungs through a small mouthpiece or mask. Although a nebulizer may take a longer time to deliver the drug to the lungs than the inhalers, the nebulizer dosage form may be more effective for some patients. See Chapter 9 for more information.

Beta-agonists should be taken exactly as prescribed and recommended dosage and frequency should be adhered to as overdosage may be life threatening. Oral sustained-released tablets should not be crushed or chewed and should be taken with food to decrease GI upset. Inhaled forms and their instructions are presented in the Patient Teaching Tips. Before, during and after therapy with these drugs, it is important to re-assess the respiratory status and breath sounds. Anticholinergic drugs used for respiratory diseases (e.g., ipratropium), should be taken daily as ordered and with appropriate use of the MDI. See patient education tips present more information on the administration of this drug but it is important to wait anywhere from 5 to 10 minutes before inhaling the second dose of the drug allowing for maximal lung penetration. Exact instructions should be included in the physician's order for the medication and may vary. Rinsing the mouth with water immediately after use of any inhaled/nebulized drug may help to prevent mucosal irritation and dryness.

The Food and Drug Administration (FDA) issued a final rule on albuterol metered-dose inhalers (MDIs) that use chlorofluorocarbon (CFC) propellants and their effect on the environment. The concern was that the CFCs that propel the medicine into the lungs via the inhaler harm the ozone layer. Under the FDA final rule, which was published in the March 31, 2005, issue of the *Federal Register* and reported in a talk paper released on the same date, these inhalers must no longer be produced, marketed, or sold in the United States after December 31, 2008. The Department of Health and Human Services (DHHS) said that sufficient supplies of two FDA-approved and environmentally friendly albuterol inhalers will be available by that date. This will allow a phasing out of other similar inhalers that are not environmentally friendly. The FDA and DHHS are encouraged that drug manufacturers are proactively implementing programs to help patients afford the costs of the non-CFC albuterol MDIs so that all patients can have access to these drugs regardless of their economic circumstances. CFC-containing MDIs used to treat respiratory diseases were previously exempted from a general ban on CFC production and importation under an international agreement established through the Montreal Protocol on Substances that Deplete the Ozone Layer and the U.S. Clean Air Act. The FDA final rule also creates the basis for the phase-out of CFC-containing albuterol products by withdrawing their "essential use" status as of December 31, 2008.

In January of 2006, the FDA also recommended a ban on some of the nonprescription inhalers containing propellants that are known to harm the ozone layer. An FDA advisory panel voted to support the removal of essential use status for these over-the-counter inhalers (e.g., Primatene Mist), and the agency may opt to begin a rule-making process that would include public comment. The American Lung Association agreed with the recommendations of the FDA. The association also expressed concern for the many individuals who use over-the-counter asthma inhalers because they lack insurance that covers prescription drug costs or have no medical insurance at all. This concern echoes the need for adequate access to health care by all Americans.

Modified from U.S. Food and Drug Administration: FDA talk paper: FDA publishes final rule on chlorofluorocarbons in metered dose inhalers. Available at www.fda.gov/cder/mdi/default.htm; further information may be obtained at www.WebMD.com and 1-888-INFO-FDA; Edelman NH, American Lung Association: Statement on FDA's recommendation to ban CFC inhalers, January 25, 2006. Available at www.lungusa.org.

Xanthine derivatives should also be given exactly as prescribed. If they are to be administered parenterally, the nurse should always determine the correct diluent and rate of administration. IV infusion pumps should be used to ensure dosage accuracy and help prevent toxicity. Too rapid an infusion may lead to profound hypotension with possible syncope, tachycardia, seizures, and even cardiac arrest. To prevent a sudden increase in drug release and the irritating effects on the gastric mucosa, timed-release preparations should not be crushed or chewed. Oral forms should be taken with food to decrease GI upset. Suppository forms of the drug should be refrigerated, and patients should notify the physician if rectal burning, itching, or irritation occurs. The patient should continue to be monitored for respiratory status and improvement in baseline condition during drug therapy.

Inhaled glucocorticoids should also be used exactly as prescribed, with cautions about overuse. The medication should be taken as ordered every day, regardless of whether the patient is feeling better or not. Often these drugs (e.g., flunisolide) are used as maintenance drugs and are taken twice daily for maximal response. An inhaled β_2-agonist may be used before the inhaled glucocorticoid to provide bronchodilation before administration of the antiinflammatory drug. The bronchodilator inhaled drug is generally taken several minutes before the glucocorticoid or corticosteroid aerosol. All equipment (inhalers or nebulizers) should be kept clean, with filters cleaned and changed (nebulizers) and in good working condition. Use of a spacer may be indicated, especially if success with inhalation is limited. Rinsing of the mouth immediately after use of the inhaler or nebulizer dosage forms of corticosteroids/glucocorticoids is recommended to help prevent overgrowth of oral fungi/oral candidiasis (thrush).

Pediatric patients may need a physician's order to have these medications on hand at school and during athletic events or physical education. Peak flow meter use is also encouraged to help patients of all ages better regulate their disease. Journaling may help in recording peak flow levels, signs and symptoms of the disease, any improvement, and any adverse effects associated with therapy. For pediatric patients, there should be concern over the use of systemic forms of glucocorticoids. Specifically, in children the use of systemic forms of the glucocorticoids may lead to suppression of the hypothalamic-pituitary-adrenal axis and subsequent growth stunting. However, benefits versus risks are considerable. Inhaled forms and use of short-term systemic therapy are often combined in pediatric patients. The nurse should continue to monitor the patient's condition during therapy with a focus on the respiratory, cardiac, and central nervous systems.

The antileukotrienes zileuton, montelukast, and zafirlukast are given orally. Of most concern are the montelukast chewable tablets, which contain aspartame and approximately 0.842 mg of phenylamine per 5-mg tablet. Patient education should emphasize that they are indicated for chronic, not acute, asthma. These drugs should be taken every night on a continuous schedule, even if symptoms improve. Fluid intake should increase, as with all the respiratory drugs, to help decrease the viscosity of secretions.

◆ EVALUATION

The therapeutic effects of any of the drugs used to improve the control of acute/chronic respiratory symptoms/diseases and treat or help prevent respiratory diseases including the following: a decrease in dyspnea, wheezing, restlessness, and anxiety; improved respiratory patterns with return to normal rate and quality; improved activity tolerance and arterial blood gas levels; improved quality of life; and decreased severity and incidence of respiratory symptoms. The therapeutic effects of bronchodilators (e.g., xanthines, β-agonists) include decreased symptoms and increased ease of breathing. Blood levels of theophylline should be between 5 and 15 mcg/mL and should be frequently monitored. Peak flow meters are easy to use and help reveal early decreases in peak flow caused by bronchospasms. They also serve as a monitor of treatment effectiveness. Other respiratory drugs should produce the therapeutic effects related to the specific drug. Adverse effects for which to monitor in all drugs in this chapter are presented in the drug profiles and drug tables. Therapeutic effects include an improvement in the control of the acute and/or chronic respiratory disease process. Achievement of goals and outcomes should also be evaluated.

Patient Teaching Tips

β-Agonists

- The patient should be sure to maintain healthy living habits, such as undergoing regular health checkups, forcing fluids, eating three balanced meals daily, and engaging in consistent exercise as tolerated and as ordered.
- With asthma, bronchitis, or COPD, the patient should be encouraged to avoid exposure to conditions or situations that may lead to bronchoconstriction and/or worsening of the disorder (e.g., allergens, stress, smoking, and/or air pollutants).
- Educate patients about precipitating events for their respiratory problems or symptoms, as well as measures to help alleviate them. Patients should receive adequate information about their medications, OTC drugs, herbals, and supplemental therapies as well as about all actions that will help prevent and/or control the patient's illness.
- The patient should be instructed in the proper use and care of MDIs, dry powder inhalers, and other such devices, as described in the Patient Teaching Tips for corticosteroids. (Also see Chapter 9 or the photo atlas for more specific information.)

Xanthines

- Educate patients about interactions between smoking and xanthines. Smoking decreases the blood concentrations of aminophylline and theophylline. Other interactions associated with xanthines include charcoal-broiled foods that may decrease serum levels of the drug.
- Make sure the patient is aware of food and beverage items that contain caffeine (e.g., chocolate, coffee, cola, cocoa, tea) because of exacerbation of CNS stimulation.
- Encourage the patient to keep follow-up appointments because of the importance in monitoring therapeutic levels of medications.
- Educate the patient to take the medication around the clock to maintain steady-state drug levels and to never chew or crush extended-release preparations. Any problems such as headaches, insomnia, restlessness, muscle twitching, nausea, vomiting, GI pain, palpitations, and seizures should be reported immediately to the health care provider.

Anticholinergics

- Educate patients that ipratropium is used prophylactically to decrease the frequency and severity of asthma and has to be taken as ordered and generally year-round for therapeutic effectiveness. This drug should not be given if there is an existing allergy to soybeans, legumes, or soy.
- Encourage forcing of fluids with use of anticholinergics and with all other respiratory drugs, unless contraindicated. Fluids decrease the thickness of secretions and help with expectoration of sputum.
- Educate the patient taking any respiratory drugs (including anticholinergics) to take the prescribed number of puffs of an inhaler and no more than two puffs with one dosing or as ordered. Educate patients about the proper use of MDIs with or without a spacer (which applies to inhaled drugs in this chapter), how to use a dry powder inhaler, and how to properly clean and store the equipment.

Corticosteroids/Glucocorticoids

- In addition to adhering to the dosing and frequency of these drugs, if inhaled forms are used, the patient should practice good oral hygiene (e.g., rinsing of the mouth) after the last inhalation. Rinsing the mouth with water is appropriate and necessary to prevent oral fungal infections.

- Educate about keeping inhalers clean, including (once a week) removing the medication canister from the plastic casing and washing the casing in warm, soapy water. Once the casing is dry, the patient can replace the canister and cap the mouthpiece.
- The patient should be taught to keep track of the doses left in the MDI as follows: The number of doses in the canister should be noted and the number of days the doses will last should be calculated. For example, assume that two puffs are taken four times a day, and the inhaler has a capacity of 200 inhalations. Two puffs four times a day equals eight inhalations per day. Eight divided into 200 yields 25; that is, the inhaler will last approximately 25 days. The MDI should be marked with the date it will be empty and a refill obtained a few days before that date. Note that using extra doses will alter the refill date.
- Encourage the patient to always check the expiration dates of all medications!
- The patient should be encouraged to keep a journal of the medications being taken, how they work, what progress is being made in alleviating the asthma or illness, and how the patient is feeling every day. Any adverse effects should also be recorded.
- Educate patients to wear a medic-alert bracelet or necklace and/or carry a medical card with their diagnoses and list of medications and allergies. Emergency contact persons and phone numbers should also be listed.
- If the patient is using an intranasal dosage form, educate him or her to be sure to clear the nasal passages before administration. The patient should tilt the head slightly forward and insert the spray tip into one nostril, pointing it toward the inflamed nasal turbinates. The medication should be pumped into the nasal passage as the patient sniffs inward while holding the other nostril closed; the procedure is then repeated in the other nostril. Any unused portion should be discarded after 3 months.
- The patient needs to be aware that excess levels of systemic corticosteroids may lead to cushingoid symptoms; even though an inhaler minimizes this problem, education about it is very important to patient safety. Signs and symptoms of cushingoid syndrome include moon face, acne, an increase in fat pads, and swelling. These signs and symptoms would be at a higher risk of occurrence if these drugs are given systemically, either orally or in parenteral dosage forms.
- In addition, Addison's crisis can occur if a systemic corticosteroid is abruptly discontinued, so any dosage forms of these drugs should be weaned prior to withdrawal of the medication. The problems that the patient may experience should be emphasized and include nausea, shortness of breath, joint pain, weakness, and fatigue. If these occur, the patient should know to contact the physician immediately.
- Patients should always check for drug interactions with any type of medication.
- Encourage patients to report to the physician any weight gain of 2 lb or more in 24 hours or 5 lb or more in 1 week.

Leukotriene Antagonists

- Educate patients about the action and purpose of leukotriene antagonists (e.g., used for maintenance therapy and not for treatment of an acute attack of bronchospasms).
- The patient should be told to report worsening of the underlying asthma or any adverse effects of drug therapy that are not tolerable.
- Educate patients to report any abdominal pain, jaundice, nausea, or vomiting to the physician.

Points to Remember

- The β-agonists may stimulate α and β receptors, β₁ and β₂ receptors, or just β₁ receptors. The β₂ stimulants are the most specific for the lungs and have the fewest adverse effects.
- Xanthines include drugs such as caffeine and theophylline and work by inhibiting phosphodiesterase. Phosphodiesterase breaks down cAMP, which is needed to relax smooth muscles.
- Theophylline is the most common xanthine; aminophylline is the parenteral form of theophylline.
- A major anticholinergic, ipratropium, is the only anticholinergic drug that is used for treatment of COPD.
- Anticholinergic drugs are used for maintenance and not for relief of acute bronchospasms; they work by blocking the bronchoconstrictive effects of ACh.
- Corticosteroids are also used for treatment of the various respiratory disorders and have many indications. The most commonly used are beclomethasone, dexamethasone, flunisolide, and triamcinolone. Corticosteroids work by stabilizing the membranes of cells that release harmful bronchoconstricting substances.
- Contraindications to β-agonist use include cardiac disease and seizure disorders. Use of anticholinergics is contraindicated in patients with benign prostatic hypertrophy or glaucoma. Use of xanthine derivatives is contraindicated in patients with a history of GI tract disorders or peptic ulcer disease.
- The antileukotriene drugs zileuton and zafirlukast are given orally. Adverse effects include headache, dizziness, insomnia, and dyspepsia.
- The nurse should be sure to give the patient proper instructions for the use of MDIs, dry powder inhalers, and other inhalant equipment. Keeping the equipment clean and in a good state of repair is important, so adequate instructions should be provided not only for their use but also for their cleaning and storage.

NCLEX Examination Review Questions

1. A patient who has a history of asthma is experiencing an acute episode of shortness of breath and needs to take a medication for immediate relief. Which medication will the nurse choose for this situation?
   a. A β-agonist, such as albuterol
   b. An antileukotriene, such as montelukast
   c. A corticosteroid, such as fluticasone
   d. An anticholinergic, such as ipatropium
2. After a nebulizer treatment with the β-agonist albuterol, the patient complains of feeling a little "shaky," with slight tremors of the hands. His heart rate is 98 beats/min, increased from the pretreatment rate of 88 beats /min. The nurse knows that this reaction is
   a. an expected adverse effect of the medication.
   b. an allergic reaction to the medication.
   c. an indication that he has received an overdose of the medication.
   d. an idiosyncratic reaction to the medication.
3. A patient has been receiving an aminophylline (xanthine derivative) infusion for 24 hours. When monitoring for adverse effects, the nurse knows to expect which of the following?
   a. CNS depression
   b. Sinus tachycardia
   c. Increased appetite
   d. Temporary urinary retention
4. During a teaching session for a patient who will be receiving a new prescription for the antileukotriene montelukast (Singulair), the nurse should tell the patient that the drug works to do which of the following?
   a. Improve the respiratory drive
   b. Loosen and remove thickened secretions
   c. Reduce inflammation in the airway
   d. Stimulate immediate bronchodilation
5. After taking a dose of an inhaled corticosteroid, such as fluticasone, what is the most important action the patient should do next?
   a. Hold the breath for 60 seconds
   b. Rinse out the mouth with water
   c. Follow the corticosteroid with a bronchodilator inhaler, if ordered
   d. Repeat the dose in 15 minutes if the patient feels short of breath

1. a, 2. a, 3. b, 4. c, 5. b.

Critical Thinking Activities

1. Your patient is taking a xanthine derivative and should not ingest xanthine-containing beverages. What are examples of these beverages, and why is it important to avoid consuming them while taking a xanthine derivative?
2. Discuss the necessary patient education regarding the use of leukotriene modifiers, especially the rationale for the emphasis on taking the medication daily as ordered.

For answers, see http://evolve.elsevier.com/Lilley.

Antiinfective and Antiinflammatory Drugs

STUDY SKILLS TIPS

- *Nursing Process*
- *Assessment*
- *Nursing Diagnoses*
- *Evaluation*

NURSING PROCESS

This study model focuses on the Nursing Process section in Chapter 37. Since there is a Nursing Process section at the end of each chapter, the discussion of the example in Chapter 37 is applicable to all chapters.

ASSESSMENT

"What is the purpose of this section?" Each time you begin to read the Nursing Process section of a chapter, you need to ask this question. What are you supposed to learn? What are you supposed to know? What are you supposed to be able to do? All these questions relate to your role as a nurse. Consider the following sentence from this section in Chapter 37.

In general, <u>before the administration</u> of any antibiotic, it is <u>crucial to assess for a history of or symptoms indicative of hypersensitivity or allergic reactions (mild reactions with rash, pruritus, or hives, to severe reactions with laryngeal edema, bronchospasms, hypotension, and possible cardiac arrest)</u>.

Assessment clearly has to do with patient care. You are assessing the patient as he or she relates to the pharmacologic interventions that this chapter discusses. I have done some underlining in this section to bring into sharper focus some of the things that you must be very aware of as you study.

First, notice the use of the word *crucial* in the first line. Something is so important at this point that it cannot be ignored. Immediately the questioning process should be activated. What is crucial? The answer follows immediately in the sentence. You must assess for history of or symptoms indicative of hypersensi-

tivity or allergic reactions. The sentence goes on to identify the kind of data that should be available, and the sentence makes it clear that it has to be done *before the administration*. Each of the data factors is important, and each relates to other parts and chapters in this text. The next data item is hypersensitivities. Some individuals are *allergic* to certain antibiotics. It would be dangerous and possibly fatal to administer an antibiotic to a patient if he or she is hypersensitive.

Another data item specifies rash, pruritus, and hives and laryngeal edema, bronchospasms, and hypotension. As you read this you should instantly think to what they refer. Then you should try to recall information from this chapter that related the specific antibiotics to these reactions. Learning is cumulative. The Nursing Process section assumes you have read and understood what was presented earlier in the chapter.

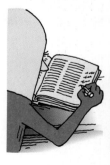

Often you may encounter standard medical abbreviations. As you read on in the Assessment section, you find this sentence:

Further assessment should include the patient's age, weight, baseline vital signs with body temperature and examination of the results of any laboratory studies that have been ordered, including liver function studies (aspartate aminotransferase [AST] level and alanine aminotransferase [ALT] level), kidney function studies (usually blood urea nitrogen and creatinine levels), cardiac function studies/tests (pertinent laboratory tests, electrocardiogram, or ultrasonography if indicated), culture and sensitivity tests, and complete blood count (CBC) with hemoglobin/hematocrit (Hgb/Hct) levels and platelet/clotting values (because of possible bleeding potential with some antibiotics).

In earlier Study Skills Tips, it has been suggested that you prepare vocabulary cards for these abbreviations to help you in a situation such as this. You need to know what *CBC*, *Hgb*, and *Hct* mean, what they measure, and how they relate to appropriate and effective administration of antibiotics. If these letters are not meaningful to you, then you will not be able to link what you know about the antibiotics with what you must know about administering them as a nurse. Many test questions on nursing examinations use the standard abbreviations, and you must know them instantly and be able to relate them to the situation covered. As you look at antibiotic administration and *CBC*, *Hgb*, and *Hct*, think what a test question might ask about these data elements in a real application in patient care? This is what the nursing process is all about.

NURSING DIAGNOSES

The same first question applies here as in every other section. What am I supposed to learn? Since the focus is on administration of antibiotics, the expectation you should bring to this is an awareness of your role in diagnosis. What should you look for in working with patients that affect the administration of antibiotics?

This same procedure should be applied to the sections on Planning, Outcome Criteria, and Implementation. Consider what each of these headings suggests about the nursing process, and read and evaluate the information, relating it to what you have already learned. Also consider the implications of the information as possible test questions that may ask you to do more than recall specific facts. As an example, consider the following case:

> Patient A, age 23, has a fever of 100.8° F. She was admitted yesterday and delivered a healthy infant 8 hours ago. She is breast feeding the newborn. What antibiotics might be administered for the fever? What specific antibiotics should be used with caution or eliminated from consideration?

This case demonstrates the need to read and think critically. You need to remember not only the specific facts from the chapter, but also be able to take a case study example and apply those facts to that specific situation.

EVALUATION

This is the final section under Nursing Process. What are you supposed to evaluate?

Evaluation should include monitoring of goals, outcome criteria, and therapeutic effects and adverse effects. Therapeutic effects of antibiotics include a decrease in the signs and symptoms of the infection; a return to normal vital signs, including temperature, and negative results on culture and sensitivity tests; normal results for CBC; and improved appetite, energy level, and sense of well-being. Evaluation for adverse effects includes monitoring for the specific drug-related adverse effects (see each drug profile).

First you should look for the positive responses (therapeutic effects) set forth in the above text sample that indicate the patient is responding favorably to the treatment. However, then you read *Evaluation for adverse effects includes...* This says your role in evaluation is to monitor the patient for negative responses and be prepared to educate the patient as to the effects he or she is experiencing and possible steps to help alleviate the symptoms.

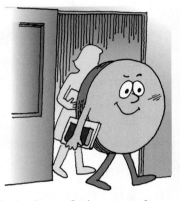

The Nursing Process section in each chapter should be read carefully and thoughtfully because it is in this section where you begin to see how the complex pharmacologic material presented earlier in the chapter fits into your role as a nurse. This material should be read with the same concern and care that you have given to the highly complex materials earlier in the chapter, as this is the section in which you must think about *application* of all you have learned. Your thinking process may be stimulated when you review this section with your study group. Each person brings his or her understanding and experience to the discussion. The insights can be richer and the learning more complete as you exchange ideas. Apply the PURR model with a study group or alone and be an active questioner and reader, and you will be successful in working with Nursing Process in each chapter.

Antibiotics Part 1

Objectives

When you reach the end of this chapter, you should be able to do the following:

1. Discuss the general principles of antibiotic therapy.
2. Explain how antibiotics work to rid the body of infection.
3. Discuss the pros and cons of antibiotic use with attention to the overuse or abuse of antibiotics and development of drug resistance.
4. Classify the various antibiotics by general category, including sulfonamides, penicillins, cephalosporins, macrolides, and tetracyclines.
5. Discuss the mechanisms of action, indications, cautions, contraindications, routes of administration, and drug interactions for the sulfonamides, penicillins, cephalosporins, macrolides, and tetracyclines.
6. Identify drug-specific adverse effects and toxic effects of each of the antibiotic classes listed earlier and cite measures to decrease their occurrence.
7. Discuss the concept of superinfection, including how it occurs and how to prevent it.
8. Develop a nursing care plan that includes all phases of the nursing process for patients receiving drugs in each of the following classes of antibiotic: sulfonamides, penicillins, cephalosporins, macrolides, and tetracyclines.

e-Learning Activities

Companion CD

- NCLEX Review Questions: see questions 328-337
- Animations
- Audio Glossary
- Category Catchers
- Medication Errors Checklists
- IV Therapy Checklists

evolve Website (http://evolve.elsevier.com/Lilley)

• Nursing Care Plans • Frequently Asked Questions • Content Updates • WebLinks • Supplemental Resources • Elsevier ePharmacology Update • Medication Administration Animations

Drug Profiles

▶ amoxicillin, p. 578
amoxicillin, p. 578
▶ azithromycin and
  clarithromycin, p. 585
aztreonam, p. 584
▶ cefazolin, p. 582
cefepime, p. 583
▶ cefoxitin, p. 582
ceftazidime, p. 582
▶ ceftriaxone, p. 582
cefuroxime, p. 582

▶ cephalexin, p. 582
demeclocycline, p. 589
▶ doxycycline, p. 589
▶ erythromycin, p. 585
▶ imipenem-cilastatin, p. 583
nafcillin, p. 578
▶ penicillin G and penicillin V
  potassium, p. 578
sulfamethoxazole-trimethoprim
  (co-trimoxazole), p. 575
telithromycin, p. 587

▶ Key drug.

Glossary

Antibiotic Having or pertaining to the ability to destroy or interfere with the development of a living organism. The term is used most commonly to refer to antibacterial drugs. (p. 570)

β-Lactam The name for a broad, major class of antibiotics that includes four subclasses: penicillins, cephalosporins, carbapenems, and monobactams. (p. 575)

β-Lactamase Any of a group of enzymes produced by bacteria that catalyze the chemical opening of the crucial β-lactam ring structures in β-lactam antibiotics. (p. 575)

β-Lactamase inhibitors Medications combined with certain penicillin drugs to block the effect of β-lactamase enzymes. (p. 575)

Bactericidal antibiotic An antibiotic that kills bacteria. (p. 576)

Bacteriostatic antibiotic An antibiotic that does not actually kill bacteria but rather inhibits their growth. (p. 574)

Empiric therapy Administration of antibiotics based on the practitioner's judgment of the pathogens most likely to be causing an apparent infection; it involves the presumptive treatment of an infection to avoid treatment delay before specific culture information has been obtained. (p. 572)

Glucose-6-phosphate dehydrogenase (G6PD) deficiency An inherited disorder in which the red blood cells are partially or completely deficient in glucose-6-phosphate dehydrogenase, a critical enzyme in the metabolism of glucose. Certain medications can cause hemolytic anemia in patients with this disorder. This is an example of a *host factor* related to drug therapy. (p. 573)

Host factors Factors that are unique to the body of a particular patient that affect the patient's susceptibility to infection and response to various antibiotic drugs. (p. 570)

Infections Invasions and multiplications of microorganisms in body tissues. (p. 570)

Microorganisms Microscopic living organisms (also called a *microbe*). (p. 570)

Prophylactic antibiotic therapy Antibiotics taken before anticipated exposure to an infectious organism in an effort to prevent the development of infection. (p. 572)

Slow acetylation A common genetic host factor in which the rate of metabolism of certain drugs is reduced. (p. 573)

Subtherapeutic Referring to antibiotic treatment that is ineffective in treating a given infection. Possible causes include inappropriate drug therapy, insufficient drug dosing, or bacterial drug resistance. (p. 572)

Superinfection (1) An infection occurring during antimicrobial treatment for another infection, resulting from overgrowth of an organism not susceptible to the antibiotic used. (2) A secondary microbial infection that occurs in addition to an earlier primary infection, often due to weakening of the patient's immune system function by the first infection. (p. 572)

Teratogens Substances that can interfere with normal prenatal development and cause one or more developmental abnormalities in the fetus. (p. 573)

Therapeutic Referring to antibiotic therapy that results in sufficient concentrations of the drug in the blood or other tissues to render it effective against specific bacterial pathogens. (p. 572)

MICROBIAL INFECTION

A person is normally able to remain healthy and resistant to infectious **microorganisms** because of the existence of certain host defenses. These defenses take various forms. They can be actual physical barriers such as intact skin or the ciliated respiratory mucosa. They can be physiologic defenses such as the gastric acid in the stomach and immune factors such as antibodies. They can also be the phagocytic cells (macrophages and polymorphonuclear neutrophils) that are part of the reticuloendothelial system.

Microorganisms are everywhere in both the external environment and many parts of the internal environment of our bodies. They can be intrinsically harmful to humans or they can be innocuous and even beneficial under normal circumstances but can become harmful when conditions are altered in some way. An example of an intrinsically harmful microorganism is *Rickettsia rickettsii*, which causes Rocky Mountain spotted fever. In contrast, certain species of *Streptococcus* are normally present on the body skin surface and usually do not cause harm. However, a common streptococcal throat infection ("strep throat") can cause endocarditis in patients whose heart valves have been damaged as a result of rheumatic fever. Rheumatic fever is a condition that is often a result of a previous streptococcal infection. Every known major class of microbes has member organisms that can infect humans. This includes bacteria, viruses,

fungi, and protozoa. The focus of this chapter is common bacterial **infections.**

Recall from microbiology that bacteria come in a number of different shapes. This property of bacteria is called their *morphology* (Figure 37-1). Bacteria may also be grouped according to other common recognizable characteristics (Figure 37-2). One of the most important ways of categorizing different bacteria is on the basis of their response to the *Gram-stain* procedure (Figure 37-3). Bacterial species that stain purple with the Gram-stain dyes are classified as gram-positive organisms. Those bacteria that stain red are classified as gram-negative organisms. This seemingly simple difference proves to be very significant in guiding the choice of **antibiotic** therapy.

Gram-positive organisms have cell walls with a much thicker constituent known as *peptidoglycan,* the name of which refers to the protein (peptido-) and sugar (-glycan) components of its chemical structure. In addition, gram-positive organisms have a thicker outer cell *capsule.* However, gram-negative organisms have a cell wall structure that is more complex, with a smaller outer capsule and peptidoglycan layer than gram-positive bacteria but with two cell membranes: an outer and an inner membrane (Figures 37-4 and 37-5). These differences usually make gram-negative bacterial infections more difficult to treat because the drug molecules have a harder time penetrating the more complex cell walls of gram-negative organisms.

When a person's normal host defenses are breached or somehow compromised, that person becomes susceptible to infection. The microorganisms invade and multiply in the body tissues, and if the infective process overwhelms the body's own defense system, the infection becomes clinically apparent. The patient then usually manifests the following classic signs and symptoms of infection: fever, chills, sweats, redness, pain and swelling, fatigue, weight loss, increased white blood cell (WBC) count, and the formation of pus. Not all patients will exhibit signs of infection. This is especially true in elderly and immunocompromised patients.

To help the body and its normal host defenses combat an infection, antibiotic therapy is often required. Antibiotics are most effective when their actions are combined with functioning bodily defense mechanisms. Before specific types of drug therapy are considered, some general principles are reviewed.

Bacterial Morphology Shapes

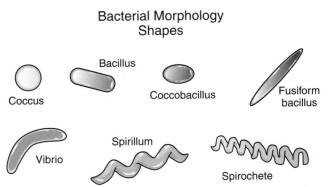

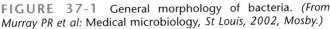

FIGURE 37-1 General morphology of bacteria. *(From Murray PR et al: Medical microbiology, St Louis, 2002, Mosby.)*

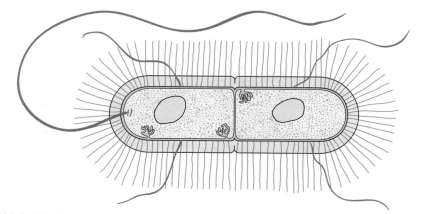

FIGURE 37-2 A dividing bacterial cell with a single flagellum, four sex pili, numerous common fibrae, a cell wall, a cytoplasmic membrane, two nuclear bodies, three mesosomes, and numerous ribosomes. *(From Greenwood D et al: Medical microbiology, ed 16, Edinburgh, 2002, Elsevier Science.)*

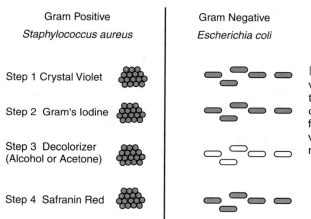

FIGURE 37-3 Gram-stain differentiation of bacteria. The crystal violet of Gram stain is precipitated by Gram iodine and is trapped in the thick peptidoglycan layer in gram-positive bacteria. The decolorizer disperses the gram-negative outer membrane and washes the crystal violet from the thin layer of peptidoglycan. Gram-negative bacteria are visualized by the red counterstain. *(From Murray PR et al: Medical microbiology, St Louis, 2002, Mosby.)*

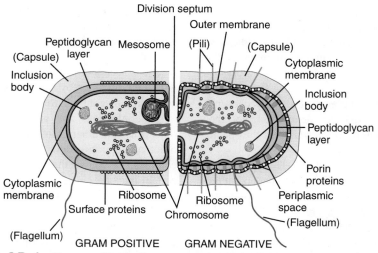

FIGURE 37-4 Gram-positive and gram-negative bacteria. A gram-positive bacterium has a thick layer of peptidoglycan *(left)*. A gram-negative bacterium has a thin peptidoglycan layer and an outer membrane *(right)*. Structures in parentheses are not found in all bacteria. *(From Murray PR et al: Medical microbiology, St Louis, 2002, Mosby.)*

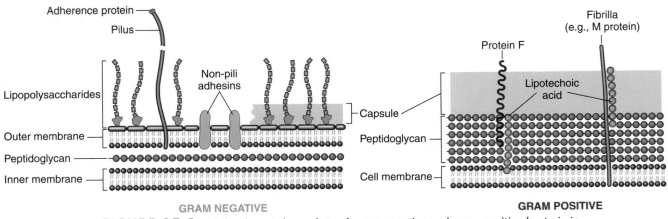

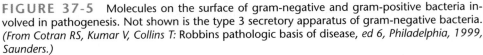

FIGURE 37-5   Molecules on the surface of gram-negative and gram-positive bacteria involved in pathogenesis. Not shown is the type 3 secretory apparatus of gram-negative bacteria. *(From Cotran RS, Kumar V, Collins T:* Robbins pathologic basis of disease, *ed 6, Philadelphia, 1999, Saunders.)*

GENERAL PRINCIPLES OF ANTIBIOTIC THERAPY

Antibiotic drug therapy should begin with a clinical assessment of the patient to determine whether he or she has the common signs and symptoms of infection previously mentioned. The patient should also be assessed during and after antibiotic therapy to evaluate the effectiveness of the drug therapy, monitor for adverse drug effects, and make sure the infection is not recurring.

Often the signs and symptoms of an infection appear long before an organism can be identified. When this happens and the risk of life-threatening or severe complications is high (e.g., suspected acute meningitis), an antibiotic is given to the patient immediately. The antibiotic selected is one that can best kill the microorganisms known to be the most common causes of infection. This is called **empiric therapy.** Before the start of empiric antibiotic therapy, specimens from suspected areas of infection should be cultured in an attempt to identify a causative organism. It must be emphasized that culture specimens should be obtained before drug therapy is initiated whenever possible. Otherwise, the presence of antibiotics in the tissues may result in misleading culture results. If an organism is identified in the laboratory, it is then tested for susceptibility to various antibiotics. The results of these tests can confirm whether the empiric therapy chosen is appropriate for eradicating the organism identified. If not, therapy can be adjusted to optimize its efficacy against the specific infectious organism(s).

Antibiotics are also given for prophylaxis. This is often the case, for example, when patients are scheduled to undergo a procedure in which the likelihood of dangerous microbial contamination is high during or after the procedure. **Prophylactic antibiotic therapy** is used to prevent an infection. However, the risk of infection varies depending on the procedure being performed. For example, the risk of infection in a patient undergoing coronary artery bypass surgery (with standard preoperative cleansing of the body) is relatively low compared with that in a person undergoing intraabdominal surgery for the treatment of injuries suffered in a motor vehicle accident. In the latter case, contamination with bacteria from the gastrointestinal (GI) tract is more likely to be present in the abdominal cavity. This would constitute a contaminated or "dirty" surgical field, and therefore the likelihood of clinically serious infection would be much higher. Antibiotic therapy would likely be required for a longer period after the procedure.

As mentioned earlier, to optimize antibiotic therapy the patient should be continuously monitored for both **therapeutic** efficacy and adverse drug effects. A therapeutic response to antibiotics is one in which there is a decrease in the specific signs and symptoms of infection compared with the baseline findings (e.g., fever, elevated WBC count, redness, inflammation, drainage, pain). Antibiotic therapy is said to be **subtherapeutic** when these signs and symptoms do not improve. This can result from use of an incorrect route of drug administration, inadequate drainage of an abscess, poor drug penetration to the infected area, insufficient serum levels of the drug, or bacterial resistance to the drug. Antibiotic therapy is considered toxic when the serum levels of the antibiotic are too high or when the patient has an allergic or other major adverse reaction to the drug. These reactions include rash, itching, hives, fever, chills, joint pain, difficulty breathing, or wheezing. Relatively minor adverse drug reactions such as GI discomfort and diarrhea are quite common with antibiotic therapy and are usually not severe enough to require drug discontinuation.

Superinfections and antibiotic interactions with food and other drugs are other problems to watch for in patients taking antibiotics. Superinfections can occur when antibiotics reduce or completely eliminate the normal bacterial flora, which consists of certain bacteria and fungi that are needed to maintain normal function in various organs. When these bacteria or fungi are killed by antibiotics, other bacteria or fungi are permitted to take over and cause infection. An example of a **superinfection** caused by antibiotics is the development of vaginal yeast infections when the normal vaginal bacterial flora is reduced by antibiotic therapy and yeast growth is no longer kept in balance.

Another type of superinfection occurs when a second infection closely follows an initial primary infection from an external source (as opposed to normal body flora), which may still be ongoing. A common example is a case in which a patient who already has a viral respiratory infection develops a secondary bacterial infection. This is likely due to weakening of the patient's immune system function by the primary viral infection. Although the viral infection will not respond to antibiotic therapy, antibiotics may be needed to treat the secondary bacterial infection. This situation calls for some diagnostic finesse on the part of prescribers (physicians or nurse practitioners), who should avoid prescribing unnecessary antibiotics for a viral infection. The presence of colored sputum (e.g., green or yellow) is one sign of a bacterial superinfection during a viral respiratory illness. Patients will often expect to receive an antibiotic prescription even when they show no signs of a bacterial superinfection. From their perspective they know they are "sick" and want "some medicine" to expedite their recovery from illness. This can create both diagnostic confusion and an emotional dilemma for the prescriber. Over the decades since antibiotics were first developed in the 1940s, many formerly very treatable bacterial infections have become increasingly resistant to antibiotic therapy. One major cause of this phenomenon is considered to be the overprescribing of antibiotics, often in the clinical situations described earlier. Antibiotic resistance is now considered one of the world's most pressing public health problems. *Emerging infections,* such as those with drug-resistant bacteria, are a major culprit. Inappropriate antibiotic prescribing has had the effect of selecting out for survival the most drug-resistant bacteria. Another factor that contributes to this problem is the tendency of many patients not to complete their antibiotic regimen. Patients should be counseled to take the entire course of prescribed antibiotic drugs, even if they feel that they are no longer ill. This increases the likelihood of a more complete bacterial kill, while reducing the chance of recurrent illness and survival of drug-resistant bacteria. The only usual exceptions are cases in which culture results indicate that the chosen antibiotic therapy is not ideal for the particular type of bacterial infection or major drug intolerance occurs. Patients should be educated as needed regarding such matters.

The chemical makeup of antibiotics can also cause the body to react in many ways. Food-drug and drug-drug interactions are common problems when antibiotics are taken. One of the more common food-drug interactions is that between milk or cheese and tetracycline, which results in decreased GI absorption of tetracycline. An example of a drug-drug interaction is that between quinolone antibiotics and antacids, which leads to decreased absorption of quinolones.

Other important factors that must be understood to use antibiotics appropriately are host-specific factors, or **host factors.** These are factors that pertain specifically to a given patient, and they can have an important bearing on the success or failure of antibiotic therapy. Some of these host factors are age, allergy history, kidney and liver function, pregnancy status, genetic characteristics, site of infection, and host defenses.

Age-related host factors are those that apply to patients at either end of the age spectrum. For example, infants and children may not be able to take certain antibiotics such as tetracyclines, which affect developing teeth or bones; fluoroquinolones, which may affect bone or cartilage development in children; and sulfonamides, which may displace bilirubin from albumin and precipitate kernicterus (hyperbilirubinemia) in neonates. The aging process affects the function of various organ systems. As people age there is a gradual decline in the function of the kidneys and liver,

the organs primarily responsible for metabolizing and eliminating antibiotics. Therefore, depending on the level of kidney or liver function of a given older adult, dosage adjustments may be necessary. Pharmacists often play a significant role in evaluating the dosages of antibiotics and other medications to ensure optimal dosing for a given patient's level of organ function.

A patient history of allergic reaction to an antibiotic plays an important role in the selection of the most appropriate antibiotic for that patient. Penicillins and sulfonamides are two broad classes of antibiotic to which many people have allergic anaphylactic reactions. The most dangerous such reaction is anaphylactic shock, in which a patient can suffocate from drug-induced respiratory arrest. Although this outcome is the most extreme, the potential for it does underscore the importance of consistently assessing patients for drug allergies and documenting any known allergies clearly in the medical record. All reported drug allergies should be taken seriously and investigated further before a final decision is made about whether to administer a given drug. Many patients will say that they are "allergic" to a medication when in fact what they had was a common mild adverse effect such as stomach upset or nausea. Patients who report drug allergies should be asked open-ended questions to elicit descriptions of prior allergic reactions so that the actual severity of the reaction can be assessed. As mentioned earlier, the most common severe reactions to any medication that need to be noted in the patient's chart include any difficulty breathing; significant rash, hives, or other skin reaction; and severe GI intolerance. Although some antibiotics are ideally taken on an empty stomach, eating a small amount of food with the medication may be sufficient to help the patient tolerate it and realize its therapeutic benefits.

Pregnancy-related host factors are also important to the selection of appropriate antibiotics because several antibiotics can pass through the placenta and cause harm to the developing fetus. Drugs that cause development abnormalities in the fetus are called **teratogens.** Their use in pregnant women can result in birth defects.

Some patients also have certain genetic abnormalities that result in various enzyme deficiencies. These conditions can adversely affect drug actions in the body. Two of the most common examples of such genetic host factors are **glucose-6-phosphate dehydrogenase (G6PD) deficiency** and **slow acetylation.** The administration of antibiotics such as sulfonamides, nitrofurantoin, and dapsone to a person with G6PD deficiency may result in the hemolysis, or destruction, of red blood cells (RBCs). Patients who are slow acetylators have a physiologic makeup that causes certain drugs to be metabolized more slowly than usual in a chemical step known as *acetylation.* This can lead to toxicity from drug accumulation. The most common example of such toxic effects is the development of peripheral neuropathy in a slow acetylator patient who is given typical adult dosages of the antituberculosis drug isoniazid (Chapter 40). Enzyme deficiencies such as G6PD deficiency are discussed in Chapter 2.

The anatomic site of the infection is another important host factor to consider when deciding not only which antibiotic to use but also the dosage, route of administration, and duration of therapy.

Consideration of these host factors helps prescribers and pharmacists to ensure optimal drug selection for each individual patient. Continued patient assessment and proper monitoring of antibiotic therapy increase the likelihood that this therapy will be safe and effective.

ANTIBIOTICS

Antibiotics are classified into many broad categories based on their chemical structure. Some of the more common of these categories are sulfonamides, penicillins, cephalosporins, macrolides, fluoroquinolones, aminoglycosides, and tetracyclines. In addition to chemical structure, the characteristics that distinguish one class of drugs from the next include antibacterial spectrum, mechanism of action, potency, toxicity, and pharmacokinetic properties. The four most common mechanisms of antibiotic action are interference with bacterial cell wall synthesis, interference with protein synthesis, interference with replication of nucleic acids (deoxyribonucleic acid [DNA] and ribonucleic acid [RNA]), and antimetabolite action that disrupts critical metabolic reactions inside the bacterial cell. Figure 37-6 portrays these mechanisms of action in combating bacterial infections and indicates which mechanism is used by several major antibiotic classes. Perhaps the greatest challenge in understanding antimicrobial therapy is remembering the types and species of microorganisms against which a given drug can act. The list of individual microorganisms against which a given drug has activity can be quite extensive and can seem daunting to the inexperienced practitioner. Most antimicrobials have activity against only one *type* of microbe (e.g., bacteria, viruses, fungi, protozoans). However, a few drugs do have activity against more than one class of organisms. The reader should recognize that his or her understanding of antimicrobial therapy will deepen with clinical experience. The field of infectious disease treatment is continually evolving, largely because of the continual emergence of resistant bacterial strains. For this reason, drug indications change frequently, often from year to year, as various bacterial species become resistant to previously effective antiinfective

therapy. It is always appropriate to check the most current reference materials or consult with colleagues (e.g., nurses, pharmacists, physicians) when questions remain.

SULFONAMIDES

Sulfonamides are a chemically related group of antibiotics that are all synthetic derivatives of sulfanilamide, the first sulfonamide to be discovered. They were one of the first groups of drugs used as antibiotics. Some of the more commonly prescribed single-drug sulfonamides are sulfadiazine, sulfamethoxazole, and sulfisoxazole. However, in most cases, the sulfonamide is combined with another antibiotic known as *trimethoprim.* Sulfasalazine, another sulfonamide, is used to treat ulcerative colitis and rheumatoid arthritis and is not used as an antibiotic.

Mechanism of Action and Drug Effects

Sulfonamides do not actually destroy bacteria but inhibit their growth. For this reason they are considered **bacteriostatic antibiotics.** They inhibit the growth of susceptible bacteria by preventing bacterial synthesis of folic acid, a B-complex vitamin that is required for the proper synthesis of *purines,* one of the chemical components of nucleic acids (DNA and RNA). Chemical components of folic acid include paraaminobenzoic acid (PABA), pteridine, and glutamic acid. Specifically, in a process known as competitive inhibition, sulfonamides compete with PABA for the bacterial enzyme *tetrahydropteroic acid synthetase,* which incorporates PABA into the folic acid molecule during biosynthesis. Because sulfonamides are capable of blocking a specific step in a biosynthetic pathway, they are also considered antimetabolites. However, those microorganisms that require exogenous folic acid (not synthesized by the bacterium itself) are not affected by sulfonamide antibiotics.

Trimethoprim, mentioned earlier, is a nonsulfonamide antibiotic that is given in combination with sulfamethoxazole in the most common type of sulfonamide therapy. The resulting combination is called co-trimoxazole and is often abbreviated as SMX-TMP to reflect the generic names of the two component drugs. Although trimethoprim is also sometimes given as a single drug, sulfamethoxazole is currently available only in the combination drug co-trimoxazole. Trimethoprim blocks the action of bacterial tetrahydrofolate reductase, another enzyme required for bacterial folic acid synthesis. The step that involves this enzyme occurs immediately after the step inhibited by sulfonamide drugs. Thus, when sulfamethoxazole and trimethoprim are given in combination, they inhibit two successive steps in the bacterial folic acid pathway. This allows for an additive antibacterial effect with greater antiinfective efficacy (e.g., against urinary tract infections [UTIs]).

Again, only microorganisms that synthesize their own folic acid are inhibited by sulfonamides. These drugs do not affect folic acid metabolism in human cells and cells of other organisms that require exogenous folic acid.

Indications

Sulfonamides have a broad spectrum of antibacterial activity, including activity against both gram-positive and gram-negative organisms. These antibiotics achieve very high concentrations in the kidneys, through which they are eliminated. In particular, co-trimoxazole is often used in the treatment of UTIs. Commonly susceptible organisms include strains of *Enterobacter* species (spp.),

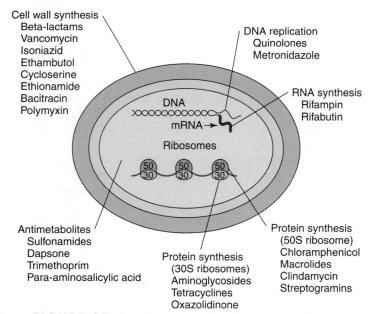

FIGURE 37-6 Basic sites of antibiotic activity. *DNA,* Deoxyribonucleic acid; *mRNA,* messenger ribonucleic acid; *RNA,* ribonucleic acid. *(From Murray PR et al: Medical microbiology, St Louis, 2002, Mosby.)*

Escherichia coli, Klebsiella spp., *Proteus mirabilis, Proteus vulgaris,* and *Staphylococcus aureus.* Unfortunately, however, resistant bacterial strains are a growing problem, as is the case with other antibiotic classes. Results of culture and sensitivity testing help to optimize drug selection in individual cases. This combination drug is also used for respiratory tract infections. However, it is now less effective than previously against streptococci infecting the upper respiratory tract and pharynx. Another specific use for co-trimoxazole is prophylaxis and treatment of opportunistic infections in patients with human immunodeficiency virus (HIV) infection, especially infection by *Pneumocystis jirovecii* (formerly known as *Pneumocystis carinii*), a common cause of HIV-associated pneumonia (Chapter 39). There are also several less common uses for co-trimoxazole. The drug is used to treat nocardiosis, a bacterial infection caused by various *Nocardia* spp. Such infection usually occurs as pneumonia but can lead to skin and brain abscesses. Co-trimoxazole is also a drug of choice for infections caused by the bacterium *Stenotrophomonas maltophilia.* Although an uncommon infection, it is associated with prolonged hospitalization.

Contraindications

Use of sulfonamides is contraindicated in cases of known drug allergy to sulfonamides or to chemically related drugs such as the sulfonylureas (used to treat diabetes; Chapter 31), thiazide and loop diuretics, carbonic anhydrase inhibitors (Chapter 25), and cyclooxygenase-2 inhibitors like celecoxib (Chapter 44). Their use is also contraindicated in pregnant women at term and in infants younger than 2 months of age.

Adverse Effects

Sulfonamide drugs are a common cause of allergic reaction. Patients will sometimes refer to this as "sulfa allergy" or even "sulfur allergy." Although immediate reactions can occur, sulfonamides typically cause delayed cutaneous reactions. These reactions frequently begin with fever followed by a rash (morbilliform eruptions, erythema multiforme, or toxic epidermal necrolysis). Photosensitivity reactions are another type of skin reaction that is induced by exposure to sunlight during sulfonamide drug therapy. In some cases, such reactions can result in severe sunburn. Such reactions are also common with the *tetracycline* class of antibiotics discussed later in this chapter, as well as with various other drug classes (see Index) and may occur immediately or have a delayed onset. Other reactions to sulfonamides include mucocutaneous, GI, hepatic, renal, or hematologic complications, all of which may be fatal in severe cases. It is believed that sulfonamide reactions are immune mediated and involve the production of reactive drug metabolites in the body. It is important to differentiate between sulfites and sulfonamides. Sulfites are commonly used as preservatives in everything from wine to food to injectable drugs. A person allergic to sulfonamide drugs may or may not also be allergic to sulfite preservatives. Reported adverse effects to the sulfonamides are listed in Table 37-1.

Interactions

Sulfonamides can have clinically significant interactions with a number of other medications. Sulfonamides can potentiate the hypoglycemic effects of sulfonylureas in diabetes, the toxic effects of phenytoin, and the anticoagulant effects of warfarin, which can lead to hemorrhage. There is also limited case-report evidence that sulfonamides can inhibit the immunosuppressant

Table 37-1   Sulfonamides: Reported Adverse Effects

Body System	Adverse Effects
Blood	Agranulocytosis, aplastic anemia, hemolytic anemia, thrombocytopenia
Gastrointestinal	Nausea, vomiting, diarrhea, pancreatitis
Integumentary	Epidermal necrolysis, exfoliative dermatitis, Stevens-Johnson syndrome, photosensitivity
Other	Convulsions, crystalluria, toxic nephrosis, headache, peripheral neuritis, urticaria

effects of cyclosporine in transplant patients and can also increase the likelihood of cyclosporine-induced nephrotoxicity. Patients receiving any of these drug combinations may require more frequent monitoring to ensure optimal drug effects. Sulfonamides may also reduce the efficacy of oral contraceptives. Patients should be advised to use additional contraceptive methods.

Dosages

For recommended dosages of selected sulfonamides, see the Dosages table on page 576.

Drug Profiles

Sulfonamides work by interfering with bacterial synthesis of the essential nutrient *folic acid.* Most sulfonamide therapy today uses the combination drug co-trimoxazole. However, a few other sulfonamide drugs remain on the market for specific uses. These include sulfadiazine, sulfacetamide, sulfadoxine (with pyrimethamine), sulfapyridine, sulfisoxazole (with and without erythromycin), mafenide, and zonisamide.

sulfamethoxazole-trimethoprim (co-trimoxazole)

Co-trimoxazole (Bactrim, Septra) is a fixed-combination drug product containing a 5:1 ratio of sulfamethoxazole to trimethoprim. It is available in both oral and injectable dosage forms.

Pharmacokinetics

Half-Life	Onset	Peak	Duration
7-12 hr	Variable	2-4 hr (plasma)	Up to 12 hr

β-LACTAM ANTIBIOTICS

The **β-lactam** antibiotics are very commonly used drugs, so named because of the β-lactam ring that is part of their chemical structure (Figure 37-7). This broad group of drugs includes four major subclasses: penicillins, cephalosporins, carbapenems, and monobactams. Some bacterial strains produce the enzyme **β-lactamase.** This enzyme provides a mechanism for bacterial resistance to these antibiotics. The enzyme can break the chemical bond between the carbon (C) and nitrogen (N) atoms in the structure of the β-lactam ring. When this happens, all β-lactam drugs lose their antibacterial efficacy. Because of this, additional drugs known as **β-lactamase inhibitors** are added to the dosage forms of several of the penicillin β-lactam antibiotics to make the drug more powerful against β-lactamase–producing bacterial strains. Each of the four classes of β-lactam antibiotics is examined in detail in the following sections.

DOSAGES

Selected Sulfonamides and Combination Drug Products

Drug (Pregnancy Category)	Pharmacologic Class	Usual Dosage Range*	Indications
sulfamethoxazole-trimethoprim (co-trimoxazole, SMX-TMP, SMZ-TMP) (Bactrim, Septra) (C)	Sulfonamide and folate antimetabolite	**Adult and pediatric** IV/PO: 8-10 mg/kg/day divided bid (dose is in terms of trimethoprim component) **Adult** PO: 160 mg TMP/800 mg SMX once daily **Pediatric** PO: 150 mg/m² TMP/750 mg/m² SMX daily × 3 consecutive days/wk	UTI, shigellosis enteritis; higher doses for nocardiosis and *Pneumocystis jirovecii* infection *P. jirovecii* prophylaxis, otitis media, acute exacerbation of chronic bronchitis
▶erythromycin-sulfisoxazole (Pediazole, Eryzole) (C)	Macrolide and sulfonamide	**Pediatric older than 2 mo only** PO: Fixed combination of erythromycin 200 mg and sulfisoxazole 600 mg/5 mL oral suspension Liquid dose range: 2.5-10 mL q6h based on weight	*Haemophilus influenzae* otitis media
sulfisoxazole (Gantrisin Pediatric) (C)	Sulfonamide	**Adult** PO: 2-4 g load, then 4-8 g/day divided q4-6h **Pediatric older than 2 mo** PO: 75 mg/kg load, then 150 mg/kg/day divided q4-6h	Otitis media, UTI, nocardiosis, toxoplasmosis (with pyrimethamine)

IV, Intravenous; *PO,* oral; *UTI,* urinary tract infection.
*Dosage ranges are typical but are not necessarily exhaustive due to space limitations. Clinical variations may occur.

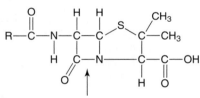

FIGURE 37-7   Chemical structure of penicillins showing the β-lactam ring. *R,* Variable portion of drug chemical structure.

PENICILLINS

The penicillins are a very large group of chemically related antibiotics that are derived from a mold fungus often seen on bread or fruit. The penicillins can be divided into four subgroups based on their structure (see Figure 37-7) and the spectrum of bacteria that they can kill: natural penicillins, penicillinase-resistant penicillins, aminopenicillins, and extended-spectrum penicillins. Examples of antibiotics in each subgroup and a brief description of their characteristics are given in Table 37-2.

Natural penicillins were first introduced in the early 1940s during World War II, and to this day they have remained very effective and safe antibiotics. They are **bactericidal antibiotics** and can kill a wide variety of gram-positive and some gram-negative bacteria. Penicillins work by inhibiting bacterial cell wall synthesis. However, some bacteria have acquired the capacity to produce enzymes capable of destroying penicillins. These enzymes are called β-*lactamases,* and they can inactivate the

penicillin molecules by opening the β-lactam ring. There are many types of β-lactamase enzymes with differing abilities to resist various β-lactam antibiotics. The β-lactamases that specifically inactivate penicillin molecules are called *penicillinases.* Bacterial strains that produce these drug-inactivating enzymes were a therapeutic obstacle until drugs were synthesized that inhibit these enzymes. Three of these β-lactamase inhibitors are clavulanic acid (also called *clavulanate*), tazobactam, and sulbactam. These drugs bind with the β-lactamase enzyme itself to prevent the enzyme from breaking down the penicillin molecule, although they are not always effective. The following are examples of currently available combinations of penicillin and β-lactamase inhibitor:

- ampicillin + sulbactam (Unasyn)
- amoxicillin + clavulanic acid (Augmentin)
- ticarcillin + clavulanic acid (Timentin)
- piperacillin + tazobactam (Zosyn)

Mechanism of Action and Drug Effects

The mechanism of action of penicillins involves the inhibition of bacterial cell wall synthesis. Once distributed by the patient's bloodstream to infected areas, penicillin molecules slide through bacterial cell walls to get to their site of action. Some penicillins, however, are too large to pass through these openings in the cell walls, and because they cannot get to their site of action they cannot kill the bacteria. On the other hand, some bacteria can make the openings in their cell walls smaller so that the penicillin cannot get through to kill them. The penicillin molecules that do gain entry into the bacterium must then find the appropriate bind-

Table 37-2   Classification of Penicillins

Subclass	Generic Drug Names	Description
Aminopenicillins	amoxicillin, ampicillin, bacampicillin	Have an amino group attached to the basic penicillin structure that enhances their activity against gram-negative bacteria compared with natural penicillins.
Extended-spectrum drugs	piperacillin, ticarcillin, carbenicillin	Have wider spectra of activity than do all other penicillins.
Natural penicillins	penicillin G, penicillin V	Although many modifications of the original natural (mold-produced) structure have been made, these are the only two in current clinical use. Penicillin G is the injectable form for IV or IM use; penicillin V is a PO dosage form (tablet and liquid).
Penicillinase-resistant drugs	cloxacillin, dicloxacillin, nafcillin, oxacillin	Stable against hydrolysis by most staphylococcal penicillinases (enzymes that normally break down the natural penicillins).

IM, Intramuscular; *IV*, intravenous; *PO*, oral.

ing sites. These are known as *penicillin-binding proteins*. By binding to these proteins, the penicillin molecules interfere with normal cell wall synthesis, causing the formation of defective cell walls that are unstable and easily broken down (see Figure 37-6). Bacterial death usually results from lysis (rupture) of the bacterial cells due to this drug-induced disruption of cell wall structure.

Indications

Penicillins are indicated for the prevention and treatment of infections caused by susceptible bacteria. The microorganisms most commonly destroyed by penicillins are gram-positive bacteria, including *Streptococcus* spp., *Enterococcus* spp., and *Staphylococcus* spp. Most penicillins have little if any ability to kill gram-negative bacteria, although some of the extended-spectrum penicillins can do so.

Contraindications

Penicillins are usually safe and well-tolerated medications. The only usual contraindication is known drug allergy.

Adverse Effects

Allergic reactions to the penicillins occur in 0.7% to 4% of treatment courses. The most common reactions are urticaria, pruritus, and angioedema. A wide variety of idiosyncratic (unpredictable) drug reactions can occur, such as maculopapular eruptions, eosinophilia, Stevens-Johnson syndrome, and exfoliative dermatitis. Maculopapular rash occurs in about 2% of treatment courses with natural penicillin and 5.2% to 9.5% with ampicillin. Anaphylactic reactions are much less common, occurring in 0.004% to 0.015% of patients. They are fatal in only 0.001% to 0.003% of cases (1 in 32,000 to 1 in 100,000 cases). Severe reactions are much more common with injected than with orally administered penicillin, as is the case with most other antibiotics that come in oral and injectable form. A very common clinical scenario is that in which a prescriber wants to administer a cephalosporin to a patient reporting a penicillin allergy. Patients who are allergic to penicillins have a fourfold to sixfold increased risk of allergy to

Table 37-3   Penicillins: Reported Adverse Effects

Body System	Adverse Effects
Central nervous	Lethargy, hallucinations, anxiety, depression, twitching, coma, convulsions
Gastrointestinal	Nausea, vomiting, diarrhea, increased AST and ALT levels, abdominal pain, colitis
Hematologic	Anemia, increased bleeding time, bone marrow depression, granulocytopenia
Metabolic	Hyperkalemia, hypokalemia, alkalosis
Other	Taste alterations; sore mouth; dark, discolored, or sore tongue; hives; rash

ALT, Alanine aminotransferase; *AST*, aspartate aminotransferase.

other β-lactam antibiotics. The incidence of cross-reactivity between cephalosporins and penicillins is reported as between 1% and 18%. Patients reporting penicillin allergy should be asked to describe their prior allergic reaction. The decision to continue with cephalosporin therapy in such cases is often a matter of clinical judgment, based on the severity of reported prior reactions to penicillin drugs, the nature of the infection and the drug susceptibility of the infective organism if known, and the availability and patient tolerance of other alternative antibiotics. Macrolide antibiotics, discussed later in this chapter, are a commonly used alternative class of medications for patients reporting allergy to penicillins or cephalosporins.

As mentioned earlier, penicillins are generally well tolerated and associated with very few adverse effects.

As with many drugs, the most common adverse effects involve the GI system. The most common adverse effects and adverse effects of the penicillins are listed in Table 37-3.

Interactions

Many drugs interact with penicillins; some have positive effects, and others have harmful effects. The most common and clinically significant drug interactions associated with penicillin use are listed in Table 37-4.

Table 37-4 Penicillins: Drug Interactions

Interacting Drug	Mechanism	Result
Aminoglycosides (IV) and clavulanic acid	Additivity	More effective killing of bacteria
Aminoglycosides (IV)	Synergism, but possible inactivation of penicillin by aminoglycosides if mixed in same IV bag	Reduced penicillin efficacy when mixed in same bag; mix drugs in separate IV bags, and, if using same IV line for both, flush line with normal saline between doses
neomycin (an oral aminoglycoside)	Reduced absorption of penicillin in GI tract when both drugs are given orally	Reduced penicillin efficacy; avoid concurrent use or consider injectable penicillin instead
Tetracyclines	Uncertain	May reduce efficacy of penicillins; avoid concurrent use
Macrolides (e.g., erythromycin)	Uncertain	Has been shown to have both synergism (which can be beneficial) and antagonism with penicillins (clinical judgment call)
Potassium supplements, table salt	Penicillin G potassium has 1.7 mEq of potassium ion per million units; penicillin G sodium has 2 mEq of sodium ion per million units	Effects unlikely for most patients, but may precipitate or worsen hyperkalemia and hypernatremia; monitor sodium and/or potassium levels as needed in at-risk patients and choose alternative drugs if indicated
NSAIDs	Compete for protein binding	More free and active penicillin (may be beneficial)
Oral contraceptives	Uncertain	May decrease efficacy of the contraceptive
probenecid	Competes for elimination	Prolongs the effects of penicillins
rifampin	Inhibition	May inhibit the killing activity of penicillins
warfarin	Reduced vitamin K from gut flora	Enhanced anticoagulant effect of warfarin

IV, Intravenous; *NSAIDs,* nonsteroidal antiinflammatory drugs.

Dosages

For dosage information for selected penicillins, see the Dosages table on page 579.

Drug Profiles

Penicillins are classified as pregnancy category B drugs. They are very safe antibiotics. Their use is contraindicated in patients with a hypersensitivity to them, but because of their relatively good adverse effects profile, there are otherwise very few contraindications to their use.

Natural Penicillins

▶ penicillin G and penicillin V potassium

Penicillin G has three salt forms: benzathine, procaine, and potassium. All of these forms are given by injection, either intravenously (IV) or intramuscularly (IM). The benzathine and procaine salts are used as longer-acting IM injections. They are formulated into a thick, white, pastelike material that is designed for prolonged dissolution and absorption from the IM site of injection. These preparations should *never* be given IV, however, because their consistency is too thick for IV administration, and such use can be fatal. The IM formulations can be especially helpful for treating the sexually transmitted disease syphilis, because often only one injection is needed, and therefore it can be given one time at a clinic that treats sexually transmitted diseases.

Penicillin V potassium is available only for oral use.

Pharmacokinetics

Half-Life	Onset	Peak	Duration
PO: 30 min	PO: Variable	PO: 30-60 min (plasma)	PO: 4-6 hr

Penicillinase-Resistant Penicillins

nafcillin

Nafcillin is one of the four currently available penicillinase-resistant penicillins; the other three are cloxacillin, dicloxacillin, and oxacillin. Nafcillin is available only in injectable form, whereas cloxacillin and dicloxacillin are available only in oral form. Oxacillin is available in both oral and injectable forms. The penicillinase-resistant penicillins are able to resist breakdown by the penicillin-destroying enzyme (penicillinase) commonly produced by bacteria such as staphylococci. For this reason they may also be referred to as *antistaphylococcal penicillins.* The chemical structure of these drugs features a large, bulky side chain near the β-lactam ring. This side chain serves as a barrier to the penicillinase enzyme, preventing it from breaking the β-lactam ring, which would inactivate the drug. There are, however, certain strains of staphylococci, specifically *Staphylococcus aureus,* that are resistant to these drugs. Such bacteria therefore require alternative antibiotic regimens.

Pharmacokinetics

Half-Life	Onset	Peak	Duration
20-30 min	Variable	30-60 min	6 hr

Aminopenicillins

There are three aminopenicillins: amoxicillin, ampicillin, and bacampicillin. They are so named because of the presence of a free amino group ($^-NH_2$) in their chemical structure. This structural feature gives aminopenicillins enhanced activity against gram-negative bacteria against which the natural and penicillinase-resistant penicillins are relatively ineffective. Amoxicillin is an analogue of ampicillin, and bacampicillin is a prodrug of ampicillin. Bacampicillin has no antibacterial activity until hydrolyzed to ampicillin in the body.

▶ amoxicillin

Amoxicillin (Amoxil, Trimox, Wymox) is a very commonly prescribed aminopenicillin. Amoxicillin is used to treat infections caused by susceptible organisms in the ears, nose, throat, genitourinary tract, skin, and skin structures. Pediatric dosages are sometimes higher than in the past because of the development of increasingly resistant *Streptococcus pneumoniae* organisms. The traditional adult dosage continues to be adequate in most cases. The drug is available only for oral use.

Pharmacokinetics

Half-Life	Onset	Peak	Duration
PO: 1-1.3 hr	PO: 0.5-1 hr	PO: 1-2 hr	PO: 6-8 hr

ampicillin

Ampicillin (Principen, Totacillin) is the prototypical aminopenicillin, and it differs from penicillin G only in that it has the amino group in its molecular structure. It is available in three different salt forms:

DOSAGES

Selected Penicillins

Drug (Pregnancy Category)	Pharmacologic Class	Usual Dosage Range	Indications
▶amoxicillin (Amoxil, Trimox, Wymox, others) (B)	Aminopenicillin	**Pediatric** PO: 40-90 mg/kg/day divided q8-12h **Adult** PO: 250-500 mg q8h	Otitis media; sinusitis; various susceptible respiratory, skin, and urinary tract infections; dental prophylaxis for bacterial endocarditis; *Helicobacter pylori* infection
ampicillin (Principen, Totacillin, others) (B)	Aminopenicillin	**Adult** PO/IV/IM: 1-12 g/day divided q4-6h **Pediatric** 50-400 mg/kg/day divided q4-6h	Primarily infection with gram-negative organisms such as *Shigella, Salmonella, Escherichia, Haemophilus, Proteus,* and *Neisseria* spp.; infection with some gram-positive organisms
nafcillin (generic only) (B)	Penicillinase-resistant penicillin	**Adult** IV: 500-1000 mg q4h **Pediatric** IV: 50-200 mg/kg divided q4-6h	Infection with penicillinase-producing staphylococci
▶penicillin V potassium (Pen-Vee K, Veetids, others) (B)	Natural penicillin	**Adult and pediatric** PO: 125-500 mg q6-8h **Adult and pediatric** IV: 150-300 mg/kg/day divided q4-6h	Primarily infection with gram-positive organisms such as *Streptococcus* (including *Streptococcus pneumoniae*) and *Staphylococcus* spp.
ticarcillin disodium (Ticar) (B)	Extended-spectrum penicillin	**Adult and pediatric** IV: 150-300 mg/kg/day divided q4-6h	Primarily infection with gram-negative organisms such as *Pseudomonas, Escherichia, Proteus,* and *Enterobacter* spp., but also infection with *Streptococcus faecalis (Enterococcus),* which is gram positive

IM, Intramuscular; *IV,* intravenous; *PO,* oral; *spp,* species.

anhydrous, trihydrate, and sodium. As with penicillin G, the different salt forms are administered by different routes. Ampicillin anhydrous and trihydrate are both administered orally, whereas ampicillin sodium is given parenterally. This drug is still currently available, although it is now used less frequently than before because many other newer drug options are being marketed to prescribers.

Pharmacokinetics

Half-Life	Onset	Peak	Duration
PO: 0.7-1.4 hr	PO: Variable	PO: 1-2 hr (serum)	PO: 4-6 hr

Extended-Spectrum Penicillins

By making a few changes in the basic penicillin structure, drug developers produced another generation of penicillins that have a wider spectrum of activity than that possessed by either of the other two classes of semisynthetic penicillins (penicillinase-resistant penicillins and aminopenicillins) or by the natural penicillins. Currently three extended-spectrum penicillins are available: carbenicillin, piperacillin, and ticarcillin. Production of one formerly available drug in this class, mezlocillin, has been discontinued.

These extended-spectrum drugs have activity against some bacteria that the other classes of penicillins cannot kill, such as *Pseudomonas* spp. They also have stability against the β-lactamase enzymes produced by *Proteus* spp. Infections with both of these bacterial genera are generally among the more difficult to treat.

Ticarcillin and piperacillin are given only by injection, usually IV, although IM doses are permitted. Carbenicillin is given only orally. Both ticarcillin and piperacillin are available in fixed-combination products that include β-lactamase inhibitors. The ticarcillin fixed-combination product (Timentin) includes clavulanate

potassium. Piperacillin is available in combination with tazobactam (a combination called Zosyn). These β-lactamase–inhibiting products allow for enhanced multiorganism coverage, especially against anaerobic organisms that are common in intestinal infections.

Pharmacokinetics

carbenicillin indanyl sodium: 382-mg film-coated tablets			
Half-Life	**Onset**	**Peak**	**Duration**
PO: 0.8-1 hr	PO: Variable	PO: 0.5-2 hr (serum)	PO: 6 hr
ticarcillin disodium: 1-, 3-, 6-, and 20-g vials for injection			
Half-Life	**Onset**	**Peak**	**Duration**
IV: 0.9-1.3 hr	IV: Variable	IV: 5 min (serum)	IV: Variable

CEPHALOSPORINS

Cephalosporins are semisynthetic antibiotic derivatives of cephalosporin C, a substance produced by a fungus but synthetically altered to yield an antibiotic. These chemically altered derivatives of the fungus are structurally and pharmacologically related to the penicillins. Like penicillins, cephalosporins are bactericidal and work by interfering with bacterial cell wall synthesis. They also bind to the same penicillin-binding proteins inside bacteria that were described earlier for the penicillins. Although there are a variety of such proteins, they are collectively referred to as *penicillin-binding* regardless of the type of β-lactam drug involved.

Cephalosporins can destroy a broad spectrum of bacteria, and this ability is directly related to the chemical changes that have been made to their basic cephalosporin structure. Modifications to this chemical structure by pharmaceutical scientists have given rise to four generations of cephalosporins. Depending on the generation, these drugs may be active against gram-positive, gram-negative, or anaerobic bacteria. They are not active against fungi and viruses. The different drugs of each generation have certain chemical similarities, and thus they can kill similar spectra of bacteria. In general, the level of gram-negative coverage increases with each successive generation. However, anaerobic coverage and gram-positive coverage are both more variable among the different generations. Cefepime, cefdinir, and cefditoren pivoxil are the only fourth-generation cephalosporins available thus far, and some references classify these with the other third-generation drugs. The currently available parenteral and oral cephalosporin antibiotics are listed in Table 37-5. As is often the case, injectable drugs produce higher serum concentrations than those administered by the oral route, and they are thus needed to treat more serious infections.

The safety profiles, contraindications, and pregnancy ratings of the cephalosporins are very similar to those of the penicillins. The most commonly reported adverse effects include mild diarrhea, abdominal cramps, rash, pruritus, redness, and edema. Because cephalosporins are chemically very similar to penicillins, a person who has had an allergic reaction to penicillin may also have an allergic reaction to a cephalosporin. This is referred to as *cross-sensitivity*. Various investigators have observed that the incidence of cross-sensitivity between penicillins and cephalosporins is between 1% and 18%. However, only those patients who have had a serious anaphylactic reaction to penicillin should definitely not be given cephalosporins. As a class the cephalosporins are very safe and effective antibiotics, and they should not be unnecessarily avoided because of overcautiousness about possible cross-sensitivity.

Penicillins and cephalosporins are practically identical in their mechanism of action, drug effects, therapeutic effects, adverse effects, and adverse effects. For that reason, this information is not repeated for the cephalosporins, and the reader is referred to the pertinent discussions in the section on the penicillin drugs. Cephalosporins of all generations are very safe drugs that are categorized as pregnancy category B drugs. Their use is contraindicated in patients who have shown a hypersensitivity to them and in any patient with a history of life-threatening allergic reaction to penicillins. Drug interactions are listed in Table 37-6. The prototypical first-, second-, third-, and fourth-generation cephalosporins are described in the following drug profiles section.

Dosages

For the recommended dosages of selected cephalosporins, see the Dosages table on page 581.

Table 37-5 Cephalosporins: Parenteral and Oral Preparations

First Generation		Second Generation		Third Generation		Fourth Generation	
IV	**PO**	**IV**	**PO**	**IV**	**PO**	**IV**	**PO**
cefazolin	cefadroxil	cefoxitin	cefaclor	cefoperazone	cefpodoxime	cefepime	cefdinir
cephradine	cephalexin	cefuroxime	cefuroxime axetil*	cefotaxime	proxetil*		cefditoren
	cephradine	cefmetazole	cefprozil	ceftizoxime	ceftibuten		pivoxil*
		cefotetan		ceftriaxone			
		loracarbef		ceftazidime			

IV, Intravenous; *PO,* oral.
*Prodrug salts that aid in drug delivery into gastrointestinal tract.

Table 37-6 Cephalosporins: Drug Interactions

Interacting Drug	Mechanism	Result
ethanol (alcohol)	Accumulation of acetaldehyde metabolite of ethanol	Acute alcohol intolerance (disulfiram-like reaction) after drinking alcoholic beverages within 72 hr of taking the following cephalosporins: cefazolin, cefmetazole, cefoperazone, and cefotetan. Symptoms include stomach cramps, nausea, vomiting, diaphoresis, pruritus, headache, and hypotension.
Aminoglycosides	Potentiation of nephrotoxic effect of aminoglycosides by cephalosporins (especially cephalothin)	Avoid concurrent use, but is a clinical judgment call. Monitor patient's renal function carefully if concurrent drug therapy indicated.
Probenecid	Reduction of clearance of cephalosporins	No toxic effects reported.
Oral contraceptives (OCs)	Enhanced OC metabolism	Increased risk for unintended pregnancy

DOSAGES

Selected Cephalosporins

Drug (Pregnancy Category)	Pharmacologic Class	Usual Dosage Range	Indications
▶cefazolin (Kefzol, Ancef) (B)	First-generation cephalosporin	**Adult** IV/IM: 500-1000 mg q6-8h **Pediatric** IV/IM: 25-50 mg/kg/day divided q6-8h	Comparable to those for cephalexin plus active against some penicillinase-producing and more gram-negative organisms; preop and postop surgical prophylaxis
cefditoren pivoxil* (Spectracef) (B)	Fourth-generation cephalosporin	**Adult and pediatric older than 12 yr** PO: 200-400 mg bid	Infections of respiratory tract and skin caused by selected gram-positive and gram-negative organisms
cefepime (Maxipime) (B)	Fourth-generation cephalosporin	**Adult** IV/IM: 250-2000 mg daily-bid **Pediatric** IV/IM: 50 mg/kg q12h	Comparable to those for cefditoren, plus provides more extensive coverage of gram-negative organisms, including those causing intraabdominal infections
▶cefoxitin (Mefoxin) (B)	Second-generation cephalosporin	**Adult** IV/IM: 3-12 g/day divided q4-6h **Pediatric** IV/IM: 80-160 mg/kg/day divided q4-6h, not to exceed 12 g/day	Less coverage of gram-positive organisms, greater coverage of gram-negative and anaerobic organisms
ceftazidime (Fortaz, Tazidime) (B)	Third-generation cephalosporin	**Adult** IV/IM: 250-2000 mg q8-12h **Pediatric** IV/IM: 30-50 mg/kg/day divided q8-12h	More extensive coverage of gram-negative organisms, including *Pseudomonas* spp.
▶ceftriaxone (Rocephin) (B)	Third-generation cephalosporin	**Adult** IV/IM: 1-2 g divided daily-bid **Pediatric** IV/IM: 50-100 mg/kg/day divided daily-bid	Comparable to those for ceftazidime; also preop surgical prophylaxis
cefuroxime (Kefurox, Zinacef); cefuroxime axetil* (Ceftin, tablet form) (B)	Second-generation cephalosporin	**Adult** PO (tabs): 125-500 mg bid **Pediatric** PO tabs: 125-250 mg bid **Pediatric** PO oral suspension: 20-30 mg/kg/day divided bid **Adult** IV/IM: 750-1500 mg q8h **Pediatric** IV/IM: 50-240 mg/kg/day, divided q6-8h	Comparable to those for cephalexin, plus provides more coverage of gram-negative organisms
▶cephalexin (Keflex, Biocef) (B)	First-generation cephalosporin	**Adult** PO: 1-4 g/day divided bid-qid **Pediatric** PO: 125-500 mg bid-qid	Infections of respiratory and GU tracts, skin, and bone; otitis media caused by various susceptible gram-positive and gram-negative organisms

GI, Gastrointestinal; *GU*, genitourinary; *IM*, intramuscular; *IV*, intravenous; *PO*, oral; *preop*, preoperative; *postop*, postoperative; *spp*, species.
*Cefuroxime axetil and cefditoren pivoxil are both prodrugs for PO use that are hydrolyzed into the active ingredient in the fluids of the gastrointestinal tract.

Drug Profiles

First-Generation Cephalosporins

First-generation cephalosporins are usually active against gram-positive bacteria and have limited activity against gram-negative bacteria. They are available both in parenteral and oral forms. Cur-

rently available first-generation cephalosporins include cefadroxil, cefazolin, cephalexin, and cephradine.

▶ *cefazolin*

Cefazolin (Ancef, Kefzol) is a prototypical first-generation cephalosporin. As with all first-generation cephalosporins, it provides excellent coverage against gram-positive bacteria but limited coverage against gram-negative bacteria. It is available only for parenteral use.

Pharmacokinetics

Half-Life	Onset	Peak	Duration
1.2-2.2 hr	Variable	1-2 hr	Variable

▶ **cephalexin**

Cephalexin (Keflex, Biocef) is a prototypical oral first-generation cephalosporin. It also provides excellent coverage against gram-positive bacteria but limited coverage against gram-negative bacteria. It is available only for oral use.

Pharmacokinetics

Half-Life	Onset	Peak	Duration
0.5-1.2 hr	Variable	1 hr	6-12 hr

Second-Generation Cephalosporins

Second-generation cephalosporins have coverage against gram-positive organisms similar to that of the first-generation cephalosporins but have enhanced coverage against gram-negative bacteria. Both parenteral and oral formulations are available. Like the first-generation drugs, second-generation cephalosporins are also excellent prophylactic antibiotics because of their favorable safety profile, the broad range of organisms they can kill, and their relatively low cost. Currently available second-generation cephalosporins include cefaclor, cefoxitin, cefuroxime, cefmetazole, cefotetan, cefprozil, and loracarbef. These drugs differ slightly with regard to their antibacterial coverage. Cefoxitin and cefotetan may have better coverage against various anaerobic bacteria such as *Bacteroides fragilis, Peptostreptococcus* spp., and *Clostridium* spp. than the other drugs in this class. Three second-generation drugs (cefoxitin, cefmetazole, and cefotetan) differ structurally from the other drugs in the class by having a methoxy group rather than a hydrogen group on the β-lactam ring of the cephalosporin nucleus. They are called cephamycins. Their unique structure enables them to kill certain bacteria known as *anaerobes* that the other second-generation drugs cannot.

▶ **cefoxitin**

Cefoxitin (Mefoxin) is a parenteral second-generation cephalosporin. It provides excellent gram-positive coverage and better gram-negative coverage than the first-generation drugs. Because it is a cephamycin it can also kill anaerobic bacteria. Cefoxitin has been used extensively as a prophylactic antibiotic in patients undergoing abdominal surgery because it can effectively kill intestinal bacteria. Normal intestinal flora include gram-positive, gram-negative, and anaerobic bacteria. Cefoxitin is available only in injectable form.

Pharmacokinetics

Half-Life	Onset	Peak	Duration
30-60 min	Variable	20-30 min	Variable

cefuroxime

Cefuroxime sodium (Kefurox, Zinacef) is the parenteral form of this second-generation cephalosporin. The oral form is a different salt of cefuroxime, cefuroxime axetil (Ceftin). Cefuroxime is a very versatile second-generation cephalosporin. It is also widely used as a prophylactic antibiotic for various surgical procedures. It has more activity against gram-negative bacteria than first-generation cephalosporins but a narrower spectrum of activity against gram-negative bacteria than third-generation cephalosporins. It differs from the cephamycins such as cefoxitin in that it does not kill anaerobic bacteria. Cefuroxime axetil is a prodrug. It has little antibacterial activity until it is hydrolyzed in the liver to its active cefuroxime form. It is available only for oral use. Cefuroxime sodium is available only in injectable form.

Pharmacokinetics

Half-Life	Onset	Peak	Duration
1.2 hr	Variable	2.2-3 hr	6-8 hr

Third-Generation Cephalosporins

The currently available third-generation cephalosporins include cefoperazone, cefotaxime, cefpodoxime, ceftazidime, ceftibuten, ceftizoxime, and ceftriaxone. These are the most potent of the first three generations of cephalosporins in fighting gram-negative bacteria, but they generally have less activity than first- and second-generation drugs against gram-positive organisms. As with all of the different classes of both penicillins and cephalosporins, slight modifications in the chemical structure have endowed specific drugs with certain advantages over the others against various bacteria.

Because of specific changes in their basic cephalosporin structure, cefoperazone and ceftazidime have significant activity against *Pseudomonas* spp. In fact, these two third-generation drugs have the best activity of all the cephalosporins against this gram-negative bacterium that is notoriously difficult to treat. Cefoperazone differs from ceftazidime in that it is principally excreted in the bile through the liver rather than the kidneys, as ceftazidime is. For this reason this drug may be a better choice for patients with renal impairment, and it provides but one example of the reason that different drugs may be selected for different patients. Cefpodoxime and ceftibuten are currently the only third-generation cephalosporins available for oral use. All the other third-generation drugs are available only in parenteral forms.

▶ **ceftriaxone**

Ceftriaxone (Rocephin) is an extremely long-acting third-generation drug that can be given only once a day in the treatment of most infections. It also has the unique characteristic of being able to pass easily through the blood-brain barrier. For this reason it is one of the few cephalosporins that is indicated for the treatment of meningitis, an infection of the meninges of the brain. Structurally it resembles other third-generation drugs such as cefotaxime and ceftizoxime, but it has an acidic enol group that distinguishes it from these other drugs. This is believed to be responsible for the long serum half-life of the drug. The spectrum of activity for ceftriaxone is similar to that of the other third-generation drugs cefotaxime and ceftizoxime. It can be given both IV and IM. In some cases of infection, one IM injection can eradicate the infection. Ceftriaxone is 93% to 96% bound to plasma protein, a proportion higher than that of many of the other cephalosporins. This drug is also unique in that its elimination is primarily hepatic. For this reason, it should not be given to hyperbilirubinemic neonates or to patients with severe liver dysfunction. This drug is only available for injection.

Pharmacokinetics

Half-Life	Onset	Peak	Duration
4.3-8.7 hr	Variable	2-4 hr	24 hr

ceftazidime

Ceftazidime (Ceptaz, Fortaz, Tazidime, Tazicef) is a parenterally administered third-generation cephalosporin with excellent activity against difficult-to-treat gram-negative bacteria such as *Pseudomonas* spp. It differs from its closest third-generation relative cefoperazone in that it is eliminated renally rather than by the hepatobiliary route. It is the third-generation cephalosporin of choice for many indications because of its excellent spectrum of activity and safety profile. It is available only in injectable form. One idiosyncrasy of this particular drug is that gas builds up in the medication vial when its powder is reconstituted with diluent. The quantity of gas produced can be so great that it expels the needle directly out of the vial. The Ceptaz product was designed to minimize this gas volume.

Pharmacokinetics

Half-Life	Onset	Peak	Duration
2 hr	Variable	1 hr	8-12 hr

Fourth-Generation Cephalosporins

There are currently three fourth-generation cephalosporins: cefdinir, cefepime, and cefditoren pivoxil. Some references classify these with the third-generation drugs. They have a broader spectrum of antibacterial activity, especially against gram-positive bacteria, than the third-generation drugs. They may also be more resistant to β-lactamase enzymes. Cefepime is available only in injectable form, whereas cefdinir and cefditoren pivoxil are both oral drugs.

cefepime

Cefepime (Maxipime) is the prototypical fourth-generation cephalosporin. Cefepime is a broad-spectrum cephalosporin that most closely resembles ceftazidime in its spectrum of activity. It differs from ceftazidime in that it has increased activity against many *Enterobacter* spp. (gram negative) as well as gram-positive organisms. Cefepime is indicated for the treatment of uncomplicated and complicated UTIs, uncomplicated skin and skin structure infections, and pneumonia.

Pharmacokinetics

Half-Life	Onset	Peak	Duration
2 hr	0.5 hr	0.5-1.5 hr	8-12 hr

CARBAPENEMS

Carbapenems have among the broadest antibacterial action of any antibiotics to date. Because of this, they are often reserved for complicated body cavity and connective tissue infections in acutely ill hospitalized patients. One hazard of carbapenem use is drug-induced seizure activity, which occurs in a relatively small percentage of patients but is obviously undesirable. This is one reason that carbapenem therapy is not normally first-line drug therapy. However, the risk of seizures can be reduced by proper dosage adjustment in truly impaired patients. Currently available carbapenems include imipenem-cilastatin, meropenem, and ertapenem.

Drug Profiles

▶ imipenem-cilastatin

Imipenem-cilastatin (Primaxin) is a fixed combination of imipenem, which is a semisynthetic carbapenem antibiotic similar to β-lactam antibiotics; and cilastatin, an inhibitor of an enzyme that breaks down imipenem. Imipenem has a wide spectrum of activity against gram-positive and gram-negative aerobic and anaerobic bacteria. Cilastatin is a unique drug in that it inhibits an enzyme in the kidneys called dehydropeptidase, which would otherwise quickly break down the imipenem. Cilastatin also blocks the renal tubular secretion of imipenem, which prevents imipenem from being excreted by the kidneys, the primary route of elimination of the drug.

Imipenem-cilastatin exerts its antibacterial effect by binding to penicillin-binding proteins inside bacteria, which in turn inhibits bacterial cell wall synthesis. It also kills bacteria and is therefore bactericidal. Unlike many of the penicillins and cephalosporins, imipenem-cilastatin is very resistant to the antibiotic-inhibiting actions of β-lactamases. Drugs with which it potentially interacts include cyclosporine, ganciclovir, and probenecid, all of which may potentiate the CNS adverse effects (including seizures) of imipenem. Concurrent use with these drugs should be avoided whenever clinically feasible. The most serious adverse effect associated with imipenem-cilastatin therapy is seizures, which have been reported in up to 1.5% of the patients receiving less than 500 mg every 6 hours. In patients receiving high dosages of the drug (more than 500 mg every 6 hours), however, there is about a 10% incidence of seizures. Seizures are more likely in elderly and renally impaired patients. Seizures have also been associated with the use of both meropenem and carbapenem, but data to date suggest that they are less likely to occur than with imipenem-cilastatin.

Imipenem-cilastatin is indicated for the treatment of bone, joint, skin, and soft tissue infections; bacterial endocarditis caused by *S. aureus;* intraabdominal bacterial infections; pneumonia; UTIs and pelvic infections; and bacterial septicemia caused by susceptible bacterial organisms. The IM form of imipenem-cilastatin contains lidocaine, and its use is therefore contraindicated in patients with a known drug allergy to lidocaine or related local anesthetics. All dosage forms contain the same number of milligrams of both imipenem and cilastatin.

Meropenem (Merrem) is the second drug in the carbapenem class of antibiotics. Compared with imipenem-cilastatin, meropenem appears to be somewhat less active against gram-positive organisms, more active against Enterobacteriaceae, and equally active against *Pseudomonas aeruginosa.* However, meropenem is the only carbapenem currently indicated for treatment of bacterial meningitis. The newest carbapenem is ertapenem (Invanz), which has a spectrum of activity comparable to that of imipenem-cilastatin, although it is not active against *Enterococcal* or *Pseudomonas* spp. Note that only imipenem is combined with the dehydropeptidase inhibitor cilastatin. Neither meropenem nor ertapenem is susceptible to this bacterial enzyme, which gives these drugs one advantage over imipenem-cilastatin. For dosage information on carbapenems, see the Dosages table on page 583.

DOSAGES

Carbapenems and Monobactams

Drug (Pregnancy Category)	Pharmacologic Class	Usual Dosage Range	Indications
▶imipenem-cilastatin (Primaxin) (C)	Carbapenem	IV: 250-500 mg q6-8h IM: 750 mg q12h	Infection with gram-positive, gram-negative, and aerobic bacteria, including *Pseudomonas aeruginosa;* includes infections of bone, joint, skin, or soft-tissue and endocarditis, pneumonia, UTI, intraabdominal and pelvic infections, and septicemia
meropenem (Merrem) (B)	Carbapenem	IV: 1000 mg q8h	Same as above
ertapenem (Invanz) (B)	Carbapenem	IV/IM: 1000 mg daily	Same as above
aztreonam (Azactam) (B)	Monobactam	IV/IM: 500-1000 mg q8-12h IV: 2 g q12h	Primarily UTI caused by gram-negative organisms, severe systemic infections

IM, Intramuscular; *IV,* intravenous; *UTI,* urinary tract infection.

Pharmacokinetics

Half-Life	Onset	Peak	Duration
2-3 hr	Variable	2 hr	6-8 hr

MONOBACTAMS

Drug Profiles

aztreonam

Aztreonam (Azactam) is the only monobactam antibiotic to be developed thus far. It is a synthetic β-lactam antibiotic that is primarily active against aerobic gram-negative bacteria, including *E. coli, Klebsiella* spp., and *Pseudomonas* spp. Aztreonam is a bactericidal antibiotic. It destroys bacteria by inhibiting bacterial cell wall synthesis, which results in lysis. Aztreonam is indicated for the treatment of moderately severe systemic infections and UTIs. It has the theoretical therapeutic advantage of preserving normal gram-positive and anaerobic flora, unlike many other β-lactam antibiotics. Aztreonam is available only in injectable form. Its use is contraindicated in patients with a known drug allergy, although it is believed to have less allergic cross-reactivity with other β-lactam antibiotics. For dosage information on monobactams, see the Dosages table on page 583.

Pharmacokinetics

Half-Life	Onset	Peak	Duration
1.5-2 hr	Variable	1 hr	6-12 hr

MACROLIDES AND KETOLIDES

The macrolides are a large group of antibiotics that first became available in the early 1950s with the introduction of erythromycin. Macrolides are considered bacteriostatic; however, in high enough concentrations they may be bactericidal to some susceptible bacteria. There are four main macrolide antibiotics: azithromycin, clarithromycin, dirithromycin, and erythromycin. Azithromycin and clarithromycin are two of the newer drugs in the class, and together with the original drug, erythromycin, are currently the most widely used of the macrolides. Although the spectra of antibacterial activity of both azithromycin and clarithromycin are similar to that of erythromycin, the former have longer durations of action than erythromycin, which allows them to be given less often. They produce fewer and milder GI tract adverse effects than erythromycin, and azithromycin is usually dosed over a shorter length of time than many of the erythromycin products. They also exhibit better efficacy in eradicating various bacteria and are capable of better tissue penetration. Because erythromycin has a bitter taste and is quickly degraded by the acidity of the stomach, several salt forms and many dosage formulations were developed to circumvent these problems. The various salts and dosage formulations and the benefits of each are briefly summarized in Table 37-7.

Mechanism of Action and Drug Effects

The mechanism of action of macrolide antibiotics is similar to that of other antibiotics. They work by inhibiting protein synthesis in susceptible bacteria. For this synthesis to occur, transfer RNA must bind to the messenger RNA ribosome. The macrolides obstruct this synthesis by binding to the portion of the ribosome called the *50S subunit* inside the cells of bacteria. This prevents the production of the bacterial protein needed for the bacteria to grow, and so they eventually die (see Figure 37-6). This action can immediately kill some susceptible strains of bacteria if the concentration of the macrolide is high enough.

Macrolides are effective in the treatment of a wide range of infections. These include various infections of the upper and lower respiratory tract, skin, and soft tissue caused by some strains of *Streptococcus* and *Haemophilus;* spirochetal infections such as syphilis and Lyme disease; gonorrhea; and *Chlamydia, Mycoplasma,* and *Corynebacterium* infections. Gonorrheal infections have become increasingly difficult to treat with macrolide monotherapy, so these drugs are sometimes used in combination with other antibiotics such as cephalosporins. Because of its GI tract–irritating properties, erythromycin affects the motility of the GI tract. This characteristic has been studied experimentally and may prove to be of benefit in increasing GI motility in conditions such as delayed gastric emptying in diabetic patients (known as *diabetic gastroparesis*). Macrolides are also somewhat unique among antibiotics in that they are especially effective against several bacterial species that often reproduce inside host cells instead of just in the bloodstream or interstitial spaces. Common examples of such bacteria, some of which were previously listed, are *Listeria, Chlamydia, Legionella* (one species of which causes Legionnaires' disease), *Neisseria* (one species of which causes gonorrhea), and *Campylobacter.*

Indications

The therapeutic effects of macrolide antibiotics are mostly limited to their antibacterial actions. Infections caused by *Streptococcus pyogenes* (group A β-hemolytic streptococci) are inhibited by macrolides, as are mild to moderate upper and lower respiratory tract infections caused by *Haemophilus influenzae.* Spirochetal infections that are treated with erythromycin and other macrolides are syphilis and Lyme disease. Various forms of gonorrhea and *Chlamydia* and *Mycoplasma* infections are also susceptible to the effects of macrolides.

Table 37-7 Erythromycin Formulations

Formulation	Benefit
Salt Forms	
Stearate salt	Developed to overcome bitter taste of erythromycin
Estolate	
Ethylsuccinate ester	Developed to overcome bitter taste and to protect erythromycin from acid degradation in the stomach
Dosage Formulation	
Film coated	
Enteric coated (pellets and particles)	
Structural Changes	
Semisynthetic Macrolides	
Azide group (azithromycin)	Developed to improve resistance to acid degradation in the stomach and increase tissue penetration to improve antibiotic efficacy
Methylation of hydroxy group (clarithromycin)	

Table 37-8 Macrolides: Reported Adverse Effects

Body System	Adverse Effects
Cardiovascular	Palpitations, chest pain
Central nervous	Headache, dizziness, vertigo, somnolence
Gastrointestinal	Nausea, hepatotoxicity, heartburn, vomiting, diarrhea, stomatitis, flatulence, cholestatic jaundice, anorexia
Integumentary	Rash, pruritus, urticaria, thrombophlebitis (intravenous site)
Other	Hearing loss, tinnitus

As previously noted, a therapeutic effect of erythromycin outside its antibiotic actions is its ability to irritate the GI tract, which stimulates smooth muscle and GI motility. This may be of benefit to patients who have decreased GI motility. It has also been shown to be helpful in facilitating the passage of feeding tubes from the stomach into the small bowel. Azithromycin and clarithromycin have both been recently approved for the treatment of *Mycobacterium avium-intracellulare complex* infections. This is a common *opportunistic infection* often associated with HIV infection/acquired immunodeficiency syndrome (AIDS) (Chapter 39). Clarithromycin also has another new indication: it has been approved for use in combination with omeprazole for the treatment of patients with active ulcer associated with *Helicobacter pylori* infection.

Contraindications

The only usual contraindication to macrolide use is known drug allergy. In fact, as indicated earlier, macrolides are often used as alternative drugs for patients with allergies to β-lactam antibiotics.

Adverse Effects

Many of the older macrolide products, primarily erythromycin formulations, have many adverse effects. Most affect the GI tract, although the two newest macrolides, azithromycin and clarithromycin, seem to be associated with a lower incidence of these GI tract complications. Reported adverse effects are listed in Table 37-8.

Interactions

There are a number of potential drug interactions with the macrolides. Examples of some especially common drugs that compete for hepatic metabolism with the macrolides are carbamazepine, cyclosporine, digoxin, theophylline, and warfarin. When these drugs are given with macrolides the results are enhanced effects and possible toxicity of the second drug. Azithromycin is not as prone to such interactions as are other macrolides because of its minimal effects on the *cytochrome P-450* enzymes in the liver. Such drug combinations should be avoided when possible. When a macrolide is given together with any of these drugs, the patient should be observed for signs of drug toxicity, and appropriate laboratory measurements (e.g., blood drug levels) should be measured as indicated. These interactions may occasionally even be beneficial by allowing smaller dosages of the interacting drugs to be given and thereby reducing the likelihood of other less desirable adverse effects. Two properties of macrolides that are the source of many of these interactions are that they are highly protein bound and they are metabolized in the liver. Drugs that are bound to protein are usually bound to albumin in the blood, which makes them inactive. When they are displaced from these binding sites on albumin and are then free and unbound, they become active. Therefore, when a patient is given two or more drugs that compete for the same binding sites on albumin in the blood, one will not bind successfully but will circulate in the blood as free drug and remain active. That drug will then have a greater effect in the body. For drugs metabolized by the liver drug, interactions commonly arise from competition between the different drugs for metabolic enzymes, specifically the enzymes known as the *cytochrome P-450 complex* mentioned earlier. Such enzymatic effects generally lead to more pronounced drug interactions than does competition for protein binding. The result is a delay in the metabolic clearance of one or more interacting drugs and thus a prolonged and possibly toxic drug effect. Macrolides can also reduce the efficacy of oral contraceptives.

Dosages

For dosage information on selected macrolide antibiotics, see the Dosages table on page 586.

Drug Profiles

Macrolide antibiotics are used to treat a variety of infections ranging from Lyme disease to Legionnaires' disease. Of the four macrolide drugs currently available, erythromycin has been available the longest and has been the mainstay of treatment for various infections for more than four decades. Azithromycin and clarithromycin have fewer adverse effects and a better pharmacokinetics profile than older drugs. Dirithromycin is less commonly used.

Macrolide use is contraindicated in patients with known drug allergy. As previously noted, because these drugs are significantly protein bound to varying degrees and are metabolized in the liver, they may interact with other drugs that are also highly protein bound or hepatically metabolized.

▶ erythromycin

Erythromycin, which goes by many product names, was for many years the most commonly prescribed macrolide antibiotic. However, other macrolides are now more commonly used. The drug is available in several different salt and dosage forms for oral use that were developed to circumvent some of the drawbacks it has chemically. (These benefits are summarized in Table 37-7.) An injectable form is also available for IV use. Erythromycin is also available in topical forms for dermatologic use (Chapter 57) and in ophthalmic dosage forms (Chapter 58). The absorption of oral erythromycin is enhanced if it is taken on an empty stomach, but because of the high incidence of stomach irritation associated with its use, many of these drugs are taken after a meal or snack. The various salt forms and dosage formulations, their strengths, and product names are listed in Table 37-9.

▶ azithromycin and clarithromycin

Azithromycin (Zithromax) and clarithromycin (Biaxin) are semisynthetic macrolide antibiotics that differ structurally from erythromycin and as a result have advantages over it. These include better adverse effect profiles, including less GI tract irritation, and more favorable pharmacokinetic properties. Both have very similar spectra of activity that differ only slightly from that of erythromycin. The two drugs are used for the treatment of both upper and lower respiratory tract and skin structure infections.

Azithromycin has excellent tissue penetration, so that it can reach high concentrations in infected tissues. It also has a long duration of action, which allows it to be dosed once daily. Taking the drug with food decreases both the rate and extent of GI absorption. The drug is available on oral and injectable forms.

DOSAGES

Selected Macrolides and Ketolides

Drug (Pregnancy Category)	Pharmacologic Class	Usual Dosage Range	Indications
▶azithromycin (Zithromax) (B)	Semisynthetic macrolide	**Adult** PO: 500 mg × 1 dose, then 250 mg daily × 4 days PO: 500 mg daily × 3 days, or 2 g × 1 dose **Pediatric** 50-100 mg × 1 dose, then 75-200 mg daily × 4 days	Comparable to those for erythromycin, but especially GU and respiratory tract infections, including MAC infections
▶clarithromycin (Biaxin) (C)	Semisynthetic macrolide	**Adult** PO: 500 mg bid **Pediatric** PO: 7.5 mg/kg bid (max 500 mg/dose)	Comparable to those for erythromycin, but especially GU and respiratory tract infections, including MAC infections
▶erythromycin (E-mycin, EryPed, Eryc, E.E.S., many others) (B)	Natural macrolide	**Adult*** PO: 250-500 mg qid **Pediatric*** 30-100 mg/kg/day divided qid	Infections of respiratory and GI tracts and skin caused by various gram-positive, gram-negative, and miscellaneous organisms
telithromycin (Ketek) (C)	Ketolide	**Adult and pediatric 13 yr and older only** PO: 800 mg once daily × 5-10 days	CAP, bacterial sinusitis, and exacerbations of chronic bronchitis

CAP, Community-acquired pneumonia; *GI*, gastrointestinal; *GU*, genitourinary; *MAC*, *Mycobacterium avium-intracellulare complex*; *PO*, oral.
*There are many dosage forms, and dosages may vary from those listed.

Table 37-9 Erythromycin Dosage Forms and Product Names

Dosage Form Name	Strength	Product Name
erythromycin base (PO)		
Capsules		
Delayed release	250 mg	Eryc
Tablets		
Delayed release (enteric-coated particles)	333 and 500 mg	PCE Dispertab
Delayed release (enteric coated)	250, 333, and 500 mg	E-Mycin, Ery-Tab, E-base
Film coated	250 and 500 mg	Erythromycin Filmtabs
erythromycin estolate (PO)		
Oral suspension	125 and 250 mg/5 mL	erythromycin estolate (generic only)
erythromycin ethylsuccinate (PO)		
Tablets		
Chewable	200 mg	EryPed
Film coated	400 mg	E.E.S. 400
Oral suspension	100 mg/2.5 mL; 200 and 400 mg/5 mL	EryPed Drops, E.E.S. 200, E.E.S. 400
Powder for oral suspension	200 and 400 mg/5 mL	EryPed 200, E.E.S. Granules, EryPed 400
erythromycin stearate (PO)		
Tablets		
Film coated	250 and 500 mg	erythromycin stearate (generic only)
erythromycin gluceptate (IV)		
IV formulation	1 g	Ilotycin Gluceptate
erythromycin lactobionate (IV)		
IV formulation	500 mg and 1 g	Erythrocin

IV, Intravenous; *PO*, oral.

Clarithromycin can be given only twice daily and is recommended for use in adults and children 12 years of age and older. Its safety and efficacy in younger patients has not been established. It is availably only for oral use.

Pharmacokinetics (azithromycin)

Half-Life	Onset	Peak	Duration
PO: 6-8 hr	PO: Variable	PO: 2.5 hr	PO: Up to 24 hr

Pharmacokinetics (clarithromycin)

Half-Life	Onset	Peak	Duration
3-7 hr	Variable	2 hr	Up to 12 hr

telithromycin

Telithromycin (Ketek) is currently the only drug in a new class known as *ketolides*. It is derived from erythromycin A and has better acid stability and better antibacterial coverage than the macrolides. Its mechanism of action is also similar to that of the macrolides—inhibition of bacterial protein synthesis by binding to the 50S ribosomal subunit. The drug is active against the majority of gram-positive bacteria, including multidrug-resistant strains of *S. pneumoniae*. It also has activity against selected gram-negative bacteria, including *H. influenzae, Moraxella catarrhalis,* and *Bordetella pertussis.* It is indicated for treatment of community-acquired pneumonia, acute bacterial sinusitis, and bacterial exacerbations of chronic bronchitis. Use of this drug is contraindicated in cases of drug allergy. It is available only for oral use. Adverse reactions are similar to those of the macrolide antibiotics and include headache, dizziness, GI discomfort, hypokalemia or hyperkalemia, and prolongation of the QT interval on the electrocardiogram. Avoidance of the drug is recommended in patients with a history of cardiac disease that already includes prolonged QT interval, bradycardia, or electrolyte disturbances, and in those receiving antidysrhythmic drugs (Chapter 22) or other drugs known to prolong the QT interval such as quinolones. There are many potential drug interactions involving liver enzyme (cytochrome P-450) effects, which can increase or decrease the concentrations (and therefore the effectiveness) of either drug. Some of the interacting drugs are benzodiazepines, calcium channel blockers, cyclosporine, statins (for hypercholesterolemia), antidepressants, protease inhibitors (for HIV), doxycycline, erythromycin, verapamil, and imatinib (an antineoplastic [Chapter 48]). In complicated cases, a clinical pharmacist will be asked to evaluate complex medication regimens and made recommendations to the prescriber regarding the safest and most effective drug combinations and dosages.

Pharmacokinetics

Half-Life	Onset	Peak	Duration
9-10 hr	Unknown	1 hr	Unknown

TETRACYCLINES

The tetracyclines are a small chemically related group of five antibiotics, three of which are naturally occurring and two of which are semisynthetic. They are derivatives of *Streptomyces* organisms. Although the tetracyclines are bacteriostatic, the body's own host defense mechanisms are helping to kill bacteria as well. The three naturally occurring tetracyclines are demeclocycline, oxytetracycline, and tetracycline. The two semisynthetic tetracyclines are doxycycline and minocycline. The available tetracycline antibiotics and brief descriptions of them are given in Table 37-10.

Tetracyclines are chemically and pharmacologically similar to one another. The most significant chemical characteristic of these

Table 37-10	Available Tetracycline Antibiotics

Generic Name	Description
Natural Tetracyclines	
demeclocycline	All chemically derived from *Streptomyces*
oxytetracycline	spp. by a fermentation process
tetracycline	
Semisynthetic Tetracyclines	
doxycycline	Chemical derivative of oxytetracycline
minocycline	Chemical derivative of tetracycline

spp., Species.

drugs is their ability to bind to (chelate) divalent (Ca^{2+}, Mg^{2+}) and trivalent (Al^{3+}) metallic ions to form insoluble complexes. Therefore, their coadministration with milk, antacids, or iron salts causes a considerable reduction in the oral absorption of the tetracycline. In addition, their strong affinity for calcium usually precludes their use in pediatric patients younger than 8 years of age because it can result in significant tooth discoloration. These drugs should also be avoided in pregnant women and nursing mothers. The drugs do pass into breast milk, and this can be another route of exposure leading to tooth discoloration in nursing children.

Tetracyclines primarily differ from one another in the following ways:

- *Oral absorption:* All are adequately absorbed, but doxycycline and minocycline are absorbed the most.
- *Body tissue penetration:* Doxycycline and minocycline possess the best penetration potential (brain and cerebrospinal fluid).
- *Half-life and resulting dosage schedule:* See the table on page 588 and pharmacokinetics information in the Drug Profiles section.

Mechanism of Action and Drug Effects

Tetracyclines work by inhibiting protein synthesis in susceptible bacteria. For this synthesis to occur, transfer RNA must bind to the messenger RNA ribosome. The tetracyclines obstruct this synthesis by binding to the portion of the ribosome called the *30S subunit* (see Figure 37-6). This is comparable to the mechanism of the macrolides, which bind to the 50S subunit as noted previously. This in turn shuts down many of the bacterium's essential functions, such as growth and repair, so that eventually the bacterium stops growing and dies.

Tetracyclines are used primarily for their antibiotic effects. They inhibit the growth of and kill a very wide range of *Rickettsia, Chlamydia,* and *Mycoplasma* organisms, as well as a variety of gram-negative and gram-positive bacteria. They are also useful in the treatment of spirochetal infections such as syphilis and Lyme disease. Demeclocycline possesses a unique drug effect in that it inhibits the action of antidiuretic hormone, which makes it useful in the treatment of the syndrome of inappropriate secretion of antidiuretic hormone (SIADH). Another drug effect of tetracyclines is their ability to cause inflammation that results in fibrosis in the lungs. This is a useful property in patients with pleural or pericardial effusions caused by metastatic tumors, thoracentesis, or thoracostomy tubes, because when instilled into the pleural space of the lungs these drugs cause scar tissue to form and thereby reduce the fluid accumulation.

Indications

Tetracyclines have a wide range of activity, and all drugs in this class are effective against essentially the same spectrum of microbes. They inhibit the growth of many gram-negative and gram-positive organisms and even of some protozoa. Traditionally used to treat acne in adolescents and adults, they are also considered the drugs of choice for the treatment of the following infections caused by susceptible organisms:

- *Chlamydia:* lymphogranuloma venereum, psittacosis, and nonspecific endocervical, rectal, and urethral infections
- *Mycoplasma: Mycoplasma* pneumonia
- *Rickettsia:* Q fever, rickettsial pox, Rocky Mountain spotted fever, scrub typhus, and typhus
- *Other bacteria:* acne, brucellosis, chancroid, cholera, granuloma inguinale, shigellosis, spirochetal relapsing fever, Lyme disease, *H. pylori* infections associated with peptic ulcer disease (used as part of the treatment regimen), syphilis (used as an alternative drug to treat patients with penicillin allergy); tetracyclines are now unreliable in treating gonorrhea due to resistant bacterial strains
- *Protozoa:* balantidiasis

In addition to being used for these antibiotic-related indications, demeclocycline is also used to treat SIADH and pleural and pericardial effusions, as previously noted.

Contraindications

The only usual contraindication is known drug allergy. However, tetracyclines should be avoided by pregnant and nursing women and should not be given to children under the age of 8 years.

Adverse Effects

All tetracyclines cause similar adverse effects. They can cause discoloration of the permanent teeth and tooth enamel hypoplasia in both fetuses and children and possibly retard fetal skeletal development if taken during pregnancy. Other clinically significant undesirable effects include photosensitivity, which is most fre-

quent in patients taking demeclocycline, and alteration of the intestinal flora, which can result in the following:

- Overgrowth of nonsusceptible organisms (superinfection), especially candidiasis and pediatric staphylococcal enteritis
- Diarrhea
- Pseudomembranous colitis

The tetracyclines can also alter the vaginal flora, which results in vaginal candidiasis; cause reversible bulging fontanelles in neonates; precipitate thrombocytopenia, possible coagulation irregularities, and hemolytic anemia; and exacerbate systemic lupus erythematosus. Other effects include gastric upset, enterocolitis, and maculopapular rash.

Interactions

There are several significant drug interactions associated with the use of tetracyclines. When tetracyclines are taken with antacids, antidiarrheal drugs, dairy products, or iron preparations, the oral absorption of the tetracycline is reduced. Tetracyclines can potentiate the effects of oral anticoagulants, which necessitates more frequent monitoring of anticoagulant effect and possible dosage adjustment. They can also antagonize the effects of bactericidal antibiotics and oral contraceptives. In addition, depending on the dosage, they can cause blood urea nitrogen levels to be increased.

Dosages

For dosage information for selected tetracyclines, see the Dosages table on this page.

Drug Profiles

Tetracyclines were one of the first classes of antibiotic capable of providing coverage against a broad spectrum of microorganisms. They are also unusual in that they are useful in the treatment of conditions other than bacterial infections. They are used for the treatment of SIADH (demeclocycline) and as sclerosing (tissue hardening) drugs in the treatment of pleural effusions. They are prescription-only drugs that, as noted earlier, are potentially harmful to children younger than 8 years of age and should not be given to pregnant women because by binding to calcium they can prevent normal bone growth and cause tooth enamel hypoplasia in the fetus. Their use is also contraindicated in patients who have had hypersen-

DOSAGES

Selected Tetracyclines

Drug (Pregnancy Category)	Pharmacologic Class	Usual Dosage Range	Indications
demeclocycline (Declomycin) (D)	Tetracycline	**Adult** PO: 150 mg qid or 300 mg bid **Pediatric older than 8 yr*** 6-12 mg/kg divided bid-qid	Broad antibacterial coverage, including treatment of skin infections and respiratory, GI, and GU tract infections
▶doxycycline (Vibramycin, Monodox, others) (D)	Tetracycline	**Adult** PO: 200 mg first day, then 100 mg daily thereafter **Pediatric older than 8 yr*** PO: 4.4 mg/kg first day followed by 2.2 mg/kg daily thereafter	Comparable to that for demeclocycline

*Use of tetracyclines is contraindicated in children younger than 8 yr and in pregnant women because of the risk of significant tooth discoloration in children.
GI, Gastrointestinal; *GU*, genitourinary; *PO*, oral.

sitivity reactions to them in the past and in lactating women. Resistance to one tetracycline implies resistance to all tetracyclines.

demeclocycline
Demeclocycline (Declomycin) is a naturally occurring tetracycline antibiotic that is derived from strains of *Streptomyces*. It is used both for its antibacterial action and for its ability to inhibit SIADH. Demeclocycline has all the characteristics of this class of tetracyclines. It is available only for oral use.

Pharmacokinetics

Half-Life	Onset	Peak	Duration
10-17 hr	Variable	3-4 hr	6-12 hr

▶ doxycycline
Doxycycline (Doryx, Doxy-Caps, Vibramycin) is a semisynthetic tetracycline antibiotic that was made by altering the naturally occurring tetracycline oxytetracycline. Doxycycline is available in two salt forms: hyclate and monohydrate. It is useful in the treatment of rickettsial infections such as Rocky Mountain spotted fever, chlamydial and mycoplasmal infections, spirochetal infections, and many infections with gram-negative organisms. Doxycycline may also be used as a sclerosing drug in the treatment of pleural effusions. It is available in both oral and injectable forms.

The remaining antibiotic classes are discussed in Chapter 38.

Pharmacokinetics

Half-Life	Onset	Peak	Duration
14-24 hr	Variable	1.5-4 hr	Up to 12 hr

◆ NURSING PROCESS

◆ ASSESSMENT
In general, before the administration of any antibiotic, it is crucial to assess for a history of or symptoms indicative of hypersensitivity or allergic reactions (mild reactions with rash, pruritus, or hives, to severe reactions with laryngeal edema, bronchospasms, hypotension, and possible cardiac arrest). Further assessment should include the patient's age, weight, baseline vital signs with body temperature and examination of the results of any laboratory studies that have been ordered, including liver function studies (aspartate aminotransferase [AST] level and alanine aminotransferase [ALT] level), kidney function studies (usually blood urea nitrogen and creatinine levels), cardiac function studies/tests (pertinent laboratory tests, electrocardiogram, or ultrasonography if indicated), culture and sensitivity tests, and complete blood count (CBC) with hemoglobin/hematocrit (Hgb/Hct) levels and platelet/clotting values. Intake and output values should also be noted (e.g., more than 30 mL/hr or 600 mL/day). A neurologic assessment is important because of possible CNS adverse effects, as is an assessment of bowel sounds and patterns because of possible drug-related GI adverse effects. Contraindications, cautions, and drug interactions should be assessed with a complete list of all medications, including OTC drugs, herbals, and dietary supplements. Cultural assessment is also important due to racial/ethnic groups and their different responses to certain drugs, as well as the use of folk remedies or alternative therapies to try to alleviate infections. Learning preparedness, willingness to learn, and educational level should be assessed because of the importance of patient education in taking these (and all) medications. There should be assessment of oral mucosa, respiratory tract, GI tract, and geni-

tourinary tract because of the risk of superinfection. Superinfections are often evidenced by fever, lethargy, mouth sores, perineal itching, and other anatomically related symptoms and have been discussed previously in the General Principles section of this chapter. Because antibiotic resistance is so prevalent, questions about long-term use, overuse, or abuse of antibiotics should be posed to the patient or caregiver. Assessment information related to each group of antibiotics is presented in the following paragraphs.

For patients taking *sulfonamides*, a careful assessment for drug allergies to sulfa-type drugs, such as the oral sulfonylureas (antidiabetic drugs), and thiazide diuretics, is critical to patient safety. A thorough skin assessment during drug therapy is also important, because Stevens-Johnson syndrome is a possible adverse effect of these drugs. Blood counts, specifically RBCs, need to be assessed before the initiation of drug therapy because of the possibility of drug-related anemias and other blood dyscrasias. Renal function should also be assessed because of the potential for drug-related crystalluria.

Because of being associated with the highest incidence of allergic reactions, *penicillins* require astute assessment of hypersensitivity. In addition, the patient must be assessed for a history of asthma, sensitivity to multiple allergens, aspirin allergy, and sensitivity to cephalosporins because these conditions place the patient at higher risk for penicillin allergy. If procaine penicillin is to be given, assessment of procaine hypersensitivity should be done. Hepatic and renal functioning should be assessed, and results of culture and sensitivity tests on any specimens should be noted. Because of possible CNS and/or GI adverse effects, a thorough neurologic, abdominal, and bowel assessment should be completed. Especially important for patients with electrolyte disturbances, cardiac disease, or renal disease is an assessment of serum sodium and potassium levels because of the high sodium and potassium ion concentrations in some penicillins. For example, penicillin G contains 1.7 mEq of potassium ion per million units and 2 mEq of sodium ion per million units (see Table 37-4). In these situations, hypernatremia and/or hyperkalemia could lead to complications such as congestive heart failure, fluid overload, or cardiac dysrhythmias. With any dosage form of the penicillins, it is important to patient safety to assess for the possibility of an immediate, accelerated, or delayed allergic reaction. It is important to remember that a small percentage of patients taking penicillins may develop serious superinfections manifested by antibiotic-associated pseudomembranous colitis; therefore, thorough bowel/GI tract assessment should be ongoing for this potential complication.

Carbapenems are similar to penicillins, and assessment for allergy to the penicillin group (see previous discussion on penicillins) is needed. Assessment for neurologic functioning, seizure disorders, and baseline hearing levels is needed because of possible CNS adverse effects such as CNS stimulation and tinnitus (ringing in the ears). GI functioning should also be assessed, because these drugs may worsen any existing diarrhea, nausea, and vomiting.

Cephalosporins require thorough assessment of allergies, including allergy to penicillins because of possible cross-sensitivity. Baseline vital sign measurements, blood count, bleeding time and clotting studies, and renal and hepatic function tests should be assessed as ordered. Assessment for signs and symptoms of pseudomembranous colitis, such as severe diarrhea, bloody stools, and abdominal pain, is needed in patients taking this group of drugs. It is also important to obtain information about the specific drug and to note the generation of cephalosporins to which it belongs, because each of the four drug generations has distinctive adverse effects and/or complications in addition to commonalities with the other groups.

With *tetracyclines,* careful assessment of culture and sensitivity reports, CBC counts, and results of renal and liver function tests is needed. There is also concern regarding the use of these drugs in patients younger than 8 years of age because of the problem of permanent mottling and discoloration of the teeth. Use of these drugs in pregnancy may also pose problems for the fetus, as previously discussed. Assessment for any whitish, sore patches on the oral mucosa (due to candidiasis or yeast infection) as well as any vaginal itching, pain, and/or cottage cheese–like discharge (due to vaginal candidiasis) is important for early identification and early treatment of superinfections (see previous discussion).

With *macrolides,* assessment of cardiac function (because of the risk of exacerbation of heart disease) and a thorough assessment of renal and liver function may help to identify adverse effects early on in therapy. Drug interactions have been discussed previously, but special note should be taken of the need to assess for concurrent prescribing or use of a macrolide and warfarin, because the interaction of these drugs can be detrimental to clotting ability and therefore platelet counts and results of clotting studies (e.g., international normalized ratio, prothrombin time, partial thromboplastin time) must be examined. In addition, there is always concern for antibiotics and their use with oral contraceptives, which may lead to contraceptive failure.

◆ NURSING DIAGNOSES

- Risk for infection related to the patient's compromised immune status before treatment due to bacterial invasion
- Risk for injury (compromised organ function) related to the adverse effects of medications (e.g., anemias, hepatic and renal toxicity) and the weakened physical state
- Acute pain related to infection and adverse reaction to medications
- Deficient knowledge related to lack of information about the disease process and the medication regimen
- Noncompliance with the treatment regimen related to lack of information and/or inability to pay for and actually obtain the necessary medication

◆ PLANNING

Goals

- Patient remains free of the signs and symptoms of infection once therapy is completed.
- Patient experiences minimal adverse effects as well as full therapeutic effects of antibiotic therapy.
- Patient remains compliant with antibiotic therapy regimen for the full duration of treatment.
- Patient experiences improvement in any discomfort or pain related to the infection.
- Patient remains informed about the drug therapy as well as about other treatment modalities and/or alternative therapies.
- Patient returns for follow-up visits to health care provider as recommended.

Outcome Criteria

- Patient states the signs and symptoms of an infection or its worsening, such as fever, pain, malaise, chills, joint pain, and increase in site-related symptoms.
- Patient describes improvement in the body's response to a resolving infection with subsequent increase in energy level and ability to carry out activities of daily living.
- Patient states the adverse effects of antibiotic therapy, such as GI upset, nausea, and diarrhea (specific to each class), and which effects to report to the physician, such as severe GI symptoms, jaundice (yellowish discoloration of skin and sclera), and severe skin rashes.
- Patient implements actions to minimize the GI distress and other adverse effects associated with antibiotic therapy, such as forcing fluids and eating dairy products like yogurt and buttermilk as appropriate.
- Patient experiences increased periods of comfort related to a resolving infectious process.
- Patient keeps all follow-up appointments and takes appropriate measures after completing antibiotic therapy, as explained by the health care provider.

◆ IMPLEMENTATION

Nursing interventions that apply to *all* antibiotics are as follows: (1) Oral antibiotics should be given within the recommended time frames and with the appropriate fluids or foods. (2) Therapy should be completed in full unless otherwise instructed by the physician. (3) Drugs should be administered around the clock to maintain effective blood levels. (4) *Avoid* giving oral antibiotics at the same time as antacids, calcium supplements, iron products, laxatives containing magnesium, or some of the antilipemic drugs (see previous discussion for a listing of drug interactions). (5) Herbal products and dietary supplements should be used only if they do not interact with the antibiotic. (6) Continual monitoring for hypersensitivity reactions past the initial assessment phase is important because immediate reactions may not occur for up to 30 minutes, accelerated reactions may occur within 1 to 72 hours, and delayed responses may occur after 72 hours. Hypersensitivity reactions may be manifested by wheezing; shortness of breath; swelling of the face, tongue, or hands; itching; or rash.

Sulfonamides should always be taken as directed and with forcing of fluids (2000 to 3000 mL/24 hr) to prevent drug-related crystalluria and to take oral dosage forms with food to minimize GI upset. It is also important to encourage patients to immediately report the following to their physician: worsening abdominal cramps, stomach pain, diarrhea, blood in the urine, severe or worsening rash, shortness of breath, and fever.

With *penicillins,* as with other antibiotics, the natural flora in the GI tract may be killed off by the antibiotic. Unaffected GI bacteria such as *Clostridium difficile* may overgrow (see earlier discussion). This process may be prevented by the consumption of probiotics, such as products containing lactobacillus, supplements, or cultured dairy products like yogurt, buttermilk, and kefir. Kefir is prepared using milk from sheep, goats, and cows, and soy milk kefirs are now commercially available. Some specific nursing considerations for various penicillin formulations include the following: (1) Oral penicillins should be taken with at least 6 oz of water (not juices), because acidic juices nullify the drug's antibacterial action. (2) Penicillin V, amoxicillin, and amoxicillin-clavulanate should be taken with water 1 hour before or 2 hours after meals to help decrease GI upset while maximizing absorption. (3) Procaine and benzathine salt penicillins are thick solutions that should be administered as ordered; they should be given IM using at least a 21-gauge needle and should be injected into a large muscle mass with rotation of sites as needed. (4) IM imipenem-cilastatin should be reconstituted in sterile saline, with plain lidocaine—as ordered and if the patient has no allergy to it—and then injected deep into a large muscle mass. (5) When IV penicillins (e.g., ampicillin) are administered, as with any IV therapy, the proper diluent should be used and the medication infused over the recommended time, IV rate and site should be checked and changed as appropriate, and the compatibility of solutions and drug(s) should be checked thoroughly. (6) IV sites should be checked for infiltration (swelling and tenderness at the IV site) as well as for irritation of the vein (phlebitis), manifested by heat, redness, and pain over the vein. (7) Should the patient experience an anaphylactic reaction to a penicillin, epinephrine and other emergency drugs should be given as ordered. Supportive treatment should be on hand (e.g., oxygen).

Orally administered *cephalosporins* should be given with food to decrease GI upset. Alcohol and alcohol-containing products should be avoided due to the potentiation of a disulfiram-like reaction associated with some of the cephalosporins. With the newer cephalosporins, as with many drug groups, the nurse must check the drug names carefully to ensure patient safety, because many drug names sound alike, and this can lead to medication errors. Cephalosporin use may also predispose the patient to pseudomembranous colitis, especially if preexisting GI disease is documented.

Tetracyclines cause photosensitivity, so precautions should be taken to avoid sun exposure and tanning bed use. Oral doses should be given with at least 8 oz of fluids and food to minimize GI upset. However, tetracyclines should *not* be given with dairy products, antacids, sodium bicarbonate, kaolin-pectin, or iron, because these chelate or bind with the antibiotic and decrease the antibiotic effect. These interacting foods and drugs may be given 2 hours before or 3 hours after the tetracycline to avoid this interaction. IV doxycycline is very irritating to the veins, and the IV infusion site should be checked frequently. Patients should be encouraged to report abdominal pain, nausea, vomiting, visual changes, and/or jaundice.

Macrolides should be administered with the same precautions as other antibiotics. Macrolides should *not* be given with or immediately before or after fruit juices to avoid interaction with the drug. The patient should be informed about the many drug interactions (discussed in the pharmacology section of this chapter), including those with over-the-counter drugs, herbal products, and dietary supplements. Patients should report severe rash, itching, hives, difficulty swallowing, jaundice, dark urine, and/or pale stools to their physician immediately.

✦ EVALUATION

Evaluation should include monitoring of goals, outcome criteria, and therapeutic effects and adverse effects. Therapeutic effects of antibiotics include a decrease in the signs and symptoms of the infection; a return to normal vital signs, including temperature, and negative results on culture and sensitivity tests; normal results for CBC; and improved appetite, energy level, and sense of well-being. Evaluation for adverse effects includes monitoring for the specific drug-related adverse effects (see each drug profile).

CASE STUDY
Antibiotic Therapy

Mr. G. has been a resident of an assisted care facility since experiencing a left-sided stroke 5 years ago. Presently his cardiovascular status and cerebrovascular status are stable. However, he has had a productive cough and a low-grade fever for 2 days. After physical assessment and chest radiographic examination, the physician diagnoses him with pneumonia of the left lower lobe of the lung. The physician orders intravenous piperacillin-tazobactam (Zosyn) 2.25 g every 8 hours and oral theophylline (Theo-Dur) 300 mg every 12 hours. Mr. G. also takes warfarin (Coumadin) 2 mg every evening. Maalox 30 mL has been ordered as needed for gastrointestinal upset, and oral ibuprofen 400 mg can be given as needed for pain.

- Explain the rationale behind the use of tazobactam with piperacillin in the Zosyn.
- What concerns or drug interactions should the nurse be aware of with the use of Zosyn and the other medications ordered for Mr. G.?
- What parameters should be monitored to determine whether the Zosyn is working? Explain your answer.

For answers, see http://evolve.elsevier.com/Lilley.

Patient Teaching Tips

- Educate the patient about foods and beverages that may interact negatively with antibiotics, such as alcohol, acidic fruit juices, and dairy products.
- The patient should be instructed to report severe adverse effects to the physician. In addition, the patient should be conscientious about follow-up visits to the health care provider because of the need to monitor the infection and its treatment. Laboratory tests may also be performed at these visits.
- The patient should be instructed to increase fluid intake to up to 3000 mL/day unless contraindicated. Reporting of the following is also important because these symptoms may indicate superinfection: fever, black hairy tongue, stomatitis, loose and/or foul-smelling stools, vaginal discharge, or cough.

- Educate about foods that may help prevent superinfections (e.g., vaginal yeast infections), such as yogurt, buttermilk, and kefir (see earlier discussion). New yogurts, termed *probiotics*, are available that help reestablish the natural flora of the GI tract.
- If the patient is taking oral contraceptives for birth control, there should be education about interactions between certain antibiotics and oral contraceptives. Effectiveness of oral contraceptives may be decreased with these antibiotics. The patient should be informed to be sure to use a backup method of contraception to avoid pregnancy.
- Encourage patients to wear a medical alert bracelet or necklace if allergic to antibiotics (or to any other medication) and to keep this information on their person at all times.

Continued

Patient Teaching Tips—cont'd

- For *sulfonamides,* inform the patient to take the antibiotic with plenty of fluids (2000 to 3000 mL/24 hr) to prevent drug-related crystalluria or precipitation in the kidneys, and to take these drugs with food. Patients should report the following to their health care provider immediately: worsening abdominal cramps, stomach pain, diarrhea, blood in the urine, severe or worsening rash, shortness of breath, or fever.
- For *penicillins,* the patient should take the medication exactly as prescribed for the full duration indicated, with doses spaced at regularly scheduled intervals. The patient should take oral dosage forms with water and should avoid taking them with caffeine-containing foods or beverages, citrus fruit, cola beverages, fruit juices, or tomato juice because the drug will be inactivated. If the patient must take a penicillin drug four times a day, the patient should set up a reminder system so that blood levels will remain steady. Reminders may be provided using a watch or even a cell phone alarm so that the patient will be sure to take the drug exactly as directed.
- For *cephalosporins,* encourage the patient to report diarrhea, flu-like symptoms, blistering or peeling of the skin, hearing loss, breathing difficulty, or seizures to the health care provider immediately. The patient should also report any foul-smelling, loose, frequent, and/or bloody stools.
- For *tetracyclines,* the patient should be advised to avoid exposure to tanning beds and direct sunlight or to use sunscreen and/or wear protective clothing because of drug-related photosensitivity. These photosensitive effects may be noticed within a few minutes to hours after taking the drug and may last up to several days after the drug has been discontinued.
- For *macrolides,* the patient should take the drug as directed and should check for interactions with other drugs being taken at the same time, especially interactions between erythromycin and other medications. For some drugs in this class (e.g., azithromycin), there are newer forms in 3-day and even 1-day dose packs rather than the 5-day dose pack. The nurse should always be sure that the patient knows the proper dosage and instructions for the drug the patient is taking.

Points to Remember

- Antibiotics can be either bacteriostatic or bactericidal. Bacteriostatic antibiotics inhibit the growth of bacteria but do not directly kill them. Bactericidal antibiotics directly kill the bacteria.
- Most antibiotics work by inhibiting bacterial cell wall synthesis in some way. Bacteria have survived over the ages because they can adapt to their surroundings. If a bacterium's environment includes an antibiotic, over time it can mutate in such a way that it can survive an attack by the antibiotic. The production of β-lactamases is one way in which bacteria can fend off the effects of antibiotics.
- Nurses need to be aware of the most common adverse effects of antibiotics, which include nausea, vomiting, and diarrhea. Nurses should inform patients that antibiotics should be taken for the prescribed length of time.
- Each class of antibiotics is associated with specific cautions, contraindications, drug interactions, and adverse effects that must be carefully assessed for and monitored by the nurse.
- Because normally occurring bacteria are killed during antibiotic therapy, superinfections may arise during treatment. These may be manifested by the following signs and symptoms: fever, perineal itching, oral lesions, vaginal irritation and discharge, cough, and lethargy.

NCLEX Examination Review Questions

1. A patient is scheduled for colorectal surgery tomorrow. He does not have sepsis, his WBC count is normal, he has no fever, and he is otherwise in good health. However, the nurse notes that there are orders to administer an antibiotic on call before he goes to surgery. What is the rationale for this antibiotic order?
   a. To provide empiric therapy
   b. To provide prophylactic therapy
   c. To treat for a superinfection
   d. To reduce the number of resistant organisms
2. A teenaged patient is taking a tetracycline drug as part of treatment for severe acne. When the nurse teaches this patient about drug-related precautions, which is the most pertinent information to convey?
   a. When the acne clears up, the medication may be discontinued.
   b. This medication should be taken with antacids to reduce GI upset.
   c. The patient should use sunscreen or avoid exposure to sunlight because this drug may cause photosensitivity.
   d. The teeth should be observed closely for signs of mottling or other color changes.
3. A newly admitted patient reports a penicillin allergy. The physician has ordered a second-generation cephalosporin as part of the therapy. Which of the nursing actions below is appropriate?
   a. Call the physician to clarify the order because of the patient's allergy.
   b. Give the medication and monitor for adverse effects.

   c. Ask the pharmacy to change the order to a first-generation cephalosporin.
   d. Administer the drug with an nonsteroidal antiinflammatory to reduce adverse effects.
4. During patient education regarding an oral macrolide such as erythromycin, which of the following points is appropriate to make?
   a. If GI upset occurs, the drug will have to be stopped.
   b. The drug should be taken with an antacid to avoid GI problems.
   c. The patient should take each dose with a sip of water.
   d. The patient may take the drug with a small snack to reduce GI irritation.
5. A woman who has been taking an antibiotic for a urinary tract infection calls the nurse practitioner to complain of severe vaginal itching. She has also noticed a thick, whitish vaginal discharge. The nurse practitioner suspects that
   a. this is an expected response to antibiotic therapy.
   b. the urinary tract infection has become worse instead of better.
   c. a superinfection has developed.
   d. the urinary tract infection is resistant to the antibiotic.

1. b, 2. c, 3. a, 4. d, 5. c.

Critical Thinking Activities

1. Explain the rationale for not taking dairy products, iron, or calcium with tetracycline. What would be recommended if these products are not omitted from the diet?
2. What symptoms would alert you to the fact that a patient is suffering from a superinfection or overgrowth of normal flora stemming from the use of an antibiotic?

3. If a person is allergic to penicillin, then is that person also allergic to cephalosporins? Explain your answer.

For answers, see http://evolve.elsevier.com/Lilley.

Antibiotics Part 2

Objectives

When you reach the end of this chapter, you should be able to do the following:

1. Review the general principles of antibiotic therapy and review all of the previously discussed antibiotics in Chapter 37 in preparation for discussion of the following antibiotics or antibiotic classes: aminoglycosides, fluoroquinolones, clindamycin, metronidazole, nitrofurantoin, vancomycin, and several other miscellaneous antibiotics.
2. Review the advantages and disadvantages associated with use of antibiotics with discussion of overuse/abuse of antibiotics, development of drug resistance, superinfections, and antibiotic-associated colitis.
3. Discuss the indications, cautions, contraindications, mechanisms of action, adverse effects, toxic effects, routes of administration, and drug interactions associated with aminoglycosides, fluoroquinolones, clindamycin, metronidazole, nitrofurantoin, vancomycin, and miscellaneous antibiotics.
4. Develop a nursing care plan that includes all phases of the nursing process for the patient receiving antibiotics.

e-Learning Activities

Companion CD
- NCLEX Review Questions: see questions 338-344
- Animations
- Audio Glossary
- Category Catchers
- Medication Errors Checklists
- IV Therapy Checklists

evolve Website (http://evolve.elsevier.com/Lilley)
- Nursing Care Plans • Frequently Asked Questions • Content Updates • WebLinks • Supplemental Resources • Elsevier ePharmacology Update • Medication Administration Animations

Drug Profiles

amikacin, p. 597
▶ ciprofloxacin, p. 600
▶ clindamycin, p. 600
dapsone, p. 601
daptomycin, p. 603
▶ gentamicin, p. 597
levofloxacin, p. 600
linezolid, p. 602

▶ metronidazole, p. 602
neomycin, p. 598
nitrofurantoin, p. 602
quinupristin and dalfopristin, p. 602
tobramycin, p. 598
▶ vancomycin, p. 602

▶ Key drug.

Glossary

Concentration-dependent killing A property of some antibiotics, especially aminoglycosides and vancomycin, of achieving a relatively high, even if brief, plasma drug concentration, results in the most effective bacterial kill (see *time-dependent killing*). (p. 595)

Facultative anaerobic metabolism A property of certain bacteria (e.g., enterococci) that allows them to adapt to low tissue oxygen concentrations, and still thrive, even though they normally thrive in oxygen-rich environments. (p. 596)

Microgram One millionth of a gram. Be careful not to confuse with milligram (one thousandth of a gram), which is a thousand times greater than one microgram. Confusion of these two units sometimes results in drug dosage errors. (p. 595)

Minimum inhibitory concentration (MIC) A laboratory measurement of the lowest drug concentration needed to kill a certain standardized amount of bacteria. (p. 595)

MRSA Originally, this abbreviation stood exclusively for methicillin-resistant *Staphylococcus aureus*, to describe an *S. aureus* species that was resistant to the beta-lactamase resistant penicillin known as methicillin. It now more commonly refers to strains of *S. aureus* that are resistant to several drug classes, and it therefore may also stand for (depending on context or health facility) multidrug-resistant *S. aureus*. (p. 599)

Nephrotoxicity Toxicity to the kidneys, often drug-induced and manifesting in compromised renal function. (p. 596)

Ototoxicity Toxicity to the ears, often drug-induced and manifesting in varying degrees of hearing loss that is more likely to be permanent than nephrotoxicity. (p. 596)

Post-antibiotic effect (PAE) A period of continued bacterial suppression that occurs after brief exposure to certain antibiotic drug classes, especially aminoglycosides and carbapenems (Chapter 37). The mechanism of this effect is uncertain. (p. 596)

Pseudomembranous colitis A necrotizing, inflammatory bowel condition that is often associated with antibiotic therapy. Some antibiotics (e.g., clindamycin) are more likely to produce it than others. A more general term that is also used is *antibiotic-associated colitis*. (p. 601)

Synergistic effect Stronger bacterial kill resulting from two antibiotics given together than with either given alone. (p. 596)

Therapeutic drug monitoring Ongoing monitoring of plasma drug concentrations and dosage adjustment based on these values as well as other laboratory indicators such as kidney and liver function tests; is often carried out by a pharmacist in collaboration with medical, nursing, and laboratory staff. (p. 595)

Time-dependent killing A property of most antibiotic classes, in contrast to concentration-dependent killing (see above) that requires prolonged high plasma drug concentrations for effective bacterial kill. (p. 595)

This chapter is a continuation of Chapter 37 and focuses on additional classes of antibiotics. In general, Chapter 38 describes the various antibiotics that are used for more serious and harder-to-treat infections. Many of the drugs in this chapter are given by the *parenteral* (injectable) route only, a route generally reserved for more treating more clinically serious infections in the hospital setting. Also included are miscellaneous drugs that are unique in their class, as well as newer drugs and drug classes. The decision to divide the antibiotics chapter from the previous edition into two new chapters was made in light of the large (and increasing) number of antibiotic drugs.

AMINOGLYCOSIDES

The aminoglycosides are a group of natural and semisynthetic antibiotics that are classified as *bactericidal* drugs (Chapter 37). They are similar to the tetracyclines in that they are derived from *Streptomyces* organisms. Although they are potent antibiotics, they have been replaced to varying degrees (depending on the institution) with fluoroquinolones, which have somewhat safer adverse effect profiles. Nonetheless, bacterial resistance may be less common than with fluoroquinolones, making aminoglycosides the better choice in particularly virulent infections. The aminoglycoside antibiotics available for clinical use are listed in Table 38-1. These drugs can be given by several different routes, but they are not given orally because of their poor oral absorption. An exception to this is the use of neomycin (see Drug Profiles). The three aminoglycosides most commonly used for the treatment of systemic infections are amikacin, gentamicin, and tobramycin. Serum levels of these drugs are routinely monitored from patients' blood samples. Dosages are then adjusted to maintain known optimal levels that maximize drug efficacy and minimize the risk for toxicity. This process is known as **therapeutic drug monitoring,** and aminoglycoside therapy is commonly monitored in this way due to its associated nephrotoxicity and ototoxicity. Most commonly, dosing is adjusted for the patient's level of renal function, based on calculated estimates of creatinine clearance from serum creatinine values. This function is often carried out by a hospital pharmacist, consulting for the prescriber. The **minimum inhibitory concentration (MIC)** for any antibiotic is a measurement of the lowest concentration of drug needed to kill a certain standard amount of bacteria. This value is determined *in vitro* (in the laboratory) for each drug. It has been shown that other classes of antibiotics, such as beta-lactams, work on **time-dependent killing,** that is, the amount of time above MIC that is crucial for maximal bacterial kill. However, aminoglycosides work primarily based on **concentration-dependent killing,** where achieving an increase in plasma concentration above MIC, but for no particular length of time, enhances the bacterial kill of the drug. For this reason, although originally given in three daily intravenous doses, the current predominant practice is *once-daily aminoglycoside dosing.* Several clinical studies have shown that once-daily dosing provides a sufficient plasma drug concentration for bacterial kill, along with equal or less risk for toxicity than multiple-daily dosage regimens. A once-daily regimen, versus the traditional three times daily regimen, also reduces the required nursing care time and often allows for outpatient or even home-based aminoglycoside drug therapy. The table below lists the *traditional* desired drug levels for these drugs. Note that *peak* (highest) levels for once-daily regimens are usually not measured, as it is assumed that the peak level for a single daily dose will be short lived and drop off within a reasonable time frame. However, *trough* (lowest) levels are routinely measured to ensure adequate renal clearance of the drug and avoid toxicity. Dosage information appears in the designated table. Dosage regimens and ranges for serum levels may vary between institutions.

The trough blood sample should be drawn at least 18 hours after completion of the dose, and closer to 24 hours afterward for

Table 38-1	Availability of Aminoglycoside Antibiotics	
Origin	**Product**	**Description**
Natural	gentamicin kanamycin neomycin paromomycin streptomycin tobramycin	All chemically derived from *Streptomyces* spp. by a fermentation process
Semisynthetic	amikacin netilmicin	Chemical derivative of kanamycin Structurally related togentamicin

Serum Drug Levels	Peak		Trough	
	Multi-daily dosing*	Once-daily dosing	Multi-daily dosing	Once-daily dosing
amikacin	15-30 mcg/mL†	Usually not measured	5-10 mcg/mL	<10 mcg/mL
gentamicin and tobramycin	4-10 mcg/mL	Usually not measured	1-2 mcg/mL	<1 mcg/mL

*q8h or q12h.

†mcg = **micrograms;** note that one microgram = 1/1,000 (one thousandth of a) milligram or 1/1,000,000 (one millionth of a) gram. Also note microgram is abbreviated *mcg,* while milligram is abbreviated *mg.*

renally impaired patients. The therapeutic goal is a trough concentration ("trough") at or below 1 mcg/mL (which is considered undetectable). This is because troughs above 2 mcg/mL are associated with greater risk for both **ototoxicity** and **nephrotoxicity**. Ototoxicity (toxicity to the ears) often manifests as some degree of temporary or permanent hearing loss. Nephrotoxicity (toxicity to the kidneys) manifests in varying degrees of reduced renal function. This is generally indicated by laboratory test results such as serum creatinine level. A rising serum creatinine suggests reduced creatinine clearance by the kidneys, and is indicative of declining renal function. Trough levels are normally monitored once every 3 days until the drug therapy is discontinued. The patient's serum creatinine should also be measured at least twice weekly as an index of renal function, and drug dosages should be adjusted as needed for any changes in renal function.

Mechanism of Action and Drug Effects

Aminoglycosides (AGs) work in a way that is similar to that of the tetracyclines in that they also bind to ribosomes and thereby prevent protein synthesis in bacteria (see Figure 37-6). Specifically, they do this by binding to a structure known as the 30S ribosomal subunit. Protein synthesis is then disrupted by genetic misreadings of messenger RNA (mRNA) molecules, leading to cell death. Often AGs are used in combination with other antibiotics such as beta-lactams or vancomycin in the treatment of various infections because the combined effect of the two antibiotics is greater than that of either drug alone. This is known as a **synergistic effect.** AGs also have a property known as **post-antibiotic effect (PAE).** This is a period of continued bacterial growth suppression that occurs *after* short-term antibiotic exposure as in once-daily AG dosing (see above). Carbapenems are another antibiotic class having a PAE. PAE is enhanced with higher peak drug concentrations, smaller bacterial inocula, and concurrent use of beta-lactam antibiotics.

As is the case with most antibiotic drug classes, there have emerged various bacterial mechanisms of resistance among both gram-positive and gram-negative species previously more susceptible to aminoglycosides. The prevalence and intensity of such resistance varies with specific drugs, organisms, patient populations, disease states, and geographic prescribing patterns. Aminoglycoside resistance is less likely to develop during the course of a given patient's drug therapy, unlike the resistance of beta-lactam drugs, especially cephalosporins. Instead, it is usually a longer process or occurs in response to an especially large bacterial *inoculum,* as is common with patients having serious burns or cystic fibrosis. In addition, concurrent use of aminoglycosides with cephalosporins does not prevent the development of resistance to the cephalosporins. In general, resistant bacterial strains produce drug-impeding enzymes. These proteins result from adaptive changes at the genetic level (DNA and/or RNA) within the bacterial cells. Such enzymes may work through chemical interactions with the drug molecules themselves, or by altering the permeability of the bacterial cell wall membrane to the drug molecules. One common example is resistance among enterococcal bacterial strains. This species has a characteristic known as **facultative anaerobic metabolism,** meaning that these bacteria can adaptively function metabolically in the absence of oxygen. When this occurs, the anaerobic biochemical reactions alter the cell membrane electrical potentials in such a way as to

make it chemically more difficult for the drug molecules to enter the cell to reach their site of action.

Indications

The toxicity associated with aminoglycosides normally limits their use to treatment of serious gram-negative infections and specific conditions involving gram-positive cocci, in which case gentamicin is usually given in combination with a penicillin. Commonly treated gram-negative infections include *Pseudomonas* spp., and several organisms belonging to the *Enterobacteriaceae* family (facultatively anaerobic gram-negative rods), including *Escherichia coli, Proteus* spp., *Klebsiella* spp., and *Serratia* spp. Such infections are often treated with a suitable aminoglycoside and an extended-spectrum penicillin, third-generation cephalosporin, or a carbapenem. Gram-positive infections may include *Enterococcus* spp., *Staphylococcus aureus,* and bacterial endocarditis, which is usually streptococcal in origin. A three-daily dose regimen is more common when treating gram-positive infections, as this often enhances synergy with other antibiotics that are used. Aminoglycosides are also used for prophylaxis in procedures involving the gastrointestinal or genitourinary tract, as such procedures are high-risk for enterococcal bacteremia. They are also commonly given in combination with either ampicillin or vancomycin (for penicillin-allergic patients) for surgical patients with a history of valvular heart disease, because diseased heart valves are also more prone to enterococcal infection.

Aminoglycosides should be administered with caution in premature and full-term neonates. Because of the renal immaturity of these patients, prolonged actions of the aminoglycosides (AGs) and a greater risk for toxicities may result. Serious pediatric infections for which AGs are commonly used include pneumonia, meningitis, and urinary tract infections. Drug selection for both pediatric and adult patients is based on the susceptibility of the causative organism. Refer to Table 38-2 for more information on the antibacterial spectra of specific aminoglycosides. A few AGs have even more specific indications. Streptomycin is active against *Mycobacterium* spp, (Chapter 40), whereas paromomycin is used to treat amebic dysentery, a protozoal intestinal disease (Chapter 42). Aminoglycosides are relatively inactive against fungi, viruses, and most anaerobic bacteria.

Contraindications

The only usual contraindication is known drug allergy. The pregnancy categories for these drugs range from C to D. Aminoglycosides have been shown to cross the placenta and cause fetal harm when administered to pregnant women. There have been several case reports of total, irreversible bilateral congenital deafness in the children of women receiving aminoglycosides during pregnancy. Therefore, aminoglycosides should be used in pregnant women only in the event of life-threatening infections when safer drugs are ineffective. These drugs are also distributed in breast milk. Their use should be avoided in lactating women to avoid risk for drug toxicity in nursing infants.

Adverse Effects

Aminoglycosides are very potent antibiotics and are capable of potentially serious toxicities, especially to the kidneys *(nephrotoxicity)* and to the ears in terms of hearing and balance functions

Table 38-2 Aminoglycosides: Comparative Spectra of Antimicrobial Activity

Aminoglycoside	Spectrum
amikacin sulfate	*Acinetobacter* spp., *Enterobacter aerogenes, Escherichia coli, Klebsiella pneumoniae, Proteus* spp., *Providencia* spp., *Pseudomonas* spp., *Serratia* spp., *Staphylococcus* infections
gentamicin sulfate	*E. aerogenes, E. coli, K. pneumoniae, Proteus* spp., *Pseudomonas* spp., *Salmonella* spp., *Serratia* spp. (nonpigmented), *Shigella* spp.
kanamycin sulfate	*Acinetobacter* spp., *E. coli, K. pneumoniae, Proteus* spp., *Serratia marcescens;* it is administered PO for the treatment of cirrhotic patients in hepatic coma caused by nitrogen-producing bacteria and for intestinal antisepsis
neomycin sulfate	Toxicity limits use to gastrointestinal tract (hepatic coma, *E. coli diarrhea,* and antisepsis) and as a topical antibacterial
netilmicin sulfate	*Citrobacter* spp., *Enterobacter* spp., *E. coli, K. pneumoniae, Proteus* spp., *Pseudomonas aeruginosa, Serratia* spp.
paromomycin sulfate	Amebic dysentery
streptomycin sulfate	Granuloma inguinale, plague, tularemia, TB, nonhemolytic *Streptococcus* endocarditis
tobramycin sulfate	*Citrobacter* spp., *Enterobacter* spp., *E. coli, Klebsiella* spp., *Proteus* spp., *Providencia* spp., *P. aeruginosa, Serratia* spp.

(ototoxicity). Duration of drug therapy should be as short as possible, using sound clinical judgment and monitoring of the patient's progress. Nephrotoxicity typically occurs in 5% to 25% of patients and is usually manifested by urinary casts (visible remnants of destroyed renal cells), proteinuria, and increased BUN and serum creatinine levels. It is usually reversible, but the patient's renal function tests should be monitored throughout therapy. In contrast, ototoxicity is less common, commonly occurs in 3% to 14% of patients, but is often not reversible. It can result in varying degrees of permanent hearing loss, depending on the dosage and duration of drug therapy. It is believed to result from damage to the eighth cranial nerve (CN VIII; *cochleovestibular nerve* or *auditory nerve*) and involves both cochlear damage (hearing loss) and vestibular damage (disrupted sense of balance). Symptoms include dizziness, tinnitus, a sense of fullness in the ears, and hearing loss. Preventive monitoring may include audiometry screenings to detect high-frequency hearing loss, assuming that the patient is mentally fit to interact with the audiologist to complete the exam. However, because aminoglycosides are often used to treat serious infections in critically ill patients, this is one example in which the risk for drug toxicity may become a secondary consideration versus the risk for death or disability from the infection itself. Other less common effects include headache, paresthesia, dizziness, vertigo, skin rash, fever, overgrowth of nonsusceptible organisms, and neuromuscular paralysis (very rare and reversible). The risk for these toxicities is greatest in patients with pre-existing renal impairment, patients already receiving other renally toxic drugs, and patients on high doses of, or prolonged, aminoglycoside therapy.

Interactions

There are several significant drug interactions associated with aminoglycoside use. The risk for nephrotoxicity can be increased with concurrent use of other nephrotoxic drugs such as vancomycin, cyclosporine, and amphotericin B. Concurrent use with loop diuretics increases the risk for otoxoticity. In addition, because aminoglycosides, like many other antibiotics, also kill intestinal bacterial flora, they also reduce the amount of vitamin K produced by these gut bacteria. These normal flora normally serve to balance the effects of oral anticoagulants such as warfarin (Coumadin). Therefore, aminoglycosides can potentiate warfarin toxicity.

Dosages

For recommended dosages of selected aminoglycosides, see the table on page 598.

Drug Profiles

Historically, the aminoglycoside antibiotics (AGs) were used primarily for gram-negative infections. However, they are now used much more commonly than before for gram-positive infections due to the increased incidence of resistant gram-positive organisms. They are normally given intravenously or intramuscularly. However, neomycin is only given orally, rectally, or topically (Chapter 57). Kanamycin has both injectable and oral dosage forms. There are also topical dosage forms of both gentamicin and tobramycin for dermatologic (Chapter 57) and ophthalmic (Chapter 58) use. Currently available AGs include amikacin, gentamicin, kanamycin, neomycin, paromomycin, streptomycin, and tobramycin. The variations in the suffixes of some of the drug names, in particular *–mycin* versus *–micin,* denote different bacterial origins of the various AGs. Dosage and other information appear in the designated table.

amikacin

Amikacin (Amikin) is a semisynthetic aminoglycoside antibiotic derived by chemically altering kanamycin, a naturally occurring aminoglycoside that is derived from *Streptomyces* spp. It is often used for infections that are resistant to gentamicin or tobramycin. It is only available in injectable form.

Pharmacokinetics

Half-Life	Onset	Peak	Duration
2-3 hr	Variable	1 hr	8-12 hr

▸ gentamicin

Gentamicin (Garamycin) is a naturally occurring aminoglycoside that is obtained from cultures of *Micromonospora* spp. It is one of the most commonly used aminoglycosides in clinical practice today. It can be given either intravenously or intramuscularly, with the dosage the same for both routes. It is indicated for the treatment of several susceptible gram-positive and gram-negative bacteria. Gentamicin is available in several dosage forms, including injections, topical ointments, and ophthalmic drops and ointments.

Pharmacokinetics

Half-Life	Onset	Peak	Duration
IV: 2 hr	IV: Variable	IV: 0.5-2 hr	IV: 8-12 hr

DOSAGES

Selected Aminoglycosides

Drug (Pregnancy Category)	Pharmacologic Class	Usual Dosage Range	Indications
amikacin (Amikin) (D)	Aminoglycoside	**Adult and pediatric** IV: 15 mg/kg/day divided bid-tid or 15-20 mg/kg once daily **Neonatal** IV: 10 mg/kg load, then 7.5 mg/kg q12h	Primarily gentamicin- and tobramycin-resistant gram-negative infections along with severe staphylococcal infections
▶gentamicin (Garamycin) (C)	Aminoglycoside	**Adult** IV/IM: 2-5 mg/kg/day divided qd-qid or 5-7 mg/kg once daily **Pediatric and neonatal** IV/IM: 2-2.5 mg/kg q8h	Primarily gram-negative infections along with severe staphylococcal infections
tobramycin (Nebcin, TOBI) (D)	Aminoglycoside	**Adult** IV/IM: 3-5 mg/kg/day divided qd-tid or 5-7 mg/kg once daily **Pediatric** IV/IM: 6-7.5 mg/kg/day divided tid-qid **Neonatal** IV/IM: 3 mg/kg q24h or 2 mg/kg q12h	Primarily gram-negative infections along with severe staphylococcal infections
neomycin (Neo-Fradin) (C)	Aminoglycoside	**Adult** PO/PR: 3000-9000 mg divided between 3-9 doses **Pediatric** PO/PR: 90 mg/kg/day q4h x 2d	Preoperative bowel cleansing; (also used with different dosage regimens for hepatic encephalopathy)

tobramycin

Tobramycin (Nebcin, TOBI) is also derived from *Streptomyces* spp. It has dosages, routes of administration, and indications that are comparable to gentamicin for generalized infections. In addition, it is commonly used to treat recurrent pulmonary infections in cystic fibrosis by both injectable and inhaled dosing. It is also available in topical and ophthalmic dosage forms.

Pharmacokinetics

Half-Life	Onset	Peak	Duration
IV: 2-3 hr	IV: Variable	IV: 30 min	IV: Up to 24 hr

neomycin

Neomycin (Neo-Fradin) is also derived from *Streptomyces* spp. It is most commonly used for bacterial decontamination of the gastrointestinal tract before surgical procedures, and it is given both orally and rectally (as an enema) for this purpose. Other uses include topical application for skin infections, bladder irrigation, treatment of *E. coli* diarrhea, hepatic encephalopathy, and eye infections. In hepatic encephalopathy, the drug helps reduce the number of ammonia-producing bacteria in the gastrointestinal tract. The subsequent reduced blood ammonia levels sometimes result in neurologic improvement from the hepatic illness. This drug is not available in injectable form, but instead is available in tablets, solutions, and powders for oral, topical, or irrigation administration. Kanamycin is another AG available in oral form and has similar indications to neomycin. However, it is also available in injectable form with indications comparable to gentamicin and tobramycin.

Pharmacokinetics

Half-Life	Onset	Peak	Duration
PO: 3 hr	PO: Variable	PO: 1-4 hr	PO: Up to 24 hr

FLUOROQUINOLONES

Fluoroquinolones are very potent, bactericidal, broad-spectrum antibiotics. The first of these drugs to come available were the original quinolones, cinoxacin and nalidixic acid. These two drugs have narrower spectra of antibacterial activity than the newer, more potent, and less toxic *fluoro*quinolones and are therefore seldom used anymore. A fluorine atom was added onto the basic quinolone structure to create these newer drugs, and this increased their antibacterial potency and spectra. However, both generations of drugs are commonly referred to as "quinolones" for brevity. Currently available quinolone antibiotics include norfloxacin, ciprofloxacin, levofloxacin, moxifloxacin, gatifloxacin, and gemifloxacin.

Mechanism of Action and Drug Effects

Quinolone antibiotics destroy bacteria by altering their DNA (see Figure 37-6). They accomplish this by interfering with the bacterial enzymes DNA gyrase and topoisomerase IV. Quinolones do not seem to affect the corresponding mammalian enzymes and therefore do not inhibit the production of human DNA.

The drug effects of quinolone antibiotics are mostly limited to their effects on bacteria. They kill susceptible strains of mostly gram-negative and some gram-positive organisms. Some quinolones are also believed to diffuse into and concentrate themselves in human neutrophils, killing such bacteria as *S. aureus, Serratia marcescens,* and *Mycobacterium fortuitum* that sometimes accumulate in these cells. Nonetheless, bacterial resistance to quinolone antibiotics has been identified among several bacterial species, including *Pseudomonas aeruginosa, S. aureus, Pneumococcus spp., Enterococcus spp.,* as well as the broad *Enterobacteriaeciae* family that includes *E. coli.* Mechanisms for such resistance include altered DNA gyrase and topoisomerase enzymes, and altered cell membrane permeability to reduce entry of drug molecules into cells and speed efflux of such molecules out of cells.

Indications

Quinolones are active against a wide variety of gram-negative and selected gram-positive bacteria. Most are primarily excreted by the kidneys, which contain a high percentage of unchanged drug. Together with the fact that they have extensive gram-negative coverage, they are suitable for treating complicated urinary tract infections. Exceptions include moxifloxacin and gemifloxacin, which are less renally excreted. They are also commonly used for respiratory, skin, gastrointestinal, bone, joint infections, and sexually transmitted diseases (STDs).

Levofloxacin is somewhat more active than older quinolones against gram-positive organisms such as *S. pneumoniae,* including penicillin-resistant strains, as well as *Enterococcus* and *S. aureus.* Gatifloxacin and moxifloxacin are also effective against *S. pneumoniae* as well as some strains of *S. aureus* and enterococci. However, multidrug-resistant *S. aureus* (**MRSA**) and vancomycin-resistant enterococci (VRE) are generally also resistant to gatifloxacin and moxifloxacin. The activity of gatifloxacin and moxifloxacin against many enteric gram-negative bacteria and *P. aeruginosa* is similar to that of levofloxacin and less than that of ciprofloxacin. Moxifloxacin often has stronger anaerobic bacterial coverage. Norfloxacin has limited oral absorption, but is only available in oral form, so its use is limited to genitourinary infections, including STDs. Quinolones are often combined with aminoglycosides to treat *P. aeruginosa.* Gatifloxacin and moxifloxacin also have some *in vitro* activity anaerobes. Gemifloxacin, the newest quinolone, is primarily indicated for gram-negative respiratory infections such as bacterial exacerbations of chronic bronchitis and community-acquired pneumonia (CAP), and is also effective against resistant strains of *S. pneumoniae.*

The use of quinolones in prepubescent children is still not generally recommended because they have been shown to affect cartilage development in laboratory animals. However, more recent evidence suggests that judicial use in children might be less of a risk than previously thought. Although there is some variance in spectra between drugs, Box 38-1 lists selected microbes commonly susceptible to quinolone therapy in general. Table 38-3 lists common indications by individual drug.

Contraindications

The most common contraindication is known drug allergy. However, quinolones also have some unique contraindications related to cardiac function. Dangerous cardiac dysrhythmias are more likely to occur when quinolones are taken by patients receiving class IA and class III antiarrhythmic drugs such as disopyramide and amiodarone. For this reason, such drug combinations should be avoided.

Adverse Effects

Fluoroquinolones are capable of causing a variety of adverse effects, the most common of which are listed in Table 38-4. Bacterial overgrowth is another possible complication of quinolone therapy, but this is more commonly associated with long-term use. More worrisome is a cardiac effect that involves prolongation of the QT interval on the electrocardiogram (ECG). There is some

---

Box 38-1	**Overview of Quinolone-Susceptible Microbial Spectra**

- Gram-positive: *Streptococcus* (including *S. pneumoniae*), *Staphylococcus,* enterococci, *Listeria monocytogenes*
- Gram-negative: *Neisseria gonorrhea, N. meningitidis, Haemophilus influenzae, H. parainfluenzae,* Enterobacteriaeciae (including *Escherichia coli, Enterobacter, Klebsiella, Proteus mirabilis, Salmonella, Shigella*), *Acinetobacter, P. aeruginosa, Pastorella multocida, Legionella, Mycoplasma pneumoniae, Chlamydia*
- Anaerobes: *Bacteroides fragilis, Peptococcus, Peptostreptococcus* (moxifloxacin strongest)
- Other: *Rickettsia* (ciprofloxacin only)

Table 38-3   Quinolones: Common Indications for Specific Drugs

Generic Name (with Brand Name and Year of FDA Approval)	Antibacterial Spectrum	Common Indications
norfloxacin (Noroxin, 1986)	Extensive gram-negative and selected gram-positive coverage	Urinary tract infections, prostatitis, STDs
ciprofloxacin (Cipro, 1987)	Comparable to norfloxacin	Anthrax (inhalational, postexposure); respiratory, skin, urinary tract, prostate, intra-abdominal, gastrointestinal, bone and joint infections; typhoid fever, STDs, selected nosocomial pneumonias
levofloxacin (Levaquin, 1996)	Comparable to norfloxacin	Respiratory and urinary tract infections; prophylaxis in various transrectal and transurethral prostate surgical procedures
moxifloxacin (Avelox, 1999)	Comparable to norfloxacin	Respiratory and skin infections; CAP caused by PRSP; plus anaerobic infections
gatifloxacin (Tequin, 1999)	Comparable to norfloxacin	Respiratory and urinary tract infections
gemifloxacin (Factive, 2003)	Comparable to norfloxacin	Acute bacterial exacerbation of chronic bronchitis; CAP

CAP, Community-acquired pneumonia; *PRSP,* penicillin-resistant streptococcal pneumonia; *STD,* sexually transmitted disease.

debate regarding this effect, but cases are still reported. Also, tendonitis and even tendon rupture has been reported. This effect is more common in elderly patients, patients with renal failure, and those on concurrent glucocorticoid therapy (e.g., prednisone).

Interactions

With the exception of norfloxacin, these antibiotics have excellent oral absorption. In many cases, the extent of oral absorption is comparable to intravenous injection. However, the concurrent use of antacids with quinolones causes their oral absorption to be greatly reduced. There are several drugs that interact with quinolones. Their use with antacids, iron, or zinc preparations, or sucralfate causes the oral absorption of the fluoroquinolone to be greatly reduced. In contrast, the presence of a quinolone can reduce the oral absorption of multivalent cations, such as calcium and magnesium, whether dietary or medicinal. Patients should take calcium and magnesium supplements at least an hour before or after taking quinolones. Probenecid can reduce the renal excretion of quinolones, and the use of some quinolones with theophylline may increase the toxicity of the bronchodilator. Nitrofurantoin, discussed later in this chapter, can antagonize the antibacterial activity of the quinolones, and oral anticoagulants should be used with caution in patients receiving quinolones because of the antibiotic-induced alteration of the intestinal flora, which affects vitamin K synthesis.

Dosages

For recommended dosages of selected fluoroquinolones, see the table on this page.

Table 38-4	Quinolones: Reported Adverse Effects
Body System	**Adverse Effects**
Central nervous	Headache, dizziness, fatigue, insomnia, depression, restlessness, convulsions
Gastrointestinal	Nausea, constipation, increased AST and ALT levels, flatulence, heartburn, vomiting, diarrhea, oral candidiasis, dysphagia, pseudomembranous colitis
Integumentary	Rash, pruritus, urticaria, photosensitivity (with lomefloxacin), flushing
Other	Fever, chills, blurred vision, tinnitus

ALT, Alanine aminotransferase; *AST,* aspartate aminotransferase.

Drug Profiles

Quinolones

Two of the most commonly prescribed quinolones include ciprofloxacin and levofloxacin. Dosage information appears in the designated table.

▸ ciprofloxacin

Ciprofloxacin (Cipro) was one of the first of the newer broad-coverage, potent *fluoroquinolones* to become available. It was first marketed in an oral form and as such has the advantage and convenience of an oral medication. Also, because of its excellent bioavailability, it can work as well as many intravenous antibiotics. It is also capable of killing a wide range of gram-negative bacteria and is even effective against traditionally difficult-to-kill gram-negative bacteria such as *Pseudomonas.* Some anaerobic bacteria as well as atypical organisms such as *Chlamydia, Mycoplasma,* and *Mycobacterium* can also be killed by ciprofloxacin. It is also a drug of choice for anthrax infection *(Bacillus anthracis).* It is available in both oral, injectable, ophthalmic (Chapter 58), and otic (Chapter 59) forms.

Pharmacokinetics			
Half-Life	**Onset**	**Peak**	**Duration**
3-4.8 hr	Variable	1-2.3 hr	Up to 12 hr

levofloxacin

Levofloxacin (Levaquin) is one of the newer quinolones. It has a broad spectrum of activity similar to ciprofloxacin, but it has the advantage of once-daily dosing, as does gatifloxacin. Levofloxacin is available in both oral and injectable form.

Pharmacokinetics			
Half-Life	**Onset**	**Peak**	**Duration**
6-8 hrs	Variable	1-2 hr	Up to 24 hr

Miscellaneous Antibiotics

There are a number of antibiotics that do not fit into any of the previously described broad categories. Most have somewhat unique indications or are especially preferred for a particular type of infection. Although they may not be used as commonly compared with drugs from the other major classes, they are still of clinical importance. Several of these drugs are described individually as follows. See the table on page 600 for dosing information.

▸ clindamycin

Clindamycin (Cleocin, Cleocin Pediatric) is a semisynthetic derivative of lincomycin, an older antibiotic. Like many semisynthetic derivatives, it was improved over its predecessor drugs through the addition of certain chemical groups to the basic structure, with the result that it is more effective and causes fewer adverse effects than its parent compound.

Clindamycin can be either bactericidal or *bacteriostatic* (Chapter 37), depending on the concentration of the drug at the site of infection and on the infecting bacteria. It inhibits protein synthesis in

DOSAGES

Selected Fluoroquinolones ("Quinolones")

Drug	Pharmacologic Class	Usual Dosage Range	Indications
▸ciprofloxacin (Cipro)	Fluoroquinolone	**Adult*** IV: 200-400 mg q12h PO: 250-750 mg q8-12h	Broad gram-positive and gram-negative coverage for infections throughout the body
levofloxacin (Levaquin)	Fluoroquinolone	**Adult only** IV/PO: 250-750 mg once daily	Various susceptible bacterial infections

*Not normally recommended for children <18 yr due to adverse musculoskeletal effects shown in studies of immature animals.

DOSAGES

Selected Miscellaneous Antibiotics

Drug (Pregnancy Category)	Pharmacologic Class	Usual Dosage Range	Indications
clindamycin (Cleocin) (B)	Lincosamide	**Adult** IV/PO: 300-900 mg bid-qid **Pediatric** IV/PO: 8-25 mg/kg/day divided tid-qid	Anaerobes; streptococcal and staphylococcal infections of bone, skin, respiratory, and GU tract
dapsone (generic only) (C)	Sulfone	**Adult and pediatric** PO: 50-300 mg once daily	Leprosy (Mycobacterium leprae); dermatitis herpetiformis
linezolid (Zyvox) (C)	Oxazolidinone	**Adults only** IV/PO: 400-600 mg q12h	VRE; skin and respiratory infections caused by various Staphylococcus and Streptococcus spp.
metronidazole (Flagyl) (B)	Nitroimidazole	**Adult*** IV/PO: 250-500 mg q6-12h	Primarily anaerobic and gram-negative infections of abdominal cavity, skin, bone, and respiratory and GU tracts
nitrofurantoin (Macrodantin, Furadantin) (B)	Nitrofuran	**Adult** PO: 50-100 mg qid **Pediatric** PO: 5-7 mg/kg/day divided qid	Primarily UTIs caused by gram-negative organisms and Staphylococcus aureus
quinupristin/dalfopristin (Synercid) (B)	Streptogramins	**Adult and pediatric** IV: 7.5 mg/kg q8-12h	VRE; skin infections caused by streptococcal and staphylococcal infections
vancomycin (Vancocin, Vancoled) (B, oral; C injection)	Tricyclic glycopeptide	**Adult** IV/PO: 500-2000 mg q12-24h **Pediatric** IV/PO: 10 mg/kg q6h	Severe staphylococcal infections, including MRSA; other serious gram-positive infections, including Streptococcus spp.
daptomycin (Cubicin) (B)	Lipopeptide	**Adult only** IV: 4 mg/kg once daily ×7-14d	Complicated skin and soft tissue infections

*Not normally used in children, except for cases of amebiasis.
GU, Genitourinary; *spp.*, species.

bacteria by binding to the 50S ribosomal subunit, the same site as erythromycin (see Figure 37-6). It is indicated for the treatment of chronic bone infections, genitourinary tract infections, intra-abdominal infections, anaerobic pneumonia, septicemia caused by streptococci and staphylococci, and serious skin and soft-tissue infections caused by susceptible bacteria. Most aerobic gram-positive bacteria, including staphylococci, streptococci, and pneumococci, are susceptible to clindamycin's actions. It also has the special advantage of being active against several anaerobic organisms and is most often used for this purpose. However, resistant strains of gram-positive, gram-negative, and anaerobic organisms do occur. Also, all Enterobacteriaecae are resistant to clindamycin.

Clindamycin is contraindicated in patients with a known hypersensitivity to it, those with ulcerative colitis or enteritis, and infants younger than 1 month old. Gastrointestinal tract adverse effects are the most common and include nausea, vomiting, abdominal pain, diarrhea, pseudomembranous colitis, and anorexia. **Pseudomembranous colitis** is a necrotizing inflammatory bowel condition that is often associated with antibiotic therapy, especially clindamycin. Clindamycin is available in oral, injectable, and topical forms (Chapter 57).

With regard to drug interactions, clindamycin has been shown in the laboratory (*in vitro*) to antagonize the antibiotic effects of both erythromycin and aminoglycoside drugs. However, this has not been confirmed *in vivo* (in people or animals). Patients receiving these drug combinations should be appropriately monitored to ascertain their clinical progress. Clindamycin is also known to have some neuromuscular blocking properties that may enhance the actions of neuromuscular drugs used in perioperative and intensive care settings (Chapter 11) such as vecuronium. Patients receiving both drugs should be monitored for excessive neuromuscular blockade and respiratory paralysis, with appropriate ventilatory support as needed.

Pharmacokinetics

Half-Life	Onset	Peak	Duration
2.4 hr	Variable	45 min	6 hr

dapsone

Dapsone (generic only) is an antibiotic of the *sulfone* class, which is structurally different from the sulfonamides described earlier. It has been used clinically for several decades. Dapsone works by competitive antagonism of a compound known as *para-aminobenzoic acid (PABA)*, which is essential to bacterial synthesis of folic acid. Bacteria die off when they cannot synthesize this vitamin compound. Its official indications include leprosy and another skin condition known as *dermatitis herpetiformis*. This is an idiopathic (cause unknown) recurring inflammatory skin condition with lesions that can resemble herpes blisters but that is not caused by a herpes virus. Leprosy is an infectious skin condition also known as *Hansen's disease*. It is characterized by disfiguring nodular skin lesions and is caused by *Mycobacterium leprae*, a bacterium of the same genus that causes tuberculosis *(Mycobacterium tuberculosis)*. Unlabeled (non–U.S. Food and Drug Administration [FDA]-approved) uses include *Pneumocystis jiroveci* pneumonia (associated with HIV/AIDS) and some rheumatic disorders. Dapsone is contraindicated in cases of drug allergy. It is currently available only in tablet form. Adverse effects include stomach pain, loss of appetite, nausea, vomiting, headache, and skin rash. More serious adverse effects include tingling of the hands or feet, dizziness, incoordination, muscle weakness, blurred vision, ringing in the ears, fever, sore throat, weakness, fatigue, jaundice, and rapid heartbeat. This medication can also cause serious anemias. Patients should have ongoing blood counts while taking this medication. With regard to drug interactions, both the antitubercular drug rifampin (Chapter 40) and the anti-HIV drug didanosine (Chapter 39) can chemically reduce the efficacy of dapsone, while the sulfonamide antibiotic trimethoprim (Chapter 37) can enhance its therapeutic effects. Dapsone can also reduce the efficacy of oral contraceptives.

Pharmacokinetics

Half-Life	Onset	Peak	Duration
10-50 hr	Unknown	4-8 hr	>3 wk

linezolid

Linezolid (Zyvox) is the first antibacterial drug in a new class of antibiotics known as oxazolidinones. This drug works by inhibiting bacterial protein synthesis by binding to bacterial ribosomal RNA subunits. Linezolid is used to treat infections associated with vancomycin-resistant *Enterococcus faecium* (VREF), more commonly referred to as VRE. VRE is a notoriously difficult infection to treat and often occurs as a *nosocomial* (acquired while hospitalized) infection. Linezolid has also received approval for treatment of hospital-acquired pneumonia, complicated skin and skin structure infections, including cases caused by MRSA, and gram-positive infections in infants and children. MRSA is another virulent nosocomial infection and stands for methicillin-resistant *S. aureus*. However, methicillin, a penicillinase-resistant penicillin, has recently been removed from the U.S. market, largely because of bacterial resistance to it. Nonetheless, MRSA is still the term used, although oxacillin is now the test drug for this organism. This bacterium is notorious for causing serious infections, especially in the hospital setting. In addition, approval was granted for treatment of community-acquired pneumonia and uncomplicated skin and skin structure infections. The most commonly reported adverse effects attributed to linezolid are headache, nausea, diarrhea, and vomiting. It has also been shown to decrease platelet count. It is contraindicated in patients with a known hypersensitivity to it. It is available in oral and injectable form. In terms of drug interactions, linezolid has the potential to strengthen the vasopressor (pro-hypertensive) effects of various vasopressive drugs (Chapter 17) such as dopamine, by an unclear mechanism. Also, there have been post-marketing case reports of this drug causing *serotonin syndrome* (Chapter 15) when used concurrently with serotonergic drugs such as the serotonin-selective reuptake inhibitors (SSRI) antidepressants (Chapter 15). Finally, tyramine-containing foods such as aged cheese or wine, soy sauce, smoked meats or fish, and sauerkraut, can interact with linezolid to raise blood pressure.

Pharmacokinetics

Half-Life	Onset	Peak	Duration
5 hr	1-2 hr	1-2 hr	12 hr

▶ metronidazole

Metronidazole (Flagyl) is an antimicrobial drug of the class *nitroimidazole*. It has especially good activity against anaerobic organisms and is widely used for intra-abdominal and gynecologic infections that are caused by such organisms. Examples of the *anaerobes* include *Peptostreptococcus* spp., *Eubacterium* spp., *Bacteroides* spp., and *Clostridium* spp. The drug is also indicated for treatment of protozoal infections such as amebiasis and trichomoniasis (Chapter 42). It works by interfering with microbial DNA synthesis, and in this regard is similar to the quinolones (see Figure 37-6). Metronidazole is contraindicated in cases of drug allergy. It is available in both oral and injectable form. It is classified as a pregnancy category B drug, although it is not recommended for use during the first trimester of pregnancy. Adverse effects include dizziness, headache, gastrointestinal discomfort, nasal congestion, and reversible neutropenia and thrombocytopenia. Drug interactions include acute alcohol intolerance when taken with alcoholic beverages, due to accumulation of acetaldehyde, the principal alcohol metabolite. Metronidazole may also increase the toxicity of lithium, benzodiazepines, cyclosporine, calcium channel blockers, various antidepressants (e.g., venlafaxine), and other drugs. In contrast, phenytoin and phenobarbital may reduce the effects of this drug. These interactions occur due to various enzymatic effects among the cytochrome P450 liver enzymes that result in altered metabolism of the various drugs listed above, when taken concurrently.

Pharmacokinetics

Half-Life	Onset	Peak	Duration
8 hr	Unknown	1-2 hr	Unknown

nitrofurantoin

Nitrofurantoin (Macrodantin, Furadantin) is an antibiotic drug of the class *nitrofuran*. It is indicated primarily for urinary tract infections caused by the following bacterial species: *E. coli, S. aureus, Klebsiella* spp., and *Enterobacter* spp. The drug is believed to work by interfering with the activity of enzymes that regulate bacterial carbohydrate metabolism and also by disrupting bacterial cell wall formation. It is contraindicated in cases of drug allergy and also in cases of significant renal function impairment because the drug concentrates in the urine. The drug is available only for oral use. Adverse effects include gastrointestinal discomfort, dizziness, headache, skin reactions (mild to severe reported), blood dyscrasias, ECG changes, possibly irreversible peripheral neuropathy, and hepatotoxicity. However, this drug is very commonly used, even in frail elderly patients, and is usually well tolerated as long as the patient is kept well hydrated, which facilitates urinary elimination of the drug. Drug interactions are few and include probenecid, which can reduce renal excretion of nitrofurantoin, and antacids, which can reduce the extent of its gastrointestinal absorption.

Pharmacokinetics

Half-Life	Onset	Peak	Duration
20-60 min*	Unknown	Unknown	Unknown

*This is the plasma half-life, depending on renal function. The primary site of drug action is in the lumen of the urinary tract, including the bladder.

quinupristin and dalfopristin

Quinupristin and dalfopristin (Synercid) are two streptogramin antibacterials marketed in a 30:70 combination. They are approved for intravenous treatment of bacteremia and life-threatening infection caused by vancomycin-resistant *Enterococcus* (VRE) and for treatment of complicated skin and skin structure infections caused by *S. aureus* and *S. pyogenes*. These two streptogramin antibacterials work synergistically on the bacterial ribosome to disrupt protein synthesis (see Figure 37-6).

Common adverse effects are arthralgias and myalgias, which may become severe. Adverse effects related to the infusion site, including pain, inflammation, edema, and thrombophlebitis, have developed in approximately 75% of patients treated through a peripheral intravenous line. The drug is contraindicated in patients with a known hypersensitivity to it. It is available only in injectable form. Drug interactions are limited, the most serious being potential increase of cyclosporine levels, which can be addressed by laboratory monitoring and dosage adjustment of cyclosporine.

Pharmacokinetics

Half-Life	Onset	Peak	Duration
1-3 hr	1-2 hr	3-4 hr	8-12 hr

▶ vancomycin

Vancomycin (Vancocin, Vancoled) is a natural bactericidal antibiotic structurally unrelated to any other commercially available antibiotics. It destroys bacteria by binding to the bacterial cell wall, producing immediate inhibition of cell wall synthesis and death (see Figure 37-6). This mechanism differs from that of beta-lactam antibiotics.

It is the antibiotic of choice for the treatment of MRSA infection and infections caused by many other gram-positive bacteria. It is not active against gram-negative bacteria, fungi, or yeast. Oral vancomycin is indicated for the treatment of antibiotic-induced pseudomembranous colitis *(Clostridium difficile)* and for the treatment of staphylococcal enterocolitis. Because the oral formulation is poorly absorbed from the gastrointestinal tract, it is used for its local effects on the surface of the gastrointestinal tract. The parenteral form is indicated for the treatment of bone and joint infections and bacterial bloodstream infections caused by *Staphylococcus* spp. Resistance to vancomycin has been noted with increasing frequency in patients with infections caused by *Enterococcus* organisms. These strains have been isolated most often from gastrointestinal tract infections but have also been isolated from skin, soft tissue, and bloodstream infections.

Vancomycin is contraindicated in patients with a known hypersensitivity to it. It should be used with caution in those with preexisting renal dysfunction or hearing loss, as well as in elderly patients and neonates. Vancomycin is similar to the aminoglycosides in that there are very specific drug levels in the blood that are safe. If the levels are too low (less than 5 mcg/mL), the dosage may be subtherapeutic with reduced antibacterial efficacy. If the blood levels are too high (over 50 mg/mL), this may cause toxicities, the two most severe of which are ototoxicity (hearing loss) and nephrotoxicity (kidney damage). Nephrotoxicity is more likely to occur with concurrent therapy with other nephrotoxic drugs such as aminoglycosides and cyclosporine. Vancomycin can also cause additive neuromuscular blocking effects with patients receiving neuromuscular blockers. The patient's respiratory function must therefore be appropriately monitored, and supported as needed. Another common adverse effect that is bothersome but usually not harmful is known as *red man syndrome*. This involves flushing and/or itching of the head, face, neck, and upper trunk area. It can usually be alleviated by slowing the rate of infusion of dose to at least 1 hour. Optimal blood levels of vancomycin should be a peak level of 18 to 50 mcg/mL and a trough level of 5 to 15 mcg/mL. Vancomycin is available in both oral and injectable forms.

Pharmacokinetics

Half-Life	Onset	Peak	Duration
4-6 hr	Variable	1 hr	Up to 12 hr

daptomycin

Daptomycin (Cubicin) is currently the only drug of the new class known as *lipopeptides*. It is a fermentation product of *Streptomyces roseosporus* bacteria. Its mechanism of action is not completely known but it binds to gram-positive cells in a calcium-dependent process and disrupts cell membrane potential. It is used to treat complicated skin and soft tissue infections caused by susceptible gram-positive bacteria. This drug is contraindicated in cases of drug allergy. It is only available in injectable form. Adverse reactions include hypo- or hypertension (low incidence for both), headache, dizziness, rash, gastrointestinal discomfort, elevated liver enzymes, local injection site reaction, renal failure, dyspnea, and fungal infection. The precise mechanisms for these reactions are uncertain, but all occur in a relatively small percentage of patients (<5%). Major drug interactions have yet to be identified.

Pharmacokinetics

Half-Life	Onset	Peak	Duration
IV: 8-9 hr	IV: Unknown	IV: 30 min	IV: Unknown

◆ NURSING PROCESS

◆ ASSESSMENT

Many of the antibiotics discussed in this chapter are the types of drugs that are often reserved for more potent infections and are mainly administered by parenteral routes (as compared to those drugs discussed in Chapter 37), thus demanding more astute and thorough assessment of the patient and about the specific drug. The groups of antibiotics in this chapter require a critical assess-

ment for any history of or current symptoms that are indicative of hypersensitivity or allergic reactions (mild reactions with rash, pruritus, hives to severe with laryngeal edema, bronchospasms, hypotension, and possible cardiac arrest). Further assessment should include a nursing physical assessment, age, weight, baseline vital signs, and body temperature. Diagnostic and laboratory studies that may be ordered include some of the following: (1) For assessing liver function: AST (aspartate aminotransferase), ALT (alanine aminotransferase), (2) for renal function: urinalysis, BUN, and serum creatinine, (3) for cardiac function: ECG, echocardiogram, ultrasound and/or cardiac enzymes, (4) for sensitivity of antibiotic to the bacteria: culture and sensitivity tests of the infected tissue/site/blood, (5) for baseline blood counts: white blood count (WBC), hemoglobin (Hgb), hematocrit (Hct), red blood cells (RBC), and platelet/clotting values. A baseline neurologic assessment should include baseline sensory and motor intactness and/or assessment of any alterations in neurologic functioning—for example, altered sensorium and level of consciousness due to potential central nervous system adverse effects. Baseline abdominal/gastrointestinal assessments are important with focus on bowel patterns and bowel sounds due to possible gastrointestinal adverse effects. Contraindications, cautions, and drug interactions should also be noted, including a complete list of the patient's medications—including over-the-counter drugs (OTCs), herbals, and dietary supplements. A cultural assessment is important because of the various responses of certain racial-ethnic groups to specific drugs as well as the potential use for alternative healing practices.

With any antibiotic, it is important for the nurse to assess for *superinfection* or a secondary infection that occurs with the destruction of "normal" flora during antibiotic therapy (Chapter 37). Fungal infections (e.g., superinfections) are evidenced by fever, lethargy, perineal itching, and other anatomically-related symptoms. The status of the patient's immune system and overall condition is important to assess because if there is a deficiency (e.g., patients with cancer, autoimmune disorders such as lupus, acquired immunodeficiency syndromes, and any chronic illness) the patient's ability to physically resist infection may be diminished. Antibiotic resistance is a continual concern with antibiotic drug therapy especially with pediatrics and in large health care institutions and long-term care facilities. This resistance to certain antibiotics should be considered when assessing patients for symptoms of infection and superinfection. Once a thorough assessment has occurred with follow-up to therapy considered, the nurse should share information about antibiotic-resistance prevention (see implementation).

With *aminoglycosides,* assessment of hypersensitivity, preexisting conditions/diseases, and other medications the patient is taking is needed because of the many cautions, contraindications, and drug interactions. The aminoglycosides are known for their ototoxicity and nephrotoxicity; therefore, baseline hearing tests with audiometry and vestibular function as well as renal function studies (BUN, urinalysis, serum and urine creatinine levels) should be performed with documentation of all results. If renal baseline functioning is decreased or abnormal, dosage amounts may need to be adjusted by the physician because of the nephrotoxicity. A thorough neuromuscular assessment should be performed because of drug-related neurotoxicity and higher risk for complications in those with impaired neurologic functioning—for example, patients with myasthenia gravis and Parkinson's disease may experience worsening of muscle weakness because of the drug's neuromuscular blockade. Neonates (because of immature nervous and renal systems) and the elderly (because of decreased neurologic and renal functioning) are at highest risk for nephrotoxicity, neurotoxicity, and ototoxicity and require careful assessment before and during drug therapy. Hydration status should also be assessed.

Fluoroquinolones, such as ciprofloxacin, require careful assessment for drug allergies. Pre-existing central nervous system disorders (e.g., seizures or history of strokes) may be exacerbated with the concurrent use of these drugs, and, therefore, a careful history is needed before administering this group of drugs. Assessment of bowel activity is necessary as well as assessment of neuromuscular functioning due to the potential for dizziness, headache, and visual changes. It is also necessary to assess the timing of medication dosing and other drugs being administered at the same time because of the interaction with antacids (see previous drug interactions) and a preferred dosing time of 2 hours after meals. It is also important to remember the many drug interactions with these antibiotics including iron, multivitamin products, and zinc. These drugs may be used but should not be given within 2 hours of the fluoroquinolones because the drug absorption is decreased. Blood glucose levels and renal/liver function tests should also be assessed and documented.

Hypersensitivity to either *clindamycin* or related compounds should be assessed and documented as well as any allergy to aspirin. Although drug interactions have been discussed previously, it is important to emphasize that these drugs should never be given at the same time as neuromuscular blocking drugs. In addition, because of the risk for antibiotic-associated colitis, blood dyscrasias, and nephrotoxicity, it is critical to patient safety to assess gastrointestinal patterns, presence of abdominal pain, frequency/consistency of stools, white blood cell counts, platelets, BUN, and serum creatinine levels.

With *vancomycin,* the patient assessment should include questioning about other medications the patient is taking, especially if the drugs are nephrotoxic and ototoxic. Vital signs should be assessed with close attention to blood pressure during infusion of the drug. Assess bowel patterns and sounds because of the risk for gastrointestinal/abdominal adverse effects. Baseline hearing status should be assessed due to risk for ototoxicity, as should urinary patterns due to risk for nephrotoxicity. Assess the color of the patient's skin because of the risk for red man syndrome. Due to multiple incompatibilities, as with several of the previously mentioned parenteral antibiotics in this chapter, always stop and assess for potential fluid/medication interactions.

With *dapsone,* the indication for its use is important in assessment because if it is used for malaria, it may be taken for 3 to 5 years versus shorter-term use with other indications (e.g., *Pneumocystis carinii* pneumonia [PCP] or what is now often referred to as *Pneumocystis jiroveci* pneumonia), thus changing the entire perspective on the focus of an assessment. Assessment of gastrointestinal status and bowel patterns is important

with notice of bowel sounds, gastrointestinal upset, nausea, and vomiting, because of the drug's adverse effects. Baseline neurologic assessment with concentration on sensory/motor functioning and any preexisting neurologic abnormalities—such as numbness, tingling, dizziness, muscle weakness, blurred vision, tinnitus (ringing in the ears)—is needed because of central nervous system–related adverse effects. Seizures may be indicative of dapsone overdose, and so it is important to assess for any past/present seizure activity. In addition, vital signs with close attention to the patient's temperature and pain status are important to establish baseline parameters against which other vital signs may be compared during therapy. This may call attention to any unusual adverse effects, including fever or sore throat. Because of the drug's potential for causing tachycardia and other cardiac adverse effects and the potential for serious anemias, assessment of pulse rate, blood pressure, and auscultation of heart sounds is important. Monitoring of complete blood counts with focus on RBCs, WBCs, Hgb, and Hct is also appropriate. Skin color should be noted because a bluish discoloration of the skin may indicate toxicity or overdosage with these drugs.

Linezolid is used for diabetic foot infections, community-acquired infections, vancomycin-resistant enterococcus faecium (VRE), nosocomial pneumonias, and other severe infections. An astute and careful assessment of the patient's underlying immune status, renal, liver, gastrointestinal, and hematologic functioning is critical to patient safety and to early identification of adverse/toxic effects. A systems-related nursing assessment would include a history of infections and response to infections and overall immune status, intake/output, bladder functioning, jaundice, liver enlargement (noted on abdominal palpation/percussion), bowel sounds, bowel patterns, and any complaints of gastrointestinal-related symptoms (e.g., nausea, vomiting, diarrhea, abdominal pain). The related laboratory or diagnostic testing would possibly include the following: (1) For immune and hematologic status: immunoglobulin levels, WBCs, RBCs, platelets, Hgb, and Hct, and (2) for renal and liver status: BUN, creatinine, urinalysis, alanine aminotransferase (ALT), aspartate aminotransferase (AST), alkaline phosphatase (AP), and gamma-glutamyltransferase (GGT). These are all very important to safe use and to the prevention of possible adverse and toxic effects and important to the patient's overall well-being. Should the patient be immune-compromised and present with renal/liver dysfunction, adverse effects may be exacerbated, leading to the potential for complications and/or toxicity.

Patients taking *metronidazole* need to be assessed for allergy to the drug and to other nitroimidazole derivatives. Culture and sensitivity reports should be known prior to starting this therapy, and there should be a baseline assessment of neurologic (assess for dizziness, numbness, tingling, and other sensory/motor abnormalities), gastrointestinal (bowel sounds, bowel problems/patterns), and genitourinary (urinary patterns, color of urine and I&O) systems. Pregnancy status, even with topical applications, is important to assess and document because these would be contraindications. In addition, assessment of concurrent intake of alcohol should be completed and subsequent information given in relation to the interaction with the drug. A disulfiram-like (Antabuse) reaction may occur, leading to flushing of the face, tachycardia, palpitations, nausea, and vomiting.

Assessment of allergies and a history of asthma (which puts a patient at risk for drug allergy) are important with *nitrofurantoin*. Renal and liver function should be assessed. Patients with a history of G6PD deficiency are of concern due to a greater risk for hemolytic anemia. Patients who are debilitated are at greater risk for peripheral neuropathies. Other medications that are neurotoxic should be avoided because of an additional risk for neurologic adverse effects (e.g., irreversible peripheral neuropathy). Make note of the patient's skin, its color, turgor, and intactness because of drug-related risk Stevens-Johnson syndrome. Assessment should also include describing respiratory patterns and breath sounds and notation of cough if present. With *quinupristin-dalfopristin*, vital signs should be assessed along with baseline liver/renal function tests and CBC. An assessment of gastrointestinal functioning is also important, with a focus on bowel patterns, bowel sounds, and abdominal pain due to drug-related antibiotic-associated colitis.

♦ NURSING DIAGNOSES

- Risk for infection related to the patient's compromised immune system status before and during treatment
- Risk for injury to self (compromised organ function) related to adverse effects of medications (e.g., ototoxicity and nephrotoxicity) and from a weakened physical state
- Pain related to infection and/or adverse reaction to medications
- Deficient knowledge related to lack of information and experience with the medication regimen
- Ineffective therapeutic regimen management related to lack of information about the proper use of antibiotics and the lack of patient's experience with the therapy

♦ PLANNING

Goals

- Patient is free of the signs and symptoms of infection once therapy is completed.
- Patient experiences minimal adverse effects of antibiotic therapy.
- Patient remains compliant with therapy.
- Patient returns for follow-up visits as recommended.
- Patient completes medical regimen of entire course of antibiotics as ordered.

Outcome Criteria

- Patient experiences increased sense of well-being related to resolving infection.
- Patient states the signs and symptoms of an infection (e.g., fever, pain, malaise) and reports them if they occur while on antibiotics.
- Patient is able to identify the adverse effects of antibiotic therapy such as gastrointestinal upset, nausea, and diarrhea (specific to each class).
- Patient experiences increased periods of comfort and improved energy levels related to a resolving infectious process and minimal adverse effects of therapy.
- Patient states the reasons for compliance with therapy (i.e., to adequately eradicate bacteria).
- Patient states the measures to take to minimize the gastrointestinal distress associated with antibiotic therapy, such as taking with yogurt or other foods, as appropriate.
- Patient keeps follow-up appointments with the physician or other health care provider to be evaluated for therapeutic effects or complications of therapy.

♦ IMPLEMENTATION

Aminoglycosides should be given exactly as ordered and with adequate hydration. Fluids should be encouraged up to 3000 mL/day unless contraindicated, especially with oral dosage forms. Parenteral dosage forms are most common. Neomycin is the only oral dosage form available. With regard to the potential of nephrotoxicity, I&O should be calculated with constant monitoring of urine specific gravity. Consumption of yogurt or buttermilk may help prevent antibiotic-induced superinfections (Chapter 37). Encourage the patient to report to the health care provider any changes in hearing, ringing in the ears (tinnitus), or a full feeling in the ears. Nausea, vomiting with motion, ataxia, nystagmus, or dizziness should also be reported immediately. Redness, burning, and itching of eyes may indicate an adverse reaction to ophthalmic forms, and redness over the skin area may indicate an adverse reaction to topical forms. Intramuscular sites should be checked for induration. If noted, it should be reported immediately to the physician, and the site should not be re-used. Intravenous sites should be checked for heat, swelling, redness, pain, or red streaking over the vein (phlebitis) as per protocol/policy.

Gentamicin sulfate comes in intrathecal, ophthalmic, topical, and parenteral dosage forms. Special considerations for each of these routes include: (1) Intramuscular: give deeply and slowly to minimize discomfort, (2) intravenous: check for other drug incompatibilites and only give clear or only slightly yellow solutions that have been diluted with either NaCl or D_5W, infusing as prescribed, (3) intrathecal: this dosage form should be "preservative" free and, as a point of information, mixed with 10% estimated cerebral spinal fluid (CSF) or NaCl and given over a period of 3 to 5 minutes, (4) ophthalmic: refer to Chapter 9 for specific instructions on administering eye drops and ointments. Additionally, it is important to assess serum levels; peak levels range from 4 to 10 mcg/mL, trough levels are at 1 to 2 mcg/mL, and *toxic* peak levels are over 10 mcg/mL. Toxic trough levels are values over 2 mcg/mL.

Neomycin, another aminoglycoside, is the only one that is given orally and also available topically as an OTC drug. Oral neomycin is generally used in special situations such as preoperative bowel preparation, diarrhea from *E. coli* and hepatic encephalopathy and should be given exactly as ordered. Another important nursing consideration for neomycin—as well as other aminoglycosides—is to constantly monitor respiratory status if these drugs are used in a patient with neuromuscular disease. Nursing considerations associated with the use of tobramycin sulfate are similar to those discussed with parenteral, ophthalmic, and topical dosage forms of gentamicin.

Fluoroquinolones should be taken exactly as prescribed and for the full course of treatment. The patient should not take antacids at the same time as oral fluoroquinolones in order to prevent inactivation of the antibiotic. It is recommended that the oral fluoroquinolone be given 2 hours before antacids or ferrous sulfate to avoid alteration in the antibiotic's absorption. Alkaline foods/fluids, such as dairy products, peanuts, and sodium bicarbonate, may lead to higher incidence of crystalluria from a more alkaline urinary pH and should be avoided. It is recommended, however, to force fluids and increase the intake of fluids/foods high in ascorbic acid (e.g., cranberry juice and citrus fruits) to prevent crystalluria. See the Patient Teaching Tips for more information.

Clindamycin should be administered as ordered whether by oral, topical, intravaginal, intravenous, or intramuscular route. Oral forms should be taken with 8 ounces of water/fluids and dosed evenly over 24 hours, as with other dosage forms. After reconstituting oral solutions, and they should *never* be refrigerated because of thickening of the solution. With topical forms, it is important to avoid simultaneous use of peeling/abrasive acne products, soaps, or alcohol-containing cosmetics so that there are no cumulative effects. Topical forms should be applied in a "thin" layer to the affected area. Intravaginal doses are usually given by applicator—for example, one full applicator at bedtime for 3 to 7 days, or one suppository at bedtime or 3 days. Bedtime use is recommended for comfort reasons, and perineal pads may be worn to catch any leakage of the medicine from the vagina. IV dosage forms should be infused by piggyback technique and as ordered. Most references state to *never* give IV push. Doses of the drug should be diluted and infused per manufacturer guidelines and as ordered. Too rapid IV infusion could lead to severe hypotension and possible cardiac arrest. IM dosage forms should be given deep IM.

Vancomycin may be used orally but is poorly absorbed; thus the reason for seeing more use of parenteral dosage forms. A powder-reconstituted dose form may be used via an NG tube, and oral solutions are only stable for 2 weeks if refrigerated. Note that powder forms for oral dosage forms are not to be used with IV administration. IV dosages should be reconstituted as recommended (e.g., with either D5W or 0.9% NaCl) and should be infused over at least 60 minutes. Too rapid of infusion or IV push vancomycin may lead to severe hypotension and serious complications. Extravasation may cause local skin irritation and damage and so frequent monitoring of the infusion and, more specifically the IV site, is needed. As noted previously, too rapid of administration by IV route may lead to red man syndrome with a subsequent decrease in blood pressure and flushing of neck, face, and upper body. Constant reminders of drug-related neurotoxicity, nephrotoxicity, ototoxity, and superinfection remain critical to patient safety. In addition, adequate hydration (at least 2 liters of fluids/24 hr unless contraindicated) is most important to prevent nephrotoxicity. With monitoring of serum drug levels, therapeutic or optimal "peak" levels range from 18 to 50 mcg/mL with a trough at 5 to 15 mcg/mL. Toxic peak levels are those above 50 mcg/mL and toxic trough levels greater than 15 mcg/mL.

Dapsone should be taken with food or milk to help with gastrointestinal upset. Alternative methods of contraception should be used if the patient is taking oral contraceptives due to a lack of effectiveness when taken with dapsone. *Linezolid* is generally given orally or IV. Oral dosages should be evenly spaced and given with food or milk to decrease possible gastrointestinal upset. Oral suspension forms should be given within 21 days of reconstitution. IV dosages should be protected from light and infused over 30 to 120 minutes and should not be mixed with any other medication. Because of risk for antibiotic-associated colitis, superinfections, and myelosupression, it is important to be constantly alerted to the occurrence of frequent, loose, and foul-smelling stools, severe genital/anal pruritus, and/or severe mouth soreness. In addition, complete blood counts should be watched closely (e.g., weekly) during therapy.

Oral forms of *metronidazole hydrochloride* should be given with food or meals to help decrease gastrointestinal upset. Intravaginal doses are recommended to be given at bedtime, and topical creams, ointments, or lotions are to be applied thinly to the affected area. Use an applicator for intravaginal dosages. Generally speaking, gloves are worn to protect from undue exposure to medication, and the nurse should always wear gloves as a means of standard precautions. Topical forms should not be applied close to the eyes to avoid irritation. IV dosage forms should be stored at room temperature and are supplied in a "ready-to-use" infusion bag.

Nitrofurantoin is available in oral forms and should be given with plenty of fluids, food, or milk to decrease gastrointestinal upset. Because of the risk for superinfection, hepatotoxicity, and peripheral neuropathy (which may be irreversible), it is necessary to document findings from the constant monitoring of their respective signs and symptoms. Superinfection has been previously discussed; however, it is important to be aware that jaundice, itching, rash, and liver enlargement may indicate toxic effects to the liver whereas numbness and tingling may occur with peripheral neuropathy. In addition, constant monitoring of breath sounds, breathing patterns, and any cough is important due to the risk for permanent lung function impairment.

For *quinupristin and dalfopristin,* IV dosage forms should be reconstituted as recommended by the drug manufacturer and are only stable for 1 hour at room temperature. A diluted infusion bag is stable for up to 6 hours and 54 hours, if refrigerated. These characteristics are important to know to help prevent untoward complications. When reconstituting the drug, use only the recommended diluents, and use a gentle swirling action to mix the drug instead of shaking it (to help minimize foaming). Infusions are generally over at least 60 minutes. Also note that 0.9% NaCl is an incompatible solution! As with other antibiotics, the same measures should be implemented with superinfection, hepatotoxicity, and antibiotic-associated colitis. It is very important to report any of the following to the physician should they occur: diarrhea with fever, abdominal pain, and mucus/blood in the stools. If these symptoms occur, make sure to monitor the patient and withhold the drug until further orders are received from the physician.

◆ EVALUATION

Evaluation of goals, outcome criteria, therapeutic effects, and adverse effects should be ongoing at the onset, during, and after antibiotic therapy. Patients should report a decrease in symptoms (e.g., infection) as well as no injury to self and a decrease in pain. Therapeutic goals would include all those previously mentioned as well as a return to normal of all complete blood counts and vital signs, negative reports of culture and sensitivity, as well as improved appetite, energy level, and sense of well-being. Signs and symptoms of the infection should be resolved and knowledge levels sufficient to enhance the success of treatment. Another aspect of evaluation includes monitoring for adverse effects of therapy such as superinfections, antibiotic associated colitis, nephrotoxicity/ototoxicity/neurotoxicity/hepatotoxicity, and other drug-specific adverse effects.

Patient Teaching Tips

Aminoglycosides

- Educate the patient about the drug, its purpose, and adverse effects, and that hearing loss may occur even after therapy has been completed. Patients need to be aware that any change in hearing must be reported immediately to the health care provider.
- Forcing fluids up to 3000 mL/day, unless contraindicated, is important with any medication, and especially with antibiotics.
- Inform patients to report any of the following to their physician: tinnitus, high-frequency hearing loss, persistent headache, nausea, and vertigo. Also educate about the signs and symptoms of superinfection—as with any antibiotic—such as diarrhea; vaginal discharge; stomatitis; glottitis; black, hairy tongue; loose and foul-smelling stools; and cough.

Fluoroquinolones

- Educate patients about avoiding exposure to sun and tanning beds. Use of sunglasses and sunscreen protection is recommended.
- Educate patients about signs and symptoms that need to be reported, including dizziness, restlessness, stomach distress, diarrhea, unusual emotional behavior, confusion and/or an irregular or rapid heart beat.
- Drug interactions occur between these antibiotics and oral anticoagulants (e.g., warfarin [Coumadin]), and patients should be educated about the need for frequent coagulation studies (INR) so that clotting ability is monitored and appropriate action can be taken as needed.

Clindamycin

- Encourage the patient not to use topical forms near the eyes or near any abraded areas to avoid irritation.
- With use of vaginal dosages, it is important to inform the patient not to engage in sexual intercourse for the duration of the therapy, and the entire course of treatment must be used as ordered for maximal therapeutic effects.
- Educate the patient that in the event of accidental contact of creams into the eyes, the eyes need to be rinsed immediately with cool tap water in copious amounts.

Vancomycin

- Patients should report any changes in hearing such as ringing in the ears, feeling of fullness in the ears as well as reporting any nausea, vomiting with motion, unsteady gait, or dizziness. Other adverse effects that should be reported immediately include a generalized "tingling" (usually after IV dosing), chills, fever, rash, and/or hives.
- Therapeutic serum levels will be monitored throughout therapy and are key to prevention of toxicity. Patients should be informed

that follow-up appointments are important for monitoring serum drug levels and possible toxicity.

Dapsone

- The physician should be contacted if the patient experiences any tingling of hands or feet, dizziness, lack of coordination, muscle weakness, blurred vision, ringing of the ears (tinnitus), fever, fatigue, jaundice, or rapid heartbeat.
- Educate the patient about if a dose is missed and remembered within a short time frame: the patient may take the dose, however, remind them NOT to take the dose if it is time for the next dose. They should not double-up on the dose to "catch" up.
- If overdose is suspected (e.g., nausea, vomiting, seizures, and a bluish discoloration to the skin) the patient should be encouraged to contact a local poison control center/emergency room immediately or if within the United States, contact the national poison hotline at 1-800-222-1222. This phone number is also important for any drug overdose.
- Backup contraception is indicated.

Linezolid

- Therapy must be taken for the full length of treatment (as with all antibiotics), and education about avoiding tyramine-containing foods (e.g., red wine, aged cheeses) should be emphasized.
- The patient should immediately report the following to their physician: severe abdominal pain, fever, severe diarrhea, and/or worsening of signs and symptoms of infection.

Metronidazole Hydrochloride

- Warn the patient about the red-brown or darker color urine that may occur with this drug and to avoid any alcohol/alcohol-containing products (e.g., cough preparations and elixirs) due to the risk for an antabuse-like reaction (e.g., severe vomiting).
- Encourage the patient to understand the purpose of the drug such as use as either an antibacterial drug or used as an antifungal drug because knowing about medications is crucial to its therapeutic effect and prevention of adverse effects.

Nitrofurantoin

- Educate patients about the fact that their urine may become dark yellow or brown with drug therapy. They should also be educated about the avoidance of exposure to the sun/ultraviolet light because of photosensitivity; and, wear protective clothing and sunscreen if being exposed to the sun.
- Encourage the patient to notify the physician/health care provider if cough, fever, chest pain, difficulty breathing, numbness/tingling of extremities and alopecia are experienced.

Points to Remember

- There are a variety of classes of antibiotics with mechanisms of actions and spectrums of activity that are also varied.
- Over the years, bacteria have developed enzymes and mechanisms to interact with antibiotics and render the antibiotic ineffective. A significant condition is methicillin-resistant *Staphylococcus aureus* (MRSA).
- The aminoglycosides are a group of natural and semisynthetic antibiotics that are classified as *bactericidal* drugs, are very potent, and are capable of potentially serious toxicities (e.g., nephrotoxicity, ototoxicity).
- Fluoroquinolones are very potent, bactericidal, broad-spectrum antibiotics and include norfloxacin, ciprofloxacin, levofloxacin, moxifloxacin, gatifloxacin, and gemifloxacin.
- Clindamycin is a semisynthetic derivative of lincomycin, an older antibiotic.
- Dapsone is an antibiotic of the *sulfone* class and structurally different from the sulfonamides.
- Linezolid (Zyvox) is an antibacterial drug used to treat infections associated with vancomycin-resistant *Enterococcus faecium* (VREF), more commonly referred to as VRE. VRE is a difficult infection to treat and often occurs as a *nosocomial* (acquired while hospitalized) infection.
- Metronidazole (Flagyl) is an antimicrobial drug of the class *nitroimidazole*, has good activity against anaerobic organisms, and is widely used for intraabdominal and gynecologic infections; it is also used to treat protozoal infections (e.g., amebiasis, trichomoniasis).
- Nitrofurantoin (Macrodantin, Furadantin) is an antibiotic drug of the class *nitrofuran*. It is indicated primarily for urinary tract infections caused by the following bacterial species: *E. coli, S. aureus, Klebsiella* spp., and *Enterobacter* spp.
- Quinupristin and dalfopristin (Synercid) are two streptogramin antibacterials approved for intravenous treatment of bacteremia and life-threatening infection caused by VRE and for treatment of complicated skin and skin structure infections caused by *S. aureus* and *S. pyogenes*.
- Daptomycin (Cubicin) is used to treat complicated skin and soft tissue infections.
- Antibiotics require a critical assessment for any history of or current symptoms that are indicative of hypersensitivity or allergic reactions (mild reactions with rash, pruritus, and hives, to severe reactions with laryngeal edema, bronchospasms, hypotension, and possible cardiac arrest). Further assessment includes a nursing physical assessment, age, weight, and baseline vital signs, especially body temperature and various laboratory studies (e.g., culture and sensitivity, renal/liver function tests, and CBC).
- With any antibiotic, it is important for the nurse to assess for *superinfection*, or a secondary infection that occurs with the destruction of "normal" flora during antibiotic therapy. Superinfections may occur in the mouth, respiratory tract, gastrointestinal and genitourinary tracts, and the skin. Fungal infections are evidenced by fever, lethargy, perineal itching, and other anatomically-related symptoms.

NCLEX Examination Review Questions

1. While assessing a woman who is receiving an antibiotic for community acquired pneumonia, the nurse notes that the patient has a thick, white vaginal discharge. The patient is also complaining about perineal itching. The nurse suspects that the patient has:
   a. Resistance to the antibiotic.
   b. An adverse effect of the antibiotic.
   c. A superinfection.
   d. An allergic reaction.
2. The nurse is preparing to administer the first dose of an aminoglycoside to a patient. In addition to assessing for allergies, which laboratory results would be of greatest concern at this time?
   a. Decreased serum creatinine level.
   b. Increased serum creatinine level.
   c. Decreased red blood cell count.
   d. Increased white blood cell count.
3. While administering vancomycin, the nurse knows that the most important assessment before giving a dose is:
   a. Renal function.
   b. White blood cell count.
   c. Liver function.
   d. Platelet count.
4. During therapy with an intravenous aminoglycoside, the patient calls the nurse and says, "I am hearing some odd sounds, like ringing, in my ears." Which is the best action of the nurse at this time?
   a. Reassure the patient that these are expected adverse effects.
   b. Reduce the rate of the intravenous infusion.
   c. Increase the rate of the intravenous infusion.
   d. Stop the infusion immediately and notify the physician.
5. When giving intravenous quinolones, the nurse needs to keep in mind that these drugs may have serious interactions with which drugs?
   a. Diuretics
   b. NSAIDs
   c. Oral anticoagulants
   d. Antihypertensives

1. c, 2. b, 3. a, 4. d, 5. c.

Critical Thinking Activities

1. During an infusion of vancomycin, a patient complains of flushing of the face and neck, and itching over those same areas. Is this an allergic reaction or is there another reason for this? Explain.
2. During therapy with the aminoglycoside tobramycin, you note that the latest trough drug level was 3 mcg/mL. This drug is given daily, and the next dose is due in 1 hour. Based on this trough drug level, should you give the drug? Explain your actions.
3. Discuss what measures are used to monitor for nephrotoxicity and ototoxicity.

For answers, see http://evolve.elsevier.com/Lilley.

Antiviral Drugs

CHAPTER 39

Objectives

When you reach the end of this chapter, you should be able to do the following:

1. Discuss the effects of the immune system with attention to the various types of immunity.
2. Describe the effects of viruses in the human body.
3. Discuss the process of immunosuppression in patients with viral infections, specifically those with HIV.
4. Discuss the stages of AIDS and various drugs used to manage/treat the illness.
5. Discuss the mechanism of action, indications, contraindications, cautions, routes, adverse effects, and toxic effects associated with the various antiviral and antiretroviral drugs.
6. Develop a nursing care plan that includes all phases of the nursing process for patients receiving antiviral and antiretroviral drugs.

e-Learning Activities

Companion CD
- NCLEX Review Questions: see questions 345-351
- Animations
- Audio Glossary
- Category Catchers
- Medication Errors Checklists
- IV Therapy Checklists

evolve Website (http://evolve.elsevier.com/Lilley)
- Nursing Care Plans • Frequently Asked Questions • Content Updates • WebLinks • Supplemental Resources • Elsevier ePharmacology Update • Medication Administration Animations

Drug Profiles

▶ acyclovir, p. 617
  amandatine and rimantadine, p. 617
  enfuvirtide, p. 625
▶ ganciclovir, p. 617
▶ indinavir, p. 625

▶ nevirapine, p. 625
  oseltamivir and zanamivir, p. 619
  ribavirin, p. 619
  tenofovir, p. 625
▶ zidovudine, p. 625

▶ Key drug.

Glossary

Acquired immune deficiency syndrome (AIDS) Infection caused by the *human immunodeficiency virus (HIV)* that weakens the host's immune system, giving rise to *opportunistic infections* by pathogens that normally co-exist in the body with minimal health affects. (p. 619)

Antibody Immunoglobulin molecules that have an antigen-specific amino acid sequence and are synthesized by the humoral immune system (antibodies produced from B-lymphocytes) in response to exposure to a specific antigen, the purpose of which is to attack and destroy molecules of this antigen. (p. 611)

Antigen A substance, usually a protein, that is foreign to a host (e.g., human) and causes the formation of an antibody and reacts specifically with that antibody. Examples of antigens include bacterial exotoxins, viruses, and allergens. An *allergen* (e.g., dust, pollen, mold) is a specific type of antigen that causes allergic reactions (Chapter 36). (p. 611)

Antiretroviral drug A more specific term for antiviral drugs that work against retroviruses such HIV (see *retrovirus*). (p. 612)

Antiviral drug A general term for any drug that destroys viruses, either directly or indirectly by suppressing their replication. (p. 611)

Cell-mediated immunity (CMI) One of two major parts of the immune system. It consists of *nonspecific* immune responses mediated primarily by T lymphocytes (T cells) and other immune system cells (e.g., monocytes, macrophages, neutrophils), but not antibody-producing cells (B-lymphocytes). (p. 611)

Deoxyribonucleic acid (DNA) A *nucleic acid* composed of *nucleotide* units that contain molecules of the sugar deoxyribose, phosphate groups, and purine and pyrimidine bases. DNA molecules transmit genetic information and are found primarily in the nuclei of cells. (Compare with *RNA*.) (p. 610)

Fusion The process by which viruses attach themselves, or *fuse* with the cell membranes of host cells, in preparation for infecting the cell for purposes of viral replication (see *replication*). (p. 610)

Genome The complete set of genetic material of any organism; may be multiple chromosomes (groups of DNA or RNA molecules) in higher organisms; a single chromosome as in bacteria, or a one- or two- DNA or RNA molecule, as in viruses. (p. 610)

Herpesvirus Any of several different types of viruses of the family *Herpesviridae* that causes any form of herpes infection. (p. 611)

Host Any organism (human, animal, or plant) that is infected with a microorganism, such as bacteria or viruses. (p. 610)

Human immunodeficiency virus (HIV)   The *retrovirus* that causes AIDS. (p. 610)

Humoral immunity   The second of two major parts of the immune system. It consists of *specific* immune responses in the form of antigen-specific antibodies produced from B lymphocytes. (p. 611)

Immunoglobulin   (Synonymous with immune globulin.) A glycoprotein (sugar protein) synthesized and used by the humoral immune system to attack and kill any substance (antigen) that is foreign to the body. An immunoglobulin with an antigen-specific amino acid sequence is called an antibody and is able to recognize and inactivate molecules of a specific antigen (see *antibody* and *antigen*). (p. 612)

Influenza virus   The virus that causes influenza, an acute viral infection of the respiratory tract. There are three types of influenza virus: A, B, and C. Currently, there are medications to treat only types A and B. (p. 612)

Nucleic acids   A general term referring to DNA and RNA. These complex biomolecules contain the genetic material of all living organisms, which is passed to future generations during reproduction. (p. 610)

Nucleoside   A structural component of nucleic acid molecules (DNA or RNA) that consists of a purine or pyrimidine base attached to a sugar molecule. (p. 612)

Nucleotide   A nucleoside that is attached to a phosphate unit, which makes up the side chain "backbone" of a DNA or an RNA molecule. (p. 612)

Opportunistic infections   Infections caused by any type of micro-organism and occurring in an *immunocompromised* host that normally would not occur in an *immunocompetent* host. (p. 612)

Protease   An enzyme that breaks down the amino acid structure of protein molecules by chemically cleaving the peptide bonds that link together the individual amino acids. (p. 619)

Replication   Any process of duplication or reproduction, such as that involved in the duplication of nucleic acid molecules (DNA or RNA) during the reproduction processes of all living organisms. This is also the term used most often to describe the entire process of viral reproduction, which only occurs inside the cells of an infected host organism. (p. 610)

Retrovirus   Any virus belonging to the family Retroviridae. These viruses contain RNA (as opposed to DNA) as their *genome* and replicate using the enzyme *reverse transcriptase*. The most clinically significant retrovirus is currently HIV. (p. 611)

Reverse transcriptase   An RNA-directed DNA-polymerase enzyme. Such an enzyme promotes the synthesis of a DNA molecule from an RNA molecule, which is the "reverse" of the usual process. HIV replicates in this manner. (p. 619)

Ribonucleic acid (RNA)   A nucleic acid composed of nucleotide units (see *nucleotide*) that contain molecules of the sugar ribose, phosphate groups, and purine and pyrimidine bases. RNA molecules transmit genetic information and are found in both the nuclei and cytoplasm of cells. (Compare with *DNA*.) (p. 610)

Virion   A mature virus particle. (p. 610)

Virus   The smallest known class of microorganisms; can only replicate inside host cells. (p. 610)

GENERAL PRINCIPLES OF VIROLOGY

Viruses are very small microorganisms, usually many times smaller than bacteria. For this reason, they are usually seen only with the strongest microscopes, such as an electron microscope. Unlike bacteria, viruses can only reproduce, or replicate, inside the cells of their **host,** which can be human, animal, plant, or even other types of microorganisms (e.g., bacteria, protozoans). In this respect, all viruses are obligate intracellular parasites. It must be emphasized that viruses are not cells, per se, but instead are particles that infect and replicate inside of cells. A mature virus particle is known as a **virion.** Compared with other organisms, virions have a relatively simple structure that consists of the following parts: the *genome*, the *capsid*, and the *envelope*. The **genome** is the inner core of the virion, which consists of single- or double-stranded deoxyribonucleic acid (DNA) or ribonucleic acid (RNA) molecules, but not both. Viruses have the simplest genome of all organisms because the cells of more complex organisms have either much larger nucleic acid strands or multiple strands, which make up *chromosomes*. The latter is the case with higher organisms, including humans. The viral capsid is a protein coat that serves to surround and protect the genome. It also plays a role in the **fusion** process between the virions and the host cells. Fusion occurs when virions attach themselves to host cells in preparation for infecting the cells. The envelope is the outermost layer of the virion and occurs in some, but not all, viruses. It has a lipoprotein (lipid and protein) structure containing viral antigens that are often chemically specific for various proteins on the surface of the host cell membranes (*cell surface proteins*). This biochemical specificity, when present, also facilitates the fusion process. The **human immunodeficiency virus (HIV),** which causes AIDS, functions in this manner.

Viruses can enter the body through at least four routes: inhalation through the respiratory tract, ingestion via the gastrointestinal tract, transplacentally via mother to infant, and inoculation via skin or mucous membranes. The inoculation route can take several forms, including sexual contact, blood transfusions, sharing of syringes or needles (as in injection drug use [IDU]), organ transplants, and animal bites (including human, animal, insect, spider, and others). As mentioned earlier, once inside the body the virus particles, or virions, begin to attach themselves to the outer membranes of host cells (*cell membranes* or *plasma membranes*) as illustrated in Figure 39-1.

The viral genome then passes through the plasma membrane into the cytoplasm of the host cell. It later enters the cell *nucleus*, where the **replication** process begins. The virion may use its own or host enzymes (or both) to direct the replication process. In the host cell nucleus, the viral genome uses the cell's own genetic material, the **nucleic acids, ribonucleic acid [RNA], and deoxyribonucleic acid [DNA],** to synthesize viral nucleic acids and proteins. These are then used to construct complete new virions, including genome, capsid, and envelope (if applicable). These new virions then exit the infected host cell by budding through the plasma membrane and go on to infect other host cells, where the replication process continues. This process is called the *cytopathic effect* and usually results in the destruction of the host cell. Repeated over time, cumulative host cell destruction gives rise to the pathologic effects of the virus, which can eventually impair or even kill the host organism.

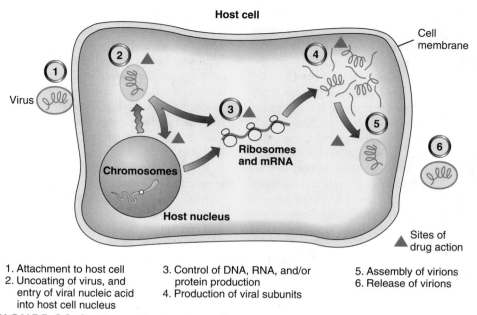

Host cell

Cell membrane

Virus

1. Attachment to host cell
2. Uncoating of virus, and entry of viral nucleic acid into host cell nucleus
3. Control of DNA, RNA, and/or protein production
4. Production of viral subunits
5. Assembly of virions
6. Release of virions

Ribosomes and mRNA

Chromosomes

Host nucleus

▲ Sites of drug action

FIGURE 39-1   *Virus replication. Some viruses integrate into host chromosome with development of latency. (Modified from Brody TM, Larner J, Minneman KP: Human pharmacology: molecular to clinical, ed 3, St Louis, 1998, Mosby.)*

Although this cytopathic effect is the most common outcome, there are other possible outcomes of viral infection. *Viral transformation* involves mutation of the host cell DNA or RNA, which can result in malignant (cancerous) host cells. Viruses that can induce cancer in this way are known as *oncogenic* viruses. More common than viral transformation is *latent,* or dormant, infection, in which the virions remain inside host cells but do not actively replicate to any significant degree. For example, HIV infection may have a lengthy dormant phase of 10 years or more before giving rise to AIDS in an infected person. HIV infection is discussed in greater detail later in this chapter in the section on retroviruses.

Viruses are said to be ubiquitous (widespread) in the environment, and most viral infections may not even be noticed before they are eliminated by the host's immune system. These are referred to as "silent" viral infections. Although the host's immune system acts to neutralize viral infection, it can become overwhelmed, depending on the strength, or *virulence,* of the virus and how rapidly it replicates inside host cells. However, in most cases, a person's immune system is able to arrest and eliminate the virus. Host immune responses to viral infections are classified as *nonspecific* or *specific.* Nonspecific immune responses include *phagocytosis* (eating) of viral particles by leukocytes (white blood cells [WBCs]) such as neutrophils, macrophages, monocytes, and T lymphocytes (T-cells). Another important nonspecific immune response is the release of *cytokines* from these leukocytes. Cytokines are biochemical substances (e.g., histamine, tumor necrosis factor) that stimulate other protective immune functions. Additionally, these *activated* immune system cells may also phagocytize infected host cells to curb the growth and spread of infection. These types of immune responses are collectively referred to as **cell-mediated immunity (CMI).** CMI is nonspecific in the sense that it does not involve **antibodies** that are specific for a given **antigen.** In contrast, *specific* immune responses include the production from B lymphocytes (B cells) of antibodies. These are immune-system proteins (immunoglobulins) that are chemically

specific for viral antigens. This type of immune response is also called **humoral immunity.** Immune system function is discussed in further detail in Chapters 44 and 47.

OVERVIEW OF VIRAL ILLNESSES AND THEIR TREATMENT

There are at least six classes of DNA viruses and at least 14 classes of RNA viruses that are known to infect humans. Some of the more prominent viral illnesses include smallpox (poxviruses), sore throat and conjunctivitis (adenoviruses), warts (papovaviruses), influenza (ortho-myxoviruses), respiratory infections (coronaviruses, rhinoviruses), gastroenteritis (rotavirus, Norwalk-like viruses), HIV/AIDS **(retroviruses),** herpes **(herpesviruses),** and hepatitis (hepadnaviruses). Effective drug therapy is currently available only for a relatively small number of active viral infections. The drug therapy for hepatitis is discussed further in Chapter 49 on immunomodulating drugs. HIV belongs to the relatively unique viral class known as *retroviruses* and is discussed in greater detail in a separate section of this chapter.

Fortunately, many viral illnesses are survivable (e.g., chickenpox), even if bothersome and uncomfortable. The incidence of some of these illnesses has been reduced by the development of effective vaccines (e.g., polio, smallpox, measles, chickenpox). Vaccines are discussed in more detail in Chapter 46. However, many other viral illnesses are either fatal or have much more severe long-term outcomes (e.g., hepatitis, HIV).

Antiviral drugs are chemicals that kill or suppress viruses by either destroying virions or inhibiting their ability to replicate. Even the best medications currently available probably never fully eradicate a virus completely from its host. However, the body's immune system has a better chance of controlling or eliminating a viral infection when the ability of the virus to replicate itself is suppressed. Drugs that actually destroy virions include various disinfectants and immunoglobulins. Disinfectants such as povidone iodine (Betadine) are *virucides* that are commonly used to disinfect medical equipment, as well as various parts of the body during invasive procedures. Such drugs are discussed further in Chapter 43.

Immunoglobulins are concentrated antibodies that can attack and destroy viruses. They are isolated and pooled from human or animal blood. They may be nonspecific (e.g., human gamma-globulin) or specific (e.g., rabies immunoglobulin, varicella-zoster immunoglobulin) in their activity. Although such substances can technically be thought of as antiviral drugs, they are more commonly thought of as immunizing drugs and are therefore also discussed in further detail in Chapter 46. A few antiviral drugs, such as the interferons, stimulate the body's immune system to kill the virions directly. These drugs are discussed in Chapter 49.

In contrast with the various types of antiviral drugs described earlier, the current antiviral drugs are all synthetic compounds that work indirectly by inhibiting viral replication as opposed to directly destroying mature virions themselves. As noted earlier, relatively few of the numerous known viruses can be controlled by current drug therapy. Some of these viruses include:

- Cytomegalovirus (CMV)
- Hepatitis viruses
- Herpes viruses
- HIV
- **Influenza viruses** ("the flu")
- Respiratory syncytial virus (RSV)

As mentioned earlier, active viral infections are usually much more difficult to eradicate than those of other microbes such as bacteria. One reason for this is that viruses can only replicate inside host cells as opposed to independently replicating in the bloodstream or other tissues. Most antiviral drugs must, therefore, enter these cells to disrupt viral replication. The need to develop antiviral drugs that are not overly toxic to host cells is historically one reason for there being relatively few effective antiviral medications on the market. However, the HIV/AIDS epidemic that began in the early 1980s strongly boosted antiviral drug research. This has resulted in more available antiviral drugs than ever before for HIV and other viral infections, such as influenza, CMV, and varicella zoster virus (VZV).

Another major reason viral illnesses are difficult to treat is that the virus has often replicated itself many thousands or even millions of times before symptoms of illness appear. This amplifies the difficulty of eradicating the virus, even with potent medications. Therefore, one goal in the field of infectious disease treatment is to be able to diagnose viral illnesses before an infecting virus has undergone widespread replication in a human host. This would theoretically allow the dual benefit of both early drug therapy and easier elimination of the virus by the host's immune system. This has happened to some degree with HIV infection, with relatively early diagnosis made possible by blood tests to screen for HIV antibodies. Of course, the patient must also be alert of the need to seek medical care before serious illness develops.

Recall that for a virus to replicate, virions must first attach themselves to host cell membranes in a process known as *fusion*. Once inside the cell, the viral genome makes use of cellular genetic processes to generate viral nucleic acids and proteins, which are then used to build new viral particles, or virions (Fig. 39-1). All virions contain a genome that consists of DNA or RNA, but not both. However, both molecules may temporarily occur simultaneously during the viral replication process. Antiviral drugs inhibit this replication process in various ways. Most antiviral drugs enter the same cells that the viruses enter. Once inside, the antiviral drugs interfere with viral nucleic acid synthesis. Other antiviral drugs work by preventing the fusion process itself. If a virion cannot fuse with and enter a host cell, it cannot replicate, and it dies.

The best responses to antiviral drug therapy are usually seen in patients with a competent immune system. Such an immune system can work synergistically with the drug to eliminate or effectively suppress viral activity. Patients who are already *immunocompromised* (have weakened immune systems) because of various illnesses are at greater risk for **opportunistic infections** (OIs) that would not normally harm an *immunocompetent* person (healthy immune system). The most common examples of such patients include cancer patients with leukemia or lymphoma, organ transplant recipients, and patients with AIDS. These patients are prone to frequent and often severe OIs of many types, including other viruses, bacteria, fungi, and protozoans. Such OIs often require long-term prophylactic anti-infective drug therapy to control the infection and prevent its recurrence because of compromised host immune functions.

Recall that there are two types of nucleic acid found in living organisms: DNA and RNA. These are also five organic bases that are major structural components of these nucleic acids. DNA consists of long chains of *deoxyribose* sugar molecules, phosphate groups, together with *purine (adenine or guanine)*, and *pyrimidine (cytosine or thymine)* bases. *RNA* consists of long chains of *ribose* sugar molecules linked to phosphate groups, together with *purine (adenine or guanine)*, and *pyrimidine (cytosine or uracil)* bases. A **nucleoside** is a single unit consisting of a base and its attached sugar molecule. Nucleosides have names similar to their bases with minor spelling modifications (e.g., adenosine, guanosine, cytidine, thymidine). A **nucleotide** is a nucleoside plus its attached phosphate molecule. Most antiviral drugs are synthetic *purine or pyrimidine* nucleoside or nucleotide analogs. These are listed in Table 39-1 along with their specific antiviral activities. In addition, several *non-nucleoside* drugs whose chemical structures are not based on DNA or RNA components are listed in Table 39-2.

Antiviral drugs are used to treat a variety of viral infections ranging from herpes to AIDS, but the effectiveness of these drugs varies widely among patients and even over time for the same patient. The specific antiviral activities for several of the currently available antiviral drugs are summarized for the different drugs in Table 39-3.

Antiviral medications are broadly subdivided into the following two major categories:

Antiviral drugs, which is now commonly used as a general term for those medications used to treat infections of viruses other than HIV.

Antiretroviral drugs, which are indicated specifically for the treatment of infections caused by HIV, the virus that causes AIDS. Although antiretroviral drugs also fall under the broader category of antiviral drugs in general, their mechanisms of action are unique to the AIDS virus, and, therefore, they are more com-

Table 39-1   Examples of Nucleoside Analog Antiviral Drugs

Drug	Nucleoside Analog of	Antiviral Activity
Purine Nucleoside Analogs		
acyclovir, valacyclovir	Guanosine	HSV-1 and -2, VZV
adefovir	Adenosine	HBV
didanosine (ddI), tenofovir	Adenosine	HIV
entecavir	Guanosine	HBV
famciclovir, penciclovir	Guanosine	HSV-1 and -2, VSV
ganciclovir (DHPG), valganciclovir	Guanosine	CMV retinitis and CMV disease
ribavirin (RTCD)	Guanosine	Influenza type A and B, RSV, LV, HV
vidarabine (Ara-A)	Adenosine	HSV, herpes zoster
Pyrimidine Nucleoside Analogs		
idoxuridine (IDU)	Thymidine	HSV
lamivudine (3TC)	Cytidine	HIV
stavudine (d4T), zidovudine (AZT)	Thymidine	HIV
trifluridine	Thymidine	HSV
zalcitabine (ddC), emtricitabine	Cytidine	HIV
Miscellaneous Nucleoside or Nucleotide Analogs		
cidofovir	Unspecified	CMV
abacavir	Unspecified	HIV

CMV, Cytomegalovirus; *HBV,* hepatitis B virus; *HIV,* human immunodeficiency virus; *HSV,* herpes simplex virus (types 1 and 2); *RSV,* respiratory syncytial virus; *VZV,* varicella zoster virus.

Table 39-2   Examples of Non-Nucleoside Analog Antiviral Drugs

Drug	Antiviral Activity
Foscarnet	CMV, HSV
amantadine	influenza A
rimantadine	influenza A
Neuraminidase Inhibitors	
zanamivir, oseltamivir	influenza A
Non-Nucleoside Reverse Transcriptase Inhibitors	
delavirdine, efavirenz, nevirapine	HIV
Protease Inhibitors	
amprenavir, atazanavir, fosamprenavir, indinavir, nelfinavir, saquinavir, ritonavir	HIV
Enfuvirtide	HIV

monly referred to by their subclassification as antiretroviral drugs.

Both classes of drugs are discussed in separate sections of this chapter. However, the indications, adverse effects, and interactions for several common antiviral drugs of both types are summarized in Table 39-3, Table 39-4, and Box 39-1, respectively. Before examining these two major drug classes in detail, we first examine, as an example, one very common viral illness.

OVERVIEW OF HERPES SIMPLEX VIRUSES AND VARICELLA-ZOSTER VIRUS INFECTION

The family of viruses known as *Herpesviridae* includes those viruses that cause any type of herpes infections. There are several specific *types* of such viruses. *Herpes simplex virus type 1 (HSV-1)* causes *mucocutaneous herpes*—usually in the form of perioral blisters ("fever blisters" or "cold sores"). *Herpes simplex virus type 2 (HSV-2)* causes genital herpes. *Human herpesvirus 3 (HHV-3)* causes both chickenpox and shingles. This virus is more commonly known as *herpes zoster virus* or *varicella zoster virus (VZV)*. *Human herpesvirus 4 (HHV-4)* is more commonly known as *Epstein-Barr virus (EBV)* and is associated with such illnesses as infectious mononucleosis ("mono") and chronic fatigue syndrome. *Human herpesvirus 5 (HHV-5) is more commonly known as cytomegalovirus (CMV)*, the cause of CMV retinitis (serious viral infection of the eye) and *CMV disease*. The latter is simply a generalized CMV infection, most often occurring in immunocompromised patients (e.g., patients who have AIDS or are receiving cancer chemotherapy or other immunosuppressive drugs; organ transplant patients). *Human herpesviruses 6 and 7* are not especially clinically significant, but may be more likely to occur in immunocompromised patients. Additionally, *human herpesvirus 8* is also known as *Kaposi's sarcoma herpesvirus* and is an *oncogenic* (cancer-causing) virus believed to cause Kaposi's sarcoma, an AIDS-associated cancer. All of these viruses occur, often asymptomatically, in varying percentages of the population. Types 3 through 7 normally do not cause diseases that require medication, except in the case of immunocompromised patients. However, the herpes simplex viruses (types 1 and 2) and the varicella zoster virus (VZV, or HHV-3) commonly cause illnesses that are now routinely treated with prescription medications. These viruses are the focus of this section.

Herpes Simplex Viruses

Although there can be anatomical overlap between the two types of herpes simplex virus (HSV). HSV-1 is most commonly associated with perioral blisters and is therefore often thought of as "oral herpes." In contrast, HSV-2 is most commonly associated with blisters on both male and female genitalia, and is therefore commonly referred to as "genital herpes." Although usually not causing serious or life-threatening illness, both infections are certainly

Table 39-3 Antiviral Drugs: Viral Spectra, Indications, and Therapeutic Effects

Drugs	Antiviral Activity	Indications and Therapeutic Effects
acyclovir, famciclovir, penciclovir, valacyclovir	HSV-1 and -2, VZV	Herpes simplex encephalitis, disseminated or CNS herpes infections in the newborn, herpes keratitis (topically), and herpes zoster. Acyclovir is used topically, PO, and IV, for treatment of herpes simplex, encephalitis, and most other significant herpes infections. Administration as soon as possible produces the best results. These drugs reduce viral shedding, decrease local symptoms, and decrease severity and duration of illness. Valacyclovir is also indicated for *herpes labialis* (perioral cold sores). Penciclovir is a topical drug for this same condition.
amantadine, rimantadine	Influenza A	Used for the treatment and prophylaxis of influenza A but ineffective against influenza B. Most effective if given before exposure or within 48 hr of development of symptoms. Reduces fever and palliates symptoms of influenza. As described in Chapter 14, amantadine is also used in the treatment of Parkinson's disease.
zanamivir, oseltamivir	Influenza A or B	Zanamivir is used for treatment only; oseltamivir for treatment or prophylaxis (13 yr-adult); usually effective only if started within 2 days of symptom onset.
cidofovir, ganciclovir, foscarnet, valganciclovir	CMV	Ganciclovir is the older and more studied of these drugs. It is available in a variety of formulations (PO, parenteral, and an ocular implant [Vitrasert]). Has been shown to be effective for not only CMV retinitis but also other CMV infections such as gastrointestinal infection and pneumonitis and for prevention of CMV in recipients of solid organ transplants and in patients with HIV infection. Primary dose-limiting toxicity of ganciclovir is bone marrow toxicity. Foscarnet and cidofovir are less toxic to the bone marrow but can cause renal failure. This can be minimized with the administration of probenecid tablets and hydration on the day of infusion. Foscarnet is also indicated for acyclovir-resistant HSV infections.
fomivirsen	CMV	For CMV retinitis only; given by intraocular injection by ophthalmologist.
delavirdine, efavirenz, nevirapine	HIV	In combination with nucleoside analogs, these 2 NNRTI are used to treat HIV-infected patients, including newly infected asymptomatic patients.
abacavir, didanosine, emtricitabine, lamivudine, stavudine, zalcitabine, zidovudine	HIV	Approved for the treatment of HIV infections. Produce a significant reduction in mortality and incidence of opportunistic infections, improve physical performance, and significantly improve T-cell counts. Lamivudine also for HBV (Epivir-HBV).
tenofovir	HIV	First and currently only nucleo*tide* reverse transcriptase inhibitor.
enfuvirtide	HIV	First and currently only fusion inhibitor.
trifluridine	HSV	Used to treat herpes simplex keratitis. Used only topically because of significant liver and bone marrow toxicity.
indinavir, ritonavir, saquinavir, nelfinavir, fosamprenavir, amprenavir, atazanavir	HIV	Newer class of drugs for the treatment of HIV infection when antiretroviral therapy is warranted. Used in combination with nucleoside analogs. Ritonavir and indinavir may be used as monotherapy. All are potent inhibitors of the HIV protease enzyme, which is critical to replication of the virus that causes AIDS.
adefovir, entecavir	HBV	Both drugs inhibit HBV nucleic acid enzymes to reduce HBV viral replication.
ribavirin, RSV immunoglobulin	HCV, RSV	Nonaerosol forms used for HCV. Severe RSV bronchopneumonia can be treated using an aerosol (ribavirin) or an IV infusion (RSV immunoglobulin). These products have been shown to improve oxygenation, decrease viral shedding, and alleviate pneumonia symptoms. Inhalation treatment with ribavirin has also been shown to be effective in influenza A and B infections.

CNS, Central nervous system; *CMV,* cytomegalovirus; *HIV,* human immunodeficiency virus; *HSV,* herpes simplex virus; *NNRTI,* non-nucleoside reverse transcriptase inhibitors; *RSV,* respiratory syncytial virus; *VZV,* varicella zoster virus.

annoying and highly transmissible through close physical contact (e.g., kissing, sexual intercourse). Outbreaks of painful skin lesions occur *intermittently* (come and go) with periods of *latency* (no sores or other symptoms) occurring between acute outbreaks. Although antiviral medications are not always clinically required and are *not* curative, they can speed up the process of remission and reduce the duration of painful symptoms. This is especially true, if the medications are started early in a given outbreak. Patients may also be prescribed an ongoing lower dose of antiviral drug for *prophylaxis* (prevention) of outbreaks. Situations in which

HSV infections can become especially serious, even life-threatening, involve immunocompromised patients and virus transmission to a newborn infant. *Neonatal herpes* is often a life-threatening infection, and babies with this disease are often treated in neonatal intensive care units (NICUs) with IV antiviral drugs. However, these treatments fail in many cases, with infant death and/or permanent disability common. Therefore, the best strategy is to *prevent* transmission of HSV to the newborn infant. For this reason, obstetricians will usually recommend delivery by cesarean section ("C-section") for any mother with active genital herpes le-

Table 39-4   Selected Antiviral Drugs: Adverse Effects

Drug	Adverse Effects
acyclovir	Most common: nausea, vomiting, diarrhea, headache, transient burning when topically applied
amantadine, rimantadine	Insomnia, nervousness, lightheadedness; gastrointestinal: anorexia, nausea; anticholinergic effects
didanosine	Gastrointestinal: pancreatitis; CNS: peripheral neuropathies, seizures
foscarnet	CNS: headache, seizures; metabolic: hypocalcemia, hypophosphatemia, hyperphosphatemia, hypokalemia; genitourinary: acute renal failure; hematologic: bone marrow suppression; gastrointestinal: nausea, vomiting, diarrhea
ganciclovir	Hematologic: bone marrow toxicity; gastrointestinal: nausea, anorexia, vomiting; CNS: headache, seizures
indinavir	Nausea, abdominal pain, headache, diarrhea, vomiting, weakness or fatigue, insomnia, flank pain, taste changes, acid regurgitation, back pain, indirect hyperbilirubinemia, nephrolithiasis
nevirapine	Rash, fever, nausea, headache, increases in liver function tests
ribavirin	Rash, conjunctivitis, anemia, mild bronchospasm
trifluridine	Burning, swelling, stinging, photophobia, pain
vidarabine	Ophthalmic effects: burning, lacrimation, keratitis, foreign body sensation, pain photophobia, uveitis, stromal edema
zalcitabine	Peripheral neuropathy, rash, ulcers
zidovudine	Bone marrow suppression, nausea, headache

Box 39-1   Selected Antiviral Drugs: Interactions

Acyclovir with the Following
- Interferon: additive antiviral effects
- Probenecid: increased acyclovir levels by decreasing renal clearance
- Zidovudine: increased risk for neurotoxicity

Amantadine with the Following
- Anticholinergic drugs: increased adverse anticholinergic effects
- CNS stimulants: additive CNS stimulant effects

Didanosine with the Following
- Antacids: increased absorption of didanosine, which is a positive effect
- Dapsone: may interfere with GI absorption of dapsone
- Itraconazole and ketoconazole: didanosine decreases their absorption; give 2 hours apart
- Quinolones: didanosine decreases absorption of some quinolone antibiotics
- Tetracyclines: decreased absorption of tetracyclines; give 2 hours before tetracyclines
- Zalcitabine: additive toxicity (peripheral neuropathies); avoid giving together
- Zidovudine: additive and synergistic effect against HIV

Ganciclovir with the Following
- Foscarnet: additive or synergistic effect against cytomegalovirus and HSV-2
- Imipenem: increased risk for seizures
- Zidovudine: increased risk for hematologic toxicity (i.e., bone marrow suppression)

Indinavir with the Following
- Drugs metabolized by the CYP3A4 hepatic microsomal enzyme system (astemizole, cisapride, triazolam, and midazolam): competition for metabolism resulting in elevated blood levels and potential toxicity
- Ketoconazole: increased plasma concentrations of ganciclovir
- Rifabutin and ketoconazole: increased plasma concentrations of rifabutin and ketoconazole
- Rifampin: increased metabolism of indinavir

Nevirapine with the Following
- Drugs metabolized by the CYP3A4 hepatic microsomal enzyme system: increased metabolism of these drugs
- Oral contraceptives: decreased plasma concentrations of oral contraceptives
- Protease inhibitors: decreased plasma concentrations of protease inhibitors
- Rifampin and rifabutin: decreased nevirapine serum concentration

Zalcitabine with the Following
- Antacids: reduced zalcitabine absorption
- Cimetidine: decreased zalcitabine renal elimination
- Drugs associated with pancreatic, peripheral neuropathy, and renal toxicities should be avoided because of additive toxicities
- Zidovudine: additive or synergistic effect against HIV

Zidovudine with the Following
- Acyclovir: increased neurotoxicity
- Beta-interferon: increased serum levels of zidovudine
- Cytotoxic drugs: increased risk for hematologic toxicity
- Didanosine and zalcitabine: additive or synergistic effect against HIV
- Ganciclovir and ribavirin: antagonize the antiviral action of zidovudine

sions. Unlike VZV (see later), there is currently no specific HSV immune globulin available for treating infected infants, so prevention is the key. The medications used for HSV are the same as those for VZV and are discussed in the section on antiviral drugs.

Varicella Zoster Virus

The latency periods associated with both HIV and HSV infections have been described. Another important and common example of latent viral infection involves the *varicella zoster virus*

(VZV). As noted earlier, this is a type of herpesvirus (HHV-3) that most commonly causes *chickenpox (varicella)* in childhood, remains dormant for many years, and can then re-emerge in later adulthood as painful *herpes zoster* lesions known as *shingles.*

Chickenpox is usually an uncomfortable but self-limiting disease of childhood. However, it is highly contagious and easily spread by either direct contact with weeping lesions or via droplet inhalation. It may also lead to significant scarring. The serious condition known as *Reye's syndrome* (fatty liver damage with encephalopathy) may also complicate varicella, as can other viral infections such as influenza. *Herpes zoster*, more commonly known as *shingles,* is caused by the reactivation of VZV from its dormant state, often decades after a case of childhood chickenpox. It is also referred to more simply as *zoster.* Its most common manifestation is in the form of skin lesions known as *dermatomes* that follow nerve tracts along the skin surface. The most common site of these lesions is around the side of the trunk, although they can appear in other areas (e.g., along trigeminal nerve dermatomes of the face). Zoster lesions are often quite painful, and some patients even require narcotics for pain control. In addition, postherpetic neuralgias (long-term nerve pain) remain following shingles outbreaks in up to 50% of elderly patients. Early administration of antiviral drugs such as acyclovir may speed recovery, but this effect is usually not dramatic. The best results are usually seen when the antiviral drug is started within 72 hours of symptom onset.

Active childhood varicella (chickenpox) infections, as mentioned earlier, are usually self-limiting and are not normally treated with antiviral drugs, except in high-risk (e.g., immunocompromised) pediatric patients. However, varicella virus vaccine was U.S. Food and Drug Administration (FDA) approved in 1995 and is now routinely recommended for healthy children older than 1 year of age who have not had chickenpox. It has even been shown effective for producing VZV immunity in HIV-positive children who are reasonably healthy. As this newly vaccinated pediatric population ages, it will become known whether the VZV vaccine also protects against shingles in adulthood. There is currently no specific vaccine for shingles. Approximately 95% of pregnant women have VZV antibodies, which protect the fetus from viral infection. However, first-time exposure to VZV infection can pose a teratogenic risk in pregnant women, especially during the first trimester. If the infection manifests in a pregnant woman within 5 days of delivery, a dose of varicella zoster immunoglobulin (VZIG) is recommended for the infant. It may also be beneficial to both mother and infant when given to the mother during pregnancy, preferably as soon as possible after diagnosis of infection. Both varicella virus vaccine and VZIG are discussed further in Chapter 46.

In a small percentage of shingles cases, skin lesions may progress beyond the usual dermatome regions, and the virus can cause solid organ infections such as pneumonitis, hepatitis, encephalitis, and optic neuritis (infection of the optic nerve). Such infections are uncommon, but elderly and immunocompromised patients (e.g., those with HIV/AIDS, organ transplants, cancer) are the most vulnerable to these more serious VZV exacerbations. These infections can also be due to first-time exposure to varicella (chickenpox). In general, these more serious infections require intravenous (IV) antiviral drugs, especially in high-risk patients. Intravenous acyclovir is the most commonly used drug with foscarnet sodium as an alternative. These intravenous antiviral medications can sometimes prevent fatalities or disability in the most serious infections. Less serious infections are usually treated orally with acyclovir, valacyclovir, or famciclovir. Topical dosage forms of some of these drugs are also available and are discussed further in Chapter 57. Although VZV reactivation is comparable in pathology to that caused by herpes simplex virus (HSV; e.g., oral or genital herpes lesions), VZV reactivation occurs much less regularly than does HSV because of a lack of reactivation genes. Because secondary bacterial infections (e.g., group A streptococcus skin infection) are common with VZV

exacerbations, antibiotics may also be needed. This is especially true in cases of ophthalmic involvement.

ANTIVIRAL DRUGS (NONRETROVIRAL)

The drugs discussed in this section include those used to treat non-HIV viral infections such as those caused by influenza viruses; HSV, VZV, and CMV. There are also antiviral drugs used for hepatitis A, B, and C viruses (HAV, HBV, and HCV). However, hepatitis treatment is discussed in further detail in Chapter 49 because it involves some additional unique drug therapy.

Mechanism of Action and Drug Effects

Most of the current antiviral drugs work by blocking the activity of a polymerase enzyme, which normally catalyzes the synthesis of new viral genomes. The result is impaired viral replication, which ideally results in viral concentrations small enough to be eliminated by the patient's immune system. If this does not occur, the virus may either enter a dormant state or remain at a low level of replication with continuous drug therapy. For some of the more serious viral infections, such as HIV or HCV, long-term drug therapy is often necessary. Pertinent information for specific drugs is also listed in Table 39-3.

Indications

Indications for several commonly used antiviral drugs, including antiretroviral drugs, are summarized in Table 39-3.

Contraindications

Most of the nonretroviral antiviral drugs are surprisingly well tolerated. The only usual contraindication for most of these drugs is known severe drug allergy, keeping in mind that the seriousness of a given patient's illness may leave few treatment options. However, there are a small number of listed contraindications for a few of the antiviral drugs. Amantadine is contraindicated in lactating women, children younger than 12 months of age, and patients with an eczematic rash. Famciclovir is contraindicated in cases of allergy to the drug itself or to a similar drug called penciclovir, which is used topically for *herpes labialis* (perioral sores). Because cidofovir has such a strong propensity for renal toxicity, it is contraindicated in cases of patients who already have severely compromised renal function as well as those receiving concurrent drug therapy with other highly nephrotoxic drugs. It is also contraindicated in cases of allergy to probenecid (a sulfa drug) or other sulfa-containing medications. As noted in Table 39-3, probenecid is recommended as concurrent drug therapy with cidofovir, to help alleviate its nephrotoxicity. Ribavirin also has additional specific contraindications besides drug allergy. Its oral dosage forms—tablets, capsules, and oral solution—are contraindicated in patients with pre-existing hemoglobinopathies such as sickle-cell anemia, because anemia is also a common adverse effect of ribavirin. This drug is also contraindicated in cases of *autoimmune* hepatitis, as it can worsen this condition. Additionally, because of the drug's teratogenic potential, it is also contraindicated in pregnant women and even their male sexual partners. The aerosol form should also not be used in pregnant women or in women who may become pregnant during exposure to the drug. This includes health providers administering the drug in aerosol form because of the potential for second-hand inhalation on the part of the health provider.

Look-Alike Drugs: Zostrix and Zovirax

An incident was reported that involved the confusion of these two similarly-named drugs. A physician prescribed Zostrix cream with the directions, "Apply to affected area qid." There were no other specific instructions for the medication. The pharmacist mistakenly entered "Zovirax" into the pharmacy computer, and the nursing staff did not catch the error. The next day, the physician saw the tube of Zovirax in the patient's room instead of Zostrix. The sound-alike drug names can be easily confused.

Zostrix is capsaicin, derived from hot chili peppers, and is used topically for the treatment of arthritic pain, muscle strains, and joint sprains. In this case, it was ordered for neuralgia pain. Zovirax 5% ointment is a topical form of acyclovir, an antiviral medication, and is used for the management of initial genital herpes.

This incident illustrates how important it is to clarify the instructions of a medication order (e.g., application to a *specific* site) and how the use of generic names can help to avoid a medication error. In addition, it shows how important it is for nurses to be familiar with the indications of the drugs they are administering.

From U.S. Pharmacopeia: *Similar drug names reported to the MER.* February 25, 2004. Available at www.usp.org/patientSafety/newsletters/practitioner ReportingNews/prn1122004-02-25.html. Accessed September 8, 2006.

Adverse Effects

The adverse effects of the antiviral drugs are as different as the drugs themselves. Each has its own specific adverse effect profile. Because viruses reproduce in human cells and therefore have many of the same features as these cells, it is hard to target a unique enzyme or other feature of the virus. Selective killing is difficult, and, as a result, many healthy human cells, in addition to virally infected cells, may be killed in the process, resulting in more serious toxicities. However, this effect is usually not as pronounced as in cancer chemotherapy, which often kills many more healthy cells. The more serious adverse effects are listed by drug in Table 39-4.

Interactions

The significant drug interactions that occur with the antiviral drugs occur most often when they are administered via systemic routes such as intravenously and orally. However, many of these drugs are also applied topically to the eye or body, and the incidence of drug interactions associated with these routes of administration is much lower. Selected common drug interactions for both antiviral and antiretroviral drugs listed in Box 39-1.

Dosages

See the corresponding dosages table for doses of all of the commonly used nonretroviral antiviral drugs. Profiles of selected drugs follow.

Drug Profiles

Nonretroviral Antiviral Drugs

Antiviral drugs are now commonly used to treat active infection with several viruses, including influenza viruses, HSV, VZV, CMV, HBV, HCV, and RSV. More effective methods of drug development have resulted in many new antiviral drugs over the past few decades.

amantadine and rimantadine

One of the earliest antiviral drugs, amantadine (Symmetrel) has a narrow antiviral spectrum in that it is only active against influenza A viruses. It is used both prophylactically and therapeutically. It has been shown to be very effective, if not lifesaving, when used prophylactically in, for instance, elderly, chronically ill, or immunocompromised patients in whom influenza A infection can be particularly devastating. It may also be used prophylactically when influenza vaccine is either not available or is contraindicated for a given patient. When used therapeutically to treat active influenza A infections, it can reduce recovery time.

Rimantadine is a structural analog of amantadine that has the same spectrum of activity, mechanism of action, and clinical indications. However, it differs from amantadine in that it has a longer half-life and causes fewer CNS adverse effects such as dizziness and blurred vision (see Chapter 14). Rimantadine has gastrointestinal adverse effects similar to those of amantadine. Both medications may be used in children. Both drugs are available only for oral use.

Pharmacokinetics

Half-Life	Onset	Peak	Duration
PO: 17 hr	PO: Unknown	PO: 1-4 hr	PO: 12-24 hr

▶ acyclovir

Acyclovir (Zovirax) is a synthetic nucleoside analog of the nucleic acid nucleoside *guanosine* that is mainly used to suppress the replication of HSV-1 and -2 and VZV. Acyclovir is considered the drug of choice for the treatment of both initial and recurrent episodes of both of these viral infections.

Acyclovir is available in oral, topical, and parenteral formulations. Its topical use is discussed in Chapter 57 (Dermatological Drugs). Other similar antiviral drugs include valacyclovir and famciclovir. However, these latter two drugs are currently available only for oral use and are indicated for the treatment of less serious infections than those requiring IV drug therapy. Note the slight inconsistencies in the spelling of these drug names. Valacyclovir is a prodrug that is metabolized to acyclovir in the body. It has the advantage of greater oral bioavailablity and less frequent dosing (three times daily vs. five times daily for acyclovir). It may also provide more effective relief of pain from zoster lesions.

Pharmacokinetics

Half-Life	Onset	Peak	Duration
PO: 2-3 hr	PO: Unknown	PO: 1.5-2 hr	PO: 10-15 hr

▶ ganciclovir

Like acyclovir, ganciclovir (Cytovene) is also a synthetic nucleoside analog of guanosine, but it has a much different spectrum of antiviral activity. The *cytomegalovirus (CMV)* is carried by up to 50% of the adult population and normally causes no harm. However, in immunocompromised patients (including premature infants), it can cause life-threatening or disabling opportunistic infections. Valganciclovir (Valcyte), foscarnet (Foscavir), and cidofovir (Vistide) are three other antiviral drugs that are used in the treatment of CMV infection. These drugs also have activity against HSV-1 and -2, Epstein-Barr virus (HSV-4), and VZV, but are not normally used for these infections because there are other effective but less toxic drugs available.

Of these three antiviral drugs, ganciclovir is the one most often used in the treatment of CMV infections. A common site of CMV infections in the immunocompromised patient involves the eye, and the result is CMV retinitis, a devastating viral infection that can lead to blindness. Ganciclovir is most commonly administered intravenously or orally. However, there is also an ophthalmic form (Vitrasert) for treating active CMV retinitis, which must be surgically inserted Fomivirsen is another anti-CMV drug used to treat CMV retinitis. It is an ocular injection that is injected directly into

DOSAGES

Antiviral Drugs (Nonretroviral)

Drug (Pregnancy Category)	Pharmacologic Class	Usual Dosage Range	Indications
acyclovir (Zovirax) (B)	Anti-herpesvirus	**Pediatric <12 yr** IV: 10-20 mg/kg q8h × 7-10 days **Pediatric 12 yr-adult** IV: 5-10 mg/kg q8h × 7-10 days PO: 200-800 mg q4h 5×/day × 7-10 days, **or** PO: 20 mg/kg (max 800 mg/dose) qid × 5 days	HSV-1 and HSV-2, including genital herpes, mucocutaneous herpes, and herpes encephalitis; herpes zoster (shingles); higher dose therapy for acute episodes; lower dose therapy for viral suppression Chickenpox (varicella)
adefovir (Hepsera) (C)	Anti-HBV	**Adult** PO: 10 mg qd	Chronic HBV infection
amantadine (Symmetrel) (C)	Anti-influenza	**Pediatric 1-9 yr** PO: 4.4-8.8 mg/kg/day divided qd or bid **Pediatric 9-12 yr** PO: 100 mg bid **Adolescent and Adult 13-64 yr** PO: 200 mg divided qd or bid **Adult >65 yr** 100 mg qd	Influenza virus type A
cidofovir (Vistide) (C)	Anti-CMV	**Adult** IV: 5 mg/kg q14d (must be given with PO probenecid)	CMV retinitis
entecavir (Baraclude) (C)	Anti-HBV	**Adult only (16 yrs+)** PO: 0.5-1 mg once daily	Chronic HBV infection
famciclovir (Famvir) (B)	Anti-herpesvirus	**Adult** PO: 125 mg bid-500 mg bid-tid × 5-7 days	Herpes zoster (shingles); recurrent genital herpes
foscarnet (Foscavir) (C)	Anti-CMV, anti-HSV	**Adult** IV: 40-120 mg/kg divided in one to three daily doses	CMV retinitis; HSV infections that are resistant to standard drug therapy
ganciclovir (Cytovene, DHPG) (C)	Anti-CMV	**Adult** IV: 5 mg/kg q12h × 1-2 wk PO: 1000 mg tid with food	CMV retinitis; prevention or treatment of other CMV infection
oseltamivir (Tamiflu) (C)	Anti-influenza	**Pediatric 1-12 yr* <15 kg** PO: 30 mg bid 15-23 kg PO: 45 mg bid 23-40 kg PO: 60 mg bid **>40 kg or 13 yr-adult** PO: 75 mg bid	Influenza A or B infection
ribavirin (Copegus, Rebetrol, Virazole) (X)	Anti-HCV; anti-RSV	**Adult and pediatric** PO: 800-1200 mg divided bid **Pediatric** Aerosol: 6 g reconstituted to 20 mg/mL via continuous aerosol 3 12-18 hr/day 3 3-7 days	Influenza A or B infection; HCV infection Severe RSV infection in hospitalized infants and toddlers
rimantadine (Flumadine) (C)	Anti-influenza	**Pediatric <10 yr** PO: 5 mg/kg once daily (max 150 mg) **10 yr-adult** PO: 100 mg bid	Influenza A infection
valacyclovir (Valtrex) (B)	Anti-herpesvirus	**Adult** PO: 500-1000 mg bid-tid × 3-10 days	Herpes zoster (shingles); genital herpes
valganciclovir (Valcyte) (C)	Anti-CMV	**Adult** PO: 900 mg bid × 3 wk with food	CMV retinitis, CMV disease prevention
zanamivir (Relenza) (C)	Anti-influenza	**Pediatric ≥7 yr-adult** Inhalation*: 10 mg (2 5-mg powder doses) bid; first day's doses must be at least 2 hr apart and q12h thereafter.	Influenza A or B infection

Use liquid oral suspension for doses <75 mg.
*Use bronchodilator inhaler first if applicable.
NOTE: Where pediatric doses are not provided, dosing guidelines for pediatric patients are not firmly established for the drug in question and should be based on the careful clinical judgment of a qualified prescriber.
CMV, Cytomegalovirus; *CNS,* central nervous system; *HBV,* hepatitis B virus; *HCV,* hepatitis C virus; *HSV,* herpes simplex virus (types 1 and 2); *RSV,* respiratory syncytial virus.

the eye by an ophthalmologist (Chapter 58). Ganciclovir is also administered to *prevent* CMV *disease* (generalized infection) in high-risk patients, such as those receiving organ transplants.

A dose-limiting toxicity of ganciclovir treatment is bone marrow suppression, whereas that of foscarnet and cidofovir is renal toxicity. These toxicities should be kept in mind when deciding which drug is more appropriate in a particular patient. For example, a heart transplant recipient who contracts CMV retinitis is immunocompromised because of immunosuppressant drug therapy and is most likely taking cyclosporine, which is nephrotoxic. Therefore, using foscarnet in this patient may be more dangerous than using ganciclovir. On the other hand, a patient who contracts a CMV infection and is immunocompromised because of a bone marrow transplant might be better treated using foscarnet.

Ganciclovir is available in oral form, injectable form, and as an ocular implant. Valganciclovir is a prodrug of ganciclovir, for oral use, that is metabolized to ganciclovir in the body. Similar to the situation described previously for valacyclovir and acyclovir, the prodrug allows greater oral bioavailability and reduced frequency of daily dosing. Cidofovir and foscarnet are available only in injectable form.

Pharmacokinetics

Half-Life	Onset	Peak	Duration
PO: 4.8 hr	PO: Unknown	PO: 24 hr	PO: Variable

oseltamivir and zanamivir

Oseltamivir (Tamiflu) and zanamivir (Relenza) belong to one of the newest classes of antiviral drugs known as *neuraminidase inhibitors*. These drugs are active against influenza virus types A and B. They are indicated for the treatment of uncomplicated acute illness caused by influenza infection in adults. They have been shown to reduce the duration of influenza infection by several days. The neuraminidase enzyme enables budding virions to escape from infected cells and spread throughout the body. Neuraminidase inhibitors are designed to stop this process in the body, speeding recovery from infection.

The most commonly reported adverse events with oseltamivir are nausea and vomiting; those with zanamivir are diarrhea, nausea, and sinusitis. Oseltamivir is only available for oral use. The drug is indicated for prophylaxis and treatment of influenza infection. Zanamivir is available in blister packets of dry powder for inhalation. It is currently indicated only for treatment of active influenza illness. Treatment with oseltamivir and zanamivir ideally should begin within 2 days of symptom onset.

Pharmacokinetics (zanamivir)

Half-Life	Onset	Peak	Duration
PO: 2.1-5 hr	PO: Unknown	PO: 1-2 hr	PO: 10-24 hr

Pharmacokinetics (oseltamivir)

Half-Life	Onset	Peak	Duration
PO: 1-3 hr	PO: Unknown	PO: 1-2 hr	PO: 5-15 hr

ribavirin

Ribavirin (Copegus, Rebetol, Virazole) is a unique antiviral drug in that it is given orally or by oral or nasal inhalation. It is a synthetic nucleoside analog of guanosine, as are many of the other antiviral drugs, but it has a spectrum of antiviral activity that is broader than that of other currently available antiviral drugs. It interferes with both RNA and DNA synthesis and as a result inhibits both protein synthesis and viral replication overall.

The inhalational form (Virazole) is used primarily in hospitalized infants for treatment of severe lower respiratory tract infections caused by RSV. This drug was first available only in inhalational form. More recently oral dosage forms have become available for use in the treatment of hepatitis C.

Pharmacokinetics

Half-Life	Onset	Peak	Duration
Inhal: 1.4-2.5 hr*	Inhal: Unknown	Inhal: End of inhalation period	Inhal: Variable
PO: 120-300 hr	PO: Unknown	PO: Up to 2 hr	PO: Unknown

*In respiratory secretions.

OVERVIEW OF HIV INFECTION AND THE AIDS PANDEMIC

The first U.S. cases of **acquired immune deficiency syndrome (AIDS)** were recognized in 1981 in 31 previously healthy homosexual men in Los Angeles and New York City. These first patients mysteriously developed *Pneumocystis carinii* pneumonia (PCP) or Kaposi's sarcoma, both normally extremely rare illnesses. (PCP is now known as *Pneumocystis jirovecii* pneumonia.) Within months, similar disease patterns were recognized in intravenous drug users and in hemophiliac patients who had been transfused with blood-derived clotting factors. Other cases began to occur in hospitalized patients transfused with a variety of blood-derived products. In 1983, the human T-cell lymphotropic virus type 3 (HTLV-3) was isolated from a patient with lymphadenopathy (swollen lymph nodes) and in 1984 was demonstrated to be the cause of AIDS. This virus was later renamed human immunodeficiency virus (HIV), a member of the retrovirus family. There are two recognized types of HIV: HIV-1 and HIV-2. Both cause AIDS, but HIV-2 is primarily localized in western Africa, with HIV-1 causing the majority of the HIV pandemic in the rest of the world. By 1985, a laboratory technique known as an *enzyme-linked immunosorbent assay* (ELISA) was developed. This technique allowed the detection of HIV exposure based on the presence of human antibodies to the virus in blood samples. This diagnostic breakthrough lead to an appreciation of the enormity of HIV prevalence both in U.S. high-risk groups and as an emerging world pandemic, especially in developing countries. This laboratory screening technique also helped to restore the safety of the transfusion blood supply, although it is not 100% reliable. In addition to HIV-1 and HIV-2, there are two other retroviruses known to infect humans: HTLV-1 and -2. HTLV-1 is an oncogenic virus capable of causing certain types of leukemia, whereas HTLV-2 is not associated with any specific disease.

The retrovirus family got its name upon discovery of a unique feature of its replication process. Retroviruses are all RNA viruses and are unique in their use of the enzyme **reverse transcriptase** during their replication process. This enzyme promotes the synthesis of complementary ("mirror image") DNA molecules from the viral RNA genome. A second enzyme, *integrase*, promotes the integration of this viral DNA into the host cell DNA. This hybrid DNA complex is known as a *provirus*. It produces new viral RNA genomes and proteins, which in turn combine to make mature HIV virions that infect other host cells. Another important enzyme is **protease,** which serves to chemically separate the new viral RNA from viral protein molecules. These components are initially synthesized into one large macromolecular strand, and the protease enzyme carefully breaks up this strand into its key components. Figure 39-2 illustrates the major structural features of the HIV virion, and Figure 39-3 illustrates the steps in its replication process. In contrast with retroviruses, nonretroviruses, on the other hand, primarily use *host* cell enzymes (DNA or RNA polymerases) to synthesize viral nucleic acids. Reverse transcriptase itself is actually an RNA-dependent DNA polymerase and is sometimes also referred to by this name. However, reverse transcriptase is not normally found in host cells—both reverse transcriptase and integrase are carried by the virus itself. This "reversal" of the usual replication processes led to the enzyme name *reverse transcriptase,* and also to the *retrovirus* name for this family of viruses. Furthermore, the fact that

retroviruses synthesize DNA from viral RNA molecules is also a reversal of the norm because in most other organisms, RNA molecules are synthesized *from* DNA molecules, as part of the reproductive process. Reverse transcriptase also differs from host cell nucleic acid polymerases in another significant way. It has a higher rate of errors when stringing together the purine and pyrimidine bases (A, T, G, C) during transcription of the viral RNA genome into a DNA molecule during the replication process. This allows more frequent genetic mutations among HIV virions and often results in viral strains that are resistant to both medications and the patient's immune system. Such mutations also hamper the development of an effective vaccine against the virus. The most common routes of transmission for HIV are sexual activity, IV drug use (IDU), and perinatally from mother to child. Heterosexual transmission is most common in Africa and Asia. In the United States, unprotected anal intercourse among male homosexuals is still the most common cause of new cases (42%), with heterosexual vaginal or anal intercourse (33%) and IDU (25%) as additional causes. In the United Kingdom in 1999, the incidence of new infections was, for the first time, greater in heterosexuals than in homosexuals. Male-to-female transmission is more common in heterosexuals. However, there are also documented cases of female-to-male sexual transmission that demonstrate the infectiousness of both vaginal secretions and menstrual blood. Cases of sexual transmission via oral mucosa are also documented. However, it should be emphasized that no solid evidence to date confirms transmission of HIV by more casual contact, including hugging; kissing; coughing; sneezing; swimming in pools; and sharing of food, water, eating utensils, or toilet facilities. HIV is also not transmitted by insect bites, unlike some

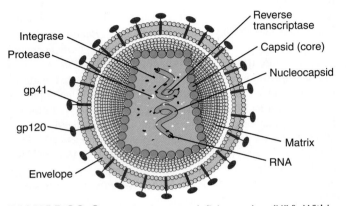

FIGURE 39-2   Human immunodeficiency virus (HIV). Within the core capsid, the diploid, single-stranded, positive-sense RNA is complexed to nucleoprotein. *(From* Dorland's illustrated medical dictionary, *ed 30, Philadelphia, 2003, Saunders.)*

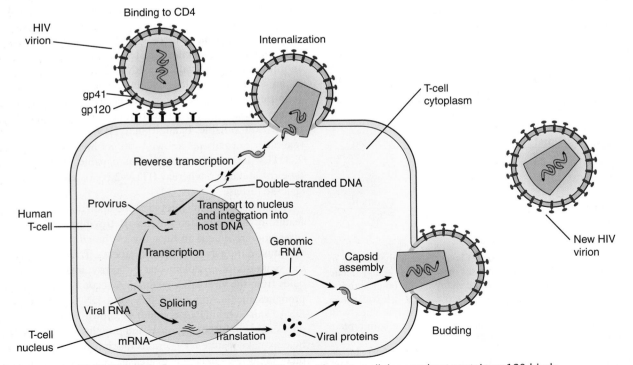

FIGURE 39-3   Life cycle of the HIV virus. The extracellular envelope protein gp120 binds to CD4 on the surface of T lymphocytes or mononuclear phagocytes, while the transmembrane protein gp41 mediates the fusion of the viral envelope with the cell membrane. *gp,* Glycoprotein. *(From* Dorland's illustrated medical dictionary, *ed 30, Philadelphia, 2003, Saunders.)*

viral illnesses. Although HIV can be isolated from almost any body fluid, including tears, sweat, saliva, and urine, its concentrations in these fluids are much lower than those in blood and genital secretions. In approximately 6% of cases, specific risk factors cannot be determined.

The risk for transmission to health care workers resulting from percutaneous (needle-stick) injuries is currently calculated at approximately 0.3%. The observance of Standard Precautions in avoiding contact with all body fluids during patient care dramatically reduces the risk for caregiver infection (see Box 9-1).

The rate of new infections is rising more rapidly in minority populations, especially among blacks and Hispanics. Worldwide, there are now more than 40 million cases of HIV/AIDS, with more than 80% occurring in developing countries. Patients in these countries often lack access to adequate drug therapy, resulting in millions of orphaned children each year. Untreated HIV-infected pregnant women transmit the virus to their infant in 15% to 30% of pregnancies. This can occur transplacentally, causing infection in utero, or during birth. When the first antiretroviral drugs were developed in the 1980s, it was feared that they would be too toxic and even teratogenic if given to pregnant women. However, prophylactic antiretroviral treatment of infected mothers has been shown to reduce infant infection by at least two thirds and is not normally harmful to either mother or infant. Medication may also be given prophylactically to the newborn infant, typically for the first 6 weeks of life. Of course, infants and children with established HIV infection must usually continue on medication indefinitely. Prescribers are encouraged to register patients with the designated Antiretroviral Pregnancy Registry (www.apregistry.com) that serves to monitor maternal and fetal outcomes of antiretroviral drug therapy. Although the website explains the purpose and processes of the registry, actual registration and follow-up occurs by phone at 800-258-4263. Breast milk can transmit the virus to the infant in 10% to 20% of cases, and, therefore, breast-feeding is contraindicated in more developed countries. In developing countries, however, breast-feeding may be the only available source of nutrition for the infant and therefore worth the risk. This is especially true if medications and other health services are lacking, as is often the case. Box 39-2 summarizes key epidemiologic concepts related to HIV/AIDS.

HIV infection that is untreated or treatment-resistant eventually leads to severe immune system failure with death occurring secondary to opportunistic infections. The infection often progresses over a period of several years. Various health organizations, including the Centers for Disease Control and Prevention (CDC) and the World Health Organization (WHO), have published classification systems describing various "stages" of this infection. In 1993, the CDC model listed five stages. A more recent WHO model lists four stages as follows:
- Stage 1: Asymptomatic infection
- Stage 2: Early, general symptoms of disease
- Stage 3: Moderate symptoms
- Stage 4: Severe symptoms, often leading to death

Stage 1 refers to the first few weeks or months after initial exposure to the virus. Patients may be asymptomatic but may show signs of *persistent generalized lymphoadenopathy (PGL)*, or swollen lymph nodes ("swollen glands"). PGL is more specifically defined as inflammation of the lymph nodes in at least

---

Box 39-2 Epidemiology of HIV Infection

Disease Viral Factors
- Developed virus is easily inactivated and must be transmitted in body fluids
- Disease has a long prodromal or incubation period
- Virus can be shed before development of identifiable symptoms

Transmission
- Virus is present in blood, semen, and vaginal secretions

Who Is At Risk?
- Intravenous drug abusers; sexually active people with many partners (homosexual and heterosexual); prostitutes; newborns of HIV-positive mothers
- Blood and organ transplant recipients and hemophiliacs: before 1985 (prescreening programs)

Geographic Factors
- There is a continuously expanding epidemic worldwide
- No particular seasonal pattern of infection (e.g., unlike influenza)

Modes of Control
- Antiviral drugs limit progression of disease
- Vaccines for prevention and treatment are in trials
- Safe, monogamous sex helps limit spread
- Sterile injection needles should be used
- Large-scale screening programs have been developed for blood for transfusions, organs for transplants, and clotting factors used by hemophiliacs

From National Institutes of Health AIDS information website. Available at www.aidsinfo.nih.gov.
CMV, Cytomegalovirus; *CNS*, central nervous system; *HIV*, human immunodeficiency virus; *HSV*, herpes simplex virus.

---

two sites outside the inguinal (groin) area that lasts for some months. During this time, the virus is present in the blood at low levels and has a low rate of replication. CD4 cell counts are usually still within normal limits at 350 cells/mm^3 of blood. *CD4* refers to the protein on the cell surface of helper T lymphocytes, to which HIV virons attach themselves. As previously described, these helper T cells normally function by releasing *cytokines*. These are chemicals that activate and modulate *cell-mediated immunity*, which is a general term for all immune system actions other than those of antibodies. Immune system function is described further in Chapter 49. Helper T lymphocytes circulate in the blood and are the primary target cells for HIV. However, HIV may also infect macrophages, which are usually stationary (noncirculating) CD4-positive cells that remain in various tissues (e.g., lungs, skin, brain) to prevent infection. But it is ultimately through widespread destruction of these helper T cells in the blood that HIV infection eventually weakens the patient's immune system.

Stage 2 involves continued lymphadenopathy along with other symptoms, including fever, rash, sore throat, night sweats, malaise, diarrhea, idiopathic thrombocytopenia, oral candidiasis, and herpes zoster (shingles). In the early years of the epidemic (early 1980s), this stage was also known as *AIDS-related complex* or *ARC*. These symptoms may actually resolve spontaneously about the time of seroconversion, which is when the patient's own antibodies to the virus (HIV antibodies) begin to appear in blood samples. Seroconversion usually occurs 3 weeks to 3 months after exposure. At this point, the patient is said to be *HIV positive*. However, the patient may not have further progression of symptoms for 1 to 10 years. During this stage, the CD4+ T-cell count begins to drop, while HIV antibody levels rise as part of an attempt by the patient's own immune system to neutralize the virus. The virus begins to multiply in the body, but does not necessarily produce disabling symptoms. This stage is often the first presenting sign of HIV infection, and stage 1 may not have been noticed or reported by the patient.

During **stage 3**, the infection progresses to a moderately symptomatic state. Continued weight loss and chronic diarrhea and fever, CD4+ count continues to drop. Opportunistic infections (OIs) begin, including oral candidiasis (thrush), severe bacterial pneumonias, and pulmonary tuberculosis (TB). Pulmonary TB is usually more severe in persons with AIDS and is currently the leading cause of death worldwide for HIV-infected patients. Dually infected patients have a greater likelihood of developing active TB and becoming infectious. OIs are so named because the destruction by HIV of the patient's immune system gives the "opportunity" for normally harmless microorganisms in the body to proliferate into serious infections. They may become life threatening or produce significant disability (e.g., blindness from CMV retinitis).

Stage 4 (formerly called *full-blown AIDS*): Viral replication increases dramatically, resulting in increasing destruction of helper T cells and a corresponding decrease in CD4 counts. At this point, there is a major decline in immune system function, and the effects of the illness begin to seriously affect the entire body. When the CD4+ count drops below 200 cells/mm^3, multiple, severe OIs often begin to occur. Fever, night sweats, and malaise resume and are now accompanied by increasingly severe *opportunistic infections (OIs)*, such as *Mycobacterium avium* complex (MAC) and *Pneumocystis jirovecii* pneumonia. Other common OIs include parasitic infections such as cryptosporidial diarrhea and toxoplasmosis encephalitis; viral infections such as HSV mouth ulcers, disseminated extrapulmonary tuberculosis, esophagitis, pneumonitis, CMV pneumonia and CMV retinitis, and fungal infections, such as candidiasis of the gastrointestinal and respiratory tracts, and invasive aspergillosis of the lungs. A similar opportunistic situation occurs with HIV-associated neo-plasms. The most common of these include Kaposi's sarcoma, and various types of lymphoma. There is also some evidence that cervical cancer is more likely to be in advanced stages upon diagnosis, in HIV-infected women. *HIV wasting syndrome* is yet another defining condition of the disease and involves major weight loss, chronic diarrhea, more frequent or even constant fever, and chronic fatigue. In addition to its attack on helper T-cells and macrophages, the HIV virus itself can also cause additional pathology in such organs as the brain (HIV-induced encephalopathy and dementia), bone marrow, lungs (recurrent pneumonia), and skin. Death is most likely when CD4+ count falls below 50 cells/mm^3. The viral load, which is measured as the number of viral RNA copies per milliliter of blood, also continues to rise uncontrollably. If this condition continues, death often ensues. All of these manifestations are said to be the *defining conditions* of AIDS. Box 39-3 lists several such conditions.

Figure 39-4 illustrates events that roughly correlate with these four stages of HIV infection. This figure refers to the hypothetical natural course of the disease, through the above states, *without* treatment. Patients who are effectively treated with drug therapy usually do not progress through all of these stages, or at least, such progression is slowed considerably (years). In fact, advances in antiretroviral drug therapy have given rise to increasingly greater numbers of long-term survivors of HIV infection. *Highly active antiretroviral therapy (HAART)* refers to combinations of antiretroviral drugs ("cocktails") that are now standard for treating HIV-infected patients. HAART is normally begun immediately upon confirmation of HIV infection. Opportunistic infections are treated with infection-specific antimicrobial drugs (see corresponding chapters) as they arise. OIs are also commonly treated prophylactically, most commonly when a patient's CD4+ count falls below 200. Opportunistic malignancies, such as Kaposi's sarcoma and lymphomas, are also treated with specific antineoplastic medications, which are discussed in Chapters 47 and 48, as well as radiation and/or surgery as indicated. *Long-term survival* is defined as living with HIV infection for at least 10 to 15 years after infection. Some particularly remarkable patients have lived for several years

---

Box 39-3   Indicator Diseases of AIDS

Opportunistic Infections

Protozoal
- Toxoplasmosis of the brain
- Cryptosporidiosis with diarrhea
- Isosporiasis with diarrhea

Fungal
- Candidiasis of the esophagus, trachea, and lungs
- *Pneumocystis jirovecii* pneumonia
- Cryptococcosis (extrapulmonary)
- Histoplasmosis (disseminated)
- Coccidioidomycosis (disseminated)

Viral
- Cytomegalovirus disease
- HSV infection (persistent or disseminated)
- Progressive multifocal leukoencephalopathy
- Hairy leukoplakia caused by Epstein-Barr virus

Bacterial
- *Mycobacterium avium complex* (MAC) (disseminated)
- Any "atypical" mycobacterial disease
- Extrapulmonary TB
- *Salmonella* septicemia (recurrent)
- Pyogenic bacterial infections (multiple or recurrent)

Opportunistic Neoplasias
- Kaposi's sarcoma
- Primary lymphoma of the brain
- Other non-Hodgkin's lymphomas

Others
- HIV wasting syndrome
- HIV encephalopathy
- Lymphoid interstitial pneumonia

From Mandell GL et al: *Principles and practices of infectious diseases,* ed 6, Philadelphia, 2005, Churchill Livingstone.
AIDS, Acquired immunodeficiency syndrome; *HIV,* human immunodeficiency virus; *HSV,* herpes simplex virus; *MAC, Mycobacterium avium intracellular* complex; *TB,* tuberculosis.

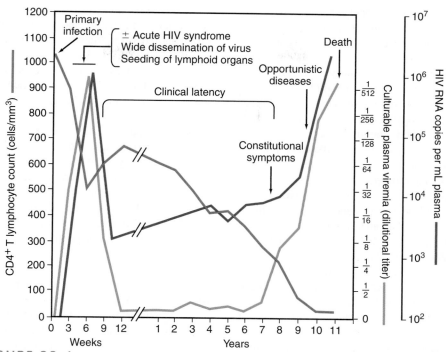

FIGURE 39-4 Natural history of HIV infection in the absence of therapy in a hypothetical patient. *(From Fauci AS, Pantaleo G, Stanley S, Weissman D: Immunopathogenic mechanisms of HIV infection.* Ann Intern Med *1996; 124:654-663. In Mandell GL, Bennett JE, Dolin R:* Principles and practice of infectious diseases, *ed 6, Philadelphia, 2005, Churchill Livingstone.)*

with CD4 counts remaining at the often fatal levels of 200 cells/mm³ or less. Improved drug therapy against both HIV and OIs is still believed to play an important role in these unusual cases. Other remarkable patients are the long-term nonprogressors. These are long-term survivors who have maintained normal CD4 counts and low HIV viral loads, despite not receiving *any* anti-HIV drug treatment! These patients are usually able to mount especially strong cell-mediated and humoral immune responses that prevent progression of the viral infection. They are also the subject of much research to identify the mechanisms of their survival and hopefully find ways to share these advantages with other patients. Research attempts to develop an effective anti-HIV vaccine are also underway throughout the world. There have been several *pre-clinical* (animal) studies using monkeys. Human clinical trials have been conducted since 1990, primarily on non-HIV-infected research volunteers. However, vaccines are also being studied in HIV-positive patients, with some data suggesting the possibility of vaccine-induced enhanced immune response that could retard disease progression. A variety of laboratory techniques have been used to manufacture the vaccines used in these research studies. Examples of these include attenuated HIV virions, HIV components (e.g., RNA alone), or other virus particles with HIV components attached (e.g., envelope proteins). Despite encouraging data regarding potential benefits, the design of an effective HIV vaccine continues to remain elusive.

ANTIRETROVIRAL DRUGS

Much has happened in medical science since the AIDS virus was first identified in the early 1980s. The increasing urgency and public awareness of the HIV epidemic has stimulated much re-search into the fields of immunology and pharmacology. This has resulted in the development of several increasingly effective antiretroviral drugs, as well as antiviral drugs in general. Although new drug combinations have definitely prolonged lives and offered hope to many people, these medications often carry significant toxicities. Furthermore, HIV/AIDS is still not normally considered to be a curable disease, although there have been some remarkable recoveries and apparent cures in a small number of individuals. There are currently five classes of antiretroviral drugs, including three distinct classes of *reverse transcriptase inhibitors (RTIs)*; the *protease inhibitors (PIs)*; and the newest class, the *fusion inhibitors*, which currently includes only one medication.

Mechanism of Action and Drug Effects

Although HIV/AIDS is a very complex illness, the mechanisms of action of the various drug classes are, fortunately, straightforward and distinct. The name of each class of medication provides a reminder of its role in suppressing the viral replication process. RTIs, therefore, work by blocking activity of the enzyme reverse transcriptase, which promotes the synthesis of new viral DNA molecules from the RNA genome of the parent virion. There are currently three subclasses of RTIs: nucleoside RTIs, or NRTIs (seven drugs); non-nucleoside RTIs, or NNRTIs (three drugs); and nucleo*tide* RTIs, or NTRTIs (one drug).

There are currently seven PIs. These drugs work by inhibiting the *protease* retroviral enzyme. This enzyme promotes the breakup of chains of protein molecules at designated points, a process necessary for viral replication. There is also one combination protease inhibitor that includes both lopinavir and ritonavir. Both medications are protease inhibitors. The ritonavir component also serves to inhibit *cytochrome P-450*–mediated enzymatic metabolism of the lopinavir component. There is currently only one fusion inhibitor. This compound works by inhibiting viral fusion. This is the process by which an HIV virion attaches (fuses with) the membrane of a host cell (T lymphocyte) before infecting it in preparation for viral replication. All of these medications are listed in the corresponding dosages table, in addition to three NRTI combination drug products.

Single-drug therapy was most common in the early years of the HIV epidemic, partly due to a lack of treatment options. However, both the development of multiple antiretroviral drugs and the emergence of resistant viral strains have given rise to combination drug therapy as the current standard of care. This is the most effective treatment to date and is referred to as *highly active antiretroviral therapy* (HAART). HAART usually includes at least three medications. The most commonly recommended drug combinations include two or three NRTIs; two NRTIs plus one or two PIs; or an NRTI plus an NNRTI with one or two PIs. Despite the effectiveness of HAART, prescribers may still need to alter a given patient's drug regimen in the case of major drug intolerance (see Adverse Effects) or drug resistance. A given patient's HIV strain can still evolve and mutate over time, allowing it to adaptively become resistant to any drug therapy, especially when used for a prolonged period of time, as is usually the case with HIV treatment. Evidence for drug resistance includes a falling $CD4^+$ count and/or increased viral load in a patient for whom a given drug regimen previously kept those symptoms under control.

All antiretroviral drugs have, to varying degrees, similar therapeutic effects. They reduce the viral load, which is the number of viral RNA copies per milliliter of blood. A viral load of less than 50 copies/mL is considered to be an undetectable viral load and is a primary goal of antiretroviral therapy. HIV-infected patients should ideally be followed by practitioners with extensive training in drug therapy for infectious diseases. These practitioners must often make careful choices and changes in drug therapy over time, based on a given patient's clinical response and severity of any drug-related toxicities. When effective, treatment leads to a significant reduction in mortality and the incidence of opportunistic infections, improves patient's physical performance, and significantly improves T-cell counts.

Indications

As indicated in Table 39-3, the only usual indication for all of the current antiretroviral drugs is active HIV infection. Prophylactic therapy is also given to individuals (e.g., health care workers and high-risk infants) with known potential exposure to HIV (e.g., via needlestick injuries in hospitals [Table 39-5]).

Contraindications

Keeping in mind the potentially fatal outcome of HIV infection, the only usual contraindication to a given medication is known severe drug allergy or other intolerable toxicity. Fortunately, the past 25 years that saw the rise of the HIV pandemic were also marked by the development of several categories of antiretroviral medications. Most of the current antiretroviral drug classes have several alternative drugs to choose from, should a patient be especially intolerant of a given drug.

Adverse Effects

Common adverse effects of selected antiretroviral drugs are listed in Table 39-4. A few key adverse effects are discussed in more detail later. It is not uncommon to need to modify drug therapy because of adverse effects. The goal is to find the regimen that will best control a given patient's infection, with as tolerable an adverse-effect profile as possible. Different patients can vary widely in their drug tolerance, and a given patient's drug tolerance may change over time. Thus, medication regimens often must be strategically individualized and evolve with the course of the patient's illness. HAART, although certainly an effective treatment against HIV infection, also has a significant downside. Approximately 25% of HIV-infected patients in the United States are also infected with hepatitis C virus (HCV), which also tends to be more severe in HIV patients. The most common route of transmission of HCV is through needle sharing, with sexual and perinatal routes much less common. HCV is the most important cause of chronic liver disease in the United States. HCV-induced liver failure is the most common reason for liver transplantation, and liver cancer may also occur secondary to HCV infection. Unfortunately, HAART, because of the pharmacologic strain that it places on the liver, is strongly correlated with increased mortality from HCV-induced liver disease. A major adverse effect of protease inhibitor involves lipid abnormalities including *lipodystrophy*, or redistribution of fat stores under the skin. This condition often results in cosmetically un-

Table 39-5	Recommendations for Occupational HIV Exposure Chemoprophylaxis		
Type of Exposure	**Source**	**Prophylaxis**	**Therapy**
Percutaneous	Blood	Recommended	Zidovudine + lamivudine + indinavir; zidovudine + lamivudine +/− indinavir
	Fluid containing visible blood or other potentially infectious fluid or tissue		
Mucous membrane	Blood	Offer	Zidovudine + lamivudine
	Fluid containing visible blood or other potentially infectious fluid or tissue	Offer	Zidovudine + lamivudine +/− indinavir
		Offer	Zidovudine +/− lamivudine
Skin (i.e., prolonged contact, extensive area, area without skin integrity)	Blood	Offer	Zidovudine + lamivudine +/− indinavir

desirable outcomes for the patient, such as a "hump" at the posterior base of the neck, and also a *skeletonized* (bony) appearance of the face. In addition, dyslipidemias such as hypertriglyceridemia, can occur, even resulting in insulin resistance and type 2 diabetes symptoms. It is reported that in these cases, switching a patient from a PI to an NNRTI such as nevirapine may help reduce such symptoms without reducing antiretroviral efficacy. With increasing long-term antiretroviral drug therapy due to prolonged disease survival, another emerging long-term adverse effect associated with these medications is bone demineralization and possible osteoporosis. When this condition occurs, it may require treatment with standard medications for osteoporosis, such as calcium, vitamin D, and bisphosphonates (Chapter 33).

Interactions

Common selected drug interactions involving both antiretrovirals and other antivirals are listed in Box 39-1.

Dosages

Dosage and other information for all of the currently available antiretroviral medications, including combination drug products, is listed in the corresponding dosages table.

Drug Profiles

enfuvirtide

Enfuvirtide (Fuzeon) is the newest medication in the newest class of antiretroviral drugs. It received accelerated approval by the FDA in March of 2003 and is classified as a *fusion inhibitor*. It works by suppressing the fusion process whereby a virion is attached to the outer membrane of a host T cell before entry into the cell and subsequent viral replication. This mechanism of action serves as yet another example of how antiretroviral drugs are strategically designed to interfere with specific steps of the viral replication process. As mentioned previously, the use of combinations of drugs that work by different mechanisms improves a patient's chances for continued survival by reducing the likelihood of viral resistance to the drug-therapy regimen. Enfuvirtide is indicated for treatment of HIV infection in combination with other antiretroviral drugs. Adult and pediatric patients have shown comparable tolerance of the drug in clinical trials thus far. Use of this drug in combination with other standard antiretroviral drugs has been associated with markedly reduced viral loads, when compared with drug regimens that did not include this drug. The drug is currently available only in injectable form.

Pharmacokinetics

Half-Life	Onset	Peak	Duration
SC: 4 hr	SC: Unknown	SC: 6 hr	SC: Unknown

▶ indinavir

Indinavir (Crixivan) belongs to the *protease inhibitor (PI)* class of antiretroviral drugs. Others include ritonavir (Norvir), saquinavir (Invirase, Fortovase), nelfinavir (Viracept), amprenavir (Agenerase), fosamprenavir (Lexiva), atazanavir (Reyataz), and the combination product lopinavir/ritonavir (Kaletra). Indinavir can be taken in combination with other anti-HIV therapies or alone. However, this drug is best dissolved and absorbed in an acidic gastric environment, and the presence of high-protein and high-fat foods reduces its absorption. Therefore, it is recommended that it is administered in a fasting state. Indinavir therapy produces increases in CD4 cell counts, an important measure of immune system function. It also produces significant reductions in viral load, or levels

of HIV in the bloodstream. PIs are commonly given in combination with two RTIs to maximize efficacy and decrease the likelihood of viral drug resistance. Indinavir is relatively well tolerated in most patients. Nephrolithiasis (kidney stones) can occur in approximately 4% of patients. Patients who take indinavir are encouraged to drink at least 48 oz of liquids every day to maintain hydration and help avoid nephrolithiasis. Indinavir and all other PIs are available only for oral use.

Pharmacokinetics

Half-Life	Onset	Peak	Duration
PO: 1.5-2.5 hr	PO: 2 wk*	PO: 0.5-1 hr	PO: 6 mo

*Therapeutic effects.

▶ nevirapine

Nevirapine (Viramune) is *a non-nucleoside reverse transcriptase inhibitor (NNRTI)*. This is the second class of antiviral drugs indicated for the treatment of HIV infection. Other currently available NNRTIs include delavirdine (Rescriptor) and efavirenz (Sustiva). These drugs are often used in combination with *nucleoside reverse transcriptase inhibitors (NRTIs)* such as zidovudine.

Nevirapine is well tolerated when compared with other therapies for HIV. The most common adverse events associated with nevirapine therapy are rash, fever, nausea, headache, and abnormal liver function tests. Nevirapine and the other NNRTIs are available only for oral use.

Pharmacokinetics

Half-Life	Onset	Peak	Duration
PO: 25-30 hr	PO: 2 hr*	PO: 2-4 hr	PO: 24 hr

*Therapeutic effects.

tenofovir

Tenofovir (Viread) is the first, and currently the only, *nucleotide reverse transcriptase inhibitor (NTRTI)*. It is an analog of adenine but has an attached phosphate group, which distinguishes this drug class from the nucleo*side* RTIs. This drug is indicated for use against HIV infection in combination with other antiretroviral drugs. It is currently available only for oral use.

Pharmacokinetics

Half-Life	Onset	Peak	Duration
PO: Unknown	PO: Unknown	PO: 1 hr	PO: Unknown

▶ zidovudine

Zidovudine (AZT, ZDV, Retrovir) is a synthetic nucleoside analog of thymidine that has had an enormous impact on the treatment and quality of life of patients infected with HIV who have AIDS. It was the very first, and for a long time the only, anti-HIV medication that offered patients with AIDS any hope in the early years of the epidemic. Other NRTIs include lamivudine (Epivir), zalcitabine (Hivid), didanosine (Videx), stavudine (Zerit), abacavir (Ziagen), and emtricitabine (Emtriva). Zidovudine, along with various other antiretroviral drugs, is given to HIV-infected pregnant women and even to newborn babies to prevent maternal transmission of the virus to the infant.

The major dose-limiting adverse effect of zidovudine is bone-marrow suppression, and this is often the reason a patient with an HIV infection has to be switched to another anti-HIV drug such as zalcitabine or didanosine. Some patients may receive a combination of two of these drugs, in lower doses, to maximize their combined actions. This strategy may reduce the likelihood of toxicity. Zidovudine is available in both oral and injectable formulations.

Pharmacokinetics

Half-Life	Onset	Peak	Duration
0.78-1.93 hr	Unknown	0.4-1.5 hr	3-5 hr

DOSAGES

Antiretroviral Drugs

Drug (Pregnancy Category)	Pharmacologic Class	Usual Dosage Range	Indications
abacavir (Ziagen) (C)	Nucleoside reverse transcriptase inhibitor	**Pediatric 3 mo-15 yr** PO: 8 mg/kg bid (max 300 mg/dose) **16 yr-adult** PO: 300 mg bid	
amprenavir (Agenerase) (C)	Protease inhibitor	**Pediatric 4-12 yr or <50 kg** PO: 20 mg/kg bid or 15 mg/kg tid **13-16 yr-adult or >50 kg** PO: 1200 mg bid	
atazanavir (Reyataz) (B)	Protease inhibitor	**Adult** PO: 300-400 mg once daily	
delavirdine (Rescriptor, DLV) (C)	Non-nucleoside reverse transcriptase inhibitor	**Pediatric 16 yr-adult** PO: 400 mg tid	
didanosine (Videx, Videx EC, ddI) (B)	Nucleoside reverse transcriptase inhibitor	**Pediatric (specific ages not listed)** PO: 120 mg/m^2 divided q12h **Adult (depending on weight)** PO: 250-400 mg qd or 125-200 mg bid	HIV infection
efavirenz (Sustiva, EFV) (C)	Non-nucleoside reverse transcriptase inhibitor	**Pediatric 3 yr-adult** PO: 200-600 mg once daily based on weight table	
emtricitabine (Emtriva) (B)	Nucleoside reverse transcriptase inhibitor	**Adult** PO: 600 mg once daily	
enfuvirtide (Fuzeon) (B)	Fusion inhibitor	**Pediatric 6-16 yr** SC: 2 mg/kg bid (max 90 mg/dose) **17 yr-adult** SC: 90 mg bid	
fosamprenavir (Lexiva) (C)	Protease Inhibitor	**Adult** PO: 700 mg bid-1400 mg qd-bid	
▶indinavir (Crixivan) (C)	Protease inhibitor	**Adult** PO: 800 mg q8h	
lamivudine (Epivir, Epivir-HBV, 3TC) (C)	Nucleoside reverse transcriptase inhibitor	**Pediatric 3 mo-15 yr** PO: 3 mg/kg once daily 16 yr-adult PO: 150 mg bid or 300 mg once daily	HIV and HBV
nelfinavir (Viracept) (B)	Protease inhibitor	**Pediatric 2-13 yr** PO: 20-30 mg/kg tid 14 yr-adult PO: 750 mg tid or 1250 mg bid	
▶nevirapine (Viramune, NVP) (C)	Non-nucleoside reverse transcriptase inhibitor	**Pediatric 2 mo-8 yr** PO: 4 mg/kg qd × 14 days, then 7 mg/kg bid **8 yr-adult** PO: 4 mg/kg qd × 14 days, then 4 mg/kg bid **Adult** PO: 200 mg qd × 14 days, then bid	
ritonavir (Norvir) (B)	Protease inhibitor	**Pediatric 2-16 yr** PO: 250-400 mg/m^2 bid (max 600 mg/dose) **Adult** PO: 300-600 mg bid	HIV infection
saquinavir (Invirase, Fortovase) (B)	Protease inhibitor	**16 yr-adult** PO (Invirase): 600 mg tid PO (Fortovase): 1200 mg tid	

*Drug should be continued either IV or PO through at least 6 wk of age.

NOTE: Where pediatric doses are not provided, dosing guidelines for pediatric patients are not firmly established for the drug in question and should be based on the careful clinical judgment of a qualified prescriber.

HBV, Hepatitis B virus; *HIV,* human immunodeficiency virus.

DOSAGES—cont'd

Antiretroviral Drugs

Drug (Pregnancy Category)	Pharmacologic Class	Usual Dosage Range	Indications
stavudine (Zerit, d4T) (C)	Nucleoside reverse transcriptase inhibitor	**Pediatric (specific ages not listed)** PO (birth-13 days): 0.5 mg/kg/dose q12h PO (14 days of age, weight, 30 kg): 1 mg/kg/dose q12h PO (weight 30 kg or greater): adult dose Adult **<60 kg** PO: 30 mg q12h **≥60 kg** PO: 40 mg q12h	
tenofovir (Viread) (B)	Nucleotide reverse transcriptase inhibitor	**Adult** PO: 300 mg once daily	
zalcitabine (Hivid, ddC) (C)	Nucleoside reverse transcriptase inhibitor	**13 yr-adult** PO: 0.75 mg q8h	
▸ zidovudine (Retrovir, AZT, ZDV) (C)	Nucleoside reverse transcriptase inhibitor	**Pediatric infants 0-3 mo*** PO: 2 mg/kg q6h starting within 12 hr after birth and through 6 wks of age IV: 1.5 mg/kg q6h **6 wks-12 yr** PO: 160 mg/m² q8h (max 200 mg/dose) **Adult** PO: 100 mg q4h round-the-clock if symptomatic; q4h while awake if asymptomatic IV: 1mg/kg over 1 hr; 5-6×/day **Pregnant women** PO: 100 mg 5×/day during pregnancy until start of labor, then give IV bolus dose of 2 mg/kg over 1 hr followed by an IV infusion of 1 mg/kg/hr until the umbilical cord is clamped	HIV infection

Combination Drug Products

abacavir/lamivudine/ zidovudine (Trizivir) (C)	Triple-drug combination nucleoside reverse transcriptase inhibitor	**Adolescent or adult ≥40 kg** PO: 1 tab bid (1 tab = 300 mg abacavir 150 mg lamivudine + 300 mg zidovudine)	
lamivudine/zidovudine (Combivir) (C)	Double-drug combination nucleoside reverse transcriptase inhibitor	**12 yr-adult** PO: 1 tab bid (1 tab = 150 mg lamivudine + 300 mg zidovudine)	
lopinavir/ritonavir (Kaletra) (C)	Double-drug combination protease-inhibitor	**Pediatric 7-14 kg** PO: 12 mg/kg bid **Pediatric 15-40 kg** PO: 10 mg/kg bid **Pediatric >40 kg or adult** PO: 3 caps or 5 mL bid (1 cap +133.3 mg lopinavir 33.3 mg ritonavir; for the oral solution, 1 mL contains = 80 mg lopinavir + 20 mg ritonavir)	

OTHER SIGNIFICANT VIRAL ILLNESSES OF RECENT CONCERN

There are numerous other viral infections that could be discussed in this chapter. However, three of recent special significance are Avian Flu, West Nile virus (WNV), and sudden acute respiratory syndrome (SARS). All three of these viral infections have resulted in significant morbidity and mortality, sometimes requiring aggressive supportive care in an intensive care unit (ICU) setting.

In 1999, the first North American cases of WNV occurred in New York City. WNV is a member of the arbovirus family and is transmitted to humans by mosquitoes. It also infects animals, primarily birds, and has been detected in horses and cows. In humans, it can lead to meningitis and encephalitis. In 2001, an epidemic occurred with more than 4000 documented human cases, including 284 deaths. Organ transplant patients constituted one of the key groups infected. The virus can also be transmitted through blood transfusions and has been detected in breast milk. It is currently being investigated for maternal–fetal transmission during pregnancy. In July 2003, national blood banks began screening blood donations for WNV using newly developed laboratory techniques. There are currently no specific antiviral medications or vaccines available for treatment of human WNV infection. In the more severe cases that involve encephalitis, aggressive supportive measures, such as monitoring and control of intracranial pressure (ICP), can be crucial. Mannitol diuresis is one method of reducing ICP. Prevention focuses on reducing mosquito reproduction by eliminating unneeded pools of water near residential environments.

November of 2002 was marked by the emergence of a new, serious viral illness known as sudden acute respiratory syndrome, or SARS. A large outbreak later occurred in Singapore in March of 2003. This outbreak was eventually traced to a traveler returning from Hong Kong. Cases later appeared in Europe and North America. The SARS illness can range from a mild to a life-threatening respiratory syndrome. The illness usually resolves on its own within 3 to 4 weeks. However, 10% to 20% of patients required mechanical ventilation and intensive care support, with an overall fatality rate of 3%. Although standard antiviral drugs were used, including oseltamivir, no specific drug therapy proved to be definitively helpful. Thanks to a global public health response coordinated by the World Health Organization, transmission of this virus was apparently halted worldwide as of July 2003. At that point, however, there had been at least 8100 cases of SARS, including more than 800 deaths. The cause of SARS was also determined to be a coronavirus, which was named the SARS coronavirus (SARS-CoV). Coronaviruses commonly cause mild-to-moderate upper respiratory illnesses in humans, including the common cold. The CDC, along with a Canadian laboratory, were able to sequence the genome of this virus.

Avian influenza or "bird flu" is an influenza virus infection that has been shown to infect birds in Europe and both birds and humans in Asia. This disease is caused by an influenza A virus known as *avian influenza A, subtype H5N1*. The virus is carried in the intestines of many wild birds worldwide, often without causing any serious illness. The most common bird symptoms include ruffled feathers and reduced egg production. However, more serious infections can be fatal and spread rapidly among an entire flock of birds. Usually, these viruses do not infect humans. However, since 1997, there have been cases of human infection, mostly following contact with infected birds or their secretions or excrement (e.g., poultry workers). Most of these cases have occurred in Europe and Asia. However, there has also been one case each documented in New York and Virginia with H7N2, another avian influenza virus subtype. Human to human transmission has been especially rare, and normally occurred no further than between two people. Interestingly, it is believed that at least some genetic parts of current human influenza A viruses originally came from birds. Human symptoms have ranged from typical flu-like symptoms such as fever, cough, sore throat, and muscle aches, to eye infections and acute respiratory illness, with even life-threatening complications. In the current outbreaks in Asia and Europe, more than half of those infected with the virus have died. Most cases have occurred in previously healthy children and young adults. This virus is resistant to amantadine and rimantadine, although it is believed (but remains to be confirmed) that zanamivir and oseltamivir would likely offer some therapeutic benefit for this condition. Vaccine trials are also in progress, but there is currently no commercially available vaccine against this virus. Many health experts fear a flu pandemic with this virus, should it mutate to a more easily transmissible form. This occurs frequently with influenza viruses in general, which is why a new seasonal flu vaccine must be developed each year. However, although no one can predict if and when such a pandemic might occur with the H5N1 virus, WHO and other health agencies, including the CDC, are continuously monitoring H5N1 activity patterns as well as its resistance to other antiviral drugs. Some countries, including the United States, have also implemented a ban on the import of birds from countries where avian influenza has been shown to be prevalent.

◆ NURSING PROCESS

◆ ASSESSMENT

Before administering an antiviral drug, the nurse should perform a thorough medical and physical assessment and medication history. This is important to ensure safe medication use. Any known allergies to the medication should be noted. It is important for the nurse to also assess the patient's nutritional status and baseline vital signs because of the profound effects viral illnesses have, especially if the patient is immunosuppressed. Contraindications, cautions, and drug interactions associated with all of the antiviral drugs have been previously discussed.

Assessment related to the use of *antivirals* includes inquiry about the patient's allergy to medications as well as a listing of any prescription and over-the-counter drugs, herbals, and dietary supplements. Assessment of energy levels, weight loss, vital signs, and the characteristics of any visible lesions should be documented for baseline comparison once therapy is initiated. Age is also important to assess, owing to the fact that safety and efficacy have not been proven in children younger than 2 years of age. Elderly patients may require dosage adjustments because of altered renal and hepatic functioning. There should be further concern for patients who are taking other medications that are nephrotoxic, and, if there is underlying dehydration or mineral and electrolyte imbalances these conditions need to be managed before therapy. Assess information about the drug being used to ensure safe use. A blood test for HIV antibodies should also be done because if there are undiagnosed and/or untreated HIV infections, there is risk for possible HIV resistance. Results of related lab testing should always be assessed, including white blood cell (WBC) count, red blood cell (RBC) count, blood urea nitrogen (BUN), creatinine clearance, and liver function studies. If drugs are being used for influenza A viral infections (e.g., amantadine hydrochloride), there should be great caution taken if there is a history of heart failure or orthostatic hypotension because of cardiovascular adverse effects. Assessment of the patient's cardiac system is important with attention to heart sounds, heart rate and blood pressure as well as the documentation of any underlying edema, such as pedal edema. Specimens from blood, feces, throat, and urine may also be ordered prior to drug therapy. With the antiviral drug, ribavirin, respiratory secretions should be obtained for diagnostic purposes and given only after baseline renal, hepatic, cardiac, and pulmonary functioning have been documented. Breath sounds, respiratory rate and patterns, cough, and sputum production should also be assessed and noted.

Antiretrovirals include a variety of drugs that fall within five different classes of drugs that were previously discussed, including cautions, contraindications, and drug interactions. These drugs are discussed by antiretroviral class, with attention to specific drugs as deemed appropriate. The PIs also fall within this category of antiretrovirals. Use of these drugs requires assessment of the patient's medical history, vital signs, baseline weight, allergies, medication history, and baseline laboratory tests such as complete blood counts and renal/hepatic studies. These laboratory tests should also be conducted, as ordered, throughout the phases of treatment. Age is an important assessment factor owing to the fact that many of the drugs (e.g., abacavir) cannot be used in pediatrics safely for those between ages 3 months and 13 years. Dosages may need to be reduced in elderly patients. With some of these drugs, specifically didanosine, the patient should be assessed for alcoholism and elevated serum triglycerides (of concern with other antiretrovirals as well). T-cell counts must also be assessed, and if these cells are less than 100 cells/mm^3, there would be concern for use of this drug. Didanoine must also be used extremely cautiously in patients who are on sodium-restricted or phenylketonuria-restricted diets because of the sodium content of the drug itself. Ritonavir requires specific attention to blood glucose levels, serum lipase, ALT and AST, serum triglyceride levels, and allergy to sulfonamide drugs due to cross sensitivity. With nevirapine, information about the patient's use of oral contraceptives is important because of decreased effectiveness of the birth control method. Combination therapy with ritonavir and nucleosides (e.g., stavudine, zalcitabine) may lead to gastrointestinal disturbances, so assessing the patient for any preexisting gastrointestinal illnesses is important. It has been recommended that ritonavir be initiated first, with the nucleosides added before completing 2 weeks of the ritonavir. Peripheral neuropathies may occur with stavudine, so a thorough neurologic assessment is also important prior to starting drug therapy. Assess baseline

complete blood cell counts with attention to RBCs, WBCs, and platelets with the use of zidovidine because of the risk for myelosuppression. These hematologic tests should continue during therapy.

With any of the drugs presented in this chapter, especially those used for treatment/management of HIV, assessment of the patient's knowledge about their illness and need for long-term and often lifelong therapy is crucial. In addition, educational level, reading level, how the patient learns best, and knowledge about community resources are important to effectively implement patient education. Assessment of mental status and emotional state is important because of the psychological impact of chronic illness. Value systems, social patterns, hobbies, values, support systems, knowledge of community resources, and spiritual beliefs should also be noted and documented. With chronic illnesses, the synthesis of this information will help ensure the development of a nursing care plan that is complete and holistic.

◆ NURSING DIAGNOSES

- Acute pain related to the signs and symptoms associated with viral infections and HIV and related illnesses
- Risk for injury related to falls due to the adverse effects of antiviral and antiretroviral medications
- Risk for injury to self, related to the immunosuppressive effects of viral disease processes and their treatment
- Deficient knowledge related to the lack of information and experience with long-term medication therapy and lack of information about viral infections, its transmission, and treatment
- Activity intolerance related to weakness secondary to decreased energy from pathology of viral infections
- Risk for impaired tissue integrity from a break in skin due to viral lesions

◆ PLANNING
Goals

- Patient is free of symptoms of viral infection once therapy is completed.
- Patient remains compliant or adheres to prescribed therapy.
- Patient experiences improved energy and appetite and improved ability to engage in activities of daily living for the duration of therapy.
- Patient states the rationale for treatment of self and for any of their active sexual partners if diagnosed with genital herpes or other viral sexually transmitted diseases.
- Patient experiences minimal adverse effects of antivirals and antiretrovirals.
- Patient states diminished signs and symptoms of viral infection with drug therapy.
- Patient states healing of lesions and restoration of intact skin integrity.
Outcome Criteria

- Patient experiences increased periods of comfort as a result of successful treatment of viral infection.
- Patient states the physical impact and effect of a viral infection on their overall state of health (e.g., compromised immune system) and the consequences and impact of the appropriate therapy with either antivirals or antiretrovirals.
- Patient states the rationale for his or her own treatment as well as for treatment of any partners with whom the patient has

been sexually active to prevent worsening of symptoms and to decrease severity of episodes related to genital herpes and other viral diseases.

- Patient identifies the possible adverse effects of the antivirals, such as diarrhea, headache, nausea, and insomnia.
- Patient identifies the possible adverse effects of the antiretrovirals such as gastrointestinal upset, peripheral neuropathies, immunosuppression, malaise, loss of energy, and loss of strength.
- Patient communicates the appropriate and recommended measures to prevent spread of viral infection as well as means of containing, prevention of spread, and promotion of healing of lesions during and after antiviral or antiretroviral therapy.

◆ IMPLEMENTATION

Nursing interventions pertinent to patients receiving *antivirals* include use of the appropriate technique of application or administration of ointment, aerosol powders, or intravenous or oral forms of medication (see Box 9-1). Wearing gloves and thorough handwashing, before and after administration of the medication, are necessary to prevent contamination of the site and spread of infection. Remember that strict adherence to standard precautions is important to the safety of both the patient and the nurse. The antivirals (and antiretrovirals) may lead to superimposed infection or superinfections and must be constantly monitored for as well as measures implemented for prevention (Chapters 37 and 38).

Oral antivirals should be given with meals to help with gastrointestinal upset. Capsules should be stored at room temperature, and they should not be crushed or broken. Topical dosage forms (e.g., acyclovir) should be applied using a finger cot or rubber glove to prevent autoinoculation. Eye contact should be avoided. IV acyclovir is stable for 12 hours at room temperature and will often precipitate when refrigerated. IV infusions should be diluted as recommended (e.g., with D₅W or 0.9% NaCl) and infused with caution. Infusions over 1 hour are suggested to avoid the renal tubular damage seen with more rapid infusions. Adequate hydration should be encouraged during and for several hours after the infusion to prevent drug-related crystalluria. Continual assessment of the IV site should occur, and any redness, heat, pain, swelling or red streaks would indicate possible phlebitis. Lesions should be documented in regard to their characteristics. Appropriate isolation for individuals with chickenpox or herpes zoster should be implemented, and analgesics should be given for comfort. Laboratory testing for renal and hepatic functioning should be ongoing with use of antivirals as well as constant monitoring of the patient's CBC. Vital signs with attention to blood pressure should be monitored throughout therapy with these medications, especially acyclovir and amantadine, because of drug-related orthostatic hypotension.

Amantadine, and other antivirals, should be taken for the entire course of therapy and if a dose is missed it is important for the patient to take the dose as soon as it is remembered or contact the health care provider for further instructions. Should dry mouth occur, sugarless candy and gum might be helpful. Daily mouth care, including the use of dental floss and regular dental preventive visits, is encouraged. Saliva substitutes may be needed, and should dry mouth continue for more than 2 weeks, the health care provider should be contacted for further management. Li-

vedo reticularis, a red-blue network mottling of skin caused by congestion of the superficial capillaries, may occur, and patient education about this is important. Discontinuation of amantadine hydrochloride will reverse this effect. It is often recommended to give the second dose of drug several hours before bedtime to prevent insomnia.

Famciclovir should be taken for the full course of therapy, and with patients who have genital herpes, the directions are usually to provide evenly spaced doses and around the clock. Ganciclovir, if given IV, should be diluted with D₅W or 0.9% NaCl and at a concentration and time frame that are noted by the physician and authoritative sources. Large veins are recommended to provide the dilution needed to minimize the risk for vein irritation. If handling the solution of ganciclovir, be sure to avoid exposure of the drug to eyes, mucous membranes, or skin and use of latex gloves and safety glasses is recommended for handling and preparation. Should there be contact of this drug to these areas, wash/rinse the affected areas thoroughly with soap and water, and rinse/flush the eyes with plain water. Ribavirin may be given by nasal or oral inhalation.

There are aerosol generators available from the drug manufacturer. Reservoir solutions should be discarded if levels are low or empty and changed every 24 hours. Patients taking ribavirin and like drugs for RSV treatment via the Viratex Small Particle Aerosol Generator (SPAG) device should be taught how to properly mix and administer the drug. It should be reconstituted (e.g., ribavirin powder) as instructed by the manufacturer guidelines. Old solutions that are residual in the equipment should be discarded before adding fresh medication. Drugs administered via Viratex SPAG equipment are usually administered 12 to 18 hours daily for up to 7 days, beginning within 3 days of the onset of symptoms. There is also much controversy about use of this drug in ventilator patients, and only those who are specially trained with this drug and its use should administer it. Any "rainout" in the tubing of ventilators should be emptied frequently, and the nurse should always monitor breath sounds in patients receiving inhaled forms of this drug whether they are ventilator-dependent or not. Zanamivir is used per inhalation using a Diskhaler device, and it is important to be sure that the patient exhales completely first, then—while holding the mouthpiece 1 inch away from the patient's lips—instruct patients to inhale deeply and then hold their breath as long as possible prior to exhaling the drug and breath. Rinsing of the mouth with water is needed to prevent irritation and dryness. In addition, during treatment with any of the antivirals, blood counts including platelets, neutrophils, and thrombocytes should be performed periodically during therapy.

Antiretrovirals include numerous drugs, and a review of "general" types of nursing actons is presented as well as specific drug-related information as appropriate. In regard to dosage forms, it is important to realize that there are special administration and handling guidelines for some of the antiretroviral drugs. Delavirdine mesylate should first be dispersed in 6 ounces of water prior to taking it. Didanosine in tablet forms should be dispersed in water, and it remains stable for 1 hour at room temperature. The oral solution remains stable for approximately 4 hours. Give the oral dosage form 1 hour before or 2 hours after meals to help with absorption of this drug. If chewable dosage forms are given, make sure that the drug is thoroughly crushed and dispersed in at least 30 mL of water before having the patient swallow the mixture. The mixture must be mixed very well and then taken immediately. DO NOT mix didanosine with any form of acidic liquid, such as fruit juice, because it will become unstable in the acidic pH. Enteric coated forms should be taken on an empty stomach if tolerated. Always check manufacturer guidelines for any specific information as listed earlier. With didanosine, lamivudine, zalcitabine, and zidovudine, it is important to continually be aware of liver-related adverse effects, such as abdominal pain, elevated serum amylase or triglycerides, nausea, and vomiting, and to report these immediately to the health care provider, as they may indicate pancreatitis. Monitoring for peripheral neuropathies during therapy is important, with attention to any restless leg syndrome or burning of the feet and/or lack of muscle coordination. If the patient should experience signs and symptoms of opportunistic infections (e.g., respiratory signs and symptoms, fever, changes in oral mucosa), the physician should be contacted immediately. Weigh patients or encourage them to weigh themselves at least 2 times a week and report a gain of 2 pounds or more in 24 hours or 5 pounds or more in 1 week. Visual or hearing changes with didanosine should be reported as well. Headaches may occur with some of these drugs, and, therefore, be sure to provide analgesia as ordered.

With some of the antiretrovirals, avoidance of high-fat meals and an altered dosage amount for elderly patients are recommended, but only as ordered. Film-coated oral dosage forms should not be altered in any way. The taste of ritonavir may be improved by mixing it with chocolate milk or a nutritional beverage within 1 hour of its dosing. Ritonavir's dosage form should be protected from light. Zidovudine's absorption of oral dosages are not interfered by simultaneous food or milk, but it is important to keep the patient upright when giving the medication, and for up to 30 minutes after, to prevent esophageal ulceration. IV dosages should only be given if clear and not containing any particulate matter, using the appropriate dosage, diluents, and infusion time. Because these drugs often come in oral dosage forms, it is usually recommended to give these drugs with food. Zidovudine and other antiretrovirals are generally given in evenly spaced intervals around the clock—as ordered—to ensure steady state levels. With all oral and parenteral dosage forms of antiretrovirals, be sure to observe for nausea and vomiting as well as any changes in weight, occurrence of anorexia, and changes in bowel activities and patterns.

Other nursing interventions associated with these drugs include the following: (1) Continual monitoring of adverse effects throughout therapies with a focus on the various organ systems such as gastrointestinal, neurologic, renal, and hepatic. (2) With oral forms of indinavir and nevirapine, patients should drink at least 48 oz of fluids every day to maintain adequate hydration and help prevent nephrolithiasis. (3) Nevirapine, zidovudine, and like drugs may be associated with a rash; however, if the rash appears on the extremities, face, or trunk part of the body and is accompanied by blistering, fever, malaise, myalgias, oral lesions, swelling/edema, and conjunctivitis, the physician should be contacted immediately. (4) If drug therapy results in worsening of peripheral neuropathies, the specific drug may be discontinued by the physician. (5) Blood cell counts with attention to CBC, Hgb, and HIV RNA levels may be required throughout and after the drug regimen. See the Patient Teaching Tips for more information on both antivirals and antiretrovirals.

♦ **EVALUATION**

The therapeutic effects of antivirals and antiretrovirals include elimination of the virus or a decrease in the symptoms of the viral infections. There may be a delayed progression of HIV infections and AIDS as well as a decrease in flulike symptoms and/or the frequency of herpetic flare-ups and other lesion breakouts. Herpetic lesions should crust over, and the frequency of recurrence should decrease. In addition, there should be constant evaluation for the occurrence of adverse effects and toxicity to specific antiviral and antiretroviral drugs. These specific adverse effects are listed in Table 39-4. Remember to always re-evaluate the nursing care plan to ensure that the goals and outcome criteria have been met. It is also the nurse's responsibility to remain constantly attentive in the evaluation of reports from the CDC, other federal/state health care agencies, and public health care agencies regarding new strains of viruses and flu syndromes (see previous discussion).

CASE STUDY

Antiviral Therapy

One of your patients, Z.K., a 33-year-old biology professor, has just begun therapy with lamivudine/zidovudine (Combivir) for an HIV infection. She has many questions about this medication therapy, and you are meeting with her to review her questions.

She asks you why there are two drugs in this particular medication. What is your explanation?

Develop a patient teaching guide for Z.K., emphasizing any specific cautions and symptoms to report to the health care provider.

At what level with platelets and white blood cells would there probably be a change or discontinuation of this drug?

Patient Teaching Tips

- Patients should be educated about taking their medication exactly as prescribed and for the full course of therapy. Alert patients to the adverse effect of dizziness and to use caution while driving or participating in activities requiring alertness.
- Patients should consult the physician before taking any other prescribed or over-the-counter (OTC) medications.
- Educate patients that are immunocompromised to avoid crowds and persons with infections.
- Standard precautions and safe sex practices should be advocated for patients with sexually transmitted viral diseases, for example, those who are HIV positive. Condom use is a necessity in prevention of these viral infections, and presence of genital herpes requires sexual abstinence.
- Educate female patients with genital herpes to have a Pap test done every 6 months or as ordered by their health care provider to monitor the virus and especially its improvement with treatment. Cervical cancer has been found to be more prevalent in women with genital herpes simplex.
- Inform the patient that oral hygiene is needed several times a day with some of these antivirals because of drug-related gingival hyperplasia, with red and swollen oral mucosa and gums, with long-term use. Encourage patients to report the following adverse reactions to their health care provider, should they occur: decrease in urinary output, changes in sensorium and central nervous system, dizziness, confusion, syncope, nausea, vomiting, and diarrhea.
- Educate patients with demonstrations and pictures or other teaching aids about special application procedures (e.g., ophthalmic drops, use of finger cots/gloved hand with application to lesions).
- Educate patients to force fluids (e.g., 3000 mL/24 hr) unless contraindicated.
- Inform the patient that touching the lesions promotes spreading, so use of gloved hand/finger cots for application/cleansing is needed.

- Encourage patients to take the medication around the clock and in evenly spaced doses as ordered.
- Educate patients that antiviral drugs provide suppression of the virus and are not a cure!
- With respiratory inhalation forms (e.g., zanamivir), be sure educational instructions are clear and simple, with demonstrations on proper use of the delivery device for the dosage form.
- Inform patients that they should start therapy with drugs such as valacylcovir (or other antivirals) at the first sign of a recurrent episode of genital herpes or herpes zoster. Additionally, explain that early treatment within 24 to 48 hours is needed for the full therapeutic results.
- Inform patients about specific drug interactions (e.g., prescription, OTC, herbals).
- Encourage patients to immediately report to their physicians any difficulty breathing, drastic changes in blood pressure, bleeding, new symptoms, worsening of infection/fever/chills, or other unusual problems. Educate about the importance of follow-up appointments.
- Educate patients about drug-specific instructions (e.g., with didanosine, avoid alcohol due to the antabuse-type reaction; patients to take indinavir with water only and without food for the most optimal effects, though a light meal, skim milk, tea, or juice are acceptable and help decrease GI adverse effects; stavudine is associated with adverse effects such as abdominal discomfort, fatigue, dyspnea, numbness, nausea, tingling, vomiting, and weakness; with zidovudine, the patient should report any bleeding from their gums, nose, or rectum and to notify the physician if there is difficulty breathing, headache, insomnia, muscle weakness, or worsening of infection).

Points to Remember

- Viruses are difficult to kill and to treat because they live inside human cells, and most antiviral drugs work by inhibiting replication of the viral cell. Antiviral drugs include synthetic purine and pyrimidine nucleoside analogs.
- Antiviral drugs "trick" the virus into thinking that they are either a purine (a human amino acid [adenine or guanine]) or a pyrimidine (another amino acid [cytosine or thymine]) so that the virus cannot replicate.
- Purine analog antiretrovirals include drugs such as acyclovir, didanosine, and ganciclovir. Pyrimidine analog antiretroviral drugs include zalcitabine and zidovudine. Protease inhibitors are also considered to be antiretrovirals.

- Antiretroviral drugs should be administered only after physician orders are read and understood and after a thorough nursing assessment that includes an examination of the patient's nutritional status, weight, baseline vital signs, renal and hepatic functioning as well as assessment of heart sounds, neurologic status, and gastrointestinal/abdominal tract functioning.
- Comfort measures and supportive nursing care should accompany drug therapy. Patients should be encouraged to drink plenty of fluids and to space medications around the clock, as ordered, for maintaining states of the blood levels of the drug.

NCLEX Examination Review Questions

1. During treatment with zidovudine, the nurse needs to monitor for which potential adverse effect?
   a. Retinitis
   b. Deep vein thromboses
   c. Kaposi's sarcomas
   d. Bone marrow suppression
2. After giving an injection to a patient with HIV infection, the nurse accidentally receives a needlestick from a too-full needle-disposal box. Recommendations for occupational HIV exposure may include the use of which of the following?
   a. Didanosine
   b. Lamivudine and enfuvirtide
   c. Zidovudine, lamivudine, and indinavir
   d. Acyclovir
3. When teaching a patient who is taking acyclovir for genital herpes, which statement by the nurse is accurate?
   a. "This drug will help the lesions to dry and crust over."
   b. "Acyclovir will eradicate the herpes virus."
   c. "This drug will prevent the spread of this virus to others."
   d. "Acyclovir does not reduce the frequency of genital herpes outbreaks."

4. A patient who has been newly diagnosed with HIV has many questions about the effectiveness of drug therapy. After a teaching session, which statement by the patient reflects a need for more education?
   a. "I will be monitored while on this medicine for adverse effects and improvements."
   b. "These drugs do not eliminate the HIV, but hopefully the amount of virus in my body will be reduced."
   c. "There is no cure for HIV."
   d. "These drugs will eventually eliminate the virus from my body."
5. During a hospitalization for dehydration, an elderly patient also is receiving several doses of amantadine. Which statement explains the rationale for this medication therapy?
   a. Amantadine is used to prevent potential exposure to the HIV virus.
   b. This medication is given prophylactically to prevent influenza A infection.
   c. The drug is given intravenously to treat shingles.
   d. Amantadine works synergistically with antibiotics to reduce superinfections.

1. d, 2. c, 3. a, 4. d, 5. b.

Critical Thinking Activities

1. A 19-year-old male transfer college student from Germany to the United States was diagnosed with HIV approximately 7 months ago. He has been going through several treatment regimens but the infectious-disease physician is going to change his medication. He has been on several anti-HIV drugs and is now being treated with didanosine. He has experienced some bone marrow depression off and on during the last few months. Which condition(s) and/or health concern(s) would most likely lead to a change to didanosine? Discuss your answer.

2. One of your young adult female patients underwent a bone marrow transplant and less than a year postoperative contracted cytomegalovirus. Are antiviral drugs problematic for pregnant patients? Tell why or why not and explain your answer.
3. Discuss the use of rimantadine and amantadine in elderly patients. Is there a benefit of one drug over the other? Explain.

For answers, see http://evolve.elsevier.com/Lilley.

Antitubercular Drugs

Objectives

When you reach the end of this chapter, you should be able to do the following:

1. Identify the various first-line and second-line drugs indicated for the treatment of tuberculosis.
2. Discuss the mechanisms of action, dosages, adverse effects, routes of administration, special dosing considerations, cautions, contraindications, and drug interactions associated with the various antitubercular drugs.
3. Develop a nursing care plan that includes all phases of the nursing process for patients receiving antitubercular drugs.
4. Develop a comprehensive teaching guide for patients and families impacted by the diagnosis and treatment of antitubercular drugs.

e-Learning Activities

Companion CD

- NCLEX Review Questions: see questions 352-356
- Animations
- Audio Glossary
- Category Catchers
- Medication Errors Checklists
- IV Therapy Checklists

evolve Website (http://evolve.elsevier.com/Lilley)

• Nursing Care Plans • Frequently Asked Questions • Content Updates • WebLinks • Supplemental Resources • Elsevier ePharmacology Update • Medication Administration Animations

Drug Profiles

ethambutol, p. 638
▶ isoniazid, p. 638
pyrazinamide, p. 639
rifabutin, p. 639

rifampin, p. 639
rifapentine, p. 640
streptomycin, p. 640

▶ Key drug.

Glossary

Aerobic   Requiring oxygen for the maintenance of life. (p. 634)

Antitubercular drugs   Drugs used to treat infections caused by *Mycobacterium* bacterial species. (p. 636)

Bacillus   Rod-shaped bacteria. (p. 634)

Granuloma   Any small nodular aggregation of inflammatory cells (e.g., macrophages, lymphocytes); usually characterized by clearly delimited boundaries, as found in *tuberculosis.* (p. 634)

Isoniazid   The primary and most commonly prescribed tuberculostatic drug. (p. 638)

Multidrug-resistant tuberculosis (MDR-TB)   Tuberculosis (TB) that demonstrates resistance to two or more drugs. (p. 635)

Slow acetylator   Someone with a genetic defect that causes a deficiency in the enzyme needed to metabolize isoniazid, the most widely used TB drug. (p. 638)

Tubercle   The characteristic lesion of *tuberculosis;* a small round grey translucent *granulomatous* lesion, usually with a *caseated* (cheesy) consistency in its interior. (See *granuloma.*) (p. 635)

Tubercle bacilli   Another common name for rod-shaped TB bacteria; essentially synonymous with *Mycobacterium tuberculosis.* (p. 635)

Tuberculosis (TB)   Any infectious disease caused by species of *Mycobacterium;* usually *M. tuberculosis* (adjectives: *tuberculous, tubercular*). (p. 634)

TUBERCULOSIS

Tuberculosis (TB) is the medical diagnosis of any infectious disease caused by a bacterial species known as *Mycobacterium.* TB is most commonly characterized by **granulomas** in the lungs. These are nodular accumulations of inflammatory cells (e.g., macrophages, lymphocytes) that are *delimited* ("walled off" with clear boundaries) and have a center that has a cheesy or *caseated* consistency. *Casein* is the name of a protein that is prevalent in cheese and milk. Although there are technically two mycobacterial species that can cause TB, *M. tuberculosis* and *M. bovis,* infections caused by *M. tuberculosis* (abbreviated MTB) are far more common. There are also several other mycobacterial species (e.g., *M. leprae,* which causes leprosy) that have varying susceptibility to different drugs used for TB. Infections with these bacteria are much less of a public health problem and hence not the focus of this chapter. MTB is an aerobic **bacillus,** which means that it is a rod-shaped microorganism (bacillus) that requires a large supply of oxygen for it to grow and flourish (**aerobic**). This bacterium's need for a highly oxygenated body site explains why *Mycobacterium* infections most commonly affect the lungs. However, other common sites of infection include the growing ends of bones, and the brain (cerebral cortex). Less common sites of infection include the kidney, liver, and genitourinary tract, as well as virtually every other tissue and organ in the body.

These **tubercle bacilli** (a common synonym for MTB) are transmitted from one of three sources: humans, cows (bovine; hence the species name *M. bovis*), or birds (avian), although bovine and avian transmission are much less common than human transmission. **Tubercle** bacilli are conveyed in droplets expelled by infected people or animals during coughing or sneezing and then inhaled by the new host. After these infectious droplets are inhaled, the infection spreads to the susceptible organ sites by means of the blood and lymphatic system. MTB is a very slow-growing organism as well, which makes it more difficult to treat than most other bacterial infections. Many of the antibiotics used to treat TB work by inhibiting growth rather than directly killing the organism. This is because microorganisms that grow more slowly are more difficult to kill because their cells are not as metabolically active compared with other faster-growing organisms. Most bactericidal (cell-killing) drugs work by disrupting critical cellular metabolic processes in the organism. Therefore, the most drug-susceptible organisms are those with faster (not slower) metabolic activity.

At the other end of the TB patient spectrum are infected persons whose host defenses have been broken down as the result of immunosuppressive drug therapy, chemotherapy for cancer, or an immunosuppressive disease such as acquired immunodeficiency syndrome (AIDS). In these persons, the disease can inflict devastating and irreversible damage. The first infectious episode is considered the *primary* TB infection; *reinfection* represents the more chronic form of the disease. However, TB does not develop in all people who are exposed to it. In some cases, the bacteria become dormant and walled off by calcified or fibrous tissues. These patients may test positive for exposure, but not necessarily be infectious because of this dormancy process.

Tuberculosis cases have been reported on a national level in the United States beginning in 1953. Since that time, the TB incidence dropped in most years until about 1985. At this point, the HIV epidemic was growing strongly, and the TB incidence began to rise for the first time in 20 years, due to TB cases in patients co-infected with HIV. Many cities were unprepared to handle this re-emergence of TB. After an 18% increase in TB incidence between 1985 and 1991, a 50% decline was recorded from 1992 through 2002, with roughly 15,000 U.S. cases reported in 2002. This is attributed to intensified public health efforts aimed at preventing, diagnosing, and treating TB as well as HIV infection, including more effective antiretroviral drug therapy (Chapter 39). In the United States, drug therapy continues to regularly reduce the number of TB cases every year. In 2005, just over 14,000 cases of TB were reported to the Centers for Disease Control and Prevention (CDC), the lowest number since national reporting began in 1953. However, the *rate* of this more recent decline in TB cases has slowed from a yearly average decrease of 7.1% (from 1993 to 2000) to 3.8% (from 2001 to 2005), roughly a 50% difference. One contributing factor: the number of **multidrug-resistant tuberculosis (MDR-TB)** has recently *increased* 13.3%, with a total of 128 cases in 2004 (up from 113 in 2003), the most recent year with complete drug susceptibility data. An upward trend in drug resistance, especially to isoniazid (INH) and rifampin, has been observed since the 1970s. As recently

as the 1990s, one third of TB cases in New York City were resistant to at least one drug, and 20% to both INH and rifampin. Fortunately, these numbers have since declined, attributed to stronger TB-related public health efforts. Nonetheless, the prevalence and growth of TB continues to be greater in the larger global community, and TB infects one third of the world's population. It is currently second only to HIV in the number of deaths caused by a single infectious organism.

Several factors have contributed to this health care crisis, but one very important source of the problem is the increasing numbers of people in groups that are particularly susceptible to the infection—homeless, undernourished or malnourished, HIV-infected, drug abusers, cancer patients, those taking immunosuppressant drugs, and those who live in crowded and poorly sanitized housing facilities. All of these factors also favor the acquisition of a drug-resistant infection. Members of racial and ethnic minority groups are at greater risk than white populations, accounting for two thirds of new cases. Asian and Hispanic immigrants are at particularly high risk, accounting for more than half of foreign-acquired U.S. TB cases in 2005. Also in 2005, more U.S. cases were reported in Hispanics than in any other ethnic population.

ANTITUBERCULAR DRUGS

The drugs used to treat infections caused by all forms of *Mycobacterium* are called antitubercular drugs, and these drugs fall into two categories: *primary* or *first-line* and *secondary* or *second-line* drugs. As these designations imply, primary drugs are those tried first whereas secondary drugs are reserved for more complicated cases, such as those resistant to primary drugs. The antimycobacterial activity, efficacy, and potential adverse and toxic effects of the various drugs determine the class to which they belong. INH is a primary antitubercular drug and is the most widely used. It can be used either as the sole drug in the prophylaxis of TB or in combination with other antitubercular drugs. The various first- and second-line antibiotic drugs are listed in Box 40-1. There are also two miscellaneous TB-related injections, one diagnostic, the other a vaccine. These are described in Box 40-2.

Box 40-1 First- and Second-Line Antitubercular Drugs

First-Line Drugs
ethambutol
isoniazid
pyrazinamide (PZA)
rifabutin
rifampin
rifapentine
streptomycin

Second-Line Drugs
amikacin
capreomycin
cycloserine
ethionamide
kanamycin
levofloxacin
ofloxacin
para-aminosalicylic acid (PAS)

An important consideration during drug selection is the relative likelihood of drug-resistant organisms and drug toxicity. Following are other key elements that are important to the planning and implementation of effective therapy:

- Drug-susceptibility tests should be performed on the first *Mycobacterium* sp. that is isolated from a patient specimen (to prevent the development of MDR-TB).
- Before the results of the susceptibility tests are known, the patient should be started on a four-drug regimen consisting of isoniazid, rifampin, pyrazinamide (PZA), and ethambutol or streptomycin, which together are 95% effective in combating the infection. The use of multiple medications reduces the possibility of the organism becoming drug-resistant.
- Once drug susceptibility results are available, the regimen should be adjusted accordingly.

Box 40-2   Miscellaneous TB-Related Injections

Purified protein derivative (PPD): This is a diagnostic injection used intradermally in doses of 5 tuberculin units (0.1 mL) to detect TB exposure. It is composed of a protein precipitate derived from TB bacteria. A positive result is actually indicated by induration (not erythema) at the site of injection and is also known as the *Mantoux* reaction, named for a physician who described it.
Bacillus Calmette-Guérin (BCG): This is a vaccine injection derived from an inactivated strain of *Mycobacterium bovis*. Although it is not normally used in the United States because the risk is not as high, it is used in much of the world to vaccinate young children against tuberculosis. Although it does not prevent infection, evidence indicates that it reduces active TB by 60% to 80%, and is even more effective at preventing more severe cases that involve disseminated infection throughout the body.

TB, Tuberculosis.

- Patient compliance with, and the adverse effects of, the prescribed drug therapy should be monitored closely because the incidence of both patient noncompliance and adverse effects is high.
- Despite all of the drugs available to combat TB and the efforts mounted to detect and treat victims of the disease, treatment has been made difficult by two problems previously mentioned: patient nonadherence with therapy and the growing incidence of drug-resistant organisms.

Mechanism of Action and Drug Effects

The mechanisms of action of the various antitubercular drugs vary depending on the drug. These drugs act on *M. tuberculosis* in one of the following ways: they inhibit either protein synthesis or cell wall synthesis or they work by various other mechanisms. The **antitubercular drugs** are listed in Table 40-1 by their mechanism of action. The major effects of drug therapy include reduction of cough, and therefore infectiousness, of the patient. This normally occurs within 2 weeks of starting drug therapy, assuming that the patient's TB strain is drug-sensitive.

Indications

Antitubercular medications are indicated for TB infections, including both pulmonary and extrapulmonary TB. Most antitubercular drug effects have not been fully tested in pregnant women. However, the combination of isoniazid and ethambutol has been used to treat pregnant women with clinically apparent TB without teratogenic complications. Rifampin is another drug that is usually safe during pregnancy, and is a more likely choice for more advanced disease.

Besides being used for the initial treatment of TB, antitubercular drugs have also proved effective in the management of treatment

---

Table 40-1   Antitubercular Drugs: Mechanisms of Action

Drugs	Description
Inhibit Protein Synthesis amikacin, kanamycin, capreomycin, rifabutin, rifampin, rifapentine, streptomycin	Streptomycin and kanamycin work by interfering with normal protein synthesis and production of faulty proteins. Rifampin and capreomycin act at different points in the protein synthesis pathway from streptomycin and kanamycin. Rifampin inhibits RNA synthesis and may also inhibit DNA synthesis. Human cells are not as sensitive as the mycobacterial cells and are not affected by rifampin except at high drug concentrations. Capreomycin inhibits protein synthesis by preventing translocation on ribosomes.
Inhibit Cell Wall Synthesis cycloserine, ethionamide, isoniazid	Cycloserine acts by inhibiting the amino acid (D-Alanine) involved in the synthesis of cell walls. Isoniazid and ethionamide also act at least partly to inhibit the synthesis of wall components, but the mechanisms of these two drugs are still not clearly understood.
Other Mechanisms ethambutol, ethionamide, isoniazid, PAS, PZA	Other proposed mechanisms of action for isoniazid exist. Isoniazid is taken up by mycobacteria cells and undergoes hydrolysis to isonicotinic acid, which reacts with cofactor NAD to form a defective NAD that is no longer active as a coenzyme for certain life-sustaining reactions in the *Mycobacterium tuberculosis* organism. Ethionamide directly inhibits mycolic acid synthesis, which eventually has the same deleterious effects on the TB organism as isoniazid. Ethambutol affects lipid synthesis, resulting in the inhibition of mycolic acid incorporation into the cell wall, thus inhibiting protein synthesis. PAS acts as a competitive inhibitor of para-aminobenzoic acid in the synthesis of folate. The mechanism of action of PZA in the inhibition of TB is unknown. It can be either bacteriostatic or bactericidal, depending on the susceptibility of the particular *Mycobacterium* organism and the concentration of the drug attained at the site of infection.

NAD, Nicotinamide adenine; *PAS,* para-aminosalicylic acid; *PZA,* pyrazinamide; *TB,* tuberculosis.

failures and relapses. Infection with species of *Mycobacterium* other than *M. tuberculosis* (MOTT) and atypical mycobacterial infections have also been successfully treated with these drugs. Nontuberculous mycobacteria (NTM) may also be susceptible to antitubercular drugs. However, in general, antitubercular drugs are not as effective against other species of *Mycobacterium* as they are against *M. tuberculosis*. Some of these other species that may be of particular concern in immunocompromised patients such as AIDS patients are *Mycobacterium avium-intracellulare, Mycobacterium flavescens, Mycobacterium marinum,* and *Mycobacterium kansasii.* Additional *Mycobacterium* infections that may respond to antitubercular drugs are those caused by *Mycobacterium fortuitum, Mycobacterium chelonae, Mycobacterium smegmatis, Mycobacterium xenopi,* and *Mycobacterium scrofulaceum.* Treatment regimens for these non-TB mycobacterial infections often include the macrolide antibiotics clarithromycin or azithromycin (Chapter 37), either alone or in combination with one or more antitubercular drugs.

In summary, antitubercular drugs are primarily used for the prophylaxis or treatment of TB. The effectiveness of these drugs depends on the type of infection, adequate dosing, sufficient duration of treatment, drug compliance, and the selection of an effective drug combination. The indications of the different antitubercular drugs are listed in Table 40-2.

Contraindications

Contraindications to the use of various antitubercular drugs include severe drug allergy and major renal or liver dysfunction. However, it must be recognized that the urgency of treating a potentially fatal infection may have to be balanced against any prevailing contraindications. In extreme cases, patients are sometimes given a drug to which they have some degree of allergy with supportive care that enables them to at least tolerate the medication. Examples of such supportive care might include antipyretic (e.g., acetaminophen), antihistamine (e.g., diphenhydramine), or even corticosteroid (e.g., prednisone, methylprednisolone) therapy.

Reported contraindications that are specific to cycloserine include epilepsy and significant mental illness. One relative contraindication to ethambutol is optic neuritis. Chronic alcohol use, especially when associated with major liver damage, may also be a contraindication to any antitubercular drug therapy, keeping in mind the caveats mentioned earlier. Other contraindications for specific drugs, if any, may be found in the drug profiles below.

Adverse Effects

Antitubercular drugs are fairly well-tolerated. Isoniazid, one of the mainstays of treatment, is noted for causing pyridoxine deficiency and liver toxicity. For this reason, supplements of pyridoxine (vitamin B_6; Chapter 54) are often given concurrently with isoniazid with a common oral dose of 50 mg daily. The most problematic drugs and their associated adverse effects are listed in Table 40-3.

Interactions

The drugs that can interact with antitubercular drugs can cause significant effects. See Table 40-4 for a listing of selected interactions. Besides these drug interactions, isoniazid can cause false-positive urine glucose test (e.g., Clinitest) readings and an increase in the serum levels of the liver function enzymes alanine aminotransferase (ALT) and aspartate aminotransferase (AST).

Table 40-2	Antitubercular Drugs: Indications
Drug	**Indications**
amikacin, kanamycin	Used in combination with other antitubercular drugs in treatment of clinical TB. Not intended for long-term use.
capreomycin	Used with other antitubercular drugs for treatment of pulmonary TB caused by *Mycobacterium tuberculosis* after first-line drugs fail, drug resistance appears, or drug toxicity occurs.
cycloserine	Used with other antitubercular drugs for treatment of active pulmonary and extrapulmonary TB after failure of first-line drugs.
ethambutol	Indicated as a first-line drug for treatment of TB.
ethionamide	Used with other antitubercular drugs in treatment of clinical TB after failure of first-line drugs and for treatment of other types of mycobacterial infections.
isoniazid	Used alone or in combination with other antitubercular drugs in treatment and prevention of clinical TB.
para-aminosalicylate sodium	Used in combination with other antitubercular drugs for treatment of pulmonary and extrapulmonary *M. tuberculosis* infection after failure of first-line drugs.
pyrazinamide	Used with other antitubercular drugs in treatment of clinical TB.
rifabutin	Used to prevent or delay development of *M. avium*-intracellulare bacteremia and disseminated infections in patients with advanced HIV infection.
rifampin	Used with other antitubercular drugs in treatment of clinical TB.
	Used in treatment of diseases caused by mycobacteria other than *M. tuberculosis.*
	Used for preventive therapy in patients exposed to isoniazid-resistant *M. tuberculosis.*
	Used to eliminate meningococci from the nasopharynx of asymptomatic *Neisseria meningitidis* carriers when risk for meningococcal meningitis is high.
	Used for chemoprophylaxis in contacts of patients with HiB infection.
	Used with at least one other antiinfective drug in treatment of leprosy.
	Used in treatment of endocarditis caused by methicillin-resistant staphylococci, chronic staphylococcal prostatitis, and multiple-antiinfective–resistant pneumococci.
rifapentine	Used with other antitubercular drugs in the treatment of clinical TB.
streptomycin	Used in combination with other antitubercular drugs in the treatment of clinical TB and other mycobacterial diseases.

HiB, Haemophilus influenzae type B; *TB,* tuberculosis.

Table 40-3   Antitubercular Drugs: Common Adverse Effects

Drug	Adverse Effects
amikacin, kanamycin	Ototoxicity, nephrotoxicity
capreomycin	Ototoxicity, nephrotoxicity
cycloserine	Psychotic behavior, seizures
ethambutol	Retrobulbar neuritis, blindness
ethionamide	GI tract disturbances, hepatotoxicity
isoniazid	Peripheral neuritis, hepatotoxicity, optic neuritis and visual disturbances, hyperglycemia, red-orange-brown discoloration of bodily secretions (e.g. urine, sweat, tears, sputum)
levofloxacin, ofloxacin	Dizziness, headache, gastrointestinal disturbances, visual disturbances, insomnia
para-aminosalicylate sodium	GI tract disturbances, hepatotoxicity
pyrazinamide	Hepatotoxicity, hyperuricemia
rifabutin	GI tract disturbances; rash; neutropenia; red-orange-brown discoloration of urine, feces, saliva, sputum, sweat, tears, skin
rifampin	Hepatitis; hematologic disorders; red-orange-brown discoloration of urine, tears, sweat, sputum
rifapentine	GI upset; red-orange-brown discoloration of tears, sweat, skin, teeth, tongue, sputum, saliva, urine, feces, CSF
streptomycin	Ototoxicity, nephrotoxicity, blood dyscrasias

CSF, Cerebrospinal fluid; *GI,* gastrointestinal.

Table 40-4   Antitubercular Drugs: Drug Interactions

Drug	Mechanism	Results
Aminosalicylate		
probenecid	Reduces excretion	Increased aminosalicylate levels
salicylates	Additive effects	Aminosalicylate toxicity
Isoniazid		
antacids	Reduces absorption	Decreased isoniazid levels
cycloserine, ethionamide, rifampin	Additive effects	Increased CNS and hepatic toxicity
phenytoin+carbamazepine	Decreases metabolism	Increased phenytoin and carbamazepine effects
Streptomycin		
nephrotoxic and neurotoxic drugs		Increased toxicity
oral anticoagulants	Alter intestinal flora	Increased bleeding tendencies
Rifampin		
β-blockers		
benzodiazepines		
cyclosporine, oral anticoagulants, oral antidiabetics, oral contraceptives, phenytoin, quinidine, theophylline	Increased metabolism	Decreased therapeutic effects of these drugs

CNS, Central nervous system.

Dosages

For the recommended dosages of selected antitubercular drugs, see the Dosages table on page 639.

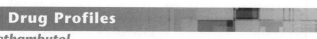

Drug Profiles

ethambutol

Ethambutol (Myambutol) is a first-line bacteriostatic drug used in the treatment of TB that is believed to work by diffusing into the mycobacteria and suppressing ribonucleic acid (RNA) synthesis, thereby inhibiting protein synthesis. Ethambutol is included with isoniazid, streptomycin, and rifampin in many TB combination-drug therapies. It may also be used to treat other mycobacterial diseases. It is contraindicated in patients with known optic neuritis as it can both exacerbate and cause this condition, resulting in varying degrees of vision loss. It is also contraindicated in children younger than 13 years of age. It is available only in oral form.

Pharmacokinetics

Half-Life	Onset	Peak	Duration
PO: 3.3 hr	PO: Variable	PO: 2-4 hr	PO: Up to 24 hr

▶ isoniazid

Isoniazid (INH) is not only the mainstay in the treatment of TB but also the most widely used antitubercular drug. It may be given either as a single drug for prophylaxis or in combination with other antitubercular drugs for the treatment of active TB. It is a bactericidal drug that kills the mycobacteria by disrupting cell-wall synthesis and essential cellular functions. INH is metabolized in the liver through a process called acetylation, which requires a certain enzymatic pathway to break down the drug. However, some people have a genetic deficiency of the liver enzymes needed for this to occur. Such people are called **slow acetylators.** When INH is taken by slow acetylators, the INH accumulates because there is not enough of the enzymes to break down the INH. Therefore, the dosages of INH may need to be adjusted downward in these patients.

DOSAGES

Selected Antitubercular Drugs

Drug (Pregnancy Category)	Pharmacologic Class	Usual Dosage Range	Indications
ethambutol (Myambutol) (B)	Synthetic first-line antimycobacterial	**Adult and pediatric** PO: 15-25 mg/kg/day; may also be divided in 2×/wk and 3×/wk dosage regimens with higher doses; no maximum dose listed	
isoniazid (INH) (C)	Synthetic first-line antimycobacterial	**Adult** PO: 5 mg/kg daily (max 300 mg) or 15 mg/kg 1-3×/wk (max 900 mg/dose) **Pediatric** PO: 10-20 mg/kg/day (max 300 mg) or 20-40 mg/kg 2-3×/wk (max 900 mg/dose)	
pyrazinamide (generic only) (C)	Synthetic first-line antimycobacterial	**Adult and pediatric** PO: 15-30 mg/kg/day (max 2 g) or 50-70 mg/kg 2-3×/wk (max 3-4 g/dose)	Active TB
rifabutin (Mycobutin) (B)	Semisynthetic first-line antimycobacterial antibiotic	**Adult only** PO: 300 mg once daily	
rifampin (Rifadin, Rimactane) (C)	Semisynthetic first-line antimycobacterial antibiotic	**Adult** PO/IV: 600 mg once daily. **Pediatric** PO/IV*: 10-20 mg/kg/day or 2-3×/wk (max 600 mg/dose for all regimens)	
rifapentine (Priftin) (C)	Semisynthetic first-line antimycobacterial antibiotic	**Adult only** PO: 600 mg twice weekly for first 2 months; then once weekly for 4 months	
streptomycin (generic only) (D)	Antimycobacterial aminoglycoside antibiotic	**Adult and pediatric** IM/IV:15-40 mg/kg 1-3×/wk (max 1-1.5 g/dose)	

*Use of intramuscular (IM) and subcutaneous (SC) injections is contraindicated due to soft tissue toxicity.
TB, Tuberculosis.

INH is most commonly used in oral form, although an injection is available. There is also a combination oral formulation of both INH and rifampin (Rifamate). Another combination drug product, Rifater, contains rifampin, INH, and pyrazinamide. INH is contraindicated in those with previous INH-associated hepatic injury or any acute liver disease.

Pharmacokinetics

Half-Life	Onset	Peak	Duration
PO: 1-4 hr	PO: Variable	PO: 1-2 hr	PO: Up to 24 hr

pyrazinamide

Pyrazinamide is an antitubercular drug that can be either bacteriostatic or bactericidal, depending on its concentration at the site of infection and the particular susceptibility of the mycobacteria. It is commonly used in combination with other antitubercular drugs for the treatment of TB. Its mechanism of action is unknown, but it is believed to work by inhibiting lipid and nucleic acid synthesis in the mycobacteria. Pyrazinamide is available only in generic oral form. It is contraindicated in patients with severe hepatic disease or acute gout. It is also not normally used in pregnant patients in the United States, due to a lack of teratogenicity data, although it is often used in pregnant patients in other countries.

Pharmacokinetics

Half-Life	Onset	Peak	Duration
PO: 9-10 hr	PO: Variable	PO: 2 hr	PO: Up to 24 hr

rifabutin

Rifabutin is the second of three currently available rifamycin antibiotics, following rifampin. Although it is considered a first-line TB drug by some clinicians, it is more commonly used to treat infections caused by *Mycobacterium avium* complex (MAC), which includes several non-TB mycobacterial species. This is also the case with the two other rifamycin-derived drugs, rifampin and rifapentine. A notable adverse effect of rifabutin is that it can turn urine, feces, saliva, skin, sputum, sweat, and tears a red-orange-brown color. Rifabutin is currently available only for oral use.

Pharmacokinetics

Half-Life	Onset	Peak	Duration
PO: 16-69 hr	PO: Variable	PO: 2-4 hr	PO: 1 to several days

rifampin

Rifampin (Rifadin, Rimactane) is the first of the *rifamycin* class of synthetic macrocyclic antibiotics, which also includes rifabutin and rifapentine. The term macrocyclic connotes the very large and complex hydrocarbon ring structure included in all three of the rifamycin compounds. Rifampin has activity against many *Mycobacterium* spp., as well as against meningococcus, *Haemophilus influenzae* type B, and leprosy. It is a broad-spectrum bactericidal drug that kills the offending organism by inhibiting protein synthesis. Rifampin is used either alone in the prevention of TB or in combination with other antitubercular drugs in its treatment. Rifampin is available in both oral and parenteral formulations and, as previously mentioned, in combination with isoniazid (Rifamate). Rifampin is available in both oral and injectable form. Rifampin is contraindicated in patients with known drug allergy to it or any other rifamycin (i.e., rifabutin, rifapentene).

Pharmacokinetics

Half-Life	Onset	Peak	Duration
PO: 3 hr	PO: Variable	PO: 2-4 hr	PO: Up to 24 hr

rifapentine

Rifapentine (Priftin) is a derivative of rifampin. It offers advantages over rifampin in that it has a much longer duration of action and possibly better efficacy. It has been shown to have greater antimycobacterial efficacy and macrophage penetration. Its accumulation into tissue macrophages allows it to work synergistically against bacterial cells that are ingested by the macrophage during phagocytosis ("cell eating"). Rifapentine is available only for oral use.

Pharmacokinetics

Half-Life	Onset	Peak	Duration
PO: 14-17 hr	PO: Unknown	PO: 5-6 hr	PO: 1 to several days

streptomycin

Streptomycin is an aminoglycoside antibiotic currently available in only generic form. Introduced in 1944, it was the very first drug available that could effectively treat TB. Because of its toxicities it is used most commonly today in combination-drug regimens for the treatment of MDR-TB infections. Streptomycin is currently available only in injectable form. It is usually not given to pregnant patients due to risk of fetal harm.

Pharmacokinetics

Half-Life	Onset	Peak	Duration
IM: 2-3 hr	IM: Variable	IM: 1-2 hr	IM: Up to 24 hr

◆ NURSING PROCESS

◆ ASSESSMENT

Before administering any of the antitubercular drugs and to ensure the safe and effective use of these medications, the nurse should obtain a thorough medical history, medication profile, and nursing history on the patient as well as perform a complete head-to-toe physical assessment. Noting any specific history of diagnoses or symptoms of tuberculosis is important as well their last PPD (purified protein derivative) tuberculin skin test with assessment of the reaction at the site of the intradermal injection. The most recent chest x-ray and results should also be noted. Liver function studies (e.g., bilirubin, liver enzymes, and blood urea nitrogen [BUN]) need to be noted, because a contraindication—as noted earlier—is severe liver dysfunction. Not only are these values important for assessing liver function, they also provide a comparative baseline throughout therapy. Because of some drugs leading to peripheral neuropathies, baseline neurologic functioning should also be noted prior to therapy. Hearing status should be noted especially with use of streptomycin because of its drug-related ototoxicity.

Assessment of age is also important because of the increased likelihood of adverse reactions or toxicity with liver dysfunction in the elderly and safety of use in children 13 years of age or younger has not been established. It is also important for the nurse to check the patient's complete blood count (CBC) before administering INH because of drug-related hematologic disorders. Renal studies, such as the serum creatinine and BUN, as well as urinalysis should be performed both at the start of antituberculin therapy and throughout, as ordered. Uric acid baseline levels should be noted because there may be an increase in these values and precipitation of gout. Sputum specimens are usually ordered, as well, to help in the determination of the appropriate drug regimen. Baseline eye function and exams should be performed prior to therapy with INH and ethambutol. Pyrazinamide

requires careful assessment of allergic reactions to other antitubercular drugs due to close cross-sensitivity. Contraindications, cautions, and drug interactions have been previously discussed.

◆ NURSING DIAGNOSES

- Risk for injury related to neurologic adverse effects of antitubercular drugs, noncompliance to drug therapy and to an overall status of poor health
- Ineffective therapeutic regimen management of TB related to poor compliance to therapy and lack of knowledge/experience about long-term therapies
- Ineffective family therapeutic regimen management related to poor compliance and poor housing and living conditions
- Deficient knowledge related to the disease process and treatment protocol

◆ PLANNING

Goals

- Patient experiences minimal adverse effects of drug therapy for TB.
- Patient takes medication regularly and for the length of time prescribed.
- Patient remains free of injury related to adverse effects (e.g., peripheral neuropathies) and drug interactions with the antitubercular drugs.
- Patient remains free of drug-related toxic effects and states the importance of reporting any symptoms of toxic effects to the physician immediately.
- Patient remains compliant with the drug therapy.

Outcome Criteria

- Patient reports therapeutic effects (improved signs and symptoms) and possible adverse effects (neuropathies, gastrointestinal upset) of drug regimens.
- Patient takes medication as ordered and regularly with acknowledgement of more effective therapy and prevention of complications, relapses, or recurrences.
- Patient states the drugs that interact with antitubercular drug such as salicylates, antacids, and anticoagulants and maintains drug safety.
- Patient reports toxic effects such as jaundice, renal problems, hearing loss, severe neuropathies, and/or blindness to the physician—should they occur.
- Patient shows improvement of disease state with drug adherence and shows a decrease in cough, fever, and sputum production as well as a return of normal laboratory values.

◆ IMPLEMENTATION

Because drug therapy is the mainstay of treatment of TB and often lasts for up to 24 months, patient education is critical, with a special emphasis on adherence. Simple, clear, and concise instructions should be given to the patient with appropriate use of audiovisuals and take-home information. This should include the fact that multiple drugs are often used to improve cure rates. All antitubercular drugs should be taken exactly as ordered and at the same time every day. Consistent use and dosing around the clock are critical to maintaining steady blood levels and for minimizing the chances of resistance to the drug therapy. Instructions to the patient should always emphasize the need for strict compliance/adherence to the therapeutic regimen.

Although many drugs are to be given without food for maximum absorption, antitubercular drugs may need to be taken with food to minimize gastrointestinal upset. There should be constant monitoring of any signs and symptoms of liver dysfunction such as fatigue, jaundice, nausea, vomiting, dark urine, and anorexia, with reporting of any of these to the physician. If vision changes occur (e.g., altered color perception, changes in visual acuity), in particular with ethambutol, these changes should be reported immediately to the physician. Uric acid levels will need to be monitored during therapy, as will symptoms of gout such as hot, painful, or swollen joints of the big toe, knee, or ankle. In addition, the physician should be notified if there are signs and symptoms of peripheral neuropathy (e.g., numbness, burning, and tingling of extremities). Pyridoxine (vitamin B$_6$) may be beneficial with INH-induced peripheral neuropathy. If the physician has ordered sputum collections for acid-fast bacilli, it is best to collect early in the morning. The most common order is for three consecutive morning specimens, with a repeat several weeks later. All drugs should be taken as ordered and without any omission of doses for maximal therapeutic results.

Follow-up visits to the health care provider are important in the monitoring of therapeutic effects and to look for adverse effects and toxicity. If intravenous (IV) dosing of an antitubercular drug is ordered, be sure to use the appropriate diluent and infuse over the recommended time. The IV site should be monitored every hour during the infusion for extravasation with possible tissue inflammation (e.g., redness, heat, and swelling at the IV site). See the Patient Teaching Tips for more information on antitubercular drugs.

Cultural considerations associated with these drugs include the fact that patients with active tuberculosis require thorough patient teaching of all family members and that some family members may need prophylactic therapy for up to 1 full year. Because some cultural practices include living in close-knit communities/living quarters, this teaching is critical to making sure there is adequate prevention of the spread of this highly communicable disease. Make sure that all family members or those in close contact with the patient receive the same thorough instructions about maintaining health while taking their medications appropriately, with emphasis on adherence.

◆ EVALUATION

The nurse should always document patient responses, or lack of them, to therapy. The therapeutic response to antitubercular therapy is reflected by a decrease in the symptoms of tuberculosis, such as cough and fever, and by weight gain. The results of laboratory studies (culture and sensitivity tests) and the chest x-ray findings should confirm the clinical findings of resolution of the infection. Meeting of goals and outcome criteria should also be evaluated to see if the infection is being adequately treated and that the drug therapy is providing therapeutic relief without complications or toxicity and with minimal adverse effects. Patients also need to be monitored for the occurrence of adverse reactions to antitubercular drugs, such as fatigue, nausea, vomiting, fever, loss of appetite, depression, jaundice, numbness/tingling/burning of extremities, abdominal pain, changes in vision, and easy bruising. Because of the need for long-term therapy and possible treatment of family or those in close contact, further evaluation of the home setting is also needed.

CASE STUDY

Tuberculosis

For a project that received new funding, you and five of your community-health nursing peers have been asked to give some mini-presentations to various large work settings in the community. One place is in your health department with the nurses who work in the adult clinic.

1. What are some key Internet resources you can share with the staff regarding TB infections, control guidelines, and OSHA recommendations?
2. What information could then be used or shared with patients in the adult clinic?
3. What conditions in the community are considered high-risk for transmission of diseases such as TB?

For answers, see http://evolve.elsevier.com/Lilley.
OSHA, Occupational Safety & Health Administration; *TB*, tuberculosis.

Patient Teaching Tips

- Patients should take medications exactly as directed by the physician, with attention to long-term therapy and strict adherence. Ineffective treatment may occur if drugs are taken intermittently or stopped once the patient begins to feel better.
- Encourage patients to keep all follow-up appointments with the physician so that the infection may be closely monitored.
- Educate patients to avoid alcohol while taking antitubercular drugs and to check with the physician before taking any other type of medication.
- Inform patients that they will most likely be taking pyridoxine (vitamin B$_6$) to prevent INH-precipitated peripheral neuropathies and avoid numbness/tingling/burning of extremities.
- Educate patients taking INH or rifampin to report the following adverse effects to the physician immediately should they occur: fever, nausea, vomiting, loss of appetite, unusual bleeding, numbness, and tingling of extremities.
- Encourage patients to wear sunscreen and protective clothing and avoid ultraviolet light exposure or prevent exposure to the sun due to drug-related photosensitivity reactions.

- Encourage patients to report any flu-like symptoms, gastrointestinal upset, or rash to the physician immediately.
- Women taking oral contraceptives who are prescribed rifampin must be switched to another form of birth control because oral contraceptives become ineffective when given with rifampin.
- Educate patients about preventing spread of the infection, and that during the initial period of the illness and its diagnosis, they should make every effort to wash their hands and cover their mouths when coughing or sneezing. They should also be careful about disposal of secretions.
- Educate patients about the need for rest, good sleep habits, adequate nutrition, and maintenance of general health and emphasize the fact that these and other medications should be kept away from children.
- Encourage patients to wear a medical alert tag or bracelet with a list of allergies, drugs being taken, and medical conditions. Written information should also be kept on their person at all times too.

Continued

Patient Teaching Tips—cont'd

- Inform patients about the importance of reporting to their health care provider any increase in fatigue, cough, sputum production, bloody sputum, chest pain, unusual bleeding, yellow skin and/or yellow eyes.
- Patients taking rifampin, rifabutin, or rifapentine may experience red-orange-brown discoloration of the skin, sweat, tears, urine, feces, sputum, saliva, cerebrospinal fluid, and tongue as an adverse effect of the drug. The discoloration reverses with discontinuation of the drug; however, contact lenses may be permanently stained.

Points to Remember

- All drug therapeutic regimens should be taken exactly as prescribed, with emphasis on adherence and long-term dosing combined with healthy living practices.
- Therapeutic effects include resolving of pulmonary and extrapulmonary *M. tuberculosis* infections.
- Vitamin B_6 is needed to combat peripheral neuritis associated with isoniazid.
- Women taking oral contraceptive therapy who are prescribed rifampin should be counseled on other forms of birth control because of the ineffectiveness of oral contraception while on rifampin.
- Educate patients about the importance of strict compliance to the drug regimen for improvement of condition or cure. Education about drug interactions and the need to avoid alcohol while taking any of these medications should be provided in written and oral formats.

NCLEX Examination Review Questions

1. When teaching a patient who is starting antitubercular therapy with rifampin, which of the following adverse effects would the nurse expect to see?
   a. Headache and neck pain
   b. Glaucoma and gynecomastia
   c. Reddish-brown urine
   d. Numbness or tingling of extremities
2. During antitubercular therapy with isoniazid, the patient received another prescription for pyridoxine. Which statement by the nurse best explains the rationale for this second medication?
   a. "This vitamin will help to improve your energy levels."
   b. "This helps to prevent neurologic adverse effects."
   c. "It works to protect your heart from toxic effects."
   d. "This drug works to reduce gastrointestinal adverse effects."
3. When counseling a woman who is beginning antitubercular therapy with rifampim, which statement by the nurse is most important regarding potential drug interactions?
   a. "If you are taking birth control pills, you will need to switch to another form of birth control."
   b. "Your birth control pills will remain effective while you are taking rifampin."
   c. "You will need to switch to a stronger brand of oral contraceptive while on rifampin."
   d. "You can take the birth control pills with the rifampin without problems, but it may cause your urine to turn reddish-orange.
4. When counseling a patient who has a new diagnosis of tuberculosis, the nurse should make sure that the patient realizes that he or she is contagious:
   a. during all phases of the illness.
   b. any time up to 18 months after therapy.
   c. during the postictal phase of TB.
   d. during the initial period of the illness and its diagnosis.
5. While monitoring a patient, the nurse knows that a therapeutic response to antitubercular drugs would be:
   a. The patient states that he or she is feeling much better.
   b. The patient's labwork reflects a lower white blood cell count.
   c. The patient reports a decrease in cough and night sweats.
   d. There is a decrease in symptoms, along with improved chest x-ray and sputum culture results.

1. c, 2. b, 3. a, 4. d, 5. d.

Critical Thinking Activities

1. What is considered a therapeutic response to antitubercular drugs?
2. Is there any concern for the female taking oral contraceptives while taking rifampin? Explain your answer.
3. What parameters should be assessed while a patient is taking antitubercular drugs and why?

For answers, see http://evolve.elsevier.com/Lilley.

CHAPTER

Antifungal Drugs

41

Objectives

When you reach the end of this chapter, you should be able to do the following:

1. Identify the various antifungal drugs.
2. Describe the mechanisms of action, indications, contraindications, routes of administration, adverse and toxic effects, and drug interactions associated with the use of the various antifungal drugs.
3. Develop a nursing care plan that includes all phases of the nursing process for patients receiving antifungal drugs.

e-Learning Activities

Companion CD

- NCLEX Review Questions: see questions 357-361
- Animations
- Audio Glossary
- Category Catchers
- Medication Errors Checklists
- IV Therapy Checklists

evolve Website (http://evolve.elsevier.com/Lilley)
- Nursing Care Plans • Frequently Asked Questions • Content Updates • WebLinks • Supplemental Resources • Elsevier ePharmacology Update • Medication Administration Animations

Drug Profiles

▸ amphotericin B, p. 646
caspofungin, p. 646
▸ fluconazole, p. 646

nystatin, p. 646
terbinafine, p. 646
voriconazole, p. 649

▸ Key drug.

Glossary

Antimetabolite A drug or other substance that is a either a receptor antagonist or that resembles a normal human metabolite and interferes with its function in the body, usually by competing for the metabolite's usual receptors or enzymes. (p. 644)

Dermatophyte One of several fungi, often found in soil, that infect skin, nails, or hair of humans. (p. 643)

Ergosterol An unsaturated hydrocarbon of the vitamin D group isolated from yeast, mushrooms, ergot, and other fungi; the main sterol in fungal membranes. (p. 645)

Fungi A very large, diverse group of eukaryotic microorganisms that require an external carbon source and that form a plant structure known as a *thallus*. Fungi consist of yeasts and molds. (p. 643)

Molds Multicellular fungi characterized by long, branching filaments called *hyphae*, which entwine to form a complex branched structure known as a *mycelium*. (p. 643)

Mycosis The general term for any fungal infection. (p. 643)
Pathologic fungi Fungi that cause mycoses. (p. 643)
Sterol The substance in the cell membranes of fungi to which polyene antifungal drugs bind. (p. 645)
Yeasts Single-celled fungi that reproduce by *budding*. (p. 643)

FUNGAL INFECTIONS

Fungi are a very large and diverse group of microorganisms that include all yeasts and molds. **Yeasts** are single-celled fungi that reproduce by *budding* (where a daughter cell forms by pouching out of and breaking off from a mother cell). These organisms have common practical uses in baking of breads and in the preparation of alcoholic beverages. **Molds** are multicellular and are characterized by long, branching filaments called *hyphae,* which entwine to form a "mat" called a *mycelium.* Some fungi are part of the normal flora of the skin, mouth, intestines, and vagina.

The infection caused by a fungus is also called a **mycosis.** There are a variety of fungi that can cause clinically significant infections or *mycoses.* These are called **pathologic fungi,** and the infections they cause range in severity from being mild infections with annoying symptoms (e.g., athlete's foot) to systemic mycoses that can become life-threatening. These infections are acquired by various routes: they can be ingested orally; they can grow on or in the skin, hair, or nails, and, if the fungal spores are airborne, they can be inhaled. There are four general types of mycotic infections: *systemic, cutaneous, subcutaneous,* and *superficial.* The latter three describe various layers of *integumentary* (skin, hair, or nail) infections. Fungi that cause integumentary infections are known as **dermatophytes,** and such infections are known as *dermatomycoses.* The most severe systemic fungal infections generally afflict people whose host immune defenses are compromised. Commonly, these are patients who have received organ transplants and are on immunosuppressive drug therapy, cancer patients who are immunocompromised as the result of their chemotherapy, and patients with AIDS. In addition, the use of antibiotics, antineoplastics, or immunosuppressants such as corticosteroids may result in colonization of *Candida*

643

Table 41-1   Mycotic Infections

Mycosis	Fungus	Endemic Location	Reservoir	Transmission	Primary Tissue Affected
Systemic Infection					
Aspergillosis	*Aspergillus* spp.	Universal	Soil	Inhalation	Lungs
Blastomycosis	*Blastomyces dermatitidis*	North America	Soil, animal dropping	Inhalation	Lungs
Coccidioidomycosis	*Coccidioides immitis*	Southwestern United States	Soil, dust	Inhalation	Lungs
Cryptococcosis	*Cryptococcus neoformans*	Universal	Soil, bird and chicken dropping	Inhalation	Lungs/meninges of brain
Histoplasmosis	*Histoplasma capsulatum*	Universal		Inhalation	Lungs
Cutaneous Infection					
Candidiasis	*Candida albicans*	Universal	Humans	Direct contact, nonsusceptible antibiotic overgrowth	Mucous membrane/skin disseminated (may be systemic)
Dermatophytes, tinea	*Epidermophyton* spp., *Microsporum* spp., *Trichophyton* spp.	Universal	Humans	Direct and indirect contact with infected persons	Scalp, skin (e.g., groin, feet)
Superficial Infection					
Tinea versicolor	*Malassezia furfur*	Universal	Humans	Unknown*	Skin

*Malassezia spp. are a usual part of the normal human flora and appear to cause infection in only select individuals.

albicans, followed by the development of a systemic infection. When this affects the mouth, it is referred to as *oral candidiasis,* or *thrush.* It is common in newborns and immunocompromised patients. Vaginal candidiasis, commonly called a *yeast infection,* often afflicts pregnant women, women with diabetes mellitus, women taking antibiotics, and women taking oral contraceptives. The characteristics of some of the systemic, cutaneous, and superficial mycotic infections are summarized in Table 41-1.

ANTIFUNGAL DRUGS

The drugs used to treat fungal infections are called antifungal drugs. Systemic mycotic infections and some cutaneous or subcutaneous mycoses are treated with oral or parenteral drugs, but these constitute a fairly small group of drugs, only three or four of which are commonly used. There are few such drugs because the fungi that cause these infections have proved to be very difficult to kill, and research into new and improved drugs has occurred at a slow pace, with relatively few important advances yielded so far. One difficulty that has slowed the development of new drugs is that often the chemical concentrations required for these experimental drugs to be effective cannot be tolerated by human beings. Those drugs that have met with success in the treatment of systemic mycoses as well as severe dermatomycoses, include amphotericin B, caspofungin, fluconazole, flucytosine, griseofulvin, itraconazole, ketoconazole, micafungin, nystatin, terbinafine, and voriconazole. These drugs are the focus of this chapter.

Topical antifungal drugs are by far the most commonly used drugs in this class and are most often used without prescription for the treatment of dermatomycoses as well as oral and vaginal

mycoses. Although topical drug therapy is usually sufficient for these conditions, systemic oral medications are also sometimes used, especially for more severe or recurrent cases. Antifungal drugs available for topical use are discussed further in Chapter 57. There is also a single antifungal drug (natamycin) for ophthalmic use (Chapter 58).

Two antifungal drugs, flucytosine and griseofulvin, are individually listed and not specifically classified according to their chemical structures. The remaining drugs currently include four specific chemical classes: *polyenes* (amphotericin B and nystatin), *imidazoles* (ketoconazole), *triazoles* (fluconazole, itraconazole, and voriconazole), and the *echinocandins* (caspofungin and micafungin). The imidazoles and triazoles are sometimes referred to by the more general term *azole antifungals.* Also included in some of these classes are drugs for topical use, which again are described further in Chapter 57.

Mechanism of Action and Drug Effects

The mechanisms of action of the various antifungal drugs vary between drug subclasses. Flucytosine, also known as *5-fluorocytosine* (5-FC), acts in much the same way as the antiviral drugs. It is an **antimetabolite,** which is a drug that is taken up into critical cellular metabolic pathways of the fungal cell. Once inside a susceptible fungal cell, the drug is deaminated by the enzyme *cytosine deaminase* to 5-fluorouracil (5-FU). Because human cells do not have this enzyme, they are not harmed by this antimetabolite. Once the 5-FU is generated inside the fungal cell, it interferes with fungal DNA synthesis, resulting in both inhibition of cell growth and reproduction and cell death. 5-FU is also available as an antineoplastic (anticancer) drug and is discussed in more detail in Chapter 48.

Griseofulvin, like flucytosine, is one of the older types of antifungal drugs. It works by preventing susceptible fungi from reproducing. It enters the fungal cell through an energy-dependent transport system and inhibits fungal mitosis (cell division) by binding to key structures known as *microtubules*. This in turn disrupts the *mitotic spindle* structure, which arrests the metaphase of cell division. It has also been proposed that griseofulvin causes the production of defective DNA, which is then unable to replicate. Although both griseofulvin and flucytosine are still currently available on the U.S. market, their clinical use has largely been supplanted by the newer antifungal drug classes.

The polyenes act by binding to **sterols** in the cell membranes of fungi, the main sterol in fungal membranes being **ergosterol.** Human cell membranes have cholesterol instead of ergosterol. Because polyene antifungals have a strong chemical affinity for ergosterol instead of cholesterol, they do not bind to human cell membranes and therefore do not kill human cells. Once the polyene drug molecule binds to the ergosterol, a channel forms in the fungal cell membrane that allows potassium and magnesium ions to leak out of the fungal cell. This loss of ions causes fungal cellular metabolism to be altered, leading to death of the cell.

Imidazoles and triazoles act as either fungistatic or fungicidal drugs, depending on their concentration in the fungus. They are most effective in combating rapidly growing fungi and work by inhibiting fungal cell cytochrome P-450 enzymes. These enzymes are needed to produce ergosterol. The allylamine terbinafine is also believed to act by a similar mechanism. When the production of ergosterol is inhibited, other sterols called *methylsterols* are produced instead. This results in a similar problem caused by the polyene antifungals, namely a leaky cell membrane that allows needed electrolytes to escape. The fungal cells die because they cannot carry on cellular metabolism.

The echinocandins caspofungin and micafungin act by preventing the synthesis of *glucans,* essential components of fungal cell walls that are not present in mammalian cells. This also contributes to fungal cell death. Some of the fungi that are susceptible to these drugs are the pathogens involved in the various mycoses listed in Box 41-1.

Indications

Indications for the use of the various antifungal drugs are specific to both the drug and type of infection being treated. The adverse effects of the newer antifungals are fewer and less serious than those of the older drugs. However, the drug of choice for the treatment of many severe systemic fungal infections remains one of the oldest antifungals, amphotericin B, which often does have major adverse effects. Amphotericin B is effective against a wide range of fungi. It is given with flucytosine in the treatment of *Candida* and cryptococcal infections because of the synergy of the two drugs. Amphotericin B is also effective for treating aspergillosis, blastomycosis, candidiasis, coccidioidomycosis, cryptococcosis, fungal endocarditis, histoplasmosis, zygomycosis, fungal septicemia, and many other systemic fungal infections. The activity of nystatin is similar to that of amphotericin B, but its usefulness is limited because of its toxic effects when given in the doses required to accomplish the same antifungal actions as those of amphotericin B. It is also not available in a parenteral form. Nystatin is most commonly used for treating oropharyngeal candidiasis, commonly referred to as *thrush.*

Fluconazole and itraconazole are synthetic imidazole antifungals, as are all of the drugs with an "-azole" suffix. Fluconazole can pass into the cerebrospinal fluid (CSF) and inhibit cryptococcal fungi. This makes it effective in the treatment of cryptococcal meningitis. Both drugs are active against oropharyngeal and esophageal *Candida* infections. Itraconazole, on the other hand, is capable of only poor CSF penetration but can be widely distributed throughout other areas of the body. It is indicated for the treatment of fungal infections in immunocompromised and non-immunocompromised patients with disseminated candidiasis, histoplasmosis, blastomycosis, and aspergillosis. The other systemic imidazole, ketoconazole, inhibits many dermatophytes and fungi that cause systemic mycoses, but it is not active against *Aspergillus* organisms or *Phycomycetes* (common molds) such as *Mucor* spp. Fortunately the newest imidazole antifungal drug, voriconazole, does have activity against some of these more tenacious fungal infections, including invasive aspergillosis, *Scedosporium* spp., and *Fusarium* spp.

Of the imidazoles, fluconazole is the most effective for combating infections with *Candida, Cryptococcus, Blastomyces,* and *Histoplasma* organisms. Fluconazole is also very effective against vaginal candidiasis. One dose of 150 mg of fluconazole can cure many vaginal candidal infections.

Flucytosine inhibits *Cryptococcus neoformans, Candida albicans,* and many *Cladosporium* and *Phialophora* spp. It does not inhibit *Aspergillus, Sporothrix, Blastomyces,* or *Histoplasma* spp. or *Coccidioides immitis.*

Griseofulvin inhibits dermatophytes of *Microsporum, Trichophyton,* and *Epidermophyton* spp. It has no effect on filamentous

---

Box 41-1   Fungal Species That Are Susceptible to Current Antifungal Drugs

Cutaneous and Subcutaneous Mycoses
Epidermophyton spp.
Malassezia furfur (causes tinea versicolor)
Microsporum spp.
Sporothrix spp.
Trichophyton spp.

Systemic Mycoses
Absidia spp.
Aspergillus spp.
Basidiobolus spp.

Blastomyces dermatitidis
Candida spp.
Coccidioides immitis
Conidiobolus spp.
Cryptococcus neoformans
Histoplasma capsulatum
Mucor spp.
Rhizopus spp.
Scedosporium apiospermum

Spp., Species.

fungi such as *Aspergillus,* yeasts such as *Candida* spp., or dimorphic species such as *Histoplasma*. Terbinafine is a synthetic allylamine derivative used in a systemic oral form for treatment of onychomycoses—fungally infected fingernails or toenails. The imidazole itraconazole is also sometimes used for this purpose. Topical forms of terbinafine are also used for various skin infections (Chapter 57).

Contraindications

Drug allergy, liver failure, kidney failure, and porphyria (griseofulvin) are the most common contraindications for antifungal drugs. Itraconazole should not be used for treating onychomycoses in patients with severe cardiac problems. Voriconazole can cause fetal harm in pregnant women.

Adverse Effects

The major adverse effects and clinical problems with antifungal drugs are encountered most commonly in conjunction with amphotericin B treatment. Drug interactions and hepatotoxicity are the primary concerns in patients receiving other antifungal drugs, but the intravenous (IV) administration of amphotericin B is associated with a multitude of adverse effects. The most common and problematic of the adverse effects of the various antifungal drugs are listed in Table 41-2. With amphotericin B treatment in particular, prescribers commonly order various premedications (including antiemetics, antihistamines, antipyretics, and corticosteroids) to prevent or minimize infusion-related reactions. The likelihood of such reactions can also be reduced by using longer-than-average drug infusion times (i.e., 2 to 6 hours) with this particular drug.

Interactions

There are many important drug interactions associated with the use of antifungal drugs, some of which can be life threatening. A common underlying source of the problem is that many of the antifungal drugs, as well as other drugs, are metabolized by a greatly used enzyme system in the liver called the *cytochrome P-450 system*. The result of the coadministration of two drugs that are both broken down by this system is that they compete for the limited amount of enzymes, and one of the drugs ends up accumulating. Key drug interactions with systemic antifungal drugs are summarized in Table 41-3.

Dosages

For the recommended dosages of selected antifungal drugs, see the table on page 648.

Drug Profiles

▶ amphotericin B

As previously mentioned, amphotericin B (Amphocin, Fungizone) remains the drug of choice for the treatment of severe systemic mycoses. It may be given with flucytosine in the treatment of many types of fungal infections because the two drugs work synergistically. The main drawback of amphotericin B therapy is that the drug causes many adverse effects. Almost all patients given the drug intravenously experience fever, chills, hypotension, tachycardia, malaise, muscle and joint pain, anorexia, nausea and vomiting, and headache. For this reason, pretreatment with an antipyretic (acetaminophen), antihistamines, and antiemetics may be given to decrease the severity of this infusion-related reaction.

Lipid formulations of amphotericin B have been developed in an attempt to decrease the incidence of its adverse effects and increase its efficacy. There are currently three lipid preparations of amphotericin B: amphotericin B lipid complex (ABLC, or Abelcet), amphotericin B cholesteryl complex (Amphotec), and liposomal amphotericin B (AmBisome). These lipid dosage forms have a much higher cost than conventional amphotericin B and for this reason are often used only when patients are intolerant of or refractory to nonlipid amphotericin B.

Amphotericin B is a prescription-only drug that is available in parenteral, topical, and oral dosage forms. It is contraindicated in patients who have shown hypersensitivity reactions to it and in those suffering from severe bone marrow suppression or renal impairment. However, patients who have life-threatening fungal infections may still be treated with this drug if cultures indicate that no other drug will kill the infection. The drug is available in injectable, oral, and topical preparations. Often a 1-mg test dose is given over 20 to 30 minutes to see if the patient will tolerate the amphotericin. It has been used as a local irrigant (bladder irrigation) for the treatment of candidal cystitis and has been used intrapleurally and intraperitoneally for the treatment of fungal infections in those body cavities.

*Pharmacokinetics**

Half-Life	Onset	Peak	Duration
IV: 1-15 days	IV: Variable	IV: 1 hr	IV: 18-24 hr

*For conventional (nonlipid) injection; lipid formulations have shorter half-lives.

caspofungin

Caspofungin (Cancidas) was the first echinocandin antifungal drug, approved in 2001. It is used for treating severe *Aspergillus* infection (invasive aspergillosis) in patients who are intolerant of or refractory to other drugs. It is only available in injectable form. In 2005, a second echinocandin known as micafungin (Mycamine) was approved.

Pharmacokinetics

Half-Life	Onset	Peak	Duration
IV: 9-50 hr	IV: Unknown	IV: Unknown	IV: Unknown

▶ fluconazole

Fluconazole (Diflucan) has proved to represent a significant improvement in the area of antifungal treatment. It has a much better adverse effect profile than that of amphotericin B, and it also has excellent coverage against many fungi. In fact, it is often preferred to amphotericin B because of these qualities. Oral fluconazole has excellent bioavailability, which means that almost the entire dose administered is absorbed into the circulation. Fluconazole is available in both oral and injectable forms.

Pharmacokinetics

Half-Life	Onset	Peak	Duration
PO: 22-30 hr	PO: <1 hr	PO: 1-2 hr	PO: Variable

nystatin

Nystatin (Nilstat, Mycostatin, Nystex) is a polyene antifungal drug that is often applied topically for the treatment of candidal diaper rash, taken orally as prophylaxis against candidal infections during periods of neutropenia in patients receiving immunosuppressive therapy, and used for the treatment of oral and vaginal candidiasis. It is not available in a parenteral form but does come in several oral and topical formulations. It is currently available for oral, topical, and vaginal use.

Pharmacokinetics

Half-Life	Onset	Peak	Duration
PO: Unknown	PO: 2 hr	PO: Unknown	PO: Unknown

terbinafine

Terbinafine (Lamisil) is classified as an allylamine antifungal drug and is currently the only drug in its class. It is available in a topical cream, gel, and spray for treating superficial dermatologic infections, including tinea pedis (athlete's foot), tinea cruris (jock itch), and tinea corporis (ringworm). A tablet form is also available for sys-

Table 41-2   Selected Antifungal Drugs: Common Adverse Effects and Cautions

Body System	Adverse Effects	Cautions
Amphotericin B		Recheck dosage and type of amphotericin B being administered
Cardiovascular	Cardiac dysrhythmias	
Central nervous	Neurotoxicity; visual disturbances; hand or feet numbness, tingling, or pain; convulsions	
Kidneys	Renal toxicity, potassium loss, hypomagnesemia	
Pulmonary	Pulmonary infiltrates, other respiratory difficulties	
Other (infusion-related)	Fever, chills, headache, malaise, nausea, occasionally hypotension	
Fluconazole		Use with caution in patients with renal or hepatic dysfunction
Gastrointestinal	Nausea, vomiting, diarrhea, stomach pain	
Other	Increased AST and ALT levels	
Flucytosine		Use with caution in patients with renal dysfunction or bone marrow depression
Central nervous	Headache, confusion, dizziness, sedation, vertigo	
Gastrointestinal	Nausea, vomiting, anorexia, diarrhea, abdominal distension, cramps, enterocolitis	
Hematologic	Bone marrow suppression: thrombocytopenia, agranulocytosis, anemia, leukopenia, pancytopenia	
Other	Increased BUN, creatine, ALT, and AST levels; rash; increased alkaline phosphatase activity	
Griseofulvin		Avoid during pregnancy
Central nervous	Headache, peripheral neuritis, paresthesias, confusion, dizziness, fatigue, insomnia, psychosis	
Ears, eyes, nose, and throat	Blurred vision, oral candidiasis, furry tongue, transient hearing loss	
Gastrointestinal	Nausea, vomiting, anorexia, diarrhea, cramps, dry mouth, flatulence, increased thirst, dysgeusia	
Genitourinary	Proteinuria, precipitate porphyria	
Hematologic	Leukopenia, granulocytopenia, neutropenia, monocytosis	
Integumentary	Rash, urticaria, photosensitivity, angioedema, systemic lupus erythematosus	
Itraconazole		Can trigger rare episodes of serious cardiovascular adverse effects
Central nervous	Headache, dizziness, insomnia, somnolence, depression	
Gastrointestinal	Nausea, vomiting, anorexia, diarrhea, cramps, abdominal pain, flatulence, gastrointestinal bleeding, hepatotoxicity	
Genitourinary	Gynecomastia, impotence, decreased libido	
Integumentary	Pruritus, fever, rash	
Other	Edema, fatigue, malaise, hypertension, hypokalemia, tinnitus, hypertriglyceridemia, adrenal insufficiency	
Ketoconazole		Avoid contact with eyes
Central nervous	Headache, dizziness, somnolence, SIADH	
Gastrointestinal	Nausea, vomiting, anorexia, diarrhea, abdominal pain, hepatotoxicity	
Genitourinary	Gynecomastia, impotence, vaginal burning	
Hematologic	Thrombocytopenia, leukopenia, hemolytic anemia	
Integumentary	Pruritus, fever, chills, photophobia, rash, dermatitis, purpura, urticaria	
Other	Hypoadrenalism, hyperuricemia, hypothyroidism	
Nystatin		Local irritation may occur
Gastrointestinal	Nausea, vomiting, anorexia, diarrhea, cramps	
Integumentary	Rash, urticaria	
Terbinafine		Rarely causes irritation
Central nervous	Headache, dizziness	
Gastrointestinal	Nausea, vomiting, diarrhea	
Integumentary	Rash, pruritus	
Other	Alopecia, fatigue	

ALT, Alanine aminotransferase; *AST,* aspartate aminotransferase; *BUN,* blood urea nitrogen; *Hct,* hematocrit; *SIADH,* syndrome of inappropriate antidiuretic hormone.

Table 41-3   Antifungal Drugs: Drug Interactions

Drug	Possible Effects
Amphotericin B	
Digitalis glycosides	Amphotericin B–induced hypokalemia may increase the potential for digitalis toxicity
Nephrotoxic drug	Additive nephrotoxicity
Thiazide diuretics	Severe hypokalemia or decreased adrenal cortex response to corticotrophin
Fluconazole, Itraconazole	
cyclosporine, phenytoin	Increased plasma concentrations of both drugs
Oral anticoagulants	Increased effects of anticoagulants seen as increases in PT
Oral hypoglycemics	Reduced metabolism of hypoglycemic drugs
Griseofulvin	
Oral anticoagulants	Decreased effects of anticoagulants seen as decreases in PT
Oral contraceptives, estrogen-containing products	Decreased effectiveness of these drugs
Ketoconazole	
Alcohol and other hepatotoxic drugs	Increased risk of hepatotoxicity
Antacids, anticholinergics, H$_2$ blockers, omeprazole	Increased gastrointestinal tract pH, which can reduce absorption of ketoconazole
cyclosporine	Increased cyclosporine levels and potential for nephrotoxicity
isoniazid, rifampin	Decreased serum levels of ketoconazole
Voriconazole	
quinidine	Prolongation of QT interval on ECG

ECG, Electrocardiograph; *PT,* prothrombin time.

DOSAGES

Selected Antifungal Drugs

Drug (Pregnancy Category)	Pharmacologic Class	Usual Dosage Range	Indications
▶amphotericin B (Amphocin, Fungizone) (B)	Polyene antifungal	IV: Initial daily dose, 0.25 mg/kg; titrate up to 1-1.5 mg/kg/day	Broad spectrum of systemic fungal infections
		Topical: apply cream or lotion bid-qid	Topical candidiasis
amphotericin B lipid complex (ABLC); doses vary with product as follows:	Polyene antifungal	**Adult and pediatric**	Systemic fungal infections
Abelcet (B)		IV: 5 mg/kg once daily, infused at 2.5 mg/kg/hr	
Amphotec (B)		IV: 3-4 mg/kg/day, infused at 1 mg/kg/hr	
AmBisome (B)		IV: 3-5 mg/kg/day, infused over 1-2 hr	
caspofungin (Cansidas) (C)	Echinocandin antifungal	**Adult only** IV: 70 mg loading dose on day 1, followed by 50 mg/day thereafter; infuse doses over 1 hour	Invasive aspergillosis in patients intolerant of or refractory to other drugs
▶fluconazole (Diflucan) (C)	Synthetic triazole antifungal	**Adult** PO: 150 mg in a single dose	Vaginal candidiasis
		Adult IV/PO: 100-400 mg/day × 2-5 wk (dose and duration depending on severity of infection) **Pediatric** IV/PO: 3-12 mg/kg, same guidelines as for adult	Oropharyngeal and esophageal candidiasis, systemic candidiasis
		Adult IV/PO: 200-400 mg/day × 10-12 wk after negative CSF cultures **Pediatric** Titrate pediatric doses as for adult	Cryptococcal meningitis

DOSAGES

Selected Antifungal Drugs—cont'd

Drug (Pregnancy Category)	Pharmacologic Class	Usual Dosage Range	Indications
micafungin (Mycamine) (C)	Echinocandin antifungal	**Adult** IV: 50-150 mg daily over 1 hr	Esophageal candidiasis; Candida prophylaxis in patients receiving hematopoietic stem cell transplants.
nystatin (Nilstat, Mycostatin, Nystex) (C)	Polyene antifungal	**Infant** PO: 200,000 units (2 mL) oral suspension in oral cavity qid **Adult and pediatric** PO: 400,000-600,000 units (4-6 mL) oral suspension in oral cavity qid **Adult and pediatric** PO (troche): 200,000-400,000 units (1-2 troches dissolved in mouth) 4-5 × day **Adult only** PO (tab): 500,000-1,000,000 units (1-2 tabs) tid Topical (cream, lotion, or powder): apply 2-3×/day Vaginal: Insert one vaginal tablet once daily × 2 wk	Oral candidiasis Intestinal candidiasis Topical candidiasis Vaginal candidiasis
terbinafine (Lamisil) (B)	Synthetic allylamine antifungal	**Adult only** PO: 250 mg qd × 6 wk (fingernail); × 12 wk (toenail) Topical cream or solution: apply bid to affected area × 1-4 wk	Onychomycosis (fungal infection of finger- or toenails) Athlete's foot (tinea pedis), jock itch (tinea cruris), or ringworm (tinea corporis)
voriconazole (Vfend) (D)	Synthetic triazole antifungal	**Adult only** PO: 100-300 mg q12h, titrated with higher doses for patients >40 kg IV: 200-mg vial diluted to 5 mg/mL and infused up to 3 mg/kg/hr over 1-2 hr	Invasive aspergillosis; other major fungal infections in patients who do not tolerate or respond to other antifungal drugs

temic use and is used primarily to treat onychomycoses of the fingernails or toenails.

Pharmacokinetics

Half-Life	Onset	Peak	Duration
PO: 22-26 hr	PO: Unknown	PO: 1-2 hr	PO: Unknown

voriconazole

Voriconazole (Vfend) is also a newer antifungal drug, approved by the U.S. Food and Drug Administration (FDA) in 2002. It is used for treating severe fungal infections caused by *Aspergillus* spp. (invasive aspergillosis). It is also used for a variety of other severe fungal infections, such as those caused by *Scedosporium* and *Fusarium* spp. Voriconazole is contraindicated in patients with known drug allergy to it and when coadministered with certain other drugs metabolized by the cytochrome P-450 enzyme CYP3A4 (e.g., quinidine) because of the risk for inducing serious cardiac dysrhythmias. It is also the only antifungal drug contraindicated in pregnancy. The drug is available in oral and injectable form.

Pharmacokinetics

Half-Life	Onset	Peak	Duration
PO: Unknown due to nonlinear kinetics	PO: Unknown	PO: 1-2 hr	PO: Unknown

◆ NURSING PROCESS

◆ ASSESSMENT

Although topical dosage forms are to be discussed in detail in Chapter 57, it is still very important to discuss these forms and related nursing process issues. Vital signs, weight, hemoglobin (Hgb), hematocrit (Hct), red blood cell counts (RBCs), complete blood counts (CBCs) with differential, liver and renal function tests, and confirmation of culture/sensitivity test results should all be assessed and noted prior to beginning antifungal therapy. Before administering amphotericin B (or any other antifungal drug), it is important for the nurse to identify any contraindications, cautions, and drug interactions, which have been previously discussed. Allergy to amphotericin B and/or sulfites should be noted and considered a contraindication, and any other nephrotoxic drugs need to be avoided if at all possible. Baseline renal function studies would be warranted in this situation. There is a risk for severe adverse reactions with intravenous antifungal administration (e.g., amphotericin B), so assessment of any special pre-medication orders for use of antiemetics, antihistamines, antipyretics, and antiinflammatory drugs, should be completed. Caspofungin and other antifungals require recording of baseline vital signs, liver function tests, and CBCs. Patients receiving griseofulvin should be assessed thoroughly for allergy to penicillin due to possible higher risk for allergic reactions to the antifungal. Griseofulvin may also precipitate severe blood dyscrasias, and therefore, baseline CBCs are needed. Patients who are to receive ketoconazole should have their liver function assessed because of drug-related hepatotoxicity. Miconazole use is associated with adverse cardiovascular effects; therefore, pulse, blood pressure, and electrocardiogram (ECG) interpretation should be noted, as should any history of cardiac disease. Nystatin lozenges should be avoided in children under the age of 5 years. Terbinafine requires close monitoring of liver function tests, especially in patients receiving treatment for longer than 6 weeks, and the drug voriconazole should be given only after baseline liver and kidney function tests have been noted. Voriconazole is contraindicated if the patient is taking drugs such as quinidine and other drugs metabolized in the same pathway. The reason for this is that voriconazole undergoes metabolism by the cytochrome P-450 enzyme CYP3A4 and could induce serious cardiac dysrhythmias.

◆ NURSING DIAGNOSES
- Acute pain related to symptoms of the infectious process
- Deficient knowledge related to lack of information and experience with the antifungal drug therapy
- Risk for injury related to adverse effects of the medication treatment regimen

◆ PLANNING
Goals
- Patient states the rationale for adherence/compliance with antifungal therapy.
- Patient states the common adverse effects and ways to prevent injury to self associated with antifungal drug therapy.
- Patient exhibits relief of the symptoms previously associated with the fungal infection.
- Patient states the importance of follow-up appointments.

Outcome Criteria
- Patient is free of the complications or suffers minimal adverse effects of the antifungal drug therapy for the duration of treatment (e.g., nausea, vomiting, gastrointestinal upset).
- Patient remains compliant with the medication regimen without omissions/skipping of doses and experiences relief of infection with a return to normal vital signs and normal culture and sensitivity reports after full course of therapy.
- Patient experiences improved appetite, energy level, and physical strength/stamina after taking the antifungal drugs for the prescribed period.
- Patient returns to the physician regularly as recommended by the health care provider for constant monitoring of the infection and of drug therapy with various blood tests (e.g., CBC with differential, RBC, Hgb, Hct, renal and liver function tests).

◆ IMPLEMENTATION
The nursing interventions appropriate to patients receiving antifungal drugs vary depending on the particular drug. It is often necessary for the nurse to check the vital signs of patients receiving any of the antifungals for at least every 15 to 30 minutes during infusion, or as needed. It is important for the nurse to monitor the intake and output amounts, urinalysis results, liver/kidney function tests, and CBCs during therapy. It is also important for the nurse to weigh patients weekly (or encourage this at home) and document

weights (even if in the home setting), because a gain of 2 lb or more in a 24-hour period or 5 lb or more in 1 week may indicate possible medication-induced renal damage, with the need for prompt medical attention. Follow manufacturer guidelines and the physician's order for specific solutions and rates of intravenous administration. With intravenous amphotericin B, avoid use of solutions that are cloudy or with precipitates. Intravenous infusion pumps are recommended. Monitoring of vital signs should be done every 15 minutes or as needed to assess for adverse reactions, with notation of abdominal pain, anorexia, chills, fever, nausea, shaking, and vomiting. Should these adverse effects or a severe reaction occur, the infusion should be discontinued (while closely monitoring the patient) and the physician contacted. The IV site should be monitored for signs of phlebitis (e.g., heat, pain, and redness over the site/vein). Intake and output should be monitored and the skin checked for burning, itching, and irritation. See the Patient Teaching Tips for further information.

Use only clear solutions of caspofungin, and dilute doses with NaCl and continue to monitor liver function studies over the duration of therapy. Liver function studies should be monitored closely. Fluconazole may be given either orally or intravenously, with intravenous dosage forms used if there is a specific indication or if the oral dosage forms are poorly tolerated. Intravenous dosage forms should be used only if clear, and no other medication should be added to the solution. Itching or a rash should be reported immediately, and there should also be monitoring of the patient's temperature, bowel activity, and stool consistency. Griseofulvin is associated with photosensitivity, and patient instructions should include proper use of sunscreen and protective clothing; however, avoiding exposure to sun is preferred. Monitoring the patient for complaints of headaches should continue, with treatment and oral dosage forms given with food to minimize gastrointestinal upset. Oral dosages of itraconazole should be given with food to minimize gastrointestinal upset. Intravenous itraconazole should be administered using only an IV bag and tubing equipment provided by the manufacturer, with infusions usually ordered for over 60 minutes. Nystatin given orally may be in the form of lozenges or troches that are to be slowly and completely dissolved in the mouth for optimal effects; these should not be chewed or swallowed whole. If a suspension is used, make sure that the patient "swishes" the medication solution thoroughly in the mouth for as long as possible prior to swallowing. Terbinafine may be given orally or topically. Local skin reactions that need to be reported include blistering, itching, oozing, redness, and swelling. Oral dosing of voriconazole should be given 1 hour before or 1 hour after a meal, and intravenous doses may be diluted with D_5W or NaCl and the accurate dosage infused over the recommended time frame. Visual acuity must be monitored with this drug (especially if ordered for longer than 28 days) and any changes reported to the health care provider.

◆ EVALUATION
The therapeutic effects of antifungals include improvement and eventual resolution of the signs and symptoms of the fungal infection if the patient has remained totally compliant/adherent with the therapy. Improved energy levels and overall improvement in sense of well-being with a baseline normal temperature and vital signs also indicate a therapeutic response. Specific adverse effects for which to monitor in patients receiving these drugs are listed in Table 41-2. Goals and outcome criteria should be evaluated in the context of the nursing care plan.

Patient Teaching Tips

- Female patients taking antifungal medications for the treatment of vaginal infections should abstain from sexual intercourse until the treatment is completed and the infection is resolved and should be told to continue to take the medication even if actively menstruating. Patients should notify the physician if symptoms persist past the treatment after treatment is completed.
- Some patients receiving amphotericin B may need long-term treatment (i.e., over weeks to months). If so, adverse effects include tinnitus, blurred vision, burning and itching at the infusion site, headache, rash, fever, chills, hypokalemia, gastrointestinal upset, and various anemias. Patients should weigh themselves weekly and notify the physician if they gain more than 2 lb in a 24-hour period or 5 pounds or more in 1 week. Muscle weakness may occur due to hypokalemia, so there is a need for monitoring of serum potassium.
- For patients taking caspofungin, any problems with shortness of breath, itching, facial swelling, and/or a rash must be reported immediately to the appropriate physician/health care provider.
- Fluconazole may cause dizziness, and, therefore, driving may be halted until adverse effects are resolved. Good hygiene should be recommended.
- Griseofulvin is to be taken exactly as prescribed and usually over weeks and months. Patients should be educated about the interaction with alcohol with resultant flushing of the face and tachycardia. Photosensitivity may occur and so appropriate measures implemented (see previous discussion). Patients should be informed about foods high in fat (e.g., milk, ice cream) because they reduce gastrointestinal upset and encourage drug absorption.
- Educate patients about proper dosing instructions related to nystatin; they should be fully informed about how to apply the drug. If vaginal troches are used, the appropriate applicator should be used with a gloved hand and inserted high into the vagina, then followed with handwashing. Educate patients to avoid sexual intercourse until treatment is completed. Oral lozenges should be dissolved and used as ordered (e.g., swish and swallow); the physician's order and manufacturer guidelines should be followed.
- Itraconazole capsules should be taken with food, and, if therapy lasts 3 months or longer, the patient should receive careful instructions to avoid extreme frustration. The patient should report anorexia, dark orange urine, nausea, vomiting, yellow skin, or unusual fatigue.
- Ketoconazole requires "acidic" environment. If patients take antacids, anticholinergics, or H_2 receptor blockers, they should take the ketoconazole 2 hours after dosing. Shampoo forms should be applied to wet hair, massaged for a full minute, rinsed thoroughly, and re-applied for 3 minutes, as ordered, followed by rinsing. Topical dosing should be applied carefully with prevention of contact to eyes, mucous membranes, and mouth. If there are new symptoms or if the patient develops dark orange urine, irritation at topical site, onset of new symptoms or pale stool or yellow skin/eyes, the physician should be contacted immediately.
- Encourage patients to keep "affected" body areas clean and dry and to wear light and cool clothing. Patients should avoid contact of the topical dosage form with their eyes, mouth, nose, or other mucous membranes. Educate patients to report any adverse effects such as skin irritation and diarrhea.
- Voriconazole should be taken 1 hour before or 1 hour after meals. Encourage patients to avoid driving at night due to visual changes, for example, blurred vision and/or photophobia. Patients should be encouraged to avoid direct sunlight and to use effective contraception.

Points to Remember

- Fungi are a very large and diverse group of microorganisms and consist of yeast and molds. Yeasts are single-celled fungi that may be harmful (e.g., causing infections) or helpful (e.g., when baking or brewing beer). Molds are multicellular and characterized by long, branching filaments called *hyphae*.
- Candidiasis is an opportunistic fungal infection caused by *Candida albicans* and occurs in patients taking broad-spectrum antibiotics, antineoplastics, or immunosuppressants, as well as in immunocompromised persons. When candidiasis occurs in the mouth, it is commonly called *oral candidiasis* or *thrush*. It is more commonly seen in newborns or immunocompromised persons.
- Vaginal candidiasis is a yeast infection and occurs mostly in patients with diabetes mellitus, women taking oral contraceptives, and pregnant women.
- Antifungals may be administered either systemically or topically. Some of the most common systemic antifungals are amphotericin B, fluconazole, itraconazole, and ketoconazole; some of the most common topical antifungals are clotrimazole, miconazole, and nystatin. Several chemical categories of antifungals include both topical and systemic drugs, each with its own unique way of killing fungi.
- Before administering antifungals, the nurse must thoroughly assess for allergies as well as other drugs patients are taking, including prescription drugs, OTC drugs, and herbals.
- Amphotericin B must be properly diluted according to the manufacturer's guidelines and administered using an intravenous infusion pump. Tissue extravasation of fluconazole at the intravenous infusion site leads to tissue necrosis; therefore, the site should be checked hourly and the assessment documented.

NCLEX Examination Review Questions

1. The nurse is assessing a patient who is about to receive antifungal drug therapy. Which problem would be of most concern?
   a. Endocrine disease
   b. Hepatic disease
   c. Cardiac disease
   d. Pulmonary disease
2. While monitoring a patient who is receiving intravenous amphotericin B, the nurse expects to see which adverse effect?
   a. Hypertension
   b. Bradycardia
   c. Fever and chills
   d. Diarrhea and stomach cramps
3. Which of the following is a common underlying source of many of the drug interactions with antifungals?
   a. Polyuria
   b. Gallbladder metabolism
   c. Bone distribution
   d. Cytochrome P-450 enzyme system

4. When monitoring the patient who is receiving griseofulvin, the nurse should look for which potentially serious adverse effect?
   a. Blood dyscrasias
   b. Hypotension
   c. Cardiac palpitations
   d. Gastrointestinal bleeding
5. When instructing a patient who is taking Nystatin lozenges for oral candidiasis, which instruction by the nurse is correct?
   a. "Chew the lozenge carefully before swallowing."
   b. "Dissolve the lozenge slowly and completely in your mouth."
   c. "Dissolve the lozenge until it is half the original size, then swallow it."
   d. "These lozenges should be swallowed whole with a glass of water."

1. b, 2. c, 3. d, 4. a, 5. b.

Critical Thinking Activities

1. What laboratory data and other assessment data should be considered before administering any of the systemic antifungals? Specify the data, and identify the reason for their importance.
2. Explain the rationale for giving doses of antipyretics, antihistamines, and antiemetics to a patient who is receiving an amphotericin B infusion. When are these drugs given?

3. What instructions should accompany a prescription of ketoconazole?

For answers, see http://evolve.elsevier.com/Lilley.

Antimalarial, Antiprotozoal, and Anthelmintic Drugs

Objectives

When you reach the end of this chapter, you should be able to do the following:

1. Briefly discuss the infection process associated with malaria, protozoal infestations, and helminths.
2. Compare the signs and symptoms associated with malaria, protozoal, and helminthic infection processes.
3. Identify the more commonly used antimalarial, antiprotozoal, and anthelmintic drugs.
4. Discuss the mechanisms of action, indications, cautions, contraindications, adverse effects, dosages, and routes of administration associated with each antimalarial, antiprotozoal, and anthelmintic drug.
5. Develop a nursing care plan that includes all phases of the nursing process for patients receiving antimalarial, antiprotozoal, or anthelmintic drugs.

e-Learning Activities

Companion CD

- NCLEX Review Questions: see questions 362-365
- Animations
- Audio Glossary
- Category Catchers
- Medication Errors Checklists
- IV Therapy Checklists

evolve Website (http://evolve.elsevier.com/Lilley)

• Nursing Care Plans • Frequently Asked Questions • Content Updates • WebLinks • Supplemental Resources • Elsevier ePharmacology Update • Medication Administration Animations

Drug Profiles

atovaquone, p. 659
▶ chloroquine and hydroxychloroquine, p. 656
diethylcarbamazine, p. 663
iodoquinol, p. 659
▶ mebendazole, p. 664
mefloquine, p. 656

▶ metronidazole, p. 661
paromomycin, p. 661
pentamidine, p. 661
praziquantel, p. 664
▶ primaquine, p. 656
pyrantel, p. 664
pyrimethamine, p. 658

▶ Key drug.

Glossary

Anthelmintic A drug that destroys or prevents the development of parasitic worm (helminthic) infections. Also called *antihelmintic* or *vermicide*; notice that the terms for the drug categories are spelled with only one "h," which appears only in the second syllable of the term, whereas the term for worm infection *(helminthic)* is spelled with two "h's," appearing in both the second and third syllables of the term. (p. 661)

Antimalarial drug A drug that destroys or prevents the development of the malaria parasite (*Plasmodium* sp.) in human hosts. Antimalarial drugs are a subset of the antiprotozoal drugs, a broader drug category. (p. 655)

Antiprotozoal A drug that destroys or prevents the development of protozoa in human hosts. (p. 658)

Helminthic infection A parasitic worm infection. (p. 662)

Malaria A widespread protozoal infectious disease caused by four species of the genus *Plasmodium*. (p. 654)

Parasite Any organism that feeds on another living organism (known as a *host*) in a way that results in varying degrees of harm to the host organism. (p. 653)

Parasitic protozoa Harmful protozoa that live on or in human beings or animals and cause disease in the process. (p. 653)

Protozoa Single-celled organisms that are the smallest and simplest members of the animal kingdom. (p. 653)

There are also more than 28,000 known types of **protozoa,** which are single-celled organisms. Those that live on or in humans are called **parasitic protozoa.** Billions of people worldwide are infected with these organisms, and, as a result, these infections are considered a serious public health problem. Some of the more common protozoal infections are malaria, leishmaniasis, trypanosomiasis, amebiasis, giardiasis, and trichomoniasis. They are relatively uncommon in the United States but are becoming increasingly prevalent among immunocompromised persons, including those with AIDS. Protozoal diseases are especially prevalent among people living in tropical climates because it is easier for protozoa to survive and be transmitted in these year-round warm and humid environments. Although the population of the United States is relatively free of many of these protozoal infections, international travel and the immigration of people from other countries where such infections are endemic are providing opportunities for increased exposure.

MALARIA

The most significant protozoal disease in terms of morbidity and mortality is **malaria.** Worldwide, it is estimated that 250 to 500 million people are infected, resulting in an annual death rate of 750,000 to 2 million people. In Africa alone, it accounts for more than 1 million infant deaths a year. The most prevalent geographic areas are sub-Saharan Africa, Southeast Asia, and Latin America. It is caused by a particular genus of protozoa called *Plasmodium,* and there are four species of organisms within this genus, each with its own characteristics and its own ability to resist being killed by antimalarial drugs. These four species are *Plasmodium vivax, P. falciparum, P. malariae, and P. ovale.* Although *P. vivax* is the most widespread of the four, *P. falciparum* is nearly as widespread and causes greater problems with drug resistance. The two remaining species are much less common and more geographically limited in their occurrence, but they can still cause serious malarial infections. Most commonly, malaria is transmitted by the bite of an infected female *anopheline* mosquito. This type of mosquito is endemic to many tropical regions of the earth. Malaria can also be transmitted by blood transfusions, congenitally from mother to infant via an infected placenta, or through the use of contaminated needles by drug abusers. Despite the combined efforts of many countries to eradicate malaria, it remains one of the most devastating infectious diseases in the world. As is also the case with tuberculosis (Chapter 40) and AIDS (Chapter 39), many lives are lost to malaria, and the cost of treating and preventing the disease imposes a tremendous economic burden on the often poor countries where the disease is prevalent.

The *Plasmodium* life cycle is quite complex and involves many stages. It has two interdependent life cycles: the *sexual cycle,* which takes place inside the mosquito, and the *asexual cycle,* which occurs in the human host. In addition, the asexual cycle of the **parasite** consists of a phase outside the erythrocyte (primarily in liver tissues) called the *exoerythrocytic phase* (also called the *tissue phase*) and a phase inside the erythrocyte called the *erythrocytic phase* (also called the *blood phase*). The malarial parasite undergoes many changes during these two phases (Figure 42-1). Malaria signs and symptoms are often described in terms of the *classic malaria paroxysm.* A paroxysm is a sudden recurrence or intensification of symptoms. Symptoms include chills and rigors, followed by fevers up to 104° F, diaphoresis, often leading to extreme fatigue and prolonged sleep. This syndrome often repeats itself periodically in 48- to 72-hour cycles. Other common symptoms include headache, nausea, and joint pain.

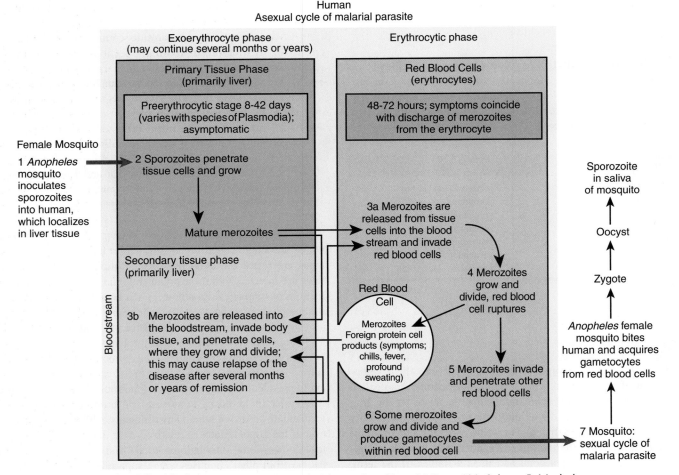

FIGURE 42-1 Life cycle of the malarial parasite. *(From McKenry LM, Salerno E: Mosby's pharmacology in nursing—revised and updated, ed 21, St Louis, 2003, Mosby.)*

ANTIMALARIAL DRUGS

Antimalarial drugs administered to humans cannot affect the parasite during its sexual cycle when it resides in the mosquito. Instead, these drugs work against the parasite during its asexual cycle, which takes place within the human body. Often these drugs are given in various combinations to achieve an additive or synergistic antimalarial effect. One example is the combination of the two antiprotozoal drugs atovaquone and proguanil (Malarone). The antibiotic combination of pyrimethamine and sulfadoxine (Fansidar) is also commonly used, especially in drug-resistant cases of malaria.

Mechanism of Action and Drug Effects

The mechanisms of action of the various antimalarial drugs differ depending on the chemical family of drugs to which they belong. The *4-aminoquinoline derivatives* (chloroquine and hydroxychloroquine) work by inhibiting DNA and RNA polymerase, an enzyme essential to DNA and RNA synthesis by the parasite cells. Parasite protein synthesis is also disrupted because protein synthesis is dependent on proper nucleic acid (DNA and RNA) function. These drugs are also believed to raise the pH within the parasite, which has the effect of interfering with the parasite's ability to metabolize and use erythrocyte hemoglobin and is one reason these drugs are ineffective during the exoerythrocytic phase (tissue phase) of infection. All of these actions contribute to the destruction of the parasite. Quinine, quinidine, and mefloquine are thought to be similar to the 4-aminoquinoline derivatives in their actions in that both are also believed to raise the pH within the parasite.

The *diaminopyrimidines* (pyrimethamine and trimethoprim [Chapter 37]) work by inhibiting dihydrofolate reductase, an enzyme that is needed for the production of certain vital substances in malarial parasites. Specifically, inhibiting this enzyme blocks the synthesis of tetrahydrofolate, a precursor of purines and pyrimidines (nucleic acid components), and certain amino acids (protein components) essential for the growth and survival of plasmodia parasites. These two drugs are also only effective during the erythrocytic phase and are often used with a sulfonamide (sulfadoxine, Chapter 37) or sulfone (dapsone, Chapter 38) because of the resulting synergistic effects exerted by such drug combinations. Tetracyclines (Chapter 37) such as doxycycline, and lincomycins (Chapter 37) such as clindamycin may also be used in combination with some of the other antimalarial drugs described earlier, again because of the synergistic effects resulting from these drug combinations.

Primaquine, an *8-aminoquinoline* that is structurally similar to the 4-aminoquinolines mentioned above, has the ability to bind to and alter parasitic DNA and is one of the few drugs that is effective in the exoerythrocytic phase. Atovaquone-proguanil also works by interference with nucleic acid synthesis.

The drug effects of the antimalarial drugs are mostly limited to their ability to kill parasitic organisms, most of which are *Plasmodium* spp. Some of these drugs do, however, have other drug effects. Chloroquine and hydroxychloroquine also have antiinflammatory effects and are sometimes used in the treatment of rheumatoid arthritis and systemic lupus erythematosus. Quinine and quinidine, two plant alkaloids from the bark of the South American cinchona tree, can also decrease the excitability of both cardiac and skeletal muscles. Quinidine is still currently used to treat certain types of cardiac dysrhythmias (Chapter 22).

Indications

Antimalarial drugs are used to kill *Plasmodium* organisms, the parasites that cause malaria. As already mentioned, different antimalarial drugs work during different phases of the parasite's growth inside the human. Those antimalarials exerting the greatest effect on all four *Plasmodium* organisms during the erythrocytic or blood phase are chloroquine, hydroxychloroquine, and pyrimethamine. Other drugs that are known to work in the blood phase include quinine, quinidine, halofantrine, and mefloquine. Halofantrine is not generally available in the United States. Because these drugs are ineffective during the exoerythrocytic phase, however, they cannot *prevent* infection. The most effective antimalarial drug for eradicating the parasite during the exoerythrocytic or tissue phase is primaquine, which actually works during both phases However, it is indicated specifically for *P. vivax*. Chloroquine and hydroxychloroquine (4-aminoquinolines) remain the drugs of choice for the treatment of susceptible strains of malarial parasites. They are highly toxic to all *Plasmodium* spp., except in resistant cases of *P. falciparum*, which is commonly resistant to the 4-aminoquinolines. Such resistant cases occur in many areas of the world, including Asia, Africa, and South America.

Quinine is indicated for chloroquine-resistant *P. falciparum*, which can cause a type of malaria that affects the cerebral hemispheres. Quinine can be used alone but is more commonly used in combination with pyrimethamine, a sulfonamide, or a tetracycline (such as doxycycline). Pyrimethamine is another antimalarial antibiotic that is commonly used in combination with the sulfonamide antibiotic sulfadoxine (Fansidar) for the prophylaxis of chloroquine-resistant *P. falciparum* and *P. vivax*. However, drug resistance in most locations has reduced its use for this purpose. Other antimalarial drugs are usually preferred for treatment of active disease. Mefloquine is a newer antimalarial drug that may also be used for both prophylaxis and treatment of malaria caused by *P. falciparum* or *P. vivax*. The drug combination atovaquone and proguanil (Malarone) is also used for prevention and treatment of *P. falciparum* infection.

Contraindications

Contraindications to various antimalarial drugs include drug allergy, tinnitus (ear ringing), and pregnancy (quinine). Severe renal, hepatic, or hematologic dysfunction may also be contraindicative to the use of antimalarial drugs. Other drug-specific contraindications are noted in the drug profiles below.

Adverse Effects

Antimalarial drugs cause diverse adverse effects, and these are listed for each drug in Table 42-1.

Interactions

Some common drug interactions associated with antimalarial drugs are listed in Table 42-2.

Dosages

For the recommended dosages for selected antimalarial drugs, see the Dosages table on page 657.

Table 42-1 Antimalarial Drugs: Common Adverse Effects

Body System	Adverse Effects
Chloroquine and Hydroxychloroquine	
Gastrointestinal	Diarrhea, anorexia, nausea, vomiting, abdominal distress
CNS	Dizziness, anxiety, headache, reduced seizure threshold
Other	Alopecia, rash, pruritus
Mefloquine	
Central nervous	Headache, dizziness, insomnia, visual disturbances, increased anxiety, convulsions, depression, psychosis
Gastrointestinal	Stomach pain, anorexia, nausea, vomiting
Primaquine	
Gastrointestinal	Nausea, vomiting, abdominal distress
Other	Headaches, pruritus, dark discoloration of urine, hemolytic anemia due to G6PD deficiency
Pyrimethamine	
Gastrointestinal	Anorexia; vomiting; taste disturbances; soreness, redness, swelling, or burning of tongue; diarrhea; throat pain; swallowing difficulties; sores, ulcerations, or white spots in mouth; sore throat
Other	Fever, increased bleeding, increased weakness, rash, hemolytic anemia resulting from G6PD deficiency, severe hypersensitivity reactions
Quinine	
Central nervous	Visual disturbances, dizziness, severe headaches, tinnitus, hearing loss
Gastrointestinal	Diarrhea, nausea, vomiting, abdominal pain or discomfort
Other	Rash, pruritus, hives, respiratory difficulties, wheezing

G6PD, Glucose-6-phosphate dehydrogenase.

Table 42-2 Antimalarial Drugs: Drug Interactions

Drug	Mechanism	Result
Chloroquine		
divalproex, valproic acid	Decreased serum levels of valproic acid	Loss of seizure control
Mefloquine		
Beta-blockers, CCBs, quinidine, quinine	Unknown	Increased risk of dysrhythmia, cardiac arrest, seizures
Primaquine		
Other hemolytic drugs	Unknown	Increased risk for myelotoxic effects (monitor for muscle weakness)

CCB, Calcium channel blocker.

Drug Profiles

The dosing instructions for several of the antimalarial drugs can be confusing because tablet strengths on the medication packaging often indicate the strength of the tablet in terms of the entire salt form of the drug, not just the active ingredient itself, which is referred to as the *base ingredient.* However, dosing guidelines often list recommended dosages in terms of the base ingredient and not the entire salt. For example, as described later in the drug profile for chloroquine, the tablets come in 250- and 500-mg strengths of the salt form of the drug, but these tablets actually only have 150 and 300 mg, respectively, of the active ingredient or base. The reader is advised to be mindful of these distinctions.

▸ chloroquine and hydroxychloroquine

Chloroquine (Aralen) is a synthetic antimalarial drug that is chemically classified as a 4-aminoquinoline derivative. It is also indicated for treatment of other parasitic infections, such as amebiasis. Hydroxychloroquine is another synthetic 4-aminoquinoline derivative that differs from chloroquine by only one hydroxyl group ($^-$OH). Its efficacy in treating malaria is comparable to that of quinine. Both medications also possess antiinflammatory actions and have been used to treat rheumatoid arthritis and systemic lupus erythematosus since the 1950s. However, hydroxychloroquine is considered to be preferable to quinine for treating these inflammatory illnesses because of its reduced risk for causing ocular toxicity at the high doses required.

Contraindications include visual field changes, optic neuritis, and psoriasis, keeping in mind that sound clinical judgment may still warrant the use of the medication in urgent clinical situations.

Chloroquine is available in both an injectable and an oral (PO) formulation. Hydroxychloroquine is available only for oral use. Both drugs are classified as pregnancy category C drugs but it is recommended that use in pregnant women should occur only in truly urgent clinical situations. These drugs are also distributed into breast milk, with one study demonstrating about one third the level of chloroquine in breast milk as in the mother's bloodstream.

Pharmacokinetics

Chloroquine

Half-Life	Onset	Peak	Duration
PO: 3-5 days	PO: 8-10 hr	PO: 2 hr	PO: Variable

Hydroxychloroquine

Half-Life	Onset	Peak	Duration
PO: 32-50 days	PO: Several hr*	PO: Few hr*	PO: Variable
	PO: 4-6 wk†	PO: Several mo†	

*For malaria.
†For rheumatic diseases.

mefloquine

Mefloquine (Lariam) is an analog of quinine that is indicated for the management of mild-to-moderate acute malaria and for the prevention and treatment of chloroquine-resistant malaria and multidrug-resistant strains of *P. falciparum,* which, as already noted, is a very difficult species of *Plasmodium* to kill. The drug is commonly used prophylactically by travelers to prevent malarial infection while visiting malaria-endemic areas. The tetracycline antibiotic doxycycline (Chapter 37) is also commonly used for this purpose. It is available only for oral use.

Pharmacokinetics

Half-Life	Onset	Peak	Duration
PO: Days to weeks	PO: <24 hr	PO: 7-24 hr	PO: Variable

▸ primaquine

Primaquine is similar in chemical structure and antimalarial activity to the 4-aminoquinolines, but it is classified as an 8-aminoquinoline. However, as previously noted, it is one of the few antimalarial drugs that can destroy the malarial parasites while they are in their exoerythrocytic phase (tissue phase). It is indicated for curative therapy

DOSAGES

Selected Antimalarial Drugs

Drug (Pregnancy Category)	Pharmacologic Class	Usual Dosage Range	Indications
►chloroquine (Aralen) (C)	Synthetic antimalarial and antiamebic	**Adult*** PO: 300 mg base weekly, beginning 1-2 wk before and continuing for 4 wk after visiting endemic area	Malaria prophylaxis
		PO: 600 mg base day 1, followed by 300 mg 6 hr later and qd days 2 and 3	Malaria treatment
		IM: 160-200 mg base when PO therapy not feasible; repeat in 6 hr if necessary but switch to PO therapy ASAP and continue × 3 days for a total base dose of at least 1.5 g	
►hydroxychloroquine (Plaquenil) (C)	Synthetic antimalarial	**Adult*** PO: 310 mg base weekly, beginning 1-2 wk before and continuing through 4 wk after visiting endemic area	Malaria treatment
		PO: 620 mg base day 1, followed by 310 mg 6 hr later and qd days 2 and 3	Malaria prophylaxis
mefloquine (Lariam) (C)	Synthetic antimalarial	**Adult*** PO: 250 mg weekly beginning 1-2 wks before travel and continuing until 4 wk after visiting endemic area	Malaria treatment
		Pediatric PO: Weekly dosing as above based on weight as follows: 15-19 kg = ¼ tab 20-30 kg = ½ tab 31-45 kg = ¾ tab >45 kg = 1 tab (250 mg)	
		Adult PO: 1250 mg (5 tabs) as single dose	Malaria prophylaxis
		Pediatric PO: 15-25 mg/kg in a single dose, not to exceed 1250 mg	
►primaquine (generic only) (C)	Synthetic antimalarial	**Adult** PO: 15 mg base qd3 × 14 days **Pediatric** 0.3 mg base/kg/day qd3 × 14 days	For cure or relapse prevention of malaria infection with *Plasmodium vivax;* may also be used for *P. vivax* in patients intolerant of chloroquine or if chloroquine is not available
pyrimethamine (Daraprim) (C)	Folic acid antagonist, antimalarial, antitoxoplasmotic drug	**Adult and pediatric >10 yr** PO: 25 mg weekly **Pediatric 4-10 yr** PO: 12.5 mg weekly **Pediatric infant-3 yr** PO: 6.25 mg weekly	Malaria prophylaxis
		Adult and pediatric >10 yr PO: 50 mg qd3 × 32 days **Pediatric 4-10 yr** PO: 25 mg qd3 × 2 days	Malaria treatment

*Only adult doses are given. Pediatric doses range from 5-10 mg/kg but should not exceed adult doses.

Table 42-3 Types of Protozoal Infections and Common Drug Therapy

Protozoal Infection	Description	Antiprotozoal Drug
Amebiasis	Infection that mainly resides in the large intestine but can also migrate to other parts of the body, such as the liver. Produced by the protozoal parasite *Entamoeba histolytica.* Usually transmitted in contaminated food or water.	chloroquine, metronidazole, paromomycin, iodoquinol, tinidazole
Giardiasis	Caused by *Giardia lamblia.* The most common intestinal protozoal infection, usually residing in the intestinal mucosa (most commonly the duodenum). May cause diarrhea, bloating, and foul-smelling stools. Transmitted by contaminated food or water or by contact with stool from infected persons.	metronidazole, nitazoxanide, quinacrine, furazolidone, albendazole, paromomycin, tinidazole
Pneumocystosis	Pneumonias caused by *Pneumocystis jirovecii* that occur exclusively in immunocompromised people. Always fatal if left untreated.	trimethoprim–sulfamethoxazole, dapsone, atovaquone, primaquine, pentamidine, clindamycin, trimetrexate
Toxoplasmosis	Caused by *Toxoplasma gondii.* Can produce systemic infection in both immunocompetent and immunocompromised hosts. Domesticated animals, usually cats, serve as intermediate host for parasites, passing infective oocysts in their feces.	sulfonamides with pyrimethamine, clindamycin, metronidazole
Trichomoniasis	Sexually transmitted disease caused by *Trichomonas vaginalis.*	metronidazole, tinidazole

in acute cases of *P. vivax, P. ovale,* and to a lesser degree, *P. falciparum* infection.

Primaquine is contraindicated in patients with anemia, lupus erythematosus, methemoglobinemia, porphyria, rheumatoid arthritis, methemoglobin reductase deficiency, and G6PD deficiency. It is available only for oral use.

Pharmacokinetics			
Half-Life	**Onset**	**Peak**	**Duration**
PO: >4-10 hr	PO: <2 hr	PO: 1-3 hr	PO: 24 hr

pyrimethamine

Pyrimethamine (Daraprim) is a synthetic antimalarial drug that is structurally related to trimethoprim (Chapter 37). Both drugs are chemically subclassified as *diaminopyrimidines.* Fansidar is a commonly used fixed-combination drug product that contains 500 mg of sulfadoxine and 25 mg of pyrimethamine. Pyrimethamine is contraindicated in patients with megaloblastic anemia caused by folate deficiency. It is available only for oral use.

Pharmacokinetics			
Half-Life	**Onset**	**Peak**	**Duration**
PO: 4 days	PO: <6 hr	PO: 2-6 hr	PO: Up to 2 wk

OTHER PROTOZOAL INFECTIONS

Although malaria is the most common, there are several other common protozoal infections. These include amebiasis, giardiasis, pneumocystosis, toxoplasmosis, and trichomoniasis. Like malaria, these are also more prevalent in tropical regions. The corresponding protozoal parasites that most often cause each of these infections are, respectively, *Entamoeba histolytica, Giardia lamblia, Pneumocystis jirovecii* (formerly *P. carinii*), *Toxoplasma gondii,* and *Trichomonas vaginalis.*

These protozoal infections can be transmitted in a number of ways: from person to person (e.g., via sexual contact), through the ingestion of contaminated water or food, through direct contact with the parasite, or by the bite of an insect (mosquito or tick). These infections can be systemic and occur throughout the body or they can be localized to a specific region. For example, amebiasis most commonly affects the gastrointestinal tract (e.g., amoebic dysentery), whereas pneumocystosis is predominantly a pulmonary infection.

The more common protozoal infections are listed in Table 42-3, along with a brief description of the infection and the **antiprotozoal** drugs commonly used in their treatment. Only selected drugs are discussed here. Patients whose immune system is compromised, such as those with leukemia, those with transplanted organs who are on immunosuppressive drugs, and those with AIDS, are at particular risk for acquiring a protozoal infection. Often such infections are fatal in these patients.

ANTIPROTOZOAL DRUGS

Several drugs are used to treat nonmalarial protozoal infections. Some of these (chloroquine, primaquine, pyrimethamine, and atovaquone) are also used in malaria treatment, as previously noted. Other antiprotozoal drugs normally used for nonmalarial parasites include iodoquinol, metronidazole, paromomycin, and pentamidine.

Mechanism of Action and Drug Effects

Antiprotozoal drugs work by several different mechanisms. The mechanisms of action of the antiprotozoal drugs are varied. The most commonly used of these drugs together with a brief description of their mechanisms of action are given in Table 42-4. Pyrimethamine and chloroquine were discussed earlier in this

Table 42-4 Selected Antiprotozoal Drugs: Mechanisms of Action

Antiprotozoal Drug	Mechanism of Action
atovaquone	Atovaquone selectively inhibits mitochondrial electron transport, reducing ATP synthesis (required for cellular energy). Also inhibits nucleic acid synthesis.
eflornithine	Inhibits the enzyme ornithine decarboxylase, hindering protozoal nucleic acid and protein synthesis.
iodoquinol	Called a *luminal* or *contact amebicide* because it acts primarily in the intestinal lumen of the infected host and directly kills the protozoa.
metronidazole	Bactericidal, amebicidal, and trichomonacidal. Can also kill anaerobic bacteria, which it accomplishes by disrupting nucleic acid synthesis.
paromomycin	Also a luminal or contact amebicide. A direct-acting drug and kills by inhibiting protein synthesis in susceptible bacteria by binding to the 30S ribosomal subunit.
pentamidine	Inhibits production of much-needed substances such as DNA and RNA. Can bind to and aggregate ribosomes. Is directly lethal to *Pneumocystis jirovecii* by inhibiting glucose metabolism, protein and RNA synthesis, and intracellular amino acid transport.
tinidazole	Possibly reaction involving a nitrogen free radical.

DNA, Deoxyribonucleic acid; *RNA*, ribonucleic acid.

chapter in the section on malaria. The drug effects of these antiprotozoal drugs are primarily limited to their ability to kill various forms of protozoal parasites.

Indications

Antiprotozoal drugs are used to treat various protozoal infections, ranging from intestinal amebiasis to pneumocystosis. Indications for selected drugs are also summarized in Table 42-5. Atovaquone and pentamidine are used for the treatment of *P. jirovecii* infection. Iodoquinol, metronidazole, and paromomycin are all used to treat intestinal amebiasis, the usual causative organism being *Entamoeba histolytica*. Metronidazole is also effective against several forms of bacteria, including anaerobic bacteria (Chapter 37), as well as against protozoa and helminths (parasitic worms). Worm infection (helminthiasis) is discussed later in this chapter.

Contraindications

Contraindications to the use of antiprotozoal drugs include known drug allergy. Additional contraindications may include serious renal, liver, or other illnesses, weighing the seriousness of the infection against the patient's overall condition.

Table 42-5 Indications for Selected Antiprotozoal Drugs

Antiprotozoal Drugs	Indications
atovaquone	Used for treatment of acute mild to moderately severe *Pneumocystis jirovecii* pneumonia in patients who cannot tolerate cotrimoxazole
eflornithine	Indicated for meningoencephalitic stage of *Trypanosoma brucei gambiense* infection ("sleepy sickness")
iodoquinol	Indicated for treatment of intestinal amebiasis in asymptomatic carriers of *Entamoeba histolytica;* also has been used for treatment of *Giardia lamblia* and *Trichomonas vaginalis* infections
metronidazole	An antibacterial (including anaerobes), anti-protozoal, and anthelmintic drug
paromomycin	Indicated for treatment of acute and chronic intestinal amebiasis and as adjunct therapy in management of hepatic coma
pentamidine	Used for treatment of pneumonia caused by *P. jirovecii*
tinidazole	Indicated for giardiasis, trichomoniasis, and amebiasis

Adverse Effects

The adverse effects of antiprotozoal drugs vary greatly depending on the drug, and those specific to various common antiprotozoal drugs are listed in Table 42-6.

Interactions

The common drug and laboratory test interactions associated with the use of antiprotozoal drugs are listed in Table 42-7. Some of these interactions can result in severe toxicities, and it is therefore important to know of them and to understand the mechanism involved.

Dosages

For dosage information on selected antiprotozoal drugs, see the Dosages table on page 661.

Drug Profiles

atovaquone

Atovaquone (Mepron) is a synthetic antiprotozoal drug indicated for the treatment of mild-to-moderate *P. jirovecii* pneumonia in patients who cannot tolerate cotrimoxazole (trimethoprim/sulfamethoxazole) (Chapter 36). It is only available for oral use.

Pharmacokinetics

Half-Life	Onset	Peak	Duration
PO: 2-3 days	PO: 8-24 hr	PO: 24-96 hr	PO: Unknown

iodoquinol

Iodoquinol (Yodoxin) is considered to be a *luminal* or *contact* amebicide (killer of intestinal protozoa infections) because it acts primarily in the intestinal lumen. It is indicated for the treatment of intestinal amebiasis.

Table 42-6 Adverse Effects for Selected Antiprotozoal Drugs

Body System	Side/Adverse Effects
Atovaquone	
Cardiovascular	Hypotension
Hematologic	Anemia
Integumentary	Pruritus, urticaria, rash, oral candidiasis
Gastrointestinal	Anorexia, increased AST and ALT levels, acute pancreatitis, nausea, vomiting, diarrhea, constipation, abdominal pain
Central nervous	Dizziness, headache, anxiety
Metabolic	Hyperkalemia, hyperglycemia, hyponatremia
Other	Sweating, cough
Iodoquinol	
Hematologic	Agranulocytosis
Integumentary	Rash; pruritus; discolored skin, hair, nails
Central nervous	Headache, agitation, peripheral neuropathy
Eyes, ears, nose, and throat	Blurred vision, sore throat, optic neuritis
Gastrointestinal	Anorexia, gastritis, abdominal cramps, nausea, vomiting, diarrhea, anal itching
Other	Fever, chills, vertigo, weakness, dysesthesia
Metronidazole	
Central nervous	Headache, dizziness, confusion, fatigue, convulsions, peripheral neuropathy
Eyes, ears, nose, and throat	Blurred vision, sore throat, dry mouth, metallic taste, glossitis
Gastrointestinal	Abdominal cramps, pseudomembranous colitis, nausea, vomiting, diarrhea
Genitourinary	Darkened urine, dysuria
Hematologic	Leukopenia, bone marrow depression
Integumentary	Rash, pruritus, urticaria, flushing
Paromomycin	
Gastrointestinal	Stomach cramps, nausea, vomiting, diarrhea
Central nervous	Hearing loss, dizziness, tinnitus
Pentamidine	
Cardiovascular	Hypotension, dysrhythmias
Hematologic	Anemia, leukopenia, thrombocytopenia
Integumentary	Pain at injection site, pruritus, urticaria, rash
Genitourinary	Acute renal failure
Gastrointestinal	Increased AST and ALT levels, acute pancreatitis, metallic taste, nausea, vomiting, diarrhea
Central nervous	Disorientation, hallucinations, dizziness, confusion
Respiratory	Cough, shortness of breath, bronchospasm
Metabolic	Hyperkalemia, hypocalcemia, hypoglycemia followed by hyperglycemia
Other	Fatigue, chills, night sweats

AST, Aspartate aminotransferase; *ALT*, alanine aminotransferase.

Table 42-7 Antiprotozoal Drugs: Drug and Laboratory Test Interactions

Antiprotozoal Drug	Mechanism	Result
atovaquone	Compete for binding on protein, resulting in free, active atovaquone	Highly protein-bound drugs (e.g., warfarin, phenytoin); may increase atovaquone drug concentrations and risk of adverse reactions
iodoquinol	Increases protein-bound serum iodine concentrations, reflecting a decrease in iodine 131 uptake	May interfere with certain thyroid function test results
metronidazole	Increased plasma acetaldehyde concentration after ingestion of alcohol by decreasing the absorption of vitamin K from the intestines by eliminating the bacteria needed to absorb vitamin K	Alcohol: causes a disulfiram-like reaction; warfarin: may increase action of warfarin (increased bleeding risk)
paromomycin	Additive nephrotoxic effects	Use with an aminoglycoside, amphotericin B, colistin, cisplatin, methoxyflurane, polymyxin B, or vancomycin may result in nephrotoxicity
pentamidine		

DOSAGES

Selected Antiprotozoal Drugs

Drug (Pregnancy Category)	Pharmacologic Class	Usual Dosage Range	Indications
atovaquone (Mepron) (C)	Synthetic antipneumocystis drug	**Adult and adolescents 13-16 yr** PO: 750 mg bid with meal × 21 days	Prophylaxis of PJP Treatment of active PJP
Iodoquinol (Yodoxin) (C)	Amebicide	**Adult** PO: 650 mg tid × 20 days **Pediatric** 40 mg/kg (max 650 mg/dose) tid × 20 days	Intestinal amebiasis
▶metronidazole (Flagyl) (X, first trimester; B, 2nd and 3rd trimesters)	Amebicide, antibacterial, trichomonacide	**Adult** PO: 500-750 mg tid × 5-10 days **Pediatric** PO: 35-50 mg/kg (max 750 mg/dose) tid × 5-10 days	Amebiasis, including amebic liver abscess
		Adult only 1-day treatment PO: 2 g × 1 dose or 1 g bid **Adult 7-day treatment** PO: 250 mg tid × 7 days **Pediatric 7-day treatment** PO: 5 mg/kg tid × 7 days	Trichomoniasis, giardiasis
paromomycin (Humatin) (C)	Antiamebic aminoglycoside antibiotic (also has antibacterial properties, but is not normally used for this purpose)	**Adult and pediatric** PO: 25-30 mg/kg/day divided tid with meals × 5-10 days	Acute and chronic intestinal amebiasis (also used in much higher doses for hepatic coma)
pentamidine (NebuPent, Pentam 300) (C)	Synthetic antipneumocystis drug	**Adult and pediatric** Inhalation aerosol: 300 mg q4wk IV/IM: 4 mg/kg qd × 14 days	Prophylaxis of PJP Treatment of active PJP

A combination product containing atovaquone and the drug proguanil is also used against malaria.
PJP, Pneumocystis jirovecii pneumonia.

It is contraindicated in patients with allergy to other iodine-containing preparations, and in patients with severe liver dysfunction. Iodoquinol is available only for oral use. Pregnancy safety information has not been established, but some references classify iodoquinol as a pregnancy category C drug. As with any medication, the drug should be given to pregnant women only when clearly needed or when the expected benefits of administration outweigh fetal risk.

Pharmacokinetics

Half-Life	Onset	Peak	Duration
PO: Unknown	PO: Unknown	PO: Unknown	PO: Unknown

▶ metronidazole

Metronidazole (Metric 21, Protostat, Flagyl) is an antiprotozoal drug that also has fairly broad antibacterial activity as well as **anthelmintic** activity. The therapeutic uses of metronidazole are many and varied and range from the treatment of trichomoniasis, amebiasis, and giardiasis to that of anaerobic bacterial infections and antibiotic-induced pseudomembranous colitis (Chapters 37 and 38). However, it can sometimes also cause this latter condition. It is believed to directly kill protozoa by causing free-radical reactions that damage their DNA and other vital biomolecules. Tinidazole (Tindamax) is a newer, similar drug.

Contraindications to metronidazole include first-trimester of pregnancy. It is available in both oral and injectable form.

Pharmacokinetics

Half-Life	Onset	Peak	Duration
PO: 8-12 hr	PO: <1.5 hr	PO: 1-2 hr	PO: Variable

paromomycin

Paromomycin (Humatin) is an aminoglycoside antibiotic that is used for the treatment of intestinal amebiasis. It directly kills intestinal protozoa when it comes in contact with them. Its bactericidal activity appears to be related to its ability to inhibit protein synthesis in susceptible organisms by binding to the 30S ribosomal subunit. Contraindications include gastrointestinal obstruction. The drug is only available for oral use.

Pharmacokinetics

Half-Life	Onset	Peak	Duration
PO: Unknown	PO: Unknown	PO: Unknown	PO: Unknown

pentamidine

Pentamidine (NebuPent, Pentam 300) is an antiprotozoal drug that is used mainly for the management of *P. jirovecii* pneumonia, although it is sometimes used for treating various other protozoal infections. It works by inhibiting protein and nucleic acid synthesis. It is used for the treatment of active pneumocystosis and for prophylaxis of *Pneumocystis jirovecii* pneumonia (PJP) in patients at high risk for initial or recurrent PJP infection, such as patients with HIV/AIDS.

Hypersensitivity to the drug, especially when administered by inhalation, is normally the only contraindication to its use. However, even if a given patient does not tolerate inhaled forms of the drug, intramuscular (IM) or intravenous (IV) injection may still be necessary, given the seriousness of PJP infection, and there are no absolute contraindications to the injectable routes of administration. The drug should also be used with caution in patients with blood dyscrasias, hepatic or renal disease, diabetes mellitus, cardiac disease, hypocalcemia, or hypertension. Pentamidine is available as an oral inhalational solution and also in injectable form.

Pharmacokinetics

Half-Life	Onset	Peak	Duration
Inhalation: 6-9 hr	Inhalation: 0.5-1 hr	Inhalation: <1 hr	Inhalation: Variable

HELMINTHIC INFECTIONS

Parasitic **helminthic infections** (worm infections) are a worldwide problem. No country is spared. It has been estimated that one third of the world's population is infected with these parasites, but persons living in undeveloped countries where sanitary conditions are often poor are by far the most common victims. The incidence of worm infections in the inhabitants of developed countries where sewage treatment is adequate is much lower, and usually only a few select helminthic diseases are the source of the problem. The most prevalent helminthic infection in the United States is enterobiasis, caused by one genus of roundworm, namely *Enterobius*.

Helminths that are parasitic in humans are classified in the following way:
- Platyhelminthes (flatworms)
- Cestodes (tapeworms)
- Trematodes (flukes)
- Nematoda (roundworms)

The characteristics of a few of the most common of the many helminthic infections are summarized in Table 42-8. There are essentially three types of helminths: cestodes (tapeworms), trematodes (flukes), and nematodes (roundworms). These usually start with and reside in the intestines of their host but can sometimes also migrate to other tissues.

ANTHELMINTIC DRUGS

Unlike protozoa, which are the single-celled members of the animal kingdom, helminths are larger and have complex multicellular structures. Anthelmintic drugs (also spelled *antihelmintic*) work to destroy these organisms by disrupting their structures. The currently available anthelmintic drugs are very specific in the worms that they can kill. For this reason, the causative worm in an infected host should be accurately identified before the start of treatment. However, there are some scenarios in which the "suspected" worm will be treated. This can usually be done by analyzing samples of feces, urine, blood, sputum, or tissue from the infected host for the presence of the particular parasite ova or larvae.

There are over a half dozen anthelmintics that are commercially available in the United States. These include:
- albendazole (Albenza)
- diethylcarbamazine (Hetrazan)
- ivermectin (Stromectol)
- mebendazole (Vermox)
- praziquantel (Biltricide)
- pyrantel (Antiminth, Reese's Pinworm)
- thiabendazol (Mintezol)

Other drugs, such as niclosamide and piperazine, may either be available in other countries or by special request from the Centers for Disease Control and Prevention (CDC). As previously mentioned, anthelmintics are very specific in their actions. Albendazole and mebendazole can be used to treat both tapeworms and roundworms. Praziquantel is a drug that can kill flukes (trematodes). The most commonly used anthelmintics and the specific class of worms they can effectively kill are summarized in Table 42-9.

Table 42-8   Helminthic Infections

Infection	Organism and Other Facts
Nematoda (Various Intestinal And Tissue Roundworms)	
Ascariasis	Caused by *Ascaris lumbricoides* (giant roundworm); resides in small intestine; treated with pyrantel, mebendazole, or albendazole
Enterobiasis	Caused by *Enterobius vermicularis* (pinworm); resides in large intestine; treated with pyrantel, mebendazole, or albendazole
Platyhelminthes (Intestinal Tapeworm Or Flatworms)	
Diphyllobothriasis	Caused by *Diphyllobothrium latum* (fishworm); acquired from fish; treated with niclosamide,* paromomycin, praziquantel, or albendazole
Hymenolepiasis	Caused by *Hymenolepis nana* (dwarf tapeworm); treated with niclosamide, paromomycin, praziquantel, or albendazole
Taeniasis	Caused by *Taenia saginata* (beef tapeworm); acquired from beef; treated with niclosamide, paromomycin, praziquantel, or albendazole
	Caused by *Taenia solium* (pork tapeworm); acquired from pork; treated with niclosamide, paromomycin, praziquantel, or albendazole

*Niclosamide is not available in the United States.

Table 42-9   Anthelmintics: Class of Worms Killed

Anthelmintic Drug	Cestodes	Nematodes	Trematodes
albendazole	Yes	Yes	Yes
diethylcarbamazine and thiabendazole	No	Yes (tissue and some intestinal)	No
ivermectin	No	Yes	No
mebendazole	Yes	Yes	No
niclosamide	Yes	No	No
oxamniquine	No	No	Yes
piperazine and pyrantel	No	Yes (giant worm and pin worm)	No
praziquantel	Yes	No	Yes

Mechanism of Action and Drug Effects

The mechanisms of action of the various anthelmintics vary greatly from drug to drug, although there are some similarities among the drugs used to kill similar types of worms. The various anthelmintic drugs and their respective mechanisms of action are listed in Table 42-10. The drug effects of the anthelmintic drugs are limited to their ability to kill various forms of worms and flukes.

Indications

Anthelmintic drugs are used to treat roundworm, tapeworm, and fluke infection. Anthelmintic drugs and the particular helminthic infections they are used to treat are listed in Table 42-11.

Contraindications

The only usual contraindication to a specific anthelmintic drug product is known drug allergy. Pyrantel is contraindicated in patients with liver disease. Praziquantel is also contraindicated in patients with *ocular cysticercosis* (tapeworm infection of the eye).

Adverse Effects

The anthelmintic drugs show a remarkable diversity in their drug-specific adverse effects. Common effects are listed in Table 42-12.

Interactions

The concurrent use of pyrantel with piperazine is not recommended, and it should be used cautiously in patients with hepatic impairment. Pyrantel has also been shown to raise blood levels of theophylline in pediatric patients. The presence of the anticonvulsants (Chapter 13) carbamazepine and phenytoin may reduce the blood levels of mebendazole. Thiabendazole may raise the blood levels of xanthines such as theophylline. The presence of dexamethasone (Chapter 44), cimetidine (Chapter 51), as well as the anthelmintic praziquantel, may all raise blood levels of albendazole. Histamine H_2-antagonists (e.g., cimetidine, ranitidine) may also raise blood levels of praziquantel.

Dosages

For dosage information for selected anthelmintic drugs, see the table on page 665.

Drug Profiles

Anthelmintics are available only as oral preparations and, with the exception of pyrantel, all require a prescription. As illustrated in Table 42-11, different drugs are selected to treat infection with different helminthic species.

diethylcarbamazine

Diethylcarbamazine (Hetrazan) is an anthelmintic drug indicated primarily for the treatment of tissue infection with roundworms. It is contraindicated in patients with a known hypersensitivity to it, and its pregnancy safety has not been established. It is generally not recommended for use in pregnant women. It is available only for oral use on a *compassionate-use* basis directly from the manufacturer at no charge.

Pharmacokinetics

Half-Life	Onset	Peak	Duration
PO: 8 hr	PO: <1 hr	PO: 1-2 hr	PO: Variable

Table 42-10	Anthelmintics: Mechanisms of Action
Anthelmintic Drug	**Mechanism of Action**
albendazole	Intestinal and segmental cells of intestinal larvae and tissue-dwelling larvae are selectively destroyed by degenerating cytoplasmic microtubules. This in turn causes secretory substances to accumulate intracellularly, which leads to impaired cholinesterase secretion and glucose. Glycogen becomes depleted, leading to decreased ATP production and energy depletion, which immobilizes and kills the worm.
diethylcarbamazine	Inhibits the rate of embryogenesis of nematodes.
ivermectin	Potentiates inhibitory signals in the CNS of nematodes, leading to their paralysis.
mebendazole	Selectively and irreversibly inhibits the uptake of glucose and other nutrients. Results in the depletion of endogenous glycogen stores, eventual autolysis of the parasitic worm, and death.
niclosamide	Inhibits mitochondrial oxidative phosphorylation; also decreases generation of ATP by inhibiting the uptake of glucose. Cestodes are then dislodged from the GI wall. The worm is digested in the intestine and subsequently expelled from the GI tract by normal peristalsis.
oxamniquine and praziquantel	Increased permeability of the cell membrane of susceptible worms to calcium, resulting in the influx of calcium loss. This causes the worms to be dislodged from their usual site of residence in the mesenteric veins to the liver; here they are killed by host tissue reactions. Dislodgement of worms is the result of contraction and paralysis of their musculature and subsequent immobilization of their suckers, which causes the worms to detach from the blood vessel wall and be passively dislodged by normal blood flow.
pyrantel	Blocks ACh at the neuromuscular junction, resulting in paralysis of the worm. The paralyzed worms are then expelled from the GI tract by normal peristalsis.
thiabendazole	Inhibits the helminth-specific enzyme, fumarate reductase.

ACh, Acetylcholine; *ATP*, adenosine triphosphate; *CNS*, central nervous system; *GI*, gastrointestinal.

Table 42-11 Anthelmintics: Indications

Anthelmintic Drug	Indications
diethylcarbamazine	Bancroft's filariasis, loiasis, onchocerciasis, topical eosinophilia
albendazole	Neurocysticercosis, hydatid disease
ivermectin	Nondisseminated intestinal *Strongyloides* (threadworms)
mebendazole	Trichuriasis (whipworm), enterobiasis, ascariasis, *Ancylostoma* infection (common hookworm), *Necator* infection (American hookworm)
niclosamide	*Taenia saginata* infection, diphyllobothriasis, hymenolepiasis
oxamniquine	Schistosomiasis (blood fluke)
praziquantel	Schistosomiasis, opisthorchiasis (liver fluke), clonorchiasis (Chinese or Oriental liver fluke), fishworm, dwarf tapeworm, neurocysticercosis
pyrantel	Ascariasis, enterobiasis, other helminthic infections
thiabendazole	Cutaneous larva migrans (creeping eruption), strongyloidiasis, trichinosis

Table 42-12 Anthelmintics: Common Adverse Effects

Body System	Adverse Effects
Mebendazole	
Gastrointestinal	Diarrhea, abdominal pain
Hematologic	Myelosuppression
Niclosamide	
Central nervous system	Headache, drowsiness
Dermatologic	Skin rash
Gastrointestinal	Nausea, vomiting, diarrhea, rectal bleeding, anal pruritus
Other	Weakness
Primaquine	
Gastrointestinal	Nausea, vomiting, abdominal distress
Other	Headaches, pruritus, dark discoloration of urine, hemolytic anemia due to G6PD deficiency
Piperazine	
Central nervous system	Headache, electroencephalogram (EEG) changes, vertigo, paresthesia, seizures
Dermatologic	Hives, erythema multiforme
Ocular	Blurred vision, cataracts
Respiratory	Bronchospasm
Pyrantel	
Central nervous system	Headache, dizziness, insomnia
Dermatologic	Skin rash
Gastrointestinal	Anorexia, abdominal cramps, diarrhea, nausea, vomiting
Praziquantel	
Central nervous system	Dizziness, headache, drowsiness
Gastrointestinal	Abdominal pain, nausea
Other	Malaise

▶ mebendazole

Mebendazole (Vermox) is a synthetic anthelmintic drug that may be used in the treatment of many types of roundworm and a few types of tapeworm infections. It is available only for oral use.

Pharmacokinetics

Half-Life	Onset	Peak	Duration
PO: 6-12 hr	PO: <2 hr	PO: 2-4 hr	PO: Variable

praziquantel

Praziquantel (Biltricide) is one of the primary anthelmintic drugs used for the treatment of various fluke infections. It is also useful against many species of tapeworm. It is contraindicated in patients with ocular worm infestation *(ocular cysticercosis)*. It is available only for oral use.

Pharmacokinetics

Half-Life	Onset	Peak	Duration
PO: 4-5 hr	PO: <1 hr	PO: 1-3 hr	PO: Variable

pyrantel

Pyrantel (Antiminth, Reese's Pinworm) is a pyrimidine-derived anthelmintic drug that is indicated for the treatment of infection with intestinal roundworms, including ascariasis, enterobiasis, and other helminthic infections. It is the only anthelmintic available in the United States without a prescription. It is available only for oral use.

Pharmacokinetics

Half-Life	Onset	Peak	Duration
PO: Unknown	PO: <1 hr	PO: 1-3 hr	PO: Unknown

DOSAGES

Selected Anthelmintic Drugs

Drug (Pregnancy Category)	Pharmacologic Class	Usual Dosage Range	Indications
albendazole (Albenza) (C)	Cestode anthelmintic	**Based on weight:** <60 kg 400 mg bid with meals <60 kg 15 mg/kg/day divided bid (max 400 mg/dose); all regimens are usually dosed × 8-30 days	Tapeworm infections
diethylcarbamazine (Hetrazan) (not listed)	General anthelmintic	**Adult** PO: approx 13 mg/kg qd × 7 days **Pediatric (no age specified)** PO: 6-10 mg/kg tid × 7-10 days	Variety of worm infections
▶mebendazole (Vermox) (C)	General anthelmintic	**Adult and pediatric** PO: 100 mg bid × 3 days PO: 100 mg in a single dose	Variety of worm infections *Enterobius* spp.
praziquantel (Biltricide) (B)	Trematode anthelmintic	**Adult and pediatric** PO: approx 20-25 mg/kg tid × 1 day	Fluke infections
pyrantel (Antiminth, Reese's Pinworm, Pin-Rid, Pin-X) (C)	Nematode anthelmintic	**Adult and pediatric** PO: 11 mg/kg in a single dose (max dose 1 g)	Roundworm infections

◆ NURSING PROCESS

◆ ASSESSMENT

Before beginning treatment with an antimalarial drug, the nurse should obtain a thorough medication history, head-to-toe physical assessment, and vital signs. There should be special attention (and documentation) to any of the manifestations of malaria (e.g., chills, profound sweating, headache, nausea, joint aching, and fatigue to exhaustion). Other signs and symptoms include periodic diaphoresis and a remittent fever as high as 104° to 105° F (40° C to 40.5° C). Baseline visual acuity, renal function tests, gastrointestinal status, and electrocardiogram (ECG) are also important to assess and document because of drug-related adverse effects of cranial nerve VIII involvement (quinine and chloroquine), renal impairment (quinine), and cardiovascular problems (quinine). Contraindications, cautions, and drug interactions should be assessed for and noted prior to use of any of the antimalarials, antiprotozoals, or anthelmintics.

Antiprotozoal drugs and their contraindications, cautions, and drug interactions have been previously discussed and, in addition to these, the patient should be assessed for renal, cardiac, liver dysfunction, and/or thyroid diseases. The patient's baseline visual acuity should be determined and documented prior to initiation of therapy. Metronidazole should be given only after there has been assessment of allergy to any of the nitroimidazole derivatives and to parabens with the topical dosage forms. Appropriate specimens should be obtained prior to treatment. Patients with blood dyscrasias, central nervous system disorders, and liver dysfunction require thorough assessment prior to use of these drugs. Atovaquone requires astute assessment for gastrointestinal problems, nausea and vomiting, skin assessment, and noting of pre-drug hemoglobin levels as well as assessment of renal/liver function studies.

With any of the anthelmintic drugs, a thorough history of foods eaten, especially meat and fish, and their means of preparation should be obtained. Other individuals in the family household should also be assessed for helminth infestation. Stool specimens are also indicated. Assessment of the patient's energy level, activities of daily living, weight, appetite, and any other symptoms should also be noted. Along with contraindications and cautions, the nurse should assess for possible drug interactions (see Tables 42-2 and 42-7).

◆ NURSING DIAGNOSES

- Risk for injury related to medication adverse effects
- Risk for impaired tissue integrity related to infestation-related lesions
- Risk for infection related to a break in skin integrity from infestation-related lesion
- Imbalanced nutrition, less than body requirements, related to the disease process and adverse effects of medication
- Deficient knowledge related to the infection and its drug treatment
- Ineffective therapeutic regimen management related to poor compliance to treatment and lack of knowledge about the infection and its treatment

◆ PLANNING

Goals

- Patient is free of self-injury related to the adverse effects of medication.
- Patient remains free of infection during duration of therapy.
- Patient remains injury free throughout the prescribed drug regimen.
- Patient maintains normal body weight during drug therapy.
- Patient remains compliant with drug therapy for prescribed length of time.
- Patient experiences minimal body image changes related to disease.

- Patient states adverse effects of medication, as well as symptoms or adverse reactions to report to the physician.

Outcome Criteria

- Patient states measures to take to minimize self-injury related to the adverse effects of medication, such as dosing, time of day, and drug interactions.
- Patient states various measures to prevent worsening of lesions and minimize tissue injury such as washing hands thoroughly, reporting worsening of lesions and/or drainage, fever, joint pain, and taking medication as prescribed.
- Patient lists foods according to the food guide pyramid to be included in his or her diet to improve overall health.
- Patient states the symptoms of the infection, such as fever, lethargy, and loss of appetite.
- Patient understands the rationale for treatment for prescribed length of time.
- Patient states the symptoms to report to the physician, such as worsening of infection, anorexia, and fever.
- Patient verbalizes feelings about altered body image openly with health care professional.
- Patient states the importance of complying with therapy and returning for follow-up visits to the physician to monitor progress and for adverse reactions.

◆ IMPLEMENTATION

With antimalarials, be sure to monitor—or have patient monitor—urinary output (more than 600 mL/day). Liver function with attention to liver enzymes should also be done as ordered throughout the drug regimen. Antimalarials will concentrate in the liver first; therefore, baseline liver functions and subsequent blood tests should be done. This is especially true if the patient has a history of alcohol abuse or drinks a considerable amount of alcohol. Chloroquine and hydroxychloroquine are administered orally and should be given exactly as prescribed. Dosaging with specific attention to the loading doses, subsequent doses, prophylactic dosing, cautions, contraindications, and drug interactions should be followed as prescribed (see previous information in the pharmacology section of this chapter). Antimalarials should be taken with sufficient amounts of fluids, that is, 6 to 8 oz with each dose as well as forcing fluids throughout the day. See patient education tips for further information.

Most of the antiprotozoal drugs (e.g., atovaquone, metronidazole) should be given with food when given orally. Quinine sulfate, an antiprotozoal, must be administered intact because it is very irritating to the gastrointestinal mucosa. Oral dosage forms of metronidazole should be given with food to decrease gastrointestinal upset. IV infusions should infuse over more than 30 to 60 minutes and should never be given as IV bolus. During use of this drug, changes in neurologic status should be reported to the health care provider. All anthelmintic drugs should be administered as ordered and for a prescribed length of time. Patients should be warned that thiabendazole, an anthelmintic, may give the urine an asparagus-like odor or the skin an unusual odor. Any syrup forms of these drugs should be stored in tight and closed containers to prevent chemical changes in the drug. Stool specimens, if indicated with the anthelmintics or other antiparasitic drugs, should be collected with use of a clean container, and the stool should not be in contact with water, urine, or chemicals because of possible risk for destroying the parasitic worms. See patient education tips for more information on these drugs.

◆ EVALUATION

The nurse should monitor the patient for the therapeutic effects of the antimalarials, antiprotozoals, and anthelmintic drugs such as improved energy levels, decrease in and/or eventual resolution of all symptoms. Evaluation of proper hygiene and prevention of spread of the infestation is also important. With these three groups of drugs, it will be important to also evaluate for the adverse effects associated with each of the drug groups: gastrointestinal upset, liver problems, anemias, thrombocytopenia, cardiac irregularities, or visual changes, including the risk for retinal damage, which may be irreversible. The antimalarial drugs may precipitate hemolysis in patients with G6PD deficiency (mostly black patients and those of Mediterranean ancestry); therefore, such patients should be closely monitored for this complication during the treatment protocol. With antiprotozoal drugs, the patient should be monitored for visual disturbances, gastrointestinal distress, blurred vision, and altered hearing and for those patients being treated with anthelmintics, there should be evaluation of adverse effects such as pallor, anorexia, and sudden decrease in red blood cells (RBCs), white blood cells (WBCs), and hemoglobin (Hgb).

Patient Teaching Tips

- Antimalarials are known to cause GI upset; however, this may be decreased if the medication is taken with food. Patients should be encouraged to contact their health care provider if they experience prolonged nausea, vomiting, profuse diarrhea, or abdominal pain. Patients should also be encouraged to report any visual disturbances, dizziness, jaundice/yellowing of skin or sclera of the eye or pruritus.
- Educate patients about the need for prophylactic doses, once prescribed, of antimalarials before visiting malaria-infested countries as well as having appropriate treatment upon return.
- Educate patients to report any changes in vision to their physician immediately.
- With antimalarials, patients should be advised to avoid consuming alcohol.
- Like all medications, antimalarials, should be kept out of the reach of children.
- The patient should be informed about the adverse effects associated with quinine-containing drugs such as dizziness, visual blurring, or yellow discoloration of the skin (often referred to as

"cinchonism". Patients should be instructed to take the entire course of medication.
- Antiprotozoals should be taken exactly as prescribed, and the importance of compliance should be emphasized, as with any of the three groups of drugs.
- Encourage the patient to take metronidazole with food. Alcohol should be avoided when taking this drug and any cough syrups or elixirs (they contain alcohol) should also be avoided.
- Inform patients to avoid activities that require mental alertness or quick motor responses while on this drug until their neurological responses have been determined to be back within normal limits.
- Patients taking metronidazole for sexually transmitted disease should avoid sexual intercourse until the physician states otherwise. Emphasize the importance of this in prevention of transmission of the disease.
- With the patients who are taking metronidazole for "amebiasis", instructions should include how to check stool samples correctly and safely with proper disposal.

Patient Teaching Tips—cont'd

- Topical forms of the drug should be applied with a finger-cot or gloved hand, and inform patients to avoid contact with the eyes. Inform patients that they can apply makeup/cosmetics after topical drug application.
- If the patient has rosacea, instructions should include avoiding alcohol, exposure to sunlight and to hot/cold temperatures and hot/spicy foods.

- Metronidazole may precipitate dizziness, so encourage patients to be cautious with all activities until a response to the drug is noted and consistent.
- Anthelmintics should be taken exactly as prescribed, and the importance of compliance should be emphasized. Patients should also be encouraged to notify the physician immediately if they experience fatigue; fever; pallor; anorexia; darkened urine; or abdominal, leg, or back pain, which could indicate a sudden decrease in RBCs, Hgb, or WBCs.

Points to Remember

- Malaria is caused by *Plasmodium,* a particular genus of protozoa, and is transmitted by the bite of an infected female mosquito. The drug primaquine attacks the parasite when it is outside the RBC (exoerythrocytic phase).
- Other common protozoal infections are amebiasis, giardiasis, pneumocystosis, toxoplasmosis, and trichomoniasis. The most toxic protozoal infections are those caused by *Cryptosporidium* spp., *Isospora belli, P. jirovecii,* and *Toxoplasma gondii.* Protozoa are parasites that are transmitted by the following: person-to-person contact, ingestion of contaminated water or food, direct contact with the parasite, and the bite of an insect (mosquito or tick).
- Antiprotozoals include atovaquone and pentamidine and they are commonly used to treat *P. jirovecii* infections. Metronidazole is an antibacterial, antiprotozoal, and anthelmintic. The drugs iodoquinol and paromomycin directly kill protozoa such as *Entamoeba histolytica.*

- Anthelmintics are drugs used to treat parasitic worm infections caused by cestodes (tapeworms), nematodes (roundworms), and trematodes (flukes).
- Nursing considerations include assessment of contraindications, cautions, and drug interactions with the use of any of the antimalarials, antiprotozoals, and anthelmintics. Contraindications related to antimalarials include pregnancy, psoriasis, porphyria, G6PD deficiency, and a history of drug allergy; contraindications to the use of antiprotozoals include hypersensitivity; underlying renal, cardiac, thyroid, or liver disease; and pregnancy and contraindications to the use of anthelmintics include a history of hypertension; hypersensitivity; visual difficulty; intestinal obstruction; inflammatory bowel disease; malaria; severe hepatic, renal, or cardiac disease; and pregnancy.

NCLEX Examination Review Questions

1. The nurse is reviewing the medication history of a patient who is taking chloroquine. However, the patient's history does not reveal a history of malaria or travel out of the country. The patient is most likely taking this medication for:
   a. Plasmodium
   b. Thyroid disorders
   c. Roundworms
   d. Rheumatoid arthritis
2. Which teaching point would be appropriate to include when the nurse is informing patients about the adverse effects of antimalarials?
   a. Skin may turn "blotchy" while the patient is on these medications.
   b. They may leave a metallic taste in the patient's mouth and cause anorexia.
   c. These drugs may cause increased urinary output
   d. The patient may experience periods of diaphoresis, chills, and fever.

3. When teaching a patient about the potential drug interactions with antimalarials, the nurse should include information about:
   a. acetaminophen
   b. warfarin
   c. decongestants
   d. antibiotics
4. Before administering antiprotozoal drugs, the nurse should review which baseline assessment?
   a. Prothrombin time
   b. Serum magnesium
   c. Hemoglobin level
   d. Arterial blood gas
5. Antimalarial drugs are used to treat patients with infections caused by which genus and species of protozoa?
   a. *Plasmodium* spp.
   b. *Candida albicans*
   c. *Pneumocystis jirovecii*
   d. *Mycobacterium tuberculosis*

1. d, 2. b, 3. b, 4. c, 5. a.

Critical Thinking Activities

1. One of your patients has been taking the antiprotozoal drug metronidazole (Flagyl) for intestinal amebiasis. What life-threatening reaction is related to the use of this drug? What can the nurse monitor for in this patient related to the occurrence of this reaction? What drug-food interaction is important to warn the patient about during therapy with this drug?

2. Your roommate is traveling to a country where there is high risk for malaria infection. She asks you what you think the physician will order for her, if anything at all. After researching this, what would you most likely tell her that the physician will do or suggest?
3. A patient with a history of AIDS has a severe *Pneumocystis jirovecii* pneumonia. Discuss the treatment options for this infection.

For answers, see http://evolve.elsevier.com/Lilley.

Objectives

When you reach the end of this chapter, you should be able to do the following:

1. Identify the differences between antiseptics and disinfectants.
2. List the most commonly used and prescribed antiseptics and disinfectants.
3. Develop a nursing care plan that includes all phases of the nursing process related to the administration of antiseptics and disinfectants.

e-Learning Activities

Companion CD

- NCLEX Review Questions: see questions 366-368
- Animations
- Audio Glossary
- Category Catchers
- Medication Errors Checklists
- IV Therapy Checklists

evolve Website (http://evolve.elsevier.com/Lilley)

- Nursing Care Plans • Frequently Asked Questions • Content Updates • WebLinks • Supplemental Resources • Elsevier ePharmacology Update • Medication Administration Animations

Drug Profiles

Acid agents, p. 671
Alcohol agents, p. 671
Aldehyde agents, p. 671
Biguanide agents, p. 671
Chlorine compounds, p. 671
Dyes, p. 671

Iodine compounds, p. 672
Mercurial agents, p. 672
Oxidizing agents, p. 672
Phenolic compounds, p. 673
Surface-active agents, p. 673

Glossary

Acid A compound that yields hydrogen ions when dissociated in solution. (p. 671)

Aldehyde Any of a large category of organic compounds derived from a corresponding alcohol by the removal of two hydrogen atoms, as in the conversion of ethyl alcohol to acetaldehyde (p. 671)

Antiseptic One type of *topical antimicrobial* agent; a chemical that can be applied to the surfaces of both living tissue and nonliving objects that inhibits the growth and reproduction of microorganisms without necessarily killing them. Antiseptics are also called static agents. (p. 669)

Community-acquired infection An infection acquired from the environment, including infections acquired indirectly through the use of medications. (p. 668)

Disinfectant A second type of *topical antimicrobial* agent; a chemical applied to nonliving objects to kill microorganisms. Also called *cidal agents*. (p. 669)

Nosocomial infection An infection acquired at least 72 hours after hospitalization, often caused by *Candida albicans, Escherichia coli*, hepatitis viruses, herpes zoster virus, *Pseudomonas* organisms, or *Staphylococcus* spp.; also called *hospital-acquired infection*. (p. 668)

Spore (1) A fastidious (hard to kill), dormant structure formed by certain bacterial species (e.g., *Bacillus* spp.). (2) The reproductive structure of certain lower microorganisms, including protozoa and fungi. (p. 670)

Topical antimicrobials A substance applied to any surface that either kills microorganisms or inhibits their growth or replication. (p. 669)

COMMUNITY-ACQUIRED AND NOSOCOMIAL INFECTIONS

Infectious organisms—bacteria, fungi, and viruses—can be acquired from a number of different sources, such as hospitals, workplace, nursing homes, and home. These can, however, be categorized into two main sites of origin: the community and the hospital. **Community-acquired infections** are defined as those infections that are contracted either in the home or any place in the community outside of a health care facility. Hospital-acquired infections, more commonly known as **nosocomial infections,** are defined as those that are contracted in a hospital or institutional setting such as a nursing home and that were not present or incubating in the patient on admission to the hospital.

Of the two types of infections, nosocomial infections are much more difficult to treat, and there are several reasons for this. The primary reason is that these causative microorganisms have been exposed to many strong antibiotics in the past, and those that are left alive in the hospital or institutional setting, are the most drug resistant and the most virulent. The particular organisms that cause these infections have changed over time. These various pathogens and the reasons for their prevalence are summarized by different time periods in Table 43-1.

Table 43-1	**Changing Prevalence of Nosocomial Pathogens**	
Period	**Cause for Change**	**Pathogen**
Before 1940	No antibiotics	Group A streptococci
Mid-1950s	Antibiotic era	Coagulase-positive *Staphylococcus aureus*
Today	New antibiotics	Gram-negative bacilli (*Pseudomonas* spp.), fungi or yeast *(Candida albicans),* herpes virus, MRSA, VRE spp.

MRSA, Multidrug-resistant *Staphylococcus aureus; spp.,* species; *VRE,* vancomycin-resistant *Enterococcus.*

Nosocomial infections develop in 5% to 10% of hospitalized patients, and the cost of treating them because of the extra hospitalization required amounts to nearly $5 billion annually. Most of these infections (70% or more) are either urinary tract infections (UTIs) or postoperative wound infections. Often they are acquired from various devices, such as mechanical ventilators, intravenous (IV) infusion lines, catheters, and dialysis equipment. Areas of the hospital where the risk for acquiring a nosocomial infection is particularly high are the critical care, dialysis, oncology, transplant, and burn units. This is because the host defenses of the patients in these areas are typically compromised, making them more vulnerable to infection.

TOPICAL ANTIMICROBIALS

Topical antimicrobials are agents that can be used to reduce the risk for nosocomial infections. They are substances that are applied to any surface for the purpose of either inhibiting or killing as many microorganisms as possible in a given pathogen population. There are two categories of these agents: antiseptics and disinfectants. **Disinfectants** are able to kill organisms and are used only on nonliving objects to destroy organisms that may be present on them. They are sometimes called *cidal agents.* **Antiseptics** generally only inhibit the growth of microorganisms but do not necessarily kill them and are applied exclusively to living tissue. They are also called *static agents.* The differences between disinfectants and antiseptics in a clinical sense are summarized in Table 43-2. Some antiseptic agents differ from disinfectants in their chemical makeup; others may simply be a diluted version of a disinfectant. Table 43-3 contains a list of these agents classified according to their chemical structure.

Mechanism of Action and Effects of Antiseptics and Disinfectants

Antimicrobial agents either inhibit the growth of microorganisms or destroy them, but the extent to which they do this depends on the number and type of microorganisms present, the concentration of the agent, the patient's body temperature, and the time of exposure to the agent. The mechanisms of action of the various antiseptics and disinfectants are summarized in Table 43-4.

Table 43-2	**Antiseptics Versus Disinfectants**	
	Antiseptics	**Disinfectants**
Where used	Living tissue	Nonliving objects
Toxic?	No	Yes
Potency	Less	More
Activity against organisms	Primarily inhibits growth (bacteriostatic)	Kills (bactericidal)

Table 43-3	**Disinfectants and Antiseptics: Chemical Categories**	
Agent	**Antiseptic**	**Disinfectant**
Acids		
Acetic	X	X
Benzoic	X	
Boric	X	
Lactic	X	
Alcohols		
Ethanol	X	X
Isopropanol	X	X
Aldehydes		
Formaldehyde		X
Glutaraldehyde		X
Biguanides		
Chlorhexidine gluconate	X	
Dyes		
Gentian violet	X	
Carbol-fuchsin	X	
Halogens		
Chlorine Compounds		
Sodium hypochlorite	X	X
Halazone		X
Iodine Compounds		
Iodine (tincture and solution)	X	X
Iodophors (povidone)	X	
Mercurials		
Merbromin	X	
Thimerosal	X	
Yellow mercuric oxide	X	
Silver		
Silver nitrate	X	
Nitrofurazone	X	
Oxidizing Agents		
Benzoyl peroxide	X	
Hydrogen peroxide	X	X
Potassium permanganate	X	
Phenolic Compounds		
Cresol		X
Hexachlorophene	X	
Hexylresorcinol	X	
Resorcinol	X	
Surface-Active Agents		
Benzalkonium chloride	X	
Cetylpyridinium chloride	X	

Table 43-4   Antiseptics and Disinfectants: Mechanisms of Action

Agent	Mechanism of Action	Comments
Alcohols	Denature or essentially destroy the microorganism's protein; some may directly lyse the microorganism.	60%-70% concentration, most effective; >90% or <60% concentration → ↓ bactericidal activity
Aldehydes	Act via alkylation, inhibiting the formation of the essential amino acid methionine.	Bacteriostatic or bactericidal depending on concentration
Biguanides	Disrupt bacterial cytoplasmic membranes and inhibit membrane-bound ATPase (inhibit cell wall synthesis).	Chlorhexidine
Halogens	Precipitate protein and oxidize essential enzymes by binding to and changing structure of proteins.	Iodine compounds: bactericidal; mercurials: bacteriostatic; chlorine compounds: bactericidal
Oxidizing agents	Attack membrane lipids, DNA, and other essential components of the cell.	3%-6% concentration: bactericidal and virucidal; 10%-25% concentration: sporicidal
Phenolic compounds	Interrupt bacterial electron transport (cellular respiration of microorganisms) and inhibit other membrane-bound enzymes; high concentrations rupture bacterial membranes.	Bacteriostatic or bactericidal depending on concentration
Surface-active agents	Denature or essentially destroy the microorganism's protein, cell membrane, and cytoplasm components.	↓ Concentrations → bacteriostatic; ↑ concentrations: bactericidal and fungicidal

ATPase, Adenosine triphosphatase.

Table 43-5   Antiseptics and Disinfectants: Therapeutic Effects

Agent	Therapeutic Effects				
	Bacteria	**Tubercle**	**Fungi**	**Viruses**	**Spores**
Alcohols	X	X	X	X	
Aldehydes	X	X	X	X	X
Chlorhexidine	X		X		
Chlorine compounds	X	X	X	X	
Dyes	X				
Iodine compounds	X	X	X	X	O
Mercurial compounds	O				
Oxidizing agents	X			X	O
Phenolic compounds	X	X	X	X	
Silver Compounds	X				
Surface-active	X		X	O	

O, Some activity if high concentrations of agent and lengthy exposure; *X,* static or cidal activity.

Indications

Living tissue such as skin and mucous membranes cannot be sterilized. However, the risk for infection can be minimized by reducing the number of microorganisms on such tissues. Antiseptics are applied to these living tissues to inhibit the growth of the microorganisms that typically reside on the tissue surfaces (normal flora) and that can do harm if they get into the body through an incision in the skin or by means of an injection. For example, these agents are contained in the presurgical scrubs (soaps) used by members of surgical teams to wash their hands in preparation for surgery. They are also applied to the patient's skin before the incision is made. The degerming action is only temporary, however, and is limited to the skin surface. Chapter 37 also describes how systemic antibiotic drugs (e.g., cefazolin, 1 g intravenously preop) are often administered to surgical patients as prophylaxis against infection. Antimicrobial agents, including antiseptics, are also commonly used to irrigate body cavities either directly during surgery or through various transdermal catheter devices that are designed for irrigation purposes. Antiseptics are also contained in ointments, mouthwashes, and douches.

Inanimate objects such as tabletops and surgical equipment may be treated with disinfectants, as well as by autoclaving, radiation, heat, and so on. These instruments acquire these microbes by being placed on or inserted into anatomic sites in patients where many organisms naturally dwell (e.g., thermometers, which are placed orally, rectally, or under the axilla, and colonoscopies, which are used in examinations of the lower gastrointestinal tract [colonoscopy]). Before their use in other patients, the bacteria, fungi, viruses, and **spores** (dormant, hard-to-kill microbial reproductive structures) that may have been acquired from the previous patient's tissues must be removed from the instrument surfaces to prevent their transmission to others. The therapeutic effects of the antiseptics and disinfectants are listed in Table 43-5.

Table 43-6 Antiseptic and Disinfectant Agents: Adverse Effects

Body System	Adverse Effects
Alcohols	
Integumentary	Excessive dryness of the skin.
Aldehydes	
Integumentary	Burns to skin or mucous membranes
Chlorhexidine Gluconate	
Central nervous	Use as a preoperative scrub or as a wash for neonates and burn patients has been stopped because absorption from the skin into systemic circulation has resulted in serious CNS toxicity.
Hexylresorcinol	
Hepatic	Toxicity resulting from systemic absorption from the skin.
Cardiovascular	Myocardial toxicity resulting from systemic absorption from the skin.
Integumentary	May produce burns on skin or mucous membranes.
Iodine Compounds	
Integumentary	*Iodine* at concentrations >3% may produce skin blistering. Burns may appear with *tincture of iodine* when the treated area is covered with an occlusive dressing. It may stain skin and cause irritation and pain at wound sites.
Surface-Active Agents	
Integumentary	Chemical burns if left in contact with skin for too long, as in wet packs for occlusive dressings.

CNS, Central nervous system.

Contraindications

The only usual contraindication to the use of a particular antiseptic agent is known patient allergy to a specific product.

Adverse Effects

Antiseptics and disinfectants are normally very safe agents, with the most common adverse effects, if any at all, being mild skin irritation. Although quite uncommon, other adverse effects are summarized in Table 43-6.

Interactions

There are very few drugs that interact with the antiseptics, although other topical agents that also irritate the skin may produce an additive effect when given in combination with one of them. Two topical agents used together may also increase one another's rate of absorption, raising the risk for systemic toxicity, and should be administered separately when possible.

Dosages

For information on the recommended dosages and concentrations for selected antimicrobial agents, see the Dosages table on page 672.

Drug Profiles

Following are descriptions of the various chemical categories of antimicrobials.

Acid Agents

Acetic (vinegar), benzoic, boric, and lactic acid are all members of the **acid** family of antiseptic and disinfectant agents. They are very commonly used because of their practicality, availability, and low cost. All of these acid agents either kill microorganisms or inhibit their growth by creating an acidic environment for organisms that require a neutral or alkaline medium to live and grow. Acetic acid in a 5% solution kills many organisms. In this concentration, it is used as a vaginal douche for antisepsis and as a mild antiseptic–deodorant for the collection containers of indwelling urinary drainage catheters, for bladder irrigation, and for diaper soaks. The 1% solution may be used as a topical antiseptic for certain surgical wounds and burns.

Alcohol Agents

Isopropanol (isopropyl alcohol) and ethanol are both members of the alcohol category of antiseptics. The alcohol solutions are most effective at a concentration of 60% to 70%; at a concentration of more than 95% or less than 60% their "cidal" activity dramatically decreases. These agents kill microorganisms by either denaturing their cellular proteins or directly lysing their cell membranes. Both isopropyl and ethyl alcohol are able to kill bacteria, tubercle bacilli, fungi, and viruses.

Aldehyde Agents

Formaldehyde and glutaraldehyde are members of the **aldehyde** category of agents. These disinfectants act by means of alkylation, inhibiting the formation of the essential amino acid methionine. This either kills organisms or inhibits their growth, depending on the concentration of the solution. The aldehydes, such as formaldehyde and glutaraldehyde, are active against all types of microorganisms, including bacteria, tubercle bacilli, fungi, viruses, and spores. Because these agents are somewhat caustic, they can cause burns to the skin or mucous membranes if used as antiseptics. For this reason they are used mostly as disinfectants. Formaldehyde comes as formalin in a 37% concentration, and glutaraldehyde (Cidex) comes in a 2% solution. Both agents are commonly used as disinfectants for instruments. Cidex is used in particular to disinfect and sterilize surgical equipment.

Biguanide Agents

Chlorhexidine gluconate (Hibiclens) is a biguanide agent with antiseptic activity. Biguanides act by disrupting bacterial cytoplasmic membranes and inhibiting membrane-bound adenosine triphosphatase (ATPase), which results in the inhibition of cell wall synthesis. Chlorhexidine is active against both gram-positive and gram-negative bacteria. It is used as a bactericidal skin cleansing solution and is useful as a surgical scrub, a handwashing agent for health care personnel, and a skin wound cleanser. It may also be used to treat aphthous ulcers of the mouth and for the prevention of dental caries, and is available in a prescription mouthwash for this purpose.

Dyes

Gentian violet, crystal violet, methyl violet, brilliant green, and fuchsin are all rosaniline dyes. These are basic dyes that are currently used only occasionally as antiseptic or antiprotozoal agents. Gentian violet is typically used only topically as a 1% to 2% preparation, and it has both antibacterial and antifungal activity.

Chlorine Compounds

Chlorine compounds actively kill bacteria, tubercle bacilli, and viruses but are only partially active against fungi. They have no activity against spores. Dilute sodium hypochlorite (Dakin's solution) is one of the chlorine compounds that is commonly used clinically as an antiseptic irrigation. Its antibacterial action is due to the hypochlorous acid that forms when chlorine reacts with water. Hypochlorous acid is rapidly antibacterial.

DOSAGES

Selected Antiseptic and Disinfectant Agents

Agent	Pharmacologic Class	Usual Concentration or Dosage Range	Indications
acetic acid (otic: Domeboro, Vosol Otic; irrigation solution)	Antibacterial, antifungal acid antimicrobial	Otic solution: 2%; 4-7 gtt tid-qid Irrigation solution: 0.25%; 500-1500 mL/24 hr	Antibacterial, antifungal Bladder irrigation
benzalkonium chloride (Zephiran)	Broad-spectrum cationic detergent, surface-active antimicrobial	Solution concentrate: 17% for preparing dilutions from 1:750 to 1:40,000 Tincture/spray: 1:750	Skin cleanser, antiseptic irrigation solution, instrument storage
carbolic acid (phenol; Chloraseptic)	Phenolic antiseptic	Spray: 0.5% Gargle: 1.4%	Oral antiseptic Topical anesthetic
Cresol	Phenolic disinfectant	Solution: 2%, 5%, 50%	Concurrent/terminal disinfectant
chlorhexidine gluconate (Hibiclens)	Broad-spectrum biguanide antimicrobial	Liquid: 4%	Cleanser, surgical scrub
formaldehyde (formaldehyde-10, Lazer Formalyde)	Broad-spectrum aldehyde antimicrobial	Solution: 37% Solution/spray: 1%	General disinfectant Skin-drying agent
Gentian violet (crystal violet)	Antibacterial/antifungal dye	Solution: 1%, 2%; apply qd-bid	Topical antiinfective
hydrogen peroxide	Oxidizing agent	Solution: 3%	Wound cleansing, antiseptic
iodine (iodine topical, Lugol's solution, iodine tincture, strong iodine tincture)	Broad-spectrum iodine antimicrobial	Solution/spray/tincture: 2%, 5%, 7% apply qd-bid	Topical antiseptic
isopropanol (isopropyl alcohol)	General alcohol antiseptic/disinfectant/astringent	Solution 70%	Skin astringent, cleansing, utensil disinfectant
povidone-iodine (Betadine)	Broad-spectrum iodine antimicrobial	Aerosol: 5% Solution: 10% Mouthwash: 0.5% Surgical scrub: 7.5%	Topical antiseptic
sodium hypochlorite (Dakin's solution)	Broad-spectrum antimicrobial	Solution: 0.25%, 0.5%	Topical antiseptic
thimerosal (Merthiolate)	Organic mercurial antiseptic	Solution/spray/tincture: 1:1000; apply qd-tid	Topical antiseptic

Sodium hypochlorite in a 5% solution is commonly used to disinfect utensils, walls, furniture, floors, and swimming pools; in a 0.5% solution, it is used on skin surfaces for the treatment of fungus infections such as athlete's foot (tinea pedis). The strength of most household bleach solutions is 5.25% sodium hypochlorite. Intravenous drug users, who frequently share needles and are at increased risk for acquiring HIV, are being given small bottles of bleach by various public health outreach programs to use as a disinfectant for their injection equipment to hopefully prevent the spread of the HIV and other dangerous microbes.

Halazone is a chloramine compound. Chloramines are chlorine-related compounds but are more stable, less irritating, and slower and more prolonged in their action than their chlorine cousins. Halazone is the only chloramine product used in the United States. It is available in tablet form for sanitizing drinking water. Adding 1 or 2 tablets to a liter of water can kill water-borne pathogens within 30 to 60 minutes.

Mercurial Agents

Topical mercurial antiseptics are relatively weak in their actions. They are primarily bacteriostatic agents whose effectiveness is enhanced by the vehicle in which they are contained. Inorganic mercury compounds such as ammoniated mercury ointment owe their effectiveness primarily to these vehicles, which sustain the bacteriostatic action of the agent. Organic mercurial agents such as thimerosal (Merthiolate) are more bacteriostatic, less irritating, and less toxic than inorganic mercurials. Other examples of mercury com-

pounds that are used as topical antiinfectives are merbromin, yellow mercuric oxide, and triclosan (Septisol).

Mercurial antiseptics probably act by inhibiting bacterial sulfhydryl enzymes, but they may also inhibit tissue enzymes as well, which reduces their usefulness. Ammoniated mercury is used for the treatment of psoriasis, impetigo, dermatomycoses, pediculosis pubis (crabs), seborrheic dermatitis, and superficial pyodermias (pus-producing skin infections). Skin irritations, as well as hypersensitivity to the agents, have been reported as adverse effects of these compounds.

Iodine Compounds

Iodine (tincture and solution) is a nonmetallic element that readily forms salts when combined with many other elements. Although it is a nonmetallic element, it has a bluish black metallic luster and a characteristic odor. It is only slightly soluble in water but is completely soluble in alcohol and in aqueous solutions of sodium iodide and potassium iodide. Iodine tincture and solution are both active against and kill all forms of microorganisms: bacteria, tubercle bacilli, fungi, viruses, and spores. Their activity against spores depends on the concentration and the timing of administration. There are actually many forms of iodine, some of which are listed in Table 43-7.

Oxidizing Agents

Hydrogen peroxide is one of three members of the oxidizing family of antiseptic agents, the other agents being benzoyl peroxide and potassium permanganate. Oxidizing agents work by attacking membrane lipids, DNA, and other essential components of the microorganism's cell. In concentrations of 3% to 6%, they are bactericidal and virucidal; at 10% to 25% they are sporicidal.

The use of hydrogen peroxide as a solution to irrigate wounds is controversial. Its use may be detrimental to wounds in that it can destroy newly forming cells as well as bacteria.

Phenolic Compounds

Cresol, carbolic acid (phenol), and Lysol are all phenolic compounds that are used primarily as disinfectants. Because these agents cause burning and possibly blistering, they should not be allowed to come in contact with the skin in concentrations stronger than 2% and never in contact with areas where the skin is broken.

Phenolic compounds work by interrupting bacterial electron transport (cellular respiration of microorganisms) and inhibiting other membrane-bound enzymes. At high concentrations, they rupture bacterial membranes. Depending on the concentration of the phenolic compound, they can be either static or cidal in their actions. The phenolic compounds are active against bacteria, tubercle, fungi, and viruses, but not spores. Hexachlorophene and resorcinol are two other phenolic compounds. Hexachlorophene is available by prescription only and is used as a surgical scrub as well as a bacteriostatic skin cleanser. Its use should be avoided in infants because they are particularly susceptible to transdermal absorption of this agent, with the risk for such serious neurotoxic effects as seizures. Resorcinol is bactericidal and fungicidal and is about one third as effective as carbolic acid. It is used to treat acne, ringworm, eczema, psoriasis, seborrheic dermatitis, and similar skin lesions.

Surface-Active Agents

Benzalkonium chloride (Zephiran) and cetylpyridinium chloride are surface-active agents. They work by denaturing the microorganism or essentially destroying its protein, cell membrane, and cytoplasm components. At low concentrations, they are bacteriostatic, and at high concentrations, they are bactericidal and fungicidal. These agents are used to treat bacteria, fungi, and some viral topical infections.

Certain substances, when used in combination with surface-acting agents, will absorb the active ingredient and thereby weaken the surface-acting agent. Substances such as organic matter, soaps, anionic detergents, and tap water that contains metallic ions are a few examples.

◆ NURSING PROCESS

◆ ASSESSMENT

When any type of topical medication such as an antiseptic is to be administered, the concentration of the medication, length of exposure to the skin, condition of the skin, size of area affected, and hydration status of the skin must be taken into consideration because they have a significant influence on the action of the medication. Before applying any topical medication, it is important for the nurse to question the patient about any drug allergies or any previous sensitivity to antiseptics, disinfectants, related compounds, and/or any additive within the solution, ointment, or other topical dosage form. If the drug is iodine-based, for example, povidone-iodine, the nurse should question the patient about allergies to iodine or seafood (due to iodine concentrations), because these are contraindications to the use of these drugs. Patients being treated with peroxide and other antiseptics and disinfectants should be questioned thoroughly about any previous allergic and local reaction to any of these drugs and their ingredients. Allergies to alcohol/chlorine/mercurial and phenolic compounds should be noted and the drugs or ingredients avoided. It is also important to understand that there is a higher risk to reactions of antiseptics/disinfectants if there has been an allergic reaction to antibacterial topical drugs. Should a patient have an allergy to a particular type of antibacterial drug, that specific drug/ingredient should not be used at all, regardless of the dosage form. Culture and sensitivity reports will identify appropriate therapy with antiseptics or disinfectants. In addition, specific compounds within an antiseptic or disinfectant are used for particular bacteria or viruses based on "known" sensitivity.

◆ NURSING DIAGNOSES

- Risk for infection related to compromised skin integrity
- Risk for infection related to skin trauma or injury resulting from adverse reactions to the topical agent
- Deficient knowledge related to topical agents and their proper use

Table 43-7   Iodine Formulations

Iodine Formulation	Composition	Uses
Aqueous solution	5% Iodine and 10% potassium iodide	These forms of iodine are used preoperatively to disinfect the skin. They are applied topically for their antimicrobial effects against bacteria, fungi, viruses, protozoa, and yeasts.
Iodine topical solution	2% Iodine	
Iodine tincture	2% Iodine in alcohol solution	
Strong iodine solution	7% Iodine in alcohol	
Strong iodine tincture		
Povidone-iodine (Betadine, Operand, Pharmadine)	Iodine with polyvinylpyrrolidone	Used as a 10% applicator solution or as a 2% scrub, spray, foam, vaginal gel, ointment, mouthwash, perineal wash, or whirlpool concentrate.
Tincture of iodine	2% Iodine and 2.4% sodium iodide in 46% ethyl alcohol	For cutaneous infections caused by bacteria and fungi. Even a 1% tincture will kill almost an entire bacterial population in 1.5 min. Three drops in 1 qt ($\approx$1 L) of drinking water will reduce ameba and bacteria counts in 15 min without impairing palatability.
Iodophors (Betadine, Prepodyne)	Iodine compounds with a carrier that acts as a sustained-release pool of iodine	Widely used as antiseptics.

♦ PLANNING

Goals

- Patient remains free of adverse reactions to the agent when used for the treatment of skin injury or infection.
- Patient shows evidence of resolution of infection.
- Patient is compliant with the medication regimen.
- Patient experiences minimal to no adverse reactions to medication.
- Patient returns for follow-up visits with physician.

Outcome Criteria

- Patient experiences minimal discomfort (such as stinging, itching, burning) resulting from the use of the agent in the treatment of a skin injury or infection.
- Patient experiences maximal therapeutic effects of medication once therapy is complete, with resolution of symptoms such as intact skin, no redness, or no drainage.
- Patient demonstrates proper technique for applying topical antiseptic with applicator, tongue blade, gloved hand, and proper handwashing technique.
- Patient states those situations (adverse reactions to medication or worsening of symptoms of infection) when the physician should be notified immediately.

♦ IMPLEMENTATION

Before applying any topical agent, the nurse should check the physician's order to validate the order, route of administration, equipment needed, and application procedure. Standard Precautions should be followed with any situation requiring direct contact with a patient or possible exposure situations (see Chapter 9). If the skin is intact and it is not otherwise indicated, the nurse should wear nonsterile gloves; however, if the skin is not intact or the nurse judges it appropriate, sterile gloves and sterile technique should be used. Often there are specific directions regarding the application of the antiseptic/disinfectant. The order may specify that the agent be applied with a tongue depressor or sterile cotton-tipped applicator or that an occlusive dressing be placed. The nurse should follow if within standards of care. As with any procedure, the nurse should always be aware and ensure patient privacy, dignity, and level of comfort. The skin site should be thoroughly cleansed and any other specific directions, such as removing water- or alcohol-based topicals with soap and water or normal saline (NS), should be followed. Before application or administration of additional doses of the antiseptic or disinfectant, the site should be cleansed of any debris (e.g., pus, drainage) and of any residual medication. If using an antiseptic or disinfectant for preparing the skin, exact instructions should be followed. Remember to always avoid cross-contamination through adherence to technique and handwashing. For dressing of the wound, follow the physician's order or wound care protocol (e.g., use of occlusive, wet, or wet-to-dry dressings). The nurse should make sure to document the site of application and any drainage from the site, whether there is any swelling, the temperature and color of the site, and any painful or other sensations that may occur.

Before and after the use of the medication, nurses should wash their hands thoroughly, dispose of contaminated dressings, and record the nature of the procedure and findings while maintaining asepsis. Biohazardous waste bags are usually red and should be used. The nurse should encourage the patient to follow instructions closely, if at home and caring for the site, make sure that the patient knows to follow directions closely and to avoid self-harm/injury. Patient Teaching Tips for antiseptic agents are presented below. If the nurse is using the antiseptic or disinfectant for handwashing or preparation of skin, always follow the instructions related to each specific agent.

♦ EVALUATION

When antiseptics are used, the patient's therapeutic response may be manifested by improved healing of the affected area; decreased symptoms of inflammation or infection; or even prevention of infection for which the agent was ordered, such as preoperative. In addition, when using these agents on inanimate objects the nurse must be sure to constantly monitor for patient safety from exposure to the agent. It is also important for the nurse to evaluate patients for any adverse effects (see Table 43-6) and to evaluate self for any reaction to the compound used for handwashing.

Patient Teaching Tips

- Patients using antiseptics should be instructed to wash their hands before and after applying any topical medication. Handwashing technique should also be emphasized and demonstrated.
- Educate patients about proper application of medication and dressings and to provide hands-on demonstrations. Along with oral instructions, be sure to provide written instructions, pamphlets, and any other aids to reinforce the importance of the procedure. Make sure patients have all the supplies needed for at-home care. A tongue blade, cotton-tipped applicator, or gloved finger may be used to apply the medication. Encourage handwashing and noting of any unusual color of the skin, odor, or drainage.
- Encourage patients to report any increase in redness, drainage, pain, swelling, and fever.

Points to Remember

- Topical antimicrobials (antiseptics and disinfectants) are used to reduce the risk for nosocomial infections and are applied to topical surfaces to inhibit or kill as many microorganisms as possible.
- Disinfectants are antimicrobials that are used only on nonliving objects, and they kill any organisms on these objects. They are *not* the same as antiseptics.
- Antiseptics are defined as antimicrobials that are used only on living tissues and primarily inhibit growth and reproduction of microorganisms.

- Antiseptics and disinfectants are categorized by their chemical makeup and include such agents as alcohols, aldehydes, phenolic compounds, biguanides, surface-active agents, acid agents, dyes, oxidizing agents, chlorine, mercurial, and iodine.
- Nurses should always observe standard precautions whenever applying antiseptics or disinfectants and apply these drugs to clean, dry skin unless otherwise ordered or specified, as well as ensure that patients receive adequate instructions about their medication, its application, and handwashing technique.

NCLEX Examination Review Questions

1. Which of the following statements best describes the purpose of disinfectants?
   a. Bacteriocidal function and used in open wounds
   b. Applied to nonliving objects to kill microorganisms
   c. Used to inhibit growth of microorganisms on the skin surface
   d. Used to sterilize the skin before surgery
2. Which of the following is considered to be a property of an antiseptic agent?
   a. Useful on nonliving tissues
   b. More potent than a disinfectant
   c. Bacteriostatic
   d. Bacteriocidal
3. Which patient is most susceptible to a nosocomial infection?
   a. A teenager who has a sports injury
   b. An elderly patient admitted for cataract surgery
   c. A woman who has delivered her baby via vaginal delivery
   d. A middle-aged woman who has had two courses of chemotherapy for cancer

4. Which statement most correctly describes Dakin's solution?
   a. Used as a topical antiseptic for wound care
   b. Sterilize all surfaces
   c. A 5.25% concentration used for skin surfaces
   d. Contains the same active ingredient as vinegar
5. During a health history, a patient cites an allergy to iodine. Which antiseptic preparation would be contraindicated for this patient?
   a. Isopropyl alcohol
   b. Betadine solution
   c. Dakin's solution
   d. Chlorhexidine gluconate (Hibiclens)

1. c, 2. c, 3. d, 4. a, 5. b.

Critical Thinking Activities

1. What is the main purpose of using antiseptics and disinfectants?
2. Can disinfectants and antiseptics be used interchangeably? Why or why not?

3. For a patient who is receiving an antiseptic as part of wound care, how would you know that a patient is having a therapeutic response to the antiseptic?

For answers, see http://evolve.elsevier.com/Lilley.

Antiinflammatory, Antirheumatic, and Related Drugs

Objectives

When you reach the end of this chapter, you should be able to do the following:

1. Discuss the inflammatory response and the part it plays in the generation of pain.
2. Compare the various disease processes that are often identified as inflammatory in nature, such as rheumatoid arthritis, osteoarthritis, degenerative joint disorders, and gout.
3. Compare the various nonsteroidal antiinflammatory drugs (NSAIDs), antigout drugs, and antiarthritic drugs in relation to their mechanisms of action, indications, adverse effects, dosage ranges, routes of administration, cautions, contraindications, drug interactions, and toxicities.
4. Develop a nursing care plan that includes all phases of the nursing process for the patient receiving NSAIDs, antigout drugs, antiarthritic drugs, and other antiinflammatory drugs.

e-Learning Activities

Companion CD
- NCLEX Review Questions: see questions 369-379
- Animations
- Audio Glossary
- Category Catchers
- Medication Errors Checklists
- IV Therapy Checklists

evolve Website (http://evolve.elsevier.com/Lilley/)
• Nursing Care Plans • Frequently Asked Questions • Content Updates • WebLinks • Supplemental Resources • Elsevier ePharmacology Update • Medication Administration Animations

Drug Profiles

▶ allopurinol, p. 684
▶ aspirin, p. 682
auranofin, p. 685
aurothioglucose and gold
   sodium thiomalate, p. 685
▶ celecoxib, p. 683
colchicine, p. 685

▶ ibuprofen, p. 683
▶ indomethacin, p. 683
▶ ketorolac, p. 683
leflunomide, p. 685
probenecid and sulfinpyrazone,
   p. 685

▶ Key drug.

Glossary

Arthritis   Inflammation of one or more joints. (p. 684)

Disease-modifying antirheumatic drugs (DMARDs)   Medications used in the treatment of rheumatic diseases that have the potential to arrest or slow the actual disease process as opposed to, like the nonsteroidal antiinflammatory drugs (NSAIDs), only providing antiinflammatory and analgesic effects. (p. 685)

Done nomogram   A standard plot of graphic data, originally published in 1960 in the journal *Pediatrics,* for rating the sever-

ity of aspirin toxicity following overdose. Serum salicylate levels are plotted against time elapsed after ingestion. (p. 680)

Gout   Hyperuricemia (elevated uric acid); the arthritis caused by tissue build-up of uric acid crystals. (p. 679)

Inflammation   A localized protective response stimulated by injury to tissues that serves to destroy, dilute, or wall off (sequester) both the injurious agent and the injured tissue. (p. 676)

Nonsteroidal antiinflammatory drugs (NSAIDs)   A large and chemically diverse group of drugs that possess analgesic, antiinflammatory, antirheumatic, and antipyretic (fever-reducing) activity. (p. 676)

Rheumatism   General term for any of several disorders characterized by inflammation, degeneration, or metabolic derangement of connective tissue structures, especially joints and related structures. (p. 676)

Salicylism   The syndrome of salicylate toxicity, including such symptoms as tinnitus (ringing sound in the ears), nausea, and vomiting. (p. 680)

Nonsteroidal antiinflammatory drugs (NSAIDs) are among the most commonly prescribed drugs. Every year, approximately 70 million prescriptions are written for these drugs. This represents more than 5% of all prescriptions. There are currently more than 23 different NSAIDs available in the United States. Some of these are used much more commonly than others, and a given patient may respond better to some NSAIDs than others, both in terms of symptom relief and adverse effect profile. **Inflammation** is defined as a localized protective response stimulated by injury to tissues, which serves to destroy, dilute, or wall off (sequester) both the injurious agent and the injured tissue. Classic signs and symptoms of inflammation include pain, fever, loss of function, redness, and swelling. These symptoms result from arterial, venous, and capillary dilation; enhanced blood flow and vascular permeability; exudation of fluids, including plasma proteins; and leukocyte migration into the inflammatory focus. **Rheumatism** is a general term for any of several disorders characterized by inflammation, degeneration, or metabolic derangement of connective tissue structures, especially joints and related structures such as muscles, tendons, bursae, fibrous tissue, and ligaments. Rheumatic symptoms are similar to and often concurrent with inflammatory symptoms and include pain, stiffness, and reduced range of motion.

NSAIDs comprise a large and chemically diverse group of drugs that possess analgesic, antiinflammatory, antirheumatic, and antipyretic (antifever) activity. They are also used for the relief of mild-to-moderate headaches, myalgia, neuralgia, and arthralgia; alleviation of postoperative pain; inhibition of platelet aggregation; relief of the pain associated with arthritic disorders such as rheumatoid arthritis, juvenile arthritis, ankylosing spondylitis, and osteoarthritis; and treatment of *gout* and *hyperuricemia* (discussed later in this chapter). Steroidal antiinflammatory drugs (e.g., prednisone, dexamethasone) are also used for similar purposes, and were discussed in Chapter 32. NSAIDs have a generally more favorable adverse effect profile than steroidal antiinflammatory drugs.

In 1899, acetylsalicylic acid (ASA; aspirin) was marketed and rapidly became the most widely used drug in the world. The success of aspirin established the importance of drugs with antipyretic, analgesic, antiinflammatory, and antirheumatic properties—the properties that all NSAIDs share. However, the widespread use of aspirin also yielded evidence of its potential for causing some major adverse effects. Gastrointestinal intolerance, bleeding, and renal impairment became major factors limiting its long-term administration. As a result, efforts were mounted to develop drugs that did not have the adverse effects of aspirin. This led to the discovery of other NSAIDs, which in general are associated with a lower incidence of and less serious adverse effects and are often better tolerated than aspirin in patients with chronic diseases.

Before getting into the in-depth discussion of the NSAID drugs, it is first important to explain the body's arachidonic acid metabolic pathway. The beneficial effects of NSAIDs are thought to result primarily from their inhibition of this pathway.

ARACHIDONIC ACID PATHWAY

The inflammatory response is mediated by a host of endogenous compounds, including proteins of the complement system, histamine, serotonin, bradykinin, leukotrienes, and prostaglandins, the latter two being major contributors to the symptoms of inflammation.

Arachidonic acid is released from phospholipids in cell membranes in response to a triggering event (e.g., an injury). It is metabolized by either the *prostaglandin (PG) pathway* or the *leukotriene (LT) pathway*, both of which are branches of the arachidonic acid pathway, as shown in Figure 44-1. Both of these pathways result in inflammation, edema, headache, and other pain characteristic of the body's response to injury or inflammatory illnesses such as arthritis. Such symptoms are also observed when research subjects are injected with PG compounds.

In the PG pathway, arachidonic acid is converted by the enzyme *cyclooxygenase (COX)* into various PGs such as *prostacyclin (PGI$_2$)*, as well as into *thromboxane A$_2$ (TXA$_2$)*. PGs indirectly mediate and perpetuate inflammation by inducing vasodilation and enhancing vasopermeability. These effects in turn potentiate the action of proinflammatory substances, such as histamine and bradykinin, in the production of edema and pain. These symptoms arise as a result of PG-induced hyperalgesia (excessive motor sensitivity). In this situation stimuli that would normally not be painful, such as simply moving a joint through its natural range of motion, become painful because of the inflammatory process at work. Fever results when PGE$_2$ is synthesized in the preoptic hypothalamic region, the area of the brain that regulates temperature.

The LT pathway utilizes lipoxygenases to metabolize the arachidonic acid and convert it into various LTs. Although LTs are more newly discovered than PGs and not as well studied, they are also mediators of inflammation, promoting vasoconstriction, bronchospasms, and increased vascular permeability with resultant edema.

NONSTEROIDAL ANTIINFLAMMATORY DRUGS

As a single class of drugs, NSAIDs constitute an exceptional variety of drugs, and they are used for an equally wide range of indications. Box 44-1 lists these drugs among seven distinct chemical classes. The carboxylic acid drugs are more commonly called *salicylates* and, as previously noted, were the first NSAIDs to be isolated and used therapeutically.

Currently, at least one NSAID has been approved for each of the therapeutic indications listed in Box 44-2, and an NSAID is considered the drug of choice for the treatment of most of these conditions. Almost all NSAIDs are used for the treatment of rheumatoid arthritis and degenerative joint disease (osteoarthritis). Several of these drugs are available in sustained-release formulations, allowing for once- or twice-daily dosing, which is known to improve patients' adherence to prescribed drug therapy regimens.

Mechanism of Action and Drug Effects

NSAIDs work through inhibition of the LT pathway, the PG pathway, or both. More specifically, NSAIDs relieve pain, headache, and inflammation by blocking the chemical activity of either or both of the enzymes COX (PG pathway) and leukotriene

---

> ### CASE STUDY
>
> #### Postoperative Pain
>
> One of your postoperative abdominal surgery patients is complaining of abdominal pain, nausea, and breakthrough pain after receiving the pain protocol for Dilaudid PCA and ketorolac (Toradol) intramuscularly. She has received ketorolac for some 15 days and in multiple doses. A gastrointestinal ulcer is now diagnosed and has been attributed to the ketorolac; however, the patient has a history of gastritis and reflux disease and a 5-year history of ulcer disease.
>
> - What is the action of the ketorolac, and its purpose in this case?
> - What could have been done to prevent the gastrointestinal bleeding and ulcer formation?
> - What concerns would you have regarding the history of gastrointestinal disorders, and how could you have handled this potential risk to the patient?

For answers, see http://evolve.elsevier.com/Lilley.
GI, Gastrointestinal.

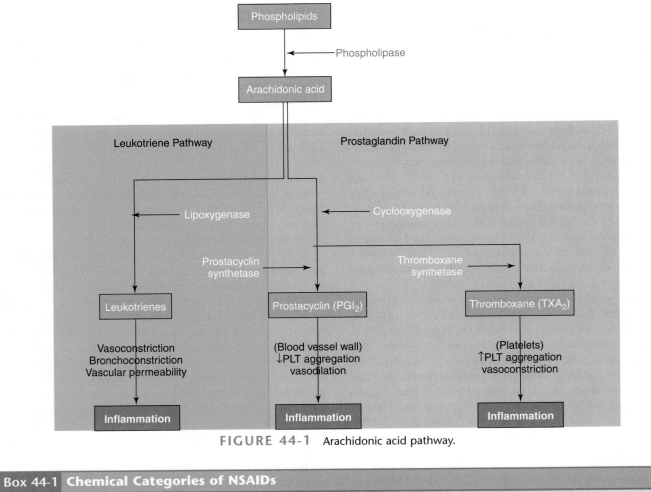

FIGURE 44-1 Arachidonic acid pathway.

Box 44-1 **Chemical Categories of NSAIDs**

Acetic Acids
diclofenac sodium (Voltaren)
diclofenac potassium (Cataflam)
indomethacin (Indocin)
sulindac (Clinoril)
tolmetin (Tolectin)

Carboxylic Acids
Acetylated
aspirin (many brands)
etodolac (Lodine)
choline salicylate (Arthropan)
diflunisal (Dolobid)

Nonacetylated
ketorolac (Toradol)
magnesium salicylate (Magan, others)
salsalate (Salsitab, others)
sodium salicylate (generic only)
sodium thiosalicylate (Rexolate)

COX-2 Inhibitors
celecoxib (Celebrex)

Fenamic Acids
meclofenamate (generic only)
mefenamic acid (Ponstel)

Napthylalkanones (Nonacidic)
nabumetone (Relafen)

Oxicams
meloxicam (Mobic)
piroxicam (Feldene)

Propionic Acids
fenoprofen (Nalfon)
flurbiprofen (Ansaid)
ibuprofen (Motrin, Advil, others)
ketoprofen (Orudis KT)
naproxen (Naprosyn, Aleve)
oxaprozin (Daypro)

COX, Cyclooxygenase; *NSAID,* nonsteroidal antiinflammatory drug.

(LT) pathway. Both of these mechanisms differ from that of the opioids, which relieve pain by interfering with its recognition of pain signals in the brain. Furthermore, it is now recognized that there are at least two types, or isoforms, of COX. COX-1 is the isoform of the enzyme that promotes the synthesis of homeostatic PGs, which have primarily beneficial effects on various body functions. One example is their role in maintaining an in-

tact gastrointestinal mucosa. In contrast, the COX-2 isoform promotes the synthesis of PGs that are involved in inflammatory processes. In 1998, the newest class of NSAIDs, the COX-2 inhibitors, appeared on the U.S. market. These NSAIDs work by specifically inhibiting the COX-2 isoform of cyclooxygenase and theoretically have limited or no COX-1 effects. Previous NSAID groups functioned nonspecifically by inhibiting both COX-1 and

Box 44-2 NSAIDs: FDA-Approved Indications

Acute gout
Acute gouty arthritis
Acute painful shoulder
Ankylosing spondylitis
Bursitis
Fever
Juvenile rheumatoid arthritis
Mild-to-moderate pain
Osteoarthritis
Primary dysmenorrhea
Rheumatoid arthritis
Tendinitis
Various ophthalmic uses

FDA, Food and Drug Administration; *NSAID,* nonsteroidal antiinflammatory drug.

Table 44-1 Suggested NSAIDs for Patients with Various Medical Conditions

Medical Condition	Recommended NSAID
Ankylosing spondylitis	indomethacin, diclofenac
Diabetic neuropathy	sulindac
Dysmenorrhea	Fenamates, naproxen, ibuprofen
Gout	indomethacin, naproxen, sulindac
Headaches	aspirin, naproxen. ibuprofen
Hepatotoxicity	tolmetin, naproxen, ibuprofen, piroxicam, fenamates
History of aspirin or NSAID allergy	Avoid if possible; if deemed necessary, consider a nonacetylated salicylate
Hypertension	sulindac, nonacetylated salicylate, ibuprofen, etodolac
Osteoarthritis	diclofenac, oxaprozin, indomethacin
Risk for gastrointestinal toxicity	All COX-2 inhibitors: celecoxib, nonacetylated salicylate, enteric-coated aspirin, diclofenac, nabumetone, etodolac, ibuprofen, oxaprozin
Risk for nephrotoxicity	sulindac, nonacetylated salicylate, nabumetone, etodolac, diclofenac, oxaprozin
Warfarin therapy	sulindac, tolmetin, naproxen, ibuprofen, oxaprozin

COX, Cyclooxygenase; *NSAID,* nonsteroidal antiinflammatory drug.

COX-2 activity. The greater enzyme specificity of the COX-2 inhibitors allows for the beneficial antiinflammatory effects associated with all other NSAIDs while reducing the prevalence of adverse effects, such as gastrointestinal ulceration, associated with the anti–COX-1 activity of the more nonspecific NSAIDs.

The LT pathway is inhibited by some antiinflammatory drugs, but not by salicylates. Several antiinflammatory drugs block both the PG pathway and the LT pathway, whereas others only weakly inhibit COX but primarily inhibit lipoxygenase.

The main drug effects of NSAIDs are those of analgesic, antiinflammatory, and antipyretic effects. NSAIDs reduce fever by inhibiting PGE_2, specifically by inhibiting its biosynthesis within the preoptic hypothalamic region of the brain, which regulates body temperature. One notable effect of the salicylates, especially aspirin, is their inhibition of platelet aggregation, also known as its *antiplatelet activity.* Although all NSAIDs can be ulcerogenic and induce gastrointestinal bleeding, as mentioned earlier, most of these effects are due to drug activity against tissue COX-1. Aspirin has the unique property among NSAIDs of being an irreversible inhibitor of COX-1 receptors within the platelets themselves. This in turn results in reduced formation by the platelets of TXA_2, a substance that normally promotes platelet aggregation. For this reason, aspirin is often used both prophylactically and following myocardial infarction (MI) to aid in the prevention of platelet aggregation, which unopposed, could lead to fibrin clot formation and and reinfarction.

Indications

Some of the more noted therapeutic uses of this broad class of drugs are listed in Table 44-1, but they are primarily used for their analgesic, antigout, antiinflammatory, and antipyretic effects; for the relief of vascular headaches; and for platelet inhibition.

NSAIDs are also widely used for the treatment of rheumatoid arthritis and osteoarthritis, as well as other inflammatory conditions, rheumatic fever, and mild-to-moderate pain. They also have proved beneficial as adjunctive pain relief medications in patients with chronic pain syndromes, such as pain from bone cancer and chronic back pain. For the relief of pain they are sometimes combined with an opioid. They also do not cause many of the undesirable effects of opioids, mainly respiratory depression. However, unlike opioids, their effectiveness is limited by a ceiling effect in that any further increase in the dose beyond a certain level in-

creases the risk for adverse effects without a corresponding increase in the therapeutic effect. In contrast, opioid doses may be titrated almost indefinitely to increasingly higher levels, especially for terminally ill patients with severe pain.

As noted earlier, salicylates also have the additional beneficial property of opposing the aggregation properties of platelets. For this reason, they are commonly used for both prophylaxis and treatment of arterial, and possibly venous, thrombosis. This is known as the *antithrombotic effect* of aspirin. This antiplatelet action has made aspirin, along with thrombolytic drugs (Chapter 27), a primary drug in the treatment of acute MI and many other thromboembolic disorders. Other NSAIDs generally lack these antiplatelet effects. However, they can be ulcerogenic, with possible blood loss, by inhibition of the synthesis of protective PGs, which normally function to protect the gastrointestinal mucosa. Other NSAIDs are commonly used in the treatment of **gout,** which is caused by the overproduction of uric acid or decreased uric acid excretion, or by both processes. This can often result in hyperuricemia (too much uric acid in the blood), a condition that causes joint pain as a result of the deposition of needlelike crystals of urate precipitate in tissues and the joints.

The appropriate selection of an NSAID is a clinical judgment based on consideration of the patient's history, including any previous medical conditions; the intended use of the drug; the patient's previous experience with NSAIDs; the patient's preference; and the cost.

Contraindications

Contraindications to NSAIDs include known drug allergy and conditions that place the patient at risk for bleeding. These conditions include rhinitis (risk for epistaxis [nosebleed]), vitamin K deficiency, and peptic ulcer disease. NSAIDs are also not advised during pregnancy, especially during the last trimester, because of the risk for maternal bleeding and possible miscarriage. Other common contraindications apply to most drugs and include severe renal or hepatic disease. All NSAIDs are generally rated as pregnancy category C drugs for use during the first two trimesters of pregnancy, but are rated pregnancy category D (not recommended) during the third trimester. This is because NSAID use has been associated with both excessive maternal bleeding and neonatal NSAID toxicity during the perinatal period. Because the ongoing presence of NSAIDs may hinder the desired natural synthesis of PGs in an infant's body, these drugs are also not recommended for nursing mothers as they are known to be excreted into human milk.

Adverse Effects

One of the more common complaints and potentially serious adverse effects of the NSAIDs is gastrointestinal distress. This can range from mild symptoms such as heartburn to the most severe gastrointestinal complication, gastrointestinal bleeding. In fact, the adverse effects of salicylates mainly involve the gastrointestinal tract and, besides bleeding, include symptomatic gastrointestinal disturbances and mucosal lesions (e.g., erosive gastritis, gastric ulcer). The potential adverse effects of NSAIDs listed in Table 44-2 do not necessarily apply to all drugs, but they do apply to many of them.

Many of the adverse effects and adverse effects of NSAIDs are secondary to their inactivation of protective PGs that help maintain the normal integrity of the stomach lining. However, a drug known as misoprostol (Cytotec) has proved successful in preventing the gastric ulcers and hence gastrointestinal bleeding that can occur in patients receiving NSAIDs. It is a synthetic PGE_1 analog that potently inhibits gastric acid secretion, which it does by directly inhibiting the function of *parietal cells* in the stomach that secrete its acid content. It also has a cytoprotective component, although the mechanism responsible for this action is unclear. This drug also has abortifacient properties, which were discussed in Chapter 33.

Renal function depends partly on PGs, which stimulate vasodilation and increased renal blood flow. Disruption of this PG function by NSAIDs is sometimes strong enough to precipitate acute or chronic renal failure, depending on the patient's current level of renal function. Elderly patients are at greater risk for this adverse drug reaction.

Toxicity and Management of Overdose

There are both chronic and acute manifestations of salicylate toxicity. *Chronic salicylate intoxication* is also known as **salicylism** and results from either short-term high doses or prolonged therapy with high or even lower doses. The most common signs and symptoms of acute or chronic salicylate intoxication are listed in Table 44-3.

The most common manifestations of chronic intoxication in adults are tinnitus and hearing loss. Those in children are hyperventilation and central nervous system (CNS) effects such as dizziness, drowsiness, and behavioral changes. These effects usually arise when serum salicylate concentrations exceed 40 to 60 mg/dL. A deciliter is equivalent to one tenth of a liter, or 100 mL. Metabolic complications such as metabolic acidosis and respiratory alkalosis often occur to varying degrees in cases of chronic salicylate intoxication. Metabolic acidosis can also occur with acute intoxication, but it is usually less severe than that in patients with chronic intoxication. Hypoglycemia may also occur and can be life threatening.

The treatment of chronic intoxication is based on the presenting symptoms. Serum salicylate concentrations may be determined but are not as useful in estimating the severity because severe intoxication can occur with a concentration as low as 150 mg/dL.

The signs and symptoms of *acute salicylate toxicity* are similar to those of chronic intoxication, but the effects are often more pronounced and occur more quickly. Acute salicylate overdose usually results from the ingestion of a single toxic dose, and its severity can be estimated based on the estimated amount (in mg/kg of body weight) ingested, as follows:

- Little or no toxicity: <150 mg/kg
- Mild to moderate toxicity: 150-300 mg/kg
- Severe toxicity: 300-500 mg/kg
- Life-threatening toxicity: >500 mg/kg

It should be noted, however, that even doses lower than 150 mg/kg have resulted in fatal toxicity, whereas some patients have survived aspirin overdoses as high as 130 g. A serum salicylate concentration measured 6 hours or more after the ingestion may be used in conjunction with the **Done nomogram** to estimate the severity of intoxication and help guide treatment. The

Table 44-2	**NSAIDs: Adverse Effects**
Body System	**Adverse Effects**
Cardiovascular	Moderate-to-severe noncardiogenic pulmonary edema
Gastrointestinal	Most frequent: dyspepsia, heartburn, epigastric distress, nausea
	Less frequent: vomiting, anorexia, abdominal pain, gastrointestinal bleeding, mucosal lesions (erosions or ulcerations)
Hematologic	Altered hemostasis through effects on platelet function
Hepatic	Acute reversible hepatotoxicity
Renal	Reduction in creatinine clearance, acute tubular necrosis with renal failure
Other	Skin eruption, sensitivity reactions, tinnitus, hearing loss

NSAID, Nonsteroidal antiinflammatory drug.

Table 44-3	**Acute or Chronic Salicylate Intoxication: Signs and Symptoms**
Body System	**Signs and Symptoms**
Cardiovascular	Increased heart rate
Central nervous	Tinnitus, hearing loss, dimness of vision, headache, dizziness, mental confusion, lassitude, drowsiness
Gastrointestinal	Nausea, vomiting, diarrhea
Metabolic	Sweating, thirst, hyperventilation, hypo- or hyperglycemia

Done nomogram is a graphic plot of serum salicylate levels (in milligrams per deciliter [mg/dL]) as a function of elapsed time following salicylate ingestion. It was first published in a 1960 issue of the journal *Pediatrics* and is still widely used today for gauging salicylate toxicity. However, this nomogram is only intended for estimating the severity of acute intoxications and not that of chronic salicylate intoxication. Table 44-4 describes, in general terms, treatment for cases of varying severity.

Treatment goals include removing salicylate from the gastrointestinal tract and/or preventing its further absorption; correcting fluid, electrolyte, and acid-base disturbances; and implementing measures to enhance salicylate elimination. This is summarized in Table 44-5.

An acute overdose of nonsalicylate NSAIDs (e.g., ibuprofen) causes effects similar to those of salicylate overdose, but they are generally not as extensive or as dangerous. These symptoms include CNS toxicities such as drowsiness, lethargy, mental confusion, paresthesias (abnormal touch sensations), numbness, aggressive behavior, disorientation, seizures, and gastrointestinal toxicities such as nausea, vomiting, and gastrointestinal bleeding. Intense headache, dizziness, cerebral edema, cardiac arrest, and death have also been known to occur in extreme cases. Treatment should consist of the immediate removal of the ingested drug by inducing emesis with gastric lavage. This should be followed by the administration of activated charcoal, with supportive and symptomatic treatment initiated thereafter. Unlike the case with salicylates, hemodialysis appears to be of no value in enhancing the elimination of NSAIDs.

Interactions

The drug interactions associated with the use of salicylates and other NSAIDs can result in significant complications and morbidity. Some of the more common of these are listed in Table 44-6.

These drugs can also interfere with laboratory test results. Specifically, salicylates can cause what are usually minor and transient elevations in liver enzymes (ALT, AST), but cases of severe hepatotoxicity are rare. Hematocrit, hemoglobin, and

Table 44-4	Acute Salicylate Intoxication: Treatment
Severity	**Treatment**
Mild	1. Dosage reduction or discontinuation of salicylates
	2. Symptomatic and supportive therapy
Severe	1. Discontinuation of salicylates
	2. Intensive symptomatic and supportive therapy
	3. Dialysis if: high salicylate levels, unresponsive acidosis (pH <7.1), impaired renal function or renal failure, pulmonary edema, persistent CNS symptoms (e.g., seizures, coma), progressive deterioration despite appropriate therapy

CNS, Central nervous system.

Table 44-5 Acute Salicylate Intoxication: Treatment Goals	
Treatment Goal	**Measure**
Reduce salicylate absorption	Gastric lavage*
	Activated charcoal
Treat fluid and electrolyte imbalance	Appropriate fluid replacement and electrolyte therapy should be implemented promptly, based on fluid, acid–base, and electrolyte status. Therefore, arterial pH and blood gases and electrolytes, serum creatinine, BUN, and blood glucose should be determined.
Enhance salicylate elimination	Alkaline diuresis: intravenous administration of sodium bicarbonate to alkalinize the urine to a pH of ≥7.5 with sufficient urine flow.
	Hemodialysis: the same considerations as those that apply to chronic intoxication.
Provide symptomatic and supportive measures	Hypotension and/or hemorrhagic complications: fluids and transfusions, along with possible vitamin K injections.
	Respiratory depression: may require assisted pulmonary ventilation and oxygen.
	Seizures: intravenous administration of a benzodiazepine or short-acting barbiturate.

*Effective up to 3 to 4 hr after acute ingestion and may be up to 10 hr after ingestion in the event of massive overdose.
BUN, Blood urea nitrogen.

Table 44-6 Salicylates and Other NSAIDs: Drug Interactions		
Drug	**Mechanism**	**Result**
Alcohol	Additive effect	Increased gastrointestinal bleeding
Anticoagulants	Platelet inhibition, hypoprothrombinemia	Increased bleeding tendencies
Aspirin and other salicylates with NSAIDs	Reduce NSAID absorption, additive gastrointestinal toxicities	Increased gastrointestinal toxicity with no therapeutic advantage
Corticosteroids and other ulcerogenic drugs	Additive toxicities	Increased ulcerogenic effects
Cyclosporine	Inhibits renal PG synthesis	May increase the nephrotoxic effects of cyclosporine
Diuretics and ACE inhibitors	Inhibit PG synthesis	Reduced hypotensive and diuretic effects
Protein-bound drugs	Compete for binding	More pronounced drug actions
Uricosurics	Antagonism	Decreased uric acid excretion

NSAID, Nonsteroidal antiinflammatory drug; *PG*, prostaglandin.

DOSAGES

Most Commonly Used NSAIDs

Drug (Pregnancy Category)	Pharmacologic Class	Usual Dosage Range	Indications
aspirin (ASA; many product names) (C/D)	Salicylate	**Adult** PO/PR: 25-1000 mg 4-6 × day (max 4 g/day) PO/PR: 3.2-6 g/day divided q4-6h PO/PR: 30-325 mg/day; 300 or 325 mg/day PO: 81-325 mg once daily **Pediatric** PO/PR: 10-15 mg/kg q4-6h PO/PR: 10-18 mg/kg divided q6-8h	Fever, pain Arthritis Fever, pain Arthritis Thromboprevention, (e.g., post-MI or other risk factors for MI, stroke, or DVTs)
celecoxib (Celebrex) (C/D)	COX-2 inhibitor	**Adult and adolescent >15 yr** PO: 100-200 mg once daily PO: 400 mg bid	Arthritis, acute pain, primary dysmenorrhea Reduction of number of heredity colon polyps in FAP
ibuprofen (Motrin, Advil, others) (C/D)	Propionic acid	**Adult** 1200-3200 mg/day divided tid-qid **Pediatric** 20-40 mg/kg/day divided tid-qid	Arthritis, fever, pain, dysmenorrhea
indomethacin (Indocin, Indocin SR) (C/D)	Acetic acid	**Adult** PO/PR: 25-50 mg bid-tid (max 200 mg/day) **Pediatric** PO/PR: 1-4 mg/kg/day divided bid-qid (max 200 mg/day)	Arthritis, including acute gouty arthritis, acute painful shoulder due to bursitis or tendonitis
ketorolac (Toradol) (C/D)	Pyrrolizine carboxylic acid	**Adult*** PO: 10 mg q4-6h (max 40 mg/day) IV/IM: 15-60 mg q6-12h (max 120 mg/day if <65 yr; max 60 mg/day if >65 yr)	Acute painful conditions that would otherwise require opioid level analgesia; PO form is recommended only when transitioning from injectable form to oral form

*Pediatric dosing guidelines are not as well established, but the recommended range for IV, IM, or PO use is 0.4-1 mg/kg as a single dose for acute conditions (e.g., sports injury).
ASA, Acetylsalicylic acid; *COX,* cyclooxygenase; *DVT,* deep vein thrombosis; *FAP,* familial adenomatous polyposis; *MI,* myocardial infarction; *NSAID,* nonsteroidal antiinflammatory drug.
Pregnancy categories: C/D = C, first trimester; D, third trimester.

RBC levels can drop if any drug-induced gastrointestinal bleeding does occur. There can also be NSAID-induced hyperkalemia or hyponatremia.

Dosages

For the recommended dosages of various NSAIDs, see the Dosages table on this page.

Drug Profiles

Nonsteroidal Antiinflammatory Drugs

Chemically speaking, the broad drug category of NSAIDs includes four major categories of carboxylic acids (acetic acids, propionic acids, pyranocarboxylic acids, and pyrrolizine carboxylic acids) along with the newest class of NSAIDs, the COX-2 inhibitors.

Acetic Acids

Salicylates are chemically classified as carboxylic acids. Although aspirin is the most commonly used of all these drugs, the others have many of the same beneficial effects as aspirin. Although aspirin is available without prescription, many of the other salicylate drugs do require a prescription. These include diflunisal (Dolobid),

choline magnesium trisalicylate (Trilisate), and salsalate (Salsitab). Magnesium salicylate comes in both nonprescription (e.g., Bayer Select Maximum Strength Backache) and prescription (Magan) products, even though both are of comparable medication strength. Salicylates are most commonly used in solid oral dosage forms (i.e., tablets, capsules). Other available dosage forms include a topical cream (Aspercreme), rectal suppositories, and oral liquids. Sodium thiosalicylate (Rexolate) is currently the only commercially available injectable salicylate and requires a prescription. Aspirin is also contained in many combination products, including aspirin, acetaminophen, and caffeine combinations such as Excedrin, and aspirin/antacid combinations (e.g., Bufferin). Aspirin also is available in special dosage forms, such as enteric-coated aspirin (Ecotrin), designed to protect the stomach mucosa by dissolving in the duodenum.

Indomethacin (Indocin) is one of the six commonly used acetic acid or *acetylated* NSAIDs, the others being aspirin, diflunisal (Dolobid), diclofenac (Voltaren, Cataflam), etodolac (Lodine), sulindac (Clinoril), and tolmetin (Tolectin). There is debate in the literature over whether acylated or nonacetylated NSAIDs provide better pain relief. However, patients vary in their drug responses, and it is usually a matter of clinical trial and error to find the ideal drug(s) for a given patient.

▶ *aspirin*

Aspirin is known chemically as acetylsalicylic acid (ASA). It is the prototype salicylate and NSAID and is the most widely used drug in the world. First introduced in the late 1800s, it remains a mainstay of many drug treatment regimens. A daily aspirin tablet (81 mg or 325 mg) is now routinely recommended as prophylactic therapy for adults who have strong risk factors for developing coronary artery disease or stroke, even if they have no previous history of such an event. Both the 81 mg (which is traditionally thought of as "children's" aspirin) and the 325-mg strengths appear to be equally beneficial for the prevention of thrombotic events. For this reason, the lower strength is often chosen for patients who have any elevated risk for bleeding, such as those with previous stroke history or history of peptic ulcer disease and those taking the anticoagulant warfarin (Coumadin). Aspirin is also often used to treat the pain associated with headache, neuralgia, myalgia, and arthralgia, as well as other pain syndromes resulting from inflammation. These include arthritis, pleurisy, and pericarditis. Patients with systemic lupus erythematosus may also benefit from aspirin therapy because of its antirheumatic effects.

Aspirin and other salicylates all have one very specific contraindication to their use. This drug class is contraindicated children with flulike symptoms, as their use has been strongly associated with Reye's syndrome. This is an acute and potentially life-threatening condition involving progressive neurologic deficits that can lead to coma, and may also involve liver damage. It is believed to be triggered by viral illnesses such as influenza, and also by salicylate therapy itself, in the presence of a viral illness. Survivors of this condition may or may not suffer permanent neurologic damage.

Pharmacokinetics

Half-Life	Onset	Peak	Duration
PO: 5-9 hr	PO: 15-30 min	PO: 1-2 hr	PO: 4-6 hr

▶ *indomethacin*

Like the other NSAIDs, indomethacin (Indocin) has analgesic, antiinflammatory, antirheumatic, and antipyretic properties. Its therapeutic actions are of particular use in the treatment of rheumatoid arthritis, osteoarthritis, acute bursitis or tendinitis, ankylosing spondylitis, and acute gouty arthritis. The drug is available for both oral and rectal use. An injectable form of the drug is also used intravenously (IV) to promote closure of patent ductus arteriosus (PDA), a heart defect that sometimes occurs in premature infants.

Pharmacokinetics

Half-Life	Onset	Peak	Duration
PO: 1.5-2 hr	PO: <30 min	PO: 0.5-3 hr	PO: 4-6 hr

Propionic Acids
▶ *ibuprofen*

Ibuprofen (Motrin, Advil) is the prototype NSAID in the propionic acid category, which also includes fenoprofen, flurbiprofen, ketoprofen, naproxen, and oxaprozin. Ibuprofen is the most commonly used of the propionic acid drugs because of the numerous indications for its use and because of its relatively safe adverse effect profiles. It is often used for rheumatoid arthritis, osteoarthritis, primary dysmenorrhea, gout, dental pain, and musculoskeletal disorders. Naproxen is the second most commonly used NSAID with a somewhat improved reported adverse effect profile over ibuprofen, including fewer drug interactions with angiotensin-converting enzyme inhibitors for hypertension. Evidence indicates that ibuprofen is more likely to interact with these drugs to hinder their desired hypotensive effects than is naproxen. Both drugs are available only for oral use in both over the counter (OTC) and prescription strengths.

Pharmacokinetics

Half-Life	Onset	Peak	Duration
PO: <30 min	PO: 0.5-2 hr	PO: 1-2 hr	PO: 4-6 hr

Pyrrolizine Carboxylic Acids
▶ *ketorolac*

Ketorolac (Toradol) is classified as a pyrrolizine carboxylic acid and is currently the only drug in this category, having a somewhat unique chemical structure. Although it does have some antiinflammatory activity, it is used primarily for its powerful analgesic effects, which are comparable to those of narcotic drugs such as morphine. It is indicated for the treatment of moderate to severe acute pain such as that resulting from orthopedic injuries. The opioid-level analgesic potential of the drug can make it a particularly desirable choice for opiate-addicted patients who have acute pain control needs because ketorolac lacks the addictive properties of the true opioids. Ketorolac is the only NSAID that can be given orally, or by injection, and there is also a dosage form for ophthalmic use (Chapter 58).

Ketorolac is available only by prescription. It is indicated for the short-term (up to 5 days) management of moderate-to-severe acute pain that requires analgesia at the opioid level. It is not indicated for minor or chronic painful conditions. Ketorolac is a very potent NSAID with many contraindications.

Pharmacokinetics

Half-Life	Onset	Peak	Duration
IV/IM: 5-7 hr	IV/IM: 0.5 hr	IV/IM: 1-2 hr	IV/IM: 4-6 hr

COX-2 Inhibitors

COX-2 inhibitors have little effect on platelet function. These drugs were designed primarily to cause fewer gastrointestinal adverse effects relative to other NSAIDs because of their COX-2 selectivity. However, they are not totally devoid of gastrointestinal toxicity. Gastritis and upper gastrointestinal bleeding have been reported with their use, although much less frequently than with older NSAIDs. Specific adverse effects of this NSAID subclass include fatigue, dizziness, lower extremity edema, and hypertension.

▶ *celecoxib*

Celecoxib (Celebrex) was the first COX-2 inhibitor, approved in December of 1998. It is indicated for the treatment of osteoarthritis, rheumatoid arthritis, acute pain symptoms, and primary dysmenorrhea. More recently, this drug has also been approved for reduction of colon polyps in patients with an inherited condition known as *familial adenomatous polyposis*. It is available only for oral use. Since 1998, two other COX-2 inhibitors were marketed and have since been recalled. These are rofecoxib (Vioxx), recalled by Merck in 2004, and valdecoxib (Bextra), recalled by Pfizer in 2005. These two drugs were recalled following several case reports indicating an increased risk for adverse cardiovascular events, including blood clots during medical and surgical procedures, MI, cardiovascular accident, and death. Valdexocib has also been associated with severe skin reactions known as *toxic epidermal necrolysis* and Stevens-Johnson syndrome. There is also evidence that celecoxib may pose similar risks. However, it currently remains on the U.S. market, although its use is now being monitored more closely by the U.S. Food and Drug Administration (FDA).

Pharmacokinetics

Half-Life	Onset	Peak	Duration
PO: 11 hr	PO: 0.75-1 hr	PO: 3 hr	PO: 4-8 hr

ENOLIC ACIDS, FENAMIC ACIDS, AND NONACIDIC COMPOUNDS

The last three chemical categories of NSAIDs consist of the smallest number of drugs, and the indications for their use are more limited, as is their actual clinical use. The drugs are profiled briefly here. Pregnancy category information is essentially the same as other NSAIDs. Both piroxicam (Feldene) and meloxicam (Mobic) belong to the enolic acid family of NSAIDs. These compounds are more commonly called *oxicams*. They are very potent drugs that have been observed to produce severe gastrointestinal toxicities. They are commonly used in the treatment of mild-to-moderate osteoarthritis, rheumatoid arthritis, and gouty arthritis. Both are available only in oral dosage formulations and have contraindications similar to those of the other NSAIDs.

Meclofenamate (Meclomen) and mefenamic acid (Ponstel) are fenamic acid NSAIDs that are also older drugs and not used as commonly as the other NSAIDs. They are indicated for the treatment of mild-to-moderate pain, osteoarthritis, and rheumatoid arthritis.

Nabumetone (Relafen) is a relatively newer NSAID that is better tolerated than some of the others in terms of gastrointestinal adverse effects. It is classified as a naphthylalkanone and is currently the only drug in its class. It is relatively nonacidic compared with most of the other NSAIDs, which probably accounts for its improved gastrointestinal tolerance. Currently it is indicated only for the treatment of osteoarthritis and rheumatoid arthritis.

ANTIRHEUMATIC DRUGS

As previously emphasized in this chapter, all NSAIDs have some antirheumatic activity. As defined at the beginning of this chapter, *rheumatic* illnesses involve inflammation, degeneration, or metabolic derangement of joints and other connective tissue structures, with symptoms including pain, stiffness, and reduced range of motion. The most common rheumatic illnesses include gout and rheumatoid arthritis. There are several non-NSAID medications recognized primarily for their antirheumatic properties, as opposed to the analgesic, antiinflammatory, and antipyretic properties that are associated with NSAIDs. These drugs are referred to here as *antirheumatic* drugs, and they are further subdivided into the *antigout* and *antirheumatoid arthritis* drugs. Although some of these drugs have additional medical uses, they are commonly used to treat the very prevalent rheumatic conditions known as gout and arthritis. Gout was described previously as a build-up of uric acid crystals in the tissues that often causes painful deposits into joint spaces known as *gouty arthritis*. Gout results from inappropriate uric acid metabolism. Persons with gout either overproduce or underexcrete uric acid, an end-product of purine metabolism. Purines are part of the normal dietary intake and are used to make the essential nucleoside and nucleotide structural units of DNA and RNA. During their metabolism, they are converted from hypoxanthine to xanthine and eventually to uric acid. The normal pathway for the purine metabolism is depicted in Figure 44-2. This pathway is overactive in pa-

tients with gout, and is reduced by antigout drug therapy. **Arthritis** is a general term that can include numerous identified subtypes. The most common of these, in addition to gout, are *rheumatoid arthritis* and *osteoarthritis*. Osteoarthritis tends to simply be an age-related degeneration of joint tissues resulting in pain and reduced function in terms of strength and range of motion. It is commonly exacerbated by comorbid obesity. Rheumatoid arthritis involves similar inflammatory symptoms, but can occur as early as childhood. It is believed to be an autoimmune disorder, possibly triggered by a viral infection. As noted earlier throughout the chapter, NSAIDs are commonly used for the pain and inflammatory symptoms of all three of these conditions. However, the drugs described below that have specific designation as *antirheumatic* drugs have characteristics that make them different from NSAIDs, and are used primarily for gout and rheumatoid arthritis. Because each is unique in its mechanism of action, these drugs are not described in grouped format. Additional antirheumatic drugs are discussed in Chapter 49 because of their even more distinct mechanisms of action.

Drug Profiles

Antigout Drugs
When the body contains too much uric acid, deposits of uric acid crystals collect in tissues and joints. This causes the pain of gout because these crystals are like small needles that jab and stick into sensitive tissues and joints. Antigout drugs include such drugs as allopurinol (Zyloprim), colchicine, probenecid (Benemid), and sulfinpyrazone (Anturane). They are targeted at the underlying defect in uric acid metabolism, which causes either overproduction or underexcretion of uric acid (Figure 44-2). Both of these pathologic processes lead to tissue accumulations of uric acid crystalline deposits *(gouty deposits)* and symptoms of gout. Although not all gouty deposits occur within joints, gouty arthritis is the condition of one or more inflamed joints resulting from gouty deposits that collect inside the joint anatomy. This is also called *articular gout*, whereas gout that occurs in tissues outside of the joints is called *abarticular gout*.

▸ allopurinol
The beneficial effect of allopurinol (Zyloprim) in the relief of gout is the inhibition of the enzyme xanthine oxidase, which thereby prevents uric acid production. Allopurinol is indicated for patients whose gout is caused by the excess production of uric acid (hyperuricemia). Oxypurinol, a metabolite of allopurinol, also prevents uric acid production. Oxypurinol is available as an orphan drug for patients with hyperuricemia who are intolerant to allopurinol therapy.

Allopurinol is contraindicated in patients with a hypersensitivity to it. Significant adverse effects to the drug include agranulocytosis, aplastic anemia, and serious and potentially fatal skin conditions such as exfoliative dermatitis, Stevens-Johnson syndrome,

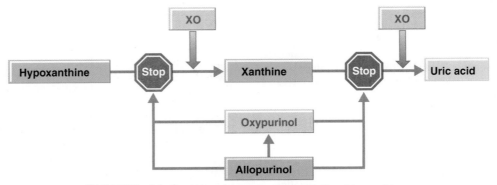

FIGURE 44-2   Uric acid production. *XO,* Xanthine oxidase.

and toxic epidermal necrolysis. Azathioprine and mercaptopurine both interact with allopurinol, and because of the important interactions that can result, their doses may have to be adjusted. Allopurinol is available only for oral use. The recommended adult dosage is 200 to 600 mg/day, to a maximum of 800 mg/day. Pregnancy category C.

colchicine

Colchicine is an antigout medication that has weak antiinflammatory activity, no effect on the urinary excretion of uric acid, and no analgesic activity. It appears to be effective in the treatment of gout by reducing the inflammatory response to the deposits of urate crystals in joint tissue. There are many possible explanations for its ability to do this, but the one most favored is that it inhibits polymorphonuclear leukocyte metabolism, mobility, and *chemotaxis* (chemical attraction of these cells to the site of inflammation, that worsens an inflammatory response).

Colchicine is a powerful inhibitor of cell mitosis and can cause short-term leukopenia. For this reason it is generally used for the treatment of acute attacks of gout. Its more severe adverse effects can include bleeding into the gastrointestinal or urinary tracts, and the drug should be stopped should such effects appear. Colchicine can also cause renal failure. There is no specific antidote for colchicine poisoning. Hypersensitivity is the only contraindication to its use. The drug is available in both oral and injectable form. The usual adult dosage is an initial dose of 1 to 1.2 mg, then 0.5 to 1.2 mg every 1 to 2 hours until the gout pain disappears or until nausea, vomiting, or diarrhea develops. Pregnancy category D.

probenecid and sulfinpyrazone

The beneficial effect of probenecid (Benemid) in the treatment of gout is the increased excretion of uric acid in the urine by inhibiting its reabsorption by the kidney. Drugs that promote uric acid excretion are known as *uricosurics*. In patients whose gout is due to the underexcretion of uric acid, urate crystals form because uric acid is not being excreted in the urine in sufficient quantities. Instead, most of the uric acid is being reabsorbed from the renal tubules back into the bloodstream and then conveyed throughout the body. Probenecid works by preferentially binding to the special transporter protein in the proximal convoluted renal tubule that takes uric acid from the urine and places it back into the blood. The probenecid is then reabsorbed back into the bloodstream while the uric acid remains in the urine and is excreted. Besides its use for the treatment of the hyperuricemia associated with gout and gouty arthritis, it also has the ability to delay the renal excretion of penicillin, thus increasing the serum levels of penicillin and prolonging its effect (Chapter 37). Probenecid is available as a 500-mg oral tablet. The usual adult dosage is 250 mg twice a day with food, milk, or antacids for 1 week, followed by 500 mg twice daily thereafter. This dose may be adjusted as needed to maintain desirable serum uric acid levels. Contraindications include peptic ulcer disease. Pregnancy category B. Sulfinpyrazone (Anturane) works similarly to probenecid. It is also a uricosuric drug. Despite its generic name, it is not a sulfonamide drug per se, but is chemically related to phenylbutazone, an early NSAID, which is no longer available on the U.S. market. Like other NSAIDs, however, sulfinpyrazone can be ulcerogenic and is therefore contraindicated in patients with peptic ulcer disease. Sulfinpyrazone is available only for oral use. The usual adult dosage is 100 to 200 mg twice a day for 1 week. The subsequent adjusted maintenance dosage can range from 200 to 800 mg daily. Pregnancy category C (category D during the third trimester).

Antirheumatoid Arthritis Drugs

Antirheumatoid arthritis drugs suppress the specific types of inflammation associated with rheumatoid arthritis (hereafter referred to as *arthritis*) and are therefore used in its treatment. These drugs are considered to be more powerful than the NSAIDs in that they do not merely provide antiinflammatory and analgesic effects but can actually arrest or slow the disease processes associated with arthritis. For these reasons, this class of medications is also referred to as the **disease-modifying antirheumatic drugs (DMARDs).** DMARDs

often have a slow onset of action of several weeks, versus minutes to hours for NSAIDs. For this reason, DMARDs are sometimes also referred to as *slow-acting antirheumatic drugs (SAARDs)*. They are also commonly thought of as second-line drugs for the treatment of arthritis because they can have much more toxic adverse effects than the NSAIDs. However, the use of the term *second-line drugs* can be misleading because DMARDs may be appropriately used as first-line drug therapy, in spite of their greater toxicity, for more severe cases of arthritis as diagnosed by a rheumatologist. Grading of the severity of a given case of arthritis often depends on careful evaluation by the prescriber of such factors as radiographic (X-ray) evidence and various laboratory indicators such as serum *rheumatoid factor* and *antinuclear antibody*. Less severe cases of arthritis are the more common clinical picture, however, and in such cases DMARDs are in fact used as second-line therapy, usually only after a patient has failed at least a 3-month trial of NSAID therapy. DMARDs exhibit antiinflammatory, antiarthritic, and immunomodulating effects and work by inhibiting the movement of various cells into an inflamed, damaged area, such as a joint. These cells (neutrophils, monocytes, and macrophages) are responsible for causing many of the deleterious effects of chronic rheumatoid arthritis. By preventing the accumulation of these inflammatory cells in the area of the diseased joint, antiarthritic drugs prevent progression of the disease. One of these drugs, hydroxychloroquine (Plaquenil), is also used to treat malaria, and was discussed in Chapter 42. Another, sulfasalazine (Azulfidine), is used for colitis and is discussed in Chapter 51. Some additional DMARDs, such as the newer drug etanercept (Enbrel), are designed and known especially for their immunomodulating effects. These drugs are discussed in Chapter 49.

auranofin

Auranofin (Ridaura) is an orally active antiarthritic drug. Twenty-nine percent of it is gold, and like all DMARDs, it has antiinflammatory, antiarthritic, and immunomodulating effects. It is poorly absorbed orally—only about 25% of the medication is absorbed from the gastrointestinal tract into the blood. Auranofin is contraindicated in patients with a history of gold-induced necrotizing enterocolitis, pulmonary fibrosis, exfoliative dermatitis, bone marrow aplasia, or other types of blood dyscrasia. It is available only for oral use. The normal recommended adult dosage is 6 mg once per day or 3 mg twice per day. The dosage can be increased to 9 mg after 6 months of therapy if the response is inadequate. Pregnancy category C.

aurothioglucose and gold sodium thiomalate

Aurothioglucose (Solganal) and gold sodium thiomalate (Aurolate) are parenterally administered antiarthritic drugs. Both are approximately 50% gold, and both are currently available only in an injectable form of 50 mg/mL. These products are made by complexing gold with thioglucose and thiomalate via a sulfur linkage. Both drugs are also dosed similarly by the intramuscular (IM) route only with weekly injections ranging from 10 to 50 mg for aurothioglucose and 10 to 100 mg for gold sodium thiomalate. Both require regular monitoring with either dose reduction or discontinuation if symptoms of toxicity appear as detected by complete blood count (CBC), urinalysis, and kidney and liver function tests.

leflunomide

Leflunomide (Arava) is a new drug indicated for the treatment of active rheumatoid arthritis. It modulates or alters the response of the immune system to rheumatoid arthritis. It has antiproliferative, antiinflammatory, and immunosuppressive activity. Its most common adverse effects are diarrhea, respiratory tract infection, alopecia, elevated liver function tests, and rash. It is contraindicated in women who are or may become pregnant and should not be used by nursing mothers or those with a hypersensitivity to it. Leflunomide is most commonly given by a loading dose of 100 mg daily for 3 days, then a maintenance dose of 20 mg daily. Aspirin, NSAIDs, and/or low-dose corticosteroids may be continued during leflunomide therapy. It is available only for oral use. Pregnancy category X.

◆ NURSING PROCESS

◆ ASSESSMENT

Before administering any of the antiinflammatory, antirheumatoid, and related drugs, it is critical to patient safety and drug effectiveness to assess for drug allergies, contraindications, cautions, and drug interactions associated with each drug within each of these major groups of drugs. This specific information has been discussed previously in the pharmacology section of this chapter as well as in various tables and drug profiles. Each of the major drug categories are presented in this nursing process section, with attention to specific drugs as deemed appropriate. A thorough head-to-toe physical assessment, vital signs, assessment, and a thorough medication history with noting of prescription, over-the-counter, and herbal/alternative drugs that the patient is taking. Laboratory tests reflecting hematologic, renal, and hepatic functioning should be analyzed, including RBCs; Hgb, Hct, WBCs, platelets, BUN, and liver enzymes, before NSAIDs, antigout, DMARDs, and other drugs in these categories are used. In addition, laboratory studies that assess the status inflammatory-type diseases may be ordered, with attention to rheumatoid factors, sedimentation rate values, and immunoglobulin levels.

With aspirin, NSAIDs, and other drugs in this chapter, it is important for the nurse to assess the duration, onset, location, and type of inflammation and/or pain the patient is experiencing with documentation of precipitating/exacerbating and relieving factors as well as interference with activities of daily living (ADLs). Inspection of all joints with attention to deformities, immobility, or limitations in mobility, overlying skin condition, and any heat or swelling over the joint should be noted. Age is important to assess as well because drugs, such as celecoxib and aspirin, are not to be used in children and teenagers due to the increased risk for Reye's syndrome. Assessing the odor of aspirin is also important because a vinegary smell is associated with a chemical breakdown of the drug. With aspirin, there is also the importance of assessing for a history of asthma, wheezing, or other respiratory problems because of increased incidence of allergic reactions to aspirin in these individuals. With aspirin, it is also important to assess for patients who have been diagnosed with "aspirin triad," which includes asthma, nasal polyps, and rhinitis because of the risk for reactions to aspirin. Other contraindications, cautions, and drug interactions have been previously discussed for aspirin and NSAIDs. It is still very important to remember that salicylic acid/aspirin and NSAIDs have antiinflammatory, antipyretic, analgesic, and antiplatelet activity as well as risk for ulcerogenic and bleeding tendencies. NSAIDs require close assessment not only for gastrointestinal upset but also for any pre-existing peripheral edema. Baseline CBC, blood chemistries with electrolytes, BUN, creatinine, liver function tests and bleeding/clotting times should also be noted prior to initiation of drug therapy. Ketorolac requires assessment of the "drug" order as well because it is important to be sure that the order is for a short-term (e.g., no more than 5 days) and ordered for patients experiencing severe acute pain. Assessment of underlying signs of infection should be done prior to use of indomethacin because it may mask them with its use.

With *antigout* drugs, it is necessary to obtain a history of gastrointestinal distress, ulcers, and cardiac/renal/liver disease as well as an assessment of baseline hydration status. Serum uric acid levels are generally done prior to therapy for baseline comparisons, as ordered. Urinary output should also be closely assessed prior to and during the drug therapy to ensure at least 30 to 60 mL/hour output. BUN, serum creatinine, alkaline phosphatase (ALP), aspartate aminotransferase (AST), alanine aminotransferase (ALT), and lactate dehydrogenase (LDH) are some of the more common blood tests done prior to therapy for baseline comparisons. Also worthy of mentioning with *antigout drugs* (e.g., allopurinol, colchicine, probenicid) is that these drugs are indicated for either acute, chronic, or both actions. For example, it is important to assess the presence of an acute versus chronic gout because use of colchicine is initiated only after an acute attack has subsided. Therefore, it is important to assess the order and indication of the antigout drug so that the patient is receiving the appropriate treatment. Contraindications, cautions, and drug interactions for *DMARDs* have been previously discussed. Administration of *auranofin* (29% gold) and *gold products* require assessment for pregnancy status prior to beginning therapy as well as results of CBC, BUN, Hct, Hgb, platelets, serum alkaline phosphatase, creatinine, AST, and ALT tests. After injections of gold products, it is common practice to continue to assess the patient for possible hypersensitivity/allergic reactions with the first and/or second injection. This reaction would most commonly occur within 10 to 15 minutes after the injection of the gold.

◆ NURSING DIAGNOSES

- Acute pain related to disease process or injury to joints and injury/disease-affected areas
- Activity intolerance related to the disorder, condition, or disease process causing the pain
- Risk for injury to self related to the influence of the disease and even its treatment on mobility and performance of ADLs
- Ineffective health maintenance related to lack of knowledge about pharmacologic and nonpharmacologic measures of treatment
- Deficient knowledge related to first-time drug therapy for treatment of a disease process

◆ PLANNING
Goals

- Patient is able to describe the use of the medication as it relates to the relief of inflammation and pain.
- Patient experiences pain relief or relief of symptoms within expected period or timeframe.
- Patient uses nonpharmacologic measures to enhance drug therapy in order to decrease inflammation so that he or she can increase ADLs, including walking.
- Patient reports adverse effects to the physician as indicated.
- Patient remains compliant with medication therapy.

Outcome Criteria

- Patient states that pain and changes in joints and mobility are characteristic of inflammation, injury, or related disease processes and will decrease with an effective therapy.
- Patient identifies factors that aggravate or alleviate pain, such as movement, activity, exercising, change in weather/atmosphere, etc.
- Patient states nonpharmacologic measures to use to promote comfort, increase joint function/mobility, and ADLs (e.g., biofeedback, imagery, massage, hot or cold packs, physical therapy, and relaxation therapy).
- Patient states adverse effects associated with the specific group of drugs.
- Patient discusses symptoms to report to the physician immediately.
- Patient states the importance of correct dosing and of consistency in the self-administration of medication.
- Patient returns for follow-up visits with the physician and states the importance of returning for monitoring success of treatment and/or for side/toxic effects.

◆ IMPLEMENTATION

If aspirin is used oral dosage forms should be given with food, milk, or meals. Sustained-released or enteric coated tablets should not be crushed or broken. Aspirin rectal suppositories should be refrigerated prior to use. Serum levels of aspirin should be monitored if aspirin therapy is used for its antiarthritic effect. Serum aspirin levels are also important to monitor for determining mild versus moderate to severe toxicity. Although aspirin therapy is not generally recommended or used because of its toxicity, it is important to remain current about its possible use. More information about it is discussed in the pharmacology section. It is important to be alert to signs of toxicity such as bleeding, gastric ulcers, and gastric bleeding and report to the physician for immediate treatment. If used as an antipyretic, the patient's temperature should begin to decrease within 1 hour. For more information, see the Patient Teaching Tips.

Lifespan Considerations: The Pediatric Patient
Reye's Syndrome

Reye's syndrome is associated with the administration of aspirin in children and teenagers and is a potentially life-threatening illness. Encephalopathy and liver damage are a few of the serious complications resulting from Reye's syndrome that usually occurs after a viral infection, such as chickenpox or influenza B, during which time aspirin is often given for fever. To reduce the risk for Reye's syndrome, aspirin or medications that contain aspirin should not be given to children or teenagers to treat viral illnesses or fever. Other names for aspirin include acetylsalicylic acid, acetylsalicylate, salicylic acid, and salicylate. Other drugs that can be used include acetaminophen and/or ibuprofen to reduce fever and relieve pain. Check the label on any medication you are going to give your child, because aspirin may be in many over-the-counter drugs, for example, Alka-Seltzer, some Excedrin products, and Pepto-Bismol.

Signs and Symptoms
- Altered liver function
- Causes encephalopathy and fatty degeneration of the viscera, primarily in children and teenagers
- Changes in level of consciousness
- Coma, flaccid paralysis, loss of deep tendon reflexes
- Hypoglycemia
- Linked with the use of salicylates and often occurs after a viral illness
- Seizures
- Vomiting

Medical Management
- Supportive treatment in ICU
- Maintain life functions, regain metabolic balance, and control cerebral edema
- Intravenous glucose (10% or higher) for treatment of hypoglycemia
- Monitor blood sugars; insulin may be needed
- Vitamin K for clotting problems
- Fresh-frozen plasma may be needed if there is significant bleeding
- Prophylactic AEDs
- Monitor ICP
- Cautious fluid administration
- Osmotic diuretics may be needed with steroids for cerebral edema

Nursing Management
- Critical care setting often indicated
- Assess neurologic status, vital signs, and arterial and central venous pressures
- Monitor blood gases and ICP as ordered
- Control temperature to prevent elevations and increased O_2 demands
- Elevate HOB
- I&O
- Hyperventilation may be needed with intubation to reduce ICP by lowering CO_2 levels and increasing O_2 levels
- Quiet environment
- Handle gently
- Monitor for seizure activity
- Family support
- Physical and emotional support for child and family with recovery
- Spiritual care
- Educate the public about Reye's syndrome and the life-threatening complications.

Modified from Mayo Foundation for Medical Education and Research (MFMER), November 17, 2005, #DS00142.

AED, Antiepileptic drug; *HOB,* head of bed; *ICP,* intracranial pressure; *ICU,* intensive care unit; *I&O,* intake and output.

NSAIDs may come in enteric coated/sustained-release preparations and should not be crushed or chewed. These drugs in oral dosage forms—including ketorolac—may be taken with antacids or food to decrease gastrointestinal upset or irritation. Moderate-to-severe gastrointestinal upset, dyspepsia with nausea, vomiting, abdominal pain, and blood in the stool or emesis should be reported to the physician immediately. Other ulcerogenic substances (e.g., alcohol, prednisone, aspirin-containing products, other NSAIDs) should be avoided to help minimize risk for gastrointestinal mucosal breakdown. During therapy with NSAIDs, bowel patterns, stool consistency, and the occurrence of dizziness should be constantly monitored and documented as well as monitoring of CBC and BUN levels, platelet, bilirubin, serum alkaline phosphatase, and AST and ALT levels. Additionally, with indomethacin, suppository use should be administered with instructions similar to those for aspirin suppositories (see earlier). Other dosage forms include powder for IV injection and oral liquid/suspension. IV dosages should be clear and administered as per manufacturer guidelines for dilutional solutions/infusion rates or over 5 to 10 seconds. Safe ambulation should always be emphasized with NSAIDs. With ketorolac, it is important to understand that dosing should "not" exceed a 5-day time period with either the oral, IM (deep IM and slowly injected into a large muscle mass), or IV (infused over at least 15 seconds) dosage forms. Cyclooxygenase (COX-2) inhibitors should be given/taken only as ordered with the same concern for avoiding alcohol, aspirin, other NSAIDs, and over-the-counter drugs containing these drugs (e.g., NSAIDs, aspirin, salicylates). Any stomach or abdominal pain, gastrointestinal problems, unusual bleeding, blood in the stool or emesis, chest pain, and/or palpitations should be reported immediately to the physician.

The antigout drugs are somewhat different from the NSAIDs and have some different types of nursing considerations. Colchicine should be taken on an empty stomach for more complete absorption, which means 1 hour before meals or 2 hours after meals. Intravenous colchicine should be administered as recommended per the guidelines and over the recommended time frame. Increase the patient's fluid intake unless contraindicated up to 2 to 3 L/24 hours. Alcohol and any over-the-counter cold-relief products that contain alcohol should be avoided while taking this medication. In addition, patients with gout must be instructed that compliance with the entire medical regimen is critical to successful treatment. Allopurinol should be given with meals to try to prevent the occurrence of gastrointestinal symptoms (nausea, vomiting, anorexia). If the allopurinol is being administered in conjunction with chemotherapy (in an attempt to decrease hyperuricemia associated with the malignancy and cell death from successful treatment), it is recommended that it be given a few days before the antineoplastic therapy. Patients taking allopurinol should be informed to increase fluid intake to 3 L/day, avoid hazardous activities if dizziness or drowsiness occurs with the medication, avoid the use of alcohol and caffeine because these drugs will increase uric acid levels, and decrease the levels of allopurinol.

DMARDs, specifically gold sodium thiomalate, should never be given intravenously and when given intramuscularly, it should be given into deep muscle. It is important for the patient to remain recumbent for at least 10 minutes after the injection, and, in addition, special precautions should be taken for the patient with bleeding disorders or thrombocytopenia. Perform daily checks of the patient's skin for pruritis, purpura, rash, and/or ecchymoses as well as examinations of the oral mucosa, palate, pharynx, and borders of the tongue for any ulcerations. Be attentive to any complaints of a metallic taste in the mouth as this may indicate stomatitis. With any drugs used for rheumatoid arthritis, the patient should be constantly watched and questioned about improved mobility, increased grip strength and joint flexibility, and a decrease in joint pain/stiffness/swelling. Fluids should be forced, as ordered, and only if not contraindicated. Leflunomide may be given with meals or food to minimize gastrointestinal upset should it occur. See the Patient Teaching Tips for more information on these drugs.

◆ EVALUATION

Aspirin and NSAIDs may vary in their potency and antiinflammatory and analgesic effects. Therapeutic responses to NSAIDs include the following: decrease in acute pain; decrease in swelling, pain, stiffness/ tenderness of a joint or muscle area, improved ability to conduct ADLs, improved muscle grip/strength, reduction in fever, return to normal of laboratory values (CBC, RBC, Hgb level, Hct, and sedimentation rates); and return to a less inflamed state as evidenced by improved sedimentation rates, X-ray examination, computed tomography (CT) scan, or magnetic resonance imaging (MRI). COX-II inhibitors should also result in improved joint function and fewer inflammation-based signs and symptoms. Patients should begin to show improvement in ADLs and mobility with any of these drugs but within the time frame, which may be up to 2 to 3 months, depending on the drug. Monitoring for the occurrence of adverse effects and toxicity is essential to the safe and effective use of aspirin, NSAIDs, antigout drugs, and COX-II inhibitors (see Table 44-2).

Evaluating therapeutic responses to all other antiarthritics/DMARDs includes monitoring for the increased ability to move joints with less discomfort and an overall increased sense of improvement in the condition. Toxicity to gold products is evident by a decreased Hgb level, a white blood cell (WBC) count of less than 4000/mm^3, platelets less than 150,000/mm^3, hematuria, severe diarrhea, itching, and proteinuria. Toxicity to DMARDs is evident by an elevation of ALT level (if more than 2 but less than or equal to 3 a liver biopsy may be needed). A therapeutic response to antigout drugs (e.g., colchicines) includes decreased pain in affected joints and increased sense of well-being. The patient should be monitored closely for or should report to the physician the occurrence of increased pain, blood in the urine, excessive fatigue and lethargy, and chills or fever. A therapeutic response to allopurinol, another antigout drug, includes a decrease in pain in the joints, a decrease in uric acid levels, and a decrease of stone formation in the kidneys.

Patient Teaching Tips

- Educate patients to not crush or chew any sustained-release or enteric-coated aspirin and to report ringing in the ears or any persistent gastrointestinal or abdominal pain and any easy bruising or bleeding. Make sure a patient knows that the antiinflammatory effect of the drug may take up to 1 to 3 weeks.
- Educate patients that they need to inform other health care professionals and dentists that they are taking aspirin or NSAIDs prior to any treatment, specifically if they are taking high doses of aspirin or have been taking aspirin for prolonged periods. Aspirin and NSAIDs should also be discontinued, as per physician's orders, 3 to 7 days prior to surgery, including oral/dental surgery.
- Aspirin and other drugs should be kept out of the reach of children, but if a child (or adult) has consumed large or unknown quantities of aspirin or NSAIDs, the poison control center should be contacted immediately and/or emergency medical attention sought out immediately. Children and teenagers should not be taking aspirin due to the risk of Reye's syndrome. Acetaminophen is usually preferred in the recommended dosage range.
- Educate patients about adverse effects of aspirin such as gastrointestinal upset, flushing of the face, dizziness, tinnitus, drowsiness, visual changes, seizures, gastrointestinal bleeding, heartburn, and any bleeding tendencies or easy bruising. Any black/tarry stools, bleeding around the gums, petechiae (very small red-brown spots), ecchymosis (easy bruising), and purpura (large red spots) should be reported to the physician immediately.
- Patients should understand that NSAIDs are used for the treatment of pain, injuries, or inflammatory disease-related process and work by decreasing the inflammation that leads to pain.

- Educate about the most common adverse effects of the NSAIDs, which include the following: heartburn, gastrointestinal upset, ulcers, nausea, vomiting, hemorrhage, hemolytic anemias, epistaxis, blurred vision, rash, leukopenia, blurred vision, vertigo, and tinnitus. Also educate patients to take NSAIDs with food, milk, or antacids to help minimize gastrointestinal distress. Include education about the many drug interactions with NSAIDs, including anticoagulants, aspirin, steroids, corticosteroids, salicylates, oral antidiabetic drugs, insulin, penicillin, sulfonamides, and barbiturates. In addition, it is important to educate about the difference between the onset of action of the medication for the relief of acute pain as opposed to its more delayed effect when used for the relief of arthritis pain; in the latter case, the therapeutic effects may not be realized for 3 to 4 weeks. In addition, NSAIDs (as well as salicylates and other drugs) come in enteric-coated dosage forms and should not be crushed or chewed.
- With gold injections, be sure to encourage patients to report any adverse effects such as headache, local pain at the injection site, lethargy, and joint pain. Gold sodium thiomalate is usually given once weekly, as ordered.
- Inform the patient that it may take 3 to 6 months for the full therapeutic response to DMARDs.
- Educate patients about the adverse effects of gold products, such as pruritic dermatitis, stomatitis, ulcers of the oral mucus membranes, sore throat, diarrhea, and abdominal pain; if these occur, they should be reported to the physician.

Points to Remember

- NSAIDs are one of the most commonly prescribed categories of drugs.
- The first drug in this category to be synthesized was salicylic acid or aspirin. Aspirin is often identified and included within discussion of antiinflammatory drugs. NSAIDs have analgesic, antiinflammatory, antipyretic activity; aspirin also has antiplatelet activity. NSAIDs are often used in the treatment of gout, osteoarthritis, juvenile arthritis, rheumatoid arthritis, dysmenorrhea, and musculoskeletal injuries such as strains and sprains.
- The three main adverse effects of NSAIDs are gastrointestinal intolerance, bleeding (often gastrointestinal bleeding), and renal impairment. Misoprostol (Cytotec) may be given to prevent gastrointestinal intolerance and ulcers resulting from NSAIDs. It is classified as a PG (prostaglandin) analog. There are also many contraindications to the use of NSAIDs, such as gastrointestinal tract lesions, peptic ulcers and bleeding disorders.
- Most NSAIDs are better tolerated orally if taken with food to minimize gastrointestinal upset.

- Patients on NSAIDs should be closely monitored for the occurrence of bleeding, such as blood in the stools or emesis. When NSAIDs are used to decrease inflammation in the joints of arthritis patients, therapeutic effects usually take up to 3 to 4 weeks.
- Antigout drugs are indicated for either acute or chronic/prophylactic gout. Diarrhea and abdominal pain are common adverse effects. Antigout drugs are often used in patients with cell death during cancer chemotherapy to avoid gout-like syndromes and pain.
- DMARDs alter or modify the disease process of rheumatoid arthritis but are not curative. It may take up to 3 to 6 months for the full therapeutic effects, depending on the specific drug used. Because a stepped approach to treating rheumatoid arthritis is no longer emphasized, it is important to emphasize the individualization of each treatment protocol for patients with this disease. DMARDs include aranofin, gold sodium thiomalate, leflunomide, and sulfasalazine.

NCLEX Examination Review Questions

1. When a patient is receiving long-term NSAID therapy, which drug may be given to prevent the serious gastrointestinal adverse effects of NSAIDs?
   a. misoprostol (Cytotec)
   b. metoprolol (Lopressor)
   c. metoclopramide (Reglan)
   d. magnesium sulfate (MgSO$_4$)
2. The nurse recognizes that manifestations of NSAID toxicity would include:
   a. Constipation
   b. Nausea and vomiting
   c. Tremors
   d. Urinary retention
3. During a teaching session about antigout drugs, the nurse would tell the patient that antigout drugs work by which mechanism?
   a. Increasing blood oxygen levels
   b. Decreasing leukocytes and platelets
   c. Increasing protein and rheumatoid factors
   d. Decreasing serum uric acid levels
4. When teaching about antigout drugs, which statement by the nurse is accurate?
   a. "Drink only limited amounts of fluids with the drug."
   b. "This drug may cause limited movements of your joints."
   c. "There are very few drug interactions with these medications."
   d. "Colchicine is best taken on an empty stomach."
5. A mother calls the clinic to ask about what medication to give her 5-year-old child for a fever during a bout of chicken pox. The nurse's best response would be:
   a. "Since your child is 5 years old, it would be okay to use children's aspirin to treat his fever.
   b. "Start with acetaminophen or ibuprofen, but if those do not work, then you can try aspirin"
   c. "You can use children's dosages of acetaminophen or ibuprofen, but aspirin is not recommended."
   d. "It is best to wait to let the fever break on its own without medication."

1. a, 2. b, 3. d, 4. d, 5. c.

Critical Thinking Activities

1. Is the following statement true or false? Acetaminophen is an NSAID and exerts antiinflammatory, antipyretic, analgesic, and antiplatelet effects. Explain your answer.
2. What are the drug interactions for NSAIDs? What problems may occur if these drugs are used with NSAIDs?
3. Describe the protocol for treating salicylate intoxication of a chronic nature.

For answers, see http://evolve.elsevier.com/Lilley.

Immune and Biologic Modifiers and Chemotherapeutic Drugs

STUDY SKILLS TIPS

- *Time Management*
- *Evaluate Prior Performance*
- *Anticipate the Test*
- *Plan for Distributed Study*

TIME MANAGEMENT

The first step in preparing for a chapter or part exam is to plan for the time needed. Let us begin by assuming that the next test you have will cover the chapters in Part Eight. First examine the material to determine just how much there is to cover. Look at the objectives, the glossary, and the number of pages of text in each chapter. This will help you determine just how big a task you face. As you are doing this, also consider how much study time you have been devoting to these chapters in the days before the exam. If you have been doing regular study with frequent review sessions, then the demand on your time in the day or two just before the exam will be less than if you have to do a major "cram" session to try to catch up on study that has been put off. The basic question to answer here is a simple one. "How much time do I need to schedule for exam preparation?" The answer varies with each student. Some will need 6, 8, or more hours of preparation time in the 2 to 3 days before the exam. Others will find that 3, 4, or 5 hours will be adequate. You must assess your own learning and prior success to determine what time is necessary for you, but you must set time aside and use it effectively.

There is one thing that should play a major role in helping you determine the time you will need to set aside. Evaluate your performance on prior exams. How have you been doing? How much time have you been spending to achieve that level?

If you are not achieving according to your capabilities, then you should certainly consider spending more time preparing for the next exam. If you are achieving at a satisfactory level, then plan on devoting about the same amount of time to test preparation.

The next step in preparing for an exam is to organize the time. Write down what you are going to study and when, as well as how much time you will spend. Consider the following example based on the materials in Chapters 47 and 49:

1. Review Chapter 47 objectives. Monday, 4:00 to 4:30 PM. Note objectives that are unclear for further review.
2. Question and Answer review, Monday, 4:30 to 5:15 PM.
3. Self-test, Chapter 47 glossary. Monday, 6:30 to 7:00 PM. Note terms that need further review for mastery.
4. Review Chapter 49 objectives. Monday, 7:00 to 7:30 PM.
5. Question and Answer review, Monday, 7:30 to 8:00 PM.
6. Self-test, Chapter 49 glossary. Monday, 8:00 to 8:30 PM.

The advantage to this test preparation model is that you now know where you must focus in the days before the exam.

EVALUATE PRIOR PERFORMANCE

As you begin preparing to review for any exam, take some time to look back at previous exams. Evaluate your performance, and use that evaluation to improve on subsequent tests. As you look at prior tests, consider the following factors.

691

What Type of Errors Did I Make?

As students we often find that there are certain question types or forms that are missed consistently. Assess your errors and try to pinpoint any recurring patterns in your mistakes. Did you miss questions that contained an exemption in the multiple-choice stem? Question stems that state "All of the following except" and "Which of the following would not be..." are exemption questions. Questions like 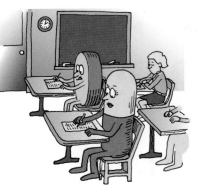 this are often missed because they contain too many apparently correct responses. Remember that an exemption stem means you are looking for the one response choice that is "wrong." The stem asks you to identify the inappropriate response, and it is the best choice.

Did I Have Trouble with Questions That Required Mastery of Terminology?

As part of the evaluation of prior tests, also look at questions that demanded mastery of the terms from the chapters. If you missed more than one or two questions of that type, then you know you need to spend more time in review of terminology.

Did I Miss Concept Questions?

If the question asked you to apply a principle, evaluate a drug response, or in some other way apply knowledge from the course, you are dealing with concepts rather than facts. If you missed a number of concept questions, then you should spend more of your review time studying applications and principles than memorizing facts and terms. Working with a study group may help to improve your response to concept questions.

Did I Make Errors Because I Did not Know the Material?

This question focuses on the quality of your learning. If you miss one or two questions on an exam because you did not learn (or did not remember) the material, it is not a major problem. There will almost always be one or two questions that we do not remember. If you are analyzing past performance and find that there are several questions on which you guessed because you did not recall any information that seemed relevant to the question, it may be necessary to put more time into review. This may involve doing more oral rehearsal so that the material is stored in long-term memory. Whatever the cause it is essential that you acknowledge to yourself that you have missed questions because you did not know the material. Once you have acknowledged the problem, take steps to correct it.

ANTICIPATE THE TEST

Do not wait until exam time to find out what you should know. As you do your review, try to think like the instructor. Generate questions that you think might be a part of the test. This does not mean you need to try to write multiple-choice stems and choices, but you should be trying to focus your review in a way that will facilitate learning and long-term memory. The process of working with a study group to anticipate test questions and to quiz each other can help move concepts from short-term memory to long-term memory.

Here are some examples of questioning that you might use based on material found in Chapter 49.
1. What are biologic response modifiers (BRMs)?
2. What is the role of BRMs in the care of patients with cancer?
3. What is the role of the immune system in treating cancer?

These sample questions were drawn from just the first few pages of the chapter. These questions focus on literal comprehension and are relatively easy to generate. Being able to answer them is important, but if all of your questions are literal in nature, it may be difficult to answer questions that require application of principles and concepts. For that reason, it is essential that some questions require analysis, synthesis, and/or evaluation of the material. A study group is helpful in creating this more compli- 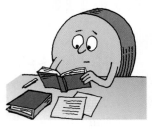 cated type of question. The process of discussion can generate ideas you may not develop on your own. Question 3 is an example of this type of question. Answers to these questions require the learner to put together the literal information and relate the terms to the concepts being explained.

PLAN FOR DISTRIBUTED STUDY

One of the major problems that many students encounter when trying to review for a test is waiting too long to begin the review, which forces students into a review pattern of long hours of intensive study all packed into the last day or two before the exam. This is known as "cramming," and although cramming does work to some degree, it is not the most effective way to learn. A better model is to distribute the review over a period of several days with short, 30-minute to 1-hour study sessions several times each day. Distributing practice in this way allows time for you to think about what you have been learning, and it fosters long-term memory. Studying with a group adds variety to your study time and provides another method of receiving and processing information.

One important consideration is spending more of the review time doing oral rehearsal ("ask and answer" sessions) and not simply rereading material. Oral rehearsal encourages active learning, which enhances your ability to concentrate, improves comprehension and memory, and thus improves test performance. Oral rehearsals work well in study groups, but if you are satisfied with the tests results you get by reviewing alone, keep doing what works for you.

Immunosuppressant Drugs

Objectives

When you reach the end of this chapter, you should be able to do the following:

1. Discuss the role of immunosuppressive therapy in organ transplant recipients and in the treatment of autoimmune diseases.
2. Discuss the mechanisms of action, contraindications, cautions, adverse effects, routes of administration, drug interactions, and toxicity associated with the most commonly used immunosuppressants.
3. Develop a nursing care plan that includes all phases of the nursing process for the patient receiving immunosuppressants for either an organ transplant or for the treatment of autoimmune diseases.

e-Learning Activities

Companion CD

- NCLEX Review Questions: see questions 380-385
- Animations
- Audio Glossary
- Category Catchers
- Medication Errors Checklists
- IV Therapy Checklists

evolve Website (http://evolve.elsevier.com/Lilley)

• Nursing Care Plans • Frequently Asked Questions • Content Updates • WebLinks • Supplemental Resources • Elsevier ePharmacology Update • Medication Administration Animations

Drug Profiles

▶ azathioprine and mycophenolate mofetil, p. 696
basiliximab and daclizumab, p. 697

▶ cyclosporine, p. 697
glatiramer acetate, p. 697
▶ muromonab-CD3, p. 697
sirolimus and tacrolimus, p. 697

▶ Key drug.

Glossary

Autoimmune diseases A large group of diseases characterized by the subversion or alteration of the function of the immune system wherein the immune response is directed against normal tissue(s) of the body, resulting in pathologic conditions. (p. 693)

Graft The term used for a transplanted tissue or organ. (p. 693)

Immune-mediated diseases A large group of diseases that result when the cells of the immune system react to a variety of situations, such as transplanted organ tissue or drug-altered cells. (p. 693)

Immunosuppressant A drug that decreases or prevents an immune response. (p. 693)

Immunosuppressive therapy A drug treatment used to suppress the immune system. (p. 693)

Murine antibodies Monoclonal immunoglobulins. Monoclonal refers to a protein from a single clone of cells; all molecules of the protein are identical. Murine refers to the family Muridae, to which mice belong. An antibody is a protective protein that counters the actions of antigens, substances that cause sensitivity, or an allergic response. Thus, murine antibodies are protective proteins obtained from mice. Muromonab-CD3 is a murine antibody used to reverse graft rejection. (p. 697)

IMMUNOSUPPRESSANT DRUGS

The human body is under constant attack by invading microorganisms, but it possesses several mechanisms with which to fight off these foreign invaders; one is the *immune system.* This system defends the body against invading pathogens, foreign antigens, and its own cells that become cancerous, or neoplastic. Besides performing this beneficial function, however, this highly sophisticated system can also sometimes attack itself and cause what are known as **autoimmune diseases** or **immune-mediated diseases.** It also participates in hypersensitivity, or anaphylactic, reactions, which can be life threatening. The rejection of kidney, liver, and heart (whole organ) transplants is directed by the immune system as well. From this it is easy to see that the immune system is capable of having many beneficial and detrimental effects.

Drugs that decrease or prevent an immune response, and hence suppress the immune system, are known as **immunosuppressants.** Treatment with such drugs is referred to as **immunosuppressive therapy,** and it is used to selectively eradicate certain cell lines that play a major role in the rejection of a transplanted organ. These cell lines must be targeted and selectively altered or suppressed, or organ rejection will occur. The primary immunosuppressant drugs are the corticosteroids (Chapter 32), cyclophosphamide (Chapter 47), azathioprine, cyclosporine, muromonab-CD3, tacrolimus, glatiramer acetate, daclizumab, basiliximab, and sirolimus.

Mechanism of Action and Drug Effects

All immunosuppressants have similar mechanisms of action because they all selectively suppress certain T-lymphocyte cell lines, thereby preventing their involvement in the immune response. This results in a pharmacologically immunocompromised state similar to that in a cancer patient whose bone marrow and immune cells have been destroyed as the result of chemotherapy or that in a patient with AIDS, whose immune cells have been destroyed by HIV. Each drug differs in the exact way in which it suppresses certain cell lines involved in an immune response. See Table 45-1 for pharmacologic classifications, mechanisms of action, and indications of the immunosuppressant drugs.

Indications

The therapeutic uses of immunosuppressants are multiple and vary from drug to drug, as illustrated in Table 45-1. They are primarily indicated for the prevention of organ rejection, which is the focus of this chapter. However, some are also used for other immunologic illnesses, such as rheumatoid arthritis and multiple sclerosis. Only muromonab-CD3 is indicated for treatment of organ rejection once rejection of a transplanted organ is underway. The four newer drugs (basiliximab, daclizumab, sirolimus, and mycophenolate mofetil), all immunosuppressants used in transplant patients, are indicated for organ rejection prophylaxis. Azathioprine is used as an adjunct medication to prevent the rejection of kidney transplants and to ameliorate severe rheumatoid arthritis. Cyclosporine is the primary immunosuppressant drug used in the prevention of kidney, liver, heart, and bone marrow transplant rejection. It may also have beneficial effects in the treatment of other conditions with an immunologic cause, such as certain types of arthritis, psoriasis, and irritable bowel disease.

Tacrolimus has many of the same therapeutic effects as cyclosporine but is currently indicated only for the prevention of liver

---

Table 45-1   Classification, Mechanisms of Action, and Indications for Available Immunosuppressant Drugs

Drug Name, Year of FDA Approval	Pharmacologic Class and Mechanism of Action	Indications
azathioprine (Imuran), 1980	Blocks metabolism of purines, inhibiting the synthesis of T-cell DNA, RNA, and proteins, thereby blocking immune response.	Organ rejection prevention in kidney transplantation; rheumatoid arthritis.
muromonab-CD3* (Orthoclone OKT3), 1986	Binds to CD3 glycoprotein on T-cell receptors, which blocks antigen recognition and reverses graft rejection that is already in progress.	Treatment of acute organ rejection in kidney, liver, and heart transplantation.
cyclosporine (Cyclosporin A, Sandimmune, Neoral), 1983	Inhibits activation of T-cells by blocking the production and release of the cytokine mediator IL-2.	Organ rejection prevention in kidney, liver, and heart transplantation; rheumatoid arthritis; psoriasis. Unlabeled uses† include pancreas, bone marrow, and heart/lung transplantation.
glatiramer acetate (Copaxone), 1996	Precise mechanism unknown. Believed to somehow modify immune system processes that are associated with MS symptoms.	Reduction of relapse frequency in patients with RRMS.
tacrolimus (Prograf, FK-506), 1994	Inhibits T-cell activation, possibly by binding to an intracellular protein known as FKBP-12.	Organ rejection prevention in liver transplantation. Unlabeled uses† include kidney, bone marrow, heart, pancreas, pancreatic islet cell, and small intestine transplantation; autoimmune diseases; and severe psoriasis.
mycophenolate mofetil (CellCept), 1995	Prevents proliferation of T cells by inhibiting intracellular purine synthesis.	Organ rejection prevention in kidney, liver, and heart transplantation.
daclizumab* (Zenapax), 1997	Suppresses T-cell activity by blocking the binding of the cytokine receptor IL-2 to a specific receptor.	Organ rejection prevention in kidney transplantation.
basiliximab* (Simulect), 1998	Suppresses T-cell activity by blocking the binding of the cytokine mediator IL-2 to a specific receptor.	Organ rejection prevention in kidney transplantation.
sirolimus (Rapamune), 1999	Inhibits T-cell activation by a unique mechanism: binding to an intracellular protein known as FKBP-12, creating a complex that subsequently binds to a cellular component known as the mTOR, which prevents cellular proliferation.	Organ rejection prevention in kidney transplantation.

*Note that "ab" in any drug name usually indicates that it is a monoclonal antibody synthesized using recombinant DNA technology.
†Non-FDA approved but under investigation.
DNA, Deoxyribonucleic acid; *RNA,* ribonucleic acid; *FDA,* Food and Drug Administration; *IL-2,* interleukin-2; *MS,* multiple sclerosis; *mTOR,* mammalian target of rapamycin; *RRMS,* relapsing-remitting multiple sclerosis.

transplant rejection, although it has shown promise in preventing the rejection of other transplanted organs as well.

Glatiramer acetate is the only immunosuppressant currently indicated for treatment of multiple sclerosis (MS). Specifically, it is indicated for reduction of the frequency of MS relapses (exacerbations) in a type of MS known as *relapsing-remitting multiple sclerosis* (RRMS). This is currently its sole indication.

Contraindications

The main contraindication for all immunosuppressants is known drug allergy. Relative contraindications, depending on the patient's condition, may include renal or hepatic failure, hypertension, and concurrent radiation therapy. Pregnancy is not necessarily a contraindication to these drugs, but use of immunosuppressants in pregnant women should only occur in clinically urgent situations.

Adverse Effects

Many of the adverse effects of the immunosuppressants can be devastating, especially to a transplant patient. Although not strictly an adverse effect, a heightened susceptibility to opportunistic infections is a major risk factor in immunosuppressed pa-

tients. Other adverse effects are limited to the particular drugs, and some of the most common of these are listed in Table 45-2.

Interactions

Cyclosporine, tacrolimus, and sirolimus are capable of many drug interactions, several of which can be very harmful. Drugs that may overenhance their actions are diltiazem, nicardipine, verapamil, fluconazole, itraconazole, clarithromycin, allopurinol, metoclopramide, amphotericin B, cimetidine, and ketoconazole. Grapefruit, including its juice, because of its inhibition of key metabolizing enzymes, can also have a similar effect on these three immunosuppressants. Patients who eat grapefruit or drink grapefruit juice need not avoid it entirely, but are advised to maintain a relatively regular use of this fruit. They are also advised to notify their health provider if their grapefruit consumption levels change as this may require either an increase or decrease in immunosuppressant dosage. Drug levels should be monitored as needed until stabilized. Drugs that may reduce the effects of these immunosuppressants include nafcillin, carbamazepine, phenobarbital, phenytoin, and rifampin. The mechanism for these drug interactions centers largely on the fact that some of the same cytochrome P450 metabolizing enzymes are shared among these drugs and the immunosuppressant drugs. Although these are the most significant interactions, there are many more of less significance. Cyclosporine can have a rather profound interaction with grapefruit juice. When they are taken together, there is an increase in the bioavailability of cyclosporine by 20% to 200%. The intentional administration of cyclosporine with grapefruit juice may sometimes be done to achieve therapeutic blood levels of cyclosporine with decreased doses. The manufacturer of cyclosporine does not endorse this.

It is also not recommended that azathioprine be given with allopurinol because allopurinol inhibits azathioprine's metabolism and thereby increases its effects. The coadministration of angiotensin-converting enzyme (ACE) inhibitors with azathioprine may result in severe leukopenia, whereas azathioprine may reduce the effectiveness of anticoagulants (e.g., warfarin). Azathioprine may also reduce the serum levels of cyclosporine, which may require an increase in dosage of desired immunosuppressant effects. Mycophenolate absorption may be reduced by antacids, iron preparations, and cholestyramine resins. Mycophenolate may also reduce the protein binding of both theophylline and phenytoin, increasing their free plasma levels, and it may also reduce the efficacy of oral contraceptives as well as live virus vaccines.

Because the antibodies basiliximab, daclizumab, and muromonab-CD3 are generally given in a relatively short single course of therapy, they have few recognized drug interactions. However, cases of encephalopathy have occurred in which the antiinflammatory drug indomethacin (Chapter 44) was used concurrently with muromonab-CD3.

The potential interactions between immunosuppressant drugs and herbal preparations should also not be overlooked. For example, the enzyme induction properties of St. John's Wort have been demonstrated in case reports to reduce the therapeutic levels of cyclosporine and cause organ rejection. The immunostimulant properties of cat's claw and echinacea may be similarly undesirable in transplant recipients.

Dosages

For the recommended dosages of selected immunosuppressant drugs, see the table on page 696.

Table 45-2	Selected Immunosuppressant Drugs: Common Adverse Effects
Body System	**Adverse Effects**
Azathioprine	
Hematologic	Leukopenia, thrombocytopenia
Hepatic	Hepatotoxicity is a common adverse effect
Cyclosporine	
Cardiovascular	Moderate hypertension in as many as 50% of patients
Central nervous	Neurotoxicity including tremors in about 20% of patients
Hepatic	Hepatotoxicity with cholestasis and hyperbilirubinemia
Renal	Nephrotoxicity is common and dose limiting
Other	Hypersensitivity reactions to the vehicle, gingival hyperplasia, and hirsutism
Muromonab-CD3	
Cardiovascular	Chest pain
Central nervous	Pyrexia, chills, tremors
Gastrointestinal	Vomiting, nausea, diarrhea
Respiratory	Dyspnea, wheezing, pulmonary edema
Other	Flulike symptoms, fluid retention
Tacrolimus	
Central nervous	Agitation, anxiety, confusion, hallucinations, neuropathy
Renal	Albuminuria, dysuria, acute renal failure, renal tubular necrosis
Antibody Immunosuppressants	
(basiliximab, daclizumab, and muromonab-CD3)	*Cytokine release syndrome,* which includes such immune-mediated symptoms as fever, dyspnea, tachycardia, sweating, chills, headache, nausea, vomiting, diarrhea, muscle and joint pain, and general malaise

DOSAGES

Selected Immunosuppressant Drugs

Drug (Pregnancy Category)	Pharmacologic Class	Usual Dosage Range	Indications
▶azathioprine (Imuran) (D)	Purine antagonist	**Adult and pediatric** IV/PO: 2-5 mg/kg/day to start, then 1-3 mg/kg/day maintenance **Adult** PO: 1 mg/kg/day as a single or divided dose for 6-8 wk, then may increase prn by 0.5 mg/kg/day q4wk to a maximum of 2.5 mg/kg/day	Renal transplants Rheumatoid arthritis
basiliximab (Simulect) (B)	Monoclonal antibody	**Pediatric 2-15 yr** <35 kg: IV: 10 mg within 2 hr of transplant surgery, then 4 days afterward **Adult and pediatrics 35 kg or greater** Use 20-mg doses in same regimen	Prevention of rejection of kidney transplants
▶cyclosporine (Sandimmune, Neoral) (C)	Polypeptide antibiotic	**Adult and pediatric** PO: 15 mg/kg as a single dose 4-12 hr preop; continue same dose postop for 1-2 wk, then reduce by 5%/wk to a maintenance dose of 5-10 mg/kg/day IV: 5-6 mg/kg as a single dose 4-16 hr preop and continued daily postop until patient can be switched to PO dosing	Kidney, liver, heart transplants
daclizumab (Zenapax) (C)	Monoclonal antibody	**Adult and pediatric** IV: Bolus injection of 1 mg/kg 24 hr preop and for 4 additional postop doses, spaced 14 days apart	Prevention of rejection of kidney transplants
glatiramer acetate (Copaxone) (B)	Miscellaneous biological	**Adult only** SC: 20 mg once daily	RRMS
▶muromonab-CD3 (Orthoclone OKT3) (C)	Monoclonal antibody	**Adult and pediatric** IV: 2.5-5 mg/day as a single bolus injection for 10-14 days (pediatric patients often started with 2.5 mg/day)	Treatment of active rejection of kidney transplants; treatment of active rejection of liver, heart, pancreas, and bone marrow transplants that are resistant to conventional treatment
▶mycophenolate mofetil (CellCept, Myfortic) (C)	Miscellaneous	**Adult** IV/PO: 1 gm twice daily **Pediatric** IV/PO: 400 mg/m^2 twice daily (maximum daily dose: 1440 mg or 720 mg twice daily)	Prevention of rejection of kidney transplants
sirolimus (Rapamune) (C)	Fungus-derived	**Adult and pediatric** IV/PO: 6 mg loading dose on day 1, followed by maintenance dose of 2 mg/day	Prevention of rejection of kidney transplants
tacrolimus (Prograf) (C)	Fungus-derived	**Adult and pediatric** IV: 0.03-0.05 mg/kg/day as continuous IV infusion; then PO: 0.1-0.2 mg/kg/day divided q12h	Prevention of rejection of liver and kidney transplants

RRMS, Relapsing-remitting multiple sclerosis.

Drug Profiles

As previously stated, the primary use for the immunosuppressant drugs discussed in this chapter is the prevention of organ rejection. Other immunologic disorders, such as rheumatoid arthritis and multiple sclerosis, may also be treated with these drugs. Selected immunosuppressants are described further in the drug profiles that follow.

▶ azathioprine and mycophenolate mofetil

Azathioprine (Imuran) is a chemical analog of the physiologic purines, such as adenine and guanine. It blocks T-cell proliferation by inhibiting purine synthesis, which in turn prevents deoxyribonucleic acid (DNA) synthesis. Mycophenolate mofetil (CellCept) is another immunosuppressant drug that works with a mechanism similar to azathioprine. Both are used for prophylaxis of organ rejection concurrently with other immunosuppressant drugs, such as cyclosporine and corticosteroids. Both drugs are available in both oral and injectable form.

Pharmacokinetics (azathioprine)

Half-Life	Onset	Peak	Duration
PO: 5 hr	PO: 2-4 days*	PO: 1-2 hr	PO: Unknown

*6-8 wk for rheumatoid arthritis.

Pharmacokinetics (mycophenolate mofetil)

Half-Life	Onset	Peak	Duration
PO: 18 hr	PO: Unknown	PO: 0.75-1 hr	PO: Unknown

basiliximab and daclizumab

Basiliximab (Simulect) and daclizumab (Zenapax) are both monoclonal antibodies that work by inhibiting the binding of the cytokine mediator interleukin-2 (IL-2) to what is known as the high-affinity IL-2 receptor. These drugs are used to prevent rejection of transplanted kidneys (**grafts**) and are generally used as part of a multidrug immunosuppressive regimen that includes cyclosporine and corticosteroids. They are both prone to cause the allergic-like reaction known as *cytokine release syndrome,* which can be severe and even involve anaphylaxis. Patients are often premedicated with corticosteroids (e.g., intravenous methylprednisolone) in an effort to avoid or alleviate this problem. Both drugs are available only in injectable form.

Pharmacokinetics (basiliximab)

Half-Life	Onset	Peak	Duration
IV: 7-9 days	IV: 1 day	IV: 3-4 days	IV: Unknown

Pharmacokinetics (daclizumab)

Half-Life	Onset	Peak	Duration
IV: 20 days	IV: <1 day	IV: 3-5 days	IV: Unknown

▶ cyclosporine

Cyclosporine (Sandimmune, Neoral, Gengraf) is an immunosuppressant drug that is indicated for the prevention of organ rejection. It is a very potent immunosuppressant and the principal drug in many immunosuppressive drug regimens. Like azathioprine, it may also be used for the treatment of other immunologic disorders, such as various forms of arthritis, psoriasis, and irritable bowel disease.

Cyclosporine is available in both oral and injectable forms, including three brand names as noted above. Although these three products contain the same active ingredient (cyclosporine), they cannot be used interchangeably. When changing between Neoral or Gengraf to Sandimmune, start with a 1:1 mg amount, but dosage adjustments may be necessary to account for the greater bioavailability of Neoral and Gengraf. It is recommended that cyclosporine blood concentration be monitored in patients changing from one product to another. Cyclosporine has a narrow therapeutic index and for this reason laboratory monitoring of drug levels may be used to ensure therapeutic plasma concentrations and avoid toxicity.

Pharmacokinetics*

Half-Life	Onset	Peak	Duration
PO: 1-2 hr (parent compound), then 10-27 hr (metabolites)	PO: 1-3 hr	PO: Unknown	PO: Unknown

*May vary somewhat between brand names.

glatiramer acetate

Glatiramer acetate (Copaxone) is a mixture of random polymers of four different amino acids. This mixture results in a compound that is antigenically similar to myelin basic protein. This is a protein that is found on the myelin sheath of nerves. The drug is believed to work by blocking T-cell autoimmune activity against this protein, which reduces the frequency of the neuromuscular exacerbations associated with multiple sclerosis. As this drug is mixed in the sugar

known as mannitol, it is contraindicated in patients who are allergic to that component. It is available only in injectable form.

▶ muromonab-CD3

Muromonab-CD3 (Orthoclone OKT3) is the only drug indicated for the reversal (not just the prevention) of graft rejection. It is unique in that it is a monoclonal antibody, synthesized using recombinant DNA technology, and it is very similar to the antibodies naturally produced by the body (immunoglobulin G [IgG], IgM, IgD, IgA, and IgE). It specifically targets the binding sites on the T cells that recognize foreign invaders, such as a transplanted organ. It differs from human antibodies in that it comes from mice. These types of antibodies are commonly referred to as **murine antibodies,** hence the name muromonab. "Muro" stands for murine; "mon" for monoclonal, which means they come from a single-cell clone; and "ab" for antibody. As described previously, other monoclonal antibodies used for the prevention of organ rejection are basiliximab and daclizumab. Muromonab, often called OKT3, is contraindicated in patients with a hypersensitivity to murine products and in those who are experiencing fluid overload. This is another drug that can cause cytokine release syndrome, and patients are often pre-treated with a corticosteroid as mentioned previously for basiliximab and daclizumab This drug is available only in injectable form.

Pharmacokinetics

Half-Life	Onset	Peak	Duration
IV: Unknown	IV: Very rapid	IV: ~3 days	IV: Unknown

sirolimus and tacrolimus

Sirolimus (Rapamune) is another immunosuppressant drug similar in structure to tacrolimus (Prograf). Sirolimus is a macrocyclic immunosuppressive, antifungal, and antitumor drug produced by fermentation of the fungus *Streptomyces hygroscopicus.* Other macrocyclic immunosuppressive drugs are cyclosporine and tacrolimus. Sirolimus and tacrolimus are structurally related and act through similar mechanisms. Sirolimus is available only for oral use, whereas tacrolimus is available in both oral and injectable form.

Pharmacokinetics (sirolimus)

Half-Life	Onset	Peak	Duration
PO: 60-80 hr	PO: Unknown	PO: 1-3 hr	PO: Unknown

Pharmacokinetics (tacrolimus)

Half-Life	Onset	Peak	Duration
PO: 35 hr	PO: Unknown	PO: 1.5 hr	PO: Unknown

◆ NURSING PROCESS

✦ ASSESSMENT

Before administering any of the immunosuppressants, the nurse should perform a thorough patient assessment with baseline vital signs, history of medical conditions, and documentation of pre-existing chronic diseases affecting immune status (e.g., diabetes, hypertension, cancer). Assessment should also include noting of weight; urinalysis and urinary patterns; jaundice; edema, and/or ascites; history of cardiac disease and/or dysrhythmias; chest pain or hypertension; central nervous system assessment with attention to occurrence of seizure disorders and/or alteration of motor/sensory function; paresthesias; changing levels of consciousness; occurrence of any inflammatory processes with attention to duration, location, onset, and specific type of inflammation; appearance of joints with noting of deformities; ability for full range-of-motion and performing ADLs; and the condition of skin over an inflamed joint or area. Respiratory assessment should include questioning about any complaints such as wheezing, cough, activity intolerance, and/or sputum production. In addition, the following laboratory and diagnostic tests may be ordered and the results analyzed: renal function tests with blood urea nitrogen (BUN) and creatinine levels; hepatic function tests with alkaline phosphatase, aspartate aminotransferase (AST), alanine aminotransferase (ALT), and bilirubin levels; and cardiovascular function with baseline electrocardiogram (ECG). See Table 45-2 for information on other systems affected by the immunosuppressant drugs.

As discussed, several of the immunosuppressant drugs are metabolized by cytochrome CYP3A isoenzymes and interact with a specific group of medications such as antifungals, antibiotics, and calcium channel blockers. In addition, there are several herbal drug interactions, as noted with St. John's wort and grapefruit juice, and these may interact severely with some of the immunosuppressants—thus, the importance of a thorough drug history profile and cautious concern for use of other prescription drugs, OTCs, and herbals.

Azathioprine requires assessment of platelet counts and bleeding tendencies due to related thrombocytopenia. Cyclosporine and related contraindications, cautions, and drug interactions have been previously discussed as with other drugs in this chapter; however, specific to cyclosporine is the need to know that the herbal product, St. John's Wort, may alter the absorption of the drug, and grapefruit juice may increase the absorption of cyclosporine and lead to increased risk for toxicity. It is also important to know that lovastatin, an antilipemic drug that is commonly used, may increase the risk for renal failure and rhabdomyolysis, which may both be serious complications. Nephrotoxicity and liver/renal and cardiac toxicity may occur with the related organ transplant process, and, therefore, it is critical to continue to watch for the organ function preoperatively and postoperatively with this drug and other immunosuppressants that are indicated. Serum potassium and uric acid levels should be assessed, too, for increased and toxic levels. As with most organ transplants, mild nephrotoxicity generally occurs within about 2 to 3 months, whereas severe toxicity occurs more immediately after the transplantation. Other conditions that require careful assessment include cardiac, liver or kidney impairment, and malabsorptive syndromes.

Daclizumab requires assessment of baseline vital signs with specific attention to blood pressure and pulse rate. Any immune-compromised disorders should also be noted as well as infectious disease processes. Laboratory studies (e.g., hemoglobin [Hgb] level, hematocrit [Hct] values, white blood cell [WBC], and platelet counts) should be performed and the results documented before, during (monthly), and after therapy. If the leukocyte count should drop below 3000/mm^3, the drug should be discontinued, but only after the physician is contacted.

Muromonab-CD3 should be given only after a chest x-ray is ordered within 24 hours of beginning the drug to be sure that baseline lung fields are clear and with no fluid. Weight, vital signs, and noting of any edema should also be completed.

Questioning the patient for any chickenpox, herpes zoster infection, or malignancy should be performed, as these are important cautions/concerns prior to the use of sirolimus. Baseline CBC levels and lipid profile levels should also be performed prior to administering sirolimus. See previous discussion for information about contraindications, cautions, and drug interactions with use of this drug and others in this class. Tacrolimus requires a thorough patient history and physical assessment with attention to the drug history, BUN levels, CBC, hepatic enzymes, serum creatinine, and serum electrolytes. With administration of this drug, the patient requires very close assessment for the first 30 minutes and with the first dosage of the medication. Concern for anaphylactic reaction also goes past this first 30 minutes and first dose, and it is usually important to assess the presence and functioning of resuscitative equipment because it should be readily available along with appropriate doses of epinephrine and oxygen.

◆ NURSING DIAGNOSES

- Risk for injury to self related to physiologic influence of the disease, overall weakness, and adverse effects of immunosuppressants
- Risk for injury, allergic reaction, and subsequent systemic responses, due to risk for hypersensitivity reactions with immunosuppressants
- Risk for infection related to altered immune status from chronic disease and from medication regimen with immunosuppressants
- Acute pain, myalgias, and arthralgias related to adverse effects of immunosuppressant medications
- Noncompliance related to undesired adverse effects of drug treatment and lack of knowledge

◆ PLANNING

Goals

- Patient experiences minimal complications and injuries during drug therapy.
- Patient experiences maximal comfort during drug therapy.
- Patient remains compliant with drug therapy and comes in for follow-up visits with the physician.
- Patient states symptoms of adverse reactions to therapy and of exacerbation of illness to report to physician.
- Patient states importance of reporting any signs and symptoms of allergic reactions to the nurse, physician, or other health care provider.

Outcome Criteria

- Patient states measures to help minimize unpleasant adverse effects such as taking acetaminophen for fever and joint pain, reporting unusually high blood pressure readings, and participating in relaxation therapy, massage, and biofeedback.
- Patient states an improvement in energy levels, decrease in disease-related symptoms, increased ability to perform ADLs, and overall mental status improvement.
- Patient is compliant with follow-up visits with physician and other health care professionals to monitor therapeutic effects of immunosuppressant (e.g., decreased symptomatology) as well as any adverse effects and/or toxic reactions to medication (e.g., myalgias, arthralgias).
- Patient notifies physician immediately if fever, rash, sore throat, fatigue, or other unusual problems/symptoms develop.
- Patient states measures to implement to enhance comfort while on immunosuppressant therapy (e.g., use of non-

aspirin analgesics, rest, biofeedback, therapeutic touch/massage, imagery, diversional activities, hypnosis).

- Patient notifies appropriate health care personnel—or EMS personnel if in home setting—with complaints of difficulty breathing, shortness of breath, flushing of the face, urticaria, rash/whelps, dizziness, and syncope.
- Patient states appropriate measures—after contacting physician and/or EMS personnel—to help alleviate risk for further systemic symptoms of hypersensitivity such as taking diphenhydramine or related drugs to alter allergic reaction, as ordered.

♦ IMPLEMENTATION

It is important that oral immunosuppressants are taken with food to minimize gastrointestinal upset. It is also important, considering the immunosuppressed state of patients receiving immunosuppressants, that oral forms of the drugs be used whenever possible to decrease the risk for infection associated with intramuscular (IM) injections. An oral antifungal medication may be ordered to help with treating oral candidiasis that may occur in these patients as a consequence of the treatment and the disease processes; however, there may be significant drug interactions between the immunosuppressant and antifungal drug. Therefore, this should be considered and avoided prior to giving the medications. It is also very important to make sure that supportive treatment equipment and drugs are available in case of an allergic reaction with the immunosuppressants. Nurses should be aware of the high risk for this occurrence. It is also common to see pre-medication protocols with antihistamines and antiinflammatory drugs.

Cyclosporine is now available in several oral formulations but they are not intended to be used interchangeably. Oral liquid dosage forms are available with a calibrated liquid measuring device. Oral solutions may be mixed in a glass container with chocolate milk, milk, or orange juice and served at room temperature. Once the solution is mixed, make sure the patient drinks it immediately, and avoid Styrofoam containers, because the drug has been found to adhere to the inside wall of the cup/container. If using oral solutions, be sure that they are not refrigerated.

When given intravenously, cyclosporine should be diluted as recommended in the manufacturer guidelines and given according to the standards of care and institutional policy regarding its administration. Cyclosporine is usually diluted with normal saline (NS) or 5% dextrose in water (D_5W) and infused through an IV infusion pump and over the recommended time frame. Closely monitor the patient during the infusion, especially the first 30 minutes, for any allergic reactions, such as facial flushing, urticaria, wheezing, dyspnea, and rash. Make sure to record frequent vital signs, too. It is also important to closely monitor the patient's BUN, LDH, AST, and ALT during therapy for possible renal and hepatic impairment. Oral hygiene should be performed frequently to prevent gum hyperplasia. In addition, it is important to know therapeutic serum levels of cyclosporine are found to be 50 to 300 ng/mL and toxic levels are 400 ng/mL or greater.

Intravenously administered muromonab-CD3 is usually given over 1 minute and only after the medication is withdrawn through a 0.22 low protein–binding micron filter. A sterile needle must be used after the medication is withdrawn. A premedication protocol is usually used (see previous discussion) to help minimize reactions. Both sirolimus and tacrolimus have long half-lives, so toxicity is an added concern due to possible cumulative effects. Basiliximab and daclizumab are administered parenterally. Dilutional solutions and amounts should be followed as per manufacturer guidelines and intravenous drip closely monitored. An intravenous infusion pump may help to keep the proper dosage administered. Sirolimus and tacromilus should be administered as ordered by either IV or oral routes. If IV tacrolimus is to be discontinued and maintenance dosing needed, oral tacrolimus is usually ordered to be given 8 to 12 hours after the discontinuation of the IV drug. IV solution should not be stored in polyvinyl chloride containers and should be given in appropriately designed container and tubing. Oral dosages of tacrolimus should be given on an empty stomach and in a glass container. The same concern for not using of Styrofoam and no grapefruit use within 2 hours of the drug applies (as with cyclosporine). Complete blood counts, liver enzymes, and serum potassium levels will need to be monitored throughout the duration of therapy with these drugs as well.

♦ EVALUATION

The nurse should continually evaluate and reevaluate the goals and outcome criteria as related to the nursing process and administration of drug therapy. In addition, therapeutic responses to immunosuppressants should be evaluated and may include acceptance of transplanted organ or graft and/or improved symptoms in those with autoimmune disorders. CBC levels, erythrocyte sedimentation rates (ESR), C-reactive protein levels, liver/kidney/cardiac function tests, pulmonary function, chest x-ray, and plasma levels of T-lymphocyte surface phenotyping are a few of the tests that may be evaluated during and after drug therapy. Evaluation of drug-specific adverse effects and toxicity (see Table 45-2) and specific therapeutic drug levels (as indicated) should be ongoing.

Patient Teaching Tips

- Encourage patients taking immunosuppressants to avoid crowds to minimize the risk for infection. Educate patients to report fever, sore throat, chills, joint pain, or fatigue to the physician because these may indicate severe infection and require immediate medical attention.
- For female patients receiving immunosuppressants, educate about the use of some form of contraception during treatment and for up to 12 weeks after therapy.
- Inform patients taking cyclosporine to take the drug the same time every day (as with most immunosuppressants) and that if a dosage is omitted, they should contact the physician for further instructions.

- Inform patients that blood work will be drawn during therapy, so routine follow-up appointments are to be encouraged.
- Educate patients about the adverse effects of cyclosporine, which include headache and tremor and to avoid consumption of grapefruit/grapefruit juice because of a potential for increase in blood concentrations of cyclosporine.
- Educate the patient to keep the gel caps in a cool, dry environment and avoid their exposure to light, as well as that the dosage form should be kept in its original packaging. Also, remind patients to avoid prolonged exposure to the sun and to wear sunscreen and protective clothing when outdoors.

Continued

Patient Teaching Tips—cont'd

- Patients who are to undergo transplant surgery and who are receiving cyclosporine should know that several days before surgery they may be told to take it with corticosteroids, and they may also be given an oral antifungal as prophylaxis for *Candida* infections
- Patients taking the oral form of cyclosporine should be told to take their medication with meals or mixed with milk to minimize GI upset.
- Patients taking azathioprine or muromonab-CD3 should be informed that several days before transplant surgery they should

take all their medication by the oral route if possible and avoid intramuscular injection, which carries the risk for infection.
- Patients should be informed to take sirolimus or tacrolimus exactly as ordered and at the same time every day, as well as to avoid crowds and those with infections. Educate patients about the adverse effects of chest pain, dizziness, headache, problems with urination, rash, and respiratory and/or other infections.
- Patients should be told to avoid sun exposure and grapefruit when taking sirolimus or tacrolimus. Patients should also know the importance of follow-up visits to the physician for laboratory tests.

Points to Remember

- Immunosuppressants decrease or prevent the body's immune response and include drugs such as cyclosporine, muromonoab-CD3, etanercept, sirolimus, and tacrolimus.
- Regardless of the immunosuppressants, if the recipient's immune system cannot recognize the organ as being foreign, it will not mount an immune response against it.
- Some of the indications for immunosuppressants include to suppress immunodeficiency disorders and malignancies, and to improve short-term and long-term allograft survival and outcomes in the treatment of autoimmune disease processes.
- Nursing considerations include the possible administration of oral antifungals that are usually given with these medications to

treat the oral candidiasis that occurs as a result of immunosuppression and fungal overgrowth. The nurse should inspect the oral cavity as often as necessary (at least once every shift) for any white patches on the tongue, mucous membranes, and oral pharynx. These patches may indicate oral candidiasis.
- Other nursing considerations associated with the immunosuppressants include monitoring laboratory studies (e.g., Hgb level, Hct values, WBC, and platelet count). Studies should be performed and the results documented before, during (monthly), and after therapy. Should the leukocyte count drop below 3000/mm³, the drug should be discontinued (but as ordered).

NCLEX Examination Review Questions

1. When assessing a patient who is to begin therapy with cyclosporine, the nurse recognizes that it should be used cautiously in patients with which condition?
   a. Renal dysfunction
   b. Glaucoma
   c. Anemia
   d. Myalgia
2. While assessing a patient who is to receive muromonab-CD3, the nurse knows that which condition would be a contraindication for this drug?
   a. Acute myalgia
   b. Fluid overload
   c. Polycythemia
   d. Diabetes mellitus
3. During therapy with azathioprine (Imuran), the nurse must monitor for which common adverse effect?
   a. Bradycardia
   b. Diarrhea

   c. Thrombocytopenia
   d. Vomiting
4. During a patient teaching session for a patient receiving an immunosuppressant drug, the nurse should include which statement?
   a. "It is better to use oral forms of these drugs to prevent the occurrence of thrush."
   b. "You will remain on antibiotics to prevent infections."
   c. "It is important to use some form of contraception during treatment and for up to 12 weeks after the end of therapy."
   d. "Be sure to take your medications with grapefruit juice to enhance its effects."
5. During drug therapy with basiliximab (Simulect), the nurse monitors for signs of cytokine release syndrome, which results in:
   a. Hepatotoxicity
   b. Neurotoxicity
   c. Polycythemia
   d. An allergic-type reaction

1. a, 2. b, 3. c, 4. c, 5. d.

Critical Thinking Activities

1. A 58-year-old heart transplant recipient is currently taking cyclosporine to prevent his immune system from rejecting his transplanted heart. How does cyclosporine prevent this patient's immune system from attacking his transplanted heart?
2. What type of medication may be needed with the administration of muromonab-CD3 and why?

3. Your patient is about to undergo a right lung transplant. Why are intramuscular injections to be kept at a minimal during the time before his surgery?

For answers, see http://evolve.elsevier.com/Lilley.

Immunizing Drugs and Biochemical Terrorism

Objectives

When you reach the end of this chapter, you should be able to do the following:

1. Discuss the importance of immunity as it relates to the various immunizing drugs and their use in patients of all ages.
2. Identify the diseases that are treated or prevented with toxoids or vaccines.
3. Compare the mechanisms of action, indications, cautions, contraindications, adverse effects, toxicity, and routes of administration for various toxoids and vaccines.
4. Develop a nursing care plan that includes all phases of the nursing process related to the administration of immunizing drugs across the lifespan.
5. Develop a nursing care plan covering aspects of the nursing process that relate to bioterrorism with emphasis on the nurse's role.

e-Learning Activities

Companion CD
- NCLEX Review Questions: see questions 386-390
- Animations
- Audio Glossary
- Category Catchers
- Medication Errors Checklists
- IV Therapy Checklists

evolve Website (http://evolve.elsevier.com/Lilley)
• Nursing Care Plans • Frequently Asked Questions • Content Updates • WebLinks • Supplemental Resources • Elsevier ePharmacology Update • Medication Administration Animations

Drug Profiles

diphtheria and tetanus toxoids, and acellular pertussis vaccine tetanus (adsorbed), p. 709
Haemophilus influenzae type b conjugate vaccine, p. 709
▶ hepatitis B immunoglobulin, p. 712
▶ hepatitis B virus vaccine (inactivated), p. 709
▶ immunoglobulin, p. 712
▶ influenza virus vaccine, p. 709
▶ measles, mumps, and rubella virus vaccine (live), p. 711

▶ pneumococcal vaccine, polyvalent and seven-valent, p. 712
▶ poliovirus vaccine (inactivated), p. 712
rabies immunoglobulin, p. 713
rabies virus vaccine, p. 712
Rh$_0$(D) immunoglobulin, p. 713
tetanus immunoglobulin, p. 713
▶ varicella virus vaccine, p. 712
varicella-zoster immunoglobulin, p. 713

▶ Key drug.

Glossary

Active immunization   A type of immunization that causes development of a complete and long-lasting immunity to a certain infection through exposure of the body to the associated disease antigen; it can be natural active immunization (i.e., having the disease) or artificial active immunization (i.e., receiving a vaccine or toxoid). (p. 703)

Active immunizing drugs   Toxoids or vaccines that are administered to a host (human or animal) to stimulate host production of antibodies). (p. 706)

Antibodies   Immunoglobulin molecules that have an antigen-specific amino acid sequence and are synthesized by the humoral immune system (B cells) in response to exposure to a specific antigen (foreign substance). Their purpose is to attack and destroy molecules of this antigen. (p. 702)

Antibody titer   Amount of an antibody needed to react with and neutralize a given volume or amount of a specific antigen. (p. 706)

Antigens   Substances, usually proteins and foreign to a host (human or animal), that stimulate the host to produce antibodies and react specifically with those antibodies. Examples of antigens include bacterial exotoxins and viruses. An allergen (e.g., dust, pollen, mold) is an antigen that can produce an immediate-type hypersensitivity reaction or allergy. (p. 702)

Antiserum   A serum that contains antibodies. It is usually obtained from an animal that has been immunized against a specific antigen, either by injection with the antigen or by infection with specific microorganisms that produce the antigen. (p. 706)

Antitoxin   An antiserum against a toxin (or toxoid); it is most often a purified antiserum obtained from animals (usually horses) by injection of a toxin or toxoid so that antibodies to the toxin (i.e., antitoxin) can be collected from the animals and used to provide artificial passive immunity to humans exposed to a given toxin (e.g., tetanus immunoglobulin). (p. 706)

Antivenin   An antiserum against a venom (poison produced by an animal) used to treat humans or other animals that have been envenomed (e.g., by snakebite, spider bite, or scorpion sting). (p. 706)

Biologic antimicrobial drugs Substances of biologic origin used to prevent, treat, or cure infectious diseases (e.g., vaccines, toxoids, immunoglobulins). These drugs are often simply referred to as *biologic*. However, *biologics* also refers to drugs of bioterrorism (e.g., anthrax spores, smallpox virus), depending on the context. (p. 703)

Bioterrorism The use of infectious biologic or chemical agents as weapons for human destruction. (p. 713)

Booster shot A repeat dose of an antigen, such as a vaccine or toxoid, which is usually administered in an amount smaller than that used in the original immunization. It is given to maintain the immune response of a previously immunized patient at, or return the response to, a clinically effective level. (p. 706)

Cell-mediated immune system The immune response that is mediated by T cells (as opposed to B cells, which produce antibodies). T cells mount their immune response through activities such as release of cytokines (chemicals that stimulate other protective immune functions; for example, production of nasal secretions to help eliminate pathogens via the nose), as well as direct cytotoxicity (e.g., phagocytosis of an antigen). (p. 703)

Herd immunity Resistance to a disease on the part of an entire community or population because a large proportion of its members are immune to the disease. (p. 706)

Immune response A cascade of biochemical events that occurs in response to entry into the body of an antigen (foreign substance); key processes of the immune response include phagocytosis (literally "eating of cells") of foreign microorganisms and synthesis of antibodies that react with (by chemically binding to) molecules of specific antigens to inactivate them. Immune response centers around the blood but may also involve the lymphatic system and the *reticuloendothelial system* (see below). (p. 702)

Immunization The induction of immunity by administration of a vaccine or toxoid (active immunization) or antiserum (passive immunization). (p. 703)

Immunizing biologics Toxoids, vaccines, or immunoglobulins that are targeted against specific infectious microorganisms or toxins. (p. 703)

Immunoglobulins Glycoproteins synthesized and used by the humoral immune system (B cells) to attack and kill all substances foreign to the body. More general than an antibody, an immunoglobulin is a nonspecific antibody (i.e., one that does not yet have a specific amino acid sequence that recognizes a specific antigen). The term is synonymous with *immune globulins*. (p. 702)

Passive immunization A type of immunization in which immunity to infection is conferred by bypassing the host's immune system and injecting a person with antiserum or concentrated antibodies obtained from other humans or animals that directly give the host the means to fight off an invading microorganism (artificial passive immunization). The host's immune system therefore does not have to manufacture these antibodies. This process also occurs when antibodies pass from mother to infant during breast-feeding or through the placenta during pregnancy (natural passive immunization). (p. 703)

Passive immunizing drugs Drugs containing antibodies or antitoxins that can kill or inactivate pathogens by binding to the associated antigens. These are directly injected into a person (host) and provide that person with the means to fend off infection, bypassing the host's own immune system. (p. 706)

Recombinant Relating to or containing a combination of genetic material from two or more organisms. Such genetic recombination is one of the key methods of biotechnology and is often used to make immunizing drugs and various other medications. (p. 709)

Reticuloendothelial system Specialized cells located in the liver, spleen, lymphatics, and bone marrow that remove miscellaneous particles from the circulation, such as aging antibody molecules. (p. 706)

Toxin Any poison produced by a plant, animal, or microorganism that is highly toxic to other living organisms. (p. 703)

Toxoids Bacterial exotoxins that are modified or inactivated (by chemicals or heat) so that they are no longer toxic but can still bind (to host B cells) to stimulate the formation of antitoxin; toxoids are often used in the same manner as vaccines to promote artificial active immunity in humans. They are one type of active immunizing drug (e.g., tetanus toxoid). (p. 703)

Vaccines Suspensions of live, attenuated, or killed microorganisms that can promote an artificially induced active immunity against a particular microorganism. They are another type of active immunizing drug (e.g., tetanus vaccine). (p. 703)

Venom A poison that is secreted by an animal (e.g., snake, insect, or spider). (p. 706)

IMMUNITY AND IMMUNIZATION

Centuries ago it was noticed that people who contracted certain diseases acquired an immune tolerance to the disease so that, when exposed to it again, they did not experience a second bout of illness. This basic observation prompted scientists to investigate ways of artificially producing this tolerance. Along with this came an understanding of the way in which the normal immune system functions, knowledge important to an understanding of how immunizing drugs work. Briefly, when the body first comes into contact with **antigens** (foreign proteins) from an invading organism, some specific information is imprinted into a cellular "memory bank" of the immune system so that the body can effectively fight any future invasion by that same organism by mounting an **immune response.** This cellular memory bank consists of specialized immune cells known as *memory cells.* When an antigen presents itself to a person's humoral immune system (B cells) by binding to B lymphocytes (B cells), the B cells differentiate into two other types of cells. One type is the memory cells. The second type is known as *plasma cells*, the role of which is to produce large volumes of antibodies against the antigen in question. **Antibodies** are immunoglobulin molecules that have antigen-specific amino acid sequences. **Immunoglobulins**, or *immune globulins*, are glycoprotein molecules synthesized by the humoral immune system for the purpose of destroying all substances that the body recognizes as foreign. Immunoglobulins can be general or specific. A general immunoglobulin lacks a specific amino acid sequence that allows it to recognize a specific antigen. An immunoglobulin with such a specific amino

Table 46-1   Active Versus Passive Immunization

Characteristic	Active	Passive
Artificial		
Type of immunizing drug	Toxoid or vaccine	Immunoglobulin or antitoxin
Mechanism of action	Causes an antigen-antibody response, similar to that in exposure to natural disease process	Results from direct administration of exogenous antibodies; antibody concentration will decrease over time, so if reexposure is expected, it is wise to continue passive immunizations
Use	To prevent development of active disease in the event of exposure to a given antigen in people who have at least a partially functioning immune system	To provide temporary protection against disease in people who are immunodeficient, those for whom active immunization is contraindicated, and those who have been exposed to or anticipate exposure to the disease; an antibody response is not stimulated in the host
Natural		
Mechanism of action	Production of own antibodies during actual infection	Transmission of antibodies from mother to infant through placenta or during breastfeeding

acid sequence is known as an *antibody,* as noted earlier. It is because of this process that people rarely suffer twice from certain diseases such as mumps, chickenpox, and measles. Instead they have a complete and long-lasting immunity to those infections.

In contrast to the humoral immune system, which is the focus of this chapter, the **cell-mediated immune system** is the branch of the immune system that does not synthesize antibodies. Instead, it is driven by T cells (T lymphocytes) and works by the release from these T cells of *cytokines* (chemicals that promote other immune system functions such as inflammatory responses, runny nose, etc.) and by *phagocytosis* (engulfing and destruction of the antigens by the T cells). To varying degrees, these two immune system branches work simultaneously or even interdependently, with the humoral immune system also being activated and/or driven partly by cytokines from the cell-mediated immune system.

There are two ways of cultivating immunity to certain infections: **active immunization** and **passive immunization.** Each can also be an artificial or natural process. In artificial active immunization the body is clinically exposed to a relatively harmless form of an antigen (foreign invader) that does not cause an actual infection. Information about the antigen is then imprinted into the memory of the immune system as described earlier, and the body's defenses are stimulated to resist any subsequent exposure (by producing antibodies). In contrast, natural active immunization occurs when a person acquires immunity by surviving the disease itself and producing antibodies to the disease-causing organism. Artificial passive immunization involves clinical administration of serum or concentrated immunoglobulins obtained from humans or animals, which directly gives the inoculated individual the substance needed to fight off the invading microorganism. This type of **immunization** bypasses the host's immune system. Finally, natural passive immunization occurs when antibodies are transferred from the mother to her infant in breast milk or through the bloodstream via the placenta during pregnancy. The major differences between active and passive immunization are summarized in Table 46-1 and are discussed in greater depth in the following sections.

ACTIVE IMMUNIZATION

In general, **biologic antimicrobial drugs** (also referred to simply as *biologics*) are substances such as antitoxins, antisera, toxoids, and vaccines that are used to prevent, treat, or cure infectious diseases. Toxoids and vaccines are known as **immunizing biologics,** and they target a particular infectious microorganism.

Toxoids

Toxoids are substances that contain antigens, most often in the form of bacterial (usually gram-positive bacterial) exotoxins. These substances have been detoxified or weakened (*attenuated*) with chemicals or heat, which renders them nontoxic and unable to revert back to a toxic form. Nonetheless, they remain highly antigenic and can stimulate an artificial active immune response (production of antitoxin antibodies) when injected into a host patient. These antibodies can then neutralize the same exotoxin upon any future exposure. Toxoids were first developed in 1923 at the Pasteur Institute by Ramon and his associates, and modern versions are effective against diseases such as diphtheria and tetanus caused by **toxin**-producing bacteria.

Vaccines

Vaccines are suspensions of live, attenuated (weakened), or killed (inactivated) microorganisms that can stimulate antibody production against the particular organism. As with toxoids, these slight alterations in the bacteria and viruses prevent the person injected with the vaccine from contracting the disease but are still able to promote active immunization against the organism, including an antibody response. People vaccinated with live bacteria or viruses (as well as those who recover from an actual infection) enjoy lifelong immunity against that particular disease. Only partial immunity is conferred on those vaccinated with killed bacteria or viruses, and for this reason they must be given periodic booster shots to maintain immune system protection against infection with the given organism. One exception to this is the smallpox vaccine, because it uses live cowpox virus (vaccinia virus) instead of the more virulent smallpox virus.

Edward Jenner, an English physician born in 1749, noticed that milkmaids who had suffered cowpox infections were rarely victims of smallpox and was the first to study the relationship of cowpox to smallpox immunity. His observation led to the development of the smallpox vaccine, which uses the cowpox virus. In 1796, Jenner successfully immunized a young boy against smallpox by vaccinating him with cowpox virus obtained from a cowpox vesicle on an infected cow. With the help of the modern version of this vaccine, smallpox was considered to be eradicated as of 1980. However, following the terrorist attacks in the United States on September 11, 2001, fears arose of a large-scale bioterrorism attack using the smallpox virus. By 2003, these fears had subsided somewhat, and the Centers for Disease Control and Prevention (CDC) released guidelines recommending routine early detection surveillance activities on the part of all public health agencies. These guidelines also included a plan for rapid vaccination of local populations in the event of a suspected smallpox outbreak and listed several high-priority high-risk groups, including direct health care personnel, who should be vaccinated first if a suspected outbreak occurs. Today there are more than 20 infectious diseases for which vaccines are available. New vaccines appear periodically but not with the rapidity of other types of drugs, because of the complexities of developing a safe and effective vaccine.

Most modern vaccines are produced in a laboratory by genetic engineering methods and contain some extract of the pathogen, or a synthetic extract, rather than the microbe itself. This extract gives the vaccine its ability to stimulate an antibody response in host patients against a particular bacterial or viral infection without causing active disease. Some vaccines, such as influenza vaccine, may contain actual whole or split virus particles. Most, however, contain a smaller fraction of the organism, such as the bacterial capsular polysaccharides that are used to make pneumococcal vaccine. The attenuating or killing agent is usually a chemical such as formaldehyde or a physical mechanism such as heat. Attenuation may also be accomplished by repeated passage of the microbe through some medium such as a fertile hen egg or a special tissue culture. The search for new and better drugs will never end. Current goals include finding vaccines against human immunodeficiency virus (HIV) infection/acquired immunodeficiency syndrome (AIDS) and malaria; the ultimate goal is to develop an effective vaccine against all infectious diseases. The currently available immunizing vaccines are listed in Box 46-1. Note that the drug given to prevent respiratory syncytial virus (RSV) infection is not an immunizing drug per se but is a specialized antiviral drug. It is discussed in Chapter 49. The RSV immunoglobulin is listed in Box 46-1.

The current childhood immunization schedule published by the CDC is shown in Figure 46-1. This advisory is published annually as a joint effort of the American Academy of Pediatrics, the CDC's Advisory Committee on Immunization Practices, and the American Academy of Family Physicians. The CDC also posts on its website a catch-up schedule for children who may have missed scheduled immunizations. The CDC's current adult immunization schedule can be found online at http://evolve.elsevier.com/Lilley or www.cdc.gov/nip/recs/adult-schedule.pdf. It is interesting to note that a mumps outbreak began in the Midwest in 2005 and by the time of this writing (spring of 2006) had spread to nine Midwestern states. Situations like this, although relatively uncommon, do serve as a reminder of the reality of vaccine-preventable illnesses.

PASSIVE IMMUNIZATION

As previously mentioned, in passive immunization the host's immune system is bypassed and the person is inoculated with serum containing immunoglobulins obtained from other humans or ani-

---

Box 46-1 Available Immunizing Drugs

Passively Immunizing Drugs
Antivenin, pit viper (Crotalidae) polyvalent
Crotalidae polyvalent immune Fab (for pit viper snakebite; e.g., rattlesnake, water moccasin)
Antivenin, *Latrodectus mactans* (black widow spider)
Antivenin, *Micrurus fulvius* (coral snake)
Botulism immunoglobulin
Cytomegalovirus immunoglobulin (human)
Digoxin immune Fab
Hepatitis B immunoglobulin
Immunoglobulin, intramuscular
Immunoglobulin, intravenous
Lymphocyte immunoglobulin, antithymocyte globulin
Rabies immunoglobulin (human)
Respiratory syncytial virus immunoglobulin, intravenous (human)
$Rh_0(D)$ immunoglobulin (e.g., RhoGAM)
Tetanus immunoglobulin
Vaccinia immunoglobulin
Varicella-zoster immunoglobulin (chickenpox/shingles)

Actively Immunizing Drugs
BCG (bacillus Calmette-Guérin) vaccine (tuberculosis)
Diphtheria and tetanus toxoids, adsorbed
Diphtheria and tetanus toxoids and acellular pertussis vaccine, adsorbed
Diphtheria and tetanus toxoids, acellular pertussis, and *Haemophilus influenzae* type b conjugate vaccines
Diphtheria and tetanus toxoids, acellular pertussis (adsorbed), hepatitis B (recombinant), and inactivated poliovirus vaccine combined
Haemophilus influenzae type b conjugate vaccine
Haemophilus influenzae type b conjugate vaccine with hepatitis B vaccine
Hepatitis A virus vaccine, inactivated
Hepatitis B virus vaccine, recombinant
Hepatitis A virus vaccine (inactivated) and hepatitis B virus vaccine (recombinant)
Influenza virus vaccine
Japanese encephalitis virus vaccine
Measles virus* vaccine, live attenuated
Measles, mumps, and rubella virus vaccine, live
Meningococcal bacterial vaccine
Mumps virus vaccine, live
Pneumococcal bacterial vaccine, polyvalent
Pneumococcal seven-valent conjugate vaccine
Poliovirus vaccine, inactivated
Rabies virus vaccine
Rubella virus vaccine, live
Rubella and mumps virus vaccine, live
Rubella, measles, and mumps virus vaccine, live
Smallpox virus vaccine†
Tetanus toxoid, fluid
Tetanus toxoid, adsorbed
Typhoid bacterial vaccine
Varicella virus vaccine
Yellow fever virus vaccine

*Also known as rubeola virus.
†Not currently on the U.S. market but according to the Centers for Disease Control and Prevention website may be reintroduced because of current bioterrorism threats.

---

mals. These substances give the person the means to fight off the invading organism. This is known as *artificially acquired passive immunity* and it confers temporary immunity against a particular antigen following exposure to the antigen. It differs from active immunization in that it produces a comparatively transitory

Recommended Childhood and Adolescent Immunization Schedule UNITED STATES • 2006

Vaccine ▼ Age ►	Birth	1 month	2 months	4 months	6 months	12 months	15 months	18 months	24 months	4–6 years	11–12 years	13–14 years	15 years	16–18 years
Hepatitis B[1]	HepB	HepB		HepB[1]		HepB			HepB Series					
Diphtheria, Tetanus, Pertussis[2]			DTaP	DTaP	DTaP		DTaP			DTaP	Tdap	Tdap		
Haemophilus influenzae type b[3]			Hib	Hib	Hib[3]	Hib								
Inactivated Poliovirus			IPV	IPV		IPV				IPV				
Measles, Mumps, Rubella[4]						MMR				MMR	MMR			
Varicella[5]						Varicella			Varicella					
Meningococcal[6]							Vaccines within broken line are for selected populations		MPSV4		MCV4		MCV4 / MCV4	
Pneumococcal[7]			PCV	PCV	PCV	PCV				PCV	PPV			
Influenza[8]					Influenza (Yearly)					Influenza (Yearly)				
Hepatitis A[9]									HepA Series					

This schedule indicates the recommended ages for routine administration of currently licensed childhood vaccines, as of December 1, 2005, for children through age 18 years. Any dose not administered at the recommended age should be administered at any subsequent visit when indicated and feasible. ▓ Indicates age groups that warrant special effort to administer those vaccines not previously administered. Additional vaccines may be licensed and recommended during the year. Licensed combination vaccines may be used whenever any components of the combination are indicated and other components of the vaccine are not contraindicated and if approved by the Food and Drug Administration for that dose of the series. Providers should consult the respective ACIP statement for detailed recommendations. Clinically significant adverse events that follow immunization should be reported to the Vaccine Adverse Event Reporting System (VAERS). Guidance about how to obtain and complete a VAERS form is available at www.vaers.hhs.gov or by telephone, 800-822-7967.

▓ **Range of recommended ages**   ▓ **Catch-up immunization**   ▓ **11–12 year old assessment**

1. **Hepatitis B vaccine (HepB).** *AT BIRTH:* All newborns should receive monovalent HepB soon after birth and before hospital discharge. **Infants born to mothers who are HBsAg-positive** should receive HepB and 0.5 mL of hepatitis B immune globulin (HBIG) within 12 hours of birth. **Infants born to mothers whose HBsAg status is unknown** should receive HepB within 12 hours of birth. The mother should have blood drawn as soon as possible to determine her HBsAg status; if HBsAg-positive, the infant should receive HBIG as soon as possible (no later than age 1 week). **For infants born to HBsAg-negative mothers,** the birth dose can be delayed in rare circumstances but only if a physician's order to withhold the vaccine and a copy of the mother's original HBsAg-negative laboratory report are documented in the infant's medical record. *FOLLOWING THE BIRTHDOSE:* The HepB series should be completed with either monovalent HepB or a combination vaccine containing HepB. The second dose should be administered at age 1–2 months. The final dose should be administered at age ≥24 weeks. It is permissible to administer 4 doses of HepB (e.g., when combination vaccines are given after the birth dose); however, if monovalent HepB is used, a dose at age 4 months is not needed. **Infants born to HBsAg-positive mothers** should be tested for HBsAg and antibody to HBsAg after completion of the HepB series, at age 9–18 months (generally at the next well-child visit after completion of the vaccine series).

2. **Diphtheria and tetanus toxoids and acellular pertussis vaccine (DTaP).** The fourth dose of DTaP may be administered as early as age 12 months, provided 6 months have elapsed since the third dose and the child is unlikely to return at age 15–18 months. The final dose in the series should be given at age ≥4 years.

   Tetanus and diphtheria toxoids and acellular pertussis vaccine (Tdap – adolescent preparation) is recommended at age 11–12 years for those who have completed the recommended childhood DTP/DTaP vaccination series and have not received a Td booster dose. Adolescents 13–18 years who missed the 11–12-year Td/Tdap booster dose should also receive a single dose of Tdap if they have completed the recommended childhood DTP/DTaP vaccination series. Subsequent **tetanus and diphtheria toxoids (Td)** are recommended every 10 years.

3. ***Haemophilus influenzae* type b conjugate vaccine (Hib).** Three Hib conjugate vaccines are licensed for infant use. If PRP-OMP (PedvaxHIB® or ComVax® [Merck]) is administered at ages 2 and 4 months, a dose at age 6 months is not required. DTaP/Hib combination products should not be used for primary immunization in infants at ages 2, 4 or 6 months but can be used as boosters after any Hib vaccine. The final dose in the series should be administered at age ≥12 months.

4. **Measles, mumps, and rubella vaccine (MMR).** The second dose of MMR is recommended routinely at age 4–6 years but may be administered during any visit, provided at least 4 weeks have elapsed since the first dose and both doses are administered beginning at or after age 12 months. Those who have not previously received the second dose should complete the schedule by age 11–12 years.

5. **Varicella vaccine.** Varicella vaccine is recommended at any visit at or after age 12 months for susceptible children (i.e., those who lack a reliable history of chickenpox). Susceptible persons aged ≥13 years should receive 2 doses administered at least 4 weeks apart.

6. **Meningococcal vaccine (MCV4).** Meningococcal conjugate vaccine (MCV4) should be given to all children at the 11–12 year old visit as well as to unvaccinated adolescents at high school entry (15 years of age). Other adolescents who wish to decrease their risk for meningococcal disease may also be vaccinated. All college freshmen living in dormitories should also be vaccinated, preferably with MCV4, although **meningococcal polysaccharide vaccine (MPSV4)** is an acceptable alternative. Vaccination against invasive meningococcal disease is recommended for children and adolescents aged ≥2 years with terminal complement deficiencies or anatomic or functional asplenia and certain other high risk groups (see *MMWR* 2005;54 [RR-7]:1-21); use MPSV4 for children aged 2–10 years and MCV4 for older children, although MPSV4 is an acceptable alternative.

7. **Pneumococcal vaccine.** The heptavalent **pneumococcal conjugate vaccine (PCV)** is recommended for all children aged 2–23 months and for certain children aged 24–59 months. The final dose in the series should be given at age ≥12 months. **Pneumococcal polysaccharide vaccine (PPV)** is recommended in addition to PCV for certain high-risk groups. See *MMWR* 2000; 49(RR-9):1-35.

8. **Influenza vaccine.** Influenza vaccine is recommended annually for children aged ≥6 months with certain risk factors (including, but not limited to, asthma, cardiac disease, sickle cell disease, human immunodeficiency virus [HIV], diabetes, and conditions that can compromise respiratory function or handling of respiratory secretions or that can increase the risk for aspiration), healthcare workers, and other persons (including household members) in close contact with persons in groups at high risk (see *MMWR* 2005;54[RR-8]:1-55). In addition, healthy children aged 6–23 months and close contacts of healthy children aged 0–5 months are recommended to receive influenza vaccine because children in this age group are at substantially increased risk for influenza-related hospitalizations. For healthy persons aged 5–49 years, the intranasally administered, live, attenuated influenza vaccine (LAIV) is an acceptable alternative to the intramuscular trivalent inactivated influenza vaccine (TIV). See *MMWR* 2005;54(RR-8):1-55. Children receiving TIV should be administered a dosage appropriate for their age (0.25 mL if aged 6–35 months or 0.5 mL if aged ≥3 years). Children aged ≤8 years who are receiving influenza vaccine for the first time should receive 2 doses (separated by at least 4 weeks for TIV and at least 6 weeks for LAIV).

9. **Hepatitis A vaccine (HepA).** HepA is recommended for all children at 1 year of age (i.e., 12–23 months). The 2 doses in the series should be administered at least 6 months apart. States, counties, and communities with existing HepA vaccination programs for children 2–18 years of age are encouraged to maintain these programs. In these areas, new efforts focused on routine vaccination of 1-year-old children should enhance, not replace, ongoing programs directed at a broader population of children. HepA is also recommended for certain high risk groups (see *MMWR* 1999; 48[RR-12]1-37).

The Childhood and Adolescent Immunization Schedule is approved by:
Advisory Committee on Immunization Practices www.cdc.gov/nip/acip • American Academy of Pediatrics www.aap.org • American Academy of Family Physicians www.aafp.org

FIGURE 46-1   Recommended childhood immunization schedule. *ACIP,* Advisory Committee on Immunization Practices; *DTP,* diphtheria, tetanus, and pertussis vaccine; *HBsAG,* hepatitis B surface antigen; *Tdap,* tetanus and diphtheria toxoids and acellular pertussis vaccine. *(From Centers for Disease Control and Prevention, National Immunization Program: Recommended childhood and adolescent immunization schedule: United States: 2006. Available at www.cdc.gov/nip/recs/child-schedule-color-print.pdf.)*

(short-lived) immune state and the antibodies are already prepared for the host—the host's immune system does not have to synthesize its own antibodies. This allows for more rapid prevention or treatment of disease. Important examples include immunization with tetanus immunoglobulin, hepatitis immunoglobulin, rabies immunoglobulin, and snakebite antivenin.

As noted earlier, passive immunization occurs naturally between a mother and the fetus or the nursing infant when the mother passes maternal antibodies directly, either through the placenta to the fetus or through breast milk to the nursing infant. This is called *naturally acquired passive immunity.*

As Table 46-1 indicates, there are specific populations that can benefit from passive immunization but not from active immunization. These are persons who have been rendered immunodeficient for whatever reason (e.g., by drugs or disease) and who therefore cannot mount an immune response to a toxoid or vaccine injection because their immune systems are too suppressed to do so. People who already have the diseases targeted by **passive immunizing drugs** are also candidates for these drugs, especially individuals with diseases that are rapidly harmful or fatal, such as rabies, tetanus, and hepatitis. Because these diseases can progress rapidly, the body does not have time to mount an adequate immune defense against them before death occurs. The passive immunization of such individuals confers a temporary protection that is usually sufficient to keep the invading organisms from killing them, even though it does not stimulate an antibody response.

The passive immunizing drugs are divided into three groups: antitoxins, immunoglobulins, and snake and spider antivenins. An **antitoxin** is a purified **antiserum** that is usually obtained from horses inoculated with the toxin. An immunoglobulin is a concentrated preparation containing predominantly immunoglobulin G and is harvested from a large pool of blood donors. An **antivenin,** often referred to as *antivenom,* is an antiserum containing antibodies against a **venom,** which is a poison secreted by an animal such as a reptile, insect, or arthropod (spider). Antivenins are obtained from animals (usually horses) that have been injected with the particular venom. The serum contains immunoglobulins that can neutralize the toxic effects of the venom.

IMMUNIZING DRUGS

Mechanism of Action and Drug Effects

Active immunizing drugs consist of vaccines and toxoids that may be administered either orally or intramuscularly and that work by stimulating that part of the immune system known as the humoral immune system. This system synthesizes substances called *immunoglobulins,* of which there are five distinct types, designated as M, G, A, E, and D. These immunoglobulins attack and kill the foreign substances that invade the body. In this case these foreign substances are called *antigens,* and the immunoglobulins are called *antibodies.*

Vaccines contain substances that trigger the formation of these antibodies against specific pathogens. Sometimes these substances are the actual live or attenuated (weakened) pathogen or a killed pathogen, and the amount of antibodies they cause to be produced can be measured in the blood. The **antibody titer** is the amount of an antibody that must be present in the blood to

effectively protect the body against the particular pathogen. Sometimes the levels of these antibodies decline over time. When this happens, another dose of the vaccine is given to restore the antibody titers to a level that can protect the person against the infection. This repeat dose is referred to as a **booster shot.** Toxoids are altered forms of bacterial toxins that stimulate the production of antibodies in the same way as vaccines.

Because both toxoids and vaccines rely on the immunized host to mount an immune response, the host's immune system must be intact. Therefore, patients who are immunocompromised (i.e., who cannot mount an immune response), such as those undergoing immunosuppressive cancer chemotherapy, those receiving immunosuppressive therapy to prevent the rejection of transplanted organs, and those with immunosuppressive diseases such as AIDS, may not benefit from receiving vaccines or toxoids. Instead, their clinical situations may warrant giving them passive immunizing drugs such as immunoglobulins.

As previously explained, passive immunizing drugs are the actual antibodies (immunoglobulins) that can kill or inactivate the pathogen. The process is called passive because the person's immune system does not participate in the synthesis of antibodies; they are provided by the immunizing drug. Because of this, however, immunity acquired in this way generally lasts for a much shorter time than that produced by active immunization, persisting only until the injected immunoglobulins are removed from the person's immune system by the **reticuloendothelial system.** The reticuloendothelial system is composed of specialized cells in the liver, spleen, lymphatics, and bone marrow.

Indications

Vaccines and toxoids are the active immunizing drugs that have been developed for the prevention of many illnesses caused by bacteria and their toxins, as well as those caused by various viruses. Antivenins, antitoxins, and immunoglobulins comprise the passive immunizing drugs. Such drugs can inactivate spider and snake venom, bacterial toxins (exotoxins), and potentially lethal viruses. Box 46-1 lists the currently available immunizing drugs. The successful immunization of 95% or more of a population confers protection on the entire population. This is called **herd immunity.**

Antivenins, also known as *antisera,* are used to prevent or minimize the effects of poisoning by the venoms of crotalids (rattlesnakes, copperheads, cottonmouths, water moccasins), black widow spiders, and coral snakes, some of which can be lethal. Most healthy adults do not die from the bites of spiders or snakes if they receive prompt and appropriate treatment (i.e., administration of the appropriate antivenin). However, very young children and older persons with health problems are particularly susceptible to the effects of the venom of some of these animals. In either situation, an antivenin is needed to neutralize the venom.

Certain viruses are very potent and even potentially lethal (e.g., hepatitis B virus, rabies virus). As noted earlier, they can do major harm very quickly before the infected person can mount an effective immune response against them. The passive immunization of the person with the appropriate immunoglobulin gives the individual the antibodies needed to fend off the harmful effects of the virus. Immunoglobulins are also available for protection against some bacterial infections (e.g., diphtheria, tetanus). In addition, antitoxins are used to provide active immunity against certain very harmful bacteria such as those that cause diphtheria and tetanus.

Contraindications

Contraindications to the administration of immunizing drugs include drug allergy and may also include allergy to egg products, because some vaccines are derived from such products. In the case of a potentially fatal illness such as rabies, however, the corresponding drugs may still need to be given, depending on the likelihood of actual exposure to the disease-causing organism, and any allergic reaction controlled with other medications. Administration of some immunizing drugs is best deferred until after recovery from a febrile illness or temporary immunocompromised state (e.g., following cancer chemotherapy), if possible. However, this is often a matter of clinical judgment, and the individual patient's condition and risk factors for serious illness may be arguments for or against administration of a given immunizing drug at a given time.

Adverse Effects

The undesirable effects of the various immunizing drugs can range from mild and transient to more serious and even life threatening. These are listed in Table 46-2. The minor reactions can be treated with acetaminophen and rest. More severe reactions, such as fever higher than 103° F (39.4° C), should be treated with acetaminophen and sponge baths. Serum sickness sometimes occurs after repeated injections of equine-derived immunizing drugs. The signs and symptoms consist of edema of the face, tongue, and throat; rash; urticaria; arthritis; adenopathy; fever; flushing; itching; cough; dyspnea; cyanosis; vomiting; and cardiovascular collapse. Serum sickness is best treated with analgesics, antihistamines, epinephrine, and/or corticosteroids. In these cases hospitalization may be required.

Any serious or unusual reactions to immunizing drugs should be reported to the Vaccine Adverse Event Reporting System (VAERS). This is a national vaccine safety surveillance program that is cosponsored by the Food and Drug Administration (FDA) and CDC. A report can be submitted via a toll-free telephone number: 1-800-822-7967. Alternatively, a reporting form can be printed from the websites of both the

FDA (www.fda.gov) and CDC (www.cdc.gov). These websites have extensive information describing this reporting system and the data collected by it. Such data are used to improve the quality of immunizing drugs and can even be grounds for an FDA recall of biologic drugs whose adverse effects exceed acceptable safety thresholds.

In the early 1980s, in response to vaccine-related injuries, many parents became reluctant to immunize their children against common, and even potentially fatal, childhood illnesses. Increasing numbers of legal actions were also brought by parents of injured children. In 1986, the U.S. Congress passed the Childhood Vaccine Injury Act, which in turn established the National Vaccine Injury Compensation Program (VICP). The purpose was to create a no-fault alternative to the civil tort system, which had driven many vaccine manufacturers out of the field. Serious adverse events following vaccination are very uncommon. The 2005 Vaccine Injury Table published by the Health Resources and Services Administration (Table 46-3) itemizes serious adverse events reported for vaccines that are covered under the VICP, as well as the expected time frame for such events to occur. Injured parties may file claims for VICP compensation. There has been recent controversy in the national news pertaining to an advertisement that appeared in *USA Today* linking immunizations to autism in children. The CDC, in a statement released April 6, 2006, challenged the advertisement as scientifically unsound, although it sympathized with the parents of autistic children.

Interactions

Drug interactions are not generally a problem with the majority of immunizing drugs. This is likely due partly to the fact that immunizing drugs are normally given in a single dose or a relatively small number of doses. One drug class of note that can potentially reduce the efficacy of immunizing drugs is immunosuppressive drugs such as corticosteroids, transplant antirejection drugs, and cancer chemotherapy drugs. All of these can hinder, to varying degrees, the generation of active immunity that would normally occur following vaccine or toxoid administration. The BCG (bacillus Calmette-Guérin) vaccine for tuberculosis (used mostly outside the United States in developing countries) can cause false-positive results on the tuberculin skin test (Chapter 40). Some vaccines should not be given in close temporal proximity. For example, the meningococcal vaccine, whole-cell pertussis vaccine, and typhoid vaccine together have an undesirably large bacterial endotoxin content and should not be administered simultaneously. The effectiveness of measles, mumps, and rubella vaccines may be reduced by concurrent interferon therapy. Influenza vaccine may also theoretically lose efficacy if given while antiviral influenza drugs are being taken (Chapter 39). Recommendations are to give the influenza vaccine at least 48 hours after stopping such antiviral drug therapy. In general, immunizations requiring intramuscular injection should be given with particular caution (and with appropriate monitoring) to patients receiving anticoagulant drugs such as warfarin (Chapter 27). The nurse should review the package insert for any immunizing drugs given to obtain the latest information and identify other specific drug interactions that may occur. Hepatitis B immunoglobulin interacts with live vaccines; administration of such vaccines should be deferred until 3 months after the dose of immunoglobulin is given.

Table 46-2	Immunizing Drugs: Minor and Severe Adverse Effects
Body System	**Adverse Effects**
Minor Effects	
Central nervous	Fever, adenopathy
Integumentary	Minor rash, soreness at injection site, urticaria, arthritis
Severe Effects	
Central nervous	Fever higher than 103° F (39.4° C), encephalitis, convulsions, peripheral neuropathy, anaphylactic reaction, shock, unconsciousness
Integumentary	Urticaria, rash
Respiratory	Dyspnea
Other	Cyanosis

Table 46-3 Vaccine Injury Table

Vaccine	Adverse Event	Time Interval
Tetanus toxoid–containing vaccines (e.g., DTaP, Tdap, DTP-Hib, DT, Td, TT)	Anaphylaxis or anaphylactic shock	0-4 hr
	Brachial neuritis	2-28 days
	Any acute complication or sequela (including death) of above events	NA
Pertussis antigen–containing vaccines (e.g., DTaP, Tdap, DTP, P, DTP-Hib)	Anaphylaxis or anaphylactic shock	0-4 hr
	Encephalopathy (or encephalitis)	0-72 hr
	Any acute complication or sequela (including death) of above events	NA
Measles, mumps, and rubella virus–containing vaccines in any combination (e.g., MMR, MR, M, R)	Anaphylaxis or anaphylactic shock	0-4 hr
	Encephalopathy (or encephalitis)	5-15 days
	Any acute complication or sequela (including death) of above events	NA
Rubella virus–containing vaccines (e.g., MMR, MR, R)	Chronic arthritis	7-42 days
	Any acute complication or sequela (including death) of above event	NA
Measles virus–containing vaccines (e.g., MMR, MR, M)	Thrombocytopenic purpura	7-30 days
	Vaccine-strain measles viral infection in an immunodeficient recipient	0-6 mo
	Any acute complication or sequela (including death) of above events	NA
Polio live virus–containing vaccines (OPV)	Paralytic polio	
	In a nonimmunodeficient recipient	0-30 days
	In an immunodeficient recipient	0-6 mo
	In a vaccine-associated community case	NA
	Vaccine-strain polio viral infection	
	In a nonimmunodeficient recipient	0-30 days
	In an immunodeficient recipient	0-6 mo
	In a vaccine-associated community case	NA
	Any acute complication or sequela (including death) of above events	NA
Polio inactivated virus–containing vaccines (e.g., IPV)	Anaphylaxis or anaphylactic shock	0-4 hr
	Any acute complication or sequela (including death) of above event	NA
Hepatitis B antigen–containing vaccines	Anaphylaxis or anaphylactic shock	0-4 hr
	Any acute complication or sequela (including death) of above event	NA
Haemophilus influenzae type b polysaccharide conjugate vaccines	No condition specified for compensation	NA
Varicella vaccine	No condition specified for compensation	NA
Rotavirus vaccine	No condition specified for compensation	NA
Vaccines containing live, oral, rhesus-based rotavirus	Intussusception	0-30 days
	Any acute complication or sequela (including death) of above event	NA
Pneumococcal conjugate vaccines	No condition specified for compensation	NA
Any new vaccine recommended by the Centers for Disease Control and Prevention for routine administration to children, after publication by the Secretary of DHHS of a notice of coverage*	No condition specified for compensation	NA

From Health Resources and Services Administration: *National Vaccine Injury Compensation Program fact sheet,* Atlanta, 2005, The Administration.
DHHS, Department of Health and Human Services; *DT,* diphtheria and tetanus vaccine; *DTaP,* diphtheria, tetanus, and acellular pertussis vaccine; *DTP,* diphtheria, tetanus, and pertussis vaccine; *Hib, Haemophilus influenzae* type b conjugate vaccine; *IPV,* inactivated poliovirus; *M,* measles vaccine; *MMR,* measles, mumps, and rubella vaccine; *MR,* measles and rubella vaccine; *NA,* not applicable; *OPV,* oral polio vaccine; *P,* pertussis vaccine; *R,* rubella vaccine; *Td,* tetanus and diphtheria toxoids; *Tdap,* tetanus and diphtheria toxoids and acellular pertussis vaccine; *TT,* tetanus toxoid.
*As of December 1, 2004, hepatitis A vaccines have been added to the Vaccine Injury Table under this category. As of July 1, 2005, *trivalent* influenza vaccines have been added to the table under this category. Trivalent influenza vaccines are given annually during the flu season either by needle and syringe or in a nasal spray. All influenza vaccines routinely administered in the United States are trivalent vaccines covered under this category. See *News* on the Vaccine Injury Compensation Program website for more information. Available at www.hrsa.gov/vaccinecompensation.

Dosages

For the recommended dosages of selected immunizing drugs, see the Dosages table on page 710.

Drug Profiles

Some of the more commonly used vaccines, toxoids, and immunoglobulins are described in the following sections. The immunizing drugs currently available commercially in the United States, including several combination vaccines for prevention of more than one disease, are listed in Box 46-1. Combination vaccines obviously reduce the number of injections that the patient receives, and thus their use is desirable when possible, especially for children.

Active Immunizing Drugs
diphtheria and tetanus toxoids, and acellular pertussis vaccine (adsorbed)

The active immunizing drugs include diphtheria and tetanus toxoids and the acellular pertussis vaccine (adsorbed) (Tripedia, Daptacel, Infanrix). *Adsorption* refers to the laboratory techniques used to make most vaccines and toxoids. The biologic materials (i.e., virus or toxin particles) are adsorbed (separated out of solution and dried) onto carrier media such as alum, from which they are later removed for packaging into final dosage forms. Diphtheria, tetanus, and pertussis are very different disorders, but an injection that combines all three vaccines (DTP; also commonly called DPT) was been routinely given to children since the 1940s. In 1996, a new vaccine combination called diphtheria and tetanus toxoids with *acellular* pertussis vaccine adsorbed (DTaP) was approved for the full childhood immunization series and has replaced DPT. It uses a different form of the pertussis component, known as acellular pertussis. Acellular pertussis consists of only a single weakened toxoid, whereas previous pertussis vaccines contained multiple toxoids. Experts hope that DTaP will prove over time to give rise to fewer adverse effects than DTP, particularly in older patients who are more prone to them, and that this will allow adults to receive a pertussis booster. Currently DTaP is the preferred preparation for primary and booster immunization against these diseases in children 6 weeks to 6 years of age, unless use of the pertussis component is contraindicated.

Tetanus, diphtheria, and pertussis are prevalent in the populations of many developing countries throughout the world, and as a result the risk of contracting one of these diseases may be higher elsewhere than in the United States. Full immunization against these diseases with DTP or DTaP is recommended for travelers to these areas and as well as for their inhabitants. The combination product containing only tetanus and diphtheria toxoids (Td) is administered to persons 7 years of age and older who require a primary or booster immunization against tetanus for routine wound management. Emergency booster doses of Td (for adult use) are unnecessary when the wound is clean and minor (not tetanus prone), provided that the patient has received a primary or booster immunization against tetanus within the previous 10 years.

Pertussis is much less common in children older than 7 years of age and in adults. The combination of tetanus and diphtheria toxoids adsorbed (Td) is generally given to children 7 years of age and older and to adults with functioning immune systems. It promotes immunity to diphtheria and tetanus by inducing the production of specific antitoxins (antibodies to toxin) by the patient's immune system. However, there is recent evidence that pertussis is actually recurring among adults (whose previous vaccine-induced immunity has waned), who in turn are passing it on to their children. In 2004, there were over 18,000 cases of pertussis in the United States, the largest reported number since the late 1950s. For this reason, prescribers may elect to give adults DTaP (described earlier) instead of the more traditional adult drug Td.

These toxoids are obtained from the bacteria *Clostridium tetani* and *Corynebacterium diphtheriae*. To make the drugs, diphtheria and tetanus toxins are taken from these bacteria, attenuated into toxoids, and adsorbed onto plates of carrier media such as aluminum hydroxide, aluminum phosphate, or potassium alum. From these plates of dried toxoid and carrier media, specific quantities are removed and placed in dosing containers to provide toxoids of uniform dose. The process is similar for other toxoids and vaccines. These toxoids (DTP, DTaP, and Td) are available only as parenteral preparations to be given as deep intramuscular injections. Their use is contraindicated in persons who have had a prior systemic hypersensitivity reaction or a neurologic reaction to one of the ingredients. Some manufacturers state that use is contraindicated in cases of concurrent acute or active infections but not in cases of minor illness. Although there have been very few, if any, studies documenting the safety of their use in pregnant women, it is generally considered safe to give diphtheria, tetanus, and pertussis toxoids after the first trimester.

Haemophilus Influenzae Type b conjugate vaccine

Haemophilus influenzae type b (Hib) (HibTITER, ActHIB, Liquid Pedvax HIB) vaccine is a noninfectious, bacteria-derived vaccine. It is made by extracting *H. influenzae* particles that are antigenic (cause an antigen-antibody reaction) and chemically attaching these particles to a protein carrier medium for use in injections. The vaccine is given by injection to adults and children considered at high risk for acquiring *H. influenzae* infection. Conditions that may predispose an individual to Hib infection are septicemia, pneumonia, cellulitis, arthritis, osteomyelitis, pericarditis, sickle cell anemia, an immunodeficiency syndrome, or Hodgkin's disease. Before this vaccine was developed, infections caused by Hib were the leading cause of bacterial meningitis in children 3 months to 5 years of age, and this bacterium can also cause several other serious infections in children and adults. This form of bacterial meningitis has a mortality rate of 5% to 10%. Of those who survive, 20% to 45% suffer serious morbidity in the form of neurologic deficits. All Hib vaccine products are parenteral formulations that are administered intramuscularly.

▶ hepatitis B virus vaccine (inactivated)

Hepatitis B virus vaccine inactivated (Recombivax HB, Engerix-B) is a noninfectious viral vaccine containing hepatitis B surface antigen (HBsAg). It is made from viral particles and yeast using **recombinant** deoxyribonucleic acid (DNA) technology. In this technique, DNA from two or more organisms is combined. Yeast cells then produces this viral antigenic substance in mass quantities. The substance is then attached to a carrier medium (alum) and made into a vaccine injection preparation. This antigenic HBsAg is used to promote active immunity to hepatitis B infection in persons considered at high risk for potential exposure to the hepatitis B virus or HBsAg-positive materials (e.g., blood, plasma, serum). Health care workers, for example, are persons considered at high risk.

Use of the vaccine is contraindicated in persons who are hypersensitive to yeast. Pregnancy is not considered a contraindication to use. The potential for exposure of a pregnant woman to hepatitis B virus and the potential for the development of chronic infection in the neonate are both good reasons to give the vaccine. The vaccine is administered by intramuscular injection. There are three main formulations designed for three different populations: a pediatric formulation for neonates, infants, children, and adolescents; an adult formulation for persons older than 20 years of age; and a dialysis formulation for predialysis and dialysis patients or for other immunocompromised individuals.

▶ influenza virus vaccine

The influenza virus vaccine (Fluzone, Fluvirin, FluMist) is the vaccine used to prevent influenza. Each year before the influenza season begins this vaccine should be administered to persons at high risk of contracting influenza. Such inoculation is the single most important influenza control measure.

Each year a new influenza vaccine is developed by virology researchers. It usually contains three different influenza virus strains (usually two type A and one type B strain). These strains are chosen from among the hundreds of influenza virus strains in the environ-

DOSAGES

Selected Immunizing Drugs

Drug (Pregnancy Category)	Pharmacologic Class	Usual Dosage Range*	Indications
Active Immunizing Drugs			
diphtheria, tetanus, and acellular pertussis (DTaP) (pediatric only)	Mixed toxoid/vaccine	**Pediatric only** IM: Series of three 0.5-mL injections; age of first injection 6 wk-7 yr; give second and third doses at 4-8 wk intervals	Prophylaxis against diphtheria, tetanus, and pertussis
Haemophilus influenzae type b conjugate vaccine (HibTITER) (C)	Bacterial capsular antigenic extract vaccine	**Pediatric** **Infant 2-6 mo** Give three IM injections (0.5 mL each) about 2 mo apart **Previously unvaccinated child 7-11 mo** Give two IM injections about 2 mo apart **Previously unvaccinated child 12-14 mo** Give only one IM injection	*H. influenzae* type b prophylaxis
▶hepatitis B virus vaccine, recombinant (Recombivax HB) (C)	Viral surface antigen	**Pediatric to age 10 yr** IM: 5 mcg (0.5 mL) at birth, then again at 1 mo and 6 mo **Adult** IM: Three 10 mcg (1 mL) doses: day 0, 1 mo, and 6 mo	Hepatitis B virus prophylaxis
▶influenza virus vaccine (Fluzone, FluShield, Fluvirin) (C)	Viral surface antigen	**Pediatric 6 mo-9 yr** IM: Single yearly dose (two doses of 0.25 mL at least 1 mo apart if receiving influenza vaccine for first time) **Adult** IM: Single yearly dose (0.5 mL)	Influenza prophylaxis
▶measles, mumps, and rubella virus vaccine, live (MMR II)	Live, attenuated viral vaccine	**Adult and pediatric older than 12 mo** SC: 0.5-mL single dose; booster recommended for children entering middle or high school	Prophylaxis against measles, mumps, and rubella
▶pneumococcal vaccine, polyvalent (Pneumovax 23) (C)	Bacterial capsular antigenic extract vaccine	**Adult and pediatric 2 yr and older** SC: 0.5 mL × 1	*Streptococcus pneumoniae* prophylaxis
▶poliovirus vaccine, inactivated (IPOL) (C)	Inactivated viral vaccine	**Pediatric (infant)** SC: Three 0.5-mL doses: 4-8 wk, 2-4 mo, and 6-12 mo **Adult** SC: Two 0.5-mL doses 1-2 mo apart, then a third dose 6-12 mo later	Polio prophylaxis
rabies virus vaccine (Imovax, RabAvert) (C)	Inactivated viral vaccine	**Adult and pediatric** *Postexposure prophylaxis* IM: 1 mL on days 0, 3, 7, 14, and 28 (with one dose of rabies immunoglobulin [see later] within 8 days of first vaccine dose) *Preexposure prophylaxis for those at high risk for rabies exposure (e.g., veterinarians)* IM/ID: 1 mL IM or 0.1 mL ID on days 0, 7, and once between days 21 and 28, for a total of three doses; then q2-5yr, depending on antibody titers	Rabies prophylaxis
tetanus and diphtheria toxoids, adsorbed (Td), pediatric and adult (C)	Mixed toxoid	**Adult and unvaccinated pediatric older than 7 yr** IM: 0.5 mL on day 0; second dose 4-8 wk later; third dose 6-12 mo later	Prophylaxis against diphtheria and tetanus
▶varicella virus vaccine (Varivax) (C)	Live, attenuated viral vaccine	**Adult and pediatric older than 12 yr** SC: Two 0.5-mL doses given 4-8 wk apart **Pediatric 1-12 yr** SC: One 0.5-mL dose	Prophylaxis against varicella virus (causes chickenpox and shingles)

ID, Intradermal; *IM,* intramuscular; *SC,* subcutaneous.

*NOTE: Dosages given are only for brands listed. Dosing amounts and regimens may vary for different brands. The user should always follow manufacturer's current dosing directions.

DOSAGES

Selected Immunizing Drugs—cont'd

Drug (Pregnancy Category)	Pharmacologic Class	Usual Dosage Range*	Indications
Passive Immunizing Drugs			
▶hepatitis B immunoglobulin (BayHep B, Nabi-HB) (C)	Pooled human immunoglobulin	**Infant (of mother known to be hepatitis B positive)** IM: 0.5 mL within 12 hr after birth **Adult** IM: 0.06 mg/kg after exposure and 30 days later	Passive hepatitis B prophylaxis
▶immunoglobulin intravenous (Gammar-P IV, Panglobulin NF, others) (C)	Pooled human immunoglobulin	Dosages vary widely; refer to manufacturer's current dosage information for specific indications	Therapy for many disorders, including primary immune deficiency syndrome, pediatric AIDS, idiopathic thrombocytopenic purpura, B-cell lymphocytic leukemia
rabies immunoglobulin (Imogam Rabies-HT, BayRab) (C)	Pooled human immunoglobulin	**Adult and pediatric** Single dose of 20 international units/kg; infiltrate as much of dose as possible into bite wound area and give remainder IM in gluteal region; do not give into same site as rabies vaccine	Rabies prophylaxis
Rh$_0$(D) immunoglobulin (RhoGAM, MICRhoGAM) (C)	Immunosuppressant globulin	**Adult female** IM (full dose): Inject total contents of a single vial within 72 hr after delivery IM (microdose): Inject full contents of a single vial after spontaneous or elective abortion of pregnancy of 12 wk gestation or less	Postpartum antibody suppression to prevent hemolytic disease of future newborns
tetanus immunoglobulin (BayTet) (C)	Pooled human immunoglobulin	**Adult and pediatric** IM: 250 units as a single dose IM: 3000-6000 units as a single dose	Postexposure tetanus prophylaxis Tetanus treatment

AIDS, Acquired immunodeficiency syndrome.

ment based on the latest epidemiologic data indicating which influenza viruses will most likely circulate in North America in the upcoming winter. The vaccine is made from highly purified, egg-grown viruses that have been rendered noninfectious (inactivated). Influenza is characterized by abrupt onset of fever, myalgia, sore throat, and nonproductive cough. Severe malaise may last several days. More severe illness can occur in certain populations. Older individuals, children, and adults with underlying serious health problems (e.g., HIV infection, asthma, cardiopulmonary disease, cancer, diabetes) are at increased risk for complications from influenza infection. Health care personnel are also considered a high-risk group. If such individuals become ill with influenza, they are more likely than the general population to require hospitalization. Health care personnel are also considered a high-risk group. Increased mortality results not only from influenza and pneumonia but also from cardiopulmonary and other chronic diseases that can be exacerbated by influenza. More than 90% of the deaths attributed to pneumonia and influenza occur among persons 65 years of age or older. Another fairly unusual but important risk group is children and teenagers who are receiving long-term aspirin therapy (e.g., for juvenile arthritis) and who therefore might be at risk for developing Reye's syndrome after influenza (Chapter 44).

The effectiveness of influenza vaccine in preventing illness varies. Factors that may alter its effectiveness are the age and immunocompetence of the vaccine recipient and the degree of similarity between the virus strains included in the vaccine and those that actually predominate during a given influenza season. Healthy persons younger than 65 years of age have a 70% chance of preventing ill-

ness caused by influenza virus when there is a good match between the vaccine and the circulating viruses.

Older persons, especially those residing in nursing homes, can avoid severe illness, secondary complications, and death by taking the influenza vaccine. In frail older persons, the vaccine can prevent hospitalization and pneumonia up to 50% to 60% of the time and death up to 80% of the time. Achieving a high rate of vaccination among nursing home residents can reduce the spread of infection in a facility, thus preventing disease through herd immunity.

▶ *measles, mumps, and rubella virus vaccine (live)*

The measles, mumps, and rubella vaccine (MMR II) is a virus preparation consisting of live measles, mumps, and rubella viruses that are weakened (attenuated). The vaccine promotes active immunity to these diseases by inducing the production of virus-specific immunoglobulin G and immunoglobulin M antibodies. The antibody response to initial vaccination resembles that caused by primary natural infection.

Administration of the measles vaccine or any of the combination products that includes the measles virus is contraindicated in persons with a history of anaphylactic or anaphylactoid reaction, or some other immediate reaction to egg ingestion. Use of these products is also contraindicated in persons who have had an anaphylactic reaction to topically or systemically administered neomycin, because this antibiotic is used as a preservative in some of the vaccine preparations. These vaccines should not be administered to pregnant women, and pregnancy should be avoided for 3 months after measles virus vaccination and 30 days after vaccination with a rubella-containing (measles-rubella [MR] or MMR) measles virus vaccine. This precaution is based on the theoretic risk that the live virus vaccine may cause a fetal infection.

▶ *pneumococcal vaccine, polyvalent and seven-valent*

Two forms of vaccine against pneumococcal pneumonia are available that also protect against any illness caused by *Streptococcus pneumoniae*. *Pneumococcus* is the common name for the bacterium *S. pneumoniae*, the causative organism of this common bacterial infection. The polyvalent type of vaccine (Pneumovax 23) is used primarily in adults. (The term *polyvalent* refers to the fact that the vaccine is designed to be effective against the 23 strains of pneumococcus most commonly implicated in adult cases of pneumonia.) This vaccine also may sometimes be recommended for pediatric patients at higher risk for pneumonia as a result of serious chronic illnesses, especially those who are immunocompromised. However, the seven-valent vaccine is the pneumococcal vaccine that is routinely recommended for children. Its official full name is seven-valent conjugate vaccine (diphtheria CRM197 protein, or Prevnar), and it is made using a special type of protein isolated from *C. diphtheriae*, the bacterium that causes diphtheria. The name *seven-valent* refers to the fact that the vaccine is designed to immunize against the top seven pneumococcal strains found in pediatric pneumonia cases. Contraindications to the use of either vaccine include known drug allergy to components of the vaccine itself, as well as the presence of current significant febrile illness or immunosuppressed state as a result of drug therapy (e.g., cancer chemotherapy). The vaccine may sometimes still be given in such cases, if it is felt that withholding the vaccine poses an even greater risk to the patient.

▶ *poliovirus vaccine (inactivated)*

The use of live oral polio vaccine (OPV) is no longer routine in the United States, due to case reports of vaccine-acquired polio. Since 1979 the only indigenous cases of poliomyelitis reported in the United States (44 cases) have been associated with use of the live OPV. Injected doses of inactivated polio vaccine (IPV) (brand name of IPOL) are instead recommended for routine use. The use of OPV should be reserved for the following groups: populations that are the target of mass vaccination campaigns to control outbreaks of paralytic polio, unvaccinated children who will be traveling in fewer than 4 weeks to areas in which polio is endemic, and children of parents who object to the recommended number of IPV injections.

rabies virus vaccine

Although vaccination against the rabies virus is not normally a routine immunization, situations requiring it do occur periodically in many practice settings. Rabies virus vaccine (Imovax, RabAvert) is produced using laboratory techniques involving infected human cell cultures and selected antimicrobial drugs. Rabies is a virus that can infect a variety of mammals, including skunks, foxes, raccoons, bats, dogs, and cats. The virus is usually transferred to humans by an animal bite and almost universally causes fatal brain tissue destruction if the patient is not treated with rabies vaccine and immunoglobulin (discussed later). Current recommendations call for a total of five intramuscular injections on days 0, 3, 7, 14, and 28 following an animal bite that raises concern for rabies transmission. This includes bites by any animal whose rabies immunization status is unknown or which escapes and cannot be observed for signs of rabies. This type of treatment is known as *postexposure prophylaxis*. *Preexposure prophylaxis* is recommended for persons at high risk for exposure to the rabies virus (e.g., veterinarians). The preexposure course consists of only three injections on day 0, day 7, and sometime between days 21 and 28. Periodic booster shots are also recommended for such individuals approximately every 2 to 5 years, or based on the levels of the patient's rabies virus antibody titers. Patients who have been previously immunized who have a new bite may need only two booster shots on days 0 and 3. Contraindications to the administration of rabies vaccine include a history of allergic reaction to the vaccine itself or to the drugs neomycin, gentamicin, or amphotericin B. However, given the life-threatening nature of rabies infection, treatment may still be required, with supportive therapy (e.g., epinephrine, diphenhydramine, corticosteroids) provided to minimize allergic reactions.

Patients with any kind of febrile illness should delay occupational preexposure prophylaxis treatment until the illness has subsided.

▶ *varicella virus vaccine*

The live attenuated varicella virus vaccine (Varivax) is used to prevent varicella (chickenpox) and herpes zoster (shingles). Varicella primarily occurs in children younger than 8 years of age or in individuals with compromised immune systems such as elderly or HIV-infected patients. It is estimated that only 10% of children older than 12 years of age are still susceptible to varicella. Only 2% of adults develop varicella virus infections. However, 50% of the deaths associated with varicella infections are in adults. Half of these are in immunocompromised patients.

The virus in varicella vaccine is attenuated by the passage of virus particles through human and embryonic guinea pig cell cultures. Varicella vaccine must be stored in a freezer. It should not be given to immunodeficient patients or to patients who have received high doses of systemic steroids in the previous month. It is also recommended that salicylates be avoided for 6 weeks after administration of varicella vaccine because of the possibility of Reye's syndrome (Chapter 44).

Passive Immunizing Drugs

The currently available antivenins, antitoxins, and immunoglobulins that comprise the passive immunizing drugs are listed in Box 46-1. Those that are more commonly used are described in the following profiles.

▶ *hepatitis B immunoglobulin*

Hepatitis B immunoglobulin (BayHep B, Nabi-HB) is used to provide passive immunity against hepatitis B infection in the postexposure prophylaxis and treatment of persons exposed to hepatitis B virus or HBsAg-positive materials (e.g., blood, plasma, serum). It is prepared from the plasma of human donors with high titers of antibodies to HBsAg. All donors are tested for HIV antibodies to prevent HIV transmission.

Because of the possible devastating consequences of hepatitis B infection, pregnancy is not considered a contraindication to the use of hepatitis B immunoglobulin when there is a clear need for it.

▶ *immunoglobulin*

Immunoglobulin (BayGam, Octagam) is available in both intramuscular and intravenous dosage forms. It provides passive immunity by increasing antibody titer and antigen-antibody reaction potential. Immunoglobulins are given to help prevent certain infectious diseases in susceptible persons or to ameliorate the diseases in those already infected. Immunoglobulins are pooled from the blood of at least 1000 human donors. This plasma is prepared by cold alcohol fractionation and usually washed with a detergent to destroy any harmful viruses, such as hepatitis virus or HIV. There are many FDA-approved and non–FDA-approved uses for immunoglobulins; the approved uses are listed in Box 46-2. In recent years there has been a shortage of immunoglobulin products. The supply of these drugs is dependent on donors. Because of fluctuations in supply and the unfavorable risk-benefit ratio of using products derived from human donors, product

---

Box 46-2 Current FDA-Approved Uses of Immunoglobulins*

Pediatric HIV infection
B-cell chronic lymphocytic leukemia
Bone marrow transplantation
Hepatitis A
Idiopathic thrombocytopenic purpura
Kawasaki's disease
Immunoglobulin deficiencies
Measles
Primary immunodeficiency diseases
Rubella .
Varicella

FDA, Food and Drug Administration; *HIV*, human immunodeficiency virus.
*Approved routes of administration are intramuscular and intravenous.

insurers have restricted reimbursement to force practitioners to administer the drug for FDA-approved indications only. "Off-label" or non–FDA-approved uses have been severely curtailed because of such restrictions as well as because of product shortages.

$Rh_0(D)$ immunoglobulin

$Rh_0(D)$ immunoglobulin (RhoGam, WinRho) is used to suppress the active antibody response and the formation of anti-$Rh_0(D)$ antibodies in an $Rh_0(D)$-negative person exposed to Rh-positive blood. Because an $Rh_0(D)$-negative person reacts to Rh-positive blood as if it were a foreign, "nonself" substance, an immune response develops against it and an antigen-antibody reaction occurs. This reaction can be fatal. The administration of this immunoglobulin helps to prevent the reaction and hence this dire outcome. The most common use of this product is in cases of maternal-fetal Rh incompatibility (postpartum). Only the mother is normally dosed, and the treatment objective is to prevent a harmful maternal immune response to a fetus during a future pregnancy should an Rh-negative mother become pregnant with an Rh-positive child.

$Rh_0(D)$ immunoglobulin is prepared from the plasma or serum of adults with a high titer of anti-$Rh_0(D)$ antibody to the red blood cell antigen $Rh_0(D)$. Administration of this immunoglobulin is contraindicated in persons who have been previously immunized with this drug and in $Rh_0(D)$-positive/Du-positive patients. It is normally given postpartum but is rated as a pregnancy category C drug.

rabies immunoglobulin

Rabies immunoglobulin (BayRab, Imogam Rabies-HT) is a passive immunizing drug that is used concurrently with rabies virus vaccine following suspected exposure to the rabies virus. In humans this usually occurs following an animal bite. Rabies immunoglobulin is derived from human cells that are harvested from persons who have been immunized with rabies vaccine. The only contraindication to its use is drug allergy, although an allergic patient may still need to be dosed rather than face infection with the almost universally fatal rabies virus. The decision to dose a patient in such a case is based on the probability of rabies infection given the particular circumstances surrounding the animal bite.

tetanus immunoglobulin

Tetanus immunoglobulin (BayTet) is a passive immunizing drug effective against tetanus. It contains tetanus antitoxin antibodies that neutralize the bacterial exotoxin produced by *C. tetani*, the bacterium that causes tetanus. Tetanus immunoglobulin is prepared from the plasma of adults hyperimmunized with the tetanus toxoid and is given as prophylaxis to persons with tetanus-prone wounds. It may also be used to treat active tetanus.

varicella-zoster immunoglobulin

Varicella-zoster immunoglobulin (VZIG; available only in generic form from the American Red Cross) can be used to modify or prevent chickenpox in susceptible individuals who have had recent significant exposure to the disease. VZIG should be administered within 96 hours of exposure. Candidates for therapy with VZIG are those at high risk of serious disease or complications if they become infected with the varicella-zoster virus (VZV). Two examples are newborn children, including premature infants with significant exposure, and immunocompromised adults. Healthy adults, including pregnant women, should be evaluated on a case-by-case basis. The duration of protection against infection provided by VZIG is at least 3 weeks. VZIG is prepared from the plasma of normal blood donors with high antibody titers to VZV. It is important that VZIG be given within 96 hours of exposure, preferably as soon as possible.

BIOLOGIC AND CHEMICAL TERRORISM

At the time of this writing there is heightened concern on the part of many governments regarding the potential use of infectious or otherwise toxic agents as weapons against human populations. A terrorist attack involving the use of pathogenic microorganisms or other biologic agents is referred to as **bioterrorism,** whereas an attack in which harmful chemical agents are used is called *chemical terrorism.* In June of 2002, President George W. Bush signed into law the Public Health Security and Bioterrorism Preparedness and Response Act (the Bioterrorism Act). This legislation marked the official beginning of the President's Countering Bioterrorism Initiative, which attempts to address this issue proactively as a matter of public health. The Center for Biologics Evaluation (CBER), a branch of the FDA, is an important participant in this public health initiative. Recent CBER activities include the funding of rapid development by private industry of new vaccines for the prevention of anthrax and smallpox (prepared from vaccinia virus, as mentioned earlier), as well as vaccinia immunoglobulin, to prepare for possible bioterrorist attack using these infectious organisms. Although smallpox vaccine is no longer routinely administered in the United States, supplies are maintained by the CDC in the event of a smallpox bioterrorist attack. The Department of Defense currently owns all lots of anthrax vaccine produced in the United States. Although the CDC does not currently recommend public inoculation with the anthrax vaccine, it is administered prophylactically to military personnel considered to be at higher risk of anthrax exposure because of the location and nature of their assigned duties. The Environmental Health Laboratory of the CDC's Division of Laboratory Science oversees planned responses to chemical terrorist attacks. One of its newest developments is the Rapid Toxic Screen. This laboratory test is able to analyze the blood and/or urine of multiple patients to detect 150 chemicals that could potentially be used in a terrorist attack in order to confirm exposure and direct treatment decisions. Tables 46-4 and 46-5 provide examples of microorganisms and chemical agents, respectively, believed potentially likely to be used in a terrorist attack. The chemical agents listed all have a history of prior military use. Because a small-scale attack with anthrax has already occurred in the United States, this disease is also discussed in more detail in the following section.

ANTHRAX

In October of 2001, the month following the September 11 terrorist attacks, six U.S. Postal Service workers were infected with anthrax from contaminated mail. Two of them did not survive. Anthrax is a bacterial infectious disease caused by spores of the bacterium *Bacillus anthracis.* In humans infection can occur via three routes of exposure: skin (20% mortality), gastrointestinal tract (25% to 75% mortality), and inhalation (80% or higher mortality). Antibiotics such as the fluoroquinolone ciprofloxacin are used to treat more severe cases (i.e., the inhalational form). Milder cases (i.e., cutaneous and gastrointestinal forms) are often treated with the tetracycline antibiotic doxycycline. The vaccine is developed from an attenuated strain of *B. anthracis.* It has a calculated efficacy level of 92.5% for protection against anthrax infection. Anthrax vaccination is recommended not only for selected military personnel, as mentioned earlier, but also for others considered to be at higher than average risk for exposure to the bacterium. Included are veterinarians and others who handle potentially infected animals as well as workers who process imported animal hair, which is used to manufacture various commercial products.

Table 46-4   Illnesses Caused by CDC Category "A" Possible Bioterrorism Agents*

Name of Illness	Causative Organism	Clinical Presentation	Prevention/Treatment
Anthrax	Bacterium: *Bacillus anthracis*	Inhalational form most severe and can lead to potentially fatal bacteremia	Vaccine available; treatable with antibiotics such as ciprofloxacin and dicloxacillin
Smallpox	Virus: vaccinia	Flulike symptoms followed by total-body disfiguring rash	Vaccine available and may be effective up to 3 days after exposure; antiviral drug cidofovir possibly effective
Botulism	Bacterium: *Clostridium botulinum*	Visual changes; dry mouth; muscle weakness; progressive downward paralysis, including paralysis of diaphragm	Vaccine available only for highly exposed persons; antitoxin effective if given early in disease; immunoglobulin also now available; antibiotics of no benefit
Tularemia	Bacterium: *Francisella tularensis*	Severe, potentially life-threatening respiratory illness	Vaccine still under review by FDA; treatable with antibiotics such as tetracycline and ciprofloxacin
Viral hemorrhagic fever	Viruses: several viral causes, including Ebola, Marburg, and Lassa viruses, yellow fever virus, Argentine hemorrhagic fever virus	Bleeding from body orifices and in internal organs in severe cases; possible renal failure and coma	No vaccines except for yellow fever virus and Argentine hemorrhagic fever virus; no current treatment other than supportive care; prevention focuses on rodent control
Plague	Bacterium: *Yersinia pestis*	Can occur in lungs (pneumonic plague), skin (bubonic plague—most common), or blood (septicemic plague) Death possible from respiratory failure and shock	No vaccine currently available in U.S.; antibiotics best if given within 24 hr and include gentamicin and tetracycline

Data from U.S. Agency for Healthcare Research and Quality and University of Alabama School of Medicine: CDC category "A" high-priority biological diseases. Available at www.bioterrorism.uab.edu.
CDC, Centers for Disease Control and Prevention; *FDA,* Food and Drug Administration.
*Classified as "high-priority" biologic diseases by the CDC.

Table 46-5   Possible Chemical Terrorism Agents

Agent (Classification)	Effects	Treatment
Sarin (nerve gas)	Headache, runny nose, difficulty breathing, seizures	Remove from area; provide supportive care (e.g., mechanical ventilation). Specific antidote drugs include atropine, pralidoxime, and pyridostigmine. FDA approved special pediatric atropine dosage forms in 2003.
Mustard (blistering agent)	Skin burns, pulmonary edema, ocular damage	Rinse copiously with water; remove contaminated clothing; provide airway support as needed. FDA approved special skin lotion in 2003.
Cyanide (blood agent)	Seizures, gastrointestinal hemorrhage, respiratory arrest	Remove from area; provide airway support. Specific antidote drug therapy includes the chemicals amyl nitrite (by inhalation), and sodium nitrite and sodium thiosulfate (both by injection).
Chlorine (choking agent)	Eye and respiratory irritation; pulmonary edema	Remove from area; remove contaminated clothing; provide airway support.
Radioactive elements	DNA mutations, tissue fibrosis, vascular insufficiency, bone marrow toxicity, organ failure, pneumonitis, enteritis	Several chelating drugs are used to facilitate bodily excretion of various radioactive elements. For example, in 2004, FDA approved two new drugs (pentetate calcium trisodium and pentetate zinc trisodium) for internal decontamination of various radioactive elements (plutonium, americium, curium).
Ricin (byproduct of processing castor beans for production of castor oil)	Respiratory failure, seizures, fever, cough, diarrhea	Remove from exposure; remove and dispose of contaminated clothing; provide supportive care as needed (e.g., mechanical ventilation, IV hydration).

DNA, Deoxyribonucleic acid; *FDA,* Food and Drug Administration.

◆ NURSING PROCESS

✦ ASSESSMENT

Before administering a toxoid or vaccine, the nurse should gather complete information about the patient's health history, including medications taken, present and past health status, previous reactions and responses to these types of drugs, previous allergy test results, use of any immunosuppressants, presence of autoimmune or immunosuppressive diseases or infections, pregnancy and lactation status, and any unusual reaction to other drugs, food, or other substances. When children are to receive a vaccine or toxoid, the immunization schedule and the dose ordered by the physician must be followed. The Department of Health and Human Services, and specifically the CDC, provide the latest recommendations for adult and pediatric immunizations in the United States. These recommendations are easily accessible on the Internet at www.cdc.gov and should be referred to and kept close at hand in any facility that administers these drugs. It is crucial for the nurse to stay current on immunization cautions and contraindications; this website and other published materials from the CDC on immunization are an important source of information.

Because passive immunizing drugs may precipitate serum sickness, elderly patients and those who have chronic illnesses or are debilitated must be assessed carefully before treatment (i.e., vital signs measured, intake and output recorded, and electrocardiogram and baseline assessment performed). Contraindications, cautions, and drug interactions have been thoroughly discussed in the pharmacology section of this chapter, but the need for special care when these drugs are considered for patients who have active infections or who may be immunocompromised should be reiterated.

Contraindications, cautions, and drug interactions for active immunizing drugs have also been discussed, but it is important to reemphasize the concerns regarding the use of these drugs in pregnant patients and patients with current infections (especially infections caused by the same pathogen or by organisms producing the same toxin), severe febrile illnesses (which exclude minor illnesses such as a cold, mild infection, ear infection, or low-grade fever), or a history of reactions or serious adverse effects to the drug. Patients who are already immunosuppressed (e.g., those with AIDS, elderly patients, those with chronic diseases or cancer, neonates) are at increased risk for serious adverse effects to toxoids or vaccines; therefore, cautious use of these drugs is indicated in such patients. Many adults assume that the vaccines they received as children will protect them for a lifetime. This is usually the case. However, some adults were never vaccinated as children, or newer vaccines were not available at the time they were vaccinated. In addition, immunity may fade over time, and as individuals, age they may become more susceptible to serious diseases caused by common infections such as pneumococcus infection.

Bioterrorism (and chemical terrorism) is unfortunately a reality in today's society. The nurse's role may range from contributing significantly during preparations for a biologic terrorist attack after a warning has been issued or performing triage and carrying out the nursing process during such an attack. The nurse's role may also include assessing individuals, groups, and communities and providing related education to help people understand the benefits of being informed, making plans, and maintaining a state of preparation at all times insofar as is possible. Cultural background, knowledge and educational levels, age, motor skills, cognitive abilities, awareness of extended family members and their level of preparedness, and ability to manage stress and to think during a crisis are just a few of the areas worthy of assessment in relation to bioterrorism. Nurses also have a responsibility to ensure that, regardless of the situation, they maintain a calm, reassuring, compassionate, caring, and empathic manner during the assessment phase (and all other phases of the nursing process) in the care of those in need and avoid excessively anxiety-provoking comments or actions. Just discussing the topic of terrorism or bioterrorism can evoke fear and other emotions in individuals, and so questioning and assessment must be conducted in manner that is calming and provides a sense of control.

✦ NURSING DIAGNOSES

- Risk for injury related to possible adverse effects of or allergic reactions to an immunizing drug
- Acute pain related to local and/or systemic effects of the injection of a toxoid, vaccine, or passive immunizing drug
- Deficient knowledge related to the use of toxoids, vaccines, or passive immunizing drugs
- Anxiety related to suspected risk of bioterrorism

✦ PLANNING

Goals

- Patient states the adverse effects of the medication.
- Patient experiences minimal discomfort stemming from the administration of a toxoid, vaccine, or passive immunizing drug.
- Patient remains compliant with the therapeutic regimen.
- Patient returns for follow-up injections and booster injections and for follow-up visits with the physician.
- Patient states the importance of proactive behavior and education related to the risk of bioterrorism.

Outcome Criteria

- Patient experiences minimal adverse effects of or allergic reactions to the immunizing drug, such as fever, chills, myalgias, and bronchospasms (allergic), and is able to manage these effects with the use of acetaminophen and diphenhydramine if ordered.
- Patient uses measures such as the application of cold or heat packs to the site of injection, as indicated and as ordered by the physician, to help relieve localized discomfort or alleviate any localized reactions.
- Patient remains compliant with the therapeutic regimen for the prevention of illness or disease through follow-up visits with the physician.
- Patient states any problems or concerns to report immediately to the physician, such as fever higher than 101° F (38.3° C), infection, wheezing, increasing weakness, or any other unusual reaction.
- Patient states methods of remaining well informed about the possibility of bioterrorism and specific actions for self-protection, including reading reliable sources, staying abreast of local and national news, and even having special kits in the home containing items useful in a disaster, such as hurricane preparedness kits and, even more importantly, Homeland Security bioterrorism kits.

✦ IMPLEMENTATION

When giving immunizing drugs, the nurse must always recheck the specific protocols and schedules of administration. In addition, it is important to check and follow the manufacturer's recommendations concerning storage and administration of the drug, routes and site of administration, dosage, precautions pertaining to its use, and contraindications to its use. Parents of young children must be encouraged and taught how to maintain an accurate journal of the child's immunization status, including dates of immunization and the reaction(s), if any. If the patient experiences discomfort at the injection site, use of warm compresses or acetaminophen may help. With regard to the possibility of bioterrorism, patients need to be kept well informed, but the nurse must be constantly awareness of the need to minimize anxiety. See http://evolve.elsevier.com/Lilley for more information on specific agencies, policy development issues, and online resources related to bioterrorism. Patient teaching tips are presented on page 716.

◆ EVALUATION

The therapeutic response in patients receiving immunizing drugs is the prevention or amelioration of the specific disease being targeted. Adverse reactions for which to monitor in patients receiving immunizing drugs are specific to the drug, but there may be a localized reaction including swelling, redness, discomfort, and heat at the site of injection or a more serious reaction that should be reported immediately to the physician (e.g., high fever, lymphadenopathy, rash, itching, joint pain, severe flulike symptoms, decreased level of consciousness, and/or shortness of breath). For a complete list of expected reactions or adverse effects, including minor and severe, see Table 46-2. As immunizing drugs improve and newer ones are developed, it is hoped that fewer adverse effects will occur and fewer adverse drug events and complications will be seen.

Patient Teaching Tips

- A localized reaction to the injection sometimes occurs when toxoids and vaccines are administered. Patients should be told that they can relieve the discomfort by placing warm compresses on the injection site, resting, and taking acetaminophen and/or diphenhydramine, as directed by the physician. Instructions for the care of infants or children experiencing such reactions are generally given by the child's health care provider when the immunizing drug is administered.

- Patients or parents-caregivers should notify the physician if high or prolonged fever, rash, itching, or shortness of breath occurs after the vaccination.
- Patients or parents-caregivers should always keep a double record (two copies kept in separate places) of all of the medications being taken, especially all vaccinations received.
- A vaccine adverse event reporting system is available through the FDA by calling 1-800-822-7967.

Points to Remember

- A foreign substance in the body is termed an *antigen;* the body creates a substance called an *antibody* specifically to bind to it.
- B lymphocytes (B cells), when stimulated by the binding of an antigen molecule, begin to differentiate into memory cells and plasma cells.
- Memory cells remember what that particular antigen looks like in case the body is exposed to the same antigen again in the future.
- Plasma cells manufacture the antibodies and will mass-produce clones of the antibodies upon reexposure to a particular antigen.
- The two types of immunity are active and passive immunity. Different types of drugs are used to induce each, and these drugs are indicated for different populations, as follows:
  - Active immunization involves administration of a toxoid or a vaccine that exposes the body to a relatively harmless form of the antigen (foreign invader) to imprint cellular memory and stimulate the body's defenses to fight any subsequent exposure. It provides long-lasting or permanent immunity. The recipient must have an active, functioning immune system to benefit.

- Passive immunization involves the administration of immunoglobulins, antitoxins, or antivenins. Serum or concentrated immunoglobulins are obtained from humans or animals and, after screening and testing, are injected into the patient, directly giving the individual the ability to fight off the invading microorganism. Passive immunization provides temporary protection and does not stimulate an antibody response in the host. It is used in patients who are immunocompromised or who have been exposed to, or anticipate exposure to, the disease.
- Patients who should not receive immunizing drugs include those with active infections, febrile illnesses, or a history of a previous reaction to the drug. Use of these drugs in pregnant women is also usually contraindicated.
- Patients who are immunocompromised are at greater risk of experiencing serious adverse effects from immunizing drugs.
- Parents should keep updated records of their children's and their own immunizations with any toxoids or vaccines.

NCLEX Examination Review Questions

1. When assessing a patient who will be receiving a passive immunizing drug, the nurse will consider which condition to be a possible contraindication?
   a. Anemia
   b. Pregnancy
   c. Ear infection
   d. Common cold
2. When giving a vaccination to an infant, the nurse should tell the mother to expect which adverse effect?
   a. Fever over 103° F (39.4° C)
   b. Dyspnea
   c. Soreness at the injection site
   d. Chills
3. After a suspected anthrax exposure, the individual would be given prophylactic doses of
   a. ciprofloxacin.
   b. cidofovir.
   c. immunoglobulin.
   d. antitoxin.
4. During a routine checkup, a 72-year-old patient is advised to receive an influenza vaccine injection. He questions this, saying, "I had one last year. Why do I need another one?" What is an appropriate response from the nurse?
   a. "The effectiveness of the vaccine wears off after 6 months."
   b. "Each year a new vaccine is developed based on the flu strains that are likely to be in circulation."
   c. "When you reach age 65, you need boosters on an annual basis."
   d. "Taking the flu vaccine each year allows you to build your immunity to a higher level each time."
5. A patient is in the urgent care center after stepping on a rusty tent nail. The nurse evaluates the patient's immunity status and knows that a tetanus booster is necessary if which of the following is true?
   a. It has been a year since his last booster shot.
   b. It has been 2 years since his last booster shot.
   c. It has been 5 years since his last booster shot.
   d. It has been 10 years since his last booster shot.

1. b, 2. c, 3. a, 4. b, 5. d.

Critical Thinking Activities

1. Compare and contrast active and passive immunization.
2. Within 2 hours after a tetanus booster vaccination, your patient is showing signs of a serious adverse reaction. Describe the process for reporting this adverse event after you address the patient's needs for physical care.
3. You are working as a staff nurse on a medical-surgical unit in a suburban area. In the event of a bioterrorism attack, what are your responsibilities?

For answers, see http://evolve.elsevier.com/Lilley.

47

Antineoplastic Drugs Part 1: Cancer Overview and Cell Cycle–Specific Drugs

Objectives

When you reach the end of this chapter, you should be able to do the following:

1. Briefly describe the concepts related to carcinogenesis.
2. Define the different types of malignancy.
3. Discuss the purpose and role of the various treatment modalities in the management of cancer.
4. Define *antineoplastic.*
5. Discuss the role of antineoplastic therapy in the treatment of cancer.
6. Contrast the cell cycle of normal cells and malignant cells with regard to growth, function, and response of the cell to chemotherapeutic drugs and other treatment modalities.
7. Compare the characteristics of highly proliferating normal cells (including cells of the hair follicles, gastrointestinal tract, and bone marrow) with the characteristics of highly proliferating cancerous cells.
8. Briefly describe the specific differences between cell cycle–specific and cell cycle–nonspecific antineoplastic drugs (cell cycle–nonspecific drugs and miscellaneous other antineoplastics are presented in Chapter 48).
9. Identify the drugs that are categorized as cell cycle–specific, including mitotic inhibitors, topoisomerase inhibitors, and antineoplastic enzymes.
10. Describe the common adverse effects and toxic reactions associated with the various antineoplastic drugs, including the causes for their occurrence and methods of treatment, such as antidotes for toxicity.
11. Discuss the mechanisms of action, indications, dosages, routes of administration, cautions, contraindications, and drug interactions of cell cycle–specific drugs, mitotic inhibitors, topoisomerase inhibitors, and antineoplastic enzymes.
12. Apply knowledge about the various antineoplastic drugs to the development of a comprehensive nursing care plan for patients receiving cell cycle–specific drugs, mitotic inhibitors, topoisomerase inhibitors, and antineoplastic enzymes.

e-Learning Activities

Companion CD
- NCLEX Review Questions: see questions 391-397
- Animations
- Audio Glossary
- Category Catchers
- Medication Errors Checklists
- IV Therapy Checklists

evolve Website (http://evolve.elsevier.com/Lilley)
• Nursing Care Plans • Frequently Asked Questions • Content Updates • WebLinks • Supplemental Resources • Elsevier ePharmacology Update • Medication Administration Animations

Drug Profiles

asparaginase, p. 736
capecitabine, p. 732
cladribine, p. 731
▶ cytarabine, p. 732
▶ etoposide, p. 733
fludarabine, p. 731
fluorouracil, p. 732

gemcitabine, p. 732
irinotecan, p. 735
▶ methotrexate, p. 731
▶ paclitaxel, p. 733
pegaspargase, p. 736
topotecan, p. 735
▶ vincristine, p. 734

▶ Key drug.

Glossary

Analogue A chemical compound with a structure similar to that of another compound but differing from it with respect to some component; it may have a similar or opposite metabolic or other action in the body. (p. 729)

Anaplasia The absence of the cellular differentiation that is part of the normal cellular growth process (see *differentiation;* adjective: *anaplastic*). (p. 725)

Antineoplastic drugs Drugs used to treat cancer. Also called *cancer drugs, anticancer drugs, cancer chemotherapy,* and *chemotherapy.* (p. 722)

Benign Denoting a neoplasm that is noncancerous and therefore not an immediate threat to life, even though treatment eventually may be required for health or cosmetic reasons. (p. 720)

Cancer A neoplastic disease, the natural course of which is fatal (see *neoplasm*). (p. 719)

Carcinogen Any cancer-producing substance or organism. (p. 722)

Carcinomas Malignant epithelial neoplasms that tend to invade surrounding tissue and metastasize to distant regions of the body. (p. 720)

Cell cycle–nonspecific Denoting antineoplastic drugs that are cytotoxic in any phase of the cellular growth cycle. (p. 725)

Cell cycle–specific   Denoting antineoplastic drugs that are cytotoxic during a specific phase of the cellular growth cycle. (p. 725)

Clone   A cell or group of cells that is genetically identical to a given parent cell. (p. 719)

Differentiation   An important part of normal cellular growth processes involving changes in immature cells that allow them to mature into different types of more specialized cells, each having different functions. (p. 719)

Dose-limiting adverse effects   Adverse effects that prevent an antineoplastic drug from being given in higher dosages, often restricting the effectiveness of the drug. (p. 727)

Emetic potential   The potential of a drug to irritate the cells of the stomach or stimulate the vomiting center in the central nervous system, which results in nausea and vomiting. (p. 727)

Extravasation   The leakage of any intravenously or intraarterially administered medication into the tissue space surrounding the vein or artery. Such an event can cause serious tissue injury, especially with antineoplastic drugs. (p. 727)

Growth fraction   The percentage of cells in mitosis at any given time. (p. 724)

Intrathecal   A route of drug injection through the theca of the spinal cord and into the subarachnoid space. This route is used to deliver certain chemotherapy medications to kill cancer cells in the central nervous system. (p. 731)

Leukemias   Malignant neoplasms of blood-forming tissues characterized by the diffuse replacement of normal bone marrow cells with proliferating leukocyte precursors, which, in turn, results in abnormal numbers and forms of immature white blood cells in the circulation and the infiltration of lymph nodes, spleen, and liver. (p. 720)

Lymphomas   Neoplasms of lymphoid tissue that are usually malignant but in rare cases may be benign. (p. 720)

Malignant   Tending to worsen and cause death; anaplastic, invasive, and metastatic. (p. 720)

Metastasis   The process by which a cancer spreads from the original site of growth to a new and remote part of the body (adjective: *metastatic*). (p. 719)

Mitosis   The process of cell reproduction occurring in somatic (nonsexual) cells and resulting in the formation of two genetically identical daughter cells containing the diploid (complete) number of chromosomes characteristic of the species. (p. 724)

Mitotic index   The number of cells per unit (usually 1000) undergoing mitosis during a given time. (p. 724)

Mutagen   A chemical or physical agent that induces or increases genetic mutations by causing changes in DNA or ribonucleic acid (RNA). (p. 722)

Mutation   A permanent change in cellular genetic material (DNA or RNA) that is transmissible to future cellular generations. Mutations can transform normal cells into cancer cells. (p. 719)

Myelosuppression   Suppression of bone marrow function, which can result in dangerously reduced numbers of red and white blood cells and platelets. Both cancer chemotherapy and radiation can cause this condition, as can the cancer disease process itself. Also called *bone marrow suppression* or *bone marrow depression*. (p. 727)

Nadir   Lowest point in any fluctuating value over time, such as the white blood cell count after it has been depressed by chemotherapy. In antineoplastic drug therapy, this term also refers to the time frame in which these drugs kill the greatest number of bone marrow cells. (p. 727)

Neoplasm   Any new and abnormal growth, specifically growth that is uncontrolled and progressive; a synonym for *tumor*. A *malignant* neoplasm or tumor is synonymous with *cancer*. (p. 720)

Nucleic acids   Molecules of DNA and RNA in the nucleus of every cell (hence the name *nucleic acid*). DNA makes up the cellular chromosomes and encodes all of the genes necessary for cellular reproduction. (p. 722)

Oncogenic   Giving rise to tumors, either benign or malignant; the term is applied especially to tumor-inducing viruses. (p. 722)

Paraneoplastic syndromes (PNSs)   Symptom complexes arising in patients with cancer that cannot be explained by local or distant spread of their tumors. (p. 721)

Primary lesion   The original site of growth of a tumor; opposite of a metastatic lesion. (p. 719)

Sarcomas   Malignant neoplasms of the connective tissues arising in bone, fibrous, fatty, muscular, synovial, vascular, or neural tissue, often first presenting as painless swellings. (p. 720)

Tumor   A new growth of tissue characterized by a progressive, uncontrolled proliferation of cells. Tumors can be solid (e.g., brain tumor) or circulating (e.g., leukemia or lymphoma), and *benign* (noncancerous) or *malignant* (cancerous). Circulating tumors are more precisely called *hematologic tumors* or *hematologic malignancies*. A tumor is also called a *neoplasm*. (p. 720)

Tumor lysis syndrome   A common metabolic complication of chemotherapy for rapidly growing tumors. It is characterized by the presence of excessive cellular waste products and electrolytes, including uric acid, phosphate, potassium, and by reduced serum calcium levels. (p. 729)

Cancer is a broad term encompassing a group of diseases that are characterized by cellular transformation (e.g., by genetic **mutation**), uncontrolled cellular growth, and possible invasion into surrounding tissue and metastasis to other tissues or organs distant from the original body site. This cellular growth differs from normal cellular growth in that cancerous cells do not possess a growth control mechanism. Lack of cellular **differentiation** or maturation into specialized, productive cells is also a common characteristic of cancer cells. Figure 47-1 illustrates the multiple steps involved in the development of cancer. Cancerous cells will continue to grow and invade adjacent structures, and they may break away from the original tumor mass and travel by means of the blood or lymphatic system to establish a new clone of cancer cells and create a metastatic growth elsewhere in the body. A **clone** is a cell or group of cells that is genetically identical to a given parent cell. For the remainder of this and the next chapter, the term *cancer* will generally be used to refer to any type of malignant neoplasm.

Metastasis refers to the spreading of a cancer (uncontrolled cell growth) from the original site of growth (**primary lesion**) to a new and remote part of the body (*secondary* or *metastatic*

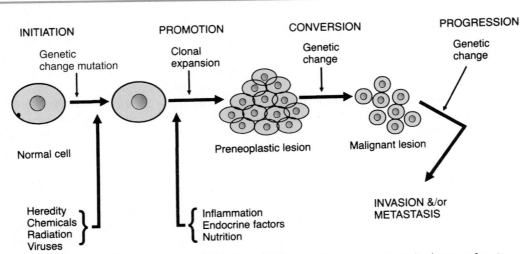

FIGURE 47-1   Schematic model of multistep carcinogenesis. *Genetic change* refers to events such as the activation of protooncogenes or drug-resistance genes or the inactivation of tumor suppressor genes, antimetastasis genes, or apoptosis (normal cell death). Genetic change may be relatively minimal, as with the translocations seen in various leukemias, or it may involve multiple sequential genetic alterations, as exemplified by the development of colon cancer. *(From Haskell CM:* Cancer treatment, *ed 5, Philadelphia, 2001, Saunders.)*

Table 47-1	Tumor Characteristics: Benign and Malignant	
Characteristic	**Benign**	**Malignant**
Potential to metastasize	No	Yes
Encapsulated	Yes	No
Similar to tissue of origin	Yes	No
Rate of growth	Slow	Unpredictable and unrestrained
Recurrence after surgical removal	Rare	Common

lesion). The terms *malignancy, neoplasm,* and *tumor* are often used as synonyms for cancer; however, each has its own meaning. A **neoplasm** ("new tissue") is a mass of new cells that exhibit uncontrolled cellular reproduction. It is another term for **tumor.** There are two types of tumors: benign and malignant. A **benign** tumor is of a uniform size and shape and displays no invasiveness (in terms of infiltrating other tissues) or metastatic properties. The terms *nonmalignant* and *benign* suggest that tumors may be harmless, which is true in most cases. However, a benign tumor can be lethal if it grows large enough to mechanically interrupt the normal function of a critical tissue or organ (e.g., brain, heart, lung). **Malignant** neoplasms typically consist of cancerous cells that invade (infiltrate) surrounding tissues at the cellular level and metastasize to other tissues and organs, where they form metastatic tumor deposits. Some of the various characteristics of benign and malignant neoplasms, or tumors, are listed in Table 47-1.

Over 100 types of cancers affect humans. They are usually classified by their primary anatomic location (organ or tissue) and the type of cell from which the cancer develops. Common body sites for the growth of such tumors include the following:

- Bladder
- Blood-producing tissue
- Breast
- Colon
- Kidney
- Liver
- Lung
- Lymphatic system
- Ovary
- Prostate gland
- Uterus
- Rectum
- Skin

Various tumor types based on tissue categories include sarcomas, carcinomas, lymphomas, leukemias, and tumors of nervous tissue origin. Examples of these common types of malignant tumors are presented in Table 47-2. It is important to know the tissue of origin because this determines the type of chemotherapy used, the likely response to therapy, and the prognosis.

Carcinomas arise from epithelial tissue, which is located throughout the body. It covers or lines all body surfaces, both inside and outside the body. Examples are the skin, the mucosal lining of the entire gastrointestinal (GI) tract, and the bronchial tree (lungs). The purpose of these epithelial tissues is to protect the body's vital organs.

Sarcomas are malignant tumors that arise primarily from connective tissues, but some sarcomas are tumors of epithelial cell origin. Connective tissue is the most abundant and widely distributed of all tissues and includes bone, cartilage, muscle, and lymphatic and vascular structures. Its purpose is to support and protect other tissues.

Lymphomas are cancers within the lymphatic tissues. **Leukemias** arise from the various types of leukocytes in the blood. These two types of tumors differ from carcinomas and sarcomas in that the cancerous cells do not form solid tumors but are interspersed throughout the lymphatic or circulatory system and interfere with the normal functioning of these systems. For this reason, they are sometimes referred to as *circulating tumors,* although *hematologic malignancy* is a more precise term.

Nerve or *neural tissue tumors* are those arising in and affecting the cells of the central or peripheral nervous systems.

Cancer patients may also experience various groups of symptoms that cannot be directly attributed to the spread of a cancerous tumor. Such symptom complexes are referred to as **paraneoplastic syndromes (PNSs).** They are estimated to occur in up to 15% of patients with cancer and may even be the first sign of malignancy, with *cachexia* (general ill health and malnutrition) being the most common such symptom complex. Examples of other common PNSs are listed in Table 47-3. These syndromes are believed to result from the effects of biologically or immunologically active substances, such as hormones and antibodies, secreted by the tumor cells. Many patients also exhibit more generalized symptoms, such as anorexia, weight loss, fatigue, and fever.

ETIOLOGY OF CANCER

The etiology of cancer remains a mystery for the most part, and cancer researchers have made slow progress toward identifying possible causes. In recent years, certain etiologic factors have come to light, however, and some of these and the cancers with which they are causally associated are listed in Table 47-4. Radiation; oncogenic viruses; and immunologic, ethnic, genetic, age-related, and sex-related characteristics are among the causative factors identified.

AGE- AND SEX-RELATED DIFFERENCES

The probability that a neoplastic disease will develop generally increases with advancing age. However, acute lymphocytic leukemia and Wilms' tumor are exceptions to this pattern, and the incidence of these disorders decreases with age. On the other hand, chronic lymphocytic and myelocytic leukemia, colon cancer, and lung cancer usually develop during middle and old age, and are rare in young children.

With the exception of cancers affecting the reproductive system, few cancers exhibit a sex-related difference in incidence. Lung and urinary cancers are more common in men than in women, but this may have more to do with exogenous factors such as smoking patterns and occupational exposure to environmental toxins than to sex-related characteristics. The incidence of colon, rectal, pancreatic, and skin cancers, as well as of leukemia, is comparable for the two sexes.

Table 47-2	Tumor Classification Based on Specific Tissue of Origin
Tissue of Origin	**Malignant Tissue**
Epithelial = Carcinomas	
Glands or ducts	Adenocarcinomas
Respiratory tract	Small and large cell carcinomas
Kidney	Renal cell carcinoma
Skin	Squamous cell, epidermoid, and basal cell carcinoma; melanoma
Connective = Sarcomas	
Fibrous tissue	Fibrosarcoma
Cartilage	Chondrosarcoma
Bone	Osteogenic sarcoma (Ewing's tumor)
Blood vessels	Kaposi's sarcoma
Synovia	Synoviosarcoma
Mesothelium	Mesothelioma
Lymphatic = Lymphomas	
Lymph tissue	Lymphomas (e.g., Hodgkin's, non-Hodgkin's)
Bone marrow	Multiple myeloma
Nerve	
Glia	Glioma
Adrenal medulla nerves	Pheochromocytoma
Blood	
White blood cells	Leukemia

Table 47-3	Paraneoplastic Syndromes Associated with Some Cancers
Paraneoplastic Syndrome	**Associated Cancer**
Hypercalcemia, sensory neuropathies, SIADH	Lung
Disseminated intravascular coagulation	Leukemia
Cushing's syndrome	Lung, thyroid, testes, adrenal
Addison's syndrome	Adrenal, lymphomas

SIADH, Syndrome of inappropriate secretion of antidiuretic hormone.

Table 47-4	Cancer: Proposed Etiologic Factors
Risk Factor	**Associated Cancer**
Environment	
Radiation (ionizing)	Leukemia, breast, thyroid, lung
Radiation (ultraviolet)	Skin, melanoma
Viruses	Leukemia, lymphoma, nasopharyngeal
Food	
Aflatoxin	Liver
Dietary factors	Colon, breast, endometrial, gallbladder
Lifestyle	
Alcohol	Esophageal, liver, stomach, laryngeal
Tobacco	Lung, oral, esophageal, laryngeal, bladder
Medical Drugs	
Diethylstilbestrol (DES)	Vaginal in offspring, breast, testicular, ovarian
Estrogens	Endometrial
Alkylating drugs	Leukemia, bladder
Occupational	
Asbestos	Lung, mesothelioma
Aniline dye	Bladder
Benzene	Leukemia
Vinyl chloride	Liver
Reproductive History	
Late first pregnancy, early menses	Breast
No children	Ovarian
Multiple sexual partners	Cervical, uterine

GENETIC AND ETHNIC FACTORS

Few cancers have been confirmed to have a hereditary basis (some types of breast, colon, and stomach cancer are exceptions). However, the understanding of tumor biology has helped guide therapy tremendously. Two such advances are determination of hormone receptor status and identification of specific gene expression in various types of tumor cells. For example, some tumor cells have been shown to express on their cell membrane surfaces either estrogen receptors or progesterone receptors, and some tumor cells express specific genes such as the HER2/neu gene. Because these indicators aid in classification of a patient's tumor, they also help in choosing appropriate drug therapy, predicting response to therapy, and anticipating prognosis. The tendency to develop tumors with identifiable gene expression patterns does often show a familial pattern of inheritance. Burkitt's lymphoma is an example of a cancer that shows a racial predilection. The disease is more common in young African children and children of African descent than in non-African children. Another example of an ethnic predisposition is the high incidence of nasopharyngeal cancer in persons of Chinese descent.

ONCOGENIC VIRUSES

Extensive research has indicated that there are cancer-causing (**oncogenic**) viruses that can affect most mammalian species. Examples include human papilloma virus, the various cat leukemia viruses, the Rous* sarcoma virus in chickens, and the Shope* papilloma virus in rabbits.

The herpes viruses are common examples of oncogenic viruses. Epstein-Barr virus is a type of herpes virus. It is most commonly recognized as the cause of infectious mononucleosis (commonly referred to as "mono" or the "kissing disease"). However, it is also associated with the development of Burkitt's lymphoma and nasopharyngeal cancer. There also seems to be a link between the development of cervical cancer and infection with the herpes simplex type 2 virus (herpes genitalis). Infection with human papilloma virus (often abbreviated as HPV) has been linked to both cervical and anal cancer.

OCCUPATIONAL AND ENVIRONMENTAL CARCINOGENS

A **carcinogen** is any substance that can induce the development of a cancer or accelerate its growth. In the nucleus of every cell are found molecules of **nucleic acids,** so named because of their location in the cell nucleus. The two types of nucleic acids are *deoxyribonucleic acid (DNA)* and *ribonucleic acid (RNA)*. DNA molecules are the master molecules of genetic material within cells. They reproduce or *replicate* by making RNA molecules, which in turn gather *amino acids* to make the protein molecules necessary for cellular reproduction. This process is discussed further in the section on alkylating drugs in Chapter 48. A **mutagen** is any substance or physical agent (e.g., radiation) that enhances the rate of genetic mutations by inducing changes in DNA molecules. Mutations in cellular genetic material (DNA) often *transform* normal cells into cancer cells whose growth is unrestrained. Thus, *mutagenicity* is associated with and often (but not always) leads to car-

cinogenicity. The U.S. Food and Drug Administration (FDA) regulations mandate that carcinogenic studies be performed before any new drug is approved for use. However, no amount of clinical testing can fully reveal all of a drug's possible carcinogenic effects. One reason for this is that testing for drug carcinogenic activity is difficult and current test methods are not very satisfactory. Besides this, there can be species-related differences in carcinogenic potential with any given drug. Carcinogenic effects may not be observed in the laboratory animals on which the drug has been tested but may become obvious only when the drugs are used in human subjects. Hopefully such effects become apparent before the medication is marketed. However, given the relatively small number of patients tested in clinical research trials, the carcinogenic potential of a given drug may not be observed until after the drug is marketed for use in the general population. If patterns of carcinogenicity begin to emerge during this period of postmarketing surveillance (or postmarketing studies), the drug may be recalled from the market. This recall can be either initiated voluntarily by the manufacturer or mandated by the FDA.

RADIATION

Radiation is a well-known and potent carcinogenic agent. There are two basic types of radiation: (1) *ionizing,* or high-energy, radiation, and (2) *nonionizing,* or low-energy, radiation. Both types can be carcinogenic. Ionizing radiation is very potent and can penetrate deeply into the body. It is called *ionizing* because it causes the formation of ions within living cells. This type of radiation (e.g., used in x-ray studies) is also applied to treat (irradiate) cancerous tumors (e.g., radium implants). Nonionizing radiation is much less potent and cannot penetrate deeply into the body. Sunlight and ultraviolet light are examples of this type of radiation. Both can cause skin cancer, although ultraviolet light is also used to treat various dermatologic conditions such as atopic dermatitis. In contrast to chemotherapy, radiation is considered to be a more localized (versus systemic) cancer treatment. Because of this, adverse effects (e.g., radiation burns; nausea with GI radiation) tend to be more localized to the site of treatment as well. Scientific specialists known as *radiation physicists* are involved in the planning of radiation treatments, including calculation of the appropriate dose (*dosimetry*).

IMMUNOLOGIC FACTORS

The immune system plays an important role in the body in terms of cancer surveillance and the elimination of neoplastic cells. Neoplastic cells are believed to develop routinely in everyone, but in healthy persons the immune system recognizes them as abnormal and eliminates them by means of cell-mediated immunity (cytotoxic T lymphocytes; Chapter 49). It has also been shown that the incidence of cancer is much higher in immunocompromised individuals. Examples include patients undergoing cancer chemotherapy, organ transplant patients receiving immunosuppressive therapy, and patients suffering from immunologic impairment or disease, including acquired immunodeficiency syndrome (AIDS). This relationship between cancer and a suppressed immune system has also been noted in cancer patients being treated with immunotherapy consisting of interferon derivatives (Chapter 49), the *bacillus Calmette-Guérin (BCG)* vaccine (used to treat bladder cancer; Chapter 48), and *lymphokines* (immune-modulating molecules; Chapter 46).

---

*Doctors P. Rous and R. Shope were early investigators of oncogenic viruses.

Table 47-5 Common Names for Selected Cell Cycle–Specific Antineoplastic Drugs

Generic Name	Trade Names	Other Names
Antimetabolites		
Folic Acid Antagonist Analogue		
methotrexate	Folex, Mexate, Rheumatrex	MTX, amethopterin
Purine Analogues		
cladribine	Leustatin	2-chlorodeoxyadenosine, 2-CdA, CdA
fludarabine	Fludara	F-AMP, NSC-312887
mercaptopurine	Purinethol	6-mercaptopurine, 6-MP
pentostatin	Nipent	deoxycoformycin, 2'-deoxycoformycin, DCF, dCF
thioguanine	Thioguanine	6-thioguanine, 6-TG, TG, thioguanine, 2-amino-6-mercaptopurine
Pyrimidine Analogues		
capecitabine	Xeloda	
cytarabine, conventional	Cytosar-U, Tarabine PFS	ara-C, cytosine arabinoside, cytosine arabinosine
cytarabine, liposomal	DepoCyt	
gemcitabine	Gemzar	2,2-difluorodeoxycytidine, dFdC
floxuridine	FUDR	fluorodeoxyuridine, FUdR
fluorouracil	Adrucil, Carac Topical, Efudex Topical, Fluoroplex Topical	5-fluorouracil, 5-FU
Natural Products		
Enzymes		
asparaginase (from *Escherichia coli* bacteria)	Elspar	L-asparaginase, *E. coli* asparaginase
pegaspargase (from *E. coli* bacteria)	Oncaspar	PEG-L-asparaginase
Camptothecin Analogues (from a Chinese Shrub)		
irinotecan	Camptosar	camptothecin-11, CPT-11
topotecan	Hycamtin	SKF-104864, NSC-609699
Epipodophyllotoxins (from Mandrake Plant or May Apple)		
etoposide	VePesid, Toposar, Etopophos	VP-16, VP-16-213
teniposide	Vumon	VM-26
Taxanes (from Yew Trees)		
paclitaxel	Taxol, Onxol	NSC-125973
docetaxel	Taxotere	
Vinca Alkaloids (from Periwinkle Plant)		
vinblastine	Velban, Alkaban-AQ	vincaleukoblastine, VLB
vincristine	Oncovin, Vincasar	VCR, leurocristine, LCR
vinorelbine	Navelbine	PM-259

CANCER DRUG NOMENCLATURE

As mentioned earlier, a more technical term for cancer is *malignant neoplasm.* Drugs used to treat cancer are therefore known as **antineoplastic drugs** but are also called *cancer drugs, anticancer drugs,* and, most commonly, *cytotoxic chemotherapy* or just *chemotherapy.* The nomenclature (naming system) of cancer drugs can be somewhat more complex and confusing than that for other drug classes. Cancer treatment is an intensively researched area in health care. Because of this there are many ongoing research protocols, and often larger numbers of new drugs are approved by the FDA for cancer treatment in any given year than are approved for treatment of other disease categories. Further complicating matters is the fact that multiple names are often used for the same drug, depending on its stage of development. The following text and Table 47-5 provide examples of the multiple names for various antineoplastic medications that may be encountered in clinical practice.

Recall from earlier chapters that medications have a chemical name, a generic name, and a trade name. This section introduces yet another name for medications, especially cancer drugs, that is often encountered in clinical practice: the *investigational* or *protocol* name. A drug's chemical name is used by the chemists who first discover and work with the drug. This is usually the very first name used to identify a particular chemical compound, often before it is classified as a "drug" with known therapeutic properties. The chemical name is based on the standard chemical nomenclature recommended by the International Union of Pure and Applied Chemists (IUPAC). For this reason, it is also often known as the *IUPAC name.* The generic name is often first assigned to a chemical compound after a pharmaceutical manufacturer has determined that it is worthy of continued clinical research because of apparent therapeutic properties. It is often at this point that the chemical compound becomes an investigational drug per se. The first evidence of therapeutic properties often appears in the laboratory setting. For example, a research scientist may discover that a given chemical compound destroys or inhibits the growth of cancer cells in a live cell culture.

Generic names are usually shorter and less complex than chemical names, and their spelling is often at least loosely based on the chemical structural features of the drug. The trade name is a marketing name used by the manufacturer of a given drug primarily to advertise the drug to prescribers and even to patients themselves. The trade name is frequently strategically chosen to be shorter and easier to pronounce and remember than the chemical, protocol, or generic name.

During the time before marketing that a given medication is undergoing clinical research, it is often referred to by its protocol name. The protocol name may be the same as the generic name, but instead it is often a code name that consists of a combination of letters and numbers separated by one or more dashes. One of the purposes of this name is to protect the code of a blinded study so that neither research staff nor study patients know who is (or is not) receiving the actual drug under investigation. This helps in distinguishing real drug effects from placebo effects when a placebo-controlled study format is used (which is not always the case). Although investigational drugs for all disease classes usually have some kind of protocol name, protocol names tend to be used more commonly in patient care settings for cancer drugs than for other drug classes. For this reason some common protocol or investigational names have been included in Table 47-5. Because chemical names are not usually encountered in patient care, they are generally not emphasized in this table, except occasionally for illustrative purposes. The following are two typical examples that illustrate these concepts:

Other Name	Generic Name	Trade Name
STI-571 (protocol name)	Imatinib	Gleevec
5-fluorouracil* (chemical name)	Fluorouracil	Adrucil

*The "5" refers to the position of a fluorine atom in the cyclic ring structure of the uracil molecule.

See Table 47-5 for additional information on the naming of cancer drugs.

CELL GROWTH CYCLE

Normal cells in the body divide (proliferate) in a controlled and organized fashion, and this growth is regulated by various mechanisms. In contrast, cancer cells lack such regulatory mechanisms and proliferate uncontrollably, although some modulation of cancer cell proliferation may occur if blood flow to the cancer is disrupted. Often the growth of cancer cells is also more constant or continuous than that of nonmalignant cells. Thus, one important growth index for malignant tumors is the time it takes for the tumor to double in size. This *doubling time* varies greatly for various types of cancers and is directly related to and important in determining the prognosis for a particular patient. Cancer treatment that cannot destroy every neoplastic cell does not prevent the regrowth of the tumor, and the time it takes for regrowth to occur depends on the doubling time of the particular cancer. For instance, Burkitt's lymphoma has an extremely short doubling time, whereas multiple myeloma has one of the longest. A cancer with a shorter doubling time is often more difficult to treat and more likely to have a poorer prognosis.

The cell growth characteristics of normal and neoplastic cells are similar. Both types of cells pass through five distinct growth phases: G_0, the *resting* phase; G_1, the first *growth* phase; S, the *synthesis* phase; G_2, the second growth phase; and M, the **mitosis** phase. During mitosis, one cell divides into two identical *daughter* cells. Mitosis is further subdivided into four distinct subphases related to the time periods before and during the alignment and separation of the chromosomes (DNA strands): *prophase, metaphase, anaphase,* and *telophase*. A complete cell cycle from one mitosis to the next is called the *generation time* (same as the doubling time), and it is different for all tumors, ranging from hours to days. The cell growth cycle and the events that occur in the various phases are summarized in Table 47-6. Figure 47-2 shows where in the general phases of the cell cycle the various cell cycle–specific chemotherapeutic drugs show their greatest proportionate kill of cancer cells.

The growth activity in a mass of tumor cells can also be characterized, and it has an important bearing on the killing power of chemotherapeutic drugs. The *percentage* of cells undergoing mitosis at any given time is called the **growth fraction** of the tumor mass. The *actual number* of cells that are in the M phase of the cell cycle is called the **mitotic index.** Chemotherapy is most effective when the greatest number of cells are dividing, that is, when both the growth fraction and mitotic index are high; a tumor in which both these indicators are high is known as a *highly proliferative* tumor.

Any cell that is a precursor to another cell is known as a *stem cell.* In the bone marrow, stem cells eventually change into more mature and specialized cells through differentiation. The level of differentiation within a tumor, whether solid or circulating, becomes especially important in the treatment of neoplasms. This is because more highly differentiated tumors generally have a better therapeutic response (tumor shrinkage) to treatments such as chemotherapy and radiation. In contrast, some cancers, such as leukemia, involve proliferation of immature white blood cells (WBCs) known as *blast cells.* Cancers with a larger proportion of such *undifferentiated* cells are often

Table 47-6	**Cell Cycle Phases**
Phase	**Description**
G_0: Resting phase	Most normal human cells exist predominantly in this phase. Cancer cells in this phase are not susceptible to the toxic effects of cell cycle–specific drugs.
G_1: First growth phase or *postmitotic* phase	Enzymes necessary for DNA synthesis are produced.
S: DNA synthesis phase	DNA synthesis takes place, from DNA strand separation to replication of each strand to create duplicate DNA molecules.
G_2: Second growth phase or *premitotic* phase	RNA and specialized proteins are made.
M: Mitosis phase	Divided into four subphases: prophase, metaphase, anaphase, and telophase; cell divides (reproduces) into two *daughter* cells.

DNA, Deoxyribonucleic acid; *RNA,* ribonucleic acid.

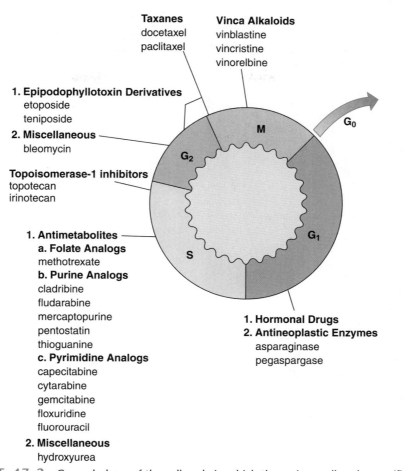

Taxanes
docetaxel
paclitaxel

Vinca Alkaloids
vinblastine
vincristine
vinorelbine

1. Epipodophyllotoxin Derivatives
etoposide
teniposide
2. Miscellaneous
bleomycin

Topoisomerase-1 inhibitors
topotecan
irinotecan

1. Antimetabolites
   a. Folate Analogs
   methotrexate
   b. Purine Analogs
   cladribine
   fludarabine
   mercaptopurine
   pentostatin
   thioguanine
   c. Pyrimidine Analogs
   capecitabine
   cytarabine
   gemcitabine
   floxuridine
   fluorouracil
2. Miscellaneous
   hydroxyurea

1. Hormonal Drugs
2. Antineoplastic Enzymes
   asparaginase
   pegaspargase

FIGURE 47-2 General phase of the cell cycle in which the various cell cycle–specific chemotherapeutic drugs have their greatest proportionate kill of cancer cells.

less responsive to chemotherapy or radiation and therefore are more difficult to treat. Lack of normal cellular differentiation is known as **anaplasia,** and such undifferentiated cells are said to be *anaplastic* cells.

DRUG THERAPY

Cancer is normally treated with one or more of three major medical approaches: surgery, radiation therapy, and chemotherapy. The term *chemotherapy* is a general term that technically can refer to chemical (drug) therapy for any kind of illness. In practice, however, this term usually refers to the pharmacologic treatment of cancer. Normal cells in the body divide (proliferate) in a controlled and organized fashion, and this growth is regulated by means of various mechanisms. In contrast, cancer cells lack regulatory mechanisms and they proliferate uncontrollably. Figure 47-3 shows what is termed the *Gompertzian tumor growth curve,* which illustrates the effects on patient clinical status of tumor growth over time. Figure 47-4 shows how various combinations of cancer treatment may succeed, or fail, over time.

Cancer chemotherapy drugs can be subdivided into two main groups based on where in the cellular life cycle they have their effects. Antineoplastic drugs that are cytotoxic (cell killing) in any phase of the cycle are called **cell cycle–nonspecific** drugs. Those drugs that are cytotoxic during a specific cell cycle phase are called **cell cycle–specific** drugs. It should be noted, however, that

these are broad categories that describe the *predominant* activity of a drug with regard to cell cycle. Individual drugs may have actions that fall into both of these categories. Cell cycle–nonspecific drugs are more effective against large, slowly growing tumors. Cell cycle–specific drugs are more effective against rapidly growing tumors. This chapter has described the various individual phases of the cell cycle and discusses the corresponding cell cycle–specific drugs. Chapter 48 focuses on cell cycle–nonspecific drugs as well as various miscellaneous antineoplastic drugs.

The ultimate goal of any anticancer regimen is to kill every neoplastic cell and produce a cure, but this goal is not achieved in most cases. One reason for this is that antineoplastic drugs are usually only cytotoxic and not tumoricidal. That is, they usually only kill a portion of the cells in a tumor, such as those that are dividing, and not all the cells in the tumor. Other factors that affect the chances of cure and the length of patient survival include the cancer stage at the time of diagnosis, type of cancer and its doubling time, efficacy of the cancer treatment, development of drug resistance, and general health of the patient. When total cure is not possible, the primary goal of therapy is to control the growth of the cancer while maintaining the best quality of life for the patient, with the least possible level of discomfort, compromise (in performing the activities of daily living), and treatment adverse effects.

It must be strongly emphasized that cancer care and treatment involve many rapidly evolving medical sciences. Cancer is an intensively researched area, with the ultimate goals being to pre-

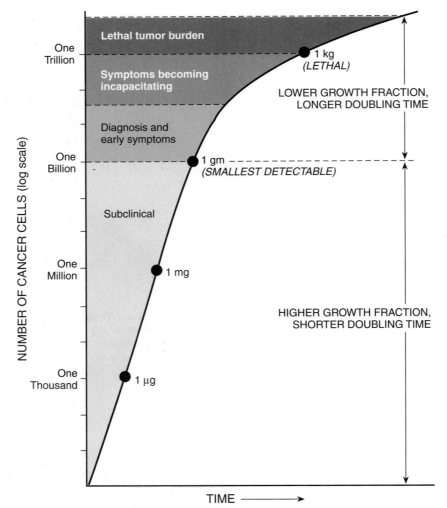

FIGURE 47-3   Gompertzian tumor growth curve showing the relationship between tumor size and clinical status. *(From Lehne RA: Pharmacology for nursing care, ed 6, St Louis, 2007, Saunders.)*

vent cancer and to prevent premature death in those diagnosed with it. Chemotherapy medications are often dosed as part of complex, specific treatment protocols that are subject to frequent revision by oncology clinicians and researchers. For these reasons the reader must recognize that the drug dosing information provided in this chapter is only intended to be representative of current cancer treatment and is not absolute or comprehensive. Oncology nursing is a highly specialized area of practice with focused ongoing continuing education requirements that may vary among state jurisdictions. Furthermore, the indications that are listed for each specific drug are the primary FDA-approved indications that are current at the time of this writing. These, too, may change unpredictably with time as a given drug is determined to be more (or less) effective for treating certain types of cancer. Also, in clinical practice, patients are often treated by their supervising oncologists with one or more antineoplastic medications for "off-label" uses; that is, the drug is not currently approved for this particular use by the FDA. This is usually a judgment call made by the attending oncologist. Such decisions may be based on case studies or simply trial and error in the final efforts to treat patients for whom other drug therapies have failed. This process is one way in which new information is dis-

covered. As noted earlier, however, only the current FDA-approved indications will generally be mentioned in this chapter.

No antineoplastic drug is effective against all types of cancer. Most cancer drugs also have a low therapeutic index, which means that a fine line exists between therapeutic and toxic levels. However, one important discovery yielded by clinical experience is that a combination of drugs is usually more effective than single-drug therapy. Because drug-resistant cells often develop in tumors as a result of the tumor's genetic instability, exposure to multiple drugs with multiple mechanisms and sites of action will destroy more subpopulations of cells. The delayed onset of resistance to a particular antineoplastic drug is thus one benefit of combination drug therapy. To be most effective, however, the drugs used in such a combination regimen should possess the following characteristics:

- Some efficacy even as single drugs in the treatment of the particular type of cancer
- Different mechanisms of action so that the cytotoxic effect is maximized; this includes differences in cell cycle specificity
- Different cytotoxic properties so that each drug in the combination can be administered in a full therapeutic dose (in other words, the drugs have no or minimal overlapping toxicities)

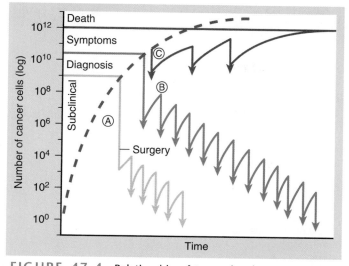

FIGURE 47-4   Relationship of tumor burden to treatment strategies and outcome with systemic chemotherapy. Human tumors grow in accordance with the Gompertz curve *(dashed line),* with a decreasing doubling time as tumor burden increases. Treatment interventions relate to tumor type and extent of disease. *A,* Surgery followed by pulse courses of adjuvant chemotherapy. Combined modality has curative potential with the addition of chemotherapy after surgery. *B,* Systemic chemotherapy for stage III Hodgkin's disease. Cure is possible with prolonged administration of combination chemotherapy. *C,* Palliative chemotherapy for advanced non–small cell cancer. The patient's tumor burden is too great, and the potency of the drugs for this specific form of cancer too inadequate because of the development of drug resistance, to allow cure. *(Modified from Salmon SE, Sartorelli AC: Cancer chemotherapy. In Katzung BG, editor: Basic and clinical pharmacology, ed 4, Norwalk, Conn, 1989, Appleton & Lange, p. 685.)*

One major drawback to the use of antineoplastic drugs is that nearly all of them cause adverse effects. Many of these effects are severe or even toxic and stem from the fact that these drugs are harmful to all rapidly proliferating cells—both harmful cancer cells and healthy, normal cells. Three types of such rapidly dividing, beneficial human cells are the cells of hair follicles, GI tract cells, and bone marrow cells. Because most of today's antineoplastic drugs still cannot differentiate between cancer cells and these healthy cells, the latter are also destroyed, and hair loss, nausea and vomiting, and bone marrow toxicity are the undesirable consequences. These effects are called **dose-limiting adverse effects** because they often prevent the antineoplastic drug from being administered in sufficiently high doses to kill the entire population of cancer cells, which would likely be curative.

Hair follicle cells are continually in a rapidly dividing state, which results in the normal growth and replacement of head and body hair. Cancer drugs that affect these cells often cause the adverse effect known as *alopecia,* or hair loss. Many patients, especially women, choose to wear wigs, hats, or scarves to disguise this adverse effect. Some antineoplastic drugs are more harmful to the epithelial cells of the stomach and intestinal tract, which often leads to nausea, vomiting, and diarrhea. The likelihood that a given drug will produce vomiting is known as its **emetic potential.** Other anticancer drugs cause nausea and vomiting by stimulating the cells of the *vomiting center* in the brain, also known as the *chemoreceptor trigger zone.* Preventing these adverse effects

entirely would likely require subtherapeutic drug dosages and more limited cancer treatment. Several antiemetic drugs are used to prevent these symptoms. These are described in Chapter 53. Box 47-1 lists the relative emetic potential of selected chemotherapy drugs. **Myelosuppression,** also known as *bone marrow suppression* or *bone marrow depression,* is another unwanted adverse effect of certain antineoplastics. It commonly results from drug- or radiation-induced destruction of certain rapidly dividing cells in the bone marrow, primarily the cellular precursors of WBCs, red blood cells (RBCs), and platelets. This can also occur secondary to the disease processes of the cancer itself. Myelosuppression, in turn, leads to leukopenia, anemia, and thrombocytopenia. The cancer patient is often at great risk for infection because of *leukopenia* (reduced WBC count) secondary to chemotherapy. Patients tend to need large quantities of antibiotics, often intravenously (IV), either to prevent or to treat bacterial infections. Drug-induced *anemia* (reduced RBC count) often leads to hypoxia and fatigue, whereas *thrombocytopenia* (reduced platelet count) makes the patient more susceptible to bleeding. The lowest level reached by bone marrow cells following a chemotherapy (or radiation) treatment is the **nadir.** The time until the nadir is reached in a given patient may become shorter and the recovery time for the bone marrow may become longer with multiple courses of antineoplastic treatment. The nadir normally occurs roughly 10 to 28 days after dosing, depending on the particular cancer drug or combinations of drugs that is used to treat the patient. Anticipation of this nadir based on known cancer drug data can be used to guide the timing of prophylactic (preventative) administration of antibiotics and blood stimulants known as *biologic response modifiers* (Chapter 49).

Common specific indications for use of drugs in the various antineoplastic classes are listed in the dosages tables provided for selected drugs in each class. Also provided in various locations in this and the next chapter are tables and boxes containing drug-specific guidelines for the treatment of **extravasation**—unintended leakage of a chemotherapy drug (with vesicant potential) into the surrounding tissues outside of the IV line used for administration.

Because of the often severe toxicity of cancer medications, a current major focus of cancer drug research is the development of *targeted* drug therapy; that is, drugs that chemically recognize and act against only cancer cells, while sparing healthy cells. One example of such targeted therapy is the newer class of cancer drugs known as *monoclonal antibodies* (Chapter 49).

Pharmacokinetic data for antineoplastic medications are especially hard to obtain. It is difficult to determine precise values for onset of action, peak effect, and duration of action when treating malignant tumors that often have erratic growth kinetics of their own. Response to therapy is usually determined by clinical evaluation of the patient, blood sampling to determine cell counts and measure the presence of various tumor marker proteins, and imaging scans (e.g., computed tomography, magnetic resonance imaging) to assess the extent of tumor response to cancer treatment. For these reasons pharmacokinetic data are not included with the drug profiles in this chapter.

In spite of their notorious toxicity, given the often fatal outcome of neoplastic diseases, most cancer drugs are only rarely considered to be absolutely contraindicated for a given patient. Even if a patient has a known allergic reaction to a given antineoplastic medication, the urgency of treating the patient's cancer may still

Box 47-1 Relative Emetic Potential of Selected Antineoplastic Drugs*

Low (Less Than 10% to 30%)
asparaginase
bleomycin
busulfan
capecitabine
chlorambucil
cladribine
cytarabine (less than 1000 mg/m²)
daunorubicin, liposomal
docetaxel
doxorubicin (less than 20 mg/m²)
doxorubicin, liposomal
estramustine
etoposide
floxuridine
fludarabine
fluorouracil (less than 1000 mg/m²)
gefitinib
gemcitabine
hydroxyurea
imatinib
melphalan
mercaptopurine
methotrexate (less than 250 mg/m²)
mitomycin
paclitaxel
pegaspargase
pentostatin
rituximab
teniposide
thioguanine
thiotepa
topotecan
trastuzumab
tretinoin

vinblastine
vincristine
vinorelbine

Moderate (30% to 60%)
altretamine
cyclophosphamide (less than 750 mg/m²)
dactinomycin
daunorubicin (less than 50 mg/m²)
doxorubicin (20 to 60 mg/m²)
epirubicin (less than 90 mg/m²)
idarubicin
ifosfamide (less than 1500 mg/m²)
irinotecan
methotrexate (250 to 1000 mg/m²)
mitoxantrone (less than 15 mg/m²)
temozolomide

High (60% to More Than 90%)
carboplatin
carmustine
cisplatin
cyclophosphamide (750 to more than 1500 mg/m²)
cytarabine (more than 1000 mg/m²)
dacarbazine
dactinomycin
daunorubicin (more than 50 mg/m²)
doxorubicin (more than 60 mg/m²)
ifosfamide (more than 1500 mg/m²)
lomustine
mechlorethamine
methotrexate (more than 1000 mg/m²)
mitoxantrone (more than 15 mg/m²)
oxaliplatin
procarbazine
streptozocin

*Drugs in this list not covered in this chapter are described in Chapter 48.

necessitate administering the medication and treating any allergic symptoms with supportive medications such as antihistamines and acetaminophen. These latter medications are often given before chemotherapy treatment with many drugs known to have potential for allergic-type reactions. For these reasons, no specific contraindications are listed for any of the drugs in this chapter.

Common relative contraindications for all cancer drugs include weakened status of the patient as manifested by indicators such as very low WBC count, any ongoing infectious process, or severe compromise in nutritional and hydration status, kidney or liver function, or the function of any other organ system that may be affected by a given drug. These are situations in which chemotherapy treatment is commonly delayed until the patient's status improves. Alternatively, dosages are often reduced for frail elderly patients or others with significantly compromised organ system function, depending on the drugs used. For these reasons, it can be assumed that all of the cancer drugs described in this chapter have no absolute contraindications. Reduction in fertility is often a major concern in postpubertal pediatric patients. Cancer also complicates 1 in 1000 pregnancies. Prepubertal patients are more resilient, however, and can have normal puberty and fertility. In the elderly, *frailty* refers to loss of most of the patient's functional reserve and limited ability to tolerate even minimal physiologic stress (e.g., chemotherapy treatment). More robust

elderly patients are certainly better candidates for cancer treatment, although frail patients often benefit as well, especially in terms of *palliative* (noncurative) symptom control. Both radiation and chemotherapy treatments can cause significant, permanent fetal harm or death. The greatest risk is during the first trimester. Chemotherapy treatment during the second- or third-trimester is more likely to improve maternal outcome without significant fetal risk. However, radiation poses great risk to the fetus throughout pregnancy and should be reserved for the postpartum period if possible. Patients are usually examined (and laboratory blood tests performed) by qualified specialists before each chemotherapy treatment. At that time a clinical judgment is made regarding each patient's fitness for receiving specific antineoplastic drugs.

CELL CYCLE–SPECIFIC ANTINEOPLASTIC DRUGS

Cell cycle–specific drug classes include antimetabolites, mitotic inhibitors, topoisomerase I inhibitors, and antineoplastic enzymes. These drugs are collectively used to treat a variety of solid and/or circulating tumors, although some drugs have much more specific indications than others. Table 47-5 shows the nomenclature for these drugs.

ANTIMETABOLITES

An **analogue** is a compound that is structurally similar to a normal cellular metabolite. Analogues may have agonist or antagonist activity relative to the corresponding cellular compounds. An antagonist analogue is also known as an *antimetabolite.*

Mechanism of Action and Drug Effects

Antineoplastic antimetabolites are cell cycle–specific analogues that work by antagonizing the actions of key cellular metabolites. More specifically, antimetabolites inhibit cellular growth by interfering with the synthesis or actions of three classes of compounds critical to cellular reproduction: the vitamin *folic acid* as well as *purines* and *pyrimidines,* the two classes of compounds that make up the bases contained in *nucleic acid* molecules (DNA and RNA). These drugs work via two mechanisms: (1) by falsely substituting for purines, pyrimidines, or folic acid, or (2) by inhibiting critical enzymes involved in the synthesis or function of these compounds. Thus, they ultimately inhibit the synthesis of DNA, RNA, and proteins, all of which are necessary for cellular reproduction. Antimetabolites work primarily in the S phase of the cell cycle, during which DNA synthesis occurs. The available antimetabolites and the metabolites they antagonize are as follows:

Folate antagonists
- methotrexate (MTX)
- pemetrexed

Purine antagonists
- cladribine
- fludarabine (F-AMP)
- mercaptopurine (6-MP)
- pentostatin
- thioguanine (6-TG)
- allopurinol
- rasburicase

Pyrimidine antagonists
- capecitabine
- cytarabine (ara-C)
- floxuridine (FUDR)
- fluorouracil (5-FU)
- gemcitabine

Folic Acid Antagonism

The antimetabolite methotrexate is an analogue of folic acid and inhibits the action of dihydrofolate reductase, an enzyme responsible for converting folic acid to a chemically reduced form that is normally used in the biosynthesis of other molecules. This inhibition prevents the formation of the folate, the reduced or anionic form of folic acid, that is needed for the synthesis of DNA and hence for cell reproduction. The result is that DNA is not produced and the cell dies. In practice, the terms *folic acid* and *folate* are often used interchangeably. Pemetrexed is the name of a newer folate antagonist with a mechanism of action similar to that of methotrexate.

Purine Antagonism

The purine bases present in DNA and RNA are adenine and guanine (see the discussion in Chapter 48), and they are required for the synthesis of the purine nucleotides that are incorporated into the nucleic acid molecules. Mercaptopurine and fludarabine are synthetic analogues of adenine, and thioguanine is a synthetic analogue of guanine. Cladribine is a more general purine antagonist, whereas pentostatin inhibits the action of the critical enzyme *adenosine deaminase.* Cladribine is unique in that it actually lacks cell cycle specificity relative to other drugs in its class. However, it is included in this section because of its similar pharmacology and mechanism of action. All of these drugs work by ultimately interrupting the synthesis of both DNA and RNA. Although allopurinol and rasburicase are chemically similar to purines, they do not disrupt DNA synthesis, unlike the other drugs in this class. Instead, both work by reducing serum and/or urinary levels of *uric acid.* Uric acid is a common waste product that often accumulates in the blood following lysis of tumor cells, part of a condition known as **tumor lysis syndrome** (see Adverse Effects).

Pyrimidine Antagonism

Of the pyrimidine bases, cytosine and thymine occur in the structure of DNA molecules, and cytosine and uracil are part of the structure of RNA molecules. These bases are essential for DNA and RNA synthesis. Floxuridine and fluorouracil are synthetic analogues of uracil, and cytarabine is a synthetic analogue of cytosine. Capecitabine is actually a prodrug of fluorouracil and is converted to that drug in the liver and other body tissues. Its prodrug form allows it to be given orally. Gemcitabine inhibits the action of two essential enzymes, *DNA polymerase* and *ribonucleotide reductase.* Overall, these drugs act in a way that is very similar to that of the purine antagonists, incorporating themselves into the metabolic pathway for the synthesis of DNA and RNA, and thereby interrupting the synthesis of both of these nucleic acids.

Indications

Antimetabolite antineoplastic drugs are used for the treatment of a variety of solid tumors and some hematologic cancers. They may also be used in combination chemotherapy regimens to enhance the overall cytotoxic effect. Methotrexate is also used to treat severe cases of psoriasis (a skin condition) as well as rheumatoid arthritis (Chapter 44). Because some of these drugs are available in both oral and topical preparations, they are sometimes used for low-dose maintenance and palliative (noncurative) cancer therapy. Allopurinol and rasburicase are both indicated for the hyperuricemia associated with tumor lysis syndrome and are usually given in anticipation of this condition during various chemotherapy regimens associated with this syndrome. Allopurinol is also used commonly in oral form to treat gout (Chapter 44). Rasburicase is used primarily in pediatric patients, and there is little published information to date regarding its use in adults. The commonly used drugs and their common specific therapeutic uses are listed in the table on page 732.

Adverse Effects

Like most antineoplastic drugs, antimetabolites can cause hair loss, nausea, vomiting, diarrhea, and myelosuppression. The relative emetic potentials for some of these drugs are listed in Box 47-1. In addition, these and other antineoplastic drug classes are also associated with other major types of toxicity including neurologic, cardiovascular, pulmonary, hepatobiliary,

Table 47-7 Common Manifestations of Antineoplastic Toxicity

Type of Toxicity	Common Manifestations
Neurologic	Fatigue, weakness, depression, agitation, euphoria, insomnia, sedation, headache, reduced libido, confusion, amnesia, hallucinations, dizziness, loss of taste or altered taste sensations, dysarthria (joint pain), polyneuropathy (e.g., numbness in extremities), neuritis, paresthesia (abnormal touch sensations), facial paralysis, migraine, tremor, hemiplegia, loss of consciousness, seizures, ataxia, stroke, encephalopathy
Cardiovascular	Hot flushes, edema, thrombophlebitis and bleeding (e.g., near infusion site), chest pain, tachycardia, bradycardia, other dysrhythmias, angina, venous or arterial thrombosis, transient ischemic attacks, heart failure, myocardial ischemia, pericarditis, pericardial effusion, pulmonary embolism, aneurysm, cardiomyopathy, myocardial infarction, stroke, cardiac arrest, sudden cardiac death
Pulmonary-respiratory	Cough, rhinorrhea (runny nose), sore throat, sinusitis, bronchitis, pharyngitis, laryngitis, epistaxis (nosebleed), abnormal breath sounds, asthma, bronchospasms, atelectasis, pleural effusion, hemoptysis, hypoxia, respiratory distress, pneumothorax, diffuse interstitial pneumonitis, fibrosis, hemorrhage, anaphylaxis and generalized allergic reactions
Hepatobiliary	Increased bilirubin and liver enzyme levels, jaundice, cholestasis, acalculic cholecystitis (inflamed gallbladder without stones), hepatitis, sclerosis, fibrosis, fatty liver changes, venoocclusive hepatic disease, cirrhosis, hepatic coma
Gastrointestinal (GI)	Dyspepsia (heartburn), hiccups, gingivitis (inflamed gums), glossitis (inflamed tongue), abdominal pain, nausea, vomiting, diarrhea, constipation, gastroenteritis, stomatitis (painful mouth sores), oral candidiasis (thrush), ulcers, proctalgia (rectal pain), hematemesis, GI hemorrhage, melena (blood in stool), toxic intestinal dilation, ileus (bowel paralysis), ascites, necrotizing enterocolitis
Genitourinary	Oliguria, nocturia, dysuria, proteinuria, crystalluria, hematuria, urinary retention, abnormal renal function test results, hemorrhagic cystitis, renal failure
Dermatologic	Rash, erythema, pruritus, ecchymosis, dryness, edema, photosensitivity, sweating, discoloration (pigmentation changes), freckling, petechiae, purpura, numbness, tingling, hypersensitivity, fissuring, scaling, seborrhea, acne, eczema, psoriasis, skin hypertrophy, subcutaneous nodules, alopecia, nail disorder including onycholysis (loss of nails), dermatitis, cellulitis, excoriation, maceration, ulceration, urticaria, abscesses, benign skin neoplasm, hemorrhage (at injection site), palmar-plantar dysesthesia-paresthesia, toxic epidermal necrolysis, Stevens-Johnson syndrome.
Ocular	Eye irritation, increased lacrimation, nystagmus, photophobia, visual changes, visual hallucinations, conjunctivitis, keratitis, dacryostenosis (narrowing of lacrimal duct)
Otic	Hearing loss, auditory hallucinations
Metabolic	Weight loss or gain, anorexia, dehydration, hypokalemia, hypocalcemia, hypomagnesemia, hypertriglyceridemia, hyperglycemia, syndrome of inappropriate secretion of antidiuretic hormone, hypoadrenalism, protein-losing enteropathy, hyperuricemia, tumor lysis syndrome
Musculoskeletal	Back pain, limb pain, bone pain, myalgia, joint stiffness, arthralgia, muscle weakness, fibromyositis

Table 47-8 Selected Antimetabolites: Common Drug-Specific Adverse Effects

Antimetabolite Drug	Adverse Effects
capecitabine	Neurologic, hepatobiliary, cardiac, GI, GU, ocular, musculoskeletal
cladribine	Neurologic, GU, GI, dermatologic, cardiac, pulmonary, musculoskeletal, metabolic
cytarabine	Hepatic, pulmonary, CV, GI, GU, neurologic, ocular
floxuridine	GI, GU, hepatic, CV, neurologic, ocular
fluorouracil	GI, GU, hepatic, CV, neurologic, ocular
fludarabine	Neurologic, pulmonary, GI, GU, CV, dermatologic, metabolic
gemcitabine	Neurologic, pulmonary, GI, GU, CV, hepatic, dermatologic toxicity
mercaptopurine	Hepatic, GI, GU
methotrexate	Hepatic, GI, CV, pulmonary, dermatologic
pentostatin	Neurologic, ocular, otic, GI, GU, hepatic, dermatologic, CV, pulmonary
thioguanine	Hepatic, GI

CV, Cardiovascular; *GI*, gastrointestinal; *GU*, genitourinary.

GI, genitourinary, dermatologic, ocular, otic, and metabolic toxicity. Common manifestations of these various toxicities are listed in Table 47-7, roughly in order of increasing severity, and are also described in general terms for each drug in Table 47-8. Note that a single drug may not cause all of the specific symptoms that are listed for each toxicity category, and actual symptoms may vary widely in severity among individual patients. The most common general symptoms are fever and malaise. Metabolic toxicity also includes tumor lysis syndrome, a common postchemotherapy condition. This syndrome is often associated with *induction* (initial) chemotherapy for rapidly growing malignancies. It may include hyperphosphatemia, hyperkalemia, and hypocalcemia. These electrolyte abnormalities are often treated with diuretics such as mannitol, IV calcium supplementation, oral or rectal potassium exchange resin (for hyperkalemia; Chapter 26), and oral aluminum hydroxide (for hyperphosphatemia; Chapter 51). Hyperuricemia can lead to nephropathy, and hemodialysis may be required in severe cases of tumor lysis syndrome.

A severe, but usually reversible, form of dermatologic toxicity is known as *palmar-plantar dysesthesia or paresthesia* (also called *hand-foot syndrome*). It can range from mild symptoms such as painless swelling and erythema to painful blistering of the patient's palms and soles. Other severe, but fortunately uncommon, dermatologic syndromes that can similarly affect the skin in more generalized regions include *Stevens-Johnson syndrome* and *toxic epidermal necrolysis*.

Table 47-9	Selected Antimetabolites: Common Drug Interactions
Antimetabolite	**Interacting Drug/Observed and Reported Effects***
capecitabine	warfarin: altered coagulation test results with potential for fatal bleeding
	phenytoin: reduced phenytoin clearance and toxicity
	leucovorin: potentiation of capecitabine with possible toxicity
cladribine	None listed
cytarabine	digoxin: reduced absorption likely due to cytarabine-induced damage to intestinal mucosa; elixir form may be better absorbed
	aminoglycoside antibiotics: reduced antibiotic efficacy against *Klebsiella pneumoniae* infections
floxuridine	None listed
fludarabine	cytarabine: reduction of fludarabine metabolism, which reduces its antineoplastic effects
	pentostatin: potentially fatal pulmonary toxicity; do not use together
fluorouracil	warfarin: enhanced anticoagulant effects
gemcitabine	None listed
mercaptopurine (6-MP)	allopurinol: inhibition of 6-MP metabolism by inhibition of xanthine oxidase enzyme, with possible enhanced 6-MP toxicity
	warfarin: 6-MP reported to both enhance and inhibit its effects
	hepatotoxic drugs: increased risk of liver toxicity
methotrexate (MTX)	Protein-bound drugs and weak organic acids (e.g., salicylates, sulfonamides, sulfonylureas, phenytoin, tetracyclines): possible displacement of MTX from protein-binding sites, enhancing its toxicity
	penicillins, NSAIDs: possible reduced renal elimination of MTX with potentially fatal hematologic and GI toxicity
	live virus vaccines: viral infection (true for any immunosuppressive drug)
	folic acid: reduced MTX efficacy (theoretical only)
	theophylline: reduced theophylline clearance
	hepatotoxic drugs: increased risk of liver toxicity
pentostatin	fludarabine: potentially fatal pulmonary toxicity
	allopurinol: reported cases of minor and reversible renal and hepatic dysfunction
thioguanine	busulfan: reports of hepatotoxicity, esophageal varices, and portal hypertension
	other cytotoxic drugs in general: reports of hepatotoxicity

GI, Gastrointestinal; *NSAIDs*, nonsteroidal antiinflammatory drugs.

*Note that not all mechanisms of these drug interactions have been clearly identified. The information in this table is based on reported clinical observations, with mention of known or theorized mechanisms when available.

Interactions

As is true for cancer drugs in general, the administration of one antimetabolite drug with another that causes similar toxicities may result in additive toxicities. Therefore, the respective risks and benefits should be weighed carefully before therapy is initiated with either another antimetabolite or any other drug possessing a similar toxicity profile. Table 47-9 lists some known common examples of drugs that cause interactions with antimetabolites.

Dosages

For information on the dosages of selected antimetabolite chemotherapeutic drugs, see the Dosages table on page 732.

Drug Profiles

Folate Antagonists
▸ **methotrexate**
Methotrexate (Trexall in tablet form) is the prototypical antimetabolite antineoplastic of the folate antagonist group and is currently one of only two antineoplastic folate antagonists used clinically. It has proved useful for the treatment of solid tumors such as breast, head and neck, and lung cancers and for the management of acute lymphocytic leukemia and non-Hodgkin's lymphomas. Methotrexate also has immunosuppressive activity because it can inhibit lymphocyte multiplication. For this reason it may be useful in the treatment of rheumatoid arthritis (Chapter 44). Its combined immunosuppressant and antiinflammatory properties also make it useful for the treatment of psoriasis.

The bone marrow suppression associated with high-dose methotrexate (doses of more than 500 mg/m^2) is always tempered with "rescue" dosing of its antidote drug *leucovorin*. Methotrexate is available in both injectable and oral (tablet) form. A preservative-free injectable formulation is required for **intrathecal** (spinal) administration, used in some cancers. Currently the only other folate antagonist is a newer drug called pemetrexed, which has an action similar to that of methotrexate. However, it is much less widely used because of its limited indications for treatment of certain types of lung cancer.

Purine Antagonists
The currently available purine antagonists are cladribine, fludarabine, mercaptopurine, pentostatin, and thioguanine. Of the five, mercaptopurine and thioguanine are administered orally. The other three are available only in injectable form. These drugs are not currently widely used. Those not profiled in the following paragraph are listed in the dosages table with their corresponding indications.
cladribine
Cladribine (Leustatin) is a newer drug first marketed in the early 1990s. It is indicated specifically for the treatment of a certain type of leukemia known as hairy cell leukemia, so named because of the appearance of its cancerous cells under the microscope.
fludarabine
Fludarabine (Fludara) was also approved by the FDA in the early 1990s. Like cladribine, it also has a very specific single indication—in this case, chronic lymphocytic leukemia.

Pyrimidine Antagonists
The currently available antimetabolite antineoplastics that are members of the pyrimidine antagonist family are capecitabine, cytarabine, floxuridine, fluorouracil, and gemcitabine. These drugs are

DOSAGES

Selected Antimetabolites

Drug (Pregnancy Category)	Pharmacologic Class	Usual Dosage Range	Indications
allopurinol (Zyloprim, Aloprim) (C)	Purine antagonist analogue	IV: 200-400 mg/m²/day PO: 300-600 mg daily	Prevention of uric acid nephropathy during chemotherapy; gout
capecitabine (Xeloda) (D)	Pyrimidine antagonist (analogue)	PO: 1250 mg/m² bid for 2 wk, followed by 1-wk rest period; this 3-wk cycle repeatable as ordered	Metastatic colorectal and breast cancer
cladribine (Leustatin) (D)	Purine antagonist analogue	IV: 0.09 mg/kg/day by continuous infusion for 7 consecutive days	Hairy cell leukemia
▶cytarabine (Cytosar-U) (D)	Pyrimidine antagonist (analogue)	IV: 100 mg/m²/day by continuous infusion × 7 days (other regimens as well)	Leukemias (several varieties), NHL
fludarabine (Fludara) (D)	Purine antagonist analogue	IV: 25 mg/m²/day for 5 consecutive days; repeatable q28d	Various acute and chronic leukemias, NHL
fluorouracil (Adrucil) (D)	Pyrimidine antagonist (analogue)	IV: 12 mg/kg once daily for 14 days initial dose; dose varies afterward depending on patient response	Colon, rectal, breast, esophageal, head and neck, cervical, and renal cancer
gemcitabine (Gemzar) (D)	Pyrimidine antagonist (analogue)	IV: 1000 mg/m² once weekly or as protocol dictates; cycle may be repeated or modified according to patient tolerance	Pancreatic, non–small cell lung, and bladder cancer
▶methotrexate (Trexall, tablet form; otherwise generic) (X)	Folate antagonist analogue	IV: 30-40 mg/m²/wk PO: 15-30 mg/day × 5 days, repeated q7d × 3-5 courses	Acute lymphocytic* leukemia; gestational choriocarcinoma; breast, head and neck, and many other cancers
pemetrexed (Alimta) (D)	Folate antagonist analogue	IV: 500-600 mg/m² on day 1 of each 21-day cycle	Malignant pleural mesothelioma, non–small cell lung cancer
rasburicase (Elitek) (C)	Purine antagonist analogue	IV: 0.15 or 0.2 mg/kg over 30 min once daily for 5 days	Prevention of uric acid nephropathy during chemotherapy

IV, Intravenous; *NHL*, non-Hodgkin's lymphoma; *PO*, oral.
*The term *lymphocytic* is synonymous in the literature with the term *lymphoblastic*.

used more commonly than the purine antagonists. They are available only in parenteral formulations except for capecitabine, which is currently available only in tablet form. Dosage and other information appear in the table on this page.

capecitabine
Capecitabine (Xeloda) was approved by the FDA in 1998. It is indicated primarily for the treatment of metastatic breast cancer.

▶ *cytarabine*
Cytarabine (Ara-C, Cytosar-U) is used primarily for the treatment of leukemias (acute myelocytic and lymphocytic and meningeal leukemia) and non-Hodgkin's lymphomas. As previously noted, it is available only in injectable form and may be given IV, subcutaneously, or intrathecally. It is also now available in a special encapsulated liposomal form for intrathecal use only in treating meningeal leukemia.

fluorouracil
Fluorouracil (5-FU) is used in a variety of treatment regimens, including the palliative treatment of cancers of the colon, rectum, stomach, breast, and pancreas.

gemcitabine
Gemcitabine (Gemzar) is an antineoplastic drug structurally related to cytarabine. Gemcitabine is believed to have antitumor activity superior to that of cytarabine. Gemcitabine was approved for marketing in 1996 by the FDA. Approved uses include first-line therapy for locally advanced or metastatic cancer of the pancreas and the treatment of non–small cell lung cancer.

MITOTIC INHIBITORS

Mitotic inhibitors include natural products obtained from the periwinkle plant (*Catharanthus roseus*, formerly called *Vinca rosea*) and semisynthetic drugs obtained from the mandrake plant (also known as the *may apple*). The periwinkle plant contains antineoplastic alkaloids. These include vinblastine, vincristine, and vinorelbine. These are also known as the *vinca alkaloids*. Etoposide and teniposide are semisynthetic derivatives of *epipodophyllotoxin*, which is obtained from the resinous extract of the mandrake plant. Two newer plant-derived drugs are the *taxanes*. These include paclitaxel, derived from the bark of the slow-growing Western (Pacific) yew tree, and docetaxel, a semisynthetic taxoid produced from the needles of the European yew tree. Docetaxel is pharmacologically similar to paclitaxel. The various mitotic inhibitors and their plant sources can be summarized as follows:

Vinca alkaloids (periwinkle)
- vinblastine
- vincristine
- vinorelbine

Epipodophyllotoxin derivatives (mandrake plant)
- etoposide
- teniposide

Taxanes
- docetaxel (European yew tree: needles)
- paclitaxel (Western yew tree: bark)
  Dosage and other information appears in the table on page 734.

Mechanism of Action and Drug Effects

Depending on the particular drug, these plant-derived compounds can work in various phases of the cell cycle (late S phase, throughout G_2 phase, and M phase), but they all work shortly before or during mitosis and thus retard cell division. Each different subclass inhibits mitosis in a unique way.

The vinca alkaloids (vincristine, vinblastine, and vinorelbine) bind to the protein *tubulin* during the metaphase of mitosis (M phase). This prevents the assembly of key structures called *microtubules*. This, in turn, results in the dissolution of other important structures known as *mitotic spindles*. Without these mitotic spindles, cells cannot reproduce properly. This results in inhibition of cell division and synthesis of DNA, RNA, and protein. The epipodophyllotoxin derivatives (etoposide and teniposide) exert their cytotoxic effects by inhibiting the enzyme *topoisomerase II*, which causes breaks in DNA strands. These drugs work during the late S phase and the G_2 phase of the cell cycle.

The yew tree derivatives (taxanes) paclitaxel and docetaxel both act in the late G_2 phase and M phase of the cell cycle. They work by causing the formation of nonfunctional microtubules, which halts mitosis during metaphase.

Indications

Mitotic inhibitors are used to treat a variety of solid tumors and some hematologic malignancies. They are often used in combination chemotherapy regimens to enhance the overall cytotoxic effect. The commonly administered drugs and some of their specific therapeutic uses are listed in the table on page 734.

Adverse Effects

Like many of their antineoplastic counterparts in other classes, mitotic inhibitor antineoplastic drugs can cause hair loss, nausea and vomiting, and myelosuppression. The emetic potential of some of these drugs is given in Box 47-1. Major adverse effects specific to mitotic inhibitors are described in general terms in Table 47-10, and in greater detail in Table 47-7 earlier in the chapter.

Table 47-10 Selected Mitotic Inhibitors: Adverse Effects

Antibiotic Drug	Adverse Effects
etoposide	GI, CV, dermatologic, neurologic
docetaxel	Neurologic, CV, GI, dermatologic, musculoskeletal
paclitaxel	Neurologic, CV, GI, GU, dermatologic, musculoskeletal, hepatic, pulmonary, ocular
vincristine	Neurologic, pulmonary, dermatologic, CV, GI, otic, metabolic

CV, Cardiovascular; *GI*, gastrointestinal; *GU*, genitourinary.

Toxicity: Management of Extravasation

Most of the mitotic inhibitor antineoplastics are administered IV, which makes extravasation of the drugs and its serious consequences a constant threat. Specific antidotes and additional measures to be taken for the treatment of extravasation of the mitotic inhibitors are given in Table 47-11.

Interactions

A variety of drug interactions are possible with most antineoplastic drugs, some more significant than others. A few basic principles should be kept in mind that apply to all antineoplastic drug classes. When a drug interacts with warfarin, resulting in enhanced anticoagulation, this can generally be assumed to be due to displacement of warfarin from its plasma protein-binding sites by the drug in question. Any drug that reduces the clearance of another drug also increases the risk of toxicity for the second drug. Also, because most antineoplastic drugs cause bone marrow depression, with increased risk of infection, it can usually be assumed that this risk is greater for patients receiving multiple antineoplastic drugs. Patients should be monitored and treated accordingly for hematologic toxicity and infections. Observed drug interactions specific for mitotic inhibitor drugs are summarized in Table 47-12.

Dosages

For information on the dosages of selected mitotic inhibitors, see the Dosages table on page 734.

Drug Profiles

▶ etoposide
Etoposide (VP-16, VePesid) is a semisynthetic epipodophyllotoxin derivative. Its structure, mechanism of action, and adverse effect profile are similar to those of teniposide. As previously noted, it is believed to kill cancer cells in the late S phase and the G_2 phase of the cell cycle. It is indicated for the treatment of small cell lung cancer and testicular cancer. It is available in both oral and injectable forms.

▶ paclitaxel
Paclitaxel (Taxol) is a natural mitotic inhibitor that is obtained from the bark of the Pacific yew tree. The European yew tree is the source for another mitotic inhibitor known as docetaxel (Taxotere). Paclitaxel is currently approved for the treatment of ovarian cancer, breast

Table 47-11 Mitotic Inhibitor Extravasation: Listed Specific Antidotes

Mitotic Inhibitor	Antidote Preparation	Method
etoposide	hyaluronidase (Wydase) 150 units/mL: add 1 mL NaCl (150 units/mL)	1. Inject 1-6 mL into the extravasated site with multiple SC injections.
teniposide		2. Repeat SC dosing over the next few hours.
vinblastine		3. Apply warm compresses.*
vincristine		4. No total dose established.

SC, Subcutaneous.
*Important: Administration of corticosteroids and topical cooling appear to worsen toxicity.

cancer, non–small cell lung cancer, and Kaposi's sarcoma, among other cancers. Paclitaxel is extremely water insoluble (hydrophobic), and for this reason it is put into a solution containing oil rather than water. The particular oil used is a type of castor oil called Cremophor EL, the same oil with which cyclosporine is formulated. Many patients cannot tolerate it and show hypersensitivity responses similar

to anaphylactic reactions. For this reason, before patients receive paclitaxel they may be premedicated with a steroid, antihistamine, and histamine-2 (H_2) antagonist (e.g., ranitidine). Paclitaxel is available only in injectable form.

▶ **vincristine**
Vincristine is an alkaloid isolated from the periwinkle plant that is indicated for the treatment of acute leukemia and other cancers. It is available only in injectable form.

Table 47-12	**Selected Mitotic Inhibitors: Common Drug Interactions**
Mitotic Inhibitor	**Interacting Drug/Observed and Reported Effects***
etoposide	warfarin: enhanced anticoagulation
	cyclosporine: reduced etoposide clearance
docetaxel	CYP3A4 inhibitors (azole antifungals, ciprofloxacin, clarithromycin, imatinib, verapamil, many others): enhanced docetaxel effect (possible toxicity)
	CYP3A4 inducers (e.g., carbamazepine, nafcillin, phenytoin): reduced docetaxel effect
paclitaxel	CNS depressants: enhanced sedation due to alcohol in paclitaxel formulation
	azole antifungals: reduced paclitaxel clearance
vincristine	phenytoin: reduced phenytoin concentrations, enhancing seizure risk
	asparaginase: reduced vincristine clearance (give vincristine 12-24 hr before asparaginase)
	mitomycin: increased risk of pulmonary toxicity
	azole antifungals: increased risk of severe neuromuscular toxicity (consider reduction of vincristine dose during azole therapy)

CNS, Central nervous system; *CYP3A4,* cytochrome P-450 liver enzyme subtype 3A4.
*Note that not all mechanisms of these drug interactions have been clearly identified. The information in this table is based on reported clinical observations, with mention of known or theorized mechanisms when available.

TOPOISOMERASE I INHIBITORS

Topoisomerase I inhibitors are a relatively new class of chemotherapy drugs. The two drugs currently available in this class are topotecan and irinotecan. Both are semisynthetic analogues of the compound camptothecin, which was originally isolated in the 1960s from *Camptotheca acuminata,* a Chinese shrub. For this reason, they are also referred to as *camptothecins.*

Mechanism of Action and Drug Effects

The Chinese shrub–derived camptothecins inhibit proper DNA function in the S phase by binding to the DNA–topoisomerase I complex. This complex normally allows DNA strands to be temporarily cleaved and then reattached *(religated)* in a critical step known as *religation.* The binding of the camptothecin drugs to this complex retards this religation process.

Indications

The two currently available topoisomerase I inhibitors are used primarily to treat ovarian and colorectal cancer. Topotecan has been shown to be effective even in cases of metastatic ovarian cancer that has failed to respond to platinum-containing regimens (e.g., cisplatin, carboplatin) and paclitaxel. Topotecan is also sometimes used to treat small cell lung cancer. Irinotecan is cur-

---

DOSAGES

Selected Mitotic Inhibitors

Drug (Pregnancy Category)	Pharmacologic Class	Usual Dosage Range*	Indications
Epipodophyllotoxin Derivative			
▶etoposide (VePesid, Toposar, Etopophos) (D)	Topoisomerase II inhibitor	IV: 50-160 mg/m²/day for 4-5 days PO: 2 × IV dose rounded to nearest 50 mg	Testicular and small cell lung cancer
Taxanes			
docetaxel (Taxotere) (D)	Mitotic spindle inhibitor	IV: 60-100 mg/m² q3wk	Breast and non–small cell lung cancer
▶paclitaxel (Taxol, Onxol) (D)	Inhibitor of tubulin depolymerization	IV: 135-250 mg/m² q3wk	Ovarian, breast, esophageal, bladder, head and neck, cervical cancer; non–small cell and small cell lung cancer; Kaposi's sarcoma
Vinca Alkaloid			
▶vincristine (Oncovin, Vincasar PFS) (D)	Inhibitor of tubulin polymerization	IV: 1.4 mg/m² q1wk; usual max dose 2 mg; fatal if given intrathecally	ALL, AML, HL, NHL, rhabdomyosarcoma, neuroblastoma, Wilms' tumor, brain tumors, small cell lung cancer, Kaposi's sarcoma

ALL, Acute lymphocytic leukemia; *AML,* acute myelocytic leukemia; *HL,* Hodgkin's lymphoma; *IV,* intravenous; *NHL,* non-Hodgkin's lymphoma; *PO,* oral.
*Note that dosages may vary widely among treatment protocols.

rently approved for the treatment of metastatic colorectal cancer, small cell lung cancer, and cervical cancer.

Adverse Effects

As with many cancer chemotherapeutic drugs, the main adverse effect of topotecan is suppression of blood cell production in the bone marrow. This bone marrow suppression is predictable, noncumulative, reversible, and manageable. Topotecan should not be given to patients with baseline neutrophil counts of less than 1500/mm³. Other adverse effects are relatively minor compared to those of the other antineoplastic drug classes. These include mild to moderate nausea, vomiting, and diarrhea; headache; rash; muscle weakness; and cough.

Irinotecan causes more severe adverse effects than topotecan. In addition to producing similar hematologic adverse effects, it has been associated with severe diarrhea known as *cholinergic diarrhea* that may occur during irinotecan infusion. It is recommended that this condition be treated with atropine unless use of that drug is strongly contraindicated. Delayed diarrhea may occur 2 to 10 days after infusion of irinotecan. This diarrhea can be severe and even life threatening. Delayed diarrhea should be treated aggressively with loperamide. Severe cardiovascular toxicity, including thrombosis, pulmonary embolism, stroke, and acute fatal myocardial infarction have been reported during irinotecan therapy. Such effects have been seen particularly when irinotecan is given with IV fluorouracil and leucovorin. Such drug combinations should be given with especially careful monitoring or avoided whenever possible. Severe nausea and vomiting are also seen with irinotecan, requiring appropriate supportive care such as IV rehydration and antiemetic drug therapy.

Interactions

The *granulocyte colony-stimulating factor* filgrastim (Chapter 49), used to enhance WBC recovery after chemotherapy, has actually been shown to worsen myelosuppression when given concurrently with topotecan. It is recommended that filgrastim be administered 24 hours after completion of the topotecan infusion. Laxatives and diuretics should not be given concomitantly with irinotecan because of the potential to worsen the dehydration resulting from the severe diarrhea that this drug can produce. Several additional recognized drug interactions occur with irinotecan, which are summarized in Table 47-13.

Dosages

For recommended dosages of selected topoisomerase I inhibitors, see the Dosages table on this page.

Table 47-13	Irinotecan: Common Drug Interactions
Interacting Drug	**Observed and Reported Effects***
CYP2B6 inhibitors (e.g., paroxetine, sertraline)	Increased effects and toxicity of irinotecan
CYP3A4 inhibitors (e.g., azole antifungals, ciprofloxacin, clarithromycin, imatinib, isoniazid, verapamil)	Increased effects and toxicity of irinotecan; concurrent use not recommended
CYP2B6 inducers (e.g., carbamazepine, phenytoin, nevirapine)	Reduced effects of irinotecan
CYP3A4 inducers (e.g., aminoglutethimide, carbamazepine, nafcillin, nevirapine, phenytoin)	Reduced effects of irinotecan
St. John's wort	Reduced effects of irinotecan; stop St. John's wort 2 wk before initiating irinotecan therapy

CYP2B6, Cytochrome P-450 liver enzyme subtype 2B6; *CYP3A4,* cytochrome P-450 subtype 3A4.

*Note that not all mechanisms of these drug interactions have been clearly identified. The information in this table is based on reported clinical observations, with mention of known or theorized mechanisms when available.

Drug Profiles

irinotecan
Irinotecan (Camptosar) is usually given with both fluorouracil and leucovorin. It is available only in injectable form.

topotecan
After initial therapy with other antineoplastics, cancer cells commonly become resistant to their effects. The use of topotecan (Hycamtin) to treat ovarian cancer and small cell lung cancer has been extensively studied. As noted earlier, it produces therapeutic responses even in cases in which powerful drugs such as cisplatin and paclitaxel have failed. It is available only in injectable form.

ANTINEOPLASTIC ENZYMES

Two antineoplastic enzymes are commercially available: asparaginase and pegaspargase. A third, *Erwinia* asparaginase, is available only by special request from the National Cancer Institute for patients who have developed allergic reactions to *Escherichia coli*–based asparaginase, which is described in the following

DOSAGES

Selected Topoisomerase I Inhibitors

Drug (Pregnancy Category)	Pharmacologic Class	Usual Dosage Range	Indications
irinotecan (Camptosar) (D)	Synthetic camptothecin	IV: 125-350 mg/m² on various days depending on protocol	Metastatic colorectal cancer, small cell lung cancer, and cervical cancer
topotecan (Hycamtin) (D)	Semisynthetic camptothecin	IV: 1.5 mg/m² once daily for 5 consecutive days on a repeatable 21-day course	Ovarian and small cell lung cancer

IV, Intravenous.

drug profile. All three drugs are synthesized from cultures of certain bacteria using recombinant DNA technology. Specifically, a critical segment of DNA that contains the genes for producing the enzyme is inserted into the genetic material of the bacteria, which then mass-produce the enzyme as the bacteria multiply in culture. The enzyme itself is then isolated from this culture using various laboratory techniques and purified for clinical use.

Indications

The antineoplastic enzymes are currently approved exclusively for the treatment of acute lymphocytic leukemia.

Adverse Effects

Of particular note for the antineoplastic enzymes is a fairly unique adverse effect of impaired pancreatic function. This can lead to hyperglycemia and severe or fatal pancreatitis. Other types of adverse effects associated with these drugs are dermatologic, hepatic, genitourinary, neurologic, musculoskeletal, GI, and cardiovascular effects.

Interactions

Commonly reported drug interactions involving the antineoplastic enzymes are summarized in Table 47-14.

Dosages

Dosages for the antineoplastic enzymes are given in the Dosages table on this page.

Table 47-14	Selected Antineoplastic Enzymes: Common Drug Interactions	
Enzyme	**Interacting Drug/Observed and Reported Effects***	
asparaginase	cyclophosphamide, mercaptopurine, vincristine: interference with efficacy or clearance	
	mercaptopurine, methotrexate, prednisone: enhanced liver toxicity	
	methotrexate: reduced antineoplastic effect when given concurrently, but possibly enhanced antineoplastic effect when given 9-10 days before or shortly after methotrexate	
	prednisone: hyperglycemia (give asparaginase after prednisone)	
	vincristine: neuropathy (give asparaginase after vincristine)	
pegaspargase	Same as above, plus the following:	
	aspirin, other NSAIDs, dipyridamole, heparin, warfarin: coagulation factor imbalances	
	cyclophosphamide: reduced clearance of cyclophosphamide	

NSAIDs, Nonsteroidal antiinflammatory drugs.
*Note that not all mechanisms of these drug interactions have been clearly identified. The information in this table is based on reported clinical observations, with mention of known or theorized mechanisms when available.

Drug Profiles

▶ asparaginase

Asparaginase (Elspar) is used for the treatment of acute lymphocytic leukemia. Its mechanism of action is slightly different from that of traditional antineoplastic drugs in that it is an enzyme that catalyzes the conversion of the amino acid asparagine to aspartic acid and ammonia. Leukemic cells are then unable to synthesize the asparagine required for the synthesis of DNA and proteins needed for cell survival.

The only commercially available asparaginase product in the United States is the Elspar product manufactured by Merck, Inc. This product is derived from the *E. coli* bacterium, and it is common for patients to develop allergic reactions to it. When this happens, one alternative is to switch to a product synthesized from a *Erwinia* bacteria. As noted earlier, this product is not sold commercially in the United States but is available by special request from the National Cancer Institute. Another treatment alternative is to use the commercially available pegaspargase product described in the following drug profile. All antineoplastic enzymes are available only in injectable form.

pegaspargase

Pegaspargase (Oncaspar) has a mechanism of action, indications, and contraindications similar to those of asparaginase. It is essentially the same enzyme that has been formulated so as to reduce its allergenic potential. This process involves chemical conjugation of the enzyme with units of a relatively inert compound known as monomethoxypolyethylene glycol. Because polyethylene glycol is abbreviated PEG, this process is known as *pegylation*. It is a relatively new process that is increasingly used in formulating various other drugs described in other chapters (e.g., Chapter 49). These drugs are recognized by the prefix *peg* in their generic names. Pegaspargase is usually prescribed for patients who have developed an allergy to asparaginase—a common occurrence, as mentioned earlier, especially with repeated treatment.

DOSAGES

Selected Antineoplastic Enzymes

Drug (Pregnancy Category)	Pharmacologic Class	Usual Dosage Range	Indications
▶asparaginase (Elspar) (C)	*Escherichia coli*–derived L-asparagine amidohydrolase enzyme	IV/IM: 200 units/kg/day to 40,000 units per dose depending on protocol	Acute lymphocytic leukemia
pegaspargase (Oncaspar) (C)	Pegylated version of asparaginase	IV/IM: 2500 international units/m^2 q14d (smaller pediatric dosages)	Acute lymphocytic leukemia (usually in patients who have developed an allergy to asparaginase)

IM, Intramuscular; *IV*, intravenous.

◆ NURSING PROCESS

◆ ASSESSMENT

A patient should undergo thorough assessment before any antineoplastic drug is administered. The assessment should include taking a complete and thorough nursing history; performing a head-to-toe physical examination; measuring height, weight, and vital signs; testing hearing and vision; taking a complete medical history and family history; and noting any food and drug allergies. A complete assessment of cultural, emotional, spiritual, sexual, and financial influences, concerns, or issues should also be carried out. Ability to perform the activities of daily living is important to assess, as are mobility and gait pattern. Assessment of bowel and bladder patterns, neurologic status, heart sounds, heart rhythm, and breath sounds and lung function should also occur. Examination of the skin and mucosa should note turgor, hydration, color, and temperature. Signs and symptoms of fear and anxiety should be assessed with attention to verbalization of feelings, insomnia, irritability, shakiness, restlessness, palpitations, and any unusual problems that could be attributed to stress and anxiety.

Contraindications, cautions, drug interactions, and drug allergies should be assessed for and documented prior to use of any antineoplastic drug. A number of laboratory tests are usually ordered, as well, and need to be reviewed. These tests may include complete blood counts, platelet counts, and bleeding times, as well as liver, kidney, and cardiac function tests and pulmonary function tests. In addition, measurement of various tumor markers and related blood work may be ordered to help monitor baseline levels and determine the impact of the disease on the patient, to help confirm the diagnosis, and/or to help determine the patient's response to different drug therapies. Further discussion of various laboratory studies specific to antineoplastic therapy is provided in the Laboratory Values Related to Drug Therapy box. Another area of importance is the information on the specific antineoplastic drug(s) being used for the treatment protocol and how the protocol is to be implemented as related to the nurse's responsibility. Many of the adverse effects and toxic effects associated with antineoplastic drugs are attributed to the killing of rapidly dividing malignant cells but also killing rapidly normal cells. See Box 47-2 for more information about the specific adverse effects associated with destruction of various populations of normal cells.

Areas of assessment related to some of the more common effects of antineoplastic therapy on normal, rapidly dividing cells include the following:

- For *altered nutritional status* and *impaired oral mucosa:* Assess for signs and symptoms of altered nutrition with a focus on weight loss, abnormal serum protein-albumin and blood urea nitrogen levels (negative nitrogen status due to low protein levels would be indicated by a decreasing blood urea nitrogen level), weakness, fatigue, lethargy, poor skin turgor, and pale conjunctiva. Assess oral mucosa for signs and symptoms of *stomatitis* such as pain or burning in the mouth, difficulty swal-

---

LABORATORY VALUES RELATED TO DRUG THERAPY

Antineoplastic Therapy: Rationales for Assessment and Monitoring of Blood Cell Counts

Because antineoplastics kill both normal and abnormal cells that are rapidly dividing cells, the bone marrow and its rapidly dividing cellular constituents are negatively impacted. Due to this characteristic of chemotherapeutic drugs, red blood cells (RBCs), white blood cells (WBCs), and platelets are suppressed and therefore require frequent monitoring. This box presents information specifically on RBCs and subsequent hemoglobin (Hgb) and hematocrit (HCT) levels as well as platelet levels. Chapter 48 presents more information on WBCs with neutrophil counts and nadir levels.

Laboratory Test	Normal Ranges	Rationale for Assessment
RBCs	M: 4.6-6.2 million cells/mm³ F: 4.2-5.4 million cells/mm³	Bone marrow suppression from antineoplastics also affects RBC values, leading to severe anemia. Red blood cells carry oxygen from the lungs—with O_2 attached to the hemoglobin—to the rest of the body. RBCs also help carry CO_2 back to the lungs for it to be exhaled. Therefore, if RBC counts are low (e.g., with anemia), the body does not get the oxygen it needs, leading to lack of energy, fatigue, intolerance for activity, shortness of breath, and hypoxemia. For the cancer patient who may already be experiencing the impact of bone marrow suppression either from the disease or the treatment, this loss of oxygen may be exacerbated, with even more of an impact on the patient with deterioration of the ability to get up and about and perform activities of daily living, and even a loss of ability to eat meals and/or visit with family and friends.
Hct	M: 40%-54%; F: 37%-47%	Hct measures the amount of space or volume of red blood cells in the blood, aso if the RBC value is low the Hct is also low. The impact of this low value is discussed with RBCs.
Hgb	M: 14-18g/dL F: 12-16 g/dL	Hgb is the major substance in red blood cells, carries oxygen, and is responsible for the blood cell color of red. With low levels of Hgb the consequence to the patient is as noted with RBCs.
Platelets	150,000-140,000/mm³	Platelets are the smallest type of blood cell and play a large role in the process of blood coagulation/clotting. When bleeding occurs, the platelets swell, clump, and form a plug that helps stop the bleeding. Therefore, if platelet levels are <100,000/mm³, the patient is at high risk for uncontrolled bleeding and/or hemorrhage.

F, Female; *M,* male.

Box 47-2 Effects of Antineoplastic Drugs on Normal Cells and Related Adverse Effects

Antineoplastic drugs are designed to kill rapidly dividing *cancer* cells, but they also kill rapidly dividing *normal* cells. Such normal cells include cells of the oral and gastrointestinal (GI) mucous membranes, hair follicles, reproductive germinal epithelium, and components of bone marrow (e.g., white blood cells [WBCs], red blood cells [RBCs], and platelets). The more common adverse effects of normal cell kill are as follows:

- Killing of normal cells of the GI mucous membranes may result in adverse effects such as *altered nutritional status, stomatitis* with inflammation and/or ulcerations of the oral mucosa and throughout the GI tract, *altered bowel function, poor appetite, nausea, vomiting* (often intractable and requiring aggressive antiemetics treatment), and *diarrhea.*
- Killing of the normal cells of hair follicles leads to *alopecia* (loss of hair).
- Killing of normal cells in the bone marrow results in dangerously low (life-threatening) blood cell counts. Because of the negative impact on these normal cells, the nurse must carefully assess the patient's WBC counts (leukocytes, neutrophils, and band neutrophils), RBC counts, hemoglobin level, hematocrit, and platelet (thrombocyte) counts (see the Laboratory Values Related to Drug Therapy box on p. 737 for discussion of *anemia, leukopenia, neutropenia,* and *thrombocytopenia*). In addition, monitoring of the patient's absolute neutrophil count (ANC) is needed (ANC is the WBC count multiplied by the percentage of neutrophils). Following the ANC values allows the nurse and other health care providers to identify the nadir (see the Laboratory Values Related to Drug Therapy box on p. 737)—the time of the lowest count when the patient is most vulnerable. An ANC of 1000/mm³ or below indicates severely impaired immune function and high risk for immunosuppression and infection.
- Killing of germinal epithelial cells (also rapidly dividing) leads to *sterility* (irreversible) in males and to *teratogenic* effects with possible fetal death as well as damage to the ovaries with *amenorrhea* in females.

lowing, taste changes, viscous saliva, dryness, cracking, and/or fissures with or without bleeding of mucosa.

- For *effects on the GI mucosa:* Assess for signs and symptoms of *diarrhea* such as frequent, loose stools (more than three stools per day), urgency, abdominal cramping, and hyperactive bowel sounds and obtain information about the presence of blood, consistency, color, odor, and amount. Assess for *nausea and vomiting* and determine whether symptoms are acute, delayed, or anticipatory; if vomiting occurs, determine the color, amount, consistency, frequency, odor, and whether blood is present. The severity of nausea and vomiting may be rated using a scale of 1 to 10 (where 10 is the worst) or using the terms *mild, moderate,* and *severe.*
- For *alopecia:* Assess the patient's views, concerns, and emotions about potential hair loss. Assess the patient's need to prepare for hair loss either by leaving the hair as it is and allowing it to fall out on its own; by having the hair cut short; or by wearing a scarf, hat, bandana, or hair wrap or purchasing a wig before the hair is actually lost so that the hairstyle is similar to that before chemotherapy.
- For *bone marrow suppression:* Assess for signs and symptoms of *anemia* (decrease in RBC, hemoglobin, and hematocrit)

such as pallor of skin, oral mucus membranes and conjunctiva, fatigue, loss of interest in activities, shortness of breath and other intolerance of activity, lethargy, and an inability to concentrate (see the Laboratory Values Related to Drug Therapy box on p. 737). Assess for signs and symptoms of *leukopenia* or *neutropenia* (decrease in WBC and an absolute neutrophils count below 1000/mm³) including fever; chills; tachycardia; abnormal breath sounds; productive cough with purulent, green, or rust-colored sputum; change in color of urine; lethargy or fatigue and acute confusion. For more information, see the Laboratory Values Related to Drug Therapy box on p. 758 in Chapter 48). Assess for signs and symptoms of *thrombocytopenia* (decrease in thrombocyte or platelet counts and abnormal clotting test results) including indications of unusual bleeding such as petechiae, purpura, ecchymosis, gingival (gum) bleeding, excessive or prolonged bleeding from puncture sites (e.g., intramuscular or IV sites or laboratory draw sites), unusual joint pain, or blood in stool, urine, or vomitus; and a decrease in blood pressure with elevated pulse rate; (see the Laboratory Values Related to Drug Therapy box on p. 737 in this chapter, as well as in Chapter 27).

- For possible *sterility, teratogenesis,* damage to ovaries with *amenorrhea:* For the adult male patient, assess baseline reproductive history with attention to sexual functioning, fathering of children, and past and current reproductive or sexual problems or concerns; for the female adult patient, inquire about reproductive history with attention to sexual functioning, fertility, childbearing history, menstrual history with focus on menstrual irregularities, and age at the onset of menses and menopause if applicable.

Assessing for *pain* is also an important part of the care of the patient with cancer. Assess for reports of oral, pharyngeal, esophageal, and/or abdominal pain; painful swallowing; epigastric or gastric pain, especially after eating spicy or acidic foods; achiness in joints or lower extremities; and numbness, tingling, and any burning or sharp pain that is general or localized. Pain should be assessed using an intensity rating scale (e.g., 0 to 10 with 0 = no pain and 10 = worse pain ever). Be sure also to note the pattern of pain, with a focus on the location, quality, onset, duration, and precipitating or alleviating factors. Also inquire about past experiences with pain and any drug, nondrug, or alternative therapies used and successes or failures in its treatment. Cultural beliefs and background as they relate to pain are important to assess because the individual's culture may affect how pain is perceived, verbalized, and treated (Chapter 10).

With *cell cycle–specific drugs,* once allergies, cautions, contraindications, and drug interactions have been documented, a baseline assessment of the patient's general health status is an important starting point in development of a care plan. A thorough baseline and physical assessment should include weight, height, vital signs including pain assessment, and a complete nursing history with attention to the hepatic, renal, gastrointestinal, male and female genitourinary systems as well as cardiac and respiratory systems.. Laboratory testing associated with these systems (e.g., uric acid level, complete blood cell counts, platelets, RBCs, hemoglobin/hematocrit, fluid/electrolyte levels, clotting studies) is generally performed before, during, and after chemotherapy (see the Laboratory Values Related to Drug Therapy box on p. 737, as well as in Chapter 27). For antimetabolites, most of the drugs do not produce severe emesis (i.e., in fewer than 10% of cases); however, pentostatin and some of the pyrimidine analogues have emetic potential and thus require assessment of baseline gastrointestinal functioning. Folate antagonists are not as likely to cause emesis but may be associated with GI abnormalities (e.g., peptic ulcer disease, ulcerative colitis, stomatitis) and genitourinary abnormalities requiring baseline assessment of bowel patterns, bowel sounds, and bladder patterns. Because these drugs are generally administered parenterally (IV), assessing peripheral access areas or central venous sites is critical to prevent possible damage to surrounding tissue, joints, and tendons.

Specific assessment features associated with use of the antimetabolite cytarabine include monitoring for the occurrence of *cytarabine syndrome*. This syndrome occurs usually within 6 to 12 hours after drug administration and is characterized by fever, myalgia, bone pain, nausea, vomiting, occasional chest pain, and rash. In addition, a thorough assessment of cardiac and breath sounds, with a complete nursing assessment of cardiac and respiratory systems, is warranted with the use of cytarabine (as well as other antimetabolites) because they may cause cardiac and/or pulmonary toxicity.

Patients receiving *mitotic inhibitors* (e.g., vinblastine, vincristine, etoposide) should undergo thorough assessment for baseline fluid and electrolyte levels and blood counts (see the Laboratory Values Related to Drug Therapy boxes on p. 737 and p. 758 in this chapter and Chapter 48). Hepatic and renal toxicities are a concern, so liver and renal function studies are performed frequently. Serum uric acid levels generally increase with cell death (related to the therapeutic effects as well as adverse effects of these drugs), and the patient should be observed for first-time appearance of gout or exacerbation of existing gout once therapy is initiated. Bowel and bladder patterns should be noted, and baseline neurologic functioning should be assessed with attention to muscle tone and reflexes. Because these drugs have multiple incompatibilities and are either irritants (irritating the IV site and vein) or vesicants (causing cell death with extravasation and necrosis with ulcerations), the nurse should know all potential solution and drug interactions and should document initial and follow-up assessments of the IV site.

Other mitotic inhibitors, docetaxel and paclitaxel, are drugs in the *taxane* family and are also associated with severe neutropenia (see the Laboratory Values Related to Drug Therapy box on p. 758 in Chapter 48); thus, blood counts must be performed before drug therapy. The patient should constantly be assessed for severe hypersensitivity reactions characterized by dyspnea, severe hypotension, angioedema, and generalized urticaria during treatments and in the home setting. Results of all blood cell counts should also be examined. The nurse should be alert to the smallest clues to a hypersensitivity reaction, which may indicate the potential for severe reactions. Levels of platelets and neutrophils are of most concern with these drugs, and thus close examination of baseline levels and assessment for a decrease in these levels with therapy are important. Drops in these blood cell counts may even occur before any clinical evidence of the actual anemia or other blood-related adverse effect. Peripheral neuropathies may occur and thus the need for thorough assessment of any abnormal sensations in the extremities or other abnormalities that are present before treatment.

Topoisomerase inhibitors are associated with hematologic adverse effects and thus the need for baseline WBC counts; spe-

cifically, topotecan may produce severe neutropenia due to bone marrow suppression. This bone marrow suppression is predictable, noncumulative, reversible, and manageable and so topotecan should not be given to patients with baseline neutrophil counts of less than 1500/mm^3. Assessment of GI functioning and bowel patterns is important with these drugs due to the related adverse effects of mild to moderate nausea, vomiting, and diarrhea. Irinotecan causes more severe adverse effects than topotecan and so related systems should be assessed with findings noted. The concern for *cholinergic diarrhea* that may occur during irinotecan infusion is of concern and requires continual assessment. This diarrhea may occur 2 to 10 days after the irinotecan infusion and require further medical treatment, especially with the occurrence of severe forms of diarrhea. Severe cardiovascular toxicity, including thrombosis, pulmonary embolism, stroke, and acute fatal myocardial infarction are related adverse effects and require cautious and astute assessment of related systems. These adverse effects have been seen particularly when irinotecan is given with intravenous fluorouracil and leucovorin. Such drug combinations should be given with especially careful monitoring or avoided whenever possible. Severe nausea and vomiting is also seen with irinotecan and should be assessed for and documented, as appropriate.

Patients being given *natural enzyme* drugs (e.g., asparaginase, pegaspargase) require assessment for allergies and gout as well as examination of the results of complete blood counts and renal and liver function tests because of the associated damage to these systems. The nurse should also determine whether the patient has a history or concurrent outbreak of chickenpox or herpes zoster, because the virus can become active and create problems for the patient. Any recent cytotoxic treatment or radiation therapy should be noted because of the potential for worsening of adverse effects and toxicity. Baseline neurologic functioning should be assessed, with a focus on any history of seizures; the presence of numbness or tingling in the extremities, nervousness, irritability, or confusion; and evaluation of level of mobility, muscle strength, and gait. Measurement of vital signs is an important aspect of assessment with these drugs, as with any drug therapy; in particular, hyperthermia may be an adverse effect. Temperature should be measured and checked frequently. Because of the risk of pancreatitis, patients should be assessed for moderate to severe abdominal pain, which often occurs in the left quadrant, and for nausea and vomiting. Coagulopathies may occur, so baseline blood cell counts are also important to assess and document (see the Laboratory Considerations Box box on p. 737 and also in Chapter 27). It is also important to assess for high serum ammonia levels and complaints of headache.

Cultural assessment should be thorough and the results should be respected by everyone involved in the care of the cancer patient, because members of different cultural groups have various interpretations of health, illness, and pain; verbalize illnesses and symptoms in different ways; and may even differ in how they respond to a given drug. Cancer and its treatment may affect the patient's body image, coping mechanisms, and emotional status, so the nurse must constantly assess mental status and support systems, and remain alert to clues that the patient may need more support before, during, and after chemotherapy. Genetic considerations are an additional area of importance in the treatment of cancer with antineoplastics as well as with all drug therapy. Individuals should be assessed for the presence of the following characteristics before chemotherapy is initiated: (1) genetic markers for oral cancers, (2) genetic determinants of testosterone or estrogen metabolism, and (3) genetically linked enzyme system abnormalities such as those involving specific cytochrome P-450 enzymes that metabolically convert nicotine to a carcinogenic substance. These genetic factors are very complex; nevertheless, the nurse should be aware of the possible influence of genetic differences and should look to those involved in drug research and administration for additional information.

◆ NURSING DIAGNOSES

- Activity intolerance related to drug-induced anemia with fatigue and lethargy caused by cell cycle–specific and related antineoplastic drugs
- Anxiety related to the unknowns of therapy and illness and the fear of death
- Disturbed body image related to drug-induced alopecia, darkening of skin, and sexual dysfunctioning
- Constipation related to the adverse effects of antineoplastic drugs
- Ineffective coping related to fears about cancer and dying
- Diarrhea related to the adverse effects of antineoplastic drugs
- Risk for infection related to drug-induced bone marrow suppression with possible leukopenia, and neutropenia
- Imbalanced nutrition, less than body requirements, related to loss of appetite, nausea, vomiting, stomatitis, and changes in taste as a result of antineoplastic therapy
- Impaired oral mucous membranes related to the adverse effects of stomatitis, leukopenia, and neutropenia
- Nausea (and vomiting) related to the adverse effects of antineoplastic therapy
- Acute pain related to the disease process and drug-induced joint pain, stomatitis, nausea and vomiting, and other discomforts associated with antineoplastic cell cycle–specific therapy (e.g., neuropathies)
- Impaired physical mobility related to drug-induced anemia and fatigue
- Disturbed self-concept related to the adverse effects of alopecia, muscle wasting, weight loss, amenorrhea, and other physical changes caused by antineoplastic therapy

◆ PLANNING

Goals

- Patient maintains levels of activity and mobility, as tolerated and without major muscle mass loss, during drug treatment.
- Patient remains calm and comfortable without moderate or severe anxiety during therapy.
- Patient maintains an intact and healthy body image and effective coping mechanisms while experiencing alopecia, skin changes, and sexual dysfunction associated with antineoplastic drugs.
- Patient experiences minimal problems due to oral and GI adverse effects—specifically stomatitis, constipation, diarrhea, nausea, and vomiting—while taking antineoplastic drugs.
- Patient experiences minimal risks for infection as well as minimal breaks in skin integrity and oral mucous membranes (possibly due to the occurrence of stomatitis) while receiving antineoplastic drugs.

- Patient remains safe and free from injury with minimal neurologic, sensory, and motor deficits due to the adverse effects of antineoplastic drugs.
- Patient's nutritional status returns to normal during the recovery period and after completion of the antineoplastic protocol.
- Patient regains normal urinary patterns during and after antineoplastic therapy.

Outcome Criteria

- Patient states measures to maximize activity levels and mobility, such as conserving energy with planned activities, seeking assistance, and maintaining range of motion daily.
- Patient uses nonpharmacologic, complementary and alternative therapies (e.g., relaxation, music therapy, pet therapy, biofeedback, massage, therapeutic touch, diversion) as well as prescribed drug therapy to control pain and discomfort related to the adverse effects of antineoplastic drugs or the disease process itself.
- Patient states measures to enhance levels of comfort during drug therapy, such as managing pain (see earlier); taking antiemetics as prescribed; keeping skin clean, dry, and moist; and maintaining range of motion daily.
- Patient openly verbalizes any anxieties, fears, concerns, or feelings of upset or depression about changes in body image and self-concept to help in coping.
- Patient states measures to assist in maintaining healthy breathing and respiratory patterns as well as measures to prevent respiratory infections such as deep breathing exercises, frequent hand washing, forcing of fluids, consumption of a well-balanced diet, avoidance of malls and other crowded places, and avoidance of persons with colds, flu, or communicable respiratory illnesses while undergoing chemotherapy.
- Patient states and demonstrates ways to minimize oral mucosal breakdown, such as performing frequent mouth care and dental hygiene measures using mild toothpaste, gentle sponge-type toothettes, and non–alcohol-based mouthwash, and taking fluid frequently while undergoing drug therapy.
- Patient demonstrates the use of various measures to enhance skin integrity while undergoing antineoplastic therapy, such as keeping skin clean, dry, and lubricated.
- Patient understands the importance of daily measures to help minimize the risk of self-injury related to the adverse effects of bone marrow suppression, such as avoiding crowds, monitoring temperature daily or as needed, not using straight razors, and avoiding venipuncture and injections if possible.
- Patient uses nonpharmacologic methods (e.g., consumption of a well-balanced diet with fiber and roughage as allotted, intake of fluids, exercise) and pharmacologic methods (e.g., use of stool softeners or bulk-forming laxatives) to regain and/or maintain normal or pre-chemotherapy bowel elimination patterns.
- Patient states ways to minimize risk for injury from neurologic adverse effects of chemotherapy by establishing a safety plan that includes removing throw rugs or furniture that may lead to falls, using assistive devices such as a walker or cane, having a bedside commode, using night lights, and instituting other measures to ease mobility.
- Patient adheres to daily regimen for increasing urinary health, such as forcing fluids, consuming fluids that minimize urinary

infections (e.g., cranberry juice), and maintaining daily hydration while undergoing antineoplastic therapy.

Note that the nursing diagnoses, goals, and outcome criteria presented here are appropriate to treatment with many antineoplastic drugs as well to specific application to the cell cycle–specific and other drugs discussed in this chapter.

♦ IMPLEMENTATION

Antineoplastic drugs are some of the most toxic medications given to patients. Because of their toxicity, serious complications and adverse effects may occur. The possibility of such adverse effects and toxicities requires that astute nursing care be based on critical thinking and careful assessment. General considerations in nursing implementation applicable to most antineoplastic drugs as well as specific aspects of implementation related to cell cycle–specific drugs are discussed here. Other nursing process information related to cell cycle–nonspecific drugs is presented in Chapter 48.

For antineoplastic therapy in general, nursing considerations related to *reducing fear and anxiety* include establishing a therapeutic relationship with the patient that begins with trust and empathy. In addition, the nurse should always maintain a calm, warm, empathic, and supportive manner while projecting confidence in providing nursing care. The nurse should give thorough yet appropriate explanations of the various tests as well as specific instructions as ordered. Collaboration with all members of the health care team is needed, and the nurse should reinforce the physician's explanations while clearing up any misconceptions about treatment protocols. The patient should be encouraged to consider relaxation techniques such as listening to music, performing yoga, or engaging in guided imagery. It may be necessary to call on other sources of support, such as social services, counseling services, or members of the patient's religious denomination or belief community while respecting the patient's emotional or other support systems. Appropriate consults with other practitioners may be necessary (e.g., clinical psychiatrist, mental health nurse, nurse practitioner, oncology nurse specialist, psychologist or psychiatrist, clergy).

A variety of interventions can assist in the management of *stomatitis* or excessive oral mucosa dryness and irritation, including the following: (1) Performing oral hygiene measures before and after eating or as needed may help provide cleanliness and comfort. Products containing lemon, glycerin, undiluted peroxide, or alcohol should be avoided because of their drying and irritating effects on the oral mucosa. (2) Use of a soft-bristle toothbrush or soft-tipped toothette or swab with solutions of diluted warm saline is recommended. Chlorhexidine gluconate (Peridex) in a spray bottle with warm saline solution can be used to mist the oral cavity as needed. (3) Dentures, if used, should be removed and cleaned frequently and, if stomatitis is severe, replaced only at mealtimes. (4) Keeping the lips moist and using sugarless candy or gum to stimulate saliva production or using over-the-counter saliva substitutes is important. (5) Spicy, acidic, or hot foods should be avoided. (6) Oral antifungal suspensions (e.g., nystatin) may be ordered if stomatitis worsens or if white patches are noted on the oral mucosa. (7) Other oral suspensions may be mixed by the pharmacy to help with the pain associated with stomatitis (e.g., lidocaine to swish and swallow). (8) Smoking, tobacco chewing, and alcohol

consumption should be avoided because of the irritation to the oral mucosa.

Nausea and vomiting occur commonly with antineoplastic drugs. Emetic potential varies depending on the drug or treatment protocol (see earlier discussion and Box 47-1). Measures to enhance comfort during times of nausea and vomiting include restricting oral intake; removing noxious odors or sights to avoid stimulating the vomiting center; performing oral hygiene measures as needed; promoting relaxation through slow, deep breathing and other techniques; consuming small, frequent meals and eating slowly; and consuming clear liquids and a bland diet. Use of intravenous fluids may be indicated if nausea and vomiting are severe. Antiemetics are also a vital part of antineoplastic therapy (see Chapter 53 for more specific drug-related information). Granisetron, ondansetron, dolasetron, and palonosetron hydrochloride are a few of the drugs used; however, H_2 antagonists, metoclopramide, prochlorperazine, methylprednisolone, or lorazepam may also be used. Dronabinol and nabilone (synthetic cannabinoids) may also be prescribed. Premedication with antiemetics 30 to 60 minutes before administration of the antineoplastic(s) is the preferred treatment protocol to help reduce nausea and vomiting, prevent dehydration and malnutrition, and promote comfort. Combination antiemetic drug therapy may be more effective than single-drug therapy. Intravenous hydration may also be helpful in preventing complications.

Diarrhea is also a common adverse effect of antineoplastic therapy, and the following nursing interventions may be helpful: (1) Restricting oral intake of irritating, spicy, and gas-producing foods; caffeine; high-fiber foods; alcohol; very hot or cold foods or beverages; and lactose-containing foods and beverages. Foods high in nonabsorbable sugars (e.g., sorbitol) may be helpful. (2) Appropriate resource personnel should be consulted, as ordered, to help the patient and family plan meals and arrange ways to meet the patient's dietary and bowel elimination needs. (3) Cheese is a constipating food and may be consumed if tolerated. (4) Opioids (e.g., paregoric) or synthetic opioids (e.g., loperamide, diphenoxylate hydrochloride) may be ordered as antidiarrheals. Adsorbents-protectants and antisecretory drugs may also help reduce GI upset and diarrhea (Chapter 52).

To address *nutritional concerns*, the meals and snacks consumed over a 24-hour period should be monitored to determine if nutritional intake is adequate. The following measures may help to improve oral intake and nutritional status: (1) Antiemetic therapy, pain management, mouth care, and hydration may reduce the adverse effects of therapy. (2) Taste alterations caused by antineoplastic drugs may be eased with consumption of mild-tasting foods and use of cold chicken, turkey, or cheese for protein sources. Consumption of iced protein drinks or protein bars may be helpful. (3) Eating meat at breakfast may be helpful for those who find meat distasteful at dinnertime. (4) Using extra honey or other sweeteners; marinating meats in bland wine, sauces, or flavorings; and serving foods cold or at room temperature may help with taste changes. (5) Plastic rather than metal utensils may be used if the patient complains of a metallic taste. (6) Difficulty in swallowing should be reported to the physician immediately, and lidocaine swish-and-swallow solutions may be prescribed. (7) The patient should be encouraged to eat foods that are easy to swallow, such as custards; gelatins; puddings; mashed white or sweet potatoes; blended drinks with crushed ice, fruit, and yogurt; nutritional supplement drinks and snacks; and frozen popsicles or lactose-free ice cream. (8) Sticky or dry foods should be avoided, whereas the use of gravy or cream sauces to moisten food items should be encouraged. (9) Small, frequent meals are recommended and should be consumed in an environment that is conducive to eating (e.g., free of odors, excess noise, etc.). (10) Appetite stimulants such as megestrol acetate or dronabinol may be prescribed. (11) The patient should be encouraged to rest before and after meals for energy conservation. (12) Snacks containing protein and extra calories (e.g., milkshakes, eggnog with cream, and commercially prepared dietary supplement shakes, ice creams, and breakfast drinks) should be used frequently.

Alopecia, a common adverse effect of antineoplastic drugs, may be disturbing to patients regardless of age or gender. Ensuring that the patient is informed is crucial to helping the patient feel in control, because the illness and its treatment take away the control a patient has over other parts of his or her life. Nursing interventions that may be helpful include the following: (1) The patient and family should know about the fact that hair loss is reversible and usually begins 7 to 10 days after treatment. New hair growth is often a different color and/or texture from the hair lost. (2) The patient should be given the option of acquiring a wig or hairpiece, or scarves or hats, before the actual hair loss; the American Cancer Society is a resource for these items and possibly for financial assistance.

Antineoplastic-induced bone marrow suppression leads to *anemias, leukopenia, neutropenia,* and *thrombocytopenia* (see previous discussions regarding myelosuppression caused by antineoplastic drugs). Anemias lead to fatigue and loss of energy and are common adverse effects of therapy and the disease process. Anemias may require blood transfusions, peripheral blood stem cell treatment, or treatment with prescribed medications such as iron preparations, folic acid, or erythropoietic growth factors (e.g., epoetin or darbepoetin alfa). These injections may be given at home, and may be administered at the first sign of a decrease in RBC levels. Other nursing measures include the following: forcing fluids to at least 2500 mL/day unless contraindicated, allowing activity as tolerated and scheduling several rest periods during the day, providing assistance with personal care, limiting the number of visitors or the length of stay, organizing the patient's personal space so that necessary items (e.g., phone, light, call bell, and personal items) are close at hand, and encouraging sleep (the use of sedative hypnotics may be needed, as ordered). Energy-saving measures should be encouraged and include, for example, using a chair or bench when showering and sitting while carrying out the activities of daily living (e.g., hair brushing, oral care).

Risk of infection from *leukopenia* or *neutropenia* and/or immunosuppression is one of the more significant adverse effects that deserves close attention. The patient and family and/or caregivers need to understand that when WBC counts are low, the patient is at high risk for infection and that defenses remain low until the counts recover. Following standard precautions and using good hand-washing technique are most important in preventing transmission of infection in the hospital and home settings. Because fever is a principal early sign of infection, oral or axillary temperature should be taken at least every 4 hours during periods in which the patient is at risk. Taking the temperature

rectally should be avoided to minimize tissue trauma, breaks in skin integrity, and thus loss of the first line of defense. Temperature elevations of 38.3° C (101° F) or above should be reported immediately to the physician so that appropriate treatment can be initiated and complications avoided. Invasive procedures such as urinary catheterization, venipunctures, and injections should be avoided if possible to prevent introduction of bacteria. IV sites should be monitored and sites and tubing changed as per policy, and all drainage systems (wound or urinary) should be kept sterile. Minimizing exposure to contagions is critical to preventing infections; therefore, if a patient is hospitalized (and some physicians avoid hospitalization because of the risk of nosocomial infections), every precaution must be taken to minimize infection. WBC and differential counts should be monitored weekly, and therapy may be postponed temporarily if WBC count is lower than 3500/mm^3 (this value may vary depending on the physician, drug, and patient). The onset of neutropenia is rapid, with the lowest neutrophil count, or nadir, reached between days 10 and 14. Recovery occurs within 3 or 4 weeks or longer depending on the drug(s) used. Delayed neutropenia may occur with some drugs in about 2 weeks, the nadir for these drugs is reached in 3 to 4 weeks, and recovery occurs in about 7 weeks. Monitoring neutrophil counts is essential to safe nursing care and prevention of infections, and normal ranges are between 2500 and 7000 cells/mm^3. Should counts fall below 500 cells/mm^3, the physician should be contacted immediately so that protective or neutropenic precautions can be instituted (see the Laboratory Values Related to Drug Therapy box on p. 758 in Chapter 48). These precautions include having nurses, health care workers, and visitors wear gloves, mask, and gown to decrease the patient's exposure to bacteria and viruses. Other interventions may include IV antibiotic therapy based on laboratory test results and culture and sensitivity reports. It is important to inform the patient and those involved in the patient's care that fever in the presence of neutropenia is a primary early sign of infection, and frequent temperature monitoring is indicated.

If needed, and ordered, administration of colony-stimulating factors may be beneficial. Filgrastim, pegfilgrastim, and sargramostim are examples of drugs given to accelerate WBC recovery during antineoplastic drug therapy. These drugs may be used to minimize neutropenia and specifically act on the bone marrow to enhance neutrophil production; help decrease the incidence, severity, and duration of neutropenia; and possibly help to decrease the incidence of hospitalization and/or the need for IV antibiotic therapy. These medications must be administered within a certain time frame and are discussed further in Chapter 49. Patients with *immune suppression* should be encouraged to do the following: (1) be aware of environments and persons to avoid, such as individuals who have been recently vaccinated (who may have a subclinical infection) or have a cold or flu or other symptoms of an infection; (2) hydrate with up to 3000 mL/day of fluid unless contraindicated and maintain adequate nutrition (see earlier); (3) adhere to a "low-microbe" diet by washing fresh fruits and vegetables and making sure foods are well cooked; (4) maintain intact oral and GI mucosa (see discussion of stomatitis); (5) turn, cough, and deep breathe to help prevent stasis of respiratory secretions; and (6) report temperatures of 38.3° C (101° F) or higher, sore throat, cough, or flulike symptoms to the health care provider immediately.

Thrombocytopenia may also be a consequence of antineoplastic therapy and puts the patient at risk for bleeding (because of a decrease in circulating platelets). Platelet counts, coagulation studies, RBC counts, hemoglobin levels, and hematocrit values should be monitored and reported if decreased (see the Laboratory Values Related to Drug Therapy box on p. 737). Injections should be avoided if possible and alternative routes of administration sought if available. If injections or venipunctures are absolutely necessary, the nurse should use the smallest gauge needle possible and apply gentle, prolonged pressure to the site. Patients undergoing bone marrow aspiration should be monitored closely after the procedure for bleeding at the aspiration site. Blood pressure monitoring should be performed only if necessary and should be done quickly without overinflation of the cuff. The nurse should monitor the patient for bleeding from the mouth, gums, and nose, and bleeding after brushing of the teeth. If bleeding occurs with oral care, then use of the nursing measures discussed earlier for stomatitis should be encouraged. Bleeding times and results of coagulation studies should be closely monitored during and after therapy. It is also important that patients know that bleeding may be increased by drugs that affect coagulation, such as anticoagulants, aspirin and other nonsteroidal antiinflammatory drugs (NSAIDs). If an analgesic is needed, a non-NSAID should be selected (e.g., acetaminophen). Dosages of acetaminophen should not exceed recommendations because of the possibility of liver toxicity. Shaving with a straight-edge razor is discouraged. The use of electric razors is encouraged for both men and women to prevent trauma, breaks in the skin, and bleeding. Rectal temperature measurement and use of rectal suppositories or enemas should be avoided to prevent trauma and bleeding. The risk for falls should be reduced. The patient should be instructed to avoid clutter in the room and to wear slippers or shoes with nonskid or nonslip soles. If ordered, platelets or estrogen-progestin preparations (to suppress any menses and bleeding) may be given or oprelvekin may be used to stimulate platelet production as ordered.

The patient should be aware that antineoplastics also have a negative impact on the reproductive tract; they cause destruction of the germinal epithelium of the testes and are associated with sterility, amenorrhea, and teratogenesis. Patients should be educated about the possibility of these adverse effects as well as the risk for decreased libido and impotence. Male patients should be counseled about the risk for sterility, which is often irreversible, and sperm banking before chemotherapy may be an option. Female patients of childbearing age who are sexually active should protect themselves against pregnancy because of the risk of embryonic death. Contraceptive measures are encouraged during chemotherapy and up to at least 8 weeks after discontinuation of therapy. With some antineoplastic therapy, patients may be instructed to use contraception for up to 2 years after completion of treatment because of the risk of genetic abnormalities. Should pregnancy occur, termination of the pregnancy may be necessary. Some antineoplastic drugs may cause reversible amenorrhea due to their effect on the ovaries, and damage to the ovaries may also lead to premature menopausal symptoms (e.g., hot flashes, decreased vaginal secretions, irritability). Water-soluble lubricants may be used during intercourse to prevent tissue trauma.

With *antimetabolites*, the physician's orders should always be followed regarding pre-medication with antiemetics and/or anti-anxiety drugs. Orders or protocol for the use of other symptom-control medication should be followed as well. Fluid intake of up to 3000 mL/24 hours should be encouraged, or IV hydration should be used as needed or as ordered. All drugs should be handled carefully and direct contact with skin, eyes, or mucous membranes avoided. All protocols for chemotherapy administration, as well as any hospital or facility policies or manufacturer guidelines, should be followed. If in doubt about any order for any drug, the nurse should stop and consult appropriate resources for further information. Drug incompatibilities are common, and the nurse should check for these before infusions are given to prevent more adverse reactions. Oral hygiene should be frequent; a soft toothbrush should be used and, if flossing, waxed dental floss should be used. Nutritional intake should be constantly monitored and weight measured daily or weekly. Generally speaking, with antimetabolites, GI adverse effects occur on about the fourth day, which requires preplanning for special medication assistance, if needed, and dietary changes to meet the patient's specific needs. Antibiotic therapy may be ordered prophylactically for infection, as well as analgesics for pain and antispasmodics for diarrhea. See earlier discussion of nursing considerations associated with stomatitis, loss of appetite, diarrhea, nausea, and vomiting as well as for the various blood disorders that may occur.

Cytarabine should also be used with extreme caution in handling and administration by the various routes (intravenous, subcutaneous, or intrathecal). Major concerns related to therapy with this drug include bone marrow suppression and cytarabine syndrome, which is manifested by fever, joint pains, chest pain, conjunctivitis, and overall malaise. If high dosages are used, cytarabine may also cause central nervous system, GI, and/or pulmonary toxicity, and so the patient must be continually monitored for these system-related adverse effects. For intrathecal administration, the drug may be reconstituted with NaCl or the physician may use the patient's spinal fluid. With fluorouracil, the solution is colorless to slightly yellow, and the drug should not be added to any other intravenous infusions—it should only be given by itself in the appropriate diluent. If an infusion port is not used, IV sites should not be over joints, tendons, or small veins, or in extremities that are edematous. Intravenous dosages should be given exactly as ordered with constant monitoring of the IV site, infusion port, and/or infusion solution and equipment. If IV infiltration occurs, the protocol for management should be followed and will most likely include the application of an ice pack. All hospital or infusion protocols should be followed without exception, because treatment of extravasation is handled differently depending on the specific drug (see discussion in the pharmacology section). If topical forms of the drug are used, the patient should be told to apply the drug exactly as ordered and to the affected area only. Gloves or finger-cots should be used to apply the topical dosage form.

Gemcitabine, an antimetabolite, is dosed based on absolute granulocyte counts and platelet nadirs and are given if the counts exceed $1500 \times 10^6/L$ and $100,000 \times 10^6/L$, respectively. Intravenous solutions should be kept at room temperature to avoid crystallization and used within 24 hours. Infusions are to be given as ordered. Antiemetics as well as antidiarrheals may be needed. Mercaptopurine comes in oral dosage forms and should not be given with meals. Finally, the antimetabolite methotrexate has numerous toxicities and adverse effects, which may be minimized by appropriate medical treatment. Preplanning for therapy includes consideration of boosting the immune status and blood cell counts before aggressive therapy is initiated. Patients must be encouraged to drink up to 2000 to 3000 mL/day if tolerated and not contraindicated. The nurse should continue to monitor creatinine clearance, as ordered, to detect any nephrotoxicity. Nutritional status may be enhanced by increasing the intake of bran, dried beans, nuts, fruits, asparagus, and other fresh vegetables (thoroughly washed and if tolerated) because these foods are high in folic acid. These food items may not be tolerated during the actual drug therapy, but their consumption is encouraged when the patient is able to tolerate them. Consumption of these foods is yet another measure to help minimize the possibility of methotrexate toxicity. Should gastrointestinal upset and/or stomatitis occur, the patient may need to decrease any sources of irritation (e.g., high-fiber food) and take the other measures noted earlier. Methotrexate is usually given orally, intramuscularly, or IV. The nurse should wear gloves when giving the drug, and if any of the powder comes in contact with the skin, the area should be washed immediately and thoroughly with soap and water. Intravenous administration of fluids should accompany therapy to insure adequate hydration. Bicarbonate may be ordered to help alkalinize the urine and encourage excretion of the drug. Intramuscular injections and other procedures that induce bleeding or trauma should be avoided until blood counts return to acceptable limits, as noted by the physician. If venipunctures are performed, pressure should be applied firmly to the site for up to 5 minutes, or longer if needed. As with many antineoplastics, there are numerous incompatibilities, and the nurse must be constantly aware of these and check for them. Methotrexate can cause life-threatening bone marrow toxicity, and a drug is available that is used as a "rescue" treatment. This drug, leucovorin, helps to limit the toxic effects of methotrexate on bone marrow cells. It is often ordered to be used within 1 hour of accidental overdosage of folic acid antagonists such as methotrexate; it may also be prescribed in conventional cytoprotective dosages. For a listing of other types of drugs that are used as antagonists to antineoplastics or are given for their cytoprotective actions, see the discussion of methotrexate in the pharmacology section.

For the *mitotic inhibitors,* including docetaxel, paclitaxel, vincristine, and vinblastine, some nursing considerations are similar to those for other antineoplastic drug categories, but others are unique to this drug class. For the taxane family of drugs, particularly docetaxel, there are generally premedication protocols that may include administration of drugs such as oral corticosteroids (e.g., dexamethasone) beginning several days before day 1 of therapy to help decrease the risk of hypersensitivity and reduce the severity of fluid retention. Solutions should be protected from light and are stable only for approximately 8 hours either at room temperature or under refrigeration. Manufacturers generally send information about diluents. Any solutions should be gently rolled to mix. During the infusion, the patient must be closely monitored for the sudden onset of bronchospasms, flushing of the face, and localized skin reactions; these may indicate a hypersensitivity response requiring immediate treatment. These symptoms may occur within just a few minutes of beginning the infusion. In addition, any dyspnea, abdominal distension, crackles in the lungs, or dependent edema during therapy should be tended to immediately by medical personnel. Cutaneous reactions may also appear during therapy and include rash on hands and feet; these also need immediate attention and treatment. With paclitaxel, the patient may also be premedicated with diphenhydramine, corticosteroids, and H_2 antagonist drugs. Nurses should wear gloves when giving these antineoplastics. Reconstituted solutions are stable for a short period of time; refer to authoritative sources for exact information. Polyvinyl chloride (PVC) plasticized tubing and equipment should not be used, and the drug should be mixed with the proper diluent and administered at the proper rate as ordered. Vital signs should be watched closely, especially during the first hour of infusion. If there is any evidence of hypersensitivity, the physician should be contacted immediately, the patient should be monitored, and treatment protocols should be initiated to prevent harm to the patient. Intramuscular injections, rectal temperature measurement and rectal administration of medications, and other traumas that might induce bleeding should be avoided. All other measures to help avoid bleeding should be implemented, including application of gentle, firm pressure to the site of any bleeding.

With *toposimase inhibitors,* irinotecan and topotecan, blood counts should be monitored closely with every treatment. A drop in blood counts and/or diarrhea (see previous discussion) may cause a temporary postponing of therapy. Extravasation of the solution should be treated immediately, and the IV site should be flushed with sterile water and ice applied. Ensuring that IV sites remain patent and without any indications of infiltration is critical to preventing damage to tissue from extravasation. Nausea and vomiting may lead to dehydration and electrolyte disturbances, so patients should be aware of the need to report these symptoms immediately before negative consequences occur (see previous discussion for specific interventions). IV incompatibilities are numerous for both these drugs and should be an area of constant concern. With topotecan, IV extravasation is usually accompanied by only a mild local reaction such as erythema or bruising and, if noted, should be managed immediately to avoid further trauma and/or risk for loss of skin integrity (the first line of defense against infection). Headaches and difficulty breathing may be more common with topotecan; therefore, the patient should be monitored closely for these symptoms with every administration. The nurse should be ready to implement appropriate interventions.

The *enzyme antineoplastics* asparaginase and pegaspargase should be handled with extreme caution and care. An intradermal test dose of asparaginase may be given before therapy has begun or when a week or longer has occurred between doses. With asparaginase, the solution and powder may be irritants to the skin, and washing is required after contact (as described later for pegaspargase). During therapy, if there are signs and symptoms of oliguria, anuria (renal failure), or pancreatitis, the drug will most likely be discontinued. Pegaspargase requires cautious handling and administration, and inhalation of its fumes should be avoided at all costs. This drug is an irritant, and should it come in contact with the skin, the area should be washed with copious amounts of water for a minimum of 15 minutes. The intramuscular route of administration is usually preferred because it carries a lower risk of clotting abnormalities, GI disorders, and renal and hepatic toxicity. If solutions are cloudy, they should not be used. If more than 2 mL is required for a dose, two injections should be used. Pancreatitis is problematic with this drug and can be serious, so close attention should be given to symptoms such as severe abdominal pain with nausea and vomiting. Serum lipase and amylase levels should be constantly monitored. If any signs or symptoms of pancreatitis occur, the drug is generally discontinued immediately. IV infusions also require close monitoring for extravasation, which is manifested by bluish discoloration of the skin around the site, burning, pain, and swelling. The infusion should be stopped and the IV catheter left in place until proper interventions are initiated.

Many of the common adverse effects associated with antineoplastic therapy are presented in earlier sections of the chapter and may be referred to for review. Use of cytoprotective drugs has been briefly discussed in the pharmacology section of this chapter, and there is further discussion in Chapter 48. In addition, extravasation is a possible complication of intravenous therapy with many antineoplastic drugs and, when it occurs, may lead to tissue irritation or severe tissue damage and sloughing. Intravenous infusions of vesicant drugs (which lead to tissue death, necrosis, and sloughing) and irritant drugs (which leads to irritation and not tissue death) should always be carefully administered via a patent IV infusion line or through an infusion port. Vesicants, if they extravasate, may lead to severe necrosis requiring surgical intervention and possibly skin grafting as compared to irritation of tissue with vesicants. The use of an infusion port helps prevent the severe tissue damage that occurs with peripheral IV infusion extravasations, and so these ports are commonly placed before therapy.

During infusions of vesicants or irritants, the site should be monitored every hour for pain, erythema, heat, swelling, and/or a bluish discoloration. If extravasation is suspected, the specific antineoplastic drug should be discontinued immediately, the IV catheter left in place, and any residual drug or blood aspirated from the IV catheter if possible and if indicated. The requisite antidote must then be prepared and instilled through the existing IV catheter, after which the needle should be removed. Antidotes and/or other substances may also be injected around the IV site to reach affected issues. A sterile occlusive dressing may be ordered to be placed on the entire area and warm or cold compresses may be indicated, depending on the extravasated drug and recommended protocol. The affected limb should then be elevated and allowed to rest to help minimize the amount of tissue damage from further spread of the drug. Appropriate and timely treatment of extravasation of vesicants may help to prevent some of the most devastating consequences of chemotherapy, such as loss of a limb or the need for multiple surgeries.

◆ EVALUATION

Evaluation of nursing care should focus on reviewing whether goals and outcomes are being met as well as monitoring for therapeutic responses and adverse effects and toxic effects of the antineoplastic therapy. Therapeutic responses may manifest as clinical improvement, decrease in tumor size, and decrease in metastatic spread. Evaluation of nursing care with reference to goals and outcomes may reveal improvements related to a decrease in adverse effects and a decrease in the impact of cancer on the patient's well-being, with increases in comfort, nutrition, hydration, energy levels, ability to carry out the activities of daily living, and quality of life. Goals and outcomes should be revisited to identify more specific areas to monitor. In addition, certain laboratory studies such as measurement of tumor markers levels, levels of carcinoembryonic antigens, and RBC, WBC, and platelet counts may be performed to aid in determining how well the treatment protocol has worked. As part of the evaluation, physicians may also order additional radiographs, computed tomographic scans, magnetic resonance images, tissue analysis, or other studies appropriate to the diagnosis both during and after antineoplastic therapy has been completed, at time intervals related to the anticipated tumor response.

CASE STUDY

Facing Chemotherapy

Mrs. D., a 48-year-old married mother of two teenaged daughters, has been diagnosed with breast cancer. She has had lumpectomy surgery to remove the tumor and is about to start chemotherapy. She states that she has "faced the facts" about her disease and the threat to her life but says, "I know this is silly, but I hate the thought of losing my hair to this disease."

1. What measures can be taken to help her deal with her hair loss?
2. Ten days after the chemotherapy, her neutrophil count drops to 2000/mm³. She has been hospitalized because she has developed a cough, and her friends have sent a fruit basket to the hospital. What actions should be taken to protect her from infection?
3. During rounds, the nurse finds Mrs. D. curled up in the bed and sobbing. Mrs. D. states that she feels "so afraid" and is worried about who will care for her family if she dies. What should the nurse do?

Patient Teaching Tips

- To help minimize GI adverse effects and decrease irritation to the oral and GI mucosa, patients should be encouraged to avoid consuming foods that are high in fiber, are spicy, contain citric acid, are hot or cold, or have a rough texture. Alcohol use and smoking are also irritating to the oral and GI mucosa and should be avoided.
- Inform patients that examining their mouth daily is important and to report any problems (e.g., sores, pain, white patches) to the health care provider immediately. They should also report, at the first sign, symptoms such as headache, fatigue, faintness, and shortness of breath (possibly indicative of anemia); bleeding and easy bruising (possibly indicative of drop in platelet count); and sore throat and fever (possibly indicative of infection). Fever and/or chills may be the first sign of an oncoming infection.
- Educate women of childbearing age that they should use nonpharmacologic forms of contraception for the duration of antineoplastic therapy and for up to several months or years after treatment. Sperm conservation through sperm donor/banking may be an option for men treated with these drugs to allow fathering a child at a later time.

Continued

Patient Teaching Tips—cont'd

- Educate the patient about medications to avoid, including aspirin, ibuprofen, and products containing these drugs while receiving antineoplastics to help prevent excessive bleeding.
- Patients receiving antineoplastics should be informed about the risk of alopecia (hair loss) before drug therapy begins. Patients should have the opportunity to discuss options for hair and scalp care, including the option of having their hair cut short before treatment and selecting and purchasing or renting a wig or hairpiece comparable to their existing hair in color, texture, length, and style, or having bandanas, scarves, or hats on hand before the hair is actually lost. Although hair loss is temporary, patients need to be informed that it will occur and should also be aware that wigs and hairpieces are available through the American Cancer Society.
- The following websites are helpful online resources for the patient and significant others: www.fda.gov, www.fda.gov/oc/oha, www.nih.gov, www.healthfinder.gov, www.who.int/en, and www.oncolink.upenn.edu.
- *With cytarabine,* patients should be encouraged to increase fluid intake to help decrease the risk of dehydration and/or hyperuricemia. The importance of reporting any signs of easy bruising, fever, infection, or unusual bleeding from any site; of not receiving vaccinations during treatment; and of avoiding individuals who have recently received a live virus vaccine should be stressed.
- *With fluorouracil and gemcitabine,* frequent oral hygiene should be encouraged, and patients should be told to report bleeding, bruising, chest pain, diarrhea, nausea or vomiting, heart palpitations, infection, or changes in vision to their physician immediately. For fluorouracil, the patient should be encouraged to avoid overexposure to sun or ultraviolet light and to wear protective clothing, sunscreen, and sunglasses when in the sun. The use of topical ointment may leave the affected area looking somewhat unsightly for several weeks after therapy, and the hands should be washed thoroughly after its application.

- *With mercaptopurine,* the patient should be advised to avoid alcohol consumption because it increases the risk of drug toxicity. The same concerns regarding vaccination and precautions for infection and bleeding apply as were noted earlier.
- *With methotrexate,* the patient should be told to notify the physician if nausea and vomiting are problematic or uncontrollable, or if fever, sore throat, muscle aches and pains, or unusual bleeding occurs. Alcohol, salicylates, NSAIDs, and exposure to sunlight or ultraviolet light should be avoided. Both male and female patients should use contraceptive measures for up to 3 months or longer after therapy.
- *With taxanes,* drug-induced alopecia is reversible, but the patient should be warned that new hair growth will most likely differ in color and/or texture from the hair lost. Hair growth usually resumes 2 to 3 months after the last dose of chemotherapy. Oral hygiene must be thorough, and patients should avoid individuals with infections or those who have received live virus vaccines. Patients should use contraceptive measures until otherwise advised by the physician. Nausea and vomiting should be reported immediately so that appropriate treatment can be rendered—especially if the patient is at home, to prevent hospitalizations. For paclitaxel, the patient should also be told to report any signs or symptoms of neuropathy (e.g., numbness or tingling of extremities).
- *With etoposide and teniposide,* patients should be cautioned to avoid individuals who have received live viral vaccines or who are ill and to avoid crowds when patient blood cell counts are low. Patients should be encouraged to contact the physician if they experience easy bleeding, bruising, difficulty breathing, fever, sore throat, or chills. Contraception should be used. Hair loss is reversible (see earlier).
- *With asparaginase and pegaspargase,* patients should be encouraged to force fluids and to report immediately to the physician any severe nausea or vomiting as well as any bleeding, excessive fatigue, or fever or other signs or symptoms of infection.

Points to Remember

- Cancers are diseases that are characterized by uncontrolled cellular growth.
- *Malignancy* refers specifically to a neoplasm that is anaplastic, invasive, and metastatic, as opposed to benign. Malignant tumors typically consist of cancerous cells that infiltrate surrounding tissues spread to other tissues and organs. Malignant growths invade surrounding tissues and migrate to other tissues and organs, where they form metastatic tumor deposits.
- Tumors are generally classified by tissue of origin, as follows: epithelial (carcinoma), connective (sarcoma), lymphatic (lymphoma), and leukocytes (leukemia).
- Antineoplastics are drugs that are used to treat malignancies. They may be either cell cycle–specific or cell cycle–nonspecific drugs or may have miscellaneous actions.
- Cell cycle–specific drugs kill cancer cells during specific phases of the cell growth cycle. Cell cycle–nonspecific drugs kill cancer cells during any phase of the cell growth cycle.
- Chemotherapy, or antineoplastic drug therapy, requires very astute nursing care, and the nurse must act prudently and make critical decisions about the nursing care of patients receiving these drugs. Knowledge is important to ensure patient safety and also to protect the nurse from the adverse effects of antineoplastic drugs.
- Cell cycle–specific drug classes include antimetabolites, mitotic inhibitors, topoisomerase I inhibitors, and antineoplastic enzymes. These drugs are collectively used to treat a variety of solid and/or

circulating tumors, although some drugs have much more specific indications than others.
- Antineoplastic antimetabolites are cell cycle–specific antagonistic analogues that work by inhibiting the actions of key cellular metabolites. They interfere with the biosynthesis of precursors essential to cellular growth by inhibiting the synthesis or actions of three classes of compounds: the vitamin folic acid, as well as purines and pyrimidines, the two classes of compounds that make up the bases contained in nucleic acid molecules (DNA and RNA).
- Two plant-derived antineoplastic drugs are the taxanes and include paclitaxel, derived from the bark of the slow-growing Western (Pacific) yew tree, and docetaxel, a semisynthetic taxoid produced from the needles of the European yew tree. Docetaxel is pharmacologically similar to paclitaxel.
- Topoisomerase I inhibitors are a relatively new class of chemotherapy drugs. The two drugs currently available in this class are topotecan and irinotecan.
- Antineoplastic enzymes include asparaginase and pegaspargase. A third, *Erwinia* asparaginase, is available only by special request from the National Cancer Institute for patients who have developed allergies to *E. coli*–based asparaginase.
- Several drugs are available that are classified as cytoprotective drugs. These medications help to reduce the toxicity of various antineoplastics. The decision regarding whether to use them is often very patient specific, as is the case with chemotherapy regimens.

NCLEX Examination Review Questions

1. Which intervention is appropriate for a patient suffering from stomatitis?
   a. Clean the mouth with a soft-bristle toothbrush and warm saline solution.
   b. Rinse the mouth with commercial mouthwash twice a day.
   c. Use lemon-glycerin swabs to keep the mouth moist.
   d. Keep dentures in the mouth between meals.
2. Which intervention is most appropriate in caring for a patient who is very nauseated during chemotherapy?
   a. Encourage light activity during chemotherapy as a distraction.
   b. Provide antiemetic medications 30 to 60 minutes before chemotherapy begins.
   c. Provide antiemetic medications only upon the request of the patient.
   d. Hold all fluids during chemotherapy to avoid vomiting.
3. The nurse monitors the patient who is experiencing thrombocytopenia from severe bone marrow suppression by looking for:
   a. Severe weakness and fatigue
   b. Elevated body temperature
   c. Decreased skin turgor
   d. Excessive bleeding and bruising
4. A patient receiving chemotherapy is experiencing severe bone marrow suppression. Which nursing diagnosis is most appropriate at this time?
   a. Activity intolerance
   b. Acute pain
   c. Disturbed body image
   d. Impaired physical mobility
5. Should extravasation of an antineoplastic medication occur, which intervention should the nurse perform first?
   a. Apply cold compresses to the site and elevate the arm.
   b. Inject subcutaneous doses of epinephrine around the IV site every 2 hours.
   c. Stop the infusion immediately while leaving the catheter in place, and notify the physician.
   d. Inject the appropriate antidote through the IV catheter after stopping the IV infusion.

1. a, 2. b, 3. d, 4. a, 5. c.

Critical Thinking Activities

1. Two broad categories of drugs used to treat cancer are cell cycle–specific drugs and cell cycle–nonspecific drugs. Explain the difference between the two categories of drugs based on their mechanisms of action.
2. Your patient is experiencing stomatitis. What kinds of foods would you encourage her to avoid? Explain your answer.
3. Your patient is taking irinotecan as part of his chemotherapy regimen. He has received the dose and is about to be discharged. Discuss a potential problem he may face at home as a result of this chemotherapy, and how it can be treated.

For answers, see http://evolve.elsevier.com/Lilley.

Antineoplastic Drugs Part 2: Cell Cycle–Nonspecific and Miscellaneous Drugs

Objectives

When you reach the end of this chapter, you should be able to do the following:

1. Review the concepts related to carcinogenesis, the types of malignancies and related terminology, and the different treatment modalities, including the use of cell cycle–nonspecific and miscellaneous antineoplastic drugs (see Chapter 47).
2. Identify the various drugs classified as cell cycle-nonspecific or hormonal, or that are considered miscellaneous drugs.
3. Discuss the common adverse effects and toxic effects of the cell cycle–nonspecific and miscellaneous antineoplastic drugs, including the reasons for their occurrence and methods of treatment, such as any antidotes.
4. Describe the mechanisms of action, indications, dosages, routes of administration, cautions, contraindications, and drug interactions of the cell cycle–nonspecific drugs, hormonal drugs, and miscellaneous antineoplastic drugs.
5. Apply knowledge about the cell cycle–nonspecific, hormonal agonist-antagonist, and other miscellaneous antineoplastic drugs and their characteristics to the development of a comprehensive nursing care plan for patients with cancer.
6. Briefly describe extravasation and other major adverse effects associated with the antineoplastics in this chapter, including discussion of protocols and antidotes.

e-Learning Activities

Companion CD
- NCLEX Review Questions: see questions 398-402
- Animations
- Audio Glossary
- Category Catchers
- Medication Errors Checklists
- IV Therapy Checklists

evolve Website (http://evolve.elsevier.com/Lilley)
- Nursing Care Plans • Frequently Asked Questions • Content Updates • WebLinks • Supplemental Resources • Elsevier ePharmacology Update • Medication Administration Animations

Drug Profiles

bevacizumab, p. 756
▶ cisplatin, p. 753
▶ cyclophosphamide, p. 753
▶ doxorubicin, p. 756
hydroxyurea, p. 756

imatinib, p. 756
▶ mechlorethamine, p. 754
mitotane, p. 756
mitoxantrone, p. 756
octreotide, p. 756

▶ Key drug.

Glossary

Alkylation   A chemical reaction in which an alkyl group is transferred from an alkylating drug. When such organic reactions occur with a biologically significant cellular constituent such as deoxyribonucleic acid (DNA), they result in interference with cell division, or *mitosis*. (p. 751)

Bifunctional   Referring to those alkylating drugs composed of molecules that have two reactive alkyl groups and that are

therefore able to alkylate two cancer cell DNA molecules per drug molecule. (p. 751)

Extravasation   The leakage of any intravenously or intraarterially administered medication into the tissue space surrounding the vein or artery. Such an event can cause serious tissue injury, especially with antineoplastic drugs. (p. 751)

Mitosis   The process of cell reproduction occurring in somatic (nonsexual) cells and resulting in the formation of two genetically identical daughter cells containing the diploid (complete) number of chromosomes characteristic of the species. (p. 751)

Polyfunctional   Referring to the action of alkylating drugs that can engage in several alkylation reactions with cancer cell DNA molecules per single molecule of drug. (p. 751)

This chapter is a continuation of Chapter 47 and focuses on additional classes of antineoplastic drugs. It was decided to create two new antineoplastic drug chapters for this edition because of the complexity of drug classes and the large and ever-increasing numbers of individual drugs. Chapter 47 describes the various antineoplastic drugs that are effective against cancer cells during specific phases in the *cell growth cycle*. In contrast, this chapter focuses on drugs that have antineoplastic activity regardless of the phase of the cell cycle. Also discussed in this chapter are drugs that are classified as *miscellaneous* antineoplastics either because of their lack of clear cell cycle specificity or their unique or *novel* (new) mechanisms of action. Table 48-1 summarizes the nomenclature for these drug classes. For a description of the cell growth cycle, see Chapter 47.

Table 48-1 Common Names for Selected Antineoplastic Drugs

Generic Name	Trade Names	Other Names
Cell Cycle–Nonspecific Drugs		
Alkylating Drugs		
Classic Alkylators		
busulfan	Myleran, Busulfex	BSF, NSC-750
chlorambucil	Leukeran	B-1348, NSC-3088
cyclophosphamide	Cytoxan, Cytoxan Lyophilized, Neosar	CPM, CTX, CYT
ifosfamide	Ifex	Z-4942, NSC-10924
mechlorethamine	Mustargen	nitrogen mustard, HN2, mustine, NSC-762
melphalan	Alkeran	L-sarcolysin, L-phenylalanine mustard, L-PAM, CB-3025, NSC-8806
Nitrosoureas		
carmustine	BiCNU, Gliadel (wafer)	BCNU, bischloronitrosourea, NSC-409962
lomustine	CeeNU	CCNU, NSC-79037
streptozocin	Zanosar	streptozotocin, SZN, U-9889, NSC-85998
Probable Alkylators		
altretamine	Hexalen	hexamethylmelamine, HMM, HXM, NSC-13875
carboplatin	Paraplatin	CBDCA, JM-8, NSC-241240
cisplatin	Platinol-AQ	cis-diamminedichloroplatinum (II), cis-DDP; CDDP
dacarbazine	DTIC-DOME	DTIC imidazole carboxamide, DIC
oxaliplatin	Eloxatin	NSC-266046
procarbazine	Matulane	N-methylhydrazine, MIH, ibenzmethyzin, NSC-77213
temozolomide	Temodar	NSC-362856
thiotepa	Thioplex	triethylenethiophosphoramide, TSPA, TESPA, thiophosphoramide, NSC-6396
Cytotoxic Antibiotics		
Anthracyclines		
daunorubicin, conventional	Cerubidine	daunomycin, rubidomycin, DNR
daunorubicin, liposomal	DaunoXome	
doxorubicin, conventional	Adriamycin, Rubex	ADR, hydroxydaunomycin, hydroxyl daunorubicin, NSC-123127
doxorubicin, liposomal	Doxil	
epirubicin	Ellence	4′-epidoxorubicin
idarubicin	Idamycin	4-demethoxydaunorubicin, 4-DMDR
valrubicin	Valstar	NSC-246131
Other Cytotoxic Antibiotics		
bleomycin	Blenoxane	BLM, Bleo, NSC-125066
dactinomycin	Cosmegen	actinomycin-D, ACT
mitomycin	Mutamycin	mitomycin-C, MTC
mitoxantrone	Novantrone	DHAD, dihydroxyanthracenedione dihydrochloride
plicamycin	Mithracin	mithramycin, aurelic acid, aureolic acid
Miscellaneous Antineoplastics (Cell Cycle Specificity Unclear)		
arsenic trioxide	Trisenox	
bortezomib	Velcade	LDP-341, MLN341, PS-341
gefitinib	Iressa	NSC-715055, ZD1839
imatinib	Gleevec	STI-571
mitotane	Lysodren	o-p′-DDD
porfimer sodium	Photofrin	
bevacizumad	Avastin	
Cytoprotective Drugs		
amifostine	Ethyol	ethiofos, gammaphos
dexrazoxane	Zinecard	
leucovorin	Wellcovorin	calcium leucovorin, leucovorin calcium, citrovorum factor, folinic acid, 5-formyl tetrahydrofolate
mesna	Mesnex	Sodium 2-mercaptoethane sulfonate
Other Toxicity Inhibitors		
allopurinol	Zyloprim, Aloprim	
rasburicase	Elitek	
Radioactive Antineoplastics		
chromic phosphate P 32	Phosphocol P 32	
samarium SM 153 lexidronam	Quadramet	samarium 153, 153SM-EDTMP
sodium iodide I 131	Iodotope	I-131
sodium phosphate P 32	Sodium Phosphate P 32	
strontium 89 Sr chloride	Metastron	strontium-89

DTIC, Dimethyltriazenoimidazolecarboxamide.

Continued

Table 48-1   Common Names for Selected Antineoplastic Drugs—cont'd

Generic Name	Trade Names	Other Names
Hormonal and Related Drugs		
Androgens		
fluoxymesterone	Halotestin	
testolactone	Teslac	
testosterone propionate		
Antiandrogens		
bicalutamide	Casodex	
flutamide	Eulexin	
nilutamide	Nilandron	
Progestins		
hydroxyprogesterone caproate	Hylutin	
megestrol acetate	Megace	
medroxyprogesterone acetate	Provera, Depo-Provera	
Estrogens		
ethinyl estradiol	Estinyl	
diethylstilbestrol	Stilphostrol	DES
Estrogen–Nitrogen Mustard Combination		
estramustine (estradiol 1 nor-nitrogen mustard)	Emcyt	
Antiestrogens		
fulvestrant	Faslodex	
tamoxifen	Nolvadex	
toremifene	Fareston	
Adrenocorticosteroids		
dexamethasone	Decadron, Hexadrol	
hydrocortisone	Cortef, Solu-Cortef, A-HydroCort	
methylprednisolone	Medrol, Solu-Medrol, A-methaPred	
prednisone	Deltasone, Orasone	
Gonadotropin-Releasing Hormone Analogues		
goserelin acetate	Zoladex	
leuprolide acetate	Lupron, Lupron Depot, Lupron for Pediatric Use, Viadur	
triptorelin pamoate	Trelstar Depot	
Aromatase Inhibitors		
aminoglutethimide	Cytadren	
anastrozole	Arimidex	
letrozole	Femara	
exemestane	Aromasin	
Miscellaneous Cell Cycle–Specific Drugs		
hydroxyurea	Hydrea, Mylocel, Droxia	hydroxycarbamide, NSC-32065

CELL CYCLE–NONSPECIFIC ANTINEOPLASTIC DRUGS

There are currently two broad classes of cell cycle–nonspecific cancer drugs: alkylating drugs and cytotoxic antibiotics.

ALKYLATING DRUGS

Records of the use of drugs to treat cancer date back several centuries. However, truly successful systemic cancer chemotherapy treatments are not documented until the 1940s. At this time, the first alkylating drugs were developed from mustard gas agents that were used for chemical warfare before and during World War I. The first drug to be developed was mechlorethamine, which is also known as *nitrogen mustard*. It is the prototypical drug of this class and is still used today for cancer treatment. Since its antineoplastic activity was discovered in the mid-twentieth century, many analogues have been synthesized for use in the treatment of cancer, and they are collectively referred to as *nitrogen mustards* also. *Alkylation* is the name of the chemical process by which these drugs work in cancer cells (see Mechanism of Action later).

The alkylating drugs commonly used in clinical practice in the United States today fall into three categories: *classic alkylators* (also called *nitrogen mustards*); *nitrosoureas*, which have a different chemical structure than the nitrogen mustards but also work by alkylation; and *probable alkylators*, which also have a different chemical structure than the nitrogen mustards but are known to work at least partially by alkylation. These drugs are used to treat a wide spectrum of malignancies. The drugs in each category are as follows:

Classic alkylators (nitrogen mustards)
- chlorambucil
- cyclophosphamide
- ifosfamide
- mechlorethamine
- melphalan
- thiotepa

Nitrosoureas
- carmustine
- lomustine
- streptozocin

Probable alkylators
- altretamine
- busulfan
- carboplatin
- cisplatin
- dacarbazine
- oxaliplatin
- procarbazine
- temozolomide

Mechanism of Action and Drug Effects

The alkylating drugs work by preventing cancer cells from reproducing, and they have a unique way of accomplishing this. Specifically, they alter the chemical structure of deoxyribonucleic acid (DNA), which is essential to the reproduction of any cell, by causing alkyl groups rather than hydrogen atoms to be attached to the nucleic acid. This process is called **alkylation.** Recall from chemistry that alkyl groups are composed of both hydrogen and carbon atoms that are linked by covalent bonds. Examples include a methyl group ($—CH_3$) and an ethyl group ($—CH_2CH_3$). DNA molecules consist of two adjacent strands, each consisting of alternating sequences of phosphate and sugar molecules (Figure 48-1). These components make up what is called the "backbone" of the DNA strands. These two strands are cross-linked to each other by the third DNA structural element: nitrogen-containing bases (adenine, guanine, thymine, and cytosine, abbreviated A, G, T, and C, respectively). These bases are bound to the sugar molecules of the DNA backbone, and two bases, linked to each other by covalent hydrogen bonds, form the molecular bridges between the two DNA strands that bring them into the double helix structure. A *nucleotide,* which consists of one molecule each of base, sugar, and phosphate that are bound together, is the structural unit of molecules of both DNA and ribonucleic acid (RNA), another nucleic acid that is important in cellular reproduction. A *nucleoside* consists of a base molecule and sugar molecule only. RNA molecules are produced by DNA molecules during the complex process of cellular reproduction. RNA molecules differ from DNA molecules in at least three ways: They are single stranded (versus double stranded), the thymine base is replaced by another base known as *uracil (U),* and the sugar molecule is *ribose,* which has a slightly different structure than the *deoxyribose* molecules of DNA.

During the normal process of reproduction, the double helix uncoils, and its two strands separate. A strand of RNA is then as-

sembled next to each single DNA strand in a process known as *transcription.* RNA strands, in turn, are involved in both protein synthesis *(translation)* and replication of the original DNA structure before cell division or **mitosis.** These processes ultimately result in the creation of a new cell with the same DNA sequence, and thus the same characteristics, as its parent cell.

Alkyl groups that are part of the chemical structure of antineoplastic alkylating drugs attach to DNA molecules by forming covalent bonds with the bases described earlier. As a result, abnormal chemical bonds form between the adjacent DNA strands, which leads to the formation of defective nucleic acids that are then unable to perform the normal cellular reproductive functions mentioned previously. This leads to cell death.

Alkylating drugs can also be characterized by the number of alkyl groups they possess and thus the number of alkylation reactions in which they can participate per single molecule of drug. **Bifunctional** alkylating drugs have two reactive alkyl groups that are able to alkylate two DNA molecules. **Polyfunctional** alkylating drugs can participate in several alkylation reactions. Figure 48-2 shows the location along the DNA double helix where the alkylating drugs work.

Indications

The most commonly used alkylating drugs today are effective against a wide spectrum of malignancies, including both solid and hematologic tumors. Common examples of the various types of cancer that different alkylating drugs are used to treat are listed in the Dosages table on page 754.

Adverse Effects

Alkylating drugs are capable of causing all of the dose-limiting adverse effects described in Chapter 47. Other adverse effects are described in Table 48-2. The relative emetic potential of the various alkylating drugs is given in Box 47-1 on page 728. The adverse effects of these drugs are important because of their severity, but they can be prevented by prophylactic measures. For instance, nephrotoxicity can often be prevented or minimized by adequately hydrating the patient with intravenous fluids. Drug **extravasation** (Box 48-1) occurs when an intravenous catheter punctures the vein and medication leaks (infiltrates) into the surrounding tissues. With cancer chemotherapy, in particular, this can cause severe tissue damage and even *necrosis* (tissue death), if the drug has vesicant properties. Extravasation antidotes for selected drugs are listed in Table 48-3.

Interactions

Only a few alkylating drugs are capable of causing significant drug interactions. The most important rule for preventing such drug interactions is to avoid administering an alkylating drug with any other drug capable of causing similar toxicities. For example, a major adverse effect of cisplatin is nephrotoxicity. Therefore, if possible, it should not be administered with a drug such as an aminoglycoside antibiotic (gentamicin, tobramycin, or amikacin) because of the resulting additive nephrotoxic effect and hence the increased likelihood of renal failure. Mechlorethamine and cyclophosphamide, both of which have significant bone marrow suppressing effects, ideally should not be administered with radiation therapy or with other drugs that suppress the bone marrow. These two drugs, as well as cisplatin, also should

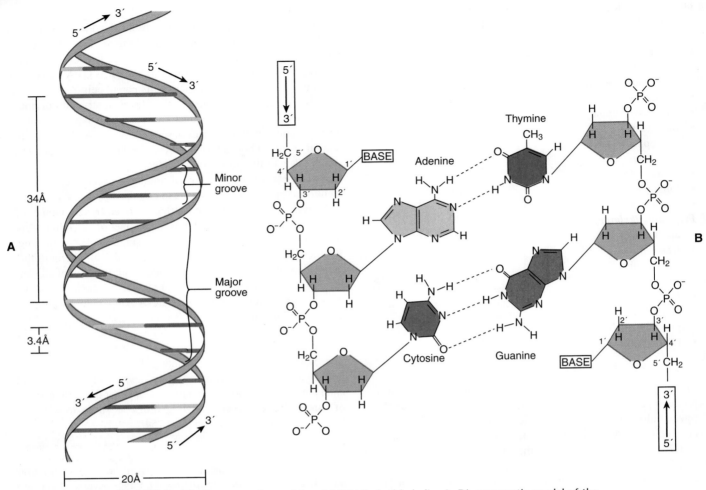

FIGURE 48-1 Deoxyribonucleic acid (DNA) double helix. **A,** Diagrammatic model of the helical structure, showing its dimensions, the major and minor grooves, the periodicity of the bases, and the antiparallel orientation of the backbone chains (represented by ribbons). The base pairs (represented by rods) are perpendicular to the axis and lie stacked one on another. **B,** The chemical structure of the backbone and bases of DNA, showing the sugar-phosphate linkages of the backbone and the hydrogen bonding between the base pairs. There are two hydrogen bonds between adenine and thymine, and three between cytosine and guanine. *(From Dorland's illustrated medical dictionary, ed 30, Philadelphia, 2003, Saunders.)*

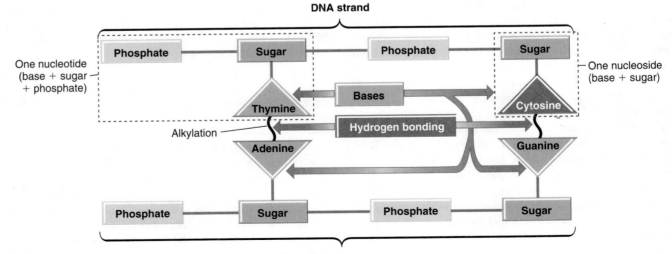

FIGURE 48-2 Organization of deoxyribonucleic acid (DNA) and site of action of alkylating drugs.

not be given with probenecid or sulfinpyrazone, both of which are *uricosuric drugs* used to treat gout. This combination can result in hyperuricemia or exacerbation of gout because of competition for renal elimination between these drugs and the molecules of normal body uric acid waste product. In general, the nurse should work with available pharmacy and oncology staff to proactively anticipate (and avoid, if possible) undesirable drug and treatment interactions.

Table 48-2	Commonly Used Alkylating Drugs: Severe Adverse Effects
Alkylating Drug	**Severe Adverse Effects**
busulfan	Pulmonary fibrosis
carboplatin	Less nephrotoxicity and neurotoxicity but more bone marrow suppression
cisplatin	Nephrotoxicity, peripheral neuropathy, ototoxicity
cyclophosphamide	Hemorrhagic cystitis

Dosages

For the recommended dosages of selected alkylating drugs, see the Dosages table on page 754.

Drug Profiles

The most widely used alkylating drugs, based on standard treatment protocols, are profiled here. Information for these as well as for some of the less commonly used drugs also appears in the Dosages table on page 754.

▶ **cisplatin**

Cisplatin (Platinol) is an antineoplastic drug that contains platinum in its chemical structure. It is classified as a probable alkylating drug because it is believed to destroy cancer cells in the same way as the classic alkylating drugs—by forming cross-links with DNA and thereby preventing its replication. It is also considered a bifunctional alkylating drug.

Cisplatin is used for the treatment of many solid tumors, such as bladder, testicular, and ovarian tumors. It is available only in injectable form.

▶ **cyclophosphamide**

Cyclophosphamide (Cytoxan, Neosar) is a nitrogen mustard derivative that was discovered during the course of research to improve mechlorethamine. It is a polyfunctional alkylating drug and is used in the

Box 48-1   Extravasation of Antineoplastics

Extravasation is one of the more devastating complications of antineoplastic therapy and may lead to extensive tissue damage, need for skin grafting, other problems to surrounding areas, and even loss of limb. Because many cell cycle–specific and cell cycle–nonspecific drugs are given intravenously (IV), there is a constant danger of extravasation of vesicants and subsequent injury, including permanent damage to nerves, tendons, and muscles. However, astute nursing care may help to prevent extravasation or to identify it early if it does occur, which can reduce the severity of tissue damage. There are important reasons for the placement of central venous IV catheters rather than peripheral catheters when long-term treatment is anticipated. Infiltration may occur with any IV catheter; it is the specific drug and its characteristics, such as irritant or vesicant properties (see discussion in Chapter 47), that poses the concern. Because peripheral veins are small and offer minimal dilution of the IV drug with blood flow, there is greater risk of severe and irreversible damage if a sub-

stance infiltrates and spreads to surrounding tissues, including muscles, tendons, ligaments. If the drug is a vesicant, extravasation may lead to massive tissue injury, whereas extravasation of an irritant results in significantly less damage. Central venous access is needed for administration of vesicants to avoid the problems associated with extravasation. Should extravasation of a vesicant be suspected, immediate action should be taken, and the antidote, if known, should be given following strict procedures. Steps to help manage extravasation include the following: (1) Stop the infusion immediately and contact the physician, but leave the IV catheter in place. (2) Usually, aspiration of any residual drug and/or blood from the catheter is performed next. (3) Consult institutional policy or guidelines or the pharmacist regarding the use of antidotes, application of hot or cold packs and/or sterile occlusive dressings, and elevation and rest of the affected limb. The extravasation incident must be thoroughly documented with attention to all phases of the nursing process related to the problem.

Data from National Cancer Institute website. Available at www.nci.hih.gov; United States Pharmacopeial Convention: *USP DI volume 1: drug information for the health care professional,* Greenwood Village, Colo, 2005, Micromedex; Internet resources for additional information: www.americancancersociety.com; www.OncoLink.com; www.hospicenet.org; www.acponline.org/public/hcare; and www.acponline.org/public/h care/7-final.htm.

Table 48-3	Alkylating Drug Extravasation: Specific Antidotes	
Alkylating Drug	**Antidote Preparation**	**Method**
carmustine	Mix equal parts 1 mEq/mL sodium bicarbonate (premixed) with sterile NS (1:1 solution); resulting solution is 0.5 mEq/mL.	1. Inject 2-6 mL IV through the existing line with multiple SC injections into the extravasated site. 2. Apply cold compresses. 3. Total dose should not exceed 10 mL of 0.5-mEq/mL solution.
mechlorethamine	Mix 4 mL 10% sodium thiosulfate with 6 mL sterile water for injection.	1. Inject 5-6 mL IV through the existing line with multiple SC injections into the extravasated site. 2. Repeat SC injections over the next few hours. 3. Apply cold compresses. 4. No total dose has been established.

IV, Intravenous; *NS,* normal saline; *SC,* subcutaneous.

DOSAGES

Selected Alkylating Drugs

Drug (Pregnancy Category)	Pharmacologic Subclass	Usual Dosage Range	Indications
altretamine (Hexalen) (D)	Methylmelamine	PO: 260 mg/m²/day, divided into 4 doses, for 14-21 consecutive days for 28-day cycles	Recurrent ovarian cancer
carmustine (BiCNU, Gliadel implantable wafer) (D)	Nitrosourea	IV: 150-200 mg/m² q6wk Implantable wafer: 8 wafers surgically implanted into resection cavity of brain tumor debulking area	Brain tumors, multiple myeloma, HL, NHL, melanoma
▶cisplatin (Platinol-AQ) (D)	Platinum coordination complex	IV: 50-100 mg/m² q4wk	Metastatic testicular, ovarian, and bladder cancer; brain tumors, esophageal, head, neck, lung, and cervical cancer
▶cyclophosphamide (Cytoxan, Neosar) (D)	Classic alkylator	IV: 3-5 mg/kg 2×/wk (many other regimens as well)	HL, NHL; leukemia, breast, ovarian, and testicular cancer; retinoblastoma; almost every solid tumor
▶mechlorethamine (Mustargen) (D)	Classic alkylator	IV: 0.4 mg/kg no more than q3wk	HL, NHL, leukemia, bronchogenic carcinoma, others
temozolomide (Temodar) (D)	Imidazotetrazine derivative	PO: 150 mg/m² once daily for 5 consecutive days per 28-day treatment cycle	Recurrent anaplastic astrocytoma
thiotepa (Thioplex) (D)	Ethylenimines	IV: 0.3-0.4 mg/kg at 1-4 wk intervals	Breast, ovarian, or bladder cancer; HL, NHL

HL, Hodgkin's lymphoma; *IV*, intravenous; *NHL*, non-Hodgkin's lymphoma; *PO*, oral.

treatment of cancers of the bone and lymph, as well as solid tumors. Various leukemias, Hodgkin's and non-Hodgkin's lymphomas, multiple myeloma, and some sarcomas may also respond to cyclophosphamide therapy. It is available in both oral and injectable dosage forms.

▶ *mechlorethamine*

Mechlorethamine (nitrogen mustard) (Mustine, Mustargen) is the prototypical alkylating drug. It is a nitrogen analogue of sulfur mustard (mustard gas) that was used for chemical warfare in World War I. As noted earlier, mechlorethamine was the very first alkylating antineoplastic drug discovered, and its beneficial effects in the treatment of various cancers were discovered after the war. Some of the cancers it is used to treat are Hodgkin's lymphoma, other lymphomas, and chronic leukemia.

Mechlorethamine is a bifunctional alkylating drug capable of forming cross-links between two DNA nucleotides, which interferes with RNA transcription and prevents cell division and protein synthesis. It is available in a parenteral form only, for administration intravenously or by an intracavitary route, such as intrapleurally or intraperitoneally.

CYTOTOXIC ANTIBIOTICS

The cytotoxic antibiotics consist of natural substances produced by the mold *Streptomyces* as well as synthetic substances not produced by this mold. Although they all have the ability to kill bacteria, and in some cases even viruses, they are normally used only for the treatment of cancer because of their toxicity. Cytotoxic antibiotics differ from other antineoplastic drugs in the toxicities they cause, but all can produce bone marrow suppression except bleomycin, which can cause pulmonary toxicity (pulmonary fibrosis and pneumonitis). Other severe toxicities associated with the use of cytotoxic antibiotics are heart failure (daunorubi-

cin) and rarely acute left ventricular failure (doxorubicin). The available cytotoxic antibiotics, categorized according to the specific subclass to which they belong, are as follows:

Anthracyclines
- daunorubicin
- doxorubicin
- epirubicin
- idarubicin
- valrubicin

Other cytotoxic antibiotics
- bleomycin (which is actually a cell cycle–specific drug)
- dactinomycin
- mitomycin
- mitoxantrone
- pentostatin*
- plicamycin

*Also classified as a purine analogue antimetabolite.

PREVENTING MEDICATION ERRORS

Sound-Alike Drugs: "Rubicins"

The anthracycline chemotherapy drugs have the same sound-alike suffix and are often nicknamed the "rubicins." These drugs include daunorubicin, doxorubicin, epirubicin, idarubicin, and valrubicin. Even though these drugs are in the same class, their use and drug effects are different. Medication errors have occurred because of mistaking one "rubicin" for another. It is important to refer to these drugs by their complete names rather than as a "rubicin."

Mechanism of Action and Drug Effects

Cytotoxic antibiotic antineoplastic drugs are primarily cell cycle–nonspecific drugs, although some, such as daunorubicin, are more active in the S phase. In most cases, however, the drugs are active during all phases of the cell cycle. Most act either through alkylation, which was explained previously, or by a process called *intercalation,* in which the drug molecule is inserted between the two strands of a DNA molecule; this process is very similar to the way in which antineoplastic antimetabolites work (Chapter 47) and ultimately blocks DNA synthesis. Specifically, the drug binds to the nucleotide base pairs of the DNA helix, causing the shape of the DNA helix to change into an unstable structure. The result is the blockade of DNA, RNA, and protein synthesis. Some cytotoxic antibiotic drugs can block all three, but others affect DNA synthesis only.

Indications

Cytotoxic antibiotics are used to treat a variety of solid tumors and some hematologic malignancies as well. Common examples of these drugs and the malignancies they are used to treat are given in the Dosages table on this page.

Adverse Effects

As with all of the antineoplastic drugs, cytotoxic antibiotics have the undesirable effects of hair loss, nausea and vomiting, and myelosuppression. The emetic potential of the various drugs in this category is given in Box 47-1. Major adverse effects specific to the cytotoxic antibiotics are listed in Table 48-4.

Toxicity and Management of Overdose

Severe cases of cardiomyopathy are associated with large cumulative doses of doxorubicin. Routine monitoring of cardiac ejection fraction with multiple-gated acquisition (MUGA) scans, cumulative dose limitations, and the use of cytoprotectant drugs such as dexrazoxane can decrease the incidence of this devastating toxicity. Box 48-2 outlines the management of doxorubicin extravasation.

Interactions

The cytotoxic antibiotics that are used in chemotherapy interact with many drugs. They all tend to produce increased toxicities when used in combination with other chemotherapeutic drugs or with radiation therapy. Some drugs, most notably bleomycin and doxorubicin, have been known to cause serum digoxin levels to increase. Patients receiving one of these drugs along with digoxin should be observed for signs of digoxin toxicity. Dosage reduction or elimination of digoxin therapy may be indicated (Chapter 21).

Dosages

For recommended dosages of selected cytotoxic antibiotic drugs, see the Dosages table on this page.

Table 48-4	Cytotoxic Antibiotics: Severe Adverse Effects
Cytotoxic Antibiotic Drug	**Severe Adverse Effects**
bleomycin	Pulmonary fibrosis, pneumonitis
dactinomycin	Liver toxicity, tissue damage in the event of extravasation, heart failure
daunorubicin	
doxorubicin	Liver and cardiovascular toxicities
idarubicin	
mitomycin	Liver, kidney, and lung toxicities
mitoxantrone	Cardiovascular toxicity
plicamycin	Tissue damage secondary to extravasation

Box 48-2	Treatment of Doxorubicin Extravasation

1. Cool the site to patient tolerance for 24 hours.
2. Elevate and rest the extremity for 24 to 48 hours, then have the patient resume normal activity as tolerated.
3. If pain, erythema, or swelling persists beyond 48 hours, discuss with the physician the need for surgical intervention or other treatment options.

DOSAGES

Selected Cytotoxic Antibiotics

Drug (Pregnancy Category)	Pharmacologic Subclass	Usual Dosage Range	Indications
Anthracycline Antibiotics			
▶doxorubicin, conventional (Adriamycin, Rubex) (D)	Anthracycline	IV: 60-75 mg/m² as a single injection given q21d	Multiple cancers, including breast, bone, and ovarian, and leukemia, neuroblastoma, HL, NHL
doxorubicin, liposomal (Doxil) (D)	Anthracycline	IV: 20 mg/m² q3wk for as long as tolerated and responsive to treatment	AIDS-related Kaposi's sarcoma when other chemotherapy drugs have failed or patient is intolerant to them; recurrent metastatic ovarian cancer
Anthracenedione Antibiotics			
mitoxantrone (Novantrone) (D)	Anthracenedione	IV: 12 mg/m² q3wk	Prostate cancer, acute myelocytic leukemia

AIDS, Acquired immunodeficiency syndrome; *HL,* Hodgkin's lymphoma; *IV,* intravenous; *NHL,* non-Hodgkin's lymphoma.

Drug Profiles

▶ *doxorubicin*

Doxorubicin (Adriamycin, Rubex) is used in many combination chemotherapy regimens. Its use is contraindicated in patients with a known hypersensitivity to it, patients with severe myelosuppression, and patients who are at risk for severe cardiac toxicity because they have already received a large cumulative dose of any of the anthracycline antineoplastics. It is available only in injectable form. Doxorubicin is also now available in a liposomal drug delivery system (Doxil). In this dosage formulation the drug is encapsulated in a lipid molecule bilayer called a *liposome*. The advantages of liposomal encapsulation are reduced systemic toxicity and increased duration of action. Liposomal encapsulation extends the biologic half-life of doxorubicin to 50 to 60 hours and increases its affinity for cancer cells. The liposomal dosage formulation is currently indicated for the treatment of Kaposi's sarcoma, which primarily affects individuals infected with the human immunodeficiency virus (HIV) that causes acquired immunodeficiency syndrome (AIDS). This formulation is available only as a 20-mg vial for injection.

mitoxantrone

Mitoxantrone (Novantrone) is indicated for the treatment of acute non-lymphocytic leukemia and prostate cancer as well as the neurologic disorder multiple sclerosis. It is available only in injectable form.

MISCELLANEOUS ANTINEOPLASTICS

The miscellaneous antineoplastic drugs are those that, because of their unique structure and mechanism of action, cannot be classified into the previously described categories. However, some drugs that are originally classified as miscellaneous drugs are later reclassified as more is learned about their mechanisms of action and other characteristics. Drugs currently in the miscellaneous category include bevacizumab, hydroxyurea, imatinib, mitotane, hormonal drugs, and radioactive and related antineoplastic drugs. Selected drugs are profiled in the following sections.

Drug Profiles

The various drugs in the miscellaneous category of antineoplastics are used to treat a wide range of neoplasms. Hydroxyurea is administered orally. Bevacizumab, imatinib, and mitotane are available only in injectable form.

bevacizumab

Bevacizumab (Avastin) is the first, and currently the only, approved antineoplastic drug in a new category—*angiogenesis inhibitors*. It was approved in February of 2004 by the U.S. Food and Drug Administration (FDA). *Angiogenesis* is the creation of new blood vessels that supply oxygen and other blood nutrients to growing tissues. In the case of malignant (and even benign) tumors, angiogenesis that occurs within the tumor mass promotes continued tumor growth. As a tumor enlarges, its central tissues gradually die off *(necrosis)*. However, its outer portion continues to grow, often to fatal proportions, with blood supplied through angiogenesis. Thus, inhibiting this process offers a promising new mechanism for antineoplastic drug action. Bevacizumab is a recombinant "humanized" monoclonal immunoglobulin G1 antibody derived from mouse antibodies. The scientific name for any compound derived from mouse tissue is *murine*. Humanization refers to the use of recombinant DNA techniques to make animal-derived antibody proteins more genetically similar to those of humans. Immunoglobulin G1 is a subtype of *immunoglobulin G*, the principal class of antibodies produced by mammalian immune systems (Chapter 46). This drug works by binding to and inhibiting the biologic activity of human *vascular endothelial growth factor (VEGF)*. VEGF is an endogenous protein that normally promotes angiogenesis in the body. Bevacizumab is available only in injectable form. The only recognized contraindication is severe drug allergy or allergy to other murine products.

Adverse reactions include those affecting the cardiovascular system (hypertension or hypotension, thrombosis), central nervous system (CNS) (pain, headache, dizziness), skin (alopecia, dry skin), metabolism (weight loss, hypokalemia), gastrointestinal (GI) tract (nausea, vomiting, diarrhea), kidneys (nephrotoxicity with proteinuria), and respiratory tract (infection). More severe effects can occur in any of these systems but are much less common than those listed. Drug interactions reported to date are limited but include potentiation of the cardiotoxic affects of the anthracycline antibiotics such as doxorubicin.

hydroxyurea

Hydroxyurea (Hydrea) most closely resembles the antimetabolite antineoplastics in its actions. It interferes with the synthesis of DNA by inhibiting the incorporation of thymidine into DNA. It works primarily in the S and G_1 phases of the cell cycle, which makes it a cell cycle–specific drug. It is indicated for the treatment of squamous cell carcinoma but may also be used to treat various types of leukemia as well as sickle cell anemia. The drug is available only in oral form. Adverse reactions include edema, drowsiness, headache, rash, hyperuricemia, nausea, vomiting, dysuria, myelosuppression, elevated liver enzyme levels, muscular weakness, peripheral neuropathy, nephrotoxicity, dyspnea, and pulmonary fibrosis. Drugs with which it interacts include the anti-HIV drugs zidovudine, zalcitabine, and didanosine (Chapter 39), all of which can actually have a synergistic effect with hydroxyurea. Concurrent use with fluorouracil increases the risk of neurotoxic symptoms. Because hydroxyurea can reduce the clearance of cytarabine, dosage reduction of cytarabine is recommended when the two are used concurrently.

imatinib

Imatinib (Gleevec) is indicated for the treatment of chronic myeloid leukemia (CML), particularly after failure of interferon alfa therapy. It is one of the newest available antineoplastic drugs, approved by the FDA in 2001. It works by inhibiting the action of a key enzyme (protein-tyrosine kinase) that plays an important role in the CML disease process. Although its name sounds similar to those of various monoclonal antibody drugs, imatinib is not a monoclonal antibody. It is available only in oral form. Common adverse reactions include fatigue, headache, rash, fluid retention, GI and hematologic effects, musculoskeletal pain, cough, and dyspnea; more severe effects occur less commonly for most body systems. Potential drug interactions are quite numerous because they primarily involve drugs metabolized by the cytochrome P-450 group of hepatic enzymes. Concurrent use of acetaminophen increases the risk of hepatotoxicity, for example. There are also many other potentially interacting drugs, too numerous to list here. Major examples include amiodarone, verapamil, warfarin, azole antifungals, antidepressants, and antibiotics. A pharmacist may be needed to review the patient's medication regimen and adjust dosages or delete medications accordingly, in collaboration with the patient's prescriber.

mitotane

Mitotane (Lysodren) is an adrenal cytotoxic drug that is indicated specifically for the treatment of inoperable adrenal corticoid carcinoma. It is available only in oral form. Adverse reactions include CNS depression, rash, nausea, vomiting, muscle weakness, and headache. Reported drug interactions include enhanced CNS depressive effects when taken concurrently with other CNS depressants (e.g., benzodiazepines). Mitotane may also increase the clearance of both warfarin and phenytoin, reducing their effects. Finally, the potassium-sparing diuretic spironolactone may negate the effects of mitotane.

octreotide

Octreotide (Sandostatin) is a unique medication used for a cancer-related condition (Chapter 29).

HORMONAL ANTINEOPLASTICS

Hormonal drugs are used in the treatment of a variety of neoplasms in both males and females. The rationale is that sex hormones act to accelerate the growth of some common types of malignant tumors, especially certain types of breast and prostate cancer. Therefore, therapy may involve administration of hormones with opposing effects (i.e., male vs. female hormones) or drugs that block the body's sex hormone receptors. These drugs are used most commonly as palliative and adjuvant therapy. For certain types of cancer they may also be used as drugs of first choice. Some of the more commonly used hormonal drugs for female-specific neoplasms such as breast cancer are anastrazole, tamoxifen, megestrol, toremifene, medroxyprogesterone, aminoglutethimide, fluoxymesterone, fulvestrant, and testolactone. For male-specific neoplasms such as prostate cancer, the following drugs are used: bicalutamide, flutamide, nilutamide, leuprolide, goserelin, and estramustine (see Table 48-1).

RADIOPHARMACEUTICALS AND RELATED ANTINEOPLASTICS

Antineoplastic drugs that are usually administered by physicians include porfimer sodium and various radioactive pharmaceuticals (radiopharmaceuticals). Porfimer sodium is used to treat esophageal or bronchial tumors that are present on the surface mucosa. The medication is given intravenously and is followed by one or more sessions of laser light therapy to the esophageal or bronchial mucosa for direct tumor lysis and manual débridement. Radiopharmaceuticals are used to treat a variety of cancers or symptoms caused by cancers. Five commonly used radiopharmaceuticals are chromic phosphate P 32 (for cancer-induced peritoneal or pleural effusions), samarium SM 153 lexidronam (for bone cancer pain), sodium iodide I 131 (for thyroid cancer and hyperthyroidism), sodium phosphate P 32 (for various leukemias and palliative treatment of bone metastases), and strontium Sr 89 chloride (for bone cancer pain). These medications are usually administered by nuclear medicine physician specialists.

CYTOPROTECTIVE DRUGS AND MISCELLANEOUS TOXICITY INHIBITORS

Several drugs are available that are classified as cytoprotective drugs. These medications help to reduce the toxicity of various antineoplastics. The decision about whether to use them is often very patient specific, as is the case with chemotherapy regimens. Such decisions are generally made by patients' oncologists. All of these drugs are normally administered intravenously with the exception of allopurinol, which may also be given orally. These medications are listed in Table 48-1 on page 749, and extravasation of irritants versus vesicants was discussed in Chapter 47. For more information related to extravasation and the handling and administration of antineoplastics, see Boxes 48-1, 48-2, and 48-3. Also see the Laboratory Values Related to Drug Therapy box on page 758.

Box 48-3   Concerns in the Handling and Administration of Vesicant Antineoplastic Drugs

The handling and administration of antineoplastic drugs is very controversial, because the nurse mixing and giving the drug may experience negative consequences. In most institutions, the pharmacy department is responsible for mixing these drugs, and preparation carried out carefully in an appropriate environment with use of a laminar airflow hood and personal protective equipment (mask, gown, gloves). Many facilities recommend taking special precautions during the care of a patient who is receiving chemotherapy, such as double-flushing the patient's bodily secretions in the commode and using special hampers for the disposal of all items that come into contact with the patient, including used personal protective equipment. Special spill kits are employed to clean up even the smallest chemotherapy spills. These precautions are necessary to protect the health care provider from the cytotoxic effects of these drugs. In addition, appropriate and updating of knowledge about these drugs is important to safe and appropriate nursing care. All nurses must be certified to administer chemotherapy and must remain current in their level of practice and competencies related to this treatment modality. All equipment and containers should be handled appropriately once the infusion is completed, and the hands and any exposed area must be washed to ensure the safety of the health care provider. The Centers for Disease Control and Prevention and the Oncology Nurses Society offer exceptional resources for individuals involved in the care of patients receiving chemotherapy.

Data from National Cancer Institute website. Available at www.nci.hih.gov; United States Pharmacopeial Convention: *USP DI volume 1: drug information for the health care professional,* Greenwood Village, Colo, 2005, Micromedex; Internet resources for additional information: www.americancancersociety.com, www.OncoLink.com, www.hopsicenet.org, www.acponline.org/public/hcare, and www.acponline.org/public/h care/7-final.htm.

◆ NURSING PROCESS

Antineoplastic drugs, as thoroughly discussed in Chapter 47, are some of the most toxic medications given to patients, and because of their toxicities, serious complications and adverse effects may occur. Nursing care must be based on a thorough knowledge of cancer and its treatment and the subsequent effects of different treatment modalities, specifically antineoplastic drug therapy, on the patient. Whereas Chapter 47 discusses the general adverse effects that occur with most antineoplastic drugs, cell cycle–specific drugs, and antineoplastic enzymes, this discussion relates to cell cycle–nonspecific, hormonal and miscellaneous drugs.

◆ ASSESSMENT

For patients receiving any of the *alkylating drugs*, such as cisplatin and cyclophosphamide, baseline fluid and electrolyte levels, renal and hepatic function test results, and complete blood cell counts should be assessed. Specific to alkylating drugs is a loss of vision for light and color, emesis, nephrotoxicity, and bone marrow suppression; therefore, assessment should include a baseline vision test and determination of any changes in near or far vision or color vision, which can be accomplished using a Snellen and/or color chart. In addition, a baseline abdominal assessment should be performed, with auscultation of bowel sounds and questioning of the patient about any problems with nausea

LABORATORY VALUES RELATED TO DRUG THERAPY

Antineoplastics

Laboratory Test	Normal Ranges	Rationale for Assessment
Leukocytes (WBCs)	5,000-10,000/mm^3	WBCs are protection against infection and when an infection develops, the WBCs attack and destroy the causative bacteria, virus or other organism. In response to the infection, WBCs increase in number dramatically. If WBCs are decreased from antineoplastic treatment and subsequent bone marrow suppression, and should they decrease to levels <3500/mm^3 (leukopenia), there is a high risk for severe infection and immunesuppression.

WBC components:
  Neutrophils
  Band neutrophils
	47%-77% or above 2000/mm^3
	0-3%
		The major types of WBCs are neutrophils, lyphocytes, monocytes, eosinophils and basophils. Immature neutrophils are called band neutrophils and—with neutrophil counts—provide a picture about the patient's immune system. If neutrophils are decreased to levels <1800-2000/mm^3 (neutropenia) then there is risk for severe infection. If band neutrophils are included in the WBC differential count, then the abnormally low value reinforces the risk for severe infection.

Nadir	See normal range of each blood cell	Nadir refers to the point in time at which bone marrow cells reach their lowest levels. This time frame may become shorter and recovery longer with successive courses of antineoplastic treatment with a general estimate of time frame between 10 and 28 days. Anticipation of the nadir allows the oncologist/health care team to develop a preventative treatment plan which may include biologic response modifiers and antibiotics.

WBCs, White blood cells.
Information on red blood cells (RBCs) and platelets is presented in Chapter 47.

and/or vomiting. Hyperactive or hypoactive to no bowel sounds are important to report, and skin turgor, moistness of mucosa, urinary output, and urine color should be noted. Loss of turgor, dryness, or cracking of the oral mucosa and lips, and decrease in urinary output and dark amber urine are indicative of dehydration as a consequence of nausea and vomiting. Baseline neurologic status should be assessed with documentation of level of consciousness, mental clarity, memory, attention, and cognition, and the patient should be questioned about any history of seizures or other CNS disorders because of the potential for drug-related seizures and neurologic changes. In addition, peripheral neuropathies are often associated with these drugs, and so the presence of any numbness or tingling of the extremities should be noted. Because of the possibility of loss of or changes in motor function, a thorough assessment of baseline motor function should be performed, with a rating of deep tendon reflexes, gait characteristics, mobility, and degree of independence in activity. Cisplatin may be ototoxic and so baseline hearing should be documented.

Alkylating drugs may have a profound impact on the patient's nutritional status, so it should be assessed (Chapter 47). Serum levels of albumin and protein as well as fluid and electrolyte values (e.g., sodium, potassium, chloride, magnesium, calcium) should be noted. The use of alkylating drugs may also result in hepatotoxicity and renal damage; therefore, the results of liver and renal function tests should be assessed. Bone marrow suppression and pulmonary toxicity may also occur, so it is important to know the patient's baseline blood cell counts and to assess for the presence of abnormal to absent breath sounds, irregular breathing patterns, difficulty breathing, cyanosis around the lips or in the fingernails, chest pain, cough with or without sputum, and any other respiratory symptoms. Because of the risk of drug-related cardiac toxicity, it is important to assess for any cardiac disease. Chest pain; abnormal heart rate and rhythm; abnormal heart sounds, including gallops or murmurs; edema;

and other signs or symptoms of cardiac disorder should be noted.

Some of the major adverse effects associated with the use of *cytotoxic antibiotics* (e.g., doxorubicin) are pulmonary fibrosis and hepatic toxicity. So that the impact of the medication on the lungs can be determined, assessment should include taking a nursing history with a focus on respiratory functioning (in the past and present); examining the results of pulmonary function studies and the values for arterial blood gas levels and partial pressures of CO_2 and O_2; evaluating breath sounds, breathing rate, rhythm, and depth; and noting the results of radiographic examination of the chest. When intravenous sites are not patent and become infiltrated due to *extravasation*—or leakage of the drug into surrounding tissues—necrosis may occur, with sloughing of the layers of skin and underlying supportive structures (e.g., muscles, ligaments). See previous discussion of extravasation in the pharmacology section, including Table 48-3 and Box 48-3. Because tissue necrosis can be severe, prevention of infiltration is critical to patient safety, and intravenous site should be assessed frequently, with attention to the patency of the intravenous line and the appearance of any redness, red streaking above the intravenous site, warmth, or swelling. Assessment of nutritional status, reproductive system, cardiac system, pulmonary system, immune system, and bone marrow functioning is needed before and during drug therapy (see previous discussion for specific information). When doxorubicin is given, patients with documented cardiac disease may need further diagnostic testing, including electrocardiograms and MUGA scans, to assess cardiac ejection fraction. These tests may also aid in evaluating the effectiveness of the cytoprotective drug dexrazoxane, which is used to help decrease the risk of life-threatening cardiac toxicities.

Hormonal antineoplastic requires a thorough assessment of very specific systems and include drugs such as corticosteroids, estrogens, estrogen-mustards, selective estrogen receptor modulators (SERMs) or estrogen antagonists (antiestrogens), progestins, androgens, androgen antagonists, gonadotropin-releasing hormone agonists, and aromatase inhibitors. Many of these drugs are discussed in Chapters 33 and 34; the use of these drugs in cancer treatment protocols and their implications for the nursing process are also presented in detail online at http://evolve.elsevier.com/Lilley.

Assessment associated with the use of *estrogen antagonists* such as fulvestrant, tamoxifen, and toremifene citrates (SERMs) often begins with the review of any tumor estrogen receptor assays, computed tomographic scans, and other x-rays. Results of complete blood cell counts, clotting studies, liver function studies, lipid profiles, and serum cholesterol and calcium levels should be noted before and during drug therapy so that drug-related changes can be identified early and any appropriate action taken. Signs and symptoms of hypercalcemia (an adverse effect) may include constipation, confusion, lethargy, weakness, and changes in urinary patterns. A neurologic assessment including assessment of sensation, motor strength, and gait is important because of the adverse effect of asthenia, or loss of strength, in the extremities. Cardiac functioning should be assessed and notation made of baseline weight and any existing edema or congestive heart failure. Patients may experience flare-ups of bone pain, so assessment for these complaints is important, including notation of severity and duration. Should these complaints continue for a prolonged period, the physician should be contacted.

Blood cell counts, hemoglobin level, hematocrit, blood pressure, and weight should be measured before and during the use of *androgens* (e.g., testosterone). Serum cholesterol level, lipid levels, and levels of electrolytes and hepatic enzymes should be measured before the initiation of therapy if ordered. Assessment of urinary patterns and any complaints should be noted. It is also important to understand the reason for the use of these hormones in cancer patients, such as the administration of androgens in cases of advanced breast cancer to promote tumor regression. The emotional turmoil that may be associated with advanced disease is, in itself, important to assess, as are the patient's feelings about treatment with a hormone that leads to masculine secondary sexual characteristics such as growth of body hair, lowering of the voice, and muscle growth in female patients (with long-term treatment). See Chapter 34 and http://evolve.elsevier.com/Lilley for more information.

Flutamide and leuprolide are *antiandrogens* and require assessment of baseline renal and liver function and blood cell counts. Flutamide may cause liver failure; thus continual assessment of nausea, vomiting, jaundice or yellowish discoloration of the skin and/or eye area, dark yellow urine, flulike symptoms, abdominal pain, extreme fatigue, and loss of appetite should occur. Weight and height are important to note as well as a nutritional assessment (Chapter 47). Urinary patterns and sexual functioning are also important to assess with attention to any existing problems or difficulties. Existing cardiac disease states and any edematous conditions should be noted because edema may occur with these drugs and the extra fluid volume could exacerbate existing disease states. Examining the patient's history for the presence of glucose-6-phosphate dehydrogenase deficiency is important, because this disorder would be a possible contraindication and cause for concern. Documentation of the use of a reliable form of birth control is important because of teratogenic effects. Male sperm production may be affected (Chapter 47) as well as a decline in sexual functioning, desire, and/or ability.

With the use of *gonadotropin-releasing hormone agonists*, such as leuprolide and goserelin, the patient must be assessed for

any allergies to the drugs. Knowing contraceptive history is important because women who are taking these drugs must use a nonhormonal contraceptive. Often the physician will order laboratory tests for serum testosterone level and prostatic acid phosphatase level for male patients before and during therapy; an increase will be noted during the initial week of therapy and then levels will return to baseline by 4 weeks. Assessment of the cardiac system should include evaluation of heart sounds, pulse rate/rhythm, blood pressure, weight, and presence of edema. Difficulty in passing urine may worsen for a short period with initiation of goserelin therapy and so documentation of urinary patterns prior to therapy is important.

Exemestane is a drug used in women whose breast cancer has progressed during treatment with tamoxifen. Baseline respiratory and cardiac function is important to document because the drug can cause cough, hoarseness, labored breathing, shortness of breath, edema of the extremities, and tightness in the chest.

For patients taking *antiadrenal drugs* (e.g., mitotane), basic assessment includes recording drug allergies, measuring vital signs, taking a medical and medication history, and identifying conditions that represent cautions or contraindications to drug use as well as possible drug interactions. Because of the common adverse effects of skin darkening, diarrhea, loss of appetite, mental depression, and nausea and vomiting, it is important to complete an assessment and to document baseline findings such as bowel sounds, skin color and turgor, results of a mental status examination, and patient 24-hour recall of dietary intake.

NURSING DIAGNOSES

- Activity intolerance related to drug-induced anemia with fatigue and lethargy
- Anxiety related to the unknowns of therapy and illness
- Disturbed body image related to drug-induced alopecia, darkening of the skin, and sexual dysfunction (such as is seen with cyclophosphamide, nitrosoureas, and other alkylating drugs)
- Decreased cardiac output related to the adverse effect of cardiotoxicity associated with cytotoxic antibiotics
- Diarrhea related to the adverse effects of antineoplastic drugs
- Disturbed sensory perception (hearing loss, optic neuritis) related to ototoxicity associated with cisplatin
- Imbalanced nutrition, less than body requirements, related to loss of appetite, nausea, vomiting, stomatitis, and changes in taste as a result of antineoplastic therapy
- Impaired urinary elimination related to the adverse effects of cyclophosphamide (hemorrhagic cystitis and nephrotoxicity)
- Ineffective breathing pattern related to the adverse effect of pulmonary toxicity associated with some antineoplastic drugs
- Risk for injury related to loss of reflexes, numbness of the hands and feet, and ataxia from cisplatin-related neurotoxicity

PLANNING
Goals

- Patient maintains as healthy a diet as possible with adequate intake of protein, vitamins, and other nutrients to increase energy and stamina and allow continued performance of the activities of daily living during antineoplastic treatment.
- Patient maintains an intact and healthy body image and effective coping mechanisms while experiencing alopecia, skin changes, and sexual dysfunction associated with antineoplastic therapy.

- Patient verbalizes concerns, fears, and anxieties associated with changes in body image.
- Patient's cardiac output remains within normal limits while the patient is taking antineoplastics.
- Patient states foods and fluids that should be avoided to prevent further GI irritation and is able to identify foods that help bulk up stool and minimize problems from diarrhea.
- Patient remains safe and free from injury with minimal neurologic, sensory, and motor deficits from the adverse effects of antineoplastic therapy.
- Patient receives consultation regarding appropriate dietary intake and fluid and electrolyte needs, help with meal planning, grocery shopping tips, and information on the use of various food groups and medications, as ordered, to prevent problems of nutritional imbalance.
- Patient regains normal urinary patterns during and after antineoplastic therapy.

Outcome Criteria
- Patient openly verbalizes any anxieties, fears, concerns, or feelings of being upset or depressed about changes in body image and self-concept and seeks out appropriate resources for help in coping, such as spiritual support, therapeutic touch, counseling, and talking with family, friends, and other individuals with cancer trained to visit cancer patients, who can be located through the American Cancer Society and community support groups.
- Patient adheres to a daily "heart-healthy" regimen of conserving energy, planning activities, and monitoring pulse rate and blood pressure in a consistent routine and asks for assistance with care and activities as needed.
- Patient adheres to a daily regimen for increasing urinary health, such as forcing fluids, consuming fluids that minimize urinary infections (e.g., cranberry juice), and maintaining daily hydration while on antineoplastic therapy.
- Patient states measures to follow for pulmonary health, including avoiding those with influenza, colds, fever, or other illnesses; avoiding smoking and exposure to second-hand smoke; coughing and performing deep breathing frequently during waking hours; forcing fluids; and taking prophylactic antibiotic therapy, if deemed necessary.
- Patient states ways to minimize risk for injury (from neurologic adverse effects) by development of a safety plan that includes ridding the home of throw rugs and furniture that may lead to falls, using assistive devices such as a walker or cane, having a bedside commode available, installing night lights, and instituting other measures to aid mobility.

See Chapter 47 for additional nursing diagnoses, goals, and outcome criteria that may be relevant to the discussion here.

♦ IMPLEMENTATION

With *alkylating* drugs, such as cisplatin and cyclophosphamide, the patient should expect problems related to bone marrow suppression, such as anemia, leukopenia, and thrombocytopenia. Stomatitis is common, as are nausea, vomiting, and diarrhea. Nursing considerations related to these adverse effects are discussed in Chapter 47; however, other interventions are associated with this group of antineoplastic drugs. Vital signs should be measured every 1 to 2 hours during infusion of these drugs (vital signs should be measured for all antineoplastic drugs). Hydration is critical to prevention of adverse effects, and if output is less than 100 mL/hr, the physician should be contacted. Patients at home

after treatment with this group of drugs should be reminded of the importance of hydration and should be told to contact the physician if they experience dry mucous membranes, very dark amber urine, or little or no urinary output or vomiting of large amounts over a period of 8 hours or less. Intravenous infusions are to be administered per guidelines and policy, and solutions must be protected from light. Any ringing or roaring in the ears or hearing loss should be reported because of the potential for ototoxicity associated with several alkylating drugs. Peripheral neuropathies may occur, and so numbness, tingling, and/or pain in the extremities should be reported immediately to prevent complications and enhance comfort. Cyclophosphamide is known to cause all of the symptoms mentioned as well as hemorrhagic cystitis. Hydration before and during therapy is important to prevent an impact on the bladder and minimize the adverse effect. Because of its possible carcinogenic, mutagenic, and teratogenic properties, the drug should be handled and administered with extreme caution.

Some alkylating drugs may be nephrotoxic, and frequent monitoring of renal function test results is required after therapy has begun. Hydration should be encouraged, with intake of up to 3000 mL/day if not contraindicated. Aluminum needles or administration sets should not be used with many of these drugs because aluminum can degrade the platinum compounds in them, and it is important that the nurse ensure that the proper infusion equipment is used. Drug-induced neuropathies may occur, so the patient should be encouraged to avoid extremely cold temperatures or the handling of cold objects during the infusion because this may exacerbate the toxicity. Other drugs in this group may be given by various routes, such as intrapericardial, intratumoral, and intravesical, so appropriate interventions will need to be performed per the manufacturer's guidelines or hospital policy. Pulmonary toxicity may occur with some of the alkylating drugs, and so the nurse should be alert to cough, shortness of breath, and abnormal breath sounds. These adverse effects should be reported immediately to the physician. Parenteral reconstitution of any of these drugs should be performed according to the manufacturer's guidelines and suggestions, because not all diluents are compatible. As with all antineoplastic drugs, the nurse should take sufficient time to discuss the protocol-therapy times, frequency, and duration of therapy with the patient, family, and/or significant others or caregivers. For example, therapy may be given at an outpatient facility for 1 day every 3 weeks, but it may take 8 hours for completion of therapy. Patient assistance with planning, transportation, and meals and/or snacks is needed for the entire protocol. This can last 3 to 6 months or even longer depending on the drug and the cancer. Community resources are available through social service departments, hospice organizations, home health services, Meals on Wheels programs, church volunteer organizations, and chapters of the American Cancer Society.

Therapy with *cytotoxic antibiotics* is also associated with bone marrow suppression, nausea, vomiting, and diarrhea, as well as with most of the other adverse effects discussed earlier for the alkylating drugs. Patients experiencing adverse effects of interstitial pneumonitis may require more frequent monitoring of pulmonary function, such as by taking chest radiographs every 1 to 2 weeks during therapy. Liver and renal function tests should be monitored throughout therapy. Hyperuricemia may occur and so provision of fluids and hydration is important to minimize this adverse effect (see previous discussion). With daunorubicin in particular, the patient should be informed that the urine may turn a reddish color for a few days after the treatment. Knowing this will help ease any fears or anxieties. Stomatitis is more severe with some of these drugs, and ulceration of the mucous membranes may occur within 2 or 3 days. See Chapter 47 for further information about stomatitis, alopecia, diarrhea, nausea, vomiting, fatigue, neutropenia, and thrombocytopenia. Cardiac toxicity may occur, so frequent checking of heart and breath sounds and daily weights should be recorded (with reporting of an increase of 2 pounds or more in 24 hours or 5 pounds or more in a week). See Chapter 47 for discussion of the common adverse effects of antineoplastic therapy such as various anemias, alopecia, nausea, vomiting, and diarrhea.

Use of *estrogens, progestins, testosterone* and hormone antagonists in the treatment of various neoplasms is somewhat common. Associated nursing interventions and patient education for the use of these hormones are discussed in depth in Chapters 33 and 34. *Corticosteroids* and related nursing considerations are presented in Chapter 32. Further information and discussion regarding the use of hormones and hormone antagonists in the treatment of patients with various types of cancer can also be found online at http://evolve.elsevier.com/Lilley.

Hydroxyurea is used in a variety of treatment protocols. When this drug is given, monitoring of platelet and leukocyte counts is important to avoid harm to the patient and should be ongoing during therapy. If platelet count falls below 100,000/mm^3 or leukocyte count falls below 2500/mm^3, therapy may need to be temporarily interrupted until counts rise toward the normal values. See earlier discussion of nursing considerations associated with anemias, fatigue, weakness, bleeding tendencies, and infection. *Etoposide* is given intravenously, so the precautions for handling and administration apply as for other antineoplastics. The drug should be given with proper diluents and at the appropriate rate. During therapy, the patient should be closely monitored for signs and symptoms of infection, anemia, bleeding tendencies, and stomatitis with appropriate interventions implemented (Chapter 47). Nursing considerations for teniposide are similar to those for the previous enzyme but the drug should be prepared and administered in containers that are glass or polyolefin and PVC containers should be avoided. Intravenous infusions should be given slowly and as ordered with supportive measures available should allergic reaction occur.

In addition to the nursing interventions discussed earlier and in Chapter 47, it is highly recommended that epinephrine, antihistamines, and antiinflammatories be kept available in case of an allergic or anaphylactic reaction. Each antineoplastic drug has its own peculiarities and its own set of cautions, contraindications, nursing implementations and toxicities. Cytoprotective drugs are useful in reducing certain toxicities (e.g., use of intravenous amifostine to reduce renal toxicity associated with cisplatin, use of intravenous or oral allopurinol to reduce hyperuricemia) (see Tables 47-7, 47-8, and 47-10 and Box 47-2). Other major concerns related to the care of patients receiving chemotherapy are the oncologic emergencies that arise because of the damage that occurs to rapidly dividing normal cells as well as rapidly dividing cancerous cells. Some of the complications that are identified as emergencies are infections, pulmonary toxicity, allergic reactions, stomatitis with severe ulcerations, bleeding, metabolic aberrations, bowel irritability with diarrhea, and renal, liver, and cardiac toxicity (Box 48-4).

◆ EVALUATION

Evaluation of nursing care should center on determining whether goals and outcomes have been met, as well as on monitoring for therapeutic responses and adverse effects or toxic effects of antineoplastic therapy. Therapeutic responses may manifest as clinical improvement, decrease in tumor size, and decrease in metastatic spread. Evaluation of nursing care with reference to goals and outcomes may reveal improvements related to a decrease in adverse effects; a decrease in the impact of cancer on the patient's well-being; an increase in comfort, nutrition, and hydration; improved energy levels and ability to carry out the activities of daily living; and improved quality of life. The goals and outcomes can be revisited to identify more specific areas to monitor. In addition, certain laboratory studies such as measurement of tumor marker levels, levels of carcinoembryonic antigens, and red blood cell, white blood cell, and platelet counts may also be used to determine how well the goals and outcomes have been met. As part of the evaluation, physicians may also order additional radiographs, computed tomographic scans, magnetic resonance images, tissue analyses, and other studies appropriate to the diagnosis during and after antineoplastic therapy, at time intervals related to anticipated tumor response.

Box 48-4	Indications of an Oncologic Emergency

Fever and/or chills with a temperature higher than 37.8° C (100° F)
New sores or white patches in the mouth or throat
Swollen tongue with or without cracks and bleeding
Bleeding gums
Dry, burning, "scratchy," or "swollen" throat
A cough that is new and persistent
Changes in bladder function or patterns
Blood in the urine
Changes in gastrointestinal or bowel patterns, including "heartburn" or nausea, vomiting, constipation, or diarrhea lasting longer than 2 or 3 days
Blood in the stools

NOTE: The patient should contact the physician immediately if any of the listed signs or symptoms occurs. If the physician is not available, the patient should seek medical treatment at the closest emergency department.

Patient Teaching Tips

- Educate the patient about avoiding aspirin, ibuprofen, or products containing these drugs to help prevent excessive bleeding.
- Educate about the risk of alopecia (hair loss) before drug therapy begins and provide the opportunity to discuss options for hair and scalp care, including the option of having their hair cut short before treatment and selecting and purchasing or renting a wig or hairpiece comparable to the existing hair in color, texture, length, and style, or having bandanas, scarves, or hats on hand before the hair is actually lost. Although hair loss is temporary, patients need to be informed that it will occur and should also be aware that wigs and hairpieces are available through the American Cancer Society.
- Encourage the patient to increase fluid intake to up to 3000 mL/day, if not contraindicated, to prevent dehydration and further weakening and, in the case of cyclophosphamide, to prevent or help manage hemorrhagic cystitis.

Continued

Patient Teaching Tips—cont'd

- Inform the patient about ways to help manage constipation or diarrhea depending on the specific antineoplastic drug given, as well as the use of certain narcotics for pain management. To help avoid constipation, forcing of fluids and consumption of a balanced diet are important; however, the oncologist generally orders either a stool softener or a mild noncramping laxative to prevent the problem. Diarrhea is generally treated by dietary restrictions and use of antidiarrheals as ordered.
- The following are helpful online resources for the patient and significant others: www.fda.gov, www.fda.gov/oc/oha, www.nih.gov, www.healthfinder.gov, www.who.int/en, and www.oncolink.upenn.edu.

Points to Remember

- Antineoplastics are drugs that are used to treat malignancies and are classified as cell cycle–specific drugs, cell cycle–nonspecific drugs, miscellaneous antineoplastics, and hormonal drugs.
- Cell cycle–specific drugs kill cancer cells during specific phases of the cell growth cycle, whereas the cell cycle–nonspecific drugs discussed in this chapter kill cancer cells during any phase of the growth cycle.
- Chemotherapy, or antineoplastic drug therapy, requires very astute nursing care, and the nurse must act prudently and make critical decisions about the nursing care of patients receiving these drugs.
- Knowledge is important to ensure patient safety and also to protect the nurse from the adverse effects of antineoplastics. Extreme caution must be exercised in the handling and administration of cell cycle–nonspecific (and cell cycle–specific drugs).
- Hormonal drugs, both agonists and antagonists and female/male hormones, are used to treat a variety of malignancies. Some of the more common hormonal drugs for the treatment of female-specific neoplasms such as breast cancer are anastrazole, tamoxifen, megestrol, toremifene, medroxyprogesterone, aminoglutethimide, fluoxymesterone, fulvestrant, and testolactone. For male-specific neoplasms such as prostate cancer, the following drugs are used: bicalutamide, flutamide, nilutamide, leuprolide, goserelin, and estramustine. More information is presented at http://evolve.elsevier.com/Lilley.
- Extravasation of vesicants may lead to severe tissue injury with complications such as permanent damage to muscles, tendons, and ligaments, and possible loss of limb.
- Oncologic emergencies occur as a consequence of cell death and may be life threatening. Astute assessment and immediate intervention may help to decrease the severity of the problem or even reduce the occurrence of such emergencies.

NCLEX Examination Review Questions

1. A patient who is receiving chemotherapy with cisplatin has developed pneumonia. The nurse would be concerned about nephrotoxicity if which type of antibiotic was ordered as treatment for the pneumonia at this time?
   a. Penicillin
   b. Sulfa drug
   c. Fluoroquinolone
   d. Aminoglycoside
2. During treatment with doxorubicin, the nurse must monitor closely for which potentially life-threatening adverse effect?
   a. Nephrotoxicity
   b. Peripheral neuritis
   c. Cardiomyopathy
   d. Ototoxicity
3. While teaching a patient who is about to receive cyclophosphamide chemotherapy, the nurse should instruct the patient to watch for potential adverse effects such as:
   a. Cholinergic diarrhea
   b. Hemorrhagic cystitis
   c. Peripheral neuropathy
   d. Ototoxicity
4. When chemotherapy with alkylating drugs is planned, which intervention may help to prevent nephrotoxicity?
   a. Hydrating the patient with intravenous fluids before chemotherapy
   b. Limiting fluids before chemotherapy
   c. Monitoring drug levels during chemotherapy
   d. Assessing creatinine clearance during chemotherapy
5. During therapy with the cytotoxic antibiotic bleomycin, which of the following must be assessed to monitor for a potentially serious adverse effect?
   a. Blood urea nitrogen and creatinine levels
   b. Cardiac ejection fraction
   c. Respiratory function
   d. Cranial nerve function

1. d, 2. c, 3. b, 4. a, 5. c.

Critical Thinking Activities

1. Compare the management of extravasation of doxorubicin and extravasation of mechlorethamine.
2. Describe bevacizumab (Avastin) and discuss the process of angiogenesis. What is different about the mechanism of action of this drug?
3. How are cytotoxic antibiotics different from regular antibiotics?

For answers, see http://evolve.elsevier.com/Lilley.

Biologic Response–Modifying Drugs

Objectives

When you reach the end of this chapter, you should be able to do the following:

1. Describe the basic anatomy, physiology, and functions of the immune system.
2. Compare the two major classes of biologic response-modifying drugs (e.g., hematopoietic drugs, immunomodulating drugs).
3. Discuss the mechanisms of action, indications, dosages, routes of administration, adverse effects, cautions, contraindications, and drug interactions of the different biologic response-modifying drugs (e.g., hematopoietic drugs, immunomodulating drugs).
4. Develop a nursing care plan that includes all phases of the nursing process for patients receiving hematopoietic drugs and/or immunomodulating drugs.

e-Learning Activities

Companion CD

- NCLEX Review Questions: see questions 403-406
- Animations
- Audio Glossary
- Category Catchers
- Medication Errors Checklists
- IV Therapy Checklists

evolve Website (http://evolve.elsevier.com/Lilley)

- Nursing Care Plans • Frequently Asked Questions • Content Updates • WebLinks • Supplemental Resources • Elsevier ePharmacology Update • Medication Administration Animations

Drug Profiles

adalimumab, p. 773
▶ aldesleukin, p. 776
alemtuzumab, p. 774
anakinra, p. 776
bevacizumab, p. 774
cetuximab, p. 774
denileukin diftitox, p. 726
▶ epoetin alfa, p. 768
▶ filgrastim, p. 769
gemtuzumab ozogamicin, p. 774
ibritumomab tiuxetan, p. 774
infliximab, p. 774
▶ interferon alfa-2a, interferon alfa-2b, interferon

alfa-n3, interferon alfacon-1, peginterferon alfa-2a, and peginterferon alfa-2b, p. 770
▶ interferon beta-1a, p. 771
interferon gamma-1b, p. 771
natalizumab, p. 774
▶ oprelvekin, p. 769
▶ rituximab, p. 774
▶ sargramostim, p. 769
tositumomab and iodine I 131
   tositumomab, p. 774
trastuzumab, p. 774

▶ Key drug.

Glossary

Adjuvant A nonspecific *immunostimulant*; that is, an immunostimulant which somehow enhances overall immune function, rather than stimulating the function of a specific immune system cell or cytokine through specific chemical reactions. An example is bacillus Calmette-Guérin vaccine. (p. 776)

Antibodies Immunoglobulin molecules (Chapter 46) having the ability to bind to and inactivate antigen molecules through formation of an antigen-antibody complex. This process ideally serves to inactivate foreign antigens that enter the body and are capable of causing disease. (p. 765)

Antigen A biologic or chemical substance that is recognized as foreign by the body's immune system. (p. 765)

B lymphocytes (B cells) Leukocytes of the humoral immune system that develop into plasma cells, which produce the antibodies that bind to and inactivate antigens. B cells are one of the two principal types of lymphocytes; *T lymphocytes* are the other. (p. 765)

Biologic response–modifying drugs A broad class of drugs that includes hematopoietic drugs and immunomodulating drugs. More commonly referred to as *biologic response modifiers (BRMs)*, these drugs alter the body's response to diseases such as cancer as well as autoimmune, inflammatory, and infectious diseases. Examples include cytokines (e.g., interleukin, interferons), monoclonal antibodies, and vaccines. Also called *biomodulators*. BRMs may be *adjuvants, immunostimulants,* or *immunosuppressants*. (p. 764)

Cell-mediated immunity Collective term for all immune responses that are mediated by T lymphocytes (T cells). Also called *cellular immunity*. Cell-mediated immunity acts in collaboration with *humoral immunity*. (p. 765)

Colony-stimulating factors (CSFs) Cytokines that regulate the growth, differentiation, and function of bone marrow stem cells. (p. 767)

Complement The collective term for about 20 different proteins normally present in plasma that assist other immune system components (e.g., B cells and T cells) in mounting an immune response. (p. 774)

Cytokines The generic term for nonantibody proteins released by specific cell populations (e.g., activated T cells) on contact with antigens. Cytokines act as intercellular mediators of an immune response. Although no cytokines are antibodies, all cytokines are proteins. (p. 766)

Cytotoxic T cells Differentiated T cells that can recognize and lyse (rupture) target cells that bear foreign antigens on their surfaces. These antigens are recognized by the corresponding specific antigen receptors that are expressed (displayed) on the cytotoxic T-cell surface. Also called *natural killer cells.* (p. 765)

Differentiation The process of cellular development from a simplified into a more complex and specialized cellular structure. In hematopoiesis, it refers to the multistep processes involved in the maturation of blood cells, in which generalized pluripotent stem cells in the bone marrow develop along different cellular paths to yield mature, specialized blood components such as erythrocytes, leukocytes, and platelets. (p. 767)

Hematopoiesis The collective term for all of the body's processes originating in the bone marrow that result in the formation of various types of blood components. It includes three main processes of *differentiation* (see above): erythropoiesis (formation of red blood cells, or erythrocytes), leukopoiesis (formation of white blood cells, or leukocytes), and thrombopoiesis (formation of platelets, or thrombocytes). (Adjective: *hematopoietic.*) (p. 764)

Humoral immunity The collective term for all immune responses that are mediated by B cells, which ultimately work through the production of antibodies against specific antigens. Humoral immunity acts in collaboration with *cell-mediated immunity* (p. 765)

Immunoglobulins Complex immune system glycoproteins that bind to and inactivate foreign antigens. The term is synonymous with *immune globulins.* (p. 765)

Immunomodulating drug Collective term for various subclasses of BRMs that specifically or nonspecifically enhance or reduce immune responses. The three major types of immunomodulators, based on mechanism of action, are adjuvants, immunostimulants, and immunosuppressants (Chapter 45). (p. 764)

Immunostimulant A drug that enhances immune response through specific chemical interactions with particular immune system components. An example is interleukin-2. (p. 776)

Immunosuppressant A drug that reduces immune response through specific chemical interactions with particular immune system components. An example is cyclosporine (Chapter 45). (p. 770)

Interferon (IFN) One type of cytokine that promotes resistance to viral infection in uninfected cells and can also strengthen the body's immune response to cancer cells. (p. 769)

Leukocytes The collective term for all subtypes of white blood cells. Leukocytes include the granulocytes (neutrophils, eosinophils, and basophils), monocytes, and lymphocytes (B cells and T cells). Some monocytes also develop into tissue macrophages. (p. 766)

Lymphokine-activated killer (LAK) cell *Cytotoxic T cells* that have been further activated by interkeukin-2 and therefore have a stronger and more specific response against cancer cells. (p. 775)

Lymphokines Cytokines that are produced by sensitized T lymphocytes on contact with antigen particles. (p. 766)

Memory cells Cells involved in the humoral immune system that remember the exact characteristics of a particular foreign invader or antigen for the purpose of expediting immune response in the event of future exposure to this antigen. (p. 765)

Monoclonal Denoting a group of identical cells or organisms derived from a single cell. (p. 765)

Plasma cells Cells derived from B cells that are found in the bone marrow, connective tissue, and blood. They produce antibodies. (p. 765)

T helper cells Cells that promote and direct the actions of various other cells of the immune system. (p. 765)

T lymphocytes (T cells) Leukocytes of the cell-mediated immune system. Unlike B cells, they are not involved in the production of antibodies but instead occur in various cell subtypes (e.g., T helper, T suppressor, and cytotoxic T cells) that act through direct cell-to-cell contact or by producing cytokines that guide the functions of other immune system components (e.g., B cells, antibodies). (p. 765)

T suppressor cells Cells that regulate and limit the immune response, balancing the effects of T helper cells. (p. 766)

Tumor antigens Chemical compounds expressed on the surfaces of tumor cells. They signal to the immune system that these cells do not belong in the body, labeling the tumor cells as foreign. (p. 765)

OVERVIEW OF IMMUNOMODULATORS

In the past, the care of patients with cancer required an understanding of only three treatment modalities: surgery, radiation, and chemotherapy. Although these are highly sophisticated methods of cancer treatment, many cancer patients still are not cured. Surgery and radiation therapy are, at best, local or regional treatments. As discussed in the preceding chapters, adjuvant drug therapy is needed to destroy undetected distant micrometastases. The advantage of cytotoxic chemotherapy with antineoplastic drugs is that these drugs attack tumor cells throughout the body. However, this advantage is also the greatest limitation, because all normal cells are exposed to the cytotoxic drug as well. This accounts for the sometimes severe adverse effects associated with chemotherapy, which often require numerous other drugs for their control (e.g., antiemetics, intravenous hydration, pain medications for drug-induced stomatitis). Antineoplastic drug dosage reduction (or discontinuation) may also be required, which unfortunately will also limit their ability to cure or arrest the cancer itself.

Over the last two decades medical technology has developed a group of drugs whose primary site of action is the immune system. This has resulted in some new additions to the class of drugs known as **biologic response–modifying drugs,** or *biologic response modifiers (BRMs).* These drugs can enhance or restrict the patient's immune response to disease, can stimulate a patient's *hematopoietic* (blood-forming) function, and can even prevent disease. **Hematopoiesis** is the collective term for all of the blood component-forming processes of the bone marrow. Two broad classes of BRMs are *hematopoietic drugs (HDs)* and **immunomodulating drugs** (IMDs); the majority of BRMs fall into the latter category. Subclasses of IMDs include *interferons, monoclonal antibodies, interleukin receptor agonists and antagonists,* and *miscellaneous IMDs.*

IMDs are defined as medications that therapeutically alter a patient's immune response. In cancer treatment, they make up the fourth type of cancer therapy, along with surgery, chemotherapy, and radiation. The human immune system is most commonly viewed as the body's natural defense against primarily pathogenic bacteria and viruses. However, it also has effective antitumor capabilities. An intact immune system can identify cells as malignant and destroy them. In contrast to chemotherapeutic drugs, a healthy immune system can distinguish between tumor cells and normal body tissues. Normal cells are recognized as "self" and are not destroyed, whereas tumor cells are recognized as "foreign" and are subject to immune system attack and destruction. It is known that people routinely develop cancerous cells in their bodies on a regular basis. Normally the immune system is able to eliminate these cells before they multiply to uncontrollable levels. It is only when the natural immune responses fail to keep pace with these initially microscopic cancer cell growths that a person develops a true "cancer" requiring clinical intervention.

With regard to action against cancer cells in particular, there are three common mechanisms by which current BRMs work. The first mechanism is enhancement or restoration of the host's immune system defenses against the tumor. The second is a direct toxic effect of the molecules of a particular BRM on the tumor cells, which causes them to *lyse*, or rupture. The third mechanism is adverse modification of the tumor's biology, which makes it harder for the tumor cells to survive and reproduce.

Some IMDs are also used to treat autoimmune, inflammatory, and infectious diseases. In these instances, the IMD ideally functions either to reduce the patient's inappropriate immune response (in the case of inflammatory and autoimmune diseases such as rheumatoid arthritis) or to strengthen the patient's immune response against microorganisms (especially viruses) and cancer cells, as noted earlier. To better understand IMDs, a review of immune system physiology is beneficial.

IMMUNE SYSTEM

The immune system is an intricate biologic defense network of cells that are capable of distinguishing an unlimited variety of substances as being either foreign ("nonself") or a natural part of the host's body ("self"). When a foreign substance such as a bacteria or virus enters the body, the cells of the immune system recognize it as being nonself and mount an immune response to eliminate or neutralize the invader. Tumors are not truly foreign substances because they arise from cells of normal tissues whose genetic material (deoxyribonucleic acid [DNA] and ribonucleic acid [RNA]) has somehow mutated, causing uncontrolled cell growth. However, tumor cells do express chemical compounds on their surfaces that signal the immune system that these cells are a threat to the body. These chemical markers, called **tumor antigens** or tumor markers, label the tumor cells as abnormal cells. An **antigen** is any substance that the body's immune system recognizes as foreign. This recognition of antigens varies among individuals, which is why some people are more prone than others to immune-related diseases such as allergies, inflammatory diseases, and cancer.

The two major components of the body's immune system are **humoral immunity,** mediated by B-cell functions (primarily through *antibody* production—see later), and **cell-mediated immunity,** which is mediated by T-cell functions. These two systems act together to recognize and destroy foreign particles and cells in the blood or other body tissues. Communication between these two divisions is vital to the success of the immune system as a whole. Attack against tumor cells by antibodies produced by the **B lymphocytes (B cells)** of the humoral immune system prepares those tumor cells for destruction by the **T lymphocytes (T cells)** of the cell-mediated immune system. This is just one example of the effective way that the two divisions of the immune system communicate with each other for a collaborative immune response.

Humoral Immune System

As mentioned, the primary functional cells of the humoral immune system are the B lymphocytes. They are also called *B cells* because they originate in the bone marrow. Antigens that enter the body send a biochemical signal to B lymphocytes when the antigen molecules bind to antigen receptors that are located on the B cells. The B cells that are capable of generating a particular antibody normally remain dormant until the corresponding antigen is detected in this manner. These B cells then mature or *differentiate* into **plasma cells,** which in turn produce antibodies. **Antibodies** are **immunoglobulins** (large glycoprotein molecules; glyco = sugar; protein = amino acid chain) that bind to specific antigens, forming an *antigen-antibody complex* that ideally inactivates disease-causing antigens.

The immune system in a healthy individual is genetically preprogrammed to be able to mount an antibody response against literally millions of different antigens. This ability results from the lifetime antigen exposure of all of a person's ancestors, and acquired immune response capability is further developed through exposure to new antigens and passed down through many generations. The antibodies that a single plasma cell makes are all identical. They are therefore called **monoclonal** antibodies, and they are active against the single specific antigen that was originally recognized by their ancestor B cell as foreign. Since the 1980s, monoclonal antibodies have also been prepared synthetically using recombinant DNA (rDNA) technology, which has resulted in newer drug therapies.

There are five major types of naturally occurring immunoglobulins in the body: immunoglobulins A, D, E, G, and M. These unique types have different structures and functions and are found in various areas of the body. During an immune response, when B lymphocytes differentiate into plasma cells, some of these B cells become **memory cells** instead. Memory cells "remember" the exact characteristics of a particular foreign invader or antigen, which allows a stronger and faster immune response in the event of reexposure to the same antigen. The cells of the humoral immune system are shown in Figure 49-1.

Cell-Mediated Immune System

The primary functional cells of the cell-mediated (as opposed to antibody-mediated) immune system are the T lymphocytes. They are also referred to as *T cells* because, although they originate in the bone marrow like their B-cell counterparts, they mature in a mediastinal gland known as the *thymus*. There are three distinct populations of T cells: cytotoxic T cells, T helper cells, and T suppressor cells. They are distinguished by the different functions that they perform. **Cytotoxic T cells** directly kill their targets by causing cell lysis or rupture. **T helper cells** are considered the

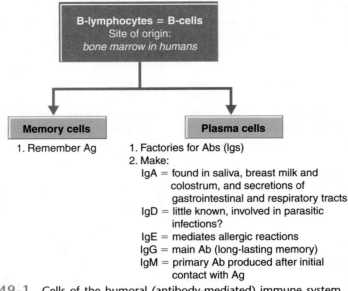

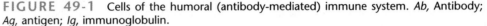

FIGURE 49-1 Cells of the humoral (antibody-mediated) immune system. *Ab,* Antibody; *Ag,* antigen; *Ig,* immunoglobulin.

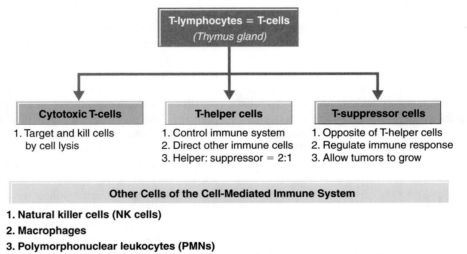

FIGURE 49-2 Cells of the cellular immune system.

master controllers of the immune system. These cells direct the actions of many other immune components, such as lymphokines and cytotoxic T cells. **Lymphokines** are a subset of a broader category of blood proteins known as cytokines. **Cytokines** are nonantibody proteins that serve as chemical mediators of a variety of physiologic functions. Lymphokines are specifically those cytokines that are released by T lymphocytes upon contact with antigens and serve as chemical mediators of the immune response. **T suppressor cells** have an effect on the immune system that is opposite to that of T helper cells and serve to limit or control the immune response. A healthy immune system has about twice as many T helper cells as T suppressor cells at any given time.

The cells of the cell-mediated immune system are believed to be the major cells involved in the destruction of cancer cells. The cancer-killing cells of the cellular immune system include macrophages (derived from monocytes), natural killer (NK) cells (another type of lymphocyte), and polymorphonuclear **leukocytes** (not lymphocytes), which are also called *neutrophils.* In

contrast, T suppressor cells have the most important negative influence on antitumor actions of the immune system. Overactive T suppressor cells may be responsible for clinically significant cancer cases by permitting tumor growth beyond immune system control. Figure 49-2 shows the components of the cellular immune system.

Therapy with BRMs combines the knowledge of several disciplines, including general biology, genetics, immunology, pharmacology, medicine, and nursing. The general therapeutic effects of BRMs are as follows:

- Enhancement of hematopoietic function (hematopoietic BRMs)
- Regulation or augmentation (enhancement) of the immune response, including cytotoxic or cytostatic activity against cancer cells
- Inhibition of metastases, prevention of cell division, or inhibition of cell maturation

Box 49-1 lists the currently available BRM drugs used in the treatment of cancer or other illnesses that have varying levels of

Box 49-1   Biologic Response Modifiers

Hematopoietic Drugs
Colony-Stimulating Factors
filgrastim G-CSF
pegfilgrastim
sargramostim GM-CSF

Other
darbepoetin alfa
epoetin alfa
oprelvekin (IL-11)

Immunomodulating Drugs
Interferons
IFN alfa-2a
IFN alfa-2b*
pegIFN alfa-2a
pegIFN alfa-2b
IFN alfacon-1
IFN alfa-n3
IFN beta-1a
IFN beta-1b
IFN gamma-1b

Monoclonal Antibodies
alemtuzumab
gemtuzumab ozogamicin
ibritumomab tiuxetan
rituximab
trastuzumab

Interleukin Receptor Agonists and Antagonists
Agonist
aldesleukin (IL-2)

Antagonists
anakinra
denileukin diftitox

Miscellaneous Immunomodulators
Tumor Necrosis Factor Receptor Antagonist
etanercept

Enzymes
pegademase bovine

Retinoid Receptor Agonists
tretinoin
bexarotene

Adjuvants (Nonspecific Immunostimulants)
BCG vaccine
leflunomide
levamisole
mitoxantrone
thalidomide

*Also available in combination with the antiviral drug ribavirin.
G-CSF, Granulocyte colony-stimulating factor; *GM-CSF,* granulocyte-macrophage colony-stimulating factor; *IFN,* interferon; *IL,* interleukin; *BCG,* bacillus Calmette-Guérin.

immune system–related pathophysiology. The drugs are classified according to their biologic effects.

HEMATOPOIETIC DRUGS

HDs include several newer medications developed over the past 10 to 15 years. Falling into this category are two erythropoietic drugs (epoetin alfa and darbepoetin alfa), three **colony-stimulating factors (CSFs)** (filgrastim, pegfilgrastim, and sargramostim), and one platelet-promoting drug (oprelvekin). All of these drugs promote the synthesis of various types of major blood components by promoting the growth, **differentiation** (development into mature specialized cells), and function of their corresponding precursor cells in the bone marrow.

Mechanism of Action and Drug Effects

All six HDs have the same basic mechanism of action. They are not directly toxic to cancer cells, but they do have beneficial effects in the treatment of cancer. They decrease the duration of chemotherapy-induced anemia, neutropenia, and thrombocytopenia and enable higher dosages of chemotherapy to be given; decrease bone marrow recovery time after bone marrow transplantation or radiation; and stimulate other cells in the immune system to destroy or inhibit the growth of cancer cells, as well as virus- or fungus-infected cells.

All of these drugs are produced by rDNA technology, which allows them to be essentially identical to their endogenously produced counterparts in the body. These substances work by binding to receptors on the surfaces of specialized *progenitor cells* in the bone marrow. These cells are responsible for the production of three particular cell lines: red blood cells [RBCs], white blood cells [WBCs], and platelets. When an HD binds to a progenitor cell surface, the progenitor cell is stimulated to mature, proliferate (reproduce itself), differentiate (transform into its respective type of specialized blood component), and become functionally active. HDs may enhance certain functions of mature cell lines as well.

Epoetin alfa is a synthetic derivative of the human hormone *erythropoietin,* which is produced primarily by the kidney. It promotes the synthesis of erythrocytes (RBCs) by stimulating RBC progenitor cells in the bone marrow. It is also called *EPO.* Darbepoetin alfa, a newer drug, is a longer-acting form of epoetin alfa. Filgrastim is a CSF that stimulates progenitor cells for the subset of WBCs (leukocytes) known as *granulocytes* (including basophils, eosinophils, and neutrophils). For this reason it is also commonly called *granulocyte colony-stimulating factor* (G-CSF). Pegfilgrastim is a newer, longer-acting form of filgrastim. Sargramostim, also a CSF, works by stimulating the bone marrow precursor cells that synthesize both granulocytes and the phagocytic (cell-eating) cells known as *monocytes,* some of which become *macrophages.* For this reason it is also called *granulocyte-macrophage colony-stimulating factor* (GM-CSF). Oprelvekin, the newest drug, is also classified as an *interleukin,* specifically interleukin-11 (IL-11). Other interleukins are discussed later in this chapter. Oprelvekin stimulates the bone marrow cells, specifically megakaryocytes, that eventually give rise to platelets.

Indications

HDs have many therapeutic uses. Neutrophils are the most important granulocytes for fighting infection. Because administration of CSFs reduces the duration of low neutrophil counts, they reduce the incidence and duration of infections. Infections normally appear in patients who have experienced destruction of bone marrow cells as a result of cytotoxic chemotherapy. CSFs stimulate these cells to grow and mature and thus directly oppose the detrimental bone marrow actions of chemotherapeutic drugs (see Interactions later). CSFs also enhance the functioning of mature cells of the immune system, such as macrophages and granulocytes. This increases the ability of the body's immune system to kill cancer cells, as well as virus- and fungus-infected cells. Ultimately these CSF properties allow patients to receive higher dosages of chemotherapy, which results in the destruction of greater numbers of cancer cells. Similar benefits occur with epoetin alfa and oprelvekin with regard to RBC and platelet counts, respectively.

The effect of HDs on the bone marrow cells also reduces their recovery time after bone marrow transplantation and radiation therapy. Bone marrow transplantation chemotherapy dosages are often much higher than those of conventional chemotherapy. Both bone marrow transplantation chemotherapy and radiation therapy are toxic to the bone marrow. When one or more HDs are administered as part of the drug therapy for bone marrow transplantation, bone marrow cell counts return to normal in a drastically shortened time. This helps to increase the likelihood of a successful bone marrow transplantation and therefore patient survival. Specific drug indications are listed in the Dosages table.

Contraindications

Contraindications for all four HDs include drug allergy. Use of epoetin and darbepoetin is contraindicated in cases of uncontrolled hypertension. Use of G-CSF, GM-CSF, and pegfilgrastim is also contraindicated in the presence of more than 10% myeloid

blasts (immature tumor cells in the bone marrow) because CSF may stimulate malignant growth of these myeloid tumor cells.

Adverse Effects

Adverse effects associated with the use of HDs are mild. The most common are fever, muscle aches, bone pain, and flushing. Table 49-1 lists additional adverse effects.

Interactions

Of the currently available HDs, G-CSF (filgrastim) and GM-CSF (sargramostim) are the only two drugs that have any significant drug interactions. The most significant drug interaction with these two drugs occurs when *myelosuppressive* (bone marrow depressant) antineoplastic drugs are given with them. G-CSF and GM-CSF are administered to enhance the production of bone marrow cells; therefore, when myelosuppressive antineoplastics are given with them, the drugs directly antagonize each other. Typically these BRMs are not given within 24 hours of administration of myelosuppressive antineoplastics. However, they are often given soon after this time to help prevent the WBC nadir from dropping to dangerous levels and also to speed WBC recovery. It is also recommended that these drugs be used with caution or not given with other medications that can potentiate their *myeloproliferative* (bone marrow–stimulating) effects. Two examples are lithium and corticosteroids.

Dosages

For the recommended dosages of HDs, see the Dosages table on this page.

Drug Profiles

▸ *epoetin alfa*

As noted earlier, epoetin alfa (Epogen, Procrit) is a biosynthetic form of the natural hormone erythropoietin, which is normally secreted by the kidneys in response to a decrease in RBCs and many other stimuli. Epoetin is synthetically manufactured in mass quantities using of rDNA technology. Although epoetin alfa is not technically classified as a CSF, its actions in promoting erythrocyte synthesis are function-

Table 49-1	Hematopoietic Drugs: Common Adverse Effects
Body System	**Adverse Effects**
Cardiovascular	Hypertension (epoetin alfa), edema
Gastrointestinal	Anorexia, nausea, vomiting, diarrhea
Integumentary	Alopecia, rash
Respiratory	Cough, dyspnea, sore throat
Other	Fever, blood dyscrasias, headache, bone pain

DOSAGES

Hematopoietic Drugs

Drug (Pregnancy Category)	Pharmacologic Class	Usual Dosage Range	Indications
▸epoetin alfa (Epogen, Procrit) (C)	Human recombinant hormone (erythropoietin) analogue	IV/SC: 2000-40,000 units 1-3 ×/wk, depending on patient weight and indication	Chemotherapy-induced anemia; anemia associated with chronic renal failure, zidovudine therapy (for HIV infection); reduction of need for blood transfusions in surgical patients
darbepoetin alfa (Aranesp) (C)	Long-acting human recombinant hormone (erythropoietin) analogue	IV/SC: 6.25-200 mcg/wk based on previous epoetin alfa dose	
▸filgrastim (Neupogen) (C)	Colony-stimulating factor	IV/SC: 5-10 mcg/kg/day	
pegfilgrastim (Neulasta) (C)	Long-acting colony-stimulating factor	SC: 6 mg once per chemotherapy cycle (not for use in children under 45 kg)	Chemotherapy-induced leukopenia
▸sargramostim (Leukine) (C)	Colony-stimulating factor	IV: 250 mcg/m²/day	
▸oprelvekin [IL-11] (Neumega) (C)	Synthetic human interleukin analogue	**Adult only** SC: 50 mcg/kg daily for up to 21 days	Chemotherapy-induced thrombocytopenia

HIV, Human immunodeficiency virus; *IL*, Interleukin; *IV*, intravenous; *SC*, subcutaneous.

ally similar to the leukocyte-enhancing functions of G-CSF and GM-CSF.

Epoetin alfa is used to correct deficiencies of endogenous erythropoietin production. These conditions are common in patients with anemia resulting from end-stage renal disease, human immunodeficiency virus (HIV) infection, and cancer. More recently, epoetin has been approved for use in both critically ill and preoperative patients to help reduce the need for blood transfusions. Epoetin causes the progenitor cells in the bone marrow to manufacture large numbers of immature RBCs and to greatly speed up their maturation. If therapy is not stopped when the hemoglobin level reaches the goal of 12 g/dL, or if the level rises too quickly, hypertension and seizures can result. This medication is also ineffective without adequate body iron stores. Pertinent laboratory values to be monitored before and during therapy include *transferrin saturation* (which should be at least 20%), and *ferritin level* (which should be at least 100 ng/mL). A newer, longer-acting form of epoetin called darbepoetin is available that reduces the required number of injections, although one cost study found that there is no significant difference in overall cost between the two. Both drugs are available for injection only.

Pharmacokinetics

Half-Life	Onset	Peak	Duration
4-13 hr	7-10 days	5-24 hr (serum)	Variable

▶ *filgrastim*

Filgrastim (Neupogen) is a synthetic analogue of human G-CSF and is commonly referred to as *G-CSF*. G-CSF promotes the proliferation, differentiation, and activation of the cells that make granulocytes. Granulocytes are the body's primary defense against bacterial and fungal infections. Filgrastim has the same pharmacologic effects as endogenous human G-CSF, which is normally secreted by specialized leukocytes known as *monocytes, macrophages,* and mature *neutrophils.* Filgrastim is indicated to prevent or treat febrile neutropenia in patients receiving myelosuppressive antineoplastics for nonmyeloid (non–bone marrow) malignancies. It should be given *before* a patient develops an infection, but not within 24 hours before or after myelosuppressive chemotherapeutic drugs, because doing so tends to cancel out the therapeutic benefits of the filgrastim. Pegfilgrastim (Neulasta) is a long-acting form of filgrastim that reduces the number of required injections. Both drugs are available for injection only.

Pharmacokinetics

Half-Life	Onset	Peak	Duration
3-5 hr	1 hr	2-6 hr	12-24 hr

▶ *sargramostim*

Sargramostim (Leukine) is a synthetic analogue of human GM-CSF and is commonly referred to as *GM-CSF*. Granulocytes are one of three major subsets of leukocytes, the other two being monocytes and lymphocytes (B cells and T cells). As noted earlier, granulocytes are further subdivided into basophils, eosinophils, and neutrophils, with neutrophils the most important in fighting infection. Macrophages are tissue-based (as opposed to circulating) cells that are derived from monocytes, which circulate in the blood. Neutrophils, monocytes, and macrophages make up the three main categories of phagocytic (cell-eating) blood cells, and they literally ingest foreign cells and other antigens as part of their immune system function. Sargramostim has the same pharmacologic effects as endogenous human GM-CSF. It stimulates the proliferation, differentiation, and activation of the cells in the bone marrow that eventually become granulocytes, monocytes, and macrophages.

Sargramostim is indicated for promoting bone marrow recovery after autologous (own marrow) or allogenic (donor marrow) bone marrow transplantation in patients with various types of leukemia and lymphoma. It is even used for bone marrow reconstitution after failure of bone marrow transplantation. This drug is available for injection only.

Pharmacokinetics

Half-Life	Onset	Peak	Duration
2 hr	4 hr*	2 hr	10 days*

*Therapeutic effect.

▶ *oprelvekin*

Oprelvekin (Neumega) is both an HD and one of the three currently available interleukins. However, its function is similar to that of the CSFs in that it enhances synthesis of a specific blood component—in this case, the platelets. It is indicated for the prevention of chemotherapy-induced severe thrombocytopenia and avoidance of the need for platelet transfusions. Its use is contraindicated in cases of drug allergy. It is available for injection only.

Pharmacokinetics

Half-Life	Onset	Peak	Duration
7 hr	5-9 days*	3 hr†	14 days

*Platelet counts begin to increase.
†Peak serum concentrations.

INTERFERONS

Before the commercial use of CSFs, **interferons (IFNs)** were the best studied and most widely used BRMs. IFNs are proteins that have three basic properties: antiviral, antitumor, and immunomodulating. Chemically they are glycoproteins. There are three different groups of IFN drugs, each with its own antigenic and biologic activity: the alfa, beta, and gamma IFNs. IFNs are most commonly used in the treatment of certain viral infections and certain types of cancer. They can be manufactured using genetically modified *Escherichia coli* bacteria with rDNA technology. In addition, IFNs are also obtained from pooled human leukocytes that have been stimulated (challenged) with various natural and synthetic inducers (antigens).

Mechanism of Action and Drug Effects

IFN drugs are recombinantly manufactured substances that are identical to the IFN cytokines that are naturally present in the human body. Therefore, they have the same properties. IFNs protect human cells from virus attack by enabling the human cells to produce proteins (enzymes) that stop virus replication and prevent viruses from penetrating healthy cells. IFNs prevent cancer cells from dividing and replicating, and IFNs also increase the activity of other cells in the immune system, such as macrophages, neutrophils, and NK cells.

Their effects on cancer cells are believed to be caused by a combination of direct inhibition of DNA and protein synthesis within cancer cells (antitumor effects) and multiple immunomodulatory effects on the host's immune system. IFNs increase the cytotoxic activity of NK cells and the phagocytic ability of macrophages. Unlike with conventional cytotoxic antineoplastics, the optimal biologic dosage of IFNs is not necessarily the maximum dosage tolerated by the patient, although some newer studies support the use of higher IFN dosages. IFNs are also believed to increase the expression of cancer cell antigens on the cell surface, which enables the immune system to recognize cancer cells more easily, specifically marking them for destruction.

Overall, IFNs have three different effects on the immune system. They can (1) restore its function if it is impaired, (2) augment (amplify) the immune system's ability to function as the body's defense, and (3) inhibit the immune system from working. This latter function may be especially useful when the immune system has become dysfunctional, causing an *autoimmune* disease. This is believed to be the case in multiple sclerosis (MS), for example, for which two IFN drugs are specifically indicated. Inhibiting the dysfunctional immune system prevents further damage to the body.

Indications

The beneficial actions of IFNs (antiviral, antineoplastic, and immunomodulatory) make them excellent drugs for the treatment of viral infections, various cancers, and some autoimmune disorders. Currently accepted indications for IFNs are listed in the dosages table.

Contraindications

Contraindications to the use of IFNs include known drug allergy and may include autoimmune disorders, hepatitis or liver failure, concurrent use of **immunosuppressant** drugs, Kaposi's sarcoma related to acquired immunodeficiency syndrome (AIDS), and severe liver disease.

Adverse Effects

The most common adverse effects can be broadly described as flulike symptoms: fever, chills, headache, malaise, myalgia, and fatigue. The major dose-limiting adverse effect of IFNs is fatigue. Patients taking high dosages become so exhausted that they are often confined to bed. Other adverse effects and adverse effects of IFNs are listed in Table 49-2.

Interactions

Drug interactions are seen with both IFN alfa-2a and IFN alfa-2b when they are used with drugs such as aminophylline that are metabolized in the liver via the cytochrome P-450 enzyme system. The combination results in decreased metabolism and increased accumulation of these drugs, which leads to drug toxicity. There is also some evidence that concomitant use of IFNs in general and antiviral drugs such as zidovudine enhances the activity of both drugs but may lead to toxic levels of zidovudine. IFNs can also interact with angiotensin-converting enzyme inhibitors to produce blood abnormalities such as anemia and diminished WBC and platelet counts. IFN beta products can enhance the anticoagulant effects of warfarin, which may be

Table 49-2 Interferons: Adverse Effects

Body System	Adverse Effects
General	Flulike syndrome, fatigue
Cardiovascular	Tachycardia, cyanosis, ECG changes, MI (rare), orthostatic hypotension
Central nervous	Mild confusion, somnolence, irritability, poor concentration, seizures, hallucinations, paranoid psychoses
Gastrointestinal	Nausea, diarrhea, vomiting, anorexia, taste alterations, dry mouth
Hematologic	Neutropenia, thrombocytopenia
Renal and hepatic	Increased BUN and creatinine levels, proteinuria, abnormal liver function test results (transaminases)

BUN, Blood urea nitrogen; *ECG,* electrocardiogram; *MI,* myocardial infarction.

undesirable and place the patient at greater risk for bleeding. Additive toxic effects to the bone marrow can occur when IFN gamma products are used with other myelosuppressive drugs.

Dosages

For the recommended dosages of IFNs, see the Dosages table on page 771.

Drug Profiles

The three major classes of IFN drugs include alfa, beta, and gamma, which are sometimes also written using the lowercase Greek letters α, β, and γ, respectively. The "alfa" designation is synonymous with the Greek letter "alpha," but "alfa" is now more commonly used clinically. The IFNs vary in their antigenic makeup, biologic actions, and pharmacologic properties. The best known IFN class is IFN alfa. As noted earlier, IFNs can be produced by *E. coli* bacteria using rDNA laboratory techniques, and some IFNs can also be collected from pooled human leukocytes. In the body, IFNs are naturally produced by activated T cells and by other cells in response to viral infection.

IFN products are BMRs that can be broadly classified as cytokines. Cytokines are immune system proteins that serve two essential functions: they direct the actions and communication between the cell-mediated and humoral divisions of the immune system, and augment or enhance the immune response. Other cytokines include tumor necrosis factor, interleukins, and CSFs. IFNs were first found to have antiviral activity in 1957. Their beneficial effects in treating cancer were discovered much later.

With the exception of the CSFs, IFNs are the most well studied and most widely used of the BRMs. Six IFN alfas, two IFN betas, and one IFN gamma are currently available.

Interferon Alfa Products

▶ *interferon alfa-2a, interferon alfa-2b, interferon alfa-n3, interferon alfacon-1, peginterferon alfa-2a, peginterferon alfa-2b*

The most commonly used IFN products are in the IFN alfa class. They are also referred to as *leukocyte IFNs* because they are produced from human leukocytes. IFN alfa-2a and IFN alfa-2b are pure clones of single IFN alfa subtypes manufactured by rDNA technology. This means that they are consistent from lot to lot. These two products differ in the sequence of two amino acids, but their therapeutic uses are very similar. Two newer types of IFN alfa include peginterferon (pegIFN) alfa-2a and pegIFN alfa-2b. The *peg* refers to the attachment of a polymer chain of the hydrocarbon polyethylene glycol (PEG). This "pegylation" process increases the size of the IFN molecule and confers upon it several advantageous properties. One is prolonged drug absorption, with increased half-life and decreased plasma clearance rate, which prolongs its therapeutic effects. In addition, pegylation is believed to reduce the immunogenicity of the IFN and thus delay its recognition and destruction by the immune system, because it is still a foreign substance to the body. This may also help to enhance and prolong its therapeutic effect. Similarly, pegfilgrastim, mentioned previously in this chapter, is a pegylated form of filgrastim and is also longer acting. The alfa-2a and alfa-2b IFNs share the following indications: chronic hepatitis C, hairy cell leukemia, and AIDS-related Kaposi's sarcoma. IFN alfa-2a (only) is also indicated for the treatment of chronic myelogenous leukemia. Additional indications unique to IFN alfa-2b are chronic hepatitis B, malignant melanoma (an often fatal form of skin cancer), follicular lymphoma (so named because its malignant cells gather in clumps called *follicles*—not to be confused with hair follicles), and condylomata acuminata (virally induced genital or venereal warts). PegIFN alfa-2b is currently indicated only for treatment of chronic hepatitis C, as is pegIFN alfa-2a.

IFN alfa-n3 is a polyclonal mixture of all IFN alfa subtypes. It is the product of pooled human leukocytes. Its only current indication

DOSAGES

Interferons

Drug (Pregnancy Category)	Pharmacologic Class	Usual Dosage Range	Indications
▶IFN alfa-2a (Roferon-A) (C)	Immunomodulator, antiviral, antineoplastic	IM/SC: 3 million units 3×/wk, depending on indication	Chronic hepatitis C, hairy cell leukemia, AIDS-related Kaposi's sarcoma, chronic myelogenous leukemia
▶IFN alfa-2b (Intron-A) (C)	Immunomodulator, antiviral, antineoplastic	IM/SC: 1-30 million units 3×/wk*	Hairy cell leukemia, malignant melanoma, follicular lymphoma, condylomata acuminata (venereal-genital warts), AIDS-related Kaposi's sarcoma, chronic hepatitis C, chronic hepatitis B
▶pegIFN alfa-2a (Pegasys) (C)	Immunomodulator, antiviral	SC: 180 mcg weekly for 48 wk	Chronic hepatitis C
▶pegIFN alfa-2b (PEG-Intron) (C)	Immunomodulator, antiviral	SC: 1 mcg/kg/wk for 1 yr†	Chronic hepatitis C
▶IFN alfa-n3 (Alferon-N) (C)	Immunomodulator, antiviral	Intralesional: 250,000 units (0.05 mL) into the base of each wart 2×/wk for up to 8 wk	Condylomata acuminata
▶IFN alfacon-1 (Infergen) (C)	Immunomodulator, antiviral	SC: 9 mcg 3×/wk for 24 wk	Chronic hepatitis C
▶IFN beta-1a (Avonex, Rebif) (C)	Immunomodulator	IM (Avonex): 30 mcg 1×/wk SC (Rebif): 44 mcg 3×/wk	Multiple sclerosis
IFN beta-1b (Betaseron) (C)	Immunomodulator	SC: 0.25 mg every other day	Multiple sclerosis
IFN gamma-1b (Actimmune) (C)	Immunomodulator	*BSA more than 0.5 m²* SC: 50 mcg/m² 3×/wk *BSA less than 0.5 m²* SC: 1.5 mcg/kg 3×/wk	Chronic granulomatous disease, osteopetrosis

*May also be given by IV infusion for melanoma. Route and dose vary depending on indication.
†Dose is 1.5 mcg/kg/wk if given with ribavirin capsules (Chapter 39).
AIDS, Acquired immunodeficiency syndrome; *BSA*, body surface area; *IFN*, interferon; *IM*, intramuscular; *pegIFN*, peginterferon; *SC*, subcutaneous.

is condylomata acuminata. IFN alfacon-1 is a purely synthetic (i.e., non–naturally occurring) recombinant product that is currently indicated only for treatment of hepatitis C.

All IFNs are most commonly given by either intramuscular or subcutaneous injection. However, IFNs have sometimes been given by intravenous and intraperitoneal routes as well. It is also important to note that some IFNs are commonly dosed in millions of units, and these doses are often abbreviated "MU." For example, a dose of 10 million units might be written as "10 MU." The nurse should always double-check to make sure that this is the correct dose, however, because the prescriber's writing of "MU" can sometimes be mistaken for "mg" or "μg" (an older abbreviation for micrograms, which is better abbreviated as "mcg"). If there is any question in the nurse's mind about the dose of any medication, he or she should double-check with the prescriber, pharmacist, or other experienced colleague before administering the medication to the patient. Although this is true for all medications, it is a special consideration for IFNs and other BRMs, because of both their potency and their dosage variability.

Interferon Beta Products
▶ interferon beta-1a

IFN beta-1a and IFN beta-1b are the two currently available IFN beta products. They interact with specific cell receptors found on the surfaces of human cells and possess antiviral and immunomodulatory activity. Both are produced by rDNA techniques and are indicated for the treatment of relapsing MS to slow the progression of physical disability and decrease the frequency of clinical exacerbations. Drug allergy, including allergy to human albumin, is currently the only contraindication. Both drugs are available for injection only.

Interferon Gamma Products
interferon gamma-1b

IFN gamma-1b (Actimmune) is another type of synthetic IFN produced by rDNA technology. It is indicated for the treatment of serious infections associated with chronic granulomatous disease, a genetic immunodeficiency, and osteopetrosis, a genetic bone disease characterized by abnormally dense bone, anemia, and frequent fractures. It is also available for injection only.

MONOCLONAL ANTIBODIES

Monoclonal antibodies (MABs) are quickly becoming standards of therapy in many areas of medicine, including treatment of cancer (Chapter 48), rheumatoid arthritis and other inflammatory diseases, MS, and organ transplantation (Chapter 45). In cancer treatment they have advantages over traditional antineoplastics in that they can specifically target cancer cells and have minimal effect on healthy cells, unlike conventional cancer treatments. This reduces many of the adverse effects traditionally associated with antineoplastic drugs. There are currently ten commercially available MABs used to treat cancer and rheumatoid arthritis. These are listed in the dosages table. Another drug, muromonab, is used in kidney transplantation and was discussed in Chapter 45. As mentioned in Chapter 45, the *mab* suffix in a drug name is usually an abbreviation for "monoclonal antibody."

Mechanism of Action, Drug Effects, and Indications

Because these drugs are so diverse, specific information for each appears in the individual drug profiles provided later in this chapter.

Contraindications

The only clear contraindication to the use of MABs reported thus far is drug allergy to a specific product. The use of MABs is also usually contraindicated in patients with known active infectious processes due to their immunosuppressive qualities. Although known drug allergy is a contraindication, depending on the urgency of the clinical situation, a given MAB may be the only viable treatment option for a seriously ill patient. In such situations allergic symptoms may be controlled with supportive medications such as diphenhydramine and acetaminophen (for fever control). Infliximab has been shown to worsen severe cases of heart failure and should be dosed at no more than 5 mg/kg and only after considering other treatment options for its indications. Use of alemtuzumab is also contraindicated in patients with active systemic infections and immunodeficiency conditions, including AIDS.

Adverse Effects

Many, if not most, patients receiving these very potent drugs manifest acute symptoms that are comparable to classic allergy or flulike symptoms, such as fever, dyspnea, and chills. The primary objective is to administer the medication and control such symptoms as well as possible. Because of their mechanisms of action, working through augmentation (or inhibition) of the human immune response, these drugs can have a variety of adverse effects, some mild, some severe, that affect several body systems. Drug-specific adverse effects with the highest reported incidence (10% to 50% or more) are listed in Table 49-3. Again, the risk of such adverse effects must be weighed against the severity of the patient's underlying illness, which itself may be fatal, especially in the case of malignancies. It should be noted that many of these adverse effects may also be associated with the patient's disease process (e.g., infections) and even with life in general (e.g., headache, depression). This is especially true for the milder effects.

Interactions

Drug interactions associated with MABs are relatively few, and there are no listed major food interactions. Administration of adalimumab with the anti–rheumatoid arthritis drug anakinra (an

---

Table 49-3 Common Adverse Effects Associated with Specific Immunomodulating Drugs

Drug	Adverse Effects
adalimumab	Localized inflammatory reaction at the injection site, infectious processes such as upper respiratory tract and urinary tract infections, and higher rates of various malignancies. Although such effects are likely related to the immunosuppressive properties of this drug, rheumatoid arthritis patients, especially those with more severe disease, are known to have higher rates of cancer.
alemtuzumab	Rash, pruritus (itching), nausea, vomiting, diarrhea, dyspnea, cough, rigors (muscle spasms), fever, fatigue, pain (especially skeletal pain), and myelosuppression.
bevacizumab	Deep vein thrombosis, hypertension, diarrhea, abdominal pain, constipation, vomiting, GI hemorrhage, leukopenia, asthenia (muscular fatigue and weakness), headache, dizziness, dry skin, proteinuria, hypokalemia, epistaxis, and weight loss.
cetuximab	Headache, insomnia, skin rash, conjunctivitis, GI discomfort, anemia, leukopenia, dehydration, edema, weight loss, dyspnea, asthenia, back pain, and fever.
gemtuzumab ozogamicin	Rash, herpes simplex outbreak of the skin, anorexia, constipation, diarrhea, nausea, vomiting, hypokalemia, cough, dyspnea, epistaxis (nosebleed), abdominal pain, asthenia, chills, fever, headache, and infection.
ibritumomab tiuxetan	Nausea, myelosuppression, asthenia, infection, and chills.
infliximab	Headache, rash, GI discomfort, dyspnea, and upper and lower respiratory tract infection.
natalizumab	Depression, fatigue, headache, GI discomfort, urinary tract infection, lower respiratory tract infection, and joint pain. Of even greater concern are four case reports from 2005 and 2006 of a rare, potentially fatal brain disorder known as *progressive multifocal leukoencephalopathy*. At the time of this writing, the drug remains on the U.S. market but is under scrutiny by the FDA.
rituximab	Fever, chills, and headache are also commonly reported with the use of rituximab. Potentially fatal infusion-related events can also occur with rituximab, including severe bronchospasm, dyspnea, hypoxia, pulmonary infiltrates, adult respiratory distress syndrome, hypotension, angioedema, *tumor lysis syndrome* (Chapter 47) with acute renal failure has also been reported. Because of these potentially fatal adverse effects, this drug should be used only after consideration of other treatment options. The drug should be stopped immediately if such a reaction appears imminent, and indicated supportive care provided.
tositumomab and iodine-131 tositumomab	Headache, rash, GI discomfort, muscle pains, dyspnea, pharyngitis, asthenia, fever, chills, and infection.
trastuzumab	Fever, chills, headache, infection, nausea, vomiting, diarrhea, dizziness, headache, insomnia, rash, GI discomfort, edema, dyspnea, rhinitis, asthenia, back pain, fever, chills, and infection.

interleukin) may increase the risk of serious infections secondary to neutropenia. The clearance of natalizumab may be reduced by concurrent use of IFN beta-1a (both used for MS). Coadministration of other anti-TNF drugs (e.g., etanercept, anakinra) with infliximab may also increase the risk of neutropenia and infections. Etanercept should also not be given concurrently with varicella-zoster immune globulin (VZIG) due to undesirable drug interactions. However, etanercept may be resumed after completion of VZIG therapy (per prescriber orders). Bevacizumab is associated with increased risk of severe diarrhea and neutropenia when given concurrently with another anti–colorectal cancer, drug irinotecan (Chapter 47). Paclitaxel (Chapter 47) has been shown to reduce the clearance of trastuzumab when the two are administered concurrently to treat breast cancer. Drug interaction data remain to be collected for other MABs.

Dosages

For the recommended dosages of the antineoplastic MABs, see the Dosages table on this page.

Drug Profiles

The design and use of pharmaceutical MABs is now considered part of the leading edge in drug therapy for several diseases, including cancer, inflammatory conditions, and MS. All of these drugs are synthesized using rDNA technology. Because of the complexities of this technology, these drugs tend to be much more expensive than most other medications, with prices in the hundreds or thousands of dollars per single dose. Because of their cost, insurance companies may refuse reimbursement for these drugs unless other, less costly medications are tried first. The majority of MABs are used to treat various forms of cancer. Their advantage is that they offer greater cell-killing specificity aimed at cancer cells instead of all body cells. Nonetheless, these drugs are all associated with significant adverse effects and therefore with risk, which must be weighed against the severity and associated risks of the patient's underlying disease using expert clinical judgment. Severe allergic inflammatory-type infusion reactions occur in varying percentages of patients. Patients may therefore be premedicated with acetaminophen or diphenhydramine to reduce such reactions. Reactions that do occur may also be treated with diphenhydramine and other drugs such as epinephrine and corticosteroids. Conventional pharmacokinetic data are not listed for the majority of these drugs because they do not follow standard pharmacokinetic models owing to their unique behavior in the body. It is known, however, that they may remain in the affected tissues for many weeks or months. The elimination half-life is listed in the following profiles when known.

adalimumab

Adalimumab (Humira) works through its specificity for human *tumor necrosis factor-α (TNF-α)*. TNF-α is a naturally occurring cytokine that is involved in normal inflammatory and immune responses. It is indicated for the treatment of severe cases of rheumatoid arthritis that have failed to respond to other medications, including methotrexate. It can be used either alone or concurrently with such medications. In patients with rheumatoid arthritis, elevated levels of TNF are found in the synovial fluid in the spaces of affected joints. In addition to preventing TNF-α molecules from binding to TNF cell-surface receptors as part of the rheumatoid arthritis disease process, adalimumab also modulates

DOSAGES

Monoclonal Antibodies

Drug (Pregnancy Category)	Pharmacologic Class	Usual Dosage Range	Indications
adalimumab (Humira) (B)	Anti-TNF-α monoclonal antibody	**Adult only** SC: 40 mg every other week; may advance to 40 mg weekly if indicated.	Severe, progressive RA for which other RA therapies have failed
alemtuzumab (Campath) (C)	Anti-glycoprotein CD52	IV: 3-10 mg daily until maximum dose is tolerated, then 30 mg 3×/wk (alternate days) for up to 12 wk	B-cell chronic lymphocytic leukemia
bevacizumab (Avastin) (C)	Anti-human vascular endothelial growth factor	IV: 5 mg/kg q14d	Metastatic colorectal cancer
cetuximab (Erbitux) (C)	Anti-human epidermal growth factor	IV: 400 mg/m² loading dose, then 250 mg/m² weekly	Metastatic colorectal cancer
gemtuzumab ozogamicin (Mylotarg) (D)	Conjugate with cytotoxic antibiotic	IV: 9 mg/m² × 2 doses 14 days apart	Acute myeloid leukemia
ibritumomab tiuxetan (Zevalin) (D)	Chelator immunoconjugate	IV: 250 mg/m² × 2 doses 7 to 9 days apart	Non-Hodgkin's lymphoma
infliximab (Remicade) (B)	Anti-TNF-α	IV: 3-5 mg/kg at 0, 2, and 6 wk, then every 6 wk	Ankylosing spondylitis, Crohn's disease, RA
natalizumab (Tysabri) (C)	Anti-α₄ integrin subunit	IV: 300 mg every 4 wk	Multiple sclerosis
▶ rituximab (Rituxan) (C)	Anti-CD20 surface antigen	IV: 375 mg/m² 1×/wk × 4 doses	Non-Hodgkin's lymphoma
tositumomab and iodine I 131 tositumomab (Bexxar) (X)	Radioactive MAB	IV: Complex dosing regimen involving both drug components—follow instructions in package insert as ordered	Non-Hodgkin's lymphoma
trastuzumab (Herceptin) (B)	Anti-HER2 protein MAB	IV: Loading dose, 4 mg/kg IV: Maintenance dose, 2 mg/kg/wk	Breast cancer

IV, Intravenous; *MAB*, monoclonal antibodies; *RA*, rheumatoid arthritis; *SC*, subcutaneous; *TNF*, tumor necrosis factor.

the inflammatory biologic responses that are induced or regulated by TNF. Use of adalimumab is contraindicated in patients with any active infectious process, whether localized or systemic, acute or chronic.

alemtuzumab

Alemtuzumab (Campath) was approved by the Food and Drug Administration (FDA) in 2001 to treat B-CLL. It is classified as a recombinant humanized antibody that is directed against the *CD52 glycoprotein* that appears on the surfaces of virtually all B and T lymphocytes. This property makes this drug useful in treating chronic lymphocytic leukemia caused by B cells (abbreviated B-CLL). It is used specifically in patients for whom other first-line chemotherapy treatments, including treatment with alkylating drugs and the antimetabolite fludarabine, have failed. Its contraindications are drug allergy; active systemic infection, and documented immunodeficiency disease such as HIV-positive status. Half-life is 10 hours to 30 days.

bevacizumab

Bevacizumab (Avastin) was approved in 2004 for the treatment of metastatic colon or rectal cancer in combination with the first-line antineoplastic drug 5-fluorouracil (Chapter 47). It is unique in that it binds to and inhibits vascular endothelial growth factor, a protein that promotes development of new blood vessels in tumors (as well as in normal body tissues). It has no listed contraindications but may complicate surgical wound healing because of its antivascular effects. Half-life is 11 to 50 days.

cetuximab

Cetuximab (Erbitux) was also approved in 2004 for the treatment of metastatic colorectal cancer. It is a recombinant MAB made from both human and mouse (*murine*) genetic material and is designed for concurrent use with the second-line antineoplastic drug irinotecan (Chapter 47). It binds to *epidermal growth factor* on the surface of tumor cells, where it hinders cell growth through interference with cell metabolism. It is used either in combination with the antineoplastic drug irinotecan (Chapter 47) or alone in patients who are intolerant of the latter drug. It has no listed contraindications but is known to cause severe infusion reactions in up to 3% of patients receiving it. Half-life is 97 to114 hours.

gemtuzumab ozogamicin

Gemtuzumab ozogamicin (Mylotarg) was approved by the FDA in 2000 as the first MAB indicated for leukemia. It is designed to treat acute myelocytic leukemia (also called *acute myelogenous* or *myeloid leukemia*). This drug is unique in that it consists of a recombinant humanized antibody that is linked ("conjugated") to a cytotoxic antineoplastic antibiotic, ozogamicin. Ozogamicin is derived from calicheamicin, the natural form of the antibiotic that is isolated from a certain bacterial species. This type of drug complex is known as an *immunoconjugate*. This particular complex binds to the CD33 cell surface antigen, which is expressed on the surface of leukemia blasts (malignant immature white cells) in more than 80% of patients with acute myelocytic leukemia. The binding of the antibody portion of the drug to the CD33 receptor leads to internalization of the drug complex by the leukemic blast. At this point the ozogamicin component is released inside the lysosomes (called *suicide sacs* in biology) of the malignant cell, which leads to DNA damage and cell death. Half-life is 40 to 100 hours.

ibritumomab tiuxetan

Ibritumomab tiuxetan (Zevalin) was approved in 2002 for treating B-cell non-Hodgkin's lymphoma. Like gemtuzumab ozogamicin, this drug is another immunoconjugate, this time consisting of the MAB ibritumomab conjugated with the metal chelator tiuxetan. This drug comes in kits that also include one of two radioactive metal isotopes (radioisotopes): indium 111 or yttrium 90. The antibody binds to the CD20 antigen that occurs on the surfaces of both normal and malignant B lymphocytes. Once the complex is bound to the cells, the tiuxetan component binds the radioisotope, which is administered as another part of the anticancer therapy. Radioactive β emission from the bound radioisotope, a unique feature of this drug, induces free radical formation and cell damage in both the cell containing the drug complex and neighboring cells.

infliximab

Infliximab (Remicade) is one of the earliest MABs, approved in 1998. It works through an anti–TNF-α action, similar to adalimumab, but it is approved for the treatment of ankylosing spondylitis, Crohn's disease, in addition to rheumatoid arthritis. It has the special contraindication of severe heart failure (grade III or IV on the New York Heart Association scale), because it may worsen this condition. It also has an FDA black box warning reporting cases of fatal tuberculosis and/or fungal infections associated with the use of this drug. It is recommended that patients be tested for latent TB before it is administered. Half-life is 8 to 9 days.

natalizumab

Natalizumab (Tysabri) was approved in late 2004 for the treatment of multiple sclerosis (MS). It is a humanized MAB derived from murine myeloma cells. *Humanization* involves the insertion of human DNA sequences during drug production to make the drug better tolerated by human patients. It works by binding to the α4 subunits of *integrins*, proteins found on leukocyte surfaces (with the exception of neutrophils). These proteins are implicated in the MS disease process, but the exact mechanism by which this drug exerts its therapeutic effects is unknown. However, the drug is known to inhibit the leukocyte adhesion that is mediated by these α4 protein subunits and which is also believed to be part of the MS disease process. Natalizumab has no listed contraindications. Half-life is 11 days.

▶ rituximab

Rituximab (Rituxan), like ibritumomab tiuxetan, specifically binds to antigen CD20. This antigen is a protein on the membranes of both normal and malignant B cells found in patients with non-Hodgkin's lymphoma. Antigen CD20 is expressed in more than 90% of B-cell non-Hodgkin's lymphomas. Once rituximab binds to these B cells, a host immune response causes lysis of the cells.Rituximab has become a standard drug for the treatment of patients with follicular low-grade non-Hodgkin's lymphoma for whom previous therapy has failed. It is recommended that patients be premedicated with acetaminophen and diphenhydramine before each infusion of the drug to reduce its well-known infusion-related adverse effects.

tositumomab and iodine I 131 tositumomab

Tositumomab and iodine I 131 tositumomab (Bexxar) were approved by the FDA in 2003 for the treatment of non-Hodgkin's lymphoma. This drug is a murine MAB with a dual radioactive and nonradioactive component. Both components bind to the CD20 antigen, a transmembrane protein that is expressed on the cell membranes of more than 90% of B-cell non-Hodgkin's lymphoma cells. Theoretical mechanisms of action include induction of *apoptosis* (programmed cell death), *complement-dependent* cytotoxicity, or antibody-dependent cytotoxicity mediated by the drug itself. **Complement** is a collective term for about 20 different proteins normally present in plasma that aid other immune system components (e.g., B cells and T cells) in mounting an immune response.

trastuzumab

Trastuzumab (Herceptin) kills tumor cells by mediating antibody-dependent cellular cytotoxicity. It accomplishes this by inhibiting proliferation of human tumor cells that overexpress HER2 protein. This protein is overexpressed in 25% to 30% of primary malignant breast tumors. It is an adverse prognostic factor for early-stage breast cancer. The overexpression of the HER2 gene has been established as an adverse prognostic factor for early-stage breast cancer. Because of the relatively selective expression of HER2 on cancer cells, it has been an appealing target for antineoplastic therapy. The combination of trastuzumab and paclitaxel has produced encouraging results. Trastuzumab has a special black box warning from the FDA reporting cases of ventricular dysfunction and heart failure associated with this drug. Patients should be monitored for signs and symptoms of heart failure and ventricular dysfunction before and during treatment. In addition, fatal hypersensitivity reactions, infusion reactions, and pulmonary events have occurred in association with it use; therefore, careful clinical judgment, risk evaluation, and informed patient consent are called for in its use. Half-life is 10 to 30 days.

INTERLEUKINS AND RELATED DRUGS

Interleukins are a natural part of the immune system and are classified as *lymphokines*. Lymphokines are soluble proteins that are released from activated lymphocytes such as NK cells. There are several known interleukins in the body (IL-2, IL-3, IL-4, IL-5, IL-6, and IL-11), and more are being identified as knowledge of the immune system increases.

The three pharmaceutical interleukin receptor agonists currently available are aldesleukin (IL-2), oprelvekin (IL-11), and denileukin diftitox. Oprelvekin was mentioned with the HDs earlier in this chapter. It has a dual classification as both an interleukin and hematologic drug. Both aldesleukin and oprelvekin are synthesized using rDNA technology and are patterned after corresponding natural interleukins in the body. Denileukin diftitox is also rDNA derived, but it contains fragments of both diphtheria toxin and aldesleukin. A fourth drug, anakinra, is actually an IL-1 receptor antagonist. It is also a recombinant product that is patterned after its natural counterpart in the body.

Mechanism of Action and Drug Effects

Interleukins cause multiple effects in the immune system, one of which is beneficial antitumor action. Aldesleukin is produced by activated T cells in response to macrophage-"processed" antigens and secreted IL-1. It was formerly called *T-cell growth factor* because, among other actions, it aids in the growth and differentiation of T lymphocytes. Aldesleukin acts indirectly to stimulate or restore immune response. Aldesleukin binds to receptor sites on T cells, which stimulates the T cells to multiply. One type of cell that results from this multiplication is the **lymphokine-activated killer (LAK) cell.** LAK cells recognize and destroy only cancer cells and ignore normal cells, which allows some of the toxic effects of standard antineoplastic drugs to be avoided. Aldesleukin is currently the most widely used of the interleukin drugs. A detailed list of its specific immunomodulating effects appears in Box 49-2.

Denileukin diftitox consists of one segment (denileukin) that is patterned after natural human IL-2 and a second segment (diftitox) that is patterned after diphtheria toxin. It is an IL-2 receptor antagonist, binding to cell-surface IL-2 receptors that are expressed on both normal and certain malignant cells. It causes cell death upon binding to these receptors through the cytocidal

activity of diphtheria toxin, which inhibits intracellular protein synthesis.

Anakinra is a recombinant form of the natural human IL-1 receptor antagonist. It competitively inhibits the binding of IL-1 to its corresponding receptor sites, which are expressed in many different tissues and organs.

Indications

Aldesleukin was previously indicated only for the treatment of metastatic renal cell carcinoma, a malignancy that originates in the kidney tissues. It is now also approved for the treatment of metastatic melanoma. Denileukin diftitox is currently indicated only as therapy for a skin-based lymphoma known as *cutaneous T-cell lymphoma,* which often metastasizes to other areas of the body. Anakinra is indicated for symptom control in patients with rheumatoid arthritis for whom other therapy has failed.

Contraindications

Contraindications to the administration of aldesleukin include drug allergy, organ transplantation, and abnormal results on thallium cardiac stress tests or pulmonary function tests. For denileukin diftitox, the only usual contraindication is drug allergy, as is also the case for anakinra.

Adverse Effects

Unfortunately, therapy with aldesleukin is commonly complicated by severe toxicity. A syndrome known as *capillary leak syndrome* is responsible for the severe toxicities of aldesleukin. As the name implies, capillary leak syndrome refers to a condition induced by interleukin therapy in which the capillaries lose their ability to retain vital colloids such as albumin, protein, and other essential components of blood. Because the capillaries are "leaky," these substances migrate into the surrounding tissues. This results in massive fluid retention (20 to 30 lb), which can lead to the life-threatening problems of respiratory distress, heart failure, dysrhythmias, and myocardial infarction. Fortunately, these are all reversible after discontinuation of the interleukin therapy. Close patient monitoring and vigorous supportive care are essential in the patient receiving aldesleukin therapy. Other adverse effects and adverse effects that may be associated with aldesleukin therapy are fever, chills, rash, fatigue, hepatotoxicity, myalgias, headaches, and eosinophilia.

The most common adverse effects associated with denileukin diftitox administration include nausea, vomiting, anorexia, diarrhea, hypoalbuminemia, elevated liver enzyme levels, edema, dyspnea, cough, fever, chills, asthenia, generalized pain, chest pain, infection, and headache. Anakinra has a much milder adverse effect profile that includes local reactions at the injection site, various respiratory tract infections, and headache.

Interactions

Aldesleukin, when given with antihypertensives, can produce additive hypotensive effects. Coadministration of corticosteroids with aldesleukin can reduce its antitumor effectiveness. The toxic effects of aldesleukin are increased when it is administered with aminoglycosteroids, indomethacin, cytotoxic chemotherapeutic drugs, methotrexate, asparaginase, and doxorubicin. No particular drug interactions have been reported to date for anakinra or denileukin diftitox.

Box 49-2 Interleukin-2: Drug Effects

Modulating Effects

Proliferation of T cells
Synthesis and secretion of cytokines
Increased production of B cells (antibodies)
Proliferation and activation of NK cells
Proliferation and activation of LAK cells

Enhancing Effects

Enhancement of killer T-cell activity
Amplification of the effects of cytokines
Enhancement of the cytotoxic actions of NK cells and LAK cells

LAK, Lymphokine-activated killer; *NK,* natural killer.

DOSAGES

Interleukins and Related Drugs

Drug (Pregnancy Category)	Pharmacologic Class	Usual Dosage Range	Indications
▶ aldesleukin [IL-2] (Proleukin) (C)	Human recombinant IL-2 analogue	IV: 600,000 international units/kg (0.037 mg/kg) q8h (14 doses)	Metastatic renal cell carcinoma or melanoma
anakinra (Kineret) (B)	IL-1 receptor antagonist	SC: 100 mg/day	Rheumatoid arthritis
denileukin diftitox (Ontak) (C)	Recombinant IL-2 and diphtheria toxin protein	IV: 9 or 18 mcg/kg/day for 5 consecutive days q21d	Cutaneous T-cell lymphoma

IL, Interleukin; *IV*, intravenous; *SC*, subcutaneous.

Dosages

For the recommended dosages of the interleukin agonists and antagonists, see the Dosages table on this page.

Drug Profiles

The interleukins are a group of naturally occurring cytokines in the body that originally were believed to be produced by and to act primarily on leukocytes (WBCs). They are now recognized as multifunctional cytokines that are produced by a variety of cells but act at least partly within the lymphatic system. As is the case with MABs, pharmacokinetic data may not have been ascertained for these drugs.

▶ aldesleukin

Aldesleukin (Proleukin) is a human IL-2 derivative that is manufactured using rDNA technology. It is a cytokine that is produced by lymphocytes and is therefore classified as a lymphokine. Aldesleukin is currently approved only for the treatment of metastatic renal cell carcinoma and metastatic melanoma, despite its activity against other cancers. Aldesleukin is contraindicated in patients with drug allergy, abnormal thallium stress test or pulmonary function tests (due to potential drug effects on cardiopulmonary function), and organ transplants (due to immunostimulating qualities of drug, which may cause organ rejection). The drug is only available for injection.

denileukin diftitox

Denileukin diftitox (Ontak) is an IL-2 receptor antagonist that is produced using rDNA technology. It is used to treat cutaneous T-cell lymphoma. Its only current contraindication is drug allergy. It is available for injection only.

anakinra

Anakinra (Kineret) is an IL-1 receptor antagonist that is also rDNA synthesized. It is used to help control symptoms of rheumatoid arthritis. Its only current contraindication is drug allergy. It is available for injection only.

MISCELLANEOUS IMMUNOMODULATING DRUGS

In addition to the drugs in the major classes discussed thus far, there are several additional medications that can be broadly classified as miscellaneous IMDs. They work by various specific and nonspecific mechanisms. A special term used for **immunostimulant** drugs that work by a nonspecific mechanism is **adjuvant.** These miscellaneous medications, including some that are classified as adjuvants, are outlined in Table 49-4.

◆ NURSING PROCESS

◆ ASSESSMENT

Before administering any of the BRMs, the nurse must assess his or her own knowledge about these medications, including (1) hematopoietic drugs, (2) IFNs, (3) MABs, (4) interleukins, and (5) miscellaneous drugs. After the nurse's knowledge base is complete, the patient must then be assessed for the presence of any contraindications, cautions, or drug interactions as well as for hypersensitivity to the drug, egg proteins, or immunoglobulin G (such patients will most likely have an allergic reaction to these drugs). Cautious use with close monitoring is recommended in pregnant and lactating women, in children, and in patients with cardiac disease, angina, heart failure, chronic obstructive pulmonary disease, diabetes mellitus, bleeding disorders, bone marrow suppression, or convulsive disorders. Therefore, the nursing history should be reviewed and analyzed. Head-to-toe examination should include thorough assessment of breath sounds with listening for any crackles in the lungs; evaluation of heart sounds and heart rate and rhythm; assessment for edema, shortness of breath, decrease in partial pressure of oxygen, or increase in partial pressure of carbon dioxide; inspection for any cyanotic discoloration around the mouth or nail beds; assessment for the presence of chest pain, hypotension, or hypertension; and evaluation of mental status and assessment for any seizure-like activity. Height, weight, uric acid levels, electrolyte levels, skin condition, ability to carry out activities of daily living, nutritional status (see Nursing Process in Chapters 47 and 48), presence or absence of underlying diseases, and symptoms and success or failure of medication regimens in the past should also be documented before therapy. In addition, baseline vital signs and complete blood count (CBC) should be determined and documented. For therapy with any of the drugs in this chapter, baseline assessment should also include gathering data about the patient's emotional status, educational level, learning needs, desire and ability to learn, past coping strategies, support systems, and self-care abilities.

For *hematopoietic* BRMs, the following assessment should be done in addition to the aforementioned: (1) For *erythropoietin* and similar drugs: The patient should be assessed for a history of hypertension, seizure activity, thrombosis, and chest pain, because these may be exacerbated by the drug. Renal

Table 49-4	Miscellaneous Immunomodulating Drugs		
Drug (Trade and Other Names)	**Classification**	**Indications**	**Mechanism of Action**
bexarotene (Targretin)	Retinoid receptor agonist	Cutaneous T-cell lymphoma	Exact mechanism unknown; binds to and activates retinoid X receptor subtypes; this regulates the expression of genes that control cellular differentiation
BCG vaccine (Pacis, TICE BCG, TheraCys)	Live virus vaccine, adjuvant	Localized bladder cancer	Promotes local inflammation and immune response in bladder mucosa
etanercept (Enbrel)	TNF receptor antagonist	RA (including juvenile) and psoriatic arthritis	Blocks effects of TNF, a major inflammatory mediator in RA
leflunomide (Arava)	Antimetabolite	RA	Exerts antiinflammatory effects via inhibition of cellular DNA synthesis
levamisole (Ergamisol)	Immunostimulant, adjuvant	Dukes' stage C colon cancer (given with fluorouracil)	Exact mechanism unclear, but may enhance the therapeutic effects of fluorouracil and have its own immunostimulatory effects
mitoxantrone (Novantrone)	Anthracycline antibiotic (also an antineoplastic drug)	MS (secondary chronic type)	Inhibits cellular DNA synthesis, which reduces neurologic disability in MS (exact mechanism unclear)
pegademase bovine (Adagen)	Immunostimulant	SCID	Modified enzyme that compensates for deficiency of the enzyme adenosine deaminase, which is associated with SCID
thalidomide (Thalomid)	Immunostimulant	Erythremia nodosum*	Exact mechanism unclear, but may have anti-TNF properties, which counter the disease process
tretinoin (Vesanoid)	Retinoid receptor agonist	Acute promyelocytic leukemia	Induces differentiation and maturation of leukemic cells, reducing proliferation of immature, disease-causing cells

*An inflammatory reaction in the subcutaneous fat, often following a bacterial infection or reaction to drugs such as oral contraceptives or sulfonamides.
BCG, Bacillus Calmette-Guérin; *DNA,* deoxyribonucleic acid; *MS,* multiple sclerosis; *RA,* rheumatoid arthritis; *SCID,* severe combined immunodeficiency disease; *TNF,* tumor necrosis factor.

function should be evaluated, because patients with chronic renal failure (and receiving these drugs) may have transient rises in blood pressure. Iron stores should be assessed by measuring transferrin saturation, which must be at least 20%, and ferritin level, which should be at 100 ng/mL. These levels allow appropriate erythropoietin stimulation. Possible subcutaneous and/or intravenous sites should be assessed and blood pressures measured before starting therapy and early in treatment. (2) For *CSFs*: CBC should be assessed; for example, with filgrastim and sargramostim, counts should be determined before therapy and throughout therapy to monitor for problems with leukocytosis and thrombocytosis. Hepatic functioning should be assessed by determining levels of liver enzymes. Potential intravenous and subcutaneous sites should be noted, and, if appropriate, chemotherapy-induced absolute neutrophil nadir (low point) should be assessed, because timing of the dose is critical in helping to boost blood cell counts. For example, with filgrastim, the drug should *not* be given within 24 hours before or after the chemotherapy (see pharmacology discussion). In addition, any existing pain, especially joint or bone pain, is important to document because of the possible adverse effect of mild, moderate, or severe bone pain with filgrastim.

Before *IFNs* (e.g., IFN alfa-2a or alfa-2b; IFN gamma-1b) are given, the patient's CBC should be documented because long-term therapy with these drugs may lead to bone marrow suppression. Other serum laboratory values such as platelet counts, BUN and creatinine levels, urinalysis results, and levels of aspartate aminotransferase and alkaline phosphatase should be checked before treatment and twice weekly during therapy or as ordered. Before aldesleukin is used, it is important for the nurse to document baseline measurements of vital signs, neurologic functioning, bowel status, and results of liver and renal studies. These laboratory and baseline assessments are important because of possible drug-related impaired renal and liver functioning. Capillary leak syndrome is also associated with interleukin drugs, so it is important to document any edema and assess baseline vital signs and baseline cardiac, respiratory, renal, and liver status. The symptoms of this potentially fatal syndrome include hypotension; reduced organ perfusion; extravasation of plasma proteins and fluid; and symptoms of angina and respiratory, renal, and liver insufficiency. Because of cardiac concerns, the interleukins may not be administered to patients with cardiac diseases or symptoms (e.g., hypotension, hypertension, angina). Any allergy to proteins of *E. coli* should be noted because of cross-sensitivity to IFN. Attention to the timing of these drugs is important, because they are not usually given at the same time as antineoplastics; instead, they are usually given at least 24 hours after chemotherapy.

Hepatic, renal, and cardiac functioning with use of trastuzumab should be assessed. Blood pressure should be monitored along with any GI signs and symptoms, fatigue, weakness, or malaise with use of the *MAB drugs* (e.g., alemtuzumab, rituximab, trastuzumab). The medication order should also be examined for timing of the dose because of different protocols. Intravenous sites should be assessed, and with rituximab, withholding antihypertensives for 12 hours before infusion may be considered, as ordered, to avoid any transient hypotensive episodes.

♦ NURSING DIAGNOSES
- Acute pain related to the adverse effects of BRMs
- Altered nutrition, less than body requirements, related to the adverse effects of BRMs
- Impaired skin integrity (rash) related to the adverse effects of BRMs
- Risk for falls related to weakness and fatigue from the disease process as well as from drug therapy
- Impaired gas exchange related to the adverse effects of the various BRMs
- Risk for caregiver role strain related to the demands of therapy and need for assistance in the care of a loved one or significant other

♦ PLANNING
Goals
- Patient experiences adequate control of pain during drug treatment.
- Patient regains prechemotherapy (and as near normal as possible) nutritional status.
- Patient experiences minimal weight loss during therapy.
- Patient maintains or regains normal bowel and bladder patterns.
- Patient's mucous membranes maintain and/or regain intactness during therapy.
- Patient is free of self-injury related to drug therapy.

LEGAL AND ETHICAL PRINCIPLES
The Nurse and Patient Care

The nurse should never neglect or be deceptive with a patient despite a conflict with the nurse's cultural, racial/ethnic, spiritual or personal belief systems. This dilemma is often encountered with various types of treatment modalities for cancer patients or those needing drugs that alter the patient's biologic response. The nurse does have the right to refuse to participate in any treatment or aspect of a patient's care that violates personal ethical principles, but it is important to understand that this refusal of care can in *no* way be through desertion or neglect of the patient. In this situation the nurse should inform the appropriate supervisory personnel about the conflict and transfer the patient to the safe care of another qualified professional before the start of nursing care by another nurse. Remember that, as detailed in the American Nurses Association Code of Ethics, nurses are bound by the profession to always remain ethical in the administration of their care to patients. This may include participation in the care of a patient who needs the nurse's care but who may be receiving treatment or care that is not "acceptable" by the nurse's own standards or ethics.

- Patient's family, caregiver, and/or significant other experiences minimal stress and anxiety and maximal rest and relaxation.

Outcome Criteria
- Patient describes nutritional needs and daily meal planning reflecting dietary needs, such as consumption of a high-calorie, low-residue, high-protein diet and forcing of fluids; patient states grocery shopping tips.
- Patient states measures to minimize GI adverse effects, such as eating small, frequent meals and avoiding spicy foods.
- Patient forces fluids up to 3000 mL/day, unless contraindicated, with creative means such as consumption of flavored water, decaffeinated iced tea, lemonade, sugar-free juices (if appropriate), and cranberry juice, with adequate urinary output noted.
- Patient's skin and mucous membranes remain intact and clean through daily bathing, skin care with moisturizing products, and daily oral hygiene with flossing as well as follow-up care with a dental professional.
- Patient states ways to minimize self-injury related to weakness and fatigue from the disease process and related BRM treatment, such as by using assistive devices and grab bars or rails; removing rugs, mats, or other obstacles in the bedroom, bathroom, and so on; maintaining muscle mass and energy; and obtaining assistance in performing the activities of daily living, if needed.
- Patient eats appropriate foods that provide high energy content through protein and "good" (complex) carbohydrates.
- Patient's family members, significant others, loved ones, and/or caregivers attend appropriate seminars or are able to obtain information and community resources designed to assist these individuals in stress management, rest, relaxation, and respite.

♦ IMPLEMENTATION
Generally speaking, BRMs should be given exactly as prescribed and in keeping with the manufacturer's guidelines to minimize all expected and untoward adverse effects. Vital signs, with special attention to temperature, should also be measured throughout drug therapy. Premedication with acetaminophen and diphenhydramine may be deemed necessary when any of the BRMs is administered. With some of the BRMs, treatment with narcotics, antihistamines, and/or antiinflammatory drugs may be required for the management of bone pain and chills should treatment with acetaminophen or diphenhydramine not be successful. Meperidine may be the narcotic of choice if the patient is in the hospital setting or in a physician's office for treatment. Antiemetics may also be needed for any drug-related nausea or vomiting and may be administered before the specific BRM is taken. Antiemetics may even need to be dosed around the clock should nausea and vomiting be problematic. The patient should be encouraged to rest when tired, not to overdo it during therapy, and to contact the physician should profound fatigue or loss of appetite be experienced. The patient should force fluids up to 3000 mL/day (unless contraindicated) to promote excretion of the byproducts of cellular breakdown. Consultation with a dietitian or nutritionist may be helpful for the patient to learn about a healthy diet (e.g., foods high in protein, complex carbohydrates, and necessary minerals, vitamins, and/or herbals) to boost health and wellness. Menu planning and grocery shopping may also be discussed, with spe-

cific suggestions provided for each individual patient care situation. Nowadays, many grocery stores support Internet food shopping with car pickup at the store on the same day, and many stores also deliver at no or minimal cost to the patient. Community resources (e.g., Meals on Wheels, respite care organizations, physical and occupational therapists) should be shared with patients as needed. A social services agency should be contacted if the patient needs assistance in covering the cost of treatments or other services.

Other nursing interventions include giving the drug at night or bedtime to decrease daytime fatigue. IFNs are administered parenterally by either subcutaneous, intravenous, or intramuscular routes, depending on the drug (e.g., IFN alfa-2a is given subcutaneously or intramuscularly). Epoetin alfa may be given intravenously or subcutaneously, and the dose may change depending on hematocrit values. If there is no response to the drug, the patient should undergo a workup for iron deficiency; underlying infection, inflammation, or malignancies; occult blood loss; hematologic disease; hemolysis; folic acid or vitamin B_{12} deficiency; and aluminum intoxication. Recommendations for the administration of epoetin alfa are to give the drug without shaking the vial and with only one use per vial; to use the smallest possible amount per injection (e.g., 1 mL or less per injection)—but always as ordered; to change the needle once the medication has been withdrawn from the vial; and to apply ice to numb the injection site. With sargramostim, only one dose

should be withdrawn per vial, and as with all vials and packages, expiration dates should be checked. Vials should not be shaken but should be rolled between the hands. Filgrastim drug vials contain single-dose only portions and should be stored in the refrigerator. Oprelvekin should not be used if any discoloration or particulate matter is noted in the vial. Treatment begins within 6 to 24 hours after completion of the antineoplastic treatment. Daily subcutaneous dosing for 14 days has been found to produce dose-dependent platelet elevations, with counts increasing within 5 to 9 days of starting injections. Once oprelvekin is discontinued, counts remain increased for about 7 days and return to baseline within 14 days. Subcutaneous sites for oprelvekin administration include the thigh, abdomen, hip, and upper arm. Drugs given subcutaneously should be done with rotation of injection sites. See the Patient Teaching Tips for more information.

♦ EVALUATION

Therapeutic responses to BRMs include a decrease in the growth of the lesion or mass, decreased tumor size, and an easing of symptoms related to the tumor or disease process. Other therapeutic effects are an improvement in WBC, RBC, and platelet counts and/or a return to normal levels, and absence of infection, anemias, and hemorrhage. Journaling may help provide health care providers with more data from which to evaluate the patient's response during and after therapy. Possible adverse effects for which to evaluate are presented in Tables 49-1 and 49-2.

Patient Teaching Tips

- Patients should avoid hazardous tasks because of the central nervous system changes noted with several BRMs. Fatigue is also a common adverse effect, so the patient should report excessive fatigue.
- Patients should report signs of infection, such as sore throat, diarrhea, vomiting, and/or a fever of 37.8° C (100° F) or higher.
- Pregnancy is discouraged while the patient is taking BRMs, and so education should include information about contraceptive choices and the need to use contraception for up to 2 years after completion of therapy.
- Patients should be told that the adverse effects associated with BRMs usually disappear within 72 to 96 hours after therapy has been discontinued. Encourage follow-up appointments.

- Interleukins may be self-administered; therefore, patients should learn self-injection technique and proper disposal of equipment (e.g., needles, syringes). A corresponding instruction sheet should be provided for patients, and patients should keep a daily journal to record the site of injection and an overall rating of how they feel.
- Bone pain and flulike symptoms often occur with some of the BRMs, and the use of nonopioid or, in some cases, opioid analgesics may be required. Some patients may find relief with ibuprofen.
- Patients should report any adverse effects (e.g., hair loss, fever, joint pain, chills, diarrhea, edema, anemia, anorexia, fatigue, hypotension, thrombocytopenia) to the physician immediately so that the dosage can be adjusted or reconsidered.

Points to Remember

- Cancer treatment has traditionally involved surgery, radiation, and chemotherapy. Surgery and radiation are usually local or regional therapies. Chemotherapy is generally systemic, but it often does not completely eliminate all of the cancer cells in the body. Adjuvant therapy is frequently used to destroy undetected distant micrometastases.
- BRMs provide another treatment option for patients who have malignancies and/or those who are receiving chemotherapy and have a need to boost blood cell counts. BRMs include hematopoietics and IMDs. IFNs, interleukins, MABs, and miscellaneous drugs are the categories of IMDs.
- In BRM therapy, the body's own immune system is used to destroy cancerous cells, and the drugs may either augment, restore, or modify host defenses against the tumor.

- The humoral and cellular immune systems act together to recognize and destroy foreign particles and cells. The humoral immune system is composed of lymphocytes that are known as B cells until they are transformed into plasma cells when they come in contact with an antigen (foreign substance). The plasma cells then manufacture antibodies to that antigen.
- Nursing management associated with the administration of BRMs focuses on the use of careful aseptic technique and other measures to prevent infection, proper nutrition, oral hygiene, monitoring of blood counts, and management of the adverse effects of BRMs, including joint and bone pain and flulike adverse effects.

NCLEX Examination Review Questions

1. Which of the following best describes the action of IFNs in the management of malignant tumors?
   a. Increase the production of specific anticancer enzymes
   b. Have antiviral and antitumor properties and strengthen the immune system
   c. Stimulate the production and activation of T lymphocytes and cytotoxic T cells
   d. Help improve the cell killing action of T cells because they are retrieved from healthy donors
2. During therapy with IFNs, the nurse must keep in mind that the major dose-limiting factor is:
   a. Fatigue
   b. Bone marrow suppression
   c. Fever
   d. Nausea and vomiting
3. Which is an appropriate nursing intervention for the patient receiving a BRM?
   a. Avoid acetaminophen products during therapy
   b. Premedicate with acetaminophen and diphenhydramine if beneficial
   c. Limit fluids to 1000 mL/day
   d. Encourage a low-protein, high-carbohydrate diet during therapy

4. In caring for a patient receiving therapy with a myelosuppressive antineoplastic drug, the nurse notes an order to begin filgrastim after the chemotherapy is completed. Which of the following statements correctly describes when the nurse should begin the filgrastim therapy?
   a. Filgrastim therapy can begin during the chemotherapy.
   b. Filgrastim therapy should begin immediately after the chemotherapy is completed.
   c. Filgrastim therapy should not be initiated until 24 hours after the chemotherapy is completed.
   d. Filgrastim therapy should not be begun until at least 72 hours after the chemotherapy is completed.
5. A patient with renal failure has severe anemia, and there is an order for darbepoetin. As the nurse assesses the patient, which condition listed below should the nurse consider a contraindication to use of this medication?
   a. Uncontrolled hypertension
   b. Diabetes mellitus
   c. Hypothyroidism
   d. Angina

1. b, 2. a, 3. b, 4. c, 5. a.

Critical Thinking Activities

1. Your patient is to receive filgrastim (Neupogen) after therapy with carmustine and radiation for treatment of a brain tumor. The patient weighs 132 lb. The protocol that the oncologist has given you states that the filgrastim should be dosed at 5 mcg/kg. Filgrastim (Neupogen) comes in both a 300-mcg/mL and a 480-mcg/0.8-mL vial. What dose should the patient receive, and what vial should be used to waste as little drug as possible?
2. What is so important about the timing of the dose of a CSF, such as filgrastim or pegfilgrastim, in the treatment of neoplasms?

3. Many medications, especially chemotherapeutic drugs, may lead to the adverse effect of bone marrow suppression of various blood cell components. What symptoms would you expect to see if your patient had diminished production of platelets? RBCs? WBCs? Explain your answers.

For answers, see http://evolve.elsevier.com/Lilley.

Gene Therapy and Pharmacogenomics

Glossary

Acquired disease Any disease acquired through external factors and not *directly* caused by a person's genes (e.g., an infectious disease, noncongenital cardiovascular diseases). (p. 782)

Alleles Any alternative forms of a gene that can occupy a specific locus (location) on a chromosome (see *chromosomes*). In humans there are two alleles for each gene, one on each of 23 paired chromosomes. One unit of each pair is supplied by the mother, the other by the father. An allele may be dominant or recessive for a given genetic trait. (p. 782)

Chromatin A collective term for all of the chromosomal material within a given cell. (p. 783)

Chromosomes Structures in the nuclei of cells that contain linear threads of deoxyribonucleic acid (DNA), which transmits genetic information, and are associated with ribonucleic acid (RNA) molecules and synthesis of protein molecules. (p. 782)

Gene The biologic unit of heredity; a segment of a DNA molecule that contains all of the molecular information required for the synthesis of a biologic product such as an RNA molecule or an amino acid chain (protein molecule). (p. 782)

Gene therapy New therapeutic technologies that directly target human genes in the treatment or prevention of illness. (p. 783)

Genetic disease Any disorder caused by a genetic mechanism. (p. 782)

Genetic material DNA or RNA molecules or portions thereof. (p. 782)

Genetic polymorphisms Allele variants that occur in the chromosomes of 1% or more of the general population (i.e., they occur too frequently to be caused by recurrent mutation). (p. 785)

Genetic predisposition The presence of certain factors in a person's genetic makeup, or *genome* (see below), that increase the individual's likelihood of eventually developing one or more diseases. (p. 782)

Genetics The study of the structure, function, and inheritance of genes. (p. 782)

Genome The complete set of genetic material of any organism. It may be contained in multiple chromosomes (groups of DNA or RNA molecules) in higher organisms; in a single chromosome, as in bacteria; or in a single DNA or RNA molecule, as in viruses. (p. 783)

Genomics The study of the structure and function of the genome, including DNA sequencing, mapping, and expression, and the way genes and their products work in both health and disease. (p. 783)

Genotype The alleles present at a given site (locus) on the chromosomes of an organism (e.g., human, animal, plant) that determine a specific genetic trait for that organism (see *phenotype*). (p. 782)

Human Genome Project (HGP)   A scientific project of the U.S. Department of Energy and National Institutes of Health to describe in detail the entire genome of a human being. This project was completed ahead of schedule in 2003. (p. 783)

Inherited diseases   Genetic diseases that result from defective alleles passed from parents to offspring. (p. 782)

Nucleic acids   Molecules of DNA and RNA in the nucleus of every cell. DNA makes up the chromosomes and encodes the genes. (p. 782)

Personalized medicine   The use of tools such as molecular-level and genetic characterizations of both disease processes and the patient for the customization of drug therapy. (p. 785)

Pharmacogenetics   A general term for the study of the genetic basis for variations in the body's response to drugs, with a focus on variations related to a single gene. (p. 784)

Pharmacogenomics   A branch of *pharmacogenetics* (see above) that involves the survey of the entire genome to detect multigenic (multiple-gene) determinants of drug response. (p. 785)

Phenotype   The expression in the body of a genetic trait that results from a person's particular genotype for that trait (see *genotype*). (p. 782)

Proteome   The entire set of proteins produced by an organism's genome. (p. 783)

Proteomics   The detailed study of the proteome, including all biologic actions of proteins. (p. 783)

Recombinant DNA (rDNA)   DNA molecules that have been artificially synthesized or modified in a laboratory setting. (p. 784)

INTRODUCTION

Genetic processes are a highly complex part of physiology and are far from being completely understood by scientists. However, genetic research is one of the most active branches of science today, involving many types of health care professionals, including nurses. Expected outcomes of this research include an increasingly deeper knowledge of the genetic influences on disease, along with the development of gene-based therapies. The practice of nursing will also increasingly require an understanding of genetic concepts, health issues, and therapeutic techniques. The goal of this chapter is to introduce some of the major concepts in this very complex and emerging branch of health science. In 1996, the *National Coalition for Health Professional Education in Genetics (NCHPEG)* was founded as a joint project of the American Medical Association, the American Nurses Association, and the National Human Genome Research Institute (www.nchpeg.org). The purpose of NCHPEG is to promote the education of health professionals and the public regarding advances in applied genetics. In February 2005, NCHPEG endorsed a revised set of core competencies for health professionals related to genetics. These guidelines continue to expand and can be viewed on the NCHPEG website at www.nchpeg.org/core/Corecomps2005.pdf. Any practicing nurse may be expected to develop these skills to varying degrees depending on the practice setting and the needs of the presenting patient population.

BASIC PRINCIPLES OF GENETIC INHERITANCE

Nucleic acids are biochemical compounds consisting of molecules of *deoxyribonucleic acid (DNA)* and *ribonucleic acid (RNA)*. It is these DNA molecules that make up the **genetic material** that is passed between all types of organisms during reproduction. In some organisms (e.g., HIV), it is actually the RNA molecules that pass the organism's genetic material between generations; however, this is an exception to the norm. A chromosome is basically a long strand of DNA that is contained in the nuclei of cells. DNA molecules, in turn, act as the template for the formation of RNA molecules, from which proteins are synthesized. Humans normally have 23 pairs of **chromosomes** in each of their *somatic cells*. Somatic cells are all the cells in the body other than the *sex cells* (sperm cells or egg cells), which have only 23 single (unpaired) chromosomes. One pair of chromosomes in each cell is called the *sex chromosomes* and is normally of the form XX for females and XY for males. One member of each pair of chromosomes comes from the father's sperm and one from the mother's egg. **Alleles** are the alternative forms of a **gene** that can vary with regard to a specific genetic trait. Genetic traits can be desirable (e.g., lack of allergies) or undesirable (e.g., predisposition toward a specific disease). Alleles are said to be dominant or recessive. Each person has two alleles for every gene-coded trait: one allele from the mother, the other from the father. The particular combination of alleles, or **genotype,** for a given trait normally determines whether or not a person manifests that trait, or the person's **phenotype.** Genetic traits that are passed on differently to male and female offspring are said to be *sex-linked traits* because they are carried on either the X or Y chromosome. For example, hemophilia genes are carried by females but manifest as a bleeding disorder only in males. This is also an example of an **inherited disease;** that is, a disease passed from parents to offspring due to genetic defects. A more general term is **genetic disease,** which is any disease caused by a genetic mechanism. Note, however, that not all genetic diseases are inherited diseases, because chromosomal abnormalities *(aberrations)* can also occur spontaneously during embryonic development. In contrast, an **acquired disease** is any disease that develops in response to external factors and is not *directly* related to a person's genetic makeup. Genetics can play an indirect role in acquired disease, however. For example, atherosclerotic heart disease is often acquired in mid or later life. Many people have certain genes in their cells that increase the likelihood of this condition. This is known as a **genetic predisposition.** In some cases, as for the example given here, a person may be able to offset his or her genetic predisposition by lifestyle choices, such as healthy diet and exercise to avoid developing heart disease.

DISCOVERY, STRUCTURE, AND FUNCTION OF DNA

A major turning point in the current understanding of **genetics** came in 1953, when Drs. James Watson and Francis Crick first reported the chemical structures of human genetic material and named the primary biochemical compound deoxyribonucleic acid (DNA). They later received a Nobel Prize for their discovery. It is now recognized that DNA is the primary molecule in the body that serves to transfer genes from parents to offspring. It exists in the nucleus of all body cells as strands in chromosomes, collectively called **chromatin.** As described in Chapter 39, DNA molecules contain four different organic bases, each of which has its own alphabetical designation: *adenine (A), guanine (G), thymine (T),* and *cytosine (C).* These bases are linked to a type of sugar molecule known as *deoxyribose.* Finally, these sugar molecules are linked to a "backbone" chain of phosphate molecules, which results in the classic *double-helix* structure of two side-by-side, spiral macromolecular chains. An important related biomolecule is RNA. RNA has a chemical structure similar to that of DNA, except that its sugar molecule is the compound *ribose* instead of deoxyribose and it contains the base *uracil (U)* in place of thymine. RNA more commonly occurs as a single-stranded molecule, although in some genetic processes it can also be double-stranded. In double-stranded nucleic acid structures, the base of each strand binds (via hydrogen bonds) to that of the other strand in the space between the two strands (see Figure 39-3). This binding is based on complementary base pairings determined by the chemistry of the base molecules themselves. Specifically, adenine can only bind with guanine, whereas cytosine can only bind with thymine or uracil.

A *nucleotide* is the structural unit of DNA and consists of a single base and its attached sugar and phosphate molecules. A *nucleoside* is the base and attached sugar without the phosphate molecule. A relatively small sequence of nucleotides is called an *oligonucleotide* (the prefix *oligo-* means "a small number"). Certain new drug therapies involve several synthetic analogues of both nucleosides and nucleotides (Chapters 39, 47, 48, and 58). One of these, the ophthalmic antiviral drug fomivirsen, is an oligonucleotide with a chemical structure that is *opposite* (complementary) to that of a critical part of the messenger RNA (mRNA) of the cytomegalovirus. For this reason it is called an *antisense oligonucleotide,* and it is the first of this new class of drugs. Other types of antisense oligonucleotide drugs are anticipated in the near future as one type of gene therapy but are not yet available in the United States as of this writing. An organism's entire DNA structure is its **genome. Genomics** is the relatively new science of determining the location *(mapping)* and structure (DNA base *sequencing*) of individual genes along the entire genome and identifying their function in both health and disease processes.

Protein Synthesis

Protein synthesis is the primary function of DNA in human cells. In the cell nuclei, the double strands of DNA uncoil and separate, and a strand of mRNA forms on each separate DNA strand through complementary base pairing as described earlier. This process is called *transcription* of the DNA. These mRNA molecules then detach from their corresponding DNA strands, leave the cell nucleus, and enter the cytoplasm, where they are then "read," or *translated,* by the *ribosomes.* Ribosomes are composed of a second type of RNA known as *ribosomal RNA* (rRNA), as well as several accessory proteins. Individual sequences of three bases at a time along the mRNA molecule serve to code for specific amino acid molecules. This translation process involves molecules of a third type of RNA, *transfer RNA* (tRNA). The tRNA molecules transport the corresponding amino acid molecules to the site of ribosomal translation along the mRNA strand in sequence according to the three-base codes

along the mRNA strand. This in turn results in the creation of chains of multiple amino acid molecules *(polypeptide chains),* which are known as protein molecules. The specificity of this code is very important for proper protein synthesis.

There are countless specific amino acid sequences (polypeptides) that result in the synthesis of many thousands of types of protein molecules. Proteins include hormones, enzymes, immunoglobulins, and numerous other biochemical molecules that regulate processes throughout the body. They are involved in both healthy (normal) physiologic processes and the pathophysiologic processes of many diseases. The biomedical literature continues to identify and describe, from both basic scientific and clinical perspectives, many proteins that are part of disease processes. Manipulation of genetic material, as in *gene therapy* (see later), can theoretically modify the synthesis of these proteins and therefore help in the treatment of disease. This emerging science continues to give rise to novel terminology. The entire set of proteins produced by a genome is now known as the **proteome. Proteomics** is the newest genetic science, taking the discovery process one step further than genomics. It is the study of the proteome, including protein expression, modification, localization, and function, as well as the protein-protein interactions that are part of biologic processes. This science is expected to provide new drug therapies in the future.

The Human Genome Project

In the mid-1980s, there was discussion in the United States of a new scientific project that would seek to map the entire DNA sequence (genome) of a human being. This project, officially begun in 1990, was known as the **Human Genome Project (HGP)** and was coordinated by the U.S. Department of Energy (DOE) and the National Institutes of Health (NIH). Sequencing was not expected to be finished until 2005 but was completed ahead of schedule in 2003. The goals of this project were to identify the estimated 30,000 genes in human DNA and to determine the roughly 3 *billion* base pairs that make up human DNA, as well as to develop new tools for genetic data analysis and storage, transfer newly developed technologies to the private sector, and address the inherent ethical, legal, and social issues involved in genetic research and clinical practice.

GENE THERAPY

One result of the availability of information from the HGP is the continued development of various types of **gene therapy.** This therapy involves the treatment or prevention of disease by transferring *exogenous* (foreign) genetic material (DNA or RNA) into the body of an individual. The main driving force of gene therapy research is the ongoing discovery of new details regarding cellular processes, including biochemical processes that occur at the molecular level. In addition, the increased understanding of allelic variation and its role in disease susceptibility can be used to guide attempts at preventive therapy based on a person's genotypic risk factors.

Currently over 300 U.S. Food and Drug Administration (FDA)–approved clinical trials using various gene therapy techniques are in progress. However, to date no gene therapy has received FDA approval for routine treatment of disease. The general goal of gene therapy is to transfer to the patient exogenous genes that will either provide a temporary substitute for, or initiate permanent changes in, the patient's own genetic functioning to treat a given disease. Originally expected to provide treatment primarily for inherited genetic diseases, gene therapy techniques are now being researched for treatment of acquired illnesses such as cancer, cardiovascular diseases, diabetes, infectious diseases, and substance abuse. In the more distant future *in utero* gene therapy may be used to prevent the development of serious diseases as part of prenatal care for the unborn infant.

During gene therapy segments of DNA are usually injected into the patient's body in a process called *gene transfer.* These DNA splices are also known as **recombinant DNA (rDNA)** and must usually be inserted into some kind of vector for the gene transfer process. Current vectors being evaluated by researchers include spherical lipid compounds known as *liposomes,* free DNA splices known as *plasmids,* DNA conjugates in which DNA splices are linked (conjugated) to either protein or gold particles, and various types of viruses. Viruses are the most widely studied rDNA vectors thus far. One commonly used group of viruses is the adenoviruses, which include the human influenza (flu) viruses. If the desired rDNA segment can be inserted into the viral genome, the virus can then be injected into the patient to therapeutically infect human cells. If this planned infectious process is successful, the viral genome will be combined with the human host cell genome and specific proteins will be produced to counter a disease process. Ideally, this would result in a permanent positive physiologic change in the host. However, viruses used in this way can also induce viral disease and be immunogenic in the human host. The proteins produced by such artificial methods can also be immunogenic. Even in the absence of significant virus-induced disease, the positive effects (e.g., supplemented protein synthesis) may only be temporary, and therefore future treatments may be required. As a result, viruses must be carefully chosen and modified in an effort to optimize therapeutic effects while minimizing undesirable adverse effects. The determination of an ideal gene transfer method remains a major challenge for gene therapy researchers. Figure 50-1 provides a clinical example of the potential use of gene therapy.

One indirect form of gene therapy is already well established. It involves the use of rDNA vectors in the laboratory to make recombinant forms of drugs, especially biologic drugs such as hormones, vaccines, antitoxins, and monoclonal antibodies (discussed in previous chapters). One of the most common examples is the use of the *Escherichia coli* bacterial genome to manufacture a recombinant form of human insulin. When the human insulin gene is inserted into the genome of the bacterial cells, the resulting culture artificially generates human insulin on a large scale. Although this insulin must be isolated and purified from its bacterial culture source, the majority of the world's medical insulin supply has been produced by this method for well over a decade.

Regulatory and Ethical Issues Regarding Gene Therapy

Gene therapy research is inherently complex, and this therapy can also carry great risks for its recipients. Research subjects who receive gene therapy often have a life-threatening illness, such as cancer, which may justify the risks involved. However, case reports of patient deaths in gene therapy trials have underscored these risks and raised the awareness of patient safety among researchers. In the 1980s the NIH Recombinant DNA Advisory Committee was assigned responsibility for oversight of gene therapy research

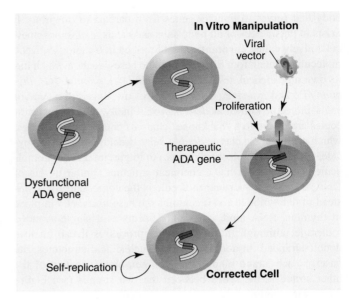

FIGURE 50-1   Gene therapy for adenosine deaminase (ADA) deficiency attempts to correct this immunodeficiency state. The viral vector containing the therapeutic gene is inserted into the patient's lymphocytes. These cells can then make the ADA enzyme. *(From Lewis SM, Heitkemper MM, Dirksen SR: Medical-surgical nursing: assessment and management of clinical problems, ed 6, St Louis, 2004, Mosby.)*

in the United States. It reviews clinical trials involving human gene transfer and schedules public forums to discuss pertinent issues. The FDA must also review and approve all human clinical gene therapy trials, as it does for any type of drug therapy.

Any institution that conducts any type of research involving human subjects must have an institutional review board, whose purpose is to protect research subjects from unnecessary risks. Also required for institutions engaging in gene therapy research is an institutional biosafety committee. The role of this committee is to ensure compliance with the *NIH Guidelines for Research Involving Recombinant DNA Molecules.*

A major ethical issue related to gene therapy techniques is the fear of *eugenics.* Eugenics is the intentional selection before birth of genotypes that are considered more desirable than others. For similar reasons, the prospect of being able to manipulate genes in human *germ cells* (sperm and eggs), even at a preembryonic stage, is also cited as a potential hazard of gene therapy experimentation. Theoretically, even cosmetic modifications could be attempted using such techniques as a part of routine family planning. Because of ethical concerns such as these, U.S. gene therapy research is limited to somatic cells only. Gene therapy in *germ-line* (reproductive) cells is currently illegal in the United States. This limitation remains despite arguments from those who believe that human germ-cell research would likely yield cures for many serious chronic illnesses and disabilities, such as Parkinson's disease and spinal paralysis.

PHARMACOGENOMICS

Pharmacogenetics is the most general term for the study of genetic variations in drug response and focuses on single-gene variations. In addition to gene therapy, a second very important emerging branch of health science that is related to the HGP is **pharmacogenomics.** This is a newer branch of pharmacogenetics and involves working with the whole genome to determine multiple individual genetic factors that influence a person's response to specific medications. For example, a given patient may be more likely to benefit from, or suffer toxicity from, a certain type of drug therapy, depending on the presence or absence of specific alleles in his or her genome. The relationship between the terms *pharmacogenetics* and *pharmacogenomics* can be intuitively difficult to understand, and they are sometimes used interchangeably in the literature.

Such individual differences in alleles are known as **genetic polymorphisms** if the alleles are common enough to occur in at least 1% of the population (i.e., they occur too frequently to be caused by recurrent mutation). Genetic polymorphisms that alter the amount or functioning of drug-metabolizing enzymes can therefore alter the body's reactions to medications. Known examples include genetic polymorphisms that affect the metabolism of certain antimalarial drugs, the antituberculosis drug isoniazid, and drugs that are metabolized by the several subtypes of cytochrome P-450 enzymes. Studying both the genome of the patient and the presenting genetic features of the disease (e.g., tumor cells, infectious organisms) before treatment could theoretically allow customized drug selection and dosing. Such analysis could permit the avoidance of drugs less likely to be effective as well as optimization of drug doses to minimize the risk of adverse drug effects for a given patient. This application of pharmacogenomics is known as **personalized medicine.** Researchers have already developed an analytical tool known as a *high-density microarray.* This technology applies methods used in computer chip manufacture to design amazingly small microchip plates that contain thousands of DNA samples. A patient's blood sample can then be screened for thousands of corresponding DNA sequences (which bind to the sequences on the chip) to determine the presence or absence of various genes, such as those related to drug metabolism. Such technology is currently used primarily in nonclinical research laboratories. However, it is expected within 5 years to become more readily available and affordable for routine use in the clinical setting. With the expanding availability of comprehensive genetic testing, proactive customization of drug therapy is expected to become increasingly more frequent over the next one to two decades. However, it is not yet a part of routine clinical practice. Most drug dosage changes are still usually made on a trial-and-error basis by monitoring patient response. Table 50-1 lists some current clinical applications of pharmacogenomics.

SUMMARY

Increasing scientific understanding of genetic processes is expected to revolutionize modern health care in many ways. The artificial manipulation and transfer of genetic material, although not yet a standard treatment for disease, is the focus of over 300 current human clinical gene therapy trials. The spectrum of diseases that may eventually be treatable by gene therapy includes inherited diseases that are present from birth, disabilities such as paralysis from spinal cord injuries, life-threatening illnesses such as cancer, and even other chronic illnesses acquired later in life for which a person may have a genetic predisposition. The science of pharmacogenomics has already identified some of the genetic nuances in how different individuals' bodies metabolize and experience benefit or harm from drugs. Continued study in this area is expected to result in proactive customization of drug therapy to promote therapeutic benefits while minimizing or eliminating toxic effects. Genetic procedures and therapeutic techniques will likely become an increasing part of nursing practice as well as of health care delivery in general. As the role and impact of genetics and genetically based drug therapy increase, so will their role in the nursing process (Box 50-1).

Table 50-1   Clinical Applications of Pharmacogenomics

Genetic Technique	Application
Genotyping for the presence of CYP2D6 isoenzyme and for the CYP2D6 alleles determining whether patients are poor, intermediate, extensive, or ultrarapid metabolizers with these enzymes (under study)	*Psychiatry* and *general medicine:* helps guide prescribing of selected medications such as anticoagulants, immunosuppressants, antidepressants, antipsychotics, anticonvulsants, β-blockers, and antidysrhythmics
Genotyping for the presence of the *p-glycoprotein* drug transport protein (under study)	*Cardiology, infectious diseases, oncology,* and other practice areas: assists in drug selection and dosing for drugs such as digoxin, antiretrovirals, and antineoplastics
Genotyping for the presence of thiopurine methyltransferase enzyme	*Oncology:* used to temper toxicity through more careful dosing of the cancer drug 6-mercaptopurine in pediatric leukemia patients
Genotyping for variations in β-adrenergic receptors (under study)	*Pulmonology:* Determines which asthma patients are more or less responsive to β-agonist therapy (e.g., albuterol) and which patients might benefit from other types of drug therapy
Genotyping for the presence of the Philadelphia chromosome	*Oncology:* identifies those patients with chronic myelogenous leukemia who can benefit from the cancer drug imatinib (Gleevec)
Genotyping for the presence of the HER2/neu proto-oncogene	*Oncology:* identifies a subset of breast cancer patients whose tumors express this gene, which indicates their suitability for treatment with the cancer drug trastuzumab (Herceptin)
Viral genotyping of hepatitis C viruses (under study)	*Infectious diseases:* can determine whether a particular infection warrants 26 versus 48 weeks of drug therapy (thereby reducing both costs and adverse drug effects)

CYP2D6, Cytochrome P-450 enzyme subtype 2D6.

Box 50-1   Application of Genetics, Genomics, and Pharmacogenomics in Nursing and Health Care

Competencies and outcome criteria for professional nursing practice are well integrated into the goals of various educational programs in nursing. The use of technology in health care is accelerating, and these defined competencies and outcomes must reflect contemporary health care practices; thus, the need for genetics and the knowledge gained through the Human Genome Project to be included in various nursing education programs. The application of human genetics to pharmacology is important to the quality care of patients and in a variety of settings. The nurse must integrate knowledge, skills, and attitudes related to genetics into everyday nursing practice with individuals, groups, and communities. Since the beginning of genetic research and the subsequent definition of core competencies in genetics for health care professionals in early 2001, the world has witnessed a number of advances in genetics and genomics, including completion of the sequencing of the human genome, the use of microarray technology to determine gene expression, the use of genetics in the treatment of selected cancers, the increasing application of pharmacogenomics in the research and development of new drugs, and the application of pharmacogenomics in treatment with drugs that are already in the market. Genetics, genomics, and—specifically with regard to the topic of this textbook—pharmacogenomics promise to transform the nursing care of patients with diseases such as diabetes, can-

cer, and mental illness. Therefore, professional nurses must remain current in their knowledge and skills related to genetics and pharmacogenomics. At some level, nurses may be involved with their patients in research and in new and experimental treatment protocols, and they should always behave in a professional, ethical, compassionate, and sensitive manner. The citations that follow represent just a few readings that relate to the current core competencies in genetics essential for nurses and other health care professionals.

Collins FS, Tabak L: A call for increased education in genetics for dental health professionals, *J Dent Educ* 68(8):807-808, 2004.

Feetham SL, Williams JK: *Nursing and 21st century genetics: leadership for global health,* Geneva, Switzerland, 2004, International Council of Nurses.

Genetics Education Medical School Objectives Project Expert Panel: *Report VI—Contemporary issues in medicine: genetics education,* Washington, DC, 2004, The Association.

Horner SD: A genetics course for advanced clinical nurse practice, *Clin Nurse Spec* 18(4):194-199, 2004.

Montana C, Northey WF: The Human Genome Project: it's all about the family, *Fam Ther Mag* 2(3):12-15, 2003.

Williams JK et al: Advancing genetic nursing knowledge, *Nurs Outlook* 52(2):73-79, 2004.

Data from Prows C: Genetics Summer Institute course, 2002-2004. Available at http://gepn.cchmc.org.

Points to Remember

- Genetic processes are a highly complex facet of human physiology, and genetics is becoming an integral part of health care that holds much promise in the form of new treatments for alterations in health.
- The HGP, spearheaded by the DOE and NIH, described in detail the entire genome of a human individual.

- Basic genetic inheritance begins with 23 pairs of chromosomes in each of the somatic cells; one pair of chromosomes in each cell is called the *sex chromosomes,* identified as XX for females and XY for males.

NCLEX Examination Review Questions

1. An indirect form of gene therapy is most appropriately seen in the creation of which of the following?
   a. Stem cells
   b. Insulin
   c. Antigen substitution
   d. Platelet inhibitors or stimulators
2. Gene therapy may be immunogenic in the human host, and should this occur it would possibly lead to:
   a. Antibody formation
   b. Biologic vaccines
   c. Only a temporary reduction of a disease process
   d. Cure of almost any type of antigen-related disease process
3. The NIH Recombinant DNA Advisory Committee has the responsibility for which of the following?
   a. Approving all forms of clinical gene therapy
   b. Identifying all major risks to the human subjects in a specific research protocol

   c. Reviewing clinical trials involving human gene transfer and scheduling public forums
   d. Analyzing genomes and determining whether they appear mutagenic
4. The presence of certain factors in a person's genetic makeup that increases the likelihood of eventually developing one or more diseases is known as a:
   a. Genetic mutation
   b. Genetic polymorphism
   c. Genetic predisposition
   d. Genotype
5. Which of the following is a commonly studied adenovirus?
   a. Hepatitis A and C
   b. Genovirum
   c. Human influenza
   d. Pallodium

1.b, 2.d, 3.b, 4.c, 5.c.

Critical Thinking Activities

1. An indirect form of gene therapy is already seen in contemporary health care practice. Explain this statement and provide examples.
2. Explain how the use of gene therapy could also be immunogenic. How would this affect patients? Give examples.
3. Analyze the process for producing human insulin and provide a few examples of how this same process could be used in other areas of health care.

For answers, see http://evolve.elsevier.com/Lilley.

Drugs Affecting the Gastrointestinal System and Nutrition

STUDY SKILLS TIPS

- *Active Questioning*
- *What Are the Right Questions?*
- *Kinds of Questions*
- *Questioning Application*

ACTIVE QUESTIONING

There is one technique for study that cannot be overemphasized: active questioning. In the PURR study model, it is critical to be able to generate questions in the Plan, Rehearsal, and Review steps. The questions you generate when applying PURR are essential in helping you maintain concentration as you study, improving your comprehension as you read assigned material, and developing your long-term memory. Active questioning is a strategy that you must practice continuously. It is a strategy that develops with practice.

WHAT ARE THE RIGHT QUESTIONS?

Some questions generated during the Plan step will be useful and will focus on exactly the right issues for maximum learning. On the other hand, sometimes the questions generated by looking at the chapter outline or accented material in the body of the text will be inappropriate. These questions seem logical and important when you are working with the limited amount of information available in the Plan step, but as you read the chap-

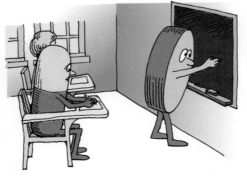

ter you will find that they miss the mark. Do not worry about whether each question you ask is perfectly focused. As you read, rehearse, and review the material, you can and should revise questions based on your growing understanding of the material. The important point is to ask many questions to help you maintain active involvement in the learning process and anticipate questions that will appear on exams. The more questions you ask, the more effective you will become both as an active questioner and as an active learner.

KINDS OF QUESTIONS

First, you must realize that there is more than one kind of question to be asked. Over the years, there have been many questioning hierarchies proposed by educators and scholars. The different kinds of questions vary from three or four to as many as seven or eight. Following is a simple approach that focuses on two types of questions.

Literal Questions

Literal questions are those that are answered directly and specifically by the text. When you were reading a story in elementary school and the teacher asked, "What did Sally do when she lost her movie money?," you were able to answer easily because the question asked for specific information that was stated clearly and directly in the story. If you were reading an American history text and found a topic heading for "The First President," an obvious question would be, "Who was the first president?" The answer is one that would be stated clearly and directly in the body of this topic. These are examples of literal questions. A literal question usually has a single correct response. The answer is stated directly in the text, and every reader will find that same information.

Interpretive Questions

Interpretive questions are more challenging questions that require the reader to interpret, synthesize, evaluate, and analyze the material. Interpretive questions require knowledge of the literal information in addition to understanding the reading material well enough to be able to select several different pieces or bits of data and put them together to formulate a response that demonstrates your understanding. In the American history example about the first president, an interpretive question might be, "Why was George Washington considered to be such an exemplary model as the first president of the new nation?" This question requires that you know not only the literal facts about Washington, but also that you are able to evaluate and judge those facts to reach a conclusion that could be supported by the literal information. Even though a question is interpretive in nature, it is possible that there will be only one correct response. However, it is equally possible that there is more than one correct response to an interpretive question. The literal information can be evaluated in a number of different ways in responding to the question, and the answers derived by different readers will vary. This is why it is a good choice to work with a study group when reviewing for interpretive questions. A study group can develop a variety of responses

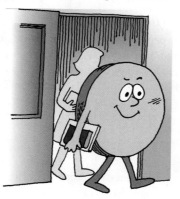

that result in a more comprehensive understanding of the course material. This depth of learning is what is necessary to pass not only your course test but also the NCLEX examination, as well as to become a competent nurse. Both literal and interpretive questions are essential in the learning process.

QUESTIONING APPLICATION

Italicization is used to gain the reader's attention and to indicate that the italicized material is especially noteworthy. Accented material should always be considered as a potential source of questions. Again, we can begin the questioning with simple, literal questions, but it is essential that interpretive questions also be asked. Your questions should require that you read for broader general understanding and not just focus on the "facts."

At the end of each chapter there is a section entitled Critical Thinking Activities. Even though this information is often stated in question form, you should consider generating additional questions of your own. The first question in Chapter 54 is, "Explain why patients with a cardiac history need a baseline ECG and serum calcium assessment performed before initiation of calcium supplemental therapy." In answering this question, some additional questions will help you focus your learning. What is serum calcium? How does calcium affect cardiac patients? Why? Is calcium supplemental therapy inappropriate for all cardiac patients? If not, what are the circumstances that might rule out supplemental calcium? Of what signs and symptoms should the caregiver be aware if calcium supplemental therapy is being administered to a cardiac patient?

The more active you become as a questioner, the easier it will become to ask the kinds of questions that are necessary for your own learning.

Acid-Controlling Drugs

Objectives

When you reach the end of this chapter, you should be able to do the following:

1. Discuss the physiologic influence of various pathologies, such as peptic ulcer disease, gastritis, spastic colon, gastroesophageal reflux disease, and hyperacidic states, on the health of patients and their gastrointestinal tracts.
2. Describe the mechanisms of action, indications, cautions, contraindications, drug interactions, adverse effects, dosages, and routes of administration for the following classes of acid-controlling drugs: antacids, histamine-2 (H_2)–blocking drugs (H_2 antagonists), proton pump inhibitors, and acid suppressants.
3. Develop a nursing care plan that includes all phases of the nursing process related to the administration of acid-controlling drugs.

e-Learning Activities

Companion CD
- NCLEX Review Questions: see questions 407-418
- Animations
- Audio Glossary
- Category Catchers
- Medication Errors Checklists
- IV Therapy Checklists

evolve Website (http://evolve.elsevier.com/Lilley)
- Nursing Care Plans • Frequently Asked Questions • Content Updates • WebLinks • Supplemental Resources • Elsevier ePharmacology Update • Medication Administration Animations

Drug Profiles

antacids, general, p. 794
▶ cimetidine, p. 796
▶ omeprazole, p. 798

misoprostol, p. 798
simethicone, p. 798
▶ sucralfate, p. 798

▶ Key drug.

Glossary

Antacids Basic compounds composed of different combinations of acid-neutralizing ionic salts. (p. 793)

Chief cells Cells in the stomach that secrete the gastric enzyme pepsinogen (a precursor to *pepsin*). (p. 791)

Gastric glands Secretory glands in the stomach containing the following cell types: parietal, chief, mucous, endocrine, and enterochromaffin. (p. 791)

Gastric hyperacidity The overproduction of stomach acid. (p. 790)

Hydrochloric acid (HCl) An acid secreted by the *parietal cells* in the lining of the stomach that maintains the environment of the stomach at a pH of 1 to 4. (p. 790)

Mucous cells Cells whose function in the stomach is to secrete mucus that serves as a protective mucous coat against

the digestive properties of HCl. Also called *surface epithelial cells.* (p. 791)

Parietal cells Cells in the stomach that produce and secrete HCl. These cells are the primary site of action for many of the drugs used to treat acid-related disorders. (p. 791)

Pepsin An enzyme in the stomach that break down proteins. (p. 791)

One of the conditions of the stomach requiring drug therapy is hyperacidity, or excessive acid production. Left untreated, hyperacidity can lead to such serious conditions as acid reflux, ulcer disease, esophageal damage, and even esophageal cancer. Overproduction of stomach acid is also referred to as **gastric hyperacidity.**

ACID-RELATED PATHOPHYSIOLOGY

For a more complete understanding of the large family of drugs used to treat acid-related disorders of the stomach, a brief overview of gastrointestinal (GI) system function and the role of **hydrochloric acid (HCl)** in digestion is beneficial. The stomach secretes several substances with various physiologic functions:

- HCl (an acid that aids digestion and also serves as a barrier to infection)
- Bicarbonate (a base that is a natural mechanism to prevent hyperacidity)
- Pepsinogen (an enzymatic precursor to pepsin, an enzyme that digests dietary proteins)
- Intrinsic factor (a glycoprotein that facilitates gastric absorption of vitamin B_{12})
- Mucus (for protection of the stomach lining from both HCl and digestive enzymes)
- Prostaglandins (PGs) (have a variety of antiinflammatory and protective functions; Chapter 44)

The stomach, although one structure, can be divided into three functional areas. Each area has specific glands with which it is associated. These glands are composed of different cells, and these cells secrete different substances. Figure 51-1 shows the three functional areas of the stomach and the distribution of the associated types of stomach glands.

The three primary types of glands in the stomach are the cardiac, pyloric, and gastric glands. These glands are named for their positions in the stomach. The cardiac glands are located around the cardiac sphincter (also known as the *gastroesophageal sphincter*); the gastric glands are in the fundus, the greater part of the body of the stomach; and the pyloric glands are in the pyloric region and in the transitional area between the pyloric and the fundic zones. The gastric glands are the most numerous and are of primary importance to the discussion of acid-related disorders and drug therapy.

The **gastric glands** are highly specialized secretory glands composed of several different types of cells: parietal, chief, mucous, endocrine, and enterochromaffin. Each cell secretes a specific substance. The three most important cell types are parietal cells, chief cells, and mucous cells. These cells are depicted in Figure 51-1.

Parietal cells produce and secrete HCl. They are the primary site of action for many of the drugs used to treat acid-related disorders. **Chief cells** secrete *pepsinogen*. Pepsinogen is a *proenzyme* (enzyme precursor) that becomes **pepsin** when activated by exposure to acid. Pepsin breaks down proteins and is therefore referred to as a *proteolytic* enzyme. **Mucous cells** are mucus-secreting cells that are also called *surface epithelial cells*. The secreted mucus serves as a protective coating against the digestive action of HCl and digestive enzymes.

These three cell types play an important role in the digestive process. When the balance of these three cells and their secretions is impaired, acid-related diseases can occur. The most harmful of these involve acid *hypersecretion* and include *peptic ulcer disease (PUD)* and *esophageal cancer*. However, the most common condition is mild to moderate hyperacidity. Many lay terms (e.g., indigestion, sour stomach, heartburn, acid stomach) have been used to describe this condition of overproduction of HCl by the parietal cells. Hyperacidity is often associated with *gastroesophageal reflux disease* (GERD). This refers to the tendency of excessive and acidic stomach contents to back up, or *reflux*, into the lower (and even upper) esophagus. Over time this condition can lead to more serious disorders such as *erosive*

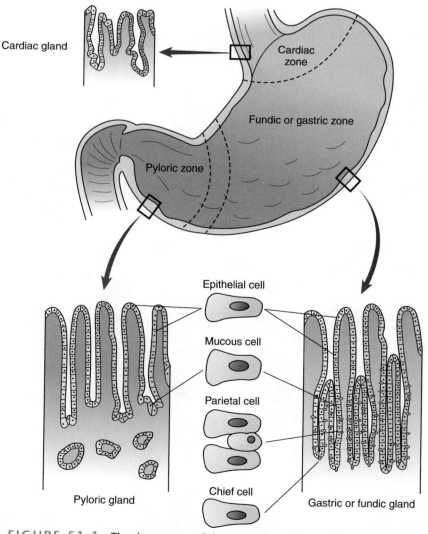

FIGURE 51-1 The three zones of the stomach and the associated glands.

esophagitis and *Barrett's esophagus*, a precancerous condition. Besides patient comfort, this is one of the major reasons for aggressively treating GERD with one or more of the medications described in this section.

HCl is an acid that, as noted earlier, is secreted by the parietal cells in the lining of the stomach. It is the primary substance secreted in the stomach that maintains the environment of the stomach at a pH of 1 to 4. This acidity aids in the proper digestion of food and also serves as one of the body's defenses against microbial infection via the GI tract. Several substances stimulate HCl secretion by the parietal cells, such as food, caffeine, chocolate, and alcohol. In moderation, any of these is usually not problematic. However, excessive consumption of large, fatty meals or alcohol, as well as emotional stress, may result in hyperproduction of HCl from the parietal cells and lead to hypersecretory disorders such as PUD.

As noted earlier, because the parietal cell is the source of HCl production, it is the primary <u>target</u> for many of the most effective drugs for the treatment of acid-related disorders. A closer look at how the parietal cell receives signals to produce and secrete HCl will enhance the understanding of the mechanism of action of many of the drugs used to treat acid-related disorders.

The wall of the parietal cell contains three types of receptors: acetylcholine (ACh), histamine, and gastrin. When any one of these is occupied by its corresponding chemical stimulant (ACh, histamine, or gastrin, which can all be considered *first messengers*), the parietal cell will produce and secrete HCl. Figure 51-2 shows the parietal cell with its three receptors. Once these receptors have become occupied, a *second messenger* is sent inside the cell. In the case of histamine receptors, occupation results in the production of adenylate cyclase. Adenylate cyclase converts adenosine triphosphate (ATP) to cyclic adenosine monophosphate (cAMP), which provides energy for the *proton pump*. The proton pump or, more precisely, the hydrogen–potassium–adenosine triphosphatase pump is a pump for the transport of hydrogen ions and is located in the parietal cells. The pump requires energy to work. If energy is present, the proton pump will be activated, and the pump will be able to transport hydrogen ions needed for the production of HCl.

In the case of both ACh and gastrin receptors on the parietal cell surfaces, the second messenger that drives the proton pump is not cAMP but is instead calcium ions. Anticholinergic drugs (Chapter 20) such as atropine block ACh receptors, which also results in decreased hydrogen ion secretion from the parietal cells. However, these drugs are now uncommonly used for this purpose and have been superseded by other drug classes discussed in this chapter. There is currently no drug to block the

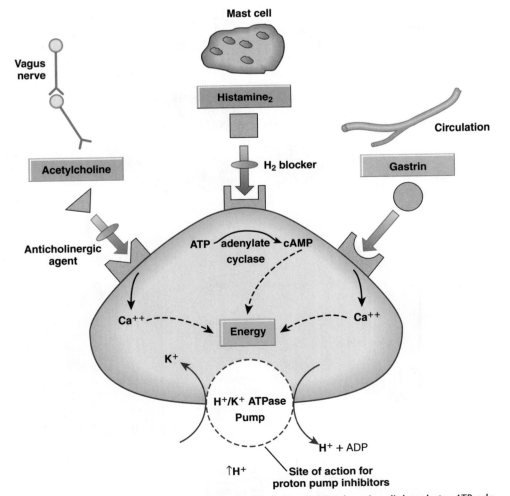

FIGURE 51-2 Parietal cell stimulation and secretion. *ADP,* Adenosine diphosphate; *ATP,* adenosine triphosphate; *ATPase,* adenosine triphosphatase; *cAMP,* cyclic adenosine monophosphate.

binding of the hormone gastrin to its corresponding receptor on the parietal cell surface.

PUD is a general term for gastric or duodenal ulcers that involve digestion of the GI mucosa by the enzyme pepsin, which normally serves to break down only food proteins. As noted earlier, pepsin is the activated form of pepsinogen, which is produced by the chief cells of the stomach in response to HCl released from the parietal cells. Again, the sight, smell, taste, and presence of food in the stomach is the primary stimulus to HCl release from the parietal cells. Because the process of ulceration is driven by the proteolytic (protein breakdown) actions of pepsin together with the caustic effects of HCl, PUD and related problems are also referred to by the more general term *acid-peptic disorders.*

In 1983 a certain gram-negative spiral bacterium, *Campylobacter pylori,* was isolated from several patients with gastritis. Over the next 6 years this bacterium was studied further, and it gradually came to be implicated in the pathophysiology of PUD. At that time the official name of this bacterium was changed to *Helicobacter pylori* because it was felt to have more characteristics of the *Helicobacter* genus. The prevalence of *H. pylori* as measured by serum antibody tests is approximately 40% to 60% for patients older than 60 years of age and only 10% for those younger than 30 years of age. The bacterium is found in the GI tracts of roughly 90% of patients with duodenal ulcers and 70% of those with gastric ulcers. However, this bacterium is also found in many patients who do not have PUD, and its presence is not associated with acute, perforating ulcers. These latter observations suggest that more than one factor is involved in ulceration. Table 51-1 lists standard treatment options for *H. pylori* infection.

Table 51-1	**Current FDA-Approved Regimens for Eradication of *Helicobacter pylori***
Regimen 1	Omeprazole 40 mg daily and clarithromycin (Chapter 37) 500 mg tid × 2 wk, then omeprazole 20 mg daily × 2 wk
Regimen 2	RBC 400 mg bid and clarithromycin 500 mg tid × 2 wk, then RBC 400 mg bid × 2 more wk
Regimen 3	Bismuth subsalicylate (Pepto-Bismol; Chapter 52) 524 mg qid and metronidazole (Chapter 38) 250 mg qid and tetracycline 500 mg qid × 2 wk, plus any H₂ antagonists as directed by physician × 4 wk
Regimen 4	Lansoprazole 30 mg bid and amoxicillin (Chapter 37) 1000 mg and clarithromycin 500 mg tid × 10 days*
Regimen 5	Lansoprazole 30 mg tid and amoxicillin 1000 mg tid × 2 wk†
Regimen 6	RBC 400 mg bid and clarithromycin 500 mg bid × 2 wk, then RBC 400 mg bid × 2 more wk
Regimen 7	Omeprazole 20 mg bid and clarithromycin 500 mg bid and amoxicillin 1000 mg bid × 10 days
Regimen 8	Lansoprazole 30 mg bid and clarithromycin 500 mg bid and amoxicillin 1000 mg bid × 10 days

FDA, Food and Drug Administration; *RBC,* ranitidine bismuth citrate.
*Although not FDA approved, amoxicillin has been substituted for tetracycline in the treatment of patients for whom tetracycline is not recommended.
†This dual-therapy regimen has restrictive labeling. It is indicated either for patients who are intolerant of clarithromycin or those infected with organisms known or suspected to be resistant to clarithromycin.

ANTACIDS

Antacids are basic compounds used to neutralize stomach acid. Most commonly they are nonprescription salts of aluminum, magnesium, calcium, and/or sodium. They have been used for centuries in the treatment of patients with acid-related disorders. The ancient Greeks used crushed coral (calcium carbonate) in the first century AD to treat patients with dyspepsia. Antacids were the principal antiulcer treatment until the introduction of the *histamine-2 (H₂) antagonists* in the late 1970s. For decades before that the classic treatment for acid-related disorders was a combination regimen that included an antacid and an anticholinergic drug such as atropine. H₂ antagonists, proton pump inhibitors, surface-protective drugs, and mucus-inducing PGs have generally replaced the anticholinergics for the treatment of acid-related GI disease. However, the antacids, especially the over-the-counter (OTC) formulations, are still used extensively. They are available in a variety of dosage forms, some including more than one antacid salt. In addition, many antacid preparations also contain the *antiflatulent* (antigas) drug simethicone (see Miscellaneous Acid-Controlling Drugs), which reduces gas and bloating.

Many aluminum- and calcium-based formulations also include magnesium, which contributes to the acid-neutralizing capacity and counteracts the constipating effects of aluminum and calcium. There are multiple salts of calcium. Calcium carbonate is the most commonly used calcium salt when calcium is used as an antacid. It is not prescribed as often as the other antacids because its use may result in kidney stones and increased gastric acid secretion. Sodium bicarbonate is a highly soluble antacid form with a quick onset but a short duration of action.

Mechanism of Action and Drug Effects

Antacids work primarily by neutralizing gastric acidity. They do nothing to prevent the overproduction of acid but instead help to neutralize acid secretions. It is also believed that antacids promote gastric mucosal defensive mechanisms, especially at lower dosages. They do this by stimulating the secretion of mucus, PGs, and bicarbonate from the cells inside the gastric glands. Mucus serves as a protective barrier against the destructive actions of HCl. Bicarbonate helps buffer the acidity of HCl. PGs prevent histamine from binding to its corresponding parietal cell receptors, thereby preventing the production of adenylate cyclase. Without adenylate cyclase, no cAMP is formed and no second messenger is available to activate the proton pump (Figure 51-2).

The primary drug effect of antacids is the reduction of the symptoms associated with various acid-related disorders, such as pain and reflux ("heartburn"). A dose of antacid that raises the gastric pH from 1.3 to 1.6 (only 0.3 point) reduces gastric acidity by 50%; acidity is reduced by 90% if the pH is raised an entire point (e.g., 1.3 to 2.3). Antacid-associated pain reduction is thought to be a result of base-mediated inhibition of the protein-digesting ability of pepsin, increase in the resistance of the stomach lining to irritation, and increase in the tone of the cardiac sphincter, which reduces reflux from the stomach.

Indications

Antacids are indicated for the acute relief of symptoms associated with peptic ulcer, gastritis, gastric hyperacidity, and heartburn.

Contraindications

The only usual contraindication to antacid use is known allergy to a specific drug product. Other contraindications may include severe renal failure or electrolyte disturbances (because of the potential toxic accumulation of electrolytes in the antacids themselves), and GI obstruction (antacids may stimulate GI motility when it is undesirable because of the presence of an obstructive process requiring surgical intervention).

Adverse Effects

The adverse effects of the antacids are limited. The magnesium preparations, especially milk of magnesia, can cause diarrhea. Both the aluminum- and calcium-containing formulations can result in constipation. Calcium products can also cause kidney stones. Excessive use of any antacid can theoretically result in systemic alkalosis. This is more common with sodium bicarbonate. Another adverse effect that is more common with the calcium-containing products is rebound hyperacidity, or acid rebound, in which the patient experiences hyperacidity when antacid use is discontinued. Long-term self-medication with antacids may mask symptoms of serious underlying disease such as bleeding ulcer or malignancy. Patients with ongoing symptoms should undergo regular medical evaluations, because additional medications or other interventions may be needed. Additionally, Box 51-1 lists several specific nursing concerns for patients taking antacids.

Interactions

Antacids are capable of causing several interactions when administered with other drugs. There are four basic mechanisms by which antacids cause these interactions. Understanding these mechanisms enhances the knowledge of interactions involving antacids. These mechanisms are (1) *adsorption* of other drugs to antacids, which reduces the ability of the other drug to be absorbed into the body; (2) chemical inactivation of other drugs by *chelation*, which produces insoluble complexes; (3) *increased stomach pH*, which increases the absorption of basic drugs and decreases the absorption of acidic drugs; and (4) *increased urinary pH*, which increases the excretion of acidic drugs and decreases the excretion of basic drugs. Most drugs are either weak acids or weak bases. Therefore, pH conditions in both the GI and urinary tracts will affect the extent to which drug molecules are ionized (charged). Ionized drug molecules are generally more water soluble and therefore more likely to be excreted (at the kidney) or not absorbed (from the GI tract). Nonionized drug molecules are more likely to be absorbed in the GI tract, because they are usually more fat soluble than their ionized counterparts. This allows them to be better absorbed through the lipid-based cell membranes of the GI tract and ultimately into the bloodstream. Common examples of drugs whose effects may be chemically enhanced by the presence of antacids (due to pH effects) include benzodiazepines, sulfonylureas (may also be reduced, depending on the drugs involved), sympathomimetics, and valproic acid. More commonly, the presence of antacids reduces efficacy of interacting drugs by interfering with their GI absorption. These drugs include allopurinol, tetracycline, thyroid hormones, captopril, corticosteroids, digoxin R, histamine antagonists, phenytoin, isoniazid, ketoconazole, methotrexate, nitrofurantoin, phenothiazines, and salicylates. Patients are advised to dose any interacting drugs at least 2 hours before or after antacids are taken.

Dosages

For information on dosages for selected antacid drugs, see the Dosages table on page 795.

Drug Profiles

Antacids, general

Some of the available aluminum, magnesium, calcium, and sodium salts that are used in many of the antacid formulations are listed in Box 51-2. There are far too many individual antacid products on the market to mention all formulations. Briefly, OTC antacid formulations are available as capsules, chewable tablets, effervescent granules and tablets, powders, suspensions, and plain tablets. This allows patients a variety of options for self-medication. Pharmacokinetic parameters are not normally listed for antacids, but these drugs are generally excreted quickly through the GI tract and/or the electrolyte homeostatic mechanisms of the kidneys. Antacids are generally considered safe for use in pregnancy if prolonged administration and high dosages are avoided. However, it is recommended that pregnant women consult their physicians before taking an antacid. Aluminum- and sodium-based antacids are often recommended for patients with renal compromise, because they are more easily excreted than other antacid categories. Calcium-containing antacids are currently advertised as an extra source of calcium. Calcium carbonate neutralization will produce gas and possibly belching. For this reason, it may be combined with an antiflatulent drug such as simethicone (see Miscellaneous Acid-Controlling Drugs). Magnesium-containing antacids commonly have a laxative effect, and frequent administration of these antacids alone often cannot be tolerated. Both calcium- and magnesium-based antacids are more likely to accumulate to toxic levels in patients with renal disease and are often avoided in this patient group.

Box 51-1 Nursing Concerns for Patients Taking Antacids

Aluminum, used to reduce gastric acid, binds to phosphate and may lead to hypercalcemia. Early hypercalcemia is characterized by constipation, headache, increased thirst, dry mouth, decreased appetite, irritability, and a metallic taste in the mouth. Later signs and symptoms of hypercalcemia include confusion, drowsiness, increase in blood pressure, irregular heart rate, nausea, vomiting, and increased urination. Use of aluminum-based antacids may also produce hypophosphatemia, which is characterized by loss of appetite, malaise, muscle weakness, and/or bone pain. The use of calcium-containing antacids (e.g., calcium carbonate) may lead to *milk-alkali syndrome*, which is associated with headache, anorexia, nausea, vomiting, and unusual tiredness. Use of sodium bicarbonate may lead to metabolic alkalosis if the drug is abused or used over the long term. Alkalosis is manifested by irritability, muscle twitching, numbness and tingling, cyanosis, slow and shallow respirations, headache, thirst, and nausea. Acid rebound occurs with the discontinuation of antacids that have high acid-neutralizing capacity and with overuse or misuse of antacid therapy. If acid neutralization is sudden and high, the result is an immediate elevation in pH to alkalinity and just as rapid a decline in pH to a more acidic state in the gut.

DOSAGES

Selected Antacid Drugs*

Drug (Pregnancy Category)	Pharmacologic Class	Usual Dosage Range	Indications
aluminum hydroxide (Amphojel) (A)	Aluminum-containing antacid	**Adult** PO: 600-1500 mg 3-6×/day	Hyperacidity (often the preferred antacid for use in renally compromised patients)
aluminum hydroxide and magnesium hydroxide (Maalox, Mylanta) (A)	Combination antacid	**Adult** 400-2400 mg 3-6×/day	Hyperacidity
calcium carbonate (Tums) (A)	Calcium-containing antacid	**Adult** PO: 0.5-1.5 g prn	Hyperacidity
magnesium hydroxide (milk of magnesia) (A)	Magnesium-containing antacid	**Adult** PO: 0.65-1.3 g prn, up to qid	Hyperacidity (more commonly used as a laxative)

PO, oral.

*Many more antacid products are available on the market than appear in this table. Dosages given are approximate dosages of active ingredients; there may be variations among different products and different dosage forms of the same product.

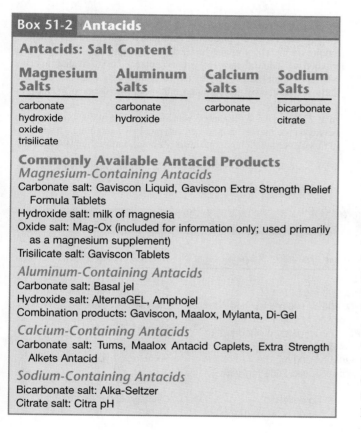

Box 51-2   Antacids

Antacids: Salt Content

Magnesium Salts	Aluminum Salts	Calcium Salts	Sodium Salts
carbonate	carbonate	carbonate	bicarbonate
hydroxide	hydroxide		citrate
oxide			
trisilicate			

Commonly Available Antacid Products

Magnesium-Containing Antacids
Carbonate salt: Gaviscon Liquid, Gaviscon Extra Strength Relief Formula Tablets
Hydroxide salt: milk of magnesia
Oxide salt: Mag-Ox (included for information only; used primarily as a magnesium supplement)
Trisilicate salt: Gaviscon Tablets

Aluminum-Containing Antacids
Carbonate salt: Basal jel
Hydroxide salt: AlternaGEL, Amphojel
Combination products: Gaviscon, Maalox, Mylanta, Di-Gel

Calcium-Containing Antacids
Carbonate salt: Tums, Maalox Antacid Caplets, Extra Strength Alkets Antacid

Sodium-Containing Antacids
Bicarbonate salt: Alka-Seltzer
Citrate salt: Citra pH

H_2 ANTAGONISTS

H_2 antagonists (HAs), also called *H_2 receptor blockers,* are the prototypical acid-secretion antagonists. These drugs reduce but do not abolish stimulated acid secretion. They have become the most popular drugs for the treatment of many acid-related disorders, including PUD. This can be attributed to their efficacy, patient acceptance, and excellent safety profile. These drugs include cimetidine, ranitidine, famotidine, and nizatidine. There is little difference among the four available HAs from the standpoint of efficacy. All are available OTC.

Mechanism of Action and Drug Effects

HAs competitively block the H_2 receptor of acid-producing parietal cells, thus rendering the cells less responsive not only to histamine but also to the stimulation of ACh and gastrin. This is shown in Figure 51-2. Up to 90% inhibition of vagal- and gastrin-stimulated acid secretion occurs when histamine is blocked. However, complete inhibition has not been shown. The drug effect of HAs is reduced hydrogen ion secretion from the parietal cells, which results in an increase in the pH of the stomach and relief of many of the symptoms associated with hyperacidity-related conditions.

Indications

H_2 antagonists have several therapeutic uses, including treatment of GERD, PUD, and erosive esophagitis; adjunct therapy in the control of upper GI tract bleeding; and treatment of pathologic gastric hypersecretory conditions such as *Zollinger-Ellison syndrome.* The latter is one form of *hyperchlorhydria,* or excessive gastric acidity.

Contraindications

The only usual contraindication to the use of H_2 antagonists is a known drug allergy. Liver and or kidney dysfunction are relative contraindications that may warrant dosage. If in doubt, the nurse should review applicable laboratory values and check with the pharmacist.

Adverse Effects

H_2 antagonists have a remarkably low incidence of adverse effects (fewer than 3% of cases). The four available H_2 antagonists are similar in many respects but have some differences in adverse effect profiles. Table 51-2 lists the adverse effects associated with these drugs. Central nervous system adverse effects occur in fewer than 1% of patients taking H_2 antagonists, but are sometimes seen in the elderly in particular, with adverse effects including confusion and disorientation. The nurse should be alert for mental status changes when giving these drugs, especially if they are new to the patient. Cimetidine may induce impotence and gynecomastia. This is the result of cimetidine's inhibition of estradiol metabolism and displacement of dihydrotestosterone from peripheral androgen-binding sites. All four H_2 antagonists may increase the secretion of prolactin from the anterior pituitary.

Interactions

Cimetidine carries a higher risk of drug interactions than the other three HAs, especially in the elderly. These may be of clinical importance. Cimetidine binds enzymes of the hepatic cytochrome P-450 microsomal oxidase system. This is a group of enzymes in the liver that metabolize many different drugs by oxidation. By inhibiting the oxidation of drugs metabolized via this pathway, cimetidine may raise the blood concentrations of these drugs. Ranitidine has only 10% to 20% of the binding action of cimetidine on the P-450 system, and nizatidine and famotidine have essentially no effect. This interaction has little clinical significance for most drugs; problems are more likely to arise with medications having a narrow therapeutic index, such as theophylline, warfarin, lidocaine, and phenytoin. All H_2 antagonists may inhibit the absorption of certain drugs, such as ketoconazole, that require an acidic GI environment for gastric absorption. Smoking has also been shown to decrease the effectiveness of H_2 antagonists. For optimal results, H_2 antagonists should be taken 1 hour before antacids.

Dosages

For dosage information for the H_2 antagonists, see the Dosages table on this page.

Drug Profiles

H_2 antagonists are the prototypical acid-secretion antagonists. These drugs reduce but do not abolish stimulated acid secretion. They are among the most commonly used drugs in the world. This can be attributed to their efficacy, patient acceptance, OTC availability, and overall excellent safety profile. However, this drug class has been partially supplanted by proton pump inhibitors (see the next section).

▸ **cimetidine**

In 1977, cimetidine (Tagamet) was the first drug in this class to be released on the market. It is the prototypical H_2 antagonist. Other drugs in this class now include ranitidine (Zantac), famotidine (Pepcid), and

Table 51-2 H_2 Antagonists: Adverse Effects

Body System	Adverse Effects
Cardiovascular	Hypotension (monitor for this effect with IV administration)
Central nervous	Headache, lethargy, confusion, depression, hallucinations, slurred speech, agitation
Endocrine	Increased prolactin secretion, gynecomastia (with cimetidine)
Gastrointestinal	Diarrhea, nausea, abdominal cramps
Genitourinary	Impotence, increased blood urea nitrogen, creatinine levels
Hepatobiliary	Elevated liver enzyme levels, jaundice
Hematologic	Agranulocytosis, thrombocytopenia, neutropenia, aplastic anemia
Integumentary	Urticaria, rash, alopecia, sweating, flushing, exfoliative dermatitis

DOSAGES

Selected H_2 Antagonists

Drug (Pregnancy Category)	Pharmacologic Class	Usual Dosage Range	Indications
▸cimetidine (Tagamet, Tagamet HB) (B)		**Adult** PO: 200 mg bid	Dyspepsia, heartburn
		PO: 300 or 400 mg qid and hs or 800 mg hs	Ulcers
		PO: 1600 mg/day divided in 2 to 4 doses	GERD
		PO/IM/IV: 300 mg qid and hs; do not exceed 2400 mg/day	Pathologic hypersecretion
famotidine (Pepcid, Pepcid AC) (B)		**Adult** PO: 10 mg daily-bid	Dyspepsia, heartburn
		PO: 40 mg daily hs or 20 mg bid	Ulcers
	H_2 antagonist	PO: 20-160 mg q6h	Pathologic hypersecretion
		IV: 20 mg q12h	
		PO: 20 mg bid	GERD
nizatidine (Axid, Axid AR) (B)		**Adult** PO: 75 mg daily-bid	Dyspepsia, heartburn
		PO: 300 mg hs or 150 mg bid	Ulcers
		PO: 150 mg daily-bid	GERD
		IV: 50 mg q8-12h	Any of the above
ranitidine (Zantac) (B)		**Adult** PO: 75 mg bid	Dyspepsia, heartburn
		PO: 150 mg daily-bid or 300 mg hs	Ulcers
		PO: 150 mg bid	Pathologic hypersecretion, GERD
		PO: 150 mg qid	Erosive esophagitis

GERD, Gastroesophageal reflux disease; *IM,* intramuscular; *IV,* intravenous; *PO,* oral.

nizatidine (Axid). All four drugs are available in oral form, and all except nizatidine are also available in parenteral dosage form.

Pharmacokinetics

Half-Life	Onset	Peak	Duration
PO: 2 hr	PO: 15-60 min	PO: 1-2 hr	PO: 4-5 hr

PROTON PUMP INHIBITORS

The newest drugs introduced for the treatment of acid-related disorders are the *proton pump inhibitors (PPIs)*. These include lansoprazole (Prevacid), omeprazole (Prilosec), rabeprazole (Aciphex), pantoprazole (Protonix), and esomeprazole (Nexium). These drugs are even more powerful than the H_2 antagonists. PPIs bind directly to the hydrogen-potassium-ATPase pump mechanism itself and irreversibly inhibit the action of this enzyme, which results in a total blockage of hydrogen ion secretion from the parietal cells.

Mechanism of Action and Drug Effects

The action of the hydrogen-potassium-ATPase pump is the final step in the acid-secretory process of the parietal cell (see Figure 51-2). If chemical energy is present to run the pump, it will transport hydrogen ions out of the parietal cell, which increases the acid content of the surrounding gastric lumen and lowers the pH. Because hydrogen ions are *protons* (positively charged hydrogen atoms), this ion pump is also called the *proton pump*. PPIs bind irreversibly to the proton pump. The binding of this enzyme prevents the movement of hydrogen ions out of the parietal cell into the stomach and thereby blocks all gastric acid secretion. Although H_2 antagonists may block close to 90% of all acid secretion, PPIs effectively stop over 90% of acid secretion over 24-hours. This makes most patients temporarily *achlorhydric* (without acid). For acid secretion to return to normal after a PPI has been stopped, the parietal cell must synthesize new hydrogen-potassium-ATPase. PPIs are specific for the proton pump. Although there are other proton pumps in the body, hydrogen-potassium-ATPase is structurally and mechanically distinct from other hydrogen-transporting enzymes and appears to exist only in the parietal cell. Thus, the action of PPIs is limited to its effects on gastric acid secretion.

Indications

PPIs are currently indicated as first-line therapy for erosive esophagitis, symptomatic GERD that is poorly responsive to other medical treatment such as therapy with H_2 antagonists, short-term treatment of active duodenal ulcers and active benign gastric ulcers, gastric hypersecretory conditions (e.g., Zollinger-Ellison syndrome), and nonsteroidal antiinflammatory drug (NSAID)–induced ulcers. Long-term therapeutic uses include maintenance of healing of erosive esophagitis and pathologic hypersecretory conditions, including both GERD and Zollinger-Ellison syndrome. Several PPIs may also be given through a nasogastric or percutaneous enterogastric (PEG) tube. This is commonly done to prevent *stress ulcers,* which may be associated with coma or other severely compromising conditions. For example, esomeprazole capsules may be opened, the granules dissolved in 50 mL of water, and given through the tube. Similar tubal administration is also listed by the manufacturer for lansoprazole capsules and omeprazole powder for oral suspension. Consult the drug packaging for drug-specific instructions.

Omeprazole, esomeprazole, and lansoprazole have been approved for the treatment of patients with *H. pylori* infections. Many treatment regimens have emerged to cure *H. pylori*–induced ulcers; these are listed in Table 51-1. *H. pylori* eradication has been shown to reduce the risk of duodenal ulcer recurrence as well. An oral suspension form of omeprazole has also been approved for reduction of the risk of upper GI tract bleeding in critically ill patients.

Contraindications

The only usual contraindication to use of the PPIs is known drug allergy.

Adverse Effects

PPIs are generally well tolerated. The frequency of adverse effects has been similar to that for placebo or H_2 antagonists. There was some early concern that long-term use of PPIs might promote malignant gastric tumors. Such has not been the case, however, and this initial concern has subsided. There are some newer concerns that these drugs may be overprescribed and may predispose patients to GI tract infections because of the reduction of the normal acid-mediated antimicrobial protection.

Interactions

Few drug interactions occur with PPIs. PPIs may increase serum levels of diazepam and phenytoin. There may be an increased chance of bleeding in patients who are taking both a PPI and warfarin. Other possible interactions include interference with ketoconazole, ampicillin, iron salts, and digoxin absorption. Sucralfate may delay absorption of PPIs. The PPI may be given 30 minutes before sucralfate to avoid this interaction.

Dosages

For recommended dosages, see the Dosages table on this page.

DOSAGES

Selected Proton Pump Inhibitors

Drug (Pregnancy Category)	Pharmacologic Class	Usual Dosage Range	Indications
▶omeprazole (Prilosec) (C)	Proton pump inhibitor	**Adult** PO: 20 mg/day for 4-8 wk PO: 60-360 mg/day divided tid	Esophagitis, duodenal ulcer Hypersecretory conditions
pantoprazole (Protonix)	Proton pump inhibitor	**Adult** PO/IV: 40-80 mg/day	GERD

GERD, gastroesophageal reflux disease; *IV*, intravenous; *PO*, oral.

Drug Profiles

▶ **omeprazole**

Omeprazole (Prilosec) was the first drug in this breakthrough class of antisecretory drugs. Omeprazole and rabeprazole are not available in injectable form, unlike the other PPIs. These include lansoprazole (Prevacid), esomeprazole (Nexium), and pantoprazole (Protonix). Orally administered PPIs (and HAs) often work best when taken 30 to 60 minutes before meals.

Pharmacokinetics

Half-Life	Onset	Peak	Duration
PO: 0.5-1 hr	PO: 2 hr*	PO: 5 days	PO: 1-5 days

*50% to 86% acid secretion reduction.

MISCELLANEOUS ACID-CONTROLLING DRUGS

There are a few other acid-controlling drugs that are unique in terms of their mechanisms and other features. These include sucralfate, misoprostol, and simethicone. They are profiled individually in the following paragraphs. Other drugs include bismuth subsalicylate (Pepto-Bismol) and metoclopramide (Chapter 53).

Drug Profiles

▶ **sucralfate**

Sucralfate (Carafate) is a drug used as a mucosal protectant in the treatment of active stress ulcerations and in long-term therapy for PUD. Sucralfate acts locally, not systemically, binding directly to the surface of an ulcer. Sucralfate has as its basic structure a sugar, sucrose. Sulfate and aluminum hydroxide groups are attached to this sugar in the places where there are normally hydroxyl groups. Once sucralfate comes into contact with the acid of the stomach, it begins to dissociate into aluminum hydroxide (an antacid) and sulfate anions. The aluminum salt stimulates secretion of both mucus and bicarbonate base. The sulfated sucrose molecules of sucralfate are attracted to and bind to positively charge tissue proteins at the bases of ulcers and erosions, forming a protective barrier that can be thought of as a liquid bandage. By binding to the exposed proteins of ulcers and erosions, sucralfate also limits the access of pepsin. This enzyme normally breaks down proteins in food but can have the same effect on GI epithelial tissue, either causing ulcers or making them worse. Sucralfate also binds and concentrates *epidermal growth factor,* present in the gastric tissues, which promotes ulcer healing. In addition, the drug also stimulates the gastric secretion of PG molecules, which serve a mucoprotective function. Despite its many beneficial actions, sucralfate has fallen out of common use because its effects are transient and multiple daily dosing (up to four times daily) is therefore needed. It is indicated for stress ulcers, esophageal erosions, and PUD. Sucralfate binds phosphates in the GI tract, it has also been used for this purpose in renal failure patients with hyperphosphatemia. However, the aluminum in the drug can also accumulate to hazardous levels in renal patients. Aluminum toxicity can result in bone disease and encephalopathy. Its use in these patients is a clinical judgment call best made by a nephrologist. The only usual contraindication to sucralfate use is drug allergy. Adverse effects are uncommon but include nausea, constipation, and dry mouth. Only minimal systemic absorption occurs, and the drug is virtually inert. Drug interactions mainly involve physical interference with the absorption of other drugs. This can be alleviated by taking other drugs at least 2 hours ahead of sucralfate. Sucralfate is also best given 1 hour before meals and at bedtime. It is a pregnancy category B drug that is normally dosed at 1 g orally four times daily.

Pharmacokinetics

Half-Life	Onset	Peak	Duration
PO: 6-20 hr	PO: 1 hr	PO: 2-4 hr	PO: 3-6 hr

▶ **misoprostol**

The use of misoprostol (Cytotec), a prostaglandin E analogue, has been shown to effectively reduce the incidence of gastric ulcers in patients taking NSAIDs. PGs have a wide variety of biologic activities. They are thought to inhibit gastric acid secretion. They are also believed to protect the gastric mucosa from injury (*cytoprotective* function), possibly by enhancing the local production of mucus or bicarbonate, by promoting local cell regeneration, and by helping to maintain mucosal blood flow. Use of misoprostol is contraindicated in patients with known drug allergy and in pregnant women (see later). Adverse effects include headache, GI distress, and vaginal bleeding. There are no major drug interactions, although antacids may reduce drug absorption.

Although some studies show that synthetic analogues of PGs promote the healing of duodenal ulcers, they must be used in dosages that usually produce more disturbing adverse effects, such as abdominal cramps and diarrhea. Thus, they are not believed to be as effective as HAs and PPIs for this indication. Misoprostol is also used for its abortifacient properties as discussed in Chapter 33. For this reason, it is a pregnancy category X drug. The usual dosage is 200 mcg four times daily with meals for the duration of NSAID therapy in patients at high risk for ulceration.

Pharmacokinetics

Half-Life	Onset	Peak	Duration
PO: 20-40 min	PO: 2 days	PO: 12 min	PO: 1-2 days

▶ **simethicone**

Simethicone (Mylicon) is used to reduce the discomforts of gastric or intestinal gas (flatulence) and aid in its release via the mouth or rectum. It is therefore classified as an *antiflatulent* drug. Gas commonly appears in the GI tract as a consequence of the swallowing of air as well as normal digestive processes. Gas in the upper GI tract is composed of swallowed air and thus consists largely of nitrogen. It is usually expelled from the body by belching. The composition of flatus, however, is determined largely by the dietary intake of carbohydrates and the metabolic activity of the bacteria in the intestines. These bacteria are anaerobic and cause fermentation with the production of hydrogen (H_2), carbon dioxide (CO_2), and methane (CH_4) gases.

Some foods, including legumes (beans) and cruciferous vegetables (e.g., cauliflower, broccoli), are well known for their gas-producing ability. Gas can also result from disorders such as diverticulitis, dyspepsia (heartburn), peptic ulcers, and spastic or irritable colon, and gaseous distention can occur postoperatively. Simethicone works by altering the elasticity of mucus-coated gas bubbles, which causes them to break into smaller ones. This reduces gas pain and facilitates the expulsion of gas via the mouth or rectum. Simethicone has no listed adverse effects, drug interactions, or pharmacokinetic parameters. It is available only for oral use. In addition, it is available in a combination product with activated charcoal, which also has antigas properties, although it is more commonly used as a GI adsorbent in oral poisonings. The usual simethicone dosage is 1 to 2 tablets four to six times daily as needed. A variety of different products are available for OTC use.

◆ NURSING PROCESS

✦ ASSESSMENT

Before administering an acid-controlling drug, the nurse should assess the patient and gather information regarding the medical history, with attention to GI tract–related illnesses and signs and symptoms of ulcer disease, GERD, and other conditions that have been mentioned earlier. Bowel patterns, any change in bowel patterns or GI tract functioning, and GI tract–related pain should also be assessed and documented. Results of baseline serum chemistry laboratory tests, as ordered, should be assessed with specific attention to hepatic function (e.g., serum alkaline phosphatase level, serum glutamic-oxaloacetic transaminase [aspartate aminotransferase] level, serum glutamic-pyruvic transaminase [alanine aminotransferase] level), as well as renal function (serum creatinine level). Contraindications, cautions, and drug interactions have already been discussed, and a thorough assessment for these should be completed. The knowledge that acid-controlling drugs have many interactions should spark close attention to all medications the patient is taking, thus underscoring the importance of a medication history with questions about prescription drugs, OTCs, and herbals. Other components of assessment include performing a physical examination and taking a thorough cardiac history with close attention to a history of heart failure, hypertension, and/or other cardiac diseases, and the presence of edema, fluid and electrolyte imbalances, or renal disease. One reason it is important to assess for these conditions is that the high sodium content of various antacids may lead to exacerbation of cardiac problems, renal dysfunction, and fluid-electrolyte problems.

When aluminum-containing antacids are taken, all other medications the patient is taking should be identified, and information about cautions and contraindications should be noted. Magnesium-containing antacids and related cautions, contraindications, and drug interactions have also been discussed previously and should be noted. It is important to note that combination products containing both magnesium and aluminum may have fewer adverse effects than either antacid by itself. For example, aluminum-containing antacids are associated with constipation, whereas magnesium-containing antacids lead to diarrhea. The net effect of a combination of these antacids is a balancing out of both adverse effects and fewer problems with altered bowel patterns. Calcium-based antacids may also be used, especially as a source of calcium; however, they carry the risks of rebound hyperacidity, milk-alkali syndrome, and changes in systemic pH, especially if the patient has abnormal renal functioning (see Box 51-1). Sodium bicarbonate is generally not recommended as an antacid because of the high risk for systemic electrolyte disturbances and alkalosis. The sodium content of sodium bicarbonate is high and also very problematic for patients who have hypertension, heart failure, or renal insufficiency.

Patients using H_2 antagonist drugs should be assessed for renal and liver function as well as level of consciousness because of drug-related adverse effects. The elderly are known to react to these drugs with more disorientation and confusion. Drugs such as cimetidine and famotidine should not be administered simultaneously with antacids. These drugs may be spaced 1 hour apart if both drugs need to be given. Patients taking nizatidine or ranitidine require assessment of baseline blood chemistry results with attention to levels of blood urea nitrogen, creatinine, alkaline phosphatase, bilirubin, alanine aminotransferase, and aspartate aminotransferase to document renal and hepatic functioning before treatment is initiated.

For PPIs (e.g., omeprazole, pantoprazole), assessment of swallowing capacity is required because of the size of some of the oral capsules. Assessment of renal and liver function and a complete blood count are also needed before initiation of long-term therapy (see earlier discussion). Drug interactions have been discussed previously in the pharmacology section and the patient's medication list should always be checked before giving this or any other type of medication. Other drugs used by patients with GI disorders include sucralfate and simethicone. The use of simethicone (an antiflatulent) and sucralfate (an ulcer-adherent) require assessment of the patient's bowel patterns and bowel sounds, and evaluation for abdominal distention and rigidity. Treatment of PUD has become focused on the use of antibiotics (to attack the *H. pylori* bacteria) with frequent dosing of other drugs as listed in Table 51-1. Assessment of the GI tract should be performed, and signs and symptoms should be noted.

✦ NURSING DIAGNOSES

- Acute pain related to gastric hyperacidity and other GI disorders such as ulcer disease
- Constipation related to the adverse effects of aluminum-containing antacids and other drugs used to treat hyperacidity
- Diarrhea related to the adverse effects of magnesium-containing antacids and other drugs used to treat hyperacidity
- Deficient knowledge related to lack of information about antacids, H_2 antagonists, or PPIs, including their use and potential adverse effects

✦ PLANNING

Goals

- Patient has minimal to no pain during therapy with antacids or other acid-controlling drugs.
- Patient experiences minimal adverse effects while using antacids or other acid-controlling drugs.
- Patient remains compliant with the therapeutic regimen.

Outcome Criteria

- Patient experiences increased comfort related to the use of these acid-controlling drugs, abdominal massage, application of heat if appropriate, and frequent repositioning.
- Patient states adverse effects of antacids, H_2 antagonists, and PPIs, including constipation, diarrhea, headache, and confusion, and seeks advice from the health care provider if adverse effects worsen or are not relieved after several days.
- Patient states the importance of compliance with the drug regimen and strict adherence to medication instructions regarding the use of acid-controlling drugs to adequately resolve symptoms of the hyperacidity or other GI disorder.

✦ IMPLEMENTATION

When giving acid-controlling drugs, the nurse should always be sure that chewable tablets are chewed thoroughly by the patient and that liquid forms are thoroughly shaken before they are taken. Antacids should be given with at least 8 oz of water to enhance absorption of the antacid in the stomach, except for newer forms that are rapid-dissolve drugs. Should constipation or diarrhea occur with single-component drugs, the nurse should suggest a combination aluminum and magnesium product to the physician and educate the patient about the adverse effects of aluminum-only or magnesium-only products. It is also recommended that antacids be given as ordered but not within 1 to 2 hours of other medications because of the effect of antacids on the absorption of oral medications. This dosing schedule can be implemented safely by the nurse without interrupting safe dosing of the other medications. The dosing will differ if the physician has ordered the drug to be given with antacids. Antacid overuse or misuse, or the rapid discontinuation of antacids with high acid-neutralizing capacity may lead to acid rebound. Therefore, antacids should be used only as prescribed or directed.

Because so many H_2 antagonists and other acid-controlling drugs are now available OTC, it is critical to patient safety that patients be educated regarding proper medication use and administration (see Patient Teaching Tips). For example, cimetidine should be taken with meals, and antacids, if also used, should be taken 1 hour before or after the cimetidine. Intravenous dosing and related mixing and infusing for cimetidine are similar to those described later for intravenous famotidine. Famotidine may be given orally in tablet or suspension form and without regard to meals or food. Famotidine RPD dissolves quickly under the patient's tongue and can be taken without water. Ranitidine should be given as ordered and, if administered with antacids, should be given 1 hour before or after the antacid. Intravenous forms of famotidine or ranitidine should be diluted with appropriate solutions and given within the documented time frame. With IV ranitidine, cardiac irregularities and hypotension may occur with rapid infusion. The nurse should refer to appropriate sources for information on other specific drugs and their intravenous administration. For all these H_2 antagonists, blood pressure readings should be monitored as needed during intravenous infusion because of the risk of hypotension. The patient should continue to be monitored for GI tract bleeding with the diagnosis of ulcers or GI irritation. Blood in the stool or the occurrence of black, tarry stool or hematemesis should be reported. The nurse should also listen to bowel sounds and examine the abdomen to assess for the effectiveness of therapy and to monitor for possible complications.

CASE STUDY

Gastroesophageal Reflux Disease

A 47-year-old attorney has just undergone an endoscopy to rule out gastroesophageal reflux disease (GERD) and gastritis secondary to stress-induced hyperacidity. The physician has prescribed omeprazole (Prilosec) 20 mg once a day and instructed the patient to stop taking so much of the liquid form of antacids.

- What laboratory studies are indicated for patients receiving omeprazole? Explain the significance of these studies. How long is treatment with this proton pump inhibitor (PPI) indicated?
- What is the rationale for the use of PPIs to treat GERD?
- Why are antacids no longer the mainstay of treatment for acid-related gastric ulcers and/or reflux disease?

For answers, see http://evolve.elsevier.com/Lilley.

Lansoprazole oral dosage forms should be given as ordered and with fluids. If the patient has difficulty swallowing these capsules, a capsule may be opened and the granules sprinkled over at least a tablespoon of applesauce, which should be swallowed immediately. The nurse should be sure to monitor for abdominal pain, distention, and abnormal bowel sounds. Omeprazole should be administered before meals, and the capsule should be taken whole and not crushed, opened, or chewed. Omeprazole may also be given with antacids if ordered. Omeprazole and most of the other PPIs are given short term, with specific patient instructions. The nurse should always double-check the names and dosages of these drugs to ensure that they are not confused with similarly named drugs. Pantoprazole may be given orally without crushing or splitting of the tablet form. Intravenous pantoprazole should be given exactly as ordered using the correct dilutional fluids and over the recommended time frame. Simethicone may also be added to the oral medication protocol with PPIs and is usually well tolerated. It is to be taken *after* meals and at bedtime. Tablets should be chewed thoroughly and suspensions shaken well before use. Sucralfate is usually given 1 hour *before* meals and at bedtime. Tablets may be crushed or dissolved in water, if needed. Antacids should be avoided for 30 minutes before or after giving sucralfate. Suggestions for patient education for these drugs are presented in Patient Teaching Tips.

◆ EVALUATION

Therapeutic response to the administration of antacids, H_2 antagonists, PPIs, and other related drugs includes the relief of symptoms associated with peptic ulcer, gastritis, esophagitis, gastric hyperacidity, or hiatal hernia (i.e., decrease in epigastric pain, fullness, and abdominal swelling). Adverse effects for which to monitor include all of those listed for each of the drug categories and range from constipation or diarrhea to nausea, vomiting, abdominal pain, hypotension, and cardiac irregularities. Milk-alkali syndrome, acid rebound, hypercalcemia, and metabolic alkalosis are known complications associated with the various antacids; the patient must also be evaluated for these adverse effects and measures taken to prevent or resolve them. Therapeutic response to all of the drugs in the various categories discussed in this chapter is also measured by evaluating whether the identified goals and outcome criteria have been met.

Patient Teaching Tips

- Patients should not take any other medications within 1 to 2 hours after taking an antacid because of their impact on the absorption of many medications in the stomach.
- Encourage patients to contact the physician immediately if they experience severe or prolonged constipation and/or diarrhea, increase in abdominal pain, abdominal distension, nausea, vomiting, hematemesis, or black tarry stools (a sign of possible GI tract bleeding).
- Inform patients that if they are taking enteric-coated medications, it is important to know that use of antacids may promote premature dissolving of the enteric coating. Enteric coatings are used to diminish the stomach upset caused by irritating medications, and if the coating is destroyed early in the stomach, gastric upset may occur.
- Encourage taking of H_2 antagonists exactly as prescribed, and patients should be informed that smoking decreases the drug's effectiveness. H_2 antagonists should not be taken within 1 hour of

antacids, and the patient should be told that occurrence of a prolonged headache with therapy should be reported to the physician immediately. Patients requiring treatment with these drugs should also be encouraged to avoid aspirin, NSAIDs, alcohol, and/or caffeine because of their ulcerogenic or GI tract–irritating effects.
- Omeprazole and other PPIs should be taken before meals, and inform patients that if taking lansoprazole, the granules may be sprinkled from the capsule in a tablespoon of applesauce if needed. If lansoprazole is taken with sucralfate, it should be taken 30 minutes before the latter drug.
- Patients should follow manufacturer's directions when taking simethicone. Chewable forms must always be chewed thoroughly; liquid preparations should be shaken thoroughly before administration. Patients with gas problems or "flatulence" should be encouraged to avoid problematic foods (e.g., spicy, gas-producing foods) and carbonated beverages.

Patient Teaching Tips—cont'd

- Sucralfate should be taken on an empty stomach, and antacids should be avoided or, if indicated, taken 2 hours before or 1 hour after sucralfate administration. Taking sips of tepid water, keeping fluids nearby, and using sugarless or sour hard candy may help relieve dry mouth.

- For patients taking the drug regimen for the treatment of *H. pylori* infection–PUD, it is important to emphasize the need to take each drug, including the antibiotics, exactly as prescribed and without fail to guarantee success in the treatment. If treatment protocols are not followed appropriately, the condition will reoccur.

Points to Remember

- The stomach secretes many substances (hydrochloric acid, pepsinogen, mucus, bicarbonate, intrinsic factor, and PGs).
- The parietal cell is responsible for the production of acid.
- In acid-related disorders there is an impairment of the balance among the substances secreted by the stomach.
- The most common impairment is hyperacidity, or the overproduction of acid. The most harmful effects are PUD and esophageal cancer. Antacids have been used for centuries and were the mainstays of antiulcer therapy until the 1970s, when other drugs were developed.
- H_2 antagonists are H_2 blockers that bind to and block histamine receptors located on parietal cells. This blockade renders these cells less responsive to stimuli and thus acid secretion. Up to 90% inhibition of acid secretion can be achieved with the H_2 antagonists.
- PPIs block the final step in the acid production pathway, the hydrogen-potassium-ATPase pump, and they block all acid secretion.
- Sucralfate is used for the treatment of PUD and stress-related ulcers. It binds to tissue proteins in the eroded area and prevents exposure of the ulcerated area to stomach acid.

- Misoprostol is a synthetic PG analogue that inhibits gastric acid secretion and is used to prevent NSAID-related ulcers.
- Cautious use of antacids is recommended in patients who have heart failure, hypertension, or other cardiac diseases or who require sodium restriction, especially if the antacid is high in sodium. Other conditions that are cautions to antacid use include fluid imbalances, dehydration, GI tract obstruction, renal disease, and pregnancy.
- Many drug interactions occur with the acid-controlling drugs, primarily because these drugs alter the absorption of other medications in the stomach. Other medications should not be taken within 1 to 2 hours after an antacid is taken. Antacids are sometimes to be avoided when other acid-controlling drugs are taken.
- Magnesium-aluminum combination antacids are used to prevent the adverse effects of constipation and diarrhea. Some of the more serious concerns with antacids include acid rebound, hypercalcemia, milk-alkali syndrome, and metabolic alkalosis.

NCLEX Examination Review Questions

1. A 30-year-old business executive is taking simethicone for excessive flatus associated with diverticulitis. Which best describes the mechanism of action by which simethicone reduces flatus?
   a. It neutralizes gastric pH, thereby preventing gas.
   b. It buffers the effects of pepsin on the gastric wall.
   c. It decreases gastric acid secretion and thereby minimizes flatus.
   d. It causes mucus-coated gas bubbles to break into smaller ones.
2. When evaluating the medication list of a patient who will be starting therapy with an H_2 antagonist, the nurse is aware that which of the following drugs would be most likely to interact with it?
   a. Codeine
   b. Penicillin
   c. Ketoconazole
   d. Acetaminophen
3. Proton pump inhibitors and antacids should not be given simultaneously. The nurse is aware that which of the following will occur if a proton pump inhibitor and an antacid are given simultaneously?
   a. Altered absorption of the antacid
   b. Altered absorption of the proton pump inhibitor

   c. Increased risk of electrolyte imbalance
   d. Enhanced action of the proton pump inhibitor
4. A patient with a history of renal problems is asking for advice about which antacid he should use. The nurse should recommend which of the following?
   a. None—antacids should not be used by patients who have renal problems
   b. Antacids that are aluminum based
   c. Antacids that are calcium based
   d. Antacids that are magnesium based
5. A patient who is taking oral tetracycline complains of heartburn and requests an antacid. The nurse should:
   a. give the tetracycline, but delay the antacid for 1 to 2 hours.
   b. give the antacid, but delay the tetracycline for at least 4 hours.
   c. administer both medications together.
   d. explain that the antacid cannot be given while the patient is taking the tetracycline.

1. d, 2. c, 3. b, 4. b, 5. a.

Critical Thinking Activities

1. What is the purpose of adding simethicone to drugs used to treat GI disorders?
2. Are there any concerns regarding the use of antacids in patients with decreased renal functioning? Explain your answer.

3. Is the following statement true or false? Explain your answer. Antacids coat the stomach and are therefore beneficial to patients with ulcers.

For answers, see http://evolve.elsevier.com/Lilley.

Antidiarrheals and Laxatives

Objectives

When you reach the end of this chapter, you should be able to do the following:

1. Discuss the anatomy and physiology of the gastrointestinal tract, including the process of peristalsis.
2. Identify the various factors affecting bowel elimination and/or bowel patterns.
3. List the various groups of drugs used to treat alterations in bowel elimination, specifically diarrhea and constipation.
4. Discuss the mechanisms of action, indications, cautions, contraindications, drug interactions, dosages, routes of administration, and adverse effects associated with the use of the various antidiarrheal and laxative drugs.
5. Develop a nursing care plan that includes all phases of the nursing process for patients taking antidiarrheals or laxatives.

e-Learning Activities

Companion CD

- NCLEX Review Questions: see questions 419-424
- Animations
- Audio Glossary
- Category Catchers
- Medication Errors Checklists
- IV Therapy Checklists

evolve Website (http://evolve.elsevier.com/Lilley)

- Nursing Care Plans • Frequently Asked Questions
- Content Updates • WebLinks • Supplemental Resources
- Elsevier ePharmacology Update • Medication Administration Animations

Drug Profiles

belladonna alkaloid
  combinations, p. 804
bismuth subsalicylate, p. 804
▶ diphenoxylate with atropine,
  p. 805
▶ docusate salts, p. 808
▶ glycerin, p. 808
Lactobacillus acidophilus, p. 806
▶ lactulose, p. 808

▶ loperamide, p. 805
magnesium salts, p. 810
methylcellulose, p. 808
mineral oil, p. 808
polyethylene glycol #3350,
  p. 810
▶ psyllium, p. 808
▶ senna, p. 810

▶ Key drug.

Glossary

Antidiarrheal drugs Drugs that counter or combat diarrhea. (p. 803)

Constipation A condition of abnormally infrequent and difficult passage of feces through the lower gastrointestinal tract. (p. 806)

Diarrhea The abnormal frequent passage of loose stools. (p. 802)

Irritable bowel syndrome (IBS) A recurring condition of the intestinal tract characterized by bloating, flatulence, and often periods of diarrhea that alternate with periods of constipation. (p. 810)

Laxatives Drugs that promote bowel evacuation, such as by increasing the bulk of the feces, softening the stool, or lubricating the intestinal wall. (p. 806)

Diarrhea and the diseases with which it is commonly associated account for 5 to 8 million deaths per year in infants and small children and are among the leading causes of death and morbidity in underdeveloped nations. Diarrheal disorders also have a financial impact on our own society. The costs of outpatient expenses and the loss of time from work because of acute infectious diarrhea have been estimated to total $23 billion per year, or $106 per person, in the United States. The key symptoms of gastrointestinal (GI) disease are abdominal pain, nausea and/or vomiting, and diarrhea. **Diarrhea** is defined as the abnormal passage of stools with increased frequency, fluidity, and weight, or with increased stool water excretion. *Acute diarrhea* refers to diarrhea of sudden onset in a previously healthy individual. It lasts from 3 days to 2 weeks and is self-limiting, resolving without sequelae. *Chronic diarrhea* lasts for longer than 3 to 4 weeks and is associated with recurrent passage of diarrheal stools, possible fever, loss of appetite, nausea, vomiting, weight reduction, and chronic weakness.

The probable cause of diarrhea should be taken into consideration when designing a drug regimen to treat it. Causes of acute diarrhea include drugs, bacteria, viruses, nutritional factors, and protozoa. Causes of chronic diarrhea include tumors, acquired immunodeficiency syndrome (AIDS), diabetes mellitus, hyperthyroidism, Addison's disease, and irritable bowel syndrome. Treatment is directed at the cessation of the increased stool frequency associated with diarrhea, alleviation of abdominal cramps, fluid resuscitation and electrolyte replacement, and prevention of weight loss and nutritional deficits from malabsorption.

ANTIDIARRHEALS

The drugs used to treat diarrhea are called **antidiarrheal drugs.** They are divided into different groups based on the specific mechanism of action: *adsorbents, antimotility drugs* (anticholinergics and opiates), and *intestinal flora modifiers* (also known as *probiotics* and *bacterial replacement drugs*). The specific classes and the drugs in each are listed in Table 52-1.

Mechanism of Action and Drug Effects

Antidiarrheal drugs have varying mechanisms of action. Having some familiarity with these gives the nurse greater insight into the treatment needs and responses of a given patient. *Adsorbents* act by coating the walls of the GI tract. They bind the causative bacteria or toxin to their adsorbent surface for elimination from the body through the stool. *Adsorption* is similar to absorption but differs in that it involves the chemical binding of substances (e.g., ions, bacterial toxins) onto the *surface of* an adsorbent. In contrast, *absorption* generally refers to the penetration of a substance into the *interior* structure of the absorbant or the uptake of a substance across a surface (e.g., the absorption of dietary nutrients into the intestinal villi). The adsorbent bismuth subsalicylate is a form of aspirin, or acetylsalicylic acid, and therefore it also has many of the same drug effects as aspirin (Chapter 44). Activated charcoal is not only helpful in coating the walls of the GI tract and adsorbing bacteria, but it is also useful in cases of overdose because of its drug-binding properties. The antilipemic drugs colestipol and cholestyramine (Chapter 28) are anion exchange resins that are sometimes prescribed as antidiarrheal adsorbents and lipid-lowering drugs. Besides binding to diarrhea-causing toxins, they have the additional benefit of decreasing cholesterol levels.

Anticholinergic drugs work to slow peristalsis by reducing the rhythmic contractions and smooth muscle tone of the GI tract. They are often used in combination with adsorbents and opiates (see later). Anticholinergics are discussed in detail in Chapter 20.

Intestinal flora modifiers are products obtained from bacterial cultures, most commonly *Lactobacillus* organisms. These make up the majority of the body's normal bacterial flora and are the organisms that are most commonly destroyed by antibiotics. Intestinal flora modifiers work by exogenously replenishing these bacteria, which helps to restore the balance of normal flora and suppress the growth of diarrhea-causing bacteria.

The primary action of *opiates* (Chapter 10) in diarrhea treatment is to reduce bowel motility. A secondary effect that make

opiates beneficial in the treatment of diarrhea is reduction of the pain associated with diarrhea by relief of rectal spasms. Because they increase the transit time of food through the GI tract, they permit longer contact of the intestinal contents with the absorptive surface of the bowel, which increases the absorption of water, electrolytes, and other nutrients from the bowel and reduces stool frequency and net volume.

Indications

Antidiarrheal drugs are indicated for the treatment of diarrhea of various types and levels of severity. Adsorbents are more likely to be used in milder cases, whereas anticholinergics and opiates tend to be used in more severe cases. Intestinal flora modifiers are often helpful in patients with antibiotic-induced diarrhea.

Contraindications

Contraindications to the use of antidiarrheals include known drug allergy and any major acute GI condition, such as intestinal obstruction or colitis, unless prescribed by the patient's physician after careful consideration of the specific case.

Adverse Effects

The adverse effects of the antidiarrheals are specific to each drug family. Most of these potential effects are minor and are not life threatening. The major adverse effects of specific drugs in each drug class are listed in Table 52-2. Intestinal flora modifiers do not have any listed adverse effects.

Interactions

Many drugs are absorbed from the intestines into the bloodstream, where they are delivered to their respective sites of action. A number of the antidiarrheals have the potential to alter this normal process, by either increasing or decreasing the absorption of these other drugs.

The adsorbents can decrease the effectiveness of many drugs when given concurrently, primarily by decreasing the absorption of these drugs. Examples include digoxin, clindamycin, quinidine, probenecid, and hypoglycemic drugs. Oral anticoagulants are more likely to cause increased bleeding times or bruising when they are coadministered with adsorbents. This is thought to be primarily because the adsorbents may bind to vitamin K, which is needed to make certain clotting factors. Vitamin K is synthesized by the normal bacterial flora in the bowel. In addition, the toxic effects of methotrexate are more likely to occur when it is given with adsorbents.

The therapeutic effects of the anticholinergic antidiarrheals can be decreased by coadministration with antacids. Amantadine, tricyclic antidepressants, monoamine oxidase inhibitors, opiates, and antihistamines, when given with anticholinergics, can result in increased anticholinergic effects. The opiate antidiarrheals have additive central nervous system (CNS) depressant effects if they are given with CNS depressants, alcohol, narcotics, sedatives-hypnotics, antipsychotics, or skeletal muscle relaxants.

Bismuth subsalicylate can lead to increased bleeding times and bruising when administered with oral anticoagulants as well as aspirin and other NSAIDs. It can also cause confusion in the elderly. Cholestyramine, when administered with glipizide, can result in decreased hypoglycemic effects.

Table 52-1	Antidiarrheals: Drug Categories and Selected Drugs	
Category	**Antidiarrheal Drugs**
Adsorbents	activated charcoal, aluminum hydroxide, attapulgite, bismuth subsalicylate, cholestyramine, kaolin-pectin, polycarbophil
Anticholinergics	atropine, hyoscyamine, hyoscine
Opiates	opium tincture, paregoric, codeine, diphenoxylate, loperamide
Intestinal flora modifiers	*Lactobacillus acidophilus*

Table 52-2 Selected Antidiarrheals: Adverse Effects

Drug	Body System	Adverse Effects
Adsorbents		
bismuth subsalicylate	Hematologic	Increased bleeding time
	Gastrointestinal	Constipation, dark stools
	Central nervous	Confusion, twitching
	Other	Hearing loss, tinnitus, metallic taste, blue gums
Anticholinergics		
atropine, hyoscyamine, hyoscine	Genitourinary	Urinary retention and hesitancy, impotence
	Central nervous	Headache, dizziness, confusion, anxiety, drowsiness
	Cardiovascular	Hypotension, hypertension, bradycardia, tachycardia
	Integumentary	Dry skin, rash, flushing
	Eye, ear, nose, throat	Blurred vision, photophobia, increased pressure in the eye
Opiates		
codeine	Central nervous	Drowsiness, sedation, dizziness, lethargy
	Gastrointestinal	Nausea, vomiting, anorexia, constipation
	Respiratory	Respiratory depression
	Cardiovascular	Bradycardia, palpitations, hypotension
	Genitourinary	Urinary retention
	Integumentary	Flushing, rash, urticaria

Life Span Considerations: The Pediatric Patient

Antidiarrheal Preparations

- Always check with the physician before administering antidiarrheal preparations to a child at home and report the symptoms in case further assessment or medical management is needed. If diarrhea is accompanied by fever, malaise, or abdominal pain, contact the physician immediately because of the possibility of excessive fluid and electrolyte loss. Dehydration and electrolyte loss occur very rapidly in the pediatric patient because of the patient's size and sensitivity to loss of fluid volume and electrolytes through the stool.
- Always contact the physician or pharmacist for the proper dosage of antidiarrheals if the child is 6 years of age or younger or if there is any doubt as to proper dosing. Never hesitate to contact the physician, pediatrician, or nurse practitioner with any concern or question regarding any medication recommended for the pediatric patient.
- Bismuth subsalicylate (Pepto-Bismol, Kaopectate) is a salicylate by chemical structure; therefore, it should be used with caution in children and teenagers because of the risk of Reye's syndrome.
- Immediately report to the physician abdominal distention, firm abdomen, painful abdomen, and worsening of or no improvement in diarrhea 24 to 48 hours after medication administration. Measurement of the amount of diarrhea by the number of soiled diapers or number of stools per day provides important information.
- Antidiarrheal preparations should always be given cautiously to the pediatric patient. If symptoms persist or dehydration occurs (e.g., no tears and decreased urine output in the child), contact the physician.
- If the patient is sluggish, lethargic, or confused or the diarrhea is bloody, contact the physician immediately or go to the closest emergency facility.

Dosages

For the recommended dosages of antidiarrheal drugs, see the Dosages table on page 805.

Drug Profiles

Drug therapy for diarrhea depends on the specific cause of the diarrhea (if known) and the antidiarrheal drug that will best combat it. All antidiarrheals are orally administered drugs available as suspensions, tablets, or capsules. Some antidiarrheals are over-the-counter (OTC) medications, whereas others require a prescription.

Adsorbents

bismuth subsalicylate

Bismuth subsalicylate (Pepto-Bismol, Kaopectate) is a salicylate by chemical structure; therefore, it should be used with caution in children and teenagers who have or are recovering from chickenpox or influenza because of the risk of Reye's syndrome (see Life Span Considerations: The Pediatric Patient box). It can also cause all of the adverse effects and adverse effects that are associated with an aspirin-based product. Two alarming but harmless adverse effects are temporary darkening of the tongue and/or stool. Bismuth subsalicylate is available OTC for oral use.

Pharmacokinetics

Half-Life	Onset	Peak	Duration
24-33 hr*	0.5-2 hr	2-5 hr	Variable

Anticholinergics

The anticholinergics atropine, hyoscyamine, and hyoscine are used either alone or in combination with other antidiarrheals because they slow GI tract motility. These drugs are commonly referred to as belladonna alkaloids and are discussed in Chapter 20. Their safety margin is not as wide as that of many of the other antidiarrheals because they can cause serious adverse effects if used inappropriately. For this reason they are available only by prescription.

belladonna alkaloid combinations

Belladonna alkaloids are used to treat many GI disorders, including diarrhea. Of the belladonna alkaloid combination products, Donnatal is the most commonly used. Use of the belladonna alkaloid preparations is contraindicated in patients who have shown a hy-

DOSAGES

Selected Antidiarrheal Drugs

Drug (Pregnancy Category)	Pharmacologic Class	Usual Dosage Range	Indications
belladonna alkaloids/phenobarbital combinations (Donnatal elixir, Donnatal capsules and tablets, Donnatal extentabs) (C to X)	Fixed-combination anticholinergic	**Adult** PO: Donnatal Elixir, 5-10 mL tid-qid 2 caps or tabs tid-qid PO: Donnatal Extentabs, 1 tab q12h	Diarrhea
bismuth subsalicylate (Pepto-Bismol) (D)	Antimicrobial, antidiarrheal	Doses repeated q30-60 min, not to exceed 8/day; all doses PO **Pediatric 3-5 yr** 5 mL or ⅓ tab **Pediatric 6-9 yr** 10 mL or ⅔ tab **Pediatric 10-12 yr** 15 mL or 1 tab	Diarrhea
Lactobacillus acidophilus (Bacid, Lactinex) (A)	Intestinal flora modifier	**Adult** PO (Bacid): 2 caps bid-qid PO (Lactinex): 1 packet granules with liquids or food tid-qid; 4 tabs tid-qid with liquid or food	Dietary supplementation,* diarrhea, need for bacterial replacement
loperamide (Imodium A-D, Pepto Diarrhea Control) (B)	Opiate antidiarrheal	**Pediatric 2-5 yr** PO: 1 mg tid (liquid only) **Pediatric 6-8 yr** PO: 2 mg bid **Pediatric 9-12 yr** PO: 2 mg tid **Adult** PO: 4 mg followed by 2 mg after each BM (not to exceed 16 mg/day)	Diarrhea

BM, Bowel movement; *PO,* oral.

*Often used to treat uncomplicated diarrhea, although this is an off-label (non–U.S. Food and Drug Administration approved) use.

persensitivity to anticholinergics and in patients with narrow-angle glaucoma, GI obstruction, myasthenia gravis, paralytic ileus, and toxic megacolon. Donnatal tablets contain a combination of four different alkaloids: atropine (0.0194 mg), hyoscyamine (0.1037 mg), phenobarbital (16.2 mg), and scopolamine (0.0065 mg). Available dosage forms of this combination include elixir, tablets, and extended-release tablets. Donnatal Extentabs contain 48.6 mg of phenobarbital and increased amounts of the other three alkaloids. Pregnancy category C to X, depending on the ingredients of the specific product.

Pharmacokinetics

Half-Life	Onset	Peak	Duration
Unknown	1-2 hr*	2-3 hr*	6-8 hr*

*Anticholinergic effects.

Opiates

There are five opiate-related antidiarrheal drugs: codeine, diphenoxylate with atropine, loperamide, paregoric, and tincture of opium. The only opiate-related antidiarrheal that is available as an OTC medication is loperamide; all others are prescription-only drugs because of the risks of respiratory depression and dependency associated with opiate use.

▸ diphenoxylate with atropine

Diphenoxylate (Logene, Lomanate, Lonox, Lomotil) is a synthetic opiate agonist that is structurally related to meperidine. It acts on smooth muscle of the intestinal tract, inhibiting GI motility and excessive GI propulsion. It has little or no analgesic activity. Diphenoxylate is combined with subtherapeutic quantities of atropine to discourage recreational opiate drug use. The amount of atropine present in the combination is too small to interfere with the conju-

gated diphenoxylate. When taken in large dosages, however, the combination results in extreme anticholinergic effects (e.g., dry mouth, abdominal pain, tachycardia, blurred vision).

Use of the combination of diphenoxylate and atropine is contraindicated in patients experiencing diarrhea associated with pseudomembranous colitis or toxigenic bacteria, because the drug's anticholinergic effects might be problematic in such conditions. This drug product is available only for oral use.

Pharmacokinetics*

Half-Life	Onset	Peak	Duration
2.5-4 hr	40-60 min	2-3 hr	3-4 hr

*Diphenoxylate component.

▸ loperamide

Loperamide (Imodium A-D) is a synthetic antidiarrheal that is similar to diphenoxylate. It inhibits both peristalsis in the intestinal wall and intestinal secretion, thereby decreasing the number of stools and their water content. Although the drug exhibits many characteristics of the opiate class, physical dependence on loperamide has not been reported. Because of its safety profile it is the only opiate antidiarrheal drug that is available as an OTC medication (as the oral liquid); the 2-mg capsule form still requires a prescription. Loperamide use is contraindicated in patients with severe ulcerative colitis, pseudomembranous colitis, and acute diarrhea associated with *Escherichia coli*.

Pharmacokinetics

Half-Life	Onset	Peak	Duration
7-15 hr	1-3 hr	4 hr	40-50 hr

Intestinal Flora Modifiers

Intestinal flora modifiers suppress the growth of diarrhea-causing bacteria and reestablish the flora that normally reside in the intestine. They are bacterial cultures of *Lactobacillus* organisms.

Lactobacillus acidophilus

Lactobacillus acidophilus (Bacid, Lactinex, Kala) is an acid-producing bacteria prepared in a concentrated, dried culture for oral administration. It is a normal inhabitant of the GI tract where, through the fermentation of carbohydrates (which produces lactic acid), it creates an unfavorable environment for the overgrowth of harmful fungi and bacteria. *L. acidophilus* has been used for more than 75 years for the treatment of uncomplicated diarrhea, particularly that caused by antibiotic therapy that destroys normal intestinal flora.

LAXATIVES

Laxatives are used for the treatment of **constipation,** which is defined as the abnormally infrequent and difficult passage of feces through the lower GI tract. Individuals may complain of constipation if they think they defecate too infrequently or with too much effort, if their stools are too hard or too small, if defecation is painful, or if they have a sense of incomplete evacuation. Constipation is a symptom, not a disease; it is a disorder of movement through the colon and/or rectum that can be caused by a variety of diseases or drugs. Some of the more common causes of constipation are noted in Table 52-3.

The GI tract is responsible for the digestive process, which involves (1) ingestion of dietary intake, (2) digestion of dietary intake into basic nutrients, (3) absorption of basic nutrients, and (4) storage and removal of fecal material via defecation.

Ingestion → Digestion → Absorption → Storage and removal

The usual time span between ingestion and defecation is 24 to 36 hours. The last segment of the GI tract, the large intestine (colon), is responsible for (1) forming the stool by removing excess water from the fecal material, (2) temporarily storing the stool until defecation, and (3) extracting essential vitamins from the intestinal bacteria (especially vitamin K).

The colon is 120 to 150 cm long and is separated from the small intestine by the ileocecal valve. The colon extends into the rectum, which terminates at the anus. The rectum is the temporary storage site for the stool, which is composed of water and unabsorbed and indigestible material. Evacuation of the rectal contents is accomplished by bowel movements.

A bowel movement (defecation) is a reflex act that involves both smooth and skeletal muscles. The entry of feces into the rectum stimulates mass peristaltic movement that results in a bowel movement. However, voluntary initiation or inhibition of defecation is also possible via skeletal muscle pathways.

Treatment of constipation must involve an understanding of the whole patient, with special attention given to the underlying causes of the constipation. Treatment should be individualized, taking into consideration the patient's age, concerns, and expectations; duration and severity of constipation; and potential contributing factors. Treatment can be either surgical (in extreme cases) or nonsurgical. Nonsurgical treatments can be separated into three broad approaches: dietary (e.g., fiber supplementation), behavioral (e.g., increased physical activity), and pharmacologic. The focus in this chapter is on pharmacologic treatment.

Laxatives are among the most misused OTC medications. Chronic and often inappropriate use of laxatives may result in laxative dependence, produce damage to the bowel, or lead to previously nonexistent intestinal problems. With the exception of the bulk-forming type, laxatives should not be used for long periods. Laxatives are divided into five major groups based on their mechanism of action: bulk-forming, emollient, hyperosmotic, saline, and stimulant laxatives. Table 52-4 lists the currently available laxative drugs by the respective drug family.

Mechanism of Action and Drug Effects

All laxatives promote bowel movements, but each class of laxative has a different mechanism of action. Laxatives may act by (1) affecting fecal consistency, (2) increasing fecal movement through the colon, and/or (3) facilitating defecation through the rectum. *Bulk-forming laxatives* act in a manner similar to that of the fiber naturally contained in the diet. They absorb water into the intestine, which increases bulk and distends the bowel to initiate reflex bowel activity, thus promoting a bowel movement.

Emollient laxatives are also referred to as stool softeners (docusate salts) and lubricant laxatives (mineral oil). Fecal softeners work by lowering the surface tension of GI fluids, so that more water and

Table 52-3	Causes of Constipation
Cause	**Examples**
Adverse drug effects	Analgesics, anticholinergics, iron supplements, aluminum antacids, calcium antacids, opiates, calcium channel blockers, vinca alkaloids
Lifestyle	Poor bowel movement habits: voluntary refusal to defecate resulting in constipation Diet: poor fluid intake and/or low-residue (low-roughage) diet or excessive consumption of dairy products Physical inactivity: lack of proper exercise, especially in elderly individuals Psychologic factors: anxiety, stress, hypochondria
Metabolic and endocrine disorders	Diabetes mellitus, hypothyroidism, pregnancy, hypercalcemia, hypokalemia
Neurogenic disorders	Autonomic neuropathy, intestinal pseudo-obstruction, multiple sclerosis, spinal cord lesions, Parkinson's disease, stroke

Table 52-4	Laxatives: Drug Categories and Selected Drugs
Category	**Laxative Drugs**
Bulk forming	psyllium, polycarbophil, methylcellulose
Emollient	docusate salts, mineral oil
Hyperosmotic	polyethylene glycol, lactulose, sorbitol, glycerin
Saline	magnesium hydroxide, magnesium sulfate, magnesium phosphate, magnesium citrate, sodium phosphate
Stimulant	caster oil, senna, anthraquinones

Table 52-5	Laxatives: Drug Effects					
Drug Effect	**Bulk**	**Emollient**	**Hyperosmotic**	**Saline**	**Stimulant**
Increases peristalsis	Y	Y	Y	Y	Y
Causes increased secretion of water and electrolytes in small bowel	Y	Y	N	Y	Y
Inhibits absorption of water in small bowel	Y	Y	N	Y	Y
Increases wall permeability in small bowel	N	Y	N	N	Y
Acts only in large bowel	N	N	Y	N	N
Increases water in fecal mass	Y	Y	Y	Y	Y
Softens fecal mass	Y	Y	Y	Y	Y

fat are absorbed into the stool and the intestines. The lubricant type of emollient laxatives works by lubricating the fecal material and the intestinal wall and preventing absorption of water from the intestines. Instead of being absorbed, this water in the bowel softens and expands the stool. This promotes bowel distension and reflex peristaltic actions, which ultimately lead to defecation.

Hyperosmotic laxatives work by increasing fecal water content, which results in distention, increased peristalsis, and evacuation. Their site of action is limited to the large intestine. *Saline laxatives* increase osmotic pressure in the small intestine by inhibiting water absorption and increasing both water and electrolyte (salt) secretions from the bowel wall into the bowel lumen. This results in a watery stool. The increased distention promotes peristalsis and evacuation. Rectal enemas of sodium phosphate, a saline laxative, produce defecation 2 to 5 minutes after administration.

As the name implies, *stimulant laxatives* stimulate the nerves that innervate the intestines, which results in increased peristalsis. They also increase fluid in the colon, which increases bulk and softens the stool. Table 52-5 summarizes the specific drug effects of the different classes of laxatives.

Indications

The various therapeutic uses of laxatives range from common constipation to bowel preparation before surgery. The therapeutic effects vary by category. Laxatives are helpful in relieving constipation, in preparing for some medical procedures, and in removing unwanted substances from the body. The following are some of the more common uses of laxatives:

- Removal of intestinal parasites
- Facilitation of bowel movements in patients with inactive colon
- Reduction of ammonia absorption in hepatic encephalopathic conditions (lactulose only)
- Treatment of drug-induced constipation
- Treatment of constipation associated with pregnancy and/or postobstetric period
- Treatment of constipation caused by reduced physical activity
- Removal of toxic substances from the body
- Treatment of constipation associated with poor dietary habits
- Facilitation of defecation in megacolon
- Preparation for colonic diagnostic procedures or surgery
- Facilitation of bowel movements with reduced pain in anorectal disorders

Table 52-6	Laxatives: Indications
Category	**Indication**
Bulk forming	Acute and chronic constipation, irritable bowel syndrome, diverticulosis
Emollient	Acute and chronic constipation, softening of fecal impaction, facilitation of bowel movements in anorectal conditions
Hyperosmotic	Chronic constipation, bowel preparation for diagnostic and surgical procedures
Saline	Constipation, removal of helminths and parasites, bowel preparation for diagnostic and surgical procedures
Stimulant	Acute constipation, bowel preparation for diagnostic and surgical procedures

See Table 52-6 for specific therapeutic indications for each laxative drug class.

Contraindications

All categories of laxatives share the same general contraindications and precautions, including drug allergy and the need for cautious use in the presence of the following: acute surgical abdomen; appendicitis symptoms such as abdominal pain, nausea, and vomiting; fecal impaction (mineral oil enemas excepted); intestinal obstruction; and undiagnosed abdominal pain.

Adverse Effects

As is true for the drug and therapeutic effects of laxatives, the adverse effects of the various drugs are specific to the laxative group. Most of the adverse effects from laxatives are confined to the intestine; however, the overuse and misuse of laxatives lead to many unwanted effects that are not expected or designed to occur with appropriate use. The major adverse effects of the laxative drugs are listed in Table 52-7.

Interactions

Many drugs are absorbed in some part of the intestine. Because laxatives alter intestinal function, they can interact with other drugs quite readily. Bulk-forming laxatives can decrease the absorption of antibiotics, digoxin, nitrofurantoin, salicylates, tetracyclines, and oral anticoagulants. Mineral oil can decrease the absorption of fat-soluble vitamins (A, D, E, and K). Hyperosmotic laxatives can cause increased CNS depression if they are given

Table 52-7   Laxatives: Adverse Effects

Category	Adverse Effects
Bulk forming	Impaction above strictures, fluid disturbances, electrolyte imbalances, gas formation, esophageal blockage, allergic reaction
Emollient	Skin rashes, decreased absorption of vitamins, lipid pneumonia, electrolyte imbalances
Hyperosmotic	Abdominal bloating, rectal irritation, electrolyte imbalances
Saline	Magnesium toxicity (with renal insufficiency), electrolyte imbalances, cramping, diarrhea, increased thirst
Stimulant	Nutrient malabsorption, skin rashes, gastric irritation, electrolyte imbalances, discolored urine, rectal irritation

with barbiturates, general anesthetics, opioids, or antipsychotics. Oral antibiotics can decrease the effects of lactulose. Stimulant laxatives decrease the absorption of antibiotics, digoxin, nitrofurantoin, salicylates, tetracyclines, and oral anticoagulants.

Dosages

For the recommended dosages of selected laxatives, see the Dosages table on page 809.

Drug Profiles

As mentioned previously, laxatives are used for the treatment of constipation. Such treatment must involve an understanding of the whole patient. Many drugs in the five major groups of laxatives are available as OTC medications, whereas others require a prescription for use. The following profiles describe the prototypical drugs in each of the laxative groups.

Bulk-Forming Laxatives

Bulk-forming laxatives are composed of water-retaining (hydrophilic) natural and synthetic cellulose derivatives. Psyllium is an example of a natural bulk-forming laxative, and methylcellulose is an example of a synthetic cellulose derivative. Other bulk-forming laxatives are malt soup extract preparations and polycarbophil preparations. Bulk-forming drugs increase water absorption, which results in greater total volume (bulk) of the intestinal contents. Unlike some of the other laxatives, bulk-forming laxatives tend to produce normal, formed stools, as opposed to liquid stools. Their action is limited to the GI tract, so there are few, if any, systemic effects. However, they should be taken with liberal amounts of water to prevent esophageal obstruction and/or fecal impaction. The bulk-forming laxatives are all OTC, are among the safest laxatives available, and are the only ones that are recommended for long-term use.

methylcellulose

Methylcellulose (Citrucel) is a synthetic bulk-forming laxative that attracts water into the intestine and absorbs excess water into the stool, stimulating the intestines and increasing peristalsis. Specific contraindications include GI obstruction and hepatitis. Methylcellulose is an oral drug available in powdered form that provides approximately 2 g of fiber per heaping tablespoon.

Pharmacokinetics

Half-Life	Onset	Peak	Duration
Unknown	12-24 hr	Unknown	Unknown

▸ *psyllium*

Psyllium (Metamucil, Fiberall) is a natural bulk-forming laxative obtained from the dried seed of the *Plantago psyllium* plant. It has many of the characteristics of methylcellulose. Psyllium use is contraindicated in patients with intestinal obstruction or fecal impaction. Its use is also contraindicated in patients experiencing abdominal pain and/or nausea and vomiting. Psyllium is available for oral use in wafer and powder form.

Pharmacokinetics

Half-Life	Onset	Peak	Duration
Unknown	12-24 hr	Unknown	Unknown

Emollient Laxatives

Emollient laxatives either directly lubricate the stool and the intestines, as with mineral oil, or act as fecal softeners. By lubricating the fecal material and the intestinal walls, lubricant emollient laxatives prevent water from moving out of the intestines, which softens and expands the stool. Stool softeners (docusate salts) work by lowering the surface tension of fluids, which allows more water and fat to be absorbed into the stool and the intestines.

▸ *docusate salts*

As noted earlier, docusate salts (calcium and sodium) are stool-softening emollient laxatives that facilitate the passage of water and lipids (fats) into the fecal mass, which softens the stool.

These drugs are used to treat constipation, soften fecal impactions, and facilitate easy bowel movements in patients with hemorrhoids and other painful anorectal conditions. In addition to the docusate salt formulations, combination products are also available. Docusate use is contraindicated in patients with intestinal obstruction, fecal impaction, or nausea and vomiting.

Pharmacokinetics

Half-Life	Onset	Peak	Duration
Unknown	1-3 days	Unknown	1-3 days

mineral oil

Mineral oil (Kondremul Plain, Fleet Mineral Oil Enema) eases the passage of stool by lubricating the intestines and preventing water from escaping the stool. Mineral oil is the only lubricant laxative in the emollient category. It is a mixture of liquid hydrocarbons derived from petroleum and is most commonly used to treat constipation associated with hard stools or fecal impaction.

Mineral oil use is contraindicated in patients with intestinal obstruction, abdominal pain, or nausea and vomiting. Mineral oil drugs are available as enemas and in products for oral use. There are also combination products that contain mineral oil, such as Haley's M-O, which contains both mineral oil and milk of magnesia (magnesium hydroxide).

Pharmacokinetics

Half-Life	Onset	Peak	Duration
Unknown	6-8 hr	Unknown	Unknown

Hyperosmotic Laxatives

The hyperosmotic laxatives glycerin, lactulose, sorbitol, and polyethylene glycol (PEG) relieve constipation by increasing the water content of the feces, which results in distention, peristalsis, and evacuation. They are most commonly used to treat constipation and to evacuate the bowels before diagnostic and surgical procedures.

▸ *glycerin*

Glycerin (Fleet Babylax, Sani-Supp) promotes bowel movement by increasing osmotic pressure in the intestine, which draws fluid into the colon. Because it is a very mild laxative, it is often used in children. Glycerin has properties similar to those of sorbitol, another hyperosmotic laxative. Glycerin use is contraindicated in patients who have shown a hypersensitivity reaction to it. It is available as a rectal solution and in both adult and pediatric suppositories.

Pharmacokinetics

Half-Life	Onset	Peak	Duration
30-45 min	16-36 min	1 hr	2-4 hr

DOSAGES

Selected Laxatives

Drug (Pregnancy Category)	Pharmacologic Class	Usual Dosage Range	Indications
▶docusate sodium (Colace, others) and docusate calcium (Surfak, others) (C)	Fecal softener, emollient laxative	**Pediatric 2-11 yr*** PO: 33-120 mg/day divided daily-tid (many products, consult product labeling) **Pediatric 12 yr and older, adult*** PO: 50-300 mg/day divided daily-qid	Facilitation of defecation (e.g., postpartum or in any condition involving painful defecation due to hardened feces) Constipation
▶glycerin (Glycerin, Sani-Supp, Colace, Fleet Babylax) (C)	Hyperosmotic laxative	**Adult and pediatric** Rectal only: Insert one adult, child, or infant suppository PR daily-bid prn; attempt to retain 15-30 min; suppository does not have to melt to induce BM	
▶lactulose (Enulose, Chronulac, others) (B)	Disaccharide, hyper-osmotic laxative	**Pediatric, infant†** PO: 2.5-10 mL/day divided bid-qid **Child-adolescent†** PO: 40-90 mL/day divided bid-qid **Adult†** PO: 30-45 mL tid-qid	Constipation; reduction of blood ammonia levels in liver failure
magnesium citrate (generic only), magnesium sulfate (Epsom salts by various manufacturers) (B)	Saline laxative	**Citrate, PO** *Pediatric younger than 6 yr* 0.5 mL/kg (max 200 mL); may repeat q4-6h until stools clear *Pediatric 6-11 yr* 100-150 mL × 1 dose *Adult* 120-300 mL × 1 dose **Sulfate, PO** *Pediatric* 0.25 g/kg q4-6h *Adult* 10-15 g in 8 oz water	Constipation; bowel cleansing before diagnostic procedure or surgery
methylcellulose (Citrucel, others) (B)	Bulk-forming laxative	**Pediatric 6-11 yr** ½ dose for pediatric 12 yr and older/adult **Pediatric 12 yr and older, adult** PO: 1 heaping tbsp in 8 oz cold water daily-tid	Constipation
mineral oil (Kondremul Plain, Fleet Oil-Retention Enema) (B)	Emollient laxative	**PO** *Pediatric 6-11 yr* 5-15 mL oil or 10-25 mL Kondremul Plain emulsion *Pediatric 12 yr and older, adult* 15-45 mL oil or 30-75 mL Kondremul Plain emulsion taken at bedtime **Rectal enema** *Pediatric 2-11 yr* PR: 59 mL × 1 *Pediatric 12 yr and older, adult* PR: 118 mL × 1	Constipation
polyethylene glycol (CoLyte, GoLYTELY, NuLytely) (C)	Emollient laxative	**Adult only** PO: 4 L solution, usually ending before procedure; patient should fast at least 4 hr before drinking solution	Bowel cleansing before diagnostic procedure or surgery
▶psyllium (Metamucil, Fiberall, others) (B)	Bulk-forming laxative	**Pediatric 6-11 yr** PO: ½ rounded tsp in water or juice daily-tid **Pediatric 12 yr and older, adult** PO: 1 rounded tsp in 8 oz water or juice daily-tid	Constipation; often used as part of a daily maintenance program
▶senna (Senokot, others) (C)	Stimulant-irritant laxative	**Pediatric 2-5 yr‡** PO (tabs): ½-¾ tab/day (max 1 tab bid) PO (liquid): ½ tsp/day (max × ½ tsp bid) **Pediatric 6-11 yr‡** PO (tabs): 1 tab daily (max × 2 tabs bid) PO (liquid): 1½-2 tsp daily (max × 1 tsp bid) **Pediatric 12 yr and older, adult‡** PO (tabs): Start with 2 tabs daily (max × 4 tabs bid) PO (liquid): 1 tbsp daily (max 2 tbsp bid)	Constipation

BM, Bowel movement; *PO,* oral; *PR,* by rectum.

*Docusate sodium is available in both capsule and liquid forms. Docusate calcium is available in capsule form only.

†Rectal route is sometimes used to reverse certain types of coma.

‡Many dosage forms; consult product labeling if in doubt. Most common dosage forms consist of 8.6 mg sennosides in tablet form and 8.8 mg/5 mL of sennosides in liquid form.

▶ *lactulose*

Lactulose (Chronulac, Duphalac, Enulose) is a disaccharide sugar containing one molecule of galactose and one molecule of fructose. It is a synthetic derivative of the natural sugar lactose, which is not digested in the stomach or absorbed in the small bowel. Instead it is passed unchanged into the large intestine, where it is metabolized. Colonic bacteria digest lactulose to produce lactic acid, formic acid, and acetic acid, which creates a hyperosmotic environment that draws water into the colon and produces a laxative effect. This drug-induced acidic environment also reduces blood ammonia levels by converting ammonia to ammonium. Ammonium is a water-soluble cation that is trapped in the intestines and cannot be reabsorbed into the systemic circulation. This has proved helpful in reducing serum ammonia levels in patients with hepatic encephalopathy. Lactulose use is contraindicated in patients on a low-galactose diet. It is available as a solution for either oral or rectal use.

Pharmacokinetics

Half-Life	Onset	Peak	Duration
Unknown	24 hr	24-48 hr	Variable

polyethylene glycol 3350

PEG-3350 is most commonly given before diagnostic or surgical bowel procedures because it is a very potent laxative that induces total cleansing of the bowel. The *3350* designation refers to the osmolality of the drug. It is usually available in a powdered dosage form that contains mixtures of electrolytes that also help stimulate bowel evacuation (e.g., Colyte). The powder is usually reconstituted in a large volume of fluid (1 gal) that is then gradually drunk by the patient on the afternoon of the day before the procedure. Use of PEG is contraindicated in patients with GI obstruction, gastric retention, bowel perforation, toxic colitis, toxic megacolon, or ileus. A common sample product composition is as follows:

- PEG-3350, 60 g/L
- Sodium chloride, 1.46 g/L
- Potassium chloride, 0.745 g/L
- Sodium bicarbonate, 1.68 g/L
- Sodium sulfate, 5.68 g/L

An oral solution of PEG-3350 and electrolytes is available for GI lavage. Diarrhea usually occurs within 30 to 60 minutes after ingestion; complete evacuation and cleansing of the bowel is accomplished within 4 hours.

Pharmacokinetics

Half-Life	Onset	Peak	Duration
Unknown	1 hr	2-4 hr	4 hr

Box 52-1 **Saline Laxatives**
Magnesium Laxatives
Sulfate
Epsom salts
Hydroxide
Milk of magnesia
Citrate
Citrate of magnesia
Sodium Laxatives
Phosphate
Fleet Phospho-Soda
Fleet enema

---

*Tegaserod was taken off the market in March 2007.

Saline Laxatives

Saline laxatives consist of various magnesium or sodium salts. They increase osmotic pressure and draw water into the colon, producing a watery stool, usually within 3 to 6 hours of ingestion. The currently available saline laxatives are listed in Box 52-1.

magnesium salts

The magnesium saline laxatives magnesium citrate, magnesium hydroxide, magnesium phosphate, and magnesium sulfate (Epsom salts) are commonly used, unpleasant tasting OTC laxative preparations. They should be used with caution in patients with renal insufficiency, because they can be absorbed enough to cause hypermagnesemia. They are most commonly used for rapid evacuation of the bowel in preparation for endoscopic examination and to help remove unabsorbed poisons from the GI tract.

Use of magnesium salts is contraindicated in patients with renal disease, abdominal pain, nausea and vomiting, obstruction, acute surgical abdomen, or rectal bleeding. Magnesium hydroxide, more commonly referred to as *milk of magnesia,* is available in oral liquid and tablet form. It is also found in a variety of combination products, such as Haley's M-O (see mineral oil profile). Other magnesium products are listed in the discussion of saline laxatives earlier in this chapter.

Pharmacokinetics

Half-Life	Onset	Peak	Duration
Unknown	0.5-3 hr	3 hr	Variable

Stimulant Laxatives

Stimulant laxatives, including natural plant products and synthetic chemical drugs, induce intestinal peristalsis. Plant-derived stimulant laxatives include bisacodyl, dicacodyl tannex, and phenolphthalein (white and yellow). The anthraquinones make up another plant-derived subgroup of the stimulant laxatives; these include drugs such as cascara sagrada, senna, aloe (casanthranol), and danthron. Their site of action is the entire GI tract. The action of the stimulant laxatives is proportional to the dose. The stimulant class is the most likely of all laxative classes to cause dependence.

▶ *senna*

Senna (Senokot) is a commonly used OTC stimulant laxative. Senna is obtained from the dried leaves of the *Cassia acutifolia* plant. It may be used for relief of acute constipation or bowel preparation for surgery or examination. Because of its stimulating action on the GI tract, it may cause abdominal pain. It can produce complete bowel evacuation in 6 to 12 hours. Senna is available in a variety of dosages as tablets, syrup, and granules. One product, Senokot-S, includes both senna and the stool softener docusate sodium.

Pharmacokinetics

Half-Life	Onset	Peak	Duration
Variable	6-24 hr	24 hr	24-36 hr

Drugs for Irritable Bowel Syndrome

Irritable bowel syndrome (IBS) is a condition of chronic intestinal discomfort, including cramps, diarrhea, and/or constipation. Patients usually cope with the symptoms by avoiding irritating foods and/or taking OTC laxatives and antidiarrheal drugs. Women are affected more often than men, and of the current prescription drugs for IBS, alosetron (Lotronex) is approved for women only. Tegaserod (Zelnorm)* is now approved for men and women. Both medications work through their interaction with various serotonin receptor subtypes in the intestinal tissue. Both are also pregnancy category B drugs, are contraindicated in patients with a history of significant non–IBS GI disorder, and are available only in oral tablet form. Dosages for IBS drugs can be found in the Dosages table on page 811.

DOSAGES

Drugs for Irritable Bowel Syndrome

Drug (Pregnancy Category)	Pharmacologic Class	Usual Dosage Range	Indications
alosetron (Lotronex)	5-HT$_3$ antagonist	**Adult females only** PO: 1 mg once daily; if symptoms not adequately controlled after 4 wk, may advance to 1 mg twice daily; if symptoms not adequately controlled after 4 wk of twice-daily dosing, drug should be discontinued	Severe diarrhea-predominant irritable bowel syndrome in women
tegaserod maleate (Zelnorm)*	5-HT$_4$ partial agonist	**Adults only** PO: 6 mg twice daily before meals for 4-6 wk; patients who respond favorably to this initial course of therapy may be given one additional 4-6 wk course of therapy	Constipation-predominant irritable bowel syndrome in men and women (short-term treatment)

5-HT$_3$, Type 3 serotonin receptor; *5-HT$_4$*, type 4 serotonin receptor.

◆ NURSING PROCESS

◆ ASSESSMENT

Before administering antidiarrheal preparations, the nurse should obtain a thorough history of bowel patterns, general state of health, and recent illness and/or dietary changes, and document this information. Abdominal assessment should include auscultation of bowel sounds in all four quadrants *after* inspection of the entire abdomen but before percussion and palpation. This avoids stimulation of peristalsis or bowel sounds that would not be there otherwise. When the frequency of bowel sounds ranges from 6 to 32 per minute, it is important to describe exactly what is heard and the amount of activity in each of the four quadrants. Terms such as *high-pitched, low-pitched, gurgling,* or *tinkling* may be used to describe the character or the sounds, whereas activity may be described as hypoactive (less than 6 per minute), normoactive (between a range of 6 to 32 sounds/minute), or hyperactive (greater than the normal range). The abdominal assessment should be performed for any patient with GI complaints, including altered bowel status. The presence of tenderness, rigidity, changes in contour, bulges, and obvious peristaltic waves across the abdomen should be noted. Frequency, consistency, amount, color, and odor (if present) of stools should be assessed and documented. In addition, it is critical to patient safety and health to be sure that the possibility of *Clostridium difficile* infection or other infectious diarrhea is ruled out.

The use of some antidiarrheals (e.g., bismuth subsalicylate, diphenoxylate, loperamide) requires assessment of the history of bowel patterns and contraindications, cautions, and drug interactions. With use of diphenoxylate there is an additional concern for use in patients with respiratory problems because of the risk for respiratory depression. Loperamide is not tolerated well in the elderly. Patients in this age group are also more susceptible to fluid and electrolyte depletion; thus, there is a need for close assessment of hydration status in addition to the abdominal and bowel pattern assessment. With any of these drugs, if an assessment shows bloody stools, abdominal rigidity, severe abdominal pain, or no bowel sounds, the drug should not be used and the physician should be contacted immediately.

CASE STUDY

Constipation

Mrs. M. is a 66-year-old retired schoolteacher. She enjoys good health and exercises three times a week with a senior citizen group in a supervised arthritis swim class at the local recreation center. She arrives at the physician's office with complaints of "constipation" and states that for the last 3 months she has had only one bowel movement every 3 days instead of one every day. In the assessment of this patient, you discover that she has been taking a laxative up to twice a day and is also now feeling "weak." She also states that she is experiencing a "lot of tummy cramping." Answer the following questions:

- What are at least five questions you, as the nurse, should ask Mrs. M.? Provide reasons for each question.
- What types of problems are generally related to chronic use of laxatives? Explain your answer.
- If you were a nurse practitioner and were to suggest an OTC drug to help prevent constipation, what would be your choice(s) and why?

For answers, see http://evolve.elsevier.com/Lilley.

Laxative use requires further assessment in addition to the abdominal assessment and bowel pattern history mentioned earlier. For example, questions should focus on changes in bowel habits or patterns, long-term use of laxatives (because patients may become laxative dependent), and dietary and fluid intake. Vital signs, especially blood pressure; daily weight measurements; intake and output; fluid and electrolyte levels; and the presence of any weakness should be assessed because of the possibility of hypotension and volume or electrolyte depletion with chronic laxative use. The type of laxative and the related mechanism of action dictate specific assessments because of differences in how strongly the patient reacts to the various laxative drugs. The bulk-forming laxatives are often used to treat chronic constipation and have few adverse effects, but they still require a basic abdominal and bowel pattern assessment and related history. Contraindications, cautions, and drug interactions should be assessed and documented. Docusate products must also be used cautiously in the elderly and require the same thorough assessment

Magnesium-based laxatives act as osmotics so assessment should include specific attention to baseline fluid and electrolyte levels to identify any deficits—before their use. All of the previously mentioned assessment data regarding abdominal examination and bowel patterns is appropriate for these drugs, but the patient should also be assessed for the presence of abdominal pain, the degree of peristalsis, history of any recent abdominal surgery, nausea, vomiting, or weight loss, and serum magnesium, blood urea nitrogen, and creatinine levels should be evaluated. The elderly react more adversely to this class of laxatives, and their use in this patient group should be avoided. Patients who have diabetes or are on a low-sodium diet should be assessed carefully because of the drug-related elevation in blood glucose and serum sodium with use of magnesium laxatives. Lactulose is also an osmotic laxative and, in addition to collecting the previous mentioned assessment data, the nurse should document baseline mental status and ammonia levels.

Assessment of patients taking cascara sagrada requires evaluation of the abdomen and bowel status. Senna should be used with caution in the elderly because of possible dehydration and electrolyte loss. Patients taking a PEG-electrolyte solution, often used for GI cleansing or preparation, should be assessed for the presence of ulcerative colitis, because the solution may be given differently and only in specific situations in these patients. The nurse should note whether other medications are to be given to the patient and, if so, they should be given 1 hour before the polyethylene solution so that absorption of the other oral medication is not decreased.

NURSING DIAGNOSES

- Constipation related to improper diet and fluid intake
- Diarrhea related to GI irritation from food, bacteria or viruses, or pathology
- Fluid volume deficit related to excessive diarrhea and loss of fluids and electrolytes through frequent, loose stools
- Risk for injury related to the adverse effects of medication
- Noncompliance related to lack of knowledge and/or experience with the medication regimen

PLANNING

Goals

- Patient regains normal bowel patterns.
- Patient remains free of fluid and electrolyte disturbances related to changes in bowel patterns and lack of proper management of bowel alterations.
- Patient is free from self-injury related to possible weakness and dizziness or the adverse effects of medications.
- Patient remains compliant with the medication regimen and nonpharmacologic measures.

Outcome Criteria

- Patient reports the signs and symptoms of constipation or diarrhea to the health care provider if recommended measures and/or medications do not correct altered bowel patterns within a specified period of time.
- Patient reports the signs and symptoms of fluid and electrolyte loss, such as weakness, lethargy, decreased urinary output, and dizziness.
- Patient states measures to take to avoid adverse effects and injuries related to change in bowel patterns, changes in fluid and electrolyte status, and/or treatment, such as changing positions slowly, increasing intake of fluids, asking for assistance with ambulation as needed, and ambulating slowly.

- Patient states methods of administration that enhance effective and safe use of the recommended drugs, including following proper dosing, taking oral doses with water or fluids as appropriate, and reporting undesired adverse effects.
- Patient states nonpharmacologic measures to relieve constipation or diarrhea, such as forcing fluids, increasing intake of fiber or bulk for constipation, removing irritating foods from the diet, and increasing bulk for diarrhea.

IMPLEMENTATION

Antidiarrheals should be taken exactly as prescribed, with strict adherence to the recommended dose, frequency, and duration of treatment. The nurse should encourage patients to be aware of their fluid intake and any dietary changes that would impact their health status or possibly exacerbate the symptoms already present. Patients should also be aware of the factors precipitating the diarrhea, and if symptoms persist, they should know to contact a physician immediately. Bowel pattern changes, weight, fluid volume status, intake and output, and mucous membrane status should be documented before, during, and after the initiation of treatment—whether for constipation or diarrhea. Bismuth subsalicylate should be taken as directed, and the patient should be aware that this medication will turn the stool black or gray. If tablets are used, they should be chewed thoroughly before swallowing with at least 6 oz. of fluid. This medication is a salicylate, and it should not be taken with other salicylates to avoid risk of toxicity. Diphenoxylate hydrochloride may be given without regard to food intake but should be given with adequate fluid. Loperamide should be taken as directed and with specific directions followed (e.g., take the specific number of tablets as recommended by the manufacturer after the first loose stool and the total number of tablets within a 24-hour time frame). Maximum amounts should not be exceeded, and if diarrhea continues or other symptoms present themselves (e.g., fever, abdominal pain, bloody stools), the health care provider should be contacted immediately. See the Patient Teaching Tips for more information.

Bulk-forming laxatives, such as methylcellulose and polycarbophil, must be administered as specified by package insert or as ordered. Methylcellulose should be taken with at least 8 oz. or 1 full glass of liquid after the powder form has been thoroughly stirred into it. The fluid must be taken immediately to avoid choking or swelling of the product in the throat or esophagus. The medication should not be taken in its dry form. Polycarbophil, used both as a bulk-forming laxative and as an antidiarrheal, should be given every half hour up to the maximum daily dosage, and it should be given with 8 oz. of liquid as directed. See the Patient Teaching Tips for more information.

Docusate is available in a variety of oral dosage forms (e.g., capsules, tablets, syrups, elixir), and all should be taken with at least 6 oz. of water or other fluid. An additional 6 to 8 glasses of water a day should be drunk to help with stool softening. Milk or fruit juices may be used to help to disguise the taste, if needed.

Bisacodyl, if ordered, should be taken on an empty stomach for faster action, and whole tablets should not be chewed or crushed. Milk, antacids, or juices should not be taken with the dose nor within 1 hour of taking the medication. Rectal suppositories, if too soft, can be placed in a medicine cup with ice to harden them before insertion. Once the wrapper is removed, a water-soluble lubricant should be applied and the suppository inserted immediately into the rectum. The patient should attempt to keep the suppository in place by lying still and on the left side for at least 15 to 30 minutes to allow the drug to dissolve. Cascara sagrada should be given with water only, because, like bisacodyl, it interacts with milk and antacids. Lactulose may be taken with juice, milk, or water to increase palatability. It is important to note that the normal color of the oral solution is pale yellow. Rectal dosage forms are administered as a retention enema with dilution as ordered and retained for 30 to 60 minutes. For a retention enema, the tip of the apparatus should be well lubricated and inserted carefully with the nozzle pointed toward the umbilicus of the patient, who should be lying on the left side. Fluid should be released gradually, and administration should be discontinued if the patient experiences severe abdominal pain. If long-term use is indicated, electrolyte levels should be monitored.

Magnesium-based laxatives should be used only as ordered and in certain situations. Fluids should be forced and other instructions followed as per the physician's order or the packaged instructions. Refrigeration may help increase the palatability of the oral solution. It is always important that this type of drug be taken exactly as prescribed for constipation, with consumption of plenty of fluids and careful attention to adverse effects. PEG-electrolyte solution should be mixed with water as directed and shaken well before taken. Chilled solutions are tolerated better, and rapid drinking is recommended.

◆ EVALUATION

Therapeutic responses to antidiarrheals and laxatives include an improvement in the GI-related signs and symptoms reported by the patient (e.g., decrease in diarrhea or constipation), return to normal bowel patterns with normal bowel sounds, and absence of abnormal findings from an assessment of the abdomen and bowel patterns. Adverse effects for which to monitor patients vary according to each drug. Goals and outcome criteria should also serve as a means to evaluate the nursing care plan related to each problem, whether it is constipation or diarrhea.

Patient Teaching Tips

- Encourage patients to take antidiarrheals exactly as prescribed, with close attention to indicated dosages and how not to exceed them. Stool frequency, consistency, and amount should be recorded for comparison and evaluation purposes. Patients should be told to contact the health care provider if they experience abdominal pain, bloody stools, fever, or abdominal distention. If diarrhea does not stop within 3 days, they should know to contact the physician.

- Remind patients that antidiarrheal drugs have sedating adverse effects, so patients should be cautious with tasks that require mental alertness or motor skills until it is clear how they are affected by the drug.

- Patients taking either antidiarrheals or laxatives should report abdominal distention, firm abdomen, pain, worsening (or no improvement) of symptoms, and other GI-related signs and symptoms to the physician immediately.

- Encourage patients to treat the adverse effect of dry mouth with frequent mouth care, fluid intake, or use of sugarless gum or candy.

- Bismuth subsalicylate may turn the stool tarry black, so patients should know this and to report any bloody stools to their physician. Encourage patients to avoid other drugs containing salicylates at this time and to always check for age-related cautions and contraindications.

- For constipation, patients should be encouraged to increase the amount of fluids; high-fiber, whole grain products; green, leafy vegetables; and fruits, as well as increase their amount of exercise and non-drug methods of treatment.

- Be sure that patients know to report rectal bleeding, abdominal pain, unrelieved constipation, or weakness to their health care provider immediately.

- Encourage patients to be honest with their health care provider in regard to their bowel elimination patterns and educate them to the fact that what is normal for one person is not normal for another.

- Warn patients to not take a laxative if they are experiencing nausea, vomiting, and/or abdominal pain. If symptoms are not resolved and worsen, the patient should contact the health care provider.

- While taking laxatives, encourage patients to contact their physician if they experience muscle weakness, cramps, or dizziness which may indicate possible fluid or electrolyte loss.

- All antidiarrheals and laxatives must be kept out of the reach of children.

- Make sure to include specific instructions for certain drugs (e.g., powder forms of methylcellulose should be thoroughly mixed with at least 6 oz of liquid, stirred, and drunk immediately to avoid esophageal or throat obstruction). Senna may turn the urine pink-red, red-violet, red-brown or yellowish brown. Patients should also be informed that other medications should not be taken within 1 hour of taking senna and that it often takes 6 to 12 hours for the laxative effect of the oral drug to occur.

- PEG solutions are more palatable if chilled and taken quickly.

Points to Remember

- Diarrhea is a leading cause of morbidity and mortality in under-developed countries.
- Drug therapy for diarrhea includes the following drugs: adsorbents, anticholinergics, opiates, and intestinal flora modifiers.
- Most acute diarrhea is self-limiting, subsiding in 3 days to 2 weeks.
- Fluid and electrolyte replacement is vital while a patient is experiencing diarrhea.
- Patients should be encouraged to check and recheck dosage instructions before taking medication and note any drug-food and drug-drug interactions.
- Anticholinergics work by decreasing GI peristalsis through their parasympathetic blocking effects. Adverse effects include urinary retention, headache, confusion, dry skin, rash, and blurred vision.
- Adsorbents work by coating the walls of the GI tract. They remain in the intestine and bind the causative bacteria or toxin to the adsorbent surface, so that it can be eliminated from the body through the stool. They may increase bleeding and cause constipation, dark stools, and black tongue.

- Intestinal flora modifiers are also used to manage diarrhea and consist of bacterial cultures of *Lactobacillus*. They reestablish normal intestinal flora destroyed by infection or antibiotics and suppress the growth of diarrhea-causing bacteria.
- Opiates are also used as antidiarrheals and help to decrease bowel motility and thus permit longer contact of intestinal contents with the absorptive surface of the bowel. Opiates also help to reduce the pain associated with rectal spasms.
- Laxatives, especially osmotic medications, may cause fluid and electrolyte loss.
- Patients must be made aware of the abuse potential and the problems associated with the misuse of laxatives and laxative dependency issues.
- Stool softeners and bulk-forming drugs are often preferred in the treatment of constipation because they are not as problematic with regard to fluid and electrolyte loss.

NCLEX Examination Review Questions

1. A patient is being prepared for a colonoscopy. Which laxative is most appropriate as preparation for this procedure?
   a. Methylcellulose
   b. Docusate sodium
   c. Polyethylene glycol (PEG)
   d. Psyllium
2. What is the major concern regarding the administration of oral methylcellulose?
   a. Dehydration
   b. Tarry stools
   c. Renal calculi
   d. Possible obstruction
3. A 45-year-old woman has been diagnosed with IBS and experiences chronic episodes of diarrhea and constipation problems. The nurse expects that which medication will be ordered for this patient?
   a. Psyllium
   b. alosetron (Lotronex)

   c. Bismuth subsalicylate (Pepto-Bismol)
   d. *Lactobacillus acidophilus* (Lactinex)
4. When the nurse teaches a patient about taking bisacodyl tablets, which instruction is correct?
   a. "Take this medication on an empty stomach."
   b. "Chew the tablet for quicker onset of action."
   c. "Take this medication with juice or milk."
   d. "Take this medication with an antacid if it upsets your stomach."
5. A patient has been on long-term antibiotic therapy as part of treatment for an infected leg wound. He tells the nurse that he has had "spells of diarrhea" for the last week. Which medication is most appropriate for him at this time?
   a. Bismuth subsalicylate
   b. *Lactobacillus acidophilus*
   c. Diphenoxylate with atropine
   d. Codeine

1. c, 2. d, 3. b, 4. a, 5. b.

Critical Thinking Activities

1. You are explaining to a group of elderly patients the importance of seeking treatment for diarrhea. During your discussion with the group, the following questions are posed to you:
   - "What are some nondrug therapies I can use once I have begun to recover from diarrhea caused by a virus or the flu?"
   - "If I have eaten something 'bad,' does it matter if I take something to stop the diarrhea?"

   Provide answers to these questions that are appropriate for this elderly population and give a rationale for each response.

2. Your pediatric patient's mother calls the clinic because her 4-month-old daughter has had diarrhea for about 8 hours. What would you recommend and why?
3. Why is it important that elderly patients be monitored closely while taking any type of bowel preparation regimen before diagnostic studies such as a colonoscopy? Explain your answer.

For answers, see http://evolve.elsevier.com/Lilley.

CHAPTER

53

Antiemetic and Antinausea Drugs

Objectives

When you reach the end of this chapter, you should be able to do the following:

1. Discuss the pathophysiology of nausea and vomiting, including specific precipitating factors and/or diseases.
2. Identify the various antiemetic and antinausea drugs and their drug classification groupings.
3. Describe the mechanisms of action, indications for use, contraindications, cautions, and drug interactions of the various categories of antiemetic and antinausea drugs.
4. Develop a nursing care plan that includes all phases of the nursing process for patients taking antiemetic and antinausea drugs.

e-Learning Activities

Companion CD
- NCLEX Review Questions: see questions 425-436
- Animations
- Audio Glossary
- Category Catchers
- Medication Errors Checklists
- IV Therapy Checklists

evolve Website (http://evolve.elsevier.com/Lilley)
- Nursing Care Plans • Frequently Asked Questions • Content Updates • WebLinks • Supplemental Resources • Elsevier ePharmacology Update • Medication Administration Animations

Drug Profiles

aprepitant, p. 821
dronabinol, p. 819
▶ meclizine, p. 819
▶ metoclopramide, p. 819
▶ ondansetron, p. 819

phosphorated carbohydrate solution, p. 821
▶ prochlorperazine, p. 819
scopolamine, p. 818

▶ Key drug.

Glossary

Antiemetic drugs Drugs given to relieve nausea and vomiting. (p. 815)
Chemoreceptor trigger zone (CTZ) The area of the brain that is involved in the sensation of nausea and the action of vomiting. (p. 815)
Emesis The forcible emptying or expulsion of gastric and, occasionally, intestinal contents through the mouth; also called *vomiting.* (p. 815)
Nausea Sensation often leading to the urge to vomit. (p. 815)
Vomiting center (VC) The area of the brain that is involved in stimulating the physiologic events that lead to nausea and vomiting. (p. 815)

NAUSEA AND VOMITING

Nausea and vomiting are two gastrointestinal (GI) disorders that not only can be extremely unpleasant but also can lead to more serious complications if not treated promptly. **Nausea** is an unpleasant feeling that often precedes vomiting. If it does not subside spontaneously or is not relieved by medication, it can lead to vomiting. Vomiting, which is also called **emesis,** is the forcible emptying or expulsion of gastric and, occasionally, intestinal contents through the mouth. A variety of stimuli can induce nausea and vomiting, including foul odors or tastes, unpleasant sights, irritation of the stomach or intestines, and certain drugs (ipecac or antineoplastic drugs).

The **vomiting center (VC)** is an area in the brain that is responsible for initiating the physiologic events that lead to nausea and, eventually, vomiting. Neurotransmitter signals are sent to the VC from the **chemoreceptor trigger zone (CTZ),** another area in the brain involved in the induction of nausea and vomiting. These signals alert these areas of the brain to the existence of nauseating substances (noxious stimuli) that need to be expelled from the body. Once the CTZ and VC are stimulated, they initiate the events that trigger the vomiting reflex. The neurotransmitters involved in this process and their respective receptors are listed in Table 53-1. The various pathways and the areas of the body that send the signals to the VC via these pathways are illustrated in Figure 53-1.

ANTIEMETIC DRUGS

The drugs used to relieve nausea and vomiting are called **antiemetic drugs.** The discovery of new drugs coupled with a better understanding of the way in which the older drugs work has had a dramatic impact on the way in which nausea and vomiting are now treated. All antiemetic drugs work at some site in the vomiting pathways. There are six categories of such drugs with varying mechanisms of action. When drugs from the various categories are combined, the antiemetic effectiveness of the resulting preparation is increased because it can then block more than just one of the pathways. Some of the more commonly used antiemetics in the various categories are listed in Table 53-2, and the sites at which some of them work in the vomiting pathway are shown in Figure 53-2.

Mechanism of Action and Drug Effects

The numerous drugs used to prevent or treat nausea and vomiting have many different mechanisms of action. Most work by blocking one of the vomiting pathways, as shown in Figure 53-2, and in doing so block the neurologic stimulus that induces vomiting. The mechanisms of action of the drugs in the six antiemetic drug categories are summarized in Table 53-3.

Anticholinergic drugs are discussed in Chapter 20 and have several uses. As antiemetics, they act by binding to and blocking acetylcholine (ACh) receptors in the vestibular nuclei, which are located deep within the brain. When ACh is prevented from binding to these receptors, nausea-inducing signals originating in this area cannot be transmitted to the CTZ. Anticholinergics also block receptors located in the reticular formation and by doing so prevent ACh from binding to these receptors, so that nausea-inducing signals originating in this area cannot be transmitted to the VC. Anticholinergics also tend to dry GI secretions and reduce

Table 53-1   Neurotransmitters Involved in Nausea and Vomiting

Neurotransmitter	Site in the Vomiting Pathway
Acetylcholine	VC in brain; vestibular and labyrinthine pathways in inner ear
Dopamine (D_2)	GI tract and CTZ in brain
Histamine (H_1)	VC in brain; vestibular and labyrinthine pathways in inner ear
Prostaglandins	GI tract
Serotonin ($5\text{-}HT_3$)	GI tract; CTZ and VC in brain

CTZ, Chemoreceptor trigger zone; D_2, dopamine-2 receptor; *GI,* gastrointestinal; H_1, histamine-1 receptor; $5\text{-}HT_3$, 5-hydroxytriptamine-3; *VC,* vomiting center.

smooth muscle spasms, both of which effects are often helpful in reducing acute GI symptoms, including nausea and vomiting.

Antihistamines (histamine-1 [H_1] receptor blockers) act by inhibiting vestibular stimulation in a manner that is very similar to the way in which anticholinergics work. Although they bind primarily to H_1 receptors, they also have potent anticholinergic activity as an adverse effect, including antisecretory and antispasmodic effects. They thus prevent cholinergic stimulation in both the vestibular and reticular systems. Nausea and vomiting occur when these systems are stimulated. Note that these drugs are not to be confused with *histamine-2 [H_2] receptor blockers* used for gastric acid control (Chapter 51). Although the latter drugs are also technically a type of antihistamine, the term *antihistamine* is usually applied to histamine H_1 blockers, often in reference to their use in treating allergy symptoms (Chapter 35).

Neuroleptic drugs, although they are traditionally used for their antipsychotic effects (Chapter 15), also prevent nausea and vomiting by blocking dopamine receptors on the CTZ. Many of the neuroleptics also have anticholinergic actions similar to those of anticholinergic drugs. In addition, neuroleptic drugs calm the central nervous system (CNS), an effect beneficial in treating the symptoms of various psychiatric disorders (anxiety, tension, and agitation).

Prokinetic drugs, in particular metoclopramide, also act as antiemetics by blocking dopamine receptors in the CTZ, which desensitizes the CTZ to impulses it receives from the GI tract. Their primary action, however, is to stimulate peristalsis in the GI tract. This enhances the emptying of stomach contents into the duodenum, as well as intestinal movements.

Serotonin blockers work by blocking serotonin receptors located in the GI tract, CTZ, and VC. There are many subtypes of serotonin receptors, and these various receptors are located throughout the body (CNS, smooth muscles, platelets, and GI tract). The receptor subtype involved in the mediation of nausea and vomiting is the 5-hydroxytryptamine-3 ($5\text{-}HT_3$) receptor. These receptors are the site of action of the serotonin blockers such as ondansetron and granisetron.

Tetrahydrocannabinol (THC), in a drug class by itself, is the major psychoactive substance in marijuana. Nonintoxicating doses in the form of the drug dronabinol are occasionally used as an antiemetic because of the drug's inhibitory effects on the reticular formation, thalamus, and cerebral cortex. These effects cause an alteration in mood and in the body's perception of its

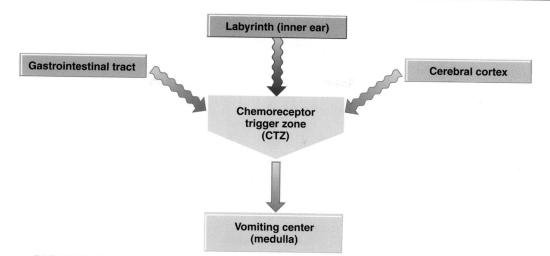

FIGURE 53-1 The various pathways and areas in the body sending signals to the vomiting center.

Table 53-2	Antiemetic Drugs: Common Drug Categories
Category	**Antiemetic Drugs**
Anticholinergics (ACh blockers)	scopolamine
Antihistamines (H₁ receptor blockers)	dimenhydrinate, diphenhydramine, meclizine, promethazine
Neuroleptics	chlorpromazine, perphenazine, prochlorperazine, promethazine, thiethylperazine, triflupromazine, trimeprazine
Prokinetics	cisapride, metoclopramide
Serotonin blockers	dolasetron, granisetron, ondansetron
Tetrahydrocannabinoids	dronabinol

ACh, Acetylcholine; *H₁,* histamine-1.

surroundings, which may be beneficial in relieving nausea and vomiting. Although this particular category of antiemetics is less commonly prescribed, there are occasionally unusual cases of nausea and vomiting that respond well to THC. Examples include nausea and vomiting in patients being treated for cancer or acquired immunodeficiency syndrome (AIDS). In such patients, dronabinol may also stimulate the appetite, and nutritional wasting syndromes are common in both diseases. The drug also demonstrates some benefit in controlling symptoms of glaucoma. There is a large, but highly controversial, political movement involving many cancer, AIDS, and glaucoma patients in favor of legalization of the marijuana plant for these uses.

Indications

The therapeutic uses of the antiemetic drugs vary depending on the drug category. There are several indications for the drugs in each class. These are listed in Table 53-4.

Contraindications

The primary contraindication for all antiemetics is known drug allergy. Other contraindications for various specific drugs are mentioned in the drug profiles.

Adverse Effects

Most of the adverse effects of the antiemetics stem from their nonselective blockade of receptors. For example, antihistamines not only bind to H₁ receptors in the vestibular nuclei and thereby prevent ACh from acting on them but also bind to histamine receptors located elsewhere in the body, thus, for instance, causing secretions to become dry. Some of the more common adverse effects associated with the various categories of antinausea drugs are listed in Table 53-5.

Interactions

The drug interactions associated with the antiemetic drugs are also specific to the individual drug categories. Anticholinergic antiemetics have additive drying effects when given with antihistamines and antidepressants. Antihistamine antiemetics, when administered with barbiturates, opioids, hypnotics, tricyclic antidepressants, or alcohol, can increase CNS depression. Neuroleptic antiemetics, when given with levodopa, may cancel the beneficial effects of the latter. Increased CNS depression can be seen when alcohol or other CNS depressants are given with neuroleptic drugs. Combining quinidine and neuroleptic drugs may result in increased adverse cardiac effects. Prokinetic drugs, when given with alcohol, can result in additive CNS depression. Anticholinergics and analgesics can block the motility effects of metoclopramide. Serotonin blockers and THC have no significant drug interactions.

Dosages

For the recommended dosages of selected antiemetic drugs, see the Dosages table on page 820.

Drug Profiles

The various antiemetics are used to treat nausea and vomiting in a variety of clinical situations. As noted earlier, some of them have other therapeutic uses as well. The ultimate goals of antiemetic therapy are minimizing or preventing fluid and electrolyte disturbances and minimizing deterioration of the patient's nutritional status. Most of the antiemetics act by blocking receptors in the CNS, but some work directly in the GI tract. As previously mentioned, there are six

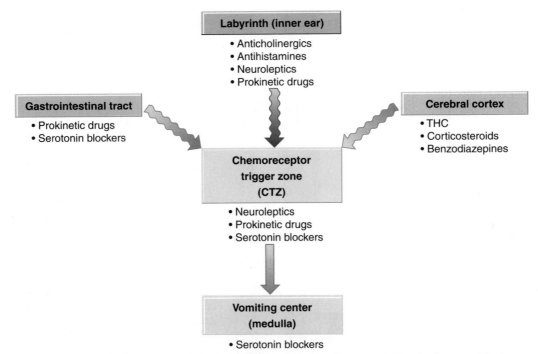

FIGURE 53-2 Sites of action of selected antinausea drugs. *THC,* Tetrahydrocannabinol.

Table 53-3	Antiemetic Drugs: Mechanisms of Action
Category	**Mechanism of Action**
Anticholinergics	Block ACh receptors in the vestibular nuclei and reticular formation
Antihistamines	Block H₁ receptors, thereby preventing ACh from binding to receptors in the vestibular nuclei
Neuroleptics	Block dopamine in the CTZ and may also block ACh
Prokinetics	Block dopamine in the CTZ or stimulate ACh receptors in the GI tract
Serotonin blockers	Block serotonin receptors in the GI tract, CTZ, and VC
Tetrahydrocannabinoids	Have inhibitory effects on the reticular formation, thalamus, and cerebral cortex

ACh, Acetylcholine; *CTZ,* chemoreceptor trigger zone; *GI,* gastrointestinal; *H₁,* histamine-1; *VC,* vomiting center.

Table 53-4	Antiemetic Drugs: Indications
Category	**Indications/Uses**
Anticholinergics	Motion sickness, secretion reduction before surgery, nausea and vomiting
Antihistamines	Motion sickness, nonproductive cough, sedation, rhinitis, allergy symptoms, nausea and vomiting
Neuroleptics	Psychotic disorders (mania, schizophrenia, anxiety), intractable hiccups, nausea and vomiting
Prokinetics	Delayed gastric emptying, gastroesophageal reflux, nausea and vomiting
Serotonin blockers	Nausea and vomiting associated with cancer chemotherapy, postoperative nausea and vomiting
Tetrahydrocannabinoids	Nausea and vomiting associated with cancer chemotherapy, anorexia associated with weight loss in patients with AIDS

AIDS, Acquired immunodeficiency syndrome.

major classes of antiemetic drugs. However, there are other drugs that may also be used to treat nausea and vomiting. These include corticosteroids such as dexamethasone (Chapter 32) and anxiolytics such as lorazepam (Chapter 15). When used in combination therapies, these latter drugs, as well as THC, are very beneficial in preventing the nausea and vomiting caused by cancer chemotherapy. Lorazepam also helps to blunt the memory of the nausea and vomiting experience (especially with cancer chemotherapy). Chemotherapy-induced nausea and vomiting and postoperative nausea and vomiting can be especially difficult to treat. The serotonin blockers have proven to be very effective in preventing these types of nausea and vomiting.

Anticholinergics
scopolamine

Scopolamine (Transderm-Scop) is the primary anticholinergic drug used as an antiemetic. It has potent effects on the vestibular nuclei, which, as previously mentioned, are located within the area of the brain that controls balance. It works by blocking the binding of ACh

to the cholinergic receptors in this region and thereby correcting an imbalance between the two neurotransmitters ACh and norepinephrine. These effects make scopolamine one of the most commonly used drugs for the treatment and prevention of the nausea and vomiting associated with motion sickness. It is also used to treat postoperative nausea and vomiting. Scopolamine use is contraindicated in patients with glaucoma. Scopolamine is available in oral, injectable, transdermal, and even ocular forms (Chapter 58). The most commonly used formulation for nausea is the 72-hour transdermal patch, which releases a total of 1 mg of the drug.

Pharmacokinetics

Half-Life	Onset	Peak	Duration
TP: 9.5 hr	TP: 1-2 hr	TP: 6-8 hr	TP: 72 hr

TP, Transdermal patch.

Table 53-5 Antinausea Drugs: Adverse Effects

Body System	Adverse Effects
Anticholinergics	
Central nervous	Dizziness, drowsiness, disorientation
Cardiovascular	Tachycardia
Ears, eyes, nose, throat	Blurred vision, dilated pupils, dry mouth
Genitourinary	Difficult urination, constipation
Integumentary	Rash, erythema
Antihistamines	
Central nervous	Dizziness, drowsiness, confusion
Ears, eyes, nose, throat	Blurred vision, dilated pupils, dry mouth
Genitourinary	Urinary retention
Neuroleptics	
Cardiovascular	Orthostatic hypotension, electrocardiographic changes, tachycardia
Central nervous	Extrapyramidal symptoms, pseudoparkinsonism, akathisia, dystonia, tardive dyskinesia, headache
Ears, eyes, nose, throat	Blurred vision, dry eyes
Genitourinary	Urinary retention
Gastrointestinal	Dry mouth, nausea and vomiting, anorexia, constipation
Prokinetics	
Cardiovascular	Hypotension, supraventricular tachycardia
Central nervous	Sedation, fatigue, restlessness, headache, dystonia
Gastrointestinal	Dry mouth, nausea and vomiting, diarrhea
Serotonin Blockers	
Central nervous	Headache
Gastrointestinal	Diarrhea, transient increased AST and ALT levels
Other	Rash, bronchospasm
Tetrahydrocannabinoids	
Central nervous	Drowsiness, dizziness, anxiety, confusion, euphoria
Ears, eyes, nose, throat	Visual disturbances
Gastrointestinal	Dry mouth

ALT, Alanine aminotransferase; *AST,* aspartate aminotransferase.

Antihistamines

Antihistamine antiemetics are some of the most commonly used and safest antiemetics. Some of the popular antihistamines are meclizine (Antivert), dimenhydrinate (Dramamine), and diphenhydramine (Benadryl). Many of the antihistamines are available over the counter (OTC), although others are prescription drugs.

▶ *meclizine*

Meclizine (Antivert, Bonine, Meni-D) is most commonly used to treat the dizziness, vertigo, and nausea and vomiting associated with motion sickness. Contraindications include shock and lactation. It is available for oral use only.

Pharmacokinetics

Half-Life	Onset	Peak	Duration
PO: 6 hr	PO: 1 hr	PO: Variable	PO: 8-24 hr

Neuroleptics

Prochlorperazine (Compazine), chlorpromazine (Thorazine), perphenazine (Prolixin), promethazine (Phenergan), thiethylperazine (Torecan), droperidol (Inapsine), and trifluoperazine (Trilafon) are antiemetics in the neuroleptic class. These drugs have antidopami-

nergic as well as antihistaminergic and anticholinergic properties. Many of these drugs are used to treat psychotic disorders such as mania and schizophrenia, their associated anxiety, and intractable hiccups, as well as nausea and vomiting.

▶ *prochlorperazine*

Prochlorperazine (Compazine), especially in the injectable form, is one of the more commonly used antiemetics in the hospital setting. Its use is contraindicated in patients with hypersensitivity to phenothiazines, those in a coma, and those suffering from seizures, encephalopathy, or bone marrow depression. It is available for both injection and oral use.

Pharmacokinetics

Half-Life	Onset	Peak	Duration
IM: 6-8 hr	IM: 30-40 min	IM: 2-4 hr	IM: 3-4 hr

Prokinetics

Prokinetic drugs promote the movement of substances through the GI tract and increase GI motility. The prokinetic drug that is also used to prevent nausea and vomiting is metoclopramide.

▶ *metoclopramide*

Metoclopramide (Reglan) is the oldest and most commonly used prokinetic drug. It is available only by prescription because it can cause some severe adverse effects if not used correctly. Metoclopramide is used for the treatment of delayed gastric emptying and gastroesophageal reflux and also as an antiemetic. Its use is contraindicated in patients with seizure disorder, pheochromocytoma, breast cancer, or GI obstruction and also in patients with a hypersensitivity to it or to procaine or procainamide. Metoclopramide is available in both oral and parenteral formulations.

Pharmacokinetics

Half-Life	Onset	Peak	Duration
PO: 2.5-5 hr	PO: 20-60 min	PO: 1-2.5 hr	PO: 3-4 hr

Serotonin Blockers

The serotonin blockers are also called *5-HT$_3$ receptor blockers* because they block the 5-HT$_3$ receptors in the GI tract, CTZ, and vomiting center. (The chemical name for serotonin is 5-hydroxytryptamine [5-HT].) Because of their specific actions, these drugs cause few adverse effects. They are indicated for the prevention of nausea and vomiting associated with cancer chemotherapy and also for the prevention of postoperative or radiation-induced nausea and vomiting. Currently there are four drugs in this category: dolasetron (Anzemet), granisetron (Kytril), ondansetron (Zofran), and palonosetron (Aloxi). Another similar drug, alosetron (Lotronex), is used for the treatment of irritable bowel syndrome. It is discussed in Chapter 52.

▶ *ondansetron*

Ondansetron (Zofran) is the prototype drug in this class. Approved in 1992, it represented a major breakthrough in treating chemotherapy-induced nausea and vomiting and, later, postoperative nausea and vomiting. Its only listed contraindication is drug allergy. It is available in both oral and injectable forms.

Pharmacokinetics

Half-Life	Onset	Peak	Duration
IV: 3-5.5 hr	IV: 15-30 min	IV: 1-1.5 hr	IV: 6-12 hr

Tetrahydrocannabinoids
dronabinol

Dronabinol (Marinol) is the only commercially available tetrahydrocannabinoid. It is a synthetic derivative of THC, the major active substance in marijuana. Dronabinol was approved by the U.S. Food and Drug Administration (FDA) in 1985 for the treatment of nausea and vomiting related to cancer chemotherapy. It is generally used as a second-line drug after treatment with other antiemetics has failed. It is also used to stimulate appetite and weight gain in patients with AIDS. Its only listed contraindication is drug allergy. It is available for oral use only.

DOSAGES

Selected Antiemetic and Antinausea Drugs

Drug (Pregnancy Category)	Pharmacologic Class	Usual Dosage Range	Indications
Anticholinergics scopolamine (Transderm-Scop) (C)	Anticholinergic, belladonna alkaloid	Apply 1 patch to hairless area behind ear q3d (starting at least 4 hr before travel)	Motion sickness prophylaxis
Antihistamines ▶meclizine (Antivert, Bonine) (B)	Anticholinergic, antihistamine	**Adult** PO: 25-50 mg 1 hr before travel and repeated daily during travel PO: 25-100 mg/day, divided daily-qid	Motion sickness prophylaxis Treatment of vertigo
Neuroleptics ▶prochlorperazine (Compazine) (C)	Phenothiazine	**Pediatric** PO/rectal: 9-13 kg: 2.5 mg daily-bid 13.5-17.5 kg: 2.5 mg bid-tid 18-38 kg: 2.5 mg tid or 5 mg bid IM: 0.132 mg/kg, no more than bid IV: 5 mg q6h **Adult** PO: 5-10 mg tid-qid IM: 5-10 mg q3-4h (max 40 mg/day) Rectal: 25 mg bid IV: 5-10 mg q6h	Antiemetic
Prokinetics ▶metoclopramide (Maxolon, Octamide, Reglan) (B)	Dopamine antagonist	**Adult** IV: 1-2 mg/kg (30 min before chemotherapy; repeat q2h × 2 doses, then q3h × 3 doses) IM: 10-20 mg × 1 dose near end of surgery	Chemotherapy antiemetic Prevention of postoperative nausea and vomiting
Serotonin Blockers ▶ondansetron (Zofran) (B)	Antiserotonergic	**Pediatric 4-11 yr** PO: 4 mg tid, 30 min before chemotherapy, repeated 4 and 8 hr after first dose **Pediatric 4-18 yr** IV: 0.15 mg/kg over 15 min, given 30 min before chemotherapy, repeated 4 and 8 hr after first dose **Adult** PO: 8 mg 30 min before chemotherapy, repeated 8 hr after first dose; followed by 8 mg q12h for 1-2 days after completion of chemotherapy **Adult** IV: 0.15 mg/kg over 15 min, given 30 min before chemotherapy, repeated 4 and 8 hr after first dose, or 1 dose of 32 mg over 15 min, given 30 min before chemotherapy IV: 4 mg over 2-5 min × 1 dose (second dose not shown to be effective in patients for whom first dose provides no relief)	Chemotherapy antiemetic Prevention and treatment of postoperative nausea

IM, Intramuscular; *IV*, intravenous; *PO*, oral.

DOSAGES

Selected Antiemetic and Antinausea Drugs—cont'd

Drug (Pregnancy Category)	Pharmacologic Class	Usual Dosage Range	Indications
Tetrahydrocannabinoids dronabinol (Marinol) (C)	Marijuana-derived antiemetic	**Adult** PO: Initially, 5 mg/m² 1-3 hr before chemotherapy, then q2-4h after chemotherapy up to 6×/day for 3 days; this dose may, if needed, be increased in 2.5-mg/m² increments to a max dose of 15 mg/m²	Chemotherapy antiemetic
		PO: 2.5-5 mg bid before lunch and before or after dinner, or 2.5 mg as single PM or hs dose for patients intolerant of 5-mg doses	Appetite stimulation in HIV/AIDS

AIDS, Acquired immunodeficiency syndrome; *HIV,* human immunodeficiency virus (infection).

Pharmacokinetics

Half-Life	Onset	Peak	Duration
PO: 19-36 hr	PO: 30-60 min	PO: 1-3 hr	PO: 4-6 hr

Miscellaneous Antinausea Drugs
phosphorated carbohydrate solution

Phosphorated carbohydrate solution (Emetrol) is a mint-flavored, pleasant-tasting oral solution used to relieve nausea. It works by direct local action on the walls of the GI tract, where it reduces cramping caused by excessive smooth muscle contraction. It can be used to control milder cases of nausea and vomiting resulting from causes such as stomach or intestinal "flu" and excessive (or unhealthy) eating or drinking. It does not have a pregnancy category rating, but one of its listed unlabeled (non–FDA-approved) uses is for treatment of morning sickness during pregnancy. It is probably not sufficient for treatment of more severe nausea symptoms such as those associated with cancer chemotherapy. Its only contraindication is drug allergy. It is available for oral use only.

aprepitant

Aprepitant (Emend) is the first in a new class of antiemetic drugs and was approved in 2003. It is an antagonist of substance P–neurokinin-1 receptors in the brain. In contrast to other antiemetics, this drug has little affinity for 5-HT₃ (serotonin) and dopamine receptors. However, studies do show that aprepitant augments the antiemetic actions of both ondansetron and the corticosteroid dexamethasone. This drug is specifically indicated for the prevention of nausea and vomiting in *highly emetogenic* cancer chemotherapy regimens, including high-dose cisplatin. Common adverse effects include dizziness, headache, insomnia, and GI discomforts, but these are generally no more common than with other standard antiemetic regimens. Aprepitant has drug interactions with warfarin (international normalized ratio should be monitored to assess the need for dosage adjustment) and steroids. Because, like aprepitant, steroids such as dexamethasone and methylprednisolone are metabolized by the cytochrome P-450 subtype 3A4 isoenzymes, aprepitant can reduce their metabolism, lowering the required steroid dosages by 25% to 50%. Pregnancy category B.

◆NURSING PROCESS

◆ ASSESSMENT

Before any antinausea or antiemetic drug is administered, a thorough nursing history and physical assessment should be completed, with attention to the following: history of the symptoms of nausea and vomiting; medical history and current medical status; medication history and drugs currently taken, including OTC drugs, herbals, prescription drugs, and social drugs (e.g., cigarettes, alcohol); and any alternative therapies used. Any factors precipitating nausea or vomiting should be identified; weight loss should be noted; baseline vital signs should be measured; intake and output should be assessed; the skin and mucous membranes should be examined, with turgor and color noted; and capillary refill (which should be less than 5 seconds) should also be noted. Once laboratory tests are ordered (e.g., serum sodium, potassium, and chloride levels; hemoglobin level; hematocrit; red and white blood cell counts; and urinalysis), the findings should be assessed and documented to establish baseline levels. The patient should be assessed for any contraindications or cautions to the use of these

CASE STUDY
Nausea and Chemotherapy

Ms. S., a 58-year-old retired seamstress, has begun outpatient chemotherapy after a recent diagnosis of breast cancer. She has recovered well from a right modified mastectomy, the incisions are well healed, and she is now physically and emotionally ready for her 3-month regimen of chemotherapy. Her premedication consists of a variety of drugs, including granisetron (Kytril). Her home medication list includes oral ondansetron (Zofran).
- What is the mechanism of action of granisetron that makes it effective in the management of chemotherapy-induced nausea and vomiting?
- What important patient teaching points should you emphasize to Ms. S. about ondansetron?
- After 2 weeks of therapy, the physician discontinues the ondansetron because Ms. S. complained that it did nothing to help her nausea and vomiting. She receives a prescription for dronabinol but expresses concern because she knows "there's marijuana in that pill!" What would you explain to her?

For answers, see http://evolve.elsevier.com/Lilley.

drugs and for drug interactions (previously discussed), as well as for any allergies. The anticholinergic drug scopolamine should be given only after careful assessment of the patient's health history and medication history. One very important concern to reemphasize with scopolamine, which is commonly administered in patch form to prevent motion sickness, is its use in patients with narrow-angle glaucoma. If the patient has a history of this disorder, then other antiemetic or antinausea drugs should be used. The same concern regarding use in patients with narrow-angle glaucoma applies to antihistamines (e.g., meclizine); in addition, antihistamines should be used cautiously in pediatric patients, who may have severe paradoxical reactions, and in the elderly, who often develop agitation, mental confusion, hypotension, and even psychotic-type reactions in response to these drugs. Other medications should be considered for patients if these reactions occur.

Neuroleptic drugs, such as prochlorperazine, should be used only after cautious assessment for signs and symptoms of dehydration and electrolyte imbalance by evaluation of skin turgor and examination of the tongue for the presence longitudinal furrows. Contraindications, cautions, and drug interactions for these drugs have been discussed earlier. Important to emphasize is the need for assessment of the psychotic patient's appearance, behavior, emotional status, responses to the environment and to others, and speech and thought content. Double-checking of the name and mechanism of action is also important so that the drug is not confused with chlorpromazine.

Prokinetic drugs (e.g., metoclopramide) are often reserved for the treatment of nausea and vomiting associated with antineoplastic drug therapy or radiation therapy and for the treatment of GI motility disturbances. The action of these drugs is decreased when they are taken with anticholinergics or opiates, and because this occurs commonly it is worthy of emphasis. Age is important to assess because of the increased risk of tardive dyskinesia in the young and the elderly. Granisetron should be given only after assessment of baseline vital signs and age (its safety in those younger

than 2 years of age has not been established). Ondansetron use requires assessment for the signs and symptoms of dehydration and electrolyte disturbances, with evaluation of skin turgor and examination for dry mucous membranes or longitudinal furrows in the tongue. Serum levels of bilirubin, aspartate aminotransferase, and alanine aminotransferase should also be assessed before initiation of therapy, especially in patients with liver dysfunction.

Dronabinol and its contraindications, cautions, and drug interactions have been discussed previously. Patients taking this drug should be assessed for signs and symptoms of dehydration with attention to low urine output, dry mucous membranes, poor skin turgor, and overall lethargy before this medication is given. A thorough assessment of hydration status is important because treatment of volume and electrolyte imbalances may be required in addition to treatment with antinausea or antiemetic drugs. In addition, motor and cognitive abilities should be assessed and a neurologic head-to-toe examination performed before and during drug therapy.

◆ NURSING DIAGNOSES

- Risk for injury related to the adverse effects of the medications (e.g., sedation and dizziness)
- Risk for falls related to weakness and dizziness from vomiting and from the adverse effects of the medications
- Risk for deficient fluid volume related to nausea and vomiting and limited oral intake
- Impaired physical mobility related to weakness from fluid and electrolyte disturbances secondary to vomiting

◆ PLANNING

Goals

- Patient remains free of injury and falls from weakness and dizziness secondary to nausea, vomiting, and/or adverse effects of medication therapy.
- Patient manages the adverse effects of medications or identifies when to seek medical care.
- Patient regains normal fluid volume status and hydration status.
- Patient regains normal levels of activity without risk of falls and injury.

Outcome Criteria

- Patient states measures to implement to prevent injury, such as obtaining assistance while ill, rising slowly, changing positions slowly, taking medications as ordered, and initiating fluid intake once nausea and/or vomiting subsides.
- Patient states adverse effects of drug therapy such as sedation, confusion, lethargy, hypotension, and CNS depression.
- Patient states measures to implement to prevent further fluid volume deficits, such as consumption of oral fluids (e.g., clear liquids) or chilled gelatin along with medications.
- Patient increases activity by 10 to 15 minutes per day with cautious rising and walking.

◆ IMPLEMENTATION

Undiluted forms of diphenhydramine should be administered intravenously at the recommended rate of 25 mg/min. Intramuscular forms should be administered into large muscles (e.g., ventral gluteal) and the sites should be rotated if repeated injections are necessary. Prochlorperazine may be given orally without regard to meals; parenteral doses should be given using the proper dilutional solutions and infusion rates. Because of the hypotensive effects of the drug, the patient should remain lying down for 30 to 60 minutes after the drug has been given parenterally, and the legs

---

HERBAL THERAPIES AND DIETARY SUPPLEMENTS

Ginger (Zingiber officinale)

Overview

Found naturally in the Asian tropics; now cultivated in other continents, including part of the United States; plant parts utilized are the rhizome and root; active ingredients include *gingerols* and *gingerdione*

Common Uses

Used as an antioxidant; also used for relief of such varied symptoms as sore throat, migraine headache, and nausea and vomiting (including that induced by cancer chemotherapy, morning sickness, and motion sickness); many other varied uses

Adverse Effects

Skin reactions, anorexia, nausea, vomiting

Potential Drug Interactions

Can increase absorption of all oral medications; may theoretically increase bleeding risk with anticoagulants (e.g., warfarin [Coumadin]) or antiplatelet drugs (e.g., clopidogrel [Plavix])

Contraindications

Contraindicated in cases of known product allergy; may worsen cholelithiasis (gallstones); anecdotal evidence of abortifacient properties—some clinicians recommend not using during pregnancy

should be elevated to help minimize the hypotensive effect. Suppository dosage forms should be moistened with water or water-soluble lubricating gel before inserting well into the rectum. Patients should be placed on the left side for suppository insertion and should remain there for several minutes and hold in the suppository as long as possible to increase its absorption. Vital signs should be taken frequently, and the patient should be monitored for extrapyramidal symptoms throughout therapy, whether at home or in the hospital. The patient should be encouraged to avoid other CNS depressants and alcohol and to limit caffeine when this drug is used, as well as to avoid driving and other activities that require mental alertness or motor coordination.

Patients taking meclizine should have their blood pressures checked frequently, especially if they are elderly. Sedation raises a concern for patient safety, with the need for cautious movement at all times. Dry mouth produced by any of these medications may be alleviated by using sugarless gum or hard candy. Metoclopramide is given orally and should be administered 30 minutes before meals and at bedtime. Intravenous dosage forms should be given over the recommended time frame. In addition, solutions for parenteral dosing should be kept for only 48 hours and protected from light. Metoclopramide should not be given in combination with any other medications, such as phenothiazines, that would lead to exacerbation of extrapyramidal reactions. Extrapyramidal reactions should be reported immediately to the physician.

The scopolamine transdermal patch should be applied behind the ear as directed. The area behind the ear should be cleansed and dried before the patch is applied. If the patch becomes dislodged, the residual drug should be washed off and a fresh patch put in place. The patient should be warned not to engage in tasks requiring mental clarity or motor skill while taking the medica-tion. Granisetron may be given intravenously or orally. Intravenous doses should be infused over the recommended time frame and diluted as appropriate. A transient taste disorder may occur, especially if the drug is taken with antineoplastic medications, but will pass with continued therapy. The patient should be encouraged to use relaxation techniques and imagery as complementary therapies. Ondansetron may be given orally, intramuscularly, or intravenously. Intramuscular doses should be injected into a large muscle mass. Intravenous push is usually given over 2 to 5 minutes and infusions over 15 minutes as ordered and as per manufacturer guidelines. Oral forms are well tolerated regardless of the relation of dosing to meals. The patient should be encouraged to avoid alcohol and other CNS depressants during this therapy and to avoid any activities requiring mental alertness or motor skill. Dronabinol, granisetron, and ondansetron are usually indicated pre-chemotherapy. Dronabinol should be administered 1 to 3 hours before antineoplastic therapy and may be taken at home before the scheduled appointment for treatment. Relief of nausea and vomiting should occur within approximately 15 minutes of oral drug administration.

◆ EVALUATION

The therapeutic effects of antiemetic and antinausea drugs range from a decrease in to the elimination of nausea and vomiting and avoidance or elimination of complications such as fluid and electrolyte imbalances and weight loss. The patient should be monitored for adverse effects such as GI upset, drowsiness, lethargy, weakness, extrapyramidal reactions, and orthostatic hypotension during the therapy. Laboratory testing (e.g., electrolyte levels, blood urea nitrogen level, urinalysis with specific gravity) may be ordered for evaluation purposes. Defined goals and outcomes may also be used to evaluate therapeutic effectiveness.

Patient Teaching Tips

- Patients taking any of the antiemetic or antinausea drugs should be warned about the drowsiness they can cause and told to avoid performing any hazardous tasks or driving while taking these medications. Patients should also be cautioned about taking antiemetic or antinausea drugs with alcohol and other CNS depressants because of the possible toxicity and CNS depression that can occur.
- Educate patients about adverse effects of ondansetron, including headache which may be relieved with a simple analgesic (e.g., acetaminophen).

- Patients taking dronabinol should be reminded to change positions slowly to prevent syncope or dizziness resulting from the hypotensive effects of the drug. They should also avoid taking any other CNS depressants with this antiemetic and should be cautious when engaging in activities that require mental alertness.
- The application sites for transdermal scopolamine patches should be rotated, and the patches should be applied to nonirritated areas behind the ear; the hands should be washed thoroughly before and after application.

Points to Remember

- Antiemetics help to control vomiting, or emesis, and are also useful in relieving or preventing nausea.
- The categories of antiemetics are anticholinergics, antihistamines, neuroleptic drugs, prokinetic drugs, and tetrahydrocannabinoid.
- Antiemetics are used to prevent motion sickness, reduce secretions before surgery, treat delayed gastric emptying, and prevent postoperative nausea and vomiting.
- Anticholinergics work by blocking ACh receptors in the vestibular nuclei and reticular formation. This blockade prevents areas in the brain from being activated by nauseous stimuli.
- Antihistamines work by blocking H_1 receptors, which has the same effect as the anticholinergics. Neuroleptic antiemetics block dopamine receptors in the CTZ and may also block ACh receptors. Prokinetic drugs also block dopamine receptors in the CTZ.
- The serotonin-blocking drugs may be highly effective antiemetics. They are most commonly used for the prevention of chemotherapy-induced nausea and vomiting and work by blocking 5-HT_3 receptors in the GI tract, CTZ, and VC.
- Antiemetics are often given ½ to 3 hours before a chemotherapy drug is administered and may also be given during the chemotherapeutic treatment.
- Most antiemetic and antinausea drugs cause drowsiness.
- Granisetron and ondansetron are successful in treating cancer chemotherapy–induced nausea and vomiting.
- Dronabinol therapy is used to prevent antineoplastic-induced nausea and vomiting and is associated with postural hypotension.
- Patients taking antiemetic or antinausea drugs should be cautioned that drowsiness and hypotension may occur and that therefore they should avoid driving and using heavy machinery while taking these medications.

NCLEX Examination Review Questions

1. Which patient teaching instruction is most appropriate for a patient who plans to use scopolamine transdermal patches during a cruise?
   a. "Apply the patch the day before traveling."
   b. "Apply the patch at least 4 hours before traveling."
   c. "The patch should be applied to the shoulder area."
   d. "The patch should be applied to the temple just above the ear."
2. A middle-aged woman is experiencing severe vertigo due to Ménière's disease. Which of the medications listed below is considered the most appropriate treatment for vertigo?
   a. Meclizine (Antivert)
   b. Prochlorperazine (Compazine)
   c. Metoclopramide (Reglan)
   d. Dronabinol (Marinol)
3. A 33-year-old patient is in the outpatient cancer center for his first round of chemotherapy. When is the best time to administer the intravenous dose of an antiemetic?
   a. Four hours before the chemotherapy begins
   b. Thirty minutes before the chemotherapy begins
   c. At the same time as the chemotherapy drugs
   d. At the first sign of nausea
4. When reviewing the various types of antinausea medications, the nurse recognizes that prokinetic drugs are also used for which of the following?
   a. Motion sickness
   b. Vertigo
   c. Delayed gastric emptying
   d. GI obstruction
5. A patient who has been receiving chemotherapy tells the nurse that he has been searching the Internet for antinausea remedies and that he found a reference to a product called Emetrol (phosphorated carbohydrate solution). He wants to know if this drug would help him. The nurse's best answer would be which of the following?
   a. "This may be a good remedy for you. Let's talk to your physician."
   b. "This drug is used only after other drugs have not worked."
   c. "This drug is used only to treat severe nausea and vomiting caused by chemotherapy."
   d. "This drug may not help the more severe nausea symptoms associated with chemotherapy."

1. b, 2. a, 3. b, 4. c, 5. d.

Critical Thinking Activities

1. Explain how ondansetron (Zofran) decreases the nausea and vomiting associated with chemotherapy. Compare its effectiveness with that of prochlorperazine for the treatment of chemotherapy-induced nausea and vomiting.
2. Explain why it is important to assess the patient's hydration status when giving antinausea and antiemetic drugs.
3. What general adverse effects of antinausea and antiemetic drugs are of the most concern, especially with elderly patients?

For answers, see http://evolve.elsevier.com/Lilley.

Vitamins and Minerals

Objectives

When you reach the end of this chapter, you should be able to do the following:

1. Discuss the importance of the various vitamins and minerals to the normal functioning of the human body.
2. Briefly describe the various disease states, conditions and acute/chronic illnesses that may lead to various imbalances with vitamins and minerals.
3. Discuss the pathologies that result from vitamin and mineral imbalances.
4. Discuss the treatment of these vitamin and mineral imbalances.
5. Identify mechanisms of action, indications, cautions, contraindications, drug interactions, dosages, recommended daily allowances (RDAs), and routes of administration associated with each of the vitamins and minerals.
6. Develop a nursing care plan related to the use of vitamins and minerals and the nursing process.

e-Learning Activities

Companion CD
- NCLEX Review Questions: see questions 437-441
- Animations
- Audio Glossary
- Category Catchers
- Medication Errors Checklists
- IV Therapy Checklists

evolve Website (http://evolve.elsevier.com/Lilley)
- Nursing Care Plans • Frequently Asked Questions • Content Updates • WebLinks • Supplemental Resources • Elsevier ePharmacology Update • Medication Administration Animations

Drug Profiles

ascorbic acid (vitamin C), p. 838
calcifediol (vitamin D), p. 831
calcitriol (vitamin D), p. 831
calcium, p. 840
cyanocobalamin (vitamin B$_{12}$), p. 837
dihydrotachysterol (vitamin D), p. 832
ergocalciferol (vitamin D), p. 832

magnesium, p. 840
niacin (vitamin B$_3$), p. 835
phosphorus, p. 841
pyridoxine (vitamin B$_6$), p. 836
riboflavin (vitamin B$_2$), p. 834
thiamine (vitamin B$_1$), p. 834
vitamin A, p. 829
vitamin E, p. 832
vitamin K$_1$, p. 833
zinc, p. 841

Glossary

Beriberi A disease of the peripheral nerves caused by an inability to assimilate thiamine (vitamin B$_1$). Symptoms are fatigue, diarrhea, appetite and weight loss, and disturbed nerve function, causing paralysis and wasting of limbs, edema, and heart failure. (p. 834)

Coenzyme A nonprotein substance that combines with a protein molecule to form an active enzyme. (p. 825)

Enzyme A specialized protein that catalyzes biochemical reactions in organic matter. (p. 825)

Fat-soluble vitamin A vitamin that can be dissolved (i.e., is soluble) in fat. (p. 826)

Mineral An inorganic substance that is ingested and attaches to enzymes or other organic molecules. (p. 825)

Pellagra A disease resulting from a niacin deficiency or a metabolic defect that interferes with the conversion of tryptophan to niacin (vitamin B$_3$). (p. 834)

Rhodopsin The purple-pigmented compound in the rods of the retina, formed by a protein, opsin, and a derivative of retinol (vitamin A). (p. 827)

Rickets A condition caused by a vitamin D deficiency. (p. 829)

Scurvy A condition resulting from an ascorbic acid (vitamin C) deficiency. (p. 838)

Tocopherols Biologically active chemicals that make up vitamin E compounds. (p. 832)

Vitamin An organic compound essential in small quantities for normal physiologic and metabolic functioning of the body. (p. 825)

Water-soluble vitamin A vitamin that can be dissolved (i.e., is soluble) in water. (p. 826)

For the body to grow and maintain itself, it needs the essential building blocks provided by carbohydrates, fats, and proteins. Vitamins and minerals are needed to efficiently utilize these nutrients. **Vitamins** are organic molecules needed in small quantities for normal metabolism and other biochemical functions, such as growth or repair of tissue. Equally important are **minerals,** inorganic elements, or salts found naturally in the earth. **Enzymes** are proteins secreted by cells; they act as catalysts to induce chemical changes in other substances, but they themselves remain chemically unchanged by the process. A **coenzyme** is a substance that enhances or is necessary for the action of enzymes. Many enzymes are totally useless without the appropriate vitamins and/or minerals that chemically bind with them and cause them to function properly. Both vitamins and minerals function primarily as coenzymes, binding to enzymes (or other organic molecules) to activate anabolic (tissue-building) processes in the body. This helps to regulate many body functions. For example, the collagen, hormone, and enzyme synthesis that is needed to heal wounds requires the presence of certain vitamins and minerals. As another example, coenzyme A (CoA) is an important carrier molecule associated with the *citric acid cycle*, one of the body's major energy-producing metabolic reactions. However, it requires pantothenic acid (vitamin B_5) to complete its function in the citric acid cycle.

Vitamins and minerals are essential in our lives, whether we are conscientious in our food choices or consume whatever we desire. Under most circumstances, daily requirements of vitamins and minerals are met by ingestion of fluids and regular, balanced meals. Ingesting food helps us maintain adequate stores of essential vitamins and minerals and serves to preserve intestinal mass and structure, provide chemicals for hormones and enzymes, and prevent harmful overgrowth of bacteria.

Various illnesses can occur that can cause acute or chronic deficiencies, including vitamins, minerals, electrolytes, and fluids. These conditions require replacement or supplementation of these nutrients. Common examples include burn patients and persons with acquired immunodeficiency syndrome (AIDS). Excessive loss of vitamins and minerals may also be the result of poor dietary intake, an inability to swallow after cancer chemotherapy or radiation, or mental disorders such as anorexia nervosa. Poor dietary absorption is also attributable to various gastrointestinal malabsorption syndromes. Drug and alcohol abuse are also frequently associated with inadequate nutritional intake that warrants vitamin and mineral supplementation.

In this chapter, we discuss both vitamins and minerals and their therapeutic effects. Deficiencies are also common in dietary protein, fat, and carbohydrates. These nutrients are discussed in Chapter 55. Because of some of their relatively distinct properties and functions in the body related to blood formation, the mineral iron and the vitamin folic acid (vitamin B_9) are discussed separately in Chapter 56.

VITAMINS

Vitamin sources occur naturally in both plant and animal foods. The human body requires vitamins in specific minimum amounts on a daily basis and can obtain them from both plant and animal food sources. In some cases, the body synthesizes some of its own vitamin supply. Supplemental amounts of vitamin B complex and vitamin K are synthesized by normal bacterial flora in the gastrointestinal tract. Vitamin D can be synthesized by the skin when exposed to sunlight.

An inadequate diet will cause various nutrition-related vitamin deficiencies. As a result of extensive food content studies, in 1941 the Food and Nutrition Board of the National Academy of Sciences (FNBNAS) published its first list of *Recommended Daily Allowances (RDAs)* of essential nutrients. A newer published standard is the list of Dietary Reference Intakes (DRIs), published by NAS and the Institute of Medicine (IOM). Whereas the RDAs represented *minimum* nutrient requirements, the DRIs are being designed to represent *optimal* nutrient requirements for

good health. Laws in the United States require detailed nutritional information to be listed on any packaged food product. The *percentage Daily Values (DVs)* are the values that appear on the mandatory labels of commercial food products and indicate what percentage of the DRI for a specific nutrient is met by a single serving of the food product. Information regarding DRIs is available at the following websites:

1. Federal Food and Nutrition Information Center: www.nal.usda.gov/fnic
2. Institute of Medicine: Dietary Reference Intakes (DRIs): Recommended intakes for individuals: www.iom.edu/?id=21381

Vitamins are classified as either fat or water-soluble. **Water-soluble vitamins** can be dissolved in water and are easily excreted in the urine. **Fat-soluble vitamins** are dissolvable in fat, and tend to be stored longer in the liver and fatty tissues. Because water-soluble vitamins (B-complex group and vitamin C) cannot be stored in the body in large amounts over long periods, daily intake is required to prevent the development of deficiencies. Conversely, fat-soluble vitamins (vitamins A, D, E, and K) do not need to be taken daily because they are stored in the liver and fatty tissues in large amounts. Deficiency in these vitamins occurs only after prolonged deprivation from an adequate supply or from disorders that prevent their absorption. Table 54-1 lists the fat-soluble and water-soluble vitamins.

One controversial topic related to vitamins is that of nutrient "megadosing," both as a strategy for health promotion and maintenance and for treating various illnesses. Some cancer patients are electing to use supplemental megadosing of specific nutrients in hopes of strengthening their body's response to more conventional cancer treatments, such as surgery, radiation, and chemotherapy. The American Dietetic Association defines megadosing as, "Doses of a nutrient that are 10 or more times the [customary] recommended amount." A related term was coined in 1968 by the Nobel prize–winning chemist Linus Pauling. He defined *orthomolecular medicine* to be "the preventive or therapeutic use of high-dose vitamins to treat disease." Probably the best-known claim of Dr. Pauling was that megadoses of vitamin C (at more than 100 times the U.S. RDA) could prevent or cure the common cold and cancer. Many studies since have not substantiated this claim. However, there are some situations in which nutrient megadosing is known to be helpful, including the following:

- When concurrent long-term drug therapy depletes vitamin stores or otherwise interferes with the function of a vitamin. A common clinical example is the use of vitamin B_6 (pyridoxine) supplementation in patients receiving the drug isoniazid (INH) for tuberculosis (TB; Chapter 40).
- For gastrointestinal malabsorption syndromes such as those seen in patients with severe colitis and cystic fibrosis (all major nutrient classes, including protein, fat, carbohydrates, vitamins, and minerals).
- For the treatment of pernicious anemia, which results from cyanocobalamin (vitamin B_{12}) deficiency. The gastrointestinal tract uses a fairly complex mechanism to drive cyanocobalamin absorption. Specifically, a glycoprotein known as *intrinsic factor* is secreted by the parietal cells of the gastric glands (Chapter 51). Intrinsic factor serves to facilitate absorption of cyanocobalamin, primarily in the intestine. When this process is compromised (e.g., by disease), megadoses of cyanocobalamin can bypass this absorption mechanism by allowing a

Table 54-1   Fat- and Water-Soluble Vitamins

Fat-Soluble			Water-Soluble	
Designation	**Name**		**Designation**	**Name**
vitamin A	retinol		vitamin B_1	thiamine
vitamin D	D_3, cholecalciferol D_2, ergocalciferol dihydrotachysterol		vitamin B_2	riboflavin
			vitamin B_3	niacin
			vitamin B_5	pantothenic acid
vitamin E	tocopherols		vitamin B_6	pyridoxine
vitamin K	K_1, phytonadione		vitamin B_9	folic acid
	K_2, menaquinone		vitamin B_{12}	cyanocobalamin
			biotin	
			vitamin C	ascorbic acid

small amount of the vitamin to diffuse on its own through the intestinal mucosa.

- When the vitamin acts as a drug when megadosed. The most common example is niacin (vitamin B_3, also called *nicotinic acid*). At doses of up to 20 mg daily, it functions as a vitamin, but at doses 50 to 100 times higher, it reduces blood levels of both triglycerides and low-density lipoprotein (LDL) cholesterol, thus acting more as a drug than a vitamin (Chapter 28).

In contrast with the above examples, there are some situations in which nutrient megadosing is known to be harmful. For example, any excess of one or more nutrients can result in deficiencies of other nutrients due to chemical "competition" for sites of absorption at the intestinal mucosa. This is more likely to be the case with mineral megadosing, such as with calcium, copper, iron, and zinc, and is less likely to result from vitamin megadosing.

Vitamin megadosing can also lead to toxic accumulations known as *hypervitaminosis,* especially with the fat-soluble vitamins A, D, and K. Vitamin E appears safer, however, even at doses 10 to 20 times the recommended DRI. Hypervitaminosis is much less likely to occur with the water-soluble vitamins (B-complex and C) because they are readily excreted through the urinary system. However, it is known that megadosing with vitamin B_6 (pyridoxine) at 50 to 100 times the DRI can cause nerve damage.

Persons with an illness may be the least able to tolerate nutrient megadosing, although megadosing regimens are often prescribed for them. For example, megadosing may be more of a strain for a gastrointestinal tract that is already weakened by illness. Megadosing can even interfere with other treatments for illness, such as drug therapy. For example, in cancer patients, many chemotherapy drugs, as well as radiation treatments, work to destroy cancer cells through oxidation processes. Nutritional supplementation with antioxidants may hinder such treatment mechanisms. Patients should be advised to share with their health care provider any unusual nutritional regimens that they plan to try, especially if they have a serious illness.

FAT-SOLUBLE VITAMINS

Because fat-soluble vitamins are not water-soluble, they are not readily excreted in the urine, in contrast to the water-soluble vitamins mentioned earlier. Thus, daily ingestion of these vitamins is not necessary to maintain good health, and in fact, is more likely to result in hypervitaminosis, as noted earlier.

The fat-soluble vitamins are A, D, E, and K. As a group they share the following characteristics:
- Present in both plant and animal foods
- Stored primarily in the liver
- Exhibit slow metabolism or breakdown
- Excreted via the feces
- Can become toxic if excessive amounts are consumed (a condition known as *hypervitaminosis*)

VITAMIN A

Vitamin A (retinol) is derived from animal fats such as those found in dairy products (butter and milk), eggs, meat, liver, and fish liver oils. The vitamin A stored in animal tissues is derived from carotenes, which are found in plants (e.g., green and yellow vegetables, yellow fruits). Therefore, vitamin A is an exogenous substance for humans because it must be obtained from either plant or animal foods.

There are more than 600 naturally occurring carotenoid compounds in plant-based foods. Of these, 40 to 50 occur commonly in the human diet. Beta-carotene is the most prevalent of these, followed by alpha-carotene and cryptoxanthin. These are known as *provitamin A carotenoids* because they are all metabolized to various forms of vitamin A in the body. The sources of vitamin A as discussed are outlined as follows:

Vitamin A (retinol) → animal source → e.g., dairy products, meat, liver

Provitamin A (carotenoids) → plant source → e.g., green and yellow vegetables, yellow fruit

Table 54-2 lists sources of several specific nutrients.

Mechanism of Action and Drug Effects

Vitamin A is essential for night vision and for normal vision because it is part of one of the major retinal pigments called **rhodopsin**. Specifically, one molecule of *beta-carotene* is metabolized in the body to two molecules of the aldehyde compound *retinaldehyde,* the name of which is often shortened to *retinal.* The *cis* isomer of retinal combines with the protein *opsin* to form *rhodopsin,* the visual pigment that is required for normal "rod vision" in the retina. This is the vision that results from stimulation (by light) of the retinal visual cells known as *rods,* enabling both black-and-white vision and peripheral vision. These are the pre-

Table 54-2   Food Sources for Selected Nutrients

Vitamins/Minerals	Food Sources
Vitamin A	Liver; fish; dairy products; egg yolks; dark green, leafy, yellow-orange vegetables and fruit
Vitamin D	Dairy products, fortified cereals and fortified orange juice, liver, fish liver oils, saltwater fish, butter, eggs
Vitamin E	Fish, egg yolks, meats, vegetable oils, nuts, fruits, wheat germ, grains, fortified cereals
Vitamin K	Cheese, spinach, broccoli, brussels sprouts, kale, cabbage, turnip greens, soybean oils
Vitamin B$_1$ (thiamine)	Yeast, liver, enriched whole-grain products, beans
Vitamin B$_2$ (riboflavin)	Meats, liver, dairy products, eggs, legumes, nuts, enriched whole-grain products, green leafy vegetables, yeast
Vitamin B$_3$ (niacin)	Liver, turkey, tuna, peanuts, beans, yeast, enriched whole-grain breads and cereals, wheat germ
Vitamin B$_6$ (pyridoxine)	Organ meats, meats, poultry, fish, eggs, peanuts, whole grain products, vegetables, nuts, wheat germ, bananas, fortified cereals
Vitamin B$_{12}$ (cyanocobalamin)	Liver, kidney, shellfish, poultry, fish, eggs, milk, blue cheese, fortified cereals
Vitamin C (ascorbic acid)	Broccoli, green peppers, spinach, Brussels sprouts, citrus fruits, tomatoes, potatoes, strawberries, cabbage, liver
Calcium	Dairy products, fortified cereals and calcium-fortified orange juice, sardines, salmon
Magnesium	Meats, seafood, milk, cheese, yogurt, green leafy vegetables, bran cereal, nuts
Phosphorus	Milk, yogurt, cheese, peas, meat, fish, eggs
Zinc	Red meats, liver, oysters, certain seafood, milk products, eggs, beans, nuts, whole grains, fortified cereals

From Medline Plus. Available at www.nlm.nih.gov/medlineplus/vitamins.html. Accessed October 20, 2006; Mahan LK, Escott-Stump S: *Krause's food, nutrition, & diet therapy,* ed 11, Philadelphia, 2004, Saunders.

Table 54-3   Vitamin A: Adverse Effects

Body System	Adverse Effects
Central nervous	Headache, increased intracranial pressure, lethargy, malaise
Gastrointestinal	Nausea, vomiting, anorexia, abdominal pain, jaundice
Integumentary	Drying of skin, pruritus, increased pigmentation, night sweats
Metabolic	Hypomenorrhea, hypercalcemia
Musculoskeletal	Arthralgia, retarded growth

dominant types of vision that are operative at night, when the colors of objects are not as visible. Other retinal cells known as *cones* are chiefly involved in color and central vision (Chapter 58).

Some of the retinal from beta-carotene is also reduced to the alcohol compound known as *retinol.* The term *vitamin A,* in the strictest sense, refers to this alcohol compound. The remainder of the retinal may be oxidized to the carboxylic acid compound retinoic acid. Unlike retinal, retinoic acid has no direct role in vision, but it is essential for normal cell growth and differentiation and for the development of the physical shapes of the body's many parts—a process known as *morphogenesis.* It is also involved in the growth and development of bones and teeth and maintaining other body processes, including reproduction, integrity of mucosal and epithelial surfaces, and cholesterol and steroid synthesis.

Indications

Supplements of vitamin A may be used to satisfy normal body requirements or an increased demand such as in infants and pregnant and nursing women. A normal diet should provide adequate amounts of vitamin A, but in cases of excessive need or inadequate dietary intake, vitamin A supplementation is indicated to avoid problems associated with deficiency. Symptoms of vitamin A deficiency include night blindness; xerophthalmia; keratomalacia (softening of the cornea); hyperkeratosis of both the stratum corneum (outermost layer) of the skin and the sclera (outermost layer of eyeball); retarded infant growth; generalized weakness; and increased susceptibility of mucous membranes to infection. Vitamin A–related compounds, such as isotretinoin, are also used to treat various skin conditions, including acne, psoriasis, and *keratosis* follicularis (Chapter 57).

Contraindications

The only usual contraindications to vitamin A supplementation include known allergy to the individual vitamin product; known current state of hypervitaminosis; and excessive supplementation beyond recommended guidelines, especially during pregnancy.

Adverse Effects

There are very few acute adverse effects associated with normal vitamin A ingestion. Only after long-term, excessive ingestion of vitamin A do symptoms appear. Adverse effects are usually noticed in bones, mucous membranes, the liver, and the skin. Table 54-3 lists some of the symptoms of long-term, excessive ingestion of vitamin A.

Toxicity and Management of Overdose

The major toxic effects of vitamin A result from ingestion of excessive amounts, which occurs most commonly in children. A few hours after administration of an excess dose of vitamin A (over 25,000 units/kg), irritability, drowsiness, vertigo, delirium, coma, vomiting, and/or diarrhea may occur. In infants, excessive amounts of vitamin A can cause an increase in cranial pressure, resulting in symptoms such as bulging fontanelles, headache, papilledema, exophthalmos (bulging eyeballs), and visual disturbances. Papilledema is the presence of edematous fluid, often including blood, in the optic disk. This is the portion of the eye in the back of the retina, where nerve fibers converge to form the optic nerve.

Over several weeks, a generalized peeling of the skin and erythema (skin reddening) may occur. These symptoms seem to disappear a few days after discontinuation of the drug, which is the only treatment necessary in situations of overdose.

Interactions

Vitamin A is absorbed to a lesser extent with the simultaneous use of lubricant laxatives and cholestyramine. In addition, the use of isotretinoin concurrently with vitamin A supplementation can result in additive effects and possibly toxicity.

Dosages

For the recommended dosages for vitamin A, see the table on page 830.

Drug Profiles

There are three forms of vitamin A: retinol, retinyl palmitate, and retinyl acetate. Medications containing vitamin A may require a prescription, but many over-the-counter (OTC) products, such as multivitamins, are also available. All vitamin A products are classified as pregnancy category A drugs and are contraindicated in patients who have a hypersensitivity to vitamin A and in those with oral malabsorption syndromes.

vitamin A

Vitamin A (Aquasol A), also known as *retinol, retinyl palmitate,* and *retinyl acetate,* is available in a variety of oral forms as well as an injectable form. Doses for vitamin A can be expressed in international units (IU) or microgram retinol equivalents (RE); one IU is approximately equal to 0.3 mcg of retinol equivalents (RE) from animal foods and about 3.6 mcg of beta-carotene from plant foods. Currently, the IU and RE standards are being replaced by a newer standard of vitamin A measurement: the *retinol activity equivalent (RAE).* One RAE is approximately equal to the following:

- 1 mcg of retinol (either dietary or supplemental)
- 2 mcg of supplemental beta-carotene
- 12 mcg of dietary beta-carotene
- 24 mcg of dietary carotenoids

Pharmacokinetics

Half-Life	Onset	Peak	Duration
PO: 50-100 days*	PO: 42 days	PO: 4 hr	PO: Unknown

*Rate of elimination of hepatic reserves upon eating a retinol-free diet.

VITAMIN D

Vitamin D, also called the *sunshine vitamin,* is responsible for the proper utilization of calcium and phosphorus in the body. The term *vitamin D* designates a group of analog steroid structural chemicals with vitamin D activity. The two most important members of the vitamin D family are vitamin D_2 (ergocalciferol) and vitamin D_3 (cholecalciferol). They have different sites of origin but similar functions in the body. Ergocalciferol (vitamin D_2) is plant vitamin D and is therefore obtained through dietary sources. The natural form of vitamin D produced in the skin by ultraviolet irradiation (sun) is chemically known as 7-dehydrocholesterol. It is more commonly referred to as *cholecalciferol* (vitamin D_3). This endogenous synthesis of vitamin D_3 usually produces sufficient amounts to meet daily requirements. Chemically, the two vitamin D compounds are different, but physiologically they produce the same effect.

$$Vitamin\ D_2 \rightarrow ergocalciferol \rightarrow plant\ vitamin\ D$$
$$Vitamin\ D_3 \rightarrow cholecalciferol \rightarrow human\ vitamin\ D$$

Vitamin D is obtained through both endogenous synthesis and through vitamin D_2-containing foods such as fish oils, salmon, sardines, and herring; fortified milk, bread, and cereals; and animal livers, tuna fish, eggs, and butter.

Mechanism of Action and Drug Effects

The basic function of vitamin D is to regulate the absorption and subsequent utilization of calcium and phosphorus. It is also necessary for the normal calcification of bone. Vitamin D in coordination with parathyroid hormone and calcitonin regulates serum calcium levels by increasing calcium absorption from the small intestine and extracting calcium from the bone when needed. As ergocalciferol and cholecalciferol, vitamin D is inactive and requires transformation into active metabolites for biologic activity. Both vitamin D_2 and vitamin D_3 are biotransformed primarily in the liver by the actions of the parathyroid hormone. The resulting compound, calcifediol, is then transported to the kidney, where it is converted to calcitriol, which is believed to be the most physiologically active vitamin D analog. Calcitriol promotes the intestinal absorption of calcium and phosphorus and the deposition of calcium and phosphorus into the structure of teeth and bones.

The drug effects of vitamin D are very similar to those of vitamin A and essentially all vitamin and mineral compounds. It is used as a supplement to satisfy normal daily requirements or an increased demand as in infants and pregnant and nursing women.

Indications

Vitamin D can be used either to supplement the current daily intake of vitamin D or to treat a deficiency of vitamin D. In the case of supplementation, it is given as a prophylactic measure to prevent deficiency-related problems. Vitamin D may also be used to treat and correct the result of a long-term deficiency that leads to such conditions as infantile rickets, tetany (involuntary sustained muscular contractions), and osteomalacia (softening of bones). **Rickets** is specifically a vitamin D deficiency state. Symptoms include soft, pliable bones, causing such deformities as bow legs and knock knees; nodular enlargement on the ends and sides of the bones; muscle pain; enlarged skull; chest deformities; spinal curvature; enlargement of the liver and spleen; profuse sweating; and general tenderness of the body when touched. Vitamin D can also help promote the absorption of phosphorus and calcium. For this reason, its use is important in preventing osteoporosis. Because of the role of vitamin D in the regulation of calcium and phosphorus, it may be used to correct deficiencies of these two elements. Other uses include dietary supplement, osteodystrophy, hypocalcemia, hypoparathyroidism, pseudohypoparathyroidism, and hypophosphatemia.

Contraindications

The only usual contraindications to vitamin D supplements are known allergy to a given vitamin product, or known hypervitaminosis D state.

Adverse Effects

As with vitamin A, very few acute adverse effects are associated with normal vitamin D ingestion. Only after long-term, excessive ingestion of vitamin D do symptoms appear. Such effects are usually noticed in the gastrointestinal tract or the central nervous system (CNS) and are listed in Table 54-4.

DOSAGES

Selected Vitamins

Drug	Pharmacologic Class	Usual Dosage Range	Indications
Vitamin D–Active Compounds			
calcifediol (hydroxyvitamin D₃, Calderol)	Fat-soluble	**Adult and pediatric >1 yr** PO: 20-100 mcg/day or up to 200 mcg qod **Infants** PO: 5-7 mcg/kg/day	Hypocalcemia in hemodialysis patients; hepatic osteodystrophy
calcitriol (dihydroxyvitamin D₃, Rocaltrol, Calcijex)	Fat-soluble	**Adult and pediatric >6 yr** PO/IV: 0.5-2 mcg/day **Pediatric 1-5 yr** PO/IV: 0.25-0.75 mcg/day	Hypoparathyroidism; hypocalcemia in patients receiving regular hemodialysis
dihydrotachysterol (DHT, Hytakerol)	Fat-soluble (a form of vitamin D)	**Adult and pediatric >12 yr** PO: 0.8-2.4 mg/day × several days, followed by 0.2-1 mg/day **Pediatric <12 yr** PO: 1-5 mg/day ×4 days, then 0.1-0.5 mg/day	Hypoparathyroidism
ergocalciferol (vitamin D₂, Drisdol, Calciferol)	Fat-soluble	**Adult** PO/IM: 10,000-60,000 IU/day **Pediatric** 3000-5000 IU/day **Adult and pediatric** PO/IM: 25,000-200,000 IU/day **Adult and pediatric** PO/IM: 4000-40,000 IU/day	Rickets Hypoparathyroidism Renal failure
Vitamin B–Active Compounds			
vitamin B₁ (thiamine, Thiamilate)	Water-soluble, B-complex group	**Adult** 1-2 mg/day **Infant/child** PO/IM/IV: 0.3-1.5 mg/day	Nutritional supplement; alcohol-induced deficiency Nutritional supplement; nutritional deficiency
vitamin B₁₂ (cyanocobalamin, Big Shot B-12, Nascobal)	Water-soluble, B-complex group	**Adult and pediatric** IM/SC: 100 mcg/mo **Adult and pediatric** PO: 50-100 mcg/day **Adult only** Intranasal gel: 500 mcg weekly	Deficiency; anemia
vitamin B₂ (riboflavin)	Water-soluble, B-complex group	**Adult** PO: 5-30 mg/day **Pediatric** 2.5-10 mg/day	Deficiency
vitamin B₃ (niacin, nicotinic acid, Nicotinex)	Water-soluble, B-complex group	**Adult** PO: 1-6 g/day PO: Up to 500 mg/day **Pediatric** PO: 50-100 mg tid	Hyperlipidemia; deficiency (pellagra)
Vitamin B₆ (pyridoxine, aminoxin, Vitelle Nestrex)	Water-soluble, B-complex group	**Adult** PO/IV: 10-20 mg/day × 3 wk **Pediatric** PO/IV: 5-25 mg/day × 3 wk, then use a pediatric multivitamin product **Adult** PO/IV: 100-200 mg/day **Pediatric** 10-50 mg/day	Dietary deficiency Drug-induced neuritis (e.g., isoniazid for TB)

DOSAGES

Selected Vitamins—cont'd

Drug	Pharmacologic Class	Usual Dosage Range	Indications
Vitamins A, C, E, and K			
vitamin A (Aquasol A, others)	Fat-soluble	**Adult and pediatric >8 yr** PO: Up to 500,000 IU/day × 3 days, then 10,000-50,000 IU/day for up to 2 mo **Pediatric 1-8 yr** PO: 5000-10,000 IU/kg/day until recovery	Deficiency
vitamin C (ascorbic acid, Vita-C, Dull-C, others)	Water-soluble	**Adult and pediatric** PO/IV/IM/SC: 100-250 mg qd-bid ×2 wk	Deficiency (scurvy)
vitamin E (d-alpha tocopherol, Aquavit E, Dry E 400, others)	Fat-soluble	**Adult and pediatric >14 yr** PO: 22.5 IU/day **Pediatric 0-14 yr** 4.5-16.5 IU/day	Nutritional supplement
vitamin K (phytonadione, Mephyton, AquaMEPHYTON)	Fat-soluble	**Adult** PO: 5-25 mg/day IM/IV: 10-25 mg single dose **Infant and pediatric** PO: 2.5-5 mg/day IM/IV: 1-2 mg single dose	Deficiency; warfarin-induced hypoprothrombinemia Deficiency; hemorrhagic disease of newborn infant

TB, Tuberculosis.

Table 54-4   Vitamin D: Adverse Effects

Body System	Adverse Effects
Cardiovascular	Hypertension, dysrhythmias
Central nervous	Fatigue, weakness, drowsiness, headache
Gastrointestinal	Nausea, vomiting, anorexia, cramps, metallic taste, dry mouth, constipation
Genitourinary	Polyuria, albuminuria, increased BUN
Musculoskeletal	Decreased bone growth, bone pain, muscle pain

BUN, Blood urea nitrogen.

Toxicity and Management of Overdose

The major toxic effects from ingesting excessive amounts of vitamin D occur most commonly in children. Discontinuation of vitamin D and reduced calcium intake reverse the toxic state. The amount of vitamin D considered to be too much varies considerably among individuals but is generally thought to be 1.25 to 2.5 mg of ergocalciferol daily in adults and 25 mcg daily in infants and children.

The toxic effects of vitamin D are those associated with hypertension, such as weakness, fatigue, headache, anorexia, dry mouth, metallic taste, nausea, vomiting, abdominal cramps, ataxia, and bone pain. If not recognized and treated, these symptoms can progress to impairment of renal function and osteoporosis.

Interactions

Reduced absorption of vitamin D occurs with the simultaneous use of lubricant laxatives and cholestyramine. Patients taking digitalis preparations can develop cardiac dysrhythmias as a result of vitamin D intake.

Dosages

For the recommended dosages for vitamin D, see the table on page 830.

Drug Profiles

There are four forms of vitamin D: calcifediol, calcitriol, dihydrotachysterol, and ergocalciferol. Vitamin D is available in OTC medications, such as a multivitamin product, or by prescription. Although various pharmaceutical manufacturers may list their individual vitamin D products as pregnancy category C, these products are generally considered to be category A or B as long as the patient is not dosed higher than the RDA of vitamin D for a pregnant woman. Contraindications to vitamin D products include known drug product allergy, hypercalcemia, renal dysfunction, or hyperphosphatemia.

calcifediol

Calcifediol (Calderol) is the 25-hydroxylated form of cholecalciferol (vitamin D_3). It is a vitamin D analog primarily used for the management of hypocalcemia in patients with chronic renal failure who are undergoing hemodialysis. Calcifediol is also used for histologic signs of hyperparathyroid disease. It is available only for oral use.

Pharmacokinetics

Half-Life	Onset	Peak	Duration
PO: 16 days	PO: Variable	PO: Unknown	PO: Unknown

calcitriol

Calcitriol (Rocaltrol, Calcijex) is the 1,25-dihydroxylated form of cholecalciferol (vitamin D_3). It is a vitamin D analog used for the management of hypocalcemia in patients with chronic renal failure who are undergoing hemodialysis. It is also used in the treatment of hypoparathyroidism and pseudohypoparathyroidism, vitamin D–dependent rickets, hypophosphatemia, and hypocalcemia in premature infants. It is available in both oral and injectable forms.

Pharmacokinetics

Half-Life	Onset	Peak	Duration
PO: 3-6 hr	PO: <3 hr	PO: 3-6 hr	PO: 3-5 days

dihydrotachysterol

Dihydrotachysterol (Hytakerol) is a vitamin D analog that is administered orally once daily for the treatment of any of the previously mentioned conditions. Intramuscular use is indicated for patients with gastrointestinal, liver, or biliary disease associated with malabsorption of vitamin D analogs. It is available only for oral use.

Pharmacokinetics

Half-Life	Onset	Peak	Duration
PO: Unknown	PO: Unknown	PO: Unknown	PO: Unknown

ergocalciferol

Ergocalciferol (Drisdol, Calciferol) is vitamin D_2. Its use is indicated for patients with gastrointestinal, liver, or biliary disease associated with malabsorption of vitamin D analogs. It is available orally and parenterally.

Pharmacokinetics

Half-Life	Onset	Peak	Duration
PO: 19 days	PO: 30 days	PO: Unknown	PO: Months to years

VITAMIN E

Four biologically active chemicals called **tocopherols** (alpha, beta, gamma, and delta) make up the vitamin E compounds. Alpha-tocopherol is the most biologically active natural form of vitamin E. The exact biologic function of vitamin E is unknown, but it is believed to act as an antioxidant.

Vitamin E → alpha-tocopherol → plant and animal sources

Mechanism of Action and Drug Effects

Although vitamin E is a powerful biologic antioxidant and an essential component of the diet, its exact nutritional function has not been fully demonstrated. The only significant deficiency syndrome for vitamin E has been recognized in premature infants. In this situation, vitamin E deficiency may result in irritability, edema, thrombosis, and hemolytic anemia.

The drug effects of vitamin E are not as well defined as those of the other fat-soluble vitamins. It is believed to protect polyunsaturated fatty acids, a component of cellular membranes. It has also been shown to hinder the deterioration of substances such as vitamin A and ascorbic acid (vitamin C), two substances that are highly oxygen sensitive and readily oxidized, thus acting as an antioxidant.

Indications

Vitamin E is most commonly used as a dietary supplement to augment current daily intake or to treat a deficiency. Those at greatest risk for complications from vitamin E deficiency are premature infants. Vitamin E has recently received much attention as an antioxidant. Preventing the oxidation of various substances prevents the formation of toxic chemicals within the body, some of which are believed to cause cancer. There is a popular but unproved theory that vitamin E has beneficial effects for patients with cancer, heart disease, premenstrual syndrome (PMS), and sexual dysfunction.

Table 54-5	Vitamin E: Adverse Effects
Body System	**Adverse Effects**
Central nervous	Fatigue, headache, blurred vision
Gastrointestinal	Nausea, diarrhea, flatulence
Genitourinary	Increased BUN
Musculoskeletal	Weakness

BUN, Blood urea nitrogen.

Contraindications

Contraindications for vitamin E include known allergy to a specific vitamin E product. There are currently no approved injectable forms for this vitamin.

Adverse Effects

As with vitamin D, very few acute adverse effects are associated with normal vitamin E ingestion because it is relatively nontoxic. Adverse effects are usually noticed in the gastrointestinal tract or CNS and are listed in Table 54-5.

Dosages

For the recommended dosages for vitamin E, see the table on page 830.

Drug Profiles

Vitamin E is available as an OTC medication. It has four forms: alpha-, beta-, gamma-, and delta-tocopherol. It is available in many multivitamin preparations and is also available by prescription. Vitamin E products are usually contraindicated only in cases of known drug allergy.

vitamin E

Vitamin E (Aquasol E) activity is generally expressed in USP or international units (IU). One unit of vitamin E equals the biologic activity of the following:

- 1 mg of DL-alpha-tocopheryl acetate
- 1.12 mg of DL-alpha-tocopheryl acid succinate
- 910 mcg of DL-alpha-tocopherol
- 735 mcg of D-alpha-tocopheryl acetate
- 830 mcg of D-alpha-tocopheryl acid succinate
- 670 mcg of D-alpha-tocopherol
- Vitamin E is available for oral and topical use.

Pharmacokinetics

Half-Life	Onset	Peak	Duration
PO: Variable	PO: Unknown	PO: Unknown	PO: Variable

VITAMIN K

Vitamin K is the last of the four fat-soluble vitamins (A, D, E, and K). There are three types of vitamin K: phytonadione (vitamin K_1), menaquinone (vitamin K_2), and menadione (vitamin K_3). The body does not store large amounts of vitamin K; however, vitamin K_2 is synthesized by the intestinal flora, thus providing an endogenous supply.

Vitamin K_1 → phytonadione → green leafy vegetables (exogenous)
Vitamin K_2 → menaquinone → intestinal flora (endogenous)

Vitamin K is essential for the synthesis of blood coagulation factors, which takes place in the liver. Vitamin K-dependent blood coagulation factors are factors II, VII, IX, and X. Other names for these clotting factors are as follows:

factor II → prothrombin
factor VII → proconvertin

Vitamin K

factor IX → Christmas factor
factor X → Stuart-Power factor

Mechanism of Action and Drug Effects

As previously mentioned, vitamin K activity is essential for effective blood clotting because it facilitates the hepatic biosynthesis of factor II *(prothrombin)*, factor VII *(convertin)*, factor IX *(Christmas factor)*, and factor X *(Stuart-Power factor)*. Vitamin K deficiency results in coagulation disorders caused by hypoprothrombinemia.

The drug effects of vitamin K are limited to its action on the vitamin K–dependent clotting factors produced in the liver (II, VII, IX, and X). Coagulation defects affecting these clotting factors can be corrected with administration of vitamin K. Vitamin K deficiency is rare because intestinal flora are normally able to synthesize sufficient amounts. If a deficiency develops, it can be corrected with vitamin K supplementation.

Indications

Vitamin K is indicated for dietary supplementation and for treating deficiency states. Although rare, deficiency states can develop with inadequate dietary intake or broad-spectrum inhibition of the intestinal flora resulting from the administration of broad-spectrum antibiotics. Deficiency states can also be seen in newborns because of malabsorption attributable to inadequate amounts of bile or selected drugs. For this reason, infants born in hospitals are often given a prophylactic intramuscular dose of vitamin K on arrival to the nursery. Vitamin K deficiency can also result from the administration and pharmacologic action of specific anticoagulants that inhibit hepatic vitamin K activity. Coumarin- and indanedione-derivative anticoagulants (e.g., warfarin) thin the blood by inhibiting vitamin K–dependent clotting factors in the liver. Administration of vitamin K overrides the mechanism by which the anticoagulants inhibit production of vitamin K–dependent clotting factors.

Contraindications

The only usual contraindication to treatment with vitamin K is known drug allergy.

Adverse Effects

Vitamin K is relatively nontoxic and thus causes very few adverse effects. Severe reactions limited to hypersensitivity or anaphylaxis have occurred rarely during or immediately after intravenous administration. Adverse effects are usually related to injection-site reactions and hypersensitivity. See Table 54-6 for a list of such major effects by body system.

Toxicity and Management of Overdose

Toxicity is primarily limited to use in the newborn. Hemolysis of red blood cells (RBCs) can occur, especially in infants with low levels of glucose-6-phosphate dehydrogenase (G6PD). In severe cases, replacement with blood products may be indicated.

Table 54-6	**Vitamin K: Adverse Effects**
Body System	**Adverse Effects**
Central nervous	Headache, brain damage (large doses)
Gastrointestinal	Nausea, decreased liver function tests
Hematologic	Hemolytic anemia, hemoglobinuria, hyperbilirubinemia
Integumentary	Rash, urticaria

Dosages

See the dosages table.

Drug Profiles

The most commonly used form of vitamin K is phytonadione (vitamin K_1). Both phytonadione and menadione (vitamin K_3) are available by prescription only in oral and parenteral forms. Menadione is classified as a pregnancy category X drug, whereas phytonadione is a category C drug. They are both contraindicated in patients who have shown a hypersensitivity reaction to them. Their use is also contraindicated during the last few weeks of pregnancy and in patients with severe hepatic disease.

vitamin K_1

Vitamin K_1 (Phytonadione, Mephyton, AquaMEPHTYON) is available for both oral and injectable use.

Pharmacokinetics			
Half-Life	**Onset**	**Peak**	**Duration**
PO: Unknown	PO: Variable	PO: 1-2 hr	PO: Unknown

WATER-SOLUBLE VITAMINS

The water-soluble vitamins include the vitamin B complex and vitamin C (ascorbic acid). They are present in a variety of plant and animal food sources. The vitamin B complex is a group of 10 vitamins that are often found together in food, although they are chemically dissimilar and have different metabolic functions. Because the B vitamins were originally isolated from the same sources, primarily liver and yeast, they were grouped together as B-complex vitamins. Vitamin C (ascorbic acid), the other principal water-soluble vitamin, is concentrated more heavily in different food sources (primarily citrus fruits) than the B-complex vitamins and thus is not classified as part of the B complex. The numeric subscripts associated with various B vitamins reflect the sequential order in which they were discovered. In clinical practice, some B vitamins are more often referred to by their "common" name, whereas others are more often referred to by their numeric designation. For example, "vitamin B_{12}" is used more often in clinical practice than its corresponding common name, "cyanocobalamin." However, "folic acid" is rarely referred to as "vitamin B_9," although this would also be correct. The most commonly used B complex vitamins, as well as vitamin C, are listed in Box 54-1. Folic acid (vitamin B_9) has a special role in hematopoiesis, and therefore is described further in Chapter 56.

Water-soluble vitamins are a chemically diverse group sharing only the characteristic of being dissolvable in water. Like fat-soluble vitamins, they act primarily as coenzymes or oxidation-reduction agents in important metabolic pathways. Unlike fat-

Box 54-1	Water-Soluble Vitamins: Alternate Names
Vitamin B complex	Vitamin B$_1$ → thiamine Vitamin B$_2$ → riboflavin Vitamin B$_3$ → niacin Vitamin B$_5$ → pantothenic acid Vitamin B$_6$ → pyridoxine Vitamin B$_9$ → folic acid Vitamin B$_{12}$ → cyanocobalamin
Vitamin C	→ ascorbic acid

soluble vitamins, water-soluble vitamins are not stored in the body in appreciable amounts. Their water-soluble properties promote urinary excretion and reduce their half-life in the body. Therefore, dietary intake must be adequate and regular or deficiency states will develop. Because these vitamins are water soluble, excess amounts are excreted in the urine. The body excretes what it does not need, which makes toxic reactions to water-soluble vitamins very rare.

VITAMIN B$_1$

A deficiency of vitamin B$_1$ results in the classic disease **beriberi** or Wernicke's encephalopathy (cerebral beriberi). Common findings in beriberi include brain lesions, polyneuropathy of peripheral nerves, serous effusions (abnormal collections of fluids in body tissues), and cardiac anatomic changes. Vitamin deficiency can result from poor diet, extended fever, hyperthyroidism, liver disease, alcoholism, malabsorption, and pregnancy and breast-feeding.

Mechanism of Action and Drug Effects

Thiamine is an essential precursor for the formation of *thiamine pyrophosphate*. When thiamine combines with *adenosine triphosphate (ATP)* the result is *thiamine pyrophosphate coenzyme*. This is required for the *Krebs cycle (citric acid cycle)*, a major part of carbohydrate metabolism, as well as several metabolic pathways. Additionally, thiamine plays a key role in the integrity of the peripheral nervous system, cardiovascular system, and the gastrointestinal tract.

Indications

The beneficial drug effects and the essential role of thiamine in so many metabolic pathways make it useful in treating a variety of metabolic disorders. These include subacute necrotizing encephalomyelopathy, maple syrup urine disease, and lactic acidosis associated with pyruvate carboxylase enzyme deficiency and hyper-β-alaninemia. Some of the deficiency states treated by thiamine are beriberi, Wernicke's encephalopathy syndrome, peripheral neuritis associated with **pellagra** (niacin deficiency)**,** and neuritis of pregnancy. Thiamine is used as a dietary supplement to prevent or treat deficiency in cases of malabsorption such as that induced by alcoholism, cirrhosis, or gastrointestinal disease. Other areas in which thiamine may have therapeutic value are the management of poor appetite, ulcerative colitis, chronic diarrhea, and cerebellar syndrome or ataxia (impaired muscular coordination). It is also used as an oral insect repellent.

Contraindications

The only usual contraindication to any of the B-complex vitamins is known allergy to a specific vitamin product.

Adverse Effects

Adverse effects are rare but include hypersensitivity reactions, nausea, restlessness, pulmonary edema, pruritus, urticaria, weakness, sweating, angioedema, cyanosis, and cardiovascular collapse. Administration by intramuscular injection can produce local tenderness, and intravenous injections can produce anaphylaxis.

Interactions

Thiamine is incompatible with alkaline- and sulfite-containing solutions.

Dosages

See the Dosages table on page 830.

Drug Profiles

thiamine

Thiamine is contraindicated only in individuals with a history of a hypersensitivity reaction. Thiamine is available for both oral use and by injection. Pregnancy category A.

Pharmacokinetics

Half-Life	Onset	Peak	Duration
Unknown	Unknown	Unknown	24 hr

VITAMIN B$_2$

A deficiency of vitamin B$_2$ (riboflavin) results in cutaneous, oral, and corneal changes that include cheilosis, seborrheic dermatitis, and keratitis.

Mechanism of Action and Drug Effects

Riboflavin serves several important functions. In the body, riboflavin is converted into two coenzymes (flavin mononucleotide [FMN] and flavin adenine dinucleotide [FAD]) that are essential for tissue respiration. Riboflavin also plays an important part in transfer reactions, especially in carbohydrate catabolism. Another B vitamin, vitamin B$_6$ (pyridoxine), requires riboflavin for activation. It is also needed to convert tryptophan into niacin and to maintain erythrocyte integrity. The drug effects of riboflavin are mainly limited to replacement therapy for deficiency states. Deficiency is rare and does not usually occur in healthy people. However, deficiency may occur as a result of malnutrition or intestinal malabsorption or because of alcoholism or other diseases or infections.

Indications

Riboflavin is primarily used as a dietary supplement and to treat deficiency states. Patients who may suffer from riboflavin deficiency include those with long-standing infections, liver disease, alcoholism, and malignancy, and those taking probenecid. Riboflavin supplementation may also be beneficial in treating microcytic anemia; acne; migraine headache; congenital methemoglobinemia (presence in the blood of an abnormal, nonfunctional hemoglobin [Hgb] pigment); muscle cramps; and Gopalan's syndrome, a symptom of suspected riboflavin [and possibly pantothenic acid (vitamin B$_5$)] deficiency that involves a sensation of tingling in the extremities. For this reason, it is also called "burning feet syndrome."

Contraindications

The only usual contraindication to riboflavin is known allergy to a given vitamin product.

Adverse Effects

Riboflavin is a very safe and effective vitamin; to date, no adverse effects or toxic effects have been reported. In large doses, riboflavin will discolor urine to a yellow-orange.

Dosages

Commonly recommended dosages for riboflavin are listed in the table on page 830.

Drug Profiles

riboflavin

Riboflavin (vitamin B_2) is needed for normal respiratory reactions. It is a safe, nontoxic water-soluble vitamin with almost no adverse effects. It is available only for oral use. Pregnancy category A.

Pharmacokinetics

Half-Life	Onset	Peak	Duration
PO: 66-84 min	PO: Unknown	PO: Unknown	PO: 24 hr

VITAMIN B_3

The body is able to produce a small amount of vitamin B_3 (niacin) from dietary tryptophan, an essential amino acid occurring in dietary proteins and some commercially available nutritional supplements.

A dietary deficiency of niacin will produce the classic symptoms known as pellagra:

- *Mental:* various psychotic symptoms
- *Neurologic:* neurasthenic syndrome
- *Cutaneous:* crusting, erythema, desquamation, scaly dermatitis
- *Mucous membrane:* inflammation in oral, vaginal, and urethral mucosa, including glossitis (inflamed tongue)
- *gastrointestinal:* diarrhea or bloody diarrhea

Mechanism of Action and Drug Effects

Generally speaking, the metabolic actions of niacin (vitamin B_3) are not due to niacin in the ingested form but rather to its metabolic product, *nicotinamide.* Nicotinamide is required for numerous metabolic reactions, including those involved in carbohydrate, protein, purine, and lipid metabolism, as well as tissue respiration (Figure 54-1). A key example involves two compounds, *nicotinamide adenosine dinucleotide (NAD) and nicotinamide adenosine dinucleotide phosphate (NADP),* both of which are necessary for the carbohydrate pathway known as *glycogenolysis* (the breakdown of stored glycogen to usable glucose). The parent compound, niacin itself, also has a pharmacologic

role as an *antilipemic* drug (Chapter 28). The doses of niacin required for this pharmacologic effect are substantially higher than those required for the nutritional and metabolic effects described earlier. Niacin lowers serum cholesterol and triglyceride levels by reducing very low-density lipoprotein (VLDL) synthesis. The principal carrier of cholesterol in the blood is LDL. Because VLDL is the precursor to LDL, reducing VLDL will result in reduction of LDL and, consequently, cholesterol.

Indications

Niacin is indicated for the prevention and treatment of pellagra, a condition caused by a deficiency of vitamin B_3 that is most commonly the result of malabsorption. As previously stated, niacin is also for certain types of hyperlipidemia (Chapter 28). It also has a beneficial effect in peripheral vascular disease.

Contraindications

Niacin, unlike certain other B-complex vitamins, has a few additional contraindications besides drug allergy. These include liver disease, severe hypotension, arterial hemorrhage, and active peptic ulcer disease.

Adverse Effects

The most frequent adverse effects associated with the use of niacin are flushing, pruritis, and gastrointestinal distress. These usually subside with continual use. They are most frequently seen when larger doses of niacin are used in the treatment of hyperlipidemia. Table 54-7 lists adverse effects and adverse effects by body system.

Dosages

Commonly recommended dosages for niacin are listed in the table on page 830.

Table 54-7 Niacin: Adverse Effects

Body System	Adverse Effects
Cardiovascular	Postural hypotension, dysrhythmias, atrial fibrillation
Central nervous	Headache, dizziness, anxiety, sensation of warmth
Gastrointestinal	Nausea, vomiting, diarrhea, peptic ulcer
Genitourinary	Hyperuricemia
Hepatic	Abnormal liver function tests, hepatitis
Integumentary	Flushing, dry skin, rash, pruritus, keratosis
Metabolic	Decreased glucose tolerance

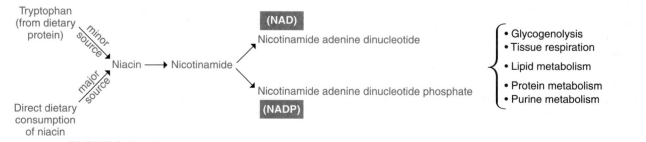

FIGURE 54-1 Niacin, once in the body, is converted to nicotinamide adenosine dinucleotide (NAD) and nicotinamide adenosine dinucleotide (NADP), which are coenzymes needed for many metabolic processes.

Drug Profiles

niacin

Niacin is used to treat pellagra, hyperlipidemias, and peripheral vascular disease. Its use should be monitored closely in patients who have a history of coronary artery disease, gallbladder disease, jaundice, liver disease, or arterial bleeding. It is available only for oral use. Pregnancy category A.

Pharmacokinetics

Half-Life	Onset	Peak	Duration
PO: 45 min	PO: Variable	PO: Serum: 45 min	PO: Variable

VITAMIN B₆

Vitamin B$_6$ (pyridoxine) is composed of three compounds: pyridoxine, pyridoxal, and pyridoxamine.

Deficiency of vitamin B$_6$ can lead to a type of anemia known as *sideroblastic anemia,* neurologic disturbances, seborrheic dermatitis, cheilosis (chapped or fissured lips), and xanthurenic aciduria (formation of xanthine crystals or "stones" in urine). It may also result in epileptiform convulsions, especially in neonates and infants; hypochromic microcytic anemia; and glossitis (inflamed tongue) and stomatitis (inflamed oral mucosa). Pyridoxine deficiency also affects the peripheral nerves, skin, mucous membranes, and the hematopoietic system. Inadequate intake or poor absorption of pyridoxine causes the development of these conditions. Vitamin B$_6$ deficiency may occur as a result of uremia, alcoholism, cirrhosis, hyperthyroidism, malabsorption syndromes, and heart failure. It may also be induced by various drugs, such as isoniazid, cycloserine, ethionamide, hydralazine, penicillamine, and pyrazinamide.

Mechanism of Action and Drug Effects

Pyridoxine, pyridoxal, and pyridoxamine are all converted in erythrocytes to the active coenzyme forms of vitamin B$_6$, *pyridoxal phosphate* and *pyridoxamine phosphate*. These compounds are necessary for many metabolic functions, such as protein, carbohydrate, and lipid utilization in the body. They also play an important part in the conversion of the amino acid tryptophan to niacin (vitamin B$_3$) and the neurotransmitter *serotonin*. They are also essential in the synthesis of gamma-aminobutyric acid (GABA), an inhibitory neurotransmitter in the CNS. They are important in the synthesis of heme and the maintenance of the hematopoietic system. Additionally, these substances are necessary for the integrity of the peripheral nerves, skin, and mucous membranes.

Indications

Pyridoxine is used to prevent and treat vitamin B$_6$ deficiency. This includes deficiency that can result from therapy with certain medications, including isoniazid (for TB), hydralazine (for hypertension), and oral contraceptives. Although deficiency of vitamin B$_6$ is rare, it can occur in conditions of inadequate intake or poor absorption of pyridoxine. Seizures that are unresponsive to usual therapy, morning sickness during pregnancy, and various metabolic disorders may respond to pyridoxine therapy.

Contraindications

The only usual contraindication to pyridoxine use is drug allergy.

Table 54-8	**Pyridoxine: Adverse Effects**
Body System	**Adverse Effects**
Central nervous	Paresthesias, flushing, warmth, headache, lethargy
Integumentary	Pain at injection site

Adverse Effects

Adverse effects with pyridoxine use are rare and usually do not occur with normal doses; high doses and chronic usage may produce adverse effects as listed in Table 54-8. Toxic effects are a result of very large doses sustained for several months. Neurotoxicity is the most likely result, but this will subside upon discontinuation of the pyridoxine.

Interactions

Pyridoxine exhibits several significant interactions with selected drugs. Pyridoxine will reduce the activity of levodopa; therefore, vitamin formulations containing B$_6$ should be avoided in patients taking levodopa. Drugs that have an antivitamin effect on pyridoxine include cycloserine, ethionamide, isoniazid, pyrazinamide, and oral contraceptives.

Dosages

Commonly recommended dosages for vitamin B$_6$ are listed in the table on page 830.

Drug Profiles

pyridoxine

Pyridoxine is a water-soluble B-complex vitamin composed of three components: pyridoxine, pyridoxal, and pyridoxamine. It has several vital roles in the body but is primarily responsible for the integrity of peripheral nerves, skin, mucous membranes, and the hematopoietic system.

It is available only for oral use. Pregnancy category A.

Pharmacokinetics

Half-Life	Onset	Peak	Duration
15-20 days	Unknown	Unknown	Unknown

VITAMIN B₁₂

Vitamin B$_{12}$ (cyanocobalamin) is a cobalt-containing (hence, its name; and "cyano-" means "blue"), water-soluble B-complex vitamin. It is synthesized by microorganisms and is present in the body as two different coenzymes: adenosylcobalamin and methylcobalamin. Cyanocobalamin is a required coenzyme for many metabolic pathways, including fat and carbohydrate metabolism and protein synthesis. It is also required for growth, cell replication, hematopoiesis, and nucleoprotein and myelin synthesis (Figure 54-2).

Vitamin B$_{12}$ deficiency results in gastrointestinal lesions, neurologic symptoms that can result in degenerative CNS lesions, and megaloblastic anemia. The major cause of cyanocobalamin deficiency is malabsorption. Other possible but less likely causes are poor diet, chronic alcoholism, and chronic hemorrhage.

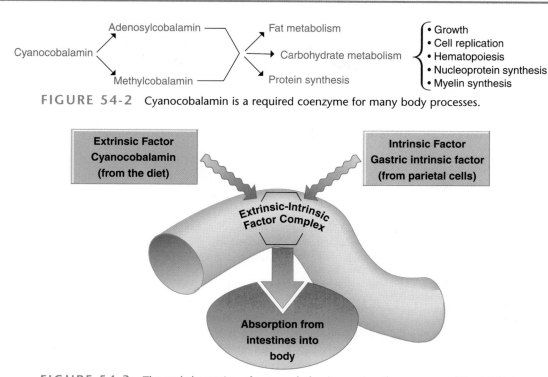

FIGURE 54-2   Cyanocobalamin is a required coenzyme for many body processes.

FIGURE 54-3   The oral absorption of cyanocobalamin requires the presence of the intrinsic factor secreted by gastric parietal cells.

Mechanism of Action and Drug Effects

Humans must have an exogenous source of cyanocobalamin because it is required for nucleoprotein and myelin synthesis, cell reproduction, normal growth, and the maintenance of normal erythropoiesis. The cells that have the greatest requirement for vitamin B_{12} are those that divide rapidly, such as epithelial cells, bone marrow, and myeloid cells.

Reduced sulfhydryl (—5H) groups are required to metabolize fats and carbohydrates and to synthesize protein. Cyanocobalamin is involved in maintaining 5H groups in the reduced form that is required by many 5H-activated enzyme systems. Cyanocobalamin deficiency can lead to neurologic damage that begins with an inability to produce myelin and is followed by gradual degeneration of the axon and nerve head.

Cyanocobalamin activity is identical to the activity of the antipernicious anemia factor present in liver extract called the *extrinsic factor* or *Castle's factor*. As previously mentioned, the oral absorption of cyanocobalamin (extrinsic factor) requires the presence of the *intrinsic factor*, which is a glycoprotein secreted by gastric parietal cells. A complex is formed between the two factors, which is then absorbed by the intestines. This is depicted in Figure 54-3.

Indications

Cyanocobalamin is used to treat deficiency states that develop because of an insufficient intake of the vitamin. It is also included in a multivitamin formulation that is used as a dietary supplement. As previously mentioned, deficiency states are most often the result of malabsorption or poor dietary intake. Poor dietary intake is most common in vegetarians because the primary source of cyanocobalamin is foods of animal origin.

The most common manifestation of untreated cyanocobalamin deficiency is pernicious anemia. The use of vitamin B_{12} to

Table 54-9	Cyanocobalamin: Adverse Effects
Body System	**Adverse Effects**
Cardiovascular	Heart failure, peripheral, vascular thrombosis, pulmonary edema
Central nervous	Flushing, optic nerve atrophy
Gastrointestinal	Diarrhea
Integumentary	Itching, rash, pain at injection site
Metabolic	Hypokalemia

treat pernicious anemia and other megaloblastic anemias results in a rapid conversion of a megaloblastic bone marrow to a normoblastic bone marrow. The preferred route of administration of vitamin B_{12} in treating megaloblastic anemias is by deep intramuscular injection. If not treated, deficiency states can lead to megaloblastic anemia and irreversible neurologic damage. Cyanocobalamin is also useful in the treatment of pernicious anemia caused by an endogenous lack of intrinsic factor.

Contraindications

The only usual contraindications to administration of extrinsic cyanocobalamin (vitamin B_{12}) are known drug product allergies. These may include sensitivity to the chemical element cobalt, which is part of the structure of cyanocobalamin, as this chemical name implies. Other contraindications include hereditary optic nerve atrophy (Leber's disease).

Adverse Effects

Vitamin B_{12} is nontoxic, and large doses must be ingested to produce adverse effects, which include itching, transitory diarrhea, and fever. Other adverse effects are listed by body system in Table 54-9.

Interactions

Use with anticonvulsants, aminoglycoside antibiotics, or long-acting potassium preparations decreases the oral absorption of vitamin B_{12}. In addition, it has been suggested that chloramphenicol antagonizes the hematologic response of vitamin B_{12}.

Dosages

Commonly recommended dosages for vitamin B_{12} are listed in the table on page 830.

Drug Profiles

cyanocobalamin

Cyanocobalamin is a water-soluble B-complex vitamin required for maintaining body fat and carbohydrate metabolism and protein synthesis. It is also needed for growth, cell replication, blood cell production, and the integrity of normal nerve function. Cyanocobalamin (vitamin B_{12}) is available both as OTC preparations and by prescription. Most of the OTC cyanocobalamin-containing products are oral multivitamin preparations, whereas many of the sole cyanocobalamin-containing products contain large doses for parenteral injection and are available by prescription only. Another available dosage form is an intranasal gel. Pregnancy category A.

Pharmacokinetics

Half-Life	Onset	Peak	Duration
PO: 6 days	PO: Unknown	PO: Plasma: 8-12 hr	PO: Unknown

VITAMIN C

Vitamin C (ascorbic acid) can be synthesized for use as a drug and is used in many therapeutic situations. Prolonged ascorbic acid deficiency results in the nutritional disease **scurvy,** which is characterized by weakness, edema, gingivitis and bleeding gums, loss of teeth, anemia, subcutaneous hemorrhage, bone lesions, delayed healing of soft tissues and bones, and hardening of leg muscles. Scurvy was recognized for several centuries, especially among sailors. In 1795, the British navy ordered the eating of limes to prevent the disease.

Mechanism of Action and Drug Effects

Vitamin C is reversibly oxidized to dehydroascorbic acid in the body, and it acts in oxidation-reduction reactions. It is required for several important metabolic activities, including collagen synthesis and the maintenance of connective tissue; tissue repair; maintenance of bone, teeth, and capillaries; and folic acid metabolism (specifically, the conversion of folic acid into its active metabolite). It is also essential for erythropoiesis. Vitamin C enhances the absorption of iron and is required for the synthesis of lipids, proteins, and steroids. It has also been shown to aid in cellular respiration and resistance to infections.

Indications

Vitamin C is used to treat diseases associated with vitamin C deficiency and as a dietary supplement. It is most beneficial in patients who require larger daily requirements because of pregnancy, lactation, hyperthyroidism, fever, stress, infection, trauma, burns, smoking, exposure to cold temperatures, and the consumption of certain drugs (e.g., estrogens, oral contraceptives, barbiturates, tetracyclines, and salicylates). Because vitamin C is an acid, it can also be used as a urinary acidifier. The benefits of other uses of vitamin C are less well documented. For example, taking vitamin C to prevent or treat the common cold is common practice. However, most large, controlled studies have shown that ascorbic acid has little or no value as a prophylactic for the common cold.

Contraindications

The only usual contraindication for vitamin C use is known allergy to a specific vitamin product.

Adverse Effects

Vitamin C is usually nontoxic unless excessive dosages are consumed. Megadoses can produce nausea, vomiting, headache, and abdominal cramps and will acidify the urine, resulting in the formation of cystine, oxalate, and urate renal stones. Furthermore, individuals who discontinue taking excessive daily doses of ascorbic acid can suffer from scurvy-like symptoms.

Interactions

Ascorbic acid has the potential to interact with many classes of drugs. However, clinical experience concerning many interactions is inconclusive. For example, it has been reported that ascorbic acid can decrease the effectiveness of oral anticoagulants. This does not always happen, but practitioners should be aware of this possibility. Coadministration with acid-labile drugs such as penicillin G or erythromycin should be avoided. As previously mentioned, vitamin C can acidify the urine. This usually requires large doses for a significant effect but can enhance the excretion of basic drugs and delay the excretion of acidic drugs. Either outcome may sometimes be desirable.

Dosages

Commonly recommended dosages for vitamin C are listed in the table on page 831.

Drug Profiles

ascorbic acid

Ascorbic acid is a water-soluble vitamin required for the prevention and treatment of scurvy. As previously explained, it is also required for erythropoiesis and the synthesis of lipids, protein, and steroids. It is available both in OTC preparations such as multivitamin products and by prescription. Ascorbic acid is available in many oral dosage forms as well as an injectable form. Pregnancy category A.

Pharmacokinetics

Half-Life	Onset	Peak	Duration
PO: Unknown	PO: Unknown	PO: Unknown	PO: Unknown

MINERALS

Minerals are essential nutrients that are classified as inorganic compounds. They act as building blocks for many body structures and thus are necessary for a variety of physiologic functions. They are also needed for intracellular and extracellular body fluid electrolytes. Iron is essential for the production of Hgb, which is necessary for oxygen transport throughout the body (Chapter 56). Minerals are required for muscle contraction, nerve transmission, and the makeup of essential enzymes.

Mineral compounds are composed of various metallic and nonmetallic elements that are chemically combined with ionic

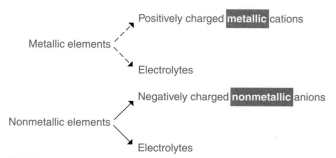

FIGURE 54-4 When mineral compounds are dissolved in water, they separate into positively charged metabolic cations or negatively charged nonmetallic anions and electrolytes.

Table 54-10 Mineral Elements

Element	Symbol	Type	Ionic/Electrolyte Form
Macrominerals			
Calcium*	Ca	Metal	Ca^{12} calcium cation
Chlorine	Cl	Nonmetal	Cl^{-1} chloride anion
Magnesium*	Mg	Metal	Mg^{+2} magnesium cation
Phosphorous*	P	Nonmetal	PO$_4$$^{-3}$ phosphate anion
Potassium	K	Metal	K^{+1} potassium cation
Sodium	Na	Metal	Na^{+1} sodium cation
Sulfur	S	Nonmetal	SO$_4$$^{-2}$ sulfate anion
Microminerals			
Chromium	Cr	Metal	Cr^{+3} chromium cation
Cobalt	Co	Metal	Co^{+2} cobalt cation
Copper	Cu	Metal	Cu^{+2} copper cation
Fluorine	F	Nonmetal	F^{+1} fluoride anion
Iodine*	I	Nonmetal	I^{+1} iodide anion
Iron*	Fe	Metal	Fe^{+2} ferrous cation
Manganese	Mn	Metal	Mn^{+2} manganese cation
Molybdenum	Mo	Metal	Mo^{+6} molybdenum cation
Selenium*	Se	Metal	Se^{+14} selenium cation
Zinc*	Zn	Metal	Zn^{+2} zinc cation

*Mineral elements that have a current recommended daily allowance (RDA).

bonds. When these compounds are dissolved in water, they separate (dissociate) into positively charged metallic cations and electrolytes or negatively charged nonmetallic anions and electrolytes (Figure 54-4).

Ingestion of mineral nutrients provides essential elements necessary for vital bodily functions. Elements that are required in larger amounts are called *macrominerals;* those required in smaller amounts are called *microminerals* or *trace elements.* Table 54-10 lists the classification of nutrient elements as either macrominerals or microminerals and as metal or nonmetal.

CALCIUM

Calcium is the most abundant mineral element in the human body, accounting for approximately 2% of the total body weight. The highest concentration of calcium is in bones and teeth. The efficient absorption of calcium requires adequate amounts of vitamin D.

Calcium deficiency results in hypocalcemia and affects many bodily functions. Causes of calcium deficiency include inadequate calcium intake and/or insufficient vitamin D to facilitate absorption; hypoparathyroidism; and malabsorption syndrome,

Table 54-11 Calcium Deficiency: Causes and Disorders

Cause	Disorder
Inadequate intake	Infantile rickets
Insufficient vitamin D	Adult osteomalacia
Hypoparathyroidism	Muscle cramps
Malabsorption syndrome	Osteoporosis

especially in older people. Calcium deficiency–related disorders include infantile rickets, adult osteomalacia, muscle cramps, osteoporosis (especially in postmenopausal females), hypoparathyroidism, and renal dysfunction. Table 54-11 lists the possible causes of calcium deficiency and the resulting disorders.

Mechanism of Action and Drug Effects

Calcium participates in a variety of essential physiologic functions and is a building block for body structures. Specifically, calcium is involved with the proper development and maintenance of teeth and skeletal bones. It is an important catalyst in many of the coagulation pathways in the blood. Calcium acts as a cofactor in clotting reactions involving the intrinsic and extrinsic pathways of thromboplastin. It is also a cofactor in the conversion of prothrombin to thrombin by thromboplastin and the conversion of fibrinogen to fibrin. Calcium is essential for the normal maintenance and function of the nervous, muscular, and skeletal systems and for cell membrane and capillary permeability. It is an important catalyst in many enzymatic reactions and is essential in many physiologic processes, including transmission of nerve impulses; contraction of cardiac, smooth, and skeletal muscles; renal function; respiration; and blood coagulation. Calcium also plays a regulatory role in the release and storage of neurotransmitters and hormones, in white blood cell (WBC) and hormone activity, in the uptake and binding of amino acids, and in intestinal absorption of cyanocobalamin (vitamin B$_{12}$) and gastrin secretion.

Indications

Calcium salts are used as a source of calcium cations for the treatment or prevention of calcium depletion in patients for whom dietary measures are inadequate. Calcium requirements are also high for growing children and for women who are pregnant or breast-feeding. Many conditions may be associated with calcium deficiency:

- Achlorhydria
- Alkalosis
- Chronic diarrhea
- Hyperphosphatemia
- Hypoparathyroidism
- Menopause
- Pancreatitis
- Pregnancy and lactation
- PMS
- Renal failure
- Sprue
- Steatorrhea
- Vitamin D deficiency

Calcium is also used to treat various manifestations of established deficiency states, including adult osteomalacia,

Table 54-12 **Calcium Salts: Calcium Content**

Calcium Salt	Calcium Content (per gram)
Phosphate tribasic	400 mg (20 mEq)
Carbonate	400 mg (20 mEq)
Phosphate dibasic anhydrous	290 mg (14.5 mEq)
Chloride	270 mg (13.5 mEq)
Acetate	253 mg (12.7 mEq)
Phosphate dibasic dihydrate	230 mg (11.5 mEq)
Citrate	211 mg (10.6 mEq)
Glycerophosphate	191 mg (9.6 mEq)
Lactate	130 mg (6.5 mEq)
Gluconate	90 mg (4.5 mEq)
Gluceptate	82 mg (4.1 mEq)
Glubionate	64 mg (3.2 mEq)

Table 54-13 **Calcium Salts: Adverse Effects**

Body System	Adverse Effects
Cardiovascular	Hemorrhage, rebound hypertension
Gastrointestinal	Constipation, obstruction, nausea, vomiting, flatulence
Genitourinary	Renal dysfunction, renal stones, renal failure
Metabolic	Hypercalcemia, metabolic alkalosis

hypoparathyroidism, infantile rickets or tetany, muscle cramps, osteoporosis, and renal insufficiency. In addition, calcium is used as a dietary supplement for women during pregnancy and lactation.

There are more than 12 different selected calcium salts available for treatment or nutritional supplementation. Each calcium salt contains a different amount of elemental calcium per gram of calcium salt. Table 54-12 lists the available salts and their associated calcium contents.

Contraindications

Contraindications for administration of exogenous calcium include hypercalcemia, ventricular fibrillation of the heart, and known allergy to a specific calcium drug product.

Adverse Effects

Although adverse effects and toxicity are rare, hypercalcemia can occur. Symptoms include anorexia, nausea, vomiting, and constipation. In addition, when calcium salts are administered by intramuscular or subcutaneous injection, mild-to-severe local reactions, including burning, necrosis and sloughing of tissue, cellulitis, and soft tissue calcification, may occur. Venous irritation may occur with intravenous administration. Other adverse effects associated with both oral and parenteral use of calcium salts are listed in Table 54-13.

Toxicity and Management of Overdose

Chronic and excessive calcium intake can result in severe hypercalcemia, which can cause cardiac irregularities, delirium, and coma. Management of acute hypercalcemia may require hemodialysis, whereas milder cases will respond to discontinuation of calcium intake.

Interactions

Calcium salts will chelate (bind) with tetracyclines to produce an insoluble complex. If hypercalcemia is present in patients taking digitalis preparations, serious cardiac dysrhythmias can occur.

Drug Profiles

calcium

Calcium salts are minerals that are primarily used in the treatment or prevention of calcium depletion in patients in whom dietary measures are inadequate. Many calcium salts are available, all with a different content of elemental calcium per gram of salt. Calcium is available in both oral and parenteral forms. There are numerous dosages and names of calcium preparations. Consult manufacturer instructions for recommended dosages. The calcium salts are available in a variety of oral and injectable dosage forms. The pharmacokinetics of calcium are highly variable and depend on individual patient physiology and the characteristics of the specific drug product used. Pregnancy category C.

MAGNESIUM

Magnesium is one of the principal cations present in the intracellular fluid. It is an essential part of many enzyme systems associated with energy metabolism. Magnesium deficiency (hypomagnesemia) is usually caused by (1) malabsorption, especially in the presence of high calcium intake; (2) alcoholism; (3) long-term intravenous feeding; (4) diuretics; and (5) metabolic disorders, including hyperthyroidism and diabetic ketoacidosis. Symptoms associated with hypomagnesemia include cardiovascular disturbances, neuromuscular impairment, and mental disturbances. Dietary intake from vegetables and other foods will usually prevent magnesium deficiency. However, magnesium is required in greater amounts in individuals with diets high in protein-rich foods, calcium, and phosphorus.

Mechanism of Action and Drug Effects

The precise mechanism for magnesium has not been fully determined. Magnesium is a known cofactor for many enzyme systems. It is required for muscle contraction and nerve physiology. Magnesium produces an anticonvulsant effect by inhibiting neuromuscular transmission for selected convulsive states.

Indications

Magnesium is used to treat magnesium deficiency and as a nutritional supplement in total parenteral nutrition (TPN) and multivitamin preparations. It is used as an anticonvulsant in magnesium deficiency–induced seizures; for complications of pregnancy, including preeclampsia and eclampsia; as a tocolytic drug for inhibition of uterine contractions in premature labor; in pediatric acute nephropathy; for various cardiac dysrhythmias; and for short-term treatment of constipation.

Contraindications

Contraindications to magnesium administration include known drug product allergy, heart block, renal failure, adrenal gland failure (Addison's disease), and hepatitis.

Adverse Effects

Adverse effects of magnesium are due to hypermagnesemia, which results in tendon reflex loss, difficult bowel movements, CNS depression, respiratory distress and heart block, and hypothermia.

Toxicity and Management of Overdose

Toxic effects are extensions of symptoms caused by hypermagnesemia, a major cause of which is the long-term use of magnesium products (especially antacids in patients with renal dysfunction). Severe hypermagnesemia is treated with a calcium salt administered intravenously in doses up to 10 mEq. The diuretic furosemide (Lasix) may also be prescribed.

Interactions

The use of magnesium with neuromuscular blocking drugs and CNS depressants produces additive effects.

Drug Profiles

magnesium

Magnesium is a mineral that has a variety of dosage forms and uses. It is an essential part of many enzyme systems. When absent or diminished in the body, cardiovascular, neuromuscular, and mental disturbances can occur. Magnesium sulfate is the most common form of magnesium used as a mineral replacement. It is available in both oral and injectable forms. Pregnancy category B.

PHOSPHORUS

Phosphorus is widely distributed in foods and thus a dietary deficiency is rare. Deficiency states are usually nondietary and are primarily due to malabsorption, extensive diarrhea or vomiting, hyperthyroidism, hepatic disease, and long-term use of aluminum or calcium antacids.

Mechanism of Action and Drug Effects

Phosphorus in the form of the phosphate group and/or anion (PO_4^{-3}) is a required precursor for the synthesis of essential body chemicals. In addition, the mineral is an important building block for body structures. Phosphorus is required as a structural unit for the synthesis of nucleic acid and the adenosine phosphate compounds (adenosine monophosphate [AMP], adenosine diphosphate [ADP], and adenosine triphosphate [ATP]) responsible for cellular energy transfer. It is also necessary for the development and maintenance of the skeletal system and teeth. The skeletal bones contain up to 85% of the phosphorus content of the body. In addition, magnesium is required for the proper utilization of many B-complex vitamins, and it is an essential component of physiologic buffering systems.

Indications

Phosphorus is used to treat deficiency states and as a dietary supplement in many multivitamin formulations.

Contraindications

Contraindications to phosphorous or phosphate administration include hyperphosphatemia and hypocalcemia.

Adverse Effects

Adverse effects are usually associated with phosphorus replacement products. Effects include diarrhea, nausea, vomiting, and other gastrointestinal disturbances. Other adverse effects include confusion, weakness, and breathing difficulties.

Toxicity and Management of Overdose

Toxic reactions to phosphorus are extremely rare and are usually restricted to the ingestion of the pure element.

Interactions

Antacids can reduce the oral absorption of phosphorus.

Drug Profiles

phosphorus

Phosphorus is a mineral that is essential to our well-being. It is needed to make energy in the form of ADP and ATP for all our bodily processes. Phosphorus is present in a large number of drug formulations and appears as a phosphate salt (PO4). Phosphorus should be used with caution in patients with renal impairment. It is available in both oral and parenteral formulations.

ZINC

The metallic element zinc is often taken orally as a mineral supplement and is available as the sulfate salt for this purpose. Normally a dietary trace element, zinc plays a crucial role in the enzymatic metabolic reactions of both proteins and carbohydrates. This serves to make it especially important for normal tissue growth and repair. It therefore also has a major role in wound repair.

◆ NURSING PROCESS

◆ ASSESSMENT

Before administering vitamins, the nurse needs to assess the patient for nutritional disorders through a survey of various laboratory tests, such as Hgb, Hct, WBC, and RBC counts as well as serum albumin and total protein levels. Assessment of the patient's dietary intake, dietary patterns, menu planning, grocery shopping, food/meal practices/habits, and cultural influences should occur prior to giving any supplemental therapy. For vitamin A deficiencies, a baseline assessment of the patient's vision, including night vision, and examination of the skin and mucous membranes should be completed and documented. Serum vitamin A levels less than 20 mcg/dL (adults) indicates a deficiency. Contraindications, cautions, and drug interactions should be noted and have been previously discussed, as with the other vitamins included in this chapter.

Patients who are deficient in vitamin D should have a baseline assessment of skeletal formation with attention to any deformities. Serum calcium levels should also be drawn as ordered. During the assessment phase with vitamin D, it is important to remember that patients with a serum calcium level less than 7.5 mg/dL may have deficient vitamin D levels. In addition, baseline inorganic phosphorous and serum citrate levels may also be helpful. Before administering vitamin E, patients should be assessed for hypoprothrombinemia because this condition may occur secondary to vitamin E deficiency. Any baseline bleeding or hematologic problems need to be documented with a thorough skin assessment noting its integrity, presence of any edema, muscle weakness, easy bruising, and/or bleeding.

The last of the fat-soluble vitamins, vitamin K, is associated with clotting function, and so, prior to its use, the patient's prothrombin time, INR, and platelet counts should be documented. Assessment of the skin for bruises, petechiae, and erythema should be completed as well as assessment of the gums for gingival bleeding. Urine and stool should also be assessed for bleeding prior to the use of this drug. Vital signs with attention to blood pressure and pulse rate should be noted. If intravenous (IV) dosage forms are used, it is important to assess baseline skin color, temperature, and vital signs because of the associated risk for facial flushing, chest pain, weak pulse rate, profuse diaphoresis, and hypotension with possible progression to shock and cardiac arrest. It is also important to remember that the fat-soluble vitamins are all stored in the body tissue when excessive quantities are consumed and may become toxic if taken in large doses, so baseline values of vitamins A, D, E, and K should always be known prior to beginning any ordered/recommended therapy.

Vitamin B₁ (thiamine) hypersensitivity may cause skin rash and wheezing; therefore, presence of any allergic reactions to vitamin B compounds needs to be documented. Because it is rare that only one vitamin B deficiency occurs, deficiencies of all forms of vitamin B must be ruled out before treatment. Baseline assessments of vital signs, mental status, and urinary thiamine levels may also be ordered (adult levels of urinary thiamine less than 27 mcg/dL indicate deficiency). Vitamin C is usually well tolerated; however, assessment should include a history of nutritional deficits or problems with dietary intake, with notation of any allergies.

With trace elements, a baseline assessment should include contraindications, cautions, and drug interactions, as well as assessment of nutritional status and nutrition-related laboratory studies (Hgb, Hct, RBC, and WBC counts; trace elemental laboratory values). Before calcium and magnesium are administered, the patient's serum levels should be obtained and recorded. Calcium interacts with many medications, so a review of previously stated interactions is important. If there is a history of cardiac disease, a baseline electrocardiogram (ECG) may be ordered prior to calcium therapy; if decreased QT wave and T wave inversion are observed, calcium may be discontinued or given in reduced dosages as ordered. Magnesium is also associated with several drug interactions and should be reviewed prior to drug therapy being initiated. Because magnesium may be given for a desired systemic effect, the patient's renal status should be assessed. It is also important to assess the physician's order for completeness and rationale for use so that it is fully understood as to why the drug is being given (e.g., replacement, antacid, or laxative purposes). In addition, it is also important to assess the order for use of trace elements (e.g., calcium, magnesium, zinc) in total parenteral nutritional infusions or hyperalimentation.

◆ NURSING DIAGNOSES

- Disturbed sensory perception (visual) related to night blindness from vitamin A deficiency
- Acute pain related to bone or skeletal deformities resulting from vitamin D deficiency
- Impaired physical mobility related to poorly developed muscles from vitamin D and/or vitamin E deficiency
- Diarrhea related to vitamin E adverse effects
- Risk for injury (e.g., bruising, bleeding) related to deficient levels of vitamin K and potential for bleeding disorders
- Disturbed thought processes related to vitamin B₁ deficiency
- Impaired physical mobility related to fatigue from poor nutrition and B vitamin deficiencies
- Acute pain in joints related to disease from vitamin C deficiency
- Impaired tissue integrity related to vitamin C deficiency and subsequent decreased healing

◆ PLANNING

Goals

- Patient maintains sensory, perceptual, and skin/mucosal membrane integrity during therapy.
- Patient experiences minimal complaints and/or adverse effects related to vitamin and mineral therapy.
- Patient regains/maintains normal bowel elimination patterns during therapy.
- Patient reports improved comfort levels during drug therapy.
- Patient reports improved thought processes and cognitive ability with therapy.
- Patient regains and maintains activity levels at expected level considered normal for age, weight, and height.

Outcome Criteria

- Patient openly verbalizes fears and anxieties about possible visual, perceptual, and bodily changes due to vitamin and mineral deficiencies with positive reports of compliance/adherence to therapies.
- Patient states measures to minimize injury/maximize intactness of skin and mucous membranes such as frequent mouth care, keeping skin clean and dry with moisturizers as needed with at least 6 to 8 glasses of water/day.
- Patient states measures to help prevent falls and injury on a daily basis (e.g., minimizing obstacles in the home; removing excess furniture or small, loose rugs; adding night lights).
- Patient uses dietary measures (e.g., increase in bulk, fiber), hydration, and progressive exercise to assist with regaining normal bowel patterns.
- Patient increases stamina/energy to enhance tolerance of performing activities of daily living and/or progressive exercise, as tolerated.

◆ IMPLEMENTATION

Before administering vitamin A, the nurse should document the patient's dietary intake for the last 24 hours. Any signs and symptoms of hypervitaminosis or hypercarotenemia (excess vitamin A; see previous discussion) should be documented. Vitamin D should be given with concurrent evaluations of renal function and serum calcium levels. The nurse should assess growth measurements in children, and all patients should be informed of signs and symptoms to report to their health care provider, such as constipation, anorexia, nausea, vomiting, metallic taste, and dry mouth. Vitamin B₁ (thiamine) therapy should be given as ordered. Niacin should be administered with milk or food to decrease gastrointestinal upset. If pyridoxine is ordered to be given intravenously, the proper infusion rate and dilutional solutions need to be verified. Cyanocobalamin should be administered orally with meals to increase its absorption. Ascorbic acid should be given orally, and oral effervescent forms should be dissolved in at least 6 oz of water or juice. If given intravenously, the proper infusion rate and dilutional solutions should be checked. Should vitamin C be used for acidification of urine, it is important for the nurse to frequently assess urinary pH.

Because of problems with venous irritation, intravenous calcium should be given via an IV infusion pump and with proper dilution. Giving intravenous calcium too rapidly may precipitate cardiac irregularities or cardiac arrest, thus prompting the need to give it slowly, as ordered, and within the manufacturer guidelines (e.g., usually less than 1 mL/min). Patients should be kept recumbent for 15 minutes after the infusion to prevent further problems. Should extravasation of the intravenous solution with calcium occur, the nurse should discontinue the infusion immediately and leave the intravenous catheter in place. The physician may then order an injection of 1% procaine and/or other antidotes/fluids to reduce vasospasm at the site and dilute the irritating effects of calcium on surrounding tissue. However, all facility policies and procedural guidelines and/or manufacturer insert information should be followed as deemed appropriate. In addition, appropriate documentation should include appearance of the IV site (e.g., erythema, swelling, and any drainage). If oral dosage forms of calcium are used, it should be given 1 to 3 hours after meals.

Magnesium should be administered according to manufacturer guidelines and as ordered. Intravenous magnesium sulfate should always be given very cautiously, with use of an infusion pump and within manufacturer guidelines for dosage and dilutional concentration. During intravenous magnesium infusion, the patient's ECG should be monitored along with vital signs and rating of patellar or knee-jerk reflexes. Reflexes are used as an indication of drug-related CNS depressant effects. CNS depression can quickly lead to respiratory and/or cardiac depression, thus requiring fre-

quent monitoring. Documentation should be complete, with recording of each set of vital signs and rating of reflexes. Should there be a decrease in strength of reflexes and/or a decrease in respirations of less than 12/min, the physician should be contacted immediately, the infusion stopped, and the patient monitored closely. Other signs that need immediate attention include confusion, irregular heart rhythm, cramping, unusual tiredness/fatigue, lightheadedness, and dizziness. Calcium gluconate should be easily accessible for use as an antidote to magnesium toxicity. Oral dosage forms of magnesium should be administered as ordered and the exact dosage given. For tips related to vitamins, minerals, and trace elements, see the Patient Teaching Tips.

◆ EVALUATION

Evaluation should always include monitoring of goals and outcome criteria as well as therapeutic responses and adverse effects of each vitamin/mineral. Therapeutic responses to vitamin A therapy include restoration of normal vision and intact skin with adverse effects of lethargy; night blindness; skin and corneal changes; and, in infancy, failure to thrive. Therapeutic responses to vitamin D include improved bone growth/formation and an intact skeleton with decreased or no pain as compared to baseline musculoskeletal deformity/weakness/discomfort. Adverse effects include constipation, anorexia, metallic taste, and dry mouth. Therapeutic responses to vitamin E include improved muscle strength, improved skin integrity, and alpha-tocopherol levels within normal limits with adverse effects including blurred vision, dizziness, drowsiness, breast enlargement, and flulike symptoms. Therapeutic responses to vitamin K include return to normal clotting with adverse effects presented in the pharmacology section of the text—as with all other vitamins/minerals in this chapter. Therapeutic response to vitamin B_1 (thiamine) includes improved mental status with less confusion. Therapeutic responses to riboflavin, niacin, pyridoxine, and cyanocobalamin include improved skin integrity; normal vision; improved mental status; and normal RBC, Hgb, and Hct levels. Therapeutic responses to vitamin C include improved capillary intactness, skin and mucous membrane integrity, healing, and energy and mental state. An adverse reaction associated with vitamin C is precipitate formation in the urine with possible stone formation. Therapeutic responses to trace elements include resolution of the deficient state and associated signs and symptoms, depending on the specific element or mineral.

CASE STUDY

Magnesium Sulfate Therapy

D.C., a 68-year-old female, was admitted to a small county hospital (100 beds with a 6-bed ICU and CCU) for exacerbation of heart failure. After 2 days of diuretic treatment with furosemide (Lasix), the physician ordered serum potassium and magnesium levels, which came back with the serum magnesium level at 0.9 mEq/L. The physician ordered magnesium sulfate 16 mEq q6h × 2 doses, with the first dose stat. The night supervisor has to retrieve the medication because the pharmacy is closed. She returns to your unit with the medication. Because you are aware of many medication errors with magnesium sulfate, you are extra cautious in checking and double checking the order. You notice that the vials are labeled 16 g, which is equal to 130 mEq, versus the 16 mEq ordered.

- What are the normal serum levels for magnesium?
- What are some of the indications for magnesium sulfate as a medication?
- What are some manifestations of overdosage with magnesium sulfate? What patients are especially prone to toxic effects of magnesium?

For answers, see http://evolve.elsevier.com/Lilley.
ICU, Intensive care unit; *CCU,* critical care unit.

Patient Teaching Tips

- Educate the patient about the best dietary sources of both water and fat-soluble vitamins (vitamins A, B, C, D, E, and K), as well as about the best sources of elements and minerals. See Table 54-2 for the nutrient content of various food items.
- Patients taking vitamins, minerals, or elements should be closely monitored for therapeutic and adverse effects. Encourage patients to monitor their own progress on how well they feel, noting any improvement in their condition/health status. Encourage intake of fluids with all vitamin and mineral therapy.
- Signs and symptoms of any related adverse effects should be shared with the patient. Vitamin E adverse effects include diarrhea, blurred vision, dizziness, and flulike symptoms.
- Patients who have had a gastrectomy, ileal resection or who have pernicious anemia should be informed of the necessity for cyanocobalamin in their diet.

- Patients taking up to 600 mg/day of vitamin C should be informed that there may be a slight increase in daily urination patterns and that diarrhea is associated with more than 1 g of vitamin C per day.
- Patients taking trace elements (e.g., zinc, copper, magnesium, iodine, chromium) must take the medication as prescribed and with adequate amounts of fluids. They should also know to call the physician if any unusual reactions occur.
- Educate the patient about calcium therapy and about food items and drugs that will chelate or bind with it. For example, calcium chelates/binds with tetracycline antibiotics and leads to a decreased or negated effect of the antibiotic.

Points to Remember

- OTC use of vitamins and minerals may lead to serious problems and adverse effects; therefore, a physician should be consulted before supplements are taken.
- Nurses must incorporate the nutritional status of patients into the nursing care plan to provide comprehensive care during medication therapy.
- The nurse's participation in health promotion and wellness includes providing information about dietary needs and the body's need for vitamins and minerals.
- Patient education as related to vitamin and mineral replacement must focus on dietary sources of the specific nutrient, drug and food interactions, and adverse effects. Patients must be instructed about when it is necessary to contact the physician.
- Vitamins and minerals can be dangerous to the patient if given without concern and caution for the patient's overall condition and underlying disease processes.
- It should never be assumed that because the drug is a vitamin or a mineral it does not have adverse reactions or toxicity. Most vitamins and minerals can become toxic.

NCLEX Examination Review Questions

1. When giving IV calcium, the nurse needs to give it slowly, keeping in mind that rapid IV administration of calcium may cause:
   a. Ototoxicity
   b. Renal damage
   c. Tetany
   d. Cardiac dysrhythmias
2. Which laboratory tests should be assessed before administration of vitamin K?
   a. Prothrombin time and INR
   b. Red and white blood cell counts
   c. Phosphorous and calcium levels
   d. Total protein and albumin levels
3. For a patient who has had severe intestinal damage due to a gastrointestinal infection, the nurse will need to assess for signs of which vitamin/mineral deficiency?
   a. Vitamin A (retinol)
   b. Vitamin B$_{12}$ (cyanocobalamin)
   c. Magnesium
   d. Vitamin E (tocopherols)

4. A patient with a stage IV pressure ulcer will probably receive which vitamin, which is known to help with wound healing?
   a. Vitamin K
   b. Vitamin B$_1$
   c. Vitamin C
   d. Vitamin D
5. While caring for a newly admitted patient who has a long history of alcoholism, the nurse anticipates that part of the patient's medication regimen will include:
   a. Vitamin B$_1$ (thiamine)
   b. Vitamin B$_6$ (pyridoxine)
   c. Vitamin C
   d. Vitamin D

1. d, 2. a, 3. b, 4. c, 5. a.

Critical Thinking Activities

1. Explain why patients with a cardiac history need a baseline ECG and serum calcium assessment performed before initiation of calcium supplemental therapy.
2. Your patient is experiencing constipation and abdominal pain since beginning calcium therapy. Your assessment reveals a distended abdomen and diminished bowel sounds. What could be occurring, and what should your nursing actions be at this time?

3. We have all heard of the use of zinc oxide as a skin protectant in cases of diaper rash or even sun exposure, but why would a patient with a surgical wound or a pressure ulcer benefit from doses of oral zinc during recovery?

For answers, see http://evolve.elsevier.com/Lilley.

Nutrition Supplements

Objectives

When you reach the end of this chapter, you should be able to do the following:

1. Describe the various pathophysiologic processes and/or disease states that may lead to nutritional deficiencies and require nutrition supplemental support.
2. Discuss the various enteral and parenteral nutrition supplements used to treat the various deficiencies, including specific ingredients.
3. Describe the nurse's role in the process of initiating and maintaining continuous or intermittent enteral feedings, total parenteral nutrition (TPN), and other forms of nutrition supplementation.
4. Compare the various enteral feeding tubes, including specific uses and the special needs for patients requiring this nutrition support.
5. Discuss the mechanisms of action, cautions, contraindications, routes of administration, drug interactions, adverse effects, and related complications associated with enteral and parenteral nutrition supplementation.
6. Develop a nursing care plan that includes all phases of the nursing process for patients receiving enteral and parenteral supplemental feedings.
7. Discuss the various laboratory values related to nutrition deficits or altered nutrition status and their impact on monitoring the therapeutic effects of the therapy.

e-Learning Activities

Companion CD

- NCLEX Review Questions: see question 442
- Animations
- Audio Glossary
- Category Catchers
- Medication Errors Checklists
- IV Therapy Checklists

evolve Website (http://evolve.elsevier.com/Lilley)

- Nursing Care Plans • Frequently Asked Questions • Content Updates • WebLinks • Supplemental Resources • Elsevier ePharmacology Update • Medication Administration Animations

Drug Profiles

amino acids, p. 850
carbohydrate formulation, p. 848
carbohydrates, p. 851
fat, p. 850

fat formulation, p. 848
lipid emulsions, p. 850
protein formulation, p. 848

Glossary

Anabolism Constructive metabolism characterized by the conversion of simple substances into the more complex compounds of living matter. (p. 846)

Casein The principal protein of milk and the basis for curd and cheese. (p. 848)

Catabolism A complex metabolic process in which energy is liberated for use in work, energy storage, or heat production by the destruction of complex substances by living cells to form simple compounds. (p. 850)

Dumping syndrome A complex bodily reaction to the rapid entry of concentrated nutrients into the jejunum of the small intestine. The patient may experience nausea, weakness, sweating, palpitations, syncope, sensations of warmth, and diarrhea. Most commonly occurs with eating following partial gastrectomy or with enteral feedings that are administered too rapidly into the stomach or jejunum via a feeding tube. (p. 847)

Enteral nutrition The provision of food or nutrients via the gastrointestinal tract, either naturally by eating or through a feeding tube in patients unable to eat. (p. 846)

Essential amino acids Those amino acids that cannot be manufactured by the body. (p. 850)

Essential fatty acid deficiency A condition that develops if fatty acids that the body cannot produce are not present in dietary or nutrition supplements. (p. 851)

Hyperalimentation Older term for parenteral nutrition; now discouraged as it may be misinterpreted as overfeeding. (p. 849)

Malnutrition Any disorder of undernutrition. (p. 846)

Multivitamin infusion (MVI) A concentrated solution containing several water- and fat-soluble vitamins and used as part of an intravenous (parenteral) nutrition source. (p. 851)

Nonessential amino acids Those amino acids that the body can produce without extracting from dietary intake. (p. 850)

Nutrient A substance that provides nourishment and affects the nutritive and metabolic processes of the body. (p. 846)

Nutrition supplements   Oral, enteral, or intravenous nutrition preparations used to provide optimal nutrients to meet the body's nutrition needs. (p. 846)

Nutrition support   Refers to the provision of nutrients orally, enterally, or parenterally for therapeutic reasons. (p. 846)

Parenteral nutrition   The administration of nutrients by a route other than through the alimentary canal, such as intravenously. (p. 846)

Semiessential amino acids   Those amino acids that can be produced by the body but not in sufficient amounts in infants and children. (p. 850)

Total parenteral nutrition (TPN)   Same as parenteral nutrition. (p. 849)

Whey   The thin serum of milk remaining after the casein and fat have been removed. It contains proteins, lactose, water-soluble vitamins, and minerals. (p. 849)

The integrity and normal function of all cells within the body require a constant supply of nutrients. **Nutrients** are dietary products that undergo chemical changes when ingested (metabolized) and cause tissue to be enhanced and energy to be liberated. Nutrients are required for cell growth and division; enzyme activity; protein, carbohydrate, and fat synthesis; muscle contraction; neurohormonal secretion (e.g., vasopressin, gastrin); wound repair; immune competence; gut integrity; and numerous other essential cellular functions. Providing for these nutrition needs is known as **nutrition support**. Adequate nutrition support is needed to prevent the breakdown of tissue proteins for use as an energy supply to sustain essential organ systems. This is what happens during starvation. Malnutrition can decrease organ size and impair the function of organ systems (e.g., cardiac, respiratory, gastrointestinal, hepatic, renal). Nutrition supplements are a means of providing adequate nutrition support to meet the body's nutrition needs.

Malnutrition is a condition in which the body's essential need for nutrients is not met by nutrient intake. The purpose of nutrition support is the successful prevention, recognition, and management of malnutrition. **Nutrition supplements** are dietary products used to provide nutrition support. Nutrition supplement products can be administered to patients in a variety of ways. They vary in their amounts and the chemical complexity of carbohydrate, protein, and fat. The electrolyte, vitamin, mineral, and osmolality of the specific product can vary as well. These nutrients may be given in a digested form, a partially digested form, or an undigested form. Nutrition supplements can also be tailored for specific disease states.

A wide variety of nutrition supplements is needed because of the wide variety of conditions for which patients require nutrition support. Patients' nutrient requirements vary according to age, gender, size or weight, physical activity, pre-existing medical conditions, nutrition status, and current medical or surgical treatment. Nutrition supplements are classified according to the method of administration. They can be classified as either enteral or parenteral. **Enteral nutrition** is the provision of food or nutrients with the gastrointestinal tract as the route of administration. Nutrition supplements may also be administered parenterally. **Parenteral nutrition** is the intravenous administration of nutrients. Its purpose is to promote anabolism (tissue building), nitrogen balance, and body weight. It is used

when the oral or enteral feeding routes cannot or should not be used (e.g., postoperative patient; patient who is cachectic from advanced cancer or AIDS). Nutrition supplements are delivered directly into the circulation by means of intravenous infusion. The selection of either enteral nutrition or parenteral nutrition and the specific nutrition composition of the product depend on the specific patient profile and the clinical situation.

Nutritional support
- Enteral nutrition → Gastrointestinal tract
- Parenteral nutrition → Circulation

ENTERAL NUTRITION

Enteral nutrition is the provision of food or nutrients through the gastrointestinal tract. The most common and least invasive route of administration is oral consumption. A feeding tube is used in the other five routes (Figure 55-1). The six routes of enteral nutrition delivery are listed in Table 55-1.

Patients who may benefit from feeding-tube delivery of nutrition supplements include those with abnormal esophageal or stomach peristalsis, altered anatomy secondary to surgery, depressed consciousness, or impaired digestive capacity. Nutrients may be administered via the enteral or parenteral routes, depending on the clinical situation. Many processes occur from the beginning of the digestive system in the mouth to the end of the digestive system in the anus. These processes have evolved over time to most effectively digest dietary nutrients. For this reason, the enteral route is considered to be the superior route of administration of nutrition supplements and should therefore be used whenever possible.

Approximately 100 different enteral formulations are available. The enteral supplements have been divided into basic groups according to the basic characteristics of the individual formulations. The enteral formulation groups are elemental, polymeric, modular, altered amino acid, and impaired glucose tolerance. These are described in Box 55-1.

Mechanism of Action and Drug Effects

The enteral formula groups provide the basic building blocks for **anabolism.** Different combinations and amounts of these drugs are used based on the individual patient's anabolic needs. After the body receives and absorbs these nutrients, it must process them into living matter. Enteral nutrition supplies complete dietary needs through the gastrointestinal tract by the normal oral route or by feeding tube.

Indications

Enteral nutrition can be used to supplement an oral diet that is currently insufficient for a patient's nutrient needs or used solely to meet all of the patient's nutrient needs. It is used for patients who are unable to consume or digest normal foods, have accelerated catabolic status, or are undernourished because of disease. Box 55-2 lists the main types of enteral nutrition supplements and their indications.

Contraindications

The usual contraindication to nutrition supplements of any kind is known drug allergy to a specific product or genetic disease that renders a patient unable to metabolize certain types of nutrients.

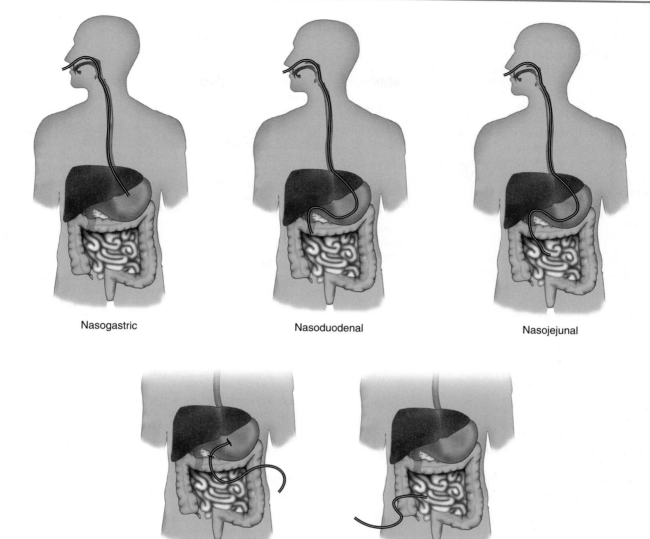

Nasogastric

Nasoduodenal

Nasojejunal

Gastrostomy

Jejunostomy

FIGURE 55-1   Tube feeding routes. *(From Beare PG, Myers JL: Adult health nursing, ed 3, St Louis, 1998, Mosby.)*

Table 55-1	**Routes of Enteral Nutrition Delivery**
Route	**Description**
Gastrostomy	Feeding tube surgically inserted directly into the stomach
Jejunostomy	Feeding tube surgically inserted into the jejunum
Nasoduodenal	Feeding tube placed from the nose to the duodenum
Nasojejunal	Feeding tube placed from the nose to the jejunum
Nasogastric	Feeding tube placed from the nose to the stomach
Oral	Nutrition supplements delivered by mouth

Adverse Effects

The most common adverse effect of nutrition supplements is gastrointestinal intolerance. The most common result of this intolerance is diarrhea. Infant nutrition formulations are most commonly associated with allergies and digestive intolerance. The other nutrition supplements are most commonly associated with osmotic diarrhea. Rapid feeding or bolus doses can result in **dumping syndrome,** which produces intestinal disturbances. In addition, tube feeding places the patient at significant risk for aspiration pneumonia. This is especially true in patients with compromised mental status, gag reflexes, and general mobility.

Interactions

Various nutrients can interact with drugs to produce significant food–drug interactions. With some exceptions, food usually delays the absorption of drugs when administered simultaneously. Chemical inactivation with high gastric acid content or prolonged emptying time can result in decreased effects of cephalosporins, erythromycin, and penicillins when given with nutrition supplements. An increased absorption rate resulting in increased therapeutic effects can be seen when corticosteroids or vitamins A and D are given with nutrition supplements. Decreased antibiotic effects of tetracyclines and quinolones are seen when they are

Box 55-1   Enteral Formulations

Elemental Formulations

Peptamen	**Contents:** dipeptides, tripeptides, or
Vital HN	crystalline amino acids, glucose oligosac-
Vivonex Plus	charides, and vegetable oil or MCTs
Vivonex TEN	**Comments:** minimum digestion; residue is
	minimal
	Indications: malabsorption, partial bowel
	obstruction, irritable bowel disease,
	radiation enteritis, bowel fistulas, and
	short bowel syndrome

Polymeric Formulations

Complete	**Contents:** complex nutrients (proteins,
Ensure	carbohydrates, and fat)
Ensure-Plus	**Indications:** preferred over elemental for
Isocal	patients with fully functional gastrointesti-
Osmolite	nal tracts and few specialized nutrient
Portagen	requirements
Precision LR	
Sustacal	

Modular Formulations

Carbohydrate	**Contents:** single nutrient formulas (protein,
Moducal	carbohydrate, or fat)
Polycose	**Indications:** can be added to a monomeric
Fat	or polymeric formulation to provide a
MCT Oil	more individualized nutrient formulation
Microlipid	
Protein	
Casec	
ProMod	
Propac	
Stresstein	

Altered Amino Acid Formulations

Amin-Aid	**Contents:** varying amounts of specific amino
Hepatic-Aid	acids
Lonalac	**Indications:** patients with diseases associ-
Stresstein	ated with altered metabolic capacities
Travasorb Renal	
Traum-Aid HBC	

Formulation for Impaired Glucose Tolerance

Glucerna	**Contents:** Protein, carbohydrate, fat,
	sodium, potassium
	Indications: patients with impaired glucose
	tolerance (e.g., diabetic patients)

Box 55-2   Enteral Nutrition Supplements: Indications

Complete Nutrition Formulations (i.e., for General Nutrition Deficiencies)
- Unable to consume or digest normal foods
- Accelerated catabolic status
- Undernourished because of disease

Incomplete Nutrition Formulations (i.e., for Specific Nutrition Deficiencies)
- Genetic metabolic enzyme deficiency
- Hepatic or renal impairment

Infant Nutrition Formulations
- Sole nutrition intake for premature and full-term infants
- Supplemental nutrition intake for older infants receiving solid foods
- Supplemental nutrition for breast-fed infants

given with nutrition supplements as a result of chemical inactivation that occurs when this drug complexes with calcium.

Dosages

Because nutrient requirements vary greatly, dosages are individualized according to patient needs.

Drug Profiles

Enteral nutrition can be provided by a variety of supplements. The individual patient characteristics determine the appropriate enteral supplement. There are four basic types of enteral formulations: elemental, polymeric, modular, and altered amino acid.

Elemental Formulations

Elemental formulations are enteral supplements that contain dipeptides, tripeptides, or crystalline amino acids. Because of the composition of elemental formulation supplements, minimal digestion is required. These supplements are indicated in patients with pancreatitis, partial bowel obstruction, irritable bowel disease, radiation enteritis, bowel fistulas, and short bowel syndrome. They are contraindicated in patients who have had hypersensitivity reactions to them. Elemental formulation supplements are available without a prescription and have no pregnancy category.

Polymeric Formulations

Polymeric formulations are enteral supplements that contain complex nutrients derived from proteins, carbohydrates, and fat. The polymeric formulations are some of the most commonly used enteral formulations because they most closely resemble normal dietary intake. They are preferred over elemental formulations in patients with fully functional gastrointestinal tracts and have no specialized nutrient needs. They are also less hyperosmolar than elemental formulations and therefore cause fewer gastrointestinal problems. They are contraindicated in patients who have had hypersensitivity reactions to them. They are available without a prescription and have no pregnancy category.

Ensure is a commonly used enteral supplement from the polymeric formulation category of enteral nutrition products. It is lactose free and also is available in a higher caloric formula called Ensure-Plus. Other polymeric formulations are Isocal, Magnacal, Meritene, Osmolite, Portagen, and Sustacal. These drugs contain complex nutrients such as **casein** and soy protein for protein, corn syrup and maltodextrins for carbohydrates, and vegetable oil or milk fat for fat. They are available in liquid formulations only.

Modular Formulations

carbohydrate formulation

Moducal and Polycose are examples of commonly used enteral supplements from the carbohydrate modular formulation category. Both are carbohydrate supplements that supply carbohydrates only. They are intended to be used as an addition to monomeric or polymeric formulations to provide a more individual specialized nutrient formulation. They are available in liquid formulations only. These products are available without a prescription, have no pregnancy category, and are contraindicated only if a patient has had a hypersensitivity reaction to them.

fat formulation

Microlipid and MCT Oil are the formulations available in the fat category. Microlipid is a fat supplement supplying solely fats. It is a concentrated source of calories and contains 4.5 kcal/mL. These drugs are used to help individualize nutrient formulations. They may be used in malabsorption and other gastrointestinal disorders and in patients with pancreatitis. They are available in liquid formulations only. These products are available without a prescription, have no pregnancy category, and are contraindicated only if a patient has had a hypersensitivity reaction to them.

protein formulation

Casec, ProMod, and Propac are examples of protein modular formulations. They are used to increase and provide additional proteins to enhance patients' protein intake. They are derived from a variety of sources such as **whey**, casein, egg whites, and amino acids. All of the available products are dried powders that have to be reconstituted with water. They may sometimes be reconstituted by placing them in enteral feedings that are already in liquid form. They are indicated for patients with increased protein needs. They are contraindicated in patients who have had hypersensitivity reactions to them. Protein formulation supplements are available without a prescription and have no pregnancy category.

Altered Amino Acid Formulations

Amin-Aid is one of the many amino acid formulation nutrition supplements available. Many of the nutrition supplements in this category are also listed as modular formulations because they can be used as both single-nutrient formulas and as nutrition formulations for patients with genetic errors of metabolism. Specialized amino acid formulations are used most commonly in patients who have metabolic disorders such as phenylketonuria, homocystinuria, and maple syrup urine disease. They are also used to supply nutrition support to patients with such illnesses as renal impairment, eclampsia, heart failure, or liver failure.

PARENTERAL NUTRITION

Parenteral nutrition supplementation (intravenous administration) is the preferred method for patients who are unable to tolerate and maintain adequate enteral or oral intake. Instead of administering partially digested nutrients into the gastrointestinal tract, vitamins, minerals, amino acids, dextrose, and lipids are administered intravenously directly into the circulatory system. This effectively bypasses the entire gastrointestinal system, eliminating the need for absorption, metabolism, and excretion. Parenteral nutrition is also called **total parenteral nutrition (TPN)** or **hyperalimentation.**

TPN can supply all of the calories, carbohydrates, amino acids, fats, trace elements, vitamins, and minerals needed for growth, weight gain, wound healing, convalescence, immunocompetence, and other health-sustaining functions.

TPN can be administered either through a peripheral vein or a central vein. Each route of delivery of TPN has specific requirements and limitations. It is generally accepted that TPN should be considered only when oral or enteral support is impossible or when the gastrointestinal absorptive or functional capacity is not sufficient to meet the nutrition needs of the patient. Some of the conditions that must be considered in the decision to place a patient on peripheral versus central TPN are listed in Table 55-2.

PERIPHERAL TOTAL PARENTERAL NUTRITION

Peripheral TPN (PPN) is one route of administration of TPN. A peripheral vein is used to deliver nutrients to the patient's circulatory system. It is usually a temporary method of administration. The long-term administration of nutrition supplements via a peripheral vein may lead to phlebitis. There are a variety of indications for peripheral TPN. PPN should be considered a temporary measure to provide adequate nutrient needs in patients with mild deficits or who are restricted from oral intake and have slightly elevated metabolic rates.

PPN is most valuable in patients who do not have large nutrition needs, can tolerate moderately large fluid loads, and need nutrition supplements only temporarily. Peripheral TPN may be used alone or in combination with oral nutrition supplements to provide the necessary fat, carbohydrate, and protein needed by the patient to maintain health.

Mechanism of Action and Drug Effects

PPN provides the basic nutrient building blocks for anabolism. Different combinations and amounts of these drugs are used based on the individual patient's anabolic needs. After the body receives these nutrients, it must process them into living matter.

Indications

PPN is used to administer nutrients to patients who need more nutrients than their current oral intake can provide or to provide entire daily nutrition. PPN is meant only as a temporary means (less than 2 weeks) of delivering TPN.

Conditions in which patients may benefit from the delivery of PPN are as follows:
- Procedures that restrict oral feedings
- Anorexia caused by radiation or cancer chemotherapy
- Gastrointestinal illnesses that prevent oral food ingestion
- After any type of surgery
- When nutrition deficits are minimal but oral nutrition will not be started for more than 5 days

Contraindications

As mentioned previously for the enteral nutrition products, the only usual contraindication to nutrition supplements of any kind is known drug allergy to a specific product or genetic disease that renders a patient unable to use certain types of nutrients.

Table 55-2 Peripheral and Central Parenteral Nutrition: Characteristics

Considerations	Characteristics	
	Peripheral	**Central**
Goal of nutrition therapy (total vs. supplemental)	Supplemental (total if moderate to low needs)	Total
Length of therapy	Short (<14 days)	Long (14 or more days)
Osmolarity	Hyperosmolar (600-900 mOsm/L)	Hyperosmolar (600-900 mOsm/L)
Fluid tolerance	Must be high	Can be fluid restricted
Dextrose	<12.5%	10%-35%
Amino acids	<3%	>3%-7%
Fats	10%-20%	10%-20%
Calories/days	<2000 kcal/day	>2000 kcal/day

Table 55-3	Amino Acids: Recommended Daily Dosage Guidelines	
Healthy		**Malnourished or Trauma/Burn, Adult**
Adult	**Infant/Child**	
0.9 g/kg	1.5-3 g/kg	Up to 2 g/kg

Adverse Effects

The most devastating adverse effect of PPN is phlebitis, which is a vein irritation or inflammation of a vein. If it is severe enough and not treated appropriately, phlebitis can lead to the loss of a limb. However, this is rare. Another potential adverse effect is fluid overload. PPN is limited to lower dextrose-concentrated solutions, generally less than 10%, to avoid sclerosing of the vein. Larger amounts of nutrition supplements are needed with lower concentrated solutions to meet a patient's daily nutrition requirements. Some patients, such as those with renal or heart failure, cannot tolerate large fluid volume. In these patients, fluid restrictions may render PPN unable to provide adequate calories.

Dosages

Dosage requirements vary from patient to patient. Age, gender, weight, and numerous other factors must be considered for proper administration of TPN. Guidelines for amino acids appear in Table 55-3.

Drug Profiles

The individual components of peripheral and central TPN are the same. The difference lies in the concentrations and amounts of the components delivered per volume of nutrition supplement. The basic components of peripheral or central TPN are amino acid, carbohydrate, lipid, trace elements, vitamins, fluids, and electrolytes. Most of the electrolyte components are discussed in Chapter 26.

Amino Acids

Amino acids have many roles in the maintenance of normal nutrition status. The primary role is protein synthesis, or anabolism. Adequate amino acids in nutrition supplements reduce the breakdown of proteins (**catabolism**) and also help to promote normal growth and wound healing.

Amino acids are commonly classified as essential or nonessential according to whether they can or cannot be produced by the body. **Nonessential amino acids** are those that the body produces and are therefore not needed in dietary intake. The body is able to manufacture, from nutrition nitrogen sources, all but eight of the available amino acids. **Essential amino acids** are those amino acids that cannot be produced by the body. Therefore, they must be included in daily dietary intake. Amino acids are used as building blocks for protein that is needed for normal growth and development. Two amino acids, histidine and arginine, are not manufactured by the body in large enough quantities during rapid growth periods such as infancy or childhood. Thus, they are referred to as **semiessential amino acids.** Box 55-3 lists the amino acids according to their categories.

amino acids

Amino acid crystalline solutions (Aminosyn 3%, 5%, and 10%, and FreAmine III 8.5% and 10%) can be used in either peripheral or central TPN. Amino acids are a source of both protein and calories. They provide 4 kcal/g. The two currently available amino acid solutions differ only in their respective concentrations. The dosage of these solutions varies depending on the patient's weight and require-

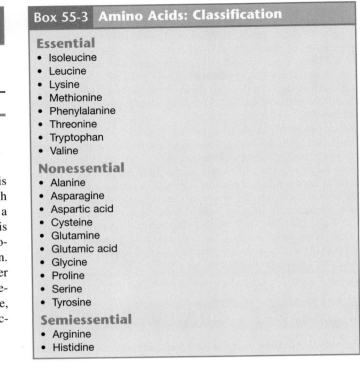

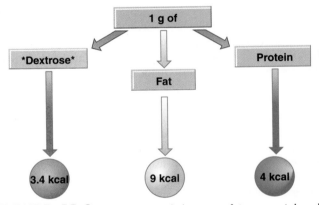

FIGURE 55-2 One gram of dextrose, fat, or protein will provide varying amounts of energy as calories.

ments. These drugs have no restrictions regarding pregnancy and have no contraindications to use. Recommended dosages for healthy and trauma patients are listed in Table 55-3.

carbohydrates

In nutrition support, carbohydrates are usually supplied to patients through dextrose. Hydrous dextrose is normally the greatest source of calories and provides 3.4 kcal/g. However, protein (amino acids) and lipids are also used as calorie sources (Figure 55-2). Concentrations of dextrose in TPN are important considerations. In peripheral TPN, dextrose concentrations are kept below 10% to decrease the possibility of phlebitis. In central TPN, dextrose concentrations can range from 10% to 50%, but they are commonly 25% to 35%. Because dextrose is a sugar, supplemental insulin may be given simultaneously in nutrition supplements. A balanced nutrition supplement that contains dextrose and lipids for caloric sources decreases the need for large amounts of insulin.

fat

The average North American diet contains 40% fat. This means that of the total calories supplied, 40% to 50% of the calories are obtained through fat grams. The ideal diet contains no more than 30%

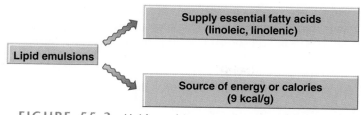

FIGURE 55-3 Lipid emulsions supply essential fatty acids and energy.

fat. Intravenous fat emulsions serve two functions: they supply essential fatty acids, and they are a source of energy or calories. As with the amino acids, certain fatty acids are essential because the body cannot produce them. Linoleic acid cannot be synthesized by the body. It is needed to produce linolenic and arachidonic acid. If these fatty acids are not present in dietary or nutrition supplements, an **essential fatty acid deficiency** may develop. Clinical signs of essential fatty acid deficiency are hair loss, scaly dermatitis, growth retardation, reduced wound healing, decreased platelets, and fatty liver (Figure 55-3).

lipid emulsions

The currently available lipid emulsions, Intralipid and Liposyn, are available as either 10%, 20%, or 30% emulsions. They differ in fat origin. Liposyn is made from safflower oil, and Intralipid is made from soybean oil.

Lipid emulsions should normally be adjusted to deliver 20% to 30% of the total daily calories, while not exceeding 60% of daily caloric intake. Fat emulsions are most beneficial when combined with dextrose solutions. The use of fat to meet caloric needs prevents potentially harmful conditions—such as hyperglycemia, hyperinsulinemia, and hyperosmolarity—that can occur when a patient's entire caloric needs are being met solely by dextrose.

TRACE ELEMENTS

Trace element solutions are available individually or in many different combinations. The following are considered trace elements:

- Chromium
- Copper
- Iodine
- Manganese
- Molybdenum
- Selenium
- Zinc

Specific dosages and frequencies depend on the individual patient's requirements. Vitamins and minerals may also be added accordingly. A common multivitamin combination is **multivitamin infusion (MVI).**

CENTRAL TOTAL PARENTERAL NUTRITION

In central TPN, a large central vein is used to deliver nutrients directly into the patient's circulation. Usually, the subclavian or internal jugular vein is used. Central TPN is generally indicated for patients who require nutrition supplements for a prolonged period, usually more than 7 to 10 days. It can also be used in the home care setting. There are a variety of indications for central TPN. The disadvantages of central TPN are the risks associated with venous catheter insertion and use and maintenance of the central vein. There is a greater potential for infection, more seri-ous catheter-induced trauma and related events, metabolic alterations, and other technical or mechanical problems than with peripheral TPN.

Mechanism of Action and Drug Effects

Central TPN is used to supply nutrients to patients who cannot ingest nutrients by mouth and cannot meet required daily nutrition needs by the enteral or peripheral parenteral routes. Like peripheral TPN, central TPN provides the basic building blocks for anabolism. However, TPN solutions for central intravenous infusion may be more concentrated, especially in terms of carbohydrate content, and may contain as much as 35% dextrose. Different combinations and amounts of liquid nutrients are used, based on the individual patient's anabolic needs. After the body receives these nutrients, it must process them into living matter. Central TPN works by delivering these essential nutrients directly into the circulation via a central vein. It provides the necessary fat, carbohydrate, and protein that the patient needs to maintain health.

Indications

TPN delivers total dietary nutrients to patients who require nutrition supplementation. Patients who may benefit from the delivery of TPN include the following:

- Patients who have large nutrition requirements (metabolic stress or hypermetabolism)
- Patients who need nutrition support for prolonged periods (more than 7 to 10 days)
- Patients who are unable to tolerate large fluid loads

Contraindications

TPN is contraindicated in patients with allergy to any of its components. Rarely, some patients who are allergic to eggs may have cross-sensitivity to lipid formulations. TPN should only be used when the gastrointestinal tract cannot or should not be used (e.g., postoperative or otherwise unable to eat or digest and absorb nutrients).

Adverse Effects

The most common adverse effects of central TPN are those surrounding the use of the central vein for delivery of the TPN. The risks associated with insertion of the infusion line, as well as the use and maintenance of the central vein for administration of TPN, can create some complications. There is a greater potential for infection, more serious catheter-induced trauma and related events, and other technical or mechanical problems than with peripheral TPN. There are larger and more concentrated volumes of nutrition supplements being delivered with central TPN and, therefore, a greater chance for metabolic complications such as hyperglycemia.

Dosages

Administration is individualized according to patient needs.

Drug Profiles

The same formulations used in peripheral TPN are used in central TPN. Often the concentrations of fluids administered through the central vein are much higher than those used in peripheral nutrition supplements. Besides these minor differences, the nutrition supplements used are identical.

◆ NURSING PROCESS

◆ ASSESSMENT

The nurse should conduct a thorough nutrition assessment with a dietary history, weekly and daily food intakes, weight and height before beginning any nutrition supplementation. A nursing history should be completed with a thorough survey of all systems, with questions about any unusual symptoms, possible nutrition concerns, nausea, vomiting, loss of appetite, and weight gain/loss. Other questions should focus on past/present medical and health history, history of any nutrition/gastrointestinal absorption/food intolerance difficulties, stressors and a complete medication profile, including a listing of all prescription, over-the-counter, herbal, and supplemental drugs. Consultation with a registered dietitian is crucial to identification of the nutrients that are missing in a particular patient's diet. Total body metabolic rate, body mass index, muscle mass, and other variables linked to nutrition status should be assessed. Laboratory studies generally include total protein, albumin, blood urea nitrogen (BUN), red blood cells (RBCs), white blood cells (WBCs), vitamin B_{12}, cholesterol, and hemoglobin (Hgb). Other laboratory studies may include cholesterol, electrolytes, total lymphocyte count, serum transferrin, iron levels, urine creatinine clearance, lipid profile, and urinalysis. Anthropometric measurements and weights may also provide much-needed data. All of the objective and subjective data will then assist the physician, nutritionist/dietician, and other members of the health care team to select the appropriate nutrition supplements for the patient.

Before beginning an enteral nutrition supplement of elemental formulations, the nurse must also determine if the patient has a history of allergic reaction to any of the contents of the solution. Contraindications, cautions, and drug interactions must also be assessed for and documented. Of most concern is the patient's cardiac and renal status and being sure that the ingredients and the amount of solution is not too taxing on these systems. In addition, because these solutions are given orally, either by mouth or per tube feedings, it is most important to assess bowel sounds, nausea, vomiting, and ability to swallow. Protein-based formulations are to be avoided in patients with allergies to egg whites and whey.

Parenteral nutrition (PN) requires assessment of allergies to any of the ordered components of the intravenous solution as well as attention to age and metabolic needs. There are usually multiple combinations of products available, thus the need for close assessment of allergies to essential proteins, amino acids, carbohydrates, trace elements, minerals, vitamins, lipids, high concentrations of dextrose, and fluids. It is important for the nurse to assess his/her knowledge base about PN and the need for infusions through a central line, peripherally inserted central lines (PICs), or peripherally inserted midline catheters. (See http://evolve.elsevier.com/Lilley for more information.) Some of the complications of PN include pneumothorax, infection, air emboli or emboli related to protein or lipid aggregation (associated with central catheter IV lines), septicemia related to the nutrient-rich solutions and invasive IV route of administration, and metabolic imbalances due to the solution/ingredients and nausea (seen with lipid administration in the PN). There must also be a baseline and thorough assessment of the following: (1) central line site, noting its patency, intactness, and appearance, (2) WBC/RBC counts and other laboratory values and parameters listed earlier, (3) vitals signs with attention to temperature, (4) serum glucose levels, and (5) cardiac rhythm with electrocardiogram readings. Other core patient variables that may be assessed other than the ones already listed include daily weights (same time, same clothing), a fractional urinary analysis, serum glucose levels every 6 to 8 hours, baseline intake and output, and neurologic status.

◆ NURSING DIAGNOSES

- Diarrhea related to a decreased tolerance to enteral feedings and their ingredients
- Ineffective airway clearance related to possible aspiration of enteral feedings
- Deficient fluid volume related to altered nutrition status
- Risk for infection, sepsis, related to parenteral infusions, and use of central venous access
- Ineffective individual therapeutic management related to lack of information about therapeutic regimen with enteral/parenteral supplementation

◆ PLANNING

Goals

- Patient remains free of complications associated with enteral feedings and parenteral supplements
- Patient regains near-normal to normal bowel patterns
- Patient remains free of injury and infection during enteral or parenteral nutrition supplementation
- Patient remains free of infection during therapy
- Patient regains normal fluid volume status
- Patient remains compliant and makes return visits to the physician as needed

Outcome Criteria

- Patient identifies measures to decrease diarrhea while receiving enteral feedings such as use of prescribed drugs to decrease motility and/or use of over-the-counter drugs or herbal products as ordered.
- Patient (or caregiver) demonstrates adequate technique for enteral tube feedings to decrease risk for aspiration, with emphasis on elevated head of bed, checking tube placement and residuals before feeding is initiated.
- Patient states measures to minimize risk for infection at PN/TPN site, such as making sure site is changed as ordered and assessed frequently for redness, swelling, drainage, or fever, and reporting these to the physician or home health care nurse immediately.
- Patient begins to show adequate fluid volume status with improved skin turgor, improved urinary output to at least 30 mL/hr, and a return to normal laboratory values.
- Patient states symptoms to report to the physician, such as increased lethargy, fever, and shortness of breath.

◆ IMPLEMENTATION

A physician's order must be complete and dated before beginning enteral, parenteral, or total parenteral supplementation. In general, monitoring the status of the patient during and after enteral feedings is crucial to safe and prudent nursing care. Tinting tube feeding solutions with blue food coloring is used at times to help detect aspiration but should not replace checking for tube placement and for residuals. Gastric residual volumes should be obtained and documented before each feeding as well as before each medication is administered. The tube feeding is usually stopped first, and stomach contents are aspirated using a syringe connected to the particular tube to detect any residual. If the volume is more than a volume that has been consistent over the previous 2 hours of continuous feeding, the nurse should return the aspirate, hold the feeding, and contact the physician while keeping the head of the bed elevated. For intermittent bolus feedings, if the residual amount is greater than 50% of the volume previously infused, the nurse should return the aspirate, withhold the feeding, and contact the physician. A reduction in the tube feeding volume will probably be ordered by the physician. Always check hospital policy.

Newer tubes for nasogastric and enteral feeding have smaller diameters and are thinner (numbers 5 through 10 French) and more pliable for better patient tolerance. However, the smaller-diameter tubes make checking for gastric aspiration more difficult. The process of medication administration through a nasogastric tube is reviewed in Chapter 9 with step-by-step guidelines.

To prevent clogging of the feeding tube, it is often helpful to flush the tube with 30 mL of cranberry juice or other designated solution (as per policy) followed by 10 mL of water. The juice may help break up the formula residue and unclog certain types of feeding tubes, and the water helps to keep the tube clean and free of residue. Percutaneous enteral gastrostomy (PEG) tubes are also commonly used in many situations but do require surgical insertion (often done under moderate sedation) by a gastroenterologist. Their care includes dressing changes in the initial time period and then progresses to checking for residuals site. Placement is not checked, but if it appears that the tube has come out of the opening and is longer in length than previously noted, stop the infusion and contact the physician.

Physician-ordered enteral feeding infusion rates and concentrations should be followed carefully. Usually the initial rate is 50 mL/hr at one-half strength, but this may be increased per patient tolerance to a rate of 25 mL/hr at three-quarter strength concentration. Although more rapid feeding increases the risk for hyperglycemia, dumping syndrome and diarrhea, the nurse should continue to increase the patient's intake because the total volume amount and amount of calories with recommended daily allowances (RDAs) is very important. Tube-feeding formulas should always be at room temperature and never administered cold or warmed. If all the necessary steps to decrease or prevent diarrhea have failed, antidiarrheal medications may be needed. Lactose-free solutions are available and should be used with patients who are lactose intolerant. Patients who suffer from lactose intolerance experience cramping, diarrhea, abdominal bloating, and flatulence with the ingestion of the enteral milk-based feeding.

Infusions of PN/TPN should be assessed every hour or as per the facility's policy and procedure. The entire infusion system and equipment as well as the condition of the patient should be documented, and it is a standard of care to examine the patient first and then check the PN/TPN insertion site, tubing, infusion pump, and solution. Tubing with PN/TPN are often ordered to be changed every 24 hours—or more frequently—to prevent infection. It is also recommended that tubing changes occur daily with the beginning of each new infusion. A 1.2 micron filter is used to trap bacteria, including *Pseudomonas* spp. The patient's temperature should be recorded every 4 hours during the infusion, and any increase in temperature over 100° F should be reported to the physician immediately. The patient should also be checked frequently for signs and symptoms of hyperglycemia, such as headache, dehydration, and weakness. IV feeding rates should never be accelerated to increase plasma volume because the rapid increase of dextrose solution may precipitate hyperglycemia and other related complications. Insulin replacement may be needed with the increase in dextrose; therefore, serum glucose levels per glucometer readings are important for immediate recognition and treatment of hyperglycemia.

Hypoglycemia is manifested by cold, clammy skin; dizziness; tachycardia; and tingling of the extremities. Hypoglycemia associated with PN/TPN may be prevented by gradual reduction of the IV feeding rate to allow the pancreas time to adapt to the changing blood glucose levels. If PN/TPN is discontinued abruptly, rebound hypoglycemia may occur. This can be prevented with providing infusions of 5% to 10% glucose in situations in which PN/TPN must be discontinued immediately. Fluid overload may also occur with PN/TPN, manifested by weak pulse, hypertension, tachycardia, confusion, decreased urine output, and pitting edema. This may be prevented by maintaining intravenous rates as ordered. If signs of fluid overload occur, the nurse should slow the infusion rate, take a set of vital signs, remain with the patient, auscultate breath and heart sounds, and contact the physician immediately. Intake and output is usually indicated in situations of use of PN/TPN and with enteral supplementation, as well. Patient Teaching Tips for nutrition supplements are found in the box on the next page. Also see http://evolve.elsevier.com/Lilley for more information about related nursing considerations associated with PN/TPN.

◆ EVALUATION

Therapeutic responses to nutrition supplementation include improved well-being, energy, strength, and performance of activities of daily living; an increase in weight; and laboratory studies that reflect a more positive nutrition status. Specific laboratory values may include some of the following: albumin, total protein, hemoglobin, hematocrit, RBC and WBC levels, blood urea nitrogen (BUN), electrolytes, blood glucose and insulin levels, and iron values. Evaluation should be ongoing and nutrition re-evaluation done periodically so that the patient's nutrition needs are met, and this may require frequent physician appointments or monitoring by a home health care nurse. Always refer to goals and outcome criteria to evaluate the effectiveness of therapy.

Patient Teaching Tips

- Because patients are often discharged with various types of tube feedings, the patient and family should receive patient education, instructions, and demonstrations about the daily care of the tube, preparation of tube feedings, and related procedures, which should be presented in a way that reflects the learning needs of the patient and those involved in their care.
- Patient/caregiver should be instructed about the need for correct placement of the tube, which should be checked prior to each tube feeding if a nasogastric tube is used. Incorrect placement of a nasogastric tube would be characterized by coughing, choking, difficulty in speaking, cyanosis, and subsequent respiratory distress. The head of the bed should remain elevated during infusions and is more critical with nasogastric tube feedings versus gastrostomy tube feedings.
- Contact names and phone numbers of physicians, home health nurse, and other resources should be made available for use by the patient/caregiver should there be any problems or concerns related to the feeding. A fever, difficulty breathing, congested lung sounds, high residual amounts, resistance against the flow of the feeding solution, or resistance against checking for residual should all be areas of "concern" and appropriate interventions implemented including seeking emergency medical care if all else fails.
- Patients who are homebound and have PN/TPN will need individualized education as well as support from home health care or related health care services. Practice is critical to acquisition of skill by the patient and/or family/caregiver and should be an integral part of patient education. All procedures for storage; cleansing and care of site; dressing changes; irrigation of the catheter; pump function and care; and changing of the bag, filters, and tubing should also be explained, demonstrated, and shown in a return demonstration by the patient before he or she is discharged. Educate the patient about the fact that PN/TPN will require home health care services by a registered nurse to help prevent complications of infection at the site, sepsis, fever, and pneumonia.
- Educate the patient about checking serum glucose levels at home as ordered by the physician if there is TPN or other infused solutions high in dextrose. The use of a glucometer should be explained and specific steps included in the demonstration to the patient/family/caregiver. Additionally, instructions in self-administration of insulin, based on sliding scale coverage, may need to be included and reinforced.
- Educate the patient/caregiver to report signs and symptoms of potential complications of PN/TPN, including fever, cough, chest pains, dyspnea, and chills, all of which are indicative of adverse reactions to lipid infusions. Restlessness, nervousness, fainting, and tachycardia are associated with hypoglycemia and should also be reported, whereas nausea, vomiting, polyuria, and polydipsia may indicate hyperglycemia (and should also be reported).

Points to Remember

- A thorough nutrition assessment and possible consultation with a registered dietitian or nutritionist are essential for adequate intervention for the malnourished patient.
- There are various enteral feedings with different nutrition content, including some that are lactose free.
- Enteral feedings may result in complications such as hyperglycemia, dumping syndrome, and aspiration of feeding.
- TPN is administered through a central venous catheter because of the hyperosmolarity of substances used and the need for dilution from a larger diameter vein as well as the larger vein and dilution preventing damage to the vein. PN given through a peripherally inserted central catheter (PICC) line is another option but uses a lower concentration of dextrose and other ingredients.
- Parenteral feedings may result in air embolism, fever, infection, fluid volume overload, hyperglycemia, or hypoglycemia. If discontinued abruptly, rebound hypoglycemia may result.
- Cautious and astute nursing care with enteral or parenteral nutrition supplementation may prevent or decrease the occurrence of associated complications.

NCLEX Examination Review Questions

1. The route of enteral nutrition delivery with a basic nasogastric feeding tube would be through which of the following?
   a. Surgical placement into the stomach
   b. Placement from the nose into the jejunum
   c. Surgical insertion directly into the jejunum
   d. Placement from the nose into the stomach
2. When administering total parenteral nutrition (TPN), the nurse is aware that a purpose of intravenous fat (lipid) emulsions is to provide:
   a. Calories
   b. Amino acids
   c. Minerals
   d. Immunoglobulins
3. When considering the various routes of administering nutrition products, the nurse is aware that an example of enteral nutrition would be:
   a. PN via a PICC line
   b. TPN via a central line
   c. Osmolite via a PEG tube
   d. Intralipid infusion
4. Peripheral parenteral nutrition would be most appropriate in which situation?
   a. Therapy that is expected to last over 2 weeks
   b. Therapy that is expected to last less than 14 days
   c. Dextrose needs of 20% concentration
   d. Nutrition need of 3000 calories per day
5. During the night shift, a patient's infusion of TPN runs out, the pharmacy is closed, and a new bag of TPN will not be available for about 6 hours. The nurse's most appropriate action at this time would be to:
   a. Hang a bottle of intralipid solution.
   b. Hang a bag of normal saline.
   c. Hang a bag of 10% dextrose.
   d. Call the physician for stat TPN orders.

1. d, 2. a, 3. c, 4. b, 5. c.

Critical Thinking Activities

1. Which nursing actions will help address the nursing diagnosis of diarrhea or diarrhea as related to enteral feedings?
2. What outcome criteria will address the nursing diagnosis of deficient fluid volume related to insufficient intake?
3. What is the concern for abrupt withdrawal of a 25% glucose TPN solution? Explain your answer.

For answers, see http://evolve.elsevier.com/Lilley.

Miscellaneous Therapeutics: Hematologic, Dermatologic, Ophthalmic, and Otic Drugs

STUDY SKILLS TIPS

- *Time Management*
- *PURR*
- *Repeat the Steps*

TIME MANAGEMENT

As you plan your study time for Part Ten, it should be very clear that Chapter 58 will take significantly more time to complete than the other chapters. Do not let the length of the chapter overwhelm you. Apply the principles of time management to this chapter and you will succeed. The most important aspect of time management to apply to this chapter is the use of clear goal statements and action plan steps to help you achieve the goals.

Goal Statements

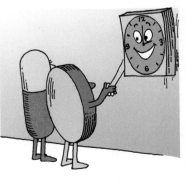

Remember the criteria for goal statements. First, they must be realistic; the statements must be things you know you can accomplish. Second, they must be specific to the task. "I will study the chapter" is not a very specific goal. Specify what you expect to accomplish. "I will master the 34 terms in the chapter glossary" is a more specific goal statement. Third, there must be a time limit. How long will you spend in achieving this goal? Set a time limit for completion of each activity for the quantity of time to be spent in each learning activity. Finally, goal statements must be measurable. In the example about studying the glossary, including the number of terms contained in Chapter 58 helps clarify the goal.

Action Planning

The second segment of time management is the use of action planning. An action plan is a series of smaller, specific activities

that you will accomplish to meet your goal statements. Your goal is to master the 34 terms. What will you do to meet that goal?

Action Steps Example

1. I will spend 1 hour from 3:00 to 4:00 PM on Monday making vocabulary drill cards for the terms found in the glossary in Chapter 58.
2. I will spend 15 minutes in rehearsal and review of these cards every day until the exam on this chapter is over.
3. Each time I cannot define and explain a term, I will put an *X* on the card to identify it as a term needing more review.
4. I will spend 1 hour the night before the exam doing a comprehensive review of the terms in Chapter 58, with special emphasis on those cards that have one or more *X* marks.

Action steps help ensure that you are spending your study time actively focusing on what you need to learn.

PURR

Prepare Example

Chapter 58, Objective 3 reads, "Discuss the mechanisms of action, indications, dosage forms with application techniques, side effects, cautions, contraindications, and drug interactions of the various ophthalmic drugs."

- Question 1: What does *ophthalmic* mean? (Literal question [LQ])
- Question 2: What are ophthalmic drugs? (LQ)
- Question 3: What is the mechanism of action of ophthalmic drugs? (LQ)
- Question 4: Is there more than one mechanism of action? (LQ)
- Question 5: If there is more than one mechanism of action, how are the mechanisms similar and how are they different? (Interpretive Question)

These questions are only suggestions of generated questions based on the chapter objectives. Many more questions can be asked about Objective 3. These questions are an essential part of the study process. Questions help make you an active reader and an active learner. The more questions you generate the easier it will be to understand the chapter.

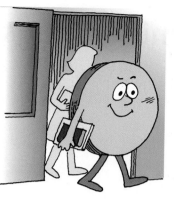

Outline Example

1. *Looking through the chapter, decide how much material is appropriate.* The section that begins with Antiglaucoma Drugs is probably too much material. Looking at the chapter headings, this section could be broken down into five blocks of material. Block one would cover the material under the heading Cholinergic Drugs. Block two would be the material under the heading Sympathomimetics. The next four blocks would be β-Adrenergic Blockers, Carbonic Anhydrase Inhibitors, Osmotic Diuretics, and Prostaglandin Agonists.

2. *Apply the Prepare step to each block.* Beginning with "Parasympathomimetics," generate some questions to guide your reading. Remember that it is important to ask questions that will focus on both literal information and questions that will help you interpret, evaluate, and analyze when you read.

3. *Read the material.* As soon as you have completed the self-questioning on the first block of material, read the material in the chapter. It is important that the reading be done immediately. Read for understanding, and as you read remember the questions you generated. This approach will help your concentration and comprehension.

4. *Take a short break.* Once you have completed the reading of this section of the chapter, give your mind a chance to reflect and consolidate the learning. Limit the time you allow for a break and use the time for something pleasurable. Give your-self 5 or 10 minutes to read the newspaper, get a snack, or just take a short walk.

5. *Rehearse.* Before going on to the next section of the chapter it is important to spend a few minutes in rehearsal. Using the questions from Step 2, go back over the material you read and try to respond to those questions. When you find yourself unable to answer a question, put a mark in the text besides the heading that caused the difficulty and move on. The mark will serve as a reminder for future review. At this point, the objective is not complete mastery of the material. The objective is to see what you have learned so that you can move smoothly into the next section. Breaking a chapter into blocks is useful, but it is imperative that the links between sections be made as you study.

6. *Review.* After completing two or three major sections of the chapter, it is time to review. Start at the beginning of the chapter. Ask your questions. Try to answer them. If you cannot formulate a clear answer, then some rereading is necessary. Also, pay attention to the marks made during the rehearsal step. Those marks indicate areas that you have already identified as needing review. When rereading, remember that the object is to read only as much of the material as needed to be able to respond to self-generated questions. There simply is not enough time to read the entire chapter a second or third time.

REPEAT THE STEPS

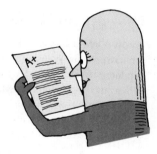

Prepare, read for understanding, take a short break, and then rehearse the material you've just read. It may seem that this process takes an excessive amount of time and involves a lot of repetition, but in the long run this process will produce better learning. The time spent in Prepare, Understand, and Rehearsal will reduce the time needed to review. Frequent review as you move through the chapter will make the final review at exam time proceed more quickly and enable you to achieve mastery of the material.

Blood-Forming Drugs

Objectives

When you reach the end of this chapter, you should be able to do the following:

1. Discuss the importance of iron, vitamin B_{12}, and folic acid to the formation of blood cells.
2. Discuss the various conditions requiring treatment with blood-forming drugs.
3. Discuss the mechanisms of action, cautions, contraindications, drug interactions, uses, dosages, special administration techniques, and measures to enhance the effectiveness of and decrease adverse effects related to the various blood-forming drugs.
4. Develop a nursing care plan that includes all phases of the nursing process related to the administration of blood-forming drugs.

e-Learning Activities

Companion CD
- NCLEX Review Questions: see questions 443-444
- Animations
- Audio Glossary
- Category Catchers
- Medication Errors Checklists
- IV Therapy Checklists

evolve Website (http://evolve.elsevier.com/Lilley)
• Nursing Care Plans • Frequently Asked Questions • Content Updates • WebLinks • Supplemental Resources • Elsevier ePharmacology Update • Medication Administration Animations

Drug Profiles

▶ ferrous fumarate, p. 862   iron dextran, p. 862
▶ folic acid, p. 863

▶ Key drug.

Glossary

Erythrocyte   Another name for red blood cell (RBC). (p. 858)

Erythropoiesis   The process of erythrocyte production. (p. 858)

Globin   Part of the *hemoglobin* molecule (see below); a protein chain of which there are four different structural chains, alpha$_1$ and alpha$_2$ and beta$_1$ and beta$_2$. (p. 859)

Hematopoiesis   The normal formation and development of all blood cell types in the bone marrow. (p. 858)

Heme   Part of the *hemoglobin* molecule; a non-protein, iron-containing pigment. (p. 859)

Hemoglobin (Hgb)   A complex protein-iron compound in the blood that carries oxygen to the cells from the lungs and carbon dioxide away from the cells to the lungs. (p. 859)

Hemolytic anemia   Any anemia resulting from excessive destruction of erythrocytes. (p. 860)

Hypochromic   Pertaining to less than normal color. The term usually describes an RBC and helps further characterize anemias associated with reduced synthesis of hemoglobin. (p. 859)

Microcytic   Pertaining to smaller-than-normal cells. (p. 859)

Pernicious anemia   A type of *megaloblastic* anemia usually seen in older adults and caused by impaired intestinal absorption of vitamin B_{12} (cyanocobalamin) due to lack of availability of *instrinsic factor*. (p. 860)

Reticulocytes   An immature erythrocyte characterized by a meshlike pattern of threads and particles at the former site of the nucleus. (p. 858)

Spherocytes   Small, globular, completely hemoglobinated erythrocytes without the usual central concavity or pallor. (p. 860)

ERYTHROPOIESIS

The formation of new blood cells is one of the primary functions of bones. This process is known as **hematopoiesis,** and it includes the production of **erythrocytes** (red blood cells or RBCs), as well as *leukocytes* (white blood cells) and *thrombocytes* (platelets). This process takes place in the *myeloid* tissue or bone marrow. This specialized tissue is located primarily in the ends, or *epiphyses*, of certain long bones, and also in the flat bones of the skull, pelvis, sternum, and ribs.

Erythropoiesis, the process of erythrocyte formation, is the focus of this chapter. This involves the maturation of a nucleated RBC precursor into a hemoglobin (Hgb)-filled, nucleus-free erythrocyte. This process is driven by the hormone *erythropoietin*, produced by the kidneys.

When RBCs are manufactured in the bone marrow by myeloid tissue, they are released into the circulation as immature RBCs called **reticulocytes.** Once in the circulation, reticulocytes undergo a 24- to 36-hour maturation process to become mature, fully functional RBCs. After this, they have a life span of about 120 days.

It is important to know the structural components of the RBC to understand how anemia develops and why certain drugs are used to correct it. More than one third of an RBC is made of hemoglobin. **Hemoglobin (Hgb)** is composed of two parts: heme and globin. **Heme** is a red pigment. Each molecule of heme contains one atom of iron. **Globin** is a protein chain that consists of four structurally different parts or globulins: alpha$_1$ and alpha$_2$ and beta$_1$ and beta$_2$ ($\alpha_1 + \alpha_2$ and $\beta_1 + \beta_2$). Together, one molecule of heme and one protein chain of globin make one Hgb molecule (Figure 56-1).

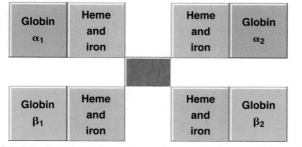

| Globin α_1 | Heme and iron | | Heme and iron | Globin α_2 |
| Globin β_1 | Heme and iron | | Heme and iron | Globin β_2 |

FIGURE 56-1   Schematic structure of a hemoglobin molecule.

TYPES OF ANEMIA

Anemias are classified into four main types based on underlying causes (Figure 56-2). Knowledge of the etiologies of anemias will help you to understand the therapies used to treat them. Anemias can be caused by maturation defects, or they can be secondary to excessive RBC destruction. Two types of maturation defects cause anemias, depending on the location of the defect within the cell: *cytoplasmic* maturation defects occur in the cell cytoplasm, and *nuclear* maturation defects occur in the cell nucleus. Factors responsible for excessive RBC destruction can be either intrinsic or extrinsic.

Figure 56-3 summarizes the types of anemias arising from cytoplasmic maturation defects. Major examples include iron deficiency anemia and genetic disorders such as *thalassemia*, which result in defective globin synthesis. The RBCs appear **hypochromic** (lighter red than normal) and **microcytic** (smaller than normal) on blood smear. Cytoplasmic maturation anemias occur as a result of reduced or abnormal Hgb synthesis. Because Hgb is synthesized from both iron and globin, a deficiency in either one can lead to a Hgb deficiency. Some common causes of

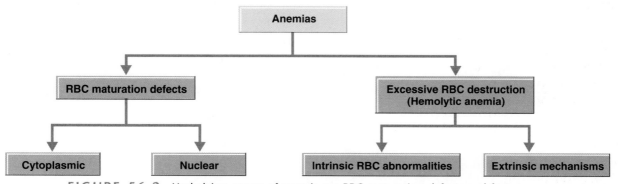

FIGURE 56-2   Underlying causes of anemia are RBC maturation defects and factors secondary to excessive RBC destruction. *RBC*, Red blood cell.

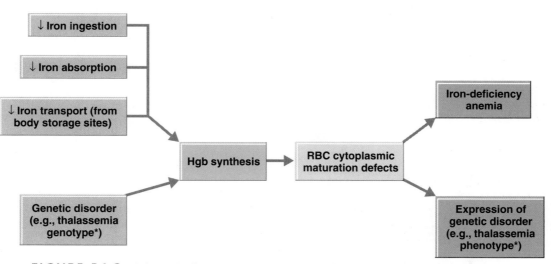

FIGURE 56-3   Schematic showing common causes and results of RBC cytoplasmic maturation defects.

iron-deficiency anemia are blood loss, surgery, childbirth, gastrointestinal bleeding, and hemorrhoids.

Figure 56-4 summarizes the types of anemias arising from nuclear maturation defects. These occur because of defects in DNA or protein synthesis. Both DNA and protein require vitamin B_{12} and folic acid to be present in normal amounts for their proper production. If either of these two vitamins is absent or deficient, anemias secondary to nuclear maturation defects may develop. RBCs in such anemias actually appear to be *normochromic* (normal in color) but are commonly *macrocytic* (larger than normal) on blood smear. One example is **pernicious anemia.** This results from a dietary deficiency of vitamin B_{12}, which is used in the formation of new RBCs. The usual underlying cause is the failure of the stomach lining to produce *intrinsic factor.*

Intrinsic factor is a gastric glycoprotein that allows vitamin B_{12} to be absorbed in the intestine (Chapter 54). Another example is the anemia caused by folic acid deficiency. Both pernicious anemia and folic acid deficiency anemia are also both known as types of *megaloblastic* anemia, as they are both characterized by large, immature RBCs. Megaloblastic anemias are usually due to poor dietary intake and are most commonly seen in infancy, childhood, and pregnancy.

Figure 56-5 summarizes the types of anemias arising from excessive RBC destruction, or **hemolytic anemias.** These can occur because of abnormalities within the RBCs themselves *(intrinsic factors)* or as a result of factors outside *(extrinsic)* to the RBCs. The erythrocytes in both cases appear on blood smear as **spherocytes,** which are small, globular erythrocytes with exces-

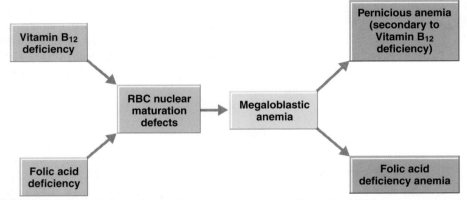

FIGURE 56-4 Schematic showing common causes and results of RBC nuclear maturation defects.

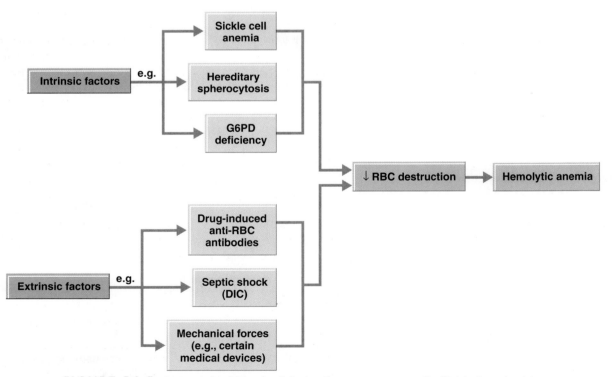

FIGURE 56-5 Increased red blood cell destruction occurs as a result of intrinsic and extrinsic factors. *DIC,* Disseminated intravascular coagulation; *G6PD,* glucose-6-phosphate dehydrogenase; *RBC,* red blood cell.

sive amounts of hemoglobin, and which, therefore, lack the central *pallor* (paleness) and concavity of normal RBCs. These RBCs also appear to be fragmented when observed on blood smear. Intrinsic RBC abnormalities are usually the result of a genetic defect. Examples include *sickle cell anemia, hereditary spherocytosis,* and *glucose-6-phosphate dehydrogenase (G6PD) deficiency.* Examples of extrinsic mechanisms for excessive RBC destruction include drug-induced *antibodies* that target and destroy RBCs, septic shock that produces *disseminated intravascular coagulation (DIC),* and mechanical forces such as *intra-aortic balloon pumps* and *ventricular assist devices,* commonly used in cardiac intensive care units.

IRON

Iron is an essential mineral for the proper function of all biologic systems in the body. It is stored in many sites throughout the body (liver, spleen, and bone marrow). It is also the principal nutrition deficiency in the United States, resulting in anemia. Individuals who require the greatest amount of iron are women (especially pregnant women) and children. They are also the individuals who are most likely to develop iron-deficiency anemia. This is partly due to ongoing menstrual blood losses, which is one reason why men are less likely to develop this disorder. In fact, most vitamin supplements for men contain little or no iron. Nonetheless, dietary iron is usually sufficient for both men and women in developed countries.

Dietary sources for iron include meats and certain vegetables and grains (see http://evolve.elsevier.com/Lilley for specific examples). These forms of iron must be converted by gastric juices before they can be absorbed. Other foods such as orange juice, veal, fish, and ascorbic acid may help with iron absorption. Conversely, eggs, corn, beans, and many cereal products containing chemicals known as *phytates* may impair iron absorption from either other iron-containing foods or iron supplements. However, it should also be noted that both beans and eggs are themselves common dietary sources of iron. Iron preparations are available as ferrous salts. See Table 56-1 for a list of the currently available iron salts and their respective iron content.

Mechanism of Action and Drug Effects

Iron is an oxygen carrier in both hemoglobin and *myoglobin* (oxygen-carrying molecule in muscle tissue), and thus is critical for tissue respiration. Iron is also a required component of a number of enzyme systems in the body and is necessary for energy transfer in the *cytochrome oxidase* and *xanthine oxidase* enzyme systems. Administration of iron corrects iron-deficiency symptoms such as anemia, dysphagia, dystrophy of the nails and skin, and fissuring of the angles of the lips, as well as maintains the bodily functions described earlier.

Indications

Supplemental iron contained in multivitamins plus iron or iron supplements alone are indicated for the prevention or treatment of iron-deficiency anemia. In all cases, an underlying cause should be identified. After identification of the cause, treatment should be aimed at attempting to correct the cause (e.g., chronic blood loss [such as from an ulcer]) rather than simply alleviate the symptoms. Iron supplementation is also used in epoetin therapy (Chapter 49) because it is essential for the production of RBCs.

Contraindications

Contraindications to the use of iron products include known drug allergy, *hemolytic anemia, hemochromatosis* (iron overload), and any anemia not associated with iron deficiency.

Adverse Effects

The most common adverse effects associated with iron preparations are nausea, vomiting, diarrhea, constipation, stomach cramps, and stomach pain. Excess iron intake can lead to accumulation and iron toxicity. See Table 56-2 for a more complete listing of the undesirable effects associated with iron preparations.

Toxicity and Management of Overdose

Iron overdose is the most common cause of pediatric poisoning deaths reported to U.S. poison control centers. Many iron supplements are enteric-coated and resemble candy. In 1991, there were 5144 cases of accidental ingestion of oral iron preparations reported; 11 of these were fatal. Toxicity from iron ingestion results from a combination of the corrosive effects on the gastrointestinal mucosa and the metabolic and hemodynamic effects caused by the presence of excessive elemental iron.

Treatment is founded on good symptomatic and supportive measures, including suction and maintenance of airway, correction of acidosis, and control of shock and dehydration with intravenous fluids or blood, oxygen, and vasopressor. Abdominal radiographs may be helpful because iron preparations are radiopaque and may be visualized on x-ray film. Serum iron concentrations may be helpful in establishing severity of ingestion. A serum iron concentration of more than 300 mcg/dL places the patient at serious risk for toxicity. The stomach should be emptied immediately by gastric lavage. Because many of the iron products are extended-release formulations that release contents in the intestines rather than the stomach, whole-gut lavage is generally believed to be superior and more effective. This should be followed by a saline cathartic or possible surgical removal of ingested iron tablets. In patients with severe symptoms of iron intoxication, such as coma, shock, or seizures, chelation therapy with deferoxamine should be initiated.

Table 56-1 **Ferrous Salts: Iron Content**	
Ferrous Salts	**Iron Content**
Ferrous fumarate	33% iron or 330 mg/g
Ferrous gluconate	12% iron or 120 mg/g
Ferrous sulfate	20% iron or 200 mg/g
Ferrous sulfate (desiccated, dried, or exsiccated)	30% iron or 300 mg/g

Table 56-2 **Iron Preparations: Adverse Effects**	
Body System	**Adverse Effects**
Gastrointestinal	Nausea, constipation, epigastric pain, black and tarry stools, vomiting, diarrhea
Integumentary	Temporarily discolored tooth enamel and eyes, pain upon injection

Interactions

The absorption of iron can be enhanced when it is given with ascorbic acid or decreased when it is given with antacids. Iron preparations can decrease the absorption of thyroid drugs, tetracyclines, and quinolone antibiotics.

Dosages

For the recommended dosages of iron preparations, see the table on this page.

Drug Profiles

Iron preparations are available by prescription and as over-the-counter (OTC) medications. They are contraindicated in patients with ulcerative colitis and regional enteritis, conditions of excessive body iron stores (e.g., *hemosiderosis, hemochromatosis*), peptic ulcer disease (PUD), hemolytic anemia, cirrhosis, gastritis, and esophagitis. Goals of therapy include maintenance of normal Hgb and hematocrit (Hct), and energy level.

▶ **ferrous fumarate**

The ferrous fumarate iron salts (Femiron) contain the largest amount of iron per gram of salt consumed. Ferrous sulfate and ferrous gluconate are two other forms of iron that are commonly used. Ferrous fumarate is 33% elemental iron; therefore, a 325-mg tablet of ferrous fumarate provides 107 mg of elemental iron. Ferrous fumarate is available only for oral use.

Pharmacokinetics

Half-Life	Onset	Peak	Duration
PO: 6 hr	PO: 3-10 days*	PO: Unknown	PO: Variable

*Increased reticulocyte values.

iron dextran

Iron dextran (InFeD, DexFerrum) is a colloidal solution of iron (as ferric hydroxide) and dextran. Sodium ferric gluconate (Ferrlecit) and iron sucrose (Venofer) are other available forms of injectable

iron. It is intended for intravenous or intramuscular use for iron deficiency. Anaphylactic reactions to iron dextran, including major orthostatic hypertension and fatal anaphylaxis, have been reported in 0.2% to 0.3% of patients. Because of this, a test dose of 25 mg of iron dextran should be administered by the chosen route before injection of the full dose. Although anaphylactic reactions usually occur within a few moments after the test dose, it is recommended that a period of at least 1 hour elapse before the remaining portion of the initial dose is given. Individual doses of 2 mL or less may be given on a daily basis until the calculated total amount required has been reached. InFeD is given undiluted at a gradual rate not to exceed 50 mg (1 mL)/min. Iron dextran is available only for injection.

Pharmacokinetics

Half-Life	Onset	Peak	Duration
IM: 5-20 hr	IM: Unknown	IM: 24-48 hr	IM: ≥3 wk

FOLIC ACID

Folic acid is a water-soluble B-complex vitamin. It is also synonymously referred to as folate, the name of its anionic form. The human body requires oral intake of folic acid. Dietary sources of folic acid include dried beans, peas, oranges, and green vegetables. Several conditions can lead to folic acid deficiency. However, because folic acid is absorbed in the upper duodenum, malabsorption syndromes are the most common cause of deficiency.

Mechanism of Action and Drug Effects

It is converted to *tetrahydrofolic acid* in the body, which is used for erythropoiesis and for synthesis of nucleic acids (DNA and RNA). Dietary ingestion of folate is required for the production of the nucleic acids DNA and RNA. It is also essential for normal

DOSAGES

Selected Iron Preparations and Folic Acid

Drug (Pregnancy Category)	Pharmacologic Class	Usual Dosage Range	Indications
▶ferrous fumarate (Feostat, Hemocyte) (A)	Oral iron salt	**Pediatric*** Infant-6 mo 10-25 mg/day in 3-4 divided doses **6 mo-2 yr** Up to 6 mg/kg/day in 3-4 divided doses **2-12 yr** 50-100 mg (1-1.5 mg/kg)/day in 3-4 divided doses **Adult*** 100-200 mg (2-3 mg/kg) qd-tid	Iron deficiency
▶folic acid (A)	Vitamin B-complex group; water-soluble B-vitamin	**Pediatric†** PO/IV/IM/SC: 0.1-0.4 mg/day **Adult†** PO/IV/IM/SC: Up to 1 mg/day	Folate deficiency; tropical sprue; nutritional supplement; pregnancy supplement
iron dextran (InFeD, DexFerrum) (C)	Parenteral iron salt	**Pediatric†** IM/IV: <5 kg, 25 mg/day (0.5 mL/day); <10 kg, 50 mg/day (1 mL/day) **Adult†** IM/IV: 100 mg/day (2 mL/day)	Iron deficiency when oral iron is unsatisfactory

*Doses are in terms of elemental iron, not the salt itself.
†Expressed in milligrams of elemental iron. Dosages are calculated for each patient's weight according to manufacturer's label. Doses are approximate.

erythropoiesis. Folic acid is not active in the ingested form. It must first be converted to tetrahydrofolic acid, which is a cofactor for reactions in the biosynthesis of purines and thymidylates of nucleic acids.

Indications

Folic acid is primarily used to prevent and treat folic acid deficiency. Anemias caused by folic acid deficiency can be treated by exogenous supplementation of folic acid. There is also much evidence to support the use of folic acid in the prevention of neural tube defects such as spina bifida, anencephaly, and encephalocele. It is recommended that administration is begun at least 1 month before pregnancy and continue through early pregnancy to reduce the risk for fetal neural tube defects. Indications for folic acid include the following:

* Folic acid deficiency anemia
* Tropical sprue
* Prophylaxis of neural tube defects in pregnant women

Contraindications

Contraindications to the use of folic acid include known allergy to a specific drug product and any anemia not related to folic acid deficiency (e.g., pernicious anemia). It should be emphasized that folic acid should not be used to treat anemias until the underlying cause and type of anemia have been determined. For example, administering folic acid to a patient with pernicious anemia may correct the hematologic changes of anemia, while deceptively masking other symptoms of pernicious anemia.

Adverse Effects

Adverse effects associated with folic acid use are rare. Allergic reaction or yellow discoloration of urine may occur.

Interactions

Oral contraceptives (Chapter 33), corticosteroids (Chapter 32), sulfonamides (Chapter 37), and dihydrofolate reductase inhibitors (including the antineoplastic drug methotrexate [Chapter 47] and the antibiotic trimethoprim [Chapter 37]) can all cause signs of folic acid deficiency. Folic acid can also lower the serum levels of phenytoin with possible breakthrough seizures.

Dosages

For recommended dosages of folic acid, see the table on page 862.

Drug Profiles

▶ folic acid

Folic acid is a water-soluble B-complex vitamin that is used primarily in the treatment and prevention of folic-acid deficiency and anemias caused by folic-acid deficiency. Folic acid is available as an OTC medication in multivitamin preparations and by prescription as a single drug. It is contraindicated in patients with anemias other than megaloblastic or macrocytic anemia. These contraindicated conditions include vitamin B_{12} deficiency anemia, and uncorrected pernicious anemia. Folic acid is available for both oral and injectable use.

Pharmacokinetics

Half-Life	Onset	Peak	Duration
PO: Unknown	PO: Unknown	PO: 60-90 min	PO: Unknown

OTHER BLOOD-FORMING DRUGS

Other drugs that may be used in the prevention and treatment of anemia are cyanocobalamin (vitamin B_{12}) and erythropoietin (Epogen, Procrit). Cyanocobalamin is discussed in detail in Chapter 54, and erythropoietin is discussed in Chapter 49.

◆ NURSING PROCESS

◆ ASSESSMENT

Before giving any blood-forming drug, it is important for the nurse to assess medical history; current condition; and medication profile, including prescription, over-the-counter, and herbal/alternative medications. Contraindications, cautions, and drug interactions should be assessed thoroughly prior to initiation of drug therapy. Laboratory studies such as Hgb, Hct, reticulocytes, bilirubin levels, and baseline levels of folate and/or B-complex vitamins should be obtained and documented. A nutritional assessment should also be performed, with concentration on the amount of iron intake in the patient's diet (a nutrition consult may be necessary) and a 24-hour recall of all food intake with serving sizes. Dietary consultation may prove beneficial if ordered.

◆ NURSING DIAGNOSES

* Activity intolerance related to fatigue and lethargy associated with anemias
* Risk for injury related to adverse effects of iron products
* Deficient knowledge related to limited exposure to use of medication
* Imbalanced nutrition, less than body requirements, related to disease process

◆ PLANNING

Goals

* Patient regains his/her normal level of activity, as ordered.
* Patient remains free of symptoms related to adverse effects of blood-forming drugs (e.g., iron products).
* Patient discusses rationale for use, adverse effects, and patient education guidelines related to use of blood-forming drugs.
* Patient attains normal nutritional status through use of pharmacologic and nonpharmacologic measures.

Outcome Criteria

* Patient is able to tolerate gradual increase in activity as ordered (e.g., performing activities of daily living, walking 10 minutes per day with increases as tolerated) while taking blood-forming drug.
* Patient uses measures to minimize occurrence of adverse effects of blood-forming drugs, such as taking with food.
* Patient takes medication exactly as prescribed to enhance its efficacy.
* Patient reports symptoms associated with increased symptomatology related to disease process or to adverse reactions to medications, such as abdominal distention, cramping, nausea, and vomiting.
* Patient keeps daily journal of dietary intake to share with health-care provider every week.
* Patient uses examples of a balanced diet for daily menu planning.

◆ IMPLEMENTATION

Liquid oral forms of iron products should be diluted per manufacturer instructions and taken through a plastic straw to avoid discoloration of tooth enamel. Oral forms should be given with juice, but not antacids or milk, or with meals for maximal absorption of the drug. Taking the oral dosages with meals/food is recommended mainly because of the high risk for gastrointestinal distress, even though the food will alter absorption. Iron dextran should be administered only after all oral iron preparations have been discontinued. A test dose of iron may be ordered, with the remaining dose to be given an hour later. Intramuscularly administered iron should be given deep in a large muscle mass using the Z-track method (Chapter 9). Intravenous iron dextran should be given after the intravenous line is flushed with 10 mL of normal saline (NS) and should be given with the recommended amount of diluent and over the recommended drip rate. Epinephrine and resuscitative equipment should always be available in case of anaphylactic reaction (to iron or any drug with a greater risk of causing anaphylaxis). In addition, it may be necessary for the patient to remain recumbent 30 minutes after the intravenous injection to prevent drug-induced orthostatic hypotension. The patient should be slow and purposeful with mobility at this time.

Ferrous salts, if given to infants, should be administered only with vitamin E to prevent the possible occurrence of hemolytic anemia. Ferrous salts are best given between meals for maximal absorption, but they are often taken with food or meals to decrease gastrointestinal upset. At least 1 to 2 hours should be allowed between intake of the ferrous drug and intake of milk or antacids. The drug should be stored in a light-resistant, airtight container. Patients should be cautioned to avoid remaining in an upright or sitting position for up to 30 minutes after taking oral dosage forms of iron, ferrous, and related products to help minimize esophageal irritation/corrosion. It is important to also inform patients that use of any iron product will turn stools from brown to a black, tarry color. Folic acid may be ordered as an additive drug for total parenteral nutrition solutions, and concerns regarding monitoring for hypotension and/or allergic reactions remain important. Teaching tips for blood-forming drugs are presented in the Patient Teaching Tips box.

◆ EVALUATION

Evaluation of therapeutic responses to blood-forming drugs should evolve around goals and outcome criteria as well as monitoring for therapeutic versus adverse effects. Therapeutic responses to iron products include improved nutrition status, increased weight, increased activity tolerance and well-being, and absence of fatigue. Adverse effects include nausea, constipation, epigastric pain, black and tarry stools, and vomiting. Toxic signs may include nausea, diarrhea (green, tarry stools), hematemesis, pallor, cyanosis, shock, and coma.

Life Span Considerations: The Elderly Patient

Iron Products

- Instructions on how to take oral forms of iron are crucial to safe administration, and all types of teaching strategies should be implemented to reinforce all verbal and/or written instructions. Make sure education is individualized and geared for the patient with alterations in sensory perception. Patients should be cautioned about making changes in their medication regimen, such as doubling doses or discontinuing without a physician's order.
- The elderly patient and spouse/caregiver should be instructed on food sources high in iron and how to include them in their menu planning. Instruct the patient to steam vegetables and not overcook them through excessive boiling. The avoidance of overcooking or boiling of vegetables/food items is important to the preservation of vitamin, mineral, and elemental content, including iron.
- Remind older patients that gastrointestinal upset may occur with many drugs, including vitamins and iron. Iron products should be taken with food or a snack to help decrease this upset.
- Always educate elderly patients, their spouses/family members/ significant others, and/or caregivers about appropriate community resources (e.g., Meals on Wheels, senior citizen community centers, public recreation centers). A list of these community resources are often made available through a city web page, social services, and other outlets.

Patient Teaching Tips

- Inform the patient to take iron products cautiously and to be aware of potential poisoning if taken at amounts greater than what is recommended. Oral dosage forms of iron should be given intact, should not be crushed or altered in any way, and should be taken with at least 4 to 6 oz of water/fluid to help minimize gastrointestinal upset and increase absorption.
- It is important to emphasize to the patient an iron product, if ordered, cannot be substituted for another because each product contains different forms of the iron salt and also come in different amounts.
- Remind patients to remain upright for up to 15 to 30 minutes and avoid reclining during this time to avoid esophageal irritation or corrosion. Inform patients that iron products may lead to the occurrence of black and tarry stools.
- Encourage patients to eat foods high in iron, such as meat; dark green, leafy vegetables; dried beans; dried fruits; and eggs (see http://evolve.elsevier.com/Lilley for more information).

Points to Remember

- Iron and folic acid are very important in the treatment of many disorders and diseases (e.g., malignancies) to achieve RBC and Hgb formation that is as adequate as possible and to help prevent nutrition deficits that can affect all body systems, especially the immune system.

- Blood-forming drugs are often used in the treatment of pernicious anemias, malabsorption syndromes, hemolytic anemias, hemorrhage, and renal and liver diseases.
- Iron products should be taken exactly as ordered. Parenteral dosage forms may cause anaphylaxis and orthostatic hypotension.

NCLEX Examination Review Questions

1. When administering oral iron tablets, the nurse should keep in mind that the most appropriate liquid, other than water, to use with these tablets is:
   a. Pudding
   b. An antacid
   c. Milk
   d. Orange juice
2. When teaching a group of patients about foods that contain iron, which foods are considered good sources of iron?
   a. Meats
   b. Citrus fruits
   c. Tomatoes
   d. Yellow vegetables
3. When administering iron dextran intramuscularly, which nursing intervention is correct?
   a. Give the entire dosage in one injection.
   b. Administer with oral iron supplements.
   c. Give via deep IM into a large muscle mass with the Z-track method.
   d. Inject intramuscularly into the deltoid muscle.

4. When assessing a patient who is to receive folic acid supplements, it is important to rule out which condition?
   a. Malabsorption syndromes
   b. Pernicious anemia
   c. Tropical sprue
   d. Pregnancy
5. A patient who is taking oral iron supplements calls the office, very upset about having "very black, shiny stools." What should the nurse's response be?
   a. "You may be bleeding and should come to the office immediately."
   b. "Are you taking this medication on an empty stomach?"
   c. "This is an unusual reaction, and you should stop the tablets immediately."
   d. "It is normal for oral iron products to change stools to a black and tarry color."

1. d, 2. a, 3. c, 4. b, 5. d.

Critical Thinking Activities

1. In your clinical area, take a 24-hour dietary intake history of any of your assigned patients. Analyze their intake for iron content while they are hospitalized. In addition, note the medications ordered to identify any supplemental vitamins or iron tablets and to identify any drug interactions. Also note any laboratory values, such as RBC, Hgb, Hct, bilirubin levels, and reticulocyte levels.

2. Discuss the importance of monitoring reticulocyte counts, Hgb, and Hct levels once oral iron therapy has been initiated.
3. Discuss teaching tips you should share with a patient who is taking oral iron supplements.

For answers, see http://evolve.elsevier.com/Lilley.

CHAPTER 57

Dermatologic Drugs

Objectives

When you reach the end of this chapter, you should be able to do the following:

1. Discuss the normal anatomy, physiology, and functions of the skin.
2. Describe the different disorders, infections, and conditions commonly affecting the skin.
3. Identify the various dermatologic drugs used to treat these disorders, infections, and conditions, with description of the various classifications.
4. Discuss the mechanisms of action, indications, contraindications, cautions, application techniques, and adverse effects associated with the various topical dermatologic drugs.
5. Develop a nursing care plan that includes all phases of the nursing process for patients using topical dermatologic drugs.

e-Learning Activities

Companion CD

- NCLEX Review Questions: see questions 445-446
- Animations
- Audio Glossary
- Category Catchers
- Medication Errors Checklists
- IV Therapy Checklists

evolve Website (http://evolve.elsevier.com/Lilley)

• Nursing Care Plans • Frequently Asked Questions • Content Updates • WebLinks • Supplemental Resources • Elsevier ePharmacology Update • Medication Administration Animations

Drug Profiles

anthralin, p. 874
▶ bacitracin, p. 869
▶ benzoyl peroxide, p. 870
calcipotriene, p. 874
clindamycin, p. 870
▶ clotrimazole, p. 871
fluorouracil, p. 875
imiquimod, p. 875
▶ isotretinoin, p. 871
▶ lindane, p. 874

miconazole, p. 871
minoxidil, p. 874
mupirocin, p. 869
neomycin and polymyxin B, p. 869
▶ pimecrolimus, p. 875
tar-containing products, p. 873
tazarotene, p. 873
tretinoin, p. 871
▶ silver sulfadiazine, p. 869

▶ Key drug.

Glossary

Acne vulgaris   A chronic inflammatory disease of the *pilosebaceous* glands of the skin, involving lesions such as *papules* and *pustules* ("pimples"); hereafter referred to as *acne*. (p. 870)

Actinic keratosis   A slowly developing, localized thickening of the outer layers of the skin resulting from long-term, prolonged exposure to the sun. Also called *solar keratosis*. (p. 875)

Atopic dermatitis   A chronic skin inflammation seen in patients with hereditary susceptibility to *pruritus*. (p. 868)

Basal cell carcinoma   The most common form of skin cancer; arises from epidermal cells known as basal cells and is rarely metastatic. (p. 868)

Carbuncle   A necrotizing infection of skin and subcutaneous tissue caused by multiple furuncles (boils). It is usually caused by the bacterium *Staphylococcus aureus*. (p. 868)

Cellulitis   An acute, diffuse, spreading infection involving the skin, subcutaneous tissue, and sometimes muscle as well. It is usually caused by a wound infected with *Streptococcus* or *Staphylococcus* spp. (p. 868)

Dermatitis   Any inflammation of the skin. (p. 868)

Dermatophyte   Any of common groups of fungi that infect skin, hair, and nails. These fungi are most commonly from the genera *Microsporum, Epidermophyton,* and *Trichophyton*. (p. 871)

Dermatosis   General term for any abnormal skin condition. (p. 868)

Dermis   The layer of the skin just below the epidermis, consisting of papillary and reticular layers and containing blood and lymphatic vessels, nerves and nerve endings, glands, and hair follicles. (p. 867)

Eczema   A pruritic, papulovesicular dermatitis occurring as a reaction to many endogenous and exogenous agents, and characterized by erythema, edema, and an inflammatory infiltrate of the dermis that includes oozing, vesiculation, crusting, and scaling. (p. 868)

Epidermis   The superficial, avascular layers of the skin, made up of an outer, dead, cornified portion and a deeper, living, cellular portion. (p. 867)

Folliculitis   Inflammation of a follicle, usually a hair follicle. A follicle is defined as any sac or pouchlike cavity. (p. 868)

Furuncle   A painful skin nodule caused by a staphylococcal infection that enters skin through the hair follicles. Also called a *boil*. (p. 868)

Impetigo   A pus-generating, contagious superficial skin infection, usually caused by staphylococci or streptococci. It usually occurs on the face and is most commonly seen in children. (p. 868)

Papule   A small circumscribed, superficial, solid elevation of the skin that is usually pink in color and less than 0.5 to 1 cm in diameter. (p. 868)

Pediculosis   An infestation with lice of the family Pediculidae. (p. 874)

Pruritus   An unpleasant cutaneous sensation that provokes the desire to rub or scratch the skin to obtain relief. (p. 871)

Psoriasis   A common, chronic squamous cell dermatosis with *polygenic* (multi-gene) inheritance and a fluctuating pattern of recurrence and remission. (p. 868)

Pustule   A visible collection of pus within or beneath the epidermis. (p. 868)

Scabies   A contagious disease caused by *S. scabiei,* the itch mite, characterized by intense itching of the skin and injury to the skin (excoriation) resulting from scratching. (p. 874)

Tinea   A group of fungal skin diseases caused by dermatophytes of several kinds and characterized by itching; scaling; and, sometimes, painful lesions. *Tinea* is a general term for infections of various dermatophytes that occur on several sites. Also called *ringworm.* (p. 871)

Vesicle   A smaller sac containing liquid; also called a *cyst.* (p. 868)

SKIN ANATOMY AND PHYSIOLOGY

The largest organ of the body is the skin. It covers the body and serves several functions, most of which we take for granted. It serves as a protective barrier for the internal organs. Without skin, harmful external forces such as microorganisms and chemicals would gain access to and damage or destroy many of our delicate internal organs. Part of this protection includes the skin's ability to maintain a surface pH of 4.5 to 5.5. This weakly acidic environment discourages the growth of microorganisms that grow at a more alkaline pH of 6 to 7.5, explaining why infected skin usually has a higher pH than noninfected skin. The skin also has the ability to sense changes in temperature (hot or cold), pressure, or pain information that is then transmitted along nerve endings. The temperature of the environment changes constantly and can be extremely hot or cold. Despite this, the body maintains an almost constant internal temperature in most environments, thanks in large part to the skin, which plays a major role in the regulation of body temperature. Heat loss and conservation are regulated in coordination with the blood vessels that supply blood to the skin and by means of perspiration. The skin is also able to excrete fluid and electrolytes through sweat glands. In addition, it stores fat, synthesizes vitamin D, and provides a site for drug absorption.

The skin is made up of two layers: the **dermis** and the epidermis (Figure 57-1). The outer skin layer, or **epidermis,** is com-

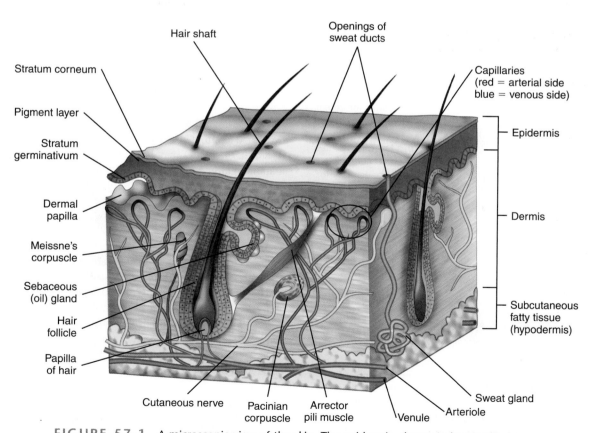

FIGURE 57-1 A microscopic view of the skin. The epidermis, shown in longitudinal section, is raised at one corner to reveal the ridges in the dermis. (*Modified from Thibodeau GA, Patton KT: Anatomy and physiology, ed 5, St. Louis, 2003, Mosby.*)

posed of four layers. From the outermost to innermost layer these are the stratum corneum, stratum lucidum, stratum granulosum, and the stratum germinativum. The respective functions of these layers are described in Table 57-1.

None of these layers has a direct blood supply of its own. Instead, its nourishment is provided through diffusion from the dermis below. The dermis lies between the epidermis and subcutaneous fat and differs from the epidermis in many ways. It is approximately 40 times thicker than the epidermis. Traversing the dermis is a rich supply of blood vessels, nerves, lymphatic tissue, elastic tissue, and connective tissue, which provide extra support and nourishment to the skin. Also contained in this layer are the exocrine glands—the eccrine, apocrine, and sebaceous glands—and the hair follicles. The functions of the various types of exocrine glands are explained in Table 57-2.

Below the dermis is a layer of loose connective tissue called the *hypodermis*. It helps make the skin flexible. It is also here that the subcutaneous fat tissue is located, which provides thermal insulation and cushioning or padding. It is also the source of nutrition for the skin.

Table 57-1   Epidermal Layers

Layer	Description
Stratum corneum ("horny layer," so named because keratin is the same protein that makes up the horns of animals)	Outermost layer consisting of dead skin cells that are made of a converted water-repellant protein known as keratin; it is the protective layer for the entire body. After it is desquamated or shed, it is replaced by new cells from below.
Stratum lucidum ("clear layer")	Layer where keratin is formed; it is translucent and contains flat cells.
Stratum granulosum ("granular layer")	Cells die in this layer; granulated cells are located here, giving this layer the appearance for which it is named.
Stratum germinativum ("germinative layer")	New skin cells are made in this layer; it contains melanocytes, which produce melanin, the skin color pigment.

Table 57-2   Exocrine Glands of the Skin

Gland	Function
Sebaceous	Large lipid-containing cells that produce oil or film that covers the epidermis; protects and lubricates skin, and is water repellent and antiseptic
Eccrine	Sweat glands that are located throughout the skin surface; help regulate body temperature and prevent skin dryness
Apocrine	Mainly in axilla, genital organs, and breast areas; emit an odor; believed to be scent or sex glands

TOPICAL DERMATOLOGIC DRUGS

Reactions or disorders of the skin are common and numerous. A **dermatosis** is any abnormal skin condition and dermatoses include a variety of types of **dermatitis** (skin inflammation). These include conditions such as **atopic dermatitis, eczema,** and **psoriasis.** In addition, there are also a variety of skin cancers, including **basal cell carcinoma,** squamous cell carcinoma, and melanoma. Drugs that are administered directly to the site are called *topical dermatologic drugs.* A variety of formulations are available that are suitable for specific indications. Each formulation has certain characteristics that make it suitable for specific indications. The formulations, their characteristics, and examples of most of these are summarized in Table 57-3. Note that the focus of this chapter is topically administered medications. Systemically administered drugs are also used to treat several skin disorders. Therefore, included in this chapter are cross-references to previous chapters where various systemic drug categories are discussed in more detail.

There are also many therapeutic categories of dermatologic drugs. Some of the most common ones are as follows:
- Antibacterial drugs
- Antifungal drugs
- Antiinflammatory drugs
- Antineoplastics
- Antipruritic drugs (for itching)
- Antiviral drugs
- Burn drugs
- Débriding drugs (promote wound healing)
- Emollients (skin softeners)
- Keratolytics (cause softening and peeling of the stratum corneum)
- Local anesthetics
- Sunscreens
- Topical vasodilators

Because there are so many drugs available, the scope of this chapter is limited to some of the most commonly used medications, and again, the focus of this chapter is topical medications. At times, the reader may be referred to other chapters for information regarding systemically administered drugs (e.g., oral, injectable) that are indicated for skin conditions.

ANTIMICROBIALS

The topical antimicrobials are antibacterial, antifungal, and antiviral drugs that, as the name implies, are applied topically. The systemically administered drugs are discussed in detail in Part Seven, where their specific pharmacologic characteristics are also described. Those with available topical dosage forms are discussed. Although they have many of the same properties as the systemic forms, there are some differences in terms of their toxicities and adverse effects. The drugs commonly used to treat acne are also covered in this section.

Drug Profiles

General Antibacterial Drugs
Common skin disorders caused by various bacteria are **folliculitis, impetigo, furuncles, carbuncles, papules, pustules, vesicles,** and **cellulitis.** The bacteria responsible are most commonly *Streptococ-*

Table 57-3   Dermatologic Formulations: Characteristics and Examples

Formulation	Characteristics	Examples
Aerosol foam	Can cover large area; useful for drug delivery into a body cavity (e.g., vagina, rectum) or hair areas	Proctofoam, Epifoam, contraceptive foams
Aerosol spray	Spreads thin liquid or powder film; covers large areas; useful when skin is tender to touch (e.g., burns)	Solarcaine, Desenex, Kenalog
Bar	Similar to a bar of soap; useful as a wash with water	PanOxyl (benzoyl peroxide)
Cleanser	Nongreasy; used as an astringent (oil remover) and/or wash with water	Zoderm
Cream	Contains water and can be removed with water; not greasy or occlusive; usually white semisolid; good for moist areas	Hydrocortisone cream, Benadryl cream
Gel/jelly	Contains water and possibly alcohol; easily removed and good lubricator; usually clear, semisolid substance; useful when lubricant properties are desirable	K-Y jelly, Saligel, Surgilube
Lotion	Contains water, alcohol, and solvents; may be a suspension, emulsion, or solution; good for large or hairy areas	Calamine lotion, Lubriderm lotion, Kwell lotion
Oil	Contains very little if any water; occlusive, liquid; not removable with water	Lubriderm bath oil
Ointment	Contains no water; not removable with water; occlusive, greasy, and semisolid; desirable for dry lesions because of occlusiveness	Petrolatum (Vaseline), zinc oxide ointment, A & D ointment
Paste	Similar properties to those of the ointments; contains more powder than ointments; excellent protectant properties	Zinc oxide paste
Pledget (pad)	Moistened pad is applied to or wiped over affected area	EryPads (erythromycin)
Powder	Slight lubricating properties; may be shaken on affected area; promotes drying of area where applied	Tinactin powder, Desenex powder
Shampoo	Soapy liquid for washing hair and/or skin	Nizoral (ketoconazole)
Solution	Nongreasy liquid; dries quickly	Erythromycin topical solution
Stick	Spreads thin chalky or viscous liquid film; often better for smaller areas	Benadryl Itch Relief
Tape	Most occlusive formulation; consistent topical drug delivery; useful when small, straight areas require drug application	Cordran tape

cus pyogenes and *Staphylococcus aureus*. Dermatologic antibacterial drugs are used to treat or prevent these skin infections, and the most commonly used drugs are bacitracin, polymyxin, and neomycin.

▶ bacitracin

Bacitracin (Baciguent) is a polypeptide antibiotic that is applied topically for the treatment or prevention of local skin infections caused by susceptible aerobic and anaerobic gram-positive organisms such as staphylococci, streptococci, anaerobic cocci, corynebacteria, and clostridia. Also available in systemic and ophthalmic (Chapter 58), it works by inhibiting bacterial cell wall synthesis, which leads to cell death. It can be either bactericidal or bacteriostatic, depending on the causative organism.

Bacitracin is active against many gram-positive organisms, including staphylococci, streptococci, anaerobic cocci, corynebacteria, and clostridia. Its antimicrobial spectrum is broadened in several available combination drug products. Most of these contain neomycin and/or polymyxin B (see later). Adverse reactions are usually minimal; however, reactions ranging from skin rash to allergic anaphylactoid reactions have occurred. If itching, burning, inflammation, or other signs of sensitivity occur, bacitracin should be discontinued. This drug is available in ointment form, and is usually applied to the affected area 1 to 3 times daily.

neomycin and polymyxin B

Neomycin and polymyxin B are two additional broad-spectrum antibiotics that are available as the popular nonprescription product known as Neosporin. Neosporin cream is a combination of these two drugs alone, whereas Neosporin ointment also contains bacitracin. Several brand-name and generic combinations of these three topical antibiotics are available, and all are commonly used as topical antiseptics for minor skin wounds. (See the Evidence-Based Practice box on p. 870 for more information on antiseptics and wound care.)

Although it is still a very popular OTC drug product, there is evidence that neomycin/polymyxin B can actually increase the likelihood of future allergic sensitivity of the skin.

mupirocin

Mupirocin (Bactroban) is another antibacterial product available only by prescription. It is used on the skin for *Staphylococcal* and *Streptococcal* impetigo. A newer indication involves intranasal use for nasal colonization with *methicillin-resistant Staphylococcal aureus* (MRSA). This drug is applied topically three times daily and intranasally twice daily. Adverse reactions are usually limited to local burning, itching, or minor pain.

▶ silver sulfadiazine

One of the concerns with burn victims is infection at the burn site, but there are two problems posed by the use of either topically or systemically administered antimicrobial drugs in this setting. Because of the increased systemic absorption of a drug that can occur in compromised skin areas such as burns, topical burn drugs must not be too potent or toxic to cause dangerous systemic effects. This is especially true for larger burned areas because the drug may be applied over a large surface area of skin and therefore absorbed in greater quantities. On the other hand, the blood supply to burned areas is often drastically reduced, such that systemically administered antibiotics either cannot reach the site or do so only in quantities too low to be effective. Therefore, the only way of applying these drugs to ensure that they reach the burn site is to do so topically. Some of the commonly used drugs that have proved both effective and safe in the prevention or treatment of infections in burns are silver sulfadiazine (Silvadene), mafenide (Sulfamylon), and nitrofurazone (Furacin).

Silver sulfadiazine is a synthetic antimicrobial drug produced when silver nitrate reacts with the chemical sulfadiazine. It appears to act on the cell membrane and cell wall of susceptible bacteria and is used as an adjunct in the prevention and treatment of infection in

EVIDENCE-BASED PRACTICE

Antiseptics and Wound Care

Review

Use of antiseptics has been long term and consisted of frequent use on wounds to prevent or treat infections. This article presented information about antiseptics and use on open wounds with discussion of relevant animal studies and clinical trials about the following drugs: iodine compounds, chlorhexidine, hydrogen peroxide, acetic acid, and silver compounds. This article examines the effects of these drugs on wound healing and the re-epithelization of wounds as well as efficacy on reducing bacterial number in wounds and incidence of wound infections. The authors of this review of research found that most antiseptics have *not* been shown to clearly impede healing, especially newer formulations like cadexomer iodine (which speeds healing) and newly designed silver delivery systems. Given the facts in this research, the role of antiseptics on wounds and their role in wound care management should be considered.

Type of Evidence and Research

The specific type of research and evidence included a review of a significant quantity of research studies with use of a variety of antiseptics. There were several categories of information "surveyed" and studied in relation to different antiseptics, and the specific authors of the studies were identified. For example, presentation of information on the disinfectant, povidone iodine, included various research studies with the authors identified and further information on wound type, species of the participant (e.g., human, rats, bacteria, pigs, etc), number of wounds being treated, control/comparison group data, effect of the antiseptic (e.g., povidone iodine/cadexomer iodine/hydrogen peroxide/acetic acid/chlorhexidine/silver compounds) on healing and the effect on the infectious process. For example, with povidone iodine, there were reviews of some 12 plus studies, with documented wounds ranging from partial thickness burn wounds/leg ulcers/contaminated lacerations with *Staphylococcus aureus* and sutured lacerations as a few examples, as well as treatment of 100 plus wounds, use of various antiseptics, and documented effects to healing and to the infection.

Results of Study

A review of the data emphasized the controversy of using antiseptics on wounds and presented findings that are worthy of consideration in this chapter. Pronounced cytotoxicity in vitro was not confirmed; however, antiseptics appeared to be safe and found *not* to negatively impact wound healing. Antimicrobial efficiency, except with hydrogen peroxide, was found to be satisfactory. In the majority of clinical trials, antiseptics appear to be safe and were not found to negatively influence wound healing. Their antimicrobial efficiency, with the exception of hydrogen peroxide, was satisfactory, as well. An overall review of these studies provides nursing with valuable information that needs to be watched, considered, and continued within the context of more research on this topic. Randomized controlled studies to evaluate the effect of each antiseptic on the different kinds of wounds (acute, venous, diabetic, or pressure ulcers) are indicated to provide more evidence on the benefits of antiseptic use on wounds. Future protocols should focus on the possibility of use of cadexomer iodine based on the fact that this research supports an acceleration of healing even in noninfected wounds and the fact that the drug does not negatively influence wound healing. Development of improved silver delivery systems would also be valuable.

Link of Evidence to Nursing Practice

Within nursing and other health care–related professions, there should be continued efforts to develop superior antiseptic formulations and document effects on wound healing and prevention/treatment of infection. One area of research for future practice could include the use of an antiseptic to see if there is a positive influence on wound healing, accelerated healing even in noninfected wounds, and treatment of infections within a wound as well as the future development of improved delivery systems. In summary, antiseptics, although controversial in today's health care arena, should remain a major component of wound care treatment and prevention in those at high risk and in other patient care situations, as deemed appropriate.

Modified from Drosou A, Falabella A, Kirsner R: Antiseptics on wounds: an area of controversy, *Wounds* 15:149-166, 2003.

second- and third-degree burns. The adverse effects of silver sulfadiazine are similar to those of other topical drugs and include pain, burning, and itching. This medication should not be used in patients who are allergic to sulfonamide drugs. It is available only as a 1% cream and should be applied topically to cleansed, débrided, burned areas once or twice daily using a sterile-gloved hand.

Anti-Acne Drugs

Other antibacterial drugs are used to treat **acne**, the most common skin infection. Its precise cause is unknown and somewhat controversial. Likely causative factors include heredity, stress, drug reactions, hormones, and bacterial infections. Common bacterial causes include staphylococcal species and *Propionibacterium acnes*. These drugs include benzoyl peroxide, clindamycin, erythromycin, meclocycline, tetracycline, isotretinoin, and the vitamin A acid known as *retinoic acid*. Many other drugs are also used in the treatment and prevention of acne, including systemic use of the antibiotics minocycline, doxycycline, and tetracycline (Chapter 37). Some practitioners also prescribe oral contraceptives (Chapter 33) for female acne patients, as beneficial estrogen effects against acne have been shown in some controlled studies. This is believed especially likely for hormone-driven acne.

▶ benzoyl peroxide

The microorganism that most commonly causes acne, *P. acnes,* is an anaerobic bacterium that needs an environment that is poor in oxygen to grow. Benzoyl peroxide (Benzac) is effective in combating such infection because it slowly and continuously liberates active

oxygen in the skin, causing antibacterial, antiseptic, drying, and keratolytic actions. These actions create an environment that is unfavorable for the continued growth of the *P. acnes* bacteria, and they soon die. Such drugs as benzoyl peroxide that soften scales and loosen the outer horny layer of the skin are referred to as *keratolytics.*

Benzoyl peroxide generally produces signs of improvement within 4 to 6 weeks. Adverse effects tend to be dose-related (including overuse) and involve peeling skin, red skin, or a sensation of warmth. Blistering or swelling of the skin is generally considered an allergic reaction to the product and is an indication to stop treatment. Overuse with this drug and also tretinoin is common with teenage patients who are attempting to quickly cure their acne. The result can be painful, reddened skin, which usually resolves upon return to use of these medications as prescribed.

Benzoyl peroxide is available in multiple topical dosage forms, including a cleansing bar, liquid, lotion, mask, cream, gel, and cleanser. It is also available in various combination drug products that include the chemical element sulfur, and the antibiotics erythromycin and clindamycin (Chapter 37). It is usually applied topically 1 to 4 times daily, depending on the dosage form and prescriber's instructions. Pregnancy category C.

▶ clindamycin

Clindamycin (Cleocin T) is a topical form of the systemic antibiotic described in Chapter 37. It is most commonly prescribed for acne. Adverse reactions are usually limited to minor, local skin reactions, including burning, itching, dryness, oiliness, and peeling. The drug is available in gel, lotion, suspension, foam, and pledget form. It is usually applied once or twice daily. Pregnancy Category B.

▶ isotretinoin

Isotretinoin (Accutane) is an oral and topical product indicated for the treatment of severe recalcitrant cystic acne. Isotretinoin inhibits sebaceous gland activity and has antikeratinizing (anti-skin hardening) and anti-inflammatory effects. Isotretinoin is one of relatively few medications that are classified as pregnancy category X drugs. This means that it is a proven human *teratogen*, or a chemical that is known to induce birth defects. It is imperative that female patients of childbearing age be counseled and agree not to become pregnant during use. For these reasons, in 2005, the U.S. Food and Drug Administration (FDA) approved more stringent guidelines regarding the prescribing and use of this medication. It is now officially required that at least two contraceptive methods be used by sexually active women during and for 1 month after completion of therapy with isotretinoin. A risk-management program of unprecedented size and scope has been designed and approved by the FDA especially for this drug. It is known as "iPLEDGE" and was fully implemented as of March 1, 2006. As a result, federal law now requires that any health provider who prescribes this drug be a registered and activated member of this program, and patients must also be qualified and registered. Drug wholesalers and pharmacists who dispense this drug are also required to be part of this program. Further information is available at the iPLEDGE call center at 866-495-0654 or online at www.ipledge-program.com. Additionally, there have been case reports of suicide and suicide attempts in patients receiving this medication. Patients should be educated to immediately report any signs of depression to their health providers. Follow-up treatment may be needed, and simply stopping the drug may be insufficient. Despite these rather severe concerns, this drug does prove to be very helpful in treating severe acne cases. Isotretinoin is available only for oral use.

tretinoin

Tretinoin (retinoic acid, vitamin A acid) (Renova, Retin-A) is a derivative of vitamin A that is used to treat acne and ameliorate the dermatologic changes (e.g., fine wrinkling, mottled hyperpigmentation, roughness) associated with photodamage (sun damage). The drug appears to act as an irritant on the skin, in particular the follicular epithelium. Specifically, it stimulates the turnover of epidermal cells, which results in skin peeling. While this is occurring, the free fatty acid levels of the skin are reduced, and horny cells of the outer epidermis cannot then adhere to one another. Without fatty acids and horny cells, acne and its comedo, or pimple, cannot exist.

Topically administered tretinoin has been shown to enhance the repair of skin damaged by ultraviolet radiation, or sunlight. It does this by increasing the formation of fibroblasts and collagen, both of which are needed to rebuild skin. The drug also may reduce collagen degradation by inhibiting the enzyme collagenase that breaks down collagen.

As with erythromycin, tretinoin's main adverse effects are local inflammatory reactions, which are reversible when therapy is discontinued. Some of the most common adverse effects are excessively red and edematous blisters, crusted skin, and temporary alterations in skin pigmentation. Tretinoin is available in many topical formulations, including creams, gels, and a liquid. Because of its potential to cause severe irritation and peeling, it may initially be applied once every 2 or 3 days, often starting with a lower-strength product.

Retin-A Micro has been approved for the treatment of acne vulgaris. This particular acne product contains tretinoin formulated inside a synthetic polymer called a *Microsponge system*. This system is made of round microscopic particles of synthetic polymer. These microspheres act as reservoirs for tretinoin, allowing the skin to absorb small amounts of the drug over time. Retin-A Micro is currently available only in gel form. All topical forms of tretinoin are rated pregnancy category C. They are not to be confused with the oral capsule form of tretinoin mentioned in Chapter 47 that is used to treat leukemia and is rated pregnancy category D. Another anti-acne retinoid is adapalene, a topical solution.

Antifungal Drugs

A few fungi produce keratinolytic enzymes, which allows them to live on the skin. Topical fungal infections are primarily caused by *Candida* spp. (candidiasis), **dermatophytes**, and *Malassezia furfur* (tinea versicolor). These fungi exist in moist, warm environments, especially in dark areas such as the feet or groin.

Candidal infections are most commonly caused by *Candida albicans*, a yeastlike opportunistic fungus present in the normal flora of the mouth, vagina, and intestinal tract. Two significant factors that commonly predispose a person to a candidal infection are broad-spectrum antibiotic therapy, which promotes an overgrowth of non-susceptible organism in the natural body florae, and immunodeficiency disorders such as those that occur in patients with cancer, acquired immunodeficiency syndrome (AIDS), or organ transplants. Because these infections favor warm, moist areas of the skin and mucous membranes, they most commonly occur orally (e.g., thrush in infants), vaginally, and cutaneously in such sites as beneath the breasts and in diapered areas. They may also cause nail infections.

Dermatophytes are a group of three closely related genera consisting of *Epidermophyton* spp., *Microsporum* spp., and *Trichophyton* spp. that use the keratin found on the skin to feed their growth. They produce superficial mycotic (fungal) infections of keratinized tissue (hair, skin, and nails). Infections caused by dermatophytes are collectively called **tinea**, or *ringworm*, infections. The name *ringworm* comes from the fact that the infection sometimes assumes a circular pattern at the site of infection. The tinea infections are further identified by the body location where they occur: tinea pedis (foot), tinea cruris (groin), tinea corporis (body), and tinea capitis (scalp). Tinea infections are also known as *athlete's foot* or *jock itch*.

Fungi usually invade the stratum corneum, which is the dead layer of desquamated (shedded) cells. Inflammation occurs when the fungi invade this layer; sensitivity (e.g., itching) occurs when they penetrate the epidermis and dermis.

Many of the fungi that cause topical infections are very difficult to eradicate. They are very slow growing, and antifungal therapy may be required for periods ranging from several weeks to as long as 1 year. However, many topical antifungal drugs are available for the treatment of both dermatophyte infections and those caused by yeast and yeastlike fungi. Some of these drugs, their dosage forms, and their uses are listed in Table 57-4. Systemically administered antifungal drugs are sometimes used for skin conditions as well. These drugs were discussed in Chapter 41.

The most commonly reported adverse effects of topical antifungals are local irritation, **pruritus,** a burning sensation, and scaling. Ciclopirox and clotrimazole are classified as pregnancy category B drugs, and econazole, ketoconazole, and miconazole are classified as pregnancy category C drugs. Hypersensitivity is the one contraindication to the use of any of these drugs.

▶ clotrimazole

Clotrimazole (Lotrimin, Mycelex-G) is available both over-the-counter (OTC) and with a prescription. It is available as a lozenge for the treatment of oropharyngeal candidiasis, commonly known as *thrush*. It also is available as a cream, lotion, or solution for the treatment of dermatophytoses (e.g., athlete's foot), superficial mycoses, and cutaneous candidiasis. Similar topical preparations are also available for intravaginal administration in the treatment of vulvovaginal candidiasis, commonly called a *yeast infection*, and vaginal trichomoniasis. Lotrimazole is available in many topical formulations: a powder; a 10-mg oral topical lozenge; a 1% cream, lotion, and solution; 1% and 2% vaginal creams; and 100- and 500-mg vaginal tablets. Different dosages and dosage forms are used for the treatment of different fungal infections. Pregnancy category B.

miconazole

Miconazole (Monistat, Micotin) is a topical antifungal drug that is available in several OTC and prescription products. It inhibits the growth of several fungi, including dermatophytes and yeast, as well as

Table 57-4   Topical Antifungal Drugs

Drug	Trade Names	Dosage Forms	Uses	Legal Status
amphotericin B	Fungizone	3% cream, lotion, and ointment	Candidiasis	Rx
butenafine	Mentax	1% cream	Tinea pedis	Rx
butoconazole	Femstat 3	2% vaginal cream	Candidiasis	OTC
ciclopirox olamine	Loprox	0.77% cream and lotion, 8% solution (for nails)	Candidiasis, dermatophytoses, tinea versicolor	Rx
clioquinol	Generic only	3% cream	Dermatophytoses	OTC
clotrimazole	Gyne-Lotrimin 3	2% vaginal cream, 100- and 200-mg vaginal tabs	Candidiasis	OTC
	Lotrimin	2% cream, 1% lotion and solution	Candidiasis, tinea versicolor	Rx
	Lotrimin AF	1% cream, lotion, and solution	Dermatophytoses	OTC
	Mycelex	1% cream and solution	Dermatophytoses	Rx
	Mycelex	10-mg troches	Oropharyngeal candidiasis	Rx
	Mycelex-7	1% vaginal cream, 100-mg vaginal tabs	Candidiasis	OTC
econazole	Spectazole	1% cream	Candidiasis, dermatophytoses	Rx
ketoconazole	Nizoral	2% cream and shampoo	Candidiasis, dermatophytoses, tinea versicolor	Rx
miconazole	Micatin	2% cream, powder, and spray	Dermatophytoses	OTC
	Monistat-Derm	2% cream	Candidiasis, dermatophytoses, tinea versicolor	Rx
naftifine	Naftin	1% cream and gel	Dermatophytoses	Rx
natamycin	Natacyn	5% ophthalmic suspension	Ocular fungal infections	Rx
nystatin	Nilstat, Mycostatin	Cream, ointment, powder	Candidiasis	Rx
oxiconazole	Oxistat	1% cream and lotion	Dermatophytoses	Rx
sulconazole	Exelderm	1% cream and solution	Dermatophytoses	Rx
terbinafine	Lamisil	1% cream and spray	Dermatophytoses	OTC
tolnaftate	Tinactin	1% cream, solution, gel, powder, and spray	Dermatophytoses	OTC
triacetin (glyceryl triacetate)	Fungoid	Solution, cream	Dermatophytoses	Rx
undecylenic acid	Cruex, Desenex, Fungoid AF	Powder, cream, solution, soap	Dermatophytoses	OTC

OTC, Available over-the-counter without prescription; *Rx,* currently available by prescription only.

gram-positive bacteria, and is commonly used to treat dermatophytoses, superficial mycoses, cutaneous candidiasis, and vulvovaginal candidiasis. It is present in many OTC remedies for athlete's foot, jock itch, and yeast infections.

For the treatment of athlete's foot, jock itch, ringworm, and other susceptible fungal infections, miconazole should be applied sparingly to the cleansed, dry, infected area twice daily, in the morning and evening. For the treatment of yeast infections, one 200-mg suppository should be inserted in the vagina once daily at bedtime for 3 consecutive days or 100 mg (one suppository or 5 g of the 2% cream) should be administered intravaginally once daily at bedtime for 7 days. The most common adverse effects of topically administered miconazole are vulvovaginal burning and itching, pelvic cramps and rash, urticaria, stinging, and contact dermatitis. It is available in a variety of topical formulations: a 2% aerosol spray and powder, a 2% powder, a 2% cream, a 2% vaginal cream, and a 100- and 200-mg vaginal suppository. It is also now available as a 1200 mg vaginal suppository for one-time dosing. Pregnancy category C.

Antiviral Drugs

Topical antivirals are now used less frequently than before in dermatology practice as systemic antiviral drug therapy has generally been shown to be superior for controlling such viral skin conditions. Nonetheless, two antiviral ointments are described here. As is the case with systemic drug therapy, these products are best used early in a viral skin lesion outbreak. Topical antivirals are more likely to be used for acute outbreaks, while systemic drugs are used for acute outbreaks as well as ongoing prophylaxis against outbreaks. As noted in Chapter 39, viral infections are very difficult to treat because they live in the body's own healthy cells and use their cell mechanisms to reproduce. The same holds true for topical viral infections. Infections caused by herpes simplex types 1 and 2, and the human papilloma virus (which causes anogenital warts) are particularly serious and are becoming more common.

The only topical antiviral drugs currently available to treat such viral infections are acyclovir (Zovirax) and penciclovir (Denavir). They work by comparable mechanisms as described for similar antiviral drugs in Chapter 39. Acyclovir and penciclovir are available as topical ointments (5% and 1%, respectively). Acyclovir is applied every 3 hours, or 6 times daily, for 1 week. Penciclovir is applied every 2 hours while awake for 4 days. A finger cot or rubber glove should be worn for the application of the ointment to prevent the spread of infection. The most common adverse effects are stinging, itching, and rash. Acyclovir is classified as a pregnancy category C drug, and penciclovir as a pregnancy category B drug.

ANESTHETIC, ANTIPRURITIC, AND ANTIINFLAMMATORY DRUGS

TOPICAL ANESTHETICS

Topical anesthetic drugs are drugs that are used to numb the skin. They accomplish this by inhibiting the conduction of nerve impulses from sensory nerves, thereby reducing or eliminating the pain or pruritus associated with insect bites, sunburn, and plant allergies such as poison ivy, as well as many other uncomfortable skin disorders. They are also used to numb the skin before a painful injection (e.g., IV insertion in a pediatric patient). Topical anesthetics are available as ointments, creams, sprays, liquids, and jellies and are discussed in Chapter 11.

TOPICAL ANTIPRURITICS

Topical antipruritic (antiitching) drugs contain antihistamines or corticosteroids. Many exert a combined anesthetic and antipruritic action when applied topically. The antihistamines and their therapeutic effects are covered in Chapter 35. New recommendations for the use of topical antihistamines state that they should not be used in the following situations because of systemic absorption and subsequent toxicity: chickenpox, widespread poison ivy, and large body surface area inducement.

Topical antiinflammatory drugs are most commonly corticosteroids (Chapter 32), and they are generally indicated for the relief of inflammatory and pruritic dermatoses. With the use of topically administered corticosteroids, many of the undesirable systemic adverse effects associated with the use of the systemically administered corticosteroids are averted. The beneficial drug effects of topically administered corticosteroids are their antiinflammatory, antipruritic, and vasoconstrictor actions.

The many different available dosage forms of the various corticosteroids vary in their relative potency, and this often guides their selection for treating various conditions. For instance, corticosteroids that are fluorinated are used for the treatment of dermatologic disorders such as psoriasis. The vehicle in which the corticosteroid is contained also has the effect of altering its vasoconstrictor properties and therapeutic efficacy. Ointments are generally the most penetrating, followed next by gels, creams, and lotions. Propylene glycol also enhances the penetration of the corticosteroid and its vasoconstrictor effects. Most corticosteroids are available in many topical formulations, thus offering a variety of options. The currently available topical corticosteroids, along with their respective potencies, are listed in Table 57-5.

Table 57-5	Commonly Used Topical Corticosteroids (in Order of Decreasing Potency)
Range of Potency	**Corticosteroid**
1. Higher-potency*	Betamethasone dipropionate (cream and ointment), clobetasol propionate, halobetasol propionate, diflorasone diacetate
2. Moderate potency*	Amcinonide, betamethasone dipropionate (cream), betamethasone benzoate, betamethasone valerate (0.1% cream, ointment, and lotion), desoximethasone (0.05% cream), desoxymetasone, fluocinolone, halcinonide, fluocinolone (cream and ointment), flurandrenolide, mometasone, triamcinolone acetonide (0.5% cream and ointment)
3. Milder potency*	Aclomethasone, desonide, fluocinolone (0.01% solution), triamcinolone (0.1% cream, lotion), hydrocortisone, dexamethasone

*Skin penetration and thus potency is enhanced by the vehicle (dosage form) containing the steroid. In decreasing order of effectiveness are ointments, gels, creams, and lotions.

Adverse effects of these drugs include skin reactions such as acne eruptions, allergic contact dermatitis, burning sensations, dryness, itching, skin fragility, hypopigmentation, purpura, hirsutism (usually facial), folliculitis, round and swollen face, and alopecia (usually of the scalp). Another adverse effect is the opportunistic overgrowth of a bacterial, fungal, or viral flora as a result of the immunosuppressive effects of this class of drugs. These drugs are also prone to *tachyphylaxis* (weakening of drug effect over time), especially with chronic use or over use. They should usually be applied no more than twice daily as a thin layer over the affected area. The usual adult dosage of these drugs is one or two applications daily, as directed. Less potent topical corticosteroids are used in children but following the same schedule. Corticosteroids are classified as pregnancy category C drugs and are contraindicated in patients with hypersensitivity to them. Because many of these products are available orally as well as topically, the potential exists for both to be administered simultaneously. This is not recommended and is potentially harmful. The combined use of topical and oral preparations of the same drug can lead to toxicity.

ANTIPSORIATIC DRUGS

Psoriasis is the name of a common, chronic skin condition involving flat, epidermal-layer skin cells known as *squamous* cells. It is a condition believed to involve *polygenic* (multi-gene) inheritance and has a characteristic fluctuating pattern of recurrence and remission. Although there are many subtypes, the most classic one is known as plaque psoriasis and typically involves large, dry, erythematous scaling patches of the skin that are often white or silver on top. Commonly affected skin areas include nails, scalp, genitals, and lower back. Various topical medications with antipsoriatic properties are profiled individually later. In addition to these topical drugs, there are also newer, systemically administered antipsoriatic drugs. A thorough discussion of these drugs is beyond the scope of this topical drug chapter, but those given by systemic injection include etanercept (Enbrel), alefacept (Amevive), and efalizumab (Raptiva). Etanercept is discussed in more detail in Chapter 49 on biologic response modifiers. In addition, the antineoplastic antimetabolite methotrexate (Chapter 47) is also used for its antipsoriatic properties.

Drug Profiles

tazarotene

Another drug in the retinoid family is tazarotene (Tazorac). Tazarotene is a receptor-selective retinoid. It is thought to normalize epidermal differentiation, reducing the influx of inflammatory cells into the skin. Synthetic retinoids are vitamin A analogs and are thought to play a role in skin cell differentiation and proliferation. It is available in gel form and is approved for the treatment of stable plaque psoriasis and mild to moderately severe facial acne vulgaris. Tazarotene is also a pregnancy category X drug, requiring appropriate counseling for female patients, as described earlier.

tar-containing products

Drug products containing actual coal tar derivatives were among the first medications used to treat psoriasis and are still used today for this purpose. Tar derivatives are known to have antiseptic, antibacterial, and *antiseborrheic* properties that serve to soften and loosen scaly or crusty areas of the skin. *Seborrhea* is excessive secretion of *sebum*, a normal skin secretion containing fat and epithelial cell debris. Tar-containing products are available in a variety of shampoo forms (for scalp psoriasis), as well as solution, oil, ointment, cream, lotion, gel, and even soap forms for bathing. These products typically contain 1% to 10% coal tar. Common product names include Zetar shampoo, Cutar Emulsion solution, Doak Tar oil, Medotar ointment, Fototar cream, PsoriGel gel, and Polytar soap. Adverse reactions usually include minor skin burning, photosensitivity, and other irritations. These products may be applied from 1 to 4 times daily or once or twice weekly as prescribed.

anthralin

Anthralin (Anthra-Derm) is a unique drug that is believed to work by inhibition of DNA synthesis and mitosis within the epidermis, to reduce psoriatic lesions. It is available in ointment and cream form and usually applied once daily. Adverse reactions are usually limited to minor skin irritation. Pregnancy Category C.

calcipotriene

Calcipotriene (Dovonex) is a synthetic vitamin D_3 analog that works by binding to vitamin D_3 receptors in skin cells known as *keratinocytes*, the abnormal growth of which contributes to psoriatic lesions. Calcipotriene helps to regulate the growth and reproduction of keratinocytes. Adverse reactions usually include minor skin irritations. However, more serious reactions can occur in some cases including worsening of psoriasis, dermatitis, skin atrophy, and folliculitis. Calcipotriene is usually applied twice daily. Pregnancy Category C.

MISCELLANEOUS DERMATOLOGIC DRUGS

There are many other topically applied drugs. Those discussed here are the topical ectoparasiticidal (scabicides and pediculicides), hair growth, antineoplastic, and antimicrobial drugs. Many of these drugs are available both OTC and by prescription. Aloe vera herbal preparations (see the Herbal Therapies and Dietary Supplements box) are also available OTC.

Drug Profiles

Ectoparasiticidal Drugs

Ectoparasites are insects that live on the outer surface of the body, and the drugs that are used to kill them are called *ectoparasiticidal drugs*. Lice are transmitted from person to person by close contact with infested people, clothing, combs, or towels. A parasitic infestation on the skin with lice is called **pediculosis,** and such infestations go by one of three different names, depending on the location of the infestation:

- Pediculosis pubis—pubic louse or "crabs," caused by *Phthirus pubis*

HERBAL THERAPIES AND DIETARY SUPPLEMENTS

Aloe (Aloe vera L.)

Overview
The dried leaves of the aloe plant contain anthranoids, which give aloe a laxative effect when taken orally. The topical application of the plant has been known for years to help aid in wound healing.

Common Uses
Wound healing, constipation

Adverse Effects
Diarrhea, nephritis, abdominal pain, dermatitis when used topically

Potential Drug Interactions
Digoxin, antidysrhythmics, diuretics, corticosteroids

Contraindications
Contraindicated in patients who are menstruating or have renal disease; can increase menstrual blood flow and also cause acute renal failure

- Pediculosis corporis—body louse, caused by *Pediculus humanus corporis*
- Pediculosis capitis—head louse, caused by *Pediculus humanus capitis*

Common findings in infested persons include itching; eggs of the lice attached to the hair shafts (called *nits*); lice on the skin or clothes; and in the case of pubic lice, sky blue macules (discolored skin patches) on the inner thighs or lower abdomen. Pediculoses are treated with a class of drugs called *pediculicides* (see later). A second common parasitic skin infection known as **scabies** is that caused by the itch mite *Sarcoptes scabiei*. Scabies is transmitted from person to person by close contact, such as by sleeping next to an infested person. The scabies mite causes irritation and itching by boring into the horny layers of skin located in cracks and folds. Itching seems to occur most commonly in the evening. The drugs used to treat these infestations are called *scabicides.*

Treatment of these parasitic infestations should begin with identification of the source of infestation to prevent reinfestation. Next, the clothing and personal articles of the infested person should be decontaminated. This is best accomplished by washing them in hot, soapy water or by dry cleaning them. All close contacts of the person should also be treated to prevent reinfestation.

Malathion (Ovide) and crotamiton (Eurax) are also ectoparasiticidal drugs.

lindane

Lindane (Kwell, Scabene) is a chlorinated hydrocarbon originally developed as an agricultural insecticide. It is both a scabicide and a pediculicide because it is effective in treating both scabies and pediculosis. It is available in two topical formulations: a 1% lotion and a 1% shampoo.

For the treatment of pubic or body lice, the cream or lotion is applied in a sufficient quantity to cover the skin and hair of the infested and surrounding areas. It is left on for 12 hours and then thoroughly washed off. A second application is seldom needed. Head lice can be treated with lindane shampoo, which should be worked into the hair and left on for 4 minutes. The hair should then be rinsed and dried, after which the nits (eggs) should be combed from the hair shafts. The treatment for scabies is similar. It involves the application of lindane over the entire body, from the neck down. It is left on for 8 to 12 hours and washed off. A similar second application is often recommended for 1 week later. The OTC products are applied in similar fashion, although details may vary between individual products. Adverse effects of lindane are an eczematous skin rash and, rarely, central nervous system (CNS) toxicity. The latter is more common in young children and in cases of overuse. For many years, lindane was the most widely used pediculocide, but its use has been superceded to some degree by permethrin. This is because of case reports of neurotoxicity, including dizziness, seizures, and deaths, with lindane. Most of the adverse events occurred on product misuse (e.g., ingestion) or overuse. Children are at higher risk of neurotoxicity due to the fact that they have a larger skin surface area to body weight ratio. As a result, lindane is still recommended as second-line therapy for lice and scabies (see later), after failure of one of the OTC preparations. However, the FDA has recommended that it be sold in smaller containers (1 to 2 ounces) with definitive patient instructions on proper use.

Hair Growth Drugs

minoxidil

Minoxidil (Rogaine) is a vasodilating drug that is administered systemically to control hypertension (Chapter 24). Topically it has the same vasodilating effect, but when used in this way it is applied to the scalp to stimulate hair growth. The vasodilation it causes is one possible explanation for how it stimulates hair growth. It may also act at the level of the hair follicle, possibly stimulating hair follicle growth directly.

Minoxidil can be used in both men and women suffering from baldness or hair thinning. Treatment involves administering the drug to the affected (balding and anticipated balding) area twice daily, usually morning and evening. It generally takes 4 months before results are seen, however. Systemic absorption of the topically applied minoxidil may occur, with possible adverse effects, including tachycardia, fluid retention, and weight gain. Local effects may include skin irritation, but the drug should not be applied to skin that is already irritated, nor should it be used concurrently with other topical medications applied to the same site. Topically administered minoxidil is available as 2% and 5% solutions. Each metered dose delivers 1 mL (20 mg or 50 mg) of the drug. The maximum recommended daily topical dose is 2 mL. Pregnancy category C. Note that the beneficial effects of this drug can be reduced by heat, including the use of a blow dryer. The systemically administered drug finasteride (Proscar, 5 mg) is used for benign prostatic hypertrophy as discussed in Chapter 34. A smaller strength version known as Propecia (1 mg) is also used for treating male pattern alopecia.

Sunscreens

Sunscreens are topical products used to protect the skin from damage caused by the ultraviolet (UV) radiation of sunlight. There are currently nearly 160 specific sunscreen products on the market. None requires a prescription for use. Each is made of typically three to five various chemical ingredients that work together to provide UV protection and, usually, a moisturizing effect as well. Common examples of these ingredients include titanium dioxide, octyl methoxycinnamate, homosalate, and parabens. Sunscreens are rated with a *sun protection factor* (SPF). This is a number ranging from 2 to 30 in order of increasing potency of UV protection. SolBar PF, Coppertone Sport, Hawaiian Tropic, and Catrix Lip Saver are just a few of the many available products. Most sunscreens come in lotion, cream, or gel form, and there are also a smaller number of lip balms available.

Antineoplastic Drugs
fluorouracil

Various premalignant skin lesions and basal cell carcinomas may be treated with the topically applied antineoplastic drug fluorouracil (Efudex). As noted in Chapter 47, this drug is an antimetabolite that acts by interfering with key cellular metabolic reactions, destroying rapidly growing cells, such as premalignant and malignant cells. It is also used topically in the treatment of *solar* or **actinic keratosis,** and superficial basal cell carcinomas of the skin—often in addition to local surgical excision. More aggressive skin cancers include *squamous cell carcinoma* and *malignant melanoma*, and these are usually treated with more aggressive surgery, radiation therapy, and/or systemic chemotherapy (Chapters 47 and 48).

The adverse effects associated with the topical use of this antineoplastic are generally limited to local inflammatory reactions such as dermatitis, stomatitis, and photosensitivity. More serious affects include swelling, scaling, pain, pruritus, burning, soreness, tenderness, suppuration, scarring, and hyperpigmentation.

Fluorouracil is available in both cream and solution form. It can be applied with a nonmetallic applicator, clean fingertips, or gloved fingers. If the fingers are used, they should be washed thoroughly immediately after application. Either a 1% or 2% fluorouracil solution should be used for the treatment of multiple actinic keratoses (AK) of the head and neck. It should be applied twice daily to the lesions. Superficial basal cell carcinoma may be treated with 5% fluorouracil, administered twice daily for at least 2 to 6 weeks. Another topical drug also used for actinic keratoses and basal cell carcinomas is the immunomodulator imiquimod, discussed later.

Immunomodulators
▶ *pimecrolimus*

The latest dermatologic drug is currently the only drug in a brand new class of medications. Pimecrolimus (Elidel) is available in a cream form for use in treating **atopic dermatitis.** This is caused by a hereditary susceptibility to **pruritus,** and is often associated with allergic rhinitis, hay fever, and asthma. This drug works through a mechanism similar to that of the anti-transplant-rejection drug tacrolimus (Prograf), which was discussed in Chapter 45 on immunosuppressant drugs. A topical form of tacrolimus (Protopic) is also used

with similar actions and indications. Adverse reactions for both drugs are usually limited to minor skin irritations.

imiquimod

Imiquimod (Aldara) is an immunomodulating drug that has demonstrated efficacy in treating AK, BCC, and anogenital warts. Its exact mechanism of action is unknown, but it is believed to somehow enhance the body's immune response to these conditions. It is applied two to five times per week, as prescribed, depending on the condition being treated. Adverse reactions range include mild skin reactions (burning, induration [hardness], irritation, pain, bleeding), which can occur both locally (at the site of medication administration) and at skin areas *remote* from the site of administration. More severe adverse skin reactions include edema, erosion/ulceration, scaling, scabbing, exudate, and vesicles. Systemic reactions, likely related to systemic immunomodulating effects, include cough, upper respiratory infection, musculoskeletal reactions (e.g., back pain), and lymphadenopathy. This drug is available only in cream form.

WOUND CARE DRUGS

Although superficial skin wounds often require minimal interventions, deeper skin wounds often require more definitive care for optimal healing. Such care includes addressing the systemic issues (e.g., body nutritional status) that are critical to tissue repair. Topical wound care medications are key to one of the fundamental steps of wound care, referred to in the literature as *preparation of the wound bed.* The concept of wound *débridement* refers to removal of nonviable tissue and removal of bacteria by suitable cleansing. Table 57-6 lists information regarding selected, currently available wound care medications.

◆ NURSING PROCESS

◆ ASSESSMENT

Before using any of the dermatologic preparations, the nurse should assess for allergies (including all ingredients such as benzoyl or peroxide), contraindications, cautions, and drug interactions (see previous discussion in the pharmacology section). Topical antibacterials are associated with a wide range of reactions because of the generalized sensitivity of patients to antibiotics, even when in a different dosage form; therefore, if a patient is allergic to a systemic antibacterial, he or she will also be allergic to topical dosage forms. The nurse should also assess the completion of an order for culture and sensitivity testing prior to use of the antibacterial to ensure appropriate identification of sensitive drugs. Before administering any type of topical medication (e.g., antimicrobial, corticosteroid, anti-acne drug), the nurse should always consider the concentration of the medication, length of exposure to the skin, condition of the skin, size of the area affected, and hydration of the skin. All of these factors have significant effects on the action of the medication.

The skin or area affected must be inspected thoroughly under an adequate lighting source, with palpation of the area with a gloved hand. In dark-skinned patients, an erythematous area may not be visible but may be palpated as an area of warmth. Should there be any possibility of systemic absorption of topical drugs—for example, tretinoin—liver function studies should be assessed prior to drug therapy. For various antibacterial drugs, the possibility of systemic absorption warrants assessment of baseline renal

Table 57-6 Selected Wound-Care Products				
Product Name	**Category**	**Advantages**	**Disadvantages**	**Contraindications**
sodium hypochlorite (Dakin's bleach solution)	Chemical, nonselective	Aids débridement; reduces microbial count	Partly toxic and irritating to healing tissue	Clean, noninfected wounds
cadexomer iodine (Iodosorb, others)	Chemical, nonselective	Slow-release; safe for viable cells; absorbs exudates; promotes wound healing	Partly toxic to fibroblast cells; stains tissue	Iodine allergy
collagenase (Santyl); papain-urea (Accuzyme); Papain-urea and chlorophyllin (Panafil)	Selective	Good for patients on antico-agulants or in whom sur-gery is contraindicated; selectively removes ne-crotic tissue; does not harm normal tissue; ok for infected wounds	Requires prescriber's order; not for use with other common wound products such as silver sulfadizaine (Silvadene; Chapter 37) or Dakin's solution; expensive; papain-urea occasionally associated with anaphylaxis	Clean, well-granulating wound; product allergies
BIAFINE Topical Emulsion	Water-based emulsion	Can be used for "tunneling" wounds as well as full-thickness wounds and radiation dermatitis	Must not be applied within 4 hours of radiation therapy	Bleeding wounds or skin rashes related to food or drug allergies

and hepatic functioning. Baseline hearing levels with drugs that are known to be ototoxic (e.g., silver sulfadiazine) should also be assessed. Physical assessment of the skin should be ac-companied with assessment of surrounding structures, includ-ing lymph nodes.

The patient's overall health status and hygiene practices should also be assessed, including whether the patient has suf-fered any trauma or if there is a history of any immunosuppres-sion. The nurse should also remember that the skin of the very young and the elderly is more fragile and permeable to certain topical dermatologic preparations. These characteristics also lead to a higher risk for systemic absorption from the skin. It is also important to note other possible situations that may result in a less than a therapeutic effect, such as the use of topical drugs over an area that is full of pus or debris. Herbal products, such as topical aloe, also require thorough assessment and noting of any allergies, contraindications, cautions, and drug interactions (see the Herbal Therapies and Dietary Supplements box on p. 874).

◆ NURSING DIAGNOSES

- Impaired skin integrity related to specific diseases, reactions, conditions, or breaks in the skin barrier
- Acute pain related to the skin condition or from adverse ef-fects of the topical drug
- Deficient knowledge related to lack of experience with and exposure to use of topical drugs
- Ineffective therapeutic regimen related to lack of information about importance of compliance/adherence and maintaining frequent dosing

◆ PLANNING

Goals

- Patient's skin remains intact and healed in appearance and integrity.
- Patient remains compliant with therapy and with its applica-tion technique.

- Patient remains free of injury to skin while on therapy.
- Patient experiences minimal to no complications of therapy.

Outcome Criteria

- Patient's skin improves daily as stated by patient with less redness, drainage, discomfort, itching, and/or rash.
- Patient states increased comfort and minimal pain and itching at site of skin disorder.
- Patient demonstrates how to apply medication as prescribed and to follow physician's orders in its application with spe-cific attention to emollient, lotion, solution, spray, cream, and ointment dosage forms.
- Patient states the rationale for treatment, adverse effects of the specific dermatologic preparation, and symptoms to report associated with the dermatologic therapy.
- Patient remains compliant with the medication therapy with resultant improved condition of skin or affected area within 2 to 4 weeks of treatment.

◆ IMPLEMENTATION

Generally speaking, before applying any topical medication, the nurse should cleanse the affected site of any debris and residual medication, making sure to follow any specific directions such as removing water or alcohol-based topical preparations with soap and water and using Standard Precautions (see Box 9-1). All dos-age forms of medication should be stored as recommended. The nurse/patient should wear gloves, not only to prevent contamina-tion from secretions but also to prevent absorption of the medica-tion through the skin. A finger-cot, tongue depressor, or cotton-tip applicator is recommended. Lotions and solutions should be shaken or mixed thoroughly before use and evenly applied. Creams, ointments, and emollients are often applied with a ster-ile cotton-tipped applicator, tongue blade, gloved hand (see ear-lier for more information and refer to Chapter 9). Be sure to wash hands not only *before* but *after* application of the medication. Any dressings should be applied as ordered, with special attention to directions concerning occlusive, wet, or wet-to-dry dressing changes. It is important to note, however, that most topical dermatologic drugs do not require a dressing once the medication is applied. The medication order may also state to avoid any sort of dressing or coverage of the area. With wound care and use of medications, there is usually a step-by-step protocol for use of a cleansing agent, possible débridement drug, rinsing solution, and final application of either antiinfective, antifungal, burn product, antiseptic—or other solution—that may have been ordered. Patient education for wound care and/or use of topical dermatologic drugs should be comprehensive. If home health care is needed for care at home, arrangements should be made and in place prior to the patient returning home. Information about the site of application, drainage (color and amount), swelling, temperature, odor, color, pain, or other sensations, as well as the type of treatment rendered and response, should be documented with each treatment or application and a "before and after" comparison assessment noted. Patients should also be encouraged to do this.

The manufacturer's guidelines regarding the use of any of the dermatologic preparations should always be followed because each medication has a different type of base solution. Specific application procedures may be required for different dosage forms. It is also important to follow any instructions or orders regarding other treatments to the affected area, such as use of an occlusive or wet dressing. Medicated areas may also need to be protected from exposure to air or sunlight. Strict adherence to the proper method of application and dosage of any dermatologic preparation is important to its effectiveness, and doubling-up of a missed dose is not recommended. After the patient or nurse has completed the medication administration process, all contaminated dressings, gloves, or equipment should be disposed of properly. Safety and comfort should be maintained at all times. See http://evolve.elsevier.com/Lilley for more information about the classifications of topical dermatologic drugs and associated nursing implications. Patient teaching tips are presented in the box below. See Table 57-6 for information about wound care, specific drugs, and their advantages and disadvantages.

◆ EVALUATION

Evaluation should always begin with monitoring of goals and outcome criteria, and, in addition, therapeutic responses to the various dermatologic preparations include improved condition of skin and healing of lesions or wounds; a decrease in the size of the lesions with eventual resolution; and a decrease in swelling, redness, weeping, itching, and burning of the area. The physician, advanced practice registered nurse, or nurse practitioner, should be notified if a therapeutic response is not noted within an appropriate time (anywhere from 48 hours to 72 hours or longer depending on the drug, disorder, skin problem, chronicity, etc.) or if signs and symptoms worsen or new ones appear. Adverse effects to evaluate for include increased severity of symptoms—for example, increased redness, swelling, pain, and drainage; fever; or any other unusual problems at the affected area. Adverse effects may range from slight irritation of the site where the topical drug has been applied to an allergic reaction to toxic systemic effects.

Patient Teaching Tips

- Instructions should include keeping the skin clean and dry and maintaining adequate general hygiene, cleanliness, adequate hydration, and proper nutrition during drug therapy. Make sure the patient understands how to prepare the skin for application of medication and to follow instructions as provided.
- Inform the patient to avoid exposure to sunlight during drug therapy and to always wear sunscreen if sun exposure is allowed.
- If indicated or ordered, dressings should be applied to the area after the medication has been applied. Proper disposal of contaminated dressings or equipment should be encouraged, too. Thorough hand-washing before and after application of medication should be emphasized and demonstrated to all those involved in the care of the patient. Compliance and its importance should also be emphasized.
- Encourage the patient to notify the physician of any unusual or adverse reactions or if the original problem/condition worsens or shows a lack of improvement within a designated period.
- All female patients of childbearing age should be counseled regarding the birth defect hazards associated with exposure to certain dermatologic drugs. All sexually active women must use contraception during treatment and for at least 1 month after use of any teratogenic medication.

Points to Remember

- Dermatologic drugs are used to treat topical infections.
- Common skin disorders caused by bacteria are folliculitis, impetigo, furuncles, carbuncles, and cellulitis.
- The bacterium most commonly responsible for acne is *Propionibacterium acnes*.
- The fungi that are responsible for causing topical fungal infections are *Candida,* dermatophytes, and *Malassezia furfur.*
- The most common topical fungal infections are *Candida* infections, for example, yeast infections.
- One of the most common topical viral infections is herpes simplex, types 1 and 2.
- Topical anesthetics are used therapeutically to topically numb the skin. Indications for topical anesthetics include insect bites, sunburn, poison ivy, and before painful injections.
- Corticosteroids are some of the most widely used topical drugs that are indicated for relief of topical inflammatory and pruritic disorders.
- Beneficial effects of corticosteroids include antiinflammatory, antipruritic, and vasoconstrictor actions.
- Adverse and toxic reactions to dermatologic drugs can and do occur; therefore, these drugs should be administered cautiously, and the physician's orders and manufacturer's guidelines followed. This is critical to ensure safe and effective treatment.
- Patient education about the medication, its administration, and its effectiveness are important to ensure compliance.

NCLEX Examination Review Questions

1. When performing wound care to a burned area with silver sulfadiazine, which method is correct?
   a. Apply cream to the wound four times a day.
   b. Use a sterile-gloved hand to apply cream to cleansed and débrided areas.
   c. Cleanse the area first, then apply with a clean-gloved hand.
   d. Do not débride the area before application of the cream.
2. When considering the variety of OTC topical corticosteroid products, the nurse is aware that which preparation is most effective?
   a. Gels
   b. Lotions
   c. Sprays
   d. Ointments
3. An allergic reaction to topical bacitracin and similar antimicrobials would be indicated by:
   a. Petecchia
   b. Thickened skin
   c. Itching and burning
   d. Purulent drainage.

4. When teaching a patient about the mechanism of action of tretinoin, which statement by the nurse is correct?
   a. "This medication acts by killing the bacteria that cause acne."
   b. "This medication actually causes skin peeling."
   c. "This medication acts by protecting your skin from UV sunlight."
   d. "This medication has antiinflammatory actions."
5. When providing wound care with Dakin's solution for a patient who has a stage III pressure ulcer, the patient exclaims, "I smell bleach! Why are you putting bleach on me?" The nurse's best explanation would be:
   a. "This is a very dilute solution and acts to reduce the bacteria in the wound so that it can heal."
   b. "This is used instead of medication to promote wound healing."
   c. "This is used to dissolve the dead tissue in your wound."
   d. "We would never use bleach on a patient!"

1. b, 2. d, 3. c, 4. b, 5. a.

Critical Thinking Activities

1. Develop a teaching plan for a 29-year-old mother who has a 6-year-old child newly diagnosed with head lice. Include an emphasis on how to prevent contaminating others and preventing future episodes.
2. Discuss the major functions of the epidermis that make its intactness so important to homeostasis.
3. A 22-year-old woman with severe acne is receiving counseling before taking isotretinoin (Accutane) therapy. She has read the online "iPLEDGE" information (see www.iPLEDGEprogram.com) and is shocked to see that two negative pregnancy tests are required before starting therapy, and a monthly test done during therapy. What can you tell her to explain these requirements?

For answers, see http://evolve.elsevier.com/Lilley.

Ophthalmic Drugs

Objectives

When you reach the end of this chapter, you should be able to do the following:

1. Discuss the anatomy and physiology of the structures of the eye and how the structures are impacted by glaucoma and other disorders and disease processes.
2. List the various classifications of ophthalmic drugs, with examples of specific drugs.
3. Discuss the mechanisms of action, indications, dosage forms with application techniques, adverse effects, cautions, contraindications, and drug interactions of the various ophthalmic drugs.
4. Develop a nursing care plan related to the nursing process for patients receiving ophthalmic drugs.

e-Learning Activities

Companion CD
- NCLEX Review Questions: see questions 447-448
- Animations
- Audio Glossary
- Category Catchers
- Medication Errors Checklists
- IV Therapy Checklists

evolve Website (http://evolve.elsevier.com/Lilley)
- Nursing Care Plans • Frequently Asked Questions • Content Updates • WebLinks • Supplemental Resources • Elsevier ePharmacology Update • Medication Administration Animations

Drug Profiles

acetylcholine, p. 886
apraclonidine, p. 887
▶ artificial tears, p. 897
▶ atropine sulfate, p. 897
azelastine, p. 897
▶ bacitracin, p. 894
▶ betaxolol, p. 888
▶ ciprofloxacin, p. 894
cromolyn, p. 897
cyclopentolate, p. 897
dapiprazole, p. 897
▶ dexamethasone, p. 896
▶ dipivefrin, p. 888
▶ dorzolamide, p. 890
▶ echothiophate and demecarium, p. 886
▶ erythromycin, p. 893

fluorescein, p. 897
flurbiprofen, p. 896
ganciclovir and fomivirsen, p. 894
▶ gentamicin, p. 893
glycerin, p. 890
ketorolac, p. 896
▶ latanoprost, p. 891
mannitol, p. 890
natamycin, p. 894
▶ pilocarpine, p. 886
▶ sulfacetamide, p. 894
tetracaine, p. 896
tetrahydrozoline, p. 897
▶ timolol, p. 889
trifluridine p. 894

▶ Key drug.

Glossary

Accommodation The adjustment of the *lens* of the eye to variation in distance. (p. 882)

Angle-closure glaucoma Glaucoma that occurs as a result of a narrowed anatomical angle between the lens and cornea. Also called closed-angle glaucoma, narrow-angle glaucoma, congestive glaucoma, and pupillary closure glaucoma. (p. 883)

Anterior chamber The bubble-like portion of the front of the eye between the *iris* and the *cornea*. (p. 882)

Aqueous humor The clear, watery fluid circulating in the *anterior* and *posterior chambers* of the eye. (p. 882)

Bactericidal Any substance that kills bacteria. (p. 893)

Bacteriostatic Any substance that stops the growth and reproduction of bacteria. (p. 894)

Canal of Schlemm A tiny circular vein at the angle of the anterior chamber of the eye through which the aqueous humor is drained and ultimately funneled into the bloodstream. Also called *Schlemm's canal*. (p. 882)

Cataract An abnormal progressive condition of the *lens* of the eye, characterized by loss of transparency, with resultant blurred vision. (p. 882)

Ciliary muscle The circular muscle between the *anterior* and *posterior* chambers behind the *iris*. It is connected to the *suspensory ligaments* that modulate the curvature of the *lens*. (p. 882)

Cones Photoreceptive (light-receiving) cells in the retina of the eye that enable a person to visualize colors and play a large role in *central* (straight-ahead) vision. (p. 882)

Cornea The convex, transparent anterior part of the eye. (p. 881)

Cycloplegia Paralysis of the *ciliary muscles*, which prevents the *accommodation* of the *lens* to variations in distance. (p. 882)

Cycloplegics Drugs that paralyze the ciliary muscles of the eye. (p. 882)

Dilator muscle A muscle that constricts the *iris* of the eye but dilates the pupil. Also called *dilator pupillae*. (p. 882)

Glaucoma   An abnormal condition of elevated pressure within an eye because of obstruction of the outflow of *aqueous humor.* (p. 883)

Intraocular pressure   The pressure of the fluids of the eye against the *tunics* (retina, choroid, and sclera). (p. 882)

Iris   A round, muscular portion of the eye that gives it its color and serves as an aperture that controls the amount of light passing through the *pupil.* (p. 882)

Lacrimal glands   Glands located at the medial corner of the eyelids that produce *tears.* (p. 881)

Lacrimal ducts   Small tubes that drain *tears* from the *lacrimal glands* into the nasal cavity. (p. 881)

Lens   The transparent, crystalline, curved structure of the eye that is located directly behind the *iris* and the *pupil* and attached to the *ciliary body* by ligaments. (p. 882)

Lysozyme   An enzyme with antiseptic actions that destroys some foreign organisms. It is normally present in tears, saliva, sweat, and breast milk. (p. 881)

Miotics   Drugs that constrict the pupil. (p. 882)

Mydriatics   Drugs that dilate the pupil. (p. 882)

Open-angle glaucoma   A type of glaucoma that is often bilateral, develops slowly, is genetically determined, and does not involve a narrow angle between the *iris* and *cornea.* (Also called *chronic glaucoma, wide-angle glaucoma,* and *simple glaucoma.*) (p. 883)

Optic nerve   A major nerve that connects the posterior end of each eye to the brain, to which it transmits visual signals. (p. 882)

Posterior chamber   The part of the eye behind the *iris* but in front of the *vitreous body.* Includes the *lens* and its suspensory ligaments, as well as *aqueous humor.* (p. 883)

Pupil   A circular opening in the *iris* of the eye, located slightly to the nasal side of the center of the iris. The pupil lies behind the *anterior chamber* of the eye and the *cornea* and in front of the *lens.* (p. 882)

Retina   The innermost layer of the eye, containing both *rods* and *cones* that receive visual stimuli and transmit them to the *optic nerve.* (p. 882)

Rod   One of the tiny cylindrical photoreceptive elements arranged perpendicularly to the surface of the retina. Rods are especially sensitive in low-intensity light and are responsible for black and white and *peripheral* ("off-to-the-side") vision. (p. 882)

Sphincter pupillae   A muscle that expands the *iris* while constricting or narrowing the diameter of the *pupil.* (p. 882)

Tears   Watery saline or alkaline fluid secreted by the *lacrimal glands* to moisten the *conjunctiva* (see Figure 58-1). (p. 881)

Uvea   The fibrous tunic beneath the sclera that includes the *iris,* the *ciliary body,* and the *choroid* of the eye (see Figure 58-1). Also called *tunica vasculosa bulbi* or *uveal tract.* (p. 882)

Vitreous humor   A transparent, semigelatinous substance contained in a thin membrane filling the cavity behind the *lens.* Also called the *corpus vitreum* or *vitreous body.* (p. 882)

OCULAR ANATOMY AND PHYSIOLOGY

To thoroughly understand the drugs used to treat disorders of the eye, it is necessary to understand the structure and normal function of the eye. The eye is the organ responsible for the sense of sight. Figure 58-1 illustrates the structures of the eye, all of which are needed for accurate eyesight. Each eyeball is nearly spherical and approximately 1 inch in diameter. Each eye is recessed into a small frontal skull cavity known as an *orbit.* The exposed anterior (front) portion of the eye is covered by three layers: the protective external layer (*cornea* and *sclera*), a vascular middle layer known as the *uvea* (includes the *choroid, iris,* and *ciliary body*), and the internal layer, known as the *retina.* All of these layers are protected by the *eyelid,* which serves as an external protection tissue.

Each eye is held in place and moved by six muscles that are controlled by cranial nerves. These muscles include the *rectus* and *oblique* muscles. There are four types of rectus muscles: *inferior, superior, medial,* and *lateral.* There are two types of oblique muscles: *inferior* and *superior.* These muscles are shown in Figure 58-2. (The medial rectus muscle is hidden from view in this figure but can be visualized to be directly across from the lateral rectus muscle.) The *levator palpebrae superioris* muscle opens the eyelid (see later). This muscle rests on top of the superior rectus muscle. There are several other important structures that are either part of or adjacent to the eye. The structures and purposes of each are as follows:

- *Eyebrow:* Rows of short hair above (superior) the upper eyelids. The eyebrow protects the eye from direct light, falling dust or other small particles, and perspiration coming from the forehead.
- *Eyelid:* The layer of muscle and skin lined interiorly by the *conjunctiva,* which also covers the outer anterior surface of the eye, which is the *convex* (outward-projecting; opposite of *concave*), transparent, anterior portion of the eye. It can be thought of as a window that sits in front of the *lens* and allows the passage of light.
  The eyelid is moveable and can open or close. It protects the eye when closed and allows vision when open. The eyelid is raised by contraction of the *levator palpebrae superioris* muscle, and is lowered by relaxation of this muscle (see Figure 58-2).
- *Eyelashes:* Two or three rows of hairs that are located on the edge (*margin*) of the eyelids. They help prevent small particles from falling into the eye when it is open.
- *Palpebral fissure:* The space between the upper and lower eyelids when the eyelids are open but relaxed.
- *Sclera:* A tough, white coat of fibrous tissue that surrounds the entire eyeball except for the cornea. It helps maintain the shape of the eye. Commonly called the *white* of the eye, the sclera is nonvascular and allows light to pass through it to the lens.
- *Choroid:* One of the middle-layer structures of the eyeball that contains the blood vessels that supply the eye, and also absorbs light.
- *Ciliary body:* The structure that supports the *ciliary muscles* that control the curvature of the lens via attached *suspensory ligaments.*
- *Conjunctiva:* The mucous membrane that lines the eyelids and also covers the exposed anterior surface of the eyeball.

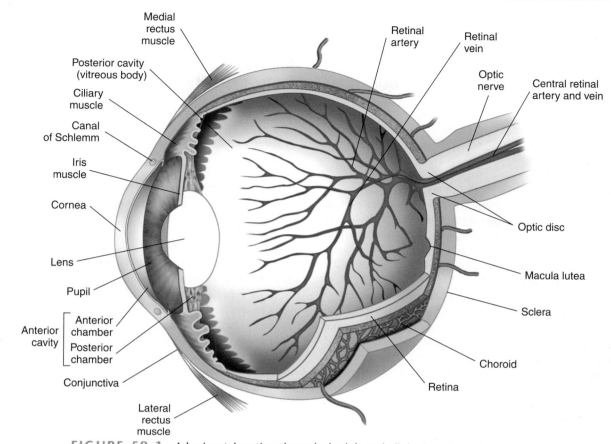

FIGURE 58-1 A horizontal section through the left eyeball, looking from the top down. *(Modified from Thibodeau GA, Patton KT: Anatomy and physiology, ed 5, St Louis, 2003, Mosby.)*

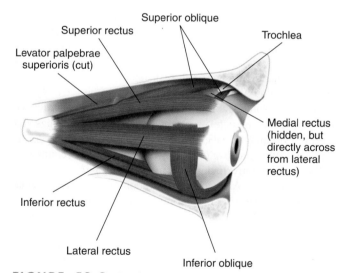

FIGURE 58-2 Extrinsic muscles of the right eye. Lateral view. *(Modified from Thibodeau GA, Patton KT: Anatomy and physiology, ed 5, St Louis, 2003, Mosby.)*

- *Iris:* The colored *(pigmented)* muscular apparatus behind the cornea.
- *Pupil:* The variable-sized opening in the center of the iris that allows light to enter into the eyeball when the eyelids are open. Its diameter changes with contraction and relaxation of the muscular fibers of the iris as the eye responds to changes

in light, emotional states, and other kinds of stimulation. The pupil is the rear portion of the window of the eye through which light passes to the lens and the retina (with the cornea as the front part of this "window").
- *Medial canthus:* The site of union near the nose for the upper and lower eyelids.
- *Lacrimal caruncle:* A small, red, rounded elevation covered by modified skin at the medial angle of the eye; the site of the *lacrimal glands* (see later).
- *Lateral canthus:* The site of union away from the nose for the upper and lower eyelids.

LACRIMAL GLANDS

The eye is kept moist and healthy by an intricate network of connected canals, ducts, and sacs that work together. The **lacrimal glands** produce tears that bathe and cleanse the exposed anterior portion of the eye. **Tears** are composed of an isotonic, aqueous solution that contains an enzyme called **lysozyme,** which acts as an antibacterial to help prevent eye infections. Tears drain into the nasal cavity through the **lacrimal ducts.**

LAYERS OF THE EYE

Overall, the eye can be conceived as having three separate anatomical layers. The fibrous *outer layer* of the eye has two parts that are continuous with each other: the *sclera* and the **cornea.**

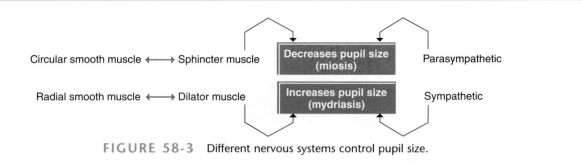

FIGURE 58-3   Different nervous systems control pupil size.

The sclera is a tough, fibrous layer that protects and maintains the shape of the eye. The cornea is a nonvascular transparent portion of the outer layer that allows light to enter the eye. It is located at the very front of the eye and is continuous with the sclera. It is pain sensitive (a protective function) and obtains nutrition from the **aqueous humor,** the clear watery fluid that circulates in the anterior and posterior chambers of the eye.

The vascular *middle layer* of the eye is composed of the **iris** (to the anterior), ciliary body, and choroid (to the posterior). These three structures are collectively called the **uvea.** The **iris** gives color to the eye and has an adjustable-sized opening in the center called the **pupil.** The main function of the iris is to regulate the amount of light that enters the eye by causing the size of the pupil to vary. Pupil size is controlled by two smooth muscles. The **sphincter pupillae** muscle is controlled by the parasympathetic nervous system and constricts *(miosis)* the diameter of the pupil (Figure 58-3). A sphincter is any circular band of muscle fibers that constricts a passage or closes a natural opening in the body (e.g., pyloric sphincter). Impulses from the parasympathetic nervous system operate this muscle. In contrast, the pupil is opened *(mydriasis)* by a radial smooth muscle called the **dilator muscle.** It is composed of radiating fibers, like spokes of a wheel, that converge from the circumference of the iris toward its center. Sympathetic nervous system impulses control this muscle (see Figure 58-3).

The anterior portions of both the retina and choroid merge to become the *ciliary body,* which produces **aqueous humor.** This is the clear, watery fluid that circulates in both the *anterior* and *posterior chambers,* and it should not be confused with *tears* (described earlier). Aqueous humor also contributes, along with *vitreous humor* (see later), to the **intraocular pressure (IOP)** of the eye. This is the internal pressure of all fluids against the *tunics* (retina, choroid, sclera) of the eye. Obviously, given the already small space of the eye, any change in the volume of aqueous humor present can lead to increased or reduced IOP. Normally, the aqueous humor is removed from the **anterior chamber** via the **canal of Schlemm** at a rate that balances out its production by the ciliary body. The ciliary body also provides a support for the suspensory ligaments that support the lens (see later). The choroid is a thin, dark layer that lines most of the internal side of the sclera. The function of the choroid is to absorb light and prevent its reflection out of the eye, and the choroid is also the major location of the network of blood vessels that supply each eye.

The **lens** is the transparent crystalline structure of the eye, located directly behind the iris and the pupil. It has a *biconvex* (oval-spherical) shape and is held in place by *suspensory ligaments* that are attached to the **ciliary muscles.** Contraction of the ciliary muscles modifies the tension of the suspensory ligaments,

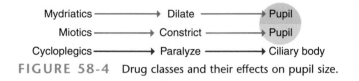

FIGURE 58-4   Drug classes and their effects on pupil size.

which changes the shape of the lens. This function is important for visual accommodation as well as the focusing of light (and visual images) onto the retina. These muscles are controlled by the parasympathetic nervous system (PSNS) through the oculomotor cranial nerve (CN-III). Accordingly, the lens divides the interior of the eyeball into posterior (rear) and anterior (forward) chambers. The larger chamber behind the lens is filled with a jelly-like fluid called the **vitreous humor.** The lens is normally transparent to easily allow the passage of light. It is composed of uniform layers of protein fibers that are encased by a clear connective-tissue capsule. A loss of lens transparency results in a visual condition called a **cataract.** This is a gray-white opacity that can be seen within the lens. If cataracts are untreated, sight may eventually be completely lost. At the onset of a cataract, vision is blurred, and may be further worsened by the glare of bright lights. *Diplopia* or double vision may also develop.

Before light images reach the retina, they are focused into a sharp image by the lens of the eye. The elasticity of the lens enables it to change its shape and focusing power. This process is called **accommodation** and is facilitated by the ciliary body. Paralysis of accommodation is called **cycloplegia. Mydriatics** are drugs that dilate the pupil (e.g., apraclonidine). Those drugs that constrict the pupil are called **miotics** (e.g., acetylcholine, pilocarpine). Drugs that paralyze the ciliary body are called **cycloplegics,** but they also have mydriatic properties (e.g., atropine, cyclopentolate) (Figure 58-4). All of these medications are used to facilitate visualization of the inner eye during ophthalmic examinations.

The third and *inner layer* of the eye is a thin delicate layer known as the **retina.** It contains light-sensitive *photoreceptors* known as **rods** and **cones.** The basic function of the retina is image formation via the rods and cones. Both types of photoreceptors are located near the surface of the retina. Rods produce black and white vision, including shades of gray, especially in low light, and cones are responsible for color vision (Figure 58-5). Additionally, rods are more active in providing peripheral (to-the-side) vision, whereas cones are more active in central (straight-ahead) vision. The posterior center part of the retina is attached to the **optic nerve.** The function of this nerve is to connect the retina with the visual center of the brain, located within the occipital lobe that extends above and behind the cerebellum. It is this location within the brain that interprets incoming visual stimuli.

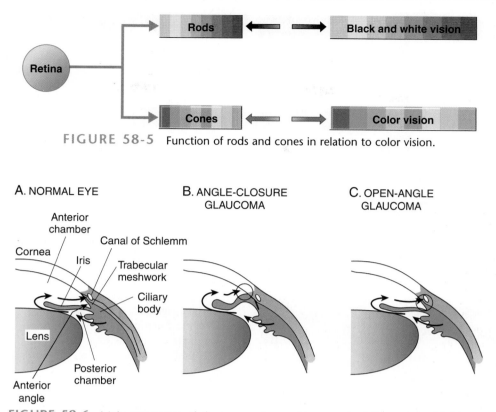

FIGURE 58-5   Function of rods and cones in relation to color vision.

FIGURE 58-6   Main structures of the eye and an enlargement of the canal of Schlemm showing an aqueous flow. **A,** Normal eye. **B,** In angle-closure glaucoma, the closure of the anterior angle prevents aqueous humor from exiting through the canal of Schlemm, leading to increased intraocular pressure. **C,** In open-angle glaucoma, the anterior angle remains open, but the canal of Schlemm is obstructed by tissue abnormalities. *(Modified from McKenry LM, Salerno E: Mosby's pharmacology in nursing—revised and updated, ed 21, St Louis, 2003, Mosby.)*

OCULAR DRUGS

In this chapter, we focus on the medications used to treat disorders of the eye, which can be divided into several major drug groups: antiglaucoma drugs, antimicrobials, antiinflammatory drugs, topical anesthetics, diagnostics, antiallergic, and lubricants and moisturizers. There are also a variety of combination drug products that include two or more medications from different subclasses. These products are not discussed further in this chapter due to space limitations and the large number of other drug classes and products that will be described in more detail. However, the reader can assume the same therapeutic indications and drug effects as those for the single-ingredient drug products that are discussed. The focus of this chapter is on commonly used therapeutic medications. A multitude of various products are also available and used in the care of contact lenses, including contact lens-cleaning enzymes, irrigating solutions, and eye washes, which, again, for space limitations, are not be discussed further in this chapter. Their use is fairly straightforward with limited risk. More exotic surgical drugs are also beyond the scope of this chapter. The reader is advised to refer to manufacturer packaging information for any unfamiliar product encountered in clinical practice.

ANTIGLAUCOMA DRUGS

As noted previously, the aqueous humor is a nourishing liquid that is produced by the ciliary body and flows from the **posterior chamber** (behind the iris) to the anterior chamber (in front of the iris). It is removed via the canal of Schlemm, which is located adjacent to the union of the sclera and cornea in the anterior chamber. When the normal flow and drainage of aqueous humor is inhibited, IOP can be raised to dangerous levels. This creates a serious ocular condition called **glaucoma.** The two major types of glaucoma for purposes of this chapter are **angle-closure glaucoma** and **open-angle glaucoma.** Figure 58-6 shows the pathophysiology of each and illustrates an enlarged view of the involved eye structures. Table 58-1 lists additional characteristic features of each. Glaucoma can be a *primary* illness (occurring on its own) or *secondary* to another eye condition or injury (e.g., post-traumatic glaucoma). Congenital glaucoma can also occur in infants. Glaucoma can also occur in the absence of increased IOP (normotensive glaucoma). There are a few other more exotic forms of glaucoma (e.g., pigmentary glaucoma, pseudoexfoliative glaucoma) that are also beyond the scope of this chapter.

In summary, glaucoma is an eye disorder characterized by excessive intraocular pressure (IOP) created by abnormally elevated

Table 58-1 Glaucoma: Types and Characteristics

	Angle-Closure	Open-Angle
Synonyms	Closed-angle glaucoma, narrow-angle glaucoma, congestive glaucoma, and pupillary closure glaucoma	Chronic glaucoma, wide-angle glaucoma, and simple glaucoma
Chronicity	Acute (can cause rapid vision loss)	Chronic
Relative incidence	Less common	More common
Nature of angle	Narrow	Larger
Most common age of onset and race	>30 yr white	>30 yr African-American
Major symptoms	Blurred vision, severe headaches, eye pain	Blurred vision, occasional headaches
Treatment	Topical or systemic drugs, surgery	Topical or systemic drugs, surgery

↑ Aqueous humor → ↑ IOP → ↑ Pressure on retina → Impaired vision

FIGURE 58-7 How increased aqueous humor can result in impaired vision. *IOP,* Intraocular pressure.

Table 58-2 Antiglaucoma Drug Effects on Aqueous Humor

Drug Class	Increased Drainage	Decreased Production
Miotics		
Direct-acting cholinergics	+ + +	0
Indirect-acting cholinergics (cholinesterase inhibitors)	+ + +	0
Mydriatics		
Sympathomimetic	+ +	+ + +
Others		
β-blockers	+	+ + +
Carbonic anhydrase inhibitors	0	+ + +
Osmotic diuretics	+ + +	0
Prostaglandin agonist	+ + +	0

0 = no effect; + = minor effect; ++ = moderate effect; +++ = pronounced effect.

levels of aqueous humor. This occurs when the aqueous humor is not drained through the canal of Schlemm as quickly as it is formed by the ciliary body. The accumulated aqueous humor creates a backward pressure that pushes the vitreous humor against the retina. Continued pressure on the retina destroys its neurons, leading to impaired vision and eventual blindness (Figure 58-7). Unfortunately, glaucoma is often without early symptoms, and, therefore, many people are not diagnosed until some permanent sight loss has occurred.

Effective treatment of glaucoma involves reducing IOP by either increasing the drainage of or decreasing the production of aqueous humor. Some drugs may do both. Effective drug therapy can delay and possibly even prevent the development of glaucoma. Drug classes used to reduce IOP include the following:

- Cholinergics, direct-acting (also called *miotics* and *parasympathomimetic drugs*)
- Cholinergics, indirect-acting (also called *miotics, cholinesterase inhibitors,* and *parasympathomimetic drugs*)
- Adrenergics (also called *mydriatics* and *sympathomimetic drugs*)
- Antiadrenergics (β-blockers; also called *sympatholytic drugs*)

- Carbonic anhydrase inhibitors
- Osmotic diuretics
- Prostaglandin agonists

See Table 58-2 for a comparison of drug effects on aqueous humor flow.

CHOLINERGIC DRUGS

There are two categories of ocular parasympathetic drugs, more concisely referred to as *cholinergic* drugs: direct-acting and indirect-acting. Directing acting cholinergics include acetylcholine, carbachol, and pilocarpine. Indirect-acting drugs, which are also called *cholinesterase inhibitors,* include echothiophate, currently the only available drug in this class. Because one primary drug effect is pupillary constriction or *miosis* (see later), these drugs are also commonly called *miotics.*

Mechanism of Action and Drug Effects

As discussed in Chapters 19 and 20, *acetylcholine (ACh)* is the endogenous neurochemical mediator of nerve impulses in the *parasympathetic nervous system (PSNS).* It stimulates parasympathetic or *cholinergic* receptors located in the brain and throughout the body along PSNS nerve branches. This results in several effects on the eye: miosis (pupillary constriction), vasodilation of blood vessels in and around the eye, contraction of ciliary muscles, drainage of aqueous humor, and reduced IOP. The ciliary muscle contraction itself promotes aqueous humor drainage by widening the space where the drainage occurs. Miosis promotes aqueous humor drainage by causing the iris to stretch, which also serves to widen this space. The action of ACh is normally short lived. It is rapidly hydrolyzed to *choline* and *acetic acid* by two *cholinesterase* enzymes known as *acetylcholinesterase (AChE)* and *pseudocholinesterase* (Figure 58-8).

Both direct- and indirect-acting miotics have effects similar to those of ACh, but their actions are more prolonged (Figure 58-9). The direct-acting miotics are able to directly stimulate ocular cholinergic receptors and actually mimic ACh. Indirect-acting miotics work by binding to and inactivating the cholinesterases (*acetylcholinesterase [AChE]* and *pseudocholinesterase),* the enzymes that break down ACh by *hydrolysis,* as noted earlier. As a result, ACh accumulates and acts longer at the cholinergic re-

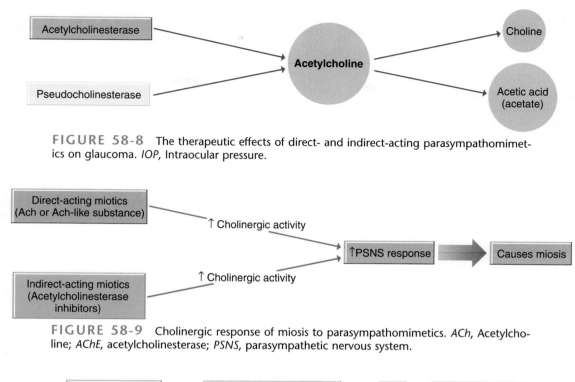

FIGURE 58-8   The therapeutic effects of direct- and indirect-acting parasympathomimetics on glaucoma. *IOP,* Intraocular pressure.

FIGURE 58-9   Cholinergic response of miosis to parasympathomimetics. *ACh,* Acetylcholine; *AChE,* acetylcholinesterase; *PSNS,* parasympathetic nervous system.

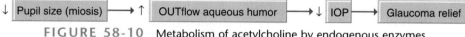

FIGURE 58-10   Metabolism of acetylcholine by endogenous enzymes.

ceptor sites. This leads to drug effects including miosis, ciliary muscle contraction, enhanced aqueous humor drainage, and reduced IOP by an average of 20% to 30% (Figure 58-10). Drug-induced miotic effects may be less pronounced in individuals with dark eyes (e.g., brown or hazel) than in those with lighter eyes (e.g., blue). This is because the pigment of the iris also absorbs the drug (reducing its therapeutic effects), and dark eyes have more pigment.

Indications

The direct- and indirect-acting miotics are used for open-angle glaucoma, angle-closure glaucoma, ocular surgery, and convergent strabismus (condition where one eye points toward the other ["cross-eye"]). They are also used to reverse the effect of mydriatic (pupil-dilating) drugs following ophthalmic examination. Specific indications may vary between drugs, as shown in Table 58-3.

Contraindications

Contraindications of miotics include known drug allergy and any serious active eye disorder with which induction of miosis might be harmful. An ophthalmologist will usually make this judgment.

Adverse Effects

Most of the adverse effects associated with the use of cholinergic and anticholinesterase drugs (miotics) are local and limited to the eye. This is an advantage of ocular drug administration. Ocular adverse effects are more likely with indirect-acting miotics as they usually have longer-lasting effects. This is because it takes more time for the ocular tissues to synthesize new cholinesterase enzymes. Effects include blurred vision, drug-induced *myopia* (nearsightedness), and accommodative spasms. Such effects are

Table 58-3	**Miotics: Indications**
Miotic Drug	**Indications**
acetylcholine	Complete and rapid miosis after cataract lens extraction, iridectomy
carbachol	Open-angle glaucoma
echothiophate	Accommodative esotropia, obstructive aqueous humor outflow, open- and angle-closure glaucoma after iridectomy
pilocarpine	Open-angle glaucoma, secondary glaucoma after iridectomy, cycloplegic reversal

secondary to contraction of the ciliary muscle, resulting in spasm (paralysis) of visual accommodation by the lens. Miotic drugs also cause vasodilation of blood vessels supplying the conjunctiva, iris, and ciliary body. This results in increased permeability of the blood-aqueous barrier, which may lead to vascular congestion and ocular inflammation. The *blood-aqueous barrier* is the anatomic barrier that normally prevents exchange of fluids between eye chambers and the blood, comparable to the blood-brain barrier mentioned in Chapter 2. Other undesirable effects include temporary stinging upon drug instillation, reduced nighttime or low-light vision, conjunctivitis, *lacrimation* (tearing), twitching eyelids *(blepharospasm),* and eye or brow pain. Prolonged use can result in iris cysts, lens opacities; and, rarely, retinal detachment.

As discussed, systemic effects are uncommon with local ocular drug administration, but are more likely to occur with cholinesterase inhibitors (indirect-acting miotics). When they do occur, they are due to generalized cholinergic stimulation apart from the eyes, as would be expected with any systemically administered cholinergic drug. Sufficient drug absorption into the general circulation must occur for systemic effects to appear. Possible systemic effects are listed in Table 58-4.

Toxicity and Management of Overdose

Occasionally, toxic effects may develop after the use of topically applied miotic drugs. Toxicity produced by miotics is an extension of their systemic effects and is more common with prolonged use of high doses. Most severe and prolonged effects are seen with long-acting anticholinesterases. Excessive PSNS effects are treated with intravenous or intramuscular atropine. Epinephrine may be used for bronchoconstriction or bradycardia.

Interactions

As with the systemic adverse effects, drug interactions are unlikely due to primarily local drug actions. Miotic drugs can, however, when given with topical adrenergic, antiadrenergic (e.g., β-blockers), and carbonic anhydrase inhibitors, have additive-lowering effects on IOP. Systemic cholinergic drugs can theoretically have additive cholinergic effects when given with miotics. Indirect-acting miotics (cholinesterase inhibitors) may also potentiate the effects of the neuromuscular blocker succinylcholine (Chapter 11), possibly even leading to cardiorespiratory arrest.

Dosages

For recommended dosages of miotic drugs, see the Dosages table on this page.

Table 58-4 Miotics: Adverse Effects	
Body System	**Adverse Effects**
Cardiovascular	Hypotension, bradycardia, or tachycardia
Central nervous	Headache
Genitourinary	Urinary incontinence
Gastrointestinal	Salivation, nausea, vomiting, abdominal cramps, diarrhea, incontinence
Respiratory	Bronchoconstriction, including asthma attacks
Dermatologic	Sweating

Drug Profiles

Direct-acting ocular cholinergics include acetylcholine (Miochol-E), carbachol (Carboptic), and pilocarpine (Pilocar). Indirect-acting drugs, which are also called *cholinesterase inhibitors,* include echothiophate (Phospholine Iodide). These drugs are used for glaucoma, as adjuncts for ocular surgery, and various other ophthalmic conditions.

Direct-Acting Miotics
acetylcholine

Acetylcholine (Miochol-E) is a direct-acting parasympathomimetic drug that is used to produce miosis during ophthalmic surgery. It is a pharmaceutical form of the naturally occurring neurotransmitter in the body. It has very quick onset and may begin to work almost immediately. When used for ophthalmic indications, acetylcholine is administered directly into the anterior chamber of the eye before and after securing one or more sutures. It is available as a 20-mg powder for intraocular use only.

Pharmacokinetics

Half-Life	Onset	Peak	Duration
Short (few minutes)	Instant	Instant	10 min

▶ pilocarpine

Pilocarpine (Pilocar) is a direct-acting parasympathomimetic drug that is used as a miotic in the treatment of glaucoma. Pilocarpine is available in many different strengths as an ocular gel and solution. One special formulation is the pilocarpine ocular insert system (Ocusert Pilo-20) that is inserted once weekly by the patient.

Pharmacokinetics (Immediate-Release Formulation)

Half-Life	Onset	Peak	Duration
Unknown	10-30 min	75 min	4-8 hr

Indirect-Acting Miotics
▶ echothiophate and demecarium

Echothiophate (Phospholine Iodide) is an indirect-acting parasympathomimetic that has an organophosphate structure and acts by phosphorylating cholinesterase enzymes. This effect is normally irreversible until new enzymes are synthesized by the body, which may take days or even weeks. For these reasons, this drug is considered to be long acting. Echothiophate is available only in ophthalmic powder form for reconstitution.

Pharmacokinetics

Half-Life	Onset	Peak	Duration
Long*	10-30 min	24 hr	7-28 days

*Exact length of half-life unclear, as drug effect is indirect and due to depleted cholinesterase levels.

DOSAGES

Selected Miotics

Drug (Pregnancy Category)	Pharmacologic Class	Usual Dosage Range	Indications
acetylcholine (Miochol-E) (C)	Direct-acting	>.0.5 to 2 mL preop	Surgical miosis
▶echothiophate (Phospholine Iodide) (C)	Indirect-acting	1 drop qd-bid	Early and advanced chronic simple glaucoma; glaucoma secondary to cataract surgery; accommodative esotropia
▶pilocarpine (Pilocar, Isopto Carpine, Akarpine, Pilopine HS) (C)	Direct-acting	Solution: 1-2 drops tid-qid Gel: 0.5 inch into lower conjunctival sac qhs (use any other eyedrops at least 5 min before gel)	Chronic open-angle and angle-closure glaucoma; acute angle-closure glaucoma; pre-op and postop intraocular hypertension; reversal of drug-induced mydriasis

SYMPATHOMIMETICS

Sympathomimetic drugs are used for the treatment of glaucoma and ocular hypertension. These drugs include the α-receptor agonists brimonidine (Alphagan P) and apraclonidine (Iopidine), as well as the α- and β-receptor agonists epinephryl (Epinal) and dipivefrin (Propine).

Mechanism of Action and Drug Effects

Because these drugs are sympathomimetic drugs, they mimic the sympathetic neurotransmitters norepinephrine and epinephrine and stimulate the dilator muscle to contract by means of α- and/or β-receptor interaction. This stimulation results in increased pupil size or *mydriasis* (Figure 58-11). Dilation is seen within minutes of instillation of the ophthalmic drops and lasts for several hours, during which time the IOP is reduced (Figure 58-12). The exact mechanism by which the sympathomimetic drugs lower IOP is unknown. However, α-receptor stimulation is known to reduce IOP by enhancing aqueous humor outflow through the canal of Schlemm. Production of aqueous humor by the ciliary body may also be reduced as another drug effect. All of these effects appear to be dose-dependent.

Indications

Both epinephrine and dipivefrin may be used to reduce elevated IOP in the treatment of chronic, open-angle glaucoma, either as initial therapy or as chronic therapy. Apraclonidine is primarily used to inhibit perioperative IOP increases. Increases in IOP during ophthalmic surgery are usually mediated via increased catecholamine stimulation of the sympathetic nervous system (SNS). Apraclonidine stimulates primarily the α$_2$ receptors, which oppose these effects, and thus corrects the surgery-induced changes in IOP. Brimonidine also has primarily α$_2$ activity but is normally used to lower IOP in patients with open-angle glaucoma or ocular hypertension.

Contraindications

Contraindications for the sympathomimetic ophthalmics include drug allergy and may include active, severe ophthalmic problems, which, in the judgment of an ophthalmologist, might be aggravated by the effects of these drugs.

Adverse Effects

The adverse effects of the sympathomimetic mydriatics are primarily limited to ocular effects and include burning, eye pain, and lacrimation. Such effects are usually temporary and may subside as the patient grows accustomed to the medication. Other ocular effects may include conjunctival hyperemia, localized melanin deposits in the conjunctiva, and released pigment granules from the iris. Although systemic effects associated with the use of sympathomimetic mydriatics are uncommon, they are theoretically possible, especially in larger doses or prolonged drug therapy. They include cardiovascular effects such as extrasystoles, tachycardia, and hypertension. Other effects that may be noticed are headache and faintness.

Toxicity and Management of Overdose

Rare toxic reactions are primarily the result of an extension of the therapeutic and adverse effects of these drugs. The most significant are cardiac dysrhythmias. Discontinuation of the drugs usually alleviates the toxic symptoms.

Interactions

With sufficient topical absorption, sympathomimetic mydriatics have the potential to react with other drugs. Cardiac dysrhythmias are potentiated when mydriatic drugs are given with halogenated anesthetics, cardiac glycosides, thyroid hormones, or tricyclic antidepressants.

Dosages

For recommended dosages of sympathomimetic drugs, see the Dosages table on page 888.

Drug Profiles

Sympathomimetic ophthalmic drugs include dipivefrin (Propine), epinephryl (Epinal), apraclonidine (Iopidine), and brimonidine (Alphagan P). These drugs are used for glaucoma, ocular hypertension, and ocular surgery.

apraclonidine

Apraclonidine (Iopidine) is structurally and pharmacologically related to the α$_2$ stimulant clonidine. It reduces IOP 23% to 39% by stimulating α$_2$ and β$_2$ receptors. It also prevents ocular vasoconstriction, which reduces ocular blood pressure as well as aqueous humor

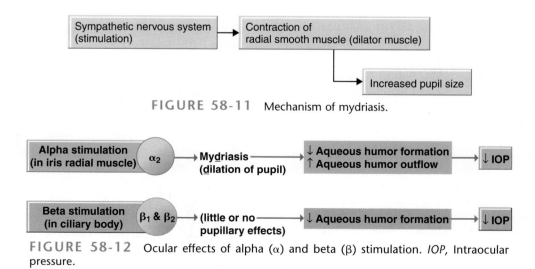

FIGURE 58-11   Mechanism of mydriasis.

FIGURE 58-12   Ocular effects of alpha (α) and beta (β) stimulation. *IOP,* Intraocular pressure.

DOSAGES

Selected Ocular Sympathomimetics

Drug (Pregnancy Category)	Pharmacologic Class	Usual Dosage Range	Indications
apraclonidine (Iopidine) (C)	Direct-acting	0.5% solution: 1-2 drops tid 1% solution: 1 drop in eye pre-op	Short-term adjunctive therapy for glaucoma not controlled with other drugs Anterior segment laser surgery
▶dipivefrin (Propine) (C)	Direct-acting	1 drop q12h	Chronic open-angle glaucoma

formation. Apraclonidine is primarily used to inhibit perioperative IOP increases, rather than for glaucoma. Brimonidine (Alphagan P) is a similar drug but is used primarily for glaucoma.

Pharmacokinetics

Half-Life	Onset	Peak	Duration
8 hr	1 hr	3-5 hr	12 hr

▶ dipivefrin

Dipivefrin (Propine) is a synthetic sympathomimetic miotic drug. It is a prodrug of epinephrine. The prodrug has little or no pharmacologic activity until hydrolyzed in the eye to two chemically modified forms of epinephrine. These chemical alterations account for the main advantage of this drug over epinephrine: It has enhanced lipophilicity (fat solubility) and can better penetrate into the tissues of the anterior chamber of the eye. This quality also reduces the likelihood of any systemic adverse effects. Dipivefrin typically reduces mean IOP approximately 15% to 25%. On a weight basis, dipivefrin is 4 to 11 times as potent as epinephrine in reducing IOP and 5 to 12 times as potent as epinephrine in terms of its mydriatic effects. Epinephryl (Epinal) is a newer drug with similar properties and uses.

Pharmacokinetics

Half-Life	Onset	Peak	Duration
1-3 hr	30 min	1 hr	12 hr

β-ADRENERGIC BLOCKERS

The antiglaucoma β-adrenergic blockers that reduce IOP include β_1-selective drugs betaxolol and levobetaxolol. Recall from Chapter 18 that β_1-selective β-blockers are also called *cardioselective*. Nonselective ocular β_1- and β_2-blockers include carteolol, levobunolol, metipranolol, and timolol.

Mechanism of Action and Drug Effects

The ophthalmic β-blockers reduce both elevated and normal IOP. They do this without affecting pupillary size, accommodation, or night vision. They appear to reduce IOP by reducing aqueous humor formation. In addition, timolol may produce a minimal increase in aqueous outflow.

Indications

Ophthalmic β-blockers are used to reduce elevated IOP in various conditions, including chronic open-angle glaucoma and ocular hypertension. They may also be used alone or in combination with a topical miotic (e.g., echothiophate iodide, pilocarpine), topical dipivefrin, and/or systemic carbonic anhydrase inhibitors (CAIs). When used in combination, these drugs may have an additive IOP-lowering effect. They may also be used to treat some forms of angle-closure glaucoma.

Contraindications

Contraindications of ophthalmic β-blockers include known drug allergy and any ocular condition where β-receptor blockade might be harmful.

Adverse Effects

The adverse effects of antiglaucoma β-blockers are primarily limited to ocular effects and limited systemic effects. The most common ocular effects are transient burning and discomfort. Other effects include blurred vision, pain, photophobia, lacrimation, blepharitis, keratitis (inflammation of the cornea), and decreased corneal sensitivity. Because these drugs are administered topically, few, if any, systemic effects are expected. Thoretical systemic effects include bradycardia, bronchospasm, headache, and dizziness as described for systemic β-blockers in Chapter 18. However, ocular β-blockers have not been shown to affect glucose metabolism.

Toxicity and Management of Overdose

Toxic reactions to β-blockers are rare and primarily involve the cardiovascular system. Symptoms include bradycardia, cardiac failure, hypotension, and bronchospasms. Treatment involves discontinuation of the drug and supportive care (e.g., adrenergic and anticholinergic drugs).

Interactions

As is the case with adverse effects, drug interactions with systemic drugs are unlikely due to the primarily localized nature of ophthalmically administered drugs. Theoretically, ophthalmic β-blockers can have additive therapeutic and/or adverse effects when given with systemically administered β-blockers or other cardiovascular drugs (e.g., calcium channel blockers), up to and including cardiorespiratory arrest.

Dosages

For recommended dosages of β-adrenergic blockers, see the Dosages table on page 889.

Drug Profiles

The currently available ophthalmic β-blocking drugs are betaxolol (Betoptic), carteolol (Ocupress), levobunolol (Betagan), levobetaxolol (Betaxon), metipranolol (Optipranolol), and timolol (Timoptic). These drugs are used for glaucoma and ocular hypertension.

▶ betaxolol

Betaxolol (Betoptic) is a β_1-selective β-blocker. It is structurally related to the systemic adrenergic β-receptor blocker metoprolol that is used primarily for cardiovascular disorders. Betaxolol is one of the most po-

DOSAGES

Selected Ocular β-Blockers

Drug (Pregnancy Category)	Pharmacologic Class	Usual Dosage Range	Indications
▶betaxolol (Betoptic, Betoptic S) (C)	Direct-acting	1-2 drops bid	Chronic open-angle glaucoma; ocular hypertension
▶timolol (Betimol, Timoptic, Timoptic-XE) (C)	Direct-acting	Solution: 1 drop bid Gel-forming solution: 1 drop qd	Open-angle glaucoma; ocular hypertension

tent and selective β-blocking drugs. Its ability to decrease aqueous humor formation and consequently IOP has made it an excellent drug for the treatment of ocular disorders such as open-angle glaucoma and ocular hypertension. Betaxolol is available only in liquid form.

Pharmacokinetics

Half-Life	Onset	Peak	Duration
Unknown	0.5-1 hr	2 hr	≥12 hr

▶ *timolol*

Timolol (Timoptic) may differ slightly from the other ophthalmic β-blockers in that it may increase the outflow of aqueous humor as well as its formation. The drug acts at both β_1 and β_2 receptors and is indicated for the treatment of open-angle glaucoma and ocular hypertension. It is available in various liquid forms, both with preservatives and preservative-free. Preservative-free products were developed due to patient allergies to benzalkonium chloride, a commonly used preservative. Timolol is also available in a gel-forming solution (with preservatives). These gel-forming products are longer acting and allow for once-daily dosing, a convenience over the twice-daily dosing that many patients require of the other timolol formulations.

Pharmacokinetics

Half-Life	Onset	Peak	Duration
Unknown	15-30 min	1-2 hr	12-24 hr

CARBONIC ANHYDRASE INHIBITORS

Ophthalmic carbonic anhydrase inhibitors (CAIs) include brinzolamide and dorzolamide. Both drugs are also sulfonamides and are therefore chemically related to the sulfonamide antibiotics (Chapter 37). These two drugs are available only in topical ophthalmic form. However, systemic CAIs for oral use are described in the chapter on diuretics (Chapter 25), and are sometimes also used as adjunct drug therapy for glaucoma.

Mechanism of Action and Drug Effects

These drugs work by inhibiting the enzyme *carbonic anhydrase*, which exists throughout the body and is involved in acid-base balance. In the eye, however, the inhibition of this enzyme results in decreased IOP by reduction of aqueous humor formation.

Indications

Ocular CAIs are used primarily for glaucoma, including both open-angle and angle-closure glaucoma, including preoperative use.

Contraindications

Contraindications for ocular CAIs include known drug allergy and any ocular condition in which they might be harmful in the judgment of an ophthalmologist.

Table 58-5	Carbonic Anhydrase Inhibitors: Adverse Effects

Body System	Adverse Effects
Central nervous	Drowsiness, confusion, paresthesias, seizures
Eyes, ears, nose, throat	Transient myopia, tinnitus
Gastrointestinal	Anorexia, vomiting, diarrhea, liver failure
Genitourinary	Polyuria, hematuria
Integumentary	Urticaria, rare photosensitivity, severe skin reactions (e.g., Stevens-Johnson syndrome)
Hematologic	Blood dyscrasias
Metabolic	Acidotic states and electrolyte imbalance with long-term therapy

Adverse Effects

Systemic absorption of these drugs occurs, and although systemic adverse effects are unlikely, the same effects listed for sulfonamide antibiotics in Chapter 37 can theoretically occur with these drugs. Patients with sulfa allergies may develop cross-sensitivities to the CAIs. Specific adverse effects are listed in Table 58-5.

Toxicity and Management of Overdose

Toxicity associated with the use of CAIs is rare. The mechanism by which these drugs work predisposes the patient to possible acidotic states and electrolyte imbalances. These toxic reactions generally require only supportive care. This may include the restoration of electrolytes, especially potassium, and the administration of bicarbonate to correct any CAI-induced acidotic state.

Interactions

The systemic use of CAIs can result in several significant drug interactions, and ocular CAIs have a theoretical (but less likely) potential for these interactions. CAIs can cause hypokalemia and increase the likelihood of digitalis toxicity. Hypokalemia is also more likely to occur when these drugs are coadministered with corticosteroids and diuretics. CAIs increase renal excretion of lithium, thereby reducing its therapeutic effects. CAIs also tend to increase the drug effects of basic drugs as a result of decreased renal excretion.

Dosages

For recommended dosages of selected CAIs, see the Dosages table on page 890.

DOSAGES

Ocular Carbonic Anhydrase Inhibitors

Drug (Pregnancy Category)	Pharmacologic Class	Usual Dosage Range	Indications
brinzolamide (Azopt) (C)	Carbonic anhydrase inhibitor	One drop tid	Open-angle glaucoma; ocular hypertension
▸dorzolamide (Trusopt) (C)	Carbonic anhydrase inhibitor	One drop tid	Open-angle glaucoma; ocular hypertension

Drug Profiles

There are currently two ocular CAIs: brinzolamide (Azopt) and dorzolamide (Trusopt). CAIs for systemic use can also be helpful in glaucoma but are discussed in Chapter 25.

▸ **dorzolamide**

Dorzolamide (Trusopt) is solely indicated for elevated IOP associated with either ocular hypertension or open-angle glaucoma. It is available only as an ophthalmic solution. The other drug in this class, brinzolamide, has comparable indications, dosage, and pharmacokinetics.

Pharmacokinetics

Half-Life	Onset	Peak	Duration
3-4 mo*	Rapid	Variable	Variable

*Due to red blood cell distribution in plasma.

OSMOTIC DIURETICS

Osmotic drugs may be administered either intravenously, orally, or topically to reduce IOP. The osmotic diuretics that are most commonly used for this purpose are glycerin and mannitol. Isosorbide and urea are two other less commonly used osmotic diuretics.

Mechanism of Action and Drug Effects

These drugs reduce ocular hypertension by causing the blood to become hypertonic in the presence of both intraocular and spinal fluids. This creates an osmotic gradient that draws water from the aqueous and vitreous humors into the bloodstream, causing a reduction of volume of intraocular fluid, which results in a decrease in IOP (Figure 58-13). Systemic (nonocular) drug effects are discussed in Chapter 25.

Indications

Ocular uses for osmotic diuretics include acute glaucoma episodes, and before or after ocular surgery to reduce IOP. Typically, glycerin is used first; if the treatment is unsuccessful, mannitol is tried. Isosorbide and urea are two other osmotic drugs that may also be used in similar situations. They are usually used after glycerin or mannitol has failed. Isosorbide may be especially beneficial for diabetic patients because it is not metabolized into sugar calories, unlike glycerin, which can cause hyperglycemia.

Contraindications

Osmotic diuretics are contraindicated in patients with known drug allergy, pronounced anuria, acute pulmonary edema, cardiac decompensation, and severe dehydration, as they can worsen all of these conditions.

Adverse Effects

The most frequent reactions to osmotic diuretic drugs are nausea, vomiting, and headache. The most significant adverse effects are fluid and electrolyte imbalance. Other effects are possible irritation and thrombosis at the injection site. A variety of other possible adverse effects are listed in Table 58-6.

Interactions

Increased lithium excretion caused by both mannitol and urea are the only significant drug interactions that have been reported.

Toxicity and Management of Overdose

Toxic reactions are primarily a result of the hyperosmolarity of the blood. The most significant toxic reactions include hypovolemia (secondary to diuresis), cardiac dysrhythmias, and hyperosmolar nonketotic coma. Treatment involves discontinuation of the drug and treatment of presenting symptoms with fluids and electrolytes.

Dosages

For recommended dosages of osmotic drugs, see the Dosages table on page 891.

Drug Profiles

Osmotic diuretics include mannitol (Osmitrol), glycerin (Osmoglyn), urea (Ureaphil), and isosorbide (Ismotic). These drugs are normally reserved for acute reduction of IOP during glaucoma crises, as well as perioperative uses in ophthalmic surgery.

glycerin

Glycerin (Osmoglyn) is an osmotic drug used orally to lower IOP or topically to reduce superficial corneal edema. Other common uses include before iridectomy to reduce IOP in individuals with acute narrow-angle glaucoma. It is also used preoperatively and/or postoperatively in conditions such as congenital glaucoma, retinal detachment, cataract extraction, and keratoplasty (corneal transplant). It may also be used in some secondary glaucomas. It is only available for oral use.

Pharmacokinetics

Half-Life	Onset	Peak	Duration
PO: 30-45 min	PO: 10-30 min	PO: 1-1.5 hr	PO: 4-5 hr

mannitol

Mannitol (Osmitrol) is used only by intravenous infusion to reduce elevated IOP when the pressure cannot be lowered by other treatments. Mannitol has been shown to be effective in the treatment of acute episodes of angle-closure, absolute, or secondary glaucoma and for lowering IOP before intraocular surgery. Mannitol does not penetrate the eye and may be used when irritation is present, unlike some of the other osmotic drugs, such as urea. This drug is normally only given by IV infusion.

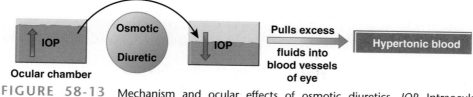

FIGURE 58-13 Mechanism and ocular effects of osmotic diuretics. *IOP,* Intraocular pressure.

Table 58-6   Osmotic Diuretics: Adverse Effects

Body System	Adverse Effects
Cardiovascular	Edema, thrombophlebitis, hypotension, hypertension, tachycardia, angina-like chest pains, fever, chills
Central nervous	Dizziness, headache, convulsions, rebound increased intracranial pressure, confusion
Electrolytes	Fluid electrolyte imbalances, acidosis, electrolyte loss, dehydration
Eyes, ears, nose, throat	Loss of hearing, blurred vision, nasal congestion
Gastrointestinal	Nausea, vomiting, dry mouth, diarrhea
Genitourinary	Marked diuresis, urinary retention, thirst

DOSAGES

Osmotic Diuretics

Drug (Pregnancy Category)	Pharmacologic Class	Usual Dosage Range	Indications
glycerin (Ophthalgan) (C)	Organic Alcohol	1-2 drops before eye exam as lubricant, more if needed during exam	Gonioscopy of edematous cornea
mannitol (Osmitrol) (C)	Organic Alcohol	IV: 1.5-2 g/kg over at least 30 min; for pre-op use give 1-1.5 hr before surgery	Acute reduction of elevated IOP

Pharmacokinetics

Half-Life	Onset	Peak	Duration
15-100 min	30-60 min	1 hr	6-8 hr

PROSTAGLANDIN AGONISTS

Latanoprost (Xalatan) is the most popular of three drugs in this newer class of ophthalmic drugs used to treat glaucoma: the prostaglandin agonists (PAs). The other two drugs are travoprost (Travatan) and bimatoprost (Lumigan).

Mechanism of Action and Drug Effects

Prostaglandins reduce IOP primarily by increasing the outflow of aqueous fluid, not by reducing its production. This is believed to occur by increasing aqueous humor outflow between the uvea and sclera in addition to the usual exit through the trabecular meshwork, a filter-like structure within the eye (see Figure 58-6). A single dose of ocular PAs lowers IOP for 20 to 24 hours, allowing a single daily dosage regimen. The drug effects of PAs are primarily limited to these ocular effects.

Indications

PAs are used in the treatment of glaucoma.

Contraindications

The only usual contraindication to the use of PAs is known drug allergy.

Adverse Effects

PAs are generally well tolerated. Adverse effects reported in clinical trials included foreign body sensation, punctate epithelial keratopathy (dotted appearance of cornea), stinging, conjunctival hyperemia ("bloodshot" eyes), blurred vision, itching, and burning. Systemic effects occur in a small percentage of patients and include skin reactions, upper respiratory infections, and headache. There is one unique adverse effect associated with all PAs. In some people with hazel, green, or bluish-brown eye color, eye color will permanently turn brown, even if they stop using the medication. This adverse effect appears to be only cosmetic with no known ill effects on the eye. This iris color change also does not affect IOP readings.

Interactions

Concurrent administration of PAs with any other eyedrops containing the preservative thimerosal may result in precipitation. It is recommended that the two medications be administered at least 5 minutes apart.

Dosages

For recommended dosages, see the table on page 892.

Drug Profiles

▶ **latanoprost**

About 3% to 10% of patients treated with latanoprost (Xalatan) have shown increased iris pigmentation after 3 to 4½ months of treatment. Latanoprost is a prodrug of a naturally occurring prostaglandin

DOSAGES

Prostaglandin Agonists

Drug (Pregnancy Category)	Pharmacologic Class	Usual Dosage Range	Indications
▶latanoprost (Xalatan) (C)	Prostaglandin	One drop every day in evening	Open-angle glaucoma and ocular hypertension in patients intolerant to or uncontrolled by other drugs

known as prostaglandin F_2-alpha. When this ester prodrug is administered, it is converted by hydrolysis (with water from ocular fluids) to the prostaglandin F_2-alpha, which in turn reduces IOP. This drug is available only in eye-drop form.

Pharmacokinetics

Half-Life	Onset	Peak	Duration
17 min	30-60 min	2 hr	24 hr

ANTIMICROBIAL DRUGS

Topical antimicrobials used for treating ocular infections include antibacterial, antifungal, and antiviral drugs. All require a prescription. Many of these drugs are also available for systemic administration for infections elsewhere in the body. The choice of a particular ophthalmic antimicrobial drug should be based on:

- Clinical experience
- Sensitivity and characteristics of the organisms most likely to cause the infection
- The disease itself
- Sensitivity and response of the patient
- Laboratory results (cultures and sensitivities)
- Some common eye infections that may require antibiotic therapy are listed in Table 58-7.

Mechanism of Action and Drug Effects

The drugs used to treat infections of the eye work in a variety of ways to destroy the invading organism. Their specific antimicrobial actions are similar to those described for systemically administered drugs. These are described in Chapters 37, 38, 39, and 41. The drug effects of the drugs used to treat ocular infections are focused on the microorganism invading the eye. Some antimicrobials destroy the causative organism, whereas others simply inhibit the organism's growth, allowing the body's immune system to fight the infection.

Indications

Indications for ocular antimicrobials are known or suspected infection with one or more specific microorganisms. Empirical treatment (without culture and sensitivity confirmation) should be based on reasonable clinical evaluation of presenting signs and symptoms. Topical use of antimicrobials helps prevent antimicrobial drug resistance that could arise from unnecessary systemic use. However, systemic antimicrobials may be used in more severe ocular infections.

Contraindications

Contraindications of antimicrobials include known drug allergy or other severe previous adverse drug reaction. Also, use of any drug class for the wrong infection (e.g., an antibacterial drug for

Table 58-7	Common Ocular Infections
Infection	**Description**
Blepharitis	Inflammation of the eyelids.
Conjunctivitis	Inflammation of the conjunctiva, which is the mucous membrane lining the back of the lids and the front of the eye except the cornea. It may be bacterial or viral in nature and is often associated with common colds. When caused by *Haemophilus* organisms, it is commonly called "pink eye." It is highly contagious but usually self-limiting.
Hordeolum (sty)	Acute localized infection of the eyelash follicles and the glands of the anterior lid; results in the formation of a small abscess or cyst.
Keratitis	Inflammation of the cornea caused by bacterial infection. Herpes simplex keratitis is caused by viral infection.
Uveitis	Infection of the uveal tract or the vascular layer of the eye, which includes the iris, ciliary body, and choroid.
Endophthalmitis	Inner eye structure inflammation caused by bacteria.

a viral infection) may obviously worsen the infection and delay treatment. This situation should be avoided whenever possible and the patient monitored for signs of progress or treatment failure.

Adverse Effects

The most common adverse effects of ocular antibiotics are local and transient inflammation, burning, stinging, urticaria, dermatitis, angioedema, and drug hypersensitivity. Other effects are listed in the profiles of specific drugs. Topical application of antimicrobial drugs may also interfere with growth of the normal bacterial flora of the eye, which may encourage growth of other more harmful organisms.

Interactions

Systemic drug interactions are unlikely due to the primarily local effects of ocular antimicrobials. One possible interaction is the concurrent use of corticosteroids (e.g., dexamethasone). Such drugs have immunosuppressive effects, which may impede the therapeutic effects of ocular antimicrobials, as is also the case with systemic antimicrobials.

Dosages

For recommended dosages of ocular antimicrobials, see the Dosages table on page 893.

DOSAGES

Selected Ocular Antimicrobials

Drug (Pregnancy Category)	Pharmacologic Class	Usual Dosage Range	Indications
Antibacterial Drugs			
▶bacitracin (AK-Tracin) (C)	Miscellaneous antibiotic	Solution: 1-2 drops q1-4h	Ocular infections
bacitracinpolymyxin B (Polysporin, AK-Poly-Bac) (C)		Ointment: 0.5-inch ribbon into lower conjunctival sacs tid-qid	
bacitracinpolymyxin B neomycin (Neosporin, AK-Spore) (C)			
▶ciprofloxacin (Ciloxan) (C)	Quinolone		
▶erythromycin (Ilotycin) (C)	Macrolide		
▶gentamicin (Genoptic, others) (C)	Aminoglycoside		
▶sulfacetamide (Bleph-10, others) (C)	Sulfonamide		
Antifungal Drug			
natamycin (Natacyn) (C)	Antifungal	1 drop into conjunctival sac q1-2h, then usually reduce after first 3-4 days to 6-8 drops/day; therapy usually continues for 14-21 days	Fungal ocular infections
Antiviral Drugs			
fomivirsen (Vitravene) (C)	DNA antimetabolite (nucleoside analog)	Intravitreal injection only (by ophthalmologist): 330 mcg q2wk for 2 initial doses, followed by 1 dose q4wk	Viral ocular infections: CMV retinitis in patients with AIDS; used after other drugs fail (second-line therapy)
ganciclovir (Vitrasert) (C)		1 surgical implant, which releases drug over 5-8 mo (inserted by ophthalmologist)	Viral ocular infections: CMV retinitis in patients with AIDS (first-line therapy)
trifluridine (Viroptic) (C)		Initially 1 drop q2h while awake (max 9 drops/day); may later decrease to 5 drops/day	Viral ocular infections: HSV type 1- and type 2-induced keratitis, keratoconjunctivitis

CMV, Cytomegalovirus; *HSV*, herpes simplex virus.

Drug Profiles

ANTIBACTERIAL DRUGS

A variety of infections can occur in the eye; many are self-limiting (i.e., the body's own immune system fights them). These infections seldom result in harm. However, some infections require the use of ocular antimicrobials to be eliminated. The most commonly used antimicrobials from the main antimicrobial drug classes are discussed here.

Aminoglycosides

Aminoglycosides (Ags; Chapter 38) are potent antimicrobials that destroy bacteria by interfering with protein synthesis in bacterial cells by binding to ribosomal subunits, which eventually leads to bacteria death. AGs used to treat ocular infections include gentamicin (Genoptic) and tobramycin (Tobrex). Adverse effects include swollen eyelids, mydriasis, and local erythema. Toxic reactions are rare because of poor topical absorption. Another possible toxic reaction is the overgrowth of nonsusceptible organisms, which can lead to eye infections that are resistant to treatment.

▶ *gentamicin*

Gentamicin (Genoptic, Garamycin) is effective against a wide variety of gram-negative and gram-positive organisms. It is particularly useful against *Pseudomonas, Proteus,* and *Klebsiella* organisms. Gram-positive organisms that are effectively destroyed by gentamicin are staphylococci and streptococci that have developed resistance to other antibiotics. Gentamicin is available as an ophthalmic ointment and a solution.

Pharmacokinetics

Half-Life	Onset	Peak	Duration
Unknown	Variable	Immediate	6-12 hr

Macrolides

Macrolide antibiotics include erythromycin, azithromycin, and other drugs (Chapter 37). Erythromycin is currently the only macrolide available for ophthalmic use.

▶ *erythromycin*

Erythromycin (Ilotycin) is a macrolide antibiotic indicated for the treatment of various ophthalmic infections. It is available only as an ophthalmic ointment. In normal concentrations, it inhibits the growth of an organism but does not destroy it. Erythromycin relies on the body's defense mechanisms to destroy the bacteria; however, in high concentrations, it becomes **bactericidal.** It is indicated for the treatment of neonatal conjunctivitis caused by *Chlamydia trachomatis* and for the prevention of eye infections in newborns that may be caused by *Neisseria gonorrhoeae* or other susceptible organisms.

Pharmacokinetics

Half-Life	Onset	Peak	Duration
Unknown	Variable	Immediate	Variable

Polypeptides

Bacitracin and polymyxin B are polypeptide antibiotics. These drugs are rarely used systemically because of their potent nephrotoxic effects. They are bactericidal antimicrobials that inhibit protein synthesis in susceptible organisms, which leads to cell death. They are most commonly used in the treatment of surface superficial infections caused by gram-positive bacteria.

Polypeptides are often used in combination with other antibiotics to broaden their spectrum of activity. For example, Neosporin ophthalmic solution is a combination of gramicidin, neomycin, and polymyxin.

▶ bacitracin

Bacitracin (AK-Tracin) is an ophthalmic antimicrobial drug used to treat various eye infections. It is available as a single-ingredient product and as a combination product with polymyxin or neomycin and polymyxin. These combinations were developed to make bacitracin a broader-spectrum antibiotic.

Bacitracin is available in ointment form.

Pharmacokinetics

Half-Life	Onset	Peak	Duration
Unknown	Variable	Immediate	Variable

Quinolones

Quinolone antibiotics are very effective broad-spectrum antibiotics. They are discussed in detail in Chapter 38. They are bactericidal, destroying a wide spectrum of organisms that are often very difficult to treat. There are currently five ophthalmic quinolones available: ciprofloxacin (Ciloxan), gatifloxacin (Zymar), moxifloxacin (Vigarox), levofloxacin (Quixin), and ofloxacin (Ocuflox).

Significant adverse effects include corneal precipitates during treatment for bacterial keratitis. Other reactions include corneal staining and infiltrates. Toxic reactions are limited because of poor topical absorption. Those that occur are usually taste disorders and nausea. There are no significant drug interactions.

▶ ciprofloxacin

Ciprofloxacin (Ciloxan) is a synthetic quinolone antibiotic. It is available in ointment and solution form. Ciprofloxacin is indicated in the treatment of bacterial keratitis and conjunctivitis caused by susceptible gram-positive and gram-negative bacteria. One notable adverse reaction to ophthalmic ciprofloxacin has been the appearance on the corneal surface of a white, crystalline precipitate occurring within any corneal lesions for which the patient was being treated. This has occurred in approximately 17% of patients, and within 1 to 7 days of starting therapy. However, all cases to date have been self-limiting, have not required drug discontinuation, and have not adversely affected clinical outcome.

Pharmacokinetics

Half-Life	Onset	Peak	Duration
1-2 hr	Variable	Immediate	Variable

Sulfonamides

Sulfonamides are synthetic **bacteriostatic** antibiotics that work by blocking the synthesis of folic acid in susceptible bacteria. Sulfacetamide sodium (Bleph-10) and sulfisoxazole (Gantrisin) are used to treat conjunctivitis and other ocular infections caused by susceptible bacteria.

The adverse effects are primarily limited to local reactions and include local irritation and stinging. Sulfonamide use can result in the overgrowth of nonsusceptible organisms. No significant topical toxic effects have been reported with their use.

▶ sulfacetamide

Sulfacetamide (Bleph-10) is the most commonly used ophthalmic sulfonamide antibacterial drug. It is available in solution and ointment form.

Pharmacokinetics

Half-Life	Onset	Peak	Duration
Unknown	Variable	Immediate	Variable

Antifungal Drugs

natamycin

Natamycin (Natacyn) is a polyene antifungal drug and therefore related to two other antifungal drugs, amphotericin B and nystatin (Chapter 41). It destroys fungi in the eye by binding to sterols in the fungal cell membrane, thus disrupting the protective capabilities of the cell, which results in cell death. Natamycin is used topically in the treatment of blepharitis, conjunctivitis, and keratitis caused by susceptible fungi (*Candida* and *Aspergillus* spp.). It is only available in suspension form.

Pharmacokinetics

Half-Life	Onset	Peak	Duration
Unknown	Variable	Immediate	Variable

ANTIVIRALS

There are three currently available antiviral ophthalmic drugs: fomivirsen (Vitravene), ganciclovir (Vitraset), and trifluridine (Viroptic). Dosages for these ophthalmic antiviral drugs appear in the Dosages table on page 893.

ganciclovir and fomivirsen

Ganciclovir (Vitracet), for treating ocular cytomegalovirus (CMV) infection, is in the form of an implant. The implant releases ganciclovir to the site of disease in the eye in which it is implanted. The implant of ganciclovir must be surgically placed in the posterior of the eye, which allows diffusion of the ganciclovir locally to the site of infection over an extended period of months. Implantation normally takes less than 1 hour, requires only local anesthesia, and is conducted in an outpatient setting. Fomivirsen is also used for treating ocular CMV infection and is administered only by an ophthalmologist via intravitreal injection (into the vitreous humor of the eye) every 2 to 4 weeks. Ocular CMV infection often presents clinically as one of the many possible opportunistic infections associated with HIV and AIDS.

trifluridine

Recall from biochemistry that the chemical bases associated with DNA and RNA structure are classified as pyrimidines and purines and that a nucleoside is a base with its attached sugar molecule from the DNA or RNA "backbone" chain (a nucleotide is a nucleoside plus its associated phosphate molecule in the "backbone" chain). Trifluridine (Viroptic, 1% ophthalmic drops) is a pyrimidine nucleoside. This medication inhibits viral replication because its metabolites block viral DNA synthesis by inhibiting viral DNA polymerase, an enzyme needed for DNA synthesis. This ophthalmic drug is used against ocular infections (keratitis and keratoconjunctivitis) caused by types 1 and 2 of the herpes simplex virus (HSV). Significant adverse effects include secondary glaucoma, corneal punctate defects, uveitis, and stromal edema (edema in the tough, fibrous, transparent portion of the cornea known as the stroma). The drugs exhibit no appreciable topical absorption, and no significant drug interactions have been reported.

ANTIINFLAMMATORY DRUGS

Many of the same antiinflammatory drug classes that are used systemically may also be used ophthalmically to treat various ocular inflammatory disorders and surgery-related pain and in-

---

Box 58-1 Ophthalmic Antiinflammatory Drugs

NSAIDs
- bromfenac (Xibrom)
- diclofenac (Voltaren)
- flurbiprofen (Ocufen)
- ketorolac (Acular)
- suprofen (Profenal)

Corticosteroids
- dexamethasone (Decadron, others)
- fluocinonide (Retisert)
- fluorometholone (Fluor-Op, others)
- loteprednol (Lotemax, others)
- medrysone (HMS)
- prednisolone (Pred Forte, others)
- rimexolone (Vexol)

NSAID, Nonsteroidal antiinflammatory drug.

flammation. These drugs include both nonsteroidal antiinflammatory drugs (NSAIDs) and corticosteroids and are listed in Box 58-1.

Mechanism of Action and Drug Effects

Corticosteroids and NSAIDs, as discussed in Chapters 32 and 44, both act to reduce inflammatory responses that arise from the body's metabolic pathway (series of biochemical reactions) for the naturally occurring biochemical arachidonic acid. Each of these two drug classes acts at different enzymatic sites of this complex metabolic pathway, as illustrated in Figure 58-14.

When tissues are damaged, their cell membranes release phospholipids as a part of the tissue-damaging process. These phospholipids are then broken down by several different enzymes within the arachidonic acid metabolic pathway. Phospholipase is one of the first enzymes involved, and it is the enzyme that is inhibited by corticosteroids. A second enzyme, cyclooxygenase, occurs farther down the pathway and is the site of action of the NSAIDs. Both drug actions reduce the production of various inflammatory mediators, such as leukotrienes, prostaglandins, and thromboxanes. This in turn reduces pain, erythema, and other inflammatory processes.

Indications

Corticosteroids and NSAIDs are applied topically for the symptomatic relief of many ophthalmic inflammatory conditions. They may be used to treat corneal, conjunctival, and scleral injuries from chemical, radiation, or thermal burns or penetration of foreign bodies. They are used during the acute phase of the injury process to prevent fibrosis and scarring that results in visual impairment. This immunosuppressant effect is more notable in corticosteroids than in NSAIDs. Consequently, NSAIDs are considered less toxic and are often preferred as initial topical therapy for such injuries. NSAIDs are also used in the symptomatic treatment of seasonal allergic conjunctivitis.

Corticosteroids and NSAIDs are used prophylactically before ocular surgery to prevent or reduce intraoperative miosis that may occur secondary to surgery-induced trauma. They are also used prophylactically after ocular surgery, such as cataract extraction, glaucoma surgery, and corneal transplants, to prevent inflammation and scarring.

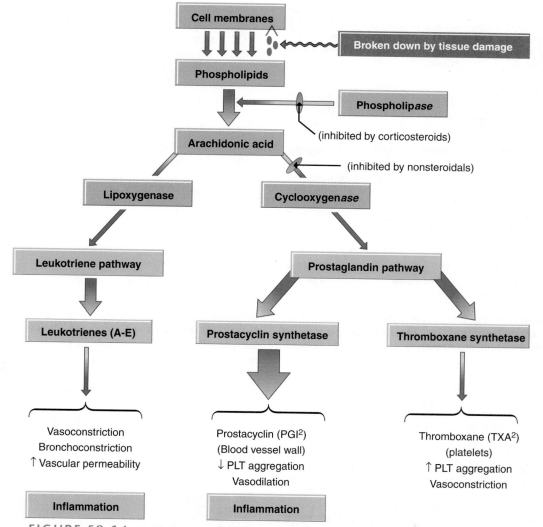

FIGURE 58-14   Antiinflammatory action of corticosteroids and nonsteroidal antiinflammatory drugs (NSAIDs).

Contraindications

Aside from known drug allergy, these drugs should not be used for minor abrasions or wounds because they may suppress the ability of the eye to resist bacterial, viral, or fungal infections. This is especially true of corticosteroids, which, as noted above, have stronger immunosuppressant effects.

Adverse Effects

The most common adverse effect of corticosteroids is transient burning or stinging on application. The extended use of corticosteroids may result in cataracts, increased IOP, and optic nerve damage.

Drug Profiles

Corticosteroids and NSAIDs that are used to treat ophthalmic inflammatory disorders are listed in Box 58-1. These ophthalmic formulations share many of the same characteristics of their systemic drug counterparts. However, the ophthalmic derivatives have limited systemic absorption. Therefore, most therapeutic and toxic effects are limited to the eye.

Corticosteroids
▶ **dexamethasone**

Dexamethasone (Decadron) is a synthetic corticosteroid that has many systemic and ophthalmic formulations. It is used to treat inflammation of the eye, eyelids, conjunctiva, and cornea, and it may also be used in the treatment of uveitis, iridocyclitis, allergic conditions, and burns and in the removal of foreign bodies. Dexamethasone is available in ointment, suspension, and solution form.

Pharmacokinetics

Half-Life	Onset	Peak	Duration
Unknown	Variable	Immediate	Variable

Nonsteroidal Antiinflammatory Drugs (NSAIDs)
flurbiprofen

Flurbiprofen (Ocufen) is an NSAID that is used to treat inflammatory ophthalmic conditions, such as postoperative inflammation after a cataract extraction. It is also used to inhibit intraoperative miosis that may be induced by operative trauma and tissue injury. It is available in solution form.

Pharmacokinetics

Half-Life	Onset	Peak	Duration
Unknown	30 min	90 min	>2 hr

ketorolac

Ketorolac (Acular) is an NSAID that is available in both oral and injectable formulations for systemic use. The ophthalmic formulation is used to reduce certain manifestations of ocular inflammation caused by trauma, such as ocular surgery, and inflammation secondary to external drugs, such as allergens and bacteria. Ketorolac is contraindicated in patients who have exhibited hypersensitivity to it. It is available in solution form. It is important to know that this drug may delay eye wound healing and lead to corneal epithelial breakdown, so constant monitoring of the eye should continue through the duration of therapy.

Pharmacokinetics

Half-Life	Onset	Peak	Duration
Unknown	Rapid	Immediate	4-6 hr

TOPICAL ANESTHETICS

Topical anesthetic ophthalmic drugs are local anesthetics that are used to alleviate eye pain. The two currently available topical anesthetics used for ophthalmic purposes are proparacaine and tetracaine.

Mechanism of Action and Drug Effects

As described in Chapter 11, local anesthetics stabilize the membranes of nerves, resulting in a decrease in the movement of ions into and out of the nerve endings. When nerves are stabilized in this way, they cannot transmit signals about painful stimuli to the brain. Usually, the application of topical anesthetic drugs to the eye results in local anesthesia in less than 30 seconds.

Indications

Ophthalmic topical anesthetic drugs are used to produce ocular anesthesia for short corneal and conjunctival procedures. They prevent pain during surgical procedures, and certain painful ophthalmic examinations. Specific examples include:
- Contact lens fitting
- Tonometry (an external measuring technique involving a puff of air used to estimate IOP)
- Minor conjunctival surgery
- Paracentesis (surgical puncture of the eye to remove fluid for diagnostic or therapeutic reasons)
- Gonioscopy (an examination technique for measuring the angle of the anterior chamber of the eye and for demonstrating ocular rotation and motility)
- Examination of painful eye injuries
- Irrigation of painful injuries
- Removal of foreign bodies
- Removal of sutures
- Corneal scraping for diagnostic purposes
- Any other uncomfortable short procedure

Contraindications

Contraindications to local ophthalmic anesthetics include known drug allergy. These medications are recommended only for short-term use and are not recommended for self-administration.

Adverse Effects

Adverse effects are rare with ophthalmic anesthetic drugs and are limited to local effects such as stinging, burning, redness, and lacrimation. Some of the more common adverse effects are allergic contact dermatitis, softening and erosion of corneal epithelium, pupillary dilation, cycloplegia, conjunctival congestion and hemorrhage, and stromal edema. These drugs also have mydriatic and cycloplegic effects because they dilate the pupil and paralyze the ciliary muscle, which prevents accommodation of vision. Systemic toxicity is rare but can theoretically lead to central nervous system (CNS) stimulation, and/or CNS or cardiovascular depression.

Interactions

Because of limited systemic absorption and short duration of action, ophthalmic anesthetic drugs have no significant drug interactions.

Drug Profiles

Topical ophthalmic anesthetic drugs are a small class of the many available ophthalmic drugs. There are currently only two drugs available for this purpose: proparacaine (Alcaine) and tetracaine (generic only). They are very similar in their indications and dosing regimens.

tetracaine

Tetracaine is a local anesthetic of the ester type (Chapter 11). It is applied as an eyedrop to numb the eye for various ophthalmic procedures as listed previously under "Indications." Tetracaine begins to work in about 25 seconds and lasts for about 30 minutes. Additional drops are applied as needed. It is currently available only in solution form.

Pharmacokinetics

Half-Life	Onset	Peak	Duration
Short	<30 sec	1-5 min	15-20 min

DIAGNOSTIC DRUGS

Drug Profiles

Cycloplegic Mydriatics
▶ **atropine sulfate**

Atropine sulfate solution and ointment are used as mydriatic and cycloplegic drugs. They dilate the pupil (mydriasis) and paralyze the ciliary muscle (cycloplegic refraction), which prevents accommodation. Such drug action may be needed for either eye examination or uveal tract inflammatory states that benefit from pupillary dilation. The usual dose for uveitis (inflammation of the choroid, iris, or ciliary body) in children and adults is 1 to 2 drops of the solution, or 0.3 to 0.5 cm of ointment, 2 to 3 times daily. The dose for eye examination is 1 drop of solution ideally 1 hour before the procedure.

cyclopentolate

Cyclopentolate solution (Cyclogyl) is used primarily as a diagnostic mydriatic and cycloplegic drug. Unlike atropine, it is not normally used to treat uveitis. The usual adult dose is 1 to 2 drops (0.5%, 1%, or 2%). This is repeated in 5 to 10 minutes if needed. The dose for children is the same as that for adults. Infants require 1 drop of the 0.5% solution. The drug effects usually subside within 24 hours. Other cycloplegic mydriatics are scopolamine (Isopto Hyoscine), homatropine (Isopto Homatropine), and tropicamide (Mydriacyl). All three are topical ophthalmic solutions with indications similar to atropine and cyclopentolate, except that tropicamide, like cyclopentolate, is generally used for diagnostic purposes only and not for inflammatory states.

Mydriatic-Reversal Drug
dapiprazole

Dapiprazole (RevEyes) is the only currently available α-adrenergic ophthalmic blocking drug. It is used to reverse the effects of mydriatic drugs and restore normal pupillary function when sustained mydriasis is not desired. Its use is contraindicated only in cases of known drug allergy, or when pupillary constriction is undesirable, as in the case of acute iritis. It is currently available only in a 25-mg vial of powder for reconstitution that comes with its own diluent and eyedropper. The recommended dosage is 2 drops in the affected eye following ophthalmologic examination. This dose is repeated once again after 5 minutes.

Ophthalmic Dye
fluorescein

Fluorescein sodium (AK-Fluor) is an ophthalmic diagnostic dye used to identify corneal defects and to locate foreign objects in the eye. It is also used in fitting hard contact lenses. After the instillation of fluorescein, various defects are highlighted. They are distinguished according to the following criteria:

- Corneal defects are colored bright green.
- Conjunctival lesions are colored yellow-orange.

- Foreign objects have a green halo around them.
- A contact lens that touches the cornea will appear black with ultraviolet light.

Fluorescein is available for use as an ophthalmic injection, solution, and in diagnostic applicator strips. Dosing and drug administration is usually carried out by an ophthalmologist.

ANTIALLERGIC DRUGS

Antihistamines
azelastine

Azelastine (Optivar) is an ocular antihistamine used to treat symptoms of allergic conjunctivitis ("hay fever"), which can be seasonal or non-seasonal. It works by competing at receptor sites of histamine, an inflammatory mediator produced by mast cells. Histamine normally produces such ocular symptoms as itching and tearing. Other ocular antihistamines include olopatadine (Patanol), emedastine (Emadine), ketotifen (Zaditor), and epinastine (Elestat). These drugs have similar mechanisms of action, therapeutic and adverse effects, and drug interactions as the systemic antihistamines described in Chapter 35, although systemic effects are less likely with ophthalmic administration. Dosages for azelastine can be found in the Dosages table on page 898.

Mast Cell Stabilizers
cromolyn

Cromolyn sodium (Crolom) is an antiallergic drug that inhibits the release of inflammation-producing mediators from sensitized inflammatory cells called *mast cells*. It is used in the treatment of vernal keratoconjunctivitis (springtime inflammation of the cornea and conjunctiva). Other mast cell stabilizers with similar effects are pemirolast (Alamast), nedocromil (Alocril), and lodoxamide (Alomide). Dosages for cromolyn can be found in the Dosages table on page 898.

Decongestants
tetrahydrozoline

Tetrahydrozoline is an ocular decongestant. It works by promoting vasoconstriction of blood vessels in and around the eye. This reduces the edema associated with allergic and inflammatory processes. It is specifically indicated to control redness, burning, and other minor irritations. Other ocular decongestants include phenylephrine (Neo-Synephrine), oxymetazoline (Visine LR), and naphazoline (Clear Eyes). Dosages for tetrahydrozoline can be found in the Dosages table on page 898.

Lubricants and Moisturizers
▶ **artificial tears**

An array of OTC products is available to use as lubrication or moisture for the eyes. This is often helpful to patients with dry or otherwise irritated eyes. Artificial tears are isotonic and contain buffers for pH control. In addition, they contain preservatives for microbial control and may contain viscosity drugs for extended ocular activity. Selected OTC brand names include Moisture Drops, Murine, Nu-Tears, Akwa Tears, and Tears Plus. There are many similar products on the market available both as a solution (eyedrop) and as a lubrication ointment. They are often dosed to patient comfort as needed. In 2002, Restasis, an ophthalmic form of the immunosuppressant drug cyclosporine (Chapter 45) was also marketed to promote tear production in the condition technically known as *keratoconjunctivitis sicca* (dry eyes). It can be used together with artificial tears, if given 15 minutes apart.

◆ NURSING PROCESS

◆ ASSESSMENT

Before administering any ophthalmic drug per the physician's orders, the nurse should perform a baseline assessment of the eye and its structures to document specific data about normal versus

DOSAGES

Ocular Antiallergics

Drug (Pregnancy Category)	Pharmacologic Class	Usual Dosage Range	Indications
azelastine (Optivar) (C)	Antihistamine	One drop into each affected eye twice daily	Allergic conjunctivitis
cromolyn (Crolom) (C)	Mast cell stabilizer	One to two drops in each eye 4-6 times daily	Vernal (springtime) conjunctivitis and/or keratitis (corneal inflammation)
tetrahydrozoline (Murine Plus, others) (C)	Decongestant	One to two drops in affected eye(s) up to four times daily	Redness, burning, or other minor irritation

abnormal findings. Any redness, swelling, pain, excessive tearing, eye drainage/discharge, decrease in visual acuity, or any other unusual symptoms should be documented. Hypersensitivity to medications or other drug- or disorder-related contraindications, cautions, and drug interactions should also be documented. Baseline vital signs and a visual acuity test (e.g., Snellen chart) should be used, and findings should be documented before, during, and after drug treatment. Loss/change in vision and loss in peripheral vision in either of both eyes should be noted. A thorough nursing history should focus on past or present systemic disease processes and exposure to any chemicals that could be topical irritants to the eye/skin/mucus membranes including occupational and environmental exposures past or present. All known drug/chemical/ingredient sensitivities should be documented, as well. The systemic effects associated with ophthalmic dosage forms are usually minimal if given as prescribed and directed. Should there be access to the circulation, adverse effects need to be anticipated.

Because of the frequency of use of the drugs in this chapter, note that content in previous chapters further explains each of the drug groups, such as sympathomimetics in Chapter 17, sympatholytics in Chapter 18, and parasympathomimetics in Chapter 19. Their pharmacologic profile and specific contraindications, cautions, and drug interactions are discussed. In addition, pharmacologic profiles and related information about antibiotics is presented in Chapter 37 and 38, antivirals in Chapter 39, and antiinflammatory drugs in Chapter 44. With antiinflammatory ophthalmic drugs, the concern about masking allergic and other reactions may be suppressed.

◆ NURSING DIAGNOSES

- Risk for infection related to eye diseases/conditions/irritation due to a lack of information about various eye problems and lack of motivation to follow directions
- Risk for injury, self (eye), related to improper use of medication and improper instillation procedures
- Acute pain related to the various eye disorder, infection, and/or inflammatory eye conditions
- Deficient knowledge related to lack of information about the eye disorder and related medication therapy

◆ PLANNING
Goals

- Patient remains free of signs and symptoms of infection/irritation of the eye.
- Patient remains compliant to therapy.
- Patient remains free from self-injury related to adverse effects of therapy.

- Patient is without eye pain related to eye disorder.

Outcome Criteria

- Patient states the signs and symptoms of infection of the eye, such as eye pain, drainage, redness, and decreased activity, and reports them immediately to the physician.
- Patient states ways to become more compliant to therapy by taking medications as prescribed including proper timing, instillation, other non-drug therapy aids such as warm or cool compresses as recommended, etc.
- Patient minimizes self-injury related to the adverse effects of therapy by creating a safe environment at home including moving out any clutter or unused rugs/furniture; putting in more lighting, especially night lights; and use of assistive devices as needed, experiencing altered vision.
- Patient minimizes eye pain related to the eye disorder by using compresses or non-aspirin analgesics as ordered.

◆ IMPLEMENTATION

Because it is important to administer only clear solutions, the nurse should shake the medication container before each use to make sure the solution has mixed well and remains clear and without particulate matter. Most important to instillation of drops/ointment is to avoid touching the eye with the tip of the dropper/container to prevent contamination of the product. Any excess medication must be removed promptly and pressure applied to the inner canthus for 1 minute (or other specified time frame) to avoid systemic adverse effects due to absorption into the vasculature. Ointments and any ophthalmic topical drug dosage form should always be applied to the conjunctival sac and never directly onto the eye itself. To facilitate the instillation, the patient needs to place their head back and look up to the ceiling during administration. Several ophthalmic drugs with different actions are often ordered, and each drug must be given exactly as ordered and within the documented time frame. Ointments may cause a temporary blurriness to the vision because of the film that bathes over the eye. This film will decrease once absorbed, and vision should become clearer. The nurse should refer to an authoritative drug source for specific instructions/guidelines about specific application techniques, length of time to apply pressure to the inner canthus, and any other specific instructions. See Chapter 9 for administration technique for ophthalmic drugs.

Directions for antiviral ophthalmic preparations should be followed closely and for the drug, ganciclovir, it is available in implant ocusert form and should be given as ordered. Other ocusert dosage forms are generally placed in the conjunctival sac and stay in place until absorption is complete. Topical anesthetics should be administered as ordered for use in foreign-body removal or treatment of eye injury. Repeated and continuous use should be avoided because of the risk for delayed wound healing, corneal perforation, permanent corneal opacification, and vision loss. When there is an injury/abrasion to the eye and appropriate medications ordered, a patch for the affected eye is recommended. This helps prevent further injury resulting from the loss of the blink reflex from overuse of topical anesthetic. Additional instructions should include any appropriate information about any change in eye color. For example, latanoprost actually turns the eye color permanently from hazel/green/bluish-brown to brown. Although this color change occurs, there is no known injury to the eye associated with this color change.

Ophthalmic ketorolac should be given as ordered. Artificial tear solutions are often used in long-term care and are available over-the-counter. Once therapy has been initiated, the physician may order intraocular pressure readings and visual field and fundoscopic examinations. The importance of these follow-up visits should be shared with the patient (see the Patient Teaching Tips). In addition, a listing of some of the ophthalmic preparations, their mechanisms of action, and related nursing considerations may be found at http://evolve.elsevier. com/Lilley.

◆ EVALUATION

Therapeutic responses to miotics include decreased aqueous humor of the eye with resultant decreased IOP and decreased signs, symptoms, and long-term effects associated with glaucoma. Possible adverse effects are included in the discussion of patient education. β-adrenergic blockers are therapeutic if there is a resultant decrease in intraocular pressure. Possible adverse effects to evaluate include weakness, depression, anxiety, nausea, confusion, eye irritation, rash, bradycardia, hypotension, and dysrhythmias. Therapeutic responses to antibiotic, antifungal, and antiviral ophthalmic drugs include elimination of the infection or condition and resolution of symptoms and prevention of complications. Therapeutic responses to ophthalmic anesthetics include healing of the eye without permanent damage and a decrease in symptoms associated with the damage. Adverse effects include CNS excitation if systemically absorbed, causing blurred vision, dizziness, tremors, nervousness, and restlessness. Drowsiness, dyspnea, and cardiac dysrhythmias may occur secondary to CNS depression. Antiinflammatory ophthalmic solutions should result in a decrease in allergic reactions, such as itching, tearing, redness, and eye discharge. Potential complications of these solutions include swelling of the conjunctiva (chemosis). Further monitoring should include re-evaluation of goals and outcome criteria.

CASE STUDY

Eye Trauma

Mr. P., a construction worker, is being seen in the emergency department because of a possible eye injury. He was working without eye protection, and a gust of wind sprayed metal shavings into his face. The physician has instilled fluorescein sodium and has noted areas in the eyeball with green halos around them.

What is the purpose of the fluorescein sodium, and what is indicated by the green halos?

He is sent to an ophthalmologist for further treatment. What eye medication do you expect will be used for the next procedure?

After the procedure, he receives a prescription for dexamethasone ocular ointment, to take three times a day. What specific patient teaching tips should be shared with Mr. P.?

For answers, see http://evolve.elsevier.com/Lilley.
IOP, Intraocular pressure.

Patient Teaching Tips

- Inform the patient taking parasympathomimetic ophthalmic drugs about the correct procedure for instilling eyedrops and for applying pressure to the inner canthus. Demonstrations and return demonstrations should be used. Solutions with eyedroppers and other equipment should be kept sterile by avoiding touching it to any surface of the eye. Long-term therapy is usually necessary and education about proper technique is important to prevent eye damage.
- Indirect parasympathomimetics should be given to patients only after they demonstrate adequate knowledge of the medication and technique for administration and after explanation of adverse effects associated with most direct- and indirect-acting drugs (e.g., blurred vision, bronchospasm, nausea, vomiting, bradycardia, hypotension, sweating). The patient should be reminded of potential adverse effects, including decreased night visual acuity, stinging sensation, dull ache, or tearing upon instillation, and also reminded that they should call the physician if these symptoms worsen. With sympathomimetic drugs, the patient needs to be reminded to report any stinging, burning, itching, lacrimation, or puffiness of the eye.
- Sympatholytic drugs should be instilled as ordered, and the patient should be cautioned to apply pressure to the inner canthus with a tissue or 2×2 gauze pad for 1 full minute or as directed. Blurred vision, difficulty breathing, wheezing, sweating, flushing, and loss of sight should be reported to the physician.

- Photosensitivity is an expected adverse effect of mydriatics, and use of sunglasses should be encouraged to help minimize eye discomfort and/or headaches while in sunlight.
- With topical anesthetics, patients should not rub or touch the eye while it is numb because of possible eye damage. They should also wear a patch to protect the eye because of loss of the blink reflex.
- The patient should always report any of the following to the health care provider immediately: increase in eye pain, discharge from the eye, fever, and loss of vision.
- Emphasize to the patient to use ophthalmic drugs as ordered and to not overuse or abuse them. The medication should not be stopped without consulting the physician because of the possibility of adverse reactions. Contact lenses should not be worn while instilling ophthalmic drugs and for the duration of therapy because the lenses may lead to further irritation.
- Patients may use a gloved hand or finger cot during application and should be encouraged to avoid touching any of the equipment (e.g., dropper tip) to the structures of the eye. Once applied, remind the patient to close the eye and apply pressure to the lacrimal sac for 1 to 2 minutes or as ordered to avoid drainage of the medication into the nose/throat and to decrease the risk of systemic adverse effects. Ophthalmic ketorolac, an antiinflammatory drug, may delay eye wound healing and lead to corneal epithelial breakdown, so any such concerns should be reported if present or suspected.

Points to Remember

- Glaucoma is a disorder of the eye caused by inhibition of the normal flow and drainage of aqueous humor and its treatment helps to reduce IOP either by increasing aqueous humor drainage or decreasing its production.
- Drugs that increase aqueous humor drainage are direct parasympathomimetics, indirect parasympathomimetics, sympathomimetics, and β-blockers.
- A large proportion of the inflammatory diseases of the eye are caused by viruses, and there are many ocular antimicrobials used to treat bacterial, viral, and fungal infections of the eye.
- Common ocular infections include conjunctivitis, hordeolum (sty), keratitis, uveitis, and endophthalmitis.

- Antiinflammatory ophthalmic drugs include corticosteroids and are used to inhibit inflammatory responses to mechanical, chemical, or immunologic drugs.
- Topical anesthetics are used to prevent pain to the eye and are beneficial during surgery, ophthalmic examinations, and the removal of foreign bodies.
- All ophthalmic preparations need to be administered exactly as ordered and into conjunctival sac. Safe and accurate application or instillation technique must be used while avoiding contact of the dropper or tube to the eye to prevent contamination of the drug.
- Patients should report any increase in symptoms, such as eye pain or drainage and fever, to the physician immediately.

NCLEX Examination Review Questions

1. The ophthalmologist has given a patient a dose of ocular atropine drops. Which statement by the nurse accurately explains to the patient the reason for these drops?
   a. "These drops will cause the surface of your eye to become numb, so that the doctor can do the examination."
   b. "These drops are used to check for any possible foreign bodies or corneal defects that may be in your eye."
   c. "These drops cause your pupils to constrict, making the eye examination easier."
   d. "These drops cause your pupils to dilate, making the eye examination easier."
2. When assessing a patient who is receiving a direct-acting sympathomimetic eyedrop as part of treatment for glaucoma, the nurse notes that the drug affects the pupil in which way?
   a. It causes mydriasis, or pupil dilation.
   b. It causes miosis, or pupil constriction.
   c. It changes the color of the pupil.
   d. It causes no change in pupil size.
3. When teaching the patient on self-administration of ophthalmic drops, which statement by the nurse is correct?
   a. "Hold the eyedrops over the cornea and squeeze out the drop."
   b. "Apply pressure against the lacrimal duct area for 5 minutes after administration."
   c. "Be sure to place the drop in the conjunctival sac of the lower eyelid."
   d. "Squeeze your eyelid closed tightly after placing the drop into your eye."

4. When providing teaching about eye medications for glaucoma, the nurse tells the patient that miotics help glaucoma by:
   a. Decreasing intracranial pressure.
   b. Decreasing intraocular pressure.
   c. Increasing tear production.
   d. Causing pupillary dilation.
5. During an assessment of a glaucoma patient who may be receiving a carbonic anhydrase inhibitor (CAI) as part of treatment, which condition would be considered a problem?
   a. Allergy to sulfa drugs
   b. Allergy to penicillins
   c. Diabetes mellitus
   d. Hypertension

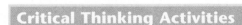

1. d, 2. b, 3. c, 4. b, 5. a.

Critical Thinking Activities

1. Describe the process of glaucoma, and explain the value of treatment to preserve vision.
2. Develop a teaching plan for the elderly patient who is already vision impaired and needs instructions for the daily administration of antiglaucoma ophthalmic drops.

3. What patient teaching tidbit is important for the patient who has a prescription for latanoprost (Xalatan) *before* the patient starts taking this medication?

For answers, see http://evolve.elsevier.com/Lilley.

Otic Drugs

Objectives

When you reach the end of this chapter, you should be able to do the following:

1. Describe the anatomy of the ear and the purposes of each structure located in the outer, middle, and inner ear.
2. Cite the various categories of ear disorders with explanation of causes and signs and symptoms.
3. List the various types of otic preparations and their indications.
4. Discuss the mechanisms of action, dosage, cautions, contraindications, drug interactions, and specific application techniques related to each of the otic drugs.
5. Develop a nursing care plan that includes all phases of the nursing process as it relates to the administration of various otic drugs.

e-Learning Activities

Companion CD

- NCLEX Review Questions: see questions 449-450
- Animations
- Audio Glossary
- Category Catchers
- Medication Errors Checklists
- IV Therapy Checklists

evolve Website (http://evolve.elsevier.com/Lilley)

• Nursing Care Plans • Frequently Asked Questions • Content Updates • WebLinks • Supplemental Resources • Elsevier ePharmacology Update • Medication Administration Animations

Drug Profiles

▶ carbamide peroxide, p. 903
Cortic (hydrocortisone/
   pramoxine/chloroxylenol),
   Acetasol HC (hydrocortisone/
   acetic acid), p. 903
Cortisporin Otic (hydrocortisone/
   neomycin/polymyxin B),

Ciprodex (ciprofloxacin),
Cipro HC Otic (ciprofloxacin/
hydrocortisone), Floxin Otic
(ofloxacin), p. 902

▶ Key drug.

Glossary

Cerumen   A yellowish or brownish waxy excretion produced by modified sweat glands in the external ear canal. Also called *earwax.* (p. 903)

Otitis externa   Inflammation or infection of the external auditory canal. (p. 902)

Otitis media   Inflammation or infection of the middle ear. (p. 902)

OVERVIEW OF EAR ANATOMY AND PATHOLOGY

The ear is made up of four parts: the external, outer, middle, and inner ears. The external ear is composed of the *pinna* (outer projecting part of the ear) and the *external auditory meatus* or opening of the ear canal. Synonyms for the pinna are *auricle* and *ala.* The outer ear refers primarily to the *external auditory canal.* This is the space between the external auditory meatus and the *tympanic membrane* (eardrum). The middle ear is composed of the *tympanic cavity,* which is the space that begins with the tympanic membrane and ends with the *oval window.* Included in the middle ear are three bony appendages of the *mastoid* bone—the *malleus* ("hammer"), *incus* ("anvil"), and *stapes* ("stirrup")—as well as the *auditory* or *eustachian tube.* The inner ear includes the *cochlea* and *semicircular canals.* The ear and its associated structures are illustrated in Figure 59-1.

Disorders of the ear can be categorized according to the portion of the ear affected. External ear (pinna) disorders are generally the result of physical trauma to the ear and consist of lacerations or scrapes to the skin and localized infection of the hair follicles that often cause the development of a boil. These disorders also tend to be self-limiting and heal with time. Other examples include contact dermatitis, seborrhea, or psoriasis as evidenced by, itching, local redness, inflammation, weeping, or drainage. These conditions usually respond to the same topical medications used for any other local skin disorders, as discussed in Chapter 59. However, symptoms such as drainage, pain, and dizziness are sometimes also the first signs of a more serious underlying condition (e.g., head trauma, meningitis) and warrant prompt medical evaluation. Medications for disorders affecting the outer (ear canal) and middle ear are the focus of this chapter. Diseases of the inner ear involve highly specialized medical practices that are beyond the scope of this chapter.

The most common disorders affecting the outer and middle ear include bacterial and fungal infections, inflammation, and earwax

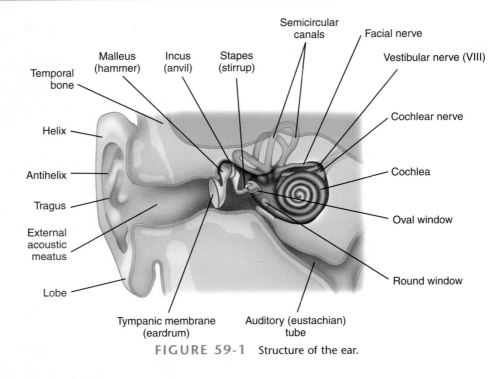

FIGURE 59-1   Structure of the ear.

accumulation. Such disorders are often self-limiting, and treatments are usually successful. However, if problems persist or are left untreated, more serious problems such as hearing loss may result. By far the most common disorder affecting the outer (ear canal) and middle ear disorder is inflammation and/or infection caused by various microorganisms. Cases affecting the ear canal are known as **otitis externa (OE),** while those affecting the middle ear are known as **otitis media (OM).** OM is a common affliction of infancy and early childhood. It is often preceded by an upper respiratory tract infection. It may also occur in adults, but it is then generally associated with trauma to the tympanic membrane. Foreign objects and infection/inflammation from water sports are the usual sources of such trauma. In adults, the condition is also more likely to manifest as otitis externa, involving the ear canal and/or external tympanic membrane. Common symptoms of both OM and OE include pain, fever, malaise, pressure, a sensation of fullness in the ears, and hearing loss. If left untreated, tinnitus (ringing in the ears), nausea, vertigo, mastoiditis, and even temporary or permanent hearing deficits may occur.

TREATMENT OF EAR DISORDERS

Some of the minor ailments that affect the outer or middle ear can be treated with over-the-counter (OTC) medications, but persistent, painful conditions generally require prescription medications. Drugs used for ear conditions are known as *otic drugs,* most of which are topically applied to the ear canal. Because of this they generally have no drug interactions. Adverse effects are uncommon but usually do not extend beyond localized irritation, and otic drugs are normally only contraindicated in cases of known drug allergy. Pertinent drug classes include:

• Antibacterials (antibiotics)
• Antifungals
• Antiinflammatory drugs

• Local analgesics
• Local anesthetics
• Steroids
• Wax emulsifiers

More serious cases of ear disorders may require treatment with systemic drug therapy such as antimicrobial drugs, analgesics, antiinflammatory drugs, and antihistamines. These medications are discussed in detail, by their respective drug classes, in previous chapters.

ANTIBACTERIAL AND ANTIFUNGAL OTIC DRUGS

Antibacterial and antifungal otic drugs are often combined with steroids to take advantage of the steroidal antiinflammatory, antipruritic, and antiallergic drug effects. These drugs are used for outer and middle ear infections (OE and OM). As they all work and are dosed very similarly, four products are profiled together below. Systemic antibiotics are also commonly prescribed for these conditions (e.g., amoxicillin; Chapter 37), either alone, or in addition to the otic drugs described in the following sections. Tables 59-1 and 59-2 list several commonly used products and their component amounts.

Drug Profiles

Antibacterial Products
Cortisporin Otic, Ciprodex, Cipro HC Otic, Floxin Otic

Cortisporin (and other brands) is a three-drug combination that includes hydrocortisone and two antimicrobials, neomycin (an *aminoglycoside;* Chapter 38) and polymyxin B. Hydrocortisone is the steroid most commonly used in otic drugs, although there is one preparation (Ciprodex) containing both ciprofloxacin (a *fluoroquinolone;* Chapter 38) with dexamethasone. In either case, the purpose of the steroid component is to reduce the inflammation and itching

Table 59-1   Common Antibacterial Otic Products

Steroid	Antibiotics	Trade Name
hydrocortisone (1%)	5 mg of neomycin and 10,000 units of polymyxin B per 10 mL bottle	Cortisporin Otic, others
hydrocortisone (1%) dexamethasone (0.1%) (none)	ciprofloxacin 2 mg/mL ciprofloxacin 3 mg/mL ofloxacin 3 mg/mL	Cipro HT Otic Ciprodex Floxin Otic

Table 59-2   Common Antifungal Otic Products

Ingredients	Trade Names
hydrocortisone, 1%; pramoxine, 1%; chloroxylenol, 0.1%; propylene glycol diacetate, 3%; and benzalkonium chloride (amount not specified)	Cortic
hydrocortisone, 1%; acetic acid, 2%; propylene glycol diacetate, 3%; sodium acetate, 0.015%; benzethonium chloride, 0.02%	Acetasol HC

associated with ear infections. Ciprofloxacin is also available in combination with hydrocortisone (Cipro HC Otic). Ofloxacin (Floxin Otic) is another fluoroquinolone available only as a single-drug product. All of these products are used for the treatment of bacterial OE or OM caused by susceptible bacteria such as *Staphylococcus aureus, Escherichia coli, Klebsiella* spp., and others. Their usual dosage is 4 drops 3 to 4 times daily, except for ofloxacin, which is 5 to 10 drops twice daily (5-drop dose for children under 12 years). With some otic drugs, it is recommended to saturate a retrievable cotton or tissue *wick* and let this wick soak inside the ear canal, as a means of dosing the drug. The wick can be periodically remoistened with additional drug, or removed with further eardrops inserted directly into the ear canal. The nurse should follow specific instructions on the drug package or as recommended by the prescriber or pharmacist.

Antifungal Products
Cortic, Acetasol HC
Although fungal infections of the ear are uncommon, otic drugs are available for their treatment. These drugs may also have antibacterial and even antiviral properties. Two commonly used preparations include Cortic and Acetasol HC. Cortic is composed of hydrocortisone (steroid), pramoxine (local anesthetic), chloroxylenol (antiseptic antifungal), propylene glycol diacetate (emulsifying drug), and benzalkonium chloride (antiseptic preservative). Acetasol HC consists of hydrocortisone, acetic acid (antifungal), propylene glycol diacetate, sodium acetate (preservative), and benzethonium chloride (antiseptic preservative). The local anesthetic components help ease both pain and itching common in ear infections.

Earwax Emsulfiers
An additional common ear problem is the accumulation and eventual *impaction* (hardening) of earwax, or **cerumen,** which can also contribute to or complicate the infectious and inflammatory conditions described earlier. Products that soften and help to eliminate earwax are referred to as *earwax emulsifiers*. Wax, or cerumen, is a natural product of the ear and is produced by modified sweat glands in the ear canal. However, it can occasionally build up and become impacted, resulting in pain and partial temporary deafness. From chemistry a nonpolar substance is one that is non–water-soluble. Such a substance is said to be *emulsified* when it is chemically and/or physically converted to a more water-soluble form. *Earwax emulsifiers*

loosen impacted cerumen, allowing it to be irrigated (with water) out of the ear canal.

▸ *carbamide peroxide*
Carbamide peroxide (Debrox) is a commonly used ear wax emulsifier. It is combined with other components (e.g., glycerin, a lubricant) that help soften and lubricate cerumen prior to irrigation. Carbamide peroxide slowly releases hydrogen peroxide and oxygen when exposed to moisture. This release of oxygen imparts a weak antibacterial action to this otic drug. In addition, the *effervescence* (foaming) resulting from the release of oxygen has the mechanical effect of emulsifying impacted cerumen from against the walls of the ear canal. Earwax emulsifiers should not be used without prescription in cases of ear drainage, tympanic membrane rupture, or significant pain or other irritation. After allowing the drug to dissolve the earwax, it can be removed by gentle flushing of the ear canal with warm water from a bulb syringe. Some earwax removal products include such a syringe in the package.

◆ NURSING PROCESS

✦ ASSESSMENT
Before administering any of the otic preparations, the nurse should ensure that the patient's baseline hearing or auditory status is evaluated—as appropriate—and the findings documented. There should also be a thorough evaluation of the patient's symptoms, and any other related medical information should be noted. Any drug or food allergies should be documented. The nurse must understand the specific indication for, or the intended use of, the medication so that it can be given exactly as ordered and without adverse effects or complications. This understanding should also extend to the specific administration technique used. A baseline understanding of the anatomy of the ear is also important, especially as it relates to patients in different age groups. Contraindications, cautions, and drug interactions to any of the drugs, chemicals, and/or solutions have been previously discussed in the pharmacology section. In addition, if there is a perforated eardrum, this is usually a contraindication to the use of these drugs.

✦ NURSING DIAGNOSES
- Impaired verbal communication related to possible hearing impairment/loss stemming from damage from long-term ear disorders/infections
- Risk for injury related to symptoms of the ear disorder and possible vestibular dysfunction
- Risk for infection related to inadequate treatment
- Disturbed sensory perception related to complications from untreated/undertreated ear infections/disorders
- Deficient knowledge related to lack of experience with otic drugs and their method of administration
- Noncompliance related to a lack of motivation for using frequent eardrops as ordered

✦ PLANNING
Goals
- Patient regains normal patterns of hearing and communicating.
- Patient is free of discomfort and symptoms related to the ear disorder.
- Patient remains free of or experiences minimal signs and symptoms of ear infection with the course of treatment.
- Patient is free of adverse reactions or adverse effects.
- Patient is free of complications associated with medication therapy.

- Patient remains compliant and adheres to recommended drug therapy as ordered.

Outcome Criteria

- Patient openly verbalizes feelings related to problems of therapy such as a decrease/loss of hearing related to ear infections/disorders or as a consequence of therapy.
- Patient reports increased hearing loss; increased symptoms of ear pain, redness, and swelling of the ear canal; and fever to the physician immediately.
- Patient states measures to take to increase the effectiveness of the medication regimen, such as accurate application or instillation, remaining supine or sitting with affected ear remaining upward.
- Patient demonstrates accurate medication administration techniques as related to age group and subsequent directions.
- Patient takes medication exactly as ordered and within the directions/guidelines for frequency and demonstrates the proper skills needed as ordered.

◆ IMPLEMENTATION

Eardrops should be instilled only after the ear has been thoroughly cleansed, all cerumen removed (by irrigation if necessary or if ordered), and the dropper cleansed with alcohol—or other drug as ordered—before use. Eardrops/solutions/ointments should be kept to room temperature before instillation. Solutions that are too cold may cause a vestibular type of reaction, with vomiting and dizziness. If the solution has been refrigerated, allow it to warm to room temperature. Higher temperatures may affect the potency of these solutions; therefore, room temperature is recommended. Generally speaking, the corticosteroid drug, antibiotic drug, corticosteroid–antibiotic combination drugs, wax emulsifiers, and/or ear-drying products should be administered according to the aforementioned guidelines and as ordered. Adults should receive eardrops while holding the pinna up and back, whereas children younger than 3 years of age need to have the pinna held down and back. Time should be allowed for adequate coverage of the ear by the medication. Gentle massage to the tragus area of the ear may also help to increase coverage of the medication. See the Patient Teaching Tips and also Chapter 9 for further information on eardrop instillation.

◆ EVALUATION

The therapeutic effects of otic drugs, as with all drugs, should be gauged by evaluation of goals and objectives. However, therapeutic effects should include less pain, redness, and swelling in the ear; a reduction in fever and the white blood cell counts; and negative culture findings if the previous culture has yielded positive findings. The ear canal should be monitored for the occurrence of rash and/or any signs of local irritation such as redness and heat at the site. Adverse effects should also be evaluated with each application/instillation and any unusual appearance of the outer ear and ear canal should be reported immediately to the physician and documented.

Patient Teaching Tips

- Patients should be instructed regarding use of eardrops. The patient should understand and repeat/specific instructions and relate further information about the frequency of dosing and the drug's mechanism of action and adverse effects. In addition, the technique of instillation should be thoroughly discussed and the instructions/technique re-demonstrated. Patients should be encouraged not to touch the dropper/tip to the ear. They should also be warned that dizziness may occur after instillation of the medication, and, therefore, they should remain supine during instillation and for a few minutes thereafter.
- Patients should be told to administer eardrops/solutions at body temperature. This may be achieved by running warm water over the bottle, but care must be taken to not allow water to get into the bottle or to damage the label so that the directions are unreadable. Patients should take care not to actually heat drops—for example, no use of microwave—because eardrops that are overheated may lose potency. If the drug is kept in a refrigerator as indicated by the pharmacy, the drug should be taken out of the refrigerator up to 1 hour before drops are to be instilled so that they can warm up to room temperature; however, otic preparations are usually stored at room temperature.
- Patients should lie on the side opposite the side of the affected ear for about 5 minutes after instillation of the drug. If the patient prefers, a small cotton ball may be inserted gently into the ear canal to keep the drug there, but it should not be forced into the ear or jammed down into the ear canal.
- Patients should be encouraged to show family members how to instill eardrops so that their assistance can be solicited if necessary.
- The eardrop solution and the placement of cotton balls in the ear may cause a seeming loss of hearing. A loss of hearing not resulting from these factors may be due to the ear disorder.

Points to Remember

- Otic drugs may include the following ingredients, either by themselves or mixed together (depending on physician's order): steroids, antibacterials, antifungals, antiinflammatory, and wax emulsifying compounds. Many of the antiinfective drugs are combined with steroids (in solution) to take advantage of their additional antiinflammatory, antipruritic, and antiallergic drug effects.
- Some ear infections require additional drug therapy with systemic dosage forms of corticosteroids, antibiotics, antifungals, and antiinflammatory drugs, so the patient may need to be reminded of oral and other dosage forms.
- Some disorders of the ear are self-limiting to a degree, but appropriate treatment is important to prevent complications to the area and/or systemic complications. However, it is necessary to understand that ear infections/disorders left untreated may lead to loss or a decrease in hearing.
- Wax, or cerumen, is a natural product of the ear and is normally produced by modified sweat glands in the auditory canal; emulsifying otic drugs (such as carbamide peroxide) loosen and help remove this wax.
- Single-drug use or combination-drug products are used to treat many ear conditions, and the nurse must know the indications and specific information about the drugs to ensure their safe use.

NCLEX Examination Review Questions

1. While teaching a patient about treatment of otitis media, the nurse should mention that untreated otitis media may lead to:
   a. Mastoiditis
   b. Throat infections
   c. Fungal ear infection
   d. Decreased cerumen production

2. During a teaching session about ear drops, the patients tells the nurse, "I know why an antibiotic is in this medicine, but why do I need to take a steroid?" The nurse's best answer would be:
   a. "The steroid will help to soften the cerumen."
   b. "The steroid reduces itching and inflammation."
   c. "The steroid also has antifungal effects."
   d. "This medication helps to anesthetize the area to decrease pain."

3. Which technique for administering eardrops is correct?
   a. Warm the solution to 106° F before using.
   b. Position the patient so that the unaffected ear is accessible.
   c. Massage the tragus before administering the eardrops.
   d. Gently insert a cotton ball into the outer ear canal after the drops are given.

4. Which statement about ear wax emulsifiers is true?
   a. These drugs are useful for treatment of ear infections.
   b. These drugs loosen impacted cerumen so that it may be removed by irrigation.
   c. These drugs are used to rinse out excessive earwax.
   d. These drugs enhance the secretion of earwax.

5. During an examination, the nurse notes that a patient has a perforated tympanic membrane. There is an order for eardrops. Which action by the nurse is most appropriate?
   a. Give the medication as ordered.
   b. Check the patient's hearing, then give the drops.
   c. Hold the medication, and check with the prescriber.
   d. Administer the drops with a cotton wick.

1. a, 2. b, 3. d, 4. b, 5. c.

Critical Thinking Activities

1. Develop a patient teaching plan for the caregiver who will be administering antibacterial and steroidal otic drops to a 2-year-old child.

2. Your pediatric patient's mother tells you that she does not understand why ear infections require treatment with antibiotics. She states, "We used home remedies when I was growing up." What information would you share with the patient's mother and why?

3. What is the indication for a wax emulsifier? Explain your answer.

For answers, see http://evolve.elsevier.com/Lilley.

Pharmaceutical Abbreviations

Abbreviation	Translation
Drug Dosage	
cc	Cubic centimeter (equivalent to 1 ml)
g or gm	Gram
gr	Grain
gtt	Drop
IU	International units
L	Liter
lb	Pound
M	Minim
MEq	Milliequivalent
Min	Minute
ml or mL	Milliliter
no	Number
os	Quantity sufficient, as much as needed
ss	One half
oz	Ounce
tbsp	Tablespoon
tsp	Teaspoon
u or U	Unit
μg or mcg	Microgram
Drug Route	
AD	Right ear
AS	Left ear
AU	Both ears
ID	Intradermal
IM	Intramuscular
IV	Intravenous
NG	Nasogastric
OD	Right eye
OS	Left eye
OU	Both eyes
PO	By mouth
SC or SQ	Subcutaneous
SL	Sublingual

Abbreviation	Translation
Drug Administration	
aa	Of each
ac	Before meals
ad lib	As desired, freely
bid	Twice a day
h or hr	Hour
hs	Hour of sleep, at bedtime
noct	Night
NPO	Nothing by mouth
pc	After meals
prn	When needed
qd	Every day, once a day
qh	Every hour
qid	Four times a day
qod	Every other day
Rx	Prescribe, take
stat	Immediately
tid	Three times a day

Note: As part of their 2004 National Patient Safety Goals, the Joint Commission on Accreditation of Healthcare Organizations (JCAHO) announced that all accredited organizations must discontinue using the following abbreviations/acronyms/symbols: U, IU, qd, qod, and MS/MSO$_4$/MgSO$_4$. Also to be discontinued are trailing zeros and lack of leading zeros. In other words, never write a zero by itself after a decimal point (1 mg instead of 1.0 mg), and always use a zero before a decimal point (0.1 mg instead of .1 mg). In addition, abbreviations for drug names should not be used because they can be misinterpreted, and the @ sign should be written out as *at*. Lastly *greater than* and *less than* should be written out instead of > and <. For more information, please see www.jointcommission.org/PatientSafety/DoNotUseList.

Bibliography

General

Abbas AK, Lichtman AH: *Basic immunology: functions and disorders of the immune system,* ed 2, Philadelphia, 2006, Saunders.

Abeloff MD et al: *Clinical oncology,* ed 3, Philadelphia, 2004, Churchill Livingstone.

Abrahams PH et al: *McMinn's color atlas of human anatomy,* ed 5, Philadelphia, 2003, Mosby.

Albanese J, Nutz P: *Mosby's 2007 nursing drug cards,* St Louis, 2007, Mosby.

American Hospital Formulary Service: *AHFS drug information 2005,* Bethesda, Md, 2005, American Society of Health-System Pharmacists.

American Nurses Association: *ANA code of ethics for nurses,* Washington, DC, 2005, American Nurses Publishing. Available at www.ana.org.

Anderson DM et al: *Dorland's illustrated medical dictionary,* ed 30, Philadelphia, 2003, Saunders.

Anderson PO, Knoben JE, Troutman WG: *Handbook of clinical drug data,* ed 10, New York, 2002, McGraw-Hill/Appleton & Lange.

Antman EM et al: *Cardiovascular therapeutics: a companion to Braunwald's heart disease,* ed 2, Philadelphia, 2002, Saunders.

Bachman KA et al: *Drug interactions handbook,* ed 1, Hudson, Ohio, 2003, Lexi-Comp.

Baddour LM, Gorbach SL: *Therapy of infectious diseases,* Philadelphia, 2003, Saunders.

Berne R, Levy M: *Principles of physiology,* ed 4, St Louis, 2006, Mosby.

Boron WF, Boulpaep EL: *Medical physiology,* Philadelphia, 2003, Saunders.

Bradley WG et al: *Neurology in clinical practice,* ed 4, Philadelphia, 2004, Butterworth-Heinemann.

Braunwald E et al: *Harrison's principles of internal medicine,* ed 15, New York, 2001, McGraw-Hill.

Brunton LL, Lazo JS, Parker KL: *Goodman and Gilman's the pharmacological basis of therapeutics,* ed 11, New York 2006, McGraw-Hill.

Capriotti, T: Changes in inhaler devices for asthma and COPD, *Medsurg Nurs* 14(3):185-194, 2005.

Clinical Pharmacology. Available at http://cp.gsm.com.

Colwell JA: *Diabetes: hot topics,* Philadelphia, 2003, Hanley & Belfus.

DeMaagd G: The pharmacologic management of coronary artery disease: a brief overview, *Pharmacy Times,* February:38-54, 2004.

Facts and Comparisons: *Drug facts and comparisons,* St Louis, updated monthly, Facts and Comparisons.

Fetrow CW, Avila JR: *The complete guide to herbal remedies,* Springhouse, Pa, 2000, Springhouse Corp.

Ford M et al: *Clinical toxicology,* ed 1, Philadelphia, 2001, Saunders.

Goldman L et al: *Cecil textbook of medicine,* ed 22, Philadelphia, 2004, Saunders.

Greenwood D et al: *Medical microbiology,* ed 16, Edinburgh, 2002, Elsevier Science.

Gupta K: Emerging antibiotic resistance in urinary tract pathogens, *Infect Dis Clin N Am* 17:243-259, 2003.

Hockenberry MJ et al: *Wong's nursing care of infants and children,* ed 7, St Louis, 2003, Mosby.

Hoffman R et al: *Hematology: basic principles and practice,* ed 4, Philadelphia, 2005, Churchill Livingstone.

Jellin JM et al: *Natural medicines comprehensive database,* Stockton, Calif, 2001, Therapeutic Research Faculty.

Johns Hopkins Hospital, Nechyba C, Gunn V: *The Harriet Lane handbook,* ed 17, St Louis, 2005, Mosby.

Joint National Committee on Detection, Evaluation, and Treatment of High Blood Pressure: *The seventh report of the Joint National Committee on Detection, Evaluation, and Treatment of High Blood Pressure (JNC-7),* National Institutes of Health, May 2003.

Katzung BG: *Basic and clinical pharmacology,* ed 8, New York, 2004, McGraw-Hill/Appleton & Lange.

Koda-Kimble M et al: *Applied therapeutics: the clinical use of drugs,* ed 8, Baltimore, 2005, Lippincott Williams & Wilkins.

Lacy C et al: *Drug information handbook,* ed 13, Hudson, Ohio, 2005, Lexi-Comp/American Pharmacists Association.

Larsen PR et al: *Williams textbook of endocrinology,* ed 10, Philadelphia, 2003, Saunders.

Mandell GL et al: *Principles and practices of infectious diseases,* ed 6, Philadelphia 2005, Churchill Livingstone.

McEvoy G et al: *AHFS drug information 2005,* Bethesda, Md, 2005, American Society of Health-System Pharmacists.

McKenry LM, Tessier E, Hogan M: *Mosby's pharmacology in nursing,* ed 22, St Louis, 2006, Mosby.

Micromedex Healthcare Series. Available at www.micromedex.com.

Miller R et al: *Miller's anesthesia,* ed 6, Philadelphia, 2005, Churchill Livingstone.

Moran GJ, Mount J: Update on emerging infections: News from the Centers for Disease Control and Prevention, *Ann Emerg Med* 41 (1), 148-151.

Mosby's drug consult 2006: the comprehensive reference for generic and brand name drugs, ed 15, St Louis, 2006, Mosby.

Murray PR et al: *Medical microbiology,* St Louis, 2002, Mosby.

Office of Disease Prevention and Health Promotion: *Healthy people 2010,* Washington, DC, 2005, U.S. Department of Health and Human Services. Available at http://odphp.osophs.dhhs.gov.

Roitt I, Brostoff J, Male D: *Immunology,* ed 6, London, 2001, Mosby.

Rubin BK, Durotoye L: How do patients determine that their metered-dose inhaler is empty?, *Chest* 126(4):1134-1137, 2004.

Skidmore-Roth L: *Mosby's handbook of herbs and natural supplements,* ed 2, St Louis, 2004, Mosby.

Skidmore-Roth L: *Mosby's 2007 nursing drug reference,* St Louis, 2007, Mosby.

Tatro DS: *Drug interaction facts 2004,* St Louis, 2004, Facts and Comparisons.

Tierney LM, McPhee SJ, Papadakis MA: *2002 Current medical diagnosis and treatment: adult ambulatory and inpatient management,* New York, 2002, McGraw-Hill.

Timbury MC et al: *Notes on medical microbiology,* Edinburgh, 2002, Churchill Livingstone.

Townsend CM et al: *Sabiston textbook of surgery,* ed 17, Philadelphia, 2004, Saunders.

U.S. Centers for Disease Control and Prevention: *Background on antibiotic resistance.* Available at www.cdc.gov/drugresistance/community.

U.S. Food and Drug Administration website. Available at www.fda.gov.

United States Pharmacopeia: *USP DI: drug information for the health care professional,* vol 1, Greenwood Village, Colo, 2005, Micromedex.

Weiner CP, Buhimschi C: *Drugs for pregnant and lactating women,* ed 1, Philadelphia 2004, Churchill Livingstone.

Wooten J, Salkind A: Superbugs: unmasking the threat, *RN* 66(3):37-43, 2003.

Zipes DP et al: *Braunwald's heart disease,* ed 7, Philadelphia, 2005, Saunders.

Zuckerman JM: Macrolides and ketolides: azithromycin, clarithromycin, telithromycin, *Infect Dis Clin N Am* 18:621-649, 2004.

Chapter 1

Hodgson BB, Kizior RJ: *Saunders nursing drug handbook 2007,* St Louis, 2005, Saunders.

Lewis SM, Heitkemper MM, Dirksen SR: *Medical-surgical nursing: assessment and management of clinical problems,* ed 6, St Louis, 2004, Mosby.

McCaffery M, Pasero C: *Pain: clinical manual,* ed 2, St Louis, 1999, Mosby.

NANDA International: *NANDA nursing diagnoses: definitions and classification 2005-2006,* Philadelphia, 2005, NANDA.

O'Connell D, Reifsteck SW: Disclosing unexpected outcomes and medical error, *J Med Pract Manage* 19(6):317-323, 2004.

Smetzer J: Take ten giant steps to medication safety, *Nursing* 31(11):49-53, 2001.

Chapter 3

Brager R, Sloand E: The spectrum of polypharmacy, *Nurse Pract* 30(6):44-50, 2005.

Burkhart PV, Rayens MK, Bowman RK: An evaluation of children's metered-dose inhaler technique for asthma medications, *Nurs Clin North Am* 40(1):167-182, 2005.

Chang CM et al: *Use of the Beers Criteria to predict adverse drug reaction among first-visit elderly outpatients.* Available at http://medscape. com/viewpublication/132 index. Accessed June 30, 2005.

DiPiro JT et al: *Pharmacotherapy: a pathophysiologic approach,* ed 6, New York, 2005, McGraw-Hill.

Fick DM et al: Updating the Beers Criteria for potentially inappropriate medication use in older adults, *Arch Intern Med* 163(22), 2003.

Miller C: The connection between drugs and falls in elders, *Geriatr Nurs* 23(2):109-110, 2002.

Molony S: *Beers Criteria for potentially inappropriate medication use in the elderly,* 2005. Available at www.medscape.com/viewpublication/ 786 index.

Sloane PD et al: Inappropriate medication prescribing in residential care/assisted living facilities, *J Am Geriatr Soc* 50:1001-1011, 2002.

Taketomo CK, Hodding JH, Kraus DM: *Pediatric dosage handbook,* ed 9, Hudson, Ohio, 2002, Lexi-Comp.

Wooten J, Glass J: Polypharmacy: keeping the elderly safe, *RN* 68(8):44-50, 2005.

Chapter 4

Munoz C, Hilgenberg C: Ethnopharmacology, *Am J Nurs* 105(8):40-49, 2005.

News Target: *FDA under scrutiny as criticisms mount,* March 26, 2005, News Target Network. Available at www.newstarget.com/005991. html.

U.S. Food and Drug Administration: *Timeline: chronology of drug regulation in the United States.* Available at www.fda.gov/cder/about/ history/time1.htm.

U.S. Food and Drug Administration: *Overview of dietary supplements,* January 2001. Available at www.cfsan.fda.gov/~dms/ds-overview. html.

U.S. Food and Drug Administration: *Dietary supplements,* July 2005. Available at www.cfsan.fda.gov/~dms/supplmnt.html.

U.S. Office of Regulatory Affairs: *Compliance policy guidelines,* sec 420.200, compendium revisions and deletions (CPG 7132.02). Available at www.fda.gov/ora/compliance ref/cpg/cpgdrg/cpg420-200.html.

Chapter 5

American Medical Association: *Physicians with disruptive behavior,* January 2005. Available at www.ama-assn.org/ama/pub/category/ 8533.html.

American Society of Health-System Pharmacists: Suggested definitions and relationships among medication misadventures, medication errors, adverse drug events, and adverse drug reactions, *Am J Health Syst Pharm* 15:165-166, 1998.

Associated Press: *Report: nursing shortage may lead to deaths; many leave nursing because of poor staffing conditions, survey says,* June 18, 2003.

Cohen M: Medication errors: reconciling medications, safeguarding transitions, *Nursing* 34(7):14-16, 2005.

DeMoro RA, American Association of Registered Nurses (AARN): A new voice for quality patient care and health care reform, *Calif Nurse,* April 2002. Available at www. calnurse.org/cna/calnurseapril02/ raded.html.

Dennison RD: Creating an organizational culture for medication safety, *Nurs Clin North Am* 40(1):1-23, 2005.

Fletcher JJ, Sorrell JM, Silva MC: Whistleblowing as a failure of organizational ethics, *Online J Issues Nurs,* December 1998. Available at http://nursingworld.org/ojin/topic8/topic8 3. htm.

Hartz AJ et al: Hospital characteristics and mortality rates, *N Engl J Med* 321(25):1720-1725, 1989.

Huckleberry Y et al: Dosage conversions as a potential cause of adverse drug events, *Am J Health Syst Pharm* 60(2):189-191, 2003.

Hughes RE, Edgerton EA: First, do no harm, *AJN* 105(5):79-89, 2005.

Institute for Safe Medication Practices: *High-reliability organizations (HROs): what they know that we don't* (part I), July 14, 2005. Available at www.ismp.org/MSAarticles/20050714.htm.

Institute for Safe Medication Practices: *High-reliability organizations (HROs): what they know that we don't* (part II), July 28, 2005. Available at www.ismp.org/MSAarticles/20050728.htm.

Intravenous Nurses Society: Medication safety (symposium summary), *J Infus Nurs* 28:42-47, 2005.

Joint Commission for the Accreditation of Healthcare Organizations: *2006 National patient safety goals.* Available at www.jcaho.org.

Kelly WN: Potential risks and prevention, part 1: fatal adverse drug events, *Am J Health Syst Pharm* 58(14):1317-1324, 2001.

Kelly WN: Potential risks and prevention, part 2: drug-induced permanent disabilities, *Am J Health Syst Pharm* 58(14):1325-1329, 2001.

Lambert BL et al: Immediate free recall of drug names: effects of similarity and availability, *Am J Health Syst Pharm* 60(2):156-168, 2003.

Lang TA et al: Nurse-patient ratios: a systematic review on the effects of nurse staffing on patient, nurse employee, and hospital outcomes, *J Nurs Adm* 34(7-8):326-337, 2004.

LaPointe NMA, Jollis JG: Medication errors in hospitalized cardiovascular patients, *Arch Intern Med* 163:1461-1466, 2003.

Manasse HR: Not too perfect: hard lessons and small victories in patient safety, *Am J Health Syst Pharm* 60(8):780-787, 2003.

Manno MS, Hayes DD: Best-practice interventions: how medication reconciliation saves lives. *Nursing* 36(3):63-64, 2006.

McCleave SH: How to respond to a formal patient complaint, *J Clin Outcomes Manage* 8(10):35-42, 2001.

Neuenschwander M: Practical guide to bar coding for patient medication safety, *Am J Health Syst Pharm* 60(8):768-779, 2003.

O'Connell D et al: Disclosing unanticipated outcomes and medical errors, *J Clin Outcomes Manage* 10(1):25-29, 2003.

Richardson WC et al: *To err is human: building a safer health system,* Washington DC, 1999, Institute of Medicine, National Academy of Sciences, National Academy Press.

Rosenstein AH: Nurse-physician relationships: impact on nurse satisfaction and retention, *Am J Nurs* 102(6):26-34, 2002.

Rosenstein AH, O'Daniel M: Disruptive behavior and clinical outcomes: perceptions of nurses and physicians, *Am J Nurs* 105(1):54-65, 2005.

Scarsi KK et al: Pharmacist participation in medical rounds reduces medication errors, *Am J Health Syst Pharm* 59(21):2089-2092, 2002.

Scott BE et al: Pharmacy-nursing shared vision for safe medication use in hospitals: executive session summary (conference proceedings), *Am J Health Syst Pharm* 60(10):1046-1052, 2003.

Smith DS, Haig K: Reduction of adverse drug events and medication errors in a community hospital setting, *Nurs Clin North Am* 40(1):25-32, 2005.

Spencer DC et al: Effect of a computerized prescriber-order-entry system on reported medication errors, *Am J Health Syst Pharm* 62(4):416-419, 2005.

Staffing survey, January 2005, American Nurses Association.

Stetina P, Groves M, Pafford L: Managing medication errors—a qualitative study, *Medsurg Nurs* 14(3):174-178, 2005.

Tamen JF: Nurses outraged by plan to strip health professionals of overtime pay, *South Florida Sun-Sentinel,* June 25, 2003.

Wager N et al: The effects on ambulatory blood pressure of working under favourably and unfavourably perceived supervisors, *Occup Environ Med* 60:468-474, 2003.

White C: Double duty: nurses put stamp on legislation in Maine, *Revolution* 3(2):14-17, 2002.

Chapter 6

Aiken L et al: Educational levels of hospital nurses and surgical patient mortality, *JAMA* 290(12):1617-1623, 2003.

Canobbio MM: *Mosby's handbook of patient teaching,* ed 3, St Louis, 2006, Mosby.

Cramer J: *Pardon me, but your medicine cabinet is speaking,* WHO Report WHO/MNC/03.01, World Health Organization, WebMD Medical News, December 10, 2003.

Cutilli CC: Do your patients understand? Determining your patient's health literacy skills, *Orthop Nurs* 24(5):372-377, 2005.

Executive summary: Side effects make therapy education tougher: difference between side effects and infection, *Patient Educ Manage,* pp 1-2, May 2003.

Kicklighter L, Trosty S (presenters): *Avoiding medication errors: saving lives, time, dollars* (audio conference CD recording), American Health Consultants.

Redman BK: *The practice of patient education,* ed 9, St Louis, 2001, Mosby.

Woods, A: How to use your medicine safely (patient education series), *Nursing* 33(12): 50-51, 2003.

Chapter 7

Berardi RR et al: *Handbook of nonprescription drugs,* ed 14, Washington, DC, 2004, American Pharmacists Association.

Bressler R: Herb-drug interactions: Interactions between ginseng and prescription medications, *Geriatrics* 60(7):16-17, 2005.

Bressler R: Herb-drug interactions: St. John's wort and prescription medications, *Geriatrics* 60(7):21-23, 2005.

Harkness R, Bratman S: Mosby's *handbook of drug-herb and drug supplement interactions,* St Louis, 2003, Mosby.

Hoblyn J: Herbal supplements in older adults, *Geriatrics* 60(2):18-23, 2005

Huang SM et al: Drug interactions with herbal products and grapefruit juice, *Clin Pharmacol Ther* 75(1):1-12, 2004.

National Center for Complementary and Alternative Medicine. Available at http://nccam.nih.gov.

Novey DW: *Clinician's complete reference to complementary and alternative medicine,* St Louis, 2000, Mosby.

U.S. Food and Drug Administration: *Kava-containing dietary supplements may be associated with severe liver injury,* March 25, 2002. Available at www.cfsan.fda.gov/~dms/addskava.html.

U.S. Food and Drug Administration: *Evidence on the safety and effectiveness of ephedra: implications for regulation,* February 23, 2003. Available at www.fda.gov/bbs/topics/NEWS/ephedra/whitepaper.html.

U.S. Food and Drug Administration: *Sales of supplements containing ephedrine alkaloids (Ephedra) prohibited,* April 12, 2004. Available at www.fda.gov/oc/initiatives/ephedra/february2004.

U.S. Food and Drug Administration: *Overview of dietary supplements,* August 17, 2005. Available at www.cfsan.fda.gov/~dms/ds-oview.html#what.

Wolinsky I, Williams L: *Nutrition in pharmacy practice,* Washington, DC, 2003, APHA Publications.

Wren KR, Norred CL: *Real world nursing survival guide: complementary and alternative therapies,* St Louis, 2003, Saunders.

Chapter 8

Anderson CE, Loomis GA: Recognition and prevention of inhalant abuse, *Am Fam Physician* 68(5):869-874, 2003.

Greenberg M: *Occupational, industrial, and environmental toxicology,* ed 2, Philadelphia 2003, Mosby.

Hamid H, El-Mallakh R, Vandeveir K: Substance abuse: medical and slang terminology, *South Med J* 98(3):350-362, 2005.

Stoll D, King LE Jr. Disulfiram-alcohol skin reaction to beer-containing shampoo, *JAMA* 244(18):2045, 1980.

U.S. Food and Drug Administration: *Dear health care professional* (letter), July 2001. Available at www.fda.gov/medwatch/safety/2001/oxycontin.htm.

U.S. Food and Drug Administration, Center for Drug Evaluation and Research: *OxyContin: questions and answers,* July 2001. Available at www.fda.gov/cder/drug/infopage/oxycontin/oxycontin-qa.htm.

Chapter 9

Burkhart PV et al: An evaluation of children's metered-dose inhaler technique for asthma medications, *NCNA* 40(1):167-182. 2003.

Ignatavicius DD: Asking the right questions about medication safety, *Nursing,* 30(9): 51-54, 2000.

Institute for Safe Medication Practices: *Hazard alert! Asphyxiation possible with syringe tip caps,* ISMP medication safety alert, August 2001. Available at www.ismp.org/hazardalerts/Hypodermic.asp. Retrieved March 10, 2006.

Karch A: Not so fast! IV push drugs can be dangerous when given too rapidly, *AJN* 103(8):71, 2003.

Karch A, Karch F: Practice errors: a hard pill to swallow, *AJN* 100(4):25, 2000.

Love GH: Clinical do's and don'ts: administering an intradermal injection, *Nursing* 36(6):20, 2005.

McConnell E: Clinical do's and don'ts: administering an intradermal injection, *Nursing* 30(2):50-52, 2000.

McConnell E: Clinical do's and don'ts: applying nitroglycerin ointment, *Nursing* 31(6):17, 2001.

McConnell E: Clinical do's and don'ts: administering medications through a gastrostomy tube, *Nursing* 32(12):22, 2002.

Miller D, Miller H: To crush or not to crush?, *Nursing* 30(2):50-52, 2000.

Moshang, J: Making a point about insulin pens, *Nursing* 35(2):46-47, 2005.

Perry A, Potter P: *Clinical nursing skills and techniques,* ed 6, St Louis, 2006, Mosby.

Pope, BA: Now to administer subcutaneous and intramuscular injections, *Nursing* 32(1): 50, 2002.

Pruitt W: Teaching your patient to use a peak flowmeter, *Nursing* 35(3):54-55, 2005.

Pullen R: Clinical do's and don'ts: administering medication by the Z-track method, *Nursing* 35(7):24, 2005.

Pullen R: Clinical do's and don'ts: managing IV patient-controlled analgesia, *Nursing* 33(7):24, 2003.

Schulmeister L: Transdermal drug patches: medicine with muscle, *Nursing* 35(1):48-52, 2005.

Stein HG: Glass ampules and filter needles: an example of implementing the sixth "r" in medication administration, *Medsurg Nurs* 15(5):290-294, 2006.

Chapter 10

Abboud, L: Narcotic Actiq's use and abuse raise concern, *Wall Street Journal*, May 17, 2004.

American Pain Society. Available at www.ampainsoc.org/advocacy/opioids2.htm.

D'Arcy Y: Conquering pain: have you tried these new techniques?, *Nursing* 35(3):36-41, 2005.

Kim HS et al: Strategies of pain assessment used by nurses on surgical units, *Pain Manag Nurs* 6(1), 2005.

National Cancer Institute: *Basic principles of cancer pain management,* November 2005. Available at www.nci.nih.gov/cancertopics/pdq/supportivecare/pain/Patient/page4.

Olson J: *Clinical pharmacology made ridiculously simple,* Miami, 2003, MedMaster, Inc.

Roman M, Cabaj T: Epidural analgesia, *Medsurg Nurs* 14(4):257-259, 2005.

U.S. Drug Enforcement Administration: *To do no harm: strategies for preventing prescription drug abuse,* DEA Congressional testimony, executive summary, February 9, 2004. Available at www.usdoj.gov/dea/pubs/cngrtest/ct020904.htm.

U.S. Food and Drug Administration: *FDA approves Actiq for marketing,* November 5, 1998. Available at www.fda.gov/bbs/topics/ANSWERS/ANS00921.html.

World Health Organization: *Pain ladder for cancer pain,* 1990. Available at www.who.int/cancer/palliative/painladder/en/print.html.

Chapter 11

Drain CB: *Perianesthesia nursing: a critical care approach,* ed 4, St Louis, 2003, Saunders.

Dripps RD et al: *Introduction to anesthesia: the principles of safe practice,* ed 7, Philadelphia, 1988, Saunders.

Litman DO, Rosenberg H: Malignant hyperthermia, *JAMA* 293:23, 2005.

Chapter 12

Anderson DM et al: *Dorland's illustrated medical dictionary,* ed 30, Philadelphia, 2003, Saunders.

Bachman KA et al: *Drug interactions handbook,* ed 1, Hudson, Ohio, 2003, Lexi-Comp.

Bradley WG et al: *Neurology in clinical practice,* ed 4, Philadelphia, 2004, Butterworth-Heinemann.

Brunton LL, Lazo JS, Parker KL: *Goodman and Gilman's the pharmacological basis of therapeutics,* ed 11, New York, 2006, McGraw-Hill.

Ford M et al: *Clinical toxicology,* ed 1, Philadelphia, 2001, Saunders.

Goldman L et al: *Cecil textbook of medicine,* ed 22, Philadelphia, 2004, Saunders.

Katzung BG: *Basic and clinical pharmacology,* ed 9, New York, 2004, Lange Medical Books/McGraw-Hill.

Koda-Kimble M et al: *Applied therapeutics: the clinical use of drugs,* ed 8, Baltimore, 2005, Lippincott Williams & Wilkins.

Kryger MH et al: *Principles and practices of sleep medicine,* ed 4, Philadelphia, 2005, Saunders.

Lacy C et al: *Drug information handbook,* ed 13, Hudson, Ohio, 2005, Lexi-Comp/American Pharmacists Association.

McEvoy G et al: *AHFS drug information 2005,* Bethesda, Md, 2005, American Society of Health-System Pharmacists.

Miller R et al: *Miller's anesthesia,* ed 6, Philadelphia, 2005, Churchill Livingstone.

Sweetman SC et al: *Martindale: the complete drug reference,* ed 34, London, 2005, Pharmaceutical Press.

Swiss Pharmaceutical Society: *Index nominum international drug directory,* Stuttgart, Germany, 2004, medpharm GmbH Scientific Publishers.

Weiner CP, Buhimschi C: *Drugs for pregnant and lactating women,* ed 1, Philadelphia 2004, Churchill Livingstone.

Chapter 13

Bergey GK. Initial treatment of epilepsy: special issues in treating the elderly, *Neurology* 63(10, suppl 4):S40-S48, 2004.

Briggs DE, French JA: Levetiracetam safety profiles and tolerability in epilepsy patients, *Expert Opin Drug Saf* 3(5):415-424, 2004.

French JA et al: Efficacy and tolerability of the new antiepileptic drugs I: treatment of new onset epilepsy: report of the Therapeutics and Technology Assessment Subcommittee and Quality Standards Subcommittee of the American Academy of Neurology and the American Epilepsy Society, *Neurology* 62(8):1252-1273, 2004.

French JA et al: Efficacy and tolerability of the new antiepileptic drugs II: treatment of refractory epilepsy: report of the Therapeutics and Technology Assessment Subcommittee and Quality Standards Subcommittee of the American Academy of Neurology and the American Epilepsy Society, *Epilepsia* 45(5):410-423, 2004.

Kaplan PW: Reproductive health effects and teratogenicity of antiepileptic drugs, *Neurology* 63(10, suppl 4):S13-S23, 2004.

Leppik IE et al: Advances in antiepileptic drug treatments: a rational basis for selecting drugs for older patients with epilepsy, *Geriatrics* 59(12):14-18, 22-24, 2004.

Manufacturer's package inserts for Gabitril, Keppra, Lamictal, Lyrica, Neurontin, Trileptal, and Zonegran.

McCorry D et al: Current drug treatment of epilepsy in adults, *Lancet Neurol* 3(12):729-735, 2004.

Omnicare: *Omnicare geriatric pharmaceutical care guidelines,* ed 10, Covington, Ky, 2003, Omnicare.

Ortinski P, Meador KJ: Cognitive side effects of antiepileptic drugs, *Epilepsy Behav* 5(suppl 1):S60-S65, 2004.

Perucca E: An introduction to antiepileptic drugs, *Epilepsia* 46(suppl 4):31-37, 2005.

Ramsay RE et al: Special considerations in treating the elderly patient with epilepsy, *Neurology* 62(5, suppl 2):S24-S29, 2004.

Sander JW. The use of antiepileptic drugs—principles and practice, *Epilepsia* 45(suppl 6):28-34, 2004.

Springhouse nurse's drug guide 2005, Philadelphia, 2005, Lippincott Williams & Wilkins.

Trinka E: Epilepsy: comorbidity in the elderly, *Acta Neurol Scand Suppl* 180:33-36, 2003.

Vigevano F: Levetiracetam in pediatrics, *J Child Neurol* 20(2):87-93, 2005.

Wilby J et al: Clinical effectiveness, tolerability and cost-effectiveness of newer drugs for epilepsy in adults: a systematic review and economic evaluation, *Health Technol Assess* 9(15):1-157, iii-iv, 2005.

Chapter 14

Brooks DJ: Safety and tolerability of COMT inhibitors, *Neurology* 62(1, suppl 1):S39-S46, 2004.

Frucht SJ: Parkinson disease: an update, *Neurologist* 10(4):185-194, 2004.

Nyholm D, Aquilonius SM: Levodopa infusion therapy in Parkinson disease: state of the art in 2004, *Clin Neuropharmacol* 27(5):245-256, 2004.

Poewe W: The role of COMT inhibition in the treatment of Parkinson's disease, *Neurology* 62(1, suppl 1):S31-S38, 2004.

Chapter 15

Buchanan RW et al: Olanzapine treatment of residual positive and negative symptoms, *Am J Psychiatry* 162(1):124-129, 2005.

Calabrese JR: A randomized, double-blind, placebo-controlled trial of quetiapine in the treatment of bipolar I or II depression, *Am J Psychiatry* 162(7):1351-1360, 2005.

Catalano G et al: Acute akathisia associated with quetiapine use, *Psychosomatics* 46(4):291-301, 2005.

Edlinger M: Trends in the pharmacological treatment of patients with schizophrenia over a 12 year observation period, *Schizophr Res* 77(1):25-34, 2005.

Gijsman HJ et al: Antidepressants for bipolar depression: a systematic review of randomized, controlled trials, *Am J Psychiatry* 161(9):1537-1547, 2004.

Grunze H: Reevaluating therapies for bipolar depression, *J Clin Psychiatry* 66(suppl 5):17-25, 2005.

Hamrin V, Scahill L: Selective serotonin reuptake inhibitors for children and adolescents with major depression: current controversies and recommendations, *Issues Ment Health Nurs* 26(4):433-450, 2005.

Hunt N: *Your questions answered: bipolar disorder,* London, 2005, Elsevier Limited.

Moore DP, Jefferson JW: *Handbook of medical psychiatry,* ed 2, Philadelphia, 2004, Mosby.

Nelson JC et al: Are there differences in the symptoms that respond to a selective serotonin or norepinephrine reuptake inhibitor?, *Biol Psychiatry* 57(12):1535-1542, 2005.

Phelan KM et al: Lithium interaction with the cyclo-oxygenase 2 inhibitors rofecoxib and celecoxib and other nonsteroidal anti-inflammatory drugs, *J Clin Psychiatry* 64:1328-1334, 2003.

Shastry BS: Genetic diversity and new therapeutic concepts, *J Hum Genet* 50:321-328, 2005.

Shastry BS: Role of SNP/haplotype in gene discovery and drug development: an overview, *Drug Dev Res* 62:143-150, 2004.

Silva de Lima M et al: Quality of life in schizophrenia: a multicenter, randomized, naturalistic, controlled trial comparing olanzapine to first-generation antipsychotics, *J Clin Psychiatry* 66(7):831-838, 2005.

Simpson GM et al: Randomized, controlled, double-blind multicenter comparison of the efficacy and tolerability of ziprasidone and olanzapine in acutely ill inpatients with schizophrenia or schizoaffective disorder, *Am J Psychiatry* 161(10):1837-1847, 2004.

Simpson GM et al: Six-month, blinded, multicenter continuation study of ziprasidone versus olanzapine in schizophrenia, *Am J Psychiatry* 162(8):1535-1538, 2005.

Talbott JA: *Yearbook of psychiatry and applied mental health 2005,* Philadelphia, 2005, Mosby.

Texas Department of State Health Services: *Algorithm for mania/hypomania.* Available at www.dshs.state.tx.us/mhprograms/timabd1algo.pdf. Accessed March 1, 2006.

Texas Department of State Health Services: *Algorithm for the treatment of depression in bipolar disorder.* Available at www.dshs.state.tx.us/mhprograms/timabd2algo.pdf. Accessed March 1, 2006.

U.S. Food and Drug Administration: *Class suicidality labeling language for antidepressants,* January 2005. Available at www.fda.gov/cder/drug/antidepressants/PI_template.pdf.

U.S. Food and Drug Administration: *List of drugs receiving a boxed warning, other product labeling changes, and a medication guide pertaining to pediatric suicidality,* January 2005. Available at www.fda.gov/cder/drug/antidepressants/MDD_alldruglist.pdf.

U.S. Food and Drug Administration: *Medication guide (for parents) about using antidepressants in children and teenagers,* January 2005. Available at www.fda.gov/cder/drug/antidepressants/MG_template.pdf.

U.S. Food and Drug Administration: *Atypical antipsychotic drugs information,* April 2005. Available at www.fda.gov/cder/drug/infopage/antipsychotics/default.htm.

U.S. Food and Drug Administration: *FDA issues public health advisory for antipsychotic drugs used for treatment of behavioral disorders in elderly patients,* April 2005. Available at www.fda.gov/bbs/topics/ANSWERS/2005/ANS01350.html.

U.S. Food and Drug Administration: *FDA public health advisory: deaths with antipsychotics in elderly patients with behavioral disturbances,* April 2005. Available at www.fda.gov/cder/drug/advisory/antipsychotics.htm.

U.S. Food and Drug Administration: *Antidepressant drugs that have healthcare professional and patient information sheets,* June 2005. Available at www.fda.gov/cder/drug/antidepressants/antidepressantList.htm.

U.S. Food and Drug Administration: *FDA public health advisory: suicidality in adults being treated with antidepressant medications,* June 2005. Available at www.fda.gov/cder/drug/advisory/SSRI200507.htm.

U.S. Food and Drug Administration: *FDA reviews data for antidepressant use in adults,* FDA talk paper, July 2005. Available at www.fda.gov/bbs/topics/ANSWERS/2005/ANS01362.html.

Vieta E: The package of care for patients with bipolar depression, *J Clin Psychiatry* 66(suppl 5):34-39, 2005.

Ward KS: New developments in antidepressant therapy, *Nurs Clin North Am* 40(1):95-105, 2005.

Yatham LN et al: Atypical antipsychotics in bipolar depression: potential mechanisms of action, *J Clin Psychiatry,* 66(suppl 5):40-48, 2005.

Zheng CJ et al: Drug ADME associated protein data base as a resource for facilitating pharmacogenomics research, *Drug Dev Res* 62:134-142, 2004.

Chapter 16

Jones HR: *Netter's neurology,* Teterboro, NJ, 2005, Icon Learning Systems.

Kenan WN et al: Phenylpropanolamine and the risk of hemorrhagic stroke, *N Engl J Med* 343(25):1826, 2000.

Kryger MH et al: *Principles and practices of sleep medicine,* ed 4, Philadelphia, 2005, Saunders.

Nutrition Action: *Caffeine: the inside scoop,* 2004. Available at www.cspinet.org/nah/caffeine/caffeine_corner.htm.

U.S. Centers for Disease Control and Prevention, National Center for Health Statistics: *Obesity still a major problem, new data show,* October 2004. Available at www.cdc.gov/nchs/pressroom/04facts/obesity.htm.

U.S. Centers for Disease Control and Prevention, National Center for Health Statistics: *Prevalence of overweight and obesity among adults: United States, 1999-2002,* December 2004. Available at www.cdc.gov/nchs/products/pubs/pubd/hestats/obese/obse99.htm.

U.S. Centers for Disease Control and Prevention: *BMI—body mass index: home,* December 2004. Available at www.cdc.gov/nccdphp/dnpa/bmi/index.htm.

U.S. Centers for Disease Control and Prevention: *Body mass index formula for adults,* July 2005. Available at www.cdc.gov/nccdphp/dnpa/bmi/bmi-adult-formula.htm.

U.S. Centers for Disease Control and Prevention: *Overweight and obesity: home,* September 2005. Available at www.cdc.gov/nccdphp/dnpa/obesity.

U.S. Centers for Disease Control and Prevention: *Overweight and obesity: defining overweight and obesity,* September 2005. Available at www.cdc.gov/nccdphp/dnpa/obesity/defining.htm.

U.S. Department of Health and Human Services: *FDA approves orlistat for obesity,* Rockville, Md, 2001. Available at www.fda.gov/bbs/topics.

U.S. Food and Drug Administration. *FDA announces plans to prohibit sales of dietary supplements containing ephedra.* Retrieved from www.fda.gov/oc/initiatives/ephedra/december2003/

U.S. Food and Drug Administration: *FDA issues public health advisory on Strattera (atomoxetine) for attention deficit disorder.* Available at www.fda.gov/bbs/topics/news/2005/new01237.html.

U.S. Food and Drug Administration: *Public health advisory: suicidal thinking in children and adolescents being treated with Strattera (atomoxetine).* Available at www.fda.gov/cder/drug/advisory/atomoxetine.htm.

U.S. Food and Drug Administration: *Talk paper: FDA approves Xyrem for cataplexy attacks in patients with narcolepsy,* July 17, 2002. Available at www.fda.gov/bbs/topics/ANSWERS/2002/ANS01157.html.

U.S. Food and Drug Administration: *FDA issues regulation prohibiting sale of dietary supplements containing ephedrine alkaloids and reiterates its advice that consumers stop using these products,* February 06, 2004. Available at www.fda.gov/bbs/topics/NEWS/2004/NEW01050.html.

U.S. Food and Drug Administration: *FDA announces rule prohibiting sale of dietary supplements containing ephedrine alkaloids effective April 12,* April 12, 2004. Available at www.fda.gov/bbs/topics/NEWS/2004/NEW01050.html.

U.S. Food and Drug Administration: *Sales of supplements containing ephedrine alkaloids (Ephedra) prohibited,* April 12, 2004. Available at www.fda.gov/oc/initiatives/ephedra/february2004.

U.S. National Institutes of Health: *Statistics related to overweight and obesity,* October 2004. Available at http://win.niddk.nih.gov/statistics/index.htm.

Chapter 18

American Heart Association, Heart Disease and Stroke Statistics — 2006 Update (At-a-Glance Version), Available at www.americanheart.org/downloadable/heart/1140534985281Statsupdate06book.pdf. Accessed February 21, 2006.

Colbert K, Greene MH: Nesiritide (Natecor): A new treatment for acute decompensated congestive heart failure, *Crit Care Nurs Q* 26(1):40, 2003.

Hobbs RE: Using BNP to diagnose, manage, and treat heart failure, *Cleve Clin J Med* 70(4):333-336, 2003.

Poole-Wilson PA et al: Comparison of carvedilol and metoprolol on clinical outcomes in patients with chronic heart failure in the Carvedilol or Metoprolol European Trial (COMET): Randomized controlled trial, *Lancet* 362(9377):7, 2003.

Riggs JM: New therapies for heart failure, *RN* 67(3):29-33, 2004.

Sauls JL, Rone T: Emerging trends in the management of heart failure: beta blocker therapy, *Nurs Clin North Am* 40(1):135-148, 2005.

Chapter 20

Murphy JL: *Monthly prescribing reference,* New York, 2005, Haymark Media Publications.

Chapter 21

Clayton BD, Stock YN: *Basic pharmacology for nurses,* ed 13, St Louis, 2004, Mosby.

Digitalis Investigation Group: The effect of digoxin on mortality and morbidity in patients with heart failure, *N Engl J Med* 336:525, 1997.

Natrecor information website (Scios, Inc.). Available at www.natrecor.com.

Turkoski BB: *Drug information handbook for nursing 1999-2000: including assessment, administration, monitoring guidelines, and patient education,* ed 2, Cleveland, Ohio, 1999, Lexi-Comp.

U.S. Food and Drug Administration: *FDA approves acute congestive heart failure treatment.* Available at www.fda.gov/bbs/topics/ANSWERS/2001/ANS01097.html. Accessed January 21, 2004.

Chapter 22

Coleman CI et al: Model of effect of magnesium prophylaxis on frequency of torsades de pointes in ibutilide-treated patients, *Am J Health Syst Pharm* 61:685-688, 2004.

Crough MA: Chronic heart failure: developments and perspectives, *Consult Pharm* 20(9):751-765, 2005.

Estes NAM et al: Use of antiarrhythmics and implantable cardioverter-defibrillators in congestive heart failure, *Am J Cardiol* 91(6A):45D-52D, 2003.

Filipecki A et al: Effectiveness of rhythm control in persistent or permanent atrial fibrillation with overdrive atrial pacing and antiarrhythmic drugs after linear right atrial catheter ablation, *Am J Cardiol* 92:1037-1044, 2003.

Goldberger AL: *Clinical electrocardiography,* ed 6, St Louis 1999, Mosby.

Goldstein RN, Stambler BS: New antiarrhythmic drugs for prevention of atrial fibrillation, *Prog Cardiovasc Dis* 48(3):193-208, 2005.

Naccarelli GV et al: Old and new antiarrhythmic drugs for converting and maintaining sinus rhythm in atrial fibrillation: comparative efficacy and results of trials, *Am J Cardiol* 91(6A):15D-26D, 2003.

Prabashni R et al: Economic analysis of intravenous plus oral amiodarone, atrial septal pacing, and both strategies to prevent atrial fibrillation after open heart surgery, *Pharmacotherapy* 24(8):1013-1019, 2004.

Raitt MH et al: Comparison of arrhythmia recurrence in patients presenting with ventricular fibrillation versus ventricular tachycardia in the Antiarrhythmics Versus Implantable Defibrillators (AVID) Trial, *Am J Cardiol* 91:812-816, 2003.

Rogers WJ et al: Preliminary report of the Cardiac Arrhythmia Suppression Trial (CAST): Effect of encainide and flecainide on mortality in a randomized trial of arrhythmia suppression after myocardial infarction, *N Engl J Med* 321(6):406-412, 1989.

Wojnowski L: Genetics of the variable expression of CYP3A in humans, *Ther Drug Monit,* 26(2):192-199.

Chapter 23

Anderson S et al: Dosage of beta-adrenergic blockers after myocardial infarction, *Am J Health Syst Pharm* 60:2471-2474, 2003.

Crouch MA: Chronic heart failure: developments and perspectives, *Consult Pharm* 20(9):751-765, 2005.

Henderson RA et al: Seven-year outcome in the RITA-2 trial: coronary angioplasty versus medical therapy, *J Am Coll Cardiol* 42(7):1161-1170, 2003.

Oparil S, Weber MA: *Hypertension: companion to Brenner & Rector's the kidney,* ed 2, Philadelphia, 2005, Saunders.

Trujillo TC, Nolan PE: Ischemic heart disease: Anginal. In M.A. Koda-Kimble et al (Eds.). *Applied therapeutics: the clinical use of drugs,* ed 9, Philadelphia, 2004, Lippincott Williams & Wilkins.

Chapter 24

American Heart Association: *An eating plan for healthy Americans,* revised 2000. Available at www.americanheart.org/presenter.jhtml?identifier=1088. Accessed May 11, 2005.

Choi HK et al: Obesity, weight change, hypertension, diuretic use, and risk of gout in men: The Health Professionals Follow-up Study, *Arch Intern Med* 165:742-748, 2005.

Flack JM, Sica DA: Therapeutic considerations in the African-American patient with hypertension: considerations with calcium channel blocker therapy, *J Clin Hypertens (Greenwich)* 7(4, suppl 1):9-14, 2005.

Inspra information website. Available at www.inspra.com.

JNC 7 Express: The *seventh report of the Joint National Committee on Detection, Evaluation, and Treatment of High Blood Pressure (JNC-7),* 2003, National Institutes of Health.

Monthly prescribing reference, 21(10), 2005, New York. Available at www.presribingref.com.

National Guideline Clearinghouse, Agency for Healthcare Research and Quality: *Essential hypertension: managing adult patients in primary care,* September 2005. Available at www.guideline.gov.

National Guideline Clearinghouse, Agency for Healthcare Research and Quality: *Medical management of adults with essential hypertension,* September 2005. Available at www.guideline.gov.

National Institute of Aging: *Exercise: A guide from the National Institute of Aging,* NIH Publication No. 01-4258, revised June 2001. Bethesda, Md. Available at www.niapublications.org/exercisebook/index.asp. Accessed May 11, 2005.

Remodulin information website. Available at www.remodulin.com.

Stewart KJ et al. Effect of exercise on blood pressure in older persons: a randomized controlled trial, *Arch Intern Med* 165:756-762, 2005.

Tracleer information website. Available at www.tracleer.com.

U.S. Food and Drug Administration: *FDA approves first oral medication for pulmonary artery hypertension,* November 20, 2001. Available at www.fda.gov/bbs/topics/ANSWERS/2001/ANS01121.html. Accessed January 21, 2004.

Van Vlaanderen E: New hypertension guidelines, *Clin Advisor* 7:13-16, 2003.

Vasan RS et al: Residual lifetime risk for developing hypertension in middle-aged women and men, *JAMA* 287:1003-1010, 2002.

Whelton PK et al: Primary prevention of hypertension: clinical and public health advisory from the national high blood pressure education program, *JAMA* 288:1882-1888, 2002.

Woods A, Moshang J: Triple threat: diabetes, hypertension, and heart disease, *Nurs Manage* 36(11):27-33, 2005.

Wright JT et al: Successful blood pressure control in the African American study of kidney disease and hypertension, *Arch Intern Med* 162:1636-1643, 2002.

Chapter 25

Bauer J: Blood pressure cuffs, *RN* 65(8), 2002. Available at www.rnweb.com.

Coleman WL, Garfield C, Committee on Psychosocial Aspects of Child and Family Health: Fathers and pediatricians: enhancing men's role in the care and development of their children, *Pediatrics,* 113:1406-1411, 2004.

Mancia G et al: *Manual of hypertension,* London, 2002, Churchill Livingstone.

Opie LH, Gersh BJ: *Drugs for the heart,* ed 6, Philadelphia, 2005, Saunders.

Chapter 27

Aronow WS: Treatment of peripheral arterial disease in the elderly person, *Ann Long-Term Care* 13(9), 2005.

Fugate S et al: Impaired warfarin response secondary to high-dose vitamin K1 for rapid anticoagulation reversal: case series and literature review, *Pharmacotherapy* 24(9):1213-1220, 2004.

Howard P et al: An update on the diagnosis, complications, and treatment of heparin-induced thrombocytopenia, *Hosp Pharmacy* 39:408-17, 2004.

Kerr JL et al: Role of clopidogrel in unstable angina and non-ST-segment elevation in myocardial infarction: From literature and guidelines to practice, *Pharmacotherapy* 24(8):1037-1049, 2004.

Manor SM et al: Clopidogrel-induced thrombotic thrombocytopenic purpura-hemolytic uremic syndrome after coronary artery stenting, *Pharmacotherapy* 24(5):664-7, 2004.

Spyropoulos AC et al: A disease management protocol for outpatient perioperative bridge therapy with enoxaparin in patients requiring temporary interruption of long-term oral anticoagulation, *Pharmacotherapy* 24(5):649-58, 2004.

Wittkowsky A et al: Effect of age on international normalized ratio at the time of major bleeding episodes in patients treated with warfarin, *Pharmacotherapy* 24(5):600-605, 2004.

Chapter 28

Bayer Corporation: *Dear healthcare professional letter regarding market withdrawal of Baycol (cerivastatin),* August 8, 2001. Available at www.fda.gov/medwatch/safety/2001/Baycol2.htm.

Briel M et al: Effects of statins on stroke prevention in patients with and without coronary heart disease, *EBN* 8:86, 2005.

Carvol JC et al: Differential effects of lipid-lowering therapies on stroke prevention: a meta-analysis of randomized trials, *Arch Intern Med* 163:669-676, 2003.

Cleveland Clinic Heart Center: *Update on cholesterol guidelines: More intensive treatment options for higher risk patients,* report endorsed by National Heart, Lung, and Blood Institute, American College of Cardiology, and American Heart Association, July 13, 2004. Available at www.clevelandclinic.org/heartcenter/pub/news/archive/2004/NCEPLDL7_13print.htm.

Expert Panel on Detection, Evaluation, and Treatment of High Blood Cholesterol in Adults (Adult Treatment Panel III): *Brief summary,* 2001, National Guideline Clearinghouse. Available at www.guideline.gov.

Expert Panel on Detection, Evaluation, and Treatment of High Blood Cholesterol in Adults (Adult Treatment Panel III): Third Report of the National Cholesterol Education Program (NCEP) Expert Panel on Detection, Evaluation, and Treatment of High Blood Cholesterol in Adults (Adult Treatment Panel III): final report, *Circulation* 106:3143-3421, 2002.

Hulley S et al: Randomized trial of estrogen plus progestin for secondary prevention of coronary heart disease in postmenopausal women, *JAMA* 280:605-613, 1998.

Jones PH: Statins as the cornerstone of drug therapy for dyslipidemia: monotherapy and combination therapy options, *Am Heart J* 148(suppl 1):S9-S13, 2004.

Ky B, Rader DJ: The effects of statin therapy on plasma markers of inflammation in patients without vascular disease, *Clin Cardiol* 28:67-70, 2005.

Malik S, Kashvap ML: Dyslipidemia treatment: current considerations and unmet needs, *Expert Rev Cardiovasc Ther* 1(1):121-134, 2003.

Mikhailidis DP et al: The use of ezetimibe in achieving low density lipoprotein lowering goals in clinical practice: position statement of a United Kingdom consensus panel, *Curr Med Res Opin* 21(6):959-69, 2005.

Natural Standard: *Red yeast rice,* monograph. Available at www.naturalstandard.com. Accessed September 1, 2005.

Spratt KA, Denke MA: Utility of currently available modes of therapy in reaching lipid goals, *J Am Osteopathic Assn* 104(suppl 9):14-16, 2004.

Stein EA: The power of statins: aggressive lipid lowering, *Clin Cardiol* 26(4, suppl 3):III25-III31, 2003.

Steinmetz KL, Schonder KS: Colesevelam: potential uses for the newest bile resin, *Cardiovasc Drug Rev* 23(1):15-30, 2005.

Talbert RL: Role of the National Cholesterol Education Program Adult Treatment Panel III guidelines in managing dyslipidemia, *Am J Health Syst Pharm* 60(2):S3-S8, 2003.

Turkoski BB: *Drug information handbook for nursing 1999-2000: including assessment, administration, monitoring guidelines, and patient education,* ed 2, Cleveland, Ohio, 1999, Lexi-Comp.

U.S. Food and Drug Administration: *FDA determines Cholestin to be an unapproved drug.* May 28, 1998. Available at www.fda.gov/cder/drug.

U.S. Food and Drug Administration: *Bayer voluntarily withdraws Baycol,* FDA talk paper, August 8, 2001. Available at www.fda.gov/bbs/topics/ANSWERS/2001/ANS01095.html.

U.S. Food and Drug Administration: *FDA public health advisory for Crestor (rosuvastatin),* June 9, 2004. Available at www.fda.gov/cder/drug/advisory/crestor.htm.

U.S. Food and Drug Administration: *FDA public health advisory on Crestor (rosuvastatin),* March 2, 2005. Available at www.fda/gov/cder/drug/advisory/crestor_3_2005.htm.

Worz CR, Bottorff M: Treating dyslipidemic patients with lipid-modifying and combination therapies, *Pharmacotherapy* 23(5):625-637, 2003.

Writing Group for the Women's Health Initiative Investigators: Risks and benefits of estrogen plus progestin in healthy postmenopausal women: principal results from the Women's Health Initiative randomized controlled trial, *JAMA* 288:321-333, 2002.

Zetia prescribing information, March 2003, Merck/Schering Plough Pharmaceuticals, North Wales, Pa. Available at www.zetia.com.

Chapter 29

Urbano FL: Signs of hypocalcemia: Chvostek's and Trousseau's signs, *Hospital Physician*, March 2000.

Chapter 30

Nazario B: *Thyroid Q&A*, WebMD Live events transcript. Available at www.webmd.com/content/chat_transcripts/1/103872.htm.

Chapter 31

American Diabetes Association: *Drug therapy for high cholesterol.* Available at www.diabetes.org/diabetes-cholesterol/drug-therapy.jsp Accessed March 1, 2006.

American Diabetes Association: *People with diabetes should use aspirin to lower heart-attack risk.* Available at www.diabetes.org/diabetes-research/summaries/persell-asprin.jsp. Accessed March 1, 2006.

American Diabetes Association: Standards of medical care for patients with diabetes mellitus, *Diabetes Care* 26(suppl 1):S33-S50, 2003.

American Diabetes Association: *Diabetes care: information for health professionals,* 26(suppl 1), January 2003. Available at www.diabetes.org.

American Diabetes Association: *Intensive diabetes control yields less nerve damage years later,* 2004. Available at www.diabetes.org/formedia/2004-press-releases/neuropathy.jsp.

Bartol TG: Treating type 2 diabetes to goal: The role of pharmacotherapy, *Am J for NP* 7(11):34-37, 2003.

Bickston TH: *Medical-surgical nursing recall,* Philadelphia, 2004, Lippincott Williams and Wilkins.

Czoski-Murray C et al: Clinical effectiveness and cost-effectiveness of pioglitazone and rosiglitazone in the treatment of type 2 diabetes: a systematic review and economic evaluation, *Health Technol Assess* 8(13):iii, ix-x, 1-91, 2004.

Davis T, Edelman SV: Insulin therapy in type 2 diabetes, *Med Clin North Am* 88(4):865-95, x, 2004.

Diabetes Control and Complications Research Trial Group: The effect of intensive treatment of diabetes on the development and progression of long-term complications of insulin-dependent diabetes mellitus, *New Engl J Med* 329:977-986, 1993.

Dow, NE: Tight insulin control: Making it work, *RN* 68(7):45-52, 2005.

Edmisson KW: Multidimensional pharmacologic strategies for diabetes, *Nurs Clin North Am* 40(1):107-117, 2005.

Evans E, Patry R: Management of gestational diabetes mellitus and pharmacists' role in patient education, *Am J Health Syst Pharm* 61(14):1460-1465, 2004.

Exubera manufacturer's website. Available at www.exubera.com.

Greenfield JR, Campbell LV: Insulin resistance and obesity, *Clin Dermatol* 22(4):289-295, 2004.

Haas L: Management of diabetes mellitus medications in the nursing home, *Drugs Aging* 22(3):209-218, 2005.

Harmel AP, Mathur R: *Davidson's diabetes mellitus: diagnosis and treatment,* ed 5, Philadelphia, 2004, Saunders.

Hirsch IR: Treatment of patients with severe insulin deficiency: what we have learned over the past 2 years, *Am J Med* 116(3A), 2004.

Lebovitz HE. Oral antidiabetic agents: 2004, *Med Clin North Am* 88(4):847-63, ix-x, 2004.

Lien LF, Bethel MA, Feinglos MN: In-hospital management of type 2 diabetes mellitus, *Med Clin North Am* 88(4):1085-105, xii, 2004.

Mitzner L: Selecting the best medication for type 2 diabetes, *Clin Advisor* 7:23-26, 2003.

National Institute of Diabetes and Digestive and Kidney Diseases: *National diabetes statistics,* 2004. Available at http://diabetes.niddk.nih.gov/dm/pubs/statistics/index.htm.

National Institute of Diabetes and Digestive and Kidney Diseases: *Diabetes control and complications trial (DCCT).* Available at http://diabetes.niddk.nih.gov/dm/pubs/control.

National Institute of Diabetes and Digestive and Kidney Diseases: *Diabetes control and complications trial (DCCT): follow-up.* Available at www.diabetes.org/for-media/2004-press-releases/neuropathy.jsp.

Odegard PS, Capoccia KL: Inhaled insulin: Exubera, *Ann Pharmacother* 39(5):843-53, 2005.

Ohkubo Y et al: Intensive insulin therapy prevents the progression of diabetic microvasuclar complications in Japanese patients with non-insulin-dependent diabetes mellitus: a randomized prospective 6-year study, *Diabetes Res Clin Pract* 28:103, 1995.

Physicians' desk reference 2005, Montvale, NJ, 2004, Thomson.

Reynolds NA, Wagstaff AJ: Insulin aspart: a review of its use in the management of type 1 or 2 diabetes mellitus, *Drugs* 64(17):1957-74, 2004.

Riddle MC: Glycemic management of type 2 diabetes: an emerging strategy with oral agents, insulins, and combinations, *Endocrinol Metab Clin N Am* 34:77-98, 2005.

Riddle MC: Making the transition from oral to insulin therapy, *Am J Med* 118(suppl 5A):14S-20S, 2005.

Stoneking K: Initiating basal insulin therapy in patients with type 2 diabetes mellitus, *Am J Health Syst Pharm* 62(5):510-518, 2005.

Turner RC et al: Intensive blood glucose control with sulphonylureas of insulin compared with conventional treatment and risk of complications in patients with type 2 diabetes (UKPDS 33), *Lancet* 352:837-853, 1998.

U.S. Food and Drug Administration: *FDA approves new drug to treat type 1 and type 2 diabetes,* 2005. Available at www.fda.gov/bbs/topics/ANSWERS/2005/ANSO1345.html.

Woods A, Moshang J: Triple threat: diabetes, hypertension, and heart disease, *Nurs Manage* 36(11):27-33, 2005.

Chapter 33

American Psychiatric Association: *Diagnostic and statistical manual of mental disorders (DSM-IV-TR),* Arlington, Va, 2000, American Psychiatric Publishing.

Anderson GL et al: Women's Health Initiative investigators. effects of estrogen plus progestin on gynecologic cancers and associated diagnostic procedures: The Women's Health Initiative randomized trial, *JAMA* 290(13):1739-1748, 2003.

Mozurkewich E et al: The MisoPROM study: A multicenter randomized comparison of oral misoprostol and Oxytocin for premature rupture of membranes at term, *Am J Obstet Gynecol* 189(4):1026-1030, 2003.

National Cancer Institute: *Women's Health Initiative study.* Available at www.cancer.gov. Accessed February 1, 2004.

National Institutes of Health: NIH asks participants in Women's Health Initiative estrogen-alone study to stop study pills, begin follow-up phase, *NIH News,* March 2, 2004. Available at www.nhlbi.nih.gov/new/press/04-03-02.htm.

New drug at a glance. Available at www.pharmacist.com/new_drug/Forteo.cfm. Accessed February 1, 2004.

NuvaRing manufacturer's website. Available at www.nuvaring.com.

Parsons LC: Osteoporosis: Incidence, prevention, and treatment of the silent killer. *Nurs Clin North Am* 40(1):119-133, 2005.

Santoro NF: Should you still prescribe hormones for menopause?, *Clin Advisor* October:18-24, 2003.

Thibodeau GA, Patton KT: *Anatomy and physiology,* ed 5, St Louis, 2003, Mosby.

U.S. Food and Drug Administration: *FDA public health advisory: sepsis and medical abortion,* November 2005. Available at www.fda.gov/cder/drug/advisory/mifeprex.htm.

U.S. Food and Drug Administration: *Estrogen and estrogen with progestin therapies,* February 2006. Available at www.fda.gov/cder/drug/infopage/estrogens_progestins/default.htm.

U.S. Food and Drug Administration: *Mifeprex (mifepristone) information,* March 2006. Available at www.fda.gov/cder/drug/advisory/mifeprex200603.htm.

U.S. National Heart, Lung, and Blood Institute (NHLBI): *Calcium and Vitamin D supplements offer modest bone improvements, no benefits for colorectal cancer,* February 2006. Available at www.nhlbi.nih. gov/new/press/06-02-15.htm.

U.S. National Heart, Lung, and Blood Institute (NHLBI): *NHLBI advisory for physicians on the WHI trial of conjugated equine estrogens versus placebo,* March 2006. Available at www.nhlbi.nih.gov/whi/e-a_advisory.htm.

U.S. National Heart, Lung, and Blood Institute (NHLBI): *Women's Health Initiative home page.* Available at www.nhlbi.nih.gov/whi. Accessed March 1, 2006.

Chapter 34

Avodart manufacturer's website. Available at www.avodart.com.

Benign prostatic hypertrophy drugs available in U.S., *Health and Medicine Week,* 83, 2003.

Gaines K: Tadalafil (Cialis) and vardenafil (Levitra): recently approved drugs for erectile dysfunction, *Urol Nurs* 24(1), 2004.

Gordon AE, Shaughness AF: Saw palmetto for prostate disorders, *Am Fam Physician* 67(6):1281-1283, 2003.

Levitra manufacturer's website. Available at www.levitra.com.

Chapter 35

Clarinex (desloratadine) professional product information and package insert, Kenilworth, NJ, 2002, Schering Corp.

Chapter 36

Albert RK et al: *Clinical respiratory medicine,* ed 2, Philadelphia, 2004, Mosby.

U.S. Food and Drug Administration: *Labeling changes for drug products that contain salmetrol,* FDA talk paper. Available at www.fda.gov/bbs/topics/ANSWERS/2003/ANS01248.html.

U.S Food and Drug Administration, Edelman NH, and American Lung Association: *Statement of support on the FDA's recommendation to ban CFC inhalers,* FDA talk paper, January 2006. Available at www.lungusa.org.

U.S. National Heart, Lung, and Blood Institute: *National Asthma Education and Prevention Program,* home page. Available at www.nhlbi.nih.gov/about/naepp/. Accessed March 1, 2006.

U.S. National Heart, Lung, and Blood Institute: *NAEPP Expert Panel Report guidelines for the diagnosis and management of asthma,* executive summary, 2002. Available at www.nhlbi.nih.gov/guidelines/asthma/execsumm.pdf. Accessed March 1, 2006.

Chapter 37

Clarithromycin (Biaxin) update. Available at www.biaxinxl.com.

Hessen MT, Kaye D: Principles of use of antibacterial agents, *Infect Dis Clin N Am* 18:435-450, 2004.

Plouffe JF, Martin DR: Re-evaluation of the therapy of severe pneumonia caused by Streptococcus pneumoniae, *Infect Dis Clin N Am* 18:963-974, 2004.

Stanley IM, Kaye KM: Beta-lactam antibiotics: newer formulations and newer agents, *Infect Dis Clin N Am* 18:603-619, 2004.

Chapter 38

American Journal of Health-System Pharmacy: New drug overview: cefditoren pivoxil, *Am J Health Syst Pharm* 59(5):414-415, 2002.

Barclay L: Linezolid treats resistant gram-positive infections in children, *Pediatr Infect Dis J* 23:677-685.

de Roux A, Lode H: Recent developments in antibiotic treatment, *Infect Dis Clin N Am* 17:739-751, 2003.

Sheff B: Multidrug-resistant microorganisms, *Nursing* 33(11):59-63, 2003.

Smith MA: Antibiotic resistance, *Nurs Clin N Am* 40(1):63-75, 2005.

Chapter 39

Associated Press Health: *Taiwan rejects China's help in SARS fight,* Taipei, Taiwan, May 25, 2003.

Coleman CI, Musial BL, Ross J: Focus on Enfuvirtide: the first fusion inhibitor for the treatment of patients with HIV-1 infection, *Formulary* 38:204-222, 2003.

DePestel DD et al: Magnitude and duration of elevated gastric pH in patients infected with human immunodeficiency virus after administration of chewable, dispersible, buffered didanosine tablets, *Pharmacotherapy* 24(11):1539-45, 2004.

Deutsch KF FNP: Hepatitis C: The silent epidemic, *Clin Advisor* 6(5):10-18, 2003.

Ellis JM et al: Fosamprenavir: A novel protease inhibitor and prodrug of amprenavir, *Formulary* 39:151-160, 2004.

Jamijan MC, McNicholl IR: Enfuvirtide: first fusion inhibitor for treatment of HIV infection, *Am J Health Syst Pharm* 61:1242-1247, 2004.

Musial BL et al: Atazanavir: a new protease inhibitor to treat HIV infection, *Am J Health Syst Pharm* 61:1365-1374, 2004.

National Institute of Allergy and Infectious Diseases (NIAID): *Course of HIV infection.* Available at www.niaid.nih.gov/publications/hivaids/9.htm. Accessed April 1, 2006.

National Institute of Allergy and Infectious Diseases (NIAID): *HIV infection and AIDS: an overview.* Available at www.niaid.nih.gov/factsheets/hivinf.htm. Accessed April 1, 2006.

National Institutes of Health: *AIDS information homepage.* Available at www.aidsinfo.nih.gov. Accessed April 1, 2006.

Qaquish RB et al: Bone disorders associated with the human immunodeficiency virus: pathogenesis and management, *Pharmacotherapy* 24(10):1331-1346, 2004.

Schiller DS: Identification, management, and prevention of adverse effects associated with highly active antiretroviral therapy, *Am J Health Syst Pharm* 61:2507-2522, 2004.

Schleicher SM, Schiffman LA: On-the-job infections, *Clin Advisor* 97-101, 2003.

Thompson JM et al: *Mosby's clinical nursing,* ed 5, St Louis, 2003, Mosby.

U.S. Centers for Disease Control and Prevention: *West Nile virus information page: treatment.* Available at www.cdc.gov/ncidod/dvbid/westnile/clinicians/treatment.htm.

U.S. Centers for Disease Control and Prevention: *Preliminary clinical description of severe acute respiratory syndrome,* March 21, 2003. Available at www.cdc.gov/mmwr/preview/mmwrhtml/mm5212a5.htm.

U.S. Centers for Disease Control and Prevention: *Fact sheet for clinicians: interpreting SARS test results from CDC,* April 9, 2003. Available at www.cdc.gov/ncidod/sars/testresultsc.htm.

U.S. Centers for Disease Control and Prevention: *CDC lab sequences genome of new Coronavirus,* April 14, 2003. Available at www.cdc.gov/od/oc/media/pressrel/r030414.htm.

U.S. Centers for Disease Control and Prevention: *Severe acute respiratory syndrome (SARS), diagnosis/evaluation,* April 30, 2003. Available at www.cdc.gov/ncidod/sars/diagnosis.htm.

U.S. Centers for Disease Control and Prevention: *Updated interim U.S. case definition of severe acute respiratory syndrome (SARS),* April 30, 2003. Available at www.cdc.gov/ncidod/sars/casedefinition.htm.

U.S. Centers for Disease Control and Prevention: *Key facts about avian influenza (bird flu) and avian influenza A (H5N1) virus,* February 2006. Available at www.cdc.gov/flu/avian/gen-info/facts.htm.

U.S. Centers for Disease Control and Prevention: *Avian influenza infection in humans,* March 2006. Available at www.cdc.gov/flu/avian/gen-info/avian-flu-humans.htm.

U.S. Centers for Disease Control and Prevention: *Avian influenza: current situation,* April 2006. Available at www.cdc.gov/flu/avian/outbreaks/current.htm.

USA Today: *Health officials gear up as West Nile virus begins assault,* May 19, 2003.

Chapter 40

American Thoracic Society: *International standards for tuberculosis treatment,* 2006. Available at www.thoracic.org/sections/about-ats/assemblies/mtpi/resources/istc-report.pdf.

American Thoracic Society: *Tuberculosis: patients' rights and responsibilities,* 2006. Available at www.thoracic.org/sections/about-ats/assemblies/mtpi/resources/istc-charter.pdf.

American Thoracic Society, Centers for Disease Control and Prevention, and Infectious Disease Society of America: Treatment of tuberculosis, *Am J Respir Crit Care Med* 167:603-672, 2003.

National Guideline Clearinghouse: *Treatment of tuberculosis,* June 2003. Available at www.guideline.gov/summary/summary.aspx?doc_id=3829&nbr=003054&string=tuberculosis.

U.S. Centers for Disease Control and Prevention: *Update: adverse event data and revised American Thoracic Society/CDC recommendations against the use of Rifampin and Pyrazinamide for treatment of latent tuberculosis infection—United States, 2003,* August 2003. Available at www.cdc.gov/mmwr/preview/mmwrhtml/mm5231a4.htm.

U.S. Centers for Disease Control and Prevention: *Emergence of Mycobacterium tuberculosis with extensive resistance to second-line drugs—worldwide, 2000-2004,* March 2006. Available at www.cdc.gov/mmwr/preview/mmwrhtml/mm5511a2.htm.

U.S. Centers for Disease Control and Prevention: *Trends in tuberculosis—United States, 2005,* March 2006. Available at www.cdc.gov/mmwr/preview/mmwrhtml/mm5511a3.htm.

U.S. Centers for Disease Control and Prevention: *Tuberculosis control activities after Hurricane Katrina—New Orleans, Louisiana, 2005,* March 2006. Available at www.cdc.gov/mmwr/preview/mmwrhtml/mm5512a2.htm.

U.S. Centers for Disease Control and Prevention: *World TB Day,* March 2006. Available at www.cdc.gov/mmwr/preview/mmwrhtml/mm5511a1.htm.

Volmink J, Matchaba P, Gainer P: Directly observed therapy and treatment adherence, *Lancet* 355:1345-1352, 2000.

Chapter 41

Brown J: Zygomycosis: an emerging fungal infection, *Am J Health Syst Pharm* 62(24): 2593-2596, 2005.

Huang CC, Nunley JR: Dermatologic look-alikes, *Clin Advisor* 6(3):95-98, 2003.

Pappas PG et al: Combating invasive fungal infections: reports from the 45th annual Interscience Conference on Antimicrobial Agents and Chemotherapy, *Contagion* 3(3, suppl 1), 2006.

Chapter 42

National Institute of Allergy and Infectious Diseases (NIAID): *International Centers for Tropical Disease Research,* September 2003. Available at www.niaid.nih.gov/factsheets/ictdr.htm.

National Institute of Environmental Health Services: *Cryptosporidiosis,* January 2004. Available at www.niehs.nih.gov/external/faq/crypto.htm.

Nogid B, Nogid A: A microscopic look at parasitic infections, *Pharmacy Times* February:34-37, 2006.

Sweetman SC et al: *Martindale: the complete drug reference,* ed 34, London, 2005, Pharmaceutical Press.

Swiss Pharmaceutical Society: *Index nominum international drug directory,* Stuttgart, Germany, 2004, medpharm GmbH Scientific Publishers.

Timbury MC et al: *Notes on medical microbiology,* Edinburgh, 2002, Churchill Livingstone.

U.S. Centers for Disease Control and Prevention: *Amebiasis fact sheet,* January 2004. Available at www.cdc.gov/ncidod/dpd/parasites/amebiasis/factsht_amebiasis.htm.

U.S. Centers for Disease Control and Prevention: *Giardiasis fact sheet,* Summer, 2004. Available at www.cdc.gov/ncidod/dpd/parasites/giardiasis/factsht_giardiasis.htm.

U.S. Centers for Disease Control and Prevention: *Treatment of malaria (guidelines for clinicians),* 2005. Available at www.cdc.gov/malaria/pdf/clinicalguidance.pdf.

U.S. Centers for Disease Control and Prevention: *Parasitic roundworm diseases,* February 2005. Available at www.niaid.nih.gov/factsheets/roundwor.htm.

U.S. Centers for Disease Control and Prevention: *Traveler's health: destinations,* July 2005. Available at www.cdc.gov/travel/destinat.htm.

U.S. Centers for Disease Control and Prevention: *Traveler's health: destinations: Mexico and Central America,* January 2006. Available at www.cdc.gov/travel/camerica.htm.

U.S. Centers for Disease Control and Prevention: *Information for health care providers: prescription drugs for malaria,* February 2006. Available at www.cdc.gov/travel/malariadrugs2.htm.

Chapter 44

Kamienski MC: Reye syndrome, *Am J Nursing* 103(7):54-57, 2003.

Pfizer Pharmaceuticals: *Pfizer statement on status of Bextra,* May 2005. Available at www.pfizer.com/pfizer/are/news_releases/2005pr/mn_2005_0510.jsp.

U.S. Food and Drug Administration: *Vioxx (rofecoxib) questions and answers,* September 2004. Available at www.fda.gov/cder/drug/infopage/vioxx/vioxxQA.htm.

U.S. Food and Drug Administration: *Bextra label updated with boxed warning concerning severe skin reactions and warning regarding cardiovascular risk,* FDA talk paper, December 2004. Available at www.fda.gov/bbs/topics/ANSWERS/2004/ANS01331.html.

U.S. Food and Drug Administration: *Questions and answers: strengthened warnings on Bextra,* December 2004. Available at www.fda.gov/cder/drug/infopage/bextra/bextraQA.htm.

U.S. Food and Drug Administration: *COX-2 selective (includes Bextra, Celebrex, and Vioxx) and non-selective non-steroidal anti-inflammatory drugs (NSAIDs),* July 2005. Available at www.fda.gov/cder/drug/infopage/COX2/default.htm.

Zanni GR: Gout: treatment considerations for the practicing pharmacist, *Pharmacy Times,* January:76-77, 2006.

Chapter 46

National Academy of Sciences/Department of Homeland Security: *Chemical attack: warfare agents, industrial chemicals and toxins,* 2004. Available at http://images.main.uab.edu/isoph/SCCPHP/Journalists/Chemical%20FS.pdf.

U.S. Centers for Disease Control and Prevention: *Mumps 2006 outbreak.* Available at www.phppo.cdc.gov/HAN/ArchiveSys/ViewMsgV.asp?AlertNum=00243.

U.S. Centers for Disease Control and Prevention: *Recommended adult immunization schedule by vaccine and age group, United States, 2005-2006.* Available at www.cdc.gov/nip/recs/adult-schedule.pdf.

U.S. Centers for Disease Control and Prevention: *Recommended child and adolescent immunization schedule, United States, 2006, and recommended immunization schedule for children and adolescents who start late or are more than one month behind.* Available at www.cdc.gov/nip/recs/child-schedule-color-print.pdf.

U.S. Centers for Disease Control and Prevention: *Tularemia case definition,* February 2001. Available at www.bt.cdc.gov/agent/tularemia/casedef.asp.

U.S. Centers for Disease Control and Prevention: *Questions and answers: smallpox vaccination program implementation: information to support public health and clinical personnel planning for smallpox vaccination,* April 2003. Available at www.bt.cdc.gov/agent/smallpox/vaccination/vaccination-program-qa.asp?type=cat&cat=Smallpox+Vaccine&subCat1=Vaccine+Candidates.

U.S. Centers for Disease Control and Prevention: *CDC vaccine contraindications,* May 2004. Available at www.cdc.gov/nip/recs/contraindications.htm.

U.S. Centers for Disease Control and Prevention: *Brucellosis case definition,* March 2005. Available at www.bt.cdc.gov/agent/brucellosis/casedef.asp.

U.S. Centers for Disease Control and Prevention: *Plague case definition,* March 2005. Available at www.bt.cdc.gov/agent/plague/casedef.asp.

U.S. Centers for Disease Control and Prevention: *Botulism case definition,* December 2005. Available at www.bt.cdc.gov/agent/botulism/casedef.asp.

U.S. Centers for Disease Control and Prevention: *Bioterrorism case definitions,* 2006. Available at www.bt.cdc.gov/bioterrorism/casedef.asp.

U.S. Centers for Disease Control and Prevention: *Mumps factsheet,* 2006. Available at www.cdc.gov/nip/diseases/mumps/vac-chart.htm.

U.S. Centers for Disease Control and Prevention: *Anthrax case definition,* February 2006. Available at www.bt.cdc.gov/agent/anthrax/anthrax-hcp-factsheet.asp.

U.S. Centers for Disease Control and Prevention: *Smallpox case definition,* February 2006. Available at www.bt.cdc.gov/agent/smallpox/diagnosis/casedefinition.asp.

U.S. Centers for Disease Control and Prevention: *CDC statement regarding autism-related advertisement in* USA Today, April 2006. Available at www.cdc.gov/od/oc/media/pressrel/s060406.htm.

U.S. Centers for Disease Control and Prevention: *Chemical terrorism,* April 2006. Available at www.cdc.gov/nceh/dls/chemical_terrorism.htm.

U.S. Centers for Disease Control and Prevention: *Chemical terrorism: rapid toxic screen,* December 2005. Available at www.cdc.gov/nceh/dls/rapid_toxic_screen.htm.

U.S. Centers for Disease Control and Prevention: *Chemical terrorism: laboratory response,* February 2006. Available at www.cdc.gov/nceh/dls/laboratory_response.htm.

U.S. Centers for Disease Control and Prevention: Smallpox vaccine Q&A, 2003. Available at www.bt.cdc.gov/agent/smallpox/vaccination/vaccination-program-qa_asp?type=cat&cat=Smallpox+Vaccine&subCat1=Vaccine+Candidates.

U.S. Centers for Disease Control and Prevention: Follow-up of deaths among U.S. Postal Service workers potentially exposed to Bacillus anthracis—District of Columbia, 2001—2002, *Mortality and Morbidity Weekly Report (MMWR),* October 2003. Available at www.cdc.gov/mmwr/preview/mmwrhtml/mm5239a2.htm.

U.S. Food and Drug Administration: *Bioterrorism Act of 2002.* Available at www.fda.gov/oc/bioterrorism/bioact.html.

U.S. Food and Drug Administration: *FDA approves pyridostigmine for nerve gas exposure,* February 2003. Available at www.fda.gov/bbs/topics/NEWS/2003/NEW00870.html.

U.S. Food and Drug Administration: *Skin lotion for chemical burns,* March 2003. www.fda.gov/bbs/topics/NEWS/2003/NEW00888.html.

U.S. Food and Drug Administration: *FDA approves pediatric doses of atropen,* June 2003. Available at www.fda.gov/bbs/topics/ANSWERS/2003/ANS01232.html.

U.S. Food and Drug Administration: *FDA approves drugs to treat internal contamination from radioactive elements,* August 2004. Available at www.fda.gov/bbs/topics/news/2004/NEW01103.html.

U.S. Food and Drug Administration, Center for Biologics Evaluation and Research: *Countering bioterrorism: frequently asked questions,* February 2005. Available at www.fda.gov/CBER/faq/cntrbfaq.htm.

U.S. Food and Drug Administration: *Drug preparedness and response to bioterrorism,* February 2006. Available at www.fda.gov/cder/drugprepare.

U.S. Department of Health and Human Services: *Vaccine adverse event reporting system,* 2004. Available at http://vaers.hhs.gov.

U.S. Department of Health and Human Services, Health Resources and Services Administration: *National Childhood Vaccine Injury Act vaccine injury table,* July 2005. Available at www.hrsa.gov/vaccinecompensation/table.htm.

U.S. Department of Justice: *National Vaccine Injury Compensation Program intro page.* Available at www.usdoj.gov/civil/torts/const/vicp/index.htm.

U.S. Department of Justice: *National Vaccine Injury Compensation Program fact sheet.* Available at www.usdoj.gov/civil/torts/const/vicp/about.htm.

U.S. Health Resources and Services Administration: *National Vaccine Injury Compensation Program fact sheet,* 2002. Available at www.hrsa.gov/osp/vicp/fact_sheet.htm.

University of Alabama: *Bioterrorism and emerging infections education,* January 2005. Available at www.bioterrorism.uab.edu.

Chapters 47 and 48

American Society of Clinical Oncology. Available at www.asco.org.

Chu E, DeVita VT Jr: *Physicians' cancer chemotherapy drug manual,* Sudbury, Mass, 2003, Jones and Bartlett.

Kaplow R: Innovations in antineoplastic therapy, *Nurs Clin North Am* 40(1), 77-94, 2005.

Lehne RA: *Pharmacology for nursing care,* ed 5, St Louis, 2004, Saunders.

Leon TG, Pase M: Essential oncology facts for the float nurse, *Medsurg Nurs* 13(3):165-171.

National Cancer Institute. Available at www.nci.hih.gov.

Sadler GR et al.: Managing the oral sequelae of cancer therapy, *Medsurg Nurs* 12(1):28-36, 2003.

Schnell FM: Chemotherapy-induced nausea and vomiting: the importance of acute antiemetic control, *Oncologist* 8(2):187-198, 2003.

Swinburne C: Looking good, *Nurs Stand* 17(39):16-17, 2003.

Ulrich P, Canale SW: *Nursing care planning guides for adults in acute, extended and home care settings,* ed 6, St Louis, 2005, Saunders.

Wilkes GM, Ingwersen K, Barton-Burke M: *Oncology nursing drug handbook,* 2003. Sudbury, Mass, Jones and Bartlett.

Chapter 49

Honeywell M et al: Product profiler: Infliximab: a chimeric monoclonal antibody against tumor necrosis factor, *P&T Journal* 30(11):section two supplement, 2005.

Kruep EJ et al: Cost-minimization analysis of darbepoetin alfa versus epoetin alfa in the hospital setting, *Am J Health Syst Pharm* 62, Dec 15, 2005.

Morrow T et al: Long-term pharmacologic management of multiple sclerosis. In Effective management of multiple sclerosis: a managed care clinician's guidebook, *Formulary,* November 2005.

Morrow T: Natalizumab: FDA is concerned—should managed care be too?, *Formulary,* April:184-189, 2006

Pell LJ et al: Epoetin alfa protocol and multidisciplinary blood-conservation program for critically ill patients, *Am J Health Syst Pharm* 62, Feb 15, 2005.

Chapter 50

Elias P: "RNA interference" making strides, *Associated Press,* July 19, 2003.

Evans WE, McLeod HL: Pharmacogenomics drug disposition, drug targets, and side effects, *N Engl J Med* 348(6):538-549, 2003.

Gates BJ et al: AmpliChip for cytochrome P-450 genotyping: the epoch of personalized prescriptions, *Hosp Pharm* 41:442-445, 2006.

Goldstein DB: Pharmacogenetics in the laboratory and the clinic, *N Engl J Med* 348(6):553-556, 2003.

Greco KE: Nursing in the genomic era: nurturing our genetic nature, *Medsurg Nurs* 12(5):307-312, 2003.

Human Genome Project Information: *Gene testing, gene therapy, pharmacogenomics,* June 11, 2003. Available at www.ornl.gov/TechResources/Human_Genome/home.html.

Kenna GA et al: Pharmacotherapy, pharmacogenomics, and the future of alcohol dependence treatment, part 2, *Am J Health Syst Pharm* 61:2380-2388, 2004.

Kirk M: *Fit for practice in the genetics era—a competence based education framework for nurses, midwives and health visitors,* 2003. Available at www.glam.ac.uk/socs/research/gpu/index.php.

Kreiner T, Buck KT: Moving toward whole-genome analysis: a technology perspective, *Am J Health Syst Pharm* 62:296-305, 2005.

Lau NC, Bartel DP: Censors of the genome, *Sci Am* 289(2):34-41, 2003.

Nicol MJ: The variation of response to pharmacotherapy: pharmacogenetics: a new perspective to "the right drug for the right person," *Medsurg Nurs* 12(4):242-249, 2003.

Nussbaum RL, McInnes RR, Willard HE: *Thompson & Thompson genetics in medicine,* ed 6, Philadelphia, 2004, Saunders.

Pauli EK: Pharmacogenomics: going down the rabbit hole, *Formulary* 30(11):667-669, 2005.

Prows C: *Genetics Summer Institute course,* 2002-2004. Available at http://gepn.cchmc.org.

Teagarden JR: Pharmacogenomics and its potential uses in managed care pharmacy, *Hosp Pharm* 41:477-481, 2006.

Turnpenny P, Ellard S: *Emery's elements of medical genetics,* ed 12, London, 2005, Churchill Livingstone.

Weinshilboum R: Inheritance and drug response, *N Engl J Med* 348(6):529-537, 2003.

Wheelwright J: Testing your future, *Discover* 24(7):33-41, 2003.

Chapter 51

Weinstein WM, Hawkey CJ, Bosh J: *Clinical gastroenterology and hepatology,* ed 1, 2005, Mosby.

Chapter 53

Oncology Nursing Society Online. Available at www.ons.org.

Chapter 54

Insel P, Turner RE, Ross D: *Discovering nutrition,* Boston, 2003, Jones and Bartlett.

Chapter 57

Beitz JM: Wound debridement: therapeutic options and care considerations, *Nurs Clin N Am* 40(2):233-249, 2005.

Doughty D: Dressings and more: guidelines for topical wound management, *Nurs Clin N Am* 40(2):217-231, 2005.

Food and Drug Administration: *FDA talk paper: FDA issues health advisory regarding labeling changes for lindane products,* March 2003. Available at www.fda.gov/bbs/topics/ANSWERS/2003/ANS01205.html.

Food and Drug Administration: *iPLEDGE update,* March 2006. Available at www.fda.gov/cder/drug/infopage/accutane/iPLEDGEupdate200603.htm.

Food and Drug Administration: *Isotretinoin (marketed as Accutane) capsule information,* March 2006. Available at www.fda.gov/cder/drug/infopage/accutane/default.htm.

Grandinetti PJ, Fowler JF: Simultaneous contact allergy to neomycin, bacitracin, and polymyxin, *J Am Acad Dermatol* 23(4, pt 1):646-647, 1990.

Lebwohl MG et al: *Treatment of skin disease: comprehensive therapeutic strategies,* ed 2, 2006, Mosby.

OrthoNeutrogena, division of Ortho-McNeil Pharmaceuticals, Inc., information website for Biafine topical emulsion. Available at www.biafine/orthoneutrogena.com/BIAFINE_PI.pdf#zoom=200. Accessed June 1, 2006.

Chapter 58

Allergan Pharmaceuticals, Department of Scientific Information and Medical Compliance: Personal e-mail regarding flurbiprofen pharmacokinetics, January 2003.

Yanoff M et al: *Ophthalmology,* ed 2, St Louis 2004, Mosby.

Index

Page numbers followed by *b, t,* or *f* indicate boxes, tables, or figures, respectively. Entries in blue indicate disorders. Boldface entries indicate generic drug names.

Special Features